# LiveAdvise
## Medical-Surgical Nursing

**Lippincott Williams & Wilkins** *offers online teaching advice and student tutoring with this textbook!*

### Students—have you ever needed:
…help studying for a test at a time your instructor was not available?

…questions answered outside of class?

…feedback on assignments before turning them in?

### Instructors—have you ever wanted to:
…get help generating classroom activities or discussion ideas from an expert in your discipline?

…ask questions about the content of your adopted textbook or ancillary package, and have someone get back to you right away?

…have your lesson plans evaluated?

If so, **Live**Advise: Medical-Surgical Nursing is the service you need!

Our tutors are handpicked educators that we train to help you. They are very familiar with the textbook you are using in class and the text's ancillary package. You can connect live to a tutor during certain hours of the week, or send e-mail style messages to which the tutor will respond quickly – often within 24 hours.

**Turn to the back of your text to obtain your access code and instructions!**

## And the best part—the service is free with the purchase of your textbook!

Instructors—to use this service, please visit http://thePoint.LWW.com/LiveAdvise

Students—see the codebook inside the front cover of this book for more details. In it you'll find instructions for using this great service, along with your own personal code to log on and get started.

# Brunner & Suddarth's Textbook of Medical-Surgical Nursing

## Eleventh Edition

**Suzanne C. Smeltzer, EdD, RN, FAAN**
Professor and Director, Center for Nursing Research
Villanova University College of Nursing
Villanova, Pennsylvania

**Brenda G. Bare, RN, MSN**
Consultant, Inova Health System
Fairfax, Virginia

**Janice L. Hinkle, PhD, RN, CNRN**
Senior Research Fellow, Acute Stroke Programme
Oxford Brookes University and John Radcliffe Hospital
Oxford, United Kingdom

**Kerry H. Cheever, PhD, RN**
Professor and Chairperson
St. Luke's Hospital School of Nursing at Moravian College
Assistant Vice President
St. Luke's Hospital & Health Network
Bethlehem, Pennsylvania

**VOLUME 1**

Philadelphia · Baltimore · New York · London
Buenos Aires · Hong Kong · Sydney · Tokyo

*Acquisitions Editor:* Pete Darcy
*Development Editor:* Melanie Cann
*Senior Production Editor:* Marian A. Bellus/Tom Gibbons
*Director of Nursing Production:* Helen Ewan
*Senior Managing Editor / Production:* Erika Kors
*Art Director, Design:* Joan Wendt
*Art Director, Illustration:* Brett MacNaughton
*Senior Manufacturing Manager:* William Alberti
*Manufacturing Coordinator:* Karin Duffield
*Indexer:* Maria Coughlin
*Compositor:* Circle Graphics
*Printer:* R. R. Donnelley-Willard

Eleventh Edition

Copyright © 2008 by Lippincott Williams & Wilkins, a Wolters Kluwer business.
Copyright © 2004, 2000 by Lippincott Williams & Wilkins. Copyright © 1996 by Lippincott-Raven Publishers. Copyright © 1992, 1988, 1984, 1980, 1975, 1970, 1964 by J. B. Lippincott Company. All rights reserved. This book is protected by copyright. No part of it may be reproduced, stored in a retrieval system, or transmitted, in any form or by any means—electronic, mechanical, photocopy, recording, or otherwise—without prior written permission of the publisher, except for brief quotations embodied in critical articles and reviews and testing and evaluation materials provided by publisher to instructors whose schools have adopted its accompanying textbook. Printed in the United States of America. For information write Lippincott Williams & Wilkins, 530 Walnut Street, Philadelphia PA 19106.

Materials appearing in this book prepared by individuals as part of their official duties as U.S. Government employees are not covered by the above-mentioned copyright.

9  8  7  6  5  4  3  2

**Library of Congress Cataloging-in-Publication Data**

Brunner & Suddarth's textbook of medical-surgical nursing. — 11th ed. / [edited by] Suzanne C. Smeltzer . . . [et al.].
    p. ; cm.
  Includes bibliographical references and index.
  ISBN-13: 978-0-7817-5978-6 (one-volume ed. : alk. paper)
  ISBN-10: 0-7817-5978-1 (one-volume ed. : alk. paper)
  ISBN-13: 978-0-7817-6695-1 (two-volume ed. : alk. paper)
  ISBN-10: 0-7817-6695-8 (two-volume ed. : alk. paper) 1. Nursing. 2. Surgical nursing.
I. Brunner, Lillian Sholtis. II. Smeltzer, Suzanne C. O'Connell. III. Title: Brunner and Suddarth's textbook of medical-surgical nursing. IV. Title: Textbook of medical-surgical nursing.
  [DNLM: 1. Nursing Care. 2. Perioperative Nursing. WY 150 B8972 2007]

RT41.T46 2007
610.73—dc22

2006026479

Care has been taken to confirm the accuracy of the information presented and to describe generally accepted practices. However, the authors, editors, and publisher are not responsible for errors or omissions or for any consequences from application of the information in this book and make no warranty, express or implied, with respect to the content of the publication.

The authors, editors, and publisher have exerted every effort to ensure that drug selection and dosage set forth in this text are in accordance with the current recommendations and practice at the time of publication. However, in view of ongoing research, changes in government regulations, and the constant flow of information relating to drug therapy and drug reactions, the reader is urged to check the package insert for each drug for any change in indications and dosage and for added warnings and precautions This is particularly important when the recommended agent is a new or infrequently employed drug.

Some drugs and medical devices presented in this publication have Food and Drug Administration (FDA) clearance for limited use in restricted research settings. It is the responsibility of the health care provider to ascertain the FDA status of each drug or device planned for use in his or her clinical practice.

LWW.com

# Contributors

**Roberta H. Baron, RN, MSN, AOCN**
Clinical Nurse Specialist
Memorial Sloan Kettering Cancer Center
New York, New York
*Chapter 48: Assessment and Management of Patients With Breast Disorders*

**Lisa Bowman, RN, MSN, CNRN, CRNP**
Nurse Practitioner
Thomas Jefferson University Hospital
Philadelphia, Pennsylvania
*Chapter 62: Management of Patients With Cerebrovascular Disorders*

**Jo Ann Brooks, DNS, RN, FAAN, FCCP**
Vice President, Quality
Clarian Health Partners Inc.
Indianapolis, Indiana
*Chapter 23: Management of Patients With Chest and Lower Respiratory Tract Disorders*
*Chapter 24: Management of Patients With Chronic Obstructive Pulmonary Disease*

**Kim Cantwell-Gab, BSN, RN, CVN, RVT, RDMS**
Clinical Nurse Specialist, Vascular Surgery
University of Washington
Seattle, Washington
*Chapter 31: Assessment and Management of Patients With Vascular Disorders and Problems of Peripheral Circulation*

**Patricia E. Casey, RN, MSN**
Director, Clinical Content, Care Management Group
Quality Department
Kaiser Permanente Mid-Atlantic States
Rockville, Maryland
*Chapter 27: Management of Patients With Dysrhythmias and Conduction Problems*

**Jill Cash, MSN, APRN, BC**
Family Nurse Practitioner
Southern Illinois OB-GYN Associates, SC
Carbondale, Illinois
*Chapter 59: Assessment and Management of Patients With Hearing and Balance Disorders*

**Kerry H. Cheever, PhD, RN**
Professor and Chairperson
St. Luke's Hospital School of Nursing at Moravian College
Assistant Vice President
St. Luke's Hospital & Health Network
Bethlehem, Pennsylvania

*Chapter 66: Assessment of Musculoskeletal Function*
*Chapter 69: Management of Patients With Musculoskeletal Trauma*

**JoAnn Coleman, RN, MS, ACNP, AOCN**
Acute Care Nurse Practitioner
Gastrointestinal Surgical Oncology
Johns Hopkins Hospital
Baltimore, Maryland
*Chapter 37: Management of Patients With Gastric and Duodenal Disorders*

**Linda Carman Copel, PhD, APRN, BC, DAPA**
Associate Professor
Villanova University College of Nursing
Villanova, Pennsylvania
*Chapter 4: Health Education and Health Promotion*
*Chapter 6: Homeostasis, Stress and Adaptation*
*Chapter 7: Individual and Family Considerations Related to Illness*

**Susanna L. Cunningham, PhD, RN, FAAN**
Professor
University of Washington School of Nursing
Department of Biobehavioral Nursing and Health Systems
Seattle, Washington
*Chapter 32: Assessment and Management of Patients With Hypertension*

**Nancy E. Donegan, RN, BSN, MPH**
Director—Infection Control
Washington Hospital Center
Washington, District of Columbia
*Chapter 70: Management of Patients With Infectious Diseases*

**Diane Dressler, RN, MSN, CCRN**
Clinical Assistant Professor
Marquette University College of Nursing
Milwaukee, Wisconsin
*Chapter 28: Management of Patients With Coronary Vascular Disorders*
*Chapter 30: Management of Patients With Complications From Heart Disease*

**Phyllis Dubendorf, RN, MSN, CS-ACNP**
Lecturer, Acute Care Nurse Practitioner Program
University of Pennsylvania, School of Nursing
Philadelphia, Pennsylvania
*Chapter 61: Neurologic Dysfunction*

**Linda S. Ehrlich-Jones, PhD, RN, CS**
Clinical Research Coordinator
Rehabilitation Institute of Chicago
Chicago, Illinois
*Chapter 54: Management of the Patient With Rheumatic Disorders*

**Susan M. Fallone, RN, MS, CNN**
Clinical Nurse Specialist, Adult and Pediatric Dialysis
Albany Medical Center
Albany, New York
*Chapter 43: Assessment of Renal and Urinary Tract Function*
*Chapter 44: Management of Patients With Kidney Disorders*
*Chapter 45: Management of Patients With Urinary Disorders*

**Catharine Farnan, RN, MS, CRRN, ONC**
Member
American Spinal Injury Association;
Association of American Spinal Cord Injury Nurses; Association of Rehabilitation Nurses
Philadelphia, Pennsylvania
*Chapter 11: Principles and Practices of Rehabilitation*

**Eleanor Fitzpatrick, RN, MSN, CCRN**
Clinical Nurse Specialist
Thomas Jefferson University Hospital
Philadelphia, Pennsylvania
*Chapter 39: Assessment and Management of Patients With Hepatic Disorders*
*Chapter 40: Assessment and Management of Patients With Biliary Disorders*

**Virginia M. Fitzsimons, RNC, EdD, FAAN**
Professor
Kean University, Department of Nursing
Union, New Jersey
*Chapter 38: Management of Patients With Intestinal and Rectal Disorders*

**Kathleen K. Furniss, RNC, MSN, DMH**
Coordinator, Women's Imaging
Mountainside Hospital
Montclair, New Jersey
Nurse Practitioner, Health Service
Drew University
Madison, New Jersey
*Chapter 46: Assessment and Management of Problems Related to Female Physiologic Processes*
*Chapter 47: Management of Patients With Female Reproductive Disorders*

# CONTRIBUTORS

**Margaret J. Griffiths, RN, MSN, AOCN, CNE**
Professor
Thomas Jefferson University
Philadelphia, Pennsylvania
*Chapter 50: Assessment of Immune Function*
*Chapter 51: Management of Patients With Immunodeficiency*

**Janice L. Hinkle, PhD, RN, CNRN**
Senior Research Fellow, Acute Stroke Programme
Oxford Brookes University and John Radcliffe Hospital
Oxford, United Kingdom
*Chapter 5: Health Assessment*
*Chapter 60: Assessment of Neurologic Function*
*Chapter 63: Management of Patients With Neurologic Trauma*
*Chapter 65: Management of Patients With Oncologic or Degenerative Neurologic Disorders*

**Joyce Y. Johnson, PhD, RN, CCRN**
Dean
College of Health Professions/Department of Nursing
Albany State University
Albany, Georgia
*Chapter 1: Health Care Delivery and Nursing Practice*
*Chapter 2: Community-Based Nursing Practice*
*Chapter 3: Critical Thinking, Ethical Decision Making, and the Nursing Process*
*Chapter 8: Perspectives in Transcultural Nursing*

**Elizabeth Keech, PhD, RN**
Assistant Professor
Villanova University College of Nursing
Villanova, Pennsylvania
*Chapter 12: Health Care of the Older Adult*

**Dale Halsey Lea, RN, MPH, CGC, APGN, FAAN**
Assistant Director
Southern Maine Regional Genetics Services
Scarborough, Maine
*Chapter 9: Genetics Perspectives in Nursing*

**Mary Beth Flynn Makic, RN, MS CNS, CCNS, CCRN**
Clinical Nurse Specialist/Senior Instructor
University of Colorado Hospital
Denver, Colorado
*Chapter 15: Shock and Multisystem Failure*

**Barbara J. Maschak-Carey, RN, MSN, CDE**
Clinical Nurse Specialist
University of Pennsylvania
Philadelphia, Pennsylvania
*Chapter 41: Assessment and Management of Patients With Diabetes Mellitus*

**Agnes Masny, RN, MPH, MSN, CRNP**
Research Associate/Nurse Practitioner
Population Science Division, Family Risk Assessment Program
Fox Chase Cancer Center
Philadelphia, Pennsylvania
*Chapter 9: Genetics Perspectives in Nursing*

**LouAnn McGinty, RN, MSN**
Part-Time Instructor
Villanova University College of Nursing
Villanova, Pennsylvania
*Chapter 64: Management of Patients With Neurologic Infections, Autoimmune Disorders, and Neuropathies*

**Carol Gullo Mest, PhD, APRN, BC**
Associate Professor
DeSales University, Department of Nursing and Health
Center Valley, Pennsylvania
*Chapter 68: Management of Patients With Musculoskeletal Disorders*

**Barbara A. Moyer, RN, EdD**
Assistant Professor
DeSales University, Department of Nursing and Health
Center Valley, Pennsylvania
*Chapter 67: Musculoskeletal Care Modalities*

**Martha A. Mulvey, MS, RN, CNS, C**
Advanced Practice Nurse, Neurology
University Hospital
University of Medicine and Dentistry of New Jersey
Newark, New Jersey
*Chapter 14: Fluid and Electrolytes: Balance and Disturbances*

**Victoria Navarro, RN, MAS, MSN**
Director of Nursing
The Wilmer Eye Institute at Johns Hopkins
Baltimore, Maryland
*Chapter 58: Assessment and Management of Patients With Eye and Vision Disorders*

**Donna Nayduch, RN, MSN, ACNP, CCRN**
Trauma Consultant
K-Force
Evans, Colorado
*Chapter 71: Emergency Nursing*
*Chapter 72: Terrorism, Mass Casualty, and Disaster Nursing*

**Kathleen Nokes, PhD, RN, FAAN**
Professor
Hunter College
New York, New York
*Chapter 52: Management of Patients With HIV Infection and AIDS*

**Janet A. Parkosewich, RN, MSN, CCRN, FAHA**
Cardiac Clinical Nurse Specialist
Yale-New Haven Hospital
New Haven, Connecticut
*Chapter 26: Assessment of Cardiovascular Function*

**Jana Perun, ARNP, AOCN**
Formerly, Nurse Practitioner
M. D. Anderson Cancer Center Orlando
Orlando, Florida
*Chapter 22: Management of Patients With Upper Respiratory Tract Disorders*
*Chapter 49: Assessment and Management of Problems Related to Male Reproductive Processes*

**Kimberly L. Quinn, RN, MSN, CCRN, ACNP, ANP**
Nurse Practitioner—Thoracic Surgery
Union Memorial Hospital
Baltimore, Maryland
*Chapter 35: Management of Patients With Oral and Esophageal Disorders*

**Patricia S. Regojo, RN, MSN**
Nurse Manager—Burn Unit
Temple University Hospital
Philadelphia, Pennsylvania
*Chapter 57: Management of Patients With Burn Injury*

**JoAnne Reifsnyder, PhD, APRN, BC-PCM**
Senior Vice President, Research
excelleRx, Inc.
Philadelphia, Pennsylvania
*Chapter 17: End-of-Life Care*

**Judith L. Reishtein, PhD, RN**
Assistant Professor
College of Nursing and Health Professions
Drexel University
Philadelphia, Pennsylvania
*Chapter 25: Respiratory Care Modalities*

**Susan Rokita, CRNP, MS**
Nurse Practitioner/Hematology Oncology
Milton S. Hershey Medical Center
Hershey, Pennsylvania
*Chapter 16: Oncology: Nursing Management in Cancer Care*

**Catherine Sackett, RN, BS, CANP**
Ophthalmic Research Nurse Practitioner
Wilmer Eye Institute
Retinal Vascular Center
The Johns Hopkins Medical Institutions
Baltimore, Maryland
*Chapter 58: Assessment and Management of Patients With Eye and Vision Disorders*

**Linda Schakenbach, MSN, RN, CNS, CCRN, CWCN, APRN, BC**
Clinical Nurse Specialist, Medical Cardiology
Inova Fairfax Hospital—Inova Heart and Vascular Institute
Falls Church, Virginia
*Chapter 29: Management of Patients With Structural, Infectious, and Inflammatory Cardiac Disorders*

**Suzanne C. Smeltzer, EdD, RN, FAAN**
Professor and Director, Center for Nursing Research
Villanova University College of Nursing
Villanova, Pennsylvania
*Chapter 10: Chronic Illness and Disability*
*Chapter 21: Assessment of Respiratory Function*
*Chapter 53: Assessment and Management of Patients With Allergic Disorders*

**Cathy Stanfield, MS, CRNP**
Acute Care Nurse Practitioner
Gastro-Intestinal Surgery Service
The John Hopkins Medical Institutions
Baltimore, Maryland
*Chapter 34: Assessment of Digestive and Gastrointestinal Function*

**Cindy Stern, RN, MSN**
Cancer Network Coordinator
University of Pennsylvania Cancer Center
University of Pennsylvania Health System
Philadelphia, Pennsylvania
*Chapter 16: Oncology: Nursing Management in Cancer Care*

**Caroline Steward, RN, MSN, APN C, CCRN, CNN**
Case Manager
Renaissance Health Care, Fresenius Medical Care North America
Broomfield, Colorado
*Chapter 43: Assessment of Renal and Urinary Tract Function*
*Chapter 44: Management of Patients With Kidney Disorders*
*Chapter 45: Management of Patients With Urinary Disorders*

**Christine Tea, RN, MSN**
Service Line Director
Main OR Perioperative Services
Inova Fairfax Hospital
Falls Church, Virginia
*Chapter 18: Preoperative Nursing Management*
*Chapter 19: Intraoperative Nursing Management*
*Chapter 20: Postoperative Nursing Management*

**Jean Smith Temple, DNS, RN**
Assistant Dean and Associate Professor
College of Nursing
Valdosta State University
Valdosta, Georgia
*Chapter 1: Health Care Delivery and Nursing Practice*

*Chapter 2: Community-Based Nursing Practice*
*Chapter 3: Critical Thinking, Ethical Decision Making, and the Nursing Process*
*Chapter 8: Perspectives in Transcultural Nursing*

**Mary Laudon Thomas, RN, MS, AOCN**
Hematology Clinical Nurse Specialist
Veterans Affairs Palo Alto Health Care System
Palo Alto, California
*Chapter 33: Assessment and Management of Patients With Hematologic Disorders*

**Renay D. Tyler, RN, MSN, ACNP, CNSN**
Acute Care Nurse Practitioner
The Johns Hopkins Hospital
Department of Surgical Nursing
Baltimore, Maryland
*Chapter 36: Gastrointestinal Intubation and Special Nutritional Modalities*

**Joan M. Webb, RN, MSN**
Instructor
Widener University, College of Nursing
Chester, Pennsylvania
*Chapter 42: Assessment and Management of Patients With Endocrine Disorders*

**Joyce S. Willens, PhD, RN, C**
Assistant Professor
Villanova University College of Nursing
Villanova, Pennsylvania
*Chapter 13: Pain Management*

**Iris Woodard, RN-CS, ANP**
Dermatology Nurse Practitioner
Kaiser Permanente
Springfield, Virginia
*Chapter 55: Assessment of Integumentary Function*
*Chapter 56: Management of Patients With Dermatologic Problems*

# Preface

As we complete the first half of the first decade of the 21st century, nursing continues to be influenced by the expansion of science and technology and by a myriad of social, cultural, economic, and environmental changes throughout the world. At the same time, today's nurses are faced with the many challenges that result from the acute shortage of nurses throughout health care settings. This worldwide nursing shortage has resulted in the need for nurses to have increasingly high levels of nursing knowledge and skills in meeting the acute care, long-term care, and health promotion needs of individuals and groups. Nurses must be particularly skilled in critical thinking and clinical decision-making as well as in consulting and collaborating with other members of the multidisciplinary health care team.

Along with the challenges that today's nurses confront, there are many opportunities for them to provide skilled, compassionate nursing care in a variety of health care settings, for patients in the various stages of illness, and for patients across the age continuum. At the same time, there are significant opportunities for fostering health promotion activities for individuals and groups; this is an integral part of providing nursing care.

This eleventh edition of *Brunner & Suddarth's Textbook of Medical-Surgical Nursing* is designed to assist nurses in preparing for their roles and responsibilities within the complex health care system. A goal of the textbook is to provide balanced attention to the art and science of adult medical-surgical nursing. The textbook focuses on physiologic, pathophysiologic, and psychosocial concepts as they relate to nursing care, and emphasis is placed on integrating a variety of concepts from other disciplines such as nutrition, pharmacology, and gerontology. Throughout the textbook particular emphasis has been placed on addressing the nursing care and health care needs of people with disabilities, identified in 2005 by the U.S. Surgeon General as a priority for the education and training of tomorrow's health care professionals. In addition, content relative to nursing research findings and evidence-based practice has been expanded to provide opportunities for the nurse to refine clinical decision-making skills.

## ORGANIZATION

*Brunner & Suddarth's Textbook of Medical-Surgical Nursing*, 11th edition, is organized into 16 units. Units 1 through 4 cover core concepts related to medical-surgical nursing practice. Units 5 through 16 discuss adult health conditions that are treated medically or surgically. Each unit covering adult health conditions is structured in the following way, to facilitate understanding:

- The first chapter in the unit covers assessment and includes a review of normal anatomy and physiology of the body system being discussed.
- The subsequent chapters in the unit cover management of specific disorders. Pathophysiology, clinical manifestations, assessment and diagnostic findings, medical management, and nursing management are presented. Special "Nursing Process" sections, provided for selected conditions, clarify and expand on the nurse's role in caring for patients with these conditions.

## FEATURES

### Practice-Oriented Features

Nurses assume many different roles when caring for patients. Many of the features in this textbook have been developed to help nurses fulfill these varied roles.

#### The Nurse as Practitioner

One of the central roles of the nurse is to provide holistic care to patients and their families, both independently and through collaboration with other health care professionals. Many features in *Brunner & Suddarth's Textbook of Medical-Surgical Nursing* are designed to assist students with clinical practice.

# PREFACE

**Nursing Process sections.** The nursing process is the basis for all nursing practice. Special sections throughout the text, organized according to the nursing process framework, clarify the nurse's responsibilities in caring for patients with selected disorders.

**Plans of Nursing Care.** These plans, provided for selected disorders, illustrate how the nursing process is applied to meet the person's health care and nursing needs.

**Applying Concepts from NANDA, NIC, and NOC.** Each unit begins with a case study and a chart presenting examples of NANDA, NIC, and NOC terminologies related to the case study. Concept maps, which provide a visual representation of the NANDA, NIC, and NOC chart for each case study, are found in Appendix C. This feature introduces the student to the NIC and NOC language and classifications and brings them to life in graphic form.

### Nursing Classifications and Languages

| NANDA Nursing Diagnoses | NIC Nursing Interventions | NOC Nursing Outcomes — Return to functional baseline status, stabilization of, or improvement in: |
|---|---|---|
| **Chronic Pain**—Unpleasant sensory and emotional experience arising from actual or potential tissue damage or described in terms of such damage; sudden or slow onset of any intensity from mild to severe, constant or recurring, without an anticipated or predictable end and a duration of greater than 6 months | **Pain Management**—Alleviation of pain or reduction in pain to a level of comfort that is acceptable to the patient | **Pain Level**—Severity of observed or reported pain |
| **Risk for Powerlessness**—At risk for perceived lack of control over a situation and/or one's ability to significantly affect an outcome | **Medication Management**—Facilitation of safe and effective use of prescribed or over-the-counter medicine | **Comfort Level**—Extent of positive perception of physical and psychological ease |
| | **Simple Relaxation Therapy**—Use of techniques to encourage and elicit relaxation for the purpose of decreasing undesirable signs and symptoms such as pain, muscle tension, or anxiety | **Pain Control**—Personal actions to control pain |
| | **Simple Guided Imagery**—Purposeful use of imagination to achieve relaxation and/or direct attention away from undesirable sensations | **Pain: Disruptive Effects**—Severity of observed or reported disruptive effects of chronic pain on daily functioning |
| | **Emotional Support**—Provision of reassurance, acceptance, and encouragement during times of stress | **Pain: Adverse Psychological Response**—Severity of observed or reported adverse responses to physical pain |
| | **Self-Esteem Enhancement**—Assisting a patient to increase his or her personal judgment of self-worth | |

NANDA International (2005). *Nursing diagnoses: Definitions & classification 2005–2006.* Philadelphia: North American Nursing Diagnosis Association.
Dochterman, J. M. & Bulechek, G. M. (2004). *Nursing interventions classification (NIC)* (4th ed.). St. Louis: Mosby.
Iowa Outcomes Project (2004). In Moorhead, S., Johnson, M. & Maas, M. (2004). *Nursing outcomes classification (NOC)* (3rd ed.). St. Louis: Mosby.
Dochterman, J. M. & Jones, D. A. (2003). *Unifying nursing languages: The harmonization of NANDA, NIC, and NOC.* Washington, D.C.: American Nurses Association.

**Assessment charts.** These charts help to focus the student's attention on data that should be collected as part of the assessment step of the nursing process.

### CHART 17-8

#### Assessing Symptoms Associated With Terminal Illness

- How is this symptom affecting the patient's life?
- What is the meaning of the symptom to the patient? To the family?
- How does the symptom affect physical functioning, mobility, comfort, sleep, nutritional status, elimination, activity level, and relationships with others?
- What makes the symptom better?
- What makes it worse?
- Is it worse at any particular time of the day?
- What are the patient's expectations and goals for managing the symptom? The family's?
- How is the patient coping with the symptom?
- What is the economic effect of the symptom and its management?

Adapted from Jacox, A., Carr, D. B., & Payne, R. (1994). *Management of cancer pain*. Rockville, MD: AHCPR.

### CHART 23-3

#### Risk Factors for Tuberculosis

- Close contact with someone who has active TB. Inhalation of airborne nuclei from an infected person is proportional to the amount of time spent in the same air space, the proximity of the person, and the degree of ventilation.
- Immunocompromised status (eg, those with HIV infection, cancer, transplanted organs, and prolonged high-dose corticosteroid therapy)
- Substance abuse (IV/injection drug users and alcoholics)
- Any person without adequate health care (the homeless; impoverished; minorities, particularly children under age 15 y and young adults between ages 15 and 44 y)
- Preexisting medical conditions or special treatment (eg, diabetes, chronic renal failure, malnourishment, selected malignancies, hemodialysis, transplanted organ, gastrectomy, jejunoileal bypass)
- Immigration from countries with a high prevalence of TB (southeastern Asia, Africa, Latin America, Caribbean)
- Institutionalization (eg, long-term care facilities, psychiatric institutions, prisons)
- Living in overcrowded, substandard housing
- Being a health care worker performing high-risk activities: administration of aerosolized pentamidine and other medications, sputum induction procedures,

**Risk Factor charts.** These charts draw the student's attention to factors that can impair health.

### CHART 25-9  Guidelines for Care of the Patient With a Tracheostomy Tube

| ACTIONS | RATIONALE |
|---|---|
| 1. Gather the needed equipment, including sterile gloves, hydrogen peroxide, normal saline solution or sterile water, cotton-tipped applicators, dressing and twill tape (and the type of tube prescribed, if the tube is to be changed). | Everything needed to care for a tracheostomy should be readily on hand for the most effective care. |
| A cuffed tube (air injected into cuff) is required during mechanical ventilation. A low-pressure cuff is most commonly used. | A cuffed tube prevents air from leaking during positive-pressure ventilation and also prevents tracheal aspiration of gastric contents. An adequate seal is indicated by the disappearance of any air leakage from the mouth or tracheostomy or by the disappearance of the harsh, gurgling sound of air coming from the throat. |
| Patients requiring long-term use of a tracheostomy tube and who can breathe spontaneously commonly | Low-pressure cuffs exert minimal pressure on the tracheal mucosa and thus reduce the danger of tracheal |

**Guidelines charts.** These charts review key nursing interventions, and the rationales for those interventions, for specific patient care situations.

**Pharmacology charts and tables.** Pharmacology charts and tables remind the student of important considerations relative to administering medications and monitoring drug therapy.

### TABLE 16-6  Antineoplastic Agents

| Drug Class and Examples | Mechanism of Action | Cell Cycle Specificity | Common Side Effects |
|---|---|---|---|
| **Alkylating Agents** | | | |
| Busulfan, carboplatin, chlorambucil, cisplatin, cyclophosphamide, dacarbazine, hexamethyl melamine, ifosfamide, melphalan, nitrogen mustard, oxaliplatin, thiotepa | Alter DNA structure by misreading DNA code, initiating breaks in the DNA molecule, cross-linking DNA strands | Cell cycle–nonspecific | Bone marrow suppression, nausea, vomiting, cystitis (cyclophosphamide, ifosfamide), stomatitis, alopecia, gonadal suppression, renal toxicity (cisplatin) |
| **Nitrosureas** | | | |
| Carmustine (BCNU), lomustine (CCNU), semustine (methyl CCNU), streptozocin | Similar to the alkylating agents; cross the blood–brain barrier | Cell cycle–nonspecific | Delayed and cumulative myelosuppression, especially thrombocytopenia; nausea, vomiting |
| **Topoisomerase I Inhibitors** | | | |
| Irinotecan, topotecan | Induce breaks in the DNA | Cell cycle–specific | Bone marrow suppression, |

**Nursing Alerts.** These special sections offer brief tips for clinical practice and red-flag warnings to help students avoid common mistakes.

**Gerontologic Considerations.** In the United States, older adults comprise the fastest-growing segment of the population. This icon  is applied to headings, charts, and tables as appropriate to highlight information that pertains specifically to the care of the older adult patient.

**Genetics in Nursing Practice charts.** These charts summarize and highlight the role that genetics play in many disorders.

**Physiology/Pathophysiology figures.** These illustrations and algorithms help students to understand normal physiologic and pathophysiologic processes.

## The Nurse as Educator

Health education is a primary responsibility of the nursing profession. Nursing care is directed toward promoting, maintaining, and restoring health; preventing illness; and helping patients and families adapt to the residual effects of illness. Teaching, in the form of patient education and health promotion, is central to all of these nursing activities.

**Patient Education charts.** These charts help the nurse to prepare the patient and family for procedures, assist them with understanding the patient's condition, and explain to them how to provide for self-care after discharge from the health care facility.

### CHART 18-4
#### Patient Education

**Preoperative Instructions to Prevent Postoperative Complications**

**DIAPHRAGMATIC BREATHING**
Diaphragmatic breathing refers to a flattening of the dome of the diaphragm during inspiration, with resultant enlargement of the upper abdomen as air rushes in. During expiration, the abdominal muscles contract.
1. Practice in the same position you would assume in bed after surgery: a semi-Fowler's position, propped in bed with the back and shoulders well supported with pillows.
2. With your hands in a loose-fist position, allow the hands to rest lightly on the front of the lower ribs, with your fingertips against lower chest to feel the movement.
3. Breathe with the diaphragm as described under "Diaphragmatic Breathing."
4. With your mouth slightly open, breathe in fully.
5. "Hack" out sharply for three short breaths.
6. Then, keeping your mouth open, take in a quick deep breath and immediately give a strong cough once or twice. This helps clear secretions from your chest. It may cause some discomfort but will not harm your incision.

**LEG EXERCISES**
1. Lie in a semi-Fowler's position and perform the following simple exercises to improve circulation.
2. Bend your knee and raise your foot—hold it a few seconds, then extend the leg and lower it to the bed.

Diaphragmatic breathing

Leg exercises

### CHART 23-8
#### HOME CARE CHECKLIST • Prevention of Recurrent Pulmonary Embolism

| At the completion of the home care instruction, the patient or caregiver will be able to: | Patient | Caregiver |
|---|---|---|
| • Describe the underlying process leading to pulmonary embolism. | ✔ | ✔ |
| • Describe the need for continued anticoagulant therapy after the initial embolism. | ✔ | ✔ |
| • Name the anticoagulant prescribed and identify dosage and schedule of administration. | ✔ | ✔ |
| • Describe potential side effects of coagulation such as bruising and bleeding and identify ways to prevent bleeding. | ✔ | ✔ |
|    • Avoid the use of sharps (razors, knives, etc.) to prevent cuts; shave with an electric shaver. | | |
|    • Use a toothbrush with soft bristles to prevent gum injury. | | |
|    • Do not take aspirin or antihistamines while taking warfarin sodium (Coumadin). | | |

**Home Care checklists.** These checklists review points that should be covered as part of patient education prior to discharge from the health care facility.

**Health Promotion charts.** These charts review important points that the nurse should discuss with the patient to prevent common health problems from developing.

### CHART 16-2
#### Health Promotion

**Reducing Cancer Risk**

- Encourage patients to increase consumption of fresh vegetables (especially those of the cabbage family) because studies indicate that roughage and vitamin-rich foods help to prevent certain kinds of cancer.
- Encourage increased fiber intake because high-fiber diets may reduce the risk for certain cancers (eg, breast, prostate, and colon).
- Recommend increased intake of vitamin A, which reduces the risk for esophageal, laryngeal, and lung cancers.
- Recommend increased intake of foods rich in vitamin C, such as citrus fruits and broccoli, which are thought to protect against stomach and esophageal
- Advise patients to reduce intake of dietary fat because a high-fat diet increases the risk for breast, colon, and prostate cancers.
- Recommend moderation in consumption of salt-cured, smoked, and nitrate-cured foods; these have been linked to esophageal and gastric cancers.
- Advise patients to stop smoking cigarettes and cigars, which are carcinogens.
- Advise patients to reduce alcohol intake because drinking large amounts of alcohol increases the risk of liver cancer. (*Note:* People who drink heavily and smoke are at greater risk for cancers of the mouth, throat, larynx, and esophagus.)

### The Nurse as Patient Advocate

Nurses advocate for patients by protecting their rights (including the right to health care) and assisting patients and their families to make informed decisions about health care.

**Ethics and Related Issues charts.** These charts present a scenario, a description of potential ethical dilemmas that could arise as a result of the scenario, and a list of questions about the scenario to stimulate thought and discussion.

### The Nurse as Researcher

Nurses identify potential research problems and questions to increase nursing knowledge and improve patient care. Use and evaluation of research findings in nursing practice are essential to further the science of nursing.

**Nursing Research Profiles.** These charts identify the implications and applications of nursing research findings for nursing practice.

**Evidence-Based Practice (EBP) questions.** This icon  appears next to critical thinking exercises that encourage the student to think about the evidence base for specific nursing interventions. A journals supplement (new to the 11th edition) offers students free on-line access to over 70 journal articles that relate to the evidence-based practice questions in the text.

---

**CHART 11-1**

### Ethics and Related Issues

**Are All Persons Entitled to Rehabilitation?**

**SITUATION**
You work in an area where many illegal aliens and uninsured residents live. Community violence often creates life-threatening and disabling conditions in members of the population. After a victim of violence has been saved and stabilized, the health care team identifies rehabilitation needs. You are concerned about your patient's inability to perform self-care and to demonstrate safe mobility skills.

**DILEMMA**
As a health care provider, you are concerned about the community as a whole; costs to the community, and the values of the community. You are also aware of client fiduciary responsibility; you recognize costs to your patient when treatment is provided or not provided.

**DISCUSSION**

---

### NURSING RESEARCH PROFILE

#### The Effect of Preoperative Teaching on Outcomes

Oetker-Black, S. L., Jones, S., Estok, P., et al. (2003). Preoperative teaching and hysterectomy outcomes. *AORN Journal, 77*(6), 1215–1231.

**Purpose**
This study used a theoretical model of self-efficacy to determine whether an efficacy-enhancing teaching protocol was effective in improving immediate postoperative behaviors and selected short- and long-term health outcomes in women who underwent abdominal hysterectomy.

**Design**
A sample of 108 women admitted to a 486-bed teaching hospital in the Midwest for total abdominal hysterectomy was obtained by convenience sampling. Data collectors used the operating room schedule to identify potential participants based on pre-determined criteria (eg, age, able to read English, alert and oriented). Those willing to participate in the 6-month study were randomly assigned to one of the study groups and received either the usual care protocol or the efficacy-enhancing teaching protocol. The efficacy-enhancing group received enhanced preoperative teaching. Sessions stressed the importance of early ambulation, included a detailed demonstration of the effective way to get out of bed, and required that participants demonstrate how to get out of bed.

**Findings**
There were no significant differences found between groups except in ambulation. Patients who received the efficacy-enhancing teaching ambulated significantly longer than those in the usual care group (330 seconds compared to a mean of 56 seconds).

**Nursing Implications**
The most common postoperative complications of hysterectomy or any major abdominal surgery are atelectasis, pneumonia, paralytic ileus, and deep vein thrombosis. Studies have previously shown that postoperative ambulation decreases or prevents all these complications. By incorporating enhanced preoperative patient instruction with return demonstrations, perioperative nurses can improve patients' postoperative ambulation.

---

### Critical Thinking Exercises

1. An 80-year-old patient with Parkinson's disease is scheduled for surgery to replace a fractured hip. Identify the considerations and associated responsibilities of the OR nurse for safe intraoperative care of this patient.

2. **ebp** A patient has a large open lower-extremity wound caused by a motorcycle accident and is undergoing emergency surgery. What resources would you use to identify the current guidelines for surgical asepsis? What is the evidence base for current patient and environmental surgical asepsis practices? Identify the criteria used to evaluate the strength of the evidence for these practices.

3. A patient develops a temperature of 38°C (100°F) and becomes tachycardic halfway through an abdominal surgery. Five minutes later, the patient's temperature is 42°C (104°F). Describe the protocol you would follow and the medication you would administer for this condition.

4. **ebp** A patient with an infected wound is undergoing an incision and drainage in the OR. Develop an evidence-based plan of care that will reduce the risk of contamination and infection.

---

## Pedagogical Features

**Learning Objectives.** Each chapter begins with a list of learning objectives. These give the student an overview of the chapter and help to focus his or her reading.

**Glossaries.** Glossaries provided at the beginning of each chapter let the student review vocabulary words before reading the chapter, and also serve as a useful reference tool while reading.

**Critical Thinking Exercises.** These questions, which appear at the end of each chapter, foster critical thinking by challenging the student to apply textbook knowledge to clinical scenarios.

**References and Selected Readings.** A list of current references cited and a bibliography are given at the end of each chapter.

**Resources.** A resource list at the end of each chapter directs the reader to sources of additional information, websites, agencies, and patient education materials.

## A COMPREHENSIVE PACKAGE FOR TEACHING AND LEARNING

To further facilitate teaching and learning, a carefully designed ancillary package is available. In addition to the usual print resources, we are pleased to present multimedia tools that have been developed in conjunction with the text.

### Resources for Students

**Interactive CD-ROM.** Packaged with the textbook at no additional charge, this CD helps students test their knowledge and enhance their understanding of medical-surgical nursing. This CD includes:

- 500 self-study questions organized by unit
- 3000 bonus NCLEX-style cross-disciplinary questions
- CONCEPTS in action ANIMATION Concepts in Action™ Animations
- Nursing in Action™ Video: Performing a Physical Examination
- Clinical Simulations
- Bonus Tutorials on fluids and electrolytes and NCLEX alternate-format items
- Spanish-English Audioglossary

**Study Guide to Accompany Smeltzer, Bare, Hinkle & Cheever: Brunner & Suddarth's Textbook of Medical-Surgical Nursing, 11th edition.** Available at student bookstores or at www.LWW.com, this study guide presents a variety of exercises to reinforce the textbook content and enhance learning.

**Handbook to Accompany Smeltzer, Bare, Hinkle & Cheever: Brunner & Suddarth's Textbook of Medical-Surgical Nursing, 11th edition.** Available at student bookstores or at www.LWW.com, this clinical reference presents need-to-know information on nearly 200 commonly encountered disorders in an easy-to-use alphabetized outline format.

### Resources for Instructors

**Instructor's Resource CD-ROM.** The instructor's resource CD contains the following items:

- A thoroughly revised and augmented test generator, containing 2100 NCLEX-style questions
- Sample syllabi for 1-semester, 2-semester, and 3-semester courses
- Strategies for effective teaching
- PowerPoint™ lectures, guided lecture notes, and prelecture quizzes
- An image bank
- Discussion topics and assignments

**Partners in Education.** This service is available to assist with faculty development, technology training, curriculum development, and more.

### Resources for Students and Instructors

**thePoint ThePoint\*** (http://thepoint.lww.com) is a web-based course and content management system that provides every resource instructors and students need in one easy-to-use site. Advanced technology and superior content combine at thePoint to allow instructors to design and deliver on-line and off-line courses, maintain grades and class rosters, and communicate with students. Students can visit thePoint to access supplemental multimedia resources to enhance their learning experience, check the course syllabus, download content, upload assignments, and join an on-line study group. ThePoint . . . where teaching, learning, and technology click!

**LiveAdvise Student Online Tutorial Service.** This service, powered by Smarthinking™, provides on-line tutoring and assistance for students and instructors. Med-Surg instructors are available Sunday through Thursday, 8:30 P.M. to 11:30 P.M., to assist with questions.

**MyPowerLearning** is a learning styles assessment and assistance service for instructors and students.

It is with pleasure that we introduce these resources—the textbook and the ancillary package—to you. One of our primary goals in creating these resources has been to help prepare nursing students to provide quality care to patients and families across health care settings and in the home. We hope that we have succeeded in that goal, and we welcome feedback from our readers.

*Suzanne C. O'Connell Smeltzer, EdD, RN, FAAN*
*Brenda G. Bare, RN, MSN*
*Janice L. Hinkle, PhD, RN, CNRN*
*Kerry H. Cheever, PhD, RN*

\*thePoint is a trademark of Wolters Kluwer Health.

# Reviewers

**Elizabeth A. (Libby) Archer, EdD, RN**
Associate Professor
Baptist College of Health Sciences
Memphis, Tennessee

**Liz Aycock, RN, BSN, MSN**
Associate Professor of Nursing
Middle Georgia College
Cochran, Georgia

**Roberta P. Bartee, MS, RNc**
Assistant Professor, Charity School of Nursing
Delgado Community College
New Orleans, Louisiana

**Barbara J. Bloink, RN, BSN, MSN**
Professor
St. Clair County Community College
Port Huron, Michigan

**Diane M. Breckenridge, PhD, RN**
Associate Professor
LaSalle University
Philadelphia, Pennsylvania
Associate Research Director
Abington Memorial Hospital
Abington, Pennsylvania

**Sandra Drozdz Burke, PhD, APRN, CDE, BC-ADM**
BroMenn Assistant Professor
Illinois State University
Mennonite College of Nursing
Normal, Illinois

**Lisa Burkhart, MPH, PhD, RN**
Assistant Professor
Marcella Niehoff School of Nursing
Loyola University Chicago
Chicago, Illinois

**Susan E. Caulkins, MSN, CS, FNP**
ADN Nursing Instructor
Central Carolina Technical College
Sumter, South Carolina

**Marty J. Chamot, MSN, RN**
Professor of Nursing
Jackson Community College
Jackson, Michigan

**Joy Churchill, RN, MSN**
Associate Professor of Nursing
Northern Kentucky University
Highland Heights, Kentucky

**Pattie Clark, RN, MSN**
Associate Professor and Nursing Outreach Coordinator
Abraham Baldwin College
Tifton, Georgia

**John D. Colbath, MSN, MBA, RNC**
Professor of Nursing and Department Chairman
New Hampshire Community Technical College
Berlin, New Hampshire

**Lora Crowe, RN, MSN, FNP**
Assistant Professor
Macon State College
Macon, Georgia

**Jan Fletcher, RN, MNSc, CEN**
Assistant Professor of Nursing
Arkansas Tech University
Russellville, Arkansas

**Mary Catherine Gebhardt, RN, PhD, CRRN**
Assistant Professor
Byrdine F. Lewis School of Nursing at Georgia State University
Atlanta, Georgia

**Bonnie Higgins, EdD, MS, BS, RN, CMSRN**
Professor
Tarrant County College
Fort Worth, Texas

**Jane Hook, RN, BSN, MSN**
Lecturer/Coordinator Medical Surgical Faculty
California State University, Los Angeles
Los Angeles, California

**Sara M. Howell, RN, MSN**
Assistant Professor of Nursing, ASN Program
Mississippi University for Woman
Columbus, Mississippi

**Brenda Jordan, RN, MSN**
Instructor in Associate Degree Nursing
South Plains College
Levelland, Texas

**Eileen Kaslatas, BSN, MSN, RN**
Professor
Macomb County Community College
Clinton Township, Michigan

**Colleen Kiberd, RN, BN, MEd, MN**
Assistant Professor
Dalhousie University
School of Nursing
Halifax, Nova Scotia

**Mary F. King, RN, BSN, MS**
Level Coordinator, Associate Degree Instructor
Phillips Community College of the University of Arkansas
West Helena, Arkansas

**Cathy MacDonald, MN**
Assistant Professor
Saint Francis Xavier University
Antigonish, Nova Scotia

**Rosemary Macy, RN, MS**
Assistant Professor
Boise State University
Boise, Idaho

**Cecilia Jane Maier, MS, RN, CCRN**
Assistant Professor
Mount Carmel College of Nursing
Columbus, Ohio

**Linda Moore, RN/MSN, CCRN**
Assistant Professor
St. Philip's College
San Antonio, Texas

**Ann Powers-Prather, PhD, RN**
Faculty, Coordinator Research and Evaluation
El Centro College
Dallas, Texas

**Miley O. Pulliam, RN, MSN**
Associate Degree Nursing Instructor
McLennan Community College
Waco, Texas

**Diane Reynolds, RN, MS, OCN, CNE**
Assistant Professor of Nursing
Long Island University
Brooklyn, New York

**Mattie L. Rhodes, PhD, RN**
Clinical Associate Professor, Nursing
State University New York at Buffalo
Buffalo, New York

**Buckie Sasser, RN, MSN**
Assistant Professor of Nursing
South Georgia College
Douglas, Georgia

**Katherine Saulnier, BScN, RN, CCNP**
Clinical Associate
Saint Francis Xavier University
Antigonish, Nova Scotia

**Donna Schutte, RN, DNSc**
Associate Professor, Nursing
Riverside Community College
Riverside, California

**Debra P. Shelton, MSN, RN, CAN, OCN**
Assistant Professor
Northwestern State University College of Nursing
Shreveport, Louisiana

**Mary B. Wiese, RN, MSEd**
Associate Professor
Ivy Tech State College
Lafayette, Indiana

**Regina L. Wright, MSN, RN, CEN**
Clinical Assistant Professor
Drexel University
Philadelphia, Pennsylvania

# Contents

## UNIT 1
## Basic Concepts in Nursing . . . . . . . . . 2

### CHAPTER 1
### Health Care Delivery and Nursing Practice  4

**THE HEALTH CARE INDUSTRY AND THE NURSING PROFESSION  5**
Nursing Defined  5
The Patient/Client: Consumer of Nursing and Health Care  5
Health Care in Transition  5
**HEALTH, WELLNESS, AND HEALTH PROMOTION  6**
Health  6
Wellness  6
Health Promotion  6
**INFLUENCES ON HEALTH CARE DELIVERY  7**
Population Demographics  7
Changing Patterns of Disease  7
Advances in Technology and Genetics  8
Economic Changes  8
Demand for Quality Health Care  8
Alternative Health Care Delivery Systems  9
**ROLES OF THE NURSE  10**
Practitioner Role  10
Leadership Role  10
Research Role  10
**MODELS OF NURSING CARE DELIVERY  11**
Primary Nursing  11
Community-Based Nursing and Community-Oriented/Public Health Nursing  11
**EXPANDED NURSING ROLES  12**
Collaborative Practice  13

### CHAPTER 2
### Community-Based Nursing Practice  15

**THE GROWING NEED FOR COMMUNITY-BASED HEALTH CARE  16**
Community-Based Care  16
Home Health Care  17
**COMMUNITY-BASED NURSING  18**
**DISCHARGE PLANNING FOR HOME CARE  18**
**COMMUNITY RESOURCES AND REFERRALS  18**
**HOME HEALTH VISITS  19**
Preparing for a Home Visit  19
Conducting a Home Visit  19

**OTHER COMMUNITY-BASED HEALTH CARE SETTINGS  21**
Ambulatory Settings  21
Occupational Health Programs  21
School Health Programs  21
Community Nurse–Managed Centers  22
Care for the Homeless  22

### CHAPTER 3
### Critical Thinking, Ethical Decision Making, and the Nursing Process  24

**CRITICAL THINKING  25**
Definition  25
Rationality and Insight  25
Components of Critical Thinking  25
Critical Thinking in Nursing Practice  26
**ETHICAL NURSING CARE  27**
Ethics Versus Morality  27
Ethics Theories  27
Approaches to Ethics  27
Moral Situations  27
Types of Ethical Problems in Nursing  29
Preventive Ethics  33
Ethical Decision Making  33
**THE NURSING PROCESS  34**
Definition  34
Using the Nursing Process  35

### CHAPTER 4
### Health Education and Health Promotion  48

**HEALTH EDUCATION TODAY  49**
Purpose of Health Education  49
**ADHERENCE TO THE THERAPEUTIC REGIMEN  50**
**THE NATURE OF TEACHING AND LEARNING  50**
Learning Readiness  51
The Learning Environment  52
Teaching Techniques  52
Teaching People With Disabilities  52
**THE NURSING PROCESS IN PATIENT TEACHING  54**
Assessment  54
Nursing Diagnosis  54
Planning  54
Implementation  55
Evaluation  56
**HEALTH PROMOTION  56**
Definition  56
Health and Wellness  57

Health Promotion Models 57
Components of Health Promotion 57
**HEALTH PROMOTION THROUGHOUT THE LIFE SPAN** 58
Children and Adolescents 58
Young and Middle-Aged Adults 59
**NURSING IMPLICATIONS** 61

## CHAPTER 5
### Health Assessment 63

**THE ROLE OF THE NURSE IN HEALTH ASSESSMENT** 64
**BASIC GUIDELINES FOR CONDUCTING A HEALTH ASSESSMENT** 64
**ETHICAL USE OF HISTORY OR PHYSICAL EXAMINATION DATA** 64
**INCREASING USE OF TECHNOLOGY** 64
**THE HEALTH HISTORY** 65
The Informant 65
Cultural Considerations 65
Content of the Health History 66
Other Health History Formats 73
**PHYSICAL ASSESSMENT** 74
Inspection 74
Palpation 75
Percussion 76
Auscultation 76
**NUTRITIONAL ASSESSMENT** 77
Body Mass Index 77
Biochemical Assessment 78
Clinical Examination 80
Dietary Data 80
Factors Influencing Nutritional Status in Various Situations 83
Analysis of Nutritional Status 83
**ASSESSMENT IN THE HOME AND COMMUNITY** 84

# UNIT 2
# Biophysical and Psychosocial Concepts in Nursing Practice....88

## CHAPTER 6
### Homeostasis, Stress, and Adaptation 90

**STRESS AND FUNCTION** 91
**DYNAMIC BALANCE: THE STEADY STATE** 91
**STRESS AND ADAPTATION** 92
**STRESS: THREATS TO THE STEADY STATE** 92
Types of Stressors 92
Stress as a Stimulus for Disease 93
Psychological Responses to Stress 93
Physiologic Response to Stress 94
Maladaptive Responses to Stress 97
Indicators of Stress 98
Nursing Implications 98
**STRESS AT THE CELLULAR LEVEL** 99
Control of the Steady State 99
Cellular Adaptation 100
Cellular Injury 101
Cellular Response to Injury: Inflammation 103

Cellular Healing 104
Nursing Implications 104
**STRESS MANAGEMENT: NURSING INTERVENTIONS** 104
Promoting a Healthy Lifestyle 105
Enhancing Coping Strategies 105
Teaching Relaxation Techniques 105
Educating About Stress Management 107
Enhancing Social Support 107
Recommending Support and Therapy Groups 108

## CHAPTER 7
### Individual and Family Considerations Related to Illness 111

**HOLISTIC APPROACH TO HEALTH AND HEALTH CARE** 112
**THE BRAIN AND PHYSICAL AND EMOTIONAL HEALTH** 113
**EMOTIONAL HEALTH AND EMOTIONAL DISTRESS** 114
**FAMILY HEALTH AND DISTRESS** 115
Nursing Implications 115
**ANXIETY** 116
Nursing Implications 116
**POSTTRAUMATIC STRESS DISORDER** 116
Nursing Implications 117
**DEPRESSION** 118
Nursing Implications 118
**SUBSTANCE ABUSE** 120
Nursing Implications 120
**LOSS AND GRIEF** 121
Nursing Implications 122
**DEATH AND DYING** 122
**SPIRITUALITY AND SPIRITUAL DISTRESS** 122
Nursing Implications 123

## CHAPTER 8
### Perspectives in Transcultural Nursing 127

**CULTURAL CONCEPTS** 128
Subcultures 128
Minorities 129
**TRANSCULTURAL NURSING** 129
Culturally Competent Nursing Care 129
Cross-Cultural Communication 130
**CULTURALLY MEDIATED CHARACTERISTICS** 131
Space and Distance 132
Eye Contact 132
Time 132
Touch 132
Observance of Holidays 133
Diet 133
Biologic Variations 133
Complementary and Alternative Therapies 134
**CAUSES OF ILLNESS** 134
Biomedical or Scientific 134
Naturalistic or Holistic 135
Magico-Religious 135
**FOLK HEALERS** 135
**CULTURAL ASSESSMENT** 135
**ADDITIONAL CULTURAL CONSIDERATIONS: KNOW THYSELF** 136
**HEALTH DISPARITIES** 136
**THE FUTURE OF TRANSCULTURAL NURSING CARE** 136

## CHAPTER 9
### Genetics Perspectives in Nursing   139

**FRAMEWORK FOR INTEGRATING GENETICS INTO NURSING PRACTICE**   141
**GENETICS CONCEPTS**   141
Genes and Their Role in Human Variation   141
Inheritance Patterns   145
Chromosomal Differences and Genetic Conditions   148
**CLINICAL APPLICATIONS OF GENETICS**   149
Genetic Testing   149
Genetic Screening   149
Testing and Screening for Adult-Onset Conditions   149
Individualizing Genetic Profiles and Pharmacogenetics   153
**APPLICATIONS OF GENETICS IN NURSING PRACTICE**   154
Genetics and Health Assessment   154
Genetic Counseling and Evaluation Services   156
**ETHICAL ISSUES**   160

## CHAPTER 10
### Chronic Illness and Disability   165

**OVERVIEW OF CHRONICITY**   166
Definition of Chronic Conditions   166
Prevalence and Causes of Chronic Conditions   167
Characteristics of Chronic Conditions   167
Implications of Managing Chronic Conditions   168
Phases of Chronic Conditions   169
**NURSING CARE OF PATIENTS WITH CHRONIC CONDITIONS**   169
Applying the Nursing Process Using the Phases of the Chronic Illness System   170
Home and Community-Based Care   172
Nursing Care for Special Populations With Chronic Illness   174
**OVERVIEW OF DISABILITY**   174
Definitions of Disability   174
Prevalence of Disability   175
Characteristics of Disability   175
Federal Legislation   176
**RIGHT OF ACCESS TO HEALTH CARE**   177
Barriers to Health Care   182
Federal Assistance Programs   182
**NURSING CARE OF PATIENTS WITH DISABILITIES**   183
Nursing Considerations During Hospitalization   183
Health Promotion and Prevention   183
Significance of "People-First" Language   184
Gerontologic Considerations   184
Disability in Medical-Surgical Nursing Practice   184
Home and Community-Based Care   185

## CHAPTER 11
### Principles and Practices of Rehabilitation   189

**AMERICANS WITH DISABILITIES ACT**   191
**PATIENTS' REACTIONS TO DISABILITY**   191
**THE REHABILITATION TEAM**   191
**AREAS OF SPECIALTY REHABILITATION**   192
**ASSESSMENT OF FUNCTIONAL ABILITY**   193
▶▶ Nursing Process: The Patient With Self-Care Deficits in Activities of Daily Living   193
▶▶ Nursing Process: The Patient With Impaired Physical Mobility   195
▶▶ Nursing Process: The Patient With Impaired Skin Integrity   207
▶▶ Nursing Process: The Patient With Altered Elimination Patterns   215
**DISABILITY AND SEXUALITY ISSUES**   218
**FATIGUE**   218
**COMPLEMENTARY AND ALTERNATIVE THERAPIES**   219
**PROMOTING HOME AND COMMUNITY-BASED CARE**   219
Teaching Patients Self-Care   219
Continuing Care   221

## CHAPTER 12
### Health Care of the Older Adult   224

**OVERVIEW OF AGING**   225
Demographics of Aging   225
Health Status of the Older Adult   226
Nursing Care of the Older Adult   226
Theories of Aging   227
**AGE-RELATED CHANGES**   228
Psychosocial Aspects of Aging   228
Physical Aspects of Aging   230
Cognitive Aspects of Aging   237
Pharmacologic Aspects of Aging   237
**MENTAL HEALTH PROBLEMS IN THE OLDER ADULT**   238
Depression   238
Delirium   240
Dementia   243
**COMMON HEALTH ISSUES OF THE OLDER ADULT**   246
Impaired Mobility   246
Dizziness   247
Falls and Falling   247
Urinary Incontinence   247
Increased Susceptibility to Infection   248
Altered Pain and Febrile Responses   248
Altered Emotional Impact   248
Altered Systemic Response   249
**OTHER ASPECTS OF HEALTH CARE OF THE OLDER ADULT**   249
Elder Neglect and Abuse   249
Social Services   249
Health Care Costs of Aging   249
Home Health Care   250
Hospice Services   250
Aging With a Disability   250
**ETHICAL AND LEGAL ISSUES AFFECTING THE OLDER ADULT**   251

# UNIT 3
# Concepts and Challenges in Patient Management . . . . . . . . . . . 256

## CHAPTER 13
### Pain Management   258

**PAIN: THE FIFTH VITAL SIGN**   259
**TYPES OF PAIN**   260
Acute Pain   260
Chronic Pain   260
Cancer-Related Pain   262

Pain Classified by Location   262
Pain Classified by Etiology   262
**HARMFUL EFFECTS OF PAIN**   263
Effects of Acute Pain   263
Effects of Chronic Pain   264
**PATHOPHYSIOLOGY OF PAIN**   264
Pain Transmission   264
Factors Influencing Pain Response   266
**NURSING ASSESSMENT OF PAIN**   270
Characteristics of Pain   270
Instruments for Assessing the Perception of Pain   273
The Nurse's Role in Pain Management   276
**PAIN MANAGEMENT STRATEGIES**   277
Pharmacologic Interventions   277
Routes of Administration   285
Nonpharmacologic Interventions   289
**NEUROLOGIC AND NEUROSURGICAL APPROACHES TO PAIN MANAGEMENT**   291
Stimulation Procedures   291
**PROMOTING HOME AND COMMUNITY-BASED CARE**   292
Teaching Patients Self-Care   292
Continuing Care   295
**EVALUATING PAIN MANAGEMENT STRATEGIES**   295

# CHAPTER 14
## Fluid and Electrolytes: Balance and Disturbances   300

**FUNDAMENTAL CONCEPTS**   301
**FLUID VOLUME DISTURBANCES: HYPOVOLEMIA**   308
**FLUID VOLUME DISTURBANCES: HYPERVOLEMIA**   313
**ELECTROLYTE IMBALANCES**   315
Sodium Imbalances   315
Potassium Imbalances   321
Calcium Imbalances   325
Magnesium Imbalances   329
Phosphorus Imbalances   331
Chloride Imbalances   333
**ACID–BASE DISTURBANCES**   334
Acute and Chronic Metabolic Acidosis (Base Bicarbonate Deficit)   335
Acute and Chronic Metabolic Alkalosis (Base Bicarbonate Excess)   336
Acute and Chronic Respiratory Acidosis (Carbonic Acid Excess)   336
Acute and Chronic Respiratory Alkalosis (Carbonic Acid Deficit)   337
Mixed Acid–Base Disorders   338
**PARENTERAL FLUID THERAPY**   338

# CHAPTER 15
## Shock and Multisystem Failure   355

**SHOCK AND ITS SIGNIFICANCE**   356
**CONDITIONS PRECIPITATING SHOCK**   356
**STAGES OF SHOCK**   358
Compensatory Stage   358
Progressive Stage   361
Irreversible Stage   363
**OVERALL MANAGEMENT STRATEGIES IN SHOCK**   364
**HYPOVOLEMIC SHOCK**   366
**CARDIOGENIC SHOCK**   368
**CIRCULATORY SHOCK**   371
**SEPTIC SHOCK**   372
**NEUROGENIC SHOCK**   375

**ANAPHYLACTIC SHOCK**   376
**MULTIPLE ORGAN DYSFUNCTION SYNDROME**   376
**PROMOTING HOME AND COMMUNITY-BASED CARE**   377

# CHAPTER 16
## Oncology: Nursing Management in Cancer Care   380

**EPIDEMIOLOGY OF CANCER**   381
**PATHOPHYSIOLOGY OF THE MALIGNANT PROCESS**   383
**DETECTION AND PREVENTION OF CANCER**   388
**DIAGNOSIS OF CANCER AND RELATED NURSING CONSIDERATIONS**   389
**MANAGEMENT OF CANCER**   391
▶▶ Nursing Process: The Patient With Cancer   423
**CANCER REHABILITATION**   434
**GERONTOLOGIC CONSIDERATIONS**   436
**CARE OF THE PATIENT WITH ADVANCED CANCER**   437
**ONCOLOGIC EMERGENCIES**   437

# CHAPTER 17
## End-of-Life Care   447

**NURSING AND END-OF-LIFE CARE**   448
**SETTINGS FOR END-OF-LIFE CARE: PALLIATIVE CARE PROGRAMS AND HOSPICE**   452
**NURSING CARE OF TERMINALLY ILL PATIENTS**   456
**NURSING CARE OF PATIENTS WHO ARE CLOSE TO DEATH**   468
**COPING WITH DEATH AND DYING: PROFESSIONAL CAREGIVER ISSUES**   473

# UNIT 4
## Perioperative Concepts and Nursing Management . . . . . . . . . 478

# CHAPTER 18
## Preoperative Nursing Management   480

**PERIOPERATIVE AND PERIANESTHESIA NURSING**   481
**SURGICAL CLASSIFICATIONS**   484
**PREPARATION FOR SURGERY**   484
**SPECIAL SITUATIONS**   491
**PREOPERATIVE NURSING INTERVENTIONS**   492
**EXPECTED PATIENT OUTCOMES**   499

# CHAPTER 19
## Intraoperative Nursing Management   502

**THE SURGICAL TEAM**   503
**THE SURGICAL ENVIRONMENT**   505
**THE SURGICAL EXPERIENCE**   508
**POTENTIAL INTRAOPERATIVE COMPLICATIONS**   516
Nausea and Vomiting   516
Anaphylaxis   516
Hypoxia and Other Respiratory Complications   516
Hypothermia   517

Malignant Hyperthermia  517
Disseminated Intravascular Coagulopathy  517
▶▶ Nursing Process: The Patient During Surgery  518

## CHAPTER 20
### Postoperative Nursing Management  523

**THE POSTANESTHESIA CARE UNIT**  524
**THE HOSPITALIZED POSTOPERATIVE PATIENT**  531
▶▶ Nursing Process: The Hospitalized Patient Recovering From Surgery  532

# UNIT 5
# Gas Exchange and Respiratory Function .......... 550

## CHAPTER 21
### Assessment of Respiratory Function  552

**ANATOMIC AND PHYSIOLOGIC OVERVIEW**  553
**ASSESSMENT**  563
**DIAGNOSTIC EVALUATION**  578

## CHAPTER 22
### Management of Patients With Upper Respiratory Tract Disorders  588

**UPPER AIRWAY INFECTIONS**  589
Rhinitis  589
Viral Rhinitis (Common Cold)  591
Acute Sinusitis  593
Chronic Sinusitis  595
Acute Pharyngitis  597
Chronic Pharyngitis  598
Tonsillitis and Adenoiditis  599
Peritonsillar Abscess  600
Laryngitis  601
▶▶ Nursing Process: The Patient With Upper Airway Infection  601
**OBSTRUCTION AND TRAUMA OF THE UPPER RESPIRATORY AIRWAY**  604
Obstruction During Sleep  604
Epistaxis (Nosebleed)  605
Nasal Obstruction  606
Fractures of the Nose  607
Laryngeal Obstruction  608
Cancer of the Larynx  608
▶▶ Nursing Process: The Patient Undergoing Laryngectomy  614

## CHAPTER 23
### Management of Patients With Chest and Lower Respiratory Tract Disorders  624

**ATELECTASIS**  625
**RESPIRATORY INFECTIONS**  628
Acute Tracheobronchitis  628
Pneumonia  628
▶▶ Nursing Process: The Patient With Pneumonia  639
Severe Acute Respiratory Syndrome  643
Pulmonary Tuberculosis  643
▶▶ Nursing Process: The Patient With Tuberculosis  648
Lung Abscess  650
**PLEURAL CONDITIONS**  652
Pleurisy  652
Pleural Effusion  652
Empyema  654
**PULMONARY EDEMA**  655
**ACUTE RESPIRATORY FAILURE**  655
**ACUTE RESPIRATORY DISTRESS SYNDROME**  656
**PULMONARY ARTERIAL HYPERTENSION**  659
**PULMONARY HEART DISEASE (COR PULMONALE)**  660
**PULMONARY EMBOLISM**  662
**SARCOIDOSIS**  667
**OCCUPATIONAL LUNG DISEASES: PNEUMOCONIOSES**  668
Silicosis  668
Asbestosis  669
Coal Worker's Pneumoconiosis  669
**CHEST TUMORS**  670
Lung Cancer (Bronchogenic Carcinoma)  670
Tumors of the Mediastinum  674
**CHEST TRAUMA**  675
Blunt Trauma  675
Penetrating Trauma: Gunshot and Stab Wounds  678
Pneumothorax  678
Cardiac Tamponade  680
Subcutaneous Emphysema  680
**ASPIRATION**  681

## CHAPTER 24
### Management of Patients With Chronic Obstructive Pulmonary Disorders  685

**CHRONIC OBSTRUCTIVE PULMONARY DISEASE**  686
▶▶ Nursing Process: The Patient With COPD  696
**BRONCHIECTASIS**  701
**ASTHMA**  709
Status Asthmaticus  717
**CYSTIC FIBROSIS**  718

## CHAPTER 25
### Respiratory Care Modalities  722

**NONINVASIVE RESPIRATORY THERAPIES**  723
Oxygen Therapy  723
Incentive Spirometry (Sustained Maximal Inspiration)  729
Mini-Nebulizer Therapy  730
Intermittent Positive-Pressure Breathing  730
Chest Physiotherapy  731
**AIRWAY MANAGEMENT**  735
Emergency Management of Upper Airway Obstruction  735
Endotracheal Intubation  735
Tracheostomy  738
**MECHANICAL VENTILATION**  739
▶▶ Nursing Process: The Patient Receiving Mechanical Ventilation  747
**THE PATIENT UNDERGOING THORACIC SURGERY**  754
▶▶ Nursing Process: The Patient Undergoing Thoracic Surgery  764

# UNIT 6

## Cardiovascular, Circulatory, and Hematologic Function . . . . . . 778

### CHAPTER 26
**Assessment of Cardiovascular Function** 780

- ANATOMIC AND PHYSIOLOGIC OVERVIEW 781
- ASSESSMENT 787
- DIAGNOSTIC EVALUATION 805
- HEMODYNAMIC MONITORING 816

### CHAPTER 27
**Management of Patients With Dysrhythmias and Conduction Problems** 822

- DYSRHYTHMIAS 823
  - ▶▶ Nursing Process: The Patient With a Dysrhythmia 840
- ADJUNCTIVE MODALITIES AND MANAGEMENT 842
  - ▶▶ Nursing Process: The Patient With an Implantable Cardiac Device 850

### CHAPTER 28
**Management of Patients With Coronary Vascular Disorders** 858

- CORONARY ARTERY DISEASE 859
  - Coronary Atherosclerosis 859
  - Angina Pectoris 867
  - ▶▶ Nursing Process: The Patient With Angina Pectoris 871
  - Myocardial Infarction (MI) 874
  - ▶▶ Nursing Process: The Patient With Myocardial Infarction 879
- INVASIVE CORONARY ARTERY PROCEDURES 885
  - Percutaneous Coronary Interventions (PCIs) 885
  - Surgical Procedures: Coronary Artery Revascularization 888
  - ▶▶ Nursing Process: The Preoperative Cardiac Surgery Patient 890
  - ▶▶ Nursing Process: The Postoperative Cardiac Surgery Patient 897

### CHAPTER 29
**Management of Patients With Structural, Infectious, and Inflammatory Cardiac Disorders** 914

- VALVULAR DISORDERS 915
  - Mitral Valve Prolapse 915
  - Mitral Regurgitation 917
  - Mitral Stenosis 918
  - Aortic Regurgitation 918
  - Aortic Stenosis 919
  - Nursing Management: Valvular Heart Disorders 920
- VALVE REPAIR AND REPLACEMENT PROCEDURES 920
  - Valvuloplasty 920
  - Valve Replacement 923
  - Nursing Management: Valvuloplasty and Replacement 924
- SEPTAL REPAIR 925
- CARDIOMYOPATHY 925
  - ▶▶ Nursing Process: The Patient With Cardiomyopathy 930
- INFECTIOUS DISEASES OF THE HEART 933
  - Rheumatic Endocarditis 933
  - Infective Endocarditis 935
  - Myocarditis 938
  - Pericarditis 939
  - ▶▶ Nursing Process: The Patient With Pericarditis 940

### CHAPTER 30
**Management of Patients With Complications From Heart Disease** 944

- CARDIAC HEMODYNAMICS 945
- HEART FAILURE 946
  - Chronic Heart Failure 947
  - ▶▶ Nursing Process: The Patient With Heart Failure 958
  - Acute Heart Failure (Pulmonary Edema) 964
- OTHER COMPLICATIONS 965
  - Cardiogenic Shock 965
  - Thromboembolism 967
  - Pericardial Effusion and Cardiac Tamponade 968
  - Cardiac Arrest 969

### CHAPTER 31
**Assessment and Management of Patients With Vascular Disorders and Problems of Peripheral Circulation** 974

- ANATOMIC AND PHYSIOLOGIC OVERVIEW 975
- ASSESSMENT AND DIAGNOSTIC EVALUATION 979
- ARTERIAL DISORDERS 983
  - Arteriosclerosis and Atherosclerosis 983
  - ▶▶ Nursing Process: The Patient With Peripheral Arterial Insufficiency of the Extremities 987
  - Peripheral Arterial Occlusive Disease 992
  - Upper Extremity Arterial Occlusive Disease 995
  - Thromboangiitis Obliterans (Buerger's Disease) 995
  - Aortitis 996
  - Aortoiliac Disease 996
  - Aneurysm 997
  - Dissecting Aorta 1001
  - Arterial Embolism and Arterial Thrombosis 1001
  - Raynaud's Disease 1003
- VENOUS DISORDERS 1004
  - Venous Thrombosis, Deep Vein Thrombosis, Thrombophlebitis, and Phlebothrombosis 1004
  - Chronic Venous Insufficiency 1010
  - Leg Ulcers 1011
  - ▶▶ Nursing Process: The Patient With Leg Ulcers 1013
  - Varicose Veins 1014
- LYMPHATIC DISORDERS 1016
  - Lymphangitis and Lymphadenitis 1016
  - Lymphedema and Elephantiasis 1016
- CELLULITIS 1017

### CHAPTER 32
**Assessment and Management of Patients With Hypertension** 1020

- HYPERTENSION 1021
  - ▶▶ Nursing Process: The Patient With Hypertension 1025
- HYPERTENSIVE CRISES 1033

### CHAPTER 33
**Assessment and Management of Patients With Hematologic Disorders** 1035

- ANATOMIC AND PHYSIOLOGIC OVERVIEW 1037
- ASSESSMENT OF HEMATOLOGIC DISORDERS 1043

CONTENTS xxi

ANEMIA 1045
Overview 1045
▶▶ Nursing Process: The Patient With Anemia 1047
Hypoproliferative Anemias 1049
Hemolytic Anemias 1055
▶▶ Nursing Process: The Patient With Sickle Cell Crisis 1058
POLYCYTHEMIA 1064
Polycythemia Vera 1065
SECONDARY POLYCYTHEMIA 1066
LEUKOPENIA 1066
Neutropenia 1066
Lymphopenia 1067
LEUKEMIA 1067
Acute Myeloid Leukemia 1071
Chronic Myeloid Leukemia 1072
Acute Lymphocytic Leukemia 1073
Chronic Lymphocytic Leukemia 1074
▶▶ Nursing Process: The Patient With Acute Leukemia 1075
AGNOGENIC MYELOID METAPLASIA 1079
LYMPHOMA 1080
Hodgkin's Disease 1080
Non-Hodgkin's Lymphomas (NHLs) 1081
MULTIPLE MYELOMA 1082
BLEEDING DISORDERS 1084
Overview 1084
Primary Thrombocythemia 1085
Secondary Thrombocytosis 1086
Thrombocytopenia 1087
Idiopathic Thrombocytopenic Purpura 1088
Platelet Defects 1089
Hemophilia 1090
Von Willebrand's Disease 1092
ACQUIRED COAGULATION DISORDERS 1092
Liver Disease 1092
Vitamin K Deficiency 1092
Complications of Anticoagulant Therapy 1093
Disseminated Intravascular Coagulation (DIC) 1093
▶▶ Nursing Process: The Patient With Disseminated Intravascular Coagulation 1094
Thrombotic Disorders 1095
Hyperhomocysteinemia 1095
Antithrombin (AT) Deficiency 1098
Protein C Deficiency 1099
Activated Protein C (APC) Resistance and Factor V Leiden Mutation 1099
Protein S Deficiency 1099
Acquired Thrombophilia 1099
THERAPIES FOR BLOOD DISORDERS 1102
PROCURING BLOOD AND BLOOD PRODUCTS 1104
TRANSFUSION 1107
PERIPHERAL BLOOD STEM CELL TRANSPLANTATION AND BONE MARROW TRANSPLANTATION 1112

# UNIT 7
# Digestive and Gastrointestinal Function......1118

## CHAPTER 34
### Assessment of Digestive and Gastrointestinal Function 1120

ANATOMIC AND PHYSIOLOGIC OVERVIEW 1121
ASSESSMENT 1126
DIAGNOSTIC EVALUATION 1129
PATHOPHYSIOLOGIC AND PSYCHOLOGICAL CONSIDERATIONS 1139

## CHAPTER 35
### Management of Patients With Oral and Esophageal Disorders 1141

DISORDERS OF THE TEETH 1142
Dental Plaque and Caries 1142
Dentoalveolar Abscess or Periapical Abscess 1145
Malocclusion 1146
DISORDERS OF THE JAW 1146
Temporomandibular Disorders 1146
Jaw Disorders Requiring Surgical Management 1147
DISORDERS OF THE SALIVARY GLANDS 1147
Parotitis 1147
Sialadenitis 1147
Salivary Calculus (Sialolithiasis) 1148
Neoplasms 1148
CANCER OF THE ORAL CAVITY 1148
▶▶ Nursing Process: The Patient With Conditions of the Oral Cavity 1149
NECK DISSECTION 1153
▶▶ Nursing Process: The Patient Undergoing a Neck Dissection 1153
DISORDERS OF THE ESOPHAGUS 1162
Achalasia 1162
Diffuse Spasm 1162
Hiatal Hernia 1163
Diverticulum 1164
Perforation 1164
Foreign Bodies 1165
Chemical Burns 1165
Gastroesophageal Reflux Disease 1165
Barrett's Esophagus 1166
Benign Tumors of the Esophagus 1166
Cancer of the Esophagus 1166
▶▶ Nursing Process: The Patient With a Condition of the Esophagus 1169

## CHAPTER 36
### Gastrointestinal Intubation and Special Nutritional Modalities 1174

GASTROINTESTINAL INTUBATION 1175
TUBE FEEDINGS WITH NASOGASTRIC AND NASOENTERIC DEVICES 1181
▶▶ Nursing Process: The Patient Receiving a Tube Feeding 1183
GASTROSTOMY 1188
▶▶ Nursing Process: The Patient With a Gastrostomy 1189
PARENTERAL NUTRITION 1193
▶▶ Nursing Process: The Patient Receiving Parenteral Nutrition 1196

## CHAPTER 37
### Management of Patients With Gastric and Duodenal Disorders 1203

GASTRITIS 1204
▶▶ Nursing Process: The Patient With Gastritis 1205
PEPTIC ULCER DISEASE 1209
▶▶ Nursing Process: The Patient With Peptic Ulcer Disease 1212

## xxii CONTENTS

**MORBID OBESITY** 1217
**GASTRIC CANCER** 1220
▶▶ Nursing Process: The Patient With Gastric Cancer 1221
**GASTRIC SURGERY** 1223
▶▶ Nursing Process: The Patient Undergoing Gastric Surgery 1223
**DUODENAL TUMORS** 1227

## CHAPTER 38
### Management of Patients With Intestinal and Rectal Disorders 1231

**ABNORMALITIES OF FECAL ELIMINATION** 1232
Constipation 1232
Diarrhea 1235
Fecal Incontinence 1236
Irritable Bowel Syndrome 1237
**CONDITIONS OF MALABSORPTION** 1238
**ACUTE INFLAMMATORY INTESTINAL DISORDERS** 1239
Appendicitis 1240
Diverticular Disease 1242
▶▶ Nursing Process: The Patient With Diverticulitis 1244
Peritonitis 1245
**INFLAMMATORY BOWEL DISEASE** 1247
Types of Chronic Inflammatory Bowel Disease 1248
Medical Management of Chronic Inflammatory Bowel Disease 1249
Nursing Management of Chronic Inflammatory Bowel Disease 1251
▶▶ Nursing Process: Management of the Patient With Inflammatory Bowel Disease 1251
**INTESTINAL OBSTRUCTION** 1263
Small Bowel Obstruction 1263
Large Bowel Obstruction 1265
Colorectal Cancer 1265
▶▶ Nursing Process: The Patient With Colorectal Cancer 1268
Polyps of the Colon and Rectum 1275
**DISEASES OF THE ANORECTUM** 1276
Anorectal Abscess 1276
Anal Fistula 1276
Anal Fissure 1276
Hemorrhoids 1277
Sexually Transmitted Anorectal Diseases 1277
Pilonidal Sinus or Cyst 1277
▶▶ Nursing Process: The Patient With an Anorectal Condition 1278

## UNIT 8
# Metabolic and Endocrine Function .......... 1282

## CHAPTER 39
### Assessment and Management of Patients With Hepatic Disorders 1284

**ANATOMIC AND PHYSIOLOGIC OVERVIEW** 1285
**ASSESSMENT** 1287
**DIAGNOSTIC EVALUATION** 1288
**MANIFESTATIONS OF HEPATIC DYSFUNCTION** 1289

Jaundice 1289
Portal Hypertension 1293
Ascites 1293
Esophageal Varices 1298
Hepatic Encephalopathy and Coma 1304
Other Manifestations of Hepatic Dysfunction 1307
**VIRAL HEPATITIS** 1308
Hepatitis A Virus 1308
Hepatitis B Virus 1312
Hepatitis C Virus 1314
Hepatitis D Virus 1315
Hepatitis E Virus 1315
Hepatitis G Virus and GB Virus-C 1315
**NONVIRAL HEPATITIS** 1315
Toxic Hepatitis 1316
Drug-Induced Hepatitis 1316
**FULMINANT HEPATIC FAILURE** 1317
**HEPATIC CIRRHOSIS** 1318
▶▶ Nursing Process: The Patient With Hepatic Cirrhosis 1320
**CANCER OF THE LIVER** 1333
Primary Liver Tumors 1333
Liver Metastases 1333
**LIVER TRANSPLANTATION** 1336
**LIVER ABSCESSES** 1340

## CHAPTER 40
### Assessment and Management of Patients With Biliary Disorders 1344

**ANATOMIC AND PHYSIOLOGIC OVERVIEW** 1345
**DISORDERS OF THE GALLBLADDER** 1347
Cholecystitis 1347
Cholelithiasis 1347
▶▶ Nursing Process: The Patient Undergoing Surgery for Gallbladder Disease 1355
**DISORDERS OF THE PANCREAS** 1358
Acute Pancreatitis 1358
▶▶ Nursing Process: The Patient With Acute Pancreatitis 1360
Chronic Pancreatitis 1363
Pancreatic Cysts 1369
Cancer of the Pancreas 1369
Tumors of the Head of the Pancreas 1370
Pancreatic Islet Tumors 1372
Hyperinsulinism 1372
Ulcerogenic Tumors 1372

## CHAPTER 41
### Assessment and Management of Patients With Diabetes Mellitus 1375

**DIABETES AND ITS CLASSIFICATION** 1377
**OVERALL MANAGEMENT OF DIABETES** 1383
**NURSING MANAGEMENT** 1402
**ACUTE COMPLICATIONS OF DIABETES** 1410
Hypoglycemia (Insulin Reactions) 1410
Diabetic Ketoacidosis (DKA) 1412
Hyperglycemic Hyperosmolar Nonketotic Syndrome (HHNS) 1415
▶▶ Nursing Process: The Patient Newly Diagnosed With Diabetes Mellitus 1416
**LONG-TERM COMPLICATIONS OF DIABETES** 1421
Macrovascular Complications 1421
Microvascular Complications 1422
Foot and Leg Problems 1427

SPECIAL ISSUES IN DIABETES CARE 1429
➤➤ Nursing Process: The Patient With Diabetes as a Secondary Diagnosis 1433

## CHAPTER 42
### Assessment and Management of Patients With Endocrine Disorders 1439

ANATOMIC AND PHYSIOLOGIC OVERVIEW 1441
ASSESSMENT 1442
DIAGNOSTIC EVALUATION 1444
THE PITUITARY GLAND 1445
Anatomic and Physiologic Overview 1445
Pathophysiology 1446
Specific Disorders of the Pituitary Gland 1446
THE THYROID GLAND 1448
Anatomic and Physiologic Overview 1448
Pathophysiology 1450
Assessment and Diagnostic Findings 1450
Specific Disorders of the Thyroid Gland 1452
➤➤ Nursing Process: The Patient With Hyperthyroidism 1463
THE PARATHYROID GLANDS 1470
Anatomic and Physiologic Overview 1470
Specific Disorders of the Parathyroid Glands 1470
THE ADRENAL GLANDS 1473
Anatomic and Physiologic Overview 1473
Specific Disorders of the Adrenal Glands 1475
➤➤ Nursing Process: The Patient With Cushing's Syndrome 1481
Corticosteroid Therapy 1484

## UNIT 9
# Renal and Urinary Tract Function ............ 1490

## CHAPTER 43
### Assessment of Renal and Urinary Tract Function 1492

ANATOMIC AND PHYSIOLOGIC OVERVIEW 1493
ASSESSMENT 1500
DIAGNOSTIC EVALUATION 1505

## CHAPTER 44
### Management of Patients With Renal Disorders 1514

FLUID AND ELECTROLYTE IMBALANCES IN RENAL DISORDERS 1515
PRIMARY GLOMERULAR DISEASES 1517
Acute Glomerulonephritis 1517
Chronic Glomerulonephritis 1518
Nephrotic Syndrome 1520
Nephrosclerosis 1521
RENAL FAILURE 1521
Acute Renal Failure 1522

Chronic Renal Failure (End-Stage Renal Disease) 1527
DIALYSIS 1531
Hemodialysis 1537
Continuous Renal Replacement Therapies 1542
Continuous Venovenous Hemofiltration 1544
Continuous Venovenous Hemodialysis 1544
Peritoneal Dialysis 1545
Special Considerations: Care of the Hospitalized Patient on Dialysis 1551
KIDNEY SURGERY 1552
Preoperative Considerations 1552
Perioperative Concerns 1553
Postoperative Management 1553
➤➤ Nursing Process: The Patient Undergoing Kidney Surgery 1553
KIDNEY TRANSPLANTATION 1560
Preoperative Management 1560
Postoperative Management 1561
RENAL CANCER 1563
RENAL TRAUMA 1565

## CHAPTER 45
### Management of Patients With Urinary Disorders 1569

INFECTIONS OF THE URINARY TRACT 1570
Lower Urinary Tract Infections 1571
➤➤ Nursing Process: The Patient With a Lower Urinary Tract Infection 1575
Upper Urinary Tract Infections 1577
ADULT VOIDING DYSFUNCTION 1578
Urinary Incontinence 1578
Urinary Retention 1581
Neurogenic Bladder 1584
UROLITHIASIS AND NEPHROLITHIASIS 1589
➤➤ Nursing Process: The Patient With Kidney Stones 1593
GENITOURINARY TRAUMA 1595
URINARY TRACT CANCERS 1596
Cancer of the Bladder 1596
URINARY DIVERSIONS 1597
Cutaneous Urinary Diversions 1598
Continent Urinary Diversions 1602
Other Urinary Diversion Procedures 1603
➤➤ Nursing Process: The Patient Undergoing Urinary Diversion Surgery 1603

## UNIT 10

# Reproductive Function ......... 1610

## CHAPTER 46
### Assessment and Management of Female Physiologic Processes 1612

ROLE OF NURSES IN WOMEN'S HEALTH 1613
ANATOMIC AND PHYSIOLOGIC OVERVIEW 1614
ASSESSMENT 1616
DIAGNOSTIC TESTING AND EVALUATION 1627
MANAGEMENT OF FEMALE PHYSIOLOGIC PROCESSES 1632
Menstruation 1632
Perimenopause 1632

Menopause 1633
Menstrual Disorders 1636
Dyspareunia 1640
Contraception 1640
Abortion 1647
Infertility 1650
Preconception/Periconception Health Care 1652
Ectopic Pregnancy 1653
▶▶ Nursing Process: The Patient With an Ectopic Pregnancy 1654

## CHAPTER 47
### Management of Patients With Female Reproductive Disorders 1660

**VULVOVAGINAL INFECTIONS 1661**
Candidiasis 1662
Bacterial Vaginosis 1662
Trichomoniasis 1664
▶▶ Nursing Process: The Patient With a Vulvovaginal Infection 1664
Human Papillomavirus 1666
Herpesvirus Type 2 Infection (Herpes Genitalis, Herpes Simplex Virus) 1667
▶▶ Nursing Process: The Patient With a Genital Herpesvirus Infection 1667
Endocervicitis and Cervicitis 1669
Pelvic Infection (Pelvic Inflammatory Disease) 1670
Human Immunodeficiency Virus Infection and Acquired Immunodeficiency Syndrome 1672
**STRUCTURAL DISORDERS 1673**
Fistulas of the Vagina 1673
Pelvic Organ Prolapse: Cystocele, Rectocele, Enterocele 1674
Uterine Prolapse 1675
**BENIGN DISORDERS 1677**
Vulvar Cysts 1677
Vulvar Dystrophy 1678
Ovarian Cysts 1678
Benign Tumors of the Uterus: Fibroids (Leiomyomas, Myomas) 1679
Endometriosis 1680
Chronic Pelvic Pain 1682
Adenomyosis 1682
Endometrial Hyperplasia 1682
**MALIGNANT CONDITIONS 1682**
Cancer of the Cervix 1682
Cancer of the Uterus (Endometrium) 1685
Cancer of the Vulva 1685
▶▶ Nursing Process: The Patient Undergoing Vulvar Surgery 1686
Cancer of the Vagina 1689
Cancer of the Fallopian Tubes 1689
Cancer of the Ovary 1689
**HYSTERECTOMY 1691**
▶▶ Nursing Process: The Patient Undergoing a Hysterectomy 1692
**RADIATION THERAPY 1694**

## CHAPTER 48
### Assessment and Management of Patients With Breast Disorders 1700

**ANATOMIC AND PHYSIOLOGIC OVERVIEW 1701**
**ASSESSMENT 1702**
**DIAGNOSTIC EVALUATION 1705**
**CONDITIONS AFFECTING THE NIPPLE 1710**
Nipple Discharge 1710
Fissure 1710
**BREAST INFECTIONS 1710**
Mastitis 1710
Lactational Abscess 1710
**BENIGN CONDITIONS OF THE BREAST 1710**
Breast Pain 1710
Cysts 1710
Fibroadenomas 1711
Benign Proliferative Breast Disease 1711
Other Benign Conditions 1711
**MALIGNANT CONDITIONS OF THE BREAST 1712**
▶▶ Nursing Process: The Patient Undergoing Surgery for Breast Cancer 1718
**DISEASES OF THE MALE BREAST 1735**
Gynecomastia 1735
Male Breast Cancer 1735

## CHAPTER 49
### Assessment and Management of Problems Related to Male Reproductive Processes 1739

**ANATOMIC AND PHYSIOLOGIC OVERVIEW 1740**
Gerontologic Considerations 1742
**ASSESSMENT 1742**
**DIAGNOSTIC EVALUATION 1744**
**DISORDERS OF MALE SEXUAL FUNCTION 1744**
Erectile Dysfunction 1744
Disorders of Ejaculation 1746
**INFECTIONS OF THE MALE GENITOURINARY TRACT 1750**
**CONDITIONS OF THE PROSTATE 1750**
Prostatitis 1750
Benign Prostatic Hyperplasia (Enlarged Prostate) 1751
Cancer of the Prostate 1752
The Patient Undergoing Prostate Surgery 1761
▶▶ Nursing Process: The Patient Undergoing Prostatectomy 1764
**CONDITIONS AFFECTING THE TESTES AND ADJACENT STRUCTURES 1769**
Orchitis 1769
Epididymitis 1769
Testicular Cancer 1770
Hydrocele 1773
Varicocele 1773
Vasectomy 1773
**CONDITIONS AFFECTING THE PENIS 1774**
Hypospadias and Epispadias 1774
Phimosis 1774
Cancer of the Penis 1774
Priapism 1775
Peyronie's Disease 1775
Urethral Stricture 1775
Circumcision 1775

# UNIT 11
# Immunologic Function ......... 1780

## CHAPTER 50
### Assessment of Immune Function 1782

**ANATOMIC AND PHYSIOLOGIC OVERVIEW 1784**
**ADVANCES IN IMMUNOLOGY 1793**

ASSESSMENT 1794
DIAGNOSTIC EVALUATION 1799

## CHAPTER 51
### Management of Patients With Immunodeficiency 1801

PRIMARY IMMUNODEFICIENCIES 1802
Phagocytic Dysfunction 1802
B-Cell Deficiencies 1805
T-Cell Deficiencies 1806
Combined B-Cell and T-Cell Deficiencies 1806
Deficiencies of the Complement System 1807
SECONDARY IMMUNODEFICIENCIES 1809
NURSING MANAGEMENT FOR PATIENTS WITH IMMUNODEFICIENCIES 1809

## CHAPTER 52
### Management of Patients With HIV Infection and AIDS 1814

HIV INFECTION AND AIDS 1815
▶▶ Nursing Process: The Patient With AIDS 1837
EMOTIONAL AND ETHICAL CONCERNS 1851

## CHAPTER 53
### Assessment and Management of Patients With Allergic Disorders 1855

ALLERGIC REACTION: PHYSIOLOGIC OVERVIEW 1856
ASSESSMENT AND DIAGNOSTIC EVALUATION 1861
ALLERGIC DISORDERS 1865
Anaphylaxis 1865
Allergic Rhinitis 1869
▶▶ Nursing Process: The Patient With Allergic Rhinitis 1873
Contact Dermatitis 1877
Atopic Dermatitis 1877
Dermatitis Medicamentosa (Drug Reactions) 1878
Urticaria and Angioneurotic Edema 1878
Hereditary Angioedema 1879
Food Allergy 1879
Serum Sickness 1880
Latex Allergy 1881

## CHAPTER 54
### Assessment and Management of Patients With Rheumatic Disorders 1886

RHEUMATIC DISEASES 1887
▶▶ Nursing Process: The Patient With a Rheumatic Disease 1897
DIFFUSE CONNECTIVE TISSUE DISEASES 1906
Rheumatoid Arthritis 1906
Systemic Lupus Erythematosus 1909
Scleroderma 1912
Polymyositis 1913
Polymyalgia Rheumatica 1913
DEGENERATIVE JOINT DISEASE (OSTEOARTHRITIS) 1914
SPONDYLOARTHROPATHIES 1917
METABOLIC AND ENDOCRINE DISEASES ASSOCIATED WITH RHEUMATIC DISORDERS 1917
Gout 1918
FIBROMYALGIA 1919

ARTHRITIS ASSOCIATED WITH INFECTIOUS ORGANISMS 1919
NEOPLASMS AND NEUROVASCULAR, BONE, AND EXTRA-ARTICULAR DISORDERS 1920
MISCELLANEOUS DISORDERS 1920

# UNIT 12
# Integumentary Function .........1924

## CHAPTER 55
### Assessment of Integumentary Function 1926

ANATOMIC AND PHYSIOLOGIC OVERVIEW 1927
ASSESSMENT 1932
CONSEQUENCES OF SELECTED SYSTEMIC DISEASES 1941
DIAGNOSTIC EVALUATION 1941

## CHAPTER 56
### Management of Patients With Dermatologic Problems 1944

SKIN CARE FOR PATIENTS WITH SKIN CONDITIONS 1945
WOUND CARE FOR SKIN CONDITIONS 1945
PRURITUS 1951
General Pruritus 1951
Perineal and Perianal Pruritus 1952
SECRETORY DISORDERS 1952
Hydradenitis Suppurativa 1952
Seborrheic Dermatoses 1953
Acne Vulgaris 1953
INFECTIOUS DERMATOSES 1956
Bacterial Skin Infections 1956
Viral Skin Infections 1958
Fungal (Mycotic) Skin Infections 1960
Parasitic Skin Infestations 1962
CONTACT DERMATITIS 1964
NONINFECTIOUS INFLAMMATORY DERMATOSES 1965
Psoriasis 1965
▶▶ Nursing Process: Care of the Patient With Psoriasis 1968
Exfoliative Dermatitis 1970
BLISTERING DISEASES 1971
Pemphigus 1971
Bullous Pemphigoid 1972
Dermatitis Herpetiformis 1972
▶▶ Nursing Process: Care of the Patient With Blistering Diseases 1972
Toxic Epidermal Necrolysis and Stevens-Johnson Syndrome 1974
▶▶ Nursing Process: Care of the Patient With Toxic Epidermal Necrolysis or Stevens-Johnson Syndrome 1975
ULCERATIONS 1977
SKIN TUMORS 1977
Benign Skin Tumors 1977
Malignant Skin Tumors 1978
▶▶ Nursing Process: Care of the Patient With Malignant Melanoma 1983
Metastatic Skin Tumors 1984
Kaposi's Sarcoma 1985
DERMATOLOGIC AND PLASTIC RECONSTRUCTIVE SURGERY 1985
Wound Coverage: Grafts and Flaps 1986
Chemical Face Peeling 1988

## CONTENTS

Dermabrasion 1988
Facial Reconstructive Surgery 1989
Face Lift 1990
**LASER TREATMENT OF CUTANEOUS LESIONS** 1991
Argon Laser 1991
Carbon Dioxide Laser 1991
Pulse-Dye Laser 1992

### CHAPTER 57
**Management of Patients With Burn Injury** 1994

**INCIDENCE OF BURN INJURY** 1995
**OUTLOOK FOR SURVIVAL AND RECOVERY** 1996
**CLASSIFICATION OF BURNS** 1997
**ELECTRICAL BURNS** 1998
**PATHOPHYSIOLOGY** 1999
**MANAGEMENT OF BURN INJURY** 2002
Emergency/Resuscitative Phase 2002
Acute/Intermediate Phase 2009
➤➤ Nursing Process: Care of the Patient During the Acute Phase 2026
Rehabilitation Phase 2031
➤➤ Nursing Process: Care of the Patient During the Rehabilitation Phase 2033
**BURN CARE IN THE HOME** 2037

## UNIT 13

# Sensorineural Function ........ 2040

### CHAPTER 58
**Assessment and Management of Patients With Eye and Vision Disorders** 2042

**ANATOMIC AND PHYSIOLOGIC OVERVIEW** 2043
**ASSESSMENT** 2046
**DIAGNOSTIC EVALUATION** 2048
**IMPAIRED VISION** 2050
Refractive Errors 2050
Low Vision and Blindness 2051
**GLAUCOMA** 2054
**CATARACTS** 2059
**CORNEAL DISORDERS** 2064
Corneal Dystrophies 2064
Keratoconus 2064
Corneal Surgeries 2064
Refractive Surgeries 2065
**RETINAL DISORDERS** 2067
Retinal Detachment 2067
Retinal Vascular Disorders 2068
Macular Degeneration 2069
**ORBITAL AND OCULAR TRAUMA** 2072
Orbital Trauma 2072
Ocular Trauma 2073
**INFECTIOUS AND INFLAMMATORY CONDITIONS** 2075
Dry Eye Syndrome 2075
Conjunctivitis 2076
Uveitis 2079
Orbital Cellulitis 2079
**ORBITAL AND OCULAR TUMORS** 2080
Benign Tumors of the Orbit 2080
Benign Tumors of the Eyelids 2080
Benign Tumors of the Conjunctiva 2080
Malignant Tumors of the Orbit 2080
Malignant Tumors of the Eyelid 2080
Malignant Tumors of the Conjunctiva 2081
Malignant Tumors of the Globe 2081
**SURGICAL PROCEDURES AND ENUCLEATION** 2081
Orbital Surgeries 2081
Enucleation 2082
**OCULAR CONSEQUENCES OF SYSTEMIC DISEASE** 2083
Diabetic Retinopathy 2083
Cytomegalovirus Retinitis 2083
Hypertension-Related Eye Changes 2084
**CONCEPTS IN OCULAR MEDICATION ADMINISTRATION** 2084
**ISSUES IN OPHTHALMOLOGY** 2087

### CHAPTER 59
**Assessment and Management of Patients With Hearing and Balance Disorders** 2092

**ANATOMIC AND PHYSIOLOGIC OVERVIEW** 2093
**ASSESSMENT** 2096
**DIAGNOSTIC EVALUATION** 2099
**HEARING LOSS** 2101
**CONDITIONS OF THE EXTERNAL EAR** 2104
Cerumen Impaction 2104
Foreign Bodies 2104
External Otitis (Otitis Externa) 2105
Malignant External Otitis 2105
Masses of the External Ear 2105
Gapping Earring Puncture 2106
**CONDITIONS OF THE MIDDLE EAR** 2106
Tympanic Membrane Perforation 2106
Acute Otitis Media 2106
Serous Otitis Media 2107
Chronic Otitis Media 2107
➤➤ Nursing Process: The Patient Undergoing Mastoid Surgery 2108
Otosclerosis 2110
Middle Ear Masses 2111
**CONDITIONS OF THE INNER EAR** 2112
Motion Sickness 2112
Ménière's Disease 2112
Tinnitus 2118
Labyrinthitis 2118
Benign Paroxysmal Positional Vertigo 2119
Ototoxicity 2119
Acoustic Neuroma 2119
**AURAL REHABILITATION** 2120

## UNIT 14

# Neurologic Function .......... 2126

### CHAPTER 60
**Assessment of Neurologic Function** 2128

**ANATOMIC AND PHYSIOLOGIC OVERVIEW** 2129
**ASSESSMENT: THE NEUROLOGIC EXAMINATION** 2143
**DIAGNOSTIC EVALUATION** 2152

### CHAPTER 61
**Management of Patients With Neurologic Dysfunction** 2160

ALTERED LEVEL OF CONSCIOUSNESS 2162
▶▶ Nursing Process: The Patient With an Altered Level of Consciousness 2163
INCREASED INTRACRANIAL PRESSURE 2169
▶▶ Nursing Process: The Patient With Increased Intracranial Pressure 2175
INTRACRANIAL SURGERY 2180
Supratentorial and Infratentorial Approaches 2180
▶▶ Nursing Process: The Patient Undergoing Intracranial Surgery 2183
Transsphenoidal Approach 2189
SEIZURE DISORDERS 2190
Seizures 2190
The Epilepsies 2191
▶▶ Nursing Process: The Patient With Epilepsy 2195
Status Epilepticus 2197
HEADACHE 2198

## CHAPTER 62
## Management of Patients With Cerebrovascular Disorders 2205

ISCHEMIC STROKE 2206
▶▶ Nursing Process: The Patient Recovering From an Ischemic Stroke 2215
HEMORRHAGIC STROKE 2223
▶▶ Nursing Process: The Patient With a Hemorrhagic Stroke 2227

## CHAPTER 63
## Management of Patients With Neurologic Trauma 2232

HEAD INJURIES 2233
BRAIN INJURY 2235
▶▶ Nursing Process: The Patient With a Traumatic Brain Injury 2240
SPINAL CORD INJURY 2250
▶▶ Nursing Process: The Patient With Acute Spinal Cord Injury 2256
▶▶ Nursing Process: The Patient With Tetraplegia or Paraplegia 2261

## CHAPTER 64
## Management of Patients With Neurologic Infections, Autoimmune Disorders, and Neuropathies 2269

INFECTIOUS NEUROLOGIC DISORDERS 2270
Meningitis 2270
Brain Abscess 2273
Herpes Simplex Virus Encephalitis 2274
Arthropod-Borne Virus Encephalitis 2274
Fungal Encephalitis 2275
Creutzfeldt-Jakob and Variant Creutzfeldt-Jakob Disease 2276
AUTOIMMUNE PROCESSES 2277
Multiple Sclerosis 2277
▶▶ Nursing Process: The Patient With Multiple Sclerosis 2281
Myasthenia Gravis 2285
Guillain-Barré Syndrome 2288
▶▶ Nursing Process: The Patient With Guillain-Barré Syndrome 2289
CRANIAL NERVE DISORDERS 2292

Trigeminal Neuralgia (Tic Douloureux) 2292
Bell's Palsy 2295
DISORDERS OF THE PERIPHERAL NERVOUS SYSTEM 2296
Peripheral Neuropathies 2296
Mononeuropathy 2297

## CHAPTER 65
## Management of Patients With Oncologic or Degenerative Neurologic Disorders 2300

ONCOLOGIC DISORDERS OF THE BRAIN AND SPINAL CORD 2301
Primary Brain Tumors 2301
Cerebral Metastases 2306
▶▶ Nursing Process: The Patient With Cerebral Metastases or Incurable Brain Tumor 2307
Spinal Cord Tumors 2309
DEGENERATIVE DISORDERS 2311
Parkinson's Disease 2311
▶▶ Nursing Process: The Patient With Parkinson's Disease 2316
Huntington's Disease 2319
Alzheimer's Disease 2320
Amyotrophic Lateral Sclerosis 2320
Muscular Dystrophies 2323
Degenerative Disk Disease 2324
Herniation of a Cervical Intervertebral Disk 2326
▶▶ Nursing Process: The Patient Undergoing a Cervical Discectomy 2326
Herniation of a Lumbar Disk 2329
Postpolio Syndrome 2331

# UNIT 15
# Musculoskeletal Function . . . . . . . 2334

## CHAPTER 66
## Assessment of Musculoskeletal Function 2336

ANATOMIC AND PHYSIOLOGIC OVERVIEW 2337
ASSESSMENT 2342
DIAGNOSTIC EVALUATION 2350
NURSING IMPLICATIONS 2352

## CHAPTER 67
## Musculoskeletal Care Modalities 2354

THE PATIENT IN A CAST 2355
▶▶ Nursing Process: The Patient in a Cast 2356
THE PATIENT WITH SPLINTS OR BRACES 2364
THE PATIENT WITH AN EXTERNAL FIXATOR 2364
THE PATIENT IN TRACTION 2365
▶▶ Nursing Process: The Patient in Traction 2369
THE PATIENT UNDERGOING ORTHOPEDIC SURGERY 2371
▶▶ Nursing Process: Preoperative Care of the Patient Undergoing Orthopedic Surgery 2376
▶▶ Nursing Process: Postoperative Care of the Patient Undergoing Orthopedic Surgery 2384

## CHAPTER 68
### Management of Patients With Musculoskeletal Disorders    2391

**ACUTE LOW BACK PAIN**    2392
- ▶▶ Nursing Process: The Patient With Acute Low Back Pain    2393

**COMMON UPPER EXTREMITY PROBLEMS**    2397
- Bursitis and Tendinitis    2397
- Loose Bodies    2397
- Impingement Syndrome    2398
- Carpal Tunnel Syndrome    2398
- Ganglion    2398
- Dupuytren's Disease    2399
- ▶▶ Nursing Process: The Patient Undergoing Surgery of the Hand or Wrist    2399

**COMMON FOOT PROBLEMS**    2400
- Plantar Fasciitis    2401
- Corn    2401
- Callus    2401
- Ingrown Toenail    2401
- Hammer Toe    2401
- Hallux Valgus    2401
- Pes Cavus    2402
- Morton's Neuroma    2402
- Flatfoot    2402
- ▶▶ Nursing Process: The Patient Undergoing Foot Surgery    2402

**METABOLIC BONE DISORDERS**    2404
- Osteoporosis    2404
- ▶▶ Nursing Process: The Patient With a Spontaneous Vertebral Fracture Related to Osteoporosis    2409
- Osteomalacia    2411
- Paget's Disease    2411

**MUSCULOSKELETAL INFECTIONS**    2413
- Osteomyelitis    2413
- ▶▶ Nursing Process: The Patient With Osteomyelitis    2414
- Septic (Infectious) Arthritis    2416

**BONE TUMORS**    2417
- Benign Bone Tumors    2417
- Malignant Bone Tumors    2417
- Metastatic Bone Disease    2417
- ▶▶ Nursing Process: The Patient With a Bone Tumor    2419

## CHAPTER 69
### Management of Patients With Musculoskeletal Trauma    2424

**CONTUSIONS, STRAINS, AND SPRAINS**    2425
**JOINT DISLOCATIONS**    2426
**SPORTS-RELATED INJURIES**    2426
**OCCUPATION-RELATED INJURIES**    2427
**SPECIFIC MUSCULOSKELETAL INJURIES**    2429
- Rotator Cuff Tears    2429
- Epicondylitis (Tennis Elbow)    2429
- Lateral and Medial Collateral Ligament Injury    2429
- Anterior and Posterior Cruciate Ligament Injury    2430
- Meniscal Injuries    2430
- Rupture of the Achilles Tendon    2430

**FRACTURES**    2431
**FRACTURE HEALING AND COMPLICATIONS**    2435
- Early Complications    2435
- Delayed Complications    2438

**FRACTURES OF SPECIFIC SITES**    2440
- Clavicle    2440
- Humeral Neck    2441
- Humeral Shaft    2442
- Elbow    2443
- Radial Head    2443
- Radial and Ulnar Shafts    2443
- Wrist    2443
- Hand    2444
- Pelvis    2444
- Femur    2446
- Femoral Shaft    2449
- Knee    2458
- Tibia and Fibula    2459
- Rib    2459
- Thoracolumbar Spine    2460

**AMPUTATION**    2460
- ▶▶ Nursing Process: The Patient Undergoing an Amputation    2462

# UNIT 16
# Other Acute Problems    2472

## CHAPTER 70
### Management of Patients With Infectious Diseases    2474

**THE INFECTIOUS PROCESS**    2475
**INFECTION CONTROL AND PREVENTION**    2480
**HOME-BASED CARE OF THE PATIENT WITH AN INFECTIOUS DISEASE**    2489
- ▶▶ Nursing Process: The Patient With an Infectious Disease    2490

**DIARRHEAL DISEASES**    2492
- ▶▶ Nursing Process: The Patient With Infectious Diarrhea    2502

**SEXUALLY TRANSMITTED DISEASES**    2504
- Human Immunodeficiency Virus    2505
- Syphilis    2505
- *Chlamydia trachomatis* and *Neisseria gonorrhoeae*    2507
- ▶▶ Nursing Process: The Patient With a Sexually Transmitted Disease    2508

**EMERGING INFECTIOUS DISEASES**    2509
- Severe Acute Respiratory Syndrome    2510
- West Nile Virus    2510
- Legionnaires' Disease    2510
- Hantavirus Pulmonary Syndrome    2511
- Viral Hemorrhagic Fevers    2511

**TRAVEL AND IMMIGRATION**    2512

## CHAPTER 71
### Emergency Nursing    2516

**SCOPE AND PRACTICE OF EMERGENCY NURSING**    2517
**PRINCIPLES OF EMERGENCY CARE**    2520
**AIRWAY OBSTRUCTION**    2522
**HEMORRHAGE**    2526
**HYPOVOLEMIC SHOCK**    2527
**WOUNDS**    2528
**TRAUMA**    2529
- Collection of Forensic Evidence    2529
- Injury Prevention    2530
- Multiple Trauma    2530

Intra-Abdominal Injuries 2530
Crush Injuries 2532
Fractures 2533
**ENVIRONMENTAL EMERGENCIES 2533**
Heat Stroke 2533
Frostbite 2534
Hypothermia 2535
Near-Drowning 2536
Decompression Sickness 2537
Anaphylactic Reaction 2537
Latex Allergy 2538
Insect Stings 2539
Snake Bites 2539
**POISONING 2540**
Ingested (Swallowed) Poisons 2541
Carbon Monoxide Poisoning 2541
Skin Contamination Poisoning (Chemical Burns) 2543
Food Poisoning 2544
**SUBSTANCE ABUSE 2544**
Acute Alcohol Intoxication 2544
Alcohol Withdrawal Syndrome/Delirium Tremens 2549
**VIOLENCE, ABUSE, AND NEGLECT 2550**
Family Violence, Abuse, and Neglect 2550
Sexual Assault 2551
**PSYCHIATRIC EMERGENCIES 2553**
Overactive Patients 2553
Violent Behavior 2553
Posttraumatic Stress Disorder 2554
Underactive or Depressed Patients 2554
Suicidal Patients 2555

# CHAPTER 72
## Terrorism, Mass Casualty, and Disaster Nursing 2558

**FEDERAL, STATE, AND LOCAL RESPONSES TO EMERGENCIES 2559**
**HOSPITAL EMERGENCY PREPAREDNESS PLANS 2560**
**PREPAREDNESS AND RESPONSE 2564**
**NATURAL DISASTERS 2565**
**WEAPONS OF TERROR 2566**

**Appendix A:** Diagnostic Studies and Interpretation 2577

**Appendix B:** Understanding Clinical Pathways 2602

**Appendix C:** Concept Maps 2614

Index I-1

# UNIT 1

# Basic Concepts in Nursing

## Case Study
### Applying Concepts from NANDA, NIC, and NOC

**The Community with an Identified Health Problem**

A **nurse** working in an urgent care clinic that serves an economically depressed urban area notes a high incidence of elderly patients with dehydration and heatstroke in the summer months. The nurse verifies the observations by accessing data about hospital admissions for dehydration and heatstroke. The nurse determines that many of the admitted patients live in the area served by the clinic and that many of the patients live alone and have other chronic illnesses. The nurse sees the need for a plan that includes a community response to this problem. The plan includes arranging an education program about the prevention of dehydration; a community support buddy system in which neighbors or volunteers call or visit homebound elders during critical periods in the summer; and economic support to air condition the senior citizens' center.

 Turn to Appendix C to see a concept map that illustrates the relationships that exist between the nursing diagnoses, interventions, and outcomes for the community's identified health problem.

## Nursing Classifications and Languages

| NANDA<br>Nursing Diagnoses | NIC<br>Nursing Interventions | NOC<br>Nursing Outcomes<br>Return to functional baseline status, stabilization of, or improvement in: |
|---|---|---|
| **Ineffective Community Therapeutic Regimen Management**—Pattern of regulating and integrating into community processes programs for treatment of illness and the sequelae of illness that are unsatisfactory for meeting health-related goals | **Community Health Development**—Assisting members of a community to identify a community's health concerns, mobilize resources, and implement solutions<br><br>**Program Development**—Planning, implementing, and evaluating a co-ordinated set of activities designed to enhance wellness, or to prevent, reduce or eliminate one or more health problems for a group or community | **Community Competence**—Capacity of a community to collectively problem solve to achieve community goals |
| **Ineffective Community Coping**—Pattern of community activities (for adaptation and problem solving) that is unsatisfactory for meeting the demands or needs of the community | **Surveillance: Community**—Purposeful and ongoing acquisition, interpretation, and synthesis of data for decision making in the community | **Community Health Status**—The general state of well-being of a community or population |
| **Readiness for Enhanced Community Coping**—Pattern of community activities for adaptation and problem solving that is satisfactory for meeting the demands or needs of the community but can be improved for management of current and future problems/stressors | **Environmental Risk Protection**—Preventing and detecting disease and injury in populations at risk from environmental hazards | |

NANDA International (2005). *Nursing diagnoses: Definitions & Classification 2005–2006*. Philadelphia: North American Nursing Diagnosis Association.
Dochterman, J. M., & Bulechek, G. M. (2004). *Nursing interventions classification (NIC)* (4th ed.). St. Louis: Mosby.
Iowa Outcomes Project (2004). In Moorhead, S., Johnson, M. & Maas, M. (2004). *Nursing outcomes classification (NOC)* (3rd ed.). St. Louis: Mosby.
Dochterman, J. M. & Jones, D. A. (2003). *Unifying nursing languages: The harmonization of NANDA, NIC, and NOC*. Washington D.C.: American Nurses Association.

"Point, click, learn! Visit thePoint for additional resources."

# CHAPTER 1

# Health Care Delivery and Nursing Practice

## Learning Objectives

*On completion of this chapter, the learner will be able to:*

1. Define health and wellness.
2. Describe factors causing significant changes in the health care delivery system and their impact on the health care field and the nursing profession.
3. Describe the practitioner, leadership, and research roles of nurses.
4. Describe nursing care delivery models.
5. Discuss expanded nursing roles.

Health care in the United States has undergone profound changes during the past several decades. Nursing, as a health care profession and a major component of the health care system, has been significantly affected by these changes. Nursing has played an important role in affecting the health care system and will continue to do so.

# The Health Care Industry and the Nursing Profession

## Nursing Defined

Since the time of Florence Nightingale, who wrote in 1858 that the goal of nursing was "to put the patient in the best condition for nature to act upon him," nursing leaders have described nursing as both an art and a science. However, the definition of nursing has evolved over time. In its Social Policy Statement (2003), the American Nurses Association (ANA) defined nursing as the diagnosis and treatment of human responses to health and illness. The ANA provides the following list of phenomena that are the focus for nursing care and research:

- Self-care processes
- Physiologic and pathophysiologic processes such as rest, sleep, respiration, circulation, reproduction, activity, nutrition, elimination, skin, sexuality, and communication
- Comfort, pain, and discomfort
- Emotions related to health and illness
- Meanings ascribed to health and illnesses
- Decision making and ability to make choices
- Perceptual orientations such as self-image and control over one's body and environments
- Transitions across the life span, such as birth, growth, development, and death
- Affiliative relationships, including freedom from oppression and abuse
- Environmental systems

Nurses have a responsibility to carry out their role as described in the Social Policy Statement, to comply with the nurse practice act of the state in which they practice, and to comply with the Code for Nurses as spelled out by the International Council of Nurses and the ANA. To obtain a foundation for examining the delivery of nursing care, it is necessary to understand the needs of health care consumers and the health care delivery system, including the forces that affect nursing and health care delivery.

## The Patient/Client: Consumer of Nursing and Health Care

The central figure in health care services is, of course, the patient. The term *patient*, which is derived from a Latin verb meaning "to suffer," has traditionally been used to describe those who are recipients of care. The connotation commonly attached to the word is one of dependence. For this reason, many nurses prefer to use the term *client*, which is derived from a Latin verb meaning "to lean," connoting alliance and interdependence. The term *patient* is used throughout this book, with the understanding that either term is acceptable.

The patient who seeks care for a health problem or problems (increasing numbers of people have multiple health problems) is also an individual person, a member of a family, and a citizen of the community. Patients' needs vary depending on their problems, associated circumstances, and past experiences. Among the nurse's important functions in health care delivery is identifying the patient's immediate needs and taking measures to address them.

### The Patient's Basic Needs

Certain needs are basic to all people. Some of these needs are more important than others. Once an essential need is met, people often experience a need on a higher level of priority. Addressing needs by priority reflects Maslow's hierarchy of needs (Fig. 1-1).

### Maslow's Hierarchy

Maslow ranked human needs as follows: physiologic needs; safety and security; sense of belonging and affection; esteem and self-respect; and self-actualization, which includes self-fulfillment, desire to know and understand, and aesthetic needs. Lower-level needs always remain, but a person's ability to pursue higher-level needs indicates movement toward psychological health and well-being. Such a hierarchy of needs is a useful framework that can be applied to the various nursing models for assessment of a patient's strengths, limitations, and need for nursing interventions.

## Health Care in Transition

Changes occurring in health care delivery and nursing are the result of societal, economic, technological, scientific,

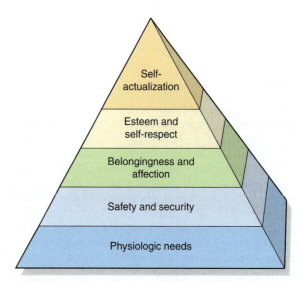

**FIGURE 1-1.** This scheme of Maslow's hierarchy of human needs shows how a person moves from fulfillment of basic needs to higher levels of needs, with the ultimate goal being integrated human functioning and health.

and political forces that have evolved throughout the 20th and into the 21st century. Among the most significant changes are shifts in population demographics, particularly the increase in the aging population and the cultural diversity of the population; changing patterns of diseases; increased technology; increased consumer expectations; higher costs of health care and changes in health care financing; and other health care reform efforts. These changes have led to institutional restructuring, staff downsizing, increased outpatient care services, decreased lengths of hospital stay, and increased health care in community and home settings. Such changes have dramatically influenced where nurses practice. These changes have influenced society's view of health and illness and affected the focus of nursing and health care.

As the proportion of the population reaching age 65 years has increased, and with the shift from acute illnesses to chronic illnesses, the traditional disease management and care focus of the health care professions has expanded. There is increasing concern about emerging infectious diseases, trauma, obesity, and bioterrorism. Thus, health care must focus more on disease prevention, health promotion, and management of chronic conditions than in previous times. This shift in focus coincides with a nationwide emphasis on cost control and resource management directed toward providing cost-efficient and cost-effective health care services to the population as a whole.

# Health, Wellness, and Health Promotion

The health care system of the United States, which traditionally has been disease-oriented, is placing increasing emphasis on health and its promotion. Similarly, a significant portion of nurses were formerly focused on the care of patients with acute conditions, but now many are directing their efforts toward health promotion and illness prevention.

## Health

How health is perceived depends on how health is defined. The World Health Organization (WHO), in the preamble to its constitution, defines *health* as a "state of complete physical, mental, and social well-being and not merely the absence of disease and infirmity" (Hood & Leddy, 2003). Although this definition of health does not allow for any variation in degrees of wellness or illness, the concept of a health–illness continuum allows for a greater range in describing a person's health status. By viewing health and illness on a continuum, it is possible to consider a person as being neither completely healthy nor completely ill. Instead, a person's state of health is ever-changing and has the potential to range from high-level wellness to extremely poor health and imminent death. Use of the health–illness continuum makes it possible to view a person as simultaneously possessing degrees of both health and illness.

The limitations of the WHO definition of health are clear in relation to chronic illness and disability. Chronically ill people do not meet the standards of health as established by the WHO definition. However, when viewed from the perspective of the health–illness continuum, people with a chronic illness or disability may be viewed as having the potential to attain a high level of wellness if they are successful in meeting their health potential within the limits of their chronic illness or disability.

## Wellness

*Wellness* has been defined as being equivalent to health. Wellness involves being proactive and involving people in efforts toward a state of physical, psychological, and spiritual well-being in which they look and feel their best (Stone, 2003). Hood and Leddy (2003) consider that wellness has four components: (1) the capacity to perform to the best of his or her ability, (2) the ability to adjust and adapt to varying situations, (3) a reported feeling of well-being, and (4) a feeling that "everything is together" and harmonious. With this in mind, it becomes evident that the goal of health care providers is to promote positive changes that are directed toward health and well-being. The sense of wellness has a subjective aspect that emphasizes the importance of recognizing and responding to patient individuality and diversity in health care and nursing.

## Health Promotion

Today, increasing emphasis is placed on health, health promotion, wellness, and self-care. Health is seen as resulting from a lifestyle oriented toward wellness. The result has been the evolution of a wide range of health promotion strategies, including multiphasic screening, genetic testing, lifetime health monitoring, environmental and mental health programs, risk reduction, and nutrition and health education. A growing interest in self-care skills is evidenced by the large number of health-related publications, conferences, and workshops designed for the lay public.

People are increasingly knowledgeable about their health and take more interest in and responsibility for their health and well-being. Organized self-care education programs emphasize health promotion, disease prevention, management of illness, self-care, and judicious use of the professional health care system. In addition, well over 500,000 self-help groups and numerous websites and chat groups promote sharing of experiences and information about self-care with others who have similar conditions, chronic diseases, or disabling conditions.

Special efforts are being made by health care professionals to reach and motivate members of various cultural and socioeconomic groups about lifestyle and health practices. Stress, improper diet, lack of exercise, smoking, use of drugs, high-risk behaviors (including risky sexual practices), and poor hygiene are all lifestyle behaviors known to affect health negatively. Health care professionals are concerned with encouraging behavior that promotes health. The goal is to motivate people to make improvements in the way they live, to modify risky behaviors, and to adopt healthy behaviors.

# Influences on Health Care Delivery

The health care delivery system is rapidly changing as the population and its health care needs and expectations change. The shifting demographics of the population, the increase in chronic illnesses and disability, the greater emphasis on health care costs, and technologic advances have resulted in changing emphases in health care delivery and in nursing.

## Population Demographics

Changes in the population in general are affecting the need for and the delivery of health care. The 2000 U.S. census data indicated that there were 281,421,906 people in the country (U.S. Bureau of the Census, 2000). Population growth is attributed in part to improved public health services and improved nutrition.

Not only is the population increasing, but the composition of the population is also changing. The decline in birth rate and the increase in life span due to improved health care have resulted in fewer school-age children and more senior citizens, most of whom are women. Much of the population resides in highly congested urban areas, with a steady migration of members of ethnic minorities to the inner cities and a migration of members of the middle class to suburban areas. The number of homeless people, including entire families, has increased significantly. The population has become more culturally diverse as increasing numbers of people from different national backgrounds enter the country.

Because of such population changes, the need for health care for specific age groups, for women, and for diverse groups of people in specific geographic locations is altering the effectiveness of traditional means of providing health care. As a result, far-reaching changes in the overall health care delivery system are necessary.

## Aging Population

The elderly population in the United States has increased significantly and will continue to grow in future years. In 2000, the 34.5 million adults who are older than 65 years of age constituted 12.7% of the U.S. population. By the year 2030, 20% of the U.S. population is expected to be older than 65 years of age. According to the U.S. Bureau of the Census (2000), the number of people 65 to 74 years of age was 8 times larger in 1999 than in 1900, and the number of people 75 to 84 years of age was 16 times larger. In addition, people 85 years of age and older constitute one of the fastest-growing segments of the population; the number was 34 times larger in 1999 than in 1900.

The health care needs of older adults are complex and demand significant investments, both professional and financial, by the health care industry. Many elderly people suffer from multiple chronic conditions that are exacerbated by acute episodes. In particular, elderly women, whose conditions are frequently underdiagnosed and undertreated, are of concern. There are approximately three women for every two men in the older population, and elderly women are expected to continue to outnumber elderly men.

### Cultural Diversity

An appreciation for the diverse characteristics and needs of people from varied ethnic and cultural backgrounds is important in health care and nursing. Some projections indicate that by 2030, racial and ethnic minority groups will constitute 40% of the population of the United States (Baldwin, 2004). With increased immigration, both legal and illegal, this figure could easily increase to more than 50% by the year 2030. As the cultural composition of the population changes, it is increasingly important to address cultural considerations in the delivery of health care. Patients from diverse sociocultural groups not only bring various health care beliefs, values, and practices to the health care setting, but they also have a variety of risk factors for some disease conditions and unique reactions to treatment. These factors significantly affect an individual's responses to health care problems or illnesses, to caregivers, and to the care itself. Unless these factors are understood and respected by health care providers, the care delivered may be ineffective, and health care outcomes may be negatively affected.

*Culture* is defined as learned patterns of behavior, beliefs, and values that are shared by a particular group of people. Included among the many characteristics that distinguish cultural groups are the manner of dress, language spoken, values, rules or norms of behavior, gender-specific practices, economics, politics, law and social control, artifacts, technology, dietary practices, and health beliefs and practices. Health promotion, illness prevention, causes of sickness, treatment, coping, caring, dying, and death are part of the health-related component of every culture. Every person has a unique belief and value system that has been shaped at least in part by his or her cultural environment. This belief and value system guides the person's thinking, decisions, and actions. It provides direction for interpreting and responding to illness and disability and to health care.

To promote an effective nurse–patient relationship and positive outcomes of care, nursing care must be culturally competent, appropriate, and sensitive to cultural differences. All attempts should be made to help each person retain his or her unique cultural characteristics. Providing special foods that have significance and arranging for special religious observances may enable a patient to maintain a feeling of wholeness at a time when he or she may feel isolated from family and community (Campinha-Bacote, 2003).

Knowing the cultural and social significance that particular situations have for each patient helps the nurse avoid imposing a personal value system when the patient has a different point of view. In most cases, cooperation with the plan of care is greatest when communication among the nurse, the patient, and the patient's family is directed toward understanding the situation or the problem and respecting each other's goals.

## Changing Patterns of Disease

During the past 50 years, the health problems of the American people have changed significantly. Although many infectious diseases have been controlled or eradicated, others, such as tuberculosis, acquired immunodeficiency syndrome (AIDS), and sexually transmitted diseases/infections, are on the rise. An increasing number of infectious agents are becoming resistant to antibiotic therapy as a result of widespread inappropriate use of antibiotics. Obesity has become a major health concern, and the multiple comorbidities that accompany it, such as hypertension, heart disease, diabetes, and cancer, add significantly to its associated mortality.

Conditions that were once easily treated have become more complex and life-threatening. The prevalence of chronic illnesses and disability is increasing because of the lengthening life span of Americans and the advances in care and treatment options for conditions such as cancer, human immunodeficiency virus (HIV) infection, and spina bifida. In addition, improvements in care for trauma and other serious acute health problems have meant that many people with these conditions live decades longer than in the past. People with chronic illness are the largest group of health care consumers in the United States (Harrison, 2003). Because the majority of health problems seen today are chronic in nature, many people are learning to maximize their health within the constraints of chronic illness and disability.

As chronic conditions increase, health care broadens from a focus on cure and eradication of disease to include the prevention or rapid treatment of exacerbations of chronic conditions. Nursing, which has always encouraged patients to take control of their conditions, plays a prominent role in the current focus on management of chronic illness and disability.

## Advances in Technology and Genetics

Advances in technology and genetics have occurred with greater frequency during the past several decades than in all other periods of civilization. Sophisticated techniques and devices have revolutionized surgery and diagnostic testing, making it possible to perform many procedures and tests on an outpatient basis. Increased knowledge and understanding of genetics have resulted in expanded screening, diagnostic testing, and treatments for a variety of conditions. The sophisticated communication systems that connect most parts of the world, with the capability of rapid storage, retrieval, and dissemination of information, have stimulated brisk change as well as swift obsolescence in health care delivery strategies. Advances in genetics and technology have resulted in many ethical issues for the health care system, health care providers, patients, families, and society.

## Economic Changes

The belief that comprehensive, quality health care should be provided for all citizens prompted governmental concern about rising health care costs and wide variations in charges among providers. In 1983, the U.S. Congress passed the most significant health legislation since the Medicare program was enacted in 1965. The federal government was no longer able to afford to reimburse hospitals for patient care that was delivered without any defined limits on costs. Therefore, it approved a prospective payment system (PPS) for hospital inpatient services. Based on diagnosis-related groups (DRGs), a PPS sets the reimbursement rates for Medicare payments for hospital services. Hospitals receive payment at a fixed rate for patients with diagnoses that fall into a specific DRG. A fixed payment has been predetermined for more than 470 possible diagnostic categories, covering the majority of medical diagnoses of patients admitted to the hospital. Hospitals receive the same payment for every patient with a given diagnosis, or DRG. If the cost of the patient's care is lower than the payment, the hospital makes a profit; if the cost is higher, the hospital incurs a loss. As a result, hospitals are placing greater emphasis on reducing costs, utilization of services, and length of patient stay.

In addition, the Balanced Budget Act of 1997 added new rate requirements for ambulatory payment classifications (APCs) to hospitals and other providers of ambulatory care services.

To qualify for Medicare reimbursement, care providers and hospitals must contract with peer review organizations (PROs) to perform quality and utilization review with the goals of cost-effectiveness and reduced costs. The PROs monitor admission patterns, lengths of stay, transfers, and quality of services, and they also validate the DRG coding. The DRG system has provided an incentive to cut costs and discharge patients as quickly as possible.

Nurses in hospitals now care for patients who are older and sicker and require more nursing services; nurses in the community are caring for patients who have been discharged earlier and need high-technology acute care services as well as long-term care. The importance of effective discharge planning, along with utilization review and quality improvement, cannot be overstated. Nurses in acute care settings must work with other health care team members to maintain quality care while facing pressures to discharge patients and decrease staffing costs. They must also work with nurses and others in community settings to ensure continuity of care.

## Demand for Quality Health Care

The general public has become increasingly interested in and knowledgeable about health care and health promotion through television, newspapers, magazines, and other communications media. Health care has become a topic of political debate. The public has also become more health conscious and subscribes to the belief that health and quality health care constitute a basic right, rather than a privilege for a chosen few.

### Quality Improvement and Evidence-Based Practice

In the 1980s, hospitals and other health care agencies implemented ongoing quality assurance (QA) programs. These programs were required for reimbursement for services and for accreditation by the Joint Commission on Accreditation of Healthcare Organizations (JCAHO). QA programs sought to establish accountability to society on the part of the health professions for the quality, appropriateness, and cost of health services provided.

In the early 1990s, it was recognized that quality of care as defined by regulatory agencies continued to be difficult to measure. QA criteria were identified as measures to ensure minimal expectations only; they did not provide mechanisms for identifying causes of problems or for determining systems or processes that needed improvement. Continuous quality improvement (CQI) was identified as a more effective mechanism for improving the quality of health care. In 1992, the revised standards of the JCAHO mandated that health care organizations implement a CQI program. Recent amendments to JCAHO standards have specified that patients have the right to health care that is considerate and preserves dignity; that respects cultural, psychosocial, and spiritual values; and that is age-specific (Krozok & Scoggins, 2002). Quality improvement efforts have focused on ensuring that the care provided meets or exceeds JCAHO standards.

Unlike QA, which focuses on individual incidents or errors and minimal expectations, CQI focuses on the processes used to provide care, with the aim of improving quality by assessing and improving those interrelated processes that most affect patient care outcomes and patient satisfaction. CQI involves analyzing, understanding, and improving clinical, financial, and operational processes. Problems that occur as more than isolated events are subject to examination, and all issues that may affect patient outcome are studied. Nurses directly involved in the delivery of care are engaged in analyzing data and refining the processes used in CQI. Their knowledge of the processes and conditions that affect patient care is critical in designing changes to improve the quality of the care provided.

As health care agencies continue to implement CQI, nurses have many opportunities to be involved in quality improvement. One such opportunity is through facilitation of evidence-based practice, which involves identifying and evaluating current literature and research, as well as incorporating the findings into care guidelines. This process has been designated as a means of ensuring quality care. Evidence-based practice includes the use of outcome assessment and standardized plans of care such as clinical guidelines, clinical pathways, or algorithms. Many of these measures are being implemented by nurses, particularly by nurse managers and advanced practice nurses, often in collaboration with other health care professionals.

### Clinical Pathways and Care Mapping

Many hospitals, managed care facilities, and home health services nationwide use clinical pathways or care mapping to coordinate care for caseloads of patients (Kinsman, 2004; Kinsman, James, & Ham, 2004). Clinical pathways are tools for tracking a patient's progress toward achieving positive outcomes within specified time frames. Clinical pathways based on current literature and clinical expertise have been developed for patients with certain DRGs (eg, open heart surgery, pneumonia with comorbidity, fractured hip), for high-risk patients (eg, those receiving chemotherapy), and for patients with certain common health problems (eg, diabetes, chronic pain). The pathways indicate key events, such as diagnostic tests, treatments, activities, medications, consultation, and education, that must occur within specified times for patients to achieve the desired and timely outcomes.

A case manager often facilitates and coordinates interventions to ensure that the patient progresses through the key events and achieves the desired outcomes. Nurses who provide direct care play an important role in the development and use of clinical pathways through their participation in researching the literature and then developing, piloting, implementing, and revising clinical pathways. In addition, nurses monitor outcome achievement and document and analyze variances. Examples of clinical pathways can be found in Appendix A.

Other evidence-based practice tools used for planning patient care are care mapping, multidisciplinary action plans (MAPs), clinical guidelines, and algorithms. These tools are used to move patients toward predetermined outcome markers. Algorithms are used more often in acute situations to determine a particular treatment based on patient information or response. Care maps, clinical guidelines, and MAPs (the most detailed of these tools) provide coordination of care and education throughout hospitalization and after discharge.

Because care mapping and guidelines are used for conditions in which a patient's progression often defies prediction, specific time frames for achieving outcomes are excluded. A patient with a highly complex condition or multiple underlying illnesses may benefit more from care mapping or guidelines than from clinical pathways, because the use of outcome markers (rather than specific time frames) is more realistic.

Through case management and the use of clinical pathways or care mapping, patients and the care they receive are continually assessed from preadmission to discharge—and in many cases after discharge in the home care and community settings. These tools are used in hospitals and other health care settings to facilitate the effective and efficient care of large groups of patients. Continuity of care, effective utilization of services, and cost containment are expected to be major benefits for society and for the health care system.

## Alternative Health Care Delivery Systems

The rising cost of health care over the past few decades has led to the use of managed health care and alternative health care delivery systems, including health maintenance organizations (HMOs) and preferred provider organizations (PPOs).

### Managed Care

Managed care is an important trend in health care. The failure of the efforts of past decades to reduce costs and the escalation of health care costs to 15% to 22% of the gross domestic product have prompted business, labor, and government to assume greater control over the financing and delivery of health care. The common features that characterize managed care include prenegotiated payment rates, mandatory precertification, utilization review, limited choice of providers, and fixed-price reimbursement. The scope of managed care has expanded from in-hospital services to HMOs or variations such as PPOs; ambulatory, long-term, and home care services; and related diagnostic and therapeutic services.

Managed care has contributed to a dramatic reduction in inpatient hospital days, continuing expansion of ambulatory care, fierce competition, and marketing strategies that appeal to consumers as well as to insurers and regulators. Hospitals are faced with declining revenues, a declining number of patients, more severely ill patients with shorter lengths of stay, and a need for cost-effective outpatient or ambulatory care services. As patients return to the community, they have more health care needs, many of which are complex. The demand for home care and community-based services is escalating. Despite their successes, managed care organizations are faced with the challenge of providing quality services under resource constraints. Case management is a strategy used by many organizations to meet this challenge.

### Case Management

Case management is a system of coordinating health care services to ensure cost-effectiveness, accountability, and quality care. It dates back to the public health programs of the early 1900s, in which public health nursing played a dominant role. The premise of case management is that the responsibility for meeting patient needs rests with one person or team whose goals are to provide the patient and family with access to required services, to ensure coordination of these services, and to evaluate how effectively these services are delivered.

Case management has gained such prominence because of decreased costs of care associated with decreased lengths of hospital stays coupled with rapid and frequent inter-unit transfers from specialty to standard care units. The case manager role, instead of focusing on direct patient care, focuses on managing the care of an entire caseload of patients and collaborating with nurses and other health care personnel who care for patients. In some settings, particularly the community setting, the focus of the nurse case manager is on managing the treatment plan of the patient with complex conditions (Schifalacqua, Ulch, & Schmidt, 2004). The caseload is usually limited in scope to patients with similar diagnoses, needs, and therapies. Case managers are experts in their specialty areas, and they coordinate the inpatient and outpatient services needed by patients. The goals of case management are quality, appropriateness, and timeliness of services as well as cost reduction. The case manager follows the patient throughout hospitalization and at home after discharge in an effort to coordinate health care services that will avert or delay rehospitalization. Evidence-based pathways or similar plans are often used in case management of similar patient populations.

## Roles of the Nurse

As stated previously, nursing is the diagnosis and treatment of human responses to health and illness and therefore focuses on a broad array of phenomena. Professional nurses who work in institutional, community-oriented, or community-based settings play three major roles: the practitioner role, which includes teaching and collaborating; the leadership role; and the research role. Although each role carries specific responsibilities, these roles are characteristic of all nursing positions and relate to one another. These roles are designed to meet the immediate and future needs of consumers who are the recipients of nursing care. Often, nurses act in a combination of roles to provide comprehensive patient care.

### Practitioner Role

The practitioner role involves those actions taken by nurses to meet the health care and nursing needs of individual patients, their families, and significant others. This role is the dominant role of nurses in primary, secondary, and tertiary health care settings and in home care and community nursing. It is achieved through use of the nursing process, the basis of all nursing practice. Nurses help patients meet their needs through direct intervention, by teaching patients and family members to perform care, and by coordinating and collaborating with other disciplines to provide needed services.

### Leadership Role

The leadership role is often perceived as a specialized role assumed by nurses who have titles that suggest leadership and who are the leaders of large groups of nurses or related health care professionals. However, because of the constant fluctuation of health care delivery demands and consumers, a broader definition of nursing leadership, one that identifies the leadership role as inherent within all nursing positions, is required. The leadership role involves those actions that nurses execute when they assume responsibility for the actions of others directed toward determining and achieving patient care goals.

Nursing leadership involves four components: decision making, relating, influencing, and facilitating. Each of these components promotes change and the ultimate outcome of goal achievement. Basic to the entire process is effective communication, which determines the success of the process and achievement of goals. Leadership in nursing is a process in which nurses use interpersonal skills to effect change in the behavior of others. The components of the leadership process are appropriate during all phases of the nursing process and in all settings.

### Research Role

The primary task of nursing research is to contribute to the scientific base of nursing practice. Studies are needed to determine the effectiveness of nursing interventions and nursing care. The science of nursing grows through research, leading to the generation of a scientifically based rationale for nursing practice and patient care. This process is the basis of evidence-based practice, with a resultant increase in the quality of patient care.

The research role is considered to be a responsibility of *all* nurses in clinical practice. Nurses must constantly be alert for nursing problems and important issues related to patient care that can serve as a basis for the identification of researchable questions. Nurses with a background in research methods can use their research knowledge and skills to initiate and implement timely, relevant studies.

Nurses directly involved in patient care are often in the best position to identify potential research problems and questions, and their clinical insights are invaluable. Nurses also have a responsibility to become actively involved in ongoing research studies. This may involve facilitating the data collection process, or it may include actual collection of data. Explaining the study to patients and their families and to other health care professionals is often of invaluable assistance to the researcher who is conducting the study.

Above all, nurses must use research findings in their nursing practice; the use, validation, replication, dissemination, and evaluation of research findings further the science of nursing. As stated previously, evidence-based practice requires the use of valid research. Nurses must continually be aware of studies that are directly related to their own area of clinical practice and critically analyze those studies to determine the applicability of their implications for specific patient populations. Relevant conclusions and implications can be used to improve patient care.

# Models of Nursing Care Delivery

Several organizational methods or models that vary greatly from one facility to another and from one set of patient circumstances to another may be used to carry out nursing care. These methods and models have changed over the years and have included functional nursing, team nursing, and, more recently, primary nursing.

## Primary Nursing

Primary nursing (not to be confused with primary health care, which pertains to first-contact general health care) refers to comprehensive, individualized care provided by the same nurse throughout the period of care. This type of nursing care allows the nurse to give direct patient care rather than manage and supervise the functions of others who care for a particular patient. This care method is too costly for many institutions because a smaller patient–nurse ratio, with a larger professional staff, is needed. However, primary nursing may provide a foundation for transition to case management in some institutions.

The primary nurse is responsible for directly involving the patient and family in all facets of care. The primary nurse accepts total 24-hour responsibility for a patient's nursing care, which is directed toward meeting the individualized needs of that patient. To promote continuity of care and collaboration directed toward quality patient care, the primary nurse communicates with other members of the health care team regarding the patient's health.

When a particular primary nurse is not working, an associate nurse or co-nurse assists in overseeing the delivery of care. This nurse implements the nursing plan of care and provides feedback to the primary nurse for evaluating the plan of care. The primary nurse retains responsibility for making appropriate referrals and for ensuring that all relevant information is provided to people involved in the patient's continuing care, including family members.

The long-term survival of primary nursing is uncertain. Although primary nursing continues to be used in many health care agencies, many variations have been developed to meet the needs of the particular agency. As cost-containment measures continue and patient acuity increases, staffing ratios of patients to nurses are increasing. Many nursing service departments and agencies are meeting the increased workload demands by modifying their approach to primary nursing or by reverting to team or functional systems of care. Others are changing their staffing mix and redesigning their practice models to accommodate nonprofessional staff. Still others are changing to more innovative systems such as case management.

## Community-Based Nursing and Community-Oriented/ Public Health Nursing

Community-based care and community-oriented/public health nursing are not new concepts in nursing. Nursing has played a vital role in the community since the middle to late 1800s, when visiting nurses provided care to the sick and poor in their homes and communities and educated patients and families. Although community health nursing, public health nursing, community-based nursing, and home health nursing may be discussed together and aspects of care in each type do overlap, these terms are distinct from one another. Confusion exists regarding the differences, and the similar settings may blur these distinctions (Stanhope & Lancaster, 2004). The central idea of community-oriented nursing practice is that nursing intervention can promote wellness, reduce the spread of illness, and improve the health status of groups of citizens or the community at large. Its emphasis is on primary, secondary, and tertiary prevention. Nurses in these settings have traditionally focused on health promotion, maternal and child health, and chronic care.

Community-based nursing occurs in a variety of settings within the community and is directed toward individuals and families (Stanhope & Lancaster, 2004). It includes home health care nursing. Most community-based and home health care is directed toward specific patient groups with identified needs, which usually relate to illness, injury, or disability, resulting most often from advanced age or chronic illness. However, both community-based and community-oriented nurses are now meeting the needs of groups of patients with a variety of problems and needs. Home health care is a major aspect of community-based care discussed throughout this text. Home health care services are provided by community-based programs and agencies for specific populations (eg, the elderly, ventilator-dependent patients), as well as by home health care agencies, hospices, independent professional nursing practices, and freestanding health care agencies.

As shortened hospital stays and increased use of outpatient health care services continue, the need for nursing care in the home and community setting increases. Because nursing services are provided outside as well as inside the hospital, nurses have a choice of practicing in a variety of health care delivery settings. These settings include acute care medical centers, ambulatory care settings, clinics, urgent care centers, outpatient departments, neighborhood health centers, home health care agencies, independent or group nursing centers, and managed care agencies.

Community nursing centers, which have emerged in the past few decades, are nurse-managed and provide primary care services such as ambulatory and outpatient care, immunizations, health assessment and screening services, and patient and family education and counseling. These centers serve varied populations that typically include a high proportion of patients who are rural, very young, very old, poor, or members of racial minorities—groups that are generally underserved.

The numbers and kinds of agencies that provide care in the home and community have increased because of the expanding needs of patients requiring care. Home health care nurses are challenged because patients are discharged from acute care institutions to their homes and communities early in the recovery process and with more complex needs. Many are elderly, and many have multiple medical and nursing diagnoses and multisystem health problems that require acute and intensive nursing care. Medical technologies such as ventilatory support and intravenous or parenteral nutrition therapy, once limited to the acute care setting, have been adapted to the home care setting.

As a result, the community-based care setting is becoming one of the largest practice areas for nursing. Home care nursing is now a specialty area that requires advanced knowledge and skills in general nursing practice, with emphasis on community health and acute medical-surgical nursing. Also required are high-level assessment skills, critical thinking, and decision-making skills in a setting where other health care professionals are not available to validate observations, conclusions, and decisions.

Home care nurses often function as acute care nurses in the home, providing "high-tech, high-touch" services to patients with acute health care needs. In addition, they are responsible for patient and family teaching and for contacting community resources and coordinating the continuing care of patients. For these reasons, the scope of medical-surgical nursing encompasses not only the acute care setting within the hospital but also the acute care setting as it expands into the community and the home. Throughout this textbook, the home health care needs of patients are addressed, with particular attention given to the teaching, self-care management, and health maintenance needs of patients and their families.

## Expanded Nursing Roles

Professional nursing is adapting to meet changing health needs and expectations. The role of the nurse has expanded in response to the need to improve the distribution of health care services and to decrease the cost of health care. Nurse practitioners (NPs), clinical nurse specialists (CNSs), certified nurse-midwives, and certified registered nurse anesthetists (CRNAs) are identified as advanced practice nurses. Nurses who function in these roles provide direct care to patients through independent practice, practice within a health care agency, or collaboration with a physician. Specialization in nursing has evolved as a result of the recent explosion of technology and knowledge.

Nurses may receive advanced education in such specialties as family care, critical care, coronary care, respiratory care, oncologic care, maternal and child health care, neonatal intensive care, rehabilitation, trauma, rural health, and gerontologic nursing. Various titles have emerged to specify the functions as well as educational preparation. In medical-surgical nursing, the most significant of these titles are *nurse practitioner* (NP) and *clinical nurse specialist* (CNS), and the more recent title of *advanced practice nurse* (APN), which encompasses both nurse practitioners and clinical nurse specialists. Most states require both nurse practitioners and clinical nurse specialists to have graduate-level education.

Nurse practitioners are prepared as generalists (eg, pediatric, geriatric) or specialists. They define their role in terms of direct provision of a broad range of primary health care services to patients and families. The focus is on providing primary health care to patients and collaborating with other health professionals. Nurse practitioners practice in both acute and non-acute care settings. The 1997 Balanced Budget Act provided for nurse practitioners to receive direct Medicare reimbursement. In addition, in some states nurse practitioners have prescriptive authority (Hales, 2002).

Clinical nurse specialists, on the other hand, are prepared as specialists who practice within a circumscribed area of care (eg, cardiovascular, oncology). They define their role as having five major components: clinical practice, education, management, consultation, and research. Studies have shown that in reality clinical nurse specialists often focus on their education and consultation roles, which involve education and counseling of patients and families, as well as education, counseling, and consultation with nursing staff. Some states have granted clinical nurse specialists prescriptive authority if they have the required educational preparation. Clinical nurse specialists practice in a variety of settings, including the community and the home, although most practice in acute care settings. Recently, clinical nurse specialists have been identified by many nursing leaders as ideal case managers. They have the educational background and the clinical expertise to organize and coordinate services and resources to meet the patient's health care needs in a cost-effective and efficient manner. The expanding role of the nurse case manager has contributed to the designation of the advanced practice nurse case manager as an advanced practice role (Hamric, Spross, & Hanson, 2005).

With advanced practice roles has come a continuing effort by professional nursing organizations to define more clearly the practice of nursing. Nurse practice acts have been amended to give nurses the authority to perform functions that were previously restricted to the practice of medicine. These functions include diagnosis (nursing), treatment, performance of selected invasive procedures, and prescription of medications and treatments. The board of nursing in each state stipulates regulations regarding these functions. In addition, the board defines the education and experience required and determines the clinical situations in which a nurse may perform these functions.

In general, initial care, ambulatory health care, palliative care, and anticipatory guidance are all becoming increasingly important in nursing practice. Advanced practice roles enable nurses to function interdependently with other health care professionals and to establish a more collegial relationship with physicians. As changes in health care continue, the role of advanced practice nurses is expected to increase in terms of scope, responsibility, and recognition.

## Collaborative Practice

This chapter has explored the changing role of nursing. Many references have been made to the significance of nurses as members of the health care team. As the unique competencies of nurses are becoming more clearly articulated, there is increasing evidence that nurses provide certain health care services distinct to the profession. However, nursing continues to recognize the importance of collaboration with other health care disciplines in meeting the needs of patients.

Some institutions use the collaborative practice model (Fig. 1-2). Nurses, physicians, and ancillary health personnel function within a decentralized organizational structure, collaboratively making clinical decisions. A joint practice committee, with representation from all care providers, may function at the unit level to monitor, support, and foster collaboration. Collaborative practice is further enhanced with integration of the health or medical record and with joint patient care record reviews.

The collaborative model, or a variation of it, should be a primary goal for nursing—a venture that promotes shared participation, responsibility, and accountability in a health care environment that is striving to meet the complex health care needs of the public.

### Critical Thinking Exercises

1. Your clinical assignment is on a rehabilitation nursing unit. Identify a patient care issue (eg, discharge planning) that could be improved. Describe the mechanism that is available within a clinical facility to address such quality improvement issues.

2. You are planning the discharge of an elderly patient who has several chronic medical conditions. A case manager has been assigned to this patient. How would you explain the role of the case manager to the patient and her husband?

3. **ebp** You are assigned to care for a hospitalized patient who is obese and newly diagnosed with diabetes. There is a diabetes clinical nurse specialist on staff at the hospital. Identify the evidence that supports the effectiveness of clinical nurse specialists in providing education to patients and promoting positive patient outcomes. What is the strength of the evidence? How might this specific patient's care be affected?

**FIGURE 1-2.** Collaborative practice model.

## REFERENCES AND SELECTED READINGS

### BOOKS

American Nurses Association. (2003). *Nursing's social policy statement* (2nd ed.). Washington, DC: Author.

American Nurses Association. (1992). *Nursing's agenda for health care reform.* Kansas City, MO: Author.

Hamric, A. B., Spross, J. A., & Hanson, C. M. (2005). *Advanced practice nursing: An integrative approach* (5th ed.). St. Louis: Elsevier.

Hood, L., & Leddy, S. K. (2003). *Leddy & Pepper's conceptual bases of professional nursing* (5th ed.). Philadelphia: Lippincott Williams & Wilkins.

Joel, L. A. (2004). *Advanced practice nursing: Essentials for role development.* Philadelphia: F. A. Davis.

Krozok, C., & Scoggins, A. (2002). *Patient rights . . . amended to comply with 2002 JCAHO standards.* Glendale, CA: CINAHL Information Systems.

Melnyk, B. M., & Fineout-Overholt, E. (2005). *Evidence-based practice in nursing & healthcare.* Philadelphia: Lippincott Williams & Wilkins.

Stanhope, M., & Lancaster, J. (2004). *Community & public health nursing.* St. Louis: Mosby-Year Book.

Stanley, J. M. (2005). *Advanced practice nursing* (2nd ed.). Philadelphia: F. A. Davis.

U.S. Bureau of the Census. (Internet release date: Jan. 13, 2000). *Profile of older Americans: 2000. Population projections of the United States by age, sex, race, and Hispanic origin: 1995–2050.* Current Population Reports, P25-1130. Washington, DC: Author.

## JOURNALS

Abrams, R. B. (2002). Rights and responsibilities for nurses: Another look. *HealthLeaders.com,* July 10, 2002.

Baldwin, D. (2003). Disparities in health and health care: Focusing efforts to eliminate unequal burdens. *Online Journal of Issues in Nursing, 8*(1). http://www.nursingworld.org/ojin/topic20/tpc20_1.htm

Campinha-Bacote, J. (2003). Many faces: Addressing diversity in health care. *Online Journal of Issues in Nursing, 8*(1).

Charlebois, D., & Wilmoth, D. (2004). Critical care of patients with obesity. *Critical Care Nurse, 24*(4), 19–27.

Hales, A. (2002). Perspectives on prescribing: Pioneer's narratives and advice. *Perspectives in Psychiatric Care, 38*(3), 79–88.

Harrison, T. (2003). Women aging with childhood onset disability: A holistic approach using the life course paradigm. *Journal of Holistic Nursing, 21*(3), 242–259.

Kinsman, L. (2004). Clinical pathway compliance and quality improvement. *Nursing Standard, 18*(18), 33–35.

Kinsman, L., James, E., & Ham, J. (2004). An interdisciplinary, evidence-based process of clinical pathway implementation increases pathway usage. *Lippincott's Case Management: Managing the Process of Patient Care, 9*(4), 184–196.

Lein, C., Collins, C., Lyles, J. S., et al. (2004). Building research relationships with managed care organizations: Issues and strategies. *Family Systems & Health, 21*(2), 205–214.

Reid Ponte, P. (2004). The American health care system at a crossroads: An overview of the American Organization of Nurse Executives Monograph. *Online Journal of Issues in Nursing, 9*(2), Manuscript 2. Available at http://www.nursingworld.org/ojin/topic24/tpc24_2.htm.

Schifalacqua, M. M., Ulch, P. O., & Schmidt, M. (2004). How to make a difference in the health care of a population, one person at a time. *Nursing Administration Quarterly, 28*(1), 29–35.

Stone, P. (September/October 2003). Wellness care for the athlete. *Today's Chiropractic,* 64–67.

Young, H. (2003). Challenges and solutions for care of frail older adults. *Online Journal of Issues in Nursing, 8*(2), Manuscript 4. Available at: http://www.nursingworld.org/ojin/topic21/tpc21_4.htm.

# CHAPTER 2

# Community-Based Nursing Practice

## Learning Objectives

*On completion of this chapter, the learner will be able to:*

1. Discuss the changes in the health care system that have increased the need for medical-surgical nurses to practice in community-based settings.
2. Compare the differences and similarities between community-based and hospital nursing.
3. Describe the discharge planning process in relation to home care preparation.
4. Explain methods for identifying community resources and making referrals.
5. Discuss how to prepare for a home health care visit and how to conduct the visit.
6. Identify personal safety precautions a home care nurse should take when making home visits.
7. Describe the various types of nursing functions provided in ambulatory care facilities, in occupational health and school nursing programs, in community nurse–managed centers, in hospice care settings, and to the homeless.

The changes that have occurred in the health care system and society in the past two decades have increased the need for care in ambulatory settings and in the home. The demand for registered nurses in ambulatory settings is likely to continue to increase, creating a demand for highly skilled and well-prepared nurses to provide community-based care (Centers for Disease Control and Prevention [CDC], 2003).

## The Growing Need for Community-Based Health Care

As described in Chapter 1, the shift in the settings for health care delivery is a result of several factors, including new population trends. The growing number of older adults in the United States increases the demand for medical and social services within the public health system. Increased life expectancy is coupled with the need for more attention to people with chronic conditions, such as hypertension, which affects more than 50 million Americans (Chobanian, Bakris, Black, et al., 2003), and decreased quality of life (Goulding, Rogers, & Smith, 2003). Increases in chronic health problems such as diabetes and obesity are at an all-time high, mandating an increased need for community health care services.

Other factors, such as changes in federal legislation, tighter insurance regulations, decreasing hospital revenues, and alternative health care delivery systems, also have affected the ways in which health care is delivered. As a result of federal legislation passed in 1983 and 1997, hospitals and other health care providers are now reimbursed at a fixed rate for patients who have the same diagnosis as defined by diagnosis-related groups (DRGs). Under this system, hospitals and other health care providers can reduce costs and earn income by carefully monitoring the types of services they provide and discharging patients as soon as possible. Consequently, patients are being discharged from acute care facilities to their homes or to residential or long-term care facilities at much earlier stages of recovery than in the past. Complex technical equipment, such as dialysis machines, intravenous lines, and ventilators, is often part of home health care (Stanhope & Lancaster, 2004). Nurses play a role in evaluating the safety and cost of technology in the home setting. In addition, "tele-health" is an emerging trend in home care that facilitates exchange of information via telephone lines between patients and nurses regarding health information such as blood glucose readings, vital signs, and cardiac parameters (Stanhope & Lancaster, 2004).

Health care systems, such as health maintenance organizations, preferred provider organizations, and managed health care systems, have also contributed to the drive to control costs and the availability of health care services. As described in Chapter 1, managed care has dramatically reduced the length of hospital stay and has led to patients being treated more frequently in ambulatory care settings and at home.

The largest group of health care professionals practicing in public health are nurses (CDC, 2003). As more health care delivery shifts into the community, more nurses are working in a variety of public health and community-based settings. These settings include public health departments, ambulatory health clinics, long-term care facilities, prenatal and well-baby clinics, hospice agencies, industrial settings (as occupational nurses), homeless shelters and clinics, nursing centers, home health agencies, urgent care centers, same-day surgical centers, short-stay facilities, and patients' homes. In these settings, nurses often deliver care without direct on-site supervision or support of other health care personnel. They must be self-directed, flexible, adaptable, and tolerant of various lifestyles and living conditions. To function effectively in community-based settings, nurses must have expertise in independent decision making, critical thinking, assessment, health education, and competence in basic nursing care (Stanhope & Lancaster, 2004).

In addition, nurses in community settings must be culturally competent. Green-Hernandez, Quinn, Denman-Vitale, et al. (2004, p. 216) underscore that "health care is the practice of care that is ethically and culturally appropriate." In working with patients and families, culture plays a role in the assignment of value priorities to health (ie, the priorities given to various aspects of health and illness from a cultural perspective) (Locsin, 2003).

## Community-Based Care

Community-based nursing is a philosophy of care of people and families in which the care is provided as patients and their families move among various service providers outside of hospitals (Stanhope & Lancaster, 2004). This nursing practice focuses on promoting and maintaining the health of individuals and families, preventing and minimizing the progression of disease, and improving quality of life (Stanhope & Lancaster, 2004). The actions of community health nurses may include providing direct care to patients and families as well as political advocacy to secure resources for aggregate populations (eg, the aged population). Community health nurses have many roles, including epidemiologist, case manager for a group of patients, coordinator of services provided to a group of patients, occupational health nurse, school nurse, visiting nurse, or parish nurse. (In parish nursing, the members of the religious community—the parish—are the recipients of care.) These roles have one element in common: a focus on community needs as well as on the needs of individual patients. Community-based care is generally focused on individuals or their families, although efforts may be undertaken to improve the health of the entire community (Fig. 2-1).

The primary concepts of community-based nursing care are self-care and preventive care within the context of culture and community. Two other important concepts are continuity of care and collaboration. Some community-based areas of nursing have become specialties in their own right, such as school health nursing and home health nursing.

Primary, secondary, and tertiary levels of preventive care are used by nurses in community-based practice. The focus of primary prevention is on health promotion and prevention of illness or disease, including interventions such as teaching about healthy lifestyles. Secondary prevention centers on health maintenance and is aimed at early detection and prompt intervention to prevent or minimize loss of

**FIGURE 2-1.** Community-based nursing takes many forms and focuses. Here the nursing focus is on wellness and the nursing setting is industry. When enlightened employers offer flu vaccines or other health services, the whole community benefits.

function and independence, including interventions such as health screening and health risk appraisal. Tertiary prevention focuses on minimizing deterioration and improving quality of life, including rehabilitation to assist patients in achieving their maximum potential by working through their physical or psychological challenges.

## Home Health Care

Home health care is becoming one of the largest practice areas for nurses. Because of the high acuity level of patients, nurses with acute care and high-technology experience are in demand in this field. Tertiary preventive nursing care, which focuses on rehabilitation and restoring maximum health function, is a major goal for home care nurses, although primary and secondary prevention are also included. Health care visits may be intermittent or periodic, and telephonic case management may be used to promote communication with home care consumers.

Home care nursing is a unique component of community-based nursing. Home care visits are made by nurses who work for home care agencies, public health agencies, and visiting nurse associations; by nurses who are employed by hospitals; and by parish nurses who voluntarily work with the members of their religious communities to promote health. Such visits may also be part of the responsibilities of school nurses, clinic nurses, or occupational health nurses. The type of nursing services provided to patients in their homes varies from agency to agency. Nurses from home care or hospice agencies make home visits to provide skilled nursing care, follow-up care, and teaching to promote health and prevent complications. Hospice nursing has become a specialty area of nursing practice in which nurses provide palliative care in patients' homes, thus promoting comfort, peace, and dignity to patients who are dying. Clinic nurses may conduct home visits as part of patient follow-up. Public health, parish, and school nurses may make visits to provide anticipatory guidance to high-risk families and follow-up care to patients with communicable diseases. Many home care patients are acutely ill, and many have chronic health problems and disabilities, requiring that nurses provide more education and monitoring to patients and families to facilitate compliance.

Holistic care is provided in the home through the collaboration of an interdisciplinary team that includes professional nurses; home health aides; social workers; physical, speech, and occupational therapists; and physicians. An interdisciplinary approach is used to provide health and social services with oversight of the total health care plan by a case manager, clinical nurse specialist, or nurse practitioner. Interdisciplinary collaboration is required if a home health agency is to receive Medicare certification (Stanhope & Lancaster, 2004).

Health care services are provided by official, publicly funded agencies; nonprofit agencies; private businesses; proprietary chains; and hospital-based agencies. Some agencies specialize in high-technology services. Most agencies are reimbursed from a variety of sources, including Medicare and Medicaid programs, private insurance, and direct patient payment. Many home health care expenditures are financed by Medicare and are affected by provisions of the Balanced Budget Act of 1997. Each funding source has its own requirements for services rendered, number of visits allowed, and amount of reimbursement the agency receives.

The elderly are the most frequent users of home care services. To be eligible for service, the patient must be acutely ill, homebound, and in need of skilled nursing services. Nursing care includes skilled assessment of the patient's physical, psychological, social, and environmental status. Nursing interventions may include IV therapy and injections (Fig. 2-2), parenteral nutrition, venipuncture, catheter

**FIGURE 2-2.** Intravenous therapy is one of many types of skilled nursing care that may be provided in the home. Courtesy Good Samaritan Certified Home Health Agency, Babylon, NY.

insertion, pressure ulcer treatment, wound care, ostomy care, and patient and family teaching. The nurse instructs the patient and family in skills and self-care strategies and in health maintenance and promotion activities (eg, nutritional counseling, exercise programs, stress management).

Medicare allows nurses to manage and evaluate patient care for seriously ill patients who have complex, labile conditions and are at high risk for rehospitalization. Nurses serve as case managers and monitor the delivery of care provided to patients in their homes.

## Community-Based Nursing

Providing nursing care in a patient's home is different from providing care in a hospital. Patients must sign a release form to stay and receive treatment in a hospital, where they have little control over what happens to them and to their environment. They are expected to comply with the hospital's rules, regulations, and schedule of activities, and they are given care, treatments, baths, and medications at times that are usually determined by institutional schedules rather than patient preference. Although hospitalized patients may select meals from a daily menu, there are limited choices in the type of food they are offered. Family members and friends may visit only during visiting hours.

In contrast, the home care nurse is considered a guest in the patient's home and must have permission to visit and give care. The nurse has minimal control over the lifestyle, living situation, and health practices of the patients he or she visits. This lack of full decision-making authority can create a conflict for the nurse and lead to problems in the nurse–patient relationship. To work successfully with patients in any setting, the nurse must be nonjudgmental and convey respect for the patient's beliefs, even if they differ sharply from the nurse's. This can be difficult when a patient's lifestyle involves activities that a nurse considers harmful or unacceptable, such as smoking, use of alcohol, drug abuse, or overeating.

The cleanliness of a patient's home may not meet the standards of a hospital. Although the nurse can provide teaching points about maintaining clean surroundings, the patient and family decide if they will implement the nurse's suggestions. The nurse must accept this possibility and deliver the care required regardless of the conditions of the setting.

The kind of equipment and the supplies or resources that usually are available in acute care settings are often unavailable in the patient's home. The nurse has to learn to improvise when providing care, such as when changing a dressing or catheterizing a patient in a regular bed that is not adjustable and lacks a bedside table (Smith-Temple & Johnson, 2005).

Infection control is as important in the home as it is in the hospital, but it can be more challenging in the home and requires creative approaches. As in any situation, it is important to clean one's hands before and after giving direct patient care, even in a home that does not have running water. If aseptic technique is required, the nurse must have a plan for implementing this technique before going to the home. This applies also to standard precautions, transmission-based precautions, and disposal of bodily secretions and excretions.

If injections are given, the nurse should use a closed container to dispose of syringes. Injectable and other medications must be kept out of the reach of children during visits and must be stored in a safe place if they are to remain in the house. Nurses who perform invasive procedures must be up to date with their immunizations, including hepatitis B and tetanus. The home environment often has more distractions than a hospital, including background noise, people, and objects. For example, a nurse may have to request that the television be turned down during the visit or that a patient move to a more private place to be interviewed.

Friends, neighbors, or family members may ask the nurse about the patient's condition. The patient has a right to confidentiality, and information should be shared only with the patient's permission. If the nurse carries a patient's medical record into a house, he or she must put it in a secure place to prevent it from being picked up by others or from being misplaced.

## Discharge Planning for Home Care

Discharge planning is an important part of making the transition from the acute to the home care setting. It is required for reimbursement from Medicare (Birmingham, 2004). Discharge planning begins with the patient's admission to prepare for early hospital discharge and the possible need for follow-up home care. Several different personnel or agencies may be involved in the planning process. In hospitals, nurses or social workers may serve as the discharge planners. Some home care agencies have liaison nurses who work with discharge planners to ensure that the patient's needs are met upon discharge from the hospital. Professionals in ambulatory health care settings may refer patients for home care services to prevent hospitalization. Public health nurses care for patients referred for anticipatory guidance with high-risk families, for case finding, and for follow-up treatment (eg, patients with communicable diseases). Parish nurses may have patients referred, or they may be contacted directly by members of the parish community who need guidance or referrals related to physical or psychosocial health needs (Carson & Koenig, 2002).

The development of a comprehensive discharge plan requires collaboration with professionals at both the referring agency and the home care agency, public health agency, or other community resource. The process involves identifying the patient's needs and developing a thorough plan to meet them. Communication with and cooperation of the patient and family are essential.

## Community Resources and Referrals

As case managers, community-based nurses may make referrals to other team members, such as home health aides and social workers. These nurses work collaboratively with the health team and the referring agency or person. Continuous coordinated care among all health care providers involved in a patient's care is essential to avoid duplication of effort by the various personnel caring for the patient.

A community-based nurse must be knowledgeable about community resources available to patients as well as services provided by local agencies, eligibility requirements, and any possible charges for the services. Most communities have directories of health and social service agencies that the nurse can consult. These directories must be continually updated as resources change. If a community does not have a resource booklet, an agency may develop one for its staff. It should include the commonly used community resources that patients need, as well as the costs of the services and eligibility requirements. The telephone book is often useful in helping patients identify the locations of grocery and drug stores, banks, health care facilities, ambulances, physicians, dentists, pharmacists, social service agencies, and senior citizens' programs. In addition, a patient's place of worship or parish may be an important resource for services.

The community-based nurse is responsible for informing the patient and family about the community resources available to meet their needs. During initial and subsequent home visits, the nurse helps the patient and family identify these community services and encourages them to contact the appropriate agencies. When appropriate, nurses may make the initial contact.

# Home Health Visits

## Preparing for a Home Visit

Most agencies have a policy manual that states the agency's philosophy and procedures and defines the services provided. Becoming familiar with these policies is essential before initiating a home visit. It is also important to know the agency's policies and the state law regarding what actions to take if the nurse finds a patient dead, encounters an abusive situation in the family, determines that a patient cannot safely remain at home, or observes a situation that possibly indicates malicious harm to the community at large.

Before making a home visit, the nurse should review the patient's referral form and other pertinent data concerning the patient. It may be necessary to contact the referring agency if the purpose for the referral is unclear or if important information is missing. The first step is to call the patient to obtain permission to visit, schedule a time for the visit, and verify the address. This initial phone conversation provides an opportunity to introduce oneself, identify the agency, and explain the reason for the visit. If the patient does not have a telephone, the nurse should see if the people who made the referral have a number where a phone message can be left for the patient. If an unannounced visit to a patient's home must be made, the nurse should ask permission to come in before entering the house. Explaining the purpose of the referral at the outset and setting up the times for future visits before leaving are also recommended.

Most agencies provide nurses with bags that contain standard supplies and equipment needed during home visits. It is important to keep the bag properly supplied and to bring any additional items that might be needed for the visit. Patients rarely have the medical supplies needed for treatment.

## Conducting a Home Visit

### Personal Safety Precautions

Community nurses must pay particular attention to personal safety, because their practice settings are often in unknown environments. Based on the principle of due diligence, agencies must inform employees of at-risk working environments. Agencies have policies and procedures concerning the promotion of safety for clinical staff, and training is provided to facilitate personal safety. Environments must be carefully assessed, and proactive measures must be taken by the individual nurse as well as the agency (Skillen, Olson, & Gilbert, 2003).

Whenever a nurse makes a home visit, the agency should know the nurse's schedule and the locations of the visits. The nurse should learn about the neighborhood and obtain directions to the destination. A plan of action should always be established in case of emergencies. If a dangerous situation is encountered during the visit, the nurse should return to the agency and contact his or her supervisor or law enforcement officials, or both. Suggested precautions to take when making a home visit are presented in Chart 2-1.

### Initial Home Visit

The first visit sets the tone for subsequent visits and is crucial in establishing the nurse–patient relationship. The situations encountered depend on numerous factors. Patients may be in pain and unable to care for themselves. Family members may be overwhelmed and doubt their ability to care for their loved ones. They may not understand why the patient was sent home from the hospital before being totally rehabilitated. They may not comprehend what home care is or why they cannot have 24-hour nursing services. It is critical that the nurse conveys an understanding of what patients and families are experiencing and how the illness is affecting their lives.

During the initial home visit, which usually lasts less than an hour, the individual patient is evaluated and a plan of care is established to be followed or modified on subsequent visits. The nurse informs the patient of the agency's practices, policies, and hours of operation. If the agency is to be reimbursed for the visit, the nurse asks for insurance information, such as a Medicare or Medicaid card.

The initial assessment includes evaluating the patient, the home environment, the patient's self-care abilities or the family's ability to provide care, and the patient's need for additional resources. Identification of possible hazards, such as cluttered walk areas, potential fire risks, air or water pollution, or inadequate sanitation facilities, is also part of the initial assessment.

Documentation considerations for home visits follow fairly specific regulations. The patient's needs and the nursing care provided are documented to ensure that the agency qualifies for payment for the visit. Medicare, Medicaid, and third-party payers require documentation of the patient's homebound status and the need for skilled professional

## CHART 2-1

### Safety Precautions in Home Health Care

- Learn or preprogram a cellular phone with the telephone numbers of the agency and police and emergency services.
- Let the agency know your daily schedule and the telephone numbers of your patients so that you can be located if you do not return when expected.
- Know where the patient lives before leaving to make the visit and carry a map for quick referral.
- Keep your car in good working order and have sufficient gas in the tank.
- Park the car near the patient's home and lock it during the visit.
- Do not drive an expensive car or wear expensive jewelry when making visits.
- Know the regular bus schedule and know the routes when using public transportation or walking to the patient's house.
- Carry agency identification and have enough change to make telephone calls in case you get lost or have problems. Most agencies provide cellular phones for their nurses so that the agency can contact the nurse, and so that the nurse can contact the agency in case of an emergency or unexpected situation.
- When making visits in high-crime areas, visit with another person rather than alone.
- Schedule visits only during daylight hours.
- Never walk into a patient's home uninvited.
- If you do not feel safe entering a patient's home, leave the area.
- Become familiar with the layout of the house, including exits from the house.
- If a patient or family member is intoxicated, hostile, or obnoxious, reschedule the visit and leave.
- If a family is having a serious argument or abusing the patient or anyone else in the household, reschedule the visit, contact your supervisor, and report the abuse to the appropriate authorities.

## Determining the Need for Future Visits

While conducting an assessment of a patient's situation, the home care nurse evaluates the need for future visits and the frequency with which those visits may need to be made. To make these judgments, the nurse should consider the questions listed in Chart 2-2. With each subsequent visit, these

## CHART 2-2

### Assessing the Need for Home Visits

**CURRENT HEALTH STATUS**
- How well is the patient progressing?
- How serious are the present signs and symptoms?
- Has the patient shown signs of progressing as expected, or does it seem that recovery will be delayed?

**HOME ENVIRONMENT**
- Are worrisome safety factors apparent?
- Are family or friends available to provide care, or is the patient alone?

**LEVEL OF SELF-CARE ABILITY**
- Is the patient capable of self-care?
- What is the patient's level of independence?
- Is the patient ambulatory or bedridden?
- Does the patient have sufficient energy, or is he or she frail and easily fatigued?

**LEVEL OF NURSING CARE NEEDED**
- What level of nursing care does the patient require?
- Does the care require basic skills or more complex interventions?

**PROGNOSIS**
- What is the expectation for recovery in this particular instance?
- What are the chances that complications may develop if nursing care is not provided?

**EDUCATIONAL NEEDS**
- How well has the patient or family grasped the teaching points made?
- Is there a need for further follow-up and retraining?
- What level of proficiency does the patient or family show in carrying out the necessary care?

**MENTAL STATUS**
- How alert is the patient?
- Are there signs of confusion or thinking difficulties?
- Does the patient tend to be forgetful or have a limited attention span?

**LEVEL OF ADHERENCE**
- Is the patient following the instructions provided?
- Does the patient seem capable of following the instructions?
- Are the family members helpful, or are they unwilling or unable to assist in caring for the patient as expected?

nursing care. The medical diagnosis and specific detailed information on the functional limitations of the patient are usually part of the documentation. The goals and the actions appropriate for attaining them must be identified. Expected outcomes of the nursing interventions must be stated in terms of patient behaviors and must be realistic and measurable. They must reflect the nursing diagnosis or the patient's problems and must specify those actions that address the patient's problems. If the documentation is inadequate, the agency may not be paid for the visit (Scala-Foley, Caruso, Ramos, et al., 2004).

same factors are evaluated to determine the continuing health needs of the patient. As progress is made and the patient, with or without the help of significant others, becomes more capable of self-care and more independent, the need for home visits may decline.

### Ending the Visit

As the visit comes to a close, it is important to summarize the main points of the visit for the patient and family and to identify expectations for future visits or patient achievements. The following points should be considered at the end of each visit:

- What are the main points the patient or family should remember from the visit?
- What positive attributes have been noted about the patient and the family that will give them a sense of accomplishment?
- What were the main points of the teaching plan or the treatments needed to ensure that the patient and family understand what they must do? A written set of instructions should be left with the patient or family, provided they can read and see (alternative formats include video or audio recordings). Printed material should be in the patient's primary language and in large print when indicated.
- Whom should the patient or family call if they need to contact someone immediately? Are current emergency telephone numbers readily available? Is telephone service available, or can an emergency cellular phone service be provided?
- What signs of complications should be reported immediately?
- How frequently will visits be made? How long will they last (approximately)?
- What is the day and time of the next visit? Will a different nurse make the visit?

## Other Community-Based Health Care Settings

### Ambulatory Settings

Ambulatory health care is provided for patients in community or hospital-based settings. The types of agencies that provide such care are medical clinics, ambulatory care units, urgent care centers, cardiac rehabilitation programs, mental health centers, student health centers, community outreach programs, and nursing centers. Some ambulatory centers provide care to a specific population, such as migrant workers or Native Americans. Neighborhood health centers provide services to patients who live in a geographically defined area. The centers may operate in freestanding buildings, storefronts, or mobile units. Agencies may provide ambulatory health care in addition to other services, such as an adult day care or health program. The kinds of services offered and the patients served depend on the agency's mission.

Nursing responsibilities in ambulatory health care settings include providing direct patient care, conducting patient intake screenings, treating patients with acute or chronic illnesses or emergency conditions, referring patients to other agencies for additional services, teaching patients self-care activities, and offering health education programs that promote health maintenance. A useful tool for community-based nurses might be the classification scheme developed by the Visiting Nurses Association of Omaha, which contains patient-focused problems in one of four domains: environmental, psychosocial, physiologic, and health-related behaviors (Barton, Clark, & Baramee, 2004).

Nurses also work as clinic managers, direct the operation of clinics, and supervise other health team members. Nurse practitioners, educated in primary care, often practice in ambulatory care settings that focus on gerontology, pediatrics, family or adult health, or women's health. Constraints imposed by federal legislation and ambulatory payment classifications require efficient and effective management of patients in ambulatory settings. Nurses can play an important part in facilitating the function of ambulatory care facilities.

### Occupational Health Programs

Federal legislation, especially the Occupational Safety and Health Act (OSHA), has had a major impact on health conditions in the workplace, with a goal of safe and healthy work conditions. It is in an employer's interest to provide a safe working environment, because decreased employee absenteeism, hospitalization, and disability are associated with reduced costs.

Occupational nurses may work in solo units in industrial settings, or they may serve as consultants on a limited or part-time basis. They may be members of an interdisciplinary team composed of a variety of personnel such as nurses, physicians, exercise physiologists, health educators, counselors, nutritionists, safety engineers, and industrial hygienists. Occupational health nurses may:

- Provide direct care to employees who become ill or injured
- Conduct health education programs for company staff members
- Set up health programs aimed at establishing specific health behaviors, such as eating properly and getting enough exercise
- Monitor employees' hearing, vision, blood pressure, or blood glucose
- Track exposure to radiation, infectious diseases, and toxic substances, reporting results to government agencies as necessary

Occupational health nurses must be knowledgeable about federal regulations pertaining to occupational health and familiar with other pertinent legislation, such as the Americans with Disabilities Act.

### School Health Programs

School health programs provide services to students and may also serve the school's community. School-age children and adolescents with health problems are at major risk for underachieving or failing in school. The leading health problems of elementary school children are injuries, infections (including influenza and pneumonia), malnutrition, dental disease, and cancer. The leading problems of high school students are alcohol and drug abuse, injuries, homicide, pregnancy, eating disorders, sexually transmitted diseases/infections, sports injuries, dental disease, and mental and emotional problems.

Ideally, school health programs have an interdisciplinary health team consisting of physicians, nurses, dentists, social workers, counselors, school administrators, parents, and students. The school may serve as the site for a family health clinic that offers primary health and mental health services to children and adolescents as well as to all family members in the community. School nurses with baccalaureate and advanced degrees are ideally suited to provide primary care in these settings. Physical examinations are performed by advanced practice nurses, who then diagnose and treat students and families for acute and chronic illnesses. These clinics are cost-effective and benefit students from low-income families who lack access to traditional health care or have no health insurance.

School nurses play a number of roles, including care provider, health educator, consultant, and counselor. They collaborate with students, parents, administrators, and other health and social service professionals regarding student health problems. School nurses perform health screenings, provide basic care for minor injuries and complaints, administer medications, monitor the immunization status of students and families, and identify children with health problems. They need to be knowledgeable about state and local regulations affecting school-age children, such as ordinances for excluding students from school because of communicable diseases or parasites such as lice or scabies.

School nurses are also health education consultants for teachers. In addition to providing information on health practices, teaching health classes, or participating in the development of the health education curriculum, school nurses educate teachers and classes when one of the students has a special problem, a disability, or a disease such as hemophilia, human immunodeficiency virus (HIV) infection, or acquired immunodeficiency syndrome (AIDS).

## Community Nurse–Managed Centers

Community nurse–managed centers are a relatively new concept in community-based nursing, having appeared only in the past 25 years. Frequently sponsored by academic centers, these centers typically are designed for the delivery of primary health care. Their services are geared toward serving people and groups who are vulnerable, uninsured, and without access to health services. Typically, community nurse–managed centers are run by advanced practice nurses and serve a large number of patients who are poor, members of minority groups, women, elderly, or homeless. The nurses provide health teaching, wellness and illness care, case management services, and psychosocial counseling (Neff, Mahama, Mohar, et al., 2003).

## Care for the Homeless

No exact figures exist on the number of homeless people in the United States, but in any given year an estimated 3.5 million people, 1.35 million of them children, are homeless (National Coalition for the Homeless, 2002; Urban Institute, 2000). Homelessness is a growing problem, and the homeless population includes growing numbers of women with children (often victims of abuse) and elderly people. The homeless are a heterogeneous group, including members of dysfunctional families, the unemployed, and those who cannot find affordable housing. A large number of homeless people are chronically mentally ill or abuse alcohol or other drugs (National Coalition for the Homeless, 2004). Some are temporarily homeless as a result of catastrophic natural disasters.

Homeless people often have limited or no access to health care. Because of numerous barriers, they seek health care late in the course of a disease and deteriorate more quickly than other patients. Many of their health problems are related in large part to their living situation. Street life exposes people to the extremes of hot and cold environments and compounds their health risks. Homeless people have high rates of trauma, tuberculosis, upper respiratory tract infections, poor nutrition and anemia, lice, scabies, peripheral vascular problems, sexually transmitted diseases/infections, dental problems, arthritis, hypothermia, skin disorders, and foot problems. Common chronic health problems also include diabetes, hypertension, heart disease, AIDS, and mental illness. These problems are made more difficult by living on the streets or being discharged to a transitory, homeless situation in which follow-up care is unlikely. Shelters frequently are overcrowded and unventilated, promoting the spread of communicable diseases such as tuberculosis.

Community-based nurses who work with homeless people must be nonjudgmental, patient, and understanding. They must be skilled in dealing with people who have a wide variety of health problems and needs and must recognize that individualized treatment strategies are required in highly unpredictable environments (Bailey, 2004). Nursing interventions are aimed at evaluating the health care needs of people who live in shelters and attempting to obtain health care services for all homeless people.

## Critical Thinking Exercises

**1** You are assisting with discharge of a homeless 20-year-old woman who has a healthy newborn 8-pound boy. What processes are needed to secure resources for follow-up care for the mother and child? What problems do you anticipate in trying to secure the services? How can you facilitate the use of community resources by this woman?

**2** **ebp** An elderly man with diabetes is being referred for home care after discharge from the hospital, and he will need glucose monitoring and teaching. He has no family at home; his wife died 3 years ago, and his only daughter lives several hundred miles away. During the nurse's initial visit to the man's home, the nurse learns that he has difficulty seeing and therefore cannot read. What is the evidence base for conducting a safety assessment of the home environment for elderly patients and for patients with visual limitations? Evaluate the strength of the evidence. What assessment criteria would you use to assess the needs of the patient's home care situation?

# REFERENCES AND SELECTED READINGS

## BOOKS

Carson, V. B., & Koenig, H. G. (2002). *Parish nursing.* Radnor, PA: Templeton Foundation Press.

Clark, M. J. (2003). *Community health nursing: Caring for populations* (4th ed). Upper Saddle River, NJ: Prentice-Hall/Pearson Education, Inc.

Smith-Temple, A. J., & Johnson, J. Y. (2005). *Nurses' guide to clinical procedures.* Philadelphia: Lippincott Williams & Wilkins.

Stanhope, M., & Lancaster, J. (2004). *Community and public health nursing* (6th ed). St. Louis: Mosby.

## JOURNALS

Bailey, S. (2004). Nursing knowledge in integrated care. *Nursing Standard, 18*(44), 38–41.

Barton, A. J., Clark, L., & Baramee J. (2004). Tracking outcomes in community-based care. *Home Health Care Management & Practice, 16*(3), 171–176.

Birmingham, J. (2004). Discharge planning: A collaboration between provider and payer case managers using Medicare's conditions of participation. *Lippincott's Case Management, 9*(3), 147–151.

Chobanian, A. V., Bakris, G. L., Black, H. R., et al. (2003). Seventh Report of the Joint National Committee on Prevention, Detection, Evaluation, and Treatment of High Blood Pressure. *Hypertension, 42*(6), 1206–1252.

Goulding, M. R., Rogers, M. E., & Smith, S. M. (2003). Public health and aging: Trends in aging, United States and worldwide. *Journal of American Medical Association, 289*(11), 1371–1373.

Green-Hernandez, C., Quinn, A., Denman-Vitale, S., et al. (2004). Making nursing care culturally competent. *Holistic Nursing Practice, 18*(4), 215–218.

Kovner, C., & Harrington, C. (2001). Counting nurses: What is community health-public health nursing? *American Journal of Nursing, 101*(1), 59–60.

Locsin, R. (2003). The integration of family health, culture, and nursing: Prescriptions and practices. *Holistic Nursing Practice, 17*(1), 8–10.

Mezey, M. (2001). CH-PH nursing and older adults. *American Journal of Nursing, 101*(1), 60–61.

Milone-Nuzzo, P. (2003). Clinical nurse specialists in home care. *Clinical Nurse Specialist, 17*(5), 234–235.

National Association for Home Care and Hospice (2004). Basic statistics about home care. Available at: http://www.nahc.org/NAHC/Research/04HPC_stats.pdf. Accessed May 3, 2006.

National Association for Home Care and Hospice (2002). Hospice facts and statistics. Available at: http://www.nahc.org/NAHC/Research/04HPC_stats.pdf. Accessed May 3, 2006.

National Coalition for the Homeless (September 2002). How many people experience homelessness? (Fact sheet #2). Available at http://www.nationalhomeless.org/numbers.html. Retrieved Sept. 29, 2004.

National Coalition for the Homeless (May 2004). Who is homeless? (Fact sheet #3). Available at: http://www.nationalhomeless.org/who.html. Retrieved Sept. 29, 2004.

Neff, D. F., Mahama, N., Mohar, D., & Kinion, E. (2003). Nursing care delivered at academic community-based nurse-managed center. *Outcomes Management, 7*(2), 84–89.

Scala-Foley, M., Caruso, J., Ramos, R., & Reinhard, S. (2004). Medicare eligibility, enrollment, and coverage: Understanding the basics of a complicated system. *American Journal of Nursing, 104*(2), 81–83.

Skillen, D. L., Olson, J. K., & Gilbert, J. A. (2003). Promoting personal safety in community health: Four educational strategies. *Nurse Educator, 28*(2), 89–94.

Urban Institute. A new look at homelessness in America. Available at: http://www.urban.org. Retrieved Sept. 29, 2004.

Centers for Disease Control and Prevention. CDC/ADSTR strategic plan for public health workforce development. Available at: http://www.phppo.cdc.gov. Accessed May 1, 2006.

## RESOURCES

Case Management Society of America (CMSA), 8201 Cantrell Road, Suite 230, Little Rock, AR 72227; 1-501-225-2229; http://www.cmsa.org. Accessed June 5, 2006.

Centers for Disease Control and Prevention (CDC), 1600 Clifton Road, Atlanta, GA 30333; 1-800-311-3435; http://www.cdc.gov. Accessed June 5, 2006.

Centers for Medicare and Medicaid Services (CMS), 7500 Security Boulevard, Baltimore, MD 21244-1850; 1-877-267-2323; http://www.cms.hhs.gov. Accessed June 5, 2006.

Joint Commission on Accreditation of Healthcare Organizations (JCAHO), One Renaissance Blvd., Oakbrook Terrace, IL 60181; 1-630-792-5000; http://www.jcaho.org. Accessed June 5, 2006.

National Association for Home Care, 228 7th Street, SE, Washington, DC 20003; 1-202-547-7424.

National Association of School Nurses, Inc., Eastern Office, P.O. Box 1300, Scarborough, ME 04070-1300; 1-877-627-6476; http://www.nasn.org. Accessed June 5, 2006.

National Guideline Clearing House (NGC): http://www.guideline.gov. Accessed June 5, 2006.

NurseLinx.com (MDLinx Inc.), 1025 Vermont Avenue, NW, Suite 810, Washington, DC 20005; 1-202-543-6544; http://www.nurselinx.com. Accessed June 5, 2006.

Urban Institute, 2100 M Street, NW, Washington, DC 20037.

# CHAPTER 3

# Critical Thinking, Ethical Decision Making, and the Nursing Process

## Learning Objectives

*On completion of this chapter, the learner will be able to:*

1. Define the characteristics of critical thinking and critical thinkers.
2. Describe the critical thinking process.
3. Define ethics and nursing ethics.
4. Identify several ethical dilemmas common to the medical-surgical area of nursing practice.
5. Specify strategies that can be helpful to nurses in ethical decision making.
6. Describe the components of the nursing process.
7. Describe the nursing process.
8. Develop a plan of nursing care for a patient using strategies of critical thinking.

In today's health care arena, nurses are faced with increasingly complex issues and situations resulting from advanced technology, greater acuity of patients in hospital and community settings, an aging population, and complex disease processes, as well as ethical issues and cultural factors. Traditionally, nurses have used a problem-solving approach in planning and providing nursing care. Today, the decision-making part of problem solving has become increasingly complex and requires critical thinking.

# Critical Thinking

## Definition

Critical thinking is a multidimensional skill, a cognitive or mental process or set of procedures. It involves reasoning and purposeful, systematic, reflective, rational, outcome-directed thinking based on a body of knowledge, as well as examination and analysis of all available information and ideas. Critical thinking leads to the formulation of conclusions and alternatives that are the most appropriate for the situation. Although many definitions of critical thinking have been offered in various disciplines, some consistent themes within those definitions are (1) a strong formal and informal foundation of knowledge; (2) willingness to pursue or ask questions; and (3) ability to develop solutions that are new, even those that do not fit the standard or current state of knowledge or attitudes. Willingness and openness to various viewpoints are inherent in critical thinking, and it is important to question the current state of a situation or knowledge (Jackson, 2004). Critical thinking includes metacognition, the examination of one's own reasoning or thought processes, to help refine thinking skills (Wilkinson, 2001). Independent judgments and decisions evolve from a sound knowledge base and the ability to synthesize information within the context in which it is presented. Nursing practice in today's society requires the use of high-level critical thinking skills within the nursing process. Critical thinking enhances clinical decision making, helping to identify patient needs and to determine the best nursing actions that will assist patients in meeting those needs.

As indicated previously, critical thinking is a conscious, outcome-oriented activity. Critical thinking is not erratic but rather is systematic and organized. Critical thinking and critical thinkers have distinctive characteristics. People who engage in critical thinking are inquisitive truth seekers who are open to the alternative solutions that might surface. Alfaro-LeFevre (2003) identified critical thinkers as individuals with the following ideal characteristics: active thinker, fair-minded, open-minded, persistent, empathic, independent in thought, good communicator, honest, organized and systematic, proactive, flexible, realistic, humble, cognizant of the rules of logic, curious and insightful, and creative and committed to excellence. The skills involved in critical thinking are developed over time, through effort, practice, and experience.

## Rationality and Insight

Skills needed in critical thinking include interpretation, analysis, evaluation, inference, explanation, and self-regulation. Critical thinking requires background knowledge and knowledge of key concepts as well as standards of logical thinking. Nurses use this disciplined process to validate the accuracy of data and the reliability of any assumptions they have made, and they then carefully evaluate the effectiveness of what they have identified as the necessary actions to take (Jackson, 2004). Nurses also evaluate the reliability of sources, being mindful of and questioning inconsistencies. Nurses use interpretation to determine the significance of data that are gathered, analysis to identify patient problems suggested by the data, and inference to draw conclusions. Explanation is the justification of actions or interventions used to address patient problems and to help patients move toward desired outcomes. Evaluation is the process of determining whether outcomes have been or are being met. Self-regulation is the process of examining the care provided and adjusting the interventions as needed.

Critical thinking is also reflective, involving metacognition, active evaluation, and refinement of the thinking process. Nurses engaged in critical thinking consider the possibility of personal bias when interpreting data and determining appropriate actions. Critical thinkers must be insightful and have a sense of fairness and integrity; the courage to question personal ethics; and the perseverance to strive continuously to minimize the effects of egocentricity, ethnocentricity, and other biases on the decision-making process (Alfaro-LeFevre, 2003).

## Components of Critical Thinking

Certain cognitive or mental activities are key components of critical thinking. Critical thinkers:

- Ask questions to determine why certain developments have occurred and to see whether more information is needed to understand the situation accurately
- Gather as much relevant information as possible to consider as many factors as possible
- Validate the information presented to make sure that it is accurate (not just supposition or opinion), that it makes sense, and that it is based on fact and evidence
- Analyze the information to determine what it means and to see whether it forms clusters or patterns that point to certain conclusions
- Draw on past clinical experience and knowledge to explain what is happening and to anticipate what might happen next, acknowledging personal bias and cultural influences
- Maintain a flexible attitude that allows the facts to guide thinking and takes into account all possibilities
- Consider available options and examine each in terms of its advantages and disadvantages
- Formulate decisions that reflect creativity and independent decision making

Critical thinking requires going beyond basic problem solving into a realm of inquisitive exploration, looking for all relevant factors that affect the issue, and being an "out-of-the-box" thinker. It includes questioning all findings until a comprehensive picture emerges that explains the phenomenon, possible solutions, and creative methods for proceeding (Wilkinson, 2001). Critical thinking in nursing practice results in a comprehensive plan of care with maximized potential for success.

## Critical Thinking in Nursing Practice

Critical thinking and decision making have been associated with improved clinical expertise (Martin, 2002). Critical thinking is at the center of the process of clinical reasoning and clinical judgment (Jackson, 2004). Using critical thinking to develop a plan of nursing care requires considering the human factors that might influence the plan. Nurses interact with patients, families, and other health care providers in the process of providing appropriate, individualized nursing care. The culture, attitude, and thought processes of nurses, patients, and others affect the critical thinking process from the data-gathering stage through the decision-making stage; therefore, aspects of the nurse–patient interaction must be considered (Wilkinson, 2001).

Nurses must use critical thinking skills in all practice settings—acute care, ambulatory care, extended care, and the home and community. Regardless of the setting, each patient situation is viewed as unique and dynamic. Key components of critical thinking behavior are withholding judgment and being open to options and explanations from one patient to another in similar circumstances (Jackson, 2004). The unique factors that patients and nurses bring to the health care situation are considered, studied, analyzed, and interpreted. Interpretation of the information then allows nurses to focus on those factors that are most relevant and most significant to the clinical situation. Decisions about what to do and how to do it are then developed into a plan of action.

In decision making related to the nursing process, nurses use intellectual skills in critical thinking. These skills include systematic and comprehensive assessment, recognition of assumptions and inconsistencies, verification of reliability and accuracy, identification of missing information, distinguishing relevant from irrelevant information, support of the evidence with facts and conclusions, priority setting with timely decision making, determination of patient-specific outcomes, and reassessment of responses and outcomes (Alfaro-LeFevre, 2003).

Because developing the skill of critical thinking takes time and practice, critical thinking exercises are offered throughout this book as a means of honing one's ability to think critically. Some of the exercises include questions that stimulate the reader to seek information about evidence-based practice relative to the clinical situation described. Additional exercises may be found in the study guide that accompanies the text. The questions listed in Chart 3-1 can serve as a guide in working through the exercises, although it is important to remember that each situation is unique and calls for an approach that fits the particular circumstances described.

In addition, much emphasis is placed on nurses basing their clinical actions on research, using evidence-based practice. Critical thinking has been associated with the

---

**CHART 3-1**

### The Inquiring Mind: Critical Thinking in Action

Throughout the critical thinking process, a continuous flow of questions evolves in the thinker's mind. Although the questions will vary according to the particular clinical situation, certain general inquiries can serve as a basis for reaching conclusions and determining a course of action.

When faced with a patient situation, it is often helpful to seek answers to some or all of the following questions in an attempt to determine those actions that are most appropriate:

- What relevant assessment information do I need, and how do I interpret this information? What does this information tell me?
- To what problems does this information point? Have I identified the most important ones? Does the information point to any other problems that I should consider?
- Have I gathered all the information I need (signs and symptoms, laboratory values, medication history, emotional factors, mental status)? Is anything missing?
- Is there anything that needs to be reported immediately? Do I need to seek additional assistance?
- Does this patient have any special risk factors? Which ones are most significant? What must I do to minimize these risks?
- What possible complications must I anticipate?
- What are the most important problems in this situation? Do the patient and the patient's family recognize the same problems?
- What are the desired outcomes for this patient? Which have the highest priority? Do the patient and I agree on these points?
- What is going to be my first action in this situation?
- How can I construct a plan of care to achieve the goals?
- Are there any age-related factors involved, and will they require some special approach? Will I need to make some change in the plan of care to take these factors into account?
- How do the family dynamics affect this situation, and will they have an effect on my actions or the plan of care?
- Are there cultural factors that I must address and consider?
- Am I dealing with an ethical issue here? If so, how am I going to resolve it?
- Has any nursing research been conducted on this subject? What are the nursing implications of this research for care of this patient?

use of research findings (Profetto-McGrath, Hesketh, Lang, et al., 2003).

# Ethical Nursing Care

In the complex modern world, we are surrounded by ethical issues in all facets of our lives. Consequently, there has been a heightened interest in the field of ethics in an attempt to gain a better understanding of how these issues influence us. Specifically, the focus on ethics in health care has intensified in response to controversial developments, including advances in technology and genetics, as well as diminished health care and financial resources.

Today, sophisticated technology can prolong life well beyond the time when death would have occurred in the past. Expensive experimental procedures, medications, equipment, and devices are available for attempting to preserve life, even when such attempts are likely to fail. The development of technologic support has influenced patients at all stages of life and also contributed to an increase in average life expectancy. For example, the prenatal period has been influenced by genetic screening, in vitro fertilization, the harvesting and freezing of embryos, and prenatal surgery. Premature infants who once would have died early in life now may survive because of technical advances. Children and adults who would have died of organ failure are living longer because of organ transplantation.

These advances in technology have been a mixed blessing. Questions have been raised about whether it is appropriate to use such technology, and if so, under what circumstances. Although many patients do achieve a better quality of life, others face extended suffering as a result of efforts to prolong life, usually at great expense. Ethical issues also surround those practices or policies that seem to allocate health care resources unjustly on the basis of age, race, gender, disability, or social mores.

The ethical dilemmas nurses may encounter in the medical-surgical nursing arena are numerous and diverse and occur in all settings. An awareness of underlying philosophical concepts helps nurses use reason to work through these dilemmas. Basic concepts related to moral philosophy, such as ethics and its terminology, theories, and approaches, are included in this chapter. Understanding the role of the professional nurse in ethical decision making helps nurses articulate their ethical positions and develop the skills needed to make ethical decisions.

## Ethics Versus Morality

The terms *ethics* and *morality* are used to describe beliefs about right and wrong and to suggest appropriate guidelines for action. In essence, ethics is the formal, systematic study of moral beliefs, whereas morality is the adherence to informal personal values. Because the distinction between the *ethics* and *morality* is slight, the two terms are often used interchangeably.

## Ethics Theories

One classic theory in ethics is teleologic theory or consequentialism, which focuses on the ends or consequences of actions. The best-known form of this theory, utilitarianism, is based on the concept of "the greatest good for the greatest number." The choice of action is clear under this theory, because the action that maximizes good over bad is the correct one. The theory poses difficulty when one must judge intrinsic values and determine whose good is the greatest. In addition, it is important to ask whether good consequences can justify any amoral actions that might be used to achieve them.

Another theory in ethics is the deontologic or formalist theory, which argues that ethical standards or principles exist independently of the ends or consequences. In a given situation, one or more ethical principles may apply. Nurses have a duty to act based on the one relevant principle, or the most relevant of several ethical principles. Problems arise with this theory when personal and cultural biases influence the choice of the most primary ethical principle.

## Approaches to Ethics

Two approaches to ethics are meta-ethics and applied ethics. An example of meta-ethics (understanding the concepts and linguistic terminology used in ethics) in the health care environment is analysis of the concept of informed consent. Nurses are aware that patients must give consent before surgery, but sometimes a question arises as to whether a patient is truly informed. Delving more deeply into the concept of informed consent would be a meta-ethical inquiry.

An example of applied ethics is for a specific discipline to identify ethical problems within that discipline's practice. Various disciplines use the frameworks of general ethical theories and principles and apply them to specific problems within their domain. Common ethical principles that apply in nursing include autonomy, beneficence, confidentiality, double effect, fidelity, justice, nonmaleficence, paternalism, respect for people, sanctity of life, and veracity. Brief definitions of these important principles can be found in Chart 3-2.

Nursing ethics may be considered a form of applied ethics because it addresses moral situations that are specific to the nursing profession and patient care. Some ethical problems that affect nursing may also apply to the broader area of bioethics and health care ethics. However, the nursing profession is a "caring" rather than a predominantly "curing" profession; therefore, it is imperative that one not equate nursing ethics solely with medical ethics, because the medical profession has a "cure" focus. Nursing has its own professional code of ethics.

## Moral Situations

Many situations exist in which ethical analysis is needed. Some are *moral dilemmas*, situations in which a clear conflict exists between two or more moral principles or competing moral claims, and nurses must choose the lesser of two evils. Other situations represent *moral problems*, in which there may be competing moral claims or principles, but one claim or principle is clearly dominant. Some situations result in *moral uncertainty*, when one cannot accurately define what the moral situation is or what moral principles apply but has a strong feeling that something is not right. Still other situations may result in *moral distress*, in which one is aware of the correct course of action but institutional constraints stand in the way of pursuing the correct action.

## CHART 3-2

## Common Ethical Principles

The following common ethical principles may be used to validate moral claims.

### AUTONOMY
This word is derived from the Greek words *autos* ("self") and *nomos* ("rule" or "law"), and therefore refers to self-rule. In contemporary discourse it has broad meanings, including individual rights, privacy, and choice. Autonomy entails the ability to make a choice free from external constraints.

### BENEFICENCE
Beneficence is the duty to do good and the active promotion of benevolent acts (eg, goodness, kindness, charity). It may also include the injunction not to inflict harm (see nonmaleficence).

### CONFIDENTIALITY
Confidentiality relates to the concept of privacy. Information obtained from an individual will not be disclosed to another unless it will benefit the person or there is a direct threat to the social good.

### DOUBLE EFFECT
This is a principle that may morally justify some actions that produce both good and evil effects.
All four of the following criteria must be fulfilled:
1. The action itself is good or morally neutral.
2. The agent sincerely intends the good and not the evil effect (the evil effect may be foreseen but is not intended).
3. The good effect is not achieved by means of the evil effect.
4. There is proportionate or favorable balance of good over evil.

### FIDELITY
Fidelity is promise keeping; the duty to be faithful to one's commitments. It includes both explicit and implicit promises to another person.

### JUSTICE
From a broad perspective, justice states that like cases should be treated alike. A more restricted version of justice is *distributive justice,* which refers to the distribution of social benefits and burdens based on various criteria that may include the following:
- Equality
- Individual need
- Individual effort
- Societal contribution
- Individual merit
- Legal entitlement

*Retributive justice* is concerned with the distribution of punishment.

### NONMALEFICENCE
This is the duty not to inflict harm as well as to prevent and remove harm. Nonmaleficence may be included within the principle of beneficence, in which case nonmaleficence would be more binding.

### PATERNALISM
Paternalism is the intentional limitation of another's autonomy, justified by an appeal to beneficence or the welfare or needs of another. Under this principle, the prevention of evil or harm takes precedence over any potential evil caused by interference with the individual's autonomy or liberty.

### RESPECT FOR PERSONS
*Respect for persons* is frequently used synonymously with *autonomy.* However, it goes beyond accepting the notion or attitude that people have autonomous choices, to treating others in such a way that enables them to make choices.

### SANCTITY OF LIFE
This is the perspective that life is the highest good. Therefore, all forms of life, including mere biologic existence, should take precedence over external criteria for judging quality of life.

### VERACITY
Veracity is the obligation to tell the truth and not to lie or deceive others.

---

For example, a patient tells a nurse that if he is dying, he wants all possible measures taken to save his life. However, the surgeon and family have made the decision not to tell the patient that he is terminally ill and not to resuscitate him if he stops breathing. From an ethical perspective, the patient should be told the truth about his diagnosis and should have the opportunity to make decisions about treatment. Ideally, this information should come from the physician, with the nurse present to assist the patient in understanding the terminology and to provide further support, if necessary. A moral problem exists because of the competing moral claims of the family and physician, who wish to spare the patient distress, and the nurse, who wishes to be truthful with the patient as the patient has requested. If the patient's competency were questionable, a moral dilemma would exist because no dominant principle would be evident. The nurse could experience moral distress if the hospital threatened disciplinary action or job termination because the information is disclosed to the patient without the agreement of the physician or the family, or both.

It is essential that nurses freely engage in dialogue concerning moral situations, even though such dialogue is difficult for everyone involved. Improved interdisciplinary communication is supported when all members of the health care team can voice their concerns and come to an understanding of the moral situation. The use of an ethics consultant or consultation team could be helpful to assist the health care team, patient, and family to identify the moral dilemma and possible approaches to the dilemma. Nurses should be familiar with agency policy supporting patient self-determination and resolution of ethical issues.

## Types of Ethical Problems in Nursing

As a profession, nursing is accountable to society. This accountability is spelled out in the American Hospital Association's Patient Care Partnership (Chart 3-3), which reflects social beliefs about health and health care. In addition to accepting this document as one measure of accountability, nursing has further defined its standards of accountability through a formal code of ethics that explicitly states the profession's values and goals. The code (Chart 3-4), established by the American Nurses Association (ANA), consists of ethical standards, each with its own interpretive statements (ANA, 2001). The interpretive statements provide guidance to address and resolve ethical dilemmas by incorporating universal moral principles (ANA's Code of Ethics Project Task Force, 2000). The code is an ideal framework for nurses to use in ethical decision making.

Ethical issues have always affected the role of professional nurses. The accepted definition of professional nursing has inspired a new advocacy role for nurses. The ANA, in *Nursing's Social Policy Statement* (2003, p. 6), defines nursing as "the protection, promotion, and optimization of health and abilities, prevention of illness and injury, alleviation of suffering through the diagnosis and treatment of human response, and advocacy in the care of individuals, families, communities, and populations." This definition supports the claim that nurses must be actively involved in the decision-making process regarding ethical concerns surrounding health care and human responses. Efforts to enact this standard may cause conflict in health care settings in which the traditional roles of nurses are delineated within a bureaucratic structure. However, if nurses learn to present ethical conflicts within a logical, systematic framework, struggles over jurisdictional boundaries may decrease. Health care settings in which nurses are valued members of the team promote interdisciplinary communication and may enhance patient care. To practice effectively in these settings, nurses must be aware of ethical issues and assist patients in voicing their moral concerns.

A basic ethical framework of the nursing profession is the phenomenon of human caring. Nursing theories that incorporate the biopsychosocial–spiritual dimensions emphasize a holistic viewpoint, with humanism or caring as the core. As the nursing profession strives to delineate its own theory of ethics, caring is often cited as the moral foundation. For nurses to embrace this professional ethos, they must be aware not only of major ethical dilemmas but also of those daily interactions with health care consumers that frequently give rise to less easily identifiable ethical challenges. Although technologic advances and diminished resources have been instrumental in raising numerous ethical questions and controversies, including life-and-death issues, nurses should not ignore the many routine sit-

---

### CHART 3-3

### The Patient Care Partnership: Understanding Expectations, Rights, and Responsibilities

When you need hospital care, your doctor and the nurses and other professionals at our hospital are committed to working with you and your family to meet your health care needs. Our dedicated doctors and staff serve the community in all its ethnic, religious, and economic diversity. Our goal is for you and your family to have the same care and attention we would want for our families and ourselves.

The sections below explain some of the basics about how you can expect to be treated during your hospital stay. They also cover what we will need from you to care for you better. If you have questions at any time, please ask them. Unasked or unanswered questions can add to the stress of being in the hospital. Your comfort and confidence in your care are very important to us.

### What to Expect During Your Hospital Stay

**High quality hospital care.** Our first priority is to provide you the care you need, when you need it, with skill, compassion, and respect. Tell your caregivers if you have concerns about your care or if you have pain. You have the right to know the identity of doctors, nurses, and others involved in your care, as well as when they are students, residents, or other trainees.

**A clean and safe environment.** Our hospital works hard to keep you safe. We use special policies and procedures to avoid mistakes in your care and keep you free from abuse or neglect. If anything unexpected and significant happens during your hospital stay, you will be told what happened and any resulting changes in your care will be discussed with you.

**Involvement in your care.** You and your doctor often make decisions about your care before you go to the hospital. Other times, especially in emergencies, those decisions are made during your hospital stay. When they take place, making decisions should include:

- *Discussing your medical condition and information about medically appropriate treatment choices.* To make informed

*continued >*

### CHART 3-3 The Patient Care Partnership: Understanding Expectations, Rights, and Responsibilities, continued

decisions with your doctor, you need to understand several things:
- The benefits and risks of each treatment.
- Whether it is experimental or part of a research study.
- What you can reasonably expect from your treatment and any long-term effects it might have on your quality of life.
- What you and your family will need to do after you leave the hospital.
- The financial consequences of using uncovered services or out-of-network providers.

Please tell your caregivers if you need more information about treatment choices.

- *Discussing your treatment plan.* When you enter the hospital, you sign a general consent to treatment. In some cases, such as surgery or experimental treatment, you may be asked to confirm in writing that you understand what is planned and agree to it. This process protects your right to consent to or refuse a treatment. Your doctor will explain the medical consequences of refusing recommended treatment. It also protects your right to decide if you want to participate in a research study.
- *Getting information from you.* Your caregivers need complete and correct information about your health and coverage so that they can make good decisions about your care. That includes:
  - Past illnesses, surgeries, or hospital stays.
  - Past allergic reactions.
  - Any medicines or diet supplements (such as vitamins and herbs) that you are taking.
  - Any network or admission requirements under your health plan.
- *Understanding your health care goals and values.* You may have health care goals and values or spiritual beliefs that are important to your well-being. They will be taken into account as much as possible throughout your hospital stay. Make sure your doctor, your family, and your care team know your wishes.
- *Understanding who should make decisions when you cannot.* If you have signed a health care power of attorney stating who should speak for you if you become unable to make health care decisions for yourself, or a "living will" or "advance directive" that states your wishes about end-of-life care, give copies to your doctor, your family, and your care team. If you or your family need help making difficult decisions, counselors, chaplains, and others are available to help.

**Protection of your privacy.** We respect the confidentiality of your relationship with your doctor and other caregivers, and the sensitive information about your health and health care that are part of that relationship. State and federal laws and hospital operating policies protect the privacy of your medical information. You will receive a Notice of Privacy Practices that describes the ways that we use, disclose and safeguard patient information and that explains how you can obtain a copy of information from our records about your care.

**Help preparing you and your family for when you leave the hospital.** Your doctor works with hospital staff and professionals in your community. You and your family also play an important role. The success of your treatment often depends on your efforts to follow medication, diet and therapy plans. Your family may need to help care for you at home.

You can expect us to help you identify sources of follow-up care and to let you know if our hospital has a financial interest in any referrals. As long as you agree we can share information about your care with them, we will coordinate our activities with your caregivers outside the hospital. You can also expect to receive information and, where possible, training about the self-care you will need when you go home.

**Help with your bill and filing insurance claims.** Our staff will file claims for you with health care insurers or other programs such as Medicare and Medicaid. They will also help your doctor with needed documentation. Hospital bills and insurance coverage are often confusing. If you have questions about your bill, contact our business office. If you need help understanding your insurance coverage or health plan, start with your insurance company or health benefits manager. If you do not have health coverage, we will try to help you and your family find financial help or make other arrangements. We need your help with collecting needed information and other requirements to obtain coverage or assistance.

While you are here, you will receive more detailed notices about some of the rights you have as a hospital patient and how to exercise them. We are always interested in improving. If you have questions, comments, or concerns, please contact _____.

Reprinted with permission of the American Hospital Association, copyright 2003.

> **CHART 3-4**
>
> ## American Nurses Association Code of Ethics for Nurses
>
> 1. The nurse, in all professional relationships, practices with compassion and respect for the inherent dignity, worth, and uniqueness of every individual, unrestricted by considerations of social or economic status, personal attributes, or the nature of health problems.
> 2. The nurse's primary commitment is to the patient, whether an individual, family, group, or community.
> 3. The nurse promotes, advocates for, and strives to protect the health, safety, and rights of the patient.
> 4. The nurse is responsible and accountable for individual nursing practice and determines the appropriate delegation of tasks consistent with the nurse's obligation to provide optimum patient care.
> 5. The nurse owes the same duties to self as to others, including the responsibility to preserve integrity and safety, to maintain competence, and to continue personal and professional growth.
> 6. The nurse participates in establishing, maintaining, and improving health care environments and conditions of employment conducive to the provision of quality health care and consistent with the values of the profession through individual and collective action.
> 7. The nurse participates in the advancement of the profession through contributions to practice, education, administration, and knowledge development.
> 8. The nurse collaborates with other health professionals and the public in promoting community, national, and international efforts to meet health needs.
> 9. The profession of nursing, as represented by associations and their members, is responsible for articulating nursing values, for maintaining the integrity of the profession and its practice, and for shaping social policy.
>
> Reprinted with permission from the American Nurses Association, *Code of Ethics for Nurses with Interpretive Statements*, © 2001, American Nurses Publishing, American Nurses Foundation/American Nurses Association, Washington, DC.

uations that involve ethical considerations. Some of the most common issues faced by nurses today include confidentiality, use of restraints, trust, refusing care, and end-of-life concerns.

## Confidentiality

All nurses should be aware of the confidential nature of information obtained in daily practice. If information is not pertinent, they should question whether it is prudent to record it in a patient's chart. In the practice setting, discussion of patients with other members of the health care team is often necessary. However, these discussions should occur in a private area where it is unlikely that the conversation will be overheard. Nurses should also be aware that the use of family members as interpreters for patients who are not fluent in the English language or who are deaf violates a patient's rights of confidentiality. Translation services should be provided for non–English-speaking patients and interpreters should be provided for those who use sign language.

Another threat to confidentiality is the widespread use of computers and the easy access people have to them. This may increase the potential for misuse of information. Because of these possibilities of maleficence (see Chart 3-2), sensitivity to the principle of confidentiality is essential.

## Restraints

The use of restraints (including physical and pharmacologic measures) is another issue with ethical overtones. It is important to weigh carefully the risks of limiting a person's autonomy and increasing the risk of injury by using restraints against the risks of not using restraints. Before restraints are used, other strategies, such as asking family members to sit with the patient, should be tried. The Joint Commission on Accreditation of Healthcare Organizations (JCAHO) and the Centers for Medicare and Medicaid Services (CMS) have designated standards for use in care of patients with restraints; these standards are available on the website listed at the end of this chapter (JCAHO, 2003).

## Trust Issues

Telling the truth (veracity) is one of the basic principles of our culture. Two ethical dilemmas in clinical practice that can directly conflict with this principle are the use of placebos (nonactive substances used to treat symptoms) and not revealing a diagnosis to a patient. Both involve the issue of trust, which is an essential element in the nurse–patient relationship. Placebos may be used in experimental research, in which a patient is involved in the decision-making process and is aware that placebos are being used in the treatment regimen. However, the use of a placebo as a substitute for an active drug to show that a patient does not have actual symptoms is deceptive, and this practice may severely undermine the nurse–patient relationship.

Informing a patient of his or her diagnosis when the family and physician have chosen to withhold information is a common ethical situation in nursing practice. The nursing staff may often use evasive comments with the patient as a means of maintaining professional relationships with other health practitioners. This area is indeed complex, because it challenges a nurse's integrity. Strategies nurses could consider include the following:

- Not lying to the patient
- Providing all information related to nursing procedures and diagnoses
- Communicating the patient's requests for information to the family and physician. The family is often unaware of the patient's repeated questions to a nurse. With a better understanding of the situation, the family members may change their perspective.

Finally, although providing the information may be the morally appropriate behavior, the manner in which the patient is told is important. Nurses must be compassionate and caring while informing patients; disclosure of information merely for the sake of patient autonomy does not convey respect for others.

## Refusing to Provide Care

Any nurse who feels compelled to refuse to provide care for a particular type of patient faces an ethical dilemma. The reasons given for refusal range from a conflict of personal values to fear of personal injury. The ethical obligation to care for all patients is clearly identified in the first statement of the Code of Ethics for Nurses. To avoid facing these moral situations, nurses can follow certain strategies. For example, when applying for a job, a nurse should ask questions regarding the patient population. If a nurse is uncomfortable with a particular situation, then not accepting the position would be an option. Denial of care, or providing substandard nursing care to some members of society, is not acceptable nursing practice.

## End-of-Life Issues

Dilemmas that center on death and dying are prevalent in medical-surgical nursing practice and frequently initiate moral discussion. Curing is paramount in health care, and this compounds the dilemmas. With advanced technology, it may be difficult to accept the fact that nothing more can be done to prolong life, or that technology may prolong life but at the expense of comfort and quality of life. Nurses are being faced with increasingly controversial dilemmas concerning patient desires to avoid prolongation of life. Many people who are terminally ill seek legal options for a peaceful and dignified death. Nurses may be in a quandary: they must choose between respect for the patient's autonomy and preservation of life (Valente, 2004).

End-of-life issues shift the focus from curative care to palliative and end-of-life care. Focusing on the caring as well as the curing role may help nurses deal with these difficult moral situations. Needs of patients and families require holistic and interdisciplinary approaches. In end-of-life care, nurses play the roles of clinician, advocate, and guide for patients and families (Norlander, 2001). End-of-life issues are discussed in detail in Chapter 17.

### PAIN CONTROL
The intent or goal of nursing interventions is to alleviate pain and suffering while promoting comfort. The administration of analgesia should be governed by the patient's needs. Patients in excruciating pain may require large doses of analgesics, and the use of opioids to alleviate the pain may present a dilemma for nurses. Fear of respiratory depression or unwarranted fear of addiction should not prevent nurses from attempting to alleviate pain in a dying patient or in a patient experiencing an episode of acute pain. For example, in the case of the terminally ill patient, the actions may be justified by the principle of double effect (see Chart 3-2). Induction of respiratory depression is not the intent of the actions and should not be used as a reason for withholding analgesia. However, the patient's respiratory status should be carefully monitored, and any signs of respiratory depression should be reported to the physician.

### "DO-NOT-RESUSCITATE" ORDERS
The "do not resuscitate" (DNR) order can result in controversy. When a patient is competent to make decisions and chooses a DNR order, this choice should be honored, according to the principles of autonomy or respect for the person. However, a DNR order is sometimes interpreted to mean that patients require less nursing care, when actually these patients may have significant medical and nursing needs, all of which demand attention. Ethically, all patients deserve and should receive appropriate nursing care, regardless of their resuscitation status.

### LIFE SUPPORT
It is important to consider the contrasting situation, in which a DNR decision has not been made by or for a dying patient. Nurses may be put in the uncomfortable position of initiating life-support measures when, because of a patient's physical condition, they appear futile. This frequently occurs when a patient is not competent to make the decision and the family (or surrogate decision maker) refuses to consider a DNR order as an option. In such cases, nurses may be told to perform a "slow code" (ie, not to rush to resuscitate the patient) or may be given a verbal order not to resuscitate the patient; both are unacceptable.

In such a situation, the best recourse for the nurse is to be aware of hospital policy related to the Patient Self-Determination Act (see the section on preventive ethics in this chapter, as well as Chapter 17) and execution of advance directives. The nurse should communicate with the physician. Discussion of the issue with the physician may lead to further communication with the family and to a reconsideration of the decision, especially if family members are afraid to let a loved one die with no further efforts at resuscitation. Finally, the nurse may find that when working with colleagues who are confronting such difficult situations, it helps to talk and listen to their concerns as a way of providing support.

### FOOD AND FLUID
In addition to requesting that no heroic measures be taken to prolong life, dying patients may request that no more food or fluid be administered. Many people think that food and hydration are basic human needs, not "invasive measures," and therefore should always be maintained. However, some consider food and hydration as means of prolonging suffering. When evaluating this issue, the nurse must take into consideration the potential harm as well

as the benefit to the patient of either administering or withdrawing sustenance.

Evaluation of harm requires a careful review of the reasons a person has requested the withdrawal of food and hydration. Although the principle of autonomy has considerable merit and is supported by the Code of Ethics for Nurses, there may be situations when the request for withdrawal of food and hydration cannot be upheld. For patients with decreased decision-making capacity, the issues are more complex. Some of these cases have reached courts of law, and different states have different case law precedents forbidding withdrawal of sustenance. Although an advance directive may provide some answers, at present there are no firm guidelines to assist nurses in this area.

## Preventive Ethics

When a nurse is faced with two conflicting alternatives, it is his or her moral decision to choose the lesser of the two evils. Various preventive strategies are available to help nurses anticipate or avoid certain kinds of ethical dilemmas.

Frequently, dilemmas occur when health care practitioners are unsure of the patient's wishes because the patient is unconscious or too cognitively impaired to communicate directly. One famous court case in this area of clinical ethics is that of Nancy Cruzan, a young woman who was involved in a car crash, after which she remained in a persistent vegetative state. Her family endured a 3-year legal battle to have her feeding tube removed so that she could be allowed to die. The U.S. Supreme Court decided that a state could require "clear and convincing evidence" of the patient's wishes before withdrawing life support. This ruling and the public response to it served as an impetus for legislation concerning advance directives, entitled the Patient Self-Determination Act, which became effective in December 1991. The intent of this legislation is to encourage people to prepare advance directives in which they indicate their wishes concerning the degree of supportive care to be provided if they become incapacitated. The regulatory language is quite broad and allows different institutions latitude in implementing a person's directives. This legislation does not require a patient to have an advance directive, but it does require that the patient be informed about advance directives by the staff of the health care facility. Consequently, this is an area in which nursing can play a significant role in patient education.

In 2005, the highly publicized case of Terri Schiavo focused national attention on the importance of advance directives. Schiavo was a young woman who suffered severe brain damage in 1990 after her heart stopped because of a chemical imbalance that was believed to have been caused by an eating disorder. Court-appointed physicians ruled she was in a persistent vegetative state with no real consciousness or chance of recovery. She left no living will or advance directive. Her husband requested that her feeding tube be removed to allow her to die, but her parents opposed this for 7 years. They involved the courts, Congress, and the President. Terri Schiavo died in 2005 after the courts ruled that her feeding tube could be removed and not replaced. This case represents an area in which nurses can play a significant role in patient education about the significance of advance directives.

### Advance Directives

Advance directives are legal documents that specify a person's wishes before hospitalization and provide valuable information that may assist health care providers in decision making. A living will is one type of advance directive. In most situations, living wills are limited to situations in which the patient's medical condition is deemed terminal. Because it is difficult to define "terminal" accurately, living wills are not always honored. Another potential drawback is that living wills are frequently written while people are in good health. It is not unusual for people to change their minds as their illness progresses; therefore, patients retain the option to nullify these documents.

Durable power of attorney for health care, in which one person identifies another person to make health care decisions on his or her behalf, is another type of advance directive. Patients may have clarified their wishes concerning a variety of medical situations. As such, the power of attorney for health care is a less restrictive type of advance directive. Laws concerning advance directives vary among state jurisdictions. However, even in states where these documents are not legally binding, they provide helpful information to determine the patient's prior expressed wishes in situations in which this information can no longer be obtained directly.

### Ethics Committees

Institutional ethics committees, which exist in many hospitals to assist practitioners with ethical dilemmas, also aid in preventive ethics. The purpose of these multidisciplinary committees varies among institutions. In some hospitals, the committees exist solely for the purpose of developing policies, whereas in others, they may have a strong educational or consultation focus. Because these committees usually are composed of people with some advanced training in ethics, they are important resources for the health care team, patient, and family. Nurses with a particular interest or expertise in the area of ethics are valuable members of ethics committees and can serve as valuable resources for staff nurses.

The heightened interest in ethical decision making has resulted in many continuing education programs, ranging from small seminars or workshops to full-semester courses offered by local colleges or professional organizations. In addition, nursing and medical journals contain articles on ethical issues, and numerous textbooks on clinical ethics or nursing ethics are available. These are valuable resources because they discuss ethical theory and dilemmas of practice in greater depth. ANA publications also assist nurses with ethical decision making.

## Ethical Decision Making

As noted in the preceding discussions, ethical dilemmas are common and diverse in nursing practice. Situations vary, and experience indicates that there are no clear solutions to these dilemmas. However, the fundamental philosophical principles are the same, and the process of moral reflection helps nurses justify their actions. The approach to ethical decision making can follow the steps of the nursing process. Chart 3-5 outlines the steps of an ethical analysis.

## CHART 3-5

### Steps of an Ethical Analysis

The following are guidelines to assist nurses in ethical decision making. These guidelines reflect an active process in decision making, similar to the nursing process detailed in this chapter.

**ASSESSMENT**

1. Assess the ethical/moral situations of the problem. This step entails recognition of the ethical, legal, and professional dimensions involved.
   a. Does the situation entail substantive moral problems (conflicts among ethical principles or professional obligations)?
   b. Are there procedural conflicts? (For example, who should make the decisions? Any conflicts among the patient, health care providers, family and guardians?)
   c. Identify the significant people involved and those affected by the decision.

**PLANNING**

2. Collect information.
   a. Include the following information: the medical facts, treatment options, nursing diagnoses, legal data, and the values, beliefs, and religious components.
   b. Make a distinction between the factual information and the values/beliefs.
   c. Validate the patient's capacity, or lack of capacity, to make decisions.
   d. Identify any other relevant information that should be elicited.
   e. Identify the ethical/moral issues and the competing claims.

**IMPLEMENTATION**

3. List the alternatives. Compare alternatives with applicable ethical principles and professional code of ethics. Choose either of the frameworks below, or other frameworks, and compare outcomes.
   a. *Utilitarian approach*: Predict the consequences of the alternatives; assign a positive or negative value to each consequence; choose the consequence that predicts the highest positive value or "the greatest good for the greatest number."
   b. *Deontological approach:* Identify the relevant moral principles; compare alternatives with moral principles; appeal to the "higher-level" moral principle if there is a conflict.

**EVALUATION**

4. Decide and evaluate the decision.
   a. What is the best or morally correct action?
   b. Give the ethical reasons for your decision.
   c. What are the ethical reasons against your decision?
   d. How do you respond to the reasons against your decision?

## The Nursing Process

### Definition

The nursing process is a deliberate problem-solving approach for meeting people's health care and nursing needs. Although the steps of the nursing process have been stated in various ways by different writers, the common components cited are assessment, diagnosis, planning, implementation, and evaluation. ANA's *Standards of Clinical Nursing Practice* (1998) includes an additional component entitled "outcome identification" and established the sequence of steps in the following order: assessment, diagnosis, outcome identification, planning, implementation, and evaluation. For the purposes of this text, the nursing process is based on the traditional five steps and delineates two components in the diagnosis step: nursing diagnoses and collaborative problems. After the diagnoses or problems have been determined, the desired outcomes are often evident. The traditional steps are defined as follows:

1. *Assessment:* The systematic collection of data to determine the patient's health status and any actual or potential health problems. (Analysis of data is included as part of the assessment. Analysis may also be identified as a separate step of the nursing process.)
2. *Diagnosis:* Identification of the following two types of patient problems:
   - *Nursing diagnoses:* Actual or potential health problems that can be managed by independent nursing interventions
   - *Collaborative problems:* "Certain physiologic complications that nurses monitor to detect onset or changes in status. Nurses manage collaborative problems using physician-prescribed and nursing-prescribed interventions to minimize the complications of the events" (Carpenito-Moyet, 2004).
3. *Planning:* Development of goals and outcomes, as well as a plan of care designed to assist the patient in resolving the diagnosed problems and achieving the identified goals and desired outcomes
4. *Implementation:* Actualization of the plan of care through nursing interventions
5. *Evaluation:* Determination of the patient's responses to the nursing interventions and the extent to which the outcomes have been achieved

Dividing the nursing process into distinct steps serves to emphasize the essential nursing actions that must be taken to address the patient's nursing diagnoses and manage any collaborative problems or complications. However, dividing the process into separate steps is artificial: the process functions as an integrated whole, with the steps being interrelated, interdependent, and recurrent (Fig. 3-1). Chart 3-6 presents an overview of the nursing activities involved in applying the nursing process.

## Using the Nursing Process

### Assessment

Assessment data are gathered through the health history and the physical assessment. In addition, ongoing monitoring is crucial to remain aware of changing patient needs and the effectiveness of nursing care.

#### HEALTH HISTORY
The health history is conducted to determine a person's state of wellness or illness and is best accomplished as part of a planned interview. The interview is a personal dialogue between a patient and a nurse that is conducted to obtain information. The nurse's approach to the patient largely determines the amount and quality of the information that is received. To achieve a relationship of mutual trust and respect, the nurse must have the ability to communicate a sincere interest in the patient. Examples of effective therapeutic communication techniques that can be used to achieve this goal are found in Table 3-1.

The use of a health history guide may help in obtaining pertinent information and in directing the course of the interview. A variety of health history formats designed to guide the interview are available, but they must be adapted to the responses, problems, and needs of the person. See Chapter 5 for further information about the health history.

#### PHYSICAL ASSESSMENT
A physical assessment may be carried out before, during, or after the health history, depending on a patient's physical and emotional status and the immediate priorities of the situation. The purpose of the physical assessment is to identify those aspects of a patient's physical, psychological, and emotional state that indicate a need for nursing care. It requires the use of sight, hearing, touch, and smell, as well as the appropriate interview skills and techniques. Physical examination techniques as well as techniques and strategies for assessing behaviors and role changes are presented in Chapters 5 and 7 and in each unit of this book.

#### OTHER COMPONENTS OF THE ASSESSMENT
Additional relevant information should be obtained from the patient's family or significant others, from other members of the health team, and from the patient's health record or chart. Depending on the patient's immediate needs, this information may have been completed before the health history and the physical assessment were obtained. Whatever the sequence of events, it is important to use all available sources of pertinent data to complete the nursing assessment.

#### RECORDING THE DATA
After the health history and physical assessment are completed, the information obtained is recorded in the patient's permanent record. This record provides a means of communication among members of the health care team and facilitates coordinated planning and continuity of care. The record fulfills other functions as well:

- It serves as the legal and business record for a health care agency and for the professional staff members who are responsible for the patient's care. A variety of systems are used for documenting patient care, and each health care agency selects the system that best meets its needs.
- It serves as a basis for evaluating the quality and appropriateness of care and for reviewing the effective use of patient care services.
- It provides data that are useful in research, education, and short- and long-range planning.

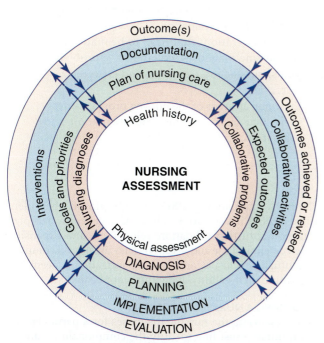

**FIGURE 3-1.** The nursing process is depicted schematically in this circle. Starting from the innermost circle, nursing assessment, the process moves outward through the formulation of nursing diagnoses and collaborative problems; planning, with setting of goals and priorities in the nursing plan of care; implementation and documentation; and, finally, the ongoing process of evaluation and outcomes.

### Diagnosis

The assessment component of the nursing process serves as the basis for identifying nursing diagnoses and collaborative problems. Soon after the completion of the health history and the physical assessment, nurses organize, analyze, synthesize, and summarize the data collected and determine the patient's need for nursing care.

## CHART 3-6 — Steps of the Nursing Process

**ASSESSMENT**
1. Conduct the health history.
2. Perform the physical assessment.
3. Interview the patient's family or significant others.
4. Study the health record.
5. Organize, analyze, synthesize, and summarize the collected data.

**DIAGNOSIS**

*Nursing Diagnosis*
1. Identify the patient's nursing problems.
2. Identify the defining characteristics of the nursing problems.
3. Identify the etiology of the nursing problems.
4. State nursing diagnoses concisely and precisely.

*Collaborative Problems*
1. Identify potential problems or complications that require collaborative interventions.
2. Identify health team members with whom collaboration is essential.

**PLANNING**
1. Assign priority to the nursing diagnoses.
2. Specify the goals.
    a. Develop immediate, intermediate, and long-term goals.
    b. State the goals in realistic and measurable terms.
3. Identify nursing interventions appropriate for goal attainment.
4. Establish expected outcomes.
    a. Make sure that the outcomes are realistic and measurable.
    b. Identify critical times for the attainment of outcomes.
5. Develop the written plan of nursing care.
    a. Include nursing diagnoses, goals, nursing interventions, expected outcomes, and critical times.
    b. Write all entries precisely, concisely, and systematically.
    c. Keep the plan current and flexible to meet the patient's changing problems and needs.
6. Involve the patient, family or significant others, nursing team members, and other health team members in all aspects of planning.

**IMPLEMENTATION**
1. Put the plan of nursing care into action.
2. Coordinate the activities of the patient, family or significant others, nursing team members, and other health team members.
3. Record the patient's responses to the nursing actions.

**EVALUATION**
1. Collect data.
2. Compare the patient's actual outcomes with the expected outcomes. Determine the extent to which the expected outcomes were achieved.
3. Include the patient, family or significant others, nursing team members, and other health care team members in the evaluation.
4. Identify alterations that need to be made in the nursing diagnoses, collaborative problems, goals, nursing interventions, and expected outcomes.
5. Continue all steps of the nursing process: assessment, diagnosis, planning, implementation, and evaluation.

## NURSING DIAGNOSIS

Nursing, unlike medicine, does not yet have a complete taxonomy, or classification system, of diagnostic labels. Nursing diagnoses, the first taxonomy created in nursing, have fostered the development of autonomy and accountability in nursing and have helped to delineate the scope of practice. Many state nurse practice acts include nursing diagnosis as a nursing function, and nursing diagnosis is included in the ANA's *Standards of Clinical Nursing Practice* and the standards of many nursing specialty organizations.

NANDA International (founded in 1982 as the North American Nursing Diagnosis Association) is the official organization that has assumed responsibility for developing the taxonomy of nursing diagnoses and formulating nursing diagnoses acceptable for study. The most commonly selected nursing diagnoses are compiled and categorized by NANDA in a taxonomy that is updated at least every 2 years (NANDA International, 2005). The diagnostic labels identified by NANDA (Chart 3-7) have been generally accepted but require further validation, refinement, and expansion based on clinical use and research. They are not yet complete or mutually exclusive, and more investigation is needed to determine their validity and clinical applicability.

## CHOOSING A NURSING DIAGNOSIS

When choosing the nursing diagnoses for a particular patient, nurses must first identify the commonalities among the assessment data collected. These common features lead to the categorization of related data that reveal the existence of a problem and the need for nursing intervention. The identified problems are then defined as specific nursing diagnoses (see Chart 3-7). Nursing diagnoses represent actual or potential health problems that can be managed by independent nursing actions.

## TABLE 3-1  Therapeutic Communication Techniques

| Technique | Definition | Therapeutic Value |
|---|---|---|
| Listening | Active process of receiving information and examining one's reactions to the messages received | Nonverbally communicates nurse's interest in patient |
| Silence | Periods of no verbal communication among participants for therapeutic reasons | Gives patient time to think and gain insights, slows the pace of the interaction, and encourages the patient to initiate conversation, while conveying the nurse's support, understanding, and acceptance |
| Restating | Repeating to the patient what the nurse believes is the main thought or idea expressed | Demonstrates that the nurse is listening and validates, reinforces, or calls attention to something important that has been said |
| Reflection | Directing back to the patient his or her feelings, ideas, questions, or content | Validates the nurse's understanding of what the patient is saying and signifies empathy, interest, and respect for the patient |
| Clarification | Asking the patient to explain what he or she means or attempting to verbalize vague ideas or unclear thoughts of the patient to enhance the nurse's understanding | Helps to clarify the patient's feelings, ideas, and perceptions and to provide an explicit correlation between them and the patient's actions |
| Focusing | Questions or statements to help the patient develop or expand an idea | Allows the patient to discuss central issues and keeps communication goal-directed |
| Broad openings | Encouraging the patient to select topics for discussion | Indicates acceptance by the nurse and the value of the patient's initiative |
| Humor | Discharge of energy through the comic enjoyment of the imperfect | Promotes insight by bringing repressed material to consciousness, resolving paradoxes, tempering aggression, and revealing new options; a socially acceptable form of sublimation |
| Informing | Providing information | Helpful in health teaching or patient education about relevant aspects of patient's well-being and self-care |
| Sharing perceptions | Asking the patient to verify the nurse's understanding of what the patient is thinking or feeling | Conveys the nurse's understanding to the patient and has the potential to clarify confusing communication |
| Theme identification | Underlying issues or problems experienced by the patient that emerge repeatedly during the course of the nurse–patient relationship | Allows the nurse to best promote the patient's exploration and understanding of important problems |
| Suggesting | Presentation of alternative ideas for the patient's consideration relative to problem solving | Increases the patient's perceived options or choices |

Adapted from Stuart, G. W., & Laraia, M. T. (2004). *Stuart and Sundeen's principles and practice of psychiatric nursing* (8th ed.). St Louis: CV Mosby.

It is important to remember that nursing diagnoses are not medical diagnoses; they are not medical treatments prescribed by the physician, and they are not diagnostic studies. Nursing diagnoses are not the equipment used to implement medical therapy, and they are not the problems that nurses experience while caring for patients. Nursing diagnoses are succinct statements in terms of specific patient problems that guide nurses in the development of the nursing plan of care.

To give additional meaning to the nursing diagnosis, the characteristics and the etiology of the problem are identified and included as part of the diagnosis. For example, the nursing diagnoses and their defining characteristics and etiology for a patient who has anemia may include the following:

- Activity intolerance related to weakness and fatigue
- Ineffective tissue perfusion related to inadequate blood volume
- Imbalanced nutrition: Less than body requirements related to fatigue and inadequate intake of essential nutrients

### COLLABORATIVE PROBLEMS

In addition to nursing diagnoses and their related nursing interventions, nursing practice involves certain situations and interventions that do not fall within the definition of nursing diagnoses. These activities pertain to potential problems or complications that are medical in origin and require collaborative interventions with the physician and other members of the health care team.

## CHART 3-7

### NANDA-Approved Nursing Diagnoses 2005–2006

This list represents the NANDA-approved nursing diagnoses for clinical use and testing.

Activity Intolerance
Activity Intolerance, Risk for
Adjustment, Impaired
Airway Clearance, Ineffective
Allergy Response, Latex
Allergy Response, Risk for Latex
Anxiety
Anxiety, Death
Aspiration, Risk for
Attachment, Risk for Impaired Parent/Infant/Child
Autonomic Dysreflexia
Autonomic Dysreflexia, Risk for
Body Image, Disturbed
Body Temperature, Risk for Imbalanced
Bowel Incontinence
Breastfeeding, Effective
Breastfeeding, Ineffective
Breastfeeding, Interrupted
Breathing Pattern, Ineffective
Cardiac Output, Decreased
Caregiver Role Strain
Caregiver Role Strain, Risk for
Communication, Impaired Verbal
Communication, Readiness for Enhanced
Conflict, Decisional (Specify)
Conflict, Parental Role
Confusion, Acute
Confusion, Chronic
Constipation
Constipation, Perceived
Constipation, Risk for
Coping, Ineffective
Coping, Defensive
Coping, Readiness for Enhanced
Coping, Ineffective Community
Coping, Readiness for Enhanced Community
Coping, Compromised Family
Coping, Disabled Family
Coping, Readiness for Enhanced Family
Death Syndrome, Risk for Sudden Infant
Denial, Ineffective
Dentition, Impaired
Development, Risk for Delayed
Diarrhea
Disuse Syndrome, Risk for
Diversional Activity, Deficient
Energy Field, Disturbed
Environmental Interpretation Syndrome, Impaired
Failure to Thrive, Adult
Falls, Risk for
Family Processes, Dysfunctional: Alcoholism
Family Processes, Interrupted
Family Processes, Readiness for Enhanced
Fatigue
Fear
Fluid Balance, Readiness for Enhanced
Fluid Volume, Deficient
Fluid Volume, Excess
Fluid Volume, Risk for Deficient
Fluid Volume, Risk for Imbalanced
Gas Exchange, Impaired
Grieving, Anticipatory
Grieving, Dysfunctional
Grieving, Risk for Dysfunctional
Growth and Development, Delayed
Growth, Risk for Disproportionate
Health Maintenance, Ineffective
Health-Seeking Behaviors (Specify)
Home Maintenance, Impaired
Hopelessness
Hyperthermia
Hypothermia
Identity, Disturbed Personal
Incontinence, Functional Urinary
Incontinence, Reflex Urinary
Incontinence, Stress Urinary
Incontinence, Total Urinary
Incontinence, Urge Urinary
Incontinence, Risk for Urge Urinary
Infant Behavior, Disorganized
Infant Behavior, Risk for Disorganized
Infant Behavior, Readiness for Enhanced Organized
Infant Feeding Pattern, Ineffective
Infection, Risk for
Injury, Risk for
Injury, Risk for Perioperative-Positioning
Intracranial Adaptive Capacity, Decreased
Knowledge, Deficient (Specify)
Knowledge, Readiness for Enhanced (Specify)
Lifestyle, Sedentary
Loneliness, Risk for
Memory, Impaired
Mobility, Impaired Bed
Mobility, Impaired Physical
Mobility, Impaired Wheelchair
Nausea
Neglect, Unilateral
Noncompliance
Nutrition, Imbalanced: Less Than Body Requirements

## CHART 3-7 NANDA-Approved Nursing Diagnoses 2005–2006, continued

- Nutrition, Imbalanced: More Than Body Requirements
- Nutrition, Readiness for Enhanced
- Nutrition, Risk for Imbalanced: More Than Body Requirements
- Oral Mucous Membrane, Impaired
- Pain, Acute
- Pain, Chronic
- Parenting, Readiness for Enhanced
- Parenting, Impaired
- Parenting, Risk for Impaired
- Peripheral Neurovascular Dysfunction, Risk for
- Poisoning, Risk for
- Post-Trauma Syndrome
- Post-Trauma Syndrome, Risk for
- Powerlessness
- Powerlessness, Risk for
- Protection, Ineffective
- Rape-Trauma Syndrome
- Rape-Trauma Syndrome: Compound Reaction
- Rape-trauma Syndrome: Silent Reaction
- Religiosity, Impaired
- Religiosity, Readiness for Enhanced
- Religiosity, Risk for Impaired
- Relocation Stress Syndrome
- Relocation Stress Syndrome, Risk for
- Role Performance, Ineffective
- Self-Care Deficit, Bathing/Hygiene
- Self-Care Deficit, Dressing/Grooming
- Self-Care Deficit, Feeding
- Self-Care Deficit, Toileting
- Self-Concept, Readiness for Enhanced
- Self-Esteem, Chronic Low
- Self-Esteem, Situational Low
- Self-Esteem, Risk for Situational Low
- Self-Mutilation
- Self-Mutilation, Risk for
- Sensory Perception, Disturbed (Specify: Visual, Auditory, Kinesthetic, Gustatory, Tactile, Olfactory)
- Sexual Dysfunction
- Sexuality Pattern, Ineffective
- Skin Integrity, Impaired
- Skin Integrity, Risk for Impaired
- Sleep Deprivation
- Sleep Pattern, Disturbed
- Sleep, Readiness for Enhanced
- Social Interaction, Impaired
- Social Isolation
- Sorrow, Chronic
- Spiritual Distress
- Spiritual Distress, Risk for
- Spiritual Well-Being, Readiness for Enhanced
- Suffocation, Risk for
- Suicide, Risk for
- Surgical Recovery, Delayed
- Swallowing, Impaired
- Therapeutic Regimen Management, Effective
- Therapeutic Regimen Management, Ineffective
- Therapeutic Regimen Management, Readiness for Enhanced
- Therapeutic Regimen Management, Ineffective Community
- Therapeutic Regimen Management, Ineffective Family
- Thermoregulation, Ineffective
- Thought Processes, Disturbed
- Tissue Integrity, Impaired
- Tissue Perfusion, Ineffective (Specify Type: Renal, Cerebral, Cardiopulmonary, Gastrointestinal, Peripheral)
- Transfer Ability, Impaired
- Trauma, Risk for
- Urinary Elimination, Impaired
- Urinary Elimination, Readiness for Enhanced
- Urinary Retention
- Ventilation, Impaired Spontaneous
- Ventilatory Weaning Response, Dysfunctional
- Violence, Risk for Other-Directed
- Violence, Risk for Self-Directed
- Walking, Impaired
- Wandering

NANDA International (2005). *Nursing diagnoses: Definitions & classification 2005–2006.* Philadelphia: Author.

---

The term *collaborative problem* is used to identify these situations.

Collaborative problems are certain physiologic complications that nurses monitor to detect changes in status or onset of complications. Nurses manage collaborative problems using physician-prescribed and nursing-prescribed interventions to minimize complications (Carpenito-Moyet, 2004). When treating collaborative problems, a primary nursing focus is monitoring patients for the onset of complications or changes in the status of existing complications. The complications are usually related to the disease process, treatments, medications, or diagnostic studies. The nurse recommends nursing interventions that are appropriate for managing the complications and implements the treatments prescribed by the physician. The algorithm in Figure 3-2 depicts the differences between nursing diagnoses and collaborative problems. After the nursing diagnoses and collaborative problems have been identified, they are recorded on the plan of nursing care.

## Planning

Once the nursing diagnoses have been identified, the planning component of the nursing process begins. This phase involves the following steps:

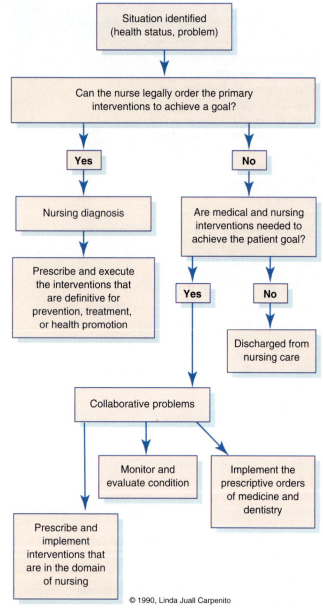

**FIGURE 3-2.** Differentiating nursing diagnoses and collaborative problems. From Carpenito-Moyet, L. J. (2004). *Nursing diagnosis: Application to clinical practice* (10th ed.). Philadelphia: Lippincott Williams & Wilkins.

1. Assigning priorities to the nursing diagnoses and collaborative problems
2. Specifying expected outcomes
3. Specifying the immediate, intermediate, and long-term goals of nursing action
4. Identifying specific nursing interventions appropriate for attaining the outcomes
5. Identifying interdependent interventions
6. Documenting the nursing diagnoses, collaborative problems, expected outcomes, nursing goals, and nursing interventions on the plan of nursing care
7. Communicating to appropriate personnel any assessment data that point to health care needs that can best be met by other members of the health care team

### SETTING PRIORITIES

Assigning priorities to the nursing diagnoses and collaborative problems is a joint effort by the nurse and the patient or family members. Any disagreement about priorities is resolved in a way that is mutually acceptable. Consideration must be given to the urgency of the problems, with the most critical problems receiving the highest priority. The Maslow hierarchy of needs provides a useful framework for prioritizing problems, with importance being given first to physical needs; once those basic needs are met, higher-level needs can be addressed.

### ESTABLISHING EXPECTED OUTCOMES

Expected outcomes of the nursing interventions are expressed in terms of the patient's behaviors and the time period in which the outcomes are to be achieved, as well as any special circumstances related to achieving the outcome (Smith-Temple & Johnson, 2005). These outcomes must be realistic and measurable. Resources for identifying appropriate expected outcomes include the Nursing-Sensitive Outcomes Classification (NOC) (Chart 3-8) and standard outcome criteria established by health care agencies for people with specific health problems. These outcomes can be associated with nursing diagnoses and interventions and can be used when appropriate. However, the NOC may need to be adapted to establish realistic criteria for the specific patient involved.

The expected outcomes that define the desired behavior of the patient are used to measure the progress made toward resolving the problem. The expected outcomes also serve as the basis for evaluating the effectiveness of the nursing interventions and for deciding whether additional nursing care is needed or whether the plan of care needs to be revised.

### ESTABLISHING GOALS

After the priorities of the nursing diagnoses and expected outcomes have been established, goals (immediate, intermediate, and long-term) and the nursing actions appropriate for attaining the goals are identified. The patient and family are included in establishing goals for the nursing actions. Immediate goals are those that can be attained within a short period. Intermediate and long-term goals require a longer time to be achieved and usually involve preventing complications and other health problems and promoting self-care and rehabilitation. For example, goals for a patient with a nursing diagnosis of impaired physical mobility related to pain and edema following total knee replacement may be stated as follows:

- Immediate goal: Stands at bedside 6 to 12 hours after surgery
- Intermediate goal: Ambulates with walker or crutches in hospital and home
- Long-term goal: Ambulates independently 1 to 2 miles each day

### DETERMINING NURSING ACTIONS

In planning appropriate nursing actions to achieve the desired goals and outcomes, the nurse, with input from the patient and significant others, identifies individualized interventions based on the patient's circumstances and

## CHART 3-8

### Nursing-Sensitive Outcomes Classification (NOC)

The NOC is a classification of patient outcomes sensitive to nursing interventions. Each outcome is a neutral statement about a variable patient condition, behavior, or perception, coupled with a rating scale. The outcome statement and scale can be used to identify baseline functioning, expected outcomes, and actual outcomes for individual patients. The following table is an example of a nursing-sensitive outcome.

**Respiratory Status: Airway Patency (0410)**

*Domain*—Physiologic Health (II)
*Class*—Cardiopulmonary (E)
*Scale(s)*—Severely compromised to Not compromised (a) and Severe to None (n)
*Definition* Open, clear tracheobronchial passages for air exchange
OUTCOME TARGET RATING:   Maintain at _____   Increase to _____

| Respiratory Status: Airway Patency Overall Rating | | Severely Compromised 1 | Substantially Compromised 2 | Moderately Compromised 3 | Mildly Compromised 4 | Not Compromised 5 | |
|---|---|---|---|---|---|---|---|
| | INDICATORS: | | | | | | |
| 041009 | Ease of breathing | 1 | 2 | 3 | 4 | 5 | NA |
| 041004 | Respiratory rate | 1 | 2 | 3 | 4 | 5 | NA |
| 041005 | Respiratory rhythm | 1 | 2 | 3 | 4 | 5 | NA |
| 041006 | Moves sputum out of airway | 1 | 2 | 3 | 4 | 5 | NA |
| 041010 | Moves blockage out of airway | 1 | 2 | 3 | 4 | 5 | NA |
| | | Severe | Substantial | Moderate | Mild | None | |
| 041002 | Anxiety | 1 | 2 | 3 | 4 | 5 | NA |
| 041011 | Fear | 1 | 2 | 3 | 4 | 5 | NA |
| 041003 | Choking | 1 | 2 | 3 | 4 | 5 | NA |
| 041007 | Adventitious breath sounds | 1 | 2 | 3 | 4 | 5 | NA |

With permission from Moorhead, S., Johnson, M., & Maas, M. (Eds.). (2004). *Nursing outcomes classification [NOC]: Iowa Outcomes Project* (3rd ed.). St. Louis: Mosby–Year Book.

---

preferences that address each outcome. Interventions should identify the activities needed and who will implement them. Determination of interdisciplinary activities is made in collaboration with other health care providers as needed.

The nurse identifies and plans patient teaching and return demonstration as needed to assist the patient in learning certain self-care activities. Planned interventions should be ethical and appropriate to the patient's culture, age, and gender. Standardized interventions, such as those found on institutional care plans or in the Nursing Interventions Classification (NIC) (Dochterman & Bulechek, 2004) can be used. Chart 3-9 describes the NIC system and provides an example of an NIC system intervention. It is important to individualize prewritten interventions to promote optimal effectiveness for each patient. Actions of nurses should be based on established standards.

### Implementation

The implementation phase of the nursing process involves carrying out the proposed plan of nursing care. The nurse assumes responsibility for the implementation and coordinates the activities of all those involved in implementation, including the patient and family, other members of the nursing team, and other members of the health care team, so that the schedule of activities facilitates the patient's recovery.

> **CHART 3-9**
>
> ## Nursing Interventions Classification (NIC)
>
> The NIC is a standardized classification of nursing treatments (interventions) that includes independent and collaborative interventions. Intervention labels are terms such as hemorrhage control, medication administration, or pain management. Listed under each intervention are multiple discrete nursing actions that together constitute a comprehensive approach to the treatment of a particular condition. Not all actions are applicable to every patient; nursing judgment will determine which actions to implement. The following is an example of a nursing intervention:
>
> **CHEST PHYSIOTHERAPY**
>
> *Definition*
> Assisting the patient to move airway secretions from peripheral airways to more central airways for expectoration and/or suctioning
>
> *Activities*
> Determine presence of contraindications for use of chest physical therapy.
> Determine which lung segment(s) needs to be drained.
> Position patient with the lung segment to be drained in uppermost position.
> Use pillows to support patient in designated position.
> Use percussion with postural drainage by cupping hands and clapping the chest wall in rapid succession to produce a series of hollow sounds.
> Use chest vibration in combination with postural drainage, as appropriate.
> Use an ultrasonic nebulizer, as appropriate.
> Use aerosol therapy, as appropriate.
> Administer bronchodilators, as appropriate.
> Monitor amount and type of sputum expectoration.
> Encourage coughing during and after postural drainage.
> Monitor patient tolerance by means of $SaO_2$, respiratory rhythm and rate, cardiac rhythm and rate, and comfort levels.
>
> With permission from Dochterman, G. M., & Bulechek, G. M. (Eds.). (2004). *Nursing interventions classification (NIC)* (4th ed.). St. Louis: Mosby.

The plan of nursing care serves as the basis for implementation, as described below:

- The immediate, intermediate, and long-term goals are used as a focus for the implementation of the designated nursing interventions.
- While implementing nursing care, the nurse continually assesses the patient and his or her response to the nursing care.
- Revisions are made in the plan of care as the patient's condition, problems, and responses change and when re-ordering of priorities is required.

Implementation includes direct or indirect execution of the planned interventions. It is focused on resolving the patient's nursing diagnoses and collaborative problems and achieving expected outcomes, thus meeting the patient's health needs. Examples of nursing interventions are assisting with hygiene care; promoting physical and psychological comfort; supporting respiratory and elimination functions; facilitating the ingestion of food, fluids, and nutrients; managing the patient's immediate surroundings; providing health teaching; promoting a therapeutic relationship; and carrying out a variety of therapeutic nursing activities. Judgment, critical thinking, and good decision-making skills are essential in the selection of appropriate evidence-based and ethical nursing interventions. All nursing interventions are patient-focused and outcome-directed and are implemented with compassion, confidence, and a willingness to accept and understand the patient's responses.

Although many nursing actions are independent, others are interdependent, such as carrying out prescribed treatments, administering medications and therapies, and collaborating with other health care team members to accomplish specific expected outcomes and to monitor and manage potential complications. Such interdependent functioning is just that—interdependent. Requests or orders from other health care team members should not be followed blindly but should be assessed critically and questioned when necessary. The implementation phase of the nursing process ends when the nursing interventions have been completed.

## Evaluation

Evaluation, the final step of the nursing process, allows the nurse to determine the patient's response to the nursing interventions and the extent to which the objectives have been achieved. The plan of nursing care is the basis for evaluation. The nursing diagnoses, collaborative problems, priorities, nursing interventions, and expected outcomes provide the specific guidelines that dictate the focus of the evaluation. Through evaluation, the nurse can answer the following questions:

- Were the nursing diagnoses and collaborative problems accurate?
- Did the patient achieve the expected outcomes within the critical time periods?
- Have the patient's nursing diagnoses been resolved?

- Have the collaborative problems been resolved?
- Do priorities need to be reordered?
- Have the patient's nursing needs been met?
- Should the nursing interventions be continued, revised, or discontinued?
- Have new problems evolved for which nursing interventions have not been planned or implemented?
- What factors influenced the achievement or lack of achievement of the objectives?
- Should changes be made in the expected outcomes and outcome criteria?

Objective data that provide answers to these questions are collected from all available sources (eg, patients, families, significant others, health care team members). These data are included in patients' records and must be substantiated by direct patient observation before the outcomes are documented.

## Documentation of Outcomes and Revision of Plan

Outcomes are documented concisely and objectively. Documentation should relate outcomes to the nursing diagnoses and collaborative problems, describe the patient's responses to the interventions, indicate whether the outcomes were met, and include any additional pertinent data. An example of an individualized plan of nursing care is given in Chart 3-10.

The plan of care is subject to change as a patient's needs change, as the priorities of needs shift, as needs are resolved, and as additional information about a patient's state of health is collected. As the nursing interventions are implemented, the patient's responses are evaluated and documented, and the plan of care is revised accordingly. A well-developed, continuously updated plan of care is the greatest assurance that the patient's nursing diagnoses and collaborative problems are addressed and his or her basic needs are met.

## Framework for a Common Nursing Language: Combining NANDA, NIC, and NOC

Various frameworks or taxonomies can be used for determining nursing diagnoses (eg, NANDA), establishing outcomes (eg, NOC), and designing interventions (eg, NIC). Ultimately a framework that uses a language common to all aspects of nursing, regardless of the classification system, is desirable. Although still controversial and in its infancy, significant efforts have been made toward accomplishing this goal of unifying the language of nursing. In 2001, a Taxonomy of Nursing Practice was developed for

---

### CHART 3-10

### Example of an Individualized Plan of Nursing Care

Mrs. Wilma Bryer, a 52-year-old court stenographer, was admitted to the nursing unit from her physician's office. She had had a gnawing pain on her right side radiating to her back for 3 days. She now describes her pain as "excruciating after eating or drinking." In the past 48 hours she has been vomiting about 2 to 3 hours after she eats. She has not had anything to eat or drink for the past 12 hours.

Mrs. Bryer stated that she had not been successful in adhering to the weight reduction diet that had been prescribed by her physician and that she had rapidly lost, then regained, weight several times in the past year and a half. She stated, "My life is just too busy—I work late hours in the court system and have to buy my meals out a lot." She indicated that in addition to her work, she and her husband share the responsibility for raising their two teenage daughters

Admission physical examination revealed BP 138/88, P 102, R 24, T 99.9°F, height 5'7", weight 270 lbs, skin warm, no jaundice. She stated that her urine has been "a strange dark-golden color" and her stools were "like putty and grayish." She was admitted with the diagnosis of acute cholecystitis. The physician's orders on admission included: monitor vital signs every 4 hours; IV of $D_5$ Ringer's lactate 125 mL per hour; 1500-calorie, low-fat liquid diet and progress to low-fat soft diet if no pain in 16 hours; morphine sulfate 2 mg IV every 2 hours as needed; notify physician for sudden increase in frequency or intensity of pain; promethazine 12.5 mg IV every 4 hours as needed for nausea or vomiting.

#### Nursing Diagnoses
- Acute pain related to distended cystic duct and inflamed or infected gallbladder
- Risk for deficient fluid volume related to vomiting and decreased intake
- Ineffective coping related to role and responsibilities at work and home
- Imbalanced nutrition: More than body requirements, related to knowledge deficit about sedentary lifestyle, poor food choices and eating pattern

*continued >*

## CHART 3-10 Example of an Individualized Plan of Nursing Care, continued

**Collaborative Problems**
- Risk for cystic duct necrosis or perforation
- Obesity

**Goals**

*Immediate:*
- Relief of pain
- Prevent fluid volume deficit and electrolyte imbalance
- Promote rest
- Early detection of any complications

*Intermediate:*
- Initiation of lifestyle alterations to decrease stress and facilitate rest

*Long-term:*
- Alteration of lifestyle to reduce emotional and environmental stressors
- Compliance with dietary regimen
- Weight reduction

| NURSING INTERVENTIONS | EXPECTED OUTCOMES | OUTCOMES |
| --- | --- | --- |
| 1. Monitor BP, pulse, temperature, and respirations every 4 hours. | 1. Vital signs within normal limits | 1. BP range 110/62–128/78 with pain relief measures; temperature 98°–98.8°F; pulse range 74–88; respirations 18–22 |
| 2. Monitor pain status with accompanying abdominal assessment every 2 hours, or more frequently, as needed.<br>  a. Assess pain characteristics every 2 hours or as needed.<br>  b. Assess abdomen every 2 hours or with pain assessment.<br>  c. Use nonpharmacologic measures (pillows, repositioning, etc.) as desired and tolerated by patient for pain relief.<br>  d. Administer analgesic at regular intervals as needed, and assess response. | 2. Experiences pain relief; abdominal assessment within normal limits | 2. Verbalized decrease in pain from severe (8) to low (2) intensity within 10 minutes after morphine administered; no pain radiation to back<br>Abdomen soft and nontender |
| 3. Monitor and support fluid and electrolyte status:<br>  a. Monitor weight.<br>  b. I&O<br>  c. Monitor skin turgor and temperature.<br>  d. Monitor serum electrolytes.<br>  e. Monitor color and consistency of urine and stool output.<br>  f. Encourage low-fat liquid intake if pain-free.<br>  g. Administer promethazine as prescribed to control or relieve vomiting. | 3. Fluid balance maintained; electrolytes within normal limits | 3. Weight 270 on admission and 269 after 2-day period<br>Urinary output adequate in relation to oral and IV intake<br>Skin warm and supple, good recoil<br>Electrolytes in normal range<br>Urine dark amber in color, no sediment; stools soft, formed, light brown<br>No vomiting reported |

## CHART 3-10 Example of an Individualized Plan of Nursing Care, continued

| NURSING INTERVENTIONS | EXPECTED OUTCOMES | OUTCOMES |
|---|---|---|
| 4. Promote atmosphere conducive to physical and mental rest:<br>   a. Encourage alternation of rest and activity.<br>   b. Encourage limitation of visitors and interactions that are stress-producing. | 4. Alternates periods of rest and activity<br>   Limits visitors to family in the evenings<br>   Avoids stress-producing interactions | 4. Rests in bed 2 hr in morning and 2 hr in afternoon; disconnects phone during rest periods.<br>   8 hours uninterrupted sleep at night; husband and daughters visit 2 hours in evening; patient calm and relaxed after visits<br>   Accurately described relationship between stress, sedentary lifestyle, and obesity |
| 5. Assist patient to alter lifestyle to decrease stress:<br>   a. Discuss relationship between emotional stress and physiologic function.<br>   b. Encourage patient to identify stress-producing stimuli.<br>   c. Encourage patient to identify adjustments necessary to reduce stress relative to the home and work setting. | 5. Describes stress, sedentary lifestyle, and obesity as precursors to alteration in physiologic functioning<br>   Identifies lifestyle factors that produce stress | 5. Identified the following stressors:<br>   Demands of job<br>   Excessive involvement in daughters' school and recreational activities |
| 6. Encourage patient to identify sedentary lifestyle, obesity, and repetitive weight loss and gain as physiologic and emotional stressors; request consultation with dietitian and reinforce instructions given. | 6. Identifies lifestyle adjustments necessary to reduce stress<br>   Discusses lifestyle adjustments with family | 6. Identified need to decrease work hours to maximum of 8 hr per day<br>   Consulted with husband and daughters; will alternate with husband in attending daughters' activities; all family members supportive |
| 7. Teach importance of maintaining low-fat liquid diet and progression toward long-term low-fat diet. Teach food and menu choices low in fat. | 7. identifies harmful effects of obesity and high-fat foods<br>   Makes plans for losing weight<br>   Makes plans for pre-planned meals<br>   Identifies foods/menu choices low in fat | 7. Accurately described effects of obesity and intake of high-fat foods on overall physical health and well-being<br>   Plans to attend Weight Watchers; has had success with this program in the past<br>   Identified that preparing low-fat lunches at home the night before work is a good preplanning option |

the harmonization of NANDA, NIC, and NOC. This three-part combination links nursing diagnoses, accompanying interventions, and outcomes, organizing them in the same way. Such organization of concepts in a common language may facilitate the process of critical thinking, because interventions and outcomes are more accurately matched with appropriately developed nursing diagnoses (Dochterman & Jones, 2003). The final taxonomic scheme identifies four clinical domains (functional, physiological, psychosocial, and environmental), which contain the 28 classes of diagnoses, outcomes, and interventions. Chart 3-11 presents the taxonomy of nursing practice.

### CHART 3-11

## Hierarchy of Taxonomy in Nursing Practice: A Unified Structure of Nursing Language

I. The **functional domain** is defined as the diagnoses, outcomes, and interventions that promote basic needs and includes the following eight classes:

   **Activity/exercise:** physical activity, including energy, conservation, and expenditure

   **Comfort:** a sense of emotional, physical, and spiritual well-being and relative freedom from distress

   **Growth and development:** physical, emotional, and social growth and developmental milestones

   **Nutrition:** processes related to taking in, assimilating, and using nutrients

   **Self-care:** ability to accomplish basic and instrumental activities of daily living

   **Sexuality:** maintenance or modification of sexual identity and patterns

   **Sleep/rest:** the quantity and quality of sleep, rest, and relaxation patterns

   **Values/beliefs:** ideas, goals, perceptions, spiritual, and other beliefs that influence choices or decisions

II. The **physiological domain** is defined as the diagnoses, outcomes, and interventions to promote optimal biophysical health and includes the following ten classes:

   **Cardiac function:** cardiac mechanisms used to maintain tissue perfusion

   **Elimination:** processes related to secretion and excretion of body wastes

   **Fluid and electrolyte:** regulation of fluid/electrolytes and acid–base balance

   **Neurocognition:** mechanisms related to the nervous system and neurocognitive functioning, including memory, thinking, and judgment

   **Pharmacological function:** effects (therapeutic or adverse) of medications or drugs and other pharmacologically active products

   **Physical regulation:** body temperature, endocrine, and immune system responses to regulate cellular processes.

   **Reproduction:** processes related to human procreation and birth

   **Respiratory function:** ventilation adequate to maintain arterial blood gases within normal limits

   **Sensation/perception:** intake and interpretation of information through the senses, including seeing, hearing, touching, tasting, and smelling

   **Tissue integrity:** skin and mucous membrane protection to support secretion, excretion, and healing

III. The **psychosocial domain** is defined as the diagnoses, outcomes, and interventions to promote optimal mental and emotional health and social functioning and includes the following seven classes:

   **Behavior:** actions that promote, maintain, or restore health

   **Communication:** receiving, interpreting, and expressing spoken, written, and nonverbal messages

   **Coping:** adjusting or adapting to stressful events

   **Emotional:** a mental state of feeling that may influence perception of the world

   **Knowledge:** understanding and skill in applying information to promote, maintain, and restore health

   **Roles/relationships:** maintenance and/or modification of expected social behaviors and emotional connectedness with others

   **Self-perception:** awareness of one's body and personal identity

IV. The **environmental domain** is defined as the diagnoses, outcomes, and interventions that promote and protect the environmental health and safety of individuals, systems, and communities and includes the following three classes:

   **Health care system:** social, political, and economic structures and processes for delivery of health care services

   **Populations:** aggregates of individuals or communities having characteristics in common

   **Risk management:** avoidance or control of identifiable health threats

From: Dochterman, J. M., & Jones, D. A. (Eds.). (2003). *Unifying nursing languages: The harmonization of NANDA, NIC, and NOC*. Washington, DC: NurseBooks.org.

## Critical Thinking Exercises

1. A patient who is in end-stage multisystem failure has just been admitted to your unit. What processes would you use to prioritize his care needs, even though he has an end-stage diagnosis? What resources facilitate critical thinking in this situation?

2. You are at the bedside of a patient who has advance directives for no resuscitation. When she codes, her son yells, "Help, save her!" What actions could be taken in this situation? What ethical and legal dilemmas exist? What other health professionals could be helpful in resolving any issues?

3. **ebp** Two patients are admitted with cardiac pain to the telemetry observation unit. One has had no pain for 2 days and is asymptomatic, and the other has had at least four episodes of pain today. How would the individualized plans of care differ for these two patients? What is the evidence base for the differences in these patients' plans of care? What criteria would you use to evaluate the strength of the evidence?

## REFERENCES AND SELECTED READINGS

### BOOKS

Alfaro-LeFevre, R. (2003). *Critical thinking in nursing: A practical approach* (3rd ed.). Philadelphia: Saunders.

American Nurses Association. (1998). *Standards of clinical nursing practice* (2nd ed.). Washington, DC: Author.

American Nurses Association. (2001). *Code of ethics for nurses with interpretive statements*. Washington, DC: American Nurses Publishing.

American Nurses Association. (2003). *Nursing's social policy statement* (2nd ed). Washington, DC: Author.

Bickley, L. S., & Fiona, R. (2004). *Bates' guide to physical examination and history taking* (8th ed.). Philadelphia: Lippincott Williams & Wilkins.

Carpenito-Moyet, L. J. (2004). *Nursing care plans and documentation* (4th ed). Philadelphia: Lippincott Williams & Wilkins.

Carpenito-Moyet, L. J. (2004). *Nursing diagnosis: Application to clinical practice* (10th ed.). Philadelphia: Lippincott Williams & Wilkins.

Dochterman, J. M., & Bulechek, G. M. (Eds.) (2004). *Nursing interventions classification (NIC)*. (4th ed.). St. Louis: Mosby-Year Book.

Dochterman, J. M., & Jones, D. A. (Eds.) (2003). *Unifying nursing languages: The harmonization of NANDA, NIC, and NOC*. Washington, DC: NursesBooks.org.

Jackson, M. (2004). Defining the concept of critical thinking. In M. Jackson, D. Ignatavicius, & B. Case (Eds.), *Conversations in critical thinking and clinical judgment* (pp. 3–17; 33–47). Pensacola, FL: Pohl Publishing.

Jameton, A. (1984). *Nursing practice: The ethical issues*. Englewood Cliffs, NJ: Prentice-Hall.

Joint Commission for Accreditation of Hospital Organizations (JCAHO). (2003). *2003 Hospital accreditation standards*. Oakbrook Terrace, IL: Author.

Moorhead, S., Johnson, M., & Maas, M. (Eds.). (2004). *Nursing outcomes classification (NOC): Iowa Outcomes Project* (3rd ed.). St. Louis: Mosby-Year Book.

NANDA International. (2005). *Nursing diagnoses: Definitions & classification 2005–2006*. Philadelphia: NANDA International.

Norlander, N. (2001). *To comfort always: A nurse's guide to end-of-life care*. Washington, DC: American Nurses Association.

Smith-Temple, J., & Johnson, J. Y. (2005). *Nurses' guide to clinical procedures* (5th ed.). Philadelphia: Lippincott Williams & Wilkins.

Stuart, G. W., & Laraia, M. T. (2004). *Stuart and Sundeen's principles and practice of psychiatric nursing* (8th ed.). St. Louis: Mosby.

Wilkinson, J. M. (2001). *Nursing process and critical thinking*. New Jersey: Prentice-Hall.

### JOURNALS

American Nurses Association's Code of Ethics Project Task Force. (2000). A code of ethics for nurses. *American Journal of Nursing, 100*(7), 69–72.

Aquilino, M. L., & Keenan, G. (2000). Having our say: Nursing's standardized nomenclatures. *American Journal of Nursing, 100*(7), 33–38.

Cody, W. K. (2002). Theoretical concerns. Critical thinking and nursing science: Judgment, or vision? *Nursing Science Quarterly, 15*(3), 184–189.

Croke, E. (2003). Nurses, negligence, and malpractice. *American Journal of Nursing, 103*(9), 54–63.

Jackson, L., & Gleason, J. (2004). Proactive management breaks the fall cycle. *Nursing Management, 35*(6), 37–38.

Kirschling, J., & Lentz, J. (2004). Infusion nurses' role in care at the end of life. *Journal of Infusion Nursing, 27*(2), 112–117.

Lunney, M. (2003). Critical thinking and accuracy of nurses' diagnoses. *International Journal of Nursing Terminologies and Classifications, 14*(3), 96–100.

Martin, C. (2002). The theory of critical thinking of nursing, *Nursing Education Perspectives, 23*(5), 243–247.

Pitorak, E. F. (2003). Care at the time of death: How nurses can make the last hours of life a richer, more comfortable experience. *American Journal of Nursing, 103*(7), 42–52.

Profetto-McGrath, J., Hesketh, K. L., Lang, S., et al. (2003). A study of critical thinking and research utilization among nurses. *Western Journal of Nursing Research, 25*(3), 322–337.

Sheehan, D. K., & Schirm, V. (2003). End-of-life care of older adults: Debunking some common misconceptions about dying in old age. *American Journal of Nursing, 103*(11), 48–58.

Trammelleo, A. D. (2000). Protecting patients' end-of-life choices. *RN, 63*(8), 75–79.

Truong, R. D., Alexandra, F., M., Brackett, S. E., et al. (2001). Recommendations for end-of-life care in the intensive care unit: The Ethics Committee of the Society of Critical Care Medicine. *Critical Care Medicine, 29*(12), 2332–2348.

Valente, S. M. (2004). End-of-life challenges: Honoring autonomy. *Cancer Nursing, 27*(4), 314–319.

### RESOURCES AND WEBSITES

American Nurses Association, Center for Ethics and Human Rights. 8515 Georgia Avenue, Suite 100; Silver Spring, MD 20910; 301 628 5000; http://www.nursingworld.org/ethics. Accessed June 5, 2006.

Centers for Medicare & Medicaid Services (CMS), 7500 Security Boulevard, Baltimore, MD 21244-1850; 877-267-2323; http://www.cms.hhs.gov. Accessed June 5, 2006.

Joint Commission on Accreditation of Healthcare Organizations (JCAHO), One Renaissance Blvd., Oakbrook Terrace, IL 60181; 630-792-5000; http://www.jcaho.org. Accessed June 5, 2006.

NANDA International, 1211 Locust St., Philadelphia, PA 19107; 215-545-8107; http://www.nanda.org. Accessed June 5, 2006.

# CHAPTER 4

# Health Education and Health Promotion

## Learning Objectives

*On completion of this chapter, the learner will be able to:*

1. Describe the purposes and significance of health education.
2. Describe the concept of adherence to a therapeutic regimen.
3. Identify variables influencing the elderly person's adherence to a therapeutic regimen.
4. Distinguish the variables that affect learning readiness.
5. Describe strategies that facilitate elderly adults' learning abilities.
6. Describe the relationship of the teaching–learning process to the nursing process.
7. Develop a teaching plan for a patient.
8. Identify modifications indicated when teaching patients with disabilities.
9. Define the concepts of health, wellness, and health promotion.
10. Discuss major health promotion theories.
11. Describe the components of health promotion: self-responsibility, nutritional awareness, stress reduction and management, and physical fitness.
12. Specify the variables that affect health promotion activities for children, young and middle-aged adults, and elderly adults.
13. Describe the role of the nurse in health promotion.

Effective **health education** lays a solid foundation for individual and **community** wellness. Teaching is an integral tool that all nurses use to assist patients and families in developing effective health behaviors and in altering lifestyle patterns that predispose people to health risks. Health education is an influential factor directly related to positive patient care outcomes.

# Health Education Today

The changes in today's health care environment mandate the use of an organized approach to health education so that patients can meet their specific health care needs. Significant factors for nurses to consider when planning patient education include the availability of health care outside the hospital setting, the use of diverse health care providers to accomplish care management goals, and the increased use of alternative strategies rather than traditional approaches to care. Careful consideration of these factors can provide patients with the comprehensive information that is essential for making informed decisions about health care. Demands from consumers for comprehensive information about their health issues throughout the life cycle accentuate the need for holistic health education to occur in every patient–nurse encounter.

Teaching, as a function of nursing, is included in all state nurse practice acts and in the *Standards of Clinical Nursing Practice* of the American Nurses Association (ANA, 2004). Health education is an independent function of nursing practice and is a primary nursing responsibility. All nursing care is directed toward promoting, maintaining, and restoring health; preventing illness; and helping people adapt to the residual effects of illness. Many of these nursing activities are accomplished through health education or patient teaching. Nurses who serve as teachers are challenged to focus on the educational needs of communities as well as to provide specific patient and family education. Health education is important to nursing care because it affects the abilities of people and families to perform important self-care activities.

Every contact an individual nurse has with a health care consumer, whether or not that person is ill, should be considered an opportunity for health teaching. Although people have a right to decide whether or not to learn, nurses have the responsibility to present information that motivates people to recognize the need to learn. Therefore, nurses must use opportunities in all health care settings to promote **wellness**. Educational environments may include homes, hospitals, community health centers, schools, places of business, service agencies, shelters, and consumer action or support groups.

## Purpose of Health Education

This emphasis on health education stems in part from the public's right to comprehensive health care, which includes up-to-date health information. It also reflects the emergence of an informed public that is asking more significant questions about health and health care. Because of the importance American society places on health and the responsibility each person has to maintain and promote his or her own health, members of the health care team, specifically nurses, are obligated to make health education consistently available. Without adequate knowledge and training in self-care skills, consumers cannot make informed decisions about their health.

People with chronic illnesses and disabilities are among those most in need of health education. As the life span of the population increases, the number of people with such illnesses also increases. People with chronic illness need health care information to participate actively in and assume responsibility for much of their own care. Health education can help those with chronic illness adapt to their illness, prevent complications, carry out prescribed therapy, and solve problems when confronted with new situations. It can also prevent crisis situations and reduce the potential for rehospitalization resulting from inadequate information about self-care. The goal of health education is to teach people to live life to its healthiest—that is, to strive toward achieving their maximum health potential.

## Glossary

**adherence:** the process of faithfully following guidelines or directions

**community:** an interacting population of individuals living together within a larger society

**feedback:** the return of information about the results of input given to a person or a system

**health education:** a variety of learning experiences designed to promote behaviors that facilitate health

**health promotion:** the art and science of assisting people to change their lifestyle toward a higher state of wellness

**learning:** the act of gaining knowledge and skill

**learning readiness:** the optimum time for learning to occur; usually corresponds to the learner's perceived need and desire to obtain specific knowledge

**nutrition:** the science that deals with food and nourishment in humans

**physical fitness:** the condition of being physically healthy as a result of proper exercise and nutrition

**reinforcement:** the process of strengthening a given response or behavior to increase the likelihood that the behavior will continue

**self-responsibility:** personal accountability for one's actions or behavior

**stress management:** behaviors and techniques used to strengthen a person's resources against stress

**teaching:** the imparting of knowledge

**therapeutic regimen:** a routine that promotes health and healing

**wellness:** a condition of good physical and emotional health sustained by a healthy lifestyle

In addition to the public's right to and desire for health education, patient education is also a strategy for promoting self-care at home and in the community, reducing health care costs by preventing illness, avoiding expensive medical treatments, decreasing lengths of hospital stays, and facilitating earlier discharge. For health care agencies, offering community wellness programs is a public relations tool for increasing patient satisfaction and for developing a positive image of the institution. Patient education is also a cost-avoidance strategy for those who believe that positive staff–patient relationships avert malpractice suits.

## Adherence to the Therapeutic Regimen

One of the goals of patient education is to encourage people to adhere to their **therapeutic regimen**. **Adherence** to treatment usually requires that a person make one or more lifestyle changes to carry out specific activities that promote and maintain health. Common examples of behaviors facilitating health include taking prescribed medications, maintaining a healthy diet, increasing daily activities and exercise, self-monitoring for signs and symptoms of illness, practicing specific hygiene measures, seeking recommended health evaluations and screening, and performing other therapeutic and preventive measures.

Many people do not adhere to their prescribed regimens; rates of adherence are generally low, especially when the regimens are complex or of long duration. Nonadherence to prescribed therapy has been the subject of many studies. For the most part, findings have been inconclusive, and no one predominant causative factor has been identified. Instead, a wide range of variables appears to influence the degree of adherence, including the following:

- Demographic variables, such as age, gender, race, socioeconomic status, and level of education
- Illness variables, such as the severity of the illness and the relief of symptoms afforded by the therapy
- Therapeutic regimen variables, such as the complexity of the regimen and uncomfortable side effects
- Psychosocial variables, such as intelligence, availability of significant and supportive people (especially family members), attitudes toward health professionals, acceptance or denial of illness, and religious or cultural beliefs
- Financial variables, especially the direct and indirect costs associated with a prescribed regimen

Nurses' success with health education is determined by ongoing assessment of the variables that affect patients' ability to adopt specific behaviors, to obtain resources, and to maintain a helpful social environment (Murray & Zentner, 2001). Teaching programs are more likely to succeed if the variables affecting patient adherence are identified and considered in the teaching plan.

The problem of nonadherence to therapeutic regimens is a substantial one that must be addressed before patients can achieve their maximum health potential. Surprisingly, patients' need for knowledge has not been found to be a sufficient stimulus for acquiring knowledge and thereby enabling complete adherence to a health regimen. Teaching directed toward stimulating patient motivation results in varying degrees of adherence. The variables of choice, establishment of mutual goals, and the quality of the patient–provider relationship directly influence the behavioral changes that can result from patient education (Rankin & Stallings, 2004). These factors are directly linked to motivation for learning.

Using a learning contract or agreement can also be a motivator for learning. Such a contract is based on assessment of patient needs; health care data; and specific, measurable goals (Redman, 2004). A well-designed learning contract is realistic and positive; it includes measurable goals, with a specific time frame and reward system for goal achievement. The learning contract is recorded in writing and contains methods for ongoing evaluation.

The value of the contract lies in its clarity, its specific description of what is to be accomplished, and its usefulness for evaluating behavioral change. In a typical learning contract, a series of goals is established, beginning with small, easily attainable objectives and progressing to more advanced goals. Frequent, positive **reinforcement** is provided as the person moves from one goal to the next. For example, incremental goals such as weight loss of 1 to 2 pounds per week are more appropriate in a weight reduction program than a general goal such as a 30-pound weight loss.

### Gerontologic Considerations

Nonadherence to therapeutic regimens is a significant problem for elderly people, leading to increased morbidity, mortality, and cost of treatment (U.S. Public Health Service, 2000). Many admissions to nursing homes and hospitals are associated with nonadherence.

Elderly people frequently have one or more chronic illnesses that are managed with numerous medications and complicated by periodic acute episodes. Elderly people may also have other problems that affect adherence to therapeutic regimens, such as increased sensitivity to medications and their side effects, difficulty in adjusting to change and stress, financial constraints, forgetfulness, inadequate support systems, lifetime habits of self-treatment with over-the-counter medications, visual and hearing impairments, and mobility limitations. To promote adherence among the elderly, all variables that may affect health behavior should be assessed (Fig. 4-1). Nurses must also consider that cognitive impairment may be manifested by the elderly person's inability to draw inferences, apply information, or understand the major teaching points (Eliopoulos, 2004). The person's strengths and limitations must be assessed to encourage use of existing strengths to compensate for limitations. Above all, health care professionals must work together to provide continuous, coordinated care; otherwise, the efforts of one health care professional may be negated by those of another.

## The Nature of Teaching and Learning

**Learning** can be defined as acquiring knowledge, attitudes, or skills. **Teaching** is defined as helping another person learn. These definitions indicate that the teaching–learning process is an active one, requiring the involvement of both

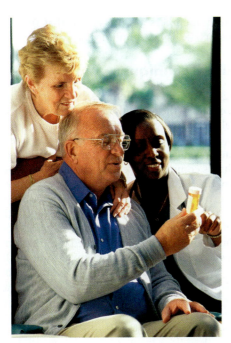

**FIGURE 4-1.** Taking time to teach patients about their medication and treatment program promotes interest and cooperation. Older adults who are actively involved in learning about their medication and treatment program and the expected effects may be more likely to adhere to the therapeutic regimen.

teacher and learner in the effort to reach the desired outcome, a change in behavior. The teacher does not simply give knowledge to the learner, but instead serves as a facilitator of learning.

In general, there is no definitive theory about how learning occurs and how it is affected by teaching. However, learning can be affected by factors such as readiness to learn, the learning environment, and the teaching techniques used (Bastable, 2003; Kreuter, Lezin, Kreuter, et al., 2003).

## Learning Readiness

One of the most significant factors influencing learning is a person's **learning readiness**. For adults, readiness is based on culture, personal values, physical and emotional status, and past experiences in learning. The "teachable moment" occurs when the content and skills being taught are congruent with the task to be accomplished (Redman, 2004).

Culture encompasses values, ideals, and behaviors, and the traditions within each culture provide the framework for solving the issues and concerns of daily living. Because people with different cultural backgrounds have different values and lifestyles, choices about health care vary. Culture is a major variable influencing readiness to learn because it affects how people learn and what information can be learned. Sometimes people do not accept health teaching because it conflicts with culturally mediated values. Before beginning health teaching, nurses must conduct an individual cultural assessment instead of relying only on generalized assumptions about a particular culture. A patient's social and cultural patterns must be appropriately incorporated into the teaching–learning interaction. Chart 4-1

> **CHART 4-1**
>
> ### Cultural Assessment Components to Consider When Formulating a Teaching Plan
>
> When formulating a teaching plan, consider the patient's beliefs about
> - Body size, shape, boundaries, and functions
> - Beauty and strength
> - Value of the mind or brain
> - Nature and function of blood
> - Diet and nutrition
> - Communication
> - Gender
> - Family and social support
> - Physical health and illness
> - Mental health and illness
> - Age-related changes
> - Pain
> - Medicine, herbs, and talismans
> - Spirituality or religion

describes cultural assessment components to consider when formulating a teaching plan.

A person's values include beliefs about behaviors that are desirable and undesirable. The nurses must know what value the patient places on health and health care. In clinical situations, patients express their values through their actions and the level of knowledge pursued (Andrews & Boyle, 2002). When the nurse is unaware of the patient's cultural values, misunderstanding, lack of cooperation, and negative health outcomes may occur (Leininger, 2001). A person's values and behaviors can be either an asset or a deficit to the readiness to learn. Therefore, patients are unlikely to accept health education unless their values and beliefs about health and illness are respected (Giger & Davidhizar, 2004).

Physical readiness is of vital importance, because until the person is physically capable of learning, attempts at teaching and learning may be both futile and frustrating. For example, a person in acute pain is unable to focus attention away from the pain long enough to concentrate on learning. Likewise, a person who is short of breath concentrates on breathing rather than on learning.

Emotional readiness also affects the motivation to learn. A person who has not accepted an existing illness or the threat of illness is not motivated to learn. A person who does not accept a therapeutic regimen, or who views it as conflicting with his or her present lifestyle, may consciously avoid learning about it. Until the person recognizes the need to learn and demonstrates an ability to learn, teaching efforts may be thwarted. However, it is not always wise to wait for the person to become emotionally ready to learn, because that time may never come unless the nurse makes an effort to stimulate the person's motivation.

Illness and the threat of illness are usually accompanied by anxiety and stress. Nurses who recognize such reactions can use simple explanations and instructions to alleviate these anxieties and provide further motivation to learn. Because learning involves behavior change, it often produces mild anxiety, which can be a useful motivating factor.

Emotional readiness can be promoted by creating a warm, accepting, positive atmosphere and by establishing realistic learning goals. When learners achieve success and a feeling of accomplishment, they are often motivated to participate in additional learning opportunities.

**Feedback** about progress also motivates learning. Such feedback should be presented in the form of positive reinforcement when the learner is successful, and in the form of constructive suggestions for improvement when he or she is unsuccessful.

Experiential readiness refers to past experiences that influence a person's ability to learn. Previous educational experiences and life experiences in general are significant determinants of a person's approach to learning. People with little or no formal education may not be able to understand the instructional materials presented. People who have had difficulty learning in the past may be hesitant to try again. Many behaviors required for reaching maximum health potential require knowledge, physical skills, and positive attitudes. In their absence, learning may be very difficult and very slow. For example, a person who does not understand the basics of normal nutrition may not be able to understand the restrictions of a specific diet. A person who does not view the desired learning as personally meaningful may reject teaching efforts. A person who is not future-oriented may be unable to appreciate many aspects of preventive health teaching. Experiential readiness is closely related to emotional readiness, because motivation tends to be stimulated by an appreciation for the need to learn and by those learning tasks that are familiar, interesting, and meaningful.

Before initiating a teaching–learning program, it is important to assess the person's physical and emotional readiness to learn, as well as his or her ability to learn what is being taught. This information then becomes the basis for establishing goals that can motivate the person. Involving learners in establishing mutually acceptable goals serves the purpose of encouraging active involvement in the learning process and shared responsibility for learning.

## The Learning Environment

Although learning can take place without teachers, most people who are attempting to learn new or altered health behaviors benefit from the services of nurses. The interpersonal interaction between the person and the nurse who is attempting to meet the person's learning needs may be formal or informal, depending on the method and techniques of teaching.

Learning may be optimized by minimizing factors that interfere with the learning process. For example, the room temperature, lighting, noise levels, and other environmental conditions should be appropriate to the learning situation. In addition, the time selected for teaching should be suited to the needs of the individual person. Scheduling a teaching session at a time of day when a patient is fatigued, uncomfortable, or anxious about a pending diagnostic or therapeutic procedure, or when visitors are present, is not conducive to learning. However, if the family is to participate in providing care, the sessions should be scheduled when family members are present so that they can learn any necessary skills or techniques.

## Teaching Techniques

Teaching techniques and methods enhance learning if they are appropriate to the patient's needs. Numerous techniques are available, including lectures, group teaching, and demonstrations, all of which can be enhanced with specially prepared teaching materials. The lecture or explanation method of teaching is commonly used but should always be accompanied by discussion. Discussion is important because it affords learners opportunities to express their feelings and concerns, to ask questions, and to receive clarification.

Group teaching is appropriate for some people because it allows them not only to receive needed information but also to feel secure as members of a group. People with similar problems or learning needs have the opportunity to identify with each other and gain moral support and encouragement. However, not everyone relates or learns well in groups or benefits from such experiences. Also, if group teaching is used, assessment and follow-up are imperative to ensure that each person has gained sufficient knowledge and skills.

Demonstration and practice are essential ingredients of a teaching program, especially when teaching skills. It is best to demonstrate the skill and then give the learner ample opportunity for practice. When special equipment is involved, such as syringes, colostomy bags, dialysis equipment, dressings, or suction apparatus, it is important to teach with the same equipment that will be used in the home setting. Learning to perform a skill with one kind of equipment and then having to change to a different kind may lead to confusion, frustration, and mistakes.

Teaching aids used to enhance learning include books, pamphlets, pictures, films, slides, audio and video tapes, models, programmed instruction, CD-ROMs, and computer-assisted learning modules. These are made available as needed for home, clinic, or hospital use, and they allow review and reinforcement of content and enhanced visual and auditory learning. Such teaching aids are invaluable when used appropriately and can save a significant amount of personnel time and related cost. However, all such aids should be reviewed before use to ensure that they meet the person's learning needs. Human interaction and discussion cannot be replaced by teaching technologies but may be enhanced by them.

Reinforcement and follow-up are important because learning takes time. Allowing ample time to learn and reinforcing what is learned are important teaching strategies; a single teaching session is rarely adequate. Follow-up sessions are imperative to promote the learner's confidence in his or her abilities and to plan for additional teaching sessions. For hospitalized patients who may not be able to transfer what they have learned in the hospital to the home setting, follow-up after discharge is essential to ensure that they have realized the full benefits of a teaching program.

## Teaching People With Disabilities

When providing health information to people with disabilities, the individual needs of each person must be assessed and incorporated into the teaching plan. Teaching techniques and the imparting of information may need to be altered. When teaching specific groups of people with physical disabilities, emotional disabilities, hearing and visual impairments, learning disabilities, and developmental disabilities, the nurse must be aware of their health promotion needs and institute new or modified approaches to teach them about their health. Table 4-1 outlines some of the teaching strategies to use when teaching people with disabilities.

## Gerontologic Considerations

Nurses caring for elderly people must be aware of how the normal changes that occur with aging affect learning abilities and how they can help elderly people adjust to these changes. Above all, it is important to recognize that just because a person is elderly does not mean that he or she cannot learn. Studies have shown that older adults *can* learn and remember if information is paced appropriately, relevant, and followed by the appropriate feedback strategies that apply to all learners (Rankin & Stallings, 2004). Because changes associated with aging vary significantly among elderly people, the nurse should conduct a thorough assessment of each person's level of physiologic and psychological functioning before beginning teaching.

Changes in cognition with age may include slowed mental functioning; decreased short-term memory, abstract thinking, and concentration; and slowed reaction time.

### TABLE 4-1 Teaching People with Disabilities

| Type of Disability | Teaching Strategy |
|---|---|
| **Physical, Emotional, or Cognitive Disability** | Adapt information to accommodate the person's cognitive, perceptual, and behavioral disabilities. |
| | Give clear written and oral information. |
| | Highlight significant information for easy reference. |
| | Avoid medical terminology. |
| **Hearing Impairment** | Use slow, directed, deliberate speech. |
| | Use sign language or interpreter services if appropriate. |
| | Position yourself so that the person can see your mouth if speech reading. |
| | Use telecommunication devices (TTY or TDD) for the hearing impaired. |
| | Use written materials and visual aids, such as models and diagrams. |
| | Use captioned videos, films, and computer-generated materials. |
| | Teach on the side of the "good ear" if unilateral deafness is present. |
| **Visual Impairment** | Use optical devices such as a magnifying lens. |
| | Use proper lighting and proper contrast of colors on materials and equipment. |
| | Use large-print materials. |
| | Use Braille materials if appropriate. |
| | Convert information to auditory and tactile formats. |
| | Obtain audiotapes and talking books. |
| | Explain noises associated with procedures, equipment, and treatments. |
| | Arrange materials in clockwise pattern. |
| **Learning Disabilities** | |
| Input disability | If visual perceptual disorder: |
| | • Explain information verbally, repeat, and reinforce frequently. |
| | • Use audiotapes. |
| | • Encourage learner to verbalize information received. |
| | If auditory perceptual disorder: |
| | • Speak slowly with as few words as possible, repeat, and reinforce frequently. |
| | • Use direct eye contact to focus person on task. |
| | • Use demonstration and return demonstration such as modeling, role playing, and hands-on experiences. |
| | • Use visual tools, written materials, and computers. |
| Output disability | Use all senses as appropriate. |
| | Use written, audiotape, and computer information. |
| | Review information and give time to interact and ask questions. |
| | Use hand gestures and motions. |
| Developmental disability | Base information and teaching on developmental stage, not chronologic age. |
| | Use nonverbal cues, gestures, signing, and symbols as needed. |
| | Use simple explanations and concrete examples with repetition. |
| | Encourage active participation. |
| | Demonstrate information and have the person perform return demonstrations. |

These changes are often accentuated by the health problems that cause the elderly person to seek health care in the first place. Effective teaching strategies include a slow-paced presentation of small amounts of material at a time; frequent repetition of information; and the use of reinforcement techniques, such as audiovisual and written materials and repeated practice sessions. Distracting stimuli should be minimized as much as possible in the teaching environment.

Sensory changes associated with aging also affect teaching and learning. Teaching strategies to accommodate decreased visual acuity include large-print and easy-to-read materials printed on nonglare paper. Because color discrimination is often impaired, the use of color-coded or highlighted materials may not be effective. To maximize hearing, teachers must speak distinctly with a normal or lowered pitch, facing the person so that speech reading can occur as needed. Visual cues often help to reinforce verbal teaching.

Family members should be involved in teaching sessions when possible. They provide another source for reinforcement of material and can help the elderly person recall instructions later. Family members can also provide valuable assessment information about the person's living situation and related learning needs.

When nurses, families, and other involved health care professionals work collaboratively to facilitate the elderly person's learning, chances of success are maximized. Successful learning for the elderly should result in improved self-care management skills, enhanced self-esteem, confidence, and a willingness to learn in the future.

# The Nursing Process in Patient Teaching

The steps of the nursing process—assessment, diagnosis, planning, implementation, and evaluation—are used when constructing a teaching plan to meet people's teaching and learning needs (Chart 4-2).

## Assessment

Assessment in the teaching–learning process is directed toward the systematic collection of data about the person's learning needs and readiness to learn, as well as the family's learning needs. All internal and external variables that affect the patient's readiness to learn are identified. A learning assessment guide may be used for this purpose. Some of the available guides are very general and are directed toward the collection of general health information, whereas others are specific to common medication regimens or disease processes. Such guides facilitate the assessment but must be adapted to the responses, problems, and needs of each person. As soon as possible after completing the assessment, the nurse organizes, analyzes, synthesizes, and summarizes the data collected and determines the patient's need for teaching.

## Nursing Diagnosis

The process of formulating nursing diagnoses makes educational goals and evaluations of progress more specific and meaningful. Teaching is an integral intervention implied by all nursing diagnoses, and for some diagnoses, education is the primary intervention. Examples of nursing diagnoses that help in planning for educational needs are Ineffective therapeutic regimen management, Ineffective home maintenance, Health-seeking behaviors, and Decisional conflict. The diagnosis "Deficient knowledge" should be used cautiously, because knowledge deficit is not a human response but a factor relating to or causing the diagnosis (eg, "Ineffective therapeutic regimen management related to a deficiency of information about wound care" is a more appropriate nursing diagnosis than "Deficient knowledge") (Carpenito-Moyet, 2003). A nursing diagnosis that relates specifically to a patient's and family's learning needs serves as a guide in the development of the teaching plan.

## Planning

Once the nursing diagnoses have been identified, the planning component of the teaching–learning process is established in accordance with the steps of the nursing process:

1. Assigning priorities to the diagnoses
2. Specifying the immediate, intermediate, and long-term goals of learning
3. Identifying specific teaching strategies appropriate for attaining goals
4. Specifying the expected outcomes
5. Documenting the diagnoses, goals, teaching strategies, and expected outcomes of the teaching plan

As in the nursing process, the assignment of priorities to the diagnoses should be a joint effort by the nurse and the patient or family members. Consideration must be given to the urgency of the patient's learning needs; the most critical needs should receive the highest priority.

After the diagnostic priorities have been established, it is important to identify the immediate and long-term goals and the teaching strategies appropriate for attaining the goals. Teaching is most effective when the objectives of both the patient and nurse are in agreement (Bastable, 2003). Learning begins with the establishment of goals that are appropriate to the situation and realistic in terms of the patient's ability and desire to achieve them. Involving the patient and family in establishing goals and in planning teaching strategies promotes their cooperation in the implementation of the teaching plan.

Expected outcomes of teaching strategies can be stated in terms of behaviors of patients, families, or both. Outcomes should be realistic and measurable, and the critical time periods for attaining them should also be identified. The desired outcomes and the critical time periods serve as a basis for evaluating the effectiveness of the teaching strategies.

During the planning phase, the nurse must consider the sequence in which the subject matter is presented in each of the teaching strategies. Critical information (eg, survival skills for a patient with diabetes) and material that the person or family identifies to be of particular importance receive high priority. An outline is often helpful for arranging the subject matter and for ensuring that all necessary information is included. In addition, appropriate teaching aids to be used in implementing teaching strategies are prepared or selected at this time.

## CHART 4-2
## A Guide to Patient Education

**ASSESSMENT**
1. Assess the person's readiness for health education.
   a. What are the person's health beliefs and behaviors?
   b. What physical and psychosocial adaptations does the person need to make?
   c. Is the learner ready to learn?
   d. Is the person able to learn these behaviors?
   e. What additional information about the person is needed?
   f. Are there any variables (eg, hearing or visual impairment, cognitive issues, literacy issues) that will affect the choice of teaching strategy or approach?
   g. What are the person's expectations?
   h. What does the person want to learn?
2. Organize, analyze, synthesize, and summarize the collected data.

**NURSING DIAGNOSIS**
1. Formulate the nursing diagnoses that relate to the person's learning needs.
2. Identify the learning needs, their characteristics, and their etiology.
3. State nursing diagnoses concisely and precisely.

**PLANNING AND GOALS**
1. Assign priority to the nursing diagnoses that relate to the individual's learning needs.
2. Specify the immediate, intermediate, and long-term learning goals established by teacher and learner together.
3. Identify teaching strategies appropriate for goal attainment.
4. Establish expected outcomes.
5. Develop the written teaching plan.
   a. Include diagnoses, goals, teaching strategies, and expected outcomes.
   b. Put the information to be taught in logical sequence.
   c. Write down the key points.
   d. Select appropriate teaching aids.
   e. Keep the plan current and flexible to meet the person's changing learning needs.
6. Involve the learner, family or significant others, nursing team members, and other health care team members in all aspects of planning.

**IMPLEMENTATION**
1. Put the teaching plan into action.
2. Use language the person can understand.
3. Use appropriate teaching aids and provide Internet resources if appropriate.
4. Use the same equipment that the person will use after discharge.
5. Encourage the person to participate actively in learning.
6. Record the learner's responses to the teaching actions.
7. Provide feedback.

**EVALUATION**
1. Collect objective data.
   a. Observe the person.
   b. Ask questions to determine whether the person understands.
   c. Use rating scales, checklists, anecdotal notes, and written tests when appropriate.
2. Compare the person's behavioral responses with the expected outcomes. Determine the extent to which the goals were achieved.
3. Include the person, family or significant others, nursing team members, and other health care team members in the evaluation.
4. Identify alterations that need to be made in the teaching plan.
5. Make referrals to appropriate sources or agencies for reinforcement of learning after discharge.
6. Continue all steps of the teaching process: assessment, diagnosis, planning, implementation, and evaluation.

---

The entire planning phase of the teaching–learning process concludes with the formulation of the teaching plan. This teaching plan communicates the following information to all members of the nursing team:

- The nursing diagnoses that specifically relate to the patient's learning needs and the priorities of these diagnoses
- The goals of the teaching strategies
- The teaching strategies, expressed in the form of teaching orders
- The expected outcomes, which identify the desired behavioral responses of the learner
- The critical time period within which each outcome is expected to be met
- The patient's behavioral responses (which are documented on the teaching plan)

The same rules that apply to writing and revising the plan of nursing care apply to the teaching plan.

## Implementation

In the implementation phase of the teaching–learning process, the patient, the family, and other members of the nursing and health care team carry out the activities outlined in the teaching plan. The nurse coordinates these activities.

Flexibility during the implementation phase of the teaching–learning process and ongoing assessment of patient responses to the teaching strategies support modification of the teaching plan as necessary. Creativity in promoting and sustaining the patient's motivation to learn is essential. New learning needs that may arise after discharge from the hospital or after home care visits have ended should also be taken into account.

The implementation phase ends when the teaching strategies have been completed and when the patient's responses to the actions have been recorded. This record serves as the basis for evaluating how well the defined goals and expected outcomes have been achieved.

## Evaluation

Evaluation of the teaching–learning process determines how effectively the patient has responded to teaching and to what extent the goals have been achieved. An evaluation must be made to determine what was effective and what needs to be changed or reinforced. It cannot be assumed that patients have learned just because teaching has occurred; learning does not automatically follow teaching. An important part of the evaluation phase addresses the question, "What can be done to improve teaching and enhance learning?" Answers to this question direct the changes to be made in the teaching plan.

A variety of measurement techniques can be used to identify changes in patient behavior as evidence that learning has taken place. These techniques include directly observing the behavior; using rating scales, checklists, or anecdotal notes to document the behavior; and indirectly measuring results using oral questioning and written tests. All direct measurements should be supplemented with indirect measurements whenever possible. Using more than one measuring technique enhances the reliability of the resulting data and decreases the potential for error from a measurement strategy.

In many situations, measurement of actual behavior is the most accurate and appropriate technique. Nurses often perform comparative analyses using patient admission data as the baseline: selected data points observed when nursing care is given and self-care is initiated are compared with the patient's baseline data. In other cases, indirect measurement may be used. Some examples of indirect measurement are patient satisfaction surveys, attitude surveys, and instruments that evaluate specific health status variables.

However, measurement is only the beginning of evaluation, which must be followed by data interpretation and value judgments about learning and teaching. These aspects of evaluation should be conducted periodically throughout the teaching–learning program, at its conclusion, and at varying periods after the teaching has ended.

Evaluation of learning after hospitalization is highly desirable, because the analysis of teaching outcomes must extend into home care. With shortened lengths of hospital stay and with short-stay and same-day surgical procedures, follow-up evaluation in the home is especially important. Coordination of efforts and sharing of information between hospital-based and community-based nursing personnel facilitate postdischarge teaching and home care evaluation.

Evaluation is not the final step in the teaching–learning process, but the beginning of a new patient assessment. The information gathered during evaluation should be used to redirect teaching actions, with the goal of improving the patient's responses and outcomes.

# Health Promotion

Health teaching and **health promotion** are linked by a common goal—to encourage people to achieve as high a level of wellness as possible so that they can live maximally healthy lives and avoid preventable illnesses. The call for health promotion has become a cornerstone in health policy because of the need to control costs and reduce unnecessary sickness and death.

The nation's first public health agenda was established in 1979 and set goals for improving the health of all Americans. Additional goals defined as the "1990 Health Objectives" identified improvements to be made in health status, risk reduction, public awareness, health services, and protective measures (U.S. Public Health Service, 2000).

Health goals for the nation were also established in the publication *Healthy People 2000*. The priorities from this initiative were identified as health promotion, health protection, and the use of preventive services. The most recent publication, *Healthy People 2010*, defines the current national health promotion and disease prevention initiative for the nation. The two essential goals from this report are (1) to increase the quality and years of healthy life for people and (2) to eliminate health disparities among various segments of the population (U.S. Public Health Service, 2000) (Chart 4-3).

## Definition

Health promotion may be defined as those activities that assist people in developing resources that maintain or enhance well-being and improve their quality of life. These

---

**CHART 4-3**

### Leading Health Indicators to be Used to Measure the Health of the Nation

1. Physical activity
2. Overweight and obesity
3. Tobacco use
4. Substance abuse
5. Responsible sexual behavior
6. Mental health
7. Injury and violence
8. Environmental quality
9. Immunization
10. Access to health care

From U.S. Department of Health & Human Services (2000). *Healthy People 2010*. Washington, DC: U.S. Government Printing Office.

activities involve people's efforts to remain healthy in the absence of symptoms and do not require the assistance of a health care team member.

The purpose of health promotion is to focus on the person's potential for wellness and to encourage appropriate alterations in personal habits, lifestyle, and environment in ways that reduce risks and enhance health and well-being. Health promotion is an active process; that is, it is not something that can be prescribed or dictated. It is up to each person to decide whether to make changes to promote a higher level of wellness. Only the individual can make these choices.

The concepts of health, wellness, health promotion, and disease prevention have been a topic of extensive discussion in the lay literature and news media as well as in professional journals. As a result, public demand for health information has increased, and health care professionals and agencies have responded by providing this information. Health promotion programs, once limited to hospital settings, have now moved into community settings such as clinics, schools, churches, and the workplace. As employers strive to reduce costs associated with absenteeism, health insurance, hospitalization, disability, excessive turnover of personnel, and premature death, the workplace has become an important site for health promotion programs.

## Health and Wellness

The concept of health promotion has evolved because of a changing definition of health and an awareness that wellness exists at many levels of functioning. Health is viewed as a dynamic, ever-changing condition that enables people to function at an optimal potential at any given time. The ideal health status is one in which people are successful in achieving their full potential, regardless of any limitations they might have.

Wellness, as a reflection of health, involves a conscious and deliberate attempt to maximize one's health. Wellness does not just happen; it requires planning and conscious commitment and is the result of adopting lifestyle behaviors for the purpose of attaining one's highest potential for well-being. Wellness is not the same for every person. The person with a chronic illness or disability may still be able to achieve a desirable level of wellness. The key to wellness is to function at the highest potential within the limitations over which there is no control.

A significant amount of research has shown that people, by virtue of what they do or fail to do, influence their own health. Today, many of the major causes of illness are chronic diseases that have been closely related to lifestyle behaviors (eg, heart disease, lung and colon cancer, chronic obstructive pulmonary diseases, hypertension, cirrhosis, traumatic injury, human immunodeficiency virus [HIV] infection, or acquired immunodeficiency syndrome [AIDS]). To a large extent, a person's health status may be reflective of his or her lifestyle.

## Health Promotion Models

Since the 1950s, many health promotion models have been constructed to identify health-protecting behaviors and to help explain what makes people engage in these preventive behaviors. A health-protecting behavior is defined as any behavior performed by people, regardless of their actual or perceived health condition, for the purpose of promoting or maintaining their health, whether or not the behavior produces the desired outcome (Downie, Fyfe, & Tannahill, 1996). One model, the health belief model, was designed to foster understanding of why some healthy people choose actions to prevent illness, whereas others refuse to engage in these protective recommendations (Becker, 1974). Another model, the resource model of preventive health behavior, addresses the ways in which people use resources to promote health (Downie, Fyfe, & Tannahill, 1996). Nurse educators can use this model to assess how demographic variables, health behaviors, and social and health resources influence health promotion.

The Canadian health promotion initiative, Achieving Health for All, builds on Lalonde's work in the 1970s, in which four determinants of health—human biology, environment, lifestyle, and the health care delivery system—were identified. Determinants of health were defined as factors and conditions that have an influence on the health of individuals and communities (Lalonde, 1977). Since the 1970s a total of 12 determinants have been identified, and this number will continue to increase as population health research progresses. Determinants of health provide a framework for assessing and evaluating the population's health.

The health promotion model developed by Becker and colleagues (1993) is based on the premise that four variables influence the selection and use of health promotion behaviors. Demographic and disease factors, the first variable, include patient characteristics such as age, gender, education, employment, severity of illness or disability, and length of illness. Barriers, the second variable, are defined as factors leading to unavailability or difficulty in gaining access to a specific health promotion alternative. Resources, the third variable, encompass such items as financial and social support. Perceptual factors, the fourth variable, consist of how the person views his or her health status, self-efficacy, and the perceived demands of the illness. Becker and colleagues demonstrated that these four variables have a positive correlation with a person's quality of life.

The health promotion model developed by Pender (2005) is based on social learning theory and emphasizes the importance of motivational factors in acquiring and sustaining health promotion behaviors. This model explores how cognitive-perceptual factors affect the person's view of the importance of health. It also examines perceived control of health, self-efficacy, health status, and the benefits and barriers to health-promoting behaviors.

These models of health promotion, along with others that can be found in the health promotion literature, can serve as an organizing framework for clinical work and research that supports the enhancement of health. Studies aim to increase understanding of the health promotion behaviors of families and communities (eg, Epple, Wright, Joish, et al., 2003; Javo, Alapack, Keyerdall, et al., 2003).

## Components of Health Promotion

There are several components of health promotion as an active process: self-responsibility, nutritional awareness, stress reduction and management, and physical fitness.

### Self-Responsibility

Taking responsibility for oneself is the key to successful health promotion. The concept of **self-responsibility** is based on the understanding that the individual controls his or her life. Each person alone must make the choices that determine how healthy his or her lifestyle is. As more people recognize that lifestyle and behavior significantly affect health, they may assume responsibility for avoiding high-risk behaviors such as smoking, alcohol and drug abuse, overeating, driving while intoxicated, risky sexual practices, and other unhealthy habits. They may also assume responsibility for adopting routines that have been found to have a positive influence on health, such as engaging in regular exercise, wearing seat belts, and eating a healthy diet.

A variety of different techniques have been used to encourage people to accept responsibility for their health, ranging from extensive educational programs to reward systems. No one technique has been found to be superior to any other. Instead, self-responsibility for health promotion is very individualized and depends on a person's desires and inner motivations. Health promotion programs are important tools for encouraging people to assume responsibility for their health and to develop behaviors that improve health.

### Nutritional Awareness

**Nutrition** as a component of health promotion has become the focus of considerable attention and publicity. A vast array of books and magazine articles address the topics of special diets; natural foods; and the hazards associated with certain substances, such as sugar, salt, cholesterol, trans fats, carbohydrates, artificial colors, and food additives. It has been suggested that good nutrition is the single most significant factor in determining health status and longevity.

Nutritional awareness involves an understanding of the importance of a healthy diet that supplies all of the essential nutrients. Understanding the relationship between diet and disease is an important facet of a person's self-care. Some clinicians believe that a healthy diet is one that substitutes "natural" foods for processed and refined ones and reduces the intake of sugar, salt, fat, cholesterol, caffeine, alcohol, food additives, and preservatives.

Chapter 5 contains further information about the assessment of a person's nutritional status. It describes the physical signs indicating nutritional status, assessment of food intake (food record, 24-hour recall), the dietary guidelines presented in the MyPyramid plan, and calculation of ideal body weight.

### Stress Reduction and Management

**Stress management** and stress reduction are important aspects of health promotion. Studies have shown the negative effects of stress on health and a cause-and-effect relationship between stress and infectious diseases, traumatic injuries (eg, motor vehicle crashes), and some chronic illnesses. Stress has become inevitable in contemporary societies in which demands for productivity have become excessive. More and more emphasis is placed on encouraging people to manage stress appropriately and to reduce stress that is counterproductive. Techniques such as relaxation training, exercise, and modification of stressful situations are often included in health promotion programs dealing with stress. Further information on stress management, including health risk appraisal and stress reduction methods such as biofeedback and the relaxation response, can be found in Chapter 6.

### Physical Fitness

**Physical fitness** is another important component of health promotion. Clinicians and researchers (Anspaugh, Hamrick, & Rosato, 2003; Leifer & Hartston, 2004; U.S. Department of Health & Human Services, 2002) who have examined the relationship between health and physical fitness have found that a regular exercise program can promote health in the following ways:

- Improve the function of the circulatory system and the lungs
- Decrease cholesterol and low-density lipoprotein levels
- Decrease body weight by increasing calorie expenditure
- Delay degenerative changes such as osteoporosis
- Improve flexibility and overall muscle strength and endurance

An appropriate exercise program can have a significantly positive effect on a person's performance capacity, appearance, and general state of physical and emotional health. An exercise program should be designed specifically for a given person, with consideration given to age, physical condition, and any known cardiovascular or other risk factors. Exercise can be harmful if it is not started gradually and increased slowly in accordance with a person's response.

# Health Promotion Throughout the Life Span

Health promotion is a concept and a process that extends throughout the life span. Studies have shown that the health of a child can be affected either positively or negatively by the health practices of the mother during the prenatal period. Therefore, health promotion starts before birth and extends through childhood, adolescence, adulthood, and old age.

Health promotion includes health screening. The American Academy of Family Physicians has developed recommendations for periodic health examinations that identify the age groups for which specific screening interventions are appropriate. Table 4-2 presents general population guidelines. Specific population standards and guidelines have also been recommended.

## Children and Adolescents

Health screening has traditionally been an important aspect of childhood health care. The goal has been to detect health problems at an early age so that they can be treated early in life. Today, health promotion goes beyond the mere screening of children for disabilities and includes extensive efforts

## TABLE 4-2  Routine Health Promotion Screening for Adults

| Type of Screening | Suggested Time Frame |
| --- | --- |
| Routine health examination | Yearly |
| Blood chemistry profile | Baseline at age 20, then as mutually determined by patient and clinician |
| Complete blood count | Baseline at age 20, then as mutually determined by patient and clinician |
| Lipid profile | Baseline at age 20, then as mutually determined by patient and clinician |
| Hemoccult screening | Yearly after age 50 |
| Electrocardiogram | Baseline at age 40, then as mutually determined by patient and clinician |
| Blood pressure | Yearly, then as mutually determined by patient and clinician |
| Tuberculosis skin test | Every 2 years or as mutually determined by patient and clinician |
| Chest x-ray film | For positive PPD results |
| Breast self-examination | Monthly |
| Mammogram | Yearly for women over 40, or earlier or more often if indicated |
| Clinical breast examination | Yearly |
| Gynecologic examination | Yearly |
| Pap test | Yearly |
| Bone density screening | Based on identification of primary and secondary risk factors (prior to onset of menopause, if indicated) |
| Nutritional screening | As mutually determined by patient and clinician |
| Digital rectal examination | Yearly |
| Colonoscopy | Every 3-5 years after age 50 or as mutually determined by patient and clinician |
| Prostate examination | Yearly |
| Prostate-specific antigen | Every 1-2 years after age 50 |
| Testicular examination | Monthly |
| Skin examination | Yearly or as mutually determined by patient and clinician |
| Vision screening | Every 2-3 years |
| Glaucoma | Baseline at age 40, then every 2-3 years until age 70, then yearly |
| Dental screening | Every 6 months |
| Hearing screening | As needed |
| Health risk appraisal | As needed |
| **Adult Immunizations** | |
| Tetanus | Boosters every 10 years |
| Diphtheria | Boosters every 10 years |
| Rubella | Given to women of childbearing age if not previously given or if titer is low |
| Pneumococcal vaccine | Given one time at age 65 or younger if chronic illness or disability is present |
| Hepatitis B (if not received as a child) | Series of three doses (now, 1 month later, then 5 months after the second date) |
| Influenza vaccine | Yearly |
| Lyme disease vaccine, if at risk | Series of three doses (now, 1 month later, and 11 months after the second dose) |

*Note:* Any of these screenings may be performed more frequently if deemed necessary by the patient or recommended by the health care provider.

to promote positive health practices at a very young age. Because health habits and practices are formed early in life, children should be encouraged to develop positive health attitudes. For this reason, more and more programs are being offered to school-age children and to adolescents to help them develop good health habits. Although the negative results of practices such as smoking, risky sexual activities, alcohol and drug abuse, and poor nutrition are explained in these educational programs, emphasis is also placed on values training, self-esteem, and healthy lifestyle practices. The projects are designed to appeal to a particular age group, with emphasis on learning experiences that are fun, interesting, and relevant.

## Young and Middle-Aged Adults

Young and middle-aged adults represent an age group that not only expresses an interest in health and health promotion but also responds enthusiastically to suggestions that show how lifestyle practices can improve health. Adults are frequently motivated to change their lifestyles in ways that are believed to enhance their health and wellness. Many adults who wish to improve their health turn to health promotion programs to help them make the desired changes in their lifestyles. Many have responded to programs that focus on topics such as general wellness, smoking cessation, exercise, physical conditioning, weight control, conflict resolution, and stress management. Because of the nationwide emphasis on health during the reproductive years, young adults actively seek programs that address prenatal health, parenting, family planning, and women's health issues.

Programs that provide health screening, such as those that screen for cancer, high cholesterol, hypertension, diabetes, abdominal aneurysm, and visual and hearing impairments, are quite popular with young and middle-aged adults. Programs that involve health promotion for people with specific chronic illnesses such as cancer, diabetes, heart disease, and pulmonary disease are also popular. It is becoming more evident that chronic disease and disability do not preclude health and wellness; rather, positive health attitudes and practices can promote optimal health for people who must live with the limitations imposed by their chronic illnesses and disabilities.

Health promotion programs can be offered almost anywhere in the community. Common sites include local clinics, elementary and high schools, community colleges, recreation centers, churches, and even private homes. Health fairs are frequently held in civic centers and shopping malls. The outreach idea for health promotion programs has served to meet the needs of many adults who otherwise would not avail themselves of opportunities to strive toward a healthier lifestyle.

The workplace has become a center for health promotion activity for several reasons. Employers have become increasingly concerned about the rising costs of health care insurance to treat illnesses related to lifestyle behaviors, and they are also concerned about increased absenteeism and lost productivity. Some employers use health promotion specialists to develop and implement these programs, and others purchase packaged programs that have already been developed by health care agencies or private health promotion corporations.

Programs offered at the workplace usually include employee health screening and counseling, physical fitness, nutritional awareness, work safety, and stress management and stress reduction. In addition, efforts are made to promote a safe and healthy work environment. Many large businesses provide exercise facilities for their employees and offer their health promotion programs to retirees. If employers can show cost-containment benefits from such programs, their dollars will be considered well spent, and more businesses will provide health promotion programs as a benefit of employment.

## Gerontologic Considerations

Health promotion is as important for the elderly as it is for other adults and children. Although 80% of people older than 65 years have one or more chronic illnesses and many are limited in their activity, the elderly as a group experience significant gains from health promotion. The elderly are very health-conscious, and most view their health positively and are willing to adopt practices that will improve their health and well-being (Ebersole, Hess, & Luggen, 2004). Although their chronic illnesses and disabilities cannot be eliminated, these adults can benefit from activities that help them maintain independence and achieve an optimal level of health.

Various health promotion programs have been developed to meet the needs of older Americans. Both public and private organizations continue to be responsive to health promotion, and more programs that serve the elderly are

---

## NURSING RESEARCH PROFILE

### Health Promotion in the Elderly

McPhee, S. D., Johnson, T. R., & Dietrich, M. S. (2004). Comparing health status with healthy habits in elderly assisted-living residents. *Family and Community Health, 27*(2), 158–170.

### Purpose
The purpose of this study was to determine the relationship between seven healthy lifestyle habits, as identified by the Health Generation Survey, and the health status of adults living in assisted-living residences. The habits studied were water consumption, tobacco use, alcohol use, hours of sleep per night, breakfast eating, healthy snack eating, and engagement in physical activity. The practice of healthy lifestyle habits and their relationships to the five most common medical conditions (arthritis, heart disease, stroke, cancer, diabetes) seen in residents of assisted-living facilities were examined.

### Design
The Health Generation Survey was distributed to the residents of several assisted-living facilities in the southeastern part of the United States. There were 1,079 adults who completed the survey within the first 6 weeks of their entrance to the facilities. This particular study was a secondary data analysis of the original data collected.

### Findings
The findings of this study revealed that older adults with a greater number of current physical health problems reported that they had more healthy lifestyle habits than older adults without health problems. People began to incorporate a greater number of healthy habits into their lifestyle after they were determined to have certain specific health problems. In addition, the study also found that residents who engaged in physical exercise and recreational activities reported a greater overall participation in other healthy lifestyle habits.

### Nursing Implications
Because older adults in assisted-living facilities tend to experience more health-related problems than older adults living within the community, nurses need to focus on the health habits examined in this study and be in a position to assess and implement strategies for healthy living. The development of appropriate educational programs and individual reinforcement of healthy habits with the residents may further increase their participation in health promotion activities.

**FIGURE 4-2.** Health promotion programs are held in community settings such as clinics, schools, churches, and the workplace. Nurses play a vital role in organizing and providing wellness services to the general public. Here, a nurse takes a student's blood pressure at a health fair held on a college campus. (Cushing Memorial Library and Archives, Texas A&M University.)

emerging. Many of these programs are offered by health care agencies, churches, community centers, senior citizen residences, and a variety of other organizations. The activities directed toward health promotion for the elderly are the same as those for other age groups: physical fitness and exercise, nutrition, safety, and stress management.

## Nursing Implications

By virtue of their expertise in health and health care and their long-established credibility with consumers, nurses play a vital role in health promotion. In many instances, they have initiated health promotion and health screening programs or have participated with other health care personnel in developing and providing wellness services in a variety of settings (Fig. 4-2).

As health care professionals, nurses have a responsibility to promote activities that foster well-being, self-actualization, and personal fulfillment. Every interaction with consumers of health care must be viewed as an opportunity to promote positive health attitudes and behaviors.

### Critical Thinking Exercises

**1** A nurse is designing a patient teaching plan for a 57-year-old woman with a history of gastrointestinal problems. This woman has been diagnosed with osteoporosis, and her physician has recommended that she begin taking alendronate sodium (Fosamax). Describe the health promotion strategies you would develop for this patient. Determine what variables may influence her willingness to follow the recommended therapy.

**2** A home health nurse is instructing a 55-year-old man with cardiovascular disease about healthy eating habits. He has recently been widowed, and his service animal (seeing-eye dog) of 15 years died last month. What physiologic and psychosocial variables would be relevant to understanding this patient's needs? How would a teaching plan be constructed to promote adequate nutrition? How would you modify the teaching plan, knowing that the patient is visually impaired?

**3** **ebp** A 72-year-old man is informed by an advanced practice nurse about a health fair being held at the local community center across the street from his home. He declines to attend, saying, "I am too old and it is too late to be concerned about health promotion. The damage to my body has already been done." What resources would you use to identify evidence of the effectiveness of health promotion activities for the elderly? Discuss the strength of the evidence. Identify the criteria used to evaluate the strength of the evidence. What information would you then include in a discussion with the patient about promoting health in the elderly?

## REFERENCES AND SELECTED READINGS

## BOOKS

Alfaro-LeFevre, R. (2004). *Critical thinking and clinical judgment*. Philadelphia: Saunders.
American Nurses Association. (2004). *Standards of clinical nursing practice*. Washington, DC: Author.
Andrews, M. M., & Boyle, J. S. (2002). *Transcultural concepts in nursing care* (4th ed.). Philadelphia: Lippincott Williams & Wilkins.
Anspaugh, D. J., Hamrick, M. H., & Rosato, F. D. (2003). *Wellness: Concepts and applications* (5th ed.). St. Louis: Mosby.
Bastable, S. B. (Ed.). (2003). *Nurse as educator: Principles of teaching and learning*. Boston: Jones & Bartlett.
Becker, M. H. (Ed.). (1974). *The health belief model and personal health behavior*. Thorofare, NJ: Charles B. Slack.
Carpenito-Moyet, L. J. (2003). *Nursing diagnosis: Application to clinical practice* (10th ed.). Philadelphia: Lippincott Williams & Wilkins.
Downie, R. S., Fyfe, C., & Tannahill, A. (1996). *Health promotion: Models and values* (2nd ed.). New York: Oxford University Press.
Doyle, E., & Ward, S. (2001). *The process of community health education and promotion*. Palo Alto, CA: Mayfield Publishing.
Ebersole, P., Hess, P. & Luggen, A. (2004). *Toward health aging: Human needs and nursing responses* (6th ed.). St. Louis: Mosby.
Eliopoulos, C. (2004). *Gerontological nursing* (6th ed.). Philadelphia: Lippincott Williams & Wilkins.
Giger, J. N., & Davidhizar, R. E. (2004). *Transcultural nursing: Assessment and intervention* (4th ed.). St. Louis: Mosby.
Glouberman, S. (2001). *Towards a new perspective on health policy*. Ottawa, Ontario: Commission on the Future of Health in Canada.
Kreuter, M. W., Lezin, M. A., Kreuter, M. W., & Green, L. W. (2003). *Community health promotion ideas that work* (2nd ed.). Sudburg, MA: Jones & Bartlett.
Insel, P. M., & Roth, W. T. (2000). *Core concepts in health*. Palo Alto, CA: Mayfield Publishing.
Lalonde, M. (1977). *New perspectives on the health of Canadians: A working document*. Ottawa, Canada: Minister of Supply and Services.

Leifer, G., & Hartston, H. (2004). Growth and Development Across the Lifespan: A Health Promotion Focus: St. Louis: Elsevier.

Leininger, M. M. (2001). *Culture care diversity and universality: A theory of nursing.* Boston: Jones & Bartlett.

Murray, R. B., & Zentner, J. P. (2001). *Nursing assessment and health promotion through the life span* (7th ed.). Englewood Cliffs, NJ: Prentice-Hall.

O'Donnell, M. P. (2001). *Health promotion in the workplace.* Albany, NY: Delmar Publishing.

Pender, N. J., Murdaugh, C., & Parsons, M. A. (2005). *Health promotion in nursing practice* (5th ed.). Upper Saddle River, NJ: Prentice-Hall Health, Inc.

Rankin, S. H., & Stallings, K. D. (2004). *Patient education in health and illness* (5th ed.). Philadelphia: Lippincott Williams & Wilkins.

Redman, B. (2004). *Advances in patient education.* New York: Springer Publishing Company.

U.S. Department of Health & Human Services (2002). *Physical activity fundamental to preventing disease.* Atlanta: U.S. Department of Health and Human Services, Centers for Disease Control and Prevention, National Center for Chronic Disease Prevention and Health Promotion.

U.S. Public Health Service. (1990). *Healthy people 2000.* Washington, DC: U.S. Government Printing Office.

U.S. Public Health Service. (1995). *Healthy people 2000: Midcourse review and 1995 revision.* Washington, DC: U.S. Government Printing Office.

U.S. Public Health Service. (2000). *Healthy people 2010: Understanding and improving health.* Washington, DC: U.S. Government Printing Office.

Whitman, T. L. (Ed.). (1999). *Life-span perspectives on health and illness.* Mahwah, NJ: Lawrence Erlbaum Associates.

Woolf, S. H., Jonas, S., & Lawrence, R. S. (1996). *Health promotion and disease prevention in clinical practice.* Baltimore: Williams & Wilkins.

## JOURNALS

*Asterisks indicate nursing research articles.*

Becker, H. A., Stuifbergen, A. K., Oh, H., et al. (1993). The self-rated abilities for health practices scale: A health self-efficacy measure. *Health Values, 17,* 42–50.

Britton, J. (2003). The use of emollients and their correct application. *Journal of Community Nursing, 17*(9), 22–25.

Cox, R. H., Carpenter, J. P., Bruce, F. A., et al. (2004). Characteristics of low-income African Americans and Caucasian adults that are important in self-management of type 2 diabetes. *Journal of Community Health, 29*(2), 155–170.

Daniel, B. T., Damato, K. L., & Johnson, J. (2004). Educational issues in oral care. *Seminars in Oncology Nursing, 20*(1), 48–52.

Duman, M., & Clark, A. (2004). Patient information: Part 4. Content and presentation. *Professional Nurse, 19*(6), 354–355.

*Enriquez, M., Gore, P. A., O'Connor, M. C., et al. (2004). Assessment of readiness for adherence by HIV-positive males who had previously failed treatment. *Journal of the Association of Nurses in AIDS Care, 15*(1), 42–49.

Epple, C., Wright, A. L., Joish, V. N., et al. (2003). The role of active family nutritional support in Navajos' type 2 diabetes mellitus control. *Diabetes Care, 26*(10), 2829–2834.

Glouberman, S. & Miller, J. (2003). Evolution of the determinants of health, health policy, and health information systems. *American Journal of Public Health, 93*(3), 388–392.

*Gyurcsik, N. C., Bray, S. R., & Brittain, D. R. (2004). Coping with barriers to vigorous physical activity during transition to university. *Family and Community Health, 27*(2), 130–143.

Hong, S., Friedman, J., & Alt, S. (2003). Modifiable risk factors for the primary prevention of heart disease in women. *Journal of the American Medical Women's Association, 58*(4), 278–284.

Javo, C., Alapack, R., Heyerdall, S., et al. (2003). Parental values and ethnic identity in indigenous Sami families: A qualitative study. *Family Process, 42*(1), 151–162.

*Jones, E. D., Kennedy-Malone, L., & Wideman, L. (2004). Early detection of type 2 diabetes among older African Americans. *Geriatric Nursing, 25*(1), 24–28.

Lai, S. C., & Cohen, M. N. (1999). Promoting lifestyle changes. *American Journal of Nursing, 99*(4), 63–67.

*Lev, E. L., & Owen, S. V. (1996). A measure of self-care self-efficacy: Strategies used by people to promote health. *Research in Nursing and Health, 19*(5), 421–429.

*Linfante, A. H., Allan, R., Smith, S. C., & Mosca, L. (2003). Psychosocial factors predict coronary heart disease, but what predicts psychosocial risk in women? *Journal of the American Medical Women's Association, 58*(4), 248–253.

Lucas, J. A., Orshan, S. A., & Cook, F. (2000). Determinants of health-promoting behaviors among women ages 65 and above living in the community. *Scholarly Inquiry for Nursing Practice, 14*(1), 77–109.

*McPhee, S. D., Johnson, T. R., & Dietrich, M. S. (2004). Comparing health status with healthy habits in elderly assisted-living residents. *Family and Community Health, 27*(2), 158–170.

*Murray, E., Lo, B., Pollack, L., Donelan, K., et al. (2003). The impact of health information on the internet on the physician–patient relationship: Patient perceptions. *Archives of Internal Medicine, 163*(14), 1727–1738.

Roberts, K. (2004). Simplify, simplify: Tackling health literacy by addressing reading literacy. *American Journal of Nursing, 104*(3), 118–119.

Robinson, A. W., & Sloan, H. L. (2000). Healthy People 2000: Heart health and old women. *Journal of Gerontological Nursing, 26*(5), 38–45.

Schank, M. J. (1999). Educational innovations—Self-health appraisal: Learning the difficulties of lifestyle change. *Journal of Nursing Education, 38*(1), 10–12.

Smeltzer, S. C., Zimmerman, V., DeSilets, L. D., et al. (2003). Accessible online health promotion information for persons with disabilities. *Online Journal of Issues in Nursing, 9*(1), 11. Available at: http://www.nursingworld.org/ojin/topic16/tpc16_5.htm.

## RESOURCES AND WEBSITES

Centers for Disease Control and Prevention, 1600 Clifton Road, Atlanta, GA 30333; 404-639-3311; http://www.cdc.gov. Accessed June 6, 2006.

Health Education Resources Exchange, Washington State Department of Health, Office of Health Promotion, P.O. Box 47833, Olympia, WA 98504; 800-525-0127; http://www.doh.wa.gov/here/Default.html. Accessed June 6, 2006.

Health Promotion for Women With Disabilities, Villanova University College of Nursing, 800 Lancaster Avenue, Villanova, PA 19085; 610-519-4900; http://www.nurseweb.villanova.edu/WomenWithDisabilities//welcom.htm. Accessed June 6, 2006.

U.S. Army Center for Health Promotion and Preventive Medicine (USACHPPM), 5158 Blackhawk Road, Aberdeen Proving Ground, MD 21010; 800-222-9698; chppm-www.apgea.army.mil/. Accessed June 6, 2006.

U.S. Department of Health and Human Services, National Institutes of Health: http://www.nih.gov/icd/. Accessed June 6, 2006.

U.S. Department of Health and Human Services, Office of Disease Prevention and Health Promotion, 1101 Wooton Parkway, Suite LL100, Rockville, MD 20852; http://www.odphp.osophs.dhhs.gov. Accessed June 6, 2006.

World Health Organization, Avenue Appia 20, 1211 Geneva 27, Switzerland; telephone: (+41 22) 791 21 11; http://www.who.int/hpr/. Accessed June 6, 2006.

# CHAPTER 5

# Health Assessment

## Learning Objectives

*On completion of this chapter, the learner will be able to:*

1. Describe the components of the health history.
2. Apply culturally sensitive interviewing skills and techniques to conduct a successful health history, physical examination, and nutritional assessment.
3. Identify modifications needed to obtain a health history and conduct a physical assessment for a person with a disability.
4. Identify genetic aspects nurses should incorporate into the health history and physical assessment.
5. Describe the physical examination techniques of inspection, palpation, percussion, and auscultation.
6. Apply the techniques of inspection, palpation, percussion, and auscultation to perform physical assessment of the major body systems of a person.
7. Discuss the techniques of measurement of body mass index, biochemical assessment, clinical examination, and assessment of food intake to assess a person's nutritional status.
8. Identify ethical considerations necessary for protecting a person's rights related to data collected in the health history and physical examination.
9. Describe factors that may contribute to altered nutritional status in high-risk groups such as adolescents and the elderly.
10. Conduct a health history and physical and nutritional assessment of a person at home.

The ability to assess patients is one of the most important skills of nursing, regardless of the practice setting. In all settings in which nurses interact with patients and provide care, eliciting a complete health history and using appropriate assessment skills are critical to identifying physical and psychological problems and concerns experienced by the patient. As the first step in the nursing process, patient assessment is necessary to obtain data that enable the nurse to make a nursing diagnosis, identify and implement nursing interventions, and assess their effectiveness.

## The Role of the Nurse in Health Assessment

In health assessment, the nurse obtains the patient's health history and performs a physical assessment, which can be carried out in a variety of settings, including the acute care setting, clinic or outpatient office, school, long-term care facility, or the home. A growing list of nursing diagnoses is used by nurses to identify and categorize patient problems that nurses have the knowledge, skills, and responsibility to treat independently (NANDA International, 2005) (see also Chapter 3, Chart 3-7). All members of the health care team—physicians, nurses, nutritionists, social workers, and others—use their unique skills and knowledge to contribute to the resolution of patient problems by first obtaining a health history and physical examination (Rasmor & Brown, 2003; Sanchez, Schreiber, Glynn, et al., 2003). Because the focus of each member of the health care team is unique, a variety of health history and physical examination formats have been developed. Regardless of the format, the information obtained by the nurse complements the data obtained by other members of the health care team and focuses on nursing's unique concerns for the patient.

## Basic Guidelines for Conducting a Health Assessment

People who seek health care for a specific problem often feel anxious. Their anxiety may be increased by fear about potential diagnoses, possible disruption of lifestyle, and other concerns. With this in mind, the nurse attempts to establish rapport, put the patient at ease, encourage honest communication, make eye contact, and listen carefully to the patient's responses to questions about health issues (Fig. 5-1).

When obtaining a health history or performing a physical examination, the nurse must be aware of his or her own nonverbal communication, as well as that of the patient. The nurse should take into consideration the patient's educational and cultural background (Flowers, 2004) as well as language proficiency. Questions and instructions to the patient are phrased in a way that is easily understandable. Technical terms and medical jargon are avoided. In addition, the nurse must take into consideration the patient's

**FIGURE 5-1.** A comfortable, relaxed atmosphere and an attentive interviewer are essential for a successful clinical interview. Photo © B. Proud.

disabilities or impairments (hearing, vision, cognitive, and physical limitations). At the end of the assessment, the nurse may summarize and clarify the information obtained and ask the patient if he or she has any questions; this gives the nurse the opportunity to correct misinformation and add facts that may have been omitted.

## Ethical Use of History or Physical Examination Data

Whenever information is elicited from a person through a health history or physical examination, the person has the right to know why the information is sought and how it will be used. For this reason, it is important to explain what the history and physical examination are, how the information will be obtained, and how it will be used (Sanchez et al., 2003). It is also important that the person be aware that the decision to participate is voluntary. A private setting for the history interview and physical examination promotes trust and encourages open, honest communication. After the history and examination are completed, the nurse selectively records the data pertinent to the patient's health status. This written record of the patient's history and physical examination findings is then maintained in a secure place and made available only to those health professionals directly involved in the care of the patient. This protects confidentiality and promotes professional conduct.

## Increasing Use of Technology

The use of technology to augment the information-gathering process has become an increasingly important aspect of obtaining a health history and physical examination. Computerization of medical records is becoming more common in private health care providers' offices as well as in medical centers. Electronic health records are thought to improve the quality of care, reduce medical errors, and help reduce health care costs. Computerized needs assessments are being used to gather family health histories (Kinzie, Cohn, Julian, et al., 2002), screen blood donors (Sanchez et al., 2003), and screen for intimate partner violence (Rhodes, Lauderdale, He, et al., 2002). Assessments can be completed and multiple aspects of health can be researched online (Eng, 2001). Nurses must be sensitive to the needs of the elderly and others who may not be comfortable with the new technology, and they may need to allow extra time and provide detailed instructions.

## The Health History

Throughout assessment, and particularly when obtaining the history, attention is focused on the impact of psychosocial, ethnic, and cultural background on a person's health, illness, and health promotion behaviors. The interpersonal and physical environments, as well as the person's lifestyle and activities of daily living, are explored in depth. Many nurses are responsible for obtaining a detailed history of the person's current health problems, past medical history, and family history and a review of the person's functional status. This results in a total health profile that focuses on health as well as illness and is more appropriately called a health history rather than a medical or a nursing history.

The format of the health history traditionally combines the medical history and the nursing assessment, although formats based on nursing frameworks, such as functional health patterns, have also become a standard. Both the review of systems and the patient profile are expanded to include individual and family relationships, lifestyle patterns, health practices, and coping strategies. These components of the health history are the basis of nursing assessment and can be easily adapted to address the needs of any patient population in any setting, institution, or agency (Rasmor & Brown, 2003). Combining the information obtained by the physician and the nurse into one health history prevents duplication of information and minimizes efforts on the part of the patient to provide this information repeatedly. This also encourages collaboration among members of the health care team who share in the collection and interpretation of the data.

Special considerations when obtaining a health history from an older adult are given in Chart 5-1.

### The Informant

The informant, or the person providing the health history, may not always be the patient, as in the case of a developmentally delayed, mentally impaired, disoriented, confused, unconscious, or comatose patient. The interviewer assesses the reliability of the informant and the usefulness of the information provided. For example, a disoriented patient is often unable to provide reliable information; people who use illicit drugs and alcohol often deny using these substances. The interviewer must make a clinical judgment about the reliability of the information (based on the context of the entire interview) and include this assessment in the record.

> **CHART 5-1**
>
> ### Health Assessment in the Older Adult
>
> A health history should be obtained from elderly patients in a calm, unrushed manner. Because of the increased incidence of impaired hearing and vision in the elderly, lighting should be adequate but not glaring, and distracting noises should be kept to a minimum. The interviewer should assume a position that enables the person to read lips and facial expressions. People who normally use a hearing aid are asked to use it during the interview. The interviewer should also recognize that there is wide diversity among the elderly and that differences exist in health practices, gender, income, and functional status (Loeb, 2004; Yarcheski, Mahon, Yarcheski, et al., 2004).
>
> Elderly people often assume that new physical problems are a result of age rather than a treatable illness. In addition, the signs and symptoms of illness in the elderly are often more subtle than those in younger people and may go unreported. Therefore, the interviewer inquires about subtle physical symptoms and recent changes in function and well-being. Special care is taken in obtaining a complete history of medications used, because many elderly people take many different kinds of prescription and over-the-counter (OTC) medications. Although elderly people may experience a decline in mental function, it should not be assumed that they are unable to provide an adequate history (Stotts & Deitrich, 2004). Nevertheless, including a member of the family in the interview process (eg, spouse, adult child, sibling, caretaker) may validate information and provide missing details. However, this should be done after obtaining the patient's permission. Further details about assessment of the older adult are provided in Chapter 12.

### Cultural Considerations

When obtaining the health history, the person's cultural background (Weber & Kelley, 2003) is taken into account. Cultural attitudes and beliefs about health, illness, health care, hospitalization, the use of medications, and use of complementary and alternative therapies, which are derived from personal experiences (Flowers, 2004), vary according to ethnic and cultural background. A person from another culture may have different views of personal health practices from those of the health care practitioner.

Similarly, people from some ethnic and cultural backgrounds will not complain of pain, even when it is severe, because outward expressions of pain are considered unacceptable. In some instances, they may refuse to take analgesics. Other cultures have their own folklore and beliefs about the treatment of illnesses. All such differences in outlook must be taken into account and accepted when caring for members of other cultures. Attitudes and beliefs about family relationships and the roles of women and elderly members of a family must be respected, even if they conflict with those of the interviewer.

## Content of the Health History

When a patient is seen for the first time by a member of the health care team, the first requirement is that baseline information be obtained (except in emergency situations). The sequence and format of obtaining data about a patient may vary, but the content, regardless of format, usually addresses the same general topics. A traditional approach includes the following:

- Biographical data
- Chief complaint
- Present health concern (or present illness)
- Past history
- Family history
- Review of systems
- Patient profile

### Biographical Data

Biographical information puts the patient's health history into context. This information includes the person's name, address, age, gender, marital status, occupation, and ethnic origins. Some interviewers prefer to ask more personal questions at this part of the interview, whereas others wait until more trust and confidence have been established or until a patient's immediate or urgent needs are first addressed. A patient who is in severe pain or has another urgent problem is unlikely to have a great deal of patience for an interviewer who is more concerned about marital or occupational status than with quickly addressing the problem at hand.

### Chief Complaint

The chief complaint is the issue that brings a person to the attention of the health care provider. Questions such as, "Why have you come to the health center today?" or "Why were you admitted to the hospital?" usually elicit the chief complaint. In the home setting, the initial question might be, "What is bothering you most today?" When a problem is identified, the person's exact words are usually recorded in quotation marks (Orient, 2005). However, a statement such as, "My doctor sent me," should be followed up with a question that identifies the probable reason why the person is seeking health care; this reason is then identified as the chief complaint.

### Present Health Concern or Illness

The history of the present health concern or illness is the single most important factor in helping the health care team arrive at a diagnosis or determine the patient's needs. The physical examination is helpful but often only validates the information obtained from the history. A careful history assists in correct selection of appropriate diagnostic tests. Although diagnostic test results can be helpful, they often support rather than establish the diagnosis.

If the present illness is only one episode in a series of episodes, the entire sequence of events is recorded. For example, a history from a patient whose chief complaint is an episode of insulin shock describes the entire course of the diabetes to put the current episode in context. The details of the health concern or present illness are described from onset until the time of contact with the health care team. These facts are recorded in chronologic order, beginning with, for example, "The patient was in good health until . . ." or "The patient first experienced abdominal pain 2 months prior to seeking help."

The history of the present illness or problem includes such information as the date and manner (sudden or gradual) in which the problem occurred, the setting in which the problem occurred (at home, at work, after an argument, after exercise), manifestations of the problem, and the course of the illness or problem. This includes self-treatment (including complementary and alternative therapies), medical interventions, progress and effects of treatment, and the patient's perceptions of the cause or meaning of the problem.

Specific symptoms (pain, headache, fever, change in bowel habits) are described in detail, along with the location and radiation (if pain), quality, severity, and duration. The interviewer also asks whether the problem is persistent or intermittent, what factors aggravate or alleviate it, and whether any associated manifestations exist.

Associated manifestations are symptoms that occur simultaneously with the chief complaint. The presence or absence of such symptoms may shed light on the origin or extent of the problem, as well as on the diagnosis. These symptoms are referred to as significant positive or negative findings and are obtained from a review of systems directly related to the chief complaint. For example, if a patient reports a vague symptom such as fatigue or weight loss, all body systems are reviewed and included in this section of the history. If, on the other hand, a patient's chief complaint is chest pain, only the cardiopulmonary and gastrointestinal systems may be included in the history of the present illness. In either situation, both positive and negative findings are recorded to define the problem further.

### Past Health History

A detailed summary of a person's past health is an important part of the health history. After determining the general health status, the interviewer should inquire about immunization status according to the recommendations of the adult immunization schedule and record the dates of immunization (if known). The Advisory Committee on Immunization Practices (ACIP), which approved the first adult immunization schedule in 2002, updates the schedule each year (ACIP, 2005). Research suggests that the health history is an economical alternative to serotesting for measles, mumps, and rubella in military recruits (Burnham, Thompson & Jackson, 2002). The interviewer should also inquire about any known allergies to medications or other substances, along with the type of allergy and adverse reactions. Other relevant material includes information, if known, about the patient's last physical examination, chest x-ray, electrocardiogram, eye examination, hearing test, dental checkup, Papanicolaou (Pap) smear and mammogram (if female), digital rectal examination of the prostate gland (if male), bone density testing, colon cancer screening, and any other pertinent tests. The interviewer then discusses previous illnesses and records negative as well as positive responses to a list of specific diseases. Dates of illness, or the age of the patient at the time, as well as the names of the primary health care provider and hospital, the diagnosis, and the treatment are noted. The interviewer elicits a history of the following areas:

- Childhood illnesses—rubeola, rubella, polio, whooping cough, mumps, measles, chickenpox, scarlet fever, rheumatic fever, strep throat
- Adult illnesses
- Psychiatric illnesses
- Injuries—burns, fractures, head injuries
- Hospitalizations
- Surgical and diagnostic procedures
- Current medications—prescription, over-the-counter (OTC), home remedies, complementary therapies
- Use of alcohol and other drugs

If a particular hospitalization or major medical intervention is related to the present illness, the account of it is not repeated; rather, the report refers to the appropriate part of the record, such as "See history of present illness" or "See HPI," on the data sheet.

## Family History

To identify diseases that may be genetic (Guttmacher, Collins & Carmona, 2004), communicable, or possibly environmental in origin, the interviewer asks about the age and health status, or the age and cause of death, of first-order relatives (parents, siblings, spouse, children) and second-order relatives (grandparents, cousins). In general, it is necessary to include the following diseases: cancer, hypertension, heart disease, diabetes, epilepsy, mental illness, tuberculosis, kidney disease, arthritis, allergies, asthma, alcoholism, and obesity. One of the easiest methods of recording such data is by using the family tree or genogram (Fig. 5-2). The results of genetic testing or screening, if known, are recorded. See Chapter 9 for a detailed discussion of genetics.

## Review of Systems

The review of systems includes an overview of general health as well as symptoms related to each body system. Questions are asked about each of the major body systems in terms of past or present symptoms. Reviewing each body system helps reveal any relevant data. Negative as well as positive answers are recorded. If a patient responds positively to questions about a particular system, the information is analyzed carefully. If any illnesses were previously mentioned or recorded, it is not necessary to repeat them in this part of the history. Instead, reference is made to the appropriate place in the health history where the information can be found.

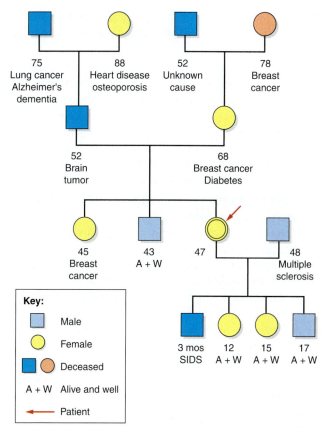

**FIGURE 5-2.** Diagram (called a genogram) used to record history of family members, including their age and cause of death or, if living, their current health status.

A review of systems can be organized in a formal checklist, which becomes a part of the health history. One advantage of a checklist is that it can be easily audited and is less subject to error than a system that relies heavily on the interviewer's memory.

## Patient Profile

In the patient profile, more biographical information is gathered. A complete composite, or profile, of the patient is critical to analysis of the chief complaint and of the person's ability to deal with the problem. A complete patient profile is summarized in Chart 5-2.

At this point in the interview, the information elicited is highly personal and subjective. People are encouraged to express feelings honestly and to discuss personal experiences. It is best to begin with general, open ended questions and to move to direct questioning when specific facts are needed. Interviews that progress from information that is less personal (birthplace, occupation, education) to information that is more personal (sexuality, body image, coping abilities) often reduce anxiety.

A general patient profile consists of the following content areas:

- Past life events related to health
- Education and occupation

# GENETICS IN NURSING PRACTICE

New and exciting discoveries emerging from human genome research are clarifying genetic aspects of health and disease and expanding health opportunities for people, families, and communities around the world. These advances call for all nurses to have a heightened awareness of genetics as the core understanding of the mechanisms of disease. Genetics concepts are central to every step of the nursing process.

## GENETIC ASPECTS OF HEALTH CARE DELIVERY AND NURSING PRACTICE

Nurses in all areas of practice carry out five main practice activities:
- Help to collect, report, and record genetics information
- Offer genetics information and resources
- Participate in the informed consent process and facilitate informed decision making
- Participate in ongoing management of patients with genetic conditions
- Evaluate and monitor the impact of genetic conditions, testing, and treatment on the individual and family

## COMMUNITY-BASED NURSING PRACTICE

Nurses providing community-based care:
- Participate in genetic screening (eg, prenatal screening and newborn screening)
- Provide health care regarding genetic risk factors and management of genetically related disorders in a way that respects the beliefs and concerns of specific ethnic communities
- Educate the public about the contribution of genetics to health and disease
- Engage in dialogue with the public about ethical, legal, and social issues related to genetics discoveries

## CRITICAL THINKING AND DECISION MAKING

Nurses use these skills in providing genetics-related health care when they:
- Assess and analyze family history data for genetic risk factors
- Identify those individuals and families in need of referral for genetic testing or counseling
- Ensure the privacy and confidentiality of genetics information

## HEALTH EDUCATION AND PROMOTION

Nurses in all settings should be prepared to:
- Inquire about patients' and families' desired health outcomes with regard to genetics-related conditions or risk factors
- Refer patients for genetics services when indicated
- Identify barriers to accessing genetics-related health services
- Offer appropriate genetics information and resources

## HEALTH ASSESSMENT

Nurses incorporate a genetics focus into the following health assessments:
- Family history—assess for genetics-related risk factors
- Cultural, social, and spiritual assessment—assess for individual and family perceptions and beliefs around genetics topics
- Physical assessment—assess for clinical features that may suggest a genetic condition is present (eg, unusually tall stature—Marfan syndrome)
- Ethnic background—since many conditions are more common in specific ethnic populations, the nurse gathers information about ethnic background (eg, Tay-Sachs disease in Ashkenazi Jewish populations or thalassemia in Southeast Asian populations)

## GENETICS RESOURCES FOR NURSES AND PATIENTS ON THE WEB

Genetic Alliance, www.geneticalliance.org—a directory of support groups for patients and families with genetic conditions

Gene Clinics, www.geneclinics.org—a listing of common genetic disorders with up-to-date clinical summaries, genetic counseling and testing information

National Organization of Rare Disorders, www.rarediseases.org—a directory of support groups and information for patients and families with rare genetic disorders

OMIM: Online Mendelian Inheritance in Man, www.ncbi.nlm.nih.gov/Omim/mimstats.html—a complete listing of inherited genetic conditions

---

- Environment (physical, spiritual, cultural, interpersonal)
- Lifestyle (patterns and habits)
- Presence of a physical or mental disability
- Self-concept
- Sexuality
- Risk for abuse
- Stress and coping response

**PAST LIFE EVENTS RELATED TO HEALTH**

The patient profile begins with a brief life history. Questions about place of birth and past places of residence help focus attention on the earlier years of life. Personal experiences during childhood or adolescence that have special significance may be elicited by asking a question such as, "Was there anything that you experienced as a child or

## CHART 5-2

### Patient Profile

**PAST EVENTS RELATED TO HEALTH**
Place of birth
Places lived
Significant childhood/adolescent experiences

**EDUCATION AND OCCUPATION**
Jobs held in past
Current position/job
Length of time at position
Educational preparation
Work satisfaction and career goals

**FINANCIAL RESOURCES**
Income
Insurance coverage

**ENVIRONMENT**
Physical—living arrangements (type of housing, neighborhood, presence of hazards)
Spiritual—extent to which religion is a part of individual's life; religious beliefs related to perception of health and illness; religious practices
Interpersonal—ethnic background (language spoken, customs and values held, folk practices used to maintain health or to cure illness); family relationships (family structure, roles, communication patterns, support system); friendships (quality of relationship)

**LIFESTYLE PATTERNS**
Sleep (time person retires, hours per night, comfort measures, awakens rested)
Exercise (type, frequency, time spent)
Nutrition (24-hour diet recall, idiosyncrasies, restrictions)
Recreation (type of activity, time spent)
Caffeine (coffee, tea, cola, chocolate)—kind, amount
Smoking (cigarette, pipe, cigar, marijuana)—kind, amount per day, number of years, desire to quit
Alcohol—kind, amount, pattern over past year
Drugs—kind, amount, route of administration

**PHYSICAL OR MENTAL DISABILITY**
Presence of a disability (physical or mental)
Effect of disability on function and health access
Accommodations needed to support functioning

**SELF-CONCEPT**
View of self in present
View of self in future
Body image (level of satisfaction, concerns)

**SEXUALITY**
Perception of self as a man or woman
Quality of sexual relationships
Concerns related to sexuality or sexual functioning

**RISK FOR ABUSE**
Physical injury in past
Afraid of partner, caregiver, or family member
Refusal of caregiver to provide necessary equipment or assistance

**STRESS AND COPING RESPONSE**
Major concerns or problems at present
Daily "hassles"
Past experiences with similar problems
Past coping patterns and outcomes
Present coping strategies and anticipated outcomes
Individual's expectations of family/friends and health care team in problem resolution

---

adolescent that would be helpful for me to know about?" The interviewer's intent is to encourage the patient to make a quick review of his or her earlier life, highlighting information of particular significance. Although many patients may not recall anything significant, others may share information such as a personal achievement, a failure, a developmental crisis, or an instance of physical, emotional, or sexual abuse.

### EDUCATION AND OCCUPATION

Inquiring about current occupation can reveal much about a person's economic status and educational preparation. A statement such as, "Tell me about your job," often elicits information about role, job tasks, and satisfaction with the position. Direct questions about past employment and career goals may be asked if the person does not provide this information.

It is important to learn about a person's educational background. Asking a person what kind of educational requirements were necessary to attain his or her present job is a more sensitive approach than asking whether he or she graduated from high school. Information about the patient's general financial status may be obtained by questions such as, "Do you have any financial concerns at this time?" or "Sometimes there just doesn't seem to be enough money to make ends meet. Are you finding this true?" Inquiries about the person's insurance coverage and plans for health care payment are also appropriate.

### ENVIRONMENT

The concept of environment includes a person's physical environment and its potential hazards, spiritual awareness, cultural background, interpersonal relationships, and support system.

**Physical Environment.** Information is elicited about the type of housing (apartment, duplex, single-family) in which the person lives, its location, the level of safety and comfort within the home and neighborhood, and the presence of environmental hazards (eg, isolation, potential fire risks, inadequate sanitation). If the patient is homeless or living in a homeless shelter or has a disability, the patient's environment assumes special importance.

**Spiritual Environment.** The term "spiritual environment" refers to the degree to which a person thinks about or contemplates his or her existence, accepts challenges in life, and seeks and finds answers to personal questions. Spirituality may be expressed through identification with a particular religion. Spiritual values and beliefs often direct a person's behavior and approach to health problems and can influence responses to sickness. Illness may create a spiritual crisis and can place considerable stress on a person's internal resources and beliefs. Inquiring about spirituality can identify possible support systems as well as beliefs and customs that need to be considered in planning care. Information is gathered about the following three areas:

- The extent to which religion is a part of the person's life
- Religious beliefs related to the person's perception of health and illness
- Religious practices related to health and illness

A spiritual assessment may involve asking the following questions:

- Is religion or God important to you?
- If yes, in what way?
- If no, what is the most important thing in your life?
- Are there any religious practices that are important to you?
- Do you have any spiritual concerns because of your present health problem?

**Interpersonal and Cultural Environment.** Cultural influences, relationships with family and friends, and the presence or absence of a support system are all part of a patient's interpersonal environment. The beliefs and practices that have been shared from generation to generation are known as cultural or ethnic patterns. They are expressed through language, dress, dietary choices, and role behaviors; in perceptions of health and illness; and in health-related behaviors. The influence of these beliefs and customs on how a person reacts to health problems and interacts with health care providers cannot be underestimated. For this reason, the health history includes information about ethnic identity (cultural and social) and racial identity (biologic) (Judd, Griffith & Faustman, 2004). The following questions may assist in obtaining relevant information:

- Where did your parents or ancestors come from? When?
- What language do you speak at home?
- Are there certain customs or values that are important to you?
- Is there anything special you do to keep in good health?
- Do you have any specific practices for treating illness?

**Family Relationships and Support System.** An assessment of family structure (members, ages, and roles), patterns of communication, and the presence or absence of a support system is an integral part of the patient profile. Although the traditional family is recognized as a mother, a father, and children, many different types of living arrangements exist within our society. "Family" may mean two or more people bound by emotional ties or commitments. Live-in companions, roommates, and close friends can all play a significant role in a person's support system.

### LIFESTYLE

The lifestyle section of the patient profile provides information about health-related behaviors. These behaviors include patterns of sleep, exercise, nutrition, and recreation, as well as personal habits such as smoking and the use of illicit drugs, alcohol, and caffeine. Although most people readily describe their exercise patterns or recreational activities, many are unwilling to report their smoking, alcohol use, and illicit drug use, and many deny or understate the degree to which they use such substances (Bridevaux, Bradley, Bryson, et al., 2004; Finfgeld-Connett, 2004). Questions such as, "What kind of alcohol do you enjoy drinking at a party?" may elicit more accurate information than, "Do you drink?" The specific type of alcohol (eg, wine, liquor, beer) and the amount ingested per day or per week (eg, 1 pint of whiskey daily for 2 years) are described.

If alcohol abuse is suspected, additional information may be obtained by using common alcohol screening questionnaires such as the CAGE (*C*utting down, *A*nnoyance by criticism, *G*uilty feelings, and *E*ye-openers), AUDIT (*A*lcohol *U*se *D*isorders *I*dentification *T*est), TWEAK (*T*olerance, *W*orry, *E*ye-opener, *A*mnesia, *K*ut down), or SMAST (*S*hort *M*ichigan *A*lcoholism *S*creening *T*est). Chart 5-3 shows the CAGE Questions Adapted to Include Drugs (CAGEAID).

---

**CHART 5-3**

### Assessing for Alcohol or Drug Use

**CAGE Questions Adapted to Include Drugs (CAGEAID)***

**Have you felt you ought to cut down on your drinking** *(or drug use)*?
____Yes ____No

**Have people annoyed you by criticizing your drinking** *(or drug use)*?
____Yes ____No

**Have you felt bad or guilty about your drinking** *(or drug use)*?
____Yes ____No

**Have you ever had a drink** *(or used drugs)* **first thing in the morning to steady your nerves or get rid of a hangover** *(or to get the day started)*?
____Yes ____No

---

* Boldface text shows the original CAGE questions; boldface italic text shows modifications of the CAGE questions used to screen for drug disorders. In a general population, two or more positive answers indicate a need for more in-depth assessment.

From Fleming, M. F., & Barry, K. L. (1992). *Addictive Disorders*. St. Louis: Mosby; and Ewing, J. A. (1984). Detecting alcoholism: The CAGE questionnaire. *Journal of the American Medical Association, 252*(14), 1905–1907.

The MAST has also been recently updated to include drug use (Westermeyer, Yargic & Thuras, 2004).

Similar questions can be used to elicit information about smoking and caffeine consumption. Questions about illicit drug use follow naturally after questions about smoking, caffeine consumption, and alcohol use. A nonjudgmental approach makes it easier for a person to respond truthfully and factually. If street names or unfamiliar terms are used to describe drugs, the person is asked to define the terms used (Bridevaux et al., 2004; Finfgeld-Connett, 2004).

Investigation of lifestyle should also include questions about complementary and alternative therapies. It is estimated that as many as 40% of Americans use some type of complementary or alternative therapies, including special diets, prayer, visualization or guided imagery, massage, meditation, herbal products, and many others (Capriotti, 2004). Marijuana is used for management of symptoms, especially pain, in a number of chronic conditions (Steinbrook, 2004).

### PHYSICAL OR MENTAL DISABILITY

The general patient profile also needs to contain questions about any hearing, vision, cognitive, or physical disability (Stotts & Deitrich, 2004). The presence of an obvious physical limitation (eg, using crutches to walk or using a wheelchair to get around) necessitates further investigation. The etiology of the disability should be elicited, and the length of time the patient has had the disability and the impact on function and health access are important to assess. Chart 5-4 presents specific issues that the nurse should consider when obtaining health histories and conducting physical assessments of patients with disabilities.

### SELF-CONCEPT

Self-concept refers to a person's view of himself or herself, an image that has developed over many years. To assess self-concept, the interviewer might ask how a person views life, using a question such as, "How do you feel about your life in general?" A person's self-concept can be threatened very easily by changes in physical function or appearance or other threats to health. The impact of certain medical conditions or surgical interventions, such as a colostomy or a mastectomy, can threaten body image. The question, "Do you have any particular concerns about your body?" may elicit useful information about self-image.

### SEXUALITY

No area of assessment is more personal than the sexual history. Interviewers are frequently uncomfortable with such questions and ignore this area of the patient profile or conduct a very cursory interview about this subject. Lack of knowledge about sexuality and anxiety about one's own sexuality may hamper the interviewer's effectiveness in dealing with this subject (Nusbaum & Hamilton, 2002).

Sexual assessment can be approached at the end of the interview, at the time interpersonal or lifestyle factors are assessed, or it may be easier to discuss sexuality as a part of the genitourinary history within the review of systems. In female patients, a discussion of sexuality would follow questions about menstruation. In male patients, a similar discussion would follow questions about the urinary system.

---

## NURSING RESEARCH PROFILE

### Predictors of Positive Health

Yarcheski, A., Mahon, N. E., Yarcheski, T. J., et al. (2004). A meta-analysis of predictors of positive health practices. *Journal of Nursing Scholarship, 36*(2) 102–108.

#### Purpose
This study was designed to identify predictors of positive health practices based on previous investigations in which the Personal Lifestyle Questionnaire (PLQ) had been used. Positive health practices were defined as exercise and relaxation activities.

#### Design
The PLQ, a 24-item, 4-point scale, has been available for more than 20 years and has proved reliable and valid for use in adolescents and adults. Quantitative meta-analysis was used to synthesize the findings of 37 studies that measured positive health practices with the PLQ. Meta-analysis was conducted on 14 predictors.

#### Results
Eight predictors had a moderate (0.30) effect size: loneliness, social support, perceived health status, self-efficacy, future time perspective, self-esteem, hope, and depression. Six predictors had a small (0.10) effect size: stress, education, marital status, age, income, and gender. Sex and income were not useful variables in predicting positive health practices.

#### Nursing Implications
During health assessment, the nurse should be aware that positive predictors of the use of exercise and relaxation involve many factors. Loneliness has a negative influence on the practice of positive health behaviors. Social support appears to influence positive health practices by increasing the information available on how to take care of oneself and prevent disease. People who take responsibility for their personal self-management and have a view toward the future also tend to practice more positive health behaviors. Further testing of these predictors is recommended.

**CHART 5-4**

# Health Assessment of People with Disabilities

## OVERVIEW

People with disabilities are entitled to the same level of health assessment and physical examination as people without disabilities. The nurse needs to be aware of the patient's disabilities or impairments (hearing, vision, cognitive, and physical limitations) and take these into consideration when obtaining a health history and conducting a physical assessment. It is appropriate to ask the patient what assistance he or she needs rather than assuming that help is needed for all activities or that, if assistance is needed, the patient will ask for it.

## HEALTH HISTORY

Communication between the nurse and the patient is essential. To ensure that the patient is able to respond to assessment questions and provide needed information, interpreters, assistive listening devices, or other alternate formats (eg, Braille, large-print forms) may be required.

When interpreters are needed, interpretation services should be arranged. Health care facilities have a responsibility to provide these services without charge to the patient. Family members (especially children) should *not* be used as interpreters, because doing so violates the patient's right to privacy and confidentiality.

The nurse should speak directly to the patient and not to family members or others who have accompanied the patient. If the patient has vision or hearing loss, normal tone and volume of the voice should be used when conducting the assessment. The patient should be able to see the nurse's face clearly during the health history, so that speech reading and nonverbal clues can be used to aid communication.

The health history should address general health issues that are important to all patients, including sexual history and risk for abuse. It should also address the impact of the patient's disability on health issues and access to care and the effect of the patient's current health problem on his or her disability.

The nurse should verify what the patient has said; if the patient has difficulty communicating verbally, the nurse should ask for clarification rather than assume that it is too difficult for the patient to do so. Most people would rather be asked to explain again than run the risk of being misunderstood.

## PHYSICAL EXAMINATION

Inaccessible facilities remain a major barrier to health care for people with disabilities. Barriers include lack of ramps and grab bars, inaccessible restrooms, small examination rooms, and examination tables that cannot be lowered to allow the patient to move himself or herself onto, or be transferred easily and safely to, the examination table. The patient may need help getting undressed for the physical examination (and dressed again), moving on and off the examination table, and maintaining positions usually required during physical examination maneuvers. It is important to ask the patient what assistance is needed.

If the patient has impaired sensory function (eg, lack of sensation, hearing or vision loss), it is important to inform the patient that you will be touching him or her. Furthermore, it is important to explain all procedures and maneuvers.

Gynecologic examinations should *not* be deferred because a patient has a disability or is assumed to be sexually inactive. Explanations of the examination are important for all women, and even more so for women with disabilities, because they may have had previous negative experiences. Slow, gentle moving and positioning of the patient for the gynecologic examination and warming the speculum before attempting insertion often minimize spasticity in women with neurologically related disabilities.

## HEALTH SCREENING AND TESTING

Many people with disabilities report that they have not been weighed for years or even decades because they are unable to stand for this measurement. Alternative methods (eg, use of wheelchair scales) are needed to monitor weight and body mass index. This is particularly important because of the increased incidence of obesity and its effects on health status and transfer of persons with disabilities (Sharts-Hopko & Sullivan, 2003).

Patients with disabilities may require special assistance if urine specimens are to be obtained as part of the visit. They are often able to suggest strategies to obtain urine specimens based on previous experience.

If it is necessary for the nurse to wear a mask during a procedure or if the patient is unable to see the face of the nurse during a procedure, it is important to explain the procedure and the expected role of the patient ahead of time. If the patient is unable to hear or is unable to communicate with the nurse or other health care provider verbally during an examination or diagnostic test, a method of communication (eg, signaling the patient by tapping his or her arm, signaling the nurse by using a bell) should be established beforehand.

Inaccessible facilities have resulted in decreased participation of people with disabilities in recommended preventive screening, including gynecologic examinations, mammograms, and bone density testing (Smeltzer, Zimmerman & Capriotti, 2005; Iezzoni, O'Day, Killeen, et al., 2001). Therefore, it is important to ask about health screening and recommendations for screening. In addition, people with disabilities should be asked about their participation in health promotion activities, because inaccessible environments may limit their participation in exercise, health programs, and other health promotion efforts.

Obtaining the sexual history provides an opportunity to discuss sexual matters openly and gives the person permission to express sexual concerns to an informed professional. The interviewer must be nonjudgmental and must use language appropriate to the patient's age and background (Nusbaum & Hamilton, 2002). The assessment begins with an orienting sentence such as, "Next, I would like to ask about your sexual health and practices." Such an opening may lead to a discussion of concerns related to sexual expression or the quality of a relationship, or to questions about contraception, risky sexual behaviors, and safer sex practices. Examples of other questions are, "Do you have one or more sexual partners?" and "Are you satisfied with your sexual relationships?"

Determining whether a person is sexually active should precede any attempts to explore issues related to sexuality and sexual function. Care should be taken to initiate conversations about sexuality with elderly patients and patients with disabilities and not to treat them as asexual people (Stotts & Deitrich, 2004). Questions are worded in such a way that the person feels free to discuss his or her sexuality regardless of marital status or sexual preference. Direct questions are usually less threatening when prefaced with such statements as, "Most people feel that . . ." or "Many people worry about. . . ." This suggests the normalcy of such feelings or behavior and encourages the person to share information that might otherwise be omitted from fear of seeming "different."

If a person answers abruptly or does not wish to carry the discussion any further, then the interviewer should move to the next topic. However, introducing the subject of sexuality indicates to the person that a discussion of sexual concerns is acceptable and can be approached again in the future if so desired. Further discussion of the sexual history is presented in Chapters 46 and 49.

**RISK FOR ABUSE**
Physical, sexual, and psychological abuse is a topic of growing importance in today's society. Such abuse occurs to people of both genders, of all ages, and from all socioeconomic, ethnic, and cultural groups. However, few patients discuss this topic unless they are asked specifically about it. In fact, one study revealed that among women currently in an abusive relationship, 92% had never told a health care provider (Rhodes et al., 2002). Therefore, it is important to ask direct questions, such as

- Is anyone physically hurting you or forcing you to have sexual activities?
- Has anyone ever hurt you physically or threatened to do so?
- Are you ever afraid of anyone close to you (your partner, caregiver, or other family members)?

Patients who are elderly or have disabilities are at increased risk for abuse and should be asked about it as a routine part of assessment. However, when elderly patients are questioned directly, they rarely admit to abuse (Fulmer, 2003). Health care professionals should assess for risk factors, such as high levels of stress or alcoholism in caregivers, evidence of violence, and emotional outbursts, as well as financial, emotional, or physical dependency.

Two additional questions have been found to be effective in uncovering specific types of abuse that may occur only in people with disabilities (McFarlane, Hughes, Nosek, et al., 2001):

- Does anyone prevent you from using a wheelchair, cane, respirator, or other assistive device?
- Does anyone you depend on refuse to help you with an important personal need, such as taking your medicine, getting to the bathroom, getting in or out of bed, bathing, dressing, or getting food or drink?

If a person's response indicates that abuse is a risk, further assessment is warranted, and efforts are made to ensure the patient's safety and provide access to appropriate community and professional resources and support systems (McFarlane et al., 2001). Further discussion of domestic violence and abuse is presented in Chapter 46.

**STRESS AND COPING RESPONSES**
Each person handles stress differently. How well people adapt depends on their ability to cope. During a health history, past coping patterns and perceptions of current stresses and anticipated outcomes are explored to identify the person's overall ability to handle stress. It is especially important to identify expectations that a person may have of family, friends, and caregivers in providing financial, emotional, or physical support.

## Other Health History Formats

The health history format discussed in this chapter is only one possible design that is useful in obtaining and organizing information about a person's health status. Some experts consider this traditional format to be inappropriate for nurses, because it does not focus exclusively on the assessment of human responses to actual or potential health problems. Several attempts have been made to develop an assessment format and database with this focus in mind. One example is the nursing database prototype based on the Unitary Person Framework of the North American Nursing Diagnosis Association and its nine human response patterns: exchanging, communicating, relating, valuing, choosing, moving, perceiving, knowing, and feeling (NANDA International, 2005). Although there is support in nursing for using this approach, no consensus for its use has been reached.

The National Center for Health Services Research of the U.S. Department of Health and Human Services (USDHHS) and other groups from the public and private sectors have focused on assessing not only biologic health but also other dimensions of health. These dimensions include physical, functional, emotional, mental, and social health. Modern efforts to assess health status have focused on the manner in which disease or disability affects a patient's functional status—that is, the ability of the person to function normally and perform his or her usual physical, mental, and social activities. An emphasis on functional assessment is viewed as more holistic than the traditional health or medical history. Instruments to assess health status in these ways may be used by nurses along with their own clinical assessment skills to determine the impact of illness, disease, disability, and health problems on functional status.

Health concerns that are not complex (eg, earache, sinusitis) and can be resolved in a short period usually do not require the depth or detail that is necessary when a person is experiencing a major illness or health problem (Stotts & Deitrich, 2004). Additional assessments that go beyond the general patient profile may be used if the patient's health problems are acute and complex or if the illness is chronic (Rosenthal & Kavic, 2004). The person should be asked about continuing health promotion and screening practices. If the person has not been involved in these practices in the past, he or she should be educated about their importance and referred to appropriate health care providers.

Regardless of the assessment format used, the focus of nurses during data collection is different from that of physicians and other health team members. However, the nursing focus complements these other approaches and encourages collaboration among the health care providers, with each member bringing his or her own expertise and focus to the situation.

## Physical Assessment

Physical assessment, or the physical examination, is an integral part of nursing assessment. The basic techniques and tools used in performing a physical examination are described in general in this chapter. The examinations of specific systems, including special maneuvers, are described in the appropriate chapters throughout the book. Because a patient's nutritional status is an important factor in overall health and well-being, a section on nutritional assessment is included in this chapter.

The physical examination is usually performed after the health history is obtained. It is carried out in a well-lighted, warm area. The patient is asked to (or helped to) undress and is draped appropriately so that only the area to be examined is exposed. The person's physical and psychological comfort are considered at all times. It is necessary to describe procedures to the patient and explain what sensations to expect before each part of the examination. The examiner's hands are washed before and immediately after the examination. Fingernails are kept short to avoid injuring the patient. If there is a possibility of coming into contact with blood or other body secretions during the physical examination, gloves should be worn.

An organized and systematic examination is the key to obtaining appropriate data in the shortest time. Such an approach encourages cooperation and trust on the part of the patient. The person's health history provides the examiner with a health profile that guides all aspects of the physical examination. Although the sequence of physical examination depends on the circumstances and on the patient's reason for seeking health care, the complete examination usually proceeds as follows:

- Skin
- Head and neck
- Thorax and lungs
- Breasts
- Cardiovascular system
- Abdomen
- Rectum
- Genitalia
- Neurologic system
- Musculoskeletal system

In clinical practice, all relevant body systems are tested throughout the physical examination, not necessarily in the sequence described (Weber & Kelley, 2003). For example, when the face is examined, it is appropriate to check for facial asymmetry and, thus, for the integrity of the fifth and seventh cranial nerves; the examiner does not need to repeat this as part of a neurologic examination. (See Chapter 60 for a full description of assessment of the cranial nerves.) When systems are combined in this manner, the patient does not need to change positions repeatedly, which can be exhausting and time-consuming.

A "complete" physical examination is not routine. Many of the body systems are selectively assessed on the basis of the presenting problem. For example, if a healthy 20-year-old college student requires an examination to play basketball and reports no history of neurologic abnormality, the neurologic assessment is brief. Conversely, a history of transient numbness and diplopia (double vision) usually necessitates a complete neurologic investigation (see Chapter 60). Similarly, a patient with chest pain receives a much more intensive examination of the chest and heart than one with an earache. In general, the health history guides the examiner in obtaining additional data for a complete picture of the patient's health.

The process of learning to perform a physical examination requires repetition and reinforcement in a clinical setting. Only after basic physical assessment techniques are mastered can the examiner tailor the routine screening examination to include thorough assessments of particular systems, including special maneuvers.

The basic tools of the physical examination are vision, hearing, touch, and smell. These human senses may be augmented by special tools (eg, stethoscope, ophthalmoscope, reflex hammer) that are extensions of the human senses; they are simple tools that anyone can learn to use well. Expertise comes with practice, and sophistication comes with the interpretation of what is seen and heard. The four fundamental techniques used in the physical examination are inspection, palpation, percussion, and auscultation (Rasmor & Brown, 2003).

### Inspection

The first fundamental technique is inspection or observation. General inspection begins with the first contact with the patient. Introducing oneself and shaking hands provide opportunities for making initial observations: Is the person old or young? How old? How young? Does the person appear to be his or her stated age? Is the person thin or obese? Does the person appear anxious or depressed? Is the person's body structure normal or abnormal? In what way, and how different from normal? It is essential to pay attention to the details in observation. Vague, general statements are not a substitute for specific descriptions based on careful observation. Consider the following examples:

- "The person appears sick." In what way does he or she appear sick? Is the skin clammy, pale, jaundiced, or cyanotic? Is the person grimacing in pain or having difficulty breathing? Does he or she have edema? What specific physical features or behavioral manifestations indicate that the person is "sick"?
- "The person appears chronically ill." In what way does he or she appear chronically ill? Does the person appear to have lost weight? People who lose weight secondary to muscle-wasting diseases (eg, acquired immunodeficiency syndrome [AIDS], malignancy) have a different appearance than those who are merely thin, and weight loss may be accompanied by loss of muscle mass or atrophy. Does the skin have the appearance of chronic illness (ie, is it pale, or does it give the appearance of dehydration or loss of subcutaneous tissue)?

These important specific observations are documented in the patient's chart or health record. Among general observations that should be noted in the initial examination of the patient are posture and stature, body movements, nutritional status, speech pattern, and vital signs.

## Posture

The posture that a person assumes often provides valuable information. Patients who have breathing difficulties (dyspnea) secondary to cardiac disease prefer to sit and may report feeling short of breath when lying flat for even a brief time. Patients with obstructive pulmonary disease not only sit upright but also may thrust their arms forward and laterally onto the edge of the bed (tripod position) to place accessory respiratory muscles at an optimal mechanical advantage. Patients with abdominal pain due to peritonitis prefer to lie perfectly still; even slight jarring of the bed causes agonizing pain. In contrast, patients with abdominal pain due to renal or biliary colic are often restless and may pace the room. Patients with meningeal irritation may experience head or neck pain on bending the head or flexing the knees.

## Body Movements

Abnormalities of body movement are of two kinds: generalized disruption of voluntary or involuntary movement and asymmetry of movement. The first category includes tremors of a wide variety; some tremors may occur at rest (Parkinson's disease), whereas others occur only on voluntary movement (cerebellar ataxia). Other tremors may exist during both rest and activity (alcohol withdrawal syndrome, thyrotoxicosis). Some voluntary or involuntary movements are fine, and others are quite coarse. At the extreme are the convulsive movements of epilepsy or tetanus and the choreiform (involuntary and irregular) movements of patients with rheumatic fever or Huntington's disease. Other aspects of body movement that are noted on inspection include spasticity, muscle spasms, and an abnormal gait.

Asymmetry of movement, in which only one side of the body is affected, may occur with disorders of the central nervous system (CNS), principally in those patients who have had a cerebrovascular accident (stroke). Patients may have drooping of one side of the face, weakness or paralysis of the extremities on one side of the body, and a foot-dragging gait. Spasticity (increased muscle tone) may also be present, particularly in patients with multiple sclerosis.

## Nutritional Status

Nutritional status is important to note. Obesity may be generalized as a result of excessive intake of calories, or it may be specifically localized to the trunk in patients who have an endocrine disorder (Cushing's disease) or who have been taking corticosteroids for long periods. Loss of weight may be generalized as a result of inadequate caloric intake, or it may be seen in loss of muscle mass with disorders that affect protein synthesis. Nutritional assessment is discussed in more detail later in this chapter.

## Speech Pattern

Speech may be slurred because of CNS disease or because of damage to cranial nerves. Recurrent damage to the laryngeal nerve results in hoarseness, as do disorders that produce edema or swelling of the vocal cords. Speech may be halting, slurred, or interrupted in flow in patients with some CNS disorders (eg, multiple sclerosis, stroke).

## Vital Signs

The recording of vital signs is a part of every physical examination (Bickley & Szilagyi, 2003). Blood pressure, pulse rate, respiratory rate, and body temperature measurements are obtained and recorded. Acute changes and trends over time are documented, and unexpected changes and values that deviate significantly from a patient's normal values are brought to the attention of the patient's primary health care provider. The "fifth vital sign," pain, is also assessed and documented, if indicated.

Fever is an increase in body temperature above normal. On average, a normal oral temperature for most people is 37.0°C (98.6°F); however, some variation is normal. Some people's temperatures are quite normal at 36.6°C (98°F) or 37.3°C (99°F). There is a normal diurnal variation of a degree or two in body temperature throughout the day; temperature is usually lowest in the morning and increases during the day to between 37.3° and 37.5°C (99° to 99.5°F), and it then decreases during the night.

## Palpation

Palpation is a vital part of the physical examination (Rasmor & Brown, 2003). Many structures of the body, although not visible, may be assessed through the techniques of light and deep palpation (Fig. 5-3). Examples include the super-

**FIGURE 5-4.** Percussion technique. The middle finger of one hand strikes the terminal phalanx of the middle finger of the other hand, which is placed firmly against the body. If the action is performed sharply, a brief, resonant tone will be produced. The clarity of the tone depends on the brevity of the action. The intensity of the tone varies with the force used. Photo © Ken Kasper.

**FIGURE 5-3.** Light palpation technique (*top*) and deep palpation (*bottom*). Photo © Ken Kasper.

ficial blood vessels, lymph nodes, thyroid gland, organs of the abdomen and pelvis, and rectum. When the abdomen is examined, auscultation is performed before palpation and percussion to avoid altering bowel sounds (Bickley & Szilagyi, 2003).

Sounds generated within the body, if within specified frequency ranges, also may be detected through touch. For example, certain murmurs generated in the heart or within blood vessels (thrills) may be detected. Thrills cause a sensation to the hand much like the purring of a cat. Voice sounds are transmitted along the bronchi to the periphery of the lung. These may be perceived by touch and may be altered by disorders affecting the lungs. The phenomenon is called *tactile fremitus* and is useful in assessing diseases of the chest. The significance of these findings is discussed in Chapters 21 and 26.

## Percussion

The technique of percussion (Fig. 5-4) translates the application of physical force into sound. It is a skill requiring practice that yields much information about disease processes in the chest and abdomen (Bickley & Szilagyi, 2003). The principle is to set the chest wall or abdominal wall into vibration by striking it with a firm object. The sound produced reflects the density of the underlying structure. Certain densities produce sounds as percussion notes. These sounds, listed in a sequence that proceeds from the least to the most dense, are tympany, hyperresonance, resonance, dullness, and flatness. Tympany is the drumlike sound produced by percussing the air-filled stomach. Hyperresonance is audible when one percusses over inflated lung tissue in a person with emphysema. Resonance is the sound elicited over air-filled lungs. Percussion of the liver produces a dull sound, whereas percussion of the thigh produces a flat sound.

Percussion allows the examiner to assess such normal anatomic details as the borders of the heart and the movement of the diaphragm during inspiration. It is also possible to determine the level of a pleural effusion (fluid in the pleural cavity) and the location of a consolidated area caused by pneumonia or atelectasis (collapse of alveoli). The use of percussion is described further with disorders of the thorax and abdomen (see Chapters 21 and 34).

## Auscultation

Auscultation is the skill of listening to sounds produced within the body created by the movement of air or fluid. Examples include breath sounds, the spoken voice, bowel sounds, heart sounds, and cardiac murmurs. Physiologic sounds may be normal (eg, first and second heart sounds) or pathologic (eg, heart murmurs in diastole, crackles in the lung). Some normal sounds may be distorted by abnormalities of structures through which the sound must travel (eg, changes in the character of breath sounds as they travel through the consolidated lung of a patient with lobar pneumonia).

Sound produced within the body, if of sufficient amplitude, may be detected with the stethoscope, which functions as an extension of the human ear and channels sound. Two end-pieces are available for the stethoscope: the bell and the diaphragm. The bell is used to assess very-low-frequency sounds such as diastolic heart murmurs. The entire surface of the bell's disk is placed lightly on the skin surface to avoid flattening the skin and reducing audible vibratory sensations. The diaphragm, the larger disk, is used to assess high-frequency sounds such as heart and lung sounds and is held in firm contact with the skin surface (Fig. 5-5). Touching the tubing or rubbing other surfaces (hair, clothing) during auscultation is avoided to minimize extraneous noises.

Sound produced by the body, like any other sound, is characterized by intensity, frequency, and quality. The *intensity*, or loudness, associated with physiologic sound is low; therefore, the use of the stethoscope is needed. The *frequency*, or pitch, of physiologic sound is in reality "noise," in that most sounds consist of a frequency spectrum, as opposed to the single-frequency sounds that we associate with music or a tuning fork. The frequency spectrum may be quite low, yielding a rumbling noise, or comparatively high, producing a harsh or blowing sound. *Quality* of sound relates to overtones that allow one to distinguish among various sounds. Sound quality enables the examiner to distinguish between the musical quality of high-pitched wheezing and the low-pitched rumbling of a diastolic murmur.

**FIGURE 5-5.** Technique for auscultating the heart.
Photo © B. Proud.

# Nutritional Assessment

Nutrition is important to maintain health and to prevent disease and death (Worthington, 2004). When illness or injury occurs, optimal nutrition is an essential factor in promoting healing and resisting infection and other complications. An in-depth nutritional assessment is often integrated into the health history and physical examination. Assessment of the patient's nutritional status provides information about obesity, weight loss, undernutrition, malnutrition, deficiencies in specific nutrients, metabolic abnormalities, the effects of medications on nutrition, and special problems affecting patients both in hospitals and in the home and other community settings.

Disorders caused by nutritional deficiency, overeating, or eating unhealthy meals are among the leading causes of illness and death in the United States today. The three leading causes of death—heart disease, cancer, and stroke—are related, in part, to consequences of unhealthy nutrition. A recent study of the fourth leading cause of death, chronic obstructive pulmonary disease (COPD), suggested that body mass index (BMI) is an important predictor of death in patients with COPD (Celli, Cote, Marin, et al., 2004). Other examples of health problems associated with poor nutrition include obesity, osteoporosis, cirrhosis, diverticulitis, and eating disorders.

Certain signs and symptoms that suggest possible nutritional deficiency, such as muscle wasting, poor skin integrity, loss of subcutaneous tissue, and obesity, are easy to note because they are specific; these should be pursued further. Other physical signs may be subtle and must be carefully assessed and pursued further (Worthington, 2004). For example, certain signs that appear to indicate nutritional deficiency may actually reflect other systemic conditions (eg, endocrine disorders, infectious disease). Others may result from impaired digestion, absorption, excretion, or storage of nutrients in the body.

The sequence of assessment of parameters may vary, but evaluation of nutritional status includes one or more of the following methods: measurement of BMI and waist circumference, biochemical measurements, clinical examination findings, and dietary data. The first two methods are discussed in this chapter.

Special considerations for nutritional assessment in the older adult are given in Chart 5-5.

## Body Mass Index

BMI is a ratio based on body weight and height. The obtained value is compared to the established standards; however, trends or changes in values over time are considered more useful than isolated or one-time measurements. BMI (Fig. 5-6) is highly correlated with body fat, but increased lean body mass or a large body frame can also increase the BMI. People who have a BMI lower than 24 (or who are 80% or less of their desirable body weight for height) are at increased risk for problems associated with poor nutritional status. In addition, a low BMI is associated with a higher mortality rate among hospitalized patients and

> **CHART 5-5**
>
>
>
> ## Nutritional Assessment in the Older Adult
>
> Nutritional screening in the elderly is a first step in maintaining adequate nutrition and replacing nutrient losses to maintain the individual's health and well being. In the United States, about 40% of hospitalized patients and 85% of those in nursing homes are estimated to be malnourished (Hogan, 2004). Elderly people who are malnourished tend to have longer and more expensive hospital stays than those who are adequately nourished; the risk of costly complications is also increased in malnourished patients (Dudek, 2006).
>
> Inadequate dietary intake in the elderly may result from physiologic changes in the gastrointestinal tract, social and economic factors, drug interactions, disease, excessive use of alcohol, and poor dentition or missing teeth. Malnutrition is a common consequence of these factors and in turn leads to illness and frailty of the elderly. Important aspects of care of the elderly in the hospital, home, outpatient setting, or extended care facility include recognizing risk factors and identifying those who are at risk for inadequate nutrition (Sabol, 2004).
>
> Many elderly people take excessive and inappropriate medications; this is referred to as polypharmacy. The number of adverse reactions increases proportionately with the number of prescribed and over-the-counter medications taken. Age-related physiologic and pathophysiologic changes may alter the metabolism and elimination of many medications. Medications can influence food intake by producing side effects such as nausea, vomiting, decreased appetite, and changes in sensorium. They may also interfere with the distribution, utilization, and storage of nutrients. Disorders affecting any part of the gastrointestinal tract can alter nutritional requirements and health status in people of any age; however, they are likely to occur more quickly and more frequently in the elderly.
>
> Nutritional problems in the elderly often occur or are precipitated by such illnesses as pneumonia and urinary tract infections. Acute and chronic diseases may affect the metabolism and utilization of nutrients, which already are altered by the aging process. Influenza and pneumonia immunizations, prompt treatment of bacterial infections, and social programs such as Meals on Wheels may reduce the risk of illness-associated malnutrition. Alcohol and substance abuse are potential factors in the elderly population that should not be overlooked (Finfgeld-Connett, 2004; Bridevaux, et al., 2004). Even the well elderly may be nutritionally at risk because of decreased odor perception, poor dental health, limited ability to shop and cook, financial hardship, and the fact that they often eat alone. Also, reduction in exercise with age without concomitant changes in carbohydrate intake places the elderly at risk for obesity.

community-dwelling elderly. Those who have a BMI of 25 to 29 are considered overweight; those with a BMI of 30 to 39, obese; and those with a BMI greater than 40, extremely obese (Dudek, 2006). In analyzing BMI, the nurse must be aware that cutoff scores for normal, overweight, and obese may differ for different ethnic groups (Wildman, Gu, Reynolds, et al., 2004).

It is important to assess for usual body weight and height and to compare these values with ideal weight (Chart 5-6). Current weight does not provide information about recent changes in weight; therefore, patients are asked about their usual body weight. Loss of height may be due to osteoporosis, an important problem related to nutrition, especially in postmenopausal women (USDHHS Public Health Service, 2004). A loss of 2 or 3 inches of height may indicate osteoporosis.

In addition to the calculation of BMI, waist circumference measurement is particularly useful for adult patients who are categorized as being of normal weight or overweight (Dudek, 2006). To measure waist circumference, a tape measure is placed in a horizontal plane around the abdomen at the level of the iliac crest. A waist circumference greater than 40 inches for men or 35 inches for women indicates excess abdominal fat. Those with a high waist circumference are at increased risk for diabetes, dyslipidemias, hypertension, cardiovascular disease, and atrial fibrillation (Wang, Parise, Levy, et al., 2004).

## Biochemical Assessment

Biochemical assessment reflects both the tissue level of a given nutrient and any abnormality of metabolism in the utilization of nutrients. These determinations are made from studies of serum (albumin and globulin, transferrin, retinol-binding protein, electrolytes, hemoglobin, vitamin A, carotene, and vitamin C) and studies of urine (creatinine, thiamine, riboflavin, niacin, and iodine). Some of these tests, while reflecting recent intake of the elements detected, can also identify below-normal levels when there are no clinical symptoms of deficiency. See Table 5-1 for guidelines for interpreting albumin and prealbumin levels.

Low serum albumin and prealbumin levels are most often used as measures of protein deficit in adults (Dudek,

## Body Mass Index

The body mass index (BMI) is used to determine who is overweight.

$$BMI = \frac{703 \times \text{weight in pounds}}{(\text{height in inches})^2} \quad OR \quad \frac{\text{weight in kilograms}}{(\text{height in meters})^2}$$

BMI score is at the intersection of height and weight. A body mass index score of 25 or more is considered overweight and 30 or more is considered obese.

**25** Overweight Limit    Overweight

| Weight | 100 | 105 | 110 | 115 | 120 | 125 | 130 | 135 | 140 | 145 | 150 | 155 | 160 | 165 | 170 | 175 | 180 | 185 | 190 | 195 | 200 | 205 |
|---|---|---|---|---|---|---|---|---|---|---|---|---|---|---|---|---|---|---|---|---|---|---|
| Height |   |   |   |   |   |   |   |   |   |   |   |   |   |   |   |   |   |   |   |   |   |   |
| 5'0" | 20 | 21 | 21 | 22 | 23 | 24 | 25 | 26 | 27 | 28 | 29 | 30 | 31 | 32 | 33 | 34 | 35 | 36 | 37 | 38 | 39 | 40 |
| 5'1" | 19 | 20 | 21 | 22 | 23 | 24 | 25 | 26 | 26 | 27 | 28 | 29 | 30 | 31 | 32 | 33 | 34 | 35 | 36 | 37 | 38 | 39 |
| 5'2" | 18 | 19 | 20 | 21 | 22 | 23 | 24 | 25 | 26 | 27 | 27 | 28 | 29 | 30 | 31 | 32 | 33 | 34 | 35 | 36 | 37 | 37 |
| 5'3" | 18 | 19 | 19 | 20 | 21 | 22 | 23 | 24 | 25 | 26 | 27 | 27 | 28 | 29 | 30 | 31 | 32 | 33 | 34 | 35 | 35 | 36 |
| 5'4" | 17 | 18 | 19 | 20 | 21 | 21 | 22 | 23 | 24 | 25 | 26 | 27 | 27 | 28 | 29 | 30 | 31 | 32 | 33 | 33 | 34 | 35 |
| 5'5" | 17 | 17 | 18 | 19 | 20 | 21 | 22 | 22 | 23 | 24 | 25 | 26 | 27 | 27 | 28 | 29 | 30 | 31 | 32 | 32 | 33 | 34 |
| 5'6" | 16 | 17 | 18 | 19 | 19 | 20 | 21 | 22 | 23 | 23 | 24 | 25 | 26 | 27 | 27 | 28 | 29 | 30 | 31 | 31 | 32 | 33 |
| 5'7" | 16 | 16 | 17 | 18 | 19 | 20 | 21 | 22 | 23 | 23 | 24 | 25 | 26 | 27 | 27 | 28 | 29 | 30 | 31 | 31 | 32 | 32 |
| 5'8" | 15 | 16 | 17 | 17 | 18 | 19 | 20 | 21 | 21 | 22 | 23 | 24 | 24 | 25 | 26 | 27 | 27 | 28 | 29 | 30 | 30 | 31 |
| 5'9" | 15 | 16 | 16 | 17 | 18 | 18 | 19 | 20 | 21 | 21 | 22 | 23 | 24 | 24 | 25 | 26 | 27 | 27 | 28 | 29 | 30 | 30 |
| 5'10" | 14 | 15 | 16 | 17 | 17 | 18 | 19 | 19 | 20 | 21 | 22 | 22 | 23 | 24 | 24 | 25 | 26 | 27 | 27 | 28 | 29 | 29 |
| 5'11" | 14 | 15 | 15 | 16 | 17 | 17 | 18 | 19 | 20 | 20 | 21 | 22 | 22 | 23 | 24 | 24 | 25 | 26 | 26 | 27 | 28 | 29 |
| 6'0" | 14 | 14 | 15 | 16 | 16 | 17 | 18 | 18 | 19 | 20 | 20 | 21 | 22 | 22 | 23 | 24 | 24 | 25 | 26 | 26 | 27 | 28 |
| 6'1" | 13 | 14 | 15 | 15 | 16 | 16 | 17 | 18 | 18 | 19 | 20 | 20 | 21 | 22 | 22 | 23 | 24 | 24 | 25 | 26 | 26 | 27 |
| 6'2" | 13 | 13 | 14 | 15 | 15 | 16 | 17 | 17 | 18 | 19 | 19 | 20 | 21 | 21 | 22 | 22 | 23 | 24 | 24 | 25 | 26 | 26 |
| 6'3" | 12 | 13 | 14 | 14 | 15 | 16 | 16 | 17 | 17 | 18 | 19 | 19 | 20 | 21 | 21 | 22 | 22 | 23 | 24 | 24 | 25 | 26 |
| 6'4" | 12 | 13 | 13 | 14 | 15 | 15 | 16 | 16 | 17 | 18 | 18 | 19 | 19 | 20 | 21 | 21 | 22 | 23 | 23 | 24 | 24 | 25 |

Source: Shape Up America. National Institutes of Health

**FIGURE 5-6.** Body mass index.

---

### CHART 5-6

## Calculating Ideal Body Weight

**WOMEN**
- Allow 100 lb for 5 feet of height.
- Add 5 lb for each additional inch over 5 feet.
- Subtract 10% for small frame; add 10% for large frame.

**MEN**
- Allow 106 lb for 5 feet of height.
- Add 6 lb for each additional inch over 5 feet.
- Subtract 10% for small frame, add 10% for large frame.

**Example**: Ideal body weight for a 5'6" adult is

|  | Female | Male |
|---|---|---|
| 5' of height | 100 lb | 106 lb |
| Per additional inch | 6" × 5 lb/inch = 30 lb | 6" × 6 lb/inch = 36 lb |
| Ideal body weight | 130 lb ± 13 lb depending on frame size | 142 lb ± 14 lb depending on frame size |

---

2006; Worthington, 2004). Albumin synthesis depends on normal liver function and an adequate supply of amino acids. Because the body stores a large amount of albumin, the serum albumin level may not decrease until malnutrition is severe; therefore, its usefulness in detecting recent protein depletion is limited. Decreased albumin levels may be caused by overhydration, liver or renal disease, or excessive protein loss due to burns, major surgery, infection, or cancer. Serial measurements of prealbumin levels are also used to assess the results of nutritional therapy (Worthington, 2004). Prealbumin, also called thyroxin-binding protein, is

**TABLE 5-1  General Guidelines for Interpreting Albumin and Prealbumin Levels**

| Interpretation | Albumin (g/dL) | Prealbumin (mg/dL) |
|---|---|---|
| Normal | 3.5–5.5 | 23–43 |
| Mild depletion | 2.8–3.4 | 10–15 |
| Moderate depletion | 2.1–2.7 | 5–9 |
| Severe depletion | <2.1 | <5 |

From Dudek, S. G. (2006). *Nutrition essentials for nursing practice* (5th ed.). Philadelphia: Lippincott Williams & Wilkins.

a more sensitive indicator of protein status than albumin, but the test is more expensive and therefore less frequently ordered (Dudek, 2006).

Additional laboratory data, such as levels of transferrin and retinol-binding protein, anergy panels, lymphocyte and electrolyte counts, are used in many institutions (Sabol, 2004). Transferrin is a protein that binds and carries iron from the intestine through the serum. Because of its short half-life, transferrin levels decrease more quickly than albumin levels in response to protein depletion. Although measurement of retinol-binding protein is not available from many laboratories, it may be a useful means of monitoring acute, short-term changes in protein status. The total lymphocyte count may be reduced in people who are acutely malnourished as a result of stress and low-calorie feeding and in those with impaired cellular immunity. Anergy, the absence of an immune response to injection of small concentrations of recall antigen under the skin, may also indicate malnutrition because of delayed antibody synthesis and response. Serum electrolyte levels provide information about fluid and electrolyte balance and kidney function. The creatinine/height index calculated over a 24-hour period assesses the metabolically active tissue and indicates the degree of protein depletion, comparing expected body mass for height with actual body cell mass. A 24-hour urine sample is obtained, and the amount of creatinine is measured and compared to normal ranges based on the patient's height and gender. Values lower than normal may indicate loss of lean body mass and protein malnutrition.

## Clinical Examination

The state of nutrition is often reflected in a person's appearance. Although the most obvious physical sign of good nutrition is a normal body weight with respect to height, body frame, and age, other tissues can serve as indicators of general nutritional status and adequate intake of specific nutrients; these include the hair, skin, teeth, gums, mucous membranes, mouth and tongue, skeletal muscles, abdomen, lower extremities, and thyroid gland (Table 5-2). Specific aspects of clinical examination that are useful in identifying nutritional deficits include oral examination and assessment of skin for turgor, edema, elasticity, dryness, subcutaneous tone, poorly healing wounds and ulcers, purpura, and bruises (Roth & Townsend, 2003; Worthington, 2004). The musculoskeletal examination also provides information about muscle wasting and weakness.

## Dietary Data

Commonly used methods of determining individual eating patterns include the food record and the 24-hour food recall, which help estimate whether food intake is adequate

### TABLE 5-2  Physical Indicators of Nutritional Status

| Indicator | Signs of Good Nutrition | Signs of Poor Nutrition |
|---|---|---|
| General appearance | Alert, responsive | Listless, appears acutely or chronically ill |
| Hair | Shiny, lustrous; firm, healthy scalp | Dull and dry, brittle, depigmented, easily plucked; thin and sparse |
| Face | Skin color uniform; healthy appearance | Skin dark over cheeks and under eyes, skin flaky, face swollen or hollow/sunken cheeks |
| Eyes | Bright, clear, moist | Eye membranes pale, dry (xerophthalmia); increased vascularity, cornea soft (keratomalacia) |
| Lips | Good color (pink), smooth | Swollen and puffy; angular lesion at corners of mouth (cheilosis) |
| Tongue | Deep red in appearance; surface papillae present | Smooth appearance, swollen, beefy-red, sores, atrophic papillae |
| Teeth | Straight, no crowding, no dental caries, bright | Dental caries, mottled appearance (fluorosis), malpositioned |
| Gums | Firm, good color (pink) | Spongy, bleed easily, marginal redness, recession |
| Thyroid | No enlargement of the thyroid | Thyroid enlargement (simple goiter) |
| Skin | Smooth, good color, moist | Rough, dry, flaky, swollen, pale, pigmented; lack of fat under skin |
| Nails | Firm, pink | Spoon-shaped, ridged, brittle |
| Skeleton | Good posture, no malformation | Poor posture, beading of ribs, bowed legs or knock knees |
| Muscles | Well developed, firm | Flaccid, poor tone, wasted, underdeveloped |
| Extremities | No tenderness | Weak and tender; edematous |
| Abdomen | Flat | Swollen |
| Nervous system | Normal reflexes | Decreased or absent ankle and knee reflexes |
| Weight | Normal for height, age, and body build | Overweight or underweight |

and appropriate. If these methods are used to obtain the dietary history, instructions must be given to the patient about measuring and recording food intake.

## Food Record

The food record is used most often in nutritional status studies. A person is instructed to keep a record of food actually consumed over a period of time, varying from 3 to 7 days, and to accurately estimate and describe the specific foods consumed. Food records are fairly accurate if the person is willing to provide factual information and able to estimate food quantities.

## 24-Hour Recall

As the name implies, the 24-hour recall method is a recall of food intake over a 24-hour period. A person is asked to recall all foods eaten during the previous day and to estimate the quantities of each food consumed. Because information does not always represent usual intake, at the end of the interview the patient is asked whether the previous day's food intake was typical. To obtain supplementary information about the typical diet, it is also necessary to ask how frequently the person eats foods from the major food groups.

## Conducting the Dietary Interview

The success of the interviewer in obtaining information for dietary assessment depends on effective communication, which requires that good rapport be established to promote respect and trust. The interviewer explains the purpose of the interview. The interview is conducted in a nondirective and exploratory way, allowing the respondent to express feelings and thoughts while encouraging him or her to answer specific questions. The manner in which questions are asked influences the respondent's cooperation. The interviewer must be nonjudgmental and avoid expressing disapproval, either by verbal comments or by facial expression.

### CHARACTER OF GENERAL INTAKE

Several questions may be necessary to elicit the information needed. When attempting to elicit information about the type and quantity of food eaten at a particular time, leading questions such as, "Do you use sugar or cream in your coffee?" should be avoided. In addition, assumptions are not made about the size of servings; instead, questions are phrased so that quantities are more clearly determined. For example, to help determine the size of one hamburger, the patient may be asked, "How many servings were prepared with the pound of meat you bought?" Another approach to determining quantities is to use food models of known sizes in estimating portions of meat, cake, or pie, or to record quantities in common measurements, such as cups or spoonfuls (or the size of containers, when discussing intake of bottled beverages).

In recording a particular combination dish, such as a casserole, it is useful to ask about the ingredients, recording the largest quantities first. When recording quantities of ingredients, the interviewer notes whether the food item was raw or cooked and the number of servings provided by the recipe. When a patient lists the foods for the recall questionnaire, it may help to read back the list of foods and ask whether anything was forgotten, such as fruit, cake, candy, between-meal snacks, or alcoholic beverages.

Additional information obtained during the interview should include methods of preparing food, sources available for food (including donated foods and food stamps), food-buying practices, use of vitamin and mineral supplements, and income range.

### CULTURAL AND RELIGIOUS CONSIDERATIONS

An individual's culture determines to a large extent which foods are eaten and how they are prepared and served. Culture and religious practices together often determine whether certain foods are prohibited and whether certain foods and spices are eaten on certain holidays or at specific family gatherings. Because of the importance of culture and religious beliefs to many individuals, it is important to be sensitive to these factors when obtaining a dietary history. It is, however, equally important not to stereotype individuals and assume that, because they are from a certain culture or religious group, they adhere to specific dietary customs. One particular area of consideration is the presence of fish and shellfish in the diet and their methods of collection and preparation. These methods may put certain populations at risk for toxicity due to contaminants (Judd, Griffith & Faustman, 2004). Culturally sensitive materials, such as the food pagoda and the Mediterranean Pyramid, are available for making appropriate dietary recommendations (U.S. Department of Agriculture, 2005; Worthington, 2004).

### EVALUATING DIETARY INFORMATION

After obtaining basic dietary information, the nurse evaluates the patient's dietary intake and communicates the information to the dietitian and the rest of the health care team for more detailed assessment and for clinical nutrition intervention. If the goal is to determine whether the patient generally eats a healthful diet, his or her food intake may be compared with the dietary guidelines outlined in the U.S. Department of Agriculture's Food Guide Pyramid (Fig. 5-7). The pyramid divides foods into five major groups (grains, vegetables, fruits, milk products, and meat and beans), plus fats and oils. Recommendations are provided for variety in the diet, proportion of food from each food group, and moderation in eating fats, oils, and sweets. A person's food intake is compared with recommendations based on various food groups for various age levels (Roth & Townsend, 2003; Stotts & Deitrich, 2004).

If nurses or dietitians are interested in knowing about the intake of specific nutrients, such as vitamin A, iron, or calcium, the patient's food intake is analyzed by consulting

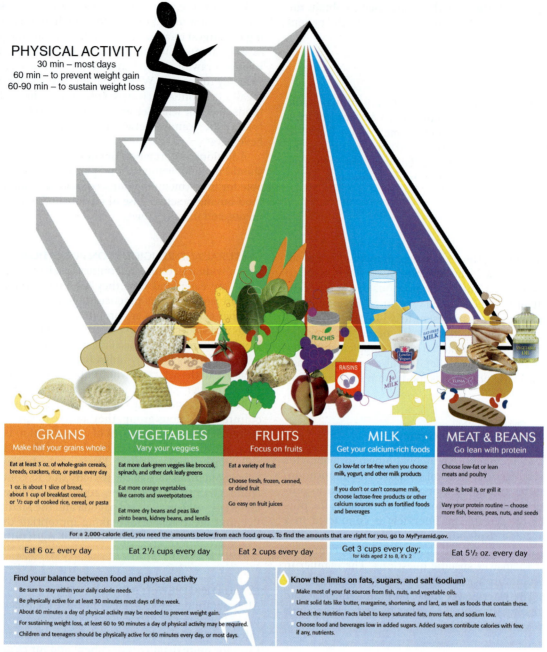

**FIGURE 5-7.** MyPyramid emphasizes foods from the five major food groups. Each of these food groups provides some, but not all, of the nutrients an adult needs. Foods in one group cannot replace those in another. No one of these major food groups is more important than another. (Source: U.S. Department of Agriculture & U.S. Department of Health and Human Services, 2005.)

a list of foods and their composition and nutrient content (Roth & Townsend, 2003). The diet is analyzed in terms of grams and milligrams of specific nutrients. The total nutritive value is then compared with the recommended dietary allowances specific for the patient's age category, gender, and special circumstances such as pregnancy or lactation (Worthington, 2004).

Fat intake and cholesterol levels are additional aspects of the nutritional assessment. Trans fats are produced when hydrogen atoms are added to monounsaturated or polyunsaturated fats to produce a semisolid product, such as margarine (Roth & Townsend, 2003). Trans fats, which are contained in many baked goods and restaurant foods, are a concern, because increased amounts of trans fats have been associated with increased risk for heart disease and stroke (Satchithanandam, Oles, Spease, et al., 2004). Effective January 2006, the Food and Drug Administration has amended food labeling regulations to require the inclusion of trans fats information on food labels (Satchithanandam et al., 2004).

## Factors Influencing Nutritional Status in Various Situations

One sensitive indicator of the body's gain or loss of protein is its nitrogen balance. An adult is said to be in nitrogen equilibrium when the nitrogen intake (from food) equals the nitrogen output (in urine, feces, and perspiration); it is a sign of health. A positive nitrogen balance exists when nitrogen intake exceeds nitrogen output and indicates tissue growth, such as occurs during pregnancy, childhood, recovery from surgery, and rebuilding of wasted tissue. A negative nitrogen balance indicates that tissue is breaking down faster than it is being replaced. In the absence of an adequate intake of protein, the body converts protein to glucose for energy. This can occur with fever, starvation, surgery, burns, and debilitating diseases. Each gram of nitrogen loss in excess of intake represents the depletion of 6.25 g of protein or 25 g of muscle tissue. Therefore, a negative nitrogen balance of 10 g/day for 10 days could mean the wasting of 2.5 kg (5.5 lb) of muscle tissue as it is converted to glucose for energy.

When conditions that result in negative nitrogen balance are combined with anorexia (loss of appetite), they can lead to malnutrition. Malnutrition interferes with wound healing, increases susceptibility to infection, and contributes to an increased incidence of complications, longer hospital stays, and prolonged confinement of patients to bed (Roth & Townsend, 2003).

Patients who are hospitalized may have an inadequate dietary intake because of the illness or disorder that necessitated the hospital stay or because the hospital's food is unfamiliar or unappealing (Worthington, 2004). Patients who are cared for at home may feel too sick or fatigued to shop and prepare food, or they may be unable to eat because of other physical problems or limitations. Limited or fixed incomes or the high costs of medications may result in insufficient money to buy nutritious foods. Patients with inadequate housing or inadequate cooking facilities are unlikely to have an adequate nutritional intake. Because complex treatments (eg, ventilators, intravenous infusions, chemotherapy), once used only in the hospital setting, are now being provided in the home and outpatient settings, nutritional assessment of patients in these settings is an important aspect of home and community-based care (Sabol, 2004; Worthington, 2004).

Many medications influence nutritional status by suppressing the appetite, irritating the oral or gastric mucosa, or causing nausea and vomiting. Others may influence bacterial flora in the intestine or directly affect nutrient absorption so that secondary malnutrition results. People who must take many medications in a single day often report feeling too full to eat. A patient's use of prescription and OTC medications and their effects on appetite and dietary intake are assessed. Many of the factors that contribute to poor nutritional status are identified in Table 5-3.

## Analysis of Nutritional Status

Physical measurements (BMI, waist circumference) and biochemical, clinical, and dietary data are used in combination to determine a patient's nutritional status. Often, these data provide more information about the patient's nutritional status than the clinical examination, which

### TABLE 5-3  Factors Associated With Potential Nutritional Deficits

| Factor | Possible Consequences |
| --- | --- |
| Dental and oral problems (missing teeth, ill-fitting dentures, impaired swallowing or chewing) | Inadequate intake of high-fiber foods |
| NPO for diagnostic testing | Inadequate caloric and protein intake; dehydration |
| Prolonged use of glucose and saline IV fluids | Inadequate caloric and protein intake |
| Nausea and vomiting | Inadequate caloric and protein intake; loss of fluid, electrolytes, and minerals |
| Stress of illness, surgery, and/or hospitalization | Increased protein and caloric requirement; increased catabolism |
| Wound drainage | Loss of protein, fluid, electrolytes, and minerals |
| Pain | Loss of appetite; inability to shop, cook, eat |
| Fever | Increased caloric and fluid requirement; increased catabolism |
| Gastrointestinal intubation | Loss of protein, fluid, and minerals |
| Tube feedings | Inadequate amounts; various nutrients in each formula |
| Gastrointestinal disease | Inadequate intake and malabsorption of nutrients |
| Alcoholism | Inadequate intake of nutrients; increased consumption of calories without other nutrients; vitamin deficiencies |
| Depression | Loss of appetite; inability to shop, cook, eat |
| Eating disorders (anorexia, bulimia) | Inadequate caloric and protein intake; loss of fluid, electrolytes, and minerals |
| Medications | Inadequate intake due to medication side effects, such as dry mouth, loss of appetite, decreased taste perception, difficulty swallowing, nausea and vomiting, physical problems that limit shopping, cooking, eating; malabsorption of nutrients |
| Restricted ambulation or disability | Inability to help self to food, liquids, other nutrients |

may not detect subclinical deficiencies unless they become so advanced that overt signs develop. A low intake of nutrients over a long period may lead to low biochemical levels and, without nutritional intervention, may result in characteristic and observable signs and symptoms (see Table 5-2). A plan of action for nutritional intervention is based on the results of the dietary assessment and the patient's clinical profile. To be effective, the plan must meet the patient's need for a healthy diet, maintain (or control) weight, and compensate for increased nutritional needs.

### Considerations in Adolescents

Adolescence is a time of critical growth and acquisition of lifelong eating habits, and therefore nutritional assessment and analysis are critical. In the past two decades, the percentage of adolescents who are overweight has almost tripled (USDHHS, 2001). Total milk consumption has decreased by 36% compared to prior years (Cavadini, Siega-Riz & Popkin, 2000), and fruit and vegetable consumption is also lower than the recommended five servings per day.

Adolescent girls are at particular nutritional risk, because iron, folate, and calcium intakes are below recommended levels. Adolescents with other nutritional disorders, such as anorexia and bulimia, have a better chance of recovery if these disorders are identified in the adolescent years rather than in adulthood (USDHHS, 2001).

## Assessment in the Home and Community

Assessment of people in community settings, including the home, consists of collecting information specific to existing health problems, including data on the patient's physiologic and emotional status, the community and home environment, the adequacy of support systems or care given by family and other care providers, and the availability of needed resources. In addition, it is important to evaluate the ability of the individual and family to cope with and address their respective needs. The physi-

---

**CHART 5-7**

### Assessing the Home Environment

**PHYSICAL FACILITIES** (check all that apply)
*Exterior*
- ☐ steps_____
- ☐ unsafe steps_____
- ☐ porch_____
- ☐ litter_____
- ☐ noise_____
- ☐ inadequate lighting_____
- ☐ other_____

*Interior*
- ☐ accessible bathroom_____
- ☐ level, safe floor surface____
- ☐ number of rooms_____
- ☐ privacy_____
- ☐ sleeping arrangements____
- ☐ refrigeration_____
- ☐ trash management_____
- ☐ animals_____
- ☐ adequate lighting_____
- ☐ steps/stairs_____
- ☐ other_____

**SAFETY HAZARDS** found in the patient's current residence (check all that apply)
- ☐ none
- ☐ inadequate floor, roof, or windows
- ☐ inadequate lighting
- ☐ unsafe gas/electric appliances
- ☐ inadequate heating
- ☐ inadequate cooling
- ☐ lack of fire safety devices
- ☐ unsafe floor coverings
- ☐ inadequate stair rails
- ☐ lead-based paint
- ☐ improperly stored hazardous material
- ☐ improper wiring/electrical cords
- ☐ other_____

**SAFETY FACTORS** (check all that apply)
- ☐ fire/smoke detectors_____
- ☐ telephone_____
- ☐ placement of electrical cords____
- ☐ emergency plan_____
- ☐ emergency phone numbers displayed____
- ☐ safe portable heaters_____
- ☐ obstacle-free paths_____
- ☐ other_____

cal assessment in the community and home consists of the same techniques used in the hospital, outpatient clinic, or office setting. Privacy is provided, and the person is made as comfortable as possible.

Before the first home visit, the nurse usually calls the patient's home to let the patient know when to expect the home care nurse; this also gives the patient's primary caregiver the opportunity to be available. During the home visit, assessment is not limited to physical assessment of the patient. Other aspects of assessment include the home environment, safety factors (eg, smoke alarms, obstacles, safety bars in the bathroom, emergency evacuation plans), adequacy of facilities required for the patient's care and recovery, accessibility if the patient has a disability, food preparation and storage facilities, bathroom facilities, access to a telephone, and the availability of family and community supports (Chart 5-7). The patient may have no family members available to assist him or her and may live alone in substandard housing or in a shelter for the homeless. Therefore the nurse must be aware of resources available in the community and methods of obtaining those resources for the patient.

## Critical Thinking Exercises

1. Identify the approach and techniques you would use to perform an admission assessment on a 58-year-old woman with metastatic lung cancer. How would your approach and technique differ if the patient has metastatic lesions to the brain and is disoriented? If the patient is disoriented and blind or hard of hearing? If the patient is from a culture with very different values from yours?

2. Your health history and physical examination of a young adult female patient with cognitive impairment alerts you to the possibility of sexual abuse. Explain how you would pursue this. What assessments are available to assist in a more comprehensive evaluation? How would you modify your assessment to evaluate the patient for other forms of abuse?

3. **ebp** You are conducting a health history on a middle-aged patient and inquire about immunizations. What resources would you use to identify the current adult immunization schedule? What is the evidence base for the use of health history questionnaires versus serotesting for immunization status? Discuss the strength of the evidence for the method you think is most effective in identifying immunization status. Identify the criteria used to evaluate the strength of the evidence for this practice.

4. **ebp** Your health assessment of a male college freshman reveals that he has a high fat intake, has minimal calcium intake, and gets little exercise. What recommendations would you make for this patient? If the patient is a vegetarian, what dietary instructions would you develop for him? What is the evidence base for the type of instructional method to use with an adolescent patient? Identify the criteria used to evaluate the strength of the evidence for this practice.

5. How would you modify your health history and physical assessment technique if your patient has the following disabilities: (1) paraplegia due to spinal cord injury, (2) profound hearing loss, (3) blindness, or (4) impaired communication due to aphasia secondary to stroke?

6. You have received a referral for home care for a 75-year-old patient who has recently had a stroke and who lives alone in a trailer. What physical and environmental factors are important to assess on the initial home visit? Identify the elements in the home that would be safety hazards and those that would be safety factors to assess.

## REFERENCES AND SELECTED READINGS

### BOOKS

Advisory Committee on Immunization Practices (ACIP). (2005). *Recommended adult immunization schedule, United States, October 2004–September 2005*. U.S. Department of Health and Human Services, Centers for Disease Control and Prevention. Available at: www.cdc.gov/nip/recs/adult-schedule.pdf (accessed May 4, 2006).

Bickley, L. S. & Szilagyi, P. G. (2003). *Bates' guide to physical examination and history taking* (8th ed.). Philadelphia: Lippincott Williams & Wilkins.

Dudek, S. G. (2006). *Nutrition essentials for nursing practice* (5th ed.). Philadelphia: Lippincott Williams & Wilkins.

Eng, T. (2001). *The eHealth landscape: A terrain map of emerging information and communication technologies in health and health care*. Princeton, NJ: Robert Wood Johnson Foundation.

Food and Nutrition Board, Institutes of Medicine. (2002). *Dietary reference intakes for energy, carbohydrates, fiber, fat, protein and amino acids (macronutrients): A report of the Panel on Micronutrients, Subcommittees on Upper Reference Levels of Nutrients and Interpretation and Uses of Dietary Reference Intakes, and the Standing Committee on the Scientific Evaluation of Dietary Reference Intakes*. Washington, DC: National Academy Press.

Klimis-Zaras, D. & Wolinsky, I. (2004). *Nutritional concerns for women* (2nd ed.). New York: CRC Press.

Melnyk, B. M. & Fineout-Overholt, E. (2005). *Evidence-based practice in nursing and healthcare: A guide to best practices*. Philadelphia: Lippincott Williams & Wilkins.

NANDA International. (2005). *Nursing diagnoses: Definitions and classification 2005–2006*. Philadelphia: North American Nursing Diagnosis Association.

Orient, J. (2005). *Sapira's art and science of bedside diagnosis* (3rd ed.). Philadelphia: Lippincott Williams & Wilkins.

Porth, C. M. (2005). *Pathophysiology: Concepts of altered health states* (7th ed.). Philadelphia: Lippincott Williams & Wilkins.

Roth, R. & Townsend, C. E. (2003). *Nutrition & diet therapy* (8th ed.). Clifton Park: Delmar Learning.

Stanley, M., Blair, K. A. & Beare, P. G. (2005). *Gerontological nursing: Promoting successful aging with older adults* (3rd ed). Philadelphia: F. A. Davis.

U.S. Department of Agriculture, Center for Nutrition Policy and Promotion. (2005). *My Pyramid: Steps to a healthier you.* April 2005. Available at: http://www.mypyramid.gov/ (accessed March 5, 2006).

U.S. Department of Agriculture & U.S. Department of Health and Human Services. (2005). *Dietary guidelines for Americans* (5th ed). Available at: http://www.healthierus.gov/dietaryguidelines/index.html (accessed March 5, 2006).

U.S. Department of Health and Human Services. (2004). *Bone health and osteoporosis: A report of the Surgeon General.* Rockville, MD: USDHHS.

U.S. Department of Health and Human Services Centers for Disease Control and Prevention. (2003). *A public health action plan to prevent heart disease and stroke.* Atlanta: USDHHS.

U.S. Department of Health and Human Services Public Health Service. (2001). *The Surgeon General's call to action to prevent and decrease overweight and obesity.* Rockville, MD: USDHHS.

Weber, J. & Kelley, J. (2003). *Health assessment in nursing* (2nd ed.). Philadelphia: Lippincott Williams & Wilkins.

Worthington, P. H. (2004). *Practical aspects of nutritional support.* Philadelphia: Saunders.

## JOURNALS

*An asterisk indicates a nursing research article.

### General Assessment

Bridevaux, I. P., Bradley, K. A., Bryson, C. L., et al. (2004). Alcohol screening results in elderly male veterans: Association with health status and mortality. *Journal of the American Geriatrics Society, 52*(9), 1510–1517.

Burnham, B. R., Thompson, D. F. & Jackson, W. G. (2002). Positive predictive value of a health history questionnaire. *Military Medicine, 167*(8), 639–642.

Capriotti, T. (2004). Any science behind the hype of natural dietary supplements? *MedSurg Nursing, 13*(5), 339–347.

Fiellin, D. A., Reid, M. C. & O'Connor, P. G. (2000). Screening for alcohol problems in primary care: A systematic review. *Archives of Internal Medicine, 160*(13), 1977–1989.

Finfgeld-Connett, D. (2004). Treatment of substance misuse in older women. *Journal of Gerontological Nursing, 30*(8), 30–37.

Flowers, D. L. (2004). Culturally competent nursing care: A challenge for the 21st century. *Critical Care Nurse, 24*(4), 48–52.

Fulmer, T. (2003). Elder abuse and neglect assessment. *Journal of Gerontological Nursing, 29*(1), 8–9.

Guttmacher, A. E., Collins, F. S. & Carmona, R. H. (2004). The family history: More important than ever. *New England Journal of Medicine, 351*(22), 2333–2336.

Iezzoni, L. I., O'Day, B. L., Killeen, M., et al. (2004). Communicating about health care: Observations from persons who are deaf or hard of hearing. *Annals of Internal Medicine, 140*(5), 356–362.

Judd, N. L., Griffith, W. C. & Faustman, E. M. (2004). Consideration of cultural and lifestyle factors in defining susceptible populations for environmental disease. *Toxicology, 198*(1–3), 121–133.

Kinzie, M. B., Cohn, W., Julian, M. F., et al. (2002). A user-centered model for web site design: Needs assessment, user interface design, and rapid prototyping. *Journal of the American Medical Informatics Association, 9*(4), 320–330.

*Loeb, S. (2004). Older men's health. *Nursing Research, 53*(3), 198–206.

McFarlane, J., Hughes, R. B., Nosek, M. A., et al. (2001). Abuse Assessment Screen—Disability (AAS-D): Measuring frequency, type, and perpetrator of abuse toward women with physical disabilities. *Journal of Women's Health and Gender-Based Medicine, 10*(9), 861–866.

Nusbaum, M. R. H. & Hamilton, C. D. (2002). The proactive sexual health history. *American Family Physician, 66*(9), 1705–1712.

Rasmor, M. & Brown, C. M. (2003). Physical examination for the occupational health nurse. *AAOHN Journal, 51*(9), 390–401.

Rhodes, K. V., Lauderdale, D., He, T., Howes, D. S. & Levinson, W. (2002). "Between me and the computer": Increased detection of intimate partner violence using a computer questionnaire. *Annals of Emergency Medicine, 40*(5), 476–484.

Rosenthal, R. A. & Kavic, S. M. (2004). Assessment and management of the geriatric patient. *Critical Care Medicine, 32*(4), S92–S105.

Sanchez, A. M., Schreiber, G., Glynn, S., et al. (2003). Blood-donor perceptions of health history screening with a computer-assisted self-administered interview. *Transfusion, 43*(2), 165–172.

Smeltzer, S. C., Zimmerman, V. & Capriotti, T. (2005). Bone mineral density and osteoporosis risks in women with disabilities. *Archives of Physical Medicine and Rehabilitation, 86*(3), 582–586.

Smeltzer, S. C., Zimmerman, V., DeSilets, L. D., et al. (2003). Accessible online health promotion information for persons with disabilities. *Online Journal of Issues in Nursing, 9*(1), 11. Available at: http://nursingworld.org/ojin/topic16/tpc16_5.htm (accessed May 5, 2006).

Steinbrook, R. (2004). Medical marijuana, physician-assisted suicide, and the Controlled Substances Act. *New England Journal of Medicine, 351*(14), 1380–1383.

Stotts, N. A. & Deitrich, C. E. (2004). The challenge to come: The care of older adults. *American Journal of Nursing, 104*(8), 40–47.

Westermeyer, J., Yargic, I. & Thuras, P. (2004). Michigan Assessment Screening Test for Alcohol and Drugs (MAST/AD): Evaluation in a clinical sample. *American Journal on Addictions, 13*(2), 151–162.

*Yarcheski, A., Mahon, N. E., Yarcheski, T. J., et al. (2004). A meta-analysis of predictors of positive health practices. *Journal of Nursing Scholarship, 36*(2), 102–108.

### Nutritional Assessment

Celli, B. R., Cote, C. G., Marin, J. M., et al. (2004). The body-mass index, airflow obstruction, dyspnea, and exercise capacity index in chronic obstructive pulmonary disease. *New England Journal of Medicine, 350*(10), 1005–1012.

Cavadini, C., Siega-Riz, A. M. & Popkin, B. M. (2000). US adolescent food intake trends from 1965 to 1996. *Archives of Disease in Childhood, 83*(1), 18–24.

Hogan, S. L. (2004). How to help wounds heal. *RN, 67*(8), 26–31.

Sabol, V. (2004). Nutritional assessment of the critically ill adult. *AACN Clinical Issues, 15*(4), 595–606.

Satchithanandam, S., Oles, C. J., Spease, C. J., et al. (2004). Trans, saturated, and unsaturated fat in foods in the United States prior to mandatory trans-fat labeling. *Lipids, 39*(1), 11–18.

Sharts-Hopko, N. C. & Sullivan, M. P. (2003). Obesity as a confounding health factor among women with mobility impairment. *Journal of the American Academy of Nurse Practitioners, 15*(10), 438–443.

Wang, T. J., Parise, H., Levy, D., et al. (2004). Obesity and the risk of new-onset atrial fibrillation. *JAMA, 292*(20), 2471–2477.

Wildman, R. P., Gu, D., Reynolds, K., et al. (2004). Appropriate body mass index and waist circumference cutoffs for categorization of overweight and central adiposity among Chinese adults. *American Journal of Clinical Nutrition, 80*(5), 1129–1136.

## RESOURCES

Advisory Committee on Immunization Practices (ACIP), Centers for Disease Control and Prevention, National Immunization Program, Division of Epidemiology and Surveillance, Mail Stop E61, 1600 Clifton Road, NE Atlanta, GA 30333; 404-639-3311; Public Inquiries: 404-639-3534 or 800-311-3435; http://www.cdc.gov/nip/recs/adult-schedule.pdf. Accessed March 5, 2006.

Alliance of Cannabis Therapeutics, P.O. Box 21210, Kalorama Station, Washington, DC 20009; 202-483-8595; http://marijuana-as-medicine.org/alliance.htm. Accessed March 5, 2006.

American Dietetic Association, 216 W. Jackson Blvd., Suite 800, Chicago, IL 60606; Consumer Nutrition Hotline: 800-366-1655; http://www.eatright.org. Accessed March 5, 2006.

American Heart Association, 7320 Greenville Ave., Dallas, TX 75231; National Center: 214-373-6300; Nutrition Information: 214-706-1179; http://www.americanheart.org. Accessed March 5, 2006.

Medical Records Institute, 425 Boylston Street, 4th Floor, Boston, MA 02116; 617-964-3923; fax 617-964-3926; http://www.medrecinst.com. Accessed March 5, 2006.

National Cancer Institute, Cancer Information Service, 9000 Rockville Pike, Bldg. 31, Room 10A-24, Bethesda, MD 20892; 1-800-4-CANCER; http://www.nci.nih.gov or http://www.cancer.gov. Accessed March 5, 2006.

Pennsylvania State Nutrition Center, The Pennsylvania State University, Ruth Building, 417 E. Calder Way, University Park, PA 16802; 814-865-6323.

# UNIT 2

# Biophysical and Psychosocial Concepts in Nursing Practice

## Case Study
### Applying Concepts from NANDA, NIC, and NOC

**A Patient with Fear Accompanied By Somatic Complaints Unsubstantiated By Physical Findings**

**Mr. Roberts** is a 40-year-old man who comes to the emergency department (ED) for treatment of high blood pressure. On his previous visit to the ED he reported chest pressure, feelings of numbness and tingling in his arms, and extreme fearfulness that he was having a heart attack. Even though a myocardial infarction was ruled out and subsequent testing revealed that he had no heart disease, Mr. Roberts continues to have feelings of chest pressure and fear that he is having a heart attack. The only abnormal finding has been an elevation of blood pressure (158/88 mm Hg). The nurse interviews Mr. Roberts, who reveals he is under intense financial pressure. The nurse assesses his compliance with his antihypertensive therapy and suggests interventions to help with Mr. Robert's anxiety.

Turn to Appendix C to see a concept map that illustrates the relationships that exist between the nursing diagnoses, interventions, and outcomes for the patient's clinical problems.

## Nursing Classifications and Languages

| NANDA<br>Nursing Diagnoses | NIC<br>Nursing Interventions | NOC<br>Nursing Outcomes<br>Return to functional baseline status, stabilization of, or improvement in: |
|---|---|---|
| **Anxiety**—Vague uneasy feeling of discomfort or dread accompanied by an autonomic response (the source often nonspecific or unknown to the individual); a feeling of apprehension caused by anticipation of danger. It is an alerting signal that warns of impending danger and enables the individual to take measures to deal with threat. | **Anxiety Reduction**—Minimizing apprehension, dread, foreboding, or uneasiness related to unidentified source of anticipated danger | **Anxiety Self-Control**—Personal actions to eliminate or reduce feelings of apprehension, tension, or uneasiness from an unidentifiable source |
| **Ineffective Coping**—Inability to form a valid appraisal of the stressors, inadequate choices of practiced responses, and/or inability to use available resources | **Coping Enhancement**—Assisting a patient to adapt to perceived stressors, changes, or threats that interfere with meeting life demands and roles<br><br>**Counseling**—Use of an interactive helping process focusing on the needs, problems, or feelings of the patient and significant others to enhance or support coping, problem-solving, and interpersonal relationships<br><br>**Support System Enhancement**—Facilitation of support to patient by family, friends, and community | **Coping**—Personal actions to manage stressors that tax an individual's resources |

NANDA International (2005). *Nursing diagnoses: Definitions & Classification 2005–2006*. Philadelphia: North American Nursing Diagnosis Association.
Dochterman, J. M. & Bulechek, G. M. (2004). *Nursing interventions classification (NIC)* (4th ed.). St. Louis: Mosby.
Iowa Outcomes Project (2004). In Moorhead, S., Johnson, M. & Maas, M. (2004). *Nursing outcomes classification (NOC)* (3rd ed.). St. Louis: Mosby.
Dochterman, J. M. & Jones, D. A. (2003). *Unifying nursing languages: The harmonization of NANDA, NIC, and NOC*. Washington D.C.: American Nurses Association.

"Point, click, learn! Visit thePoint for additional resources."

# CHAPTER 6

# Homeostasis, Stress, and Adaptation

## Learning Objectives

*On completion of this chapter, the learner will be able to:*

1. Relate the principles of internal constancy, homeostasis, stress, and adaptation to the concept of steady state.
2. Identify the significance of the body's compensatory mechanisms in promoting adaptation and maintaining the steady state.
3. Identify physiologic and psychosocial stressors.
4. Compare the sympathetic-adrenal-medullary response to stress to the hypothalamic-pituitary response to stress.
5. Describe the general adaptation syndrome as a theory of adaptation to biologic stress.
6. Describe the relationship of the process of negative feedback to the maintenance of the steady state.
7. Compare the adaptive processes of hypertrophy, atrophy, hyperplasia, dysplasia, and metaplasia.
8. Describe the inflammatory and reparative processes.
9. Assess the health patterns of a person and determine their effects on maintenance of the steady state.
10. Identify ways in which maladaptive responses to stress can increase the risk of illness and cause disease.
11. Identify measures that are useful in reducing stress.
12. Specify the functions of social networks and support groups in reducing stress.

When the body is threatened or suffers an injury, its response may involve functional and structural changes; these changes may be adaptive (having a positive effect) or maladaptive (having a negative effect). The defense mechanisms that the body uses determine the difference between adaptation and maladaptation—health and disease.

## Stress and Function

Each body system performs specific functions to sustain optimal life for an organism. Mechanisms for adjusting internal conditions promote the normal steady state of the organism and ultimately its survival. These mechanisms are compensatory in nature and work to restore balance in the body. An example of this restorative effort is the development of rapid breathing (hyperpnea) after intense exercise in an attempt to compensate for an oxygen deficit and excess lactic acid accumulated in the muscle tissue.

Pathophysiologic processes result when cellular injury occurs at such a rapid rate that the body's compensatory mechanisms can no longer make the adaptive changes necessary to remain healthy. An example of a pathophysiologic change is the development of heart failure; the body reacts by retaining sodium and water and increasing venous pressure, which worsens the condition. These pathophysiologic responses give rise to symptoms that are reported by patients or signs that are observed by patients or nurses or other health care providers. These observations, plus a sound knowledge of physiologic and pathophysiologic processes, can assist in determining the existence of a problem and can guide nurses in planning the appropriate course of action.

## Dynamic Balance: The Steady State

Physiologic mechanisms must be understood in the context of the body as a whole. Each person, as a living system, has both an internal and an external environment, between which information and matter are continuously exchanged. Within the internal environment, each organ, tissue, and cell is also a system or subsystem of the whole, each with its own internal and external environment, each exchanging information and matter (Fig. 6-1). The goal of the interaction of the body's subsystems is to produce a dynamic balance or **steady state** (even in the presence of change), so that all subsystems are in harmony with each other. Four concepts—constancy, homeostasis, stress, and adaptation—are key to the understanding of steady state.

Claude Bernard, a 19th-century French physiologist, developed the biologic principle that for life there must be a constancy or "fixity of the internal milieu" despite changes

## Glossary

**adaptation:** a change or alteration designed to assist in adapting to a new situation or environment

**adrenocorticotropic hormone (ACTH):** a hormone produced by the anterior lobe of the pituitary gland that stimulates the secretion of cortisone and other hormones by the adrenal cortex

**antidiuretic hormone (ADH):** a hormone secreted by the posterior lobe of the pituitary gland that constricts blood vessels, elevates blood pressure, and reduces the excretion of urine

**catecholamines:** any of the group of amines (such as epinephrine, norepinephrine, or dopamine) that serve as neurotransmitters

**coping:** the cognitive and behavioral strategies used to manage the stressors that tax a person's resources

**dysplasia:** a change in the appearance of a cell after exposure to chronic irritation

**glucocorticoids:** the group of steroid hormones, such as cortisol, that are produced by the adrenal cortex; they are involved in carbohydrate, protein, and fat metabolism and have anti-inflammatory properties

**gluconeogenesis:** the formation of glucose, especially by the liver from noncarbohydrate sources such as amino acids and the glycerol portion of fats

**guided imagery:** the mindful use of a word, phrase, or visual image to achieve relaxation or direct attention away from uncomfortable sensations or situations

**homeostasis:** a steady state within the body; the stability of the internal environment

**hyperplasia:** an increase in the number of new cells

**hypoxia:** inadequate supply of oxygen to the cell

**infectious agents:** biologic agents, such as viruses, bacteria, rickettsiae, mycoplasmas, fungi, protozoa, and nematodes, that cause disease in people

**inflammation:** a localized, protective reaction of tissue to injury, irritation, or infection, manifested by pain, redness, heat, swelling, and sometimes loss of function

**metabolic rate:** the speed at which some substances are broken down to yield energy for bodily processes and other substances are synthesized

**metaplasia:** a cell transformation in which a highly specialized cell changes to a less specialized cell

**negative feedback:** feedback that decreases the output of a system

**positive feedback:** feedback that increases the output of a system

**primary intention healing:** healing by fibrous adhesion, without suppuration or granulation tissue formation

**secondary intention healing:** delayed closure of two granulating surfaces

**steady state:** a stable condition that does not change over time, or when change in one direction is balanced by change in an opposite direction

**stress:** a disruptive condition that occurs in response to adverse influences from the internal or external environments

**vasoconstriction:** the narrowing of a blood vessel

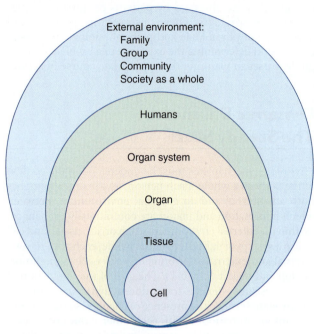

**FIGURE 6-1.** Constellation of systems. Each system is a subsystem of the larger system (suprasystem) of which it is a part. In this figure the cells represent the smallest system and are a subsystem of all other systems.

in the external environment. The internal milieu was the fluid that bathed the cells, and the constancy was the balanced internal state maintained by physiologic and biochemical processes. His principle implied a static process.

Later, Walter Cannon used the term *homeostasis* to describe the stability of the internal environment, which, he said, was coordinated by homeostatic or compensatory processes that responded to changes in the internal environment. Any change within the internal environment initiated a "righting" response to minimize the change. These biologic processes sought physiologic and chemical balance and were under involuntary control.

Rene Jules Dubos (1965) provided further insight into the dynamic nature of the internal environment with his theory that two complementary concepts, homeostasis and adaptation, were necessary for balance. Homeostatic processes occurred quickly in response to stress, rapidly making the adjustments necessary to maintain the internal environment. Adaptive processes resulted in structural or functional changes over time. Dubos also emphasized that acceptable ranges of response to stimuli existed and that these responses varied for different individuals: "absolute constancy is only a concept of the ideal." Homeostasis and adaptation were both necessary for survival in a changing world.

**Homeostasis**, then, refers to a steady state within the body. When a change or stress occurs that causes a body function to deviate from its stable range, processes are initiated to restore and maintain the dynamic balance. When these adjustment processes or compensatory mechanisms are not adequate, the steady state is threatened, function becomes disordered, and dysfunctional responses occur. This can lead to disease and may be active during disease, which is a threat to the steady state. Disease is an abnormal variation in the structure or function of any part of the body. It disrupts function and therefore limits freedom of action.

## Stress and Adaptation

**Stress** is a state produced by a change in the environment that is perceived as challenging, threatening, or damaging to a person's dynamic balance or equilibrium. The person is, or feels, unable to meet the demands of the new situation. The change or stimulus that evokes this state is the stressor. The nature of the stressor is variable; an event or change that is stressful for one person may not be stressful for another, and an event that produces stress at one time and place may not do so at another time and place. A person appraises and copes with changing situations. The desired goal is **adaptation**, or adjustment to the change so that the person is again in equilibrium and has the energy and ability to meet new demands. This is the process of **coping** with the stress, a compensatory process with physiologic and psychological components.

Adaptation is a constant, ongoing process that requires a change in structure, function, or behavior so that a person is better suited to the environment; it involves an interaction between the person and the environment. The outcome depends on the degree of "fit" between the skills and capacities of the person, the type of social support available, and the various challenges or stressors encountered. As such, adaptation is an individual process: each person has varying abilities to cope or respond. As new challenges are met, this ability to cope and adapt can change, thereby providing the person with a wide range of adaptive ability. Adaptation occurs throughout the lifespan as the person encounters many developmental and situational challenges, especially related to health and illness. The goal of these encounters is to promote adaptation. In situations of health and illness, this goal is realized by optimal wellness.

Because both stress and adaptation may exist at different levels of a system, it is possible to study these reactions at the cellular, tissue, and organ levels. Biologists are concerned mainly with subcellular components or with subsystems of the total body. Behavioral scientists, including many nurse researchers, study stress and adaptation in individuals, families, groups, and societies; they focus on how a group's organizational features are modified to meet the requirements of the social and physical environment in which the group exists. In any system, the desired goals of adaptation are survival, growth, and reproduction.

## Stress: Threats to the Steady State

### Types of Stressors

Each person operates at a certain level of adaptation and regularly encounters a certain amount of change. Such change is expected; it contributes to growth and enhances life. A stressor can upset this equilibrium. A stressor may be defined as an internal or external event or situation that creates the potential for physiologic, emotional, cognitive, or behavioral changes in an individual.

Stressors exist in many forms and categories. They may be described as physical, physiologic, or psychosocial. Physical stressors include cold, heat, and chemical agents; physiologic stressors include pain and fatigue. Examples of psychosocial stressors are fear of failing an examination, losing a job, and waiting for a diagnostic test result. Stressors can also occur as normal life transitions that require some adjustment, such as going from childhood into puberty, getting married, or giving birth.

Stressors have also been classified as (1) day-to-day frustrations or hassles; (2) major complex occurrences involving large groups, even entire nations; and (3) stressors that occur less frequently and involve fewer people. The first group, the day-to-day stressors, includes such common occurrences as getting caught in a traffic jam, experiencing computer downtime, and having an argument with a spouse or roommate. These experiences vary in effect. For example, encountering a rainstorm while you are vacationing at the beach will most likely evoke a more negative response than it might at another time. These less dramatic, frustrating, and irritating events—daily hassles—have been shown to have a greater health impact than major life events because of the cumulative effect they have over time. They can lead to high blood pressure, palpitations, or other physiologic problems (Rice, 1999).

The second group of stressors influences larger groups of people, possibly even entire nations. These include events of history, such as terrorism and war, which are threatening situations when experienced either directly, in the war zone, or indirectly, through live news coverage. The demographic, economic, and technologic changes occurring in society also serve as stressors. The tension produced by any stressor is sometimes a result not only of the change itself but also of the speed with which the change occurs.

The third group of stressors has been studied most extensively and concerns relatively infrequent situations that directly affect people. This category includes the influence of life events such as death, birth, marriage, divorce, and retirement. It also includes the psychosocial crises described by Erikson as occurring in the life cycle stages of the human experience. More enduring chronic stressors have also been placed in this category and may include having a permanent functional disability or coping with the difficulties of providing long-term care to a frail elderly parent.

Duration may also be used to categorize stressors, as in the following list:

- An acute, time-limited stressor, such as studying for final examinations
- A stressor sequence—a series of stressful events that result from an initial event such as job loss or divorce
- A chronic intermittent stressor, such as daily hassles
- A chronic enduring stressor that persists over time, such as chronic illness, a disability, or poverty

## Stress as a Stimulus for Disease

Relating life events to illness (the theoretical approach that defines stress as a stimulus) has been a major focus of psychosocial studies. This can be traced to Adolph Meyer, who in the 1930s observed a link between illnesses and critical life events in "life charts" of his patients. Subsequent research revealed that people under constant stress have a high incidence of psychosomatic disease.

Holmes and Rahe (1967) developed life events scales that assign numerical values, called life-change units, to typical life events. Because the items in the scales reflect events that require a change in a person's life pattern, and stress is defined as an accumulation of changes in one's life that require psychological adaptation, one can theoretically predict the likelihood of illness by checking off the number of recent events and deriving a total score. The Recent Life Changes Questionnaire (Tausig, 1982) contains 118 items such as death, birth, marriage, divorce, promotions, serious arguments, and vacations. The items include both desirable and undesirable events.

Sources of stress for patients have been well researched (Elder, Wollin, Hartel, et al., 2003; Erlandsson & Eklund, 2003). People typically experience distress related to alterations in their physical and emotional health status, changes in their level of daily functioning, and decreased social support or the loss of significant others. Fears of immobilization, isolation, loneliness, sensory changes, financial problems, and death or disability increase a person's anxiety level. Loss of one's role or perceived purpose in life can cause intense discomfort. Any of these identified variables, plus a myriad of other conditions or overwhelming demands, are likely to cause ineffective coping, and a lack of necessary coping skills is often a source of additional distress for the person. When a person endures prolonged or unrelenting suffering, the outcome is frequently the development of a stress-related illness. Nurses possess the skills to assist people to alter their distressing circumstances and manage their responses to stress.

## Psychological Responses to Stress

After recognizing a stressor, a person consciously or unconsciously reacts to manage the situation. This is termed the mediating process. A theory developed by Lazarus (1991a) emphasizes cognitive appraisal and coping as important mediators of stress. Appraisal and coping are influenced by antecedent variables, including the internal and external resources of the individual person.

### Appraisal of the Stressful Event

Cognitive appraisal (Lazarus, 1991a; Lazarus & Folkman, 1984) is a process by which an event is evaluated with respect to what is at stake (primary appraisal) and what might and can be done (secondary appraisal). What a person sees as being at stake is influenced by his or her personal goals, commitments, or motivations. Important factors include how important or relevant the event is to the person, whether the event conflicts with what he or she wants or desires, and whether the situation threatens the person's own sense of strength and ego identity.

Primary appraisal results in the situation being identified as either nonstressful or stressful. A nonstressful situation is irrelevant or benign (positive). A stressful situation may be one of three kinds: (1) one in which harm or loss has occurred; (2) one that is threatening, in that harm or loss is anticipated; and (3) one that is challenging, in that some opportunity or gain is anticipated.

Secondary appraisal is an evaluation of what might and can be done about the situation. Actions include assigning blame to the person responsible for a frustrating event; thinking about whether it is possible to do something about the situation (coping potential); and determining future expectancy, or whether things are likely to change for better or worse (Lazarus, 1991a, 1991c). A comparison of what is at stake and what can be done about it (a type of risk–benefit analysis) determines the degree of stress.

Reappraisal, a change of opinion based on new information, also occurs. The appraisal process is not necessarily sequential; primary and secondary appraisal and reappraisal may occur simultaneously. Information learned from an adaptational encounter can be stored, so that when a similar situation is encountered again, the entire process does not need to be repeated.

The appraisal process contributes to the development of an emotion. Negative emotions such as fear and anger accompany harm/loss appraisals, and positive emotions accompany challenge. In addition to the subjective component or feeling that accompanies a particular emotion, each emotion also includes a tendency to act in a certain way. For example, unprepared students may view an unexpected quiz as threatening. They might feel fear, anger, and resentment and might express these emotions through hostile behavior or comments.

Lazarus (1991a) expanded his former ideas about stress, appraisal, and coping into a more complex model relating emotion to adaptation. He called this model a "cognitive-motivational-relational theory," with the term *relational* "standing for a focus on negotiation with a physical and social world" (p. 13). A theory of emotion was proposed as the bridge to connect psychology, physiology, and sociology: "More than any other arena of psychological thought, emotion is an integrative, organismic concept that subsumes psychological stress and coping within itself and unites motivation, cognition, and adaptation in a complex configuration" (p. 40).

### *Coping With the Stressful Event*

Coping, according to Lazarus, consists of the cognitive and behavioral efforts made to manage the specific external or internal demands that tax a person's resources and may be emotion-focused or problem-focused. Coping that is emotion-focused seeks to make the person feel better by lessening the emotional distress. Problem-focused coping aims to make direct changes in the environment so that the situation can be managed more effectively. Both types of coping usually occur in a stressful situation. Even if the situation is viewed as challenging or beneficial, coping efforts may be required to develop and sustain the challenge—that is, to maintain the positive benefits of the challenge and to ward off any threats. In harmful or threatening situations, successful coping reduces or eliminates the source of stress and relieves the emotion it generated.

Appraisal and coping are affected by internal characteristics such as health, energy, personal belief systems, commitments or life goals, self-esteem, control, mastery, knowledge, problem-solving skills, and social skills. The characteristics that have been studied most often in nursing research are health-promoting lifestyles and hardiness. A health-promoting lifestyle buffers the effect of stressors. From a nursing practice standpoint, this outcome—buffering the effect of stressors—supports nursing's goal of promoting health. In many circumstances, promoting a healthy lifestyle is more achievable than altering the stressors.

Hardiness is the name given to a general quality that comes from having rich, varied, and rewarding experiences. It is a personality characteristic composed of control, commitment, and challenge. Hardy people perceive stressors as something they can change and therefore control. To them, potentially stressful situations are interesting and meaningful; change and new situations are viewed as challenging opportunities for growth. Some positive support has been found for hardiness as a significant variable that positively influences rehabilitation and overall improvement after an onset of an acute or chronic illness (Brooks, 2003; Ptacek & Pierce, 2003).

## Physiologic Response to Stress

The physiologic response to a stressor, whether it is physical or psychological, is a protective and adaptive mechanism to maintain the homeostatic balance of the body. When a stress response occurs, it triggers a series of neurologic and hormonal processes to be activated within the brain and body systems. The duration and intensity of the stress can cause both short-term and long-term effects. A stressor can disrupt homeostasis to the point where adaptation to the stressor fails, and a disease process results.

### *Selye's Theory of Adaptation*

Hans Selye developed a theory of adaptation that profoundly influenced the scientific study of stress. In 1936, Selye first described a syndrome consisting of enlargement of the adrenal cortex; shrinkage of the thymus, spleen, lymph nodes, and other lymphatic structures; and the appearance of deep, bleeding ulcers in the stomach and duodenum. He identified this as a nonspecific response to diverse, noxious stimuli.

#### GENERAL ADAPTATION SYNDROME

Selye then developed a theory of adaptation to biologic stress that he named the general adaptation syndrome, which has three phases: alarm, resistance, and exhaustion. During the alarm phase, the sympathetic "fight-or-flight" response is activated with release of **catecholamines** and the onset of the **adrenocorticotropic hormone** (ACTH)–adrenal cortical response. The alarm reaction is defensive and anti-inflammatory but self-limited. Because living in a continuous state of alarm would result in death, people move into the second stage, resistance. During the resistance stage, adaptation to the noxious stressor occurs, and cortisol activity is still increased. If exposure to the stressor is prolonged, the third stage, exhaustion, occurs. During the exhaustion stage, endocrine activity increases, and this has negative effects on the body systems (especially the circulatory, digestive, and immune systems) that can lead to death. Stages one and two of this syndrome are repeated, in different degrees, throughout life as the person encounters stressors.

Selye compared the general adaptation syndrome with the life process. During childhood, too few encounters with stress occur to promote the development of adaptive functioning, and children are vulnerable. During adulthood, a number of stressful events occur, and people develop resistance or adaptation. During the later years, the accumulation of life's stressors and wear and tear on the organism again decrease people's ability to adapt, resistance falls, and eventually death occurs.

### LOCAL ADAPTATION SYNDROME

According to Selye, a local adaptation syndrome also occurs. This syndrome includes the inflammatory response and repair processes that occur at the local site of tissue injury. The local adaptation syndrome occurs in small, topical injuries, such as contact dermatitis. If the local injury is severe enough, the general adaptation syndrome is activated as well.

Selye emphasized that stress is the nonspecific response common to all stressors, regardless of whether they are physiologic, psychological, or social. The many conditioning factors in each person's environment account for why different demands are experienced by different people as stressors. Conditioning factors also account for differences in the tolerance of different people for stress: some people may develop diseases of adaptation, such as hypertension and migraine headaches, whereas others are unaffected.

## Interpretation of Stressful Stimuli by the Brain

Physiologic responses to stress are mediated by the brain through a complex network of chemical and electrical messages. The neural and hormonal actions that maintain homeostatic balance are integrated by the hypothalamus, which is located in the center of the brain, surrounded by the limbic system and the cerebral hemispheres. The hypothalamus is made up of a number of nuclei and integrates autonomic nervous system mechanisms that maintain the chemical constancy of the internal environment of the body. Together with the limbic system, which contains the amygdala, hippocampus, and septal nuclei, along with other structures, the hypothalamus regulates emotions and many visceral behaviors necessary for survival (eg, eating, drinking, temperature control, reproduction, defense, aggression).

Each of these structures responds differently to stimuli, and each has its own characteristic response (Furman & Gallo, 2000). The cerebral hemispheres are concerned with cognitive functions: thought processes, learning, and memory. The limbic system has connections with both the cerebral hemispheres and the brainstem. In addition, the reticular activating system (RAS), a network of cells that forms a two-way communication system, extends from the brain stem into the midbrain and limbic system. This network controls the alert or waking state of the body.

In the stress response, afferent impulses are carried from sensory organs (eye, ear, nose, skin) and internal sensors (baroreceptors, chemoreceptors) to nerve centers in the brain. The response to the perception of stress is integrated in the hypothalamus, which coordinates the adjustments necessary to return to homeostatic balance. The degree and duration of the response varies; major stress evokes both sympathetic and pituitary adrenal responses.

Neural and neuroendocrine pathways under the control of the hypothalamus are also activated in the stress response. Initially, there is a sympathetic nervous system discharge, followed by a sympathetic-adrenal-medullary discharge. If the stress persists, the hypothalamic-pituitary system is activated (Fig. 6-2).

### SYMPATHETIC NERVOUS SYSTEM RESPONSE

The sympathetic nervous system response is rapid and short-lived. Norepinephrine is released at nerve endings that are in direct contact with their respective end organs to cause an increase in function of the vital organs and a state of general body arousal. The heart rate is increased and peripheral **vasoconstriction** occurs, raising the blood pressure. Blood is also shunted away from abdominal organs. The purpose of these responses is to provide better perfusion of vital organs (brain, heart, skeletal muscles). Blood glucose is increased, supplying more readily available energy. The pupils are dilated, and mental activity is increased; a greater sense of awareness exists. Constriction of the blood vessels of the skin limits bleeding in the event of trauma. The person is likely to experience cold feet, clammy skin and hands, chills, palpitations, and "knots" in the stomach. Typically, the person appears tense, with the muscles of the neck, upper back, and shoulders tightened; respirations may be rapid and shallow, with the diaphragm tense.

### SYMPATHETIC-ADRENAL-MEDULLARY RESPONSE

In addition to its direct effect on major end organs, the sympathetic nervous system also stimulates the medulla of the adrenal gland to release the hormones epinephrine and norepinephrine into the bloodstream. The action of these hormones is similar to that of the sympathetic nervous system and has the effect of sustaining and prolonging its actions. Epinephrine and norepinephrine are catecholamines that stimulate the nervous system and produce metabolic effects that increase the blood glucose level and increase the **metabolic rate**. The effect of the sympathetic-adrenal-medullary responses is summarized in Table 6-1. This effect is called the "fight-or-flight" reaction.

### HYPOTHALAMIC-PITUITARY RESPONSE

The longest-acting phase of the physiologic response, which is more likely to occur in persistent stress, involves the hypothalamic-pituitary pathway. The hypothalamus secretes corticotropin-releasing factor, which stimulates the anterior pituitary to produce ACTH, which in turn stimulates the adrenal cortex to produce **glucocorticoids**, primarily cortisol. Cortisol stimulates protein catabolism, releasing amino acids; stimulates liver uptake of amino acids and their conversion to glucose (**gluconeogenesis**); and inhibits glucose uptake (anti-insulin action) by many body cells but not those of the brain and heart. These cortisol-induced metabolic effects provide the body with a ready source of energy during a stressful situation. This effect has some important implications. For example, a person with diabetes who is under stress, such as that caused by an infection, needs more insulin than usual. Any patient who is under stress (eg, illness, surgery, trauma, or prolonged psychological stress) catabolizes body protein and needs

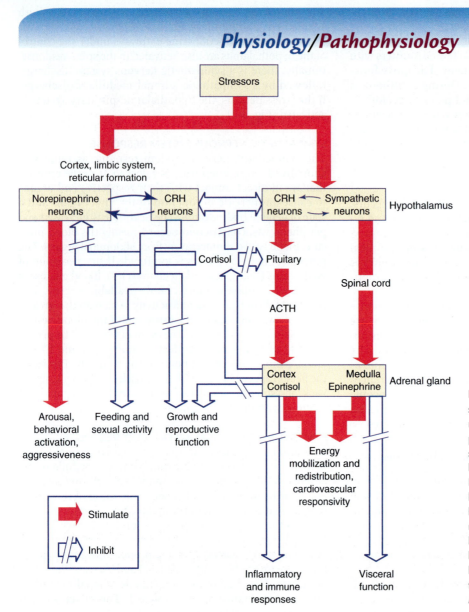

**FIGURE 6-2.** Integrated responses to stress mediated by the sympathetic nervous system and the hypothalamic–pituitary–adrenocortical axis. The responses are mutually reinforcing at both the central and peripheral levels. Negative feedback by cortisol also can limit an overresponse that might be harmful to the individual. *Colored arrows* represent stimulation, *open arrows,* inhibition. CRH, corticotropin-releasing hormone; ACTH, adrenocorticotropic hormone. Reproduced with permission from Berne, R. M., & Levy, M. N. (2003). *Physiology.* St. Louis: C. V. Mosby.

supplements. Growth is retarded in a child who has been subjected to severe stress.

The actions of the catecholamines (epinephrine and norepinephrine) and cortisol are the most important in the general response to stress. Other hormones that play a role are **antidiuretic hormone** (ADH) released from the posterior pituitary and aldosterone released from the adrenal cortex. ADH and aldosterone promote sodium and water retention, which is an adaptive mechanism in the event of hemorrhage or loss of fluids through excessive perspiration. ADH has also been shown to influence learning and may thus facilitate coping in new and threatening situations. Secretion of growth hormone and glucagon stimulates the uptake of amino acids by cells, helping to mobilize energy resources. Endorphins, which are endogenous opiates, increase during stress and enhance the threshold for tolerance of painful stimuli. They may also affect mood and have been implicated in the so-called high that long-distance runners experience. The secretion of other hormones is also affected, but their adaptive function is less clear.

### IMMUNOLOGIC RESPONSE

Research findings show that the immune system is connected to the neuroendocrine and autonomic systems. Lymphoid tissue is richly supplied by autonomic nerves capable of releasing a number of different neuropeptides that can have a direct effect on leukocyte regulation and the inflammatory response. Neuroendocrine hormones released by the central nervous system and endocrine tissues can inhibit or stimulate leukocyte function. The wide variety of stressors a person experiences may result in different alterations in autonomic activity and subtle variations in neurohormone and neuropeptide synthesis. All of these possible autonomic and neuroendocrine responses can interact to initiate, weaken, enhance, or terminate an immune response (Chiorazzi, 2003).

| TABLE 6-1 | Sympathetic–Adrenal–Medullary Response to Stress | |
|---|---|---|
| Effect | Purpose | Mechanism |
| Increased heart rate and blood pressure | Better perfusion of vital organs | Increased cardiac output due to increased myocardial contractility and heart rate; increased venous return (peripheral vasoconstriction) |
| Increased blood glucose level | Increased available energy | Increased liver and muscle glycogen breakdown; increased breakdown of adipose tissue triglycerides |
| Mental acuity | Alert state | Increase in amount of blood shunted to the brain from the abdominal viscera and skin |
| Dilated pupils | Increased awareness | Contraction of radial muscle of iris |
| Increased tension of skeletal muscles | Preparedness for activity, decreased fatigue | Excitation of muscles; increase in amount of blood shunted to the muscles from the abdominal viscera and skin |
| Increased ventilation (may be rapid and shallow) | Provision of oxygen for energy | Stimulation of respiratory center in medulla; bronchodilation |
| Increased coagulability of blood | Prevention of hemorrhage in event of trauma | Vasoconstriction of surface vessels |

The study of the relationships among the neuroendocrine system, the central and autonomic nervous systems, and the immune system and the effects of these relationships on overall health outcomes is called *psychoneuroimmunology*. Because one's perception of events and one's coping styles determine whether, and to what extent, an event activates the stress response system, and because the stress response affects immune activity, one's perceptions, ideas, and thoughts can have profound neurochemical and immunologic consequences. Multiple studies have demonstrated alteration of immune function in people who are under stress (Constantino, Secula, Rabin, et al., 2000; Norman, 2003; Robinson, Matthews, & Witek-Janusek, 2000). Other studies have identified certain personality traits, such as optimism and active coping, as having positive effects on health (Brissette, Leventhal, & Leventhal, 2003; Kennedy, 2000; Whitty, 2003). As research continues, this new field of study will likely uncover to what extent and by what mechanisms people can consciously influence their immunity.

## Maladaptive Responses to Stress

The stress response, which, as indicated earlier, facilitates adaptation to threatening situations, has been retained from humans' evolutionary past. The "fight-or-flight" response, for example, is an anticipatory response that mobilized the bodily resources of our ancestors to deal with predators and other harsh factors in their environment. This same mobilization comes into play in response to emotional stimuli unrelated to danger. For example, a person may get an "adrenaline rush" when competing over a decisive point in a ball game, or when excited about attending a party.

When the responses to stress are ineffective, they are referred to as *maladaptive*. Maladaptive responses are chronic, recurrent responses or patterns of response over time that do not promote the goals of adaptation. The goals of adaptation are somatic or physical health (optimal wellness); psychological health or having a sense of well-being (happiness, satisfaction with life, morale); and enhanced social functioning, which includes work, social life, and family (positive relationships). Maladaptive responses that threaten these goals include faulty appraisals and inappropriate coping (Lazarus, 1991a).

The frequency, intensity, and duration of stressful situations contribute to the development of negative emotions and subsequent patterns of neurochemical discharge. By appraising situations more adequately and coping more appropriately, it is possible to anticipate and defuse some of these situations. For example, frequent potentially stressful encounters (eg, marital discord) might be avoided with better communication and problem solving, or a pattern of procrastination (eg, delaying work on tasks) could be corrected to reduce stress when deadlines approach.

Coping processes that include the use of alcohol or drugs to reduce stress increase the risk of illness. Other inappropriate coping patterns may increase the risk of illness less directly. For example, people who demonstrate "type A" behaviors such as impatience, competitiveness, and achievement orientation and have an underlying hostile approach to life are more prone than others to develop stress-related illnesses. Type A behaviors increase the output of catecholamines, the adrenal-medullary hormones, with their attendant effects on the body.

Other forms of inappropriate coping include denial, avoidance, and distancing. Denial may be illustrated by the woman who feels a lump in her breast but downplays its seriousness and delays seeking medical attention. The intent of denial is to control the threat, but it may also endanger life.

Models of illness frequently cite stress and maladaptation as precursors to disease. A general model of illness, based on Selye's theory, suggests that any stressor elicits a state of disturbed physiologic equilibrium. If this state is prolonged or the response is excessive, it increases the susceptibility of the person to illness. This susceptibility, coupled with a predisposition in the person (from genetic traits, health, or age), leads to illness. If the sympathetic adrenal-medullary response is prolonged or excessive, a state of chronic arousal develops that may lead to high blood pressure, arteriosclerotic changes, and cardiovascular disease. If the production of ACTH is prolonged or excessive, behavior patterns of withdrawal and depression are seen. In addition, the immune response is decreased, and infections and tumors may develop.

Selye (1976) proposed a list of disorders that he called diseases of maladaptation: high blood pressure, diseases of the heart and blood vessels, diseases of the kidney, hypertension of pregnancy, rheumatic and rheumatoid arthritis, inflammatory diseases of the skin and eyes, infections, allergic and hypersensitivity diseases, nervous and mental diseases, sexual dysfunction, digestive diseases, metabolic diseases, and cancer.

## Indicators of Stress

Indicators of stress and the stress response include both subjective and objective measures. Chart 6-1 lists signs and symptoms that may be observed directly or reported by a person. They are psychological, physiologic, or behavioral and reflect social behaviors and thought processes. Some of these reactions may be coping behaviors. Over time, each person tends to develop a characteristic pattern of behavior during stress to warn that the system is out of balance.

Laboratory measurements of indicators of stress have helped in understanding this complex process. Blood and urine analyses can be used to demonstrate changes in hormonal levels and hormonal breakdown products. Blood levels of catecholamines, glucocorticoids, ACTH, and eosinophils are reliable measures of stress. Serum cholesterol and free fatty acid levels can also be used to measure stress. When the body experiences distress, it automatically produces adrenal hormones such as cortisol and aldosterone. As the levels of these chemicals increase, there is a simultaneous release of additional cholesterol into the general circulation. Both physical and psychological distress can trigger an elevated cholesterol level. In addition, the results of immunoglobulin assays are increased when a person is exposed to a variety of stressors, especially infections and immunodeficiency conditions. With greater attention to the field of neuroimmunology, improved laboratory measures are likely to follow.

In addition to using laboratory tests, researchers have developed questionnaires to identify and assess stressors, stress, and coping strategies. Some of these questionnaires are referenced in the work of Rice (1999), which is a compilation of information gained from research on stress, coping, and health. Some examples of the research instruments that nurses commonly use to measure levels of client distress and client functioning can be found in a variety of research reports (Cutler, Fishbain, Steele-Rosomoff, et al., 2003; Olofsson, Bengtsson, & Brink, 2003; Shapley, Jordan, & Croft, 2003). Miller and Smith (1993) provided a stress audit and a stress profile measurement tool that is available in the popular lay literature.

### CHART 6-1

### Assessing for Stress

Be on the alert for the following signs and symptoms:
- Restlessness
- Depression
- Dry mouth
- Overpowering urge to act out
- Fatigue
- Loss of interest in life activities
- Intense periods of anxiety
- Strong startle response
- Hyperactivity
- Gastrointestinal distress
- Diarrhea
- Nausea or vomiting
- Changes in menstrual cycle
- Change in appetite
- Injury-prone
- Palpitations
- Impulsive behaviors
- Emotional lability
- Concentration difficulties
- Feeling weak or dizzy
- Increased body tension
- Tremors
- Nervous habits
- Nervous laughter
- Bruxism (grinding of teeth)
- Difficulty sleeping
- Excessive perspiration
- Urinary frequency
- Headaches
- Pain in back, neck, or other parts of the body
- Increased use of tobacco
- Substance use or abuse

## Nursing Implications

It is important for nurses to realize that the optimal point of intervention to promote health is during the stage when a person's own compensatory processes are still functioning effectively. A major role of nurses is the early identification of both physiologic and psychological stressors. Nurses should be able to relate the presenting signs and symptoms of distress to the physiology they represent and identify a person's position on the continuum of function, from health and compensation to pathophysiology and disease.

For example, if an anxious middle-aged woman presented for a checkup and was found to be overweight and have a blood pressure of 150/85 mm Hg, the nurse would counsel her with respect to diet, stress management, and activity. The nurse would also encourage weight loss and discuss the woman's intake of salt (which affects fluid balance) and caffeine (which provides a stimulant effect). The patient and the nurse would identify both individual and environmental stressors and discuss strategies to decrease her lifestyle stress, with the ultimate goal being to create a healthy lifestyle and prevent hypertension and its sequelae.

## Stress at the Cellular Level

Pathologic processes may occur at all levels of the biologic organism. If the cell is considered the smallest unit or subsystem (tissues being aggregates of cells, organs aggregates of tissues, and so on), the processes of health and disease or adaptation and maladaptation can all occur at the cellular level. Indeed, pathologic processes are often described by scientists at the subcellular or molecular level.

The cell exists on a continuum of function and structure, ranging from the normal cell, to the adapted cell, to the injured or diseased cell, to the dead cell (Fig. 6-3). Changes from one state to another may occur rapidly and may not be readily detectable, because each state does not have discrete boundaries, and disease represents disruption of normal processes. The earliest changes occur at the molecular or subcellular level and are not perceptible until steady-state functions or structures are altered. With cell injury, some changes may be reversible; in other instances, the injuries are lethal. For example, tanning of the skin is an adaptive, morphologic response to exposure to the rays of the sun. However, if the exposure is continued, sunburn and injury occur, and some cells may die, as evidenced by desquamation ("peeling").

Different cells and tissues respond to stimuli with different patterns and rates of response, and some cells are more vulnerable to one type of stimulus or stressor than others. The cell involved, its ability to adapt, and its physiologic state are determinants of the response. For example, cardiac muscle cells respond to **hypoxia** (inadequate oxygenation) more quickly than do smooth muscle cells.

Other determinants of cellular response are the type or nature of the stimulus, its duration, and its severity. For example, neurons that control respiration can develop a tolerance to regular, small amounts of a barbiturate, but one large dose may result in respiratory depression and death.

## Control of the Steady State

The concept of the cell as existing on a continuum of function and structure includes the relationship of the cell to compensatory mechanisms, which occur continuously in the body to maintain the steady state. Compensatory processes are regulated primarily by the autonomic nervous system and the endocrine system, with control achieved through negative feedback.

### Negative Feedback

**Negative feedback** mechanisms throughout the body monitor the internal environment and restore homeostasis when conditions shift out of the normal range. These mechanisms work by sensing deviations from a predetermined set point or range of adaptability and triggering a response aimed at offsetting the deviation. Blood pressure, acid–base balance, blood glucose level, body temperature, and fluid and electrolyte balance are examples of functions regulated through such compensatory mechanisms.

Most of the human body's control systems are integrated by the brain and influenced by the nervous and endocrine systems. Control activities involve detecting deviations from the predetermined reference point and stimulating compensatory responses in the muscles and glands of the body. The major organs affected are the heart, lungs, kidneys, liver, gastrointestinal tract, and skin. When stimulated, these organs alter their rate of activity or the amount of secretions they produce. Because of this, they have been called the "organs of homeostasis or adjustment."

In addition to the responses controlled by the nervous and endocrine systems, local responses consisting of small feedback loops in a group of cells or tissues are possible. The cells detect a change in their immediate environment and initiate an action to counteract its effect. For example, the accumulation of lactic acid in an exercised muscle stimulates dilation of blood vessels in the area to increase blood flow and improve the delivery of oxygen and removal of waste products.

The net result of the activities of feedback loops is homeostasis. A steady state is achieved by the continuous, variable action of the organs involved in making the adjustments and by the continuous small exchanges of chemical substances among cells, interstitial fluid, and blood. For example, an increase in the carbon dioxide concentration of the extracellular fluid leads to increased pulmonary ventilation, which decreases the carbon dioxide level. On a cellular level, increased carbon dioxide raises the hydrogen ion concentration of the blood. This is detected by chemosensitive receptors in the respiratory control center of the medulla of the brain. The chemoreceptors stimulate an increase in the rate of discharge of the neurons that innervate the diaphragm and intercostal muscles, which increases the rate of respiration. Excess carbon dioxide is exhaled, the hydrogen ion concentration returns to normal, and the chemically sensitive neurons are no longer stimulated (Porth, 2005).

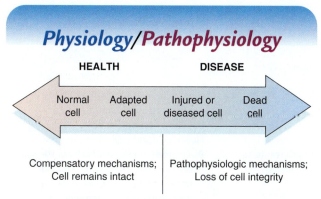

**FIGURE 6-3.** The cell on a continuum of function and structure. Changes in the cell are not as easily discerned as the diagram depicts, and the point at which compensation subsides and pathophysiology begins is not clearly defined.

## Positive Feedback

Another type of feedback, **positive feedback**, perpetuates the chain of events set in motion by the original disturbance instead of compensating for it. As the system becomes more unbalanced, disorder and disintegration occur. There are some exceptions to this; blood clotting in humans, for example, is an important positive feedback mechanism.

## Cellular Adaptation

Cells are complex units that dynamically respond to the changing demands and stresses of daily life. They possess a maintenance function and a specialized function. The maintenance function refers to the activities that the cell must perform with respect to itself; specialized functions are those that the cell performs in relation to the tissues and organs of which it is a part. Individual cells may cease to function without posing a threat to the organism. However, as the number of dead cells increases, the specialized functions of the tissues are altered, and health is threatened.

Cells can adapt to environmental stress through structural and functional changes. Some of these adaptations are hypertrophy, atrophy, hyperplasia, dysplasia, and metaplasia (Table 6-2). These adaptations reflect changes in the normal cell in response to stress. If the stress is unrelenting, cellular injury and death may occur.

Hypertrophy and atrophy lead to changes in the size of cells and hence the size of the organs they form. Compensatory hypertrophy is the result of an enlarged muscle mass and commonly occurs in skeletal and cardiac muscle that experiences a prolonged, increased workload. One example is the bulging muscles of the athlete who engages in body building.

Atrophy can be the consequence of a disease or of decreased use, decreased blood supply, loss of nerve supply, or inadequate nutrition. Disuse of a body part is often associated with the aging process and immobilization. Cell size and organ size decrease, and the structures principally affected are the skeletal muscles, the secondary sex organs, the heart, and the brain.

**Hyperplasia** is an increase in the number of new cells in an organ or tissue. As cells multiply and are subjected to increased stimulation, the tissue mass enlarges. This mitotic response (a change occurring with mitosis) is reversible when the stimulus is removed. This distinguishes hyperplasia from neoplasia or malignant growth, which continues after the stimulus is removed. Hyperplasia may be hormonally induced. An example is the increased size of the thyroid gland caused by thyroid-stimulating hormone (secreted from the pituitary gland) when a deficit in thyroid hormone occurs.

**Dysplasia** is the change in the appearance of cells after they have been subjected to chronic irritation. Dysplastic cells have a tendency to become malignant; dysplasia is seen commonly in epithelial cells in the bronchi of smokers.

**Metaplasia** is a cell transformation in which highly specialized cells change to less specialized cells. This serves a protective function, because less specialized cells are more resistant to the stress that stimulated the change. For example, the ciliated columnar epithelium lining the bronchi of smokers is replaced by squamous epithelium. The squamous cells can survive; loss of the cilia and protective mucus, however, can have damaging consequences.

### TABLE 6-2 Cellular Adaptation to Stressors

| Adaptation | Stimulus | Example |
| --- | --- | --- |
| Hypertrophy—increase in cell size leading to increase in organ size | Increased workload | Leg muscles of runner<br>Arm muscles in tennis player<br>Cardiac muscle in person with hypertension |
| Atrophy—shrinkage in size of cell, leading to decrease in organ size | Decrease in:<br>Use<br>Blood supply<br>Nutrition<br>Hormonal stimulation<br>Innervation | Secondary sex organs in aging person<br>Extremity immobilized in cast |
| Hyperplasia—increase in number of new cells (increase in mitosis) | Hormonal influence | Breast changes of a girl in puberty or of a pregnant woman<br>Regeneration of liver cells<br>New red blood cells in blood loss |
| Dysplasia—change in the appearance of cells after they have been subjected to chronic irritation | Reproduction of cells with resulting alteration of their size and shape | Alterations in epithelial cells of the skin or the cervix, producing irregular tissue changes that could be the precursors of a malignancy |
| Metaplasia—transformation of one adult cell type to another (reversible) | Stress applied to highly specialized cell | Changes in epithelial cells lining bronchi in response to smoke irritation (cells become less specialized) |

# Cellular Injury

Injury is defined as a disorder in steady-state regulation. Any stressor that alters the ability of the cell or system to maintain optimal balance of its adjustment processes leads to injury. Structural and functional damage then occurs, which may be reversible (permitting recovery) or irreversible (leading to disability or death). Homeostatic adjustments are concerned with the small changes within the body's systems. With adaptive changes, compensation occurs and a steady state is achieved, although it may be a new level. With injury, steady-state regulation is lost, and changes in functioning ensue.

Causes of disorder and injury in the system (cell, tissue, organ, body) may arise from the external or internal environment (Fig. 6-4) and include hypoxia, nutritional imbalance, physical agents, chemical agents, infectious agents, immune mechanisms, genetic defects, and psychogenic factors. The most common causes are hypoxia (oxygen deficiency), chemical injury, and infectious agents. In addition, the presence of one injury makes the system more susceptible to another injury. For example, inadequate oxygenation and nutritional deficiencies make the system vulnerable to infection. These agents act at the cellular level by damaging or destroying:

- The integrity of the cell membrane, necessary for ionic balance
- The ability of the cell to transform energy (aerobic respiration, production of adenosine triphosphate)
- The ability of the cell to synthesize enzymes and other necessary proteins
- The ability of the cell to grow and reproduce (genetic integrity)

## Hypoxia

Inadequate cellular oxygenation (hypoxia) interferes with the cell's ability to transform energy. Hypoxia may be caused by:

- A decrease in blood supply to an area
- A decrease in the oxygen-carrying capacity of the blood (decreased hemoglobin)
- A ventilation/perfusion or respiratory problem that reduces the amount of oxygen available in the blood
- A problem in the cell's enzyme system that makes it unable to use the oxygen delivered to it

The usual cause of hypoxia is ischemia, or deficient blood supply. Ischemia is commonly seen in myocardial cell injury in which arterial blood flow is decreased because of atherosclerotic narrowing of blood vessels. Ischemia also results from intravascular clots (thrombi or emboli) that may form and interfere with blood supply. Thrombi and emboli are common causes of cerebrovascular accidents (strokes, brain attacks). The length of time different tissues can survive without oxygen varies. For example, brain cells may succumb in 3 to 6 minutes, depending on the situation. If the condition leading to hypoxia is slow and progressive, collateral circulation may develop, whereby blood is supplied by other blood vessels in the area. However, this mechanism is not highly reliable.

## Nutritional Imbalance

Nutritional imbalance refers to a relative or absolute deficiency or excess of one or more essential nutrients. This may be manifested as undernutrition (inadequate consumption of food or calories) or overnutrition (caloric excess). Caloric excess to the point of obesity overloads cells in the body with lipids. By requiring more energy to maintain the extra tissue, obesity places a strain on the body and has been associated with the development of disease, especially pulmonary and cardiovascular disease.

Specific deficiencies arise when an essential nutrient is deficient or when there is an imbalance of nutrients. Protein deficiencies and avitaminosis (deficiency of vitamins) are typical examples. An energy deficit leading to cell injury can occur if there is insufficient glucose, or insufficient oxygen to transform the glucose into energy. A lack of insulin, or the inability to use insulin, may also prevent glucose from entering the cell from the blood. This occurs in diabetes mellitus, a metabolic disorder that can lead to nutritional deficiency.

## Physical Agents

Physical agents, including temperature extremes, radiation, electrical shock, and mechanical trauma, can cause injury to the cells or to the entire body. The duration of exposure and the intensity of the stressor determine the severity of damage.

### TEMPERATURE

When a person's temperature is elevated, hypermetabolism occurs and the respiratory rate, heart rate, and basal metabolic rate all increase. With fever induced by infections, the hypothalamic thermostat may be reset at a higher temperature and then return to normal when the fever abates. The increase in body temperature is achieved through physiologic mechanisms. Body temperatures greater than 41°C (106°F) indicate hyperthermia, because the physiologic function of the thermoregulatory center breaks down and

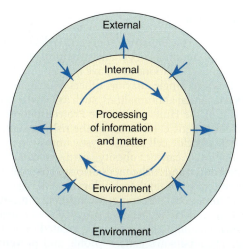

**FIGURE 6-4.** Influences leading to disorder may arise from the internal environment and the external environment of the system. Excesses or deficits of information and matter may occur, or there may be faulty regulation of processing.

the temperature soars. This physiologic condition occurs in people who have heat stroke. Eventually, the high temperature causes coagulation of cell proteins, and cells die. The body must be cooled rapidly to prevent brain damage.

The local response to thermal or burn injury is similar. There is an increase in metabolic activity, and, as heat increases, protein is coagulated, enzyme systems are destroyed, and, in the extreme, charring or carbonization occurs. Burns of the epithelium are classified as partial-thickness burns if epithelializing elements remain to support healing. Full-thickness burn wounds lack such elements and must be grafted for healing. The amount of body surface involved determines the patient's prognosis. If the injury is severe or extensive, the entire body becomes involved, and hypermetabolism develops as a pathophysiologic response.

Extremes of low temperature, or cold, cause vasoconstriction. Blood flow becomes sluggish and clots form, leading to ischemic damage in the involved tissues. With still lower temperatures, ice crystals may form, and cells may burst.

#### RADIATION AND ELECTRICAL SHOCK

Radiation is used for diagnosis and treatment of diseases. Ionizing forms of radiation may cause injury by their destructive action. Radiation decreases the protective inflammatory response of the cell, creating a favorable environment for opportunistic infections. Electrical shock produces burns as a result of the heat generated when electrical current travels through the body. It may also abnormally stimulate nerves, leading, for example, to fibrillation of the heart.

#### MECHANICAL TRAUMA

Mechanical trauma can result in wounds that disrupt the cells and tissues of the body. The severity of the wound, the amount of blood loss, and the extent of nerve damage are significant factors in the outcome.

## Chemical Agents

Chemical injuries are caused by poisons, such as lye, which have a corrosive action on epithelial tissue, or by heavy metals, such as mercury, arsenic, and lead, each of which has its own specific destructive action. Many other chemicals are toxic in certain amounts, in certain people, and in specific tissues. Excessive secretion of hydrochloric acid can damage the stomach lining; large amounts of glucose can cause osmotic shifts, affecting the fluid and electrolyte balance; and too much insulin can cause subnormal levels of glucose in the blood (hypoglycemia) and can lead to coma.

Drugs, including prescribed medications, can also cause chemical poisoning. Some people are less tolerant of medications than others and manifest toxic reactions at the usual or customary dosages. Aging tends to decrease tolerance to medications. Polypharmacy (taking many medications at one time) also occurs frequently in the aging population and is a problem because of the unpredictable effects of the resulting medication interactions.

Alcohol (ethanol) is also a chemical irritant. In the body, alcohol is broken down into acetaldehyde, which has a direct toxic effect on liver cells that leads to a variety of liver abnormalities, including cirrhosis in susceptible people. Disordered liver cell function leads to complications in other organs of the body.

## Infectious Agents

Biologic agents known to cause disease in humans are viruses, bacteria, rickettsiae, mycoplasmas, fungi, protozoa, and nematodes. The severity of the infectious disease depends on the number of microorganisms entering the body, their virulence, and the host's defenses (eg, health, age, immune responses).

Some bacteria, such as those that cause tetanus and diphtheria, produce exotoxins that circulate and create cell damage. Others, such as gram-negative bacteria, produce endotoxins when they die. Tubercle bacilli induce an immune reaction.

Viruses, the smallest living organisms known, survive as parasites of the living cells they invade. Viruses infect specific cells. Through a complex mechanism, viruses replicate within cells and then invade other cells, where they continue to replicate. An immune response is mounted by the body to eliminate the viruses, and the cells harboring the viruses can be injured in the process. Typically, an inflammatory response and immune reaction are the physiologic responses of the body to viral infection.

## Disordered Immune Responses

The immune system is an exceedingly complex system, the purpose of which is to defend the body from invasion by any foreign object or foreign cell type, such as cancerous cells. This is a steady-state mechanism, but like other adjustment processes it can become disordered, and cell injury occurs. The immune response detects foreign bodies by distinguishing non-self substances from self substances and destroying the non-self entities. The entrance of an antigen (foreign substance) into the body evokes the production of antibodies that attack and destroy the antigen (antigen–antibody reaction).

The immune system may function normally or it may be hypoactive or hyperactive. When it is hypoactive, immunodeficiency diseases occur; when it is hyperactive, hypersensitivity disorders occur. A disorder of the immune system itself can result in damage to the body's own tissues. Such disorders are labeled autoimmune diseases (see Unit 11).

## Genetic Disorders

There is intense research interest in genetic defects as causes of disease and modifiers of genetic structure. Many of these defects produce mutations that have no recognizable effect, such as lack of a single enzyme; others contribute to more obvious congenital abnormalities, such as Down syndrome. As a result of the Human Genome Project, people can be assessed for genetic conditions (or the risk for such conditions) such as sickle cell disease, cystic fibrosis, hemophilia A and B, breast cancer, obesity, cardiovascular disease, phenylketonuria, and Alzheimer's disease. The availability of genetics information and technology enables health care providers to perform screening, testing, and counseling for people with genetics concerns. Knowledge obtained from the Human Genome Project has also created opportunities for assessing a person's genetic profile and preventing or treating diseases. Diagnostic genetics and gene therapy have the potential to identify and modify genes before they begin to express traits that would lead to disease or disability. (For further information, see Chapter 9.)

## Cellular Response to Injury: Inflammation

Cells or tissues of the body may be injured or killed by any of the agents (physical, chemical, infectious) described earlier. When this happens, an inflammatory response (or inflammation) naturally occurs in the healthy tissues adjacent to the site of injury. **Inflammation** is a defensive reaction intended to neutralize, control, or eliminate the offending agent and to prepare the site for repair. It is a nonspecific response (not dependent on a particular cause) that is meant to serve a protective function. For example, inflammation may be observed at the site of a bee sting, in a sore throat, in a surgical incision, and at the site of a burn. Inflammation also occurs in cell injury events, such as strokes and myocardial infarctions.

Inflammation is not the same as infection. An infectious agent is only one of several agents that may trigger an inflammatory response. An infection exists when the infectious agent is living, growing, and multiplying in the tissues and is able to overcome the body's normal defenses.

Regardless of the cause, a general sequence of events occurs in the local inflammatory response. This sequence involves changes in the microcirculation, including vasodilation, increased vascular permeability, and leukocytic cellular infiltration (Fig. 6-5). As these changes take place, five cardinal signs of inflammation are produced: redness, heat, swelling, pain, and loss of function.

The transient vasoconstriction that occurs immediately after injury is followed by vasodilation and an increased rate of blood flow through the microcirculation to the area of tissue damage. Local heat and redness result. Next, the structure of the microvascular system changes to accommodate the movement of plasma protein from the blood into the tissues. Following this increase in vascular permeability, plasma fluids (including proteins and solutes) leak into the inflamed tissues, producing swelling. Leukocytes migrate through the endothelium and accumulate in the tissue at the site of the injury. The pain that occurs is attributed to the pressure of fluids or swelling on nerve endings and to the irritation of nerve endings by chemical mediators released at the site. Bradykinin is one of the chemical mediators suspected of causing pain. Loss of function is most likely related to the pain and swelling, but the exact mechanism is not completely known.

As blood flow increases and fluid leaks into the surrounding tissues, the formed elements (red blood cells, white blood cells, and platelets) remain in the blood, causing it to become more viscous. Leukocytes (white blood cells) collect in the vessels, exit, and migrate to the site of injury to engulf offending organisms and to remove cellular debris in a process called phagocytosis. Fibrinogen in the leaked plasma fluid coagulates, forming fibrin for clot formation, which serves to wall off the injured area and prevent the spread of infection.

### Chemical Mediators of Inflammation

Injury initiates the inflammatory response, but chemical substances released at the site induce the vascular changes. Foremost among these chemicals are histamine and kinins. Histamine is present in many tissues of the body but is concentrated in the mast cells. It is released when injury occurs and is responsible for the early changes in vasodilation and vascular permeability. Kinins increase vasodilation and vascular permeability, and they also attract neutrophils to the area. Prostaglandins, another group of chemical substances, are also suspected of causing increased permeability (Porth, 2005).

### Systemic Response to Inflammation

The inflammatory response is often confined to the site, causing only local signs and symptoms. However, systemic responses can also occur. Fever is the most common sign of a systemic response to injury, and it is most likely caused by endogenous pyrogens (internal substances that cause fever) released from neutrophils and macrophages (specialized forms of leukocytes). These substances reset the hypothalamic thermostat, which controls body temperature, and produce fever. Leukocytosis, an increase in the synthesis and release of neutrophils from bone marrow, may occur to provide the body with greater ability to fight infection. During this process, general, nonspecific symptoms develop, including malaise, loss of appetite, aching, and weakness.

### Types of Inflammation

Inflammation is categorized primarily by its duration and the type of exudate produced. It may be acute, subacute, or chronic. Acute inflammation is characterized by the local

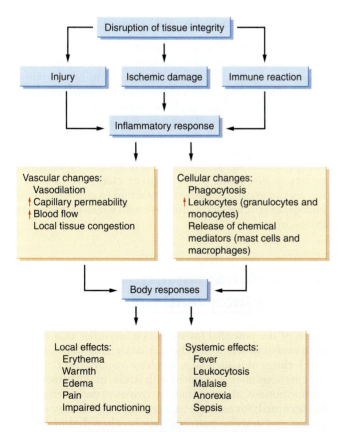

**FIGURE 6-5.** Inflammatory response.

vascular and exudative changes described earlier and usually lasts less than 2 weeks. An acute inflammatory response is immediate and serves a protective function. After the injurious agent is removed, the inflammation subsides and healing takes place with the return of normal or near-normal structure and function.

Chronic inflammation develops if the injurious agent persists and the acute response is perpetuated. Symptoms are present for many months or years. Chronic inflammation may also begin insidiously and never have an acute phase. The chronic response does not serve a beneficial and protective function; on the contrary, it is debilitating and can produce long-lasting effects. As the inflammation becomes chronic, changes occur at the site of injury and the nature of the exudate becomes proliferative. A cycle of cellular infiltration, necrosis, and fibrosis begins, with repair and breakdown occurring simultaneously. Considerable scarring may occur, resulting in permanent tissue damage.

Subacute inflammation falls between acute and chronic inflammation. It includes elements of the active exudative phase of the acute response as well as elements of repair, as in the chronic phase. The term "subacute inflammation" is not widely used.

## Cellular Healing

The reparative process begins at approximately the same time as the injury and is interwoven with inflammation. Healing proceeds after the inflammatory debris has been removed. Healing may occur by regeneration, in which gradual repair of the defect occurs by proliferation of cells of the same type as those destroyed, or by replacement, in which cells of another type, usually connective tissue, fill in the tissue defect and result in scar formation.

### Regeneration

The ability of cells to regenerate depends on whether they are labile, permanent, or stable. Labile cells multiply constantly to replace cells worn out by normal physiologic processes; these include epithelial cells of the skin and those lining the gastrointestinal tract. Permanent cells include neurons—the nerve cell bodies, not their axons. Destruction of neurons is permanent, but axons may regenerate. If normal activity is to return, tissue regeneration must occur in a functional pattern, especially in the growth of several axons. Stable cells have a latent ability to regenerate. Under normal physiologic processes, they are not shed and do not need replacement, but if they are damaged or destroyed, they are able to regenerate. These include functional cells of the kidney, liver, and pancreas.

### Replacement

Depending on the extent of damage, tissue healing may occur by primary intention or by secondary intention. In **primary intention healing**, the wound is clean and dry and the edges are approximated, as in a surgical wound. Little scar formation occurs, and the wound healing usually occurs in a week. In **secondary intention healing**, the wound or defect is larger and gaping and has necrotic or dead material. The wound fills with granulation tissue from the bottom upward. The process of repair takes longer and results in more scar formation, with loss of specialized function. For example, people who have recovered from myocardial infarction have abnormal electrocardiographic tracings because the electrical signal cannot be conducted through the connective tissue that has replaced the infarcted area.

The condition of the host, the environment, and the nature and severity of the injury affect the processes of inflammation and repair. Any of the injuries previously discussed can lead to cell death. Essentially, the cell membrane becomes impaired, resulting in a nonrestricted flow of ions. Sodium and calcium enter the cell, followed by water, which leads to edema, and energy transformation ceases. Nerve impulses are no longer transmitted; muscles no longer contract. As the cell ruptures, lysosomal enzymes that destroy tissues escape, and cell death and necrosis occur.

## Nursing Implications

In the assessment of people who seek health care, both objective signs and subjective symptoms are the primary indicators of existing physiologic processes. The following questions are addressed:

- Are the heart rate, respiratory rate, and temperature normal?
- What emotional distress may be contributing to the patient's health problems?
- Are there other indicators of steady-state deviation?
- What are the patient's blood pressure, height, and weight?
- Are there any problems in movement or sensation?
- Are there any problems with affect, behavior, speech, cognitive ability, orientation, or memory?
- Are there obvious impairments, lesions, or deformities?

Further signs of change are indicated in diagnostic studies such as computed tomography (CT), magnetic resonance imaging (MRI), and positron emission tomography (PET). Objective evidence can also be obtained from laboratory data, such as electrolytes, blood urea nitrogen, blood glucose, and urinalysis results.

In making a nursing diagnosis, the nurse must relate the symptoms or problems reported by the patient to the existing physical signs. Management of specific biologic disorders is discussed in subsequent chapters; however, nurses can assist any patient to respond to stress-inducing biologic or psychological disorders with stress-management interventions.

# Stress Management: Nursing Interventions

Stress or the potential for stress is ubiquitous; that is, it is both everywhere and anywhere. Anxiety, frustration, anger, and feelings of inadequacy, helplessness, or powerlessness are emotions often associated with stress. In the presence of these emotions, the customary activities of daily living may be disrupted; for example, a sleep disturbance may occur, eating and activity patterns may be altered, and family processes or role performance may be disrupted.

Many nursing diagnoses are possible for patients suffering from stress. One nursing diagnosis related to stress is Anxiety, which is defined as a vague, uneasy feeling, the source of which may be nonspecific or not known to the person. Stress may also be manifested as ineffective coping patterns, impaired thought processes, or disrupted relationships. These human responses are reflected in the nursing diagnoses of Impaired adjustment, Ineffective coping, Defensive coping, and Ineffective denial, all of which indicate poor adaptive responses. Other possible nursing diagnoses include Social isolation, Risk for impaired parenting, Risk for spiritual distress, Readiness for enhanced family coping, Decisional conflict, Situational low self-esteem, and Risk for powerlessness, among others. Because human responses to stress are varied, as are the sources of stress, arriving at an accurate diagnosis allows interventions and goals to be more specific and leads to improved outcomes.

Stress management is directed toward reducing and controlling stress and improving coping. Nurses might use these methods not only with their patients but also in their own lives. The need to prevent illness, improve the quality of life, and decrease the cost of health care makes efforts to promote health essential, and stress control is a significant health promotion goal. Stress reduction methods and coping enhancements can derive from either internal or external sources. For example, healthy eating habits and relaxation techniques are internal resources that help reduce stress, and a broad social network is an external resource that helps reduce stress. Goods and services that can be purchased are also external resources for stress management. It is much easier for people with adequate financial resources to cope with constraints in the environment, because their sense of vulnerability to threat is decreased.

### CHART 6-2

**Information Addressed in Health Risk Questionnaires**

Demographic data: age, gender, race, ethnic background
Personal and family history of diseases and health problems
Lifestyle choices
- Eating, sleeping, exercise, smoking, drinking, sexual activity, and driving habits
- Stressors at home and on the job
- Role relationships and associated stressors

Physical measurements
- Blood pressure
- Height, weight, body mass index (BMI)
- Laboratory analyses of blood and urine

Participation in high-risk behaviors

## Promoting a Healthy Lifestyle

A health-promoting lifestyle provides internal resources that aid in coping, and it buffers or cushions the impact of stressors. Lifestyles or habits that contribute to the risk of illness can be identified through a health risk appraisal, an assessment method designed to promote health by examining a person's habits and recommending changes when a health risk is identified.

Health risk appraisals involve the use of health risk questionnaires that estimate the likelihood that people with a given set of characteristics will become ill. It is hoped that if people are provided with this information, they will alter their activities (eg, stop smoking, have periodic screening examinations) to improve their health. Questionnaires typically address the information presented in Chart 6-2.

The personal information is compared with average population risk data, and the risk factors are identified and weighted. From this analysis, the person's risks and major health hazards are identified. Further comparisons with population data can estimate how many years will be added to a person's lifespan if the suggested changes are made. However, research has not yet demonstrated that providing people with such information ensures that they will change their habits. The single most important factor for determining health status is social class, and within a social class the research suggests that the major factor influencing health is level of education (Bastable, 2003).

## Enhancing Coping Strategies

Dochterman and Bulechek (2004, p. 264) identified "coping enhancement" as a nursing intervention and defined it as "assisting a patient to adapt to perceived stressors, changes, or threats that interfere with meeting life demands and roles" (Chart 6-3). The nurse can build on the patient's existing coping strategies, as identified in the health appraisal, or teach new strategies for coping if necessary.

The five predominant ways of coping with illness identified in a review of 57 nursing research studies were as follows (Jalowiec, 1993):

- Trying to be optimistic about the outcome
- Using social support
- Using spiritual resources
- Trying to maintain control either over the situation or over feelings
- Trying to accept the situation

Other ways of coping included seeking information, reprioritizing needs and roles, lowering expectations, making compromises, comparing oneself to others, planning activities to conserve energy, taking things one step at a time, listening to one's body, and using self-talk for encouragement.

## Teaching Relaxation Techniques

Relaxation techniques are a major method used to relieve stress. Commonly used techniques include progressive muscle relaxation, the Benson Relaxation Response, and relaxation with guided imagery. The goal of relaxation training is to produce a response that counters the stress response. When this goal is achieved, the action of the hypothalamus adjusts and decreases the activity of the sympathetic and parasympathetic nervous systems. The sequence of physiologic effects and their signs and symptoms are interrupted, and psychological stress is reduced. This is a learned response and requires practice to achieve.

## CHART 6-3

### Coping Enhancement: Nursing Interventions

**DEFINITION**

Assisting a patient to adapt to perceived stressors, changes, or threats that interfere with meeting life demands and roles

**ACTIVITIES**

Appraise a patient's adjustment to changes in body image as indicated.
Appraise the impact of the patient's life situation on roles and relationships.
Encourage the patient to identify a realistic description of change in role.
Appraise the patient's understanding of the disease process.
Appraise and discuss alternative responses to the situation.
Use a calm, reassuring approach.
Provide an atmosphere of acceptance.
Assist the patient in developing an objective appraisal of the event.
Help the patient to identify the information that he or she is most interested in obtaining.
Provide factual information concerning diagnosis, treatment, and prognosis.
Provide the patient with realistic choices about certain aspects of care.
Encourage an attitude of realistic hope as a way of dealing with feelings of helplessness.
Evaluate the patient's decision-making ability.
Seek to understand the patient's perspective of a stressful situation.
Discourage decision making when the patient is under severe stress.
Encourage gradual mastery of the situation.
Encourage patience in developing relationships.
Encourage relationships with persons who have common interests and goals.
Encourage social and community activities.
Encourage the acceptance of limitations in others.
Acknowledge the patient's spiritual/cultural background.
Encourage the use of spiritual resources if desired.
Explore the patient's previous achievements.
Explore the patient's reasons for self-criticism.
Confront the patient's ambivalent (angry or depressed) feelings.
Foster constructive outlets for anger and hostility.
Arrange situations that encourage the patient's autonomy.
Assist the patient in identifying positive responses from others.
Encourage the identification of specific life values.
Explore with the patient previous methods of dealing with life problems.
Introduce the patient to persons (or groups) who have successfully undergone the same experience.
Support the use of appropriate defense mechanisms.
Encourage verbalization of feelings, perceptions, and fears.
Discuss the consequences of not dealing with guilt and shame.
Encourage the patient to identify his or her own strengths and abilities.
Assist the patient in identifying appropriate short- and long-term goals.
Assist the patient in breaking down complex goals into small, manageable steps.
Assist the patient in examining available resources to meet the goals.
Reduce stimuli in the environment that could be misinterpreted as threatening.
Appraise the patient's needs and desires for social support.
Assist the patient to identify available support systems.
Determine the risk of the patient's inflicting self-harm.
Encourage family involvement as appropriate.
Encourage the family to verbalize their feelings about the ill family member.
Provide appropriate social skills training.
Assist the patient to identify positive strategies to deal with limitations and manage needed lifestyle or role changes.
Assist the patient to solve problems in a constructive manner.
Instruct the patient in the use of relaxation techniques as needed.
Assist the patient to grieve and to work through the losses of chronic illness and/or disability if appropriate.
Assist the patient to clarify misconceptions.
Encourage the patient to evaluate his or her own behavior.

Reproduced with permission from Dochterman, J. M., & Bulechek, G. M. (2004). *Nursing interventions classification (NIC)* (4th ed.) St. Louis: Mosby.

The different relaxation techniques share four similar elements: (1) a quiet environment, (2) a comfortable position, (3) a passive attitude, and (4) a mental device (something on which to focus one's attention, such as a word, phrase, or sound).

### Progressive Muscle Relaxation

Progressive muscle relaxation involves tensing and releasing the muscles of the body in sequence and sensing the difference in feeling. It is best if the person lies on a soft cushion, in a quiet room, breathing easily. Someone usually reads the instructions in a low tone in a slow and relaxed manner, or a recording of the instructions may be played. The person tenses the muscles in the entire body (one muscle group at a time), holds, senses the tension, and then relaxes. As each muscle group is tensed, the person keeps the rest of the body relaxed. Each time the focus is on feeling the tension and relaxation. When the exercise is completed, the entire body should be relaxed (Benson, 1993; Benson & Stark, 1996).

### Benson's Relaxation Response

Benson (1993) describes the following steps of the Benson Relaxation Response:

1. Pick a brief phrase or word that reflects your basic belief system.
2. Choose a comfortable position.
3. Close your eyes.
4. Relax your muscles.
5. Become aware of your breathing, and start using your selected focus word.
6. Maintain a passive demeanor.
7. Continue for a set period of time.
8. Practice the technique twice daily.

This response combines meditation with relaxation. Along with the repeated word or phrase, a passive demeanor is essential. If other thoughts or distractions (noises, pain) occur, Benson recommends not fighting the distraction but simply continuing to repeat the focus phrase. Time of day is not important, but the exercise works best on an empty stomach.

### Relaxation With Guided Imagery

Simple **guided imagery** is the mindful use of a word, phrase, or visual image for the purpose of distracting oneself from distressing situations or consciously taking time to relax or reenergize. A nurse can help a person select a pleasant scene or experience, such as watching the ocean or dabbling the feet in a cool stream. This image serves as the mental device in this technique. As the person sits comfortably and quietly, the nurse guides the person to review the scene, trying to feel and relive the imagery with all of the senses. A recording may be made of the description of the image, or commercial recordings for guided imagery and relaxation can be used. Other relaxation techniques include meditation, breathing techniques, massage, Reiki, music therapy, biofeedback, and the use of humor.

## Educating About Stress Management

Two commonly prescribed nursing educational interventions—providing sensory information and providing procedural information (eg, preoperative teaching)—have the goal of reducing stress and improving the patient's coping ability. This preparatory education includes giving structured content, such as a lesson in childbirth preparation to expectant parents, a review of cardiovascular anatomy to a cardiac patient, or a description of sensations a patient will experience during cardiac catheterization. These techniques may alter the person–environment relationship such that something that might have been viewed as harmful or a threat will now be perceived more positively. Giving patients information also reduces the emotional response so that they can concentrate and solve problems more effectively (Loo, Espinosa, Tyler, et al., 2003; Millio & Sullivan, 2000).

## Enhancing Social Support

The nature of social support and its influence on coping have been studied extensively. Social support has been demonstrated to be an effective moderator of life stress. Social support has been found to provide people with several different types of emotional information (Ben-Ari, 2004; Heitzman & Kaplan, 1998). The first type of information leads people to believe that they are cared for and loved. This emotional support appears most often in a relationship between two people in which mutual trust and attachment are expressed by helping one another meet their emotional needs. The second type of information leads people to believe that they are esteemed and valued. This is most effective when there is recognition demonstrating a person's favorable position in the group. Known as esteem support, this elevates the person's sense of self-worth. The third type of information leads people to feel that they belong to a network of communication and mutual obligation. Members of this network share information and make goods and services available to the members as needed.

Social support also facilitates a person's coping behaviors; however, this depends on the nature of the social support. People can have extensive relationships and interact frequently, but the necessary support comes only when there is a deep level of involvement and concern, not when people merely touch the surface of each other's lives. The critical qualities within a social network are the exchange of intimate communications and the presence of solidarity and trust.

Emotional support from family and significant others provides love and a sense of sharing the burden. The emotions that accompany stress are unpleasant and often increase in a spiraling fashion if relief is not provided. Being able to talk with someone and express feelings openly may help a person gain mastery of the situation. Nurses can provide this support; however, it is important to identify the person's social support system and encourage its use. People who are "loners," who are isolated, or who withdraw in times of stress have a high risk of coping failure.

Because anxiety can also distort a person's ability to process information, it helps to seek information and advice from others who can assist with analyzing the threat and developing a strategy to manage it. Again, this use of others helps people maintain mastery of a situation and self-esteem.

Thus, social networks assist with management of stress by providing people with:

- A positive social identity
- Emotional support
- Material aid and tangible services
- Access to information
- Access to new social contacts and new social roles

## Recommending Support and Therapy Groups

Support groups exist especially for people in similar stressful situations. Groups have been formed by parents of children with leukemia; people with ostomies; women who have had mastectomies; and people with other kinds of cancer or other serious diseases, chronic illnesses, and disabilities. There are groups for single parents, substance abusers and their family members, and victims of child abuse. Professional, civic, and religious support groups are active in many communities. There are also encounter groups, assertiveness training programs, and consciousness-raising groups to help people modify their usual behaviors in their transactions with their environment. Being a member of a group with similar problems or goals has a releasing effect on a person that promotes freedom of expression and exchange of ideas.

As previously noted, a person's psychological and biologic health, internal and external sources of stress management, and relationships with the environment are predictors of health outcomes. These factors are directly related to the person's health patterns. The nurse has a significant role and responsibility in identifying the health patterns of the patient receiving care. If those patterns are not achieving physiologic, psychological, and social balance, the nurse is obligated, with the assistance and agreement of the patient, to seek ways to promote balance.

Although this chapter has presented some physiologic mechanisms and perspectives on health and disease, the way that one copes with stress, the way one relates to others, and the values and goals held are also interwoven into those physiologic patterns. To evaluate a patient's health patterns and to intervene if a problem exists requires a total assessment of the person. Specific problems and their nursing management are addressed in greater depth in other chapters.

### Critical Thinking Exercises

1. A female patient was carjacked, raped, and left on the shoulder of the road, where she was hit by a car. She is hospitalized with injuries related to her sexual assault and hit-and-run vehicle crash. Describe the physiologic and psychological trauma she has experienced. Prioritize her needs and identify appropriate nursing interventions to alleviate the major stressors.

2. A 50-year-old woman had a myocardial infarction after being diagnosed as HIV-positive. For the past 6 months, she has been working 7 days a week to buy her immunosuppressive medications. The nurse evaluates the woman's coping style. What indications would the nurse note in her interactions and follow-up care that demonstrate that the woman uses problem-focused coping or emotion-focused coping?

3. A patient experiences a severe hemorrhage of the leg after being involved in a boating crash. Describe the manner in which homeostasis has been disrupted and the compensatory mechanisms that are evident. How does the patient's medical treatment support the compensatory mechanisms? How do you determine the nursing interventions that are appropriate for promoting the healing process?

4. **ebp** A 90-year-old man recently moved to an assisted living community, where he maintains himself on an independent and supervised unit. A nurse practitioner assesses this patient's health promotion needs. The family's health history reveals that his mother had type 2 diabetes and thyroid disease and that his father had coronary artery disease. This client has ample resources for making necessary lifestyle changes. What suggestions would the nurse practitioner initiate to promote a healthy lifestyle? What is the evidence base that supports the relationship between lifestyle and health status? Describe the strength of the evidence regarding the effectiveness of lifestyle changes in promoting health. Identify the criteria used to evaluate the strength of the evidence.

### REFERENCES AND SELECTED READINGS

### BOOKS

Bastable, S. B. (Ed.). (2003). *Nurse as educator: Principles of teaching and learning.* Boston: Jones & Bartlett.

Benson, H. (1993). The relaxation response. In D. Goleman & J. Gurin (Eds.), *Mind-body medicine: How to use your mind for better health.* Yonkers, NY: Consumer Reports Books.

Benson, H., & Proctor, W. (1984). *Beyond the relaxation response.* New York: Berkley Books.

Benson, H., & Stark, M. (1996). *Timeless healing.* New York: Scribner.

Chiorazzi, N. (2003). *Immune mechanisms and disease.* New York: New York Academy of Science.

Copel, L. C. (2000). *Nurse's clinical guide: Psychiatric and mental health care* (2nd ed.). Springhouse, PA: Springhouse.

Dochterman, J. C., & Bulechek, G. M. (Eds.). (2004). *Nursing interventions classification (NIC)* (4th ed.). St. Louis: Mosby.

Dubos, R. (1965). *Man adapting.* New Haven, CT: Yale University Press.

Evans, P., Hucklebridge, F., & Clow, A. (2000). *Mind, immunity, and health: The science of psychoimmunology.* New York: Free Association Books.

Fauci, A. (Ed.). (2001). *Harrison's principles of internal medicine* (15th ed.). New York: McGraw-Hill.

Furman, M. E., & Gallo, F. (2000). *The neurophysics of human behavior: Explorations at the interface of the brain, mind, behavior, and information.* Boca Raton, FL: CRC Press.

Guyton, A. C., & Hall, J. E. (2001). *Textbook of medical physiology* (10th ed.). Philadelphia: W. B. Saunders.

Guyton, A. C., Hall, J. E., & Schmitt, W. (1997). *Human physiology and mechanisms of disease* (6th ed.). Philadelphia: W. B. Saunders.

Jalowiec, A. (1993). Coping with illness: Synthesis and critique of the nursing literature from 1980–1990. In J. D. Barnfather & B. L. Lyon (Eds.), *Stress and coping: State of the science and implications for nursing theory, research, and practice.* Indianapolis: Sigma Theta Tau International.

Lazarus, R. S. (1991a). *Emotion and adaptation.* New York: Oxford University Press.

Lazarus, R. S. (1993). Why we should think of stress as a subset of emotion. In L. Goldberger & S. Breznitz (Eds.), *Handbook of stress: Theoretical and clinical aspects* (2nd ed.). New York: The Free Press.

Lazarus, R. S., & Folkman, S. (1984). *Stress, appraisal, and coping.* New York: Springer Publishing Co.

McPhee, S. J., Lingrappa, V. R., & Ganong, W. F. (2003). *Pathophysiology of disease: An introduction to clinical medicine* (4th ed.). New York: McGraw-Hill.

Mickler, M. (1997). *Community organizing and community building for health.* New Brunswick, NJ: Rutgers University Press.

Miller, L. H., & Smith, A. D. (1993). *The stress solution.* New York: Pocket Books.

North American Nursing Diagnosis Association. (2002). *NANDA nursing diagnoses: Definitions and classifications 2003–2004.* Philadelphia: Author.

Pearsall, P. (2003). *The Beethoven factor: The new positive psychology of hardiness, happiness, healing, and hope.* Charlottesville, VA: Hampton Roads Publishing Company.

Porth, C. M. (2005). *Pathophysiology. Concepts of altered health status.* Philadelphia: Lippincott Williams & Wilkins.

Rice, V. (1999). *Handbook of stress, coping, and health: Implications for nursing research, theory, and practice.* Thousand Oaks, CA: Sage.

Selye, H. (1976). *The stress of life.* (Rev. ed.). New York: McGraw-Hill.

Slikker, W., Andrews, R., & Trembly, B. (2003). *Neuroprotective agents.* New York: New York Academy of Science.

Sternberg, E. M., Haour, F. G., & Smith, C. C. (Eds.). (2003). *Neuroendocrine and neural regulation of autoimmune and inflammatory disease: Molecular, systems, and clinical insights.* New York: New York Academy of Science.

Zautra, A. J. (2003). *Emotions, stress, and health.* Oxford & New York: Oxford University Press.

## JOURNALS

*Asterisks indicate nursing research articles.

*al-Absi, M., Hatsukami, D., Davis, G. L., et al. (2004). Prospective examination of effects of smoking abstinence on cortisol and withdrawal symptoms of early smoking relapse. *Drug and Alcohol Dependence, 73*(3), 267–278.

*Ben-Ari, A. (2004). Sources of social support and attachment styles among Israeli-Arab students. *International Social Work, 47*(2), 187–201.

*Brissette, I., Leventhal, H., & Leventhal, E. A. (2003). Observer ratings of health and sickness: Can other people tell us anything about our health that we don't already know? *Health Psychology, 22*(5), 471–478.

Brooks, M. V. (2003). Health-related hardiness and chronic illness: A synthesis of current research. *Nursing Forum, 38*(3), 11–19.

Carter-Snell, C., & Hegadoren, K. (2003). Stress disorders and gender: Implications for theory and research. *Canadian Journal of Nursing Research, 35*(2), 35–55.

Clark, A. M. (2003). "It's like an explosion in your life"—lay perspectives on stress and myocardial infarction. *Journal of Clinical Nursing, 12*(4), 544–553.

*Constantino, R. E., Sekula, L. K., Rabin, B., et al. (2000). Negative life experiences, depression, and immune function in abused and non-abused women. *Biological Research in Nursing, 1*(3), 190–198.

Cooper, M. A., Pommering, T. L., & Koranyi, K. (2003). Primary immunodeficiencies. *American Family Physician, 68*(10), 2001–2011.

Cutler, R. B., Fishbain, D. A., Steele-Rosomoff, R., et al. (2003). Relationships between functional capacity measures and baseline psychological measures in chronic pain patients. *Journal of Occupational Rehabilitation, 13*(4), 249–258.

Donnelly, G. (2004). From surviving to thriving: The Beethoven factor. *Holistic Nursing Practice, 18*(2), 51–52.

Dosani, S. (2003). Review: Stress is a problem for mental health nurses but research on interventions is insufficient. *Evidence-Based Mental Health, 6*(4), 126.

Edwards, D., & Burnard, P. (2003). A systematic review of stress and stress management interventions for mental health nurses. *Journal of Advanced Nursing, 42*(2), 169–200.

*Elder, R., Wollin, J., Hartel, C., et al. (2003). Hassles and uplifts associated with caring for people with cognitive impairment in community settings. *International Journal of Mental Health Nursing, 12*(4), 271–278.

*Erlandsson, L., & Eklund, M. (2003). Women's experiences of hassles and uplifts in their everyday patterns of occupations. *Occupational Therapy International, 10*(2), 95–114.

*Gross, R., Brammli-Greenberg, S., & Bentur, N. (2003). Women caring for disabled parents and other relatives: Implications for social workers in the health services. *Social Work in Health Care, 37*(4), 19–37.

Hausmann, O. N. (2003). Post-traumatic inflammation following spinal cord injury. *Spinal Cord, 41*(7), 369–378.

Heitzman, C. A., & Kaplan, R. M. (1998). Assessment of methods for measuring social support. *Health Psychology, 7,* 75–109.

Holmes, T. H., & Rahe, R. H. (1967). The social readjustment rating scale. *Journal of Psychosomatic Research, 11,* 213–218.

*Kennedy, J. W. (2000). Women's inner balance: A comparison of stressors, personality traits, and health problems by age groups. *Journal of Advanced Nursing, 31*(3), 639–650.

*Kincy, J., Pratt, D., Slater, R., et al. (2003). A survey of patterns and sources of stress among medical and nursing staff in an intensive care unit setting. *Care of the Critically Ill, 19*(3), 83–87.

Lazarus, R. S. (1991b). Cognition and motivation in emotion. *American Psychologist, 46*(4), 352–367.

Lazarus, R. S. (1991c). Progress on a cognitive-motivational-relational theory of emotion. *American Psychologist, 46*(8), 819–834.

Loo, K. K., Espinosa, M., Tyler, R., et al. (2003). Using knowledge to cope with stress in the NICU: How parents integrate learning to read the physiologic and behavioral cues of the infant. *Neonatal Network: Journal of Neonatal Nursing, 22*(1), 31–37.

*Millio, M. E., & Sullivan, K. (2000). Patients with operable esophageal cancer: Their experience of information giving in a regional thoracic unit. *Journal of Clinical Nursing, 9*(2), 236–246.

Mortzer, S. A., & Hertig, V. (2004). Stress, stress response, and health. *Nursing Clinics of North America, 39*(3), 1–17.

Norman, D. (2003). The effects of stress on wound healing and leg ulceration. *British Journal of Nursing, 12*(21), 1256–1263.

*Olofsson, B., Bengtsson, C., & Brink, E. (2003). Absence of response: A study of nurses' experience of stress in the workplace. *Journal of Nursing Management, 11*(5), 351–358.

Pike, J. L., Smith, T. L., Hauger, R. L., et al. (1997). Chronic life stress alters sympathetic, neuroendocrine, and immune responsivity to an acute psychological stressor in humans. *Psychosomatic Medicine, 59*(4), 447–457.

Ptacek, J. T., & Pierce, G. R. (2003). Issues in the study of stress and coping in rehabilitation settings. *Rehabilitation Psychology, 48*(2), 113–124.

Rankin, J. A. (2004). Biological mediators of acute inflammation. *AACN Clinical Issues: Advanced Practice in Acute and Critical Care, 15*(1), 3–17.

Rider, S. H. (2004). Psychological distress: Concept analysis. *Journal of Advanced Nursing, 45*(5), 536–545.

Robinson, F. P., Matthews, H. L., & Witek-Janusek, L. (2000). Stress reduction and HIV disease: A review of intervention studies using a psycho-immunology framework. *Journal of the Association of Nurses in AIDS Care, 11*(2), 87–96.

Sansovich, D. (2003). Harm reduction, substance use and the immune system. *HIV Clinician 15*(2), 13–15.

Shapley, M., Jordan, K., & Croft, P. R. (2003). Increased vaginal bleeding and psychological distress: A longitudinal study of their relationship in the community. *International Journal of Obstetrics and Gynecology, 110*(6), 548–554.

*Tausig, M. (1982). Measuring life events. *Journal of Health and Social Behavior, 23*(1), 52–64.

*Vines, S. W., Gupta, S., Whiteside, T., et al. (2003). The relationship between chronic pain, immune function, depression, and health behaviors. *Biological Research for Nursing, 5*(1), 18–29.

Whitty, M. T. (2003). Coping and defending: Age differences in maturity of defense mechanisms and coping strategies. *Aging and Mental Health, 7*(2), 123–132.

CHAPTER 7

# Individual and Family Considerations Related to Illness

## Learning Objectives

*On completion of this chapter, the learner will be able to:*

1. Describe the holistic approach to sustaining health and well-being.
2. Discuss the concepts of emotional well-being and emotional distress.
3. Identify variables that influence the ability to cope with stress and that are antecedents to emotional disorders.
4. Explain the concepts of anxiety, posttraumatic stress disorder, depression, loss, and grief.
5. Assess the impact of illness on the patient's family and on family functioning.
6. Determine the role of the nurse in identifying substance abuse problems and in helping families to cope.
7. Explore the concept of spirituality and address the spiritual needs of patients.
8. Identify nursing actions that promote effective coping for both patients and families.

When people experience threats to their health, they seek out various care providers for the purpose of maintaining or restoring health. In recent years, both patients and families have become increasingly involved in health care and health promotion activities. At the same time, greater numbers of consumers and practitioners have recognized the interconnectedness of mind, body, and spirit in sustaining well-being and overcoming or coping with illness. This holistic approach to health and wellness and the increased consumer involvement reflect a renewed emphasis on the concepts of choice, healing, and patient–practitioner partnerships. The holistic perspective focuses not only on promoting well-being but also on understanding how a person's emotional state contributes to health and illness. By using this knowledge, people are better able to prevent the recurrence or exacerbation of health problems and to develop strategies to improve their future health status.

## Holistic Approach to Health and Health Care

Since the 1980s, holistic therapies have more frequently accompanied traditional health care. It is estimated that approximately 35% to 45% of consumers in the United States follow **holistic health** practices. More than 50% of people supplement traditional health care treatments with **complementary and alternative therapies**. In an ambulatory care setting in which human immunodeficiency virus (HIV) and acquired immunodeficiency syndrome (AIDS) are treated, 51% of patients reported discussing their complementary therapies with their health care providers (Chang, Van Servellen, & Lombardi, 2003). In all settings, it is imperative that during clinical assessments the use of these adjunct therapies be assessed. Some of the most commonly used complementary therapies are listed in Chart 7-1.

For some people, the holistic approach is viewed as a way to capitalize on personal strengths and recultivate the values and beliefs about health that were common before the age of technological innovations and the sophistication of biomedical science. A lack of focus on individual patients, families, and their environments by some health care providers has created feelings of disillusionment and depersonalization in many people. The cost of illness, especially care for chronic disease, continues to escalate and accounts for an increasing percentage of health care dollars. At the same time, patient satisfaction with health care has decreased.

Active participation by patients and families in health promotion supports the self-care model historically embraced by the nursing profession. This model is congruent with the philosophy that seeks to balance and integrate the use of crisis medicine and advanced technology with the

---

**CHART 7-1**

### Common Complementary and Alternative Therapies

- Alternative medical systems including acupuncture, Ayurveda, homeopathic medicine, and naturopathic medicine
- Mind-body interventions including meditation, certain uses of hypnosis, dance, music, art therapy, and prayer
- Biologically based therapies including herbal, special dietary, orthomolecular, and individual biological therapies
- Manipulative and body-based methods including chiropractic and osteopathy
- Energy therapies including Qi gong, Reiki, and therapeutic touch

Reprinted with permission from Dossey, B. M., Guzzetta, C., & Keegan, L. (2002). *Holistic nursing: A handbook for practice.* Gaithersburg, MD: Aspen Publications.

---

## Glossary

**anxiety:** an emotional state characterized by feelings of apprehension, discomfort, restlessness, or worry

**bereavement:** feelings, thoughts, and responses that occur after a loss

**complementary therapies:** used as an adjunct to traditional health modalities; they typically influence the effects of stress, anxiety, depression, and other physical and emotional states

**depression:** state in which a person feels sad, distressed, and hopeless, with little to no energy for normal activities

**faith:** belief and trust in a God or higher power

**family:** a group whose members are related by reciprocal caring, mutual responsibilities, and loyalties

**grief:** a universal response to any loss

**holistic health:** promotion of the total health of mind, body, and spirit

**homeopathic medicine:** a system of medicine that promotes healing of the whole person by stimulating the natural healing processes within the person

**mental disorder:** a state in which a person has deficits in functioning, has a distorted sense of self or the world, is unable to sustain relationships, or cannot handle stress or conflict effectively

**mental health:** a state in which a person can meet basic needs, assume responsibilities, sustain relationships, resolve conflicts, and grow throughout life

**posttraumatic stress disorder (PTSD):** the development of severe anxiety-type symptoms after the experience of a traumatic life event

**substance abuse:** a maladaptive pattern of drug use that causes physical and emotional harm with the potential for disruption of daily life influence of the mind and spirit on healing. A holistic approach to health reconnects the traditionally separate approaches to mind and body. Factors such as the physical environment, economic conditions, sociocultural issues, emotional state, interpersonal relationships, and support systems can work together or alone to influence health. The connections among physical health, emotional health, and spiritual well-being must be understood and considered when providing health care. It is the nurse's conceptual integration of the physiologic health condition with the emotional and social context, along with the tasks and developments of the patient's life stage, that allows for the development of a holistic plan of nursing care.

## The Brain and Physical and Emotional Health

Research on brain structure and function, neurochemical messenger systems (neurotransmitters), and brain–body connections suggests fundamental, delicate, two-way relationships between the brain's environment and mood, behavior, and resistance to disease. One focus of brain research has been to identify and integrate traditional medical and psychiatric knowledge with new psychobiologic and psychoneuroimmunologic data. Researchers in the field of psychobiology study the biologic basis of mental disturbances and have identified some relationships between mental disorders and changes in the structure and function of the brain. Researchers in the field of psychoneuroimmunology study the connections between the emotions, the central nervous system, the neuroendocrine system, and the immune system and have established compelling evidence that psychosocial variables can affect the functioning of the immune system.

As this neuroscientific research continues, data about neurotransmitters and the functioning of the brain will augment existing understanding of emotions, intelligence, memory, and many aspects of general body functioning. In the future, an accepted definition of mental illness may well include biologic information. By enhancing the biologic knowledge base about the brain and nervous system, scientists have established the foundation for breakthroughs in the treatment of both symptoms and illnesses.

These findings suggest that the health care community should place as much emphasis on emotional health as it places on physiologic health and should recognize how biologic, emotional, and societal problems combine to affect individual patients, families, and communities. Some problems that nurses and other health care providers must address include **substance abuse**, homelessness, family violence, eating disorders, trauma, and chronic **mental health** conditions such as anxiety and depression. To focus attention on these and other mental health problems, the U.S. Department of Health and Human Services initiated a mental health agenda for the nation in *Healthy People 2010* (U.S. Public Health Service, 2000). The objectives identified are summarized in Chart 7-2. Nurses in all settings encounter patients with mental health problems and can play an integral role in helping to achieve the national goals by recognizing and relieving emotional distress and promoting emotional health.

---

**CHART 7-2**

### *Major Mental Health Objectives for Healthy People in the Year 2010*

- Reduce the proportion of children and adolescents with disabilities who are reported to be sad, unhappy, or depressed.
- Reduce the proportion of adults with disabilities who report feelings such as sadness, unhappiness, or depression that prevent them from being active.
- Increase the proportion of adults with disabilities reporting sufficient emotional support.
- Increase the proportion of adults with disabilities reporting satisfaction with life.
- Reduce the suicide rate.
- Reduce the rate of suicide attempts by adolescents.
- Reduce the proportion of homeless adults who have serious mental illness.
- Increase the proportion of persons with serious mental illness who are employed.
- Reduce the relapse rates for persons with eating disorders including anorexia nervosa and bulimia nervosa.
- Increase the number of persons in primary care who receive mental health screening and assessment.
- Increase the proportion of children with mental health problems who receive treatment.
- Increase the proportion of juvenile justice facilities that screen admissions for mental health problems.
- Increase the proportion of adults with mental disorders who receive treatment.
- Increase the proportion of persons with co-occurring substance abuse and mental disorders who receive treatment for both disorders.
- Increase the number of states and the District of Columbia that track consumer satisfaction with the mental health services they receive.
- Increase the number of states, territories, and the District of Columbia with an operational mental health plan that addresses cultural competence.

U.S. Public Health Service. (2000). *Healthy people 2010: Understanding and improving health*. Washington, DC: U.S. Government Printing Office.

# Emotional Health and Emotional Distress

Emotional health involves the ability to function as comfortably and productively as possible. Typically, people who are mentally healthy are satisfied with themselves and their life situations. In the usual course of living, emotionally healthy people focus on activities geared to meet their needs and attempt to accomplish personal goals while concurrently managing everyday challenges and problems. Often, people must work hard to balance their feelings, thoughts, and behaviors to alleviate emotional distress, and much energy is used to change, adapt, or manage the obstacles inherent in daily living. A mentally healthy person accepts reality and has a positive sense of self. Emotional health is also manifested by having moral and humanistic values and beliefs, having satisfying interpersonal relationships, doing productive work, and maintaining a realistic sense of hope (Chart 7-3).

When people have unmet emotional needs or distress, they experience an overall feeling of unhappiness. As tension escalates, security and survival are threatened. How different people respond to these troublesome situations reflects their level of coping and maturity. Emotionally healthy people endeavor to meet the demands of distressing situations while still coping with the typical issues that emerge in their lives. The ways in which people respond to uncomfortable stimuli reflect their exposure to various biologic, emotional, and sociocultural experiences.

When stress interferes with a person's ability to function comfortably and inhibits the effective management of personal needs, that person is at risk for emotional problems. The use of ineffective and unhealthy methods of coping is manifested by dysfunctional behaviors, thoughts, and feelings. These behaviors are aimed at relieving the overwhelming stress, even though they may cause further problems.

Coping ability is strongly influenced by biologic or genetic factors, physical and emotional growth and development, family and childhood experiences, and learning. Typically, people revert to the strategies observed early in life that were used by family members, caregivers, and others to resolve conflicts. If these strategies were not adaptive, the person exhibits a range of painful and nonproductive behaviors. Dysfunctional behavior in one person not only seriously affects that person's emotional health but can also put others at risk for injury or death. As these destructive behaviors are repeated, a cyclic pattern becomes evident: impaired thinking, negative feelings, and more dysfunctional actions that prevent the person from meeting the demands of daily living (Chart 7-4).

No universally accepted definition of what constitutes an emotional disorder exists, but many views and theories share the idea that a number of variables can interfere with emotional growth and development and impede successful adaptation to the environment. Most clinicians have adopted the statement from the American Psychiatric Association's *Diagnostic and Statistical Manual of Mental Disorders (DSM-IV-TR)*, which defines the term **mental disorder** as a group of behavioral or psychological symptoms or a pattern that manifests itself in significant distress, impaired functioning, or accentuated risk of enduring severe suffering or possible death (American Psychiatric Association, 2000). Risk factors for mental health problems are listed in Chart 7-5.

Patients seen in medical-surgical settings often struggle with psychosocial issues of anxiety, depression, loss, and grief. Abuse, addiction, chemical dependency, body image disturbances, and eating disorders are a few examples of health situations that require extensive physical and emotional care to restore optimal functioning. The dual challenge for the health care team is to understand how the patient's emotions influence current physiologic conditions and to

---

**CHART 7-3**

## Characteristics Associated With Mental Health

- Positive sense of self
- Satisfying interpersonal relationships
- Wide range of appropriate emotions
- Love and care for self and others
- Realistic and responsible behavior
- Effective coping skills
- Ability to negotiate and resolve conflict
- Cooperative and interdependent in working with others
- Engagement in rewarding, productive work
- Adaptable to the daily challenges of life
- Finds meaning and purpose in life
- Has hopes and dreams
- Knowledge of personal strengths and areas needing improvement
- Sense of humor
- Respect for the rights and differences of others

---

**CHART 7-4**

## Characteristics Associated With Mental Disorders

- Severe anxiety
- Severe depression
- Ineffective coping mechanisms
- Extreme feelings of helplessness or powerlessness
- Maladaptive ways of dealing with stress
- Uncomfortable with self and others
- Lack of pleasure from living
- Extreme negative thoughts, feelings, and behaviors
- Disorganized or disturbed thoughts
- Inability to accept reality
- Personality traits that contribute to dysfunctional behaviors
- Desire to hurt self or others
- History of traumatic experience
- Inability to satisfy basic needs
- Lack of a support system
- Physiologic problems resulting from severe, unrelenting stress

## CHART 7-5

### Risk Factors for Mental Health Problems

**Nonmodifiable Risk Factors**
- Age
- Gender
- Genetic background
- Family history

**Modifiable Risk Factors**
- Marital status
- Family environment
- Housing problems
- Poverty or economic difficulties
- Physical health
- Nutritional status
- Stress level
- Social environment and activities
- Exposure to trauma
- Alcohol and drug use
- Environmental toxins or other pollutants
- Availability, accessibility, and cost of health services

## CHART 7-6

### Adult Developmental Tasks

Developmental stage and associated tasks can have an impact on how individuals cope with illness.

**Young Adult**
- Establish independence
- Establish lifestyle
- Develop career
- Develop intimate relationships
- Marry and start a family

**Middle Adult**
- Establish financial security
- Prepare for retirement
- Launch children
- Refocus on marital/family relationship
- Support growing children and aging parents

**Older Adult**
- Adapt to retirement and alteration in role
- Adapt to declining physical stamina
- Review life's accomplishments
- Prepare for death

identify the best care for the patient experiencing underlying emotional and spiritual distress.

## Family Health and Distress

The **family** plays a central role in the life of the patient and is a major part of the context of the patient's life. It is within families that people grow, are nurtured, acquire a sense of self, develop beliefs and values about life, and progress through life's developmental stages (Chart 7-6). Families are also the first source for socialization and teaching about health and illness. Families prepare people with strategies for balancing closeness with separateness and togetherness with individuality. A major role of families is to provide physical and emotional resources to maintain health and a system of support in times of crises, such as in periods of illness. Educating families has been shown to add to their resiliency, adaptation, and adjustment to life stressors (Friedman, Bowden, & Jones, 2003).

Health problems often affect the family's ability to function. Five family functions described by Wright and Leahey (2000) are viewed as essential to the growth of individuals and families. The first function, management, involves the use of power, decision making about resources, establishment of rules, provision of finances, and future planning—responsibilities assumed by the adults of the family. The second function, boundary setting, makes clear distinctions between the generations and the roles of adults and children within the family structure. The third function, communication, is important to individual and family growth; healthy families have a full range of clear, direct, and meaningful communication among their members. The fourth function consists of education and support, which are interrelated. Education involves modeling skills for living a physically, emotionally, and socially healthy life. Support is manifested by actions that tell family members they are cared about and loved; it promotes health and is seen as a critical factor in coping with crises and illness situations. The fifth function, socialization, involves families' transmission of culture and the acceptable behaviors needed to perform adequately in the home and in the world.

## Nursing Implications

When a family member becomes ill, injured, or disabled, all members of the family are affected. Depending on the nature of the health problem, family members may need to modify their existing lifestyles or even restructure their lives.

There are many degrees of family functioning. Nurses assess family functioning to determine how the particular family will cope with the impact of the health condition. If the family is chaotic or disorganized, promoting coping skills becomes a priority in the plan of care. The family with preexisting problems may require additional assistance before participating fully in the current health situation. In performing a family assessment, the nurse must evaluate the present family structure and function. Areas of appraisal include demographic data, developmental information (keeping in mind that different family members can be in different developmental stages simultaneously), family structure, family functioning, and coping abilities. The role that the environment plays in family health is also assessed.

Interventions with family members are based on strengthening coping skills through direct care, communication skills, and education. Healthy family communication has a strong influence on the quality of family life and can help the family make appropriate choices, consider alternative strategies, or persevere through complex circumstances. Within a family system, for example, a particular patient may be undergoing extensive surgery for cancer while the partner has cardiac disease, an adolescent has type 1 diabetes mellitus, and a child has a fractured arm. In this situation, there are multiple health concerns along with competing developmental tasks and needs. Despite the obvious concerns of the family members, both individually and collectively, a crisis may or may not be present. The family may be coping effectively, or it may be in crisis or unable to handle the situation. Ideally, the health care team conducts a careful and comprehensive family assessment, develops interventions tailored to handle the stressors, implements the specified treatment protocols, and facilitates the construction of social support systems.

The use of existing family strengths, resources, and education is augmented by therapeutic family interventions. The primary goals of the nurse are to maintain and improve the patient's present level of health and to prevent physical and emotional deterioration. Next, the nurse intervenes in the cycle that the illness creates: patient illness, stress for other family members, new illness in other family members, and additional patient stress.

Helping the family members handle the myriad stressors that bombard them daily involves working with family members to develop coping skills. Burr and associates (Burr, Klein, Burr, et al., 1984) identified seven traits that enhance coping of family members under stress. Communication skills and spirituality were the most useful traits. Cognitive abilities, emotional strengths, relationship capabilities, willingness to use community resources, and individual strengths and talents were also associated with effective coping. As nurses work with families, they must not underestimate the impact that their therapeutic interactions, educational information, positive role modeling, provision of direct care, and corrective teaching have on promoting health.

Without the active support of the family members and the health care team, the potential for maladaptive coping increases. Often, denial and blaming of individuals occur. Sometimes, physiologic illness, emotional withdrawal, and physical distancing are the results of severe family conflict, violent behavior, or addiction to drugs and alcohol. Substance abuse may develop in family members who feel unable to cope or solve problems. Frequently, people engage in these dysfunctional behaviors when faced with difficult or problematic situations.

## Anxiety

All people experience some degree of **anxiety** (a tense emotional state) as they face new, challenging, or threatening life situations. In clinical settings, fear of the unknown, unexpected news about one's health, and any impairment of bodily functions engenders anxiety. Although a mild level of anxiety can mobilize a person to take a position, act on the task that needs to be done, or learn to alter lifestyle habits, more severe anxiety can be paralyzing. Anxiety that escalates to a near panic state can be incapacitating. When patients receive unwelcome news about results of diagnostic studies, they are certain to experience anxiety. Different patients manifest physiologic, emotional, and behavioral signs and symptoms of anxiety in different ways.

### Nursing Implications

Early clinical observations of guilt or anxiety are an essential component of nursing care (Chart 7-7). A high level of anxiety in a patient will probably exacerbate physiologic distress. For example, a postoperative patient who is in pain may discover that anxiety intensifies the sensation of pain. A patient newly diagnosed with type 1 diabetes mellitus may be worried and fearful and therefore unable to focus on or complete essential self-care activities. Somatic symptoms may occur in any patient with moderate to severe anxiety.

The *DSM-IV-TR* (2000) lists general medical conditions that cause anxiety. They include endocrine diseases, such as hypothyroidism, hyperthyroidism, hypoglycemia, and hyperadrenocorticism; cardiovascular conditions, such as cardiac dysrhythmia, heart failure, and pulmonary emboli; respiratory disorders, such as pneumonia and chronic obstructive pulmonary disease; and neurologic disorders, such as multiple sclerosis, encephalitis, and neoplasms.

All nurses must be vigilant about patients who worry excessively and deteriorate in emotional, social, or occupational functioning. If participation in the therapeutic regimen (eg, administration of insulin) becomes a problem because of extreme anxiety, nursing interventions must be immediately initiated. Caring strategies emphasize ways for the patient to verbalize feelings and fears and to identify sources of anxiety. The need to teach and promote effective coping abilities and the use of relaxation techniques are the priorities of care. In some cases, antianxiety medication may be prescribed. Chart 7-8 provides a list of basic nursing principles that are useful for assisting patients to manage severe anxiety. Chapter 6 presents additional information about stress and the relaxation response.

## Posttraumatic Stress Disorder

In medical-surgical settings, especially in emergency departments, burn units, and rehabilitation centers, nurses care for extremely anxious patients who have experienced overwhelming events that are considered to be outside the range of normal human experience. Many of these patients suffer from **posttraumatic stress disorder** (PTSD), a condition that generates waves of anxiety, anger, aggression, depression, and suspicion; threatens a person's sense of self; and interferes with daily functioning. Specific examples of events that place people at risk for PTSD are rape, family violence, torture, terrorist attacks, fire, earthquake, and military combat. Patients who have experienced a traumatic event are often frequent users of the health care system, seeking treatment for the overall emotional and physical trauma that they experienced.

The physiologic responses noted in people who have been severely traumatized include increased activity of the sympa-

## NURSING RESEARCH PROFILE

### Anxiety and Coping Behaviors

Clark, A. M. (2003). "It's like an explosion in your life": Lay perspectives on stress and myocardial infarction. *Journal of Clinical Nursing, 12*(4), 544–553.

#### Purpose
Different people manifest the physiologic, emotional, and behavioral signs and symptoms of stress and anxiety in different ways. This research study explored patient reports about the nature and complexities of emotional disturbances after myocardial infarction (MI). Patients who had an MI described their views of how stress affects functioning and the relationship of stress to their MI.

#### Design
This qualitative study used a semistructured interview technique to encourage investigation of stress from patients' perspectives. Fourteen patients (eight men and six women) from a hospital in Glasgow, Scotland, participated in the study. Criteria for inclusion in the study were first MI diagnosis, conscious and not intubated, stable vital signs, no pain, and no invasive procedure other than blood work for at least 8 hours prior to data collection.

#### Findings
The participants expressed their feelings and responses related to the experience of having an MI. An example of a participant's explanation was, "It's like an explosion in your life. Everything changes, everything." Patients reflected on their emotional conceptions of the situation and focused on everyday stress as playing a major role in the development of their MI. They used words such as "worry," "fright," "anger," "panic," and "sweats." Overall, stress was conceptualized as a cause of the MI, a societal norm, a personal trait, a response to major life events, and a response to daily life events. This study confirmed that both similarities and differences exist between how laypeople and health care professionals communicate about stress related to coronary artery disease.

#### Nursing Implications
Nurses must understand patient views of stress, because this understanding can shape beneficial nursing interventions. Nurses must recognize that the word "stress" is used by patients to denote conditions ranging from the stress of daily living to the response to major life events; nurses must focus on the language that patients use and the meaning of such language. In addition, nurses must be careful not to make assumptions about patient stress. If patients view stress as beyond their control, nursing interventions to reduce stress may not be viewed as practical. If nurses have limited or inadequate knowledge about patients' perspectives of stress, nursing interventions will be less effective.

---

thetic nervous system, increased plasma catecholamine levels, and increased urinary epinephrine and norepinephrine levels. It has been postulated (Loseke, Gelles, & Cavanaugh, 2004) that people with PTSD lose the ability to control their response to stimuli. The resulting excessive arousal can increase overall body metabolism and trigger emotional reactivity. In this situation, nurses observe that patients have difficulty sleeping, have an exaggerated startle response, and are excessively vigilant.

Symptoms of PTSD can occur hours to years after the trauma is experienced. Acute PTSD is defined as the experience of symptoms for less than a 3-month period. Chronic PTSD is defined as the experience of symptoms lasting longer than 3 months. In the case of delayed PTSD, up to 6 months may elapse between the trauma and the manifestation of symptoms (American Psychiatric Association, 2000). For more information, see Chart 7-9.

### Nursing Implications

It is often thought that the incidence of PTSD is very low in the overall population. However, when high-risk groups are studied, the results indicate that more than 50% of study participants have PTSD (Cathersall, 2004). Therefore, it is important that nurses consider which of their patients are at risk for PTSD and be knowledgeable about the common symptoms associated with it. Older people are more susceptible to the physical effects of trauma and the effects of PTSD because of the neural inactivation associated with aging. It has also been speculated that people who have a preexisting tendency to become extremely anxious have an increased vulnerability for PTSD (Sharhabani-Ary, Amir, Kotler, et al., 2003).

The sensitivity and caring of the nurse creates the interpersonal relationship necessary to work with patients who have PTSD. These patients are physically compromised and are struggling emotionally with situations that are not considered part of normal human experience—situations that violate the commonly held perceptions of human social justice. Treatment of patients with PTSD includes several essential components: establishing a trusting relationship, addressing and working through the trauma experience, and providing education about the coping skills needed for recovery and self-care. The patient's progress can be influenced by the ability to cope with the various aspects of both the physical and the emotional distress.

## CHART 7-7

### Assessing for Anxiety

Be on the alert for the following signs and symptoms:

**Physiologic Indicators**
- Appetite change
- Headaches
- Muscle tension
- Fatigue or lethargy
- Weight change
- Cold and flu symptoms
- Digestive upsets
- Grinding teeth
- Palpitations
- Hypertension
- Restlessness
- Difficulty sleeping
- Skin irritations
- Injury prone
- Increased use of any alcohol or drugs

**Emotional Indicators**
- Forgetfulness
- Low productivity
- Feeling dull
- Poor concentration
- Negative attitude
- Confusion
- Whirling mind
- No new ideas
- Boredom
- Negative self-talk
- Anxiety
- Frustration
- Depression
- Crying periods
- Irritability
- Worrying
- Feeling discouraged
- Nervous laughter

**Relational Indicators**
- Isolation
- Intolerance
- Resentment
- Loneliness
- Lashing out
- "Clamming up"
- Nagging
- Distrust
- Few friends
- No intimacy
- Using people

**Spiritual Indicators**
- Emptiness
- Loss of meaning
- Doubt
- Unforgiving attitude
- Martyrdom
- Loss of direction
- Cynicism
- Apathy

## CHART 7-8

### Managing Anxiety

- Listen actively and focus on having the patient discuss personal feelings.
- Use positive remarks and focus on the positive aspects of life in the "here and now."
- Use appropriate touch (with patient permission) to demonstrate support.
- Discuss the importance of safety and the patient's overall sense of well-being.
- Explain all procedures, policies, diagnostic studies, medications, treatments, or protocols for care.
- Explore coping strategies and work with the patient to practice and use them effectively (eg, breathing, progressive relaxation, visualization, imagery).
- Use distraction as indicated to relax and prevent self from being overwhelmed.

## Depression

**Depression** is a common response to health problems and is an often underdiagnosed problem in the patient population. People may become depressed as a result of injury or illness; may be suffering from an earlier loss that is compounded by a new health problem; or may seek health care for somatic manifestations of depression.

Clinical depression is distinguished from everyday feelings of sadness by its duration and severity. Most people occasionally feel down or depressed, but these feelings are short-lived and do not result in impaired functioning. Clinically depressed people usually have had signs of a depressed mood or a decreased interest in pleasurable activities for at least a 2-week period. An obvious impairment in social, occupational, and overall daily functioning occurs in some people. Others function appropriately in their interactions with the outside world by exerting great effort and forcing themselves to mask their distress. Sometimes they are successful at hiding their depression for months or years and astonish family members and others when they finally admit that they are seriously depressed.

Many people experience depression but seek treatment for somatic complaints. The leading somatic complaints of patients struggling with depression are headache, backache, abdominal pain, fatigue, malaise, anxiety, and decreased desire or problems with sexual functioning (Varcarolis, 2004). These sensations are frequently manifestations of depression. The depression is undiagnosed about half of the time and masquerades as physical health problems (Townsend, 2003). People with depression also exhibit poor functioning and frequent absences from work and school.

Specific symptoms of clinical depression include feelings of sadness, worthlessness, fatigue, guilt, and difficulty concentrating or making decisions. Changes in appetite, weight gain or loss, sleep disturbances, and psychomotor retardation or agitation are also common. Often, patients have recurrent thoughts about death or suicide or have made suicide attempts. A diagnosis of clinical depression is made when a person presents with at least five of nine diagnostic criteria for depression (Chart 7-10). Unfortunately, only one of three depressed people is properly diagnosed and appropriately treated (American Psychiatric Association, 2000).

### Nursing Implications

Because any loss in function, change in role, or alteration in body image is a possible antecedent to depression, nurses in all settings encounter patients who are depressed or who have thought about suicide. Depression is suspected if changes in the patient's thoughts or feelings and a loss of self-esteem are noted. Chart 7-11 lists risk factors for depression. Depression can occur at any age, and it is diagnosed more frequently in women than in men. In elderly patients, nurses should be aware that decreased mental

### CHART 7-9

## Assessing for Posttraumatic Stress Disorder (PTSD)

Be on the alert for the following signs and symptoms:

### Physiologic Indicators

- Dilated pupils
- Headaches
- Sleep pattern disturbances
- Tremors
- Elevated blood pressure
- Tachycardia or palpitations
- Diaphoresis with cold, clammy skin
- Hyperventilation
- Dyspnea
- Smothering or choking sensation
- Nausea, vomiting, or diarrhea
- Stomach ulcers
- Dry mouth
- Abdominal pain
- Muscle tension or soreness
- Exhaustion

### Psychological Indicators

- Anxiety
- Anger
- Depression
- Fears or phobias
- Survivor guilt
- Hypervigilance
- Nightmares or flashbacks
- Intrusive thoughts about the trauma
- Impaired memory
- Dissociative states
- Restlessness or irritability
- Strong startle response
- Substance abuse
- Self-hatred
- Feelings of estrangement
- Feelings of helplessness, hopelessness, or powerlessness
- Lack of interest in life
- Inability to concentrate
- Difficulty communicating, caring, and expressing love
- Problems with relationships
- Sexual problems ranging from acting out to impotence
- Difficulty with intimacy
- Inability to trust
- Lack of impulse control
- Aggressive, abusive, or violent behavior, including suicide
- Thrill-seeking behaviors

Copel, L. C. (2000). *Nurse's clinical guide: Psychiatric and mental health care* (2nd ed.). Springhouse, PA: Springhouse.

### CHART 7-10

## Diagnostic Criteria for Depression Based on the DSM-IV-TR

A person experiences at least five out of nine characteristics, with one of the first two symptoms present most of the time:

1. Depressed mood
2. Loss of pleasure or interest
3. Weight gain or loss
4. Sleeping difficulties
5. Psychomotor agitation or retardation
6. Fatigue
7. Feeling worthless
8. Inability to concentrate
9. Thoughts of suicide or death

American Psychiatric Association. (2000). *Diagnostic and statistical manual of mental disorders (DSM-IV-TR)* (4th ed.). Washington, DC: Author.

alertness and withdrawal-type responses may be indicative of depression. Consultation with a psychiatric liaison nurse to assess and differentiate between dementia-like symptoms and depression is often helpful.

Talking with the patient about his or her fears, frustration, anger, and despair can help alleviate a sense of helplessness and lead to necessary treatment. Helping the patient learn to cope effectively with conflict, interpersonal problems, and grief and encouraging the patient to discuss actual and potential losses may hasten his or her recovery from depression. It may also be possible to help the patient identify and decrease negative self-talk and unrealistic expectations and show how these contribute to depression. The nurse should monitor the patient for the onset of new problems, because depression adversely affects physical health and self-care activities. All patients with depression should be evaluated to determine if they would benefit from antidepressant therapy.

### CHART 7-11

## Risk Factors for Depression

- Family history
- Stressful situations
- Female gender
- Prior episodes of depression
- Onset before age 40 years
- Medical comorbidity
- Past suicide attempts
- Lack of support systems
- History of physical or sexual abuse
- Current substance abuse

In addition to the measures previously listed, psychoeducational programs, establishment of support systems, and counseling can reduce anxiety- and depression-related distress (Mirowsky & Ross, 2003). Psychoeducational programs can help patients and their families understand depression, treatment options, and coping strategies. (In crisis situations, it is imperative that patients be referred to psychiatrists, psychiatric nurse specialists, or crisis centers.) Explaining to patients that depression is a medical illness and not a sign of personal weakness, and that effective treatment will allow them to feel better and stay emotionally healthy, is an important aspect of care (Varcarolis, 2004).

In the United States, about 15% of severely depressed people commit suicide, and two thirds of patients who have committed suicide had been seen by health care practitioners during the month before their death (U.S. Preventive Service Task Force Agency for Healthcare Research and Quality, 2004). When patients make statements that are self-deprecating, express feelings of failure, or are convinced that things are hopeless and will not improve, they may be at risk for suicide. Risk factors for suicide are listed in Chart 7-12.

# Substance Abuse

Some people use mood-altering substances in an attempt to cope with life's challenges. People who abuse substances use illegally obtained drugs, prescribed or over-the-counter medications, and alcohol alone or in combination with other drugs in ineffective attempts to cope with the pressures, strains, and burdens of life. They are unable to make healthy decisions and to solve problems effectively. Typically, they are also unable to identify and implement adaptive behaviors. Some people may respond to personal illness or the illness of a loved one by using substances to decrease emotional pain. Over time, physiologic, emotional, cognitive, and behavioral problems develop as a result of continuous substance use. These problems cause distress for people, their families, and their communities.

## Nursing Implications

**Substance abuse** is encountered in all clinical settings. Intoxication and withdrawal are two common substance abuse problems. Often, nurses see patients who have experienced trauma as a result of intoxication. Other patients who are active substance abusers enter the primary care setting with a diagnosis other than that of substance abuse. Many do not disclose the extent of their substance use. The patient's use of denial or lack of knowledge about the harmful effects of psychoactive substances can be detected by the nurse who performs a substance use assessment. Nurses can incorporate tools into the assessment to detect drug use. Examples of such instruments are the CAGE Questionnaire (Ewing, 1984), the Michigan Alcohol Screening Test (Selzer, 1971), and the Addiction Severity Index (McLellan, Kushner, Metzger, et al., 1992). The CAGE Questions Adapted to Include Drugs (CAGEAID) instrument is presented in Chapter 5, Chart 5-3. Information that is commonly addressed in substance abuse questionnaires is summarized in Chart 7-13.

Health professionals are in pivotal positions to identify substance abuse problems, institute treatment protocols, and make referrals. Because substance abuse severely affects families, nurses can help family members confront the situation, decrease enabling behaviors, and motivate the person with the substance abuse problem to obtain treatment.

Caring for codependent family members is another nursing priority. Codependent people tend to manifest unhealthy patterns in relationships with others. Codependents struggle with a need to be needed, an urge to control others, and a willingness to remain involved and suffer with a person who has a drug problem.

Families may approach the health care team to help set limits on the dysfunctional behavior of people who abuse substances. At these times, a therapeutic intervention is organized for the purpose of confronting the patient about substance use and the need to obtain drug or alcohol treatment. Nurses or other skilled addiction counselors help fam-

---

### CHART 7-12

### Risk Factors for Suicide

- Age younger than 20 or older than 45 years, especially older than 65 years
- Gender—women make more attempts, men are more successful
- Dysfunctional family—members have experienced cumulative multiple losses and possess limited coping skills
- Family history of suicide
- Severe depression
- Severe, intractable pain
- Chronic, debilitating medical problems
- Substance abuse
- Severe anxiety
- Overwhelming problems
- Severe alteration in self-esteem or body image
- Lethal suicide plan

---

### CHART 7-13

### Assessing for Substance Abuse

- Past and recurrent use of the substance
- Patient's view of substance use as a problem
- Age when substance was first used and last used
- Length and duration of use of substance
- Preferred method of use of substance
- Amount of substance used
- How substance is procured
- Effect of or reaction to substance
- Previous attempts to cease or decrease substance use

ilies present the addicted person with a realistic perspective about the problem, their concerns about and caring for the person, and a specific plan for treatment. This therapeutic intervention works on the premise that honest and caring confrontation can break through a person's denial of the addiction. If a person refuses to participate in the designed plan, the family members define the consequences and state their commitment to follow through with them. This intervention is empowering to the family and usually provides the structure needed to secure treatment.

However, even with treatment, the patient may experience relapse. The nurse works with the patient and family to prevent relapse and to be prepared if relapse occurs. Relapse is considered a part of the illness process and therefore must be viewed and addressed in the same way that chronic illness is treated.

Nurses who work with patients and families struggling with addiction must dispel the myth that addiction is a defect in character or a moral fault. Views on substance abuse vary within society. A person's background may help determine whether he or she uses drugs, what drugs are used, and when they are used (Copel, 2000). The combination of variables, such as values and beliefs, family and personal norms, spiritual convictions, and conditions of the current social environment, predisposes a person to the possibility of drug use, motivation for treatment, and continual recovery (Copel, 2000). It has also been said that a person's attitude, especially toward alcohol, reflects the overall beliefs and attitudes of that person's culture (Giger & Davidhizar, 2004).

## Loss and Grief

Loss is a part of the life cycle. All people experience loss in the form of change, growth, and transition. The experience of loss is painful, frightening, and lonely, and it triggers an array of emotional responses (Chart 7-14). People may vacillate between denial, shock, disbelief, anger, inertia, intense yearning, loneliness, sadness, loss of control, depression, and spiritual despair (Walsh & McGoldrick, 2004).

In addition to normal losses associated with life cycle stages, there are the potential losses of health, a body part, self-image, self-esteem, and even one's life. When loss is not acknowledged or there are multiple losses, anxiety, depression, and health problems may occur. Likewise, people with physical health problems, such as diabetes mellitus, HIV infection/AIDS, cardiac disorders, gastrointestinal disorders, disabilities, and neurologic impairments, tend to respond to these conditions with feelings of **grief.**

People grieve in different ways, and there is no timeline for completing the **bereavement** process. The time of griev-

---

### NURSING RESEARCH PROFILE

#### *Substance Abuse*

Zakrzewski, R. F., & Hector, M. A. (2004). The lived experience of alcohol addiction: Men of Alcoholics Anonymous. *Issues in Mental Health Nursing, 25*(1), 61–77.

#### Purpose
Alcohol is the most widely used drug in the United States, and alcohol addiction is one of the most common psychiatric disorders among the general population. Alcoholics Anonymous (AA) is the largest self-help group for alcoholics. This research study identified themes and commonalities in the experiences of alcohol addiction of male members of AA.

#### Design
An existential phenomenologic methodology was chosen for the study. The researchers sought to gain an in-depth understanding of the subjects' experiences with alcohol addiction through the use of nondirective interviews. The sample consisted of seven men who had addiction to alcohol. All participants were between 32 and 65 years of age, sober for a period of 1 to 25 years, and AA members.

#### Findings
The subjects reflected about times before, during, and after their addiction to alcohol. They spoke about their childhoods, when they started drinking, their drinking years, turning points in their lives, treatment, and the period after attaining sobriety. Four themes were identified from the men's experiences: emotions, control, awareness of others, and turning points. Telling their stories had a therapeutic effect. All the men spoke of the "high" that alcohol provided and about their perceptions that drinking was fun. They said that they drank to mask negative feelings about themselves. For these men, challenges included relearning how to live after achieving sobriety and coping with problems previously dealt with by alcohol use.

#### Nursing Implications
Nurses must recognize that people recovering from alcoholism need to understand their feelings about alcohol use and have opportunities to discuss in their own words their experiences with alcohol. Strategies are needed to assist people recovering from alcoholism to find healthy outlets for achieving positive feelings and to identify ways to have fun without using alcohol. People recovering from alcohol addiction must handle their feelings of boredom related to sobriety and develop strategies for enjoying life. Mental health professionals can help teach them ways to cope with everyday stressors and feelings that previously led to the use of alcohol.

## CHART 7-14

### Assessing for Grieving

Be on the alert for the following signs and symptoms:

**Physiologic Indicators**
- Heart rate changes
- Blood pressure alterations
- Gastrointestinal disturbances
- Chest discomfort
- Shortness of breath
- Weakness
- Appetite changes
- Sleep problems
- Vague, but distressing, physical symptoms

**Emotional Indicators**
- Sadness
- Depression
- Anger
- Social withdrawal
- Loneliness
- Apathy
- Longing for who or what was lost
- Blaming of self or others
- Questioning of beliefs

**Behavioral Indicators**
- Slow movements
- Forgetfulness
- Purposeless activity
- Crying
- Sighing
- Lack of interest
- Easily distracted from tasks

---

ing often depends on the significance of the loss, the anticipation of or preparation for the loss, the person's emotional stability and maturity, and the person's coping ability (Arnold & Boggs, 2003).

Regardless of the duration of the grieving process, there are two basic goals: (1) healing the self and (2) recovering from the loss. Other factors that influence grieving are the type of loss, life experiences with various changes and transitions, religious beliefs, cultural background, and personality type (Walsh & McGoldrick, 2004). Some patients may resort to abuse of prescription medications, illegal drugs, or alcohol if they find it difficult to cope with the loss; the grief process is then complicated by the use of addictive substances.

### Nursing Implications

Nurses identify patients and family members who are grieving and work with them to accomplish the four major tasks of the grief process: (1) acceptance of the loss, (2) acknowledgment of the intensity of the pain of the loss, (3) adaptation to life after the loss, and (4) cultivation of new relationships and activities (Worden, 2001). Nurses also assess and differentiate between grief and depression by knowing the common thoughts, feelings, physical or bodily reactions, and behaviors associated with grief compared with depression.

The physical response to grief includes the sensation of somatic distress, a tightness in the throat followed by a choking sensation or shortness of breath, the need to sigh, an empty feeling inside the abdomen, a lack of muscle power, and intense disabling distress. Grief can further debilitate already compromised patients and can have a strong impact on family functioning.

## Death and Dying

Coping with the death of a loved one or with anticipation of one's own death is considered the ultimate challenge. The idea of death is threatening and anxiety-provoking to many people. Kubler-Ross (1975, p. 1) stated, "The key to the question of death unlocks the door of life.... For those who seek to understand it, death is a highly creative force." Common fears of dying people are fear of the unknown, pain, suffering, loneliness, loss of the body, and loss of personal control.

In recent years, the experience of dying has changed as advances have been made in the care of chronically and terminally ill patients. Technologic innovations and modern therapeutic treatments have prolonged the life span, and many deaths are now the result of chronic illnesses that result in physiologic deterioration and subsequent multisystem failure. For more information on end-of-life care and death and dying, see Chapter 17.

## Spirituality and Spiritual Distress

Spirituality is defined as connectedness with self, others, a life force, or God that allows people to experience self-transcendence and find meaning in life. Spirituality helps people discover a purpose in life, understand the ever-changing qualities of life, and develop their relationship with God or a higher power. Within the framework of spirituality, people may discover truths about the self, about the world, and about concepts such as love, compassion, wisdom, honesty, commitment, imagination, reverence, and morality. Sacred texts for the major religious traditions offer guidelines for personal conduct and social and spiritual behavior. It is important that the spiritual beliefs of people and families be acknowledged, valued, and respected for the comfort and guidance they provide.

Often, spiritual behavior is expressed through sacrifice, self-discipline, and spending time in activities that focus on the inner self or the soul. Although religion and nature are two vehicles that people use to connect themselves with God or a higher power, bonds to religious institutions, beliefs, or dogma are not required to experience the spiritual sense of self. **Faith**, considered the foundation of spirituality, is a belief in something that a person cannot see. The spiritual part of a person views life as a mystery that unfolds over the lifetime, encompassing questions about meaning, hope, relatedness to God, acceptance or forgiveness, and transcendence (Hawks, 2004; Wright, 2004).

A strong sense of spirituality or religious faith can have a positive impact on health (Dunn & Horgas, 2000; Kendrick & Robinson, 2000; Phillips, 2003). Spirituality is also a component of hope, and, especially during chronic, serious, or terminal illness, patients and their families often find comfort and emotional strength in their religious traditions or spiritual beliefs. At other times, illness and loss can cause a loss of faith or meaning in life and a spiritual crisis. The nursing diagnosis of Spiritual distress is applicable to those who have a disturbance in the belief or value system that provides strength, hope, and meaning in life.

## Nursing Implications

Spiritually distressed patients (or family members) may show despair, discouragement, ambivalence, detachment, anger, resentment, or fear. They may question the meaning of suffering, life, and death and express a sense of emptiness. The nurse assesses spiritual strength by inquiring about the person's sense of spiritual well-being, hope, and peacefulness. The nurse assesses whether spiritual beliefs and values have changed in response to illness or loss. The nurse also assesses current and past participation in religious or spiritual practices and notes the patient's responses to questions about spiritual needs—grief, anger, guilt, depression, doubt, anxiety, or calmness—to help determine the patient's need for spiritual care. Another simple assessment technique is to inquire about the patient's and family's desire for spiritual support.

For nurses to provide spiritual care, they must be open to being present and supportive when patients experience doubt, fearfulness, suffering, despair, or other difficult psychological states of being. Interventions that foster spiritual growth or reconciliation include being fully present; listening actively; conveying a sense of caring, respect, and acceptance; using therapeutic communication techniques to encourage expression; suggesting the use of prayer, meditation, or imagery; and facilitating contact with spiritual leaders or performance of spiritual rituals (Hawks, 2004).

Patients with serious, chronic, or terminal illnesses face physical and emotional losses that threaten their spiritual integrity. During acute and chronic illness, rehabilitation, or the dying process, spiritual support can stimulate patients to regain or strengthen their connections with their inner selves, their loved ones, and God or a higher power to transcend suffering and find meaning. Nurses can alleviate distress and suffering and enhance wellness by meeting their patients' spiritual needs.

## Critical Thinking Exercises

1. A 55-year-old man in a hospital clinic tells the nurse that he does not want to suffer and will obtain medication for his pain when he has a colon biopsy. He states, "I am nervous about this procedure. I know that biopsies are painful, despite what the surgeon says. I'm going to get some medicine to decrease my pain and my nervousness, aren't I?" How does the nurse handle this situation? What assessment data should be collected to determine measures that will most likely allay this patient's anxiety? What complementary or alternative methods might be helpful to this patient?

2. **ebp** The night before a patient's surgery, the nurse is approached by the man's daughter. She fears that her father's daily use of alcohol may have untoward postoperative outcomes. What would you tell her? How would you approach the patient? What strategies would be useful for this patient and for the entire family? What is the evidence base for use of these strategies? Discuss the strength of the evidence. Identify the criteria used to evaluate the strength of the evidence for the strategies.

## REFERENCES AND SELECTED READINGS

### BOOKS

Aiken, L. (2000). *Dying, death, and bereavement* (4th ed.). Mahwah, NJ: Lawrence Erlbaum.

American Psychiatric Association. (2000). *Diagnostic and statistical manual of mental disorders (DSM-IV-TR)* (4th ed.). Washington, DC: Author.

Arnold, E., & Boggs, K. (2003). *Interpersonal relationships: Professional communication skills for nurses* (3rd ed.). Philadelphia: W. B. Saunders.

Boss, P., & Mulligan, C. (2003). *Family stress: Classic and contemporary readings.* Thousand Oaks, CA: Sage.

Boyd-Franklin, N., & Bry, B. H. (2001). *Reaching out in family therapy.* New York: Guilford Press.

Burr, W., Klein, S., Burr, R., et al. (1994). *Reexamining family stress: New theory and research.* Thousand Oaks, CA: Sage.

Cathersall, D. R. (2004). *The handbook of stress, trauma, and family.* New York: Brunner-Routledge.

Copel, L. C. (2000). *Nurse's clinical guide: Psychiatric and mental health care* (2nd ed.). Springhouse, PA: Springhouse.

DiClemente, C. S. (2003). *Addiction and change: How addiction develops and addicted people recover.* NY: Guilford Press.

Feldman, R. S. (2002). *Development across the life span* (3rd ed.). Upper Saddle River, NJ: Prentice Hall.

Freeman, S. (2004). *Grief and loss: Understanding the journey.* Pacific Grove, CA: Brooks/Cole.

Friedman, M. M., Bowden, V. R., & Jones, E. G. (2003). *Family nursing: Research, theory, and practice* (5th ed.). Upper Saddle River, NJ: Prentice Hall.

Gelles, R. J. (1997). *Intimate violence in families.* Thousands Oaks, CA: Sage.

Giger, J. N., & Davidhizar, R. E. (2004). *Transcultural nursing: Assessment and intervention* (4th ed.). St. Louis: C. V. Mosby.

Jeffreys, J. S. (2004). *Helping grieving people.* New York: Brunner/Routledge.

Johnson, J. (2004). *Fundamentals of substance abuse.* Pacific Grove, CA: Brooks/Cole.

Kail, R. V., & Cavanaugh, R. C. (2004). *Human development: A life span view* (3rd ed.). Pacific Grove, CA: Brooks/Cole.

Keegan, L. (2001). *Healing with complementary and alternative therapies.* Albany, NY: Delmar.

Kubler-Ross, E. (1975). *Death: The final stage of growth.* Englewood Cliffs, NJ: Prentice-Hall.

Kuhn, M. A. (1999). *Complementary therapies for health care providers.* Philadelphia: Lippincott Williams & Wilkins.

Lattanzi-Licht, M., & Doka, K. J. (2003). *Living with grief.* New York: Brunner/Routledge.

Loseke, D. R., Gelles, R. J., & Cavanaugh, M. M. (Eds.). (2004). *Current controversies on family violence.* Newbury Park, CA: Sage.

Martocchio, B. C. (1982). *Living while dying.* Bowie, MD: Robert J. Brady.

Matthews, D. A., & Larson, D. B. (1995). *The faith factor: An annotated bibliography of clinical research on spiritual subjects* (Vol. 3). Rockville, MD: National Institute for Health Care Research.

Mirowsky, J., & Ross, C. E. (2003). *Social causes of psychological distress* (2nd ed.). New York: Aldine De Gruyter.

Munoz, C., & Luckmann, J. (2005). *Transcultural communication in nursing.* Albany, NY: Delmar.

Murray, R. B., & Zentner, J. P. (2001). *Health assessment and promotion strategies through the life span* (7th ed.). Stamford, CT: Appleton & Lange.

Nowinski, J. K. (1998). *Family recovery and substance abuse.* Thousand Oaks, CA: Sage.

Palmer, S., Cooper, C., & Thomas, K. (2003). *Creating a balance: Managing stress.* London: British Library Publishing.

Rice, F. P. (2001). *Human development: A lifespan approach* (4th ed.). Upper Saddle River, NJ: Prentice Hall.

Rice, V. H. (Ed.). (2000). *Handbook of stress, coping, and health: Implications for nursing research, theory, and practice.* Thousand Oaks, CA: Sage.

Scott, M. J. (2003). *Trauma and posttraumatic stress disorder.* Thousand Oaks, CA: Sage.

Stanhope, M., & Lancaster, J. (2004). *Community and public health nursing* (6th ed.). St. Louis: C. V. Mosby.

Suls, J., & Wallston, K. (2003). *Social psychological foundations of health and illness.* Malden, MA: Blackwell Publishing.

Townsend, M. C. (2003). *Psychiatric mental health nursing: Concepts of care.* Philadelphia: F. A. Davis.

U.S. Preventive Service Task Force Agency for Healthcare Research and Quality. (2004). *Guide to clinical prevention services* (3rd ed.). (AHRQ Publication No. 04-IP003). Rockville, MD: U.S. Government Printing Office.

U.S. Public Health Service. (2000). *Healthy people 2010: Understanding and improving health.* Washington, DC: U.S. Government Printing Office.

Varcarolis, E. M. (2004). *Foundations of psychiatric mental health nursing: A clinical approach* (4th ed.). Philadelphia: Saunders.

Walsh, F., & McGoldrick, M. (2004). *Living beyond loss.* New York: Norton.

Worden, J. W. (2001). *Grief counseling and grief therapy: A handbook for the mental health practitioner* (3rd ed.). New York: Springer Publishing.

Wright, L. M. (2004). *Spirituality, suffering, and illness: Ideas for healing.* Philadelphia: Davis.

Wright, L. M., & Leahey, M. (2000). *Nurses and families: A guide to family assessment and intervention.* Philadelphia: Davis.

## JOURNALS

*Asterisks indicate nursing research articles.

### General

Hansen, A. M., Kaergaard, A., Andersen, J. H., et al. (2003). Associations between repetitive work and endocrinological indicators of stress. *Work and Stress, 17*(3), 264–276.

Litsey, T. (2003). Acupuncture vs. cancer: Re-engaging the body's immune system. *Acupuncture Today, 4*(10), 1–21.

*Marquis, R., Freegard, H., & Hoogland, L. (2004). Influences on positive family involvement in aged care: An ethnographic view. *Contemporary Nurse, 16*(3), 178–186.

Mitchell, E., & Moore, K. (2004). Stroke: Holistic care and management. *Nursing Standard, 18*(33), 43–56.

*Montbriand, M. J. (2004). Seniors' life histories and perceptions of illness. *Western Journal of Nursing Research, 26*(2), 242–260.

Robinson, F. P., Matthews, H. L., Witek-Janusek, L. (2003). Psychoendocrine-immune response to mindfulness-based stress reduction in individuals infected with the human immunodeficiency virus: A quasi-experimental study. *Journal of Alternative and Complementary Medicine, 9*(5), 683–694.

Tower, K. D. (2003). Disability through the lens of culture. *Journal of Social Work in Disability and Rehabilitation, 2*(2/3), 5–22.

### Complementary or Alternative Therapies

Burman, M. E. (2003). Complementary and alternative medicine: Core competencies for family nurse practitioners. *Journal of Nursing Education, 42*(1), 28–35.

*Chang, B. L., Van Servellen, G., & Lombardi, E. (2003). Factors associated with complementary therapy use in people living with HIV/AIDS receiving antiretroviral therapy. *Journal of Alternative and Complementary Medicine, 9*(5), 695–710.

Dorcas, A., & Yung, P. (2003). Qigong: Harmonizing the breath, the body and the mind. *Complementary Therapies in Nursing and Midwifery, 9*(4), 198–202.

*Richardson, T. (2003). Health status and health behaviors of inner city older African-Americans: Health disparities in Wellness Center participants. *Journal of Multicultural Nursing and Health, 9*(3), 62–67.

*Tsai, J., Wang, W., Chan, P., et al. (2003). The beneficial effects of Tai Chi Chuan on blood pressure and lipid profile and anxiety status in a randomized controlled trial. *Journal of Alternative and Complementary Medicine, 9*(5), 747–754.

### Coping

*Clark, A. M. (2003). "It's like an explosion in your life": Lay perspectives on stress and myocardial infarction. *Journal of Clinical Nursing, 12*(4), 544–553.

DalMonte, J., Finlayson, M., & Helfrich, C. (2003). In their own words: Coping processes among women aging with multiple sclerosis. *Occupational Therapy in Health Care, 17*(3/4), 115–137.

Diamond, H., & Precin, P. (2003). Disabled and experiencing disaster: Personal and professional accounts. *Occupational Therapy in Mental Health, 19*(3/4), 27–41.

*Diokno, A. C., Burgio, K., Fultz, N. H., et al. (2004). Medical and self-care practices reported by women with urinary incontinence. *American Journal of Managed Care, 10*(Part 1), 69–78.

Johnson, D. M., Sheahan, T. C., & Chard, K. M. (2003). Personality disorders, coping strategies, and posttraumatic stress disorder in women with histories of childhood sexual abuse. *Journal of Child Sexual Abuse, 12*(2), 19–39.

Lee, S. (2003). Effects of using a nursing crisis intervention program on psychosocial responses and coping strategies of infertile women during in vitro fertilization. *Journal of Nursing Research, 11*(3), 197–207.

*Moser, D. K., Chung, M. L., McKinley, S., et al. (2003). Critical care nursing practice regarding patient anxiety assessment and management. *Intensive and Critical Care Nursing, 19*(5), 276–288.

*Rustoen, T., Wahl, A. K., Hanestad, B. R., et al. (2004). Expression of hope in cystic fibrosis patients: A comparison with the general population. *Heart and Lung, 33*(2), 111–118.

Scott, A. (2004). Managing anxiety in ICU patients: The role of preoperative information provision. *Nursing in Critical Care, 9*(2), 72–79.

Sears, S. R., Stanton, A. L., & Danoff-Burg, S. (2003). The Yellow Brick Road and the Emerald City: Benefit finding, positive reappraisal coping, and posttraumatic growth in women with early-stage breast cancer. *Health Psychology, 22*(5), 487–497.

Stuban, S. L. (2004). Living, not dying with ALS: Confounding the predictions of Lou Gehrig disease. *American Journal of Nursing, 104*(5), 72–76.

## Depression

*Bruce, M. L., Ten-Have, T. R., Reynolds, C. F., et al. (2004). Reducing suicidal ideation and depressive symptoms in depressed older primary care patients: A randomized controlled trial. *Journal of the American Medical Association, 291*(9), 1081–1091.

*Carpenter, J. S., Elam, J. L., Ridner, S. H., et al. (2004). Sleep, fatigue, and depressive symptoms in breast cancer survivors and matched healthy women experiencing hot flashes. *Oncology Nursing Forum, 31*(3), 591–598.

*Coleman, C. L. (2004). The contribution of religious and existential well-being to depression among African American heterosexuals with infection. *Issues in Mental Heath Nursing, 25*(1), 103–110.

*Kubik, M. Y., Lytle, L. A., Birnbaum, A. S., et al. (2003). Prevalence and correlates of depressive symptoms in young adolescents. *American Journal of Health Behavior, 27*(5), 546–553.

Nelson, R. (2004). Suicide rates rise among soldiers in Iraq. *Lancet, 363*(9405), 300.

Putnam, K., & McKibben, L. (2004). Managing workplace depression: An untapped opportunity for occupational health professionals. *Journal of the American Association of Occupational Health Nursing, 52*(3), 122–131.

## Grief

Finlayson, M., & van Denend, T. (2003). Experiencing the loss of mobility: Perspectives of older adults with MS. *Disability and Rehabilitation, 25*(20), 1168–1180.

Leichtling, B. (2004). Leadership and management: Dealing with dying, death, and grief. *Caring, 23*(1), 38–39.

Murphy, M. (2003). A model to help nurses caring for patients who are terminally ill. *Professional Nurse, 19*(4), 213–215.

*Mystakidou, K., Tsilika, E., Parpa, E., et al. (2003). Greek perspective on concepts of death and expression of grief, with implications for practice. *International Journal of Palliative Care, 9*(12), 534–537.

*Rabow, M., W., Schanche, K., Petersen, J., et al. (2003). Patient perceptions of an outpatient palliative care intervention: "It had been on my mind before, but I did not know how to start talking about death . . ." *Journal of Pain and Symptom Management, 26*(5), 1010–1015.

Ramsey, A. (2003). Monitoring the dying patient in ITC: A personalized discussion. *Nursing in Critical Care, 8*(5), 209–211.

## Posttraumatic Stress Disorder

Otis, J. D., Keane, T. M., & Kerns, R. D. (2003). An examination of the relationship between chronic pain and posttraumatic stress disorder. *Journal of Rehabilitation Research and Development, 40*(5), 397–405.

*Pulcino, T., Galea, S., Ahern, J., et al. (2003). Posttraumatic stress in women after the September 11 attacks in New York City. *Journal of Women's Health, 12*(8), 809–820.

Seo, D., & Torabi, M. R. (2004). National study of emotional and perceptual changes since September 11. *American Journal of Health Education 35*(1), 37–45.

*Sharhabani-Arzy, R., Amir, M., Kotler, M., et al. (2003). The toll of domestic violence: PTSD among battered women in an Israeli sample. *Journal of Interpersonal Violence 18*(11), 1335–1346.

*Sorenson, D. S. (2003). Healing traumatizing provider interactions among women through short-term group therapy. *Archives of Psychiatric Nursing, 17*(6), 259–269.

## Spirituality

Dunn, K. S., & Horgas, A. L. (2000). The prevalence of prayer as a spiritual self-care modality in elders. *Journal of Holistic Nursing, 18*(4), 337–351.

Hawks, S. (2004). Spiritual wellness, holistic health, and the practice of health education. *American Journal of Health Education, 35*(1), 11–16.

Kendrick, K. D., & Robinson, S. (2000). Spirituality: Its relevance and purpose for clinical nursing in a new millennium. *Journal of Clinical Nursing, 9*(5), 701–705.

Lloyd, M., (2003). Innovations in care: Challenging depression: Taking a spiritually enhanced approach. *Geriaction, 21*(4), 26–29.

*Musgrave, C. F., & McFarlane, E. A. (2004). Israeli oncology nurses' religiosity, spiritual well-being, and attitudes toward spiritual care: A path analysis. *Oncology Nursing Forum, 31*(2), 321–327.

Phillips, I. (2003). Infusing spirituality into geriatric health care: Practical applications from the literature. *Topics in Geriatric Rehabilitation, 19*(4), 249–256.

## Substance Abuse

*Boyd, M. R., Phillips, K., & Dorsey, C. J. (2003). Alcohol and other drug disorders, comorbidity, and violence: Comparison of rural African American and Caucasian women. *Archives of Psychiatric Nursing, 17*(6), 249–258.

deWit, H., Soderpalm, A. H. V., Nikolayev, L., et al. (2003). Effects of acute social stress on alcohol consumption in healthy subjects. *Alcoholism: Clinical and Experimental Research, 27*(8), 1270–1277.

Ewing, J. A. (1984). Detecting alcoholism: The CAGE questionnaire. *Journal of the American Medical Association, 252*(14), 1906.

Hugh, T. (2003). Research reviews: Prevalence of alcohol. *Journal of Addictions Nursing, 14*(3), 165–167.

McLellan, A. T., Kushner, H., Metzger, D., et al. (1992). The fifth edition of the Addiction Severity Index. *Journal of Substance Abuse Treatment, 9*(3), 199–213.

Sansovich, D. (2003). HIV and substance use: Pain and the drug-seeking patient. *HIV Clinician, 15*(1), 15–16.

Selzer, M. L. (1971). The Michigan alcoholism screening test: The quest for a new diagnostic instrument. *American Journal of Psychiatry, 127,* 1653–1658.

*Tarrier, N., & Sommerfield, C. (2003). Alcohol and substance use in civilian chronic PTSD patients seeking psychological treatment. *Journal of Substance Use, 8*(4), 197–204.

*Zakrzewski, R. F., & Hector, M. A. (2004). The lived experience of alcohol addiction: Men of Alcoholics Anonymous. *Issues in Mental Health Nursing, 25*(1), 61–77.

## RESOURCES

## AGENCIES

American Holistic Nurses Association (AHNA), P.O. Box 2130, Flagstaff, AZ 86003-2130; 1-800-278-AHNA; http://www.ahna.org. Accessed June 6, 2006.

Grief Recovery Institute Education Foundation, Inc. (GRIEF), P.O. Box 6061-382, Sherman Oaks, CA 91413; 1-818-907-9600; 1-800-445-4808 (hotline); http://www.grief.net. Accessed June 6, 2006

National Hospice and Palliative Care Organization (NHO), 1901 North Moore Street, Suite 901, Arlington, VA 22209; 1-703-243-5900; http://www.nhpco.org. Accessed June 6, 2006.

## Aging

American Association of Retired Persons (AARP), 601 "E" Street NW, Washington, DC 20049-0001; 1-202-434-2277; 1-800-424-3410; http://www.aarp.org. Accessed July 6, 2006.

Children of Aging Parents, P.O. Box 167, Richboro, PA 18954; 1-800-227-7294; www.caps4caregivers.org. Accessed July 6, 2006.

National Association for Families Caring for their Elders—Eldercare America, 1141 Loxford Terrace, Silver Spring, MD 20901-1130; 1-301-593-1621

National Council on Aging, 409 3rd Street SW, Washington, DC 20024; 1-202-424-1200; 1-800-424-9046; http://www.ncoa.org. Accessed June 6, 2006.

National Office of the Gray Panthers, P.O. Box 214777, Washington, DC 20009; 1-202-466-3132; 1-800-280-5362; http://www.graypanthers.org. Accessed June 6, 2006.

### Anxiety

Anxiety Disorders Association of America, 11900 Parklawn Drive #100, Rockville, MD 20852-2624; 1-301-231-9350; http://www.adaa.org. Accessed July 6, 2006.

### Bereavement

Compassionate Friends, P.O. Box 3696, Oak Brook, IL 60522-3696; 1-630-990-0010; nationaloffice@compassionatefriends.org; http://www.compassionatefriends.org. Accessed June 6, 2006.

They Help Each Other Spiritually (THEOS), 322 Boulevard of the Allies #105, Pittsburgh, PA 15222-1919; 1-412-471-7779

Widowed Persons Service, 601 "E" Street NW, Washington, DC 20049-0001; 1-202-434-2260

### Depression

Depression Awareness, Recognition, and Treatment (D/ART), NIMH, 5600 Fishers Lane Room 10-85, Rockville, MD 20857; 1-800-421-4211; 1-301-443-4140; http://www.nmha.org. Accessed July 6, 2006.

National Alliance for the Mentally Ill, 200 N. Grebe Road #1015, Arlington, VA 22201-3062; 1-703-524-7600; 1-800-950-NAMI; http://www.nami.org. Accessed June 6, 2006.

National Mental Health Association, 1021 Prince Street, Alexandria, VA 22314-2971; 1-703-684-7722; 1-800-969-6642; 1-800-433-5959; http://www.nmha.org. Accessed June 6, 2006.

### Eating Disorders

American Anorexia Bulimia Association Inc., 293 Central Park West, New York, NY 10024; 1-212-501-8351

National Eating Disorders Association (NEDA), 603 Stewart St., Suite 803, Seattle, WA 98101;1-206-382-3587; http://www.nationaleatingdisorders.org. Accessed June 6, 2006.

### Posttraumatic Stress Disorder

National Center for PTSD, VA Medical Center (116D), White River Junction, VT 05009; 1-802-296-5132; http://www.ncptsd.org. Accessed June 6, 2006.

### Substance Abuse

Adult Children of Alcoholics, P.O. Box 3216, Torrence, CA 90510; 1-310-534-1815; http://www.adultchildren.org. Accessed June 6, 2006.

Alanon and Alateen Family Group Headquarters Inc., 1600 Corporate Landing Parkway, Virginia Beach, VA 23454-5617; 1-888-4AL-ANON (888-425-2666); http://www.al-anon.alateen.org. Accessed June 6, 2006.

Alcoholics Anonymous, Grand Central Station, P.O. Box 459, New York, NY 10163; 1-212-870-3400; http://www.aa.org. Accessed June 6, 2006.

Center for Substance Abuse Prevention Workplace, 800-WORKPLACE (1-800-967-5752)

Center for Substance Abuse Treatment, 800-662-HELP (1-800-662-4357)

Children of Alcoholics Foundation, 164 West 74th Street, New York, NY 10115; 1-800-359-2623

Co-Anon Family Groups, P.O. Box 64742-66, Los Angeles, CA 90064; 1-818-377-4317; http://www.co-anon.org. Accessed June 6, 2006.

Cocaine Anonymous, 3740 Overland Avenue Suite G, Los Angeles, CA 90034; 1-800-347-8998; http://www.ca.org. Accessed June 6, 2006.

Dual Recovery Anonymous World Services, P.O. Box 8107, Prairie Village, KS 66208; 877-883-2332; http://www.draonline.org. Accessed June 6, 2006.

Narcotics Anonymous, P.O. Box 9999, Van Nuys, CA 91409; 1-818-773-9999; http://www.na.org. Accessed June 6, 2006.

National Alcohol Hotline, Helpline: 1-800-NCA-CALL (1-800-622-2255)

National Cocaine Hotline, 1-800-COCAINE (1-800-262-2463)

Rational Recovery Systems, Box 800, Lotus, CA 95651; 1-530-621-4374; http://www.rational.org. Accessed June 6, 2006.

Secular Organizations for Sobriety (SOS), The Center for Inquiry, 5521 Grosvenor Boulevard, Los Angeles, CA 90066; 1-310-821-8430; http://www.secularhumanism.org. Accessed June 6, 2006.

# CHAPTER 8

# Perspectives in Transcultural Nursing

## Learning Objectives

*On completion of this chapter, the learner will be able to:*

1. Identify key components of cultural assessment.
2. Apply transcultural nursing principles, concepts, and theories when providing nursing care to people, families, groups, and communities.
3. Develop strategies for planning, providing, and evaluating culturally competent nursing care for patients from diverse backgrounds.
4. Critically analyze the influence of culture on nursing care decisions and actions for patients.
5. Discuss the impact of diversity and health care disparities on health care delivery.

In the health care delivery system, as in society, nurses interact with people of similar as well as diverse cultural backgrounds. People may have similar or different frames of reference and varied preferences regarding their health and health care needs. Nurses must often practice *transcultural nursing*, providing care to clients and families across cultural variations. Acknowledging and adapting to the cultural needs of patients and significant others are important components of nursing care. In addition, facilitating access to culturally appropriate health care is critical if nursing care is to be holistic. To plan and deliver culturally appropriate and competent care, nurses must understand the definitions of culture, culturally appropriate care, and cultural competence and the various aspects of culture that should be explored for each patient.

## Cultural Concepts

The concept of culture and its relationship to the health care beliefs and practices of the patient and his or her family and friends provide the foundation for transcultural nursing. This awareness of culture in the delivery of nursing care has been described in different terms and phrases, including respect for cultural diversity, culturally sensitive or comprehensive care, and culturally competent or appropriate nursing care (Giger & Davidhizar, 2004; Spector, 2004), or culturally congruent nursing care (Leininger, 2001). Two commonly discussed concepts are cultural diversity and culturally competent care.

The term *culture* was initially defined by the British anthropologist Sir Edward Tylor in 1871 as the knowledge, belief, art, morals, laws, customs, and any other capabilities and habits acquired by humans as members of society (Campinha-Bacote, 2003). During the past century, and especially during recent decades, hundreds of definitions of culture have been offered that integrate the themes stated by Tylor and the themes of ethnic variations of a population based on race, nationality, religion, language, physical characteristics, and geography (Spector, 2004). To fully appreciate the broad impact of culture, factors such as disabilities, gender, social class, physical appearance (eg, weight, height), ideologies (political views), or sexual orientation must be integrated into the definition of culture as well (Green-Hernandez, Quinn, Denman-Vitale, et al., 2004).

Madeleine Leininger, founder of the specialty called transcultural nursing, writes that culture involves learned and transmitted knowledge about values, beliefs, rules of behavior, and lifestyle practices that guide designated groups in their thinking and actions in patterned ways (2001). Giger and Davidhizar (2004) define transcultural nursing as a research-focused, client-based practice field of culturally competent nursing. Transcultural nursing addresses the differences and similarities among cultures in relation to health, health care, and illness, with consideration of patient values, beliefs, and practices. Culture develops over time as a result of exposure to social and religious structures and intellectual and artistic manifestations, and each individual person, including each nurse, is culturally unique (Giger & Davidhizar, 2004).

The concept of ethnic culture has four basic characteristics:

- It is learned from birth through language and socialization.
- It is shared by members of the same cultural group, and it includes an internal sense and external perception of distinctiveness.
- It is influenced by specific conditions related to environmental and technical factors and to the availability of resources.
- It is dynamic and ever-changing.

With the exception of the first characteristic, cultures related to age, physical appearance, lifestyle, and other less frequently acknowledged aspects also share the above characteristics.

*Cultural diversity* has also been defined in a number of ways. Often, differences in skin color, religion, and geographic area are the only elements used to identify diversity, with ethnic minorities being considered the primary sources of cultural diversity. However, there are many other possible sources of cultural diversity. To truly acknowledge the cultural differences that may influence health care delivery, the nurse must confront self-deception and bias and recognize the influence of his or her own culture and cultural heritage (Swanson, 2004).

*Culturally competent nursing care* has been defined as effective, individualized care that demonstrates respect for the dignity, personal rights, preferences, beliefs, and practices of the person receiving care, while acknowledging the biases of the caregiver and preventing these biases from interfering with the care provided. Culturally competent nursing care is a dynamic process that requires comprehensive knowledge of culture-specific information and an awareness of, and sensitivity to, the effect that culture has on the care situation. It requires that the nurse integrate cultural knowledge, awareness of his or her own cultural perspective, and the patient's cultural perspectives when preparing a plan of care (Giger & Davidhizar, 2004). Exploring one's own cultural beliefs and how they might conflict with the beliefs of the patients being cared for is a first step toward becoming culturally competent. Understanding the diversity within cultures, such as subcultures, is also important. In addition, culturally competent care involves facilitating patient access to culturally appropriate resources (Green-Hernandez et al., 2004).

## Subcultures

Although culture is a universal phenomenon, it takes on specific and distinctive features for a particular group because it encompasses all of the knowledge, beliefs, customs, and skills acquired by the members of that group. When such groups function within a larger cultural group, they are referred to as subcultures.

The term *subculture* is used for relatively large groups of people who share characteristics that enable them to be identified as a distinct entity. Examples of American subcultures based on ethnicity (ie, subcultures with common traits such as physical characteristics, language, or ancestry) include African Americans, Hispanic/Latino Americans, Asian/Pacific Islanders, and Native Americans. Each of these subcultures may be further divided; for example, Native Americans consist of American Indians and Alaska Natives, who represent more than 500 federally and state-recognized tribes in addition to an unknown number of tribes that receive no official recognition.

Subcultures may also be based on religion (more than 1,200 religions exist in the United States), occupation (eg, nurses, physicians, other members of the health care team), or disability (eg, the Deaf community) or illness. In addition, subcultures may be based on age (eg, infants, children, adolescents, adults, older adults), gender (eg, male, female), sexual orientation (eg, homosexual, bisexual, heterosexual), or geographic location (eg, Texan, Southern, Appalachian).

Nurses should also be sensitive to the interracial applications of cultural competence. Tensions between subcultures within a designated group could add to the complexity of planning culturally competent care. Some members of one ethnic subculture may be offended or angered if they are mistaken for members of a different subculture. Similarly, if the attributes of one subculture are mistakenly generalized to patients who belong to a different subculture, extreme offense could result, as well as inappropriate care planning and implementation (Flowers, 2004). Nurses must refrain from culturally stereotyping patients in an attempt to be culturally competent. Instead, patients or significant others should be consulted regarding personal values, beliefs, preferences, and cultural identification. This strategy is also applicable for members of nonethnic subcultures.

## Minorities

The term *minority* refers to a group of people whose physical or cultural characteristics differ from the majority of people in a society. At times, minorities may be singled out or isolated from others in society or treated in different or unequal ways. Although there are four generally identified minority groups—Blacks/African Americans, Hispanics, Asian/Pacific Islanders, and Native Americans (Baldwin, 2004; Sullivan Commission, 2004)—the concept of "minority" varies widely and must be understood in a cultural context. For example, men may be considered a minority within the nursing profession, but they constitute a majority within the field of medicine. In addition, Caucasians may be in the minority in some communities in the United States, but they are currently the majority group in the country (although it has been projected that by the middle to late 21st century, Caucasians will be in the minority in the United States). Because at times the term *minority* connotes inferiority, members of many racial and ethnic groups object to being identified as minorities.

## Transcultural Nursing

*Transcultural nursing,* a term sometimes used interchangeably with cross-cultural, intercultural, or multicultural nursing, refers to a research-focused practice field that focuses on patient-centered, culturally competent nursing. Transcultural nursing incorporates the care (caring) values, beliefs, and practices of people and groups from a particular culture without imposing the nurse's cultural perspective on the patient (Giger & Davidhizar, 2004). The underlying focus of transcultural nursing is to provide culture-specific and culture-universal care that promotes the well-being or health of individuals, families, groups, communities, and institutions (Giger & Davidhizar, 2004; Leininger, 2001). All people as well as the community or institution at large benefit when culturally competent care is provided. When the care is delivered beyond a nurse's national boundaries, the term *international* or *transnational nursing* is often used.

Although many nurses, anthropologists, and others have written about the cultural aspects of nursing and health care, Leininger (2001) developed a comprehensive research-based theory called Culture Care Diversity and Universality to promote culturally congruent nursing for people of different or similar cultures. This means promoting recovery from illness, preventing conditions that would limit the patient's health or well-being, or facilitating a peaceful death in ways that are culturally meaningful and appropriate. Nursing care needs to be tailored to fit the patient's cultural values, beliefs, and lifestyles.

Leininger's theory stresses the importance of providing culturally congruent nursing care (meaningful and beneficial health care tailored to fit the patient's cultural values) through culture care accommodation and culture care restructuring (Fig. 8-1). *Culture care accommodation* refers to professional actions and decisions that nurses make in their care to help people of a designated culture achieve a beneficial or satisfying health outcome. *Culture care restructuring* or repatterning refers to professional actions and decisions that help patients reorder, change, or modify their lifestyles toward new, different, or more beneficial health care patterns. At the same time, the patient's cultural values and beliefs are respected, and a better or healthier lifestyle is provided. Other terms and definitions that provide further insight into culture and health care include the following:

- *Acculturation:* the process by which members of a cultural group adapt to or learn how to take on the behaviors of another group
- *Cultural blindness:* the inability of people to recognize their own values, beliefs, and practices and those of others because of strong ethnocentric tendencies (the tendency to view one's own culture as superior to others)
- *Cultural imposition:* the tendency to impose one's cultural beliefs, values, and patterns of behavior on a person or people from a different culture
- *Cultural taboos:* activities or behaviors that are avoided, forbidden, or prohibited by a particular cultural group

## Culturally Competent Nursing Care

*Culturally competent* or *culturally congruent nursing care* refers to the delivery of interventions within the cultural context of the patient (Campinha-Bacote, 2003). It involves a complex integration of attitudes, knowledge, and skills (including assessment, decision making, judgments, critical thinking, and evaluation) that enables nurses to provide care in a culturally sensitive and appropriate manner. Agency policies are important to achieve culturally competent care. Policies that promote culturally competent care establish flexible regulations pertaining to visitors (number, frequency, and length of visits), provide translation services

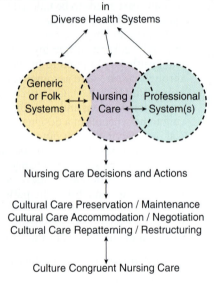

**FIGURE 8-1.** Leininger's Sunrise Model depicts her theory of cultural care diversity and universality. From Leininger, M. M. (Ed.). (2001). *Culture care diversity and university: A theory of nursing.* New York: National League for Nursing Press.

for non–English-speaking patients, and train staff to provide care for patients with different cultural values (Simpson, 2004). Culturally competent policies are developed to promote an environment in which the traditional healing, spiritual, and religious practices of patients are respected and encouraged and to recognize the special dietary practices of patients from selected cultural groups (Green-Hernandez et al., 2004).

Giger and Davidhizar (2004) created an assessment model to guide nurses in exploring cultural phenomena that might affect nursing care. They identified communication, space, time orientation, social organization, environmental control, and biologic variations as relevant phenomena. This model has been used in various patient care settings to provide data essential to the provision of culturally competent care.

## Cross-Cultural Communication

Establishment of an environment of culturally congruent care and respect begins with effective communication, which occurs not only through words, but also through body language and other cues, such as voice, tone, and loudness. Nurse–patient interactions, as well as communications among members of a multicultural health care team, are dependent on the ability to understand and be understood.

Approximately 150 different languages are spoken in the United States, with Spanish accounting for the largest percentage after English. Obviously, nurses cannot become fluent in all languages, but certain strategies for fostering effective cross-cultural communication are necessary when providing care for patients who are not fluent in English. Cultural needs should be considered when choosing an interpreter; for instance, fluency in varied dialects is beneficial (Simpson, 2004). The interpreter's voice quality, pronunciation, use of silence, use of touch, and use of nonverbal communication should also be considered (Giger & Davidhizar, 2004).

During illness, patients of all ages tend to regress, and the regression often involves language skills. Chart 8-1 summarizes suggested strategies for overcoming language

### CHART 8-1

## Overcoming Language Barriers

- Greet the patient using the last or complete name. Avoid being too casual or familiar. Point to yourself and say your name. Smile.
- Proceed in an unhurried manner. Pay attention to any effort by the patient or family to communicate.
- Speak in a low, moderate voice. Avoid talking loudly. Remember that there is a tendency to raise the volume and pitch of your voice when the listener appears not to understand. The listener may perceive that you are shouting and/or angry.
- Organize your thoughts. Repeat and summarize frequently. Use audiovisual aids when feasible.
- Use short, simple sentence structure and speak in the active voice.
- Use simple words, such as "pain" rather than "discomfort." Avoid medical jargon, idioms, and slang. Avoid using contractions, such as don't, can't, won't.
- Use nouns repeatedly instead of pronouns. *Example:* Do not say: "He has been taking his medicine, hasn't he?" Do say: "Does Juan take medicine?"
- Pantomime words (use gestures) and simple actions while verbalizing them.
- Give instructions in the proper sequence. *Example:* Do not say: "Before you rinse the bottle, sterilize it." Do say: "First, wash the bottle. Second, rinse the bottle."
- Discuss one topic at a time, and avoid giving too much information in a single conversation. Avoid using conjunctions. *Example:* Do not say: "Are you cold and in pain?" Do say (while pantomiming/gesturing): "Are you cold?" "Are you in pain?"
- Talk directly to the patient rather than to the person who accompanied him or her.
- Validate whether the person understands by having him or her repeat instructions, demonstrate the procedure, or act out the meaning.
- Use any words you know in the person's language. This indicates that you are aware of and respect the patient's primary means of communicating.
- Try a third language. Many Indo-Chinese speak French. Europeans often know three or four languages. Try Latin words or phrases, if you are familiar with the language.
- Be aware of culturally based gender and age differences and diverse socioeconomic, educational, and tribal/regional differences when choosing an interpreter.
- Obtain phrase books from a library or bookstore, make or purchase flash cards, contact hospitals for a list of interpreters, and use both formal and informal networking to locate a suitable interpreter. Although they are costly, some telecommunication companies provide translation services.

---

barriers. Nurses should also assess how well patients and families have understood what has been said. The following cues may signify lack of effective communication:

- Efforts to change the subject: This could indicate that the listener does not understand what you are saying and is attempting to talk about something more familiar.
- Absence of questions: Paradoxically, this often means that the listener is not grasping the message and therefore has difficulty formulating questions to ask.
- Inappropriate laughter: A self-conscious giggle may signal poor comprehension and may be an attempt to disguise embarrassment.
- Nonverbal cues: A blank expression may signal poor understanding. However, among some Asian Americans, it may reflect a desire to avoid overt expression of emotion. Similarly, avoidance of eye contact may be a cultural expression of respect for the speaker in some Native Americans and Asian Americans.

## Culturally Mediated Characteristics

Nurses should be aware that patients act and behave in a variety of ways, in part because of the influence of culture on behaviors and attitudes. However, although certain attributes and attitudes are frequently associated with particular cultural groups, as described in the following pages, it is important to remember that not all people from the same cultural background share the same behaviors and views. Although nurses who fail to consider patients' cultural preferences and beliefs are considered insensitive and possibly indifferent, nurses who assume that all members of any one culture act and behave in the same way run the risk of stereotyping people. As previously stated, the best way to avoid stereotyping is to view each patient as an individual and to find out the patient's cultural preferences. A thorough culture assessment using a culture assessment tool or questionnaire (see later discussion) is very beneficial.

Many aspects of care may be influenced by the diverse cultural perspectives held by health care providers, patients, families, or significant others. One example is the issue of informed consent and full disclosure. In general, nurses may argue that patients have the right to full disclosure concerning their disease and prognosis and may believe that advocacy means working to provide that disclosure. However, family members in some cultural backgrounds may believe it is their responsibility to protect and spare the patient (their loved one) knowledge about a terminal illness. Similarly, patients may in fact not want to know about their condition and may expect their family members to "take the burden" of that knowledge and related decision making. Nurses should not decide that a family or patient is simply wrong or that a patient must know all details of his or her illness regardless of the patient's preference. Similar concerns may be noted when patients refuse pain medication or treatment because of cultural beliefs regarding pain or beliefs in divine intervention or faith healing.

Determining the most appropriate and ethical approach to patient care requires an exploration of the cultural aspects of these situations. Self-examination and recognition of one's own cultural bias and world view, as discussed earlier, play a major part in helping the nurse resolve cultural and ethical conflicts. Nurses must promote open dialogue and work with patients, families, physicians, and other health care providers to reach the culturally appropriate solution for the individual patient.

## Space and Distance

People tend to regard the space in their immediate vicinity as an extension of themselves. The amount of space they need between themselves and others to feel comfortable is a culturally determined phenomenon.

Because nurses and patients usually are not consciously aware of their personal space requirements, they frequently have difficulty understanding different behaviors in this regard. For example, one patient may perceive the nurse sitting close to him or her as an expression of warmth and care; another patient may perceive the nurse's act as a threatening invasion of personal space. Research reveals that people from the United States, Canada, and Great Britain require the most personal space between themselves and others, whereas those from Latin America, Japan, and the Middle East need the least amount of space and feel comfortable standing close to others (Giger & Davidhizar, 2004).

If the patient appears to position himself or herself too close or too far away, the nurse should consider cultural preferences for space and distance. Ideally, the patient should be permitted to assume a position that is comfortable to him or her in terms of personal space and distance. The nurse should be aware that the wheelchair of a person with a disability is considered an extension of the person; therefore, the nurse should ask the person's permission before moving or touching the wheelchair. Because a significant amount of communication during nursing care requires close physical contact, the nurse should be aware of these important cultural differences and consider them when providing care (Simpson, 2004).

## Eye Contact

Eye contact is also a culturally determined behavior. Although most nurses have been taught to maintain eye contact when speaking with patients, some people from certain cultural backgrounds may interpret this behavior differently. For example, some Asians, Native Americans, Indo-Chinese, Arabs, and Appalachians may consider direct eye contact impolite or aggressive, and they may avert their own eyes when talking with nurses and others whom they perceive to be in positions of authority. Some Native Americans stare at the floor during conversations, a cultural behavior conveying respect and indicating that the listener is paying close attention to the speaker. Some Hispanic patients maintain downcast eyes as a sign of appropriate deferential behavior toward others on the basis of age, gender, social position, economic status, and position of authority (Giger & Davidhizar, 2004). If the nurse is aware that eye contact may be culturally determined, he or she can better understand the patient's behavior and provide an atmosphere in which the patient can feel comfortable.

## Time

Attitudes about time vary widely among cultures and can be a barrier to effective communication between nurses and patients. Views about punctuality and the use of time are culturally determined, as is the concept of waiting. Symbols of time, such as watches, sunrises, and sunsets, represent methods for measuring the duration and passage of time (Giger & Davidhizar, 2004; Spector, 2004).

For most health care providers, time and promptness are extremely important. For example, nurses frequently expect patients to arrive at an exact time for an appointment, although patients are often kept waiting by health care providers who are running late. Health care providers are likely to function according to an appointment system in which there are short intervals of perhaps only a few minutes. However, for patients from some cultures, time is a relative phenomenon, with little attention paid to the exact hour or minute. For example, some Hispanic people consider time in a wider frame of reference and make the primary distinction between day and night. Time may also be determined according to traditional times for meals, sleep, and other activities or events. For people from some cultures, the present is of the greatest importance, and time is viewed in broad ranges rather than in terms of a fixed hour. Being flexible in regard to schedules is the best way to accommodate these differences.

Value differences also may influence a person's sense of priority when it comes to time. For example, responding to a family matter may be more important to a patient than meeting a scheduled health care appointment. Allowing for these different views is essential in maintaining an effective nurse–patient relationship. Scolding or acting annoyed at patients for being late undermines their confidence and may result in further missed appointments or indifference to health care suggestions.

## Touch

The meaning people associate with touching is culturally determined to a great degree. In some cultures (eg, Hispanic, Arab), male health care providers may be prohibited from touching or examining certain parts of the female body. Similarly, it may be inappropriate for females to care for males. Among many Asian Americans, it is impolite to touch a person's head because the spirit is believed to reside there. Therefore, assessment of the head or evaluation of a head injury requires permission of the patient or a family member, if the patient is not able to give permission.

The patient's culturally defined sense of modesty must also be considered when providing nursing care. For example, some Jewish and Islamic women believe that modesty requires covering their head, arms, and legs with clothing.

## Observance of Holidays

People from all cultures observe certain civil and religious holidays. Nurses should familiarize themselves with major observances for members of the cultural groups they serve. Information about these observances is available from various sources, including religious organizations, hospital chaplains, and patients themselves. Routine health appointments, diagnostic tests, surgery, and other major procedures should be scheduled to avoid observances patients identify as significant. If not contraindicated, efforts should also be made to accommodate patients and families or significant others who wish to perform cultural and religious rituals in the health care setting.

## Diet

The cultural meanings associated with food vary widely but usually include one or more of the following: relief of hunger; promotion of health and healing; prevention of disease or illness; expression of caring for another; promotion of interpersonal closeness among individual people, families, groups, communities, or nations; and promotion of kinship and family alliances. Food may also be associated with solidification of social ties; celebration of life events (eg, birthdays, marriages, funerals); expression of gratitude or appreciation; recognition of achievement or accomplishment; validation of social, cultural, or religious ceremonial functions; facilitation of business negotiations; and expression of affluence, wealth, or social status.

Culture determines which foods are served and when they are served, the number and frequency of meals, who eats with whom, and who is given the choicest portions. Culture also determines how foods are prepared and served, how they are eaten (with chopsticks, hands, or fork, knife, and spoon), and where people shop (eg, ethnic grocery stores, specialty food markets). Culture also determines the impact of excess weight and obesity on self-esteem and social standing. In some cultures, physical bulk is viewed as a sign of affluence and health (eg, a healthy baby is a chubby baby).

Religious practices may include fasting (eg, Mormons, Catholics, Buddhists, Jews, Muslims), abstaining from selected foods at particular times (eg, Catholics abstain from meat on Ash Wednesday and on Fridays during Lent), and considerations for medication use (eg, Muslims may prefer to use non–pork-derived insulin). Practices may also include the ritualistic use of food and beverages (eg, Passover dinner, consumption of bread and wine during religious ceremonies). Chart 8-2 summarizes some dietary practices of selected religious groups.

Many groups tend to feast, often in the company of family and friends, on selected holidays. For example, many Christians eat large dinners on Christmas and Easter and consume other traditional high-calorie, high-fat foods, such as seasonal cookies, pastries, and candies. These culturally based dietary practices are especially significant in the care of patients with diabetes, hypertension, gastrointestinal disorders, obesity, and other conditions in which diet plays a key role in the treatment and health maintenance regimen.

### CHART 8-2
### Prohibited Foods and Beverages of Selected Religious Groups

**Hinduism**
All meats
Animal shortenings

**Islam**
Pork
Alcoholic products and beverages (including extracts, such as vanilla and lemon)
Animal shortenings
Gelatin made with pork, marshmallow, and other confections made with gelatin

**Judaism**
Pork
Predatory fowl
Shellfish and scavenger fish (eg, shrimp, crab, lobster, escargot, catfish). Fish with fins and scales are permissible.
Mixing milk and meat dishes at same meal
Blood by ingestion (eg, blood sausage, raw meat). Blood by transfusion is acceptable.
*Note:* Packaged foods will contain labels identifying kosher ("properly preserved" or "fitting") and pareve (made without meat or milk) items.

**Mormonism (Church of Jesus Christ of Latter-Day Saints)**
Alcohol
Tobacco
Beverages containing caffeine stimulants (coffee, tea, colas, and selected carbonated soft drinks)

**Seventh-Day Adventism**
Pork
Certain seafood, including shellfish
Fermented beverages
*Note:* Optional vegetarianism is encouraged.

## Biologic Variations

Along with psychosocial adaptations, nurses must also consider the physiologic impact of culture on patients' response to treatment, particularly medications. Data have been collected for many years regarding differences in the effect some medications have on people of diverse ethnic or cultural origins. Genetic predispositions to different rates of metabolism cause some patients to be prone to overdose reactions to the standard dose of a medication, whereas other patients are likely to experience a greatly reduced benefit from the standard dose of the medication. For example, an antihypertensive agent may work well for a white man within a 4-week time span but may take much longer to work or not work at all for an African-American man with hypertension. General polymorphism—biologic variation in response to medications resulting from patient age, gender, size, and body composition—has long been acknowledged by the health care community. Nurses must be aware that ethnicity and related factors such as values and beliefs regarding the use of herbal supplements, dietary intake, and genetic factors can affect the effectiveness of treatment and compliance with the treatment regimen (Giger & Davidhizar, 2004; Green-Hernandez et al., 2004).

## Complementary and Alternative Therapies

Interventions for alterations in health and wellness vary among cultures. Interventions most commonly used in the United States have been labeled as *conventional medicine* by the National Institutes of Health (NCCAM, 2004). Other names for conventional medicine are allopathy, Western medicine, regular medicine, mainstream medicine, and biomedicine. Alternative therapy used to supplement conventional medicine may be referred to as *complementary therapy*. Interest in interventions that are not an integral part of conventional medicine prompted the National Institutes of Health to create the Office of Alternative Medicine in 1992, and then to establish the National Center for Complementary and Alternative Medicine (NCCAM) in 1999.

According to a nationwide survey, 36% of adults in the United States use some form of complementary and alternative medicine. This value increases to 75% when prayer specifically for health reasons is included in the definition. Complementary and alternative interventions are classified into five main categories: alternative medical systems, mind–body interventions, biologically based therapies, manipulative and body-based methods, and energy therapies (NCCAM, 2004):

- *Alternative medical systems* are defined as complete systems of theory and practice that are different from conventional medicine. Some examples are traditional Eastern medicine (including acupuncture, herbal medicine, Oriental massage, and Qi gong); India's traditional medicine, Ayurveda (including diet, exercise, meditation, herbal medicine, massage, exposure to sunlight, and controlled breathing to restore harmony of a person's body, mind, and spirit); homeopathic medicine (including herbal medicine and minerals); and naturopathic medicine (including diet, acupuncture, herbal medicine, hydrotherapy, spinal and soft-tissue manipulation, electrical currents, ultrasound and light therapy, therapeutic counseling, and pharmacology).
- *Mind–body interventions* are defined as techniques to facilitate the mind's ability to affect symptoms and bodily functions. Some examples are meditation, dance, music, art therapy, prayer, and mental healing.
- *Biologically based therapies* are defined as natural and biologically based practices, interventions, and products. Some examples are herbal therapies (an herb is a plant or plant part that produces and contains chemical substances that act on the body), special diet therapies (such as those of Drs. Atkins, Ornish, and Pritikin), orthomolecular therapies (magnesium, melatonin, megadoses of vitamins), and biologic therapies (shark cartilage, bee pollen).
- *Manipulative and body-based methods* are defined as interventions based on body movement. Some examples are chiropractic (primarily manipulation of the spine), osteopathic manipulation, massage therapy (soft-tissue manipulation), and reflexology.
- *Energy therapies* are defined as interventions that focus on energy fields within the body (biofields) or externally (electromagnetic fields). Some examples are Qi gong, Reiki, therapeutic touch, pulsed electromagnetic fields, magnetic fields, alternating electrical current, and direct electrical current.

Patients may choose to seek an alternative to conventional medical or surgical therapies. Many of these alternative therapies are becoming widely accepted as feasible treatment options. Therapies such as acupuncture and herbal treatments may be recommended by physicians to address aspects of a condition that are unresponsive to conventional medical treatment or to minimize the side effects associated with conventional medical therapy. Physicians and advanced practice nurses may work in collaboration with herbalists or with spiritualists or shamans to provide a comprehensive treatment plan. Out of respect for the way of life and beliefs of patients from different cultures, it is often necessary that the healers and health care providers respect the strengths of each approach (NCCAM, 2004).

Complementary therapy is becoming more common as health care consumers learn what information is available in printed media and on the Internet. As patients become more informed, they are more likely to participate in a variety of therapies in conjunction with their conventional medical treatments (Barnes, Powell-Griner, McFann, et al., 2004). Nurses must assess all patients for use of complementary therapies, be alert to the danger of herb–drug interactions or conflicting treatments, and be prepared to provide information to patients about treatments that may be harmful. However, nurses must be accepting of patients' beliefs and right to control their own care. As patient advocates, nurses facilitate the integration of conventional medical, complementary, and alternative therapies.

## Causes of Illness

Three major views, or paradigms, attempt to explain the causes of disease and illness: the biomedical or scientific view, the naturalistic or holistic perspective, and the magico-religious view.

### Biomedical or Scientific

The biomedical or scientific world view prevails in most health care settings and is embraced by most nurses and other health care providers. The basic assumptions underlying the biomedical perspective are that all events in life have a cause and effect, that the human body functions much like a machine, and that all of reality can be observed and measured (eg, blood pressures, $PaO_2$ levels, intelligence tests). One example of the biomedical or scientific view is the bacterial or viral explanation of communicable diseases.

## Naturalistic or Holistic

The second way that some cultures explain the cause of illness is through the naturalistic or holistic perspective, a viewpoint that is found among many Native Americans, Asians, and others. According to this view, the forces of nature must be kept in natural balance or harmony.

One example of a naturalistic belief, held by many Asian groups, is the yin/yang theory, in which health is believed to exist when all aspects of a person are in perfect balance or harmony. Rooted in the ancient Chinese philosophy of Taoism (which translates as "The Way"), the yin/yang theory proposes that all organisms and objects in the universe consist of yin and yang energy. The seat of the energy forces is within the autonomic nervous system, where balance between the opposing forces is maintained during health. Yin energy represents the female and negative forces, such as emptiness, darkness, and cold, whereas the yang forces are male and positive, emitting warmth and fullness. Foods are classified as cold (yin) or hot (yang) in this theory and are transformed into yin and yang energy when metabolized by the body. Cold foods are eaten when a person has a hot illness (eg, fever, rash, sore throat, ulcer, infection), and hot foods are eaten when a person has a cold illness (eg, cancer, headache, stomach cramps, "cold"). The yin/yang theory is the basis for Eastern or Chinese medicine and is embraced by some Asian Americans.

Many Hispanic, African-American, and Arab groups also embrace the hot/cold theory of health and illness. The four humors of the body—blood, phlegm, black bile, and yellow bile—regulate basic bodily functions and are described in terms of temperature and moisture. The treatment of disease consists of adding or subtracting cold, heat, dryness, or wetness to restore the balance of these humors. Beverages, foods, herbs, medicines, and diseases are classified as hot or cold according to their perceived effects on the body, not their physical characteristics. According to the hot/cold theory, the person as a whole, not just a particular ailment, is significant. People who embrace the hot/cold theory maintain that health consists of a positive state of total well-being, including physical, psychological, spiritual, and social aspects of the person.

According to the naturalistic world view, breaking the laws of nature creates imbalances, chaos, and disease. People who embrace the naturalistic paradigm use metaphors such as "the healing power of nature." For example, from the perspective of many Chinese people, illness is viewed not as an intruding agent but as a part of life's rhythmic course and an outward sign of disharmony within.

## Magico-Religious

The third major way in which people view the world and explain the causes of illness is the magico-religious world view. This view's basic premise is that the world is an arena in which supernatural forces dominate and that the fate of the world and those in it depends on the action of supernatural forces for good or evil. Examples of magical causes of illness include belief in voodoo or witchcraft among some African Americans and people from Caribbean countries. Faith healing is based on religious beliefs and is most prevalent among selected Christian religions, including Christian Science, whereas various healing rituals may be found in many other religions, such as Roman Catholicism and Mormonism (Church of Jesus Christ of Latter-Day Saints).

Of course, it is possible to hold a combination of world views, and many patients offer more than one explanation for the cause of their illness. As a profession, nursing largely embraces the scientific or biomedical world view, but some aspects of holism have begun to gain popularity, including a wide variety of techniques for managing chronic pain, such as hypnosis, therapeutic touch, and biofeedback. Belief in spiritual power is also held by many nurses who credit supernatural forces with various unexplained phenomena related to patients' health and illness states. Regardless of the view held and whether the nurse agrees with the patient's beliefs in this regard, it is important to be aware of how the person views illness and health and to work within this framework to promote patient care and well-being.

## Folk Healers

People of some cultures believe in folk or indigenous healers. For example, nurses may find that some Hispanic patients may seek help from a *curandero* or *curandera*, *espiritualista* (spiritualist), *yerbo* (herbalist), or *sabador* (healer who manipulates bones and muscles). Some African-American patients may seek assistance from a *hougan* (voodoo priest or priestess), spiritualist, root doctor (usually a woman who uses magic rituals to treat diseases), or "old lady" (an older woman who has successfully raised a family and who specializes in child care and folk remedies). Native American patients may seek assistance from a shaman or medicine man or woman. Asian patients may mention that they have visited herbalists, acupuncturists, or bone setters. Several cultures have their own healers, most of whom speak the native tongue of that culture, make house calls, and cost significantly less than healers practicing in the conventional medical health care system.

People seeking complementary and alternative therapies have expanded the practices of folk healers beyond their traditional populations, so the nurse should ask the patient about use of folk healers regardless of the patient's cultural background. It is best not to disregard the patient's belief in folk healers or try to undermine trust in the healers. To do so may alienate the patient and drive him or her away from receiving the prescribed care. Nurses should make an effort to accommodate the patient's beliefs while also advocating the treatment proposed by health science.

## Cultural Assessment

*Cultural nursing assessment* refers to a systematic appraisal or examination of individuals, families, groups, and communities in terms of their cultural beliefs, values, and practices. The purpose of such an assessment is to provide culturally competent care (Giger & Davidhizar, 2004). In an effort to establish a database for determining a patient's cultural background, nurses have developed cultural assessment tools or modified existing assessment tools (Leininger, 2001; Spector, 2004) to ensure that transcultural considerations are included in the plan of care. Giger and Davidhizar's model has been used to design nursing care from health promotion to nursing skills activities (Giger & Davidhizar, 2004; Smith-Temple & Johnson, 2005). The information presented in this chapter and the general guidelines presented in Chart 8-3 can be used to direct nursing assessment of culture and its influence on a patient's health beliefs and practices.

## Additional Cultural Considerations: Know Thyself

Because the nurse–patient interaction is the focal point of nursing, nurses should consider their own cultural orientation when conducting assessments of patients and their families and friends. The following guidelines may prove useful to nurses wishing to provide culturally appropriate care:

- Know your own cultural attitudes, values, beliefs, and practices.

### CHART 8-3

### Assessing for Patients' Cultural Beliefs

- What is the patient's country of origin? How long has the patient lived in this country? What is the patient's primary language and literacy level?
- What is the patient's ethnic background? Does he or she identify strongly with others from the same cultural background?
- What is the patient's religion, and how important is it to his or her daily life?
- Does the patient participate in cultural activities such as dressing in traditional clothing and observing traditional holidays and festivals?
- Are there any food preferences or restrictions?
- What are the patient's communication styles? Is eye contact avoided? How much physical distance is maintained? Is the patient open and verbal about symptoms?
- Who is the head of the family, and is he or she involved in decision making about the patient?
- What does the patient do to maintain his or her health?
- What does the patient think caused the current problem?
- Has the advice of traditional healers been sought?
- Have complementary and alternative therapies been used?
- What kind of treatment does the patient think will help? What are the most important results he or she hopes to get from this treatment?
- Are there cultural or religious rituals related to health, sickness, or death that the patient observes?

- Regardless of "good intentions," everyone has cultural "baggage" that ultimately results in ethnocentrism.
- In general, it is easier to understand those whose cultural heritage is similar to your own, while viewing those who are unlike you as strange and different.
- Maintain a broad, open attitude. Expect the unexpected. Enjoy surprises.
- Avoid seeing all people as alike; that is, avoid cultural stereotypes, such as "all Chinese like rice" or "all Italians eat spaghetti."
- Try to understand the reasons for any behavior by discussing commonalities and differences.
- If a patient has said or done something that you do not understand, ask for clarification. Be a good listener. Most patients will respond positively to questions that arise from a genuine concern for and interest in them.
- If at all possible, speak the patient's language (even simple greetings and social courtesies are appreciated). Avoid feigning an accent or using words that are ordinarily not part of your vocabulary.
- Be yourself. There are no right or wrong ways to learn about cultural diversity.

## Health Disparities

Health disparities—higher rates of morbidity, mortality, and burden of disease in a population or community than found in the overall population—are significant in ethnic and racial minorities. Key health indicators in the United States reveal a significant gap in health status between the overall American population and people of specific ethnic backgrounds (Keltner, Kelley, & Smith, 2004). Ethnic and racial minorities are disproportionately burdened with cancer, heart disease, diabetes, human immunodeficiency virus (HIV) infection/acquired immunodeficiency syndrome (AIDS), and other conditions. They receive a lower quality of health care than non-minorities and are at a greater risk for declining health. Many reasons are cited for these disparities, including low socioeconomic status; health behaviors; limited access to health care because of poverty or disability; environmental factors; and direct and indirect manifestations of discrimination. Other causes include lack of health insurance; overdependence on publicly funded facilities; and barriers to health care such as insufficient transportation, geographic location (not enough providers in an area), cost of services, and the low numbers of minority health care providers (Baldwin, 2004; Beal, 2004; Institute of Medicine, 2003).

## The Future of Transcultural Nursing Care

By the middle of the 21st century, the average American patient will trace his or her ancestry to Africa, Asia, the Pacific Islands, or the Hispanic or Arab worlds, rather than to Europe (Giger & Davidhizar, 2004). As indicated previously, the concept of culturally competent care applies to health care institutions, which must develop culturally sensitive policies and provide a climate that fosters the provision of culturally competent care by nurses. Nurses, who reflect the multicultural complexion of our society, must learn to acknowledge and adapt to diversity among their colleagues in the workplace (Simpson, 2004).

As the population becomes more culturally diverse, efforts to increase the number of ethnic minority nurses must continue and accelerate (Sullivan Commission, 2004). Today more than 88% of all nurses are Caucasian. Progress in increasing the percentage of culturally diverse nurses has been significantly slower than the increasing percentage of ethnic minorities in the United States (Washington, Erickson, & Ditomasi, 2004). Greater efforts must be made to facilitate the recruitment and program completion of nursing students who are members of ethnic minorities. In addition, educational institutions must prepare nurses to deliver culturally competent care and must work to increase the number of ethnic minority providers in the nursing workforce. Nursing programs are exploring creative ways to promote cultural competence in nursing students, including offering multicultural health studies in their curricula (Spector, 2004).

Cultural diversity remains one of the foremost issues in health care today. With increasing frequency, nurses will be expected to provide culturally competent care for patients. Nurses must work effectively with the increasing number of patients, other nurses, and other health care team members whose ancestry reflects the multicultural complexion of contemporary society.

## Critical Thinking Exercises

1. **ebp** You are assigned to care for a hospitalized patient whose cultural background is very different from yours. What is the evidence base for use of a cultural assessment tool to ensure that cultural considerations are included in the nursing plan of care? What is the strength of that evidence? What resources are available to you to promote culturally competent care? Explain why it is important to examine your own feelings about each patient's cultural beliefs and practices.

2. An elderly Asian woman who does not speak English is hospitalized with heart failure. Her immediate family members insist on staying with her around the clock, and many extended family members visit each day, staying late into the night. They share all their meals in the waiting room. Some staff members have complained that the family members are not adhering to the hospital's established visiting hours and are disturbing other patients and visitors. How can you help the nursing staff explore the meaning of the family's behavior and understand their own negative feelings about this behavior? Devise a strategy that will help resolve this situation.

3. You have been caring for an elderly patient who does not speak English. Her family members speak only limited English. You are unable to communicate well enough with the patient and the family to provide the necessary discharge teaching. What resources would you use to assist you in providing the discharge teaching? What aspects of the patient's and family's background would you want to assess to determine the need for referral to a home health care agency?

## REFERENCES AND SELECTED READINGS

### BOOKS

American Academy of Nursing, Subpanel on Cultural Competence in Nursing. (1995). *Promoting cultural competence in and through nursing education.* New York: Author.

American Association of Colleges of Nursing. (1996). *Diversity Task Force Report, October 1996.* Washington, DC: Author.

Andrews, M. M., & Boyle, J. S. (2002). *Transcultural concepts in nursing care* (4th ed.). Philadelphia: J. B. Lippincott.

Giger, J. N., & Davidhizar, R. E. (2004). *Transcultural nursing: Assessment and intervention* (4th ed.). St. Louis: C. V. Mosby.

Institute of Medicine. (2003). *Unequal treatment: Confronting racial and ethnic disparities in healthcare.* Smedley, B. D., Stith, A. Y., & Nelson, A. R. (Eds.). Washington, DC: National Academy Press.

Leininger, M. M. (Ed.). (2001). *Culture care diversity and universality: A theory of nursing.* New York: National League for Nursing Press.

Smith-Temple, J., & Johnson, J. Y. (2005). *Nurse's guide to clinical procedures* (5th ed.). Philadelphia: Lippincott Williams & Wilkins.

Spector, R. E. (2004). *Cultural diversity in health and illness* (6th ed.). New Jersey: Prentice-Hall.

### JOURNALS

Baldwin, D. M. (2004). Disparities in health and health care: Focusing efforts to eliminate unequal burdens. *Online Journal of Issues in Nursing. 8*(1), Manuscript 1. Available at: nursingworld.org/ojin/topic20/tpc20_1.htm

Barnes, P. M., Powell-Griner, E., McFann, K., et al. (May 27, 2004). Complementary and alternative medicine use among adults: United States, 2002. *Advance Data from Vital and Health Statistics, 343.*

Beal, A. (2004). Perspective: Policies to reduce racial and ethnic disparities in child health and health care. *Health Affairs, 23*(5), 171–179.

Betancourt, S. R. (2004). Cultural competence—marginal or mainstream movement? *New England Journal of Medicine, 351*(10), 953–954.

Campinha-Bacote, J. (2003). Many faces: Addressing diversity in health care. *Online Journal of Issues in Nursing, 8*(1). Available at http://www.nursingworld.org/ojin/topics20/tpc20_2.htm

Flowers, D. (2004). Culturally competent nursing care: A challenge for the 21st century. *Critical Care Nurse, 24*(4), 48–52.

Green-Hernandez, C., Quinn, A. A., Denman-Vitale, S., et al. (2004). Making nursing care culturally competent. *Holistic Nursing Practice, 29*(4), 215–218.

Keltner, B., Kelley, F., & Smith, D. (2004). Leadership to reduce health disparities. *Nursing Administration Quarterly, 28*(3), 181–190.

Leininger, M. M. (1988). Leininger's theory of nursing: Cultural care diversity and universality. *Nursing Science Quarterly, 1*(4), 152–159.

National Institutes of Health, National Center for Complementary and Alternative Medicine (NCCAM). *Major domains of complementary and alternative medicine.* http://nccam.nih.gov (Accessed May 5, 2006).

Simpson, R. (2004). Recruit, retain, assess technology's role in diversity. *Nursing Administration Quarterly, 28*(3), 217–220.

Swanson, J. W. (2004). Diversity: Creating an environment of inclusiveness. *Nursing Administration Quarterly, 28*(3), 145–169.

Washington, D., Erikson, J. I., & Ditomassi, M. (2004). Mentoring the minority nurse leader of tomorrow. *Nursing Administration Quarterly, 28*(3), 165–169.

Watts, R. (2003). Race consciousness and the health of African Americans. *Online Journal of Issues in Nursing, 8*(1), Manuscript 3. Available at: http://nursingworld.org/ojin/topic20/tpc20_3.htm. Accessed May 5, 2006.

## RESOURCES

## ORGANIZATIONS

Asian & Pacific Islander Nurses Association, 400 N. Ingalls, Suite 3160, Ann Arbor, MI 48109; 734-998-1030

Council on Nursing and Anthropology, c/o Dr. Mildred Roberson, Nursing and Health Sciences, Salisbury State University, Salisbury, MD 21801

Language Line Services; 1-877-886-3885; http://www.languageline.com/. Accessed July 6, 2006. (Provides written and oral translation in 140 languages.)

National Black Nurses Association, 8630 Fenton St., Suite 330, Silver Spring, MD 20910; 301-589-3200; http://www.nbna.org. Accessed June 6, 2006.

National Institutes of Health, National Center for Complementary and Alternative Medicine, 6707 Democracy Blvd., Suite 2000, Bethesda, MD 20892; 1-888-644-6226; fax 1-866-464-3616; http://nccam.nih.gov. Accessed June 6, 2006.

Office of Minority Health, U.S. Department of Health and Human Services, 5600 Fisher's Lane, Room 10-49, Rockville, MD 20857; 301-443-5084; http://www.omhrc.gov. Accessed June 6, 2006.

Transcultural Nursing Society, c/o Madonna University College of Nursing and Health, 36600 Schoolcraft Road, Livonia MI 48150; 888-432-5470; http://www.tcns.org. Accessed June 6, 2006.

# CHAPTER 9

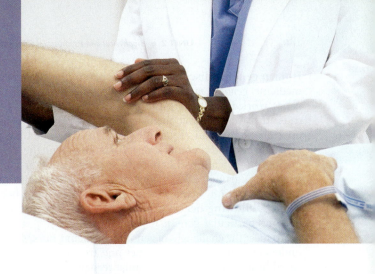

# Genetics Perspectives in Nursing

## Learning Objectives

*On completion of this chapter, the learner will be able to:*

1. Describe the role of the nurse in integrating genetics in nursing care.
2. Conduct a genetics-based assessment.
3. Identify the common patterns of inheritance of genetic disorders.
4. Identify ethical issues in nursing related to genetics.

Human **genome** discoveries have ushered in a new era of medicine, *genomic medicine*, which recognizes that multiple genes work in concert with environmental influences to cause disease. Genomic medicine aims to improve predictions about a person's susceptibility to diseases; the time of onset, extent, and eventual severity of diseases; and the treatments or medications likely to be most effective or most harmful (Varmus, 2004). New gene-based strategies for disease detection, management, and treatment have been created, allowing health professionals to tailor care to a person's particular genetic makeup.

To meet the challenges of genomic medicine, nurses must understand the new technologies and treatments of gene-based health care. Nurses also must recognize that they are a vital link between the patient and health care services; patients often turn to nurses first with questions about a family history of risk factors, genetics information, and genetic tests and interpretations. The incorporation of genetics into nursing means bringing a genetic framework to health assessments, planning, and interventions that supports identification of and response to the changing genetics-related health needs of people (Lea & Monsen, 2003).

When obtaining family and health histories, nurses must learn to recognize patterns of inheritance and understand when it is appropriate to consider new gene-based testing and treatment options. This chapter offers a foundation for the clinical application of genetics principles in medical and surgical nursing, outlines the nurse's role in genetic coun-

## Glossary

**allele:** any one of two or more alternate forms of a gene at the same location. An allele for each gene is inherited from each parent.

**autosome:** a single chromosome from any of the 22 pairs of chromosomes not involved in sex determination (XX or XY)

**carrier:** person who is heterozygous; possessing two different alleles of a gene pair

**chromosome:** microscopic structures in the cell nucleus that contain genetic information and are constant in number in a species (eg, humans have 46 chromosomes)

**deoxyribonucleic acid (DNA):** the primary genetic material in humans consisting of nitrogenous bases, a sugar group, and phosphate combined into a double helix

**diploid:** the number of chromosomes normally present in somatic cells. For humans, that number is 46

**dominant:** a genetic trait that is normally expressed when a person has a gene mutation on one of a pair of chromosomes and the "normal" form of the gene is on the other chromosome

**genetics:** the scientific study of heredity; how specific traits or predispositions are transmitted from parents to offspring

**genome:** the total genetic complement of an individual genotype

**genomics:** the study of the human genome, including gene sequencing, mapping, and function

**genotype:** the genes and the variations therein that a person inherits from his or her parents

**haploid:** the number of chromosomes present in egg or sperm (gametes); in humans, this is 23

**Human Genome Project:** an international research effort aimed at identifying and characterizing the order of every base in the human genome

**meiosis:** the reduction division of diploid egg or sperm (germ cells) resulting in haploid gametes (having 23 chromosomes each)

**mitosis:** cell division occurring in somatic cells that normally results in daughter cells with the same number of chromosomes—46 (diploid)

**monosomy:** missing one of a chromosome pair in normally diploid cells (for example, 45,X females have only one X chromosome)

**mutation:** a heritable alteration in the genetic material

**nondisjunction:** the failure of a chromosome pair to separate appropriately during meiosis, resulting in abnormal chromosome numbers in reproductive cells (gametes)

**nucleotide:** a nucleic acid "building block" composed of a nitrogenous base, a five-carbon sugar, and a phosphate group

**pedigree:** a diagrammatic representation of a family history

**penetrance:** the percentage of individuals known to carry the gene for a trait who actually manifest the condition. For example, a trait with 90% penetrance will not be manifested by 10% of persons possessing the gene.

**phenotype:** a person's entire physical, biochemical, and physiologic makeup, as determined by the person's genotype and environmental factors

**polymorphism:** a genetic variation with two or more alleles that is maintained in a population

**population screening:** the application of a test or inquiry to a group to determine if persons in the group have an increased likelihood of a genetic condition or a mutation in a specific gene (eg, cholesterol screening for hypercholesterolemia)

**predisposition testing:** testing that is used to determine the likelihood that a healthy person with or without a family history of a condition will develop the disorder. Having the gene mutation would indicate that the person has an increased susceptibility to the disorder, but this is not a diagnosis. One example is DNA mutation testing for hereditary breast/ovarian cancer.

**prenatal screening:** testing that is used to identify whether a fetus is at risk for a birth defect such as Down syndrome or spina bifida (eg, multiple marker maternal serum screening in pregnancy)

**presymptomatic testing:** genetic testing that is used to determine whether persons with a family history of a disorder, but no current symptoms, have the gene mutation. An example of this would be Huntington disease.

**recessive:** a genetic trait that is expressed only when a person has two copies of a mutant autosomal gene or a single copy of a mutant X-linked gene in the absence of another X chromosome

**transcription:** the process of transforming information from DNA into new strands of messenger RNA

**trisomy:** the presence of one extra chromosome in an otherwise diploid chromosome complement—for example, trisomy 21 (Down syndrome)

**variable expression:** variation in the degree to which a trait is manifested; clinical severity

**X-linked:** located on the X chromosome

seling and evaluation, addresses important ethical issues, and provides genetics resources for nurses and patients.

# Framework for Integrating Genetics Into Nursing Practice

The unique contribution of nursing to genomic medicine is its philosophy of holism. Nurses are ideally positioned to incorporate genetics into the care of patients at all ages and stages of life and in all settings. The holistic view that characterizes nursing takes into account each person's intellectual, physical, spiritual, social, cultural, biopsychologic, ethical, and esthetic experiences while addressing genetic information, gene-based testing, diagnosis, and treatment. Thus, knowledge of genetics is basic to nursing practice (Olsen, Feetham, Jenkins, et al., 2003).

A framework for integrating genetics into nursing practice includes a philosophy of care that recognizes when genetic factors are playing a role or could play a role in a person's health. This means using family history and the results of genetic tests effectively, informing patients about genetics concepts, understanding the personal and societal impact of genetics information, and valuing the privacy and confidentiality of genetics information.

A person's response to genetics information, genetic testing, or genetics-related conditions may be either empowering or disabling. Genetics information may stigmatize people if it affects how they view themselves or how others view them. Nurses can help individuals and families learn how genetic traits and conditions are passed on within families and how genetic and environmental factors influence health and disease (Greco, 2003).

Nurses facilitate communication among family members, the health care system, and community resources, and they offer valuable support by virtue of their continuity of care with patients and families. All nurses should be able to recognize when a patient is asking a question related to genetics information and should know how to obtain genetics information by gathering family and health histories and conducting physical and developmental assessments. Being able to recognize a genetics concern allows nurses to provide appropriate genetics resources and support to patients and families (Lea & Monsen, 2003).

Essential to a genetic framework in nursing is the awareness of one's attitudes, experience, and assumptions about genetics concepts and how these are manifested in one's own practice. Chart 9-1 offers insights on how nurses can conduct periodic self-assessments.

# Genetics Concepts

Scientists and philosophers have long speculated about heredity and developed theories to explain how traits are transmitted to offspring. Developments in technology and research have increased understanding of genetics, resulting in better understanding of relatively rare diseases such as phenylketonuria (PKU) or hemophilia that are related to mutations of a single gene inherited in families. New technologies and tools allow scientists to characterize inherited metabolic variations that interact over time and lead to common diseases such as cancer, heart disease, and dementia. This transition from **genetics** to **genomics** highlights how understanding of single genes and their individual functions has evolved to understanding how multiple genes act and control biologic processes. Most health conditions are now believed to be the result of a combination of genetic and environmental influences (Guttmacher & Collins, 2004).

## Genes and Their Role in Human Variation

Genes are central components of human health and disease. Work on the **Human Genome Project** (an international research effort to map and sequence the human genome) has shown how basic human genetics is to human development, health, and disease. Knowledge that specific genes are associated with specific genetic conditions makes diagnosis possible, even in the unborn. Research demonstrates that many common conditions have genetic causes. Many more associations between genetics, health, and disease are likely be identified with refinement of human genome mapping and sequencing.

### Genes and Chromosomes

A person's unique genetic constitution, called a **genotype**, is made up of some 30,000 to 40,000 genes (Guttmacher & Collins, 2004). A person's **phenotype**, the observable characteristics of his or her genotype, includes physical appearance and other biologic, physiologic, and molecular traits. Environmental influences modify every person's phenotype, even phenotypes with a major genetic component.

Human growth, development, and disease occur as a result of both genetic and environmental influences and interactions. The contribution of genetic factors may be large or small. For example, in a person with cystic fibrosis or PKU, the genetic contribution is significant. In contrast, the genetic contribution underlying a person's response to infection may be less important.

A single gene is conceptualized as a unit of heredity. A gene is composed of a segment of **deoxyribonucleic acid (DNA)** that contains a specific set of instructions for making the protein or proteins needed by body cells for proper functioning. Genes regulate both the types of proteins made and the rate at which proteins are produced. The structure of the DNA molecule is referred to as the double helix. The essential components of the DNA molecule are sugar–phosphate molecules and pairs of nitrogenous bases. Each **nucleotide** contains a sugar (deoxyribose), a phosphate group, and one of four nitrogenous bases: adenine (A), cytosine (C), guanine (G), and thymine (T). DNA is composed of two paired strands, each made up of a number of nucleotides. The strands are held together by hydrogen bonds between pairs of bases (Fig. 9-1).

Genes are packaged and arranged in a linear order within **chromosomes**, which are located in the cell nucleus. In humans, 46 chromosomes occur in pairs in all body cells except oocytes (eggs) and sperm, which each contain only 23 chromosomes. Twenty-two pairs of chromosomes, called **autosomes**, are the same in females and males.

## CHART 9-1

### Examining Our Own Attitudes, Experiences, and Assumptions

Self-knowledge is one of the cornerstones to providing quality nursing care, and as practitioners, our attitudes and experiences have an impact on clinical practice. These attitudes emerge from social, cultural, and religious experiences in one's personal life. Awareness of our own values, beliefs, and cultural perceptions not only is important to the nurse–patient relationship but is also the first step in developing a genetics framework.

Periodic self-assessment can help maintain an effective framework as nurses update genetics knowledge and practice. Nurses can develop an awareness of their own attitudes, experiences, and assumptions about genetics concepts by considering the following:

- *One's family's beliefs or values about health.* What are your family, religious, or cultural beliefs about the cause of illness? How have your values or biases influenced your understanding of genetics conditions?
- *One's philosophical, theologic, cultural, and ethical perspectives related to health.* How would these attitudes influence your own use of genetics information or services? What experiences have you had with people from different social, cultural, religious, or ethnic groups? How would you deliver genetics information to individuals from different social, cultural, or ethnic groups? Can you recognize when personal values or biases may affect or interfere with the delivery of genetics information?
- *One's level of genetics expertise.* Can you recognize the limitations of your own experience in genetics and know when to refer patients for further genetic workup?
- *One's experience with birth defects, chronic illnesses, and genetic conditions.* Do you have a family member or friend who has a genetic condition or disorder? Has your experience been that genetic disorders are disabling or empowering? Do you view a parent as being "at fault" for having a baby born with a birth defect or genetic condition? Do you advocate for fair access and other rights for individuals who have birth defects, genetic conditions, or other disabilities?
- *One's view of DNA (the most basic concept of who we are, since our genetic makeup is unlike that of any other person except an identical twin).* What are your assumptions about DNA? For example, do you assume that the genetic component of "the self" is a defective self? As another example, healthy carriers of genetic alterations that predispose them to develop certain diseases in the future now belong to a new class of "at risk" individuals. A person who is "at risk" is not ill at present but may not remain well as long as the "average" person. Is it good to know that you are "at risk", or is this information that should not be identified or revealed because of the risk of potential discrimination?
- *One's beliefs about reproductive options.* What are your beliefs regarding reproductive options such as prenatal diagnosis and pregnancy termination? How might these influence your care of a patient who holds different beliefs?
- *One's view of genetic testing and engineering.* Do you see genetic testing and engineering—the ability to eliminate or enhance certain traits—as a way to create an "ideal genetic self"?
- *One's approach to patients with disabilities.* How are your attitudes made apparent in your practice and practice settings? For example, do you have access to TTY machines and/or interpreters for those who have hearing impairment? Are your intake procedures adapted to meet the needs of an individual with disabilities?

Adapted from National Coalition of Health Professional Education in Genetics. (2001). *Core competencies*; http://www.nchpeg.org; Kenan, R. (1996). The at-risk health status and technology: A diagnostic invitation and the gift of knowing. *Social Science and Medicine, 42*(11), 1545–1553; Peters, J. A., Djurdjinovic, L. & Baker, D. (1999). The genetic self: The Human Genome Project, genetic counseling and family therapy. *Families, Systems & Health, 17*(1), 5–25.

---

The 23rd pair is referred to as the sex chromosomes. A female has two X chromosomes, whereas a male has one X and one Y chromosome. At conception, each parent normally gives one chromosome of each pair to his or her children. As a result, children receive half of their chromosomes from their father and half from their mother (Fig. 9-2).

Careful examination of DNA sequences from many people shows that these sequences have multiple versions in a population. These different versions, or sequence variations, are called **alleles**. Sequences found in many forms are said to be polymorphic, meaning that there are at least two common forms of a particular gene.

## Cell Division

The human body grows and develops as a result of the process of cell division. Mitosis and meiosis are two distinctly different types of cell division.

**Mitosis** is involved in cell growth, differentiation, and repair. During mitosis, the chromosomes of each cell du-

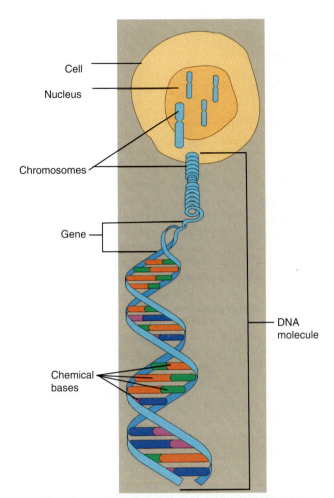

**FIGURE 9-1.** DNA carrying the instructions that allows cells to make proteins is made up of four chemical bases. Tightly coiled strands of DNA are packaged in units called chromosomes, which are housed in the cell's nucleus. Working subunits of DNA are known as genes. (From the National Institutes of Health and National Cancer Institute. [1995]. *Understanding gene testing* [NIH Pub. No. 96-3905]. Washington, DC: U.S. Department of Human Services.)

**FIGURE 9-2.** Each human cell contains 23 pairs of chromosomes, which can be distinguished by size and by their unique banding patterns. This set is from a male, because it contains a Y chromosome. Females have two X chromosomes. (From the National Institutes of Health and National Cancer Institute. [1995]. *Understanding gene testing* [NIH Pub. No. 96-3905]. Washington, DC: U.S. Department of Human Services.)

plicate. The result is two cells, called daughter cells, which each contain the same number of chromosomes as the parent cell. The daughter cells are said to be **diploid** because they contain 46 chromosomes in 23 pairs. Mitosis occurs in all cells of the body except oocytes (eggs) and sperm.

**Meiosis**, in contrast, occurs only in reproductive cells and is the process by which oocytes and sperm are formed. During meiosis, a reduction in the number of chromosomes takes place, resulting in oocytes or sperm that contain half the usual number, or 23 chromosomes. Oocytes and sperm are referred to as **haploid** because they contain a single copy of each chromosome, compared to the usual two copies in all other body cells. During the initial phase of meiosis, as the paired chromosomes come together in preparation for cell division, portions cross over, and an exchange of genetic material occurs before the chromosomes separate. This event, called recombination, creates greater diversity in the makeup of oocytes and sperm.

During meiosis, a pair of chromosomes may fail to separate completely, creating a sperm or oocyte that contains either two copies or no copy of a particular chromosome. This sporadic event, called **nondisjunction**, can lead to either a trisomy or a monosomy. Down syndrome is an example of **trisomy**. People with Down syndrome have three copies of chromosome number 21. Turner syndrome is an example of **monosomy**. Girls with Turner syndrome usually have a single X chromosome, causing them to have short stature and infertility (Rimoin, Connor, Pyeritz, et al., 2002).

## Gene Mutations

Within each cell, many intricate and complex interactions regulate and express human genes. Gene structure and function, **transcription** and translation, and protein synthesis are all involved. Alterations in gene structure and function and the process of protein synthesis may influence a person's health. Changes in gene structure, called **mutations**, permanently change the sequence of DNA, which in turn can alter the nature and type of proteins made (Fig. 9-3).

Some gene mutations have no significant effect on the protein product, whereas others cause partial or complete changes. How a protein is altered and its importance to proper body functioning determine the impact of the mutation. Gene mutations may occur in hormones, enzymes, or other important protein products, with significant implications for health and disease. Sickle cell anemia is an example of a genetic condition caused by a small gene mutation that affects protein structure, producing hemoglobin S. A person who inherits two copies of the hemoglobin S gene

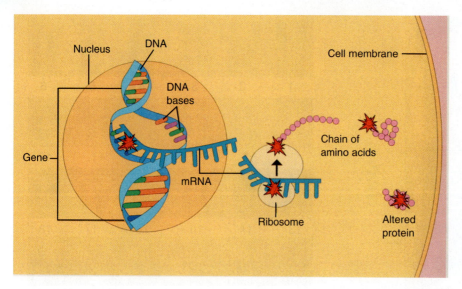

**FIGURE 9-3.** When a gene contains a mutation, the protein encoded by that gene will be altered. Some protein changes are insignificant, and others are disabling. (From the National Institutes of Health and National Cancer Institute. [1995]. *Understanding gene testing* [NIH Pub. No. 96-3905]. Washington, DC: U.S. Department of Human Services.)

mutation has sickle cell anemia and experiences the symptoms of severe anemia and thrombotic organ damage resulting from hypoxia (Rimoin et al., 2002).

Other gene mutations may be larger, such as a deletion (loss), insertion (addition), duplication (multiplication), or rearrangement (translocation) of a longer DNA segment. Duchenne muscular dystrophy, an inherited form of muscular dystrophy, is an example of a genetic disorder caused by structural gene mutations such as deletions or duplications in the dystrophin gene. Another type of gene mutation, called a triplet or trinucleotide repeat, involves expansion to more than the usual number of copies of a triplet repeat sequence within a gene. Myotonic dystrophy, Huntington disease, and fragile X syndrome are examples of conditions caused by this type of gene mutation.

Gene mutations may be inherited or acquired. Inherited or germline gene mutations are present in the DNA of all body cells and are passed on in reproductive cells from parent to child. Germline mutations are passed on to all daughter cells when body cells replicate (Fig. 9-4). The gene that causes Huntington disease is one example of a germline mutation.

Spontaneous mutations take place in individual oocytes or sperm at the time of conception. These mutations are not inherited in other family members. However, a person who carries the new "spontaneous" mutation may pass on the mutation to his or her children. Achondroplasia, Marfan syndrome, and neurofibromatosis type 1 are examples of genetic conditions that may occur in a single family member as a result of spontaneous mutation.

Acquired mutations take place in somatic cells and involve changes in DNA that occur after conception, during a person's lifetime. Acquired mutations develop as a result of cumulative changes in body cells other than reproductive cells (Fig. 9-5). Somatic gene mutations are passed on to the daughter cells derived from that particular cell line.

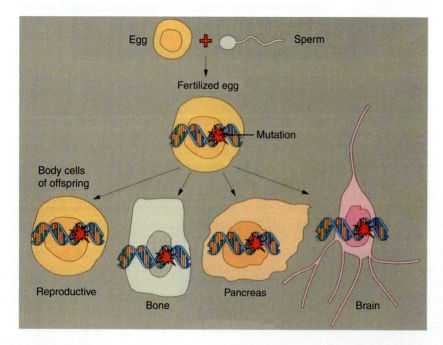

**FIGURE 9-4.** Hereditary mutations are carried in the DNA of the reproductive cells. When reproductive cells containing mutations combine to produce offspring, the mutation is present in all of the offspring's body cells. (From the National Institutes of Health and National Cancer Institute. [1995]. *Understanding gene testing* [NIH Pub. No. 96-3905]. Washington, DC: U.S. Department of Human Services.)

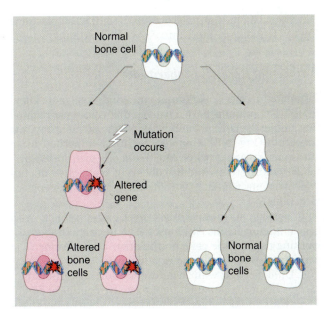

**FIGURE 9-5.** Acquired mutations develop in DNA during a person's lifetime. If the mutation arises in a body cell, copies of the mutation will exist only in the descendants of that particular cell. (From the National Institutes of Health and National Cancer Institute. [1995]. *Understanding gene testing* [NIH Pub. No. 96-3905]. Washington, DC: U.S. Department of Human Services.)

Gene mutations occur in the human body all the time. Cells have built-in mechanisms by which they can recognize mutations in DNA, and in most situations they correct the changes before they are passed on by cell division. However, over time, body cells may lose their ability to repair damage from gene mutations, causing an accumulation of genetic changes that may ultimately result in diseases such as cancer and possibly other conditions of aging, such as Alzheimer disease (Lea, 2000).

## Genetic Variation

Research is ongoing to sort out the genetic components of complex conditions (eg, heart disease, diabetes, common cancers, psychiatric disorders) that result from the interaction of environment, lifestyle, and genetic effects. New studies of genetic variation in humans are underway to develop a map of common DNA variants. Genetic variations occur among people of all populations. **Polymorphisms** and single nucleotide polymorphisms (SNPs, or "snips") are the terms used for common genetic variations that occur most frequently throughout the human genome. Some SNPs may contribute directly to a trait or disease expression by altering function. SNPs are becoming increasingly important for the discovery of DNA sequence variations that affect biologic function. Such knowledge allows clinicians to subclassify diseases and adapt therapies to individual patients (Collins & McKusick, 2001; Guttmacher & Collins, 2004). For example, a polymorphism or SNP can alter protein or enzyme activity, and thereby affect drug efficacy and safety, if it occurs in proteins that are targets of medication regimens or that are involved in drug transport or drug metabolism (Evans & McLeod, 2003).

## Inheritance Patterns

Nursing assessment of the patient's health includes obtaining and recording family history information. Evaluation of family history in the form of a **pedigree** is a first step in establishing the pattern of inheritance. Nurses must be familiar with mendelian patterns of inheritance and pedigree construction and analysis to help identify patients and families who may benefit from further genetic counseling, testing, and treatment (Jenkins & Lea, 2004).

Mendelian conditions, named after Gregor Mendel, are genetic conditions that are inherited in fixed proportions among generations. They result from gene mutations that are present on one or both chromosomes of a pair. A single gene inherited from one or both parents can cause a mendelian condition. Mendelian conditions are classified according to their pattern of inheritance: autosomal dominant, autosomal recessive, and **X-linked**. The terms **dominant** and **recessive** refer to the trait, genetic condition, or phenotype but not to the genes or alleles that cause the observable characteristics (Nussbaum, McGinnis & Willard, 2001).

### Autosomal Dominant Inheritance

Autosomal dominant inherited conditions affect female and male family members equally and follow a vertical pattern of inheritance in families (Fig. 9-6). A person who has an autosomal dominant inherited condition carries a gene mutation for that condition on one chromosome of a pair. Each of that person's offspring has a 50% chance of inheriting the gene mutation for the condition and a 50% chance of inheriting the normal version of the gene (Fig. 9-7). Offspring who do not inherit the gene mutation for the dominant condition do not develop the condition and do not have an increased chance for having children with the same condition. Table 9-1 presents characteristics and examples of different patterns of inherited conditions.

Autosomal dominant conditions often manifest with varying degrees of severity among affected people. Some may have significant symptoms, whereas others may have only mild ones. This characteristic is referred to as **variable**

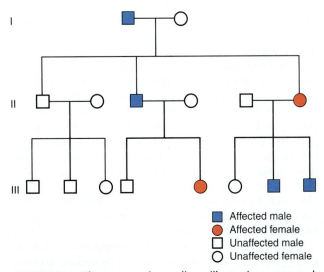

**FIGURE 9-6.** Three-generation pedigree illustrating autosomal dominant inheritance.

**FIGURE 9-7.** In dominant genetic disorders, if one affected parent has a disease-causing allele that dominates its normal counterpart, each child in the family has a 50% chance of inheriting the disease allele and the disorder. (From the National Institutes of Health and National Cancer Institute. [1995]. *Understanding gene testing* [NIH Pub. No. 96-3905]. Washington, DC: U.S. Department of Human Services.)

expression; it results from the influences of genetic and environmental factors on clinical presentation.

Another phenomenon observed in autosomal dominant inheritance is **penetrance,** or the percentage of persons known to have a particular gene mutation who actually show the trait. Almost complete penetrance is observed in conditions such as achondroplasia, in which nearly 100% of people with the gene mutation typically display traits of the disease. In some conditions, however, the presence of a gene mutation does not invariably mean that a person will have or develop an autosomal inherited condition. For example, a woman who has the BRCA1 hereditary breast cancer gene mutation has a lifetime risk for breast cancer as high as 80%, not 100%. This quality, known as incomplete penetrance, indicates the probability that a given gene will produce disease. In other words, a person may inherit the gene mutation that causes an autosomal dominant condition but may not have any of the observable physical or developmental features of that condition. However, this person carries the gene mutation and still has a 50% chance of passing the gene for the condition to each of his or her children.

One of the effects of incomplete penetrance is that the gene appears to "skip" a generation, thus leading to errors in interpreting family history and in genetic counseling. Examples of other genetic conditions with incomplete penetrance include otosclerosis (40%) and retinoblastoma (80%) (Nussbaum, McGinnis & Willard, 2001).

### Autosomal Recessive Inheritance

Compared to autosomal dominant conditions, autosomal recessive conditions have a pattern that is more horizontal than vertical; relatives of a single generation tend to have the condition (Fig. 9-8). Genetic conditions inherited in an autosomal recessive pattern are frequently seen among particular ethnic groups and usually occur more often in children of parents who are related by blood, such as first cousins (see Table 9-1).

In autosomal recessive inheritance, each parent carries a gene mutation on one chromosome of the pair and a normal working copy of the gene on the other chromosome. The parents are said to be **carriers** of the particular gene mutation. Unlike people with an autosomal dominant condition, carriers of a gene mutation for a recessive condition do not have symptoms of the genetic condition. When carriers have children together, there is a 25% chance that each child may inherit the gene mutation from both parents and have the condition (Fig. 9-9). Gaucher's disease is one example of a condition inherited in an autosomal recessive manner (Enderlin, Vogel & Conway, 2003). Other examples include cystic fibrosis, sickle cell anemia, and PKU.

### X-Linked Inheritance

X-linked conditions may be inherited in recessive or dominant patterns (see Table 9-1). In both, the gene mutation is located on the X chromosome. All males inherit an X chromosome from their mothers and a Y chromosome from their fathers for a normal sex constitution of 46,XY. Because males have only one X chromosome, they do not have a counterpart for its genes, as do females. This means that a gene mutation on the X chromosome of a male is expressed even though it is present in only one copy. Females, on the other hand, inherit one X chromosome from each parent for a normal sex constitution of 46,XX. A female may be an unaffected carrier of a gene mutation, or she may be affected if the condition results from a gene mutation causing a X-linked dominant condition. Either the X chromosome that she received from her mother or the X chromosome she received from her father may be passed on to each of her offspring, and this is a random occurrence.

The most common pattern of X-linked inheritance is that in which a female is a carrier for a gene mutation on one of her X chromosomes. This is referred to as X-linked recessive inheritance. In X-linked recessive conditions, a female carrier has a 50% chance of passing on the gene mutation to a son, who would be affected, or to a daughter, who would be a carrier like her mother (Fig. 9-10). Examples of X-linked recessive conditions include factor VIII and factor IX hemophilia, severe combined immunodeficiency, and Duchenne muscular dystrophy.

### Nontraditional Inheritance

Although mendelian conditions manifest with a specific pattern of inheritance in some families, many diseases

## TABLE 9-1  Patterns of Mendelian Inheritance

| Characteristics | Examples |
|---|---|
| **Autosomal Dominant Inherited Conditions** | |
| Vertical transmission in families | Hereditary breast/ovarian cancer syndrome |
| Males and females equally affected | Familial hypercholesterolemia |
| Variable expression among family members and others with condition | Hereditary non-polyposis colorectal cancer |
| | Huntington disease |
| Reduced penetrance (in some conditions) | Marfan syndrome |
| Advanced paternal age associated with sporadic cases | Neurofibromatosis |
| **Autosomal Recessive Inherited Conditions** | |
| Horizontal pattern of transmission seen in families | Cystic fibrosis |
| Males and females equally affected | Galactosemia |
| Associated with consanguinity (genetic relatedness) | Phenylketonuria |
| Associated with particular ethnic groups | Sickle cell anemia |
| | Tay-Sachs disease |
| | Canavan disease |
| **X-Linked Recessive Inherited Conditions** | |
| Vertical transmission in families | Duchenne muscular dystrophy |
| Males predominantly affected | Hemophilia A and B |
| | Wiscott-Aldrich syndrome |
| | Protan and Deutran forms of color blindness |
| **Multifactorial Inherited Conditions** | |
| Occur as a result of combination of genetic and environmental factors | Congenital heart defects |
| | Cleft lip and/or palate |
| May recur in families | Neural tube defects (anencephaly and spina bifida) |
| Inheritance pattern does not demonstrate characteristic pattern of inheritance seen with other mendelian conditions | Diabetes mellitus |
| | Osteoarthritis |
| | High blood pressure |

Adapted from Lea, D. H., Jenkins, J. F., & Francomano, C. A. (1998). *Genetics in clinical practice: New directions for nursing and health care.* Sudbury, MA: Jones & Bartlett; Lea, D. H. (2002). Genetics. In Maher, A. B., Salmond, S. W., & Pellino, T. A. (Eds.) *Orthopaedic nursing.* Philadelphia: W. B. Saunders.

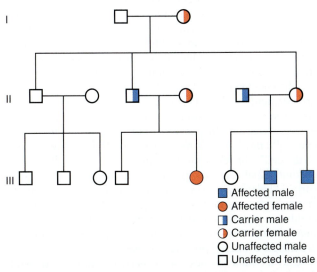

**FIGURE 9-8.** Three-generation pedigree illustrating autosomal recessive inheritance.

and traits do not follow these simple patterns. A variety of factors influence how a gene performs and is expressed. Different mutations in the same gene can produce variable symptoms in different people, as in cystic fibrosis. Different mutations in several genes can lead to identical outcomes, as in Alzheimer disease. Some traits involve simultaneous mutation in two or more genes. A recently observed phenomenon, imprinting, can determine which of a pair of genes (the mother's or the father's) is silenced or activated. This form of inheritance has been observed in Angelman syndrome, a severe form of mental retardation and ataxia (Nussbaum, McGinnis & Willard, 2001).

## Multifactorial Inheritance and Complex Genetic Conditions

Many birth defects and common health conditions such as heart disease, high blood pressure, cancer, osteoarthritis, and diabetes occur as a result of interactions of multiple gene mutations and environmental influences. Thus, they are called multifactorial or complex conditions (see Table 9-1). Other examples of multifactorial genetic conditions include

**FIGURE 9-9.** In diseases associated with altered recessive genes, both parents—although disease-free themselves—carry one normal allele and one altered allele. Each child has one chance in four of inheriting two abnormal alleles and developing the disorder; one chance in four of inheriting two normal alleles; and two chances in four of inheriting one normal and one altered allele, and therefore being a carrier like both parents.

neural tube defects such as spina bifida and anencephaly. Multifactorial conditions may cluster in families, but they do not always result in the characteristic pattern of inheritance seen in families who have mendelian inherited conditions (Fig. 9-11).

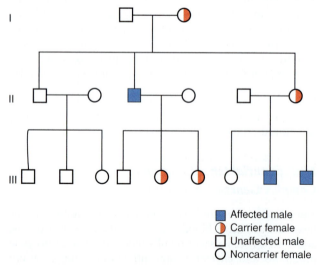

■ Affected male
◐ Carrier female
□ Unaffected male
○ Noncarrier female

**FIGURE 9-10.** Three-generation pedigree illustrating X-linked recessive inheritance.

□ Unaffected male
○ Unaffected female
■ Affected male

**FIGURE 9-11.** Three-generation pedigree illustrating multifactorial conditions.

## Chromosomal Differences and Genetic Conditions

Differences in the number or structure of chromosomes are a major cause of birth defects, mental retardation, and malignancies. Chromosomal differences are present in approximately 1 of every 160 liveborn infants and are the cause of greater than 50% of all spontaneous first-trimester pregnancy losses (Rimoin et al., 2002). Chromosomal differences most commonly involve an extra or missing chromosome; this is called aneuploidy. Whenever there is an extra or missing chromosome, there is always associated mental or physical disability to some degree.

Down syndrome, or trisomy 21, is a common chromosomal condition that occurs with greater frequency in pregnancies of women who are 35 years of age or older. A person who has trisomy 21 Down syndrome has a complete extra chromosome 21, which causes a particular facial appearance and increased risk for congenital heart defects, thyroid and vision problems, and mental retardation. Other examples of chromosomal differences include trisomy 13 and trisomy 18, both more severe than Down syndrome, and conditions involving extra or missing sex chromosomes, such as Turner syndrome, in which a female has only one X chromosome instead of the usual two (Rimoin et al., 2002).

Chromosomal differences may also involve a structural rearrangement within or between chromosomes. These are less common than chromosomal conditions in which there is an extra or missing chromosome, but they still occur in 1 of every 500 newborns (Rimoin et al., 2002). People who carry "balanced" chromosome rearrangements have all of their chromosomal material, but it is rearranged. Women who carry a "balanced" chromosomal rearrangement have an increased risk for spontaneous pregnancy loss and for having children with an unbalanced chromosomal arrangement that may result in physical or mental disabilities. Known carriers are therefore offered prenatal counseling and testing.

Chromosome studies may be needed at any age, depending on the indication. Two common indications are a suspected diagnosis such as Down syndrome and a history of two or more unexplained pregnancy losses. Chromosome studies are accomplished by obtaining a tissue sample (eg, blood, skin, amniotic fluid), preparing and staining the chromosomes, and analyzing them under a microscope. The microscopic study of chromosomes, called cytogenetics, is an area that is rapidly evolving. Today, cytogenetics is used with new molecular techniques such as fluorescent in situ hybridization (FISH), which permits more detailed examination of chromosomes. FISH is useful to detect small abnormalities and to characterize chromosomal rearrangements (Rimoin et al., 2002).

# Clinical Applications of Genetics

One of the most immediate applications of new genetic discoveries is the development of genetic tests that can be used to detect a trait, diagnose a genetic condition, and identify people who have a genetic predisposition to a disease such as cancer or heart disease. Another emerging application is pharmacogenetics, which involves the use of genetic testing to identify genetic variations that relate to the safety and efficacy of medications and gene-based treatments, so that individualized treatment and management plans can be developed. Future applications may include the use of gene chips to map a person's individual genome for genetic variations that may lead to disease. Nurses will be involved in caring for patients who are undergoing genetic testing and gene-based treatments. Knowledge of the clinical applications of modern genetic technologies will prepare nurses to inform and support patients and to provide high-quality genetics-related health care.

## Genetic Testing

Genetic tests provide information leading to the diagnosis of inherited conditions or other conditions with a known genetic contribution. Genetic testing involves the use of specific laboratory analyses of chromosomes, genes, or gene products (eg, enzymes, proteins) to learn whether a genetic alteration related to a specific disease or condition is present. This testing may be DNA-based, chromosomal, or biochemical.

Genetic testing can be used for a variety of purposes in prenatal, pediatric, and adult populations (Burke, 2004). Prenatal testing is widely used for **prenatal screening** and diagnosis of such conditions as Down syndrome. Carrier testing is used to determine carrier status—that is, to discover whether a person carries a recessive allele for an inherited condition (eg, cystic fibrosis, sickle cell anemia, Tay-Sachs disease) and therefore risks passing it on to his or her children. Genetic testing is also used widely in newborn screening. In the United States, it is made available for an increasing number of genetic conditions (eg, PKU, galactosemia). Diagnostic testing is used to detect the presence or absence of a particular genetic alteration or allele to identify or confirm a diagnosis of a disease or condition (eg, myotonic dystrophy, fragile X syndrome). Increasingly, genetic tests are being used to predict drug response and to design specific and individualized treatment and management plans. For example, genetic testing is used to identify specific gene variants that can predict therapeutic success of treatments

for human immunodeficiency virus (HIV) infection and the use of tacrine for Alzheimer disease (Weinshilboum, 2004). Examples of current uses of genetic tests are shown in Table 9-2.

Nurses are increasingly participating in genetic testing, especially in the area of patient education. In addition, they contribute by ensuring informed health choices and consent, advocating for privacy and confidentiality with regard to genetic test results, and helping patients understand the complex issues involved (Lea & Williams, 2002).

## Genetic Screening

Genetic screening, in contrast to genetic testing, is a broader concept and applies to testing of populations or groups independent of a positive family history or symptom manifestation. Genetic screening, as defined in 1975 by the Committee for the Study of Inborn Errors of Metabolism of the National Academy of Sciences (Secretary's Advisory Committee on Genetic Testing, 2000), has several major aims. The first aim is to improve management—that is, to identify people with treatable genetic conditions that could prove dangerous to their health if left untreated. For example, newborns are screened for an increasing number of conditions, including PKU, congenital hypothyroidism, and galactosemia. The second aim is to provide reproductive options to people with a high probability of having children with severe, untreatable diseases and for whom genetic counseling, prenatal diagnosis, and other reproductive options could be helpful and of interest. For example, people of Ashkenazi Jewish descent are screened for conditions such as Tay-Sachs disease and Canavan disease. The third aim is to screen pregnant women using multiple marker screening to detect birth defects such as neural tube defects and Down syndrome. Genetic screening may also be used for public health purposes to determine the incidence and prevalence of a birth defect or to investigate the feasibility and value of new genetic testing methods.

Most commonly, genetic screening occurs in prenatal and newborn programs that involve nurses in various roles and settings. In the future, population-based (widespread) genetic screening will be used to help identify people who are predisposed to conditions such as breast and colon cancer, diabetes, and heart disease. Nurses will be expected to participate in explaining risk and genetic predisposition, supporting informed health decisions and opportunities for prevention and early intervention, and protecting patients' privacy (Lea & Williams, 2002). Table 9-3 gives examples of genetic screening.

## Testing and Screening for Adult-Onset Conditions

Adult-onset conditions are disorders with a genetic basis that are manifested in later life. Often clinical signs or symptoms occur only in late adolescence or adulthood, and disease is clearly observed to run in families. Some of these conditions are attributed to specific genetic mutations and follow either an autosomal dominant or an autosomal recessive inheritance pattern. However, the majority of adult-onset condi-

## TABLE 9-2    Genetic Tests: Examples of Current Uses

| Purpose of Genetic Test | Type of Genetic Test |
|---|---|
| **Carrier Testing** | |
| Cystic fibrosis | DNA analysis |
| Tay-Sachs disease | Hexosaminidase A activity testing and DNA analysis |
| Canavan disease | DNA analysis |
| Sickle cell anemia | Hemoglobin electrophoresis |
| Thalassemia | Complete blood count and hemoglobin electrophoresis |
| **Prenatal Diagnosis**—amniocentesis is often performed when there is a risk for a chromosomal or genetic disorder: | |
| Risk for Down syndrome | Chromosomal analysis |
| Risk for cystic fibrosis | DNA analysis |
| Risk for Tay-Sachs disease | Hexosaminidase A activity testing and/or DNA analysis |
| Risk for open neural tube defect | Protein analysis |
| **Diagnosis** | |
| Down syndrome | Chromosomal analysis |
| Fragile X syndrome | DNA analysis |
| Myotonic dystrophy | DNA analysis |
| **Presymptomatic Testing** | |
| Huntington disease | DNA analysis |
| Myotonic dystrophy | DNA analysis |
| **Susceptibility Testing** | |
| Hereditary breast/ovarian cancer | DNA analysis |
| Hereditary non-polyposis colorectal cancer | DNA analysis |

tions are considered to be multifactorial (polygenetic); examples include heart disease, diabetes, and arthritis. Multifactorial influences involve the interactions among several genes (gene–gene interaction) and between genes and the environment (gene–environment interactions) (Guttmacher & Collins, 2004).

Nursing assessment for adult-onset conditions is based on family history, personal and medical risk factors, and identification of associated diseases or clinical manifestations. Knowledge of adult-onset conditions and their genetic bases (ie, mendelian versus multifactorial conditions) influences the nursing considerations for genetic testing and health promotion. Table 9-4 describes selected adult-onset conditions, their age of onset, pattern of inheritance, and risk factors, both genetic and environmental.

If a single gene accounts for an adult-onset condition in a symptomatic person, diagnostic testing is used to confirm a diagnosis to assist in the plan of care and management. Diagnostic testing for adult-onset conditions is most frequently used with autosomal dominant conditions, such

## TABLE 9-3    Applications for Genetic Screening

| Timing of Screening | Purpose | Examples |
|---|---|---|
| Preconception screening | For autosomal recessive inherited genetic conditions that occur with greater frequency among individuals of certain ethnic groups | Cystic fibrosis—all couples, but especially Northern European Caucasian, and Ashkenazi Jewish<br>Tay-Sachs disease—Ashkenazi Jewish<br>Sickle cell anemia—African American, Puerto Rican, Mediterranean, Middle Eastern<br>Alpha-thalassemia—Southeast Asian, African American |
| Prenatal screening | For genetic conditions that are common and for which prenatal diagnosis is available when a pregnancy is identified at increased risk | Neural tube defects—spina bifida, anencephaly<br>Down syndrome<br>Other chromosomal abnormalities—trisomy 18 |
| Newborn screening | For genetic conditions for which there is specific treatment | Phenylketonuria (PKU)<br>Galactosemia<br>Homocystinuria<br>Biotinidase deficiency |

## TABLE 9-4  Adult-Onset Disorders

| Clinical Description | Age of Onset (y) | Inheritance | Risk Factors |
|---|---|---|---|
| **Neurologic Conditions** | | | |
| **Early-Onset Familial Alzheimer Disease** | | | |
| Progressive dementia, memory failure, personality disturbance, loss of intellectual functioning associated with cerebral cortical atrophy, beta-amyloid plaque formation, intra-neuronal neurofibrillary tangles | <60–65 and often before 55 | A.D. <2% | Mutations on preslin 1, preslin 2 and/or beta-amyloid precursor protein<br>Carriers of apolipoprotein E4 |
| **Late-Onset Familial Alzheimer Disease** | | | |
| Progressive dementia, cognitive decline | >60–65 | A.D. ~25%<br>M.F. ~75% | Gene–gene interactions<br>Diabetes<br>Hypercholesterolemia<br>Cerebrovascular or cardiovascular disease |
| **Huntington Disease** | | | |
| Widespread degenerative brain change with progressive motor loss, both voluntary and involuntary disability, cognitive decline, chorea (involuntary movements) at later stage, psychiatric disturbances | 35–44 (mean) | A.D. 100% | HD gene |
| **Hematologic Conditions** | | | |
| **Hereditary Hemochromatosis (HHC)** | | | |
| High absorption of iron by gastrointestinal mucosa, resulting in excessive iron storage in liver, skin, pancreas, heart, joints, and testes<br>Early symptoms of abdominal pain, weakness, lethargy, weight loss<br>Possible pigmentation, diabetes mellitus, hepatic fibrosis or cirrhosis, heart failure, and arrhythmias or arthritis in untreated people | 40–60 in males; after menopause in females | A.R. ~60–90%<br>M.F. ~10–30% | Carrier or sibling of carrier of HFE gene mutations<br>Liver disease such as alcoholic liver disease, acute viral hepatitis, or chronic hepatitis C<br>Iron overload resulting from ingested iron in foods, cookware, and medicines, as well as parenteral iron from iron injections or transfusions for a chronic anemia such as beta-thalassemia or sickle cell disease |
| **Factor V Leiden Thrombophilia** | | | |
| Poor anticoagulant response to activated protein C with increased risk for venous thrombosis and risk for increased fetal loss during pregnancy | 30s; during pregnancy in females | A.D. | Carriers or relatives of individuals known to have factor V Leiden mutations<br>Families with high rates of venous thromboembolism, deep venous thrombosis, or pulmonary embolism, especially if age <50 y<br>Women with recurrent pregnancy loss or venous thromboembolism during pregnancy or who use oral contraceptives |
| **Diabetes Mellitus Type 2** | | | |
| Insulin resistance, impaired glucose tolerance | Variable onset; most often >30 | M.F. | Gene–gene interactions<br>Obesity<br>Hypertension<br>Hyperlipidemia<br>High intake of refined carbohydrates |

*continued >*

## TABLE 9-4  Adult-Onset Disorders (Continued)

| Clinical Description | Age of Onset (y) | Inheritance | Risk Factors |
|---|---|---|---|
| **Cardiovascular Disease** | | | |
| Familial hypercholesterolemia<br>Elevated LDL levels leading to coronary artery disease, xanthomas, and corneal arcus | 35–50 | A.D. | Family or personal history of coronary heart disease at <45 y in women or <40 y in men<br>Elevated LDL |
| **Oncology Conditions** | | | |
| *Multiple Endocrine Neoplasia* | | | |
| Familial medullary thyroid cancer, pheochromocytoma, and parathyroid abnormalities | Early adulthood;<br>40–50 y | A.D. | Carrier or relative of carrier of a *RET* mutation<br>Family history of medullary thyroid cancer, pheochromocytoma, and parathyroid abnormalities |
| *Breast Cancer* | | | |
| BRCA1 and BRCA2 hereditary breast/ovarian cancer<br>Breast, ovarian, and prostate (BRCA1)<br>Breast, ovarian, and other cancer (BRCA2) | 30–70; often <50 | A.D. ~5–10% of breast and ovarian cancers<br>M.F. >75% | Mutations in BRCA1, BRCA2<br>Older age<br>Early menses (<11 y)<br>Nulliparity<br>Family history<br>Breast biopsies |
| *Hereditary Non-polyposis Colorectal Cancer (HNPCC)* | | | |
| Colorectal, ovarian, endometrial, bladder, gastric, biliary, and renal cell cancers | <50 | A.D. ~1–3% of colorectal colon cancer; ~1% of endometrial cancers<br>M.F. >75% | Mutations in family of repair genes<br>Older age<br>Personal or family history of colon cancer or adenomas<br>High-fat, low-fiber diet<br>Inflammatory bowel disease |

A.D., autosomal dominant; A.R., autosomal recessive; LDL, low-density lipoprotein; M.F., multifactorial.

From Brandi, M. L., Gagel, R. F., Angeli, A., et al. (2001). Guidelines for diagnosis and therapy of MEN type 1 and type 2. *Journal of Clinical Endocrinology and Metabolism, 86*:5658–5671; Burt, M. J., George, P. M., Upton, J. D., et al. (1998). The significance of haemochromatosis gene mutations in the general population: Implications for screening. *Gut, 43*, 830–836; Campion, D., Dumanchin, C., Hannequin, D., et al. (1999). Early-onset autosomal dominant Alzheimer disease: prevalence, genetic heterogeneity, and mutation spectrum. *American Journal of Human Genetics, 65*(3), 664–670; Colditz, G. A., Rosner, B. A. & Speizer, F. E. (1996). Risk factors for breast cancer according to family history of breast cancer. For the Nurses' Health Study Research Group. *Journal of the National Cancer Institute, 88*(6), 365–371; Cunningham, J. M., Kim, C. Y., Christensen, E. R., et al. (2001). The frequency of hereditary defective mismatch repair in a prospective series of unselected colorectal carcinomas. *American Journal of Human Genetics, 69*, 780–790; Grody, W. W., Griffin, J. H., Taylor, A. K., et al. (2001). American College of Medical Genetics Consensus statement on factor V Leiden mutation testing. *Genetics in Medicine, 3*(2), 139–148.

as Huntington disease or factor V Leiden thrombophilia, and with autosomal recessive conditions such as hemochromatosis. In families with known adult-onset conditions or with a confirmed genetic mutation in an affected family member, **presymptomatic testing** provides asymptomatic people with information about the presence of a genetic mutation and about the likelihood of developing the disease. Huntington disease has served as the model for presymptomatic testing because the presence of the genetic mutation predicts disease onset and progression. Although preventive measures are not yet available for Huntington disease, the genetics information enables health care providers to develop a clinical, supportive, and psychological plan of care. Presymptomatic testing is considered for people in families with a known adult-onset condition in which either a positive or a negative test result indicates an increased or reduced risk for developing the disease, affects medical management, or allows earlier treatment of a condition.

The foremost factor that may influence the development and severity of disease is a person's genetic makeup. However, in the absence of a single disease-causing gene, it is thought that multiple genes and other environmental factors are related to the onset of most adult diseases. For some diseases, the interactions among several genes and other environmental or metabolic events affect disease onset and progression. Specific gene–gene interactions or SNPs can confer susceptibility to disease. Most susceptibility testing is conducted in the research setting to identify candidate genes for diseases such as Alzheimer disease, psychiatric conditions, heart disease, hypertension, and hypercholesterolemia. Susceptibility testing helps distinguish variations within the same disease or response to treatment. For example, no single gene is associated with osteoporosis. Several polymorphisms on candidate genes related to the vitamin D receptor, estrogen and androgen receptors, and cytokine production and its associated stimulation of osteoclasts are under study to predict bone mineral density and fracture risk (Ralston, 2004). Some susceptibility genes may predict treatment response. For example, people may present with similar clinical signs and symptoms of asthma but have different responses to treatment. Susceptibility testing helps classify people with asthma as sensitive or resistant to treatment with corticosteroids (Cookson, 2002).

**Population screening**, the use of genetic testing for large groups or whole populations, to identify late-onset conditions is under development. For a test to be considered for population screening, there must be (1) sufficient information about gene distribution within populations, (2) accurate prediction about the development and progression of disease, and (3) appropriate medical management for asymptomatic people with a mutation (Burke, Coughlin, Lee, et al., 2001). Currently, population screening is offered in some ethnic groups to identify cancer-predisposing genes. For example, Ashkenazi Jews (Jews of Eastern European origin) have a greater chance of having a specific genetic mutation in the BRCA1 or BRCA2 gene. People with one of these BRCA mutations have approximately an 80% risk for breast cancer, a 40% to 65% risk for ovarian cancer (BRCA1 carriers), a 20% risk for ovarian cancer (BRCA2 carriers) (King, Marks, Mandell, et al., 2003), and a 16% risk for prostate cancer (Kirchhoff, Kauff, Mitra, et al., 2004). The identification of one of these mutations gives patients options for cancer screening as well as chemoprevention or prophylactic mastectomy or oophorectomy in carriers. Population screening is being explored for other adult-onset conditions such as type 2 diabetes and hereditary hemochromatosis (iron overload disorder).

Nurses must be alert for family histories indicating that multiple generations (autosomal dominant inheritance) or multiple siblings (autosomal recessive inheritance) are affected with the same condition or that onset of disease is earlier than expected (eg, multiple generations with early-onset hyperlipidemia). Possible adult-onset conditions are discussed with other members of the health care team for appropriate resources and referral. When a family history of disease is identified, the nurse must be responsible for making the patient aware that this is a risk factor for disease. Regardless of whether a particular patient pursues a genetic testing workup, risk information for the disease should be explained. For example, if a 45-year-old woman presents for her annual gynecology visit and has a family history showing colon cancer in multiple paternal relatives, including her father, the nurse discusses the family history with the gynecologist. In addition, the woman is alerted to the risk for colon cancer based on the family history, and she is given information about possible genetic testing and referral for a colonoscopy.

If the existence of a mutation for an adult-onset condition in a family is identified, at-risk family members can be referred for **predisposition testing**. If the patient is found to be a carrier of the mutation, the nurse provides him or her with information about the risk to other family members. In that discussion, the nurse assures the patient that the test results are private and confidential and will not be shared with others, including family members, without the patient's permission. If the patient is an unaffected family member, the nurse discusses inheritance and the risk for developing the disease, provides support for the decision-making process, and offers referral for genetics services.

## Individualizing Genetic Profiles and Pharmacogenetics

Information about genes and their variations is helping researchers identify genetic differences that predispose certain people or groups to disease and affect their responses to treatment. The use of individualized genetics data to predict predisposition to common diseases will take considerable time to develop. Genetic tests that identify the role of genetic variations in drug response are currently under study. Drug metabolism involves genetically controlled enzyme activity for absorption, distribution, drug–cell interaction, inactivation, and excretion. Polymorphisms (genetic variations in populations) most often affect enzyme activity in the drug metabolism pathways. Pharmacogenetics, the study of the role of genetic variation in drug response and toxicity, involves methods that rapidly identify which genetic variations influence a drug's effect (Goetz, Ames, & Weinshilboum, 2004).

Variations in genes activated for enzyme activity can cause either decreased or increased drug metabolism. Genetic testing for these variations is providing a genetic profile, classifying patients according to their drug metabolism. Four classes of metabolic variations have been identified: (1) poor metabolizers, who lack enzyme function; (2) intermediate metabolizers, who have reduced enzyme activity; (3) extensive metabolizers, who have normal or expected enzyme activity; and (4) ultrarapid metabolizers, who have increased enzyme activity. The cytochrome P450 (CYP) family of enzymes has long been known for its involvement in drug metabolism. Three CYP enzymes—CYP2C9, CYP2C19, and CYP2D6—are active in about 40% of CYP-mediated drug responses (Ingelman-Sundberg, 2004). People with genetic variations in these enzymes are more likely to experience adverse drug reactions or poor response. Table 9-5 shows examples of differences in drug response for poor versus ultrarapid metabolizers. Reduced enzyme activity in poor metabolizers results in higher blood levels of active drug, predisposing them to adverse drug reactions. Ultrarapid metabolizers have increased enzyme activity with rapid breakdown and excretion of drug compounds, which results in lower blood levels of active drug and poor treatment response.

Nurses have traditionally monitored and reported drug response and drug adverse effects. In the near future, pharmacogenetic testing for CYP activity will give patients more

### TABLE 9-5 Clinical Effects of Cytochrome P450 Enzyme Variations

| Enzyme | Drug | Effects | |
|---|---|---|---|
| | | Poor metabolizer | Ultrarapid metabolizer |
| CYP2C9 | Warfarin | Bleeding | Longer treatment time to achieve stable dosing |
| | Phenytoin | Ataxia | |
| | Tolbutamide | Hypoglycemia | |
| CYP2C19 | Diazepam | Sedation | Poor response |
| CYP2D6 | Tricyclic antidepressants | Cardiotoxicity | No response to recommended dose; need 10-fold increase in dose |
| | Selective serotonin reuptake inhibitors | Nausea | |
| | Antipsychotics | Parkinson-like effects | Longer treatment time and higher drug costs |

From Ingelman-Sundberg, M. (2004). Pharmacogenetics of cytochrome P450 and its applications in drug therapy: The past, present and future. *Trends in Pharmacological Science, 25*(4), 193–200.

information about drug dosage, time to achieve response, and risk for adverse effects. Nurses will be expected to provide education about a particular patient's profile for drug metabolism and explain the rationale for the recommended dosage and likelihood of adverse effects. Although genetic profiles will add to individualized drug treatment plans, nurses will continue to incorporate information about gender differences, food interactions, and drug compliance into patient education (Nicol, 2003; Prows & Prows, 2004).

## Applications of Genetics in Nursing Practice

Nurses in genetics-related health care blend the principles of human genetics with nursing care in collaboration with other professionals, including genetic specialists, to foster improvement, maintenance, and restoration of patients' health. In all nursing practice settings, nurses have five main tasks: (1) help collect and interpret relevant family and medical histories, (2) identify patients and families who need further genetics evaluation and counseling and refer them to appropriate genetics services, (3) offer genetics information and resources to patients and families, (4) collaborate with genetics specialists, and (5) participate in the management and coordination of care of patients with genetic conditions. Genetics-related nursing practice involves the care of people who have genetic conditions, those who may be predisposed to develop or pass on genetic conditions, and those who are seeking genetics information and referral for additional genetics services (Jenkins & Lea, 2004).

Nurses support patients and families with genetics-related health concerns by ensuring that their health choices are informed ones and by advocating for the privacy and confidentiality of genetics information and for equal access to genetic testing and treatments. *The Scope and Standards of Genetics Clinical Nursing Practice,* developed by the International Society of Nurses in Genetics (ISONG, 1998) and published by the American Nurses Association, delineates roles and responsibilities for nurses in providing genetics-related health care.

## Genetics and Health Assessment

Assessment of a person's genetics-related health status is an ongoing process. Nurses collect information that can help identify individuals and families who have actual or potential genetics-related health concerns or who may benefit from further genetics information, counseling, testing, and treatment. This process can begin before conception and continue throughout the lifespan. Nurses evaluate family and past medical histories, including prenatal history, childhood illnesses, developmental history, adult-onset conditions (in adults), past surgeries, treatments, and medications; this information may relate to the genetic condition at hand or to a condition being considered. (See Chapter 5 for more information on assessing past medical history.) Nurses also identify the patient's ethnic background and conduct a physical assessment to gather pertinent genetics information. The assessment also includes information about culture, spiritual beliefs, and ancestry. Genetics-related health assessment always includes determining a patient's or family's understanding of actual or potential genetics-related health concerns and awareness of how these issues are communicated within a family (ISONG, 1998; Jenkins & Lea, 2004; Williams & Lea, 2003).

### Family History Assessment

Nurses in any practice setting continuously assess families' genetics histories to identify the presence of a genetic trait, inherited condition, or predisposition. Targeted questions are used to identify genetic conditions for which further information, education, testing, or treatment can be offered (Chart 9-2). In consultation and collaboration with other health care providers and specialists, nurses can then determine whether further genetic testing and evaluation should be offered for the trait or condition in question. A well-documented family history is a tool used by the health care team to make a diagnosis, identify testing strategies, and establish a pattern of inheritance. The family history should include at least three generations, as well as information about the current and past health status of all family members, including the age at onset of any illnesses, cause of death, and age at death. Nurses also inquire about medical conditions that are known to have a heritable com-

## CHART 9-2

### Genetics Family History: An Essential Tool for All Nurses

A well-documented family history is a tool for
- Making a medical diagnosis
- Deciding on testing strategies
- Establishing pattern of inheritance
- Identifying family members at increased risk
- Calculating risks
- Determining reproductive options
- Distinguishing genetic from other risk factors
- Making decisions about management or surveillance
- Developing patient rapport
- Educating patients

Key questions to ask about each family member include
- What is the current age or what was the age at death?
- What is the ethnic background (some genetic conditions are more common in certain ethnic groups)?
- Is there a history of
  - multiple pregnancy losses/stillbirths?
  - unexplained infertility?
  - birth defects?
  - medical problems in children whose parents are closely related (second cousins or closer)?
  - developmental delay/mental retardation?
  - learning disabilities or behavioral problems?
  - congenital or juvenile blindness, cataracts, hearing loss/deafness?
  - very short or very tall stature?
  - several close relatives with the same or related conditions (eg, breast cancer, colon cancer)?
  - occurrence of a common condition with earlier age at onset than is typical (eg, breast cancer, colon cancer, hearing loss, dementia, heart disease)?

From American Medical Association (2004). Family Medical History in Disease Prevention. Available at: www.ama-assn.org/ama/pub/category/2380.html (accessed March 3, 2006).

---

ponent and for which genetic testing may be available. Nurses obtain information about the presence of birth defects, mental retardation, familial traits, or similarly affected family members (Williams & Lea, 2003).

Nurses also consider the presence of genetic relatedness (consanguinity) among family members when assessing the risk for genetic conditions in couples or families. For example, when obtaining a preconception or prenatal family history, the nurse asks if the prospective parents have common ancestors (ie, are they first cousins?). This is important to know, because people who are related have more genes in common than those who are unrelated, thus increasing their chance for having children with an autosomal recessive inherited condition such as cystic fibrosis. The number of shared genes depends on the degree of relationship. For example, a parent and child share one half of their genes, whereas first cousins share one eighth of their genes. Ascertaining genetic relatedness gives nurses the opportunity to offer additional genetic counseling and evaluation. It may also serve as an explanation for parents who have a child with a rare autosomal recessive inherited condition or for a person who is similarly affected.

When the assessment of family history reveals that a patient has been adopted, genetics-based health assessment becomes more challenging. The nurse and the health care team should make all efforts to help the patient obtain as much information as possible about his or her biologic parents, including their ethnic backgrounds.

Questions regarding reproductive history (eg, history of miscarriage or stillbirth) are included in genetics family history health assessments to identify possible chromosomal conditions. Nurses also inquire about any history of family members with inherited conditions or birth defects; maternal health conditions such as type 1 diabetes, seizure disorders, or PKU, which may increase the risk for birth defects in children, and about exposure to alcohol or other drugs during pregnancy. Maternal age is also noted; women who are 35 years of age or older who are considering pregnancy and childbearing or who are already pregnant should be offered prenatal diagnosis (eg, testing through amniocentesis) because of the association between advanced maternal age and chromosomal abnormalities such as Down syndrome (Williams & Lea, 2003).

### Physical Assessment

Physical assessment may provide clues that a particular genetic condition is present in a person and family. Family history assessment may offer initial guidance regarding the particular area for physical assessment. For example, a family history of familial hypercholesterolemia would alert the nurse to assess family members for symptoms of hyperlipidemias (xanthomas, corneal arcus, abdominal pain of unexplained origin). As another example, a family history of neurofibromatosis type 1, an inherited condition involving tumors of the central nervous system, would prompt the nurse to carry out a detailed assessment of closely related family members. Skin findings such as *café-au-lait* spots, axillary freckling, or tumors of the skin (neurofibromas) would warrant referral for further evaluation, including genetic evaluation and counseling (Lea & Smith, 2003).

If a genetic condition is suspected as a result of a family history or physical assessment, the nurse, in collaboration with the health care team, may initiate further discussion and evaluation. Providing genetics information, offering and discussing genetic tests, and suggesting a referral to a geneticist are part of the nurse's role (Chart 9-3).

### Ancestry, Cultural, Social, and Spiritual Assessment

When collecting and discussing genetics information, nurses assess the ancestry of patients and families, as well as their ethnic, cultural, social, and spiritual orientation. Assessment of ancestry and ethnicity helps identify individual patients and groups who could benefit from genetic testing for carrier identification, prenatal diagnosis, and

> **CHART 9-3**
>
> ## Indications for Making a Genetics Referral
>
> **PREPREGNANCY AND PRENATAL**
> - Maternal age of 35 years or greater at expected time of delivery
> - Previous child with a chromosome problem
> - Positive alpha-fetoprotein profile screening test
> - Previous child with a birth defect or family history of birth defects
> - Pregnancy history of two or more unexplained miscarriages
> - Maternal conditions such as diabetes, epilepsy, or alcoholism
> - Exposures to certain medications or drugs during pregnancy
> - Family history of mental retardation
>
> **PEDIATRIC**
> - Positive newborn screening test
> - One or more major birth defects
> - Unusual (dysmorphic) facial features
> - Developmental delay/mental retardation
> - Suspicion of a metabolic disorder
> - Unusually tall or short stature, or growth delays
> - Known chromosomal abnormality
>
> **ADULT**
> - Mental retardation without a known cause
> - Unexplained infertility or multiple pregnancy losses
> - A personal or family history of thrombotic events
> - Adult-onset conditions such as hemochromatosis, hearing loss, visual impairment
> - Family history of an adult-onset neurodegenerative disorder (eg, Huntington disease)
> - Features of a genetic condition such as neurofibromatosis (*café-au-lait* spots, neurofibromas on the skin), Marfan syndrome (unusually tall stature, dilation of the aortic root), others
>
> **CANCER HISTORY**
> - A personal or family history of cancer with a known or suspected inherited predisposition (eg, early-onset breast cancer, colon cancer, ovarian cancer, retinoblastoma)
> - Several family members affected by cancer
> - A family member with cancer at an unusually young age
> - A family member with an unusual type of cancer

susceptibility testing. For example, carrier testing for sickle cell anemia is routinely offered to people of African American descent, and carrier testing for Tay-Sachs disease and Canavan disease is offered to people of Ashkenazi Jewish descent. Professional organizations such as the American College of Obstetrics and Gynecology (ACOG) recommend that members of at-risk racial and ethnic populations be offered carrier testing (ACOG, 2001). ACOG and the American College of Medical Genetics (ACMG) recommend that all couples, particularly those of Northern European and Ashkenazi Jewish ancestry, be offered carrier screening for cystic fibrosis (ACOG, 2001). Ideally, carrier testing is offered before conception to allow people who are carriers to make decisions about reproduction. Prenatal diagnosis is offered and discussed when both partners of a couple are found to be carriers.

It is also important to inquire about the patient's ethnic backgrounds when assessing for susceptibilities to adult-onset conditions such as hereditary breast or ovarian cancer. For example, a BRCA1 cancer-predisposing gene mutation seems to occur more frequently in women of Ashkenazi Jewish descent. Therefore, asking about ethnicity can help identify people with an increased risk for cancer gene mutations (American Medical Association, 2004).

The nurse also should consider the patient's views about the significance of a genetic condition and its effect on self-concept, as well as the patient's perception of the role of genetics in health and illness, reproduction, and disability. The patient's social and cultural backgrounds determine his or her interpretations and values about information obtained from genetic testing and evaluation and thus influence his or her perceptions of health, illness, and risk. Family structure and decision making and educational background contribute in the same way (Jenkins & Lea, 2004; Lea & Smith, 2003).

Assessment of the patient's beliefs, values, and expectations regarding genetic testing and genetics information helps the nurse provide appropriate information about the specific genetics topic. For example, in some cultures, people believe that health means the absence of symptoms and that the cause of illness is supernatural. Patients with these beliefs may initially reject suggestions for presymptomatic or carrier testing. However, by including resources such as family, cultural, and religious community leaders when providing genetics-related health care, nurses can help ensure that patients receive information in a way that transcends social, cultural, and economic barriers (Tranin, Masny & Jenkins, 2003).

### Psychosocial Assessment

Psychosocial assessment is an essential nursing component of the genetics health assessment (Chart 9-4). After conducting an initial psychosocial assessment, nurses become aware of the potential impact of new genetics information on the patient and family and how they may cope with this information.

## Genetic Counseling and Evaluation Services

People seek genetic counseling for a variety of reasons and at different stages of life. Some are seeking preconception or prenatal information, others are referred after the birth of a child with a birth defect or suspected genetic condition, and still others are seeking information for themselves or their families because of the presence of, or a family history

## CHART 9-4

### Assessing for Psychosocial Genetics Health

The nurse assesses:
- Educational level and understanding of the genetic condition or concern in the family.
- Desired goals and health outcomes in relation to genetic condition or concern.
- Family rules regarding disclosure of medical information (eg, some families may not reveal a history of diseases such as cancer or mental illness during the family history assessment).
- Family rules, boundaries, and cultural practices as well as personal preferences about knowing medical information.
- Past coping mechanisms and social support.
- Ability to make an informed decision (eg, is the patient under stress from family situations, acute or chronic illness, or medications that may impair the ability to make an informed decision)

---

of, a genetic condition. Regardless of the timing or setting, genetic counseling is offered to all people who have questions about genetics and their health. In collaboration with the health care team, nurses consider referral for genetic counseling for any patient who belongs to a family with a hereditary condition and who asks questions such as, "What are my chances for having this condition? Is there a genetic test that will tell me? Is there a gene-based treatment or cure? What are my options?" (Lea & Smith, 2003).

As the contribution of genetics to the health–illness continuum is recognized, the process of genetic counseling is expected to become a responsibility of all health care professionals in clinical practice. Nurses are obvious and natural providers of genetics services because they are often aware of the patient's personal and family history. Nurses assess the patient's health and make referrals for specialized diagnosis and treatment. They offer anticipatory guidance by explaining the purpose and goals of a referral. They collaborate with primary healthcare providers and specialists in giving supportive and follow-up counseling. They coordinate follow-up and case management.

### Genetics Services

Genetics services provide genetic information, education, and support to patients and families with genetics-related health concerns. Genetics professionals, including medical geneticists, genetics counselors, and advanced practice nurses in genetics, provide specific genetics services to patients and families who are referred by their primary health care providers. A team approach is often used by genetics specialists to obtain and interpret complex family history information, evaluate and diagnose genetic conditions, interpret and discuss complicated genetic test results, support patients throughout the evaluation process, and offer resources for additional professional and family support. Patients participate as team members and decision-makers throughout the process. Overall, genetics services are an evaluation and communication process by which patients and their families come to learn and understand relevant aspects of genetics, to make informed health decisions, and to receive support as they integrate personal and family genetics information into daily living (Tranin et al., 2003).

Genetic counseling may take place over an extended period and may entail more than one counseling session, which may include other family members. This allows patients and families to learn and understand genetics information, to receive support and guidance in decision-making, and to obtain comprehensive and coordinated care if they have specific genetic conditions or concerns. The components of genetic counseling are outlined in Chart 9-5. Although genetic counseling may be offered at any point during the lifespan, counseling issues are often relevant to the life stage in which counseling is sought. Some examples are presented in Chart 9-6 (Lea & Smith, 2003).

### Nursing Care and Interventions in Genetic Counseling

The process of genetic counseling and evaluation often involves additional genetic testing and procedures as well as decisions by patients and families with regard to reproduction, fertility, testing of children, and management options such as prophylactic surgery. Nurses have responsibilities in each of these areas for assessment and for providing psychosocial interventions and accurate information as family members consider their genetic testing and treatment options. In all of these areas, nurses consider individual patients in the context of the family.

When patients or family members are considering genetic testing, nurses provide accurate information as patients consider their options. For prenatal testing, this includes information and support for subsequent decisions regarding the pregnancy in the event of diagnosis of a genetic condition in the fetus. When a diagnosis such as Down syndrome or hereditary breast or ovarian cancer is made, families need information about the range and severity of potential problems, the proportion of people with milder aspects of the condition, management options, support organizations, and current understanding of the long-term prognosis (Williams & Lea, 2003).

Decision-making support is an important nursing intervention in many genetic counseling situations. Examples include consideration of pregnancy termination, presymptomatic testing for conditions such as Huntington disease, or predisposition testing for a hereditary cancer. Nurses help patients and families acquire information about options, identify the "pros" and "cons" of each option, and explore their values and beliefs. In addition, nurses help patients respect each person's right to receive or not to receive information and help them explain their decision to others (Dochterman & Bulechek, 2004).

Other essential components of nursing care and genetic counseling include teaching and an intervention known as "coping enhancement." For example, teaching is needed

## CHART 9-5 · Components of Genetic Counseling

**INFORMATION AND ASSESSMENT SOURCES**
- Reason for referral
- Family history
- Medical history/records
- Relevant test results and other medical evaluations
- Social and emotional concerns
- Relevant cultural, educational, and financial factors

**ANALYSIS OF DATA**
- Family history
- Physical examination as needed
- Additional laboratory testing and procedures (eg, echocardiogram, ophthalmology or neurologic examination)

**COMMUNICATION OF GENETIC FINDING**
- Natural history of disorder
- Pattern of inheritance
- Reproductive and family health issues and options
- Testing options
- Management and treatment issues

**COUNSELING AND SUPPORT**
- Identify individual and family questions and concerns
- Identify existing support systems
- Provide emotional and social support
- Refer for additional support and counseling as indicated

**FOLLOW-UP**
- Written summary to referring primary care providers and family
- Coordination of care with primary care providers and specialists
- Additional discussions of test results or diagnosis

From Lea, D. H., Jenkins, J. F., & Francomano, C. A. (1998). *Genetics in clinical practice: New directions for nursing and health care*. Sudbury, MA: Jones & Bartlett.

---

when a new genetics diagnosis is made. Patients and families need information about the range of possible health outcomes, treatment options, and, in the case of prenatal diagnosis of a genetic condition, management options regarding continuing or ending the pregnancy. Coping enhancement involves helping people adapt to perceived stressors or changes that interfere with daily living and functioning (Dochterman & Bulechek, 2004). Coping enhancement is essential throughout the entire genetic counseling, evaluation, and testing process. Indicators of patient knowledge, decision making, and coping outcomes have been developed (Dochterman & Bulechek, 2004), and nurses can use these indicators when documenting nursing care provided to families and its effectiveness.

### Specific Nursing Roles in Genetic Counseling

Nurses refer patients, collaborate with genetics specialists, and participate in genetic counseling when they carry out the following activities:

- Provide appropriate genetics information before, during, and in follow-up to genetic counseling
- Help gather relevant family and medical history information
- Offer support to patients and families throughout the genetic counseling process
- Coordinate genetics-related health care with relevant community and national support resources

These activities are carried out in collaboration with patients and families and help ensure that they receive the most benefit from genetic counseling (Lea & Monsen, 2003).

### RESPECTING PATIENTS' RIGHTS

Respecting the patient's right to self-determination—that is, supporting decisions that reflect the patient's personal beliefs, values, and interests—is a central principle directing how nurses provide genetics information and counseling. Genetics specialists and nurses participating in genetic counseling make every attempt to respect the patient's ability to make autonomous decisions. A first step in providing such nondirective counseling is recognizing one's own values (see Chart 9-1) and how communication of genetics information may be influenced by those values.

Confidentiality of genetics information and respect for privacy are other essential principles underlying genetic counseling. Patients have the right to have testing without having the results divulged to anyone, including insurers or physicians. Some patients pay for testing themselves so that insurers will not learn of the test, and others use a different name for testing to protect their privacy. The Health Insurance Portability and Accountability Act (HIPAA) of 1996 prohibits the use of genetics information to establish insurance eligibility. However, HIPAA does not prohibit group plans from increasing premiums, excluding coverage for a specific condition, or imposing a lifetime cap on benefits. The National Human Genome Research Institute, Policy and Public Affairs and Legislative Activities Branch has a summary of each state's legislation on employment and insurance discrimination (see the resources list at the end of this chapter).

All genetics specialists, including nurses who participate in the genetic counseling process and those with access to people's genetics information, must honor a patient's desire for confidentiality. Genetics information should be kept from family members, insurance companies, employers,

## CHART 9-6

### Genetic Counseling Across the Lifespan

**PRENATAL ISSUES**
- Understanding prenatal screening and diagnosis testing
- Implications of reproductive choices
- Potential for anxiety and emotional distress
- Effects on partnership, family, and parental–fetal bonding

**NEWBORN ISSUES**
- Understanding newborn screening results
- Potential for disrupted parent–newborn relationship on diagnosis of a genetic condition
- Parental guilt
- Implications for siblings and other family members
- Coordination and continuity of care

**PEDIATRIC ISSUES**
- Caring for children with complex medical needs
- Coordination of care
- Potential for impaired parent–child relationship
- Potential for social stigmatization

**ADOLESCENT ISSUES**
- Potential for impaired self-image and decreased self-esteem
- Potential for altered perception of family
- Implications for lifestyle and family planning

**ADULT ISSUES**
- Potential for ambiguous test results
- Identification of a genetic susceptibility or diagnosis without an existing cure ("therapeutic gap")
- Effect on marriage, reproduction, parenting, and lifestyle
- Potential impact on insurability and employability

From Lea, D. H., Jenkins, J. F., & Francomano, C. A. (1998). *Genetics in clinical practice: New directions for nursing and health care.* Sudbury, MA: Jones & Bartlett.

---

and schools if the patient so desires, even if keeping the information confidential is difficult. A nurse may want to disclose genetics information to family members who could experience significant harm if they do not know such information. However, the patient may have other views and may wish to keep this information from the family, resulting in an ethical dilemma for both patient and nurse. The nurse must honor the patient's wishes, while explaining to the patient the potential benefit this information may have for other family members (ISONG, 2002).

### PROVIDING PRECOUNSELING INFORMATION

Preparing the patient and family, promoting informed decision making, and obtaining informed consent are essential in genetic counseling. Nurses assess the patient's capacity and ability to give voluntary consent. This includes assessment of factors that may interfere with informed consent, such as hearing loss, language differences, cognitive impairment, and the effects of medication. Nurses make sure that a person's decision to undergo testing is not affected by coercion, persuasion, or manipulation. Because information may need to be repeated over time, nurses offer follow-up discussion as needed (Tranin et al., 2003).

The genetics service to which a nurse refers a patient or family for genetic counseling will ask the nurse to provide background information for evaluation. Genetics specialists need to know the reason for referral, the patient's or family's reason for seeking genetic counseling, and potential genetics-related health concerns. For example, a nurse may refer a family with a new diagnosis of hereditary breast or ovarian cancer to obtain more information or counseling or to discuss the likelihood of developing the disease and the implications for other family members. The family may have concerns about confidentiality and privacy. Using the nursing assessment, the genetics specialist tailors the genetic counseling to respond to these concerns.

With the patient's permission, nurses may also provide genetics specialists with the relevant test results and medical evaluations. Nurses need to obtain permission from the patient and, if applicable, from other family members to retrieve, review, and transfer medical records that document the genetic condition of concern. In some situations, evaluation of more than one family member may be necessary to establish a diagnosis of a genetic disorder. Nurses can prepare the family for this assessment by explaining that the medical information and evaluation are necessary to ensure that appropriate information and counseling (including risk interpretation) are provided.

Nurses will be asked to provide information about the emotional and social status of the patient and family. Genetics specialists will want to know the coping skills of patients and families who have recently learned of the diagnosis of a genetic disorder and will want to know what type of genetics information is being sought. Nurses help identify cultural and other issues that may influence how information is provided and by whom. For example, for patients with hearing loss, a sign interpreter's services may have to be arranged. For those with vision loss, alternative forms of communication may be necessary. Genetics professionals prepare for the genetic counseling and evaluation with these relevant issues in mind (Lea & Smith, 2003).

### PREPARING PATIENTS FOR GENETICS EVALUATION

Before a genetic counseling appointment, the nurse discusses with the patient and family the type and nature of family history information that will be collected during the consultation. Family history collection and analysis are comprehensive and focus on information that may be relevant to the genetics-related concern in question. Although targeted to each genetic counseling situation, such analysis always includes assessment for any other potentially inherited conditions for which testing and preventive and treatment measures may be available.

A physical examination performed by the medical geneticist may be needed to identify specific clinical features that are diagnostic of a genetic condition. The examination also helps determine whether additional laboratory tests are needed to clarify the diagnosis of a genetic disorder. The detailed physical examination generally involves assessment of all body systems, with a focus on specific physical characteristics considered for diagnosis. The nurse describes the diagnostic evaluations that are part of a genetics consultation and explains their purposes (Lea & Smith, 2003).

### COMMUNICATING GENETICS INFORMATION TO PATIENTS

After the family history and physical examination are completed, the genetics team reviews the information gathered before beginning genetic counseling with the patient and family. The genetics specialists meet with the patient and family to discuss their findings. If information from family and medical histories and examination confirms the presence of a genetic condition in a family, genetics specialists discuss with the patient the natural history of the condition, the pattern of inheritance, and the implications of the condition for reproductive and general health. When appropriate, the specialists also discuss relevant testing and management options. The nurse assesses the patient's understanding of the genetics consultation and clarifies information given by specialists.

### PROVIDING SUPPORT

The genetics team provides support throughout the counseling session and makes every effort to elicit personal and family concerns. Genetics specialists use principles of active listening to interpret patient concerns and emotions, seek and provide feedback, and demonstrate understanding of those concerns. When necessary, genetics specialists suggest referral for additional social and emotional support. Genetics specialists discuss pertinent patient and family concerns and needs with nurses and primary health care teams so that they can provide additional support and guidance (Lea & Smith, 2003). The nurse assesses the patient's understanding of the information given during the counseling session, clarifies information, answers questions, assesses patient reactions, and identifies support systems.

### *Follow-Up After Genetic Evaluation*

As follow-up to genetic evaluation and counseling, genetics specialists prepare a written summary of the evaluation and counseling session and, with the patient's permission, send this summary to the primary health care provider as well as all other providers and participants in the patient's care, as identified by the family. The consultation summary outlines the results of the family history and physical and laboratory assessments, provides a discussion of the specific diagnosis (if made), reviews the inheritance and associated risk of recurrence for the patient and family, presents reproductive and general health options, and makes recommendations for further testing and management. The summary is also sent to the patient, and a copy is retained in the patient's medical records. The nurse plays an important role in reviewing the summary with the patient and family and identifying information, education, and counseling for which follow-up genetic counseling may be useful (Lea & Smith, 2003; Lea & Williams, 2002).

Follow-up genetic counseling is always offered to patients and families, because some people may need more time to understand and discuss the specifics of a genetic test or diagnosis, or they may wish to review reproductive options again later, when pregnancy is being considered. Follow-up genetic counseling is also offered to patients when further evaluation and counseling of extended family members is recommended (Lea & Smith, 2003).

As part of follow-up, nurses can educate patients about where to find information about genetics issues. Some resources that provide the most up-to-date and reliable genetics information are available on the Internet; several of these are listed at the end of this chapter.

## Ethical Issues

With the recent advances in genetics, nurses must consider their responsibilities in handling genetics information and potential ethical issues such as informed decision-making, privacy and confidentiality of genetics information, and access to and justice in health care. The ethical principles of autonomy, fidelity, and veracity are also important (American Nurses Association, 2001).

Ethical questions relating to genetics occur in various settings and at all levels of nursing practice. At the level of direct patient care, nurses participate in providing genetics information, testing, and gene-based therapeutics. They offer patient care based on the values of self-determination and personal autonomy. The American Nurses Association (2001) states that patients should be as fully involved as possible in the planning and implementation of their own health care. To do so, patients need appropriate, accurate, and complete information given at such a level and in such a form that they and their families can make well-informed personal, medical, and reproductive health decisions. Nurses, as the most accessible health care professionals, are invaluable in the informed consent process. They can help patients clarify values and goals, assess understanding of information, protect patients' rights, and support their decisions. Nurses can advocate for patient autonomy in health decisions. ISONG's position statements, "Informed Decision-Making and Consent" (2000) and "Genetic Counseling of Vulnerable Populations" (2002), support and guide nurses who help patients considering genetic counseling and testing. Other nursing societies have also issued position statements to guide nursing practice in genetic counseling and testing. Chart 9-7 provides a list of position statements of selected genetics professional societies.

Nurses need to ensure the privacy and confidentiality of genetics information derived from such sources as the family history, genetic tests, and other genetics-based interventions. Many Americans are increasingly concerned about threats to their personal privacy. Nurses must be aware of the potential ethical issues related to the privacy and confidentiality of genetics information, including conflicts between the patient's privacy and the family's need for genetics information. ISONG's position statement, "Privacy and Confidentiality of Genetic Information" (2005), is a useful resource.

An ethical foundation provides nurses with a holistic framework for handling ethical issues with integrity. It also supplies the basis for communicating genetics information

## CHART 9-7 Genetics Resources for Nurses

**INTERNATIONAL SOCIETY OF NURSES IN GENETICS, INC. (ISONG)**
Web site: www.isong.org
ISONG is an international nursing specialty organization dedicated to fostering the scientific and professional growth of nurses in human genetics. ISONG members represent the United States, Australia, Canada, England, Japan, Israel, Korea, Ireland, and New Zealand. Members practice in diverse health care settings, including reproductive, prenatal, pediatric, and adult settings. ISONG serves as a forum for education and support for nurses who provide genetics-related health care, and promotes integration of the nursing process into the delivery of genetics-related health care services. Major goals of ISONG are incorporation of the principles of human genetics into all levels of nursing education, promotion of the development of standards of practice for nurses in human genetics, and advancement of nursing research in human genetics.

Documents created by ISONG
- Scope and Standards of Genetics Clinical Nursing Practice (published in 1998 and currently being revised): developed, written, and published in conjunction with the American Nurses Association. This document delineates competencies expected for nurses practicing at the basic level, as well as enhanced competencies for nurses practicing at the advanced level.

Position statements (available on the Web site)
- Informed Decision-Making and Consent: The Role of Nursing (approved September 30, 2000; revised April 4, 2005)
- Privacy and Confidentiality of Genetic Information: The Role of the Nurse (approved August 8, 2005)
- Genetic Counseling for Vulnerable Populations: The Role of Nursing (approved October 10, 2002)
- Access to Genomic Healthcare: The Role of the Nurse (approved September 9, 2003).

**ONCOLOGY NURSING SOCIETY (ONS)**
Web site: www.ons.org
ONS is a professional organization of more than 30,000 registered nurses and other health care providers dedicated to excellence in patient care, education, research, and administration in oncology nursing. It is the largest professional oncology association in the world.

Position statements (available on the Web site)
- Cancer Predisposition Genetic Testing and Risk Assessment Counseling
- The Role of the Oncology Nurse in Cancer Genetic Counseling

Cancer genetics resources
- ONS Genetics Short Course for Cancer Nurses
- ONS Genetics and Cancer Care Tool Kit (available on the Web site)
- Internet Resources in Genetics for Cancer Nurses (includes evidence-based practice resource center available on the Web site)
- Tranin, A., Masny, A. & Jenkins, J. (2003). *Genetics in Oncology Practice: Cancer Risk Assessment.* PA: Oncology Nursing Press.

**ASSOCIATION OF WOMEN'S HEALTH AND NEONATAL NURSES (AWHONN)**
Web site: www.awhonn.org
AWHONN is the leading professional association for nurses who specialize in the care of women and newborns. Members include neonatal nurses, advanced practice nurses, women's health nurses, obstetrics/gynecology and labor and delivery nurses, nurse scientists, nurse executives and managers, childbirth educators, and nurse practitioners.

Position statements
- The Role of the Registered Nurse as Related to Genetic Testing (available on the Web site)

**AMERICAN NURSES ASSOCIATION (ANA)**
Web site: www.ana.org

*Online Journal of Issues in Nursing:* The Genetic Revolution: What, Why, How? (Available at: nursingworld.org/ojin/admin/topics.htm) (accessed March 3, 2006).

---

to a patient, a family, other care providers, community agencies and organizations, and society as a whole. In addition, it provides support for nurses facing clinical situations that involve ethical dilemmas. Principle-based ethics offers moral guidelines that nurses can use to justify their nursing practice. The emphasis is on ethical principles of beneficence (to do good) and nonmaleficence (to do no harm), as well as autonomy, justice, fidelity, and veracity, to help solve ethical dilemmas that may arise in clinical care. Respect for people is the ethical principle underlying all nursing care. Using an ethical foundation based on these principles that incorporates the values of caring, nurses can promote the kind of thoughtful discussions that are useful when patients and families are facing genetics-related health and reproductive decisions and consequences (ISONG, 2000; Tranin et al., 2003).

## Critical Thinking Exercises

1. A 42-year-old man has just been diagnosed with colon cancer. He tells you that he is not surprised, because his father died from colon cancer when he was 45 years of age, and he has a paternal aunt who died in her late 40s from colon cancer. A paternal uncle was treated for colon cancer when he was 39 years of age, and the patient's maternal grandmother died from uterine cancer. What pattern of inheritance is suggested in this family? What genetics information would you provide to this patient?

2. **ebp** A 28-year-old woman is admitted to the medical unit with deep venous thrombosis (DVT). Your nursing assessment reveals that she has had three miscarriages, and her only child was born prematurely due to placental problems. Her mother had DVT at 32 years of age when she was pregnant with your patient. A maternal uncle had a pulmonary embolism when he was 45 years of age. What adult-onset condition does this history suggest? What nursing actions would you take? What is the evidence base for the nursing actions that you have identified? Explain how you would determine the strength of the evidence.

3. A 45-year-old woman has been admitted to your nursing unit with a new diagnosis of type 2 diabetes mellitus. She has a history of obesity and hypertension. In obtaining her family history, you learn that her 50-year-old sister and 70-year-old mother also have type 2 diabetes mellitus. Your patient has three daughters, and her 15-year-old daughter has a history of obesity. Your patient tells you, "I was afraid that I would get the diabetes, and now I have. I am so worried about my daughters. What is causing this in our family? What can we do?" How might you respond to the patient? What are the counseling issues that are important for this family? What other clinical resources could you make available to them?

## REFERENCES AND SELECTED READINGS

### BOOKS

American College of Obstetricians and Gynecologists (ACOG). (2001). *Preconception and prenatal carrier screening for cystic fibrosis: Clinical and laboratory guidelines.* Washington, DC: Author.

American Medical Association. (2001). *Identifying and managing hereditary risk for breast and ovarian cancer.* Chicago: Author.

American Nurses Association. (2001). *Code for nurses with interpretive statements.* Washington, DC: Author.

Burke, W. (2004). Genetic testing. In Guttmacher, A. E., Collins F. S. & Drazen, J. M. (Eds). *Articles from the New England Journal of Medicine: Genomic medicine.* Baltimore, MD: The Johns Hopkins University Press.

Dochterman, J. M. & Bulechek, G. M. (Eds.). (2004). *Nursing interventions classification (NIC): Iowa Intervention Project* (4th ed.). St. Louis: C. V. Mosby.

Gardiner, R. R. M. & Sutherland, G. R. (1996). *Chromosome abnormalities and genetic counseling* (2nd ed.). New York: Oxford University Press.

Guttmacher, A. E. & Collins, F. S. (2004). Genomic medicine: A primer. In Guttmacher, A. E., Collins, F. S. & Drazen, J. M. (Eds.). *Articles from the New England Journal of Medicine: Genomic medicine.* Baltimore, MD: The Johns Hopkins University Press.

International Society of Nurses in Genetics (ISONG). (1998). *Statement on the scope and standards of genetics clinical nursing practice.* Washington, DC: American Nurses Association.

Jenkins, J. & Lea, D. H. (2004). *Nursing care in the genomic era: A case-based approach.* Sudbury, MA: Jones & Bartlett.

Lea, D. H. (2002). Genetics. In Maher, A. B., Salmond, S. W. & Pellino, T. A. (Eds.). *Orthopaedic nursing.* Philadelphia: W. B. Saunders.

Lea, D. H., Jenkins, J. F. & Francomano, C. A. (1998). *Genetics in clinical practice: New directions for nursing and health care.* Sudbury, MA: Jones & Bartlett.

Lea, D. H. & Smith, R. S. (2003). *The genetics resource guide: A handy reference for public health nurses.* Scarborough, ME: Foundation for Blood Research.

Moorhead, S., Johnson, M. & Maas, M. L. (Eds.). (2004). *Nursing interventions classification* (2nd ed.) St. Louis: C. V. Mosby.

NANDA International. (2005). *Nursing diagnoses: Definitions and classification 2005–2006* (5th ed.). Philadelphia: North American Nursing Diagnosis Association.

National Academy of Sciences, Committee for the Study of Inborn Errors of Metabolism. (1975). *Genetic screening.* Washington, DC: National Academy of Sciences.

National Institutes of Health, National Cancer Institute. (1995). *Understanding gene testing.* NIH Pub. No. 9603905. Washington, DC: U.S. Department of Health and Human Services.

Nussbaum, R. L., McInnes, R. R. & Willard, H. F. (2001). *Thompson and Thompson's genetics in medicine* (6th ed.). Philadelphia: W. B. Saunders.

Rimoin, D. L., Connor, M. J., Pyeritz, R. E., et al. (2002). *Emery and Rimoin's principles and practice of medical genetics* (4th ed.). London: Churchill Livingstone.

Roesser, K. A. & Mullineaux, L. G. (2005). *Genetic testing and hereditary cancer: Implications for nurses.* Pittsburgh, PA: Oncology Education Services.

Secretary's Advisory Committee on Genetic Testing (SACGT). (2000). *A public consultation of oversight of genetic tests.* Bethesda, MD: National Institutes of Health. Available at: www4.od.nih.gov/oba/sacgt.htm (accessed March 5, 2006).

Tranin, A. S., Masny, A. & Jenkins, J. (Eds.). (2003). *Genetics in oncology practice: Cancer risk assessment.* Pittsburgh, PA: Oncology Nursing Society.

U.S. Preventive Services Task Force. (2004). *Guide to clinical preventive services.* Baltimore: Williams & Wilkins.

Varmus, H. (2004). Getting ready for gene-based medicine. In Guttmacher, A. E., Collins, F. S. & Drazen, J. M. (Eds.). *Articles from the New England Journal of Medicine: Genomic medicine.* Baltimore, MD: The Johns Hopkins University Press.

Weinshilboum, R. (2004). Genomic medicine: Inheritance and drug response. In Guttmacher, A. E., Collins, F. S. & Drazen, J. M. (Eds.). *Articles from the New England Journal of Medicine: Genomic medicine.* Baltimore, MD: The Johns Hopkins University Press.

Williams, J. K. & Lea, D. H. (2003). *Genetic issues for perinatal nurses* (2nd ed.). White Plains, NY: March of Dimes.

### JOURNALS

American Academy of Pediatrics, Committee on Genetics. (1999). Folic acid for the prevention of neural tube defects. *Pediatrics, 104*(2 Pt 1), 325–327.

American College of Medical Genetics/American Society of Human Genetics Huntington Disease Genetic Testing Working Group. (1998). ACMG/ASHG statement: Laboratory guidelines for Huntington disease genetic testing. *American Journal of Human Genetics, 62*(5), 1243–1247.

American College of Obstetrics and Gynecology, Committee on Genetics. (1996). Screening for Tay-Sachs disease. *International Journal of Gynaecology and Obstetrics, 52*(3), 311–312.

American College of Obstetrics and Gynecology, Committee on Genetics. (1999). Screening for Canavan disease. *International Journal of Gynaecology and Obstetrics, 65*(1), 91–92.

American College of Obstetrics and Gynecology, Committee on Genetics. (2001). Genetic screening for hemoglobinopathies. *International Journal of Gynaecology and Obstetrics, 74*(3), 309–310.

American Medical Association (2004). *Family medical history in disease prevention.* Es26:03-503:25M:6/04. Available at: www.ama-assn.org/go/genetics (accessed March 5, 2006).

American Society of Clinical Oncology. (2003). Policy statement update: Genetic testing for cancer susceptibility. *Journal of Clinical Oncology, 21*(12), 2397–2406.

Anderson, G., Monsen, R. B., Prows, C. A., et al. (2000). Preparing the nursing profession for participation in a genetic paradigm in health care. *Nursing Outlook, 48*(1), 23–27.

Bartsch, H., Nair, U., Risch, A., et al. (2000). Genetic polymorphism of CYP genes, alone or in combination, as a risk modifier of tobacco-related cancers. *Cancer Epidemiology, Biomarkers and Prevention, 9*(1), 3–28.

Billings, P. R. (2000). Applying advances in genetic medicine: Where do we go from here? *Healthplan, 41*(6), 32–35.

Brookes, A. J. (1999). The essence of SNPs. *Gene, 234*(2), 177–186.

Burke, W., Coughlin, S. S., Lee, N. C., et al. (2001). Applications of population screening principles to genetic screening for adult-onset conditions. *Genetic Testing, 5*(3), 201–211.

Burke, W., Thomson, E., Khoury, M. J., et al. (1998). Hereditary hemochromatosis: Gene discovery and its implications for population-based screening. *Journal of American Medical Association, 280*(2), 172–178.

Cashion, A. (2002). Genetics in transplantation. *MedSurg Nursing 11*(2), 91–94.

Collins, F. S. (1999). Medical and societal consequences of the Human Genome Project. *New England Journal of Medicine, 341*(1), 28–37.

Collins, F. S., & McKusick, V. A. (2001). Implications of the Human Genome Project for medical science. *Journal of American Medical Association, 285*(5), 540–544.

Conley, Y. P. & Gorin, M. B. (2003). The genetics of age-related macular degeneration. *MedSurg Nursing 12*(4), 238–241, 259.

Cookson, W. O. (2002). Asthma genetics. *Chest, 121*(Suppl), 7S–13S.

Cox, N. J., Frigge, M., Nicolae, D. L., et al. (1999). Loci on chromosomes 2 (NIDDM1) and 15 interact to increase susceptibility to diabetes in Mexican Americans. *Nature Genetics, 21*(2), 213–215.

Enderlin, C., Vogel, R. & Conaway, P. (2003). Gaucher disease. *American Journal of Nursing 102*(12), 50–60.

Evans, W. E. & McLeod, H. L. (2003). Drug therapy: Pharmacogenomics—Drug disposition, drug targets, and side effects. *New England Journal of Medicine, 348*(6), 538–549.

Evans, W. E. & Relling, M. V. (1999). Pharmacogenomics: Translating functional genomics into rational therapeutics. *Science, 286*(5439), 487–491.

Feetham, S. (1999). Families and the genetic revolution: Implications for primary healthcare, education, and research. *Families, Systems and Health, 17*(1), 27–43.

FitzGerald, M. G., MacDonald, D. J., Krainer, M., et al. (1996). Germ-line BRCA1 mutations in Jewish and non-Jewish women with early-onset breast cancer. *New England Journal of Medicine, 334*(3), 143–149.

Fleisher, L. K. & Cole, J. (2001). Health Insurance Portability and Accountability Act is here: What price privacy? *Genetics in Medicine, 3*(4), 286–289.

Ghosh, S., Watanabe, R. M., Valle, T. T., et al. (2000). The Finland-United States Investigation of Non-insulin-dependent Diabetes Mellitus Genetics (FUSION) Study. I. An autosomal genome scan for genes that predispose to type 2 diabetes. *American Journal of Human Genetics, 67*(5), 1174–1185.

Glassford, B. (2003). A case study in caring: Trisomy 18 syndrome. *American Journal of Nursing 103*(7), 81–83.

Goetz, M. P., Ames, M. M., & Weinshilboum, R. M. (2004). Primer on medical genomics. Part XII. Pharmacogenomics—General principles with cancer as a model. *Mayo Clinic Proceedings, 79*(3), 376–384.

Greco, K. E. (2003). Nursing in the genomic era: Nurturing our genetic nature. *MedSurg Nursing, 12*(5), 307–312.

Hetteberg, C. & Prows, C. A. (2004). A checklist to assist in the integration of genetics into nursing curricula. *Nursing Outlook 52*(2), 85–88.

Horner, S. D., Abel, E., Taylor, K., et al. (2004). Using theory to guide the diffusion of genetics content in nursing curricula. *Nursing Outlook 52*(2), 80–84.

Houfek, J. F. & Atwood, J. R. (2003). Genetic susceptibility to lung cancer: Implications for smoking cessation. *MedSurg Nursing 12*(1), 45–49.

Ingelman-Sundberg, M. (2004). Pharmacogenetics of cytochrome P450 and its applications in drug therapy: The past, present and future. *Trends in Pharmacological Sciences, 25*(4), 193–200.

International Society of Nurses in Genetics (ISONG). (2000). Position statement. Informed decision-making and consent: The role of nursing. *International Society of Nurses in Genetics Newsletter, 11*(3), 7–8. Available at: www.isong.org/about/ps_consent.cfm (accessed March 3, 2006).

International Society of Nurses in Genetics (ISONG). (2002). Position statement. Genetic counseling for vulnerable populations: The role of nursing. *MedSurg Nursing, 11*(6), 305. Available at: www.isong.org/about/ps_vulnerable.cfm (accessed March 3, 2006).

International Society of Nurses in Genetics. (2003). Position statement. Access to genomic healthcare: The role of the nurse. Available at: www.isong.org/abut/ps_genomic.cfm (accessed March 7, 2006).

International Society of Nurses in Genetics (ISONG). (2005). Position statement. Privacy and confidentiality of genetic information: The role of the nurse. *MedSurg Nursing, 11*(2), 103. Available at: www.isong.org/about/ps_privacy.cfm (accessed March 3, 2006).

Khoury, M. J. & Jones, S. L. (2004). The confluence of two clinical specialties: Genetics and assisted reproductive technologies. *MedSurg Nursing, 13*(2), 114–121.

King, M. C., Marks, J. H., Mandell, J. B. & New York Breast Cancer Study Group. (2003). Breast and ovarian cancer risks due to inherited mutations in BRCA1 and BRCA2. *Science, 302*(5645), 643–646.

Kirchhoff, T., Kauff, N. D., Mitra, N., et al. (2004). BRCA mutations and risk of prostate cancer in Ashkenazi Jews. *Clinical Cancer Research, 10*(9), 2918–2921.

Lea, D. H. (2000). A clinician's primer in human genetics: What nurses need to know. *Nursing Clinics of North America, 35*(3), 583–614.

Lea, D. H., Anderson, G., & Monsen, R. B. (1998). A multiplicity of roles for genetic nursing: Building toward holistic practice. *Holistic Nursing Practice, 12*(3), 77–87.

Lea, D. H. & Monsen, R. B. (2003). Preparing nurses for a 21st century role in genomics-based health care. *Nursing Education Perspectives, 24*(2), 75–80.

Lea, D. H. & Williams, J. K. (2002). Genetic testing and screening. *American Journal of Nursing, 102*(7), 36–50.

Lea, D. H., Williams, J. K., Jenkins, J., et al. (2000). Genetic health care: Creating interdisciplinary partnerships with nursing in clinical practice. *National Academies of Practice Forum, 2*(3), 177–186.

McCabe, L. L., & McCabe, E. R. B. (2003). Population screening in the age of genomic medicine. *New England Journal of Medicine, 348*(1), 50–58.

McCarthy, J. J. & Hilfiker, R. (2000). The use of single-nucleotide polymorphism maps in pharmacogenomics. *Nature Biotechnology, 18*(5), 505–508.

McKinnon, W. C., Baty, B. J., Bennett, R. L., et al. (1997). Predisposition genetic testing for late-onset disorders in adults. A position paper of the National Society of Genetic Counselors. *Journal of the American Medical Association, 278*(15), 1217–1220.

Nebert, D. W. & Dieter, M. Z. (2000). The evolution of drug metabolism. *Pharmacology, 61*(3), 124–135.

Nicol, M. J. (2003). The variation of response to pharmacotherapy: Pharmacogenetics—A new perspective to "the right drug for the right person." *MedSurg Nursing, 12*(4), 242–249.

Norton, R. M. (2001). Clinical pharmacogenomics: Applications in pharmaceutical R&D. *Drug Discovery Today, 6*(4), 180–185.

Olsen, S. J., Feetham, S. L., Jenkins, J., et al. (2003). Creating a nursing vision for leadership in genetics. *MedSurg Nursing, 12*(3), 177–183.

Parker, A., Meyer, J., Lewitzky, S., et al. (2001). A gene conferring susceptibility to type 2 diabetes in conjunction with obesity is located on chromosome 18p11. *Diabetes, 50*(3), 675–680.

Pasacreta, J. V., Jacobs, L. & Cataldo, J. K. (2002). Genetic testing for breast and ovarian cancer risk: The psychosocial issues. *American Journal of Nursing, 102*(12), 40–47.

Phillips, M. (2003). Genetics of hearing loss. *MedSurg Nursing, 12*(6), 386–390, 411.

Prows, C. A. & Prows, D. R. (2004). Medication selection by genotype. *American Journal of Nursing, 104*(5), 60–70.

Peters, J. L., Djurdjinovic, L. & Baker, D. (1999). The genetic self: The Human Genome Project, genetic counseling and family therapy. *Families, Systems and Health, 17*(1), 5–25.

Ralston, S. (2004). Genetic control of susceptibility to osteoporosis. *Journal of Clinical Endocrinology and Metabolism, 87*(6), 2460–2466.

Sachidanandam, R., Weissman, D., Schmidt, S. C., et al. (2001). A map of human genome sequence variation containing 1.42 million single nucleotide polymorphisms. *Nature, 409*(6822), 928–933.

Struewing, J. P., Abeliovich, D., Peretz, T. et al. (1996). The carrier frequency of the BRCA1 185delAG mutation is approximately 1 percent in Ashkenazi Jewish individuals. *Nature Genetics, 12*(1), 198–200.

Subramanian, G., Adams, D., Venter, C., et al. (2001). Implications of the Human Genome for understanding human biology and medicine. *Journal of the American Medical Association, 286*(18), 2296–2307.

Williams, J. K., Tripp-Reimer, T., Schutte, D., et al. (2004). Advancing genetic nursing knowledge. *Nursing Outlook 52*(2), 73–79.

Wung, S.-F. (2002). Genetic advances in coronary artery disease. *MedSurg Nursing, 11*(6), 296–300.

## RESOURCES

Association of Women's Health, Obstetric and Neonatal Nurses, 2000 L. Street NW, Suite 740, Washington, DC 20036; 202-261-2400 or 800-673-8499; fax 202-728-0575; http://www.awhonn.org. Accessed March 3, 2006.

Gene Tests, Children's Hospital and Regional Medical Center, P.O. Box 5371, Seattle, WA 98105; 206-527-5742; fax 206-527-5743; e-mail: genetests@genetests.org.

Genetic Alliance, Inc., 4301 Connecticut Ave. NW, Suite 404, Washington, DC 20008; 202-966-5557; e-mail: info@geneticalliance.org; http://www.geneticalliance.org. Accessed March 3, 2006.

Genetic and Rare Diseases Information Center; P.O. Box 8126, Gaithersburg, MD 20898; 888-205-2311; fax 240-632-9164; e-mail: GARDinfo@nih.gov; http://www.genome.gov/Health/GARD. Accessed May 2, 2006.

Genetics Nursing Credentialing Commission. http://www.geneticnurse.org/. Accessed March 5, 2006.

International Society of Nurses in Genetics, Inc. (ISONG), 2593 W. 15th Street, Newton, IA 50208; 641-831-9230; fax 956-581-3108; http://www.isong.org. Accessed March 3, 2006.

National Cancer Institute (NCI), Public Inquiries Office, Building 31, Room 10A03, 31 Center Drive, MSC 2580, Bethesda, MD 20892-2580; 301-435-3848; http://www.nci.nih.gov. Accessed March 5, 2006.

National Coalition for Health Professional Education in Genetics (NCHPEG), 2630 W. Joppa Rd., Suite 320, Lutherville, MD 21093; 410-583-0600; http://www.nchpeg.org. Accessed March 5, 2006.

National Human Genome Research Institute, Policy and Public Affairs and Legislative Activities Branch [summary of each state's legislation on employment and insurance discrimination], http://www.genome.gov/PolicyEthics/LegDatabase/pubsearch.cfm. Accessed May 2, 2006.

National Organization for Rare Disorders, Inc. (NORD), 55 Kenosia Avenue, PO Box 1968, Danbury, CT 06813; 203-744-0100; voicemail 800-999-6673, TDD 203-797-9590, fax 203-798-2291; e-mail: orphan@rarediseases.org; http://www.rarediseases.org. Accessed March 3, 2006.

Online Mendelian Inheritance in Man (OMIM), National Center for Biotechnology Information, National Library of Medicine, Building 38A, Room 8N805, Bethesda, MD 20894; 301-496-2475; fax 301-480-9241; http://www.ncbi.nlm.nih.gov/Omim. Accessed March 3, 2006.

# CHAPTER 10

# Chronic Illness and Disability

## Learning Objectives

*On completion of this chapter, the learner will be able to:*

1. Define "chronic conditions."
2. Identify factors related to the increasing incidence of chronic conditions.
3. Describe characteristics of chronic conditions and implications for people with chronic conditions and for their families.
4. Describe advantages and disadvantages of various models of disability.
5. Describe implications of disability for nursing practice.

Chronic illness and disability affect people of all ages—the very young, the middle-aged, and the very old. Chronic illnesses and disability are found in all ethnic, cultural, and racial groups, although some disorders occur more frequently in some groups than in others (Centers for Disease Control and Prevention [CDC], 2004; Robert Wood Johnson Foundation [RWJF], 2001). Chronic diseases account for 7 of the 10 leading causes of death in the United States, including the three most frequently occurring diseases that result from preventable causes (tobacco use, improper diet and physical inactivity, and alcohol use). Chronic disease occurs in all socioeconomic groups, but people who have low incomes and disadvantaged backgrounds are more likely to report poor health (RWJF, 2001). Factors such as poverty and inadequate health insurance decrease the likelihood that people with chronic illness or disability receive health care and health screening measures such as mammography, cholesterol testing, and routine checkups (United States Department of Health and Human Services [USDHHS], 2005).

Many people with chronic health conditions and disability function independently with only minor inconvenience to their everyday lives; others require frequent and close monitoring or placement in long-term care facilities. Certain conditions require advanced technology for survival, as in the late stages of amyotrophic lateral sclerosis or end-stage renal disease, or intensive care for periods of weeks or months. People with disorders such as these have been described as chronically critically ill (Carson & Bach, 2002). Some chronic conditions have little effect on quality of life, but others have a considerable effect because they result in disability. However, not all disabilities are a result of chronic illness, and not all chronic illnesses cause disability. In this chapter, chronic illness is discussed, followed by a discussion of disability and the implications for nursing practice.

## Overview of Chronicity

Although each chronic condition has its own specific physiologic characteristics, chronic conditions do share common features. Many chronic conditions, for example, have pain and fatigue as associated symptoms. Some degree of disability is usually present in severe or advanced chronic illness, limiting the patient's participation in many activities. Many chronic conditions require therapeutic regimens to keep them under control. Unlike the term "acute," which implies a curable and relatively short disease course, the term "chronic" describes a long disease course and conditions that may be incurable. This often makes managing chronic conditions difficult for those who must live with them.

Psychological and emotional reactions of patients to acute and chronic conditions and changes in their health status are described in detail in Chapter 7. People who develop chronic conditions or disabilities may react with shock, disbelief, depression, anger, resentment, or a number of other emotions. How people react to and cope with chronic illness is usually similar to how they react to other events in their lives, depending, in part, on their understanding of the condition and their perceptions of its potential impact on their own and their family's lives. Adjustment to chronic illness (and disability) is affected by various factors:

- Suddenness, extent, and duration of lifestyle changes necessitated by the illness
- Family and individual resources for dealing with stress
- Stages of individual/family life cycle
- Previous experience with illness and crises
- Underlying personality characteristics
- Unresolved anger or grief from the past

Psychological, emotional, and cognitive reactions to chronic conditions are likely to occur at their onset and to recur if symptoms worsen or recur after a period of remission. Symptoms associated with chronic health conditions are often unpredictable and may be perceived as crisis events by patients and their families, who must contend with both the uncertainty of chronic illness and the changes it brings to their lives. These possible effects of chronic conditions can guide nursing assessment and interventions for the patient who has a chronic illness.

## Definition of Chronic Conditions

**Chronic conditions** are often defined as medical conditions or health problems with associated symptoms or disabilities that require long-term management (3 months or longer). Chronic conditions can also be defined as illnesses or diseases that have a prolonged course, that do not resolve spontaneously, and for which complete cures are rare (McKenna, Taylor, Marks, et al., 1998). The specific condition may be a result of illness, genetic factors, or injury; it may be a consequence of conditions or unhealthy behaviors that began

## Glossary

**chronic conditions:** medical or health problems with associated symptoms or disabilities that require long-term management (3 months or longer)

**disability:** restriction or lack of ability to perform an activity in a normal manner; the consequences of impairment in terms of an individual's functional performance and activity. Disabilities represent disturbances at the level of the person (eg, bathing, dressing, communication, walking, grooming).

**impairment:** loss or abnormality of psychological, physiologic, or anatomic structure or function at the organ level (eg, dysphagia, hemiparesis); an abnormality of body structure, appearance, and organ or system function resulting from any cause.

**secondary conditions or disorders:** preventable physical, mental, or social disorders resulting directly or indirectly from an initial disabling condition during childhood and young adulthood. Management of chronic conditions includes learning to live with symptoms or disabilities and coming to terms with identity changes resulting from having a chronic condition. It also consists of carrying out the lifestyle changes and regimens designed to control symptoms and to prevent complications. Although some people assume what might be called a "sick role" identity, most people with chronic conditions do not consider themselves to be sick or ill and try to live as normal a life as possible. Only when complications develop or symptoms interfere with activities of daily living (ADLs) do most people with chronic health conditions think of themselves as being sick or disabled (Nijhof, 1998).

## Prevalence and Causes of Chronic Conditions

Chronic conditions occur in people of every age group, socioeconomic level, and culture. In 1995, an estimated 99 million people in the United States had chronic conditions, and it has been projected that by the year 2050, about 167 million people will be affected (RWJF, 2001). As the incidence of chronic illnesses increases, the costs associated with these illnesses (ie, hospital costs, equipment, medications, supportive services) also increase. Expenditures for health care for people with chronic conditions exceed billions of dollars every year (Table 10-1). Chronic disease is associated with 70% of health care costs in the United States (CDC, 2004).

Although some chronic health conditions cause little or no inconvenience, others are severe enough to cause major activity limitations. When people with activity limitations are unable to meet their needs for health care and personal services, they may be unable to carry out their therapeutic regimens or have their prescriptions filled on time, may miss appointments and office visits with their health care providers, and may be unable to carry out their ADLs.

Chronic disease is a global issue that affects both rich and poor nations (Mascie-Taylor & Karim, 2003). Chronic conditions have become the major cause of health-related problems in developed countries and are increasing in incidence in the developing countries, which are also trying to cope with new and emerging infectious diseases. Causes of the increasing number of people with chronic conditions include the following:

- A decrease in mortality from infectious diseases, such as smallpox, diphtheria, and other serious conditions
- Longer lifespans because of advances in technology and pharmacology, improved nutrition, safer working conditions, and greater access (for some people) to health care
- Improved screening and diagnostic procedures, enabling early detection and treatment of diseases
- Prompt and aggressive management of acute conditions, such as myocardial infarction and acquired immunodeficiency syndrome (AIDS)–related infections
- The tendency to develop chronic illnesses with advancing age
- Lifestyle factors, such as smoking, chronic stress, and sedentary lifestyle, that increase the risk for chronic health problems such as respiratory disease, hypertension, cardiovascular disease, and obesity

Consequences of unhealthy lifestyles include an alarming increase in the incidence of diabetes, hypertension, obesity, and cardiac and chronic respiratory disorders (Juarbe, 1998; McKenna et al., 1998; USDHHS, 2001; Wing, Goldstein, Acton, et al., 2001). Physiologic changes in the body often occur before the appearance of symptoms of chronic disease. Therefore, the goal of emphasizing healthy lifestyles early in life is to improve overall health status and slow the development of such disorders.

## Characteristics of Chronic Conditions

Sometimes it is difficult for people who are disease-free to understand the often profound effect of chronic illness on the lives of patients and their families. It is easy for health professionals to focus on the illness or disability itself while overlooking the person who has the disorder. In all illnesses, but even more so with chronic conditions, the illness cannot be separated from the person. People with chronic illness must contend with it daily. To relate to what people must cope with or to plan effective interventions, nurses must understand what it means to have a chronic illness (Cumbie, Conley & Burman, 2004). Characteristics of chronic illness include the following:

- Managing chronic illness involves more than managing medical problems. Associated psychological and social problems must also be addressed, because living for long periods with illness symptoms and disability can threaten identity, bring about role changes, alter body image, and disrupt lifestyles. These changes require continuous adaptation and accommodation, depending on age and situation in life. Each decline in functional ability requires physical, emotional, and social adaptation for patients and

| TABLE 10-1 | Estimated Number of People and Direct Medical Costs for People With Chronic Conditions, Selected Years, 1995–2050 | | | | | | | |
|---|---|---|---|---|---|---|---|---|
| | 1995 | 2000 | 2005 | 2010 | 2020 | 2030 | 2040 | 2050 |
| People (millions) | 99 | 105 | 112 | 120 | 134 | 148 | 158 | 167 |
| Dollar costs (billions) | $470 | $503 | $539 | $582 | $685 | $798 | $864 | $906 |

With permission from Robert Wood Johnson Foundation. (1996). *Chronic care in America: A 21st century challenge*. Princeton, NJ: Robert Wood Johnson Foundation.

their families (Corbin, 2003; Williams, Williams, Graff, et al., 2002).
- Chronic conditions usually involve many different phases over the course of a person's lifetime. There can be acute periods, stable and unstable periods, flare-ups, and remissions. Each phase brings its own set of physical, psychological, and social problems, and each requires its own regimens and types of management.
- Keeping chronic conditions under control requires persistent adherence to therapeutic regimens. Failing to adhere to a treatment plan or to do so consistently increases the risks of developing complications and accelerating the disease process. However, the realities of daily life, including the impact of culture, values, and socioeconomic factors, affect the degree to which people adhere to a treatment regimen. Managing a chronic illness takes time, requires knowledge and planning, and can be uncomfortable and inconvenient. It is not unusual for patients to stop taking medications or alter dosages because of side effects that are more disturbing or disruptive than symptoms of the illness, or to cut back on regimens they consider overly time-consuming, fatiguing, or costly (Corbin, 2003).
- One chronic disease can lead to the development of other chronic conditions. Diabetes, for example, can eventually lead to neurologic and vascular changes that may result in visual, cardiac, and kidney disease and erectile dysfunction (CDC, 2004). The presence of a chronic illness also contributes to a higher risk of morbidity and mortality in patients admitted to the intensive care unit with acute health conditions (Johnston, Wagner, Timmons, et al., 2002).
- Chronic illness affects the entire family. Family life can be dramatically altered as a result of role reversals, unfilled roles, loss of income, time required to manage the illness, decreases in family socialization activities, and the costs of treatment. Stress and caretaker fatigue are common with severe chronic conditions, and the entire family rather than just the patient may need care (Fisher & Weiks, 2000). However, some families are able to master the treatment regimen and changes that accompany chronic illness as well as make the treatment regimen a routine part of life. Furthermore, they are able to keep the chronic illness from becoming the focal point of family life (Knafl & Gilliss, 2002).
- The day-to-day management of illness is largely the responsibility of people with chronic disorders and their families. As a result, the home, rather than the hospital, is the center of care in chronic conditions. Hospitals, clinics, physicians' offices, nursing homes, nursing centers, and community agencies (home care services, social services, and disease-specific associations and societies) are considered adjuncts or backup services to daily home management.
- The management of chronic conditions is a process of discovery. People can be taught how to manage their conditions. However, each person must discover how his or her own body reacts under varying circumstances—for example, what it is like to be hypoglycemic, what activities are likely to bring on angina, and how these or other conditions can best be prevented and managed.
- Managing chronic conditions must be a collaborative process that involves many different health care professionals working together with patients and their families to provide the full range of services that are often needed for management at home. The medical, social, and psychological aspects of chronic health problems are often complex, especially in severe conditions.
- The management of chronic conditions is expensive (see Table 10-1). Many of the expenses incurred by an individual patient (eg, costs for hospital stays, diagnostic tests, equipment, medications, supportive services) may be covered by health insurance and by federal and state agencies. However, the cost increases affect society as a whole as insurance premiums increase to cover these costs. Cost increases at the government level decrease resources that might benefit society. In addition, many out-of-pocket expenses are not reimbursed. Many people with chronic disorders, including the elderly and people who are working, are uninsured or underinsured and may be unable to afford the high costs of care often associated with chronic illnesses (Mold, Fryer, & Thomas, 2004). Absence from work because of chronic disorders may jeopardize job security and income.
- Chronic conditions raise difficult ethical issues for patients, health care professionals, and society. Problematic questions include how to establish cost controls, how to allocate scarce resources (eg, organs for transplantation), and what constitutes quality of life and when life support should be withdrawn.
- Living with chronic illness means living with uncertainty (Bailey, Mishel, Belyea, et al., 2004; Mishel, 1999; Mishel, Germino, Belyea, et al., 2003). Although health care providers may be aware of the usual progression of a chronic disease such as Parkinson's disease, no one can predict with certainty a person's illness course because of individual variation. Even when a patient is in remission or symptom-free, he or she often fears that the illness will reappear.

## Implications of Managing Chronic Conditions

Chronic conditions have implications for everyday living and management for people and their families as well as for society at large. Most importantly, individual efforts should be directed at preventing chronic conditions, because many chronic illnesses or disorders are linked to unhealthy lifestyles or behaviors such as smoking and overeating. Therefore, changes in lifestyle can prevent some chronic disorders, or at least delay onset until a later age. Because most people resist change, bringing about alterations in people's lifestyles is a major challenge for nurses today.

Once a chronic condition has occurred, the focus shifts to managing symptoms, avoiding complications (eg, eye complications in a person with diabetes), and avoiding the development of other acute illnesses (eg, pneumonia in a person with chronic obstructive lung disease). Quality of life, often overlooked by health professionals in their approach to people with chronic conditions, is also important. Health-promoting behaviors, such as exercise, are essential to quality of life even in people who have chronic illnesses and disabilities, because they help to maintain functional status (Stuifbergen & Rogers, 1997).

Although coworkers, extended family, and health care professionals are affected by chronic illnesses, the problems of living with chronic conditions are most acutely experienced by patients and their immediate families. They experience the greatest impact, with lifestyle changes that directly affect quality of life. Nurses provide direct care, especially during acute episodes, but they also provide the teaching and secure the resources and other supports that enable people to integrate their illness into their lives and to have an acceptable quality of life despite the illness. To understand what nursing care is needed, it is important to recognize and appreciate the issues that people with chronic illness and their families contend with and manage, often on a daily basis. The challenges of living with chronic conditions include the need to accomplish the following:

- Alleviate and manage symptoms
- Psychologically adjust to and physically accommodate disabilities
- Prevent and manage crises and complications
- Carry out regimens as prescribed
- Validate individual self-worth and family functioning
- Manage threats to identity
- Normalize personal and family life as much as possible
- Live with altered time, social isolation, and loneliness
- Establish the networks of support and resources that can enhance quality of life
- Return to a satisfactory way of life after an acute debilitating episode (eg, another myocardial infarction or stroke) or reactivation of a chronic condition
- Die with dignity and comfort

Many people with chronic illness must face an additional challenge: the need to deal with more than one chronic illness at a time. The symptoms or treatment of a second chronic condition may aggravate the first chronic condition (Bayliss, Steiner, Fernald, et al., 2003). Patients need to be able to deal with their various chronic conditions separately as well as in combination. Some Medicare beneficiaries have five or more chronic conditions, see an average of 13 physicians per year, and fill an average of 50 prescriptions per year (Anderson, 2005). Furthermore, the effects of increasing longevity among Americans are likely to increase health care costs in the future (Rice & Fineman, 2004).

Even more challenging for many people with chronic illness is the need to hire and oversee caregivers who come into their homes to assist with ADLs and instrumental activities of daily living (IADLs). It is difficult for many people to be in a position of hiring, supervising, and sometimes firing people who may provide them with intimate physical care. The need to balance the role of recipient of care and oversight of the person providing care may lead to blurring of role boundaries (Allen & Ciambrone, 2003).

The challenges of living with and managing a chronic illness are well known, and people with chronic illnesses often report receiving inadequate care, information, services, and counseling (Chart 10-1). This provides an opportunity for nurses to assume a more active role in addressing many of the issues experienced, coordinating care, and serving as an advocate for patients who need additional assistance to manage their illness while maintaining a quality of life that is acceptable to them.

## Phases of Chronic Conditions

Chronic conditions can pass through different phases, as described in Table 10-2. However, this course may be too uncertain to predict with any degree of accuracy. The course of an illness can be thought of as a trajectory that can be managed or shaped over time, to some extent, through proper illness management strategies (Corbin, 1998; Robinson, Bevil, Arcangelo, et al., 2001). It is important to keep in mind that not all phases occur in all patients; some phases do not occur at all, and some phases may recur. Each phase is characterized by different medical and psychosocial issues. For example, the needs of a patient with a stroke who is a good candidate for rehabilitation are very different from those of a patient with terminal cancer. By thinking in terms of phases and individual patients within a phase, nurses can target their care more specifically to each person. Not every chronic condition is necessarily life-threatening, and not every patient passes through each possible phase of a chronic condition in the same order.

Using the trajectory model enables the nurse to put the present situation into the context of what might have happened to the patient in the past—that is, the life factors and understandings that might have contributed to the present state of the illness. In this way, the nurse can more readily address the underlying issues and problems.

# Nursing Care of Patients With Chronic Conditions

Nursing care of patients with chronic conditions is varied and occurs in a variety of settings. Care may be direct or supportive. Direct care may be provided in the clinic or physician's office, the hospital, or the patient's home, depending on the status of the illness. Examples of direct care include assessing the patient's physical status, providing wound care, managing and overseeing medication regimens, and performing other technical tasks. The availability of this type of nursing care may allow the patient to remain at home and return to a more normal life after an acute episode of illness.

Because much of the day-to-day responsibility for managing chronic conditions rests with the patient and family, nurses often provide supportive care at home. Supportive care may include ongoing monitoring, teaching, counseling, serving as an advocate for the patient, making referrals, and case-managing. Giving supportive care is just as important as giving technical care. For example, through ongoing monitoring either in the home or in a clinic, a nurse might detect early signs of impending complications and make a referral (ie, contact the physician or consult the medical protocol in a clinic) for medical evaluation, thereby preventing a lengthy and costly hospitalization.

Working with people with chronic illness or disability requires not just dealing with the medical aspects of their dis-

## CHART 10-1

### Characteristics of Patients With Chronic Illness in America, 2001

A representative sample of 24,053 people with one of six chronic health conditions (arthritis, asthma, hypertension, cardiovascular disease, depression, type 2 diabetes) or family caregivers of people with chronic illness were invited to participate in an online survey.

A total of 6,447 people (4013 patients and 2434 family caregivers) completed the online survey. The findings reveal that people with chronic illnesses

- Experience greater gaps in economic and cultural access to the health care system than those without chronic illness
- Report having increasing difficulty affording health care
- Have high rates of unmet needs for support services, including home care and transportation, rehabilitation services, referral, and counseling
- Lack financial access to health care and to insurance coverage and affordability, as well as physical access
- Report poorer quality of life, fewer visits to health care providers, less knowledge about how to manage their illness, poorer relationships with their physicians, and less complete benefit from modern standards of care if they are uninsured or underinsured when compared with those who have adequate insurance
- Do not receive the information and services needed to manage their illness successfully
- Are infrequently advised by their physicians to make healthy behavior choices
- Do not receive recommended condition-specific tests and treatments about one half of the time
- Are at high risk for having unmet health-related needs
- Are less likely to receive appropriate levels of care, information, and attention from their physicians if they are members of minority groups, especially Hispanics, are poor, or are younger than 25 years of age
- Report that they do not receive adequate information and counseling about self-care from their physician, including information about medication therapy needed to avoid complications
- Report being confused about self-care activities even if they receive counseling about self-care from their physicians
- Report that treatment options and their pros and cons are not discussed with them by their physicians
- Report that their preferences regarding treatment are not taken into account and they do not feel that their physicians collaborate with them about management of their illness
- Do not feel fully involved in decisions about their own care and do not feel a sense of confidence about managing their illness
- Report that they were never advised or are confused about how to manage their illness
- Report having little sense of control over their lives and their illness
- Report infrequently receiving information or recommendations from their physicians about healthy behaviors (eg, exercise, weight control, smoking avoidance, misuse of alcohol, healthy eating)

Adapted from Robert Wood Johnson Foundation. (2001). *A portrait of the chronically ill in America, 2001.* Report from the Robert Wood Johnson Foundation National Strategic Indicator Survey. Princeton, NJ: Robert Wood Johnson Foundation.

---

order, but also working with the whole person—physically, emotionally, and socially. This holistic approach to care requires nurses to draw on their knowledge and skills, including knowledge from the social sciences and psychology in particular. People often respond to illness, health teaching, and regimens in ways that differ from the expectations of health care providers. Although quality of life is usually affected by chronic illness, especially if the illness is severe, patients' perceptions of what constitutes quality of life often drive their management behaviors or affect how they view advice about health care. Nurses and other health care professionals need to recognize this, even though it may be difficult to see patients make unwise choices and decisions about lifestyles and disease management. People have the right to receive care without fearing ridicule or refusal of treatment, even if their behaviors (eg, smoking, substance abuse, overeating, failure to follow health care providers' recommendations) may have contributed to their chronic disorder.

## Applying the Nursing Process Using the Phases of the Chronic Illness System

The focus of care for patients with chronic conditions is determined largely by the phase of the illness and is directed by the nursing process, which includes assessment, diagnosis, planning, implementation, and evaluation.

### Step 1: Identifying Specific Problems and the Trajectory Phase

The first step is assessment of the patient to determine the specific problems identified by the patient, family, nurse, and other health care providers. Assessment enables the nurse to identify the specific medical, social, and psychological problems likely to be encountered in a phase. For instance, the problems of a patient with an acute myocardial infarction are very different from those likely to occur with

| TABLE 10-2 | Phases in the Trajectory Model of Chronic Illness | |
|---|---|---|
| **Phase** | **Description** | **Focus of Nursing Care** |
| Pretrajectory | Genetic factors or lifestyle behaviors that place a person or community at risk for a chronic condition | Refer for genetic testing and counseling if indicated; provide education about prevention of modifiable risk factors and behaviors |
| Trajectory onset | Appearance or onset of noticeable symptoms associated with a chronic disorder; includes period of diagnostic workup and announcement of diagnosis; may be accompanied by uncertainty as patient awaits a diagnosis and begins to discover and cope with implications of diagnosis | Provide explanations of diagnostic tests and procedures and reinforce information and explanations given by primary health care provider; provide emotional support to patient and family |
| Stable | Illness course and symptoms are under control as symptoms, resulting disability and everyday life activities are being managed within limitations of illness; illness management centered in the home | Reinforce positive behaviors and offer ongoing monitoring; provide education about health promotion and encourage participation in health promoting activities and health screening |
| Unstable | Characterized by an exacerbation of illness symptoms, development of complications, or reactivation of an illness in remission | Provide guidance and support; reinforce previous teaching |
| | Period of inability to keep symptoms under control or reactivation of illness; difficulty in carrying out everyday life activities | |
| | May require more diagnostic testing and trial of new treatment regimens or adjustment of current regimen, with care usually taking place at home | |
| Acute | Severe and unrelieved symptoms or the development of illness complications necessitating hospitalization, bed rest, or interruption of the person's usual activities to bring illness course under control | Provide direct care and emotional support to the patient and family members |
| Crisis | Critical or life-threatening situation requiring emergency treatment or care and suspension of everyday life activities until the crisis has passed | Provide direct care, collaborate with other health care team members to stabilize patient's condition |
| Comeback | Gradual recovery after an acute period and learning to live with or to overcome disabilities and return to an acceptable way of life within the limitations imposed by the chronic condition or disability; involves physical healing, limitations stretching through rehabilitative procedures, psychosocial coming-to-terms, and biographical reengagement with adjustments in everyday life activities | Assist in coordination of care; rehabilitative focus may require care from other health care providers; provide positive reinforcement for goals identified and accomplished |
| Downward | Illness course characterized by rapid or gradual worsening of a condition; physical decline accompanied by increasing disability or difficulty in controlling symptoms; requires biographical adjustment and alterations in everyday life activities with each major downward step | Provide home care and other community-based care to help patient and family adjust to changes and come to terms with these changes; assist patient and family to integrate new treatment and management strategies; encourage identification of end-of-life preferences and planning |
| Dying | Final days or weeks before death; characterized by gradual or rapid shutting down of body processes, biographical disengagement and closure, and relinquishment of everyday life interests and activities | Provide direct and supportive care to patients and their families through hospice programs |

Adapted from Corbin, J. M. (1998). The Corbin and Strauss Chronic Illness Trajectory Model: An update. *Scholarly Inquiry for Nursing Practice, 12*(1), 33–41.

the same patient, 10 years later, dying at home of heart failure. The types of direct care, referrals, teaching, and emotional support needed in each situation are different as well. Because complementary and alternative therapies are often used by people with chronic illness, it is important to determine whether a patient with a chronic illness is using these regimens.

## Step 2: Establishing and Prioritizing Goals

Once the phase of illness has been identified for a specific patient, along with the specific medical problems and related social and psychological problems, the nurse helps prioritize problems and establish the goals of care. Identification of goals must be a collaborative effort, with the patient, family, and nurse working together, and the goals must be consistent with the abilities, desires, motivations, and resources of those involved.

## Step 3: Defining the Plan of Action to Achieve Desired Outcomes

Once goals have been established, it is necessary to identify a realistic and mutually agreed-on plan for achieving them, including specific criteria that will be used to assess the patient's progress. The identification of the person responsible for each task in the action plan is also essential.

In addition, identification of the environmental, social, and psychological factors that might interfere with or facilitate achieving the desired outcome is an important part of planning.

## Step 4: Implementing the Plan and Interventions

This step addresses implementation of the plan. Possible nursing interventions include providing direct care, serving as an advocate for the patient, teaching, counseling, making referrals, and case-managing (eg, arranging for resources). Nurses can help patients implement the actions that allow patients to live with the symptoms and therapies associated with chronic conditions, thus helping them to gain independence. The nurse works with each patient and family to identify the best ways to integrate treatment regimens into their ADLs to accomplish two tasks: (1) adhering to regimens to control symptoms and keep the illness stable, and (2) dealing with the psychosocial issues that can hinder illness management and affect quality of life. Helping patients and their families to understand and implement regimens and to carry out ADLs within the limits of the chronic illness or disability is an important aspect of nursing care for patients with chronic disorders and disabilities and their families.

## Step 5: Following Up and Evaluating Outcomes

The final step involves following up to determine if the problem is resolving or being managed and if the patient and family are adhering to the plan. This follow-up may uncover the existence of new problems resulting from the intervention, problems that interfere with the ability of the patient and family to carry out the plan, or previously unexpected problems. Maintaining the stability of the chronic condition while preserving the patient's control over his or her life and the patient's sense of identity and accomplishment is a primary goal. Based on the follow-up and evaluation, consideration of alternative strategies or revision of the initial plan may be warranted.

Helping the patient and family to integrate changes into their lifestyle is an important part of the process. Change takes time, patience, and creativity and often requires encouragement from the nurse. Validation by the nurse for each small increment toward goal accomplishment is important for enhancing self-esteem and reinforcing behaviors. Success may be defined as making some progress toward a goal when a patient is unable to implement rapid and dramatic changes in his or her life. If no progress is made, or if progress toward goals seems too slow, it may be necessary to redefine the goals, the intervention, or the time frame. The nurse must realize and accept that some people will not change. Patients share responsibility for management of their conditions, and outcomes are as much related to their ability to accommodate the illness and carry out regimens as they are to nursing intervention.

# Home and Community-Based Care

## Teaching Patients Self-Care

Because chronic conditions are so costly to people, families, and society, one of the major goals of nursing today should be the prevention of chronic conditions and the care of people with them. This requires promoting healthy lifestyles and encouraging the use of safety and disease-prevention measures, such as wearing seat belts and obtaining immunizations. Prevention should also begin early in life and continue throughout life. Self-care teaching may need to address interactions among the patient's chronic conditions as well as skills necessary to care for the individual diseases and their interactive effects (Bayliss et al., 2003).

Patient and family teaching is an important nursing role that may make the difference in the ability of the patient and family to adapt to chronic conditions. Well-informed, educated patients are more likely than uninformed patients to be concerned about their health and to do what is necessary to maintain it. They are also more likely to manage symptoms, recognize the onset of complications, and seek health care early. Knowledge is the key to making informed choices and decisions during all phases of the chronic illness trajectory.

Despite the importance of teaching the patient and family, the nurse must recognize that patients recently diagnosed with serious chronic conditions and their families may need time to understand the significance of their condition and its effect on their lives. Teaching must be planned carefully so that it is not overwhelming. Furthermore, it is important to assess the impact of a new diagnosis of chronic illness on a patient's life and the meaning of self-management to the patient (Kralik, Koch, Price, et al., 2004).

The nurse who cares for patients with chronic conditions in the hospital, clinic, or home should assess each patient's knowledge about his or her illness and its management; the nurse cannot assume that a patient with a long-standing chronic condition has the knowledge necessary to manage the condition. Learning needs change as the trajectory phase and the patient's personal situation changes. The nurse must also recognize that patients may know how their body responds under certain conditions and how best to manage their symptoms (Gallo & Knafl, 1998). Contact with patients in the hospital, clinic, home, or long-term care facility offers nurses the ideal opportunity to reassess patients' learning needs and to provide additional teaching about an illness and its management.

Teaching strategies and teaching materials should be adapted to the individual patient, so that the patient and family can understand and follow recommendations from health care providers. For instance, teaching materials should be tailored for people with low literacy levels and available

## NURSING RESEARCH PROFILE

### Chronic Illness Self-Management: The Patient's Perspective

Kralik, D., Koch, T., Price, K., et al. (2004). Chronic illness self-management: Taking action to create order. *Journal of Clinical Nursing, 13*(2), 259–267.

### Purpose
Although self-management is widely considered essential to successful coping with chronic illness, what self-management means to people with chronic illness is not well described. The purpose of this study was to explore the ways in which people who live with chronic illness view the notion of self-management. Participants in this study had arthritis, but the focus was on the meaning of self-management rather than the experience of living with the symptoms of arthritis.

### Design
Nine community-dwelling adults with arthritis participated in this qualitative study. The sample included six women and three men between 48 years and 75 years of age (mean, 60 years) who had lived with arthritis for 4 years to 52 years (mean, 17 years). Those who agreed to participate were asked to record or write an autobiography about their lives and experiences of coping with a chronic illness. Two telephone interviews were conducted with each participant. The first interview introduced the study and provided an opportunity for participants to ask questions. The second interview was conducted using probing questions and lasted for an average of 85 minutes. Examples of questions used included the following: What have you experienced when you sought medical help? How do you live with arthritis? How has life changed for you (since diagnosis)? One participant requested a face-to-face interview that was conducted in the person's home. Notes were taken during the interviews and transcribed as soon as possible. After preliminary analysis of the data, the participants and their partners attended a dinner meeting to discuss and provide feedback on the preliminary research findings. The discussion was recorded and transcribed.

### Findings
The constant-comparative method of analysis of the three sources of data (autobiography, telephone interview transcripts, and group discussion transcripts) revealed that self-management is a complex, multi-dimensional process that people use to create order from the disorder imposed by illness. The researchers identified four themes:
- *Recognizing and monitoring boundaries.* Boundaries are created by pain and by the disorder and disruption it creates. The existence of pain serves as a constant reminder of the boundaries and dependencies created by illness.
- *Mobilizing resources.* This involves identifying, understanding, and making the most of the psychological, physical, and material resources available to help people live well. The desire to maintain independence influences use of available resources, and the availability of resources also influences the desire to maintain independence. Use of resources involves balancing self-protective behaviors without burdening others.
- *Managing the shift in self-identify.* The experience of learning to live with chronic illness involves a process of shifts in self-identity as a result of disruption in work and family relationships and future plans. Some participants experience a profound loss of self and shifts in identity.
- *Balancing, pacing, planning, and prioritizing.* Daily activities need to be paced so that patients are able to tolerate pain or not aggravate it and to balance the undesired side effects of medication against the benefits of pain reduction.

At times, self-management is predictable and certain, and at other times it requires management of a crisis. Planning and prioritizing are closely linked to accepting and managing the action needed for change and determining what is most important to the participant.

### Nursing Implications
The findings of this study revealed that self-management is perceived by people with chronic illness in ways that differ from the views of health care providers. Nurses must consider that self-management is not perceived as involving education about the illness or adherence to medical treatment regimens. Self-management should be viewed from the perspective of the person who is living with the chronic illness. The illness as well as its consequences and self-management are both a structure and a process. Although self-management interventions have been identified for chronic illness, these have often been developed from the viewpoint of the health care provider or health care system rather than from an understanding of what it is like to live with and cope with a chronic illness. Strategies to empower and support people to manage chronic illness successfully are essential for effective nursing care.

in several languages and in various alternative formats (eg, Braille, large print, audiotapes). It may be necessary to provide sign interpreters.

### Continuing Care

Chronic illness management is a collaborative process between the patient, family, nurse, and other health care providers. Collaboration extends to all settings and throughout the illness trajectory (Corbin & Cherry, 2001). Keeping an illness stable over time requires careful monitoring of symptoms and attention to management regimens. Detecting problems early and helping patients develop appropriate management strategies can make a significant difference in outcomes.

Most chronic conditions are managed in the home. Therefore, care and teaching during hospitalization should focus on essential information about the condition so that management can continue once the patient is discharged home. Nurses in all settings should be aware of the resources and services available in a community and should make the arrangements (before hospital discharge, if the patient is hospitalized) that are necessary to secure those resources and services. When appropriate, home care services are contacted directly. The home care nurse reassesses how the patient and family are adapting to the chronic condition and its treatment and continues or revises the plan of care accordingly.

Because chronic conditions occur worldwide and the world is increasingly interconnected, nurses should think beyond the personal level to the community and global levels. In terms of illness prevention and health promotion, this entails wide-ranging efforts to assess people for risks of chronic illness (eg, blood pressure and diabetes screening, stroke risk assessments) and group teaching related to illness prevention and management.

In addition, nurses should also remind patients with chronic illnesses or disabilities and their families about the need for ongoing health promotion and screening recommended for all people, because chronic illness and disability are often considered the main concern while other health-related issues are ignored.

### Nursing Care for Special Populations With Chronic Illness

When providing care and teaching, the nurse must consider a variety of factors (eg, age, gender, culture and ethnicity, cognitive status, the presence of physical and sensory limitations) that influence susceptibility to chronic illness and the ways patients respond to chronic disorders. Certain populations, for example, tend to be more susceptible to certain chronic conditions. Populations at high risk for specific conditions can be targeted for special teaching and monitoring programs. People of different cultures and genders tend to respond to illness differently, and being aware of these differences is essential (Bates, Rankin-Hill & Sanchez-Ayendez, 1997; Becker, Beyene, Newsom, et al., 1998; Thorne, McCormick & Carty, 1997). For cultures in which patients rely heavily on the support of their families, families must be involved and made part of the nursing care plan. As the United States becomes more multicultural and ethnically diverse, and as the general population ages, nurses need to be aware of how a person's culture and age affect chronic illness management and prepared to adapt their care accordingly (Becker et al., 1998; Jennings, 1999; Rehm, 1999).

It is also important to consider the effect of a preexisting disability, or a disability associated with recurrence of a chronic condition, on the patient's ability to manage ADLs, self-care, and the therapeutic regimen. These issues are discussed in the following section.

## Overview of Disability

### Definitions of Disability

A person is considered to have a disability such as a limitation in performance or function in everyday activities if he or she has difficulty talking, hearing, seeing, walking, climbing stairs, lifting or carrying objects, performing ADLs, doing school work, or working at a job. A severe disability is present if a person is unable to perform one or more activities, uses an assistive device for mobility, or needs help from another person to accomplish basic activities. People are also considered severely disabled if they receive federal benefits because of an inability to work.

The World Health Organization (WHO) once defined a disability as a limitation in a person's abilities (eg, mobility, personal care, communication, behavior), an **impairment** as a body system or function affected (eg, neurologic, respiratory, urologic), and a **handicap** as a disadvantage experienced by a person in his or her environment (eg, workplace, economic sufficiency, independence) (Lollar & Crews, 2003; WHO, 1980). In an effort to change the focus from a classification based on *disease* to one based on *health*, these definitions were revised in 2001. According to the WHO, *disability* is an umbrella term for impairments, activity limitations, participation restrictions, and environmental factors, and *impairment* is a loss or abnormality in body structure or physiologic function, including mental function. A person's functioning or disability is viewed as a dynamic interaction between health conditions (ie, diseases, disorders, injuries, trauma) and contextual factors (ie, personal and environmental factors).

The term "handicap" is no longer included in the revised WHO classification system: *International Classification of Functioning, Disability and Health—ICF* (WHO, 2001). The term was used previously to identify those circumstances in which the environment played a role in limiting the participation of people with disabilities in activities. The term *societal participation* is used in the revised WHO classification system in place of handicap, to acknowledge the fact that the environment is always interacting with people to either assist or hinder participation in life activities. The revision of the classification system acknowledges that the environment may have a greater impact on the ability of an individual to participate in life activities than does the physical, mental, or emotional condition (Lollar & Crews, 2003).

Federal legislation uses more than 50 definitions of disability, which illustrates how difficult it is to define the term

(Lollar & Crews, 2003). However, the Americans With Disabilities Act of 1990 (ADA; discussed later) defines a person with a **disability** as one who (1) has a physical or mental impairment that substantially limits one or more major life activities, (2) has a record of such an impairment, or (3) is regarded as having such an impairment. Other terms that are used to describe people with disability but are not universally accepted or understood are "people who are physically challenged," and "people with special needs."

Another approach to disability is described by Lutz and Bowers (2005), who stated that none of the existing definitions adequately addresses disability in everyday life. They defined disability as a multifaceted, complex experience that is integrated into the lives of people with disabilities. The degree of the integration is influenced by three disability-related factors: (1) the effects of the disabling condition, (2) others' perceptions of disability, and (3) the need for and use of resources by the person with a disability.

## Prevalence of Disability

It is estimated that there are 54 to 60 million people in the United States with disabilities (U.S. Census Bureau, 2003). This number is expected to increase over time as people with early-onset disabilities, chronic disorders, and severe trauma survive and have normal or near-normal lifespans (Vandenakker & Glass, 2001). In addition, changes in the demographic profile are resulting in an increased number of older people with chronic illnesses and disabilities. As the population ages, the prevalence of disability is expected to increase. Although disability is often perceived as being associated only with old age, national data demonstrate that disability occurs across the lifespan; however, its incidence increases with age (U.S. Census Bureau, 2003; USDHHS, 2005).

The most recent United States Census, conducted in 2000, indicates that 20% of people have a disability and 10% have a severe disability. More than 46% of people with one disability have other disabilities. More than 50% of people with a disability are women. Although the prevalence of disability is higher in males than in females for people younger than 65 years of age, the prevalence is higher in women than in men for people older than 65 years of age. Among people 65 years of age and older, almost 60% of those with disabilities are women (U.S. Census Bureau, 2003).

Currently, more than 10 million people need personal assistance with one or more ADLs, which include bathing, dressing, feeding, and toileting, or IADLs, which include grocery shopping, meal preparation, housekeeping, transportation, and managing finances. In addition, more than 9.3 million people have sensory disabilities that affect hearing or vision. About 5 million people use a cane, more than 2 million use a wheelchair, and at least 1 million use crutches or a walker.

Among all people 21 to 64 years of age (the prime employable years), approximately 33% of people with a severe disability and 77% of those with a nonsevere disability are employed, compared with 82% of people without a disability. However, employed people with a disability earn less money than people without disabilities (U.S. Census Bureau, 2003). Furthermore, 17.5% of people with disabilities live in poverty. Many people with disabilities who are unemployed want to work; however, they are often unable to do so because of the limited access to work settings, lack of accommodations in the workplace, reluctance of employers to hire them, and financial risk if their income exceeds eligibility limits to qualify for disability benefits.

## Characteristics of Disability

### Categories and Types of Disability

Disabilities can be categorized as developmental disabilities, acquired disabilities, and age-associated disabilities. Developmental disabilities are those that occur any time from birth to 22 years of age and result in impairment of physical or mental health, cognition, speech, language, or self-care. Examples of developmental disabilities are spina bifida, cerebral palsy, Down syndrome, and muscular dystrophy. Acquired disabilities may occur as a result of an acute and sudden injury (eg, traumatic brain injury, spinal cord injury, traumatic amputation), acute nontraumatic disorders (eg, stroke, myocardial infarction), or progression of a chronic disorder (eg, arthritis, multiple sclerosis, chronic obstructive pulmonary disease, blindness due to diabetic retinopathy). Age-related disabilities are those that occur in the elderly population and are thought to be due to the aging process. Examples of age-related disabilities include osteoarthritis, osteoporosis, and hearing loss. Because people with disabilities, including those with severe developmental disabilities, are surviving longer than ever before, there is a growing number of young, middle-aged, and elderly adults with disabilities, including developmental disabilities.

Types of disability include sensory disabilities that affect hearing or vision; learning disabilities that affect the ability to learn, remember, or concentrate; disabilities that affect the ability to speak or communicate; and disabilities that affect the ability to work, shop, care for oneself or obtain health care (U.S. Census Bureau, 2003). Many disabilities are visible, but invisible disabilities are often as disabling as those that can be seen. Some disabilities affect only IADLs, whereas others affect ADLs. People can be temporarily disabled because of an injury or acute exacerbation of an chronic disorder but later return to full functioning; this definition of disability may not apply for legal purposes.

Although different impairments may result from different types of disabilities, there are some similarities across disabilities. People with disabilities are often considered by society to be dependent and needing to be cared for by others; however, many people with disabilities are highly functioning, independent, productive people who are capable of caring for themselves and others, having children and raising families, holding a full-time job, and making significant and major contributions to society (Fig. 10-1). Like other people, those with disabilities often prefer to live in their own homes with family members. Most people with disabilities are able to live at home independently. Some patients live alone in their own homes and use home care services. However, alternative living arrangements may be necessary; these include assisted living facilities, long-term care facilities, and group homes.

**FIGURE 10-1.** Many people with disabilities lead full, productive lives. (**A**) A woman works at a retail store in Hawaii. (**B**) A man plays tennis. **A** and **B**, © Index Stock Imagery, Inc.

## Models of Disability

Several models of disability have been used to address or explain the issues encountered by people with disabilities (Lollar & Crews, 2003). These include the medical and rehabilitation models, the social model, the biopsychosocial model, and the interface model. Chart 10-2 briefly describes these models of disability. Of these, the interface model (Goodall, 1995) may be the most appropriate for use by nurses to provide care that is empowering rather than care that promotes dependency. The interface model does not ignore the disabling condition or its disabling effects; instead, it promotes the view that people with disabilities are capable, responsible people who are able to function effectively despite having a disability. The interface model can serve as a basis for the role of nurses as advocates for removal of barriers to health care and for examination of how society and health care professionals contribute to discrimination by viewing disability as an abnormal state.

## Disability Versus Disabling Disorders

Regardless of which definition or model of disability is adopted, it is important to realize that it is possible to understand the pathophysiology of a disabling condition or injury or be very knowledgeable about the physical changes resulting from a disorder without understanding the concept of disability. The nurse caring for patients with preexisting disabilities or new disabilities must recognize the implications of the existence of a disability on current and future health and well-being, ability to participate in self-care or self-management, and ability to obtain required health care and health screening. Nursing management, from assessment through evaluation of the effectiveness of nursing interventions, must be examined to determine whether appropriate modifications have been made to ensure that people with disabilities receive health care equal to that of people without disabilities. Furthermore, nurses as well as other health care providers need to examine their facilities and procedures to ensure that the needs of people with a variety of disabilities can be adequately addressed. Although the health care needs of people with disabilities generally do not differ from those of the general population, some disabilities create special needs and necessitate the use of special accommodations. Chart 10-3 reviews specific areas of assessment when caring for people with disabilities.

## Federal Legislation

Because of widespread discrimination against people with disabilities, the United States Congress has enacted legislation to address health care disparities in this population. This legislation includes the Rehabilitation Act of 1973 and the ADA. Health care in people with disabilities has received further national attention through the first-time inclusion of specific national objectives that address health care for people with disabilities in *Healthy People 2010* (USDHHS, 2000). In 2005, the United States Surgeon General called for action to improve the health and wellness of people with disabilities (USDHHS, 2005).

The Rehabilitation Act of 1973 is a law that protects people from discrimination based on their disability. The act applies to employers and organizations that receive financial assistance from any federal department or agency; this includes many hospitals, long-term care facilities, mental health centers, and human service programs. It forbids organizations from excluding or denying people with disabilities equal access to program benefits and services. It also prohibits discrimination related to availability, accessibility, and delivery of services, including health care services.

The ADA, passed by the U.S. Congress in 1990, took effect in 1992. It mandates that people with disabilities have access to job opportunities and to the community. According to the ADA, employers must evaluate an applicant's ability to perform the job and not discriminate on the basis of a disability. The act stipulates that communities must provide public transportation that is accessible to people

> **CHART 10-2**
>
> ## Models of Disability
>
> **MEDICAL MODEL**
> This model equates disabled people with their disabilities and views disability as a problem of the person, directly caused by disease, trauma, or other health condition, which requires medical care provided in the form of individual treatment by professionals. Health care providers, rather than people with disabilities, are viewed as the experts or authorities. Management of the disability is aimed at cure or the person's adjustment and behavior change. The model is viewed as promoting passivity and dependency. People with disabilities are viewed as tragic (Goodall, 1995; Scullion, 1999b, 2000; World Health Organization, 2001; Lollar & Crews, 2003).
>
> **REHABILITATION MODEL**
> The rehabilitation model emerged from the medical model. It regards disability as a deficiency that requires a rehabilitation specialist or other helping professional to fix the problem. People with disabilities are often perceived as having failed if they do not overcome the disability (Lollar & Crews, 2003).
>
> **SOCIAL MODEL**
> The social model, which is also referred to as the barriers or disability model, views disability as socially constructed and as a political issue that is a result of social and physical barriers in the environment. Its perspective is that disability can be overcome by removal of these barriers (French, 1992; Richardson, 1997; Shakespeare & Watson, 1997; World Health Organization, 2001).
>
> **BIOPSYCHOSOCIAL MODEL**
> The biopsychosocial model integrates the medical and social models to address perspectives of health from a biologic, individual, and social perspective (World Health Organization, 2001; USDHHS, 2005). Critiques of this model have suggested that the disabling condition, rather than the person and the experience of the person with a disability, remains the defining construct of the biopsychosocial model (Lutz & Bowers, 2005).
>
> **INTERFACE MODEL**
> The interface model is based on the life experience of the person with a disability and views disability at the intersection (ie, interface) of the medical diagnosis of a disability and environmental barriers. It considers rather than ignores the diagnosis. The person with a disability, rather than others, defines the problems and seeks or directs solutions (Goodall, 1995).

with disabilities. The law requires that "reasonable accommodations" be provided to facilitate employment of a person with a disability. Facilities used by the public must be accessible and accommodate those with disabilities. Examples of reasonable accommodations in health care settings include accessible facilities and equipment (eg, adjustable examination tables, access ramps, grab bars, elevated toilet seats) and alternative communication methods (eg, telecommunication devices and sign interpreters for use by people who are deaf).

Although the ADA was enacted in 1992, compliance has been slow because the provisions mandating reasonable accommodation "without undue hardship" have enabled facilities to continue with inaccessible conditions. However, all new construction and modifications of public facilities must address access for people with disabilities. Examples of modifications that should be considered if one is to provide equal access to health care to people with disabilities are identified in Chart 10-3.

## Right of Access to Health Care

People with disabilities have the right of access to health care that is equal in quality to that of other people. For years, people with disabilities have been discriminated against in employment, public accommodations, and public and private services, including health care. The needs of the people with disabilities in health care settings produce many challenges to health care providers: how to communicate effectively if there are communication deficits, the additional physical requirements for mobility, and time required to provide assistance with self-care routines during hospitalization. Health care providers, including nurses, may not be aware of the specific needs of people with disabilities and may fail to provide appropriate care and services for them. However, it is essential that health care providers, including nurses, realize that people with disabilities have a legally mandated right to accessible health care facilities for all medical care and screening procedures. Furthermore, people with disabilities have the right to health care provided by professionals who are knowledgeable about and sensitive to the effects of disability on access to health care, including care that addresses their reproductive issues and sexuality. Reasonable accommodations are mandated by law and are the financial responsibility of the health care provider or facility. People with disabilities should not be expected to provide their own accommodations (eg, sign interpreters, assistants). Family members should not be expected to serve as interpreters because of concern for the patient's privacy and confidentiality and the risk for errors in interpreting information by either the patient or the health care provider. Chart 10-4 identifies strategies to communicate effectively with people with disabilities.

*(text continues on page 182)*

### CHART 10-3 Strategies to Ensure Quality Health Care for People With Disabilities

**COMMUNICATION STRATEGIES**
- Does the patient with a disability require or prefer accommodations (eg, a sign interpreter) to ensure full participation in conversations about his or her own health care?
- Are accommodations made to communicate with the patient?
- Are efforts made to direct all conversations to the patient rather than to others who have accompanied the patient to the health care facility?

**ACCESSIBILITY OF THE HEALTH CARE FACILITY**
- Are clinics, hospital rooms, offices, restrooms, and laboratories accessible to people with disabilities, as legally required by the Americans with Disabilities Act and Rehabilitation Act?
- Has accessibility been verified by a person with a disability?
- Is a sign interpreter other than family member available to assist in obtaining a patient's health history and in conducting a physical assessment?
- Does the facility include appropriate equipment to permit people with disabilities to obtain health care (including mammography, gynecologic examination and care, dental care) in a dignified and safe manner?

**ASSESSMENT**

*Usual Health Considerations*
- Does the health history address the same issues that would be included when obtaining a history from a person without disabilities, including sexuality, sexual function, and reproductive health issues?

*Disability-Related Considerations*
- Does the health history address the patient's specific disability and the effect of disability on the patient's ability to obtain health care, manage self-care activities, and obtain preventive health screening and follow-up care?
- What physical modifications and positioning are needed to ensure a thorough physical examination, including pelvic or testicular and rectal examination?

*Abuse*
- Is the increased risk for abuse (physical, emotional, financial, and sexual) by a variety of people (family, paid care providers, strangers) addressed in the assessment?
- If abuse is detected, are men and women with disabilities who are survivors of abuse directed to appropriate resources, including accessible shelters and hotlines?

*Depression*
- Is the patient experiencing depression? If so, is treatment offered just as it would be to a patient without a disability, without assuming that depression is normal and a result of having a disability?

*Aging*
- What concerns does the patient have about aging with a preexisting disability?
- What effect has aging had on the patient's disability and what effect has the disability had on the patient's aging?

*Secondary Conditions*
- Does the patient have secondary conditions related to his or her disability or its treatment?
- Are strategies in place to reduce the risk for secondary conditions or to treat existing secondary conditions?

*Accommodations in the Home*
- What accommodations does the patient have at home to encourage or permit self-care?
- What additional accommodations does the patient need at home to encourage or permit self-care?

**COGNITIVE STATUS**
- Is it assumed that the patient is able to participate in discussion and conversation rather than assuming that he or she is unable to do so because of a disability?
- Are appropriate modifications made in written and verbal communication strategies?

**MODIFICATIONS IN NURSING CARE**
- Are modifications made during hospital stays, acute illness or injury, and other health care encounters to enable a patient with disability to be as independent as he or she prefers?
- Is "person-first language" used in referring to a patient with disability, and do nurses and other staff talk directly to the patient rather than to those who accompanied the patient?
- Are all staff informed about the activities of daily living (ADLs) for which the patient will require assistance?
- Are accommodations made to enable the patient to use his or her assistive devices (hearing/visual aids, prostheses, limb support devices, ventilators, service animals)?
- If a patient with disability is immobilized because of surgery, illness, injury, or treatments, are risks of immobility addressed and strategies implemented to minimize those risks?

## CHART 10-3 Strategies to Ensure Quality Health Care for People With Disabilities, continued

- Is the patient with a disability assessed for other illnesses and health issues (eg, other acute or chronic illness, depression, psychiatric/mental health and cognitive disorders) not related to his or her primary disability?

### PATIENT TEACHING
- Are accommodations and alternative formats of teaching materials (large print, Braille, visual materials, audiotapes) provided for patients with disabilities?
- Does patient teaching address the modifications (eg, use of assistive devices) needed by patients with disabilities to enable them to adhere to recommendations?
- Are modifications made in teaching strategies to address learning needs, cognitive changes, and communication impairment?

### HEALTH PROMOTION AND DISEASE PREVENTION
- Are health promotion strategies discussed with people with disabilities along with their potential benefits: improving quality of life and preventing secondary conditions (health problems that result because of preexisting disability)?
- Are patients aware of accessible community-based facilities (eg, health care facilities, imaging centers, public exercise settings, transportation) to enable them to participate in health promotion?

### INDEPENDENCE VERSUS DEPENDENCE
- Is independence, rather than dependence, of the person with a disability the focus of nursing care and interaction?
- Are care and interaction with the patient focused on empowerment rather than promoting dependence of the patient?

### INSURANCE COVERAGE
- Does the patient have access to the health insurance coverage and other services for which he or she qualifies?
- Is the patient aware of various insurance and other available programs?
- Would the patient benefit from talking to a social worker about eligibility for Medicaid, Medicare, Disability Insurance, and other services?

## CHART 10-4 Interacting and Communicating With People With Disabilities

Patients will feel most comfortable receiving health care if you consider the following suggestions.

### GENERAL CONSIDERATIONS
- Do not be afraid to make a mistake when interacting and communicating with someone with a disability or chronic medical condition. Keep in mind that a person with a disability is a person first, and is entitled to the dignity, consideration, respect, and rights you expect for yourself.
- Treat adults as adults. Address people with disabilities by their first names only if extending the same familiarity to all others present. Never patronize people by patting them on the head or shoulder.
- Relax. If you do not know what to do, allow the person who has a disability to identify how you may be of assistance and to put you at ease.
- If you offer assistance and the person declines, do not insist. If your offer is accepted, ask how you can best help, and follow directions. Do not take over.
- If someone with a disability is accompanied by another individual, address the person with a disability directly rather than speaking through the accompanying companion.
- Be considerate of the extra time it might take for a person with a disability to get things done or said. Let the person set the pace.
- Do not be embarrassed to use common expressions such as, "See you later," or "Got to be running," that seem to relate to the person's disability.
- Use person-first language: refer to "a person with a disability" rather than "a disabled person," and avoid referring to people by the disability they have (eg, "the diabetic").

### MOBILITY LIMITATIONS
- Do not make assumptions about what a person can and cannot do.
- Do not push a person's wheelchair or grab the arm of someone walking with difficulty without first ask-

*continued >*

## CHART 10-4 Interacting and Communicating With People With Disabilities, continued

ing if you can be of assistance and how you can assist. Personal space includes a person's wheelchair, scooter, crutches, walker, cane, or other mobility aid.
- Never move someone's wheelchair, scooter, crutches, walker, cane, or other mobility aid without permission.
- When speaking for more than a few minutes to a person who is seated in a wheelchair, try to find a seat for yourself, so that the two of you are at eye level.
- When giving directions to people with mobility limitations, consider distance, weather conditions, and physical obstacles such as stairs, curbs, and steep hills.
- It is appropriate to shake hands when introduced to a person with a disability. People who have limited hand use or who wear an artificial limb do shake hands.

### VISION LOSS (LOW VISION AND BLINDNESS)
- Identify yourself when you approach a person who has low vision or blindness. If a new person approaches, introduce him or her.
- It is appropriate to touch the person's arm lightly when you speak so that he or she knows to whom you are speaking before you begin.
- Face the person and speak directly to him or her. Use a normal tone of voice.
- Do not leave without saying you are leaving.
- If you are offering directions, be as specific as possible, and point out obstacles in the path of travel. Use specifics such as, "Left about twenty feet," or "Right two yards." Use clock cues, such as, "The door is at 10 o'clock."
- When you offer to assist someone with vision loss, allow the person to take your arm. This will help you to guide rather than propel or lead the person. When offering seating, place the person's hand on the back or arm of the seat.
- Alert people with low vision or blindness to posted information.
- Never pet or otherwise distract a canine companion or service animal unless the owner has given you permission.

### HEARING LOSS (HARD OF HEARING, DEAF, DEAF-BLIND)
- Ask the person how he or she prefers to communicate.
- If you are speaking through a sign language interpreter, remember that the interpreter may lag a few words behind—especially if there are names or technical terms to be fingerspelled—so pause occasionally to allow the interpreter time to translate completely and accurately.
- Talk directly to the person who has hearing loss, not to the interpreter. However, although it may seem awkward to you, the person who has hearing loss will look at the interpreter and may not make eye contact with you during the conversation.
- Before you start to speak, make sure you have the attention of the person you are addressing. A wave, a light touch on the arm or shoulder, or other visual or tactile signals are appropriate ways of getting the person's attention.
- Speak in a clear, expressive manner. Do not over-enunciate or exaggerate words. Unless you are specifically requested to do so, do not raise your voice. Speak in a normal tone; do not shout.
- To facilitate lip reading, face the person and keep your hands and other objects away from your mouth. Maintain eye contact. Do not turn your back or walk around while talking. If you look away, the person might assume the conversation is over.
- Avoid talking while you are writing a message for someone with hearing loss, because the person cannot read your note and your lips at the same time.
- Try to eliminate background noise.
- Encourage feedback to assess clear understanding.
- If you do not understand something that is said, ask the person to repeat it or to write it down. The goal is communication; do not pretend to understand if you do not.
- If you know any sign language, try using it. It may help you communicate, and it will at least demonstrate your interest in communicating and your willingness to try.

### SPEECH DISABILITIES OR SPEECH DIFFICULTIES
- Talk to people with speech disabilities as you would talk to anyone else.
- Be friendly; start up a conversation.
- Be patient; it may take the person a while to answer. Allow extra time for communication. Do not speak for the person.
- Give the person your undivided attention.
- Ask the person for help in communicating with him or her. If the person uses a communication device such as a manual or electronic communication board, ask the person how best to use it.
- Speak in your regular tone of voice.
- Tell the person if you do not understand what he or she is trying to say. Ask the person to repeat the message, spell it, tell you in a different way, or write it down. Use hand gestures and notes.
- Repeat what you understand. The person's reactions will clue you in and guide you to understanding.
- To obtain information quickly, ask short questions that require brief answers or a head nod. However,

## CHART 10-4 Interacting and Communicating With People With Disabilities, continued

try not to insult the person's intelligence with over-simplification.
- Keep your manner encouraging rather than correcting.

**INTELLECTUAL/COGNITIVE DISABILITIES**
- Treat adults with intellectual/cognitive disabilities as adults.
- Try to be alert to the individual's responses so that you can adjust your method of communication as necessary. For example, some people may benefit from simple, direct sentences or from supplementary visual forms of communication, such as gestures, diagrams, or demonstrations.
- Use concrete rather than abstract language. Be specific, without being too simplistic. When possible, use words that relate to things you both can see. Avoid using directional terms such as right, left, east, or west.
- Be prepared to give the person the same information more than once in different ways.
- When asking questions, phrase them to elicit accurate information. People with intellectual/cognitive disabilities may be eager to please and may tell you what they think you want to hear. Verify responses by repeating the question in a different way.
- Give exact instructions. For example, "Be back for lab work at 4:30," not "Be back in 15 minutes."
- Too many directions at one time may be confusing.
- The person may prefer information provided in written or verbal form. Ask the person how you can best relay the information.
- Using humor is fine, but do not interpret a lack of response as rudeness. Some people may not grasp the meaning of sarcasm or other subtleties of language.
- People with brain injuries may have short-term memory deficits and may repeat themselves or require information to be repeated.
- People with auditory perceptual problems may need to have directions repeated and may take notes to help them remember directions or the sequence of tasks. They may benefit from watching a task demonstrated.
- People with perceptual or "sensory overload" problems may become disoriented or confused if there is too much to absorb at once. Provide information gradually and clearly. Reduce background noise if possible.

- Repeat information using different wording or a different communication approach if necessary. Allow time for the information to be fully understood.
- Do not pretend to understand if you do not. Ask the person to repeat what was said. Be patient, flexible, and supportive.
- Some people who have an intellectual disability are easily distracted. Try not to interpret distraction as rudeness.
- Do not expect all people to be able to read well. Some people may not read at all.

**PSYCHIATRIC DISABILITIES**
- Speak directly to the person. Use clear, simple communication.
- Offer to shake hands when introduced. Use the same good manners in interacting with a person who has a psychiatric disability that you would with anyone else.
- Make eye contact and be aware of your own body language. Like others, people with psychiatric disabilities will sense your discomfort.
- Listen attentively and wait for the person to finish speaking. If needed, clarify what the person has said. Never pretend to understand.
- Treat adults as adults. Do not patronize, condescend, or threaten. Do not make decisions for the person or assume that you know the person's preferences.
- Do not give unsolicited advice or assistance. Do not panic or summon an ambulance or the police if a person appears to be experiencing a mental health crisis. Calmly ask the person how you can help.
- Do not blame the person. A person with a psychiatric disability has a complex, biomedical condition that is sometimes difficult to control. They cannot just "shape up." It is rude, insensitive, and ineffective to tell or expect a person to do so.
- Question the accuracy of media stereotypes of psychiatric disabilities: movies and media often sensationalize psychiatric disabilities. Most people never experience symptoms that include violent behavior.
- Relax. Be yourself. Do not be embarrassed if you happen to use common expressions that seem to relate to a psychiatric disability.
- Recognize that beneath the symptoms and behaviors of psychiatric disabilities is a person who has many of the same wants, needs, dreams, and desires as anyone else. If you are afraid, learn more about psychiatric disabilities.

This material is adapted and based in part on *Achieving Physical and Communication Accessibility*, a publication of the National Center for Access Unlimited; *Community Access Facts*, an Adaptive Environments Center publication; and *The Ten Commandments of Interacting with People with Mental Health Disabilities*, a publication of The Ability Center of Greater Toledo.

## Barriers to Health Care

Many people with disabilities encounter barriers to full participation in life, including health care, health screening, and health promotion (Becker & Stuifbergen, 2004). Some of these barriers are structural and make certain facilities inaccessible. Examples of structural barriers include stairs, lack of ramps, narrow doorways that do not permit entry of a wheelchair, and restroom facilities that cannot be used by people with disabilities (eg, restrooms that lack grab bars and larger restroom stalls designed for people using wheelchairs).

Structural barriers to accessibility are most easily identified and eliminated. Other, less visible barriers include negative and stereotypic attitudes (eg, believing that all people with disabilities have a poor quality of life and are dependent and nonproductive) on the part of the public. Health care providers with similar negative attitudes make it difficult for people with disabilities to obtain health care equal in quality to that of people without disabilities. The Rehabilitation Act and the ADA were enacted more than 30 and 15 years ago, respectively, to ensure equal access to people with disabilities, but people with disabilities continue to encounter and report multiple barriers to health care facilities and providers (Nosek & Center for Research on Women with Disabilities, 2004). This legislation and the United States Surgeon General's call to improve the health and wellness of people with disabilities (USDHHS, 2005) are examples of efforts to eliminate barriers encountered by people with disabilities.

People with disabilities have reported that they often encounter barriers that prevent them from obtaining recommended health care screening and care. They have also reported lack of access to information, transportation difficulties, inability to pay because of limited income, difficulty finding a health care provider knowledgeable about their particular disability, previous negative health care encounters, reliance on caretakers, and the demands of coping with the disability itself (Nosek, Howland, Rintala, et al., 1997). These issues affect both men and women with severe disabilities; however, women appear to be at higher risk for receiving a lower level of health care than men. Women with disabilities are significantly less likely to receive pelvic examinations than women without disabilities; the more severe the disability, the less frequent the examination. In particular, minority women and older women with disabilities are less likely to have regular pelvic examinations and Papanicolaou (Pap) tests. Reasons given by women for not having regular pelvic examinations are difficulty transferring onto the examination table, belief that they do not need pelvic examinations because of their disability, difficulty in accessing the office or clinic, and difficulty finding transportation (Coyle & Santiago, 2002; Odette, Yoshida, Israel, et al., 2003; Schopp, Sanford, Hagglund, et al., 2002). Health care providers may underestimate the effect of disabilities on women's ability to access health care, including health screening and health promotion, and may focus on women's disabilities while ignoring their general health issues and concerns. Furthermore, women with disabilities have also reported lack of knowledge about disability and insensitivity on the part of health care providers (Nosek et al., 1997).

Because of the persistence of these barriers, it is essential that nurses and other health care providers take steps to ensure that clinics, offices, hospitals, and other health care facilities are accessible to people with disabilities. This includes removal of structural barriers by the addition of ramps, designation of accessible parking spaces, and modification of restrooms to make them usable by people with disabilities. Alternative communication methods (eg, sign interpreters, TTY devices, assistive listening devices) and types of patient education (eg, audiotapes, large print, Braille) are essential to provision of appropriate health-related information to people with disabilities (Fig. 10-2). These reasonable accommodations are mandated by the ADA, which requires their provision without cost to the patient.

## Federal Assistance Programs

Lack of financial resources, including health insurance, is an important barrier to health care for people with chronic illness and disabilities. However, several federal assistance programs provide financial assistance for health-related expenses for people with some chronic illnesses, acquired disabling acute and chronic diseases, and disabilities from childhood (Mold et al., 2004).

Medicare is a federal health insurance program that is available to most people 65 years of age and older, people with permanent renal failure, and qualified people with disabilities. Title II of the Social Security Disability Insurance program pays benefits to those people who meet medical criteria for disability, who have worked long enough (40 quarters of covered employment) to qualify, and who have paid Social Security taxes. Title II also provides benefits to people disabled since childhood (younger than 22 years of age) who are dependents of a deceased insured parent or a parent entitled to disability or retirement benefits, and disabled widows or widowers, 50 years to 60 years of age, if their de-

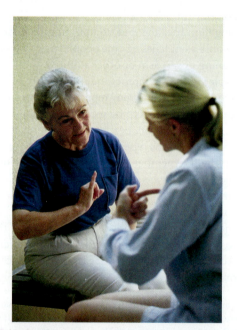

**FIGURE 10-2.** Alternative communication methods and types of patient education are essential to provision of appropriate health-related information to people with disabilities. © Will & Deni McIntyre/Photo Researchers, Inc.

ceased spouse was insured under Social Security. Title XVI of the Social Security Disability Insurance program provides supplemental security income (SSI) payments to people who are disabled and have limited income and resources.

Medicaid provides home and community-based services to people with disabilities and long-term illnesses to enable them to lead meaningful lives in their families and communities (USDHHS, 2005). (See Resources at the end of the chapter for more information about these benefits.)

Despite the availability of these federal programs, people with disabilities often have health-related costs and other expenses related to disability that result in low incomes. Furthermore, people must undergo a disability determination process to establish eligibility for benefits, and the process can be prolonged and cumbersome for those who may need assistance in establishing their eligibility.

# Nursing Care of Patients With Disabilities

As active members of society, people with disabilities are no longer an invisible minority. An increased awareness of the needs of people with disabilities will bring about changes to improve their access and accommodate their needs. Modification of the physical environment permits access to public and private facilities and services, including health care, and nurses can serve as advocates for people with disabilities to eliminate discriminatory practices (Clingerman, Stuifbergen & Becker, 2004).

## Nursing Considerations During Hospitalization

During hospitalization, as well as during periods of acute illness or injury or while recovering from surgery, patients with preexisting disabilities may require assistance with carrying out ADLs that they could otherwise manage at home independently and easily. Patients should be asked preferences about approaches to carrying out their ADLs, and assistive devices they require should be readily available. Careful planning with patients to ensure that the hospital room is arranged with their input enables them to manage as independently as possible. For example, patients who have paraplegia may be able to transfer independently from bed to wheelchair; however, if the bed is left in an elevated position, they may be unable to do so. If patients usually use service animals to assist them with ADLs, it is necessary to make arrangements for the accommodation of these animals. When patients with hearing loss or communication impairments are hospitalized, it is essential to establish effective communication strategies. Alternative methods for these patients to communicate with the health care team must be put in place and used, and all staff members must be aware that some patients are not able to respond to the intercom or telephone.

## Health Promotion and Prevention

Health care providers often neglect health promotion concerns of people with disabilities, who may be unaware of these concerns. For example, people who have had hearing loss since childhood may lack exposure to information about AIDS through radio and television. People with lifelong disabilities may not have received information about general health issues as children, and people with new-onset as well as lifelong disabilities may not receive encouragement to participate in health promotion activities. Therefore, nurses should take every opportunity to emphasize the importance of participation, both in health promotion activities (eg, healthy diet, exercise, social interactions) and in preventive health screening.

The management of some disabilities increases the risk for illness, and in some people, health screening (eg, bone density testing, gynecologic examinations, mammography) may be required earlier in life or more frequently (Smeltzer, 2006; Smeltzer & Sharts-Hopko, 2005). Referrals by nurses to accessible sites for screening may be needed, because many imaging centers are inaccessible. In addition, nursing consultation with physical therapists may be needed to identify creative ways of enabling people with disabilities to exercise safely, because exercise facilities are also often inaccessible for people with disabilities.

General health promotion strategies and health screening recommendations for all men and women also apply to those with disabilities. Although physical limitations, cognitive impairments, and structural and attitudinal barriers existing in clinical facilities may make it difficult for some men and women to obtain health care and preventive health screening, the presence of a disability should not be used as a reason or excuse to defer recommended screening. Rather, the presence of a disability may increase the risk for **secondary conditions** that require screening and follow-up. Just as people without disabilities should have regular screening tests, such as mammography or testicular and prostate examinations, so should people with disabilities (Kinne, Patrick & Doyle, 2003; USDHHS, 2005). Nurses are often in a position to influence decisions about how equipment and procedures can be adapted to meet the special needs of their patients, whether these needs are cognitive, motor, or communicative.

The effect of the disabling condition on health risks should be considered. For example, the risk for osteoporosis may be increased in women and men whose disabilities limit their ability to participate in weight-bearing exercise or who use medications that contribute to bone loss (Smeltzer, Zimmerman & Capriotti, 2005). Although people with disabilities have an increased risk for osteoporosis at a younger age than people without disabilities, little attention is given to prevention, detection, and treatment of osteoporosis, despite the increased risk for falls associated with disabling disorders (Smeltzer, 2006).

Nurses can provide expert health promotion education classes that are targeted to people with disabilities and refer them to accessible online resources (Smeltzer, Zimmerman, DeSilets, et al., 2003). Classes on nutrition and weight management are extremely important to people who are wheelchair users and need assistance with transfers. Safer sex classes are needed by adolescents and young adults who have spinal cord injury, traumatic brain injury, or developmental disabilities, because the threats of sexually transmitted diseases (STDs) and unplanned pregnancy exist for these populations just as they do for the population in general.

Other healthy behaviors about which people with neurologic disabilities need education include avoiding alcohol and nonprescription medications while taking antispasmodic and antiseizure medications.

## Significance of "People-First" Language

It is important to all people, both those with and those without disabilities, that they not be equated with their illness or physical condition. Therefore, it is important to refer to all people using "people-first" language. Using "people-first" language means referring to the person first: "the patient with diabetes" rather than "the diabetic" or "the diabetic patient"; "the person with a disability" rather than the "disabled person"; "women with disabilities" rather than "disabled women"; and "people who are wheelchair users" rather than "the wheelchair-bound." This simple use of language conveys the message that the person, rather than the illness or disability, is of greater importance to the nurse.

### Gerontologic Considerations

Stereotypical thinking often leads to the conclusion that disability is associated only with being elderly. However, aging is an important issue that affects people with preexisting disabilities. In addition, the process of aging has been described as accelerated in people with disabilities, because they often develop changes associated with aging at a younger age than do those without disabilities (Harrison, 2003; Klingbeil, Baer & Wilson, 2004). Therefore, it is important that the nurse consider the effects of aging on a preexisting disability and in turn the effects of disability on aging. The following examples may be useful.

- People who use crutches for ambulation because of polio often experience muscle problems as they age because of long-time overuse of the upper extremities; symptoms may not occur for many years but may cause discomfort and interfere with the person's ability to perform ADLs.
- People who experienced respiratory compromise with the onset of polio decades earlier may experience increasing respiratory symptoms with aging (Bartels & Omura, 2005).
- Women with long-standing mobility limitations and lack of weight-bearing exercise may experience bone loss and osteoporosis prior to menopause (Smeltzer et al., 2005). Therefore, people with preexisting disability should be evaluated for early onset of changes related to aging.

Concern about what the future holds is common in elderly people with disabilities, who may have questions about what physical, financial, and emotional supports they will have as they age (Nosek, 2000). If their disability becomes more severe in the future, they may be concerned about placement in an assisted living facility or a long-term care facility. The nurse should recognize the concerns of people with disabilities about their future and encourage them to make suitable plans, which may relieve some of their fears and concerns about what will happen to them as they age.

Parents of adult children with developmental disabilities often fear what will happen when they are no longer available and able to care for their children. The nurse should assess the concerns and arrangements made by aging parents of adult children with disabilities to help reduce some of their fears about their children's futures.

## Disability in Medical-Surgical Nursing Practice

Disability is often considered an issue that is specific or confined to rehabilitation nursing or to gerontologic nursing. However, as noted previously, disability can occur across the lifespan, and it is encountered in all settings. Patients with preexisting disabilities due to conditions that have been present from birth or due to illnesses or injuries experienced as an adolescent or young adult often require health care and nursing care in medical-surgical settings. Although in the past many people with lifelong disabilities or adult onset of severe disabilities may have had shortened lifespans, today most can expect to have a normal or near-normal lifespan and to live a productive and meaningful life (Vandenakker & Glass, 2001). They are also at risk for the same acute and chronic illnesses that affect all people.

Because of unfavorable interactions with health care providers, including negative attitudes, insensitivity, and lack of knowledge, people with disabilities may avoid seeking medical intervention or health care services. For this reason, and because the number of people with disabilities is increasing, nurses must acquire knowledge and skills and be accessible to assist these people in maintaining a high level of wellness. Nurses are in key positions to influence the architectural design of health care settings and the selection of equipment that promotes ease of access and health. Padded examination tables that can be raised or lowered make transfers easier for people with disabilities. Birthing chairs benefit women with disability during yearly pelvic examinations and Pap smears and during urologic evaluations. Ramps, grab bars, and raised and padded toilet seats benefit many people who have neurologic or musculoskeletal disabilities and need routine physical examination and monitoring (eg, bone density measurements). When a patient is admitted to the hospital, the patient's needs for these modifications should be assessed and addressed.

Men and women with disabilities may be encountered in hospitals, clinics, offices, and nursing centers when they seek health care to address a problem related to their disability. However, they may also be encountered in these settings when they seek care for a health problem that is not related in any way to their disability. For example, a woman with spina bifida or polio might seek health care related to a gynecologic issue, such as vaginal bleeding. Although her disability should be considered in the course of assessment and delivery of health and nursing care, it should not become the overriding focus or exclusive focus of the assessment or the care that she receives. Furthermore, neither a severe physical disability that affects a woman's ability to transfer to an examination table for a gynecologic examination nor a cognitive disability should be a reason to defer a complete health assessment and physical examination, including a pelvic examination. Health care, including preventive health screening, is essential to enable people with disabilities to live the highest quality of life within the limitations imposed by their disabling conditions. Men and women with disabilities have the same needs and same rights for health care and preventive health screening as others, although in some cases, the consequences of their disability increase rather than decrease their need for health screening and for participation in health-promoting activities (Smeltzer & Sharts-Hopko, 2005). Therefore, it is essential that medical-surgical nurses be knowledgeable about disability and how it affects people across the lifespan and how to provide sensitive and quality nursing care for patients with preexisting as well as new-onset disability. In an effort to address these issues, specific information on health care of people with disabilities has been included throughout this book.

## Home and Community-Based Care

### Teaching Patients Self-Care

A major and often overlooked issue in teaching patients about a health problem, a treatment regimen, or health promotion strategies is the need for alternative formats to accommodate people with a variety of disabilities. Patients with disabilities are in need of the same information as other patients; however, they often require large print, Braille, audiotapes, or the assistance of a sign interpreter. Materials may be obtained from a variety of sources for patients who need these teaching strategies and for patients with cognitive impairments due to developmental disabilities or newly acquired disabilities.

Nurses should ensure that all people, whether or not they have disabilities, recognize the warning signs and symptoms of stroke, heart attack, and cancer, as well as how to access help. In addition, nurses should teach all patients who are stroke survivors and those with diabetes how to monitor their own blood pressure or glucose levels.

### Continuing Care

When caring for patients with disabilities and helping them plan for discharge and continuing care in the home, it is important to consider how a particular disability affects a patient's ability to adhere to recommended treatment regimens and to keep follow-up appointments. Furthermore, it is important to consider how the health issue or treatment regimen affects the disability. Although many people with disabilities are independent and able to make decisions, arrangements for transportation, and appointments to accessible facilities, others may have difficulty doing so, particularly if they are experiencing a health problem. The nurse should recognize the effect that the disability has on the patient's ability to follow-up. The nurse should ask the patient whether he or she anticipates having any difficulties arranging for follow-up care. It is important for the nurse to assist the patient with disabilities to identify unmet needs and to find and use resources (community and social resources, financial and transportation services) that enable the patient to obtain needed services while remaining in his or her home, if preferred. The nurse should have a list of accessible sites and services available and share those resources with the patient and family. In collaboration with other health care providers (occupational and physical therapists, speech therapists), the nurse can identify needed home modifications, including those that are simple and inexpensive that will enable the patient to participate in self-care at home.

## Critical Thinking Exercises

1 A 65-year-old hard-working attorney experiences a mild stroke during coronary artery bypass surgery. Assessment reveals that his neurologic function is about 68% of normal. He has been transferred to a rehabilitation center. During his stay, the nurse discusses lifestyle changes with him to reduce his risk of subsequent myocardial infarction and stroke. The patient is impatient with efforts to teach him about risks and lifestyle changes, saying that he is unlikely to have subsequent cardiac problems because his heart problem has been fixed. Develop a teaching plan for this patient with rationale for including specific content and plans to use specific teaching approaches.

2 A 28-year-old woman with two children younger than 3 years of age has recently been diagnosed with type 1 diabetes. She is very active in her community and church and states that she cannot fit learning about diabetes, treatments, or blood glucose testing into her busy life. Identify approaches you would use to establish a plan of care with her. Link your teaching to the trajectory onset phase of chronic illness. How would your teaching plan change in the acute and crisis stages of chronic illness?

3 A 40-year-old woman with spina bifida is admitted to the hospital for a pneumonectomy to treat lung cancer. What modifications are needed to make sure that this patient's needs are addressed throughout her hospital stay? What planning is needed to prepare her for hospital discharge?

4 **ebp** A 43-year-old woman experienced a spinal cord injury 4 years ago as a result of a diving mishap. She has been admitted to the hospital for treatment of a grade IV pressure ulcer. The health history reveals that the patient has not been under close care of a health care provider for the past 3 years and that she has not been following recommendations for skin care and other healthy practices, including health screening. However, she indicates that she is ready to begin to take a more active role in self-care to avoid development of further pressure ulcers. What recommendations would you make to her for self-care to prevent secondary conditions and disabilities and for health screening? What is the evidence base for your recommendations? What criteria would you use to evaluate the strength of the evidence? Develop an evidence-based plan of care for her.

## REFERENCES AND SELECTED READINGS

### BOOKS

Corbin, J. & Cherry, J. (2001). Epilogue: A proactive model of health care. In Hyman, R. & Corbin, J. (Eds.). *Chronic illness: Research and theory for nursing practice.* New York: Springer.

DePoy, E. & Gilson, S. F. (2004). *Rethinking disability: Principles for professional and social change.* Belmont, CA: Thomson/Brooks/Cole.

Falvo, D. R. (2005). *Medical and psychosocial aspects of chronic illness and disability.* Sudbury, MA: Jones & Bartlett.

Jans, L. & Stoddard, S. (1999). *Chartbook on women and disability in the United States.* Washington, DC: U.S. Department of Education, National Institutes on Disability and Rehabilitation Research.

Krahn, G. (2003). *Changing concepts of health and disability.* Portland, OR: Rehabilitation Research and Training Center, Health and Wellness Consortium.

Lubkin, I. M. (1997). *Chronic illness: Impact and interventions.* Boston: Jones & Bartlett.

McKenna, M. T., Taylor, W. R., Marks, J. S., et al. (1998). Current issues and challenges in chronic disease control. In Brownson, R. C., Remington, P. L. & Davis, J. R. (Eds.). *Chronic disease epidemiology and control.* Washington, DC: American Public Health Association.

National Center for Law and Deafness. (n.d.) *ADA questions and answers for health care providers.* Washington, DC: Gallaudet University.

Neal, L. J. & Guillett, S. E. (2004) *Care of the adults with a chronic illness or disability: A team approach.* St. Louis: Mosby.

Nehring, W. M. (2205). *Core curriculum for specializing in intellectual and developmental disability: A resource for nurses and other health care professionals.* Sudbury, MA: Jones & Bartlett.

Nosek, M. & Center for Research on Women with Disabilities (CROWD). (2004). *Improving the health and wellness of women with disabilities: A symposium to establish a research agenda (Executive summary).* Houston: Center for Research on Women with Disabilities.

Nosek, M. A., Howland, C. A., Rintala, D. H., et al. (1997). *National study of women with physical disabilities: Final report.* Houston: Center for Research on Women with Disabilities.

Robert Wood Johnson Foundation. (1996). *Chronic care in America: A 21st century challenge.* Princeton, NJ: Author.

Robert Wood Johnson Foundation. (2001). *A portrait of the chronically ill in America, 2001.* Princeton, NJ: Author.

Robinson, L., Bevil, C., Arcangelo, V., et al. (2001). Operationalizing the Corbin and Strauss Trajectory Model for elderly clients with chronic illness. In Hyman, R. & Corbin, J. (Eds.). *Chronic illness: Research and theory for nursing practice.* New York: Springer.

Rogers, J. (2006). *The disabled woman's guide to pregnancy and birth.* New York: Demos Publications.

Sipski, M. & Alexander, C. (1997). *Sexual function in people with disability and chronic illness: A health professional's guide.* Gaithersburg, MD: Aspen.

Smeltzer, S. C. (1992). Use of the trajectory model of nursing in multiple sclerosis. In Woog, P. (Ed.). *The chronic illness trajectory framework.* New York: Springer.

Smeltzer, S. C. & Sharts-Hopko, N. C. (2005). *A provider's guide for the care of women with physical disabilities and chronic health conditions.* Chapel Hill, NC: North Carolina Office on Disability and Health.

Social Security Administration (2005). *Disability evaluation under Social Security.* SSA Pub. No. 64-039 ICN 468600. Washington, DC: Social Security Administration, Office of Disability Programs.

United Spinal Association. (2004). *Understanding the Americans with Disabilities Act (ADA).* Jackson Heights, NY: United Spinal Association. Available at: www.unitedspinal.org (accessed March 10, 2006).

U.S. Census Bureau. (2003). *Disability status, 2000.* Washington, DC: U.S. Department of Commerce.

U.S. Department of Health and Human Services. (2000). *Healthy People 2010.* U.S. Washington, DC: Author.

U.S. Department of Health and Human Services. (2001). *Surgeon General's call to action to prevent and decrease overweight and obesity 2001.* Rockville, MD: Public Health Service, Office of the Surgeon General.

U.S. Department of Health and Human Services. (2005). *Surgeon General's call to action to improve the health and wellness of people with disabilities.* Rockville, MD: Public Health Service, Office of the Surgeon General.

Welner, S. L. & Haseltine, F. (2004). *Welner's guide to the care of women with disabilities.* Philadelphia: Lippincott Williams & Wilkins.

Welner, S. L. & Temple, B. (2004). General health concerns and the physical examination. In Welner, S. L. & Haseltine, F. (Eds.). *Welner's guide to the care of women with disabilities.* Philadelphia: Lippincott Williams & Wilkins.

World Health Organization. (1980). *International classification of impairments, disabilities, and handicaps.* Geneva: WHO.

World Health Organization. (2001). *International classification of functioning, disability and health. Short version.* Geneva: WHO.

### JOURNALS

*An asterisk indicates a nursing research article.

Bates, M. S., Rankin-Hill, L. & Sanchez-Ayendez, M. (1997). The effects of the cultural context of health care on treatment of and response to chronic pain and illness. *Social Science in Medicine, 45*(9), 1333–1347.

Becker, G., Beyene, Y., Newsom, E. M. & Rodgers, D. V. (1998). Knowledge and care of chronic illness in three ethnic minority groups. *Family Medicine, 30*(3), 173–178.

Gallo, A. M. & Knafl, K. A. (1998). Parents' reports of "tricks of the trade" for managing childhood chronic illness. *Journal of the Society of Pediatric Nurses, 3*(3), 93–100.

Jennings, A. (1999). The use of available social support networks by older blacks. *Journal of National Black Nurses Association, 10*(2), 4–13.

Juarbe, T. C. (1998). Risk factors for cardiovascular disease in Latina women. *Progress in Cardiovascular Nursing, 13*(2), 17–27.

Mishel, M. H. (1999). Uncertainty in chronic illness. *Annual Review of Nursing Research, 17:* 269–294.

Nijhof, G. (1998). Heterogeneity in the interpretation of epilepsy. *Qualitative Health Research, 8*(1), 95–105.

*Rehm, R. S. (1999). Religious faith in Mexican-American families dealing with chronic childhood illness. *Image: Journal of Nursing Scholarship, 31*(1), 33–38.

*Thorne, S., McCormick, J. & Carty, E. (1997). Deconstructing the gender neutrality of chronic illness and disability. *Health Care Women International, 18*(1), 1–16.

Wing, R., Goldstein, M., Acton, K., et al. (2001). Behavioral science research in diabetes: Lifestyle changes related to obesity, eating behavior, and physical activity. *Diabetes Care, 24*(1), 117–123.

### *Chronic Illness*

Anderson, G. F. (2003). Physician, public, and policymaker perspectives on chronic conditions. *Archives of Internal Medicine, 163*(4), 437–442.

Anderson, G. F. (2005). Medicare and chronic conditions. *New England Journal of Medicine, 353*(3), 305–309.

Anonymous. (2002). Many working age people with chronic conditions are among the uninsured. *Healthcare Leadership and Management Report, 10*(2),12.

*Arthur, V. & Clifford, C. (2004). Rheumatology: The expectations and preferences of patients for their follow-up monitoring care. A qualitative study to determine the dimensions of patient satisfaction. *Journal of Clinical Nursing, 13*(2), 234–242.

*Bailey, D. E., Mishel, M. H., Belyea, M., et al. (2004). Uncertainty intervention for watchful waiting in prostate cancer. *Cancer Nursing, 27*(5), 339–346.

Bayliss, E. A., Steiner, J. F., Fernald, D. H., et al. (2003). Descriptions of barriers to self-care by people with comorbid chronic diseases. *Annals of Family Medicine, 1*(1), 15–21.

*Becker, H. & Stuifbergen, A. (2004). What makes it so hard? Barriers to health promotion experienced by people with multiple sclerosis and polio. *Family and Community Health, 27*(1), 75–85.

*Brooks, M. V. (2003). Health-related hardiness and chronic illness: A synthesis of current research. *Nursing Forum, 38*(3), 11–20.

Carasa, M. & Nespoli, G. (2002). Nursing the chronically critically ill patient. *Critical Care Clinics, 18*(3), 493–507.

Carson, S. S. & Bach, P. B. (2002). The epidemiology and costs of chronic critical illness. *Critical Care Clinics, 18*(3), 461–476.

Centers for Disease Control and Prevention (CDC). (2004). Indicators for chronic disease surveillance. *Morbidity and Mortality Weekly Report: Recommendations and Reports, 53*(RR-11), 1–6.

*Clingerman, E., Stuifbergen, A. & Becker, H. (2004). The influence of resources on perceived functional limitations among women with multiple sclerosis. *Journal of Neuroscience Nursing, 36*(6), 312–321.

Corbin, J. M. (1998). The Corbin and Strauss chronic illness trajectory model: An update. *Scholarly Inquiry for Nursing Practice, 12*(1), 33–41.

Corbin, J. M. (2003). The body in health and illness. *Qualitative Health Research, 13*(2), 256–267.

Cumbie, S. A., Conley, V. M. & Burman, M. E. (2004). Advanced practice nursing model for comprehensive care with chronic illness: Model for promoting process engagement. *Advances in Nursing Science, 27*(1), 70–80.

Denny, C. H., Holtzman, D., Goins, T., et al. (2005). Disparities in chronic disease risk factors and health status between American Indian/Alaska Native and white elders: Findings from a telephone survey, 2001 and 2002. *American Journal of Public Health, 95*(5), 825–827.

*Dingley, C. & Roux, G. (2003). Inner strength in older Hispanic women with chronic illness. *Journal of Cultural Diversity, 10*(1), 11–22.

Fisher, L. & Weiks, K. L. (2000). Can addressing family relationships improve outcomes in chronic disease? Report of the National Working Group on Family-Based Interventions in Chronic Disease. *Journal of Family Practice, 49*(6), 561–566.

Frich, L. M. (2003). Nursing interventions for patients with chronic conditions. *Journal of Advanced Nursing, 44*(2), 137–153.

Goertzel, R. Z., Hawkins, K., Ozminkowski, R. J., et al. (2003). The health and productivity cost burden of the "top 10" physical and mental health conditions affecting six large U.S. employers in 1999. *Journal of Occupational and Environmental Medicine, 45*(1), 5–14.

Johnston, J. A., Wagner, D. P., Timmons, S., et al. (2002). Impact of different measures of comorbid disease on predicted mortality of intensive care unit patients. *Medical Care, 40*(10), 929–940.

*Knafl, K. A. & Gillis, C. L. (2002). Families and chronic illness: A synthesis of current research. *Journal of Family Nursing, 8*(3), 178–198.

*Kralik, D., Koch, T., Price K., et al. (2004). Chronic illness self-management: Taking action to create order. *Journal of Clinical Nursing, 13*(2), 259–267.

*Loeb, S. J., Penrod, J., Falkenstern, S., et al. (2003). Supporting older adults living with multiple chronic conditions. *Western Journal of Nursing Research, 25*(1), 8–23; discussion 23–29.

*Lorig, K. R., Ritter, P. L. & Gonzalez, V. M. (2003). Hispanic chronic disease self-management: A randomized community based outcome trial. *Nursing Research, 52*(6), 361–369.

Mack, K. A. & Ahluwalia, I. B. (2003). Observations from the CDC: Monitoring women's health in the United States—Selected chronic disease indicators, 1991–2001 BRFSS. *Journal of Women's Health, 12*(4), 309–314.

Marshall, J. G. (2004). Cancer screening in women with chronic illness: The unanswered questions. *MedSurg Nursing, 13*(2), 110–113.

Mascie-Taylor, C. G. & Karim, E. (2003). The burden of chronic disease. *Science, 302*(5652), 1921–1922.

Michels, K. B. (2003). Early life predictors of chronic disease. *Journal of Women's Health, 12*(2), 157–161.

*Mishel, M. H., Germino, B. B., Belyea, M., et al. (2003). Moderators of an uncertainty management intervention: For men with localized prostate cancer. *Nursing Research, 52*(2), 89–97.

Mold, J. W., Fryer, G. E. & Thomas, C. H. (2004). Who are the uninsured elderly in the United States? *Journal of the American Geriatrics Society, 52*(4), 601–606.

*Öhman, M., Söderberg, S. & Lundman, B. (2003). Hovering between suffering and enduring: The meaning of living with serious chronic illness. *Qualitative Health Research, 13*(4), 528–542.

Rice, D. P. & Fineman, N. (2004). Economic implications of increased longevity in the United States. *Annual Review of Public Health, 25*, 457–473.

*Stuifbergen, A. K. & Becker, H. (2001). Health promotion practices in women with multiple sclerosis: Increasing quality and years of healthy life. *Physical Medicine and Rehabilitation Clinics of North America, 12*(1), 9–22.

*Stuifbergen, A. K., Harrison, T. C., Becker, H., et al. (2004). Adaptation of a wellness intervention for women with chronic disabling conditions. *Journal of Holistic Nursing, 22*(1), 12–31.

Stuifbergen, A. K. & Rogers, S. (1997). Health promotion: An essential component of rehabilitation for persons with chronic disabling conditions. *Advances in Nursing Science, 19*(4), 1–20.

*Stuifbergen, A. K., Seraphine, A., Harrison, T., et al. (2005). An explanatory model of health promotion and quality of life for people with post-polio syndrome. *Social Science and Medicine, 60*(2), 383–393.

*Sullivan, T., Weinert, C. & Cudney, S. (2002). Management of chronic illness: Voices of rural women. *Journal of Advanced Nursing, 44*(6), 566–574.

*Williams, A. (2004). Patients with comorbidities: Perceptions of acute care services. *Journal of Advanced Nursing, 46*(1), 13–22.

Williams, P. D., Williams, A. R., Graff, J. C., et al. (2002). Interrelationships among variables affecting well siblings and mothers in families of children with a chronic illness or disability. *Journal of Behavioral Medicine, 25*(5), 411–424.

## Disabilities

Allen, S. M. & Ciambrone, D. (2003). Community care for people with disability: Blurring boundaries between formal and informal caregivers. *Qualitative Health Research, 13*(2), 207–226.

Bartels, M. N. & Omura, A. (2005). Aging in polio. *Physical Medicine and Rehabilitation Clinics of North America, 16*(1), 197–218.

Brown, A. A. & Gill, C. J. (2002). Women with developmental disabilities: Health and aging. *Current Women's Health Reports, 2*(3), 219–225.

Campbell, M. L., Sheets, D. & Strong, P. S. (1999). Secondary health conditions among middle-aged people with chronic physical disabilities: Implications for unmet needs for services. *Assistive Technology, 11*(2), 105–122.

Carson, A. R. & Hieber, K. V. (2001). Adult pediatric patients. *American Journal of Nursing, 101*(3), 46–54.

Coyle, C. P. & Santiago, M. C. (2002). Healthcare utilization among women with physical disabilities. *Medscape Women's Health eJournal, 7*(4), 2.

French, S. (1992). Simulation exercises in disability awareness training. *Disability, Handicap and Society, 7*(3), 257–266.

Goodall, C. J. (1995). Is disability any business of nurse education? *Nurse Education Today, 15*(5), 323–327.

Hahn, J. E. & Marks, B. A. (Eds.) (2003). Intellectual and developmental disabilities. *Nursing Clinics in North America, 38*(2), 185–393.

*Harrison, T. (2003). Women aging with childhood onset disability. *Journal of Holistic Nursing, 21*(3), 242–259.

*Harrison, T. & Stuifbergen, A. (2001). Barriers that further disablement: A study of survivors of polio. *Journal of Neuroscience Nursing, 33*(3), 160–166.

Honeycutt, A., Dunlap, L., Chen, H., et al. (2004). Economic costs associated with mental retardation, cerebral palsy, hearing loss, and vision impairment. *MMWR Morbidity and Mortality Weekly Report, 53*(03), 57–69.

Kinne, S., Patrick, D. L. & Doyle, D. L. (2003). Prevalence of secondary conditions among people with disabilities. *American Journal of Public Health, 94*(3), 443–445.

Klingbeil, H., Baer, H. R. & Wilson, P. E. (2004). Aging with a disability. *Archives of Physical Medicine and Rehabilitation, 85*(Suppl 3), S68–S73.

Lollar, D. J. & Crews, J. E. (2003). Redefining the role of public health in disability. *Annual Review of Public Health, 24*, 195–208.

Long, S. K. & Coughlin, T. A. & Kendall, S. J. (2002). Access to care among disabled adults on Medicaid. *Health Care Financing Review, 23*(4), 159–173.

*Lutz, B. J. & Bowers, B. J. (2005). Disability in everyday life. *Qualitative Health Research, 15*(8), 1037–1054.

*McFarlane, J., Hughes, R. B., Nosek, M. A., et al. (2001). Abuse Assessment Screen—Disability (AAS-D): Measuring frequency, type, and perpetrator of abuse toward women with physical disabilities. *Journal of Women's Health and Gender-Based Medicine, 10*(9), 861–866.

Nosek, M. A. (2000). Overcoming the odds: The health of women with physical disabilities in the United States. *Archives of Physical Medicine and Rehabilitation, 81*(2), 135–138.

Odette, F., Yoshida, K. K., Israel, P., et al. (2003). Barriers to wellness activities for Canadian women with physical disabilities. *Health Care for Women International, 24*(2), 125–134.

Richardson, M. (1997). Addressing barriers: Disabled rights and the implications for nursing of the social construct of disability. *Journal of Advanced Nursing, 25*(6), 1269–1275.

Schopp, L. H., Sanford, T. C., Hagglund, K. J., et al. (2002). Removing service barriers for women with physical disabilities: Promoting accessibility in the gynecologic care setting. *Journal of Midwifery and Women's Health, 47*(2), 74–79.

Scullion, P. (1999a). Challenging discrimination against disabled patients. *Nursing Standard, 13*(8), 37–40.

*Scullion, P. (1999b). Conceptualizing disability in nursing: Some evidence from students and their teachers. *Journal of Advanced Nursing, 29*(3), 648–657.

Scullion, P. (2000). Enabling disabled people: Responsibilities of nurse education. *British Journal of Nursing, 9*(15), 1010–1015.

Shakespeare, T. & Watson, N. (1997). Defending the social model. *Disability and Society, 12*(2), 293–300.

*Smeltzer, S. C. (2002). Reproductive decision making in women with multiple sclerosis. *Journal of Neuroscience Nursing, 34*(3), 145–157.

Smeltzer, S. C. (2006). Preventive health screening for breast and cervical cancer and osteoporosis in women with physical disabilities *Family and Community Health, 29*(1 Suppl.), 35S–43S.

*Smeltzer, S. C. & Zimmerman, V. (2005). Health promotion interests of women with disabilities. *Journal of Neuroscience Nursing, 37*(2), 80–86.

*Smeltzer, S. C., Zimmerman, V. & Capriotti, T. (2005). Osteoporosis risk and low bone mineral density in women with disabilities. *Archives of Physical Medicine and Rehabilitation, 86*(3), 582–586.

Smeltzer, S. C., Zimmerman, V., DeSilets, L. D., et al. (2003). Accessible online health promotion information for people with disabilities. *Online Journal of Issues in Nursing, 9*(1), 11. Available at: nursingworld.org/ojin/topic16/tpc16_5.htm (accessed May 6, 2006).

Vandenakker, C. B. & Glass, D. D. (2001). Menopause and aging with disability. *Physical Medicine and Rehabilitation Clinics of North America, 12*(1), 133–151.

## RESOURCES

Abledata, 8630 Fenton Street, Suite 930, Silver Spring, MD 20910; 800-227-0216; http://abledata.com. Accessed ***.

American Association of the Deaf-Blind, 8630 Fenton Street, Suite 121, Silver Spring, MD 20910; 301-495-4403; TTY: 301-495-4402; http://www.aadb.org. Accessed March 10, 2006.

American Association on Mental Retardation, 444 North Capitol Street, Suite 846, Washington, DC 20001; 800-424-3688; http://www.aamr.org. Accessed March 10, 2006.

American Foundation for the Blind, 11 Penn Plaza, Suite 300, New York, NY 10001; 800-232-5463; http://www.afb.org. Accessed March 10, 2006.

Americans With Disabilities Act Information Technology Center, 451 Hungerford Drive, Suite 607, Rockville, MD 20850; 800-949-4232; http://www.adainfo.org or http://www.adata.org/. Accessed March 10, 2006.

American Speech-Language-Hearing Association, 10801 Rockville Pike, Rockville, MD 20852; 800-498-2072, fax 301-571-0457, TTY 301-897-5700; http://www.asha.org. Accessed March 10, 2006.

Arc of the United States, 1010 Wayne Avenue, Suite 650, Silver Spring, MD 20910; 301-656-3842, fax 301-565-3843; http://www.thearc.org. Accessed March 10, 2006.

Association of Late Deafened Adults, 8038 Macintosh Lane, Rockford, IL 61107, 866-402-2532, TTY 866-402-2532; http://www.alda.org. Accessed March 10, 2006.

Centers for Medicare and Medicaid Services, 7500 Security Boulevard, Baltimore, MD 21244; 800-633-4227 or 800-MEDICARE; http://www.cms.hhs.gov. Accessed March 10, 2006.

Center for Research on Women with Disabilities (CROWD), 3440 Richmond Avenue, Houston, TX 77046; 713-960-0505; http://www.bcm.edu/crowd. Accessed March 10, 2006.

ChronicNet, http://www.chronicnet.org/chronnet/project.htm. Accessed March 10, 2006. This website provides local and national data on chronic care issues and populations.

National Aphasia Association, 7 Dey Street, Suite 600, New York, NY 10007; 800-922-4622; http://www.aphasia.org. Accessed March 10, 2006.

National Center for Learning Disabilities, 381 Park Avenue South, Suite 1401, New York, NY 10016; 212-545-7510 or toll-free 888-575-7373, fax 212-545-9665; http://www.ncld.org. Accessed March 10, 2006.

North Carolina Office on Disability and Health, Division of Public Health, 1928 Mail Service Center, Raleigh, NC 27699; 919-707-5672; http://www.fpg.unc.edu/~ncodh or http://www.wch.dhhs.state.nc.us/cay.htm. Accessed March 10, 2006.

Robert Wood Johnson Foundation, http://www.rwjf.org. Accessed March 10, 2006. This website has information about health care in the United States, including proceedings of "Patient Education and Consumer Activation in Chronic Disease," July 7, 2000.

Through the Looking Glass, 2198 Sixth Street, Suite 100, Berkeley, CA 94710; 800-644-2666, TTY 800-804-1616; http://www.lookingglass.org. Accessed March 10, 2006.

United Cerebral Palsy, 1660 L Street NW, Suite 700, Washington, DC 20036; 800-872-5827; http://www.ucp.org. Accessed March 10, 2006.

United Spinal Association, 75-20 Astoria Boulevard, Jackson Heights, NY 11370; 718-803-3782, fax 718-803-0414; http://www.unitedspinal.org. Accessed March 10, 2006.

Villanova University Health Promotion for Women with Disabilities Project, Villanova University College of Nursing, 800 Lancaster Avenue, Villanova, PA 19085; http://www.villanova.nursing.edu/WomenWithDisabilities. Accessed April 30, 2006.

# CHAPTER 11

# Principles and Practices of Rehabilitation

## Learning Objectives

*On completion of this chapter, the learner will be able to:*

1. Describe the goals of rehabilitation.
2. Discuss the interdisciplinary approach to rehabilitation.
3. Identify emotional reactions exhibited by patients with disabilities.
4. Use the nursing process as a framework for care of patients with self-care deficits, impaired physical mobility, impaired skin integrity, and altered patterns of elimination.
5. Describe nursing strategies appropriate for promoting self-care through activities of daily living.
6. Describe nursing strategies appropriate for promoting mobility and ambulation and the use of assistive devices.
7. Describe risk factors and related nursing measures to prevent development of pressure ulcers.
8. Incorporate bladder training and bowel training into the plan of care for patients with bladder and bowel problems.
9. Describe the significance of continuity of care and community re-entry from the health care facility to the home or extended care facility for patients who need rehabilitative assistance and services.

**Rehabilitation** is a dynamic, health-oriented process that helps ill people or people with physical, mental, or emotional **disabilities** (restrictions in performance or function in everyday activities) to achieve the greatest possible level of physical, mental, spiritual, social, and economic functioning. The rehabilitation process also helps patients achieve an acceptable quality of life with dignity, self-respect, and independence. During rehabilitation—sometimes called habilitation—patients adjust to disabilities by learning how to use resources and focus on existing abilities. In **habilitation**, abilities, not disabilities, are emphasized.

Rehabilitation is an integral part of nursing because every major illness or injury carries the threat of disability or **impairment**, which involves a loss of function or an abnormality. The principles of rehabilitation are basic to the care of all patients, and rehabilitation efforts should begin during the initial contact with a patient. The goal of rehabilitation is to restore the patient's ability to function independently or at a preillness or preinjury level of functioning as quickly as possible. If this is not possible, the aims of rehabilitation are to maximize independence and prevent secondary disability as well as to promote a quality of life acceptable to the patient. Realistic goals based on individual patient assessment are established with each patient to guide the rehabilitation program.

Rehabilitation services are required by more people than ever before because of advances in technology that save or prolong the lives of seriously ill and injured patients and patients with disabilities. Increasing numbers of patients who are recovering from serious illnesses or injuries are returning to their homes and communities with ongoing needs. All patients, regardless of age, gender, ethnic group, socioeconomic status, or diagnosis, have a right to rehabilitation services (Chart 11-1).

---

**CHART 11-1**

### Ethics and Related Issues

### Are All Persons Entitled to Rehabilitation?

**SITUATION**
You work in an area where many illegal aliens and uninsured residents live. Community violence often creates life-threatening and disabling conditions in members of the population. After a victim of violence has been saved and stabilized, the health care team identifies rehabilitation needs. You are concerned about your patient's inability to perform self-care and to demonstrate safe mobility skills.

**DILEMMA**
As a health care provider, you are concerned about the community as a whole; costs to the community, and the values of the community. You are also aware of client fiduciary responsibility; you recognize costs to your patient when treatment is provided or not provided.

**DISCUSSION**
1. Who determines the length of stay and level of care?
2. Who will take care of patients who need rehabilitation but who are unable to pay? Is rehabilitation a basic health care need?

---

A person is considered to have a disability, such as a restriction in performance or function in everyday activities, if he or she has difficulty talking, hearing, seeing, walking,

---

## Glossary

**activities of daily living (ADLs):** self-care activities including bathing, grooming, dressing, eating, toileting, and bowel and bladder care

**adaptive device:** a type of assistive technology that is used to change the environment or help the person to modify the environment (eg, a ramp that can be used in place of steps for someone in a wheelchair)

**assistive device:** a type of assistive technology that helps people with disabilities perform a given task (eg, a lap board with pictures that is used to assist a person who cannot talk to communicate)

**assistive technology:** any item, piece of equipment, or product system—whether acquired commercially, off the shelf, modified, or customized—that is used to improve the functional capabilities of individuals with disabilities. This term encompasses both assistive devices and adaptive devices.

**disability:** restriction or lack of ability to perform an activity in a normal manner; the consequences of impairment in terms of an individual's functional performance and activity. Disabilities represent disturbances at the level of the person (eg, bathing, dressing, communication, walking, grooming).

**habilitation:** making able; learning new skills and abilities to meet maximum potential.

**impairment:** loss or abnormality of psychological, physiologic, or anatomic structure or function at the organ level (eg, dysphagia, hemiparesis); an abnormality of body structure, appearance, and organ or system function resulting from any cause.

**instrumental activities of daily living (IADLs):** complex aspects of independence including meal preparation, grocery shopping, household management, finances, and transportation.

**pressure ulcers:** breakdown of the skin due to prolonged pressure and insufficient blood supply, usually at bony prominences.

**rehabilitation:** making able again; relearning skills or abilities or adjusting existing functions.

climbing stairs, lifting or carrying objects, performing activities of daily living, doing schoolwork, or working at a job. The disability is severe if the person cannot perform one or more activities or use an assistive device for mobility, or needs help from another person to accomplish basic activities. The goal of **assistive devices** and **adaptive devices** is to maximize independence and thereby promote access. A person is also considered severely disabled if he or she receives federal benefits because of an inability to work.

Approximately 1 in 5 Americans has some form of disability, and 1 in 10 has a severe disability (U.S. Census Bureau, 2000). Approximately 60 million are affected by some form of disability, and this number is expected to increase in the coming decades due to the aging of the population. More than half of the people with disability are women, and women with disability outnumber men in all age groups except for those 15 to 24 years of age (Jans & Stoddard, 1999). One third of women 75 years of age and older need personal assistance. Currently, more than 10 million people need personal assistance with one or more **activities of daily living** (ADLs), which include bathing, dressing, feeding, and toileting, or **instrumental activities of daily living** (IADLs), which include grocery shopping, meal preparation, housekeeping, transportation, and managing finances. About 5 million people use a cane, more than 2 million use a wheelchair, and at least 1 million use crutches or a walker. Use of these devices and other types of **assistive technology** has increased dramatically due to the aging of the population, technologic advances, public policy initiatives, and changes in the delivery and financing of health care (U.S. Census Bureau, 2000).

## Americans With Disabilities Act

For years, people with disabilities have been discriminated against in employment, public accommodations, and public and private services, including health care. In 1990, the U.S. Congress passed the Americans With Disabilities Act (ADA) (PL 101-336), which is civil rights legislation designed to provide people with disabilities with access to job opportunities and to the community. See Chapter 10 for discussion of the ADA, access to health care and health promotion, and special issues that should be addressed in providing health care to people with disabilities.

## Patients' Reactions to Disability

Disability can occur at any age and may result from an acute incident, such as stroke or trauma, or from the progression of a chronic condition, such as arthritis or multiple sclerosis. People with disabilities experience many losses, including loss of function, independence, social role, status, and income. The patient and family experience a range of emotional reactions to these losses that may progress from disorganization and confusion to denial of the disability, grief over the lost function or body part, depression, anger, and, finally, acceptance of the disability. The reactions may subside over time and may recur at a later time, especially if chronic illness is progressive and results in increasing losses. Not all patients experience all of the stages, although most do exhibit grief. Patients who exhibit grief should not be dismissed and encouraged to "cheer up." The nurse should show a willingness to listen to the patient talk about the disability and should understand that grief, anger, regret, resentment, and acceptance are all part of the healing process. Chart 11-2 lists concerns unique to older adults.

The patient's preexisting coping abilities play an important role in the adaptation process. One patient may be particularly independent and determined, whereas another may be dependent and feel powerless. One goal of rehabilitation is to help the patient gain a positive self-image through effective coping. The nurse must recognize different coping abilities and identify when a patient is not coping well or not adjusting to the disability. The patient and family may benefit from participating in a support group or talking with a mental health professional to achieve this goal. Refer to Chapter 6 for a detailed discussion of adaptive and maladaptive responses to illness.

## The Rehabilitation Team

Rehabilitation is a creative, dynamic process that requires a team of professionals working together with patients and families. The team members represent a variety of disciplines, with each health professional making a unique contribution. Each health professional assesses the patient and identifies the patient's needs within his or her discipline's domain. Rehabilitative goals are set. Team members hold frequent group sessions to collaborate, evaluate progress, and modify goals as needed to facilitate rehabilitation and to promote independence, self-respect, and an acceptable quality of life for the patient.

The patient is a key member of the rehabilitation team. The patient is the focus of the team's effort and the one who

---

**CHART 11-2**

### Concerns of Older Adults Facing Disability

- Loss of independence, which is a source of self-respect and dignity
- Increased potential for discrimination or abuse
- Increased social isolation
- Added burden on spouse, who may also have impaired health
- Less access to community services and health care
- Less access to religious institutions
- Increased vulnerability to declining health secondary to other disorders, reduced physiologic reserve, or preexisting impairments of mobility and balance
- Fears and doubts about ability to learn or relearn self-care activities, exercises, and transfer and independent mobility techniques
- Inadequate support system for successful rehabilitation

determines the final outcomes of the process. The patient participates in goal setting, in learning to function using remaining abilities, and in adjusting to living with disabilities.

The patient's family is also incorporated into the team. Families are dynamic systems; therefore, the disability of one member affects other family members. Only by incorporating the family into the rehabilitation process can the family system adapt to the change in one of its members. The family provides ongoing support, participates in problem solving, and learns to provide necessary ongoing care.

The nurse develops a therapeutic and supportive relationship with the patient and family. The nurse emphasizes the patient's assets and strengths, positively reinforcing the patient's efforts to improve self-concept and self-care abilities. During nurse–patient interactions, the nurse actively listens, encourages, and shares the patient's successes.

Using the nursing process, the nurse develops a plan of care designed to facilitate rehabilitation, restore and maintain optimal health, and prevent complications. The nurse helps the patient identify strengths and past successes and develop new goals. Coping with the disability, self-care, mobility limitations, skin care, and bowel and bladder management are areas that frequently require nursing interventions. The nurse acts as a caregiver, teacher, counselor, patient advocate, case manager, and consultant. The nurse is often responsible for coordinating the total rehabilitative plan and collaborating with and coordinating the services provided by all members of the health care team, including home care nurses, who are responsible for directing patient care after the patient returns home.

Other members of the rehabilitation team may include physicians, nurse practitioners, physiatrists, physical therapists, occupational therapists, recreational therapists, speech-language therapists, psychologists, psychiatric liaison nurses, social workers, vocational counselors, orthotists or prosthetists, and sex counselors.

# Areas of Specialty Rehabilitation

Although rehabilitation must be a component of every patient's care, specialty rehabilitation programs have been established in general hospitals, free-standing rehabilitation hospitals, and outpatient facilities. The Commission for the Accreditation of Rehabilitation Facilities (CARF) sets standards for these programs and monitors compliance with the standards.

- *Stroke recovery programs* and *traumatic brain injury rehabilitation* emphasize cognitive remediation, helping patients compensate for memory, perceptual, judgment, and safety deficits as well as teaching self-care and mobility skills. Other goals include helping patients swallow food safely and communicate effectively. Neurologic disorders treated in addition to stroke and brain injury include multiple sclerosis, Parkinson's disease, amyotrophic lateral sclerosis, and nervous system tumors.
- *Spinal cord injury rehabilitation* programs have increased in number since World War II. Integral components of the programs include understanding the effects and complications of spinal cord injury; neurogenic bowel and bladder management; sexuality and fertility enhancement; self-care, including prevention of skin breakdown; bed mobility and transfers; and driving with adaptive equipment. The programs also focus on vocational assessment, training, and reentry into employment and the community. Currently, there are 16 federally funded designated spinal cord injury centers in the United States.
- *Orthopedic rehabilitation programs* provide comprehensive services to patients with traumatic or nontraumatic amputation, patients undergoing joint replacements, and patients with arthritis. Learning to be independent with a prosthesis or a new joint is a major goal of these programs. Other goals include pain management, energy conservation, and joint protection.
- *Cardiac rehabilitation* for patients who have had myocardial infarction begins during the acute hospitalization and continues on an outpatient basis. Emphasis is placed on monitored, progressive exercise; nutritional counseling; stress management; sexuality; and risk reduction.
- *Pulmonary rehabilitation* programs may be appropriate for patients with restrictive or chronic obstructive pulmonary disease or ventilator dependency. Respiratory therapists help patients achieve more effective breathing patterns. The programs also teach energy conservation techniques, self-medication, and home ventilatory management.
- *Comprehensive pain management programs* are available for people with chronic pain, especially low back pain. These programs focus on alternative pain treatment modalities, exercise, supportive counseling, and vocational evaluation.
- *Comprehensive burn rehabilitation programs* may serve as step-down units from intensive care burn units. Although rehabilitation strategies are implemented immediately in acute care, a program focused on progressive joint mobility, self-care, and ongoing counseling is imperative for burn patients.
- *Pediatric rehabilitation programs* meet the needs of children with developmental and acquired disabilities, including cerebral palsy, spina bifida, traumatic brain injuries, and spinal cord injuries.

As in all areas of nursing practice, nurses practicing in the area of rehabilitation must be skilled and knowledgeable about the care of patients with substance abuse. For all people with disabilities, including adolescents, nurses must assess actual or potential substance abuse. Almost 15 million Americans use illicit drugs, approximately 58 million engage in binge or heavy drinking of alcohol, and about 34% of the population uses tobacco products. Parental alcoholism is one of the strongest predictors of substance abuse. Alcohol abuse rates for people with disabilities may be twice as high as in the general population. Fifty percent of spinal cord injuries are related to substance abuse, and approximately 50% of all patients with traumatic brain injury were intoxicated at the time of injury (U.S. Department of Health and Human Services, 2003).

Substance abuse is a critical issue in rehabilitation, especially for people with disabilities who are attempting to gain employment via vocational rehabilitation. Treatment for alcoholism and drug dependencies includes a thorough physical and psychosocial evaluation; detoxification; counseling; medical treatment; psychological assistance for patients and families; treatment of any coexisting psychiatric illness; and referral to community resources for social, legal, spiritual, or vocational assistance. The length of treatment and the rehabilitation process depends on the patient's needs. Self-help groups are also encouraged, although attendance at meetings of such groups (eg, Alcoholics Anonymous, Narcotics Anonymous) poses various challenges for people who have neurologic disorders, are permanent wheelchair users, or must adapt to encounters with nondisabled attendees who may not understand disability. All specialty areas of rehabilitation require implementation of the nursing process as described in this chapter.

## Assessment of Functional Ability

Comprehensive assessment of functional capacity is the basis for developing a rehabilitation program. Functional capacity is a person's ability to perform ADLs and IADLs. ADLs include activities performed to meet basic needs, such as personal hygiene, dressing, toileting, eating, and moving. IADLs include activities that are necessary for independent living, such as the ability to shop for and prepare meals, use the telephone, clean, manage finances, and travel.

The nurse observes the patient performing specific activities (eg, eating, dressing) and notes the degree of independence; the time taken; the patient's mobility, coordination, and endurance; and the amount of assistance required. The nurse also carefully assesses joint motion, muscle strength, cardiovascular reserve, and neurologic function, because functional ability depends on these factors as well. Observations are recorded on a functional assessment tool. These tools provide a way to standardize assessment parameters and include a scale or score against which improvements may be measured. They also clearly communicate the patient's level of functioning to all members of the rehabilitation team. Rehabilitation staff members use these tools to provide an initial assessment of the patient's abilities and to monitor the patient's progress in achieving independence.

One of the most frequently used tools to assess the patient's level of independence is the Functional Independence Measure (FIM™). The FIM™ is a minimum data set, measuring 18 items. The self-care items measured are eating, bathing, grooming, dressing upper body, dressing lower body, toileting, bladder management, and bowel management. The FIM™ addresses transfers and the ability to ambulate and climb stairs and also includes communication and social cognition items. A WeeFIM instrument is used for children. For both children and adults, scoring is based on a seven-point scale, with items used to assess the patient's level of independence.

Other tools used to assess the patient's functional ability include the following:

- The PULSES profile is used to assess physical condition (eg, health/illness status), upper extremity functions (eg, eating, bathing), lower extremity functions (eg, transfer, ambulation), sensory function (eg, vision, hearing, speech), bowel and bladder function (ie, control of bowel or bladder), and situational factors (eg, social and financial support). Each of these areas is rated on a scale from one (independent) to four (greatest dependency).
- The Barthel Index is used to measure the patient's level of independence in ADLs (feeding, bathing, dressing, grooming), continence, toileting, transfers, and ambulation (or wheelchair mobility). This scale does not address communicative or cognitive abilities.
- The Patient Evaluation Conference System (PECS) contains 15 categories. This comprehensive assessment scale includes such areas as medications, pain, nutrition, use of assistive devices, psychological status, vocation, and recreation.

In addition to the detailed functional assessment, the nurse assesses the patient's physical, mental, emotional, spiritual, social, and economic status. Secondary problems related to the patient's disability, such as muscle atrophy and deconditioning, are assessed, as are residual strengths unaffected by disease or disability. Other areas that require nursing assessment include potential for altered skin integrity, altered bowel and bladder control, and sexual dysfunction. Many other assessment tools are designed to evaluate function in people with specific disabling conditions.

### ◂▾▸ Nursing Process

## The Patient With Self-Care Deficits in Activities of Daily Living

ADLs are those self-care activities that the patient must accomplish each day to meet personal needs. ADLs include personal hygiene/bathing, dressing/grooming, feeding, and toileting. Many patients cannot perform such activities easily. An ADL program is started as soon as the rehabilitation process begins, because the ability to perform ADLs is frequently the key to independence, return to the home, and reentry into the community.

### Assessment

The nurse must observe and assess the patient's ability to perform ADLs to determine the level of independence in self-care and the need for nursing intervention. The activity of bathing requires obtaining bath water and items used for bathing (eg, soap, washcloth), washing, and drying the body after bathing. Dressing requires getting clothes from the closet, putting on and taking off clothing, and fastening the clothing. Self-feeding requires using utensils to bring food to the mouth, and chewing and swallowing the food. The activity of toileting includes removing clothing to use the toilet, cleansing oneself, and readjusting clothing. Grooming activities include combing hair, brushing one's teeth, shaving or applying makeup, and handwashing. Patients who can sit up and raise their hands to their head can begin self-care activities. Assistive devices are often essential in achieving some level of independence in ADL.

In addition, the nurse should be aware of the patient's medical conditions or other health problems, the effect that they have on the ability to perform ADLs, and the family's involvement in the patient's ADLs. This information is valuable in setting goals and developing the plan of care to maximize self-care.

## Nursing Diagnosis

Based on the assessment data, major nursing diagnoses may include the following:

- Self-care deficit: bathing/hygiene, dressing/grooming, feeding, toileting

## Planning and Goals

The major goals include bathing/hygiene independently or with assistance, using adaptive or assistive devices as appropriate; dressing/grooming independently or with assistance, using adaptive or assistive devices as appropriate; feeding independently or with assistance, using adaptive or assistive devices as appropriate; and toileting independently or with assistance, using adaptive or assistive devices as appropriate. Another goal is patient expression of satisfaction with the extent of independence in self-care activities.

## Nursing Interventions

### Fostering Self-Care Abilities

To learn methods of self-care effectively, the patient must be motivated. An "I'd rather do it myself" attitude is encouraged. The nurse must also help the patient identify the safe limits of independent activity; knowing when to ask for assistance is particularly important.

The nurse teaches, guides, and supports the patient who is learning or relearning how to perform self-care activities. Consistency in instructions and assistance given by health care providers facilitates the learning process. Recording the patient's performance provides data for evaluating progress and may be used as a source for motivation and morale building. Guidelines for teaching about ADLs are given in Chart 11-3.

Often, a simple maneuver requires concentration and the exertion of considerable effort on the part of the patient with a disability; therefore, self-care techniques need to be adapted to accommodate the lifestyle of individual patients. There is usually more than one way to accomplish a self-care activity, and common sense and a little ingenuity may promote increased independence. For example, a person who cannot quite reach his or her head may be able to do so by leaning forward. Encouraging the patient to participate in a support group may also help the patient discover creative solutions to self-care problems.

### Recommending Assistive and Adaptive Devices

If the patient has difficulty performing an ADL, an adaptive or assistive device (self-help device) may be useful. A large variety of adaptive devices are available commercially or can be constructed by the nurse, occupational therapist, patient, or family. The nurse

---

### CHART 11-3

### Teaching About Activities of Daily Living

1. Define the goal of the activity with the patient. Be realistic. Set short-term goals that can be accomplished in the near future.
2. Identify several approaches to accomplish the task (eg, there are several ways to put on a given garment).
3. Select the approach most likely to succeed.
4. Specify the approach on the patient's plan of care and the patient's level of accomplishment on the progress notes.
5. Identify the motions necessary to accomplish the activity (eg, to pick up a glass, extend arm with hand open; place open hand next to glass; flex fingers around glass; move arm and hand holding glass vertically; flex arm toward body).
6. Focus on gross functional movements initially, and gradually include activities that use finer motions (eg, buttoning clothes, eating with a fork).
7. Encourage the patient to perform the activity up to maximal capacity within the limitations of the disability.
8. Monitor the patient's tolerance.
9. Minimize frustration and fatigue.
10. Support the patient by giving appropriate praise for effort put forth and for acts accomplished.
11. Assist the patient to perform and practice the activity in real-life situations and in a safe environment.

should be alert to "gadgets" coming on the market and evaluate their potential usefulness. The nurse must exercise professional judgment and caution in recommending devices, because in the past, unscrupulous vendors have marketed unnecessary, overly expensive, or useless items to patients.

A wide selection of computerized devices is available, or devices can be designed to help individual patients with severe disabilities to function more independently. The ABLEDATA project (see Resources list at the end of this chapter) offers a computerized listing of commercially available aids and equipment for patients with disabilities.

### Helping Patients Accept Limitations

If the patient has a severe disability, independent self-care may be an unrealistic goal; in this situation, the nurse teaches the patient how to direct his or her own care. The patient may require a personal attendant to perform ADLs. Family members may not be appropriate for providing bathing/hygiene, dressing/grooming, feeding, and toileting assistance, and spouses may have difficulty providing bowel and bladder care for patients and maintaining the role of sexual partners. If a personal caregiver is necessary, the patient and family members must learn how to manage an employee effectively. The nurse helps the patient accept self-care dependency. Independence in other areas, such as social interaction, should be emphasized to promote positive self-concept.

## Evaluation

### Expected Patient Outcomes

Expected patient outcomes may include:

1. Demonstrates independent self-care in bathing/hygiene or with assistance, using adaptive devices as appropriate
   a. Bathes self at maximal level of independence
   b. Uses adaptive devices effectively
   c. Reports satisfaction with level of independence in bathing/hygiene
2. Demonstrates independent self-care in dressing/grooming or with assistance, using adaptive devices as appropriate
   a. Dresses/grooms self at maximal level of independence
   b. Uses adaptive devices effectively
   c. Reports satisfaction with level of independence in dressing/grooming
   d. Demonstrates increased interest in appearance
3. Demonstrates independent self-care in feeding or with assistance, using adaptive and assistive devices as appropriate
   a. Feeds self at maximal level of independence
   b. Uses adaptive and assistive devices effectively
   c. Demonstrates increased interest in eating
   d. Maintains adequate nutritional intake
4. Demonstrates independent self-care in toileting or with assistance, using adaptive and assistive devices as appropriate
   a. Toilets self at maximal level of independence
   b. Uses adaptive and assistive devices effectively
   c. Indicates positive feelings regarding level of toileting independence
   d. Experiences adequate frequency of bowel and bladder elimination
   e. Does not experience incontinence, constipation, urinary tract infection, or other complications

## ◂◂▾▸▸ Nursing Process

## The Patient With Impaired Physical Mobility

Problems commonly associated with immobility include weakened muscles, joint contracture, and deformity. Each joint of the body has a normal range of motion; if the range is limited, the functions of the joint and of the muscles that move the joint are impaired, and painful deformities may develop. The nurse must identify patients at risk for such complications. The nurse needs to assess, plan, and intervene to prevent complications of immobility.

Another problem frequently seen in rehabilitation nursing is an altered ambulatory/mobility pattern. Patients with disabilities may be either temporarily or permanently unable to walk independently and unaided. The nurse assesses the mobility of the patient and designs care that promotes independent mobility within the prescribed therapeutic limits.

If a person cannot exercise and move his or her joints through their full range of motion, contractures may develop. A contracture is a shortening of the muscle and tendon that leads to deformity and limits joint mobility. When the contracted joint is moved, the patient experiences pain; in addition, more energy is required to move when joints are contracted.

### Assessment

At times, mobility is restricted because of pain, paralysis, loss of muscle strength, systemic disease, an immobilizing device (eg, cast, brace), or prescribed limits to promote healing. Assessment of mobility includes positioning, ability to move, muscle strength and tone, joint function, and the prescribed mobility limits. The nurse may need to collaborate with physical therapists or other team members to assess mobility.

During position change, transfer, and ambulation activities, the nurse assesses the patient's abilities, the extent of disability, and residual capacity for physiologic adaptation. The nurse observes for orthostatic hypotension, pallor, diaphoresis, nausea, tachycardia, and fatigue.

In addition, the nurse assesses the patient's ability to use various assistive devices that promote mobility. If the patient cannot ambulate without assistance, the nurse assesses the patient's ability to balance, transfer, and use assistive devices (eg, crutches, walker). Crutch walking requires high energy expenditure and produces considerable cardiovascular stress; therefore, people with reduced exercise capacity, decreased arm strength, and problems with balance because of aging or multiple diseases may be unable to use them. A walker is more stable and may be a better choice for such patients. If the patient uses an orthosis (an external appliance that provides support, prevents or corrects joint deformities, and improves function), the nurse monitors the patient for effective use and potential problems associated with its use.

## Nursing Diagnosis

Based on the assessment data, major nursing diagnoses may include the following:

- Impaired physical mobility
- Activity intolerance
- Risk for injury
- Risk for disuse syndrome
- Impaired walking
- Impaired wheelchair mobility
- Impaired bed mobility

## Planning and Goals

The major goals may include absence of contracture and deformity, maintenance of muscle strength and joint mobility, independent mobility, increased activity tolerance, and prevention of further disability.

## Nursing Interventions

### Positioning to Prevent Musculoskeletal Complications

Deformities and contractures can often be prevented by proper positioning. Maintaining correct body alignment when the patient is in bed is essential regardless of the position selected. During each patient contact, the nurse evaluates the patient's position and assists the patient to achieve and maintain proper positioning and alignment. The most common positions that patients assume in bed are supine (dorsal), side-lying (lateral), and prone. The nurse helps the patient assume these positions and uses pillows to support the body in correct alignment (Chart 11-4). At times, a splint (eg, wrist or hand splint) may be made by the occupational therapist to support a joint and prevent deformity. The nurse must ensure proper use of the splint and provide skin care.

#### PREVENTING EXTERNAL ROTATION OF THE HIP
The patient who is in bed for an extended period of time may develop external rotation deformity of the hip because the ball-and-socket joint of the hip tends to rotate outward when the patient lies on his or her back. A trochanter roll extending from the crest of the ilium to the midthigh prevents this deformity; with correct placement, it serves as a mechanical wedge under the projection of the greater trochanter.

#### PREVENTING FOOTDROP
Footdrop is a deformity in which the foot is plantarflexed (the ankle bends in the direction of the sole of the foot). If the condition continues without correction, the patient will not be able to hold the foot in a normal position and will be able to walk only on his or her toes, without touching the ground with the heel of the foot. The deformity is caused by contracture of both the gastrocnemius and soleus muscles. Damage to the peroneal nerve or loss of flexibility of the Achilles tendon may also result in footdrop.

### NURSING ALERT

**Prolonged bed rest, lack of exercise, incorrect positioning in bed, and the weight of bedding that forces the toes into plantar flexion contribute to footdrop.**

To prevent this disabling deformity, the patient is positioned to sit at 90 degrees in a wheelchair with his or her feet on the footrests or flat on the floor. When the patient is supine in bed, padded splints or protective boots are used to keep the patient's feet at right angles to the legs. Frequent skin inspection of the feet must also be performed to determine whether positioning devices have created any unwanted pressure areas.

The patient is encouraged to perform the following ankle exercises several times each hour: dorsiflexion and plantar flexion of the feet, flexion and extension (curl and stretch) of the toes, and eversion and inversion of the feet at the ankles. The nurse provides frequent passive range-of-motion exercises if the patient cannot perform active exercises.

### Maintaining Muscle Strength and Joint Mobility

Optimal function depends on the strength of the muscles and joint motion, and active participation in ADLs promotes maintenance of muscle strength and joint mobility. Range-of-motion exercises and specific therapeutic exercises may be included in the nursing plan of care.

#### PERFORMING RANGE-OF-MOTION EXERCISES
Range of motion involves moving a joint through its full range in all appropriate planes (Chart 11-5). To maintain or increase the motion of a joint, range-of-motion exercises are initiated as soon as the patient's

### CHART 11-4

## Positioning a Patient in Bed

### Supine (Dorsal) Position
1. Align the head with the spine, both laterally and anteroposteriorly.
2. Position the trunk to minimize hip flexion.
3. Flex the arms at the elbow and rest the hands against the abdomen.
4. Extend the legs with a small, firm support under the popliteal area.
5. Support the heels off the mattress with a small pillow or towel roll at the ankles.
6. Point the toes straight up using protective boots to prevent footdrop.
7. Place trochanter rolls under the greater trochanters to prevent external rotation of the hip.

### Side-Lying (Lateral Position)
1. Align the head with the spine, and support it with a pillow.
2. Properly align the body; avoid twisting at the shoulders, waist, or hips.
3. Flex shoulders and elbows and support the upper arm with a pillow.
4. Position the uppermost hip joint slightly forward and support the leg in a position of slight abduction by a pillow.
5. Place and support the feet in neutral dorsiflexion.
6. Support the back with a pillow.

### Prone (on Abdomen) Position
1. Turn the head laterally and align it with the rest of the body.
2. Abduct and externally rotate the arms at the shoulder joint; flex the elbows.
3. Place a small, flat support under the pelvis, extending from the level of the umbilicus to the upper third of the thigh.
4. Maintain the lower extremities in a neutral position.
5. Suspend the toes over the edge of the mattress.

*Note:* Side rails of bed are down for photographic purposes; they should remain raised if the patient is at risk for falling.

condition permits. The exercises are planned for individual patients to accommodate the wide variation in the degrees of motion that people of varying body builds and age groups can attain (Chart 11-6).

Range-of-motion exercises may be active (performed by the patient under the supervision of the nurse), assisted (with the nurse helping if the patient cannot do the exercise independently), or passive (performed by the nurse). Unless otherwise prescribed, a joint should be moved through its range of motion three times, at least twice a day. The joint to be exercised is supported, the bones above the joint are stabilized, and the body part distal to the joint is moved through the range of motion of the joint. For

## CHART 11-5

### Range-of-Motion Terminology

**Abduction:** movement away from the midline of the body
**Adduction:** movement toward the midline of the body
**Flexion:** bending of a joint so that the angle of the joint diminishes
**Extension:** the return movement from flexion; the joint angle is increased
**Rotation:** turning or movement of a part around its axis
**Internal:** turning inward, toward the center
**External:** turning outward, away from the center
**Dorsiflexion:** movement that flexes or bends the hand back toward the body or the foot toward the leg
**Palmar flexion:** movement that flexes or bends the hand in the direction of the palm
**Plantar flexion:** movement that flexes or bends the foot in the direction of the sole
**Pronation:** rotation of the forearm so that the palm of the hand is down
**Supination:** rotation of the forearm so that the palm of the hand is up
**Opposition:** touching the thumb to each fingertip on same hand
**Inversion:** movement that turns the sole of the foot inward
**Eversion:** movement that turns the sole of the foot outward

example, the humerus must be stabilized while the radius and ulna are moved through their range of motion at the elbow joint.

A joint should not be moved beyond its free range of motion; the joint is moved to the point of resistance and stopped at the point of pain. If muscle spasms are present, the joint is moved slowly to the point of resistance. Gentle, steady pressure is then applied until the muscle relaxes, and the motion is continued to the joint's final point of resistance.

To perform assisted or passive range-of-motion exercises, the patient must be in a comfortable supine position with the arms at the sides and the knees extended. Good body posture is maintained during the exercises. The nurse also uses good body mechanics during the exercise session.

### PERFORMING THERAPEUTIC EXERCISES

Therapeutic exercises are prescribed by the physician and performed with the assistance and guidance of the physical therapist or nurse. The patient should have a clear understanding of the goal of the prescribed exercise. Written instructions about the frequency, duration, and number of repetitions, as well as simple line drawings of the exercise, help ensure adherence to the exercise program. Return demonstration of the exercises also helps the patient and family to follow the instructions correctly.

When performed correctly, exercise assists in maintaining and building muscle strength, maintaining joint function, preventing deformity, stimulating circulation, developing endurance, and promoting relaxation. Exercise is also valuable in helping restore motivation and the well-being of the patient. Weight-bearing exercises may slow the bone loss that occurs with disability. There are five types of exercise: passive, active-assistive, active, resistive, and isometric. The description, purpose, and action of each of these exercises are summarized in Table 11-1.

### Promoting Independent Mobility

When the patient's condition stabilizes and his or her physical condition permits, the patient is assisted to sit up on the side of the bed and then to stand. Tolerance of this activity is assessed. Orthostatic (postural) hypotension may develop when the patient assumes a vertical position. Because of inadequate vasomotor reflexes, blood pools in the splanchnic (visceral) area and in the legs, resulting in inadequate cerebral circulation. If indicators of orthostatic hypotension (eg, drop in blood pressure, pallor, diaphoresis, nausea, tachycardia, dizziness) are present, the activity is stopped, and the patient is assisted to a supine position in bed.

Some disabilities, such as spinal cord injury, acute brain injury, and other conditions that require extended periods in the recumbent position, prevent the patient from assuming an upright position at the bedside. Several strategies can be used to help the patient assume a 90-degree sitting position. A reclining wheelchair with elevating leg rests allows a slow and controlled progression from a supine position to a 90-degree sitting position. A tilt table (a board that can be tilted in 5- to 10-degree increments from a horizontal to a vertical position) may also be used. The tilt table promotes vasomotor adjustment to positional changes and helps patients with limited standing balance and limited weight-bearing activities avoid the decalcification of bones and low bone mass associated with disuse syndrome and lack of weight-bearing exercise. Physical therapists may use a tilt table for patients who have not been upright due to illness or disability. Gradual elevation of the head of the bed may help. When getting patients with spinal cord injury out of bed, it is important to gradually raise the head of the bed to a 90-degree angle; this may take approximately 10 to 15 minutes.

Elastic compression stockings are used to prevent venous stasis. For some patients, a compression garment (leotard) or snug-fitting abdominal binder and elastic compression bandaging of the legs are needed to prevent venous stasis and orthostatic hypotension. When the patient is standing, the feet are protected with a pair of properly fitted shoes. Extended periods of standing are avoided because of venous pooling

**CHAPTER 11** • *Principles and Practices of Rehabilitation*

### CHART 11-6

## Performing Range-of-Motion Exercises

Abduction of shoulder. Move arm from side of body to above the head, then return arm to side of body or neutral position (adduction).

Forward flexion of shoulder. Move arm forward and upward until it is alongside of head.

Flexion of elbow. Bend elbow, bringing forearm and hand toward shoulder, then return forearm and hand to neutral position (arm straight).

Internal rotation of shoulder. With arm at shoulder height, elbow bent at a 90-degree angle, and palm toward feet, turn upper arm until palm and forearm point backward.

Pronation of forearm. With elbow at waist and bent at a 90-degree angle, turn hand so that palm is facing down.

Wrist extension.

External rotation of shoulder. With arm at shoulder height, elbow bent at a 90-degree angle, and palm toward feet, turn upper arm until the palm and forearm point forward.

Supination of forearm. With elbow at waist and arm bent at a 90-degree angle, turn hand so that palm is facing up.

Flexion of wrist. Bend wrist so that palm is toward forearm. Straighten to a neutral position.

*continued >*

## CHART 11-6 Performing Range-of-Motion Exercises, continued

Ulnar deviation. Move hand sideways so that the side of hand on which the little finger is located moves toward forearm.

Extension of fingers.

Internal-external rotation of hip. Turn leg in an inward motion so that toes point in. Turn leg in an outward motion so that toes point out.

Radial deviation. Move hand sideways so that side of hand on which thumb is located moves toward forearm.

To perform abduction-adduction of hip, move leg outward from the body as far as possible, as shown. Return leg from abducted position to neutral position and across the other leg as far as possible.

Hyperextension of hip. Place the patient in a prone position, and move leg backward from the body as far as possible.

Thumb opposition. Move thumb out and around to touch little finger.

Flexion of the hip and the knee. Bend hip by moving the leg forward as far as possible. Return leg from the flexed position to the neutral position.

Dorsiflexion of foot. Move foot up and toward the leg. Then move the foot down and away from the leg (plantar flexion).

## CHART 11-6 Performing Range-of-Motion Exercises, continued

Inversion and eversion of foot. Move foot so that sole is facing outward (eversion). Then move foot so that sole is facing inward (inversion).

Flexion of toes. Bend the toes toward the ball of foot.

Extension of toes. Straighten toes and pull them toward the leg as far as possible.

and pressure on the soles of the feet. The nurse monitors the patient's blood pressure and pulse and observes for signs and symptoms of orthostatic hypotension and cerebral insufficiency (eg, the patient reports feeling faint and weak), which suggest intolerance of the upright position. If the patient does not tolerate the upright position, the nurse should return the patient to the reclining position and elevate his or her legs.

### ASSISTING PATIENTS WITH TRANSFER

A transfer is movement of the patient from one place to another (eg, bed to chair, chair to commode, wheelchair to tub). As soon as the patient is permitted out

### TABLE 11-1 Therapeutic Exercises

|  | Description | Purposes | Action |
|---|---|---|---|
| *Passive* | An exercise carried out by the therapist or the nurse without assistance from the patient | To retain as much joint range of motion as possible; to maintain circulation | Stabilize the proximal joint and support the distal part; move the joint smoothly, slowly, and gently through its full range of motion; avoid producing pain. |
| *Active-assistive* | An exercise carried out by the patient with the assistance of the therapist or the nurse | To encourage normal muscle function | Support the distal part, and encourage the patient to take the joint actively through its range of motion; give no more assistance than is necessary to accomplish the action; short periods of activity should be followed by adequate rest periods. |
| *Active* | An exercise accomplished by the patient without assistance; activities include turning from side to side and from back to abdomen and moving up and down in bed | To increase muscle strength | When possible, active exercise should be performed against gravity; the joint is moved through full range of motion without assistance; make sure that the patient does not substitute another joint movement for the one intended. |
| *Resistive* | An active exercise carried out by the patient working against resistance produced by either manual or mechanical means | To provide resistance to increase muscle power | The patient moves the joint through its range of motion while the therapist resists slightly at first and then with progressively increasing resistance; sandbags and weights can be used and are applied at the distal point of the involved joint; the movements should be performed smoothly. |
| *Isometric or muscle setting* | Alternately contracting and relaxing a muscle while keeping the part in a fixed position; this exercise is performed by the patient | To maintain strength when a joint is immobilized | Contract or tighten the muscle as much as possible without moving the joint, hold for several seconds, then let go and relax; breathe deeply. |

of bed, transfer activities are started. The nurse assesses the patient's ability to participate actively in the transfer and determines, in conjunction with occupational therapists or physical therapists, the adaptive equipment required to promote independence and safety. A lightweight wheelchair with brake extensions, removable and detachable arm rests, and leg rests minimizes structural obstacles during the transfer. Tub seats or benches make transfers in and out of the tub easier and safer. Raised, padded commode seats may also be warranted for patients who must avoid flexing the hips greater than 90 degrees when transferring to a toilet. It is important that the nurse teach the patient hip precautions (ie, no adduction past the midline, no flexion greater than 90 degrees, and no internal rotation); abduction pillows can be used to keep the hip in correct alignment if precautions are warranted.

It is important that the patient maintain muscle strength and, if possible, perform push-up exercises to strengthen the arm and shoulder extensor muscles. The push-up exercise requires the patient to sit upright in bed; a book is placed under each of the patient's hands to provide a hard surface, and the patient is instructed to push down on the book, raising the body. The nurse should encourage the patient to raise and move the body in different directions by means of these push-up exercises.

The nurse or physical therapist teaches the patient how to transfer. There are several methods of transferring from the bed to the wheelchair when the patient cannot stand, and the technique chosen should take into account the patient's abilities and disabilities. It is helpful for the nurse to demonstrate the technique. If the physical therapist is involved in teaching the patient to transfer, the nurse and physical therapist must collaborate so that consistent instructions are given to the patient. During transfer, the nurse assists and coaches the patient. Figure 11-1 shows weight-bearing and non–weight-bearing transfer.

If the patient's muscles are not strong enough to overcome the resistance of body weight, a polished lightweight board (transfer board, sliding board) may be used to bridge the gap between the bed and the chair. The patient slides across on the board with or without assistance from a caregiver. This board may also be used to transfer the patient from the chair to the toilet or bathtub bench. It is important to avoid

**FIGURE 11-1.** Methods of patient transfer from the bed to a wheelchair. The wheelchair is in a locked position. Colored areas indicate non–weight-bearing body parts. (**A**) Weight-bearing transfer from bed to chair. The patient stands up, pivots until his back is opposite the new seat, and sits down. (**B**) (*Left*) Non–weight-bearing transfer from chair to bed. (*Right*) With legs braced. (**C**) (*Left*) Non–weight-bearing transfer, combined method. (*Right*) Non–weight-bearing transfer, pull-up method. One of the wheelchair arms is removed to make getting in and out of the chair easier.

the effects of shear on the patient's skin while sliding across the board. The nurse should make sure that the patient's fingers do not curl around the edge of the board during the transfer, because the patient's body weight can crush his or her fingers as he or she moves across the board. Safety is a primary concern during a transfer, and the following guidelines are recommended:

- Wheelchairs and beds must be locked before transfer begins.
- Detachable arm and foot rests are removed to make getting in and out of the chair easier.
- One end of the transfer board is placed under the buttocks and the other end on the surface to which the transfer is being made (eg, the chair).
- The patient is instructed to lean forward, push up with his or her hands, and then slide across the board to the other surface.

Nurses frequently assist weak and incapacitated patients out of bed. The nurse supports and gently assists the patient during position changes, protecting the patient from injury. The nurse avoids pulling on a weak or paralyzed upper extremity to prevent dislocation of the shoulder. The patient is assisted to move toward the stronger side (Chart 11-7).

In the home setting, getting in and out of bed and performing chair, toilet, and tub transfers are difficult for patients with weak muscles and loss of hip, knee, and ankle motion. A rope attached to the headboard of the bed enables the patient to pull himself or herself toward the center of the bed, and the use of a rope attached to the footboard facilitates getting in and out of bed. The height of a chair can be raised with cushions on the seat or with hollowed-out blocks placed under the chair legs. Grab bars can be attached to the wall near the toilet and tub to provide leverage and stability.

### PREPARING FOR AMBULATION

Regaining the ability to walk is a prime morale builder. However, to be prepared for ambulation—whether with brace, walker, cane, or crutches—the patient must strengthen the muscles required. Therefore, exercise is the foundation of preparation. The nurse and physical therapist instruct and supervise the patient in these exercises.

For ambulation, the quadriceps muscles, which stabilize the knee joint, and the gluteal muscles are strengthened. To perform quadriceps-setting exercises, the patient contracts the quadriceps muscle by attempting to push the popliteal area against the mattress and at the same time raising the heel. The patient maintains the muscle contraction for a count of five and relaxes for a count of five. The exercise is repeated 10 to 15 times hourly. Exercising the quadriceps muscles prevents flexion contractures of the knee.

In gluteal setting, the patient contracts or "pinches" the buttocks together for a count of five, relaxes for a count of five; the exercise is repeated 10 to 15 times hourly. If assistive devices (ie, walker, cane, crutches) will be used, the muscles of the upper extremities are exercised and strengthened. Push-up exercises are especially useful. While in a sitting position, the patient raises the body by pushing the hands against the chair seat or mattress. The patient should be encouraged to do push-up exercises while in a prone position also.

---

### CHART 11-7

## Assisting the Patient Out of Bed

### Technique for Moving the Patient to the Edge of the Bed

1. Move head and shoulders of patient toward the edge of the bed.
2. Move feet and legs to the edge of the bed. (The patient is now in a crescent position, which gives good range of motion to the lateral trunk muscles.)
3. Place both arms well under the patient's hips. Next, tighten (set) the muscles of your back and abdomen.
4. Straighten your back while moving the patient toward you.

### Technique for Sitting Patient on the Edge of the Bed

1. Place arm and hand under the patient's shoulders.
2. Instruct the patient to push into the bed with the elbow while you lift the patient's shoulders with one arm and swing the legs over the edge of the bed with the other. (Gravity pulls the legs downward, which aids in raising the patient's trunk.)

### Technique for Assisting Patient to Stand

1. Position the patient's feet so that they will be well grounded.
2. Face the patient while firmly grasping each side of the patient's rib cage with your hands.
3. Push your knee against one knee of the patient.
4. Rock the patient forward to a standing position. (Your knee is pushed against the patient's knee as he or she comes to the standing position.)
5. Ensure that the patient's knees are "locked" (in full extension) while standing. ("Locking" the patient's knees is a safety measure for those who are weak or have been in bed for some time.)
6. Give the patient enough time to establish balance.
7. Pivot the patient into a sitting position in the chair.

Pull-up exercises done on a trapeze while lifting the body are also effective for conditioning. The patient is taught to raise the arms above the head and then lower them in a slow, rhythmic manner while holding weights. Gradually, the weight is increased. The hands are strengthened by squeezing a rubber ball.

Typically, the physical therapist designs exercises to help the patient develop the sitting and standing balance, stability, and coordination needed for ambulation. After sitting and standing balance is achieved, the patient is able to use parallel bars. Under the supervision of the physical therapist, the patient practices shifting weight from side to side, lifting one leg while supporting weight on the other, and then walking between the parallel bars.

A patient who is ready to begin ambulation must be fitted with the appropriate assistive device, instructed about the prescribed weight-bearing limits (eg, non–weight-bearing, partial weight-bearing ambulation), and taught how to use the device safely. The nurse continually assesses the patient for stability and adherence to weight-bearing precautions and protects the patient from falling. The nurse provides contact guarding by holding on to a gait belt that the patient wears around the waist. The patient should wear sturdy, well-fitting shoes and be advised of the dangers of wet or highly polished floors and throw rugs. The patient should also learn how to ambulate on inclines, uneven surfaces, and stairs.

## *Ambulating With Crutches*

A patient who is prescribed partial weight-bearing or non–weight-bearing ambulation may use crutches. The nurse or physical therapist should determine whether crutches are appropriate for the patient, because good balance, adequate cardiovascular reserve, strong upper extremities, and erect posture are essential for crutch walking. Ambulating a functional distance (at least the length of a room or house) or maneuvering stairs on crutches requires significant arm strength, because the arms must bear the patient's weight. Muscle groups important for crutch walking include the following:

- Shoulder depressors—to stabilize the upper extremity and prevent shoulder hiking
- Shoulder adductors—to hold the crutch top against the chest wall
- Arm flexors, extensors, and abductors (at the shoulder)—to move crutches forward, backward, and sideways
- Forearm extensors—to prevent flexion or buckling; important in raising the body for swinging gait
- Wrist extensors—to enable weight bearing on the hand-piece
- Finger and thumb flexors—to grasp the hand-piece

### PREPARING PATIENTS TO WALK WITH CRUTCHES

Preparatory exercises are prescribed to strengthen the shoulder girdle and upper extremity muscles. Meanwhile, crutches need to be adjusted for the patient before he or she begins ambulating. To determine the approximate crutch length, the patient is measured standing or lying down. Standing patients are positioned against the wall with the feet slightly apart and away from the wall. Then a distance of 5 cm (2 inches) is marked on the floor, out to the side from the tip of the toe; 15 cm (6 inches) is measured straight ahead from the first mark, and this point is marked on the floor. Next, 5 cm (2 inches) is measured below the axilla to the second mark for the approximate crutch length.

If the patient must be measured while lying down, he or she is measured from the anterior fold of the axilla to the sole of the foot, and then 5 cm (2 inches) are added. If the patient's height is used, 40 cm (16 inches) is subtracted to obtain the approximate crutch length. The hand-piece should be adjusted to allow 20 to 30 degrees of flexion at the elbow. The wrist should be extended and the hand dorsiflexed. A foam rubber pad on the underarm piece is used to relieve the pressure of the crutch on the upper arm and thoracic cage. For safety, crutches should have large rubber tips, and the patient should wear firm-soled shoes that fit well.

### TEACHING CRUTCH WALKING

The nurse or physical therapist explains and demonstrates to the patient how to use the crutches. The patient learns standing balance by standing on the unaffected leg by a chair. To help the patient maintain balance, the nurse holds the patient near the waist or uses a transfer belt.

The patient is taught to support his or her weight on the hand-pieces. (For patients who cannot support their weight through the wrist and hand because of arthritis or fracture, platform crutches that support the forearm and allow the weight to be borne through the elbow are available.) If weight is borne on the axilla, the pressure of the crutch can damage the brachial plexus nerves, producing "crutch paralysis."

For maximum stability, the patient first assumes the tripod position by placing the crutches about 20 to 25 cm (8 to 10 inches) in front and to the side of his or her toes (Fig. 11-2). (This base of support is adjusted according to the height of the patient; a tall person requires a broader base of support than does a short person.) In this position, the patient learns how to shift weight and maintain balance. Before teaching crutch walking, the nurse or therapist determines which gait is best for the patient. The more common gaits are the four-point, the three-point, the two-point, and the swinging-to and swinging-through gaits. The sequence of movements for each of these gaits is depicted in Chart 11-8.

The selection of crutch gait depends on the type and severity of the patient's disability and on the patient's physical condition, arm and trunk strength, and body balance. The patient should be taught two gaits so that he or she can change from one to another. Shifting crutch gaits relieves fatigue, because each gait requires the use of a different combination of muscles (if a muscle is forced to contract steadily

FIGURE 11-2. Crutch walking. The tripod position for basic crutch stance.

without relaxing, the circulation of the blood to that part is decreased). A faster gait can be used when walking an uninterrupted distance, and a slower gait can be used for short distances or in crowded places.

The nurse walks with the patient who is just learning how to ambulate with crutches, holding the patient at the waist as needed for balance. During this time, the nurse protects the patient from falls and continually assesses the patient's stability and stamina, because prolonged periods of bed rest and inactivity affect strength and endurance. Sweating and shortness of breath are indications that crutch-walking practice should be stopped and the patient permitted to rest.

**TEACHING MANEUVERING TECHNIQUES**

Before the patient is considered to be independent in crutch walking, he or she should learn to sit in a chair, stand from sitting, and go up and down stairs using the crutches.

*To sit down:*

1. Grasp the crutches at the hand-pieces for control.
2. Bend forward slightly while assuming a sitting position.
3. Place the affected leg forward to prevent weight bearing and flexion.

*To stand up:*

1. Move forward to the edge of the chair with the strong leg slightly under the seat.
2. Place both crutches in the hand on the side of the affected extremity.
3. Push down on the hand-piece while raising the body to a standing position.

*To go down stairs:*

1. Walk forward as far as possible on the step.
2. Advance crutches to the lower step. The weaker leg is advanced first and then the stronger one. In this way, the stronger extremity shares with the arms the work of raising and lowering the body weight.

*To go up stairs:*

1. Advance the stronger leg first up to the next step.
2. Advance the crutches and the weaker extremity. Note that the strong leg goes up first and comes down last. A memory device for patients is, "Up with the good, down with the bad."

### Ambulating With a Walker

A walker provides more support and stability than a cane or crutches. There are two types of walkers: pick-up walkers and rolling walkers. A pick-up walker (one that has to be picked up and moved with each step forward) does not permit a natural walking pattern and is useful for patients who have poor balance or limited cardiovascular reserve or who cannot use crutches. A rolling walker allows automatic walking and is used by patients who cannot lift or who inappropriately carry a pick-up walker. The height of the walker is adjusted to the individual patient. The patient's arms should exhibit 20 to 30 degrees of flexion at the elbows when his or her hands are resting on the walker's hand grips. The patient should wear sturdy, well-fitting shoes. The nurse walks with the patient, holds him or her at the waist as needed for balance, continually assesses the patient's stability, and protects the patient from falls.

Patients are instructed to ambulate with a pick-up walker as follows:

1. Push off a chair or bed to come to a standing position. Never pull yourself up using the walker.
2. Hold the walker on the hand grips for stability.
3. Lift the walker, placing it in front of you while leaning your body slightly forward.
4. Walk into the walker, supporting your body weight on your hands when advancing your weaker leg, permitting partial weight bearing or non–weight bearing as prescribed.
5. Balance yourself on your feet.
6. Lift the walker, and place it in front of you again. Continue this pattern of walking.
7. Remember to look up as you walk.

### Ambulating With a Cane

A cane helps the patient walk with greater balance and support and relieves the pressure on weight-bearing joints by redistributing weight. Quad canes (four-footed canes) provide more stability than straight canes. To fit a patient for a cane, the patient is instructed to flex the elbow at a 30-degree angle, hold

### CHART 11-8

## Crutch Gaits

Shaded areas are weight-bearing. Arrow indicates advance of foot or crutch. (Read chart from bottom, starting with beginning stance.)

| 4-POINT GAIT | 2-POINT GAIT | 3-POINT GAIT | SWING-TO | SWING-THROUGH |
|---|---|---|---|---|
| • Partial weight bearing both feet<br>• Maximal support provided<br>• Requires constant shift of weight | • Partial weight bearing both feet<br>• Provides less support<br>• Faster than a 4 point gait | • Non-weight bearing<br>• Requires good balance<br>• Requires arm strength<br>• Faster gait<br>• Can use with walker | • Weight bearing both feet<br>• Provides stability<br>• Requires arm strength<br>• Can use with walker | • Weight bearing<br>• Requires arm strength<br>• Requires coordination/balance<br>• Most advanced gait |
| 4. Advance right foot | 4. Advance right foot and left crutch | 4. Advance right foot | 4. Lift both feet/swing forward/land feet next to crutches | 4. Lift both feet/swing forward/land feet in front of crutches |
| 3. Advance left crutch | 3. Advance left foot and right crutch | 3. Advance left foot and both crutches | 3. Advance both crutches | 3. Advance both crutches |
| 2. Advance left foot | 2. Advance right foot and left crutch | 2. Advance right foot | 2. Lift both feet/swing forward/land feet next to crutches | 2. Lift both feet/swing forward/land feet in front of crutches |
| 1. Advance right crutch | 1. Advance left foot and right crutch | 1. Advance left foot and both crutches | 1. Advance both crutches | 1. Advance both crutches |
| Beginning stance | Beginning stance | Beginning stance | Beginning stance | Beginning stance |

the handle of the cane about level with the greater trochanter, and place the tip of the cane 15 cm (6 inches) lateral to the base of the fifth toe. Adjustable canes make individualization easy. The cane should be fitted with a gently flaring tip that has flexible, concentric rings; the tip with its concentric rings provides optimal stability, functions as a shock absorber, and enables the patient to walk with greater speed and less fatigue.

The cane is held in the hand opposite the affected extremity. In normal walking, the opposite leg and arm move together (reciprocal motion); this motion is to be carried through in walking with a cane. Patients are taught to ambulate with a cane as follows:

*Cane–foot sequence:*

1. Hold the cane in the hand opposite the affected extremity to widen the base of support and to reduce the stress on the involved extremity. If the patient cannot use the cane in the opposite hand for some reason, the cane may be used on the same side.
2. Advance the cane at the same time the affected leg is moved forward.
3. Keep the cane fairly close to the body to prevent leaning.
4. Bear down on the cane when the unaffected extremity begins the swing phase.

*To go up and down stairs using the cane:*

1. Step up on the unaffected extremity.
2. Place the cane and affected extremity up on the step.
3. Reverse this procedure for descending steps ("up with the good, down with the bad").

As with all patients beginning ambulation with an assistive device, the nurse continually assesses the patient's stability and protects the patient from falls. The nurse accompanies the patient, holding him or her at the waist as needed for balance. The patient is assessed for tolerance of walking, and rest periods are provided as needed.

### Assisting Patients with an Orthosis or Prosthesis

Orthoses and prostheses are designed to facilitate mobilization and to maximize the patient's quality of life. An orthosis is an external appliance that provides support, prevents or corrects deformities, and improves function. Orthoses include braces, splints, collars, corsets, and supports that are designed and fitted by orthotists or prosthetists. Static orthoses (no moving parts) are used to stabilize joints and prevent contractures. Dynamic orthoses are flexible and are used to improve function by assisting weak muscles. A prosthesis is an artificial body part; it may be internal, such as an artificial knee or hip joint, or external, such as an artificial leg or arm.

In addition to learning how to apply and remove the orthosis and maneuver the affected body part correctly, rehabilitation patients must learn how to properly care for the skin that comes in contact with the appliance. Skin problems or **pressure ulcers** may develop if the device is applied too tightly or too loosely, or if it is adjusted improperly. The nurse instructs the patient to clean and inspect the skin daily, to make sure the brace fits snugly without being too tight, to check that the padding distributes pressure evenly, and to wear a cotton garment without seams between the orthosis and the skin.

If the patient has had an amputation, the nurse promotes tissue healing, uses compression dressings to promote residual limb shaping, and minimizes contracture formation. A permanent prosthetic limb cannot be fitted until the tissue has healed completely and the residual limb shape is stable and free of edema. The nurse also helps the patient cope with the emotional issues surrounding loss of a limb and encourages acceptance of the prosthesis. The prosthetist, nurse, and physician collaborate to provide instructions related to skin care and care of the prosthesis.

## Evaluation

### Expected Patient Outcomes

Expected patient outcomes may include:

1. Demonstrates improved physical mobility
    a. Maintains muscle strength and joint mobility
    b. Does not develop contractures
    c. Participates in exercise program
2. Transfers safely
    a. Demonstrates assisted transfers
    b. Performs independent transfers
3. Ambulates with maximum independence
    a. Uses ambulatory aid safely
    b. Adheres to weight-bearing prescription
    c. Requests assistance as needed
4. Demonstrates increased activity tolerance
    a. Does not experience episodes of orthostatic hypotension
    b. Reports absence of fatigue with ambulatory efforts
    c. Gradually increases distance and speed of ambulation

## ◄◄►► Nursing Process

## The Patient With Impaired Skin Integrity

An estimated 1.5 to 3 million patients develop pressure ulcers annually (Morrison, 2001). Both prevention and treatment of pressure ulcers are costly in terms of health care dollars and quality of life for patients at risk. All possible efforts to prevent skin breakdown should be made.

Pressure ulcers are localized areas of infarcted soft tissue that occur when pressure applied to the skin over time is greater than normal capillary closure pressure, which is about 32 mm Hg. Critically ill patients have a lower capillary closure pressure and a greater risk of pressure ulcers. Patients confined to bed for long periods, those with motor or sensory dysfunction, and those who experience muscular atrophy and reduction of padding between the overlying skin and the underlying bone are prone to pressure ulcers. The initial sign of pressure is erythema (redness of the skin) caused by reactive hyperemia, which normally resolves in less than 1 hour. Unrelieved pressure results in tissue ischemia or anoxia. The cutaneous tissues become broken or destroyed, leading to progressive destruction and necrosis of underlying soft tissue, and the resulting pressure ulcer is painful and slow to heal.

## Assessment

Immobility, impaired sensory perception or cognition, decreased tissue perfusion, decreased nutritional status, friction and shear forces, increased moisture, and age-related skin changes all contribute to the development of pressure ulcers.

### Immobility

When a person is immobile and inactive, pressure is exerted on the skin and subcutaneous tissue by objects on which the person rests, such as a mattress, chair seat, or cast. The development of pressure ulcers is directly related to the duration of immobility: if pressure continues long enough, small vessel thrombosis and tissue necrosis occur, and a pressure ulcer results. Weight-bearing bony prominences are most susceptible to pressure ulcer development because they are covered only by skin and small amounts of subcutaneous tissue. Susceptible areas include the sacrum and coccygeal areas, ischial tuberosities (especially in people who sit for prolonged periods), greater trochanter, heel, knee, malleolus, medial condyle of the tibia, fibular head, scapula, and elbow (Fig. 11-3).

### Impaired Sensory Perception or Cognition

Patients with sensory loss, impaired level of consciousness, or paralysis may not be aware of the discomfort associated with prolonged pressure on the skin and therefore may not change their position themselves to relieve the pressure. This prolonged pressure impedes blood flow, reducing nourishment of the skin and underlying tissues. A pressure ulcer may develop in a short period of time.

### Decreased Tissue Perfusion

Any condition that reduces the circulation and nourishment of the skin and subcutaneous tissue (altered

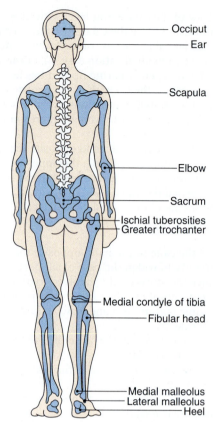

**FIGURE 11-3.** Areas susceptible to pressure ulcers.

peripheral tissue perfusion) increases the risk of pressure ulcer development. Patients with diabetes mellitus experience an alteration in microcirculation. Similarly, patients with edema have impaired circulation and poor nourishment of the skin tissue. Obese patients have large amounts of poorly vascularized adipose tissue, which is susceptible to breakdown.

### Decreased Nutritional Status

Nutritional deficiencies, anemias, and metabolic disorders also contribute to development of pressure ulcers. Anemia, regardless of its cause, decreases the blood's oxygen-carrying ability and predisposes the patient to pressure ulcers. Patients who have low protein levels or who are in a negative nitrogen balance experience tissue wasting and inhibited tissue repair. Serum albumin is a sensitive indicator of protein deficiency; serum albumin levels of less than 3 g per mL are associated with hypoalbuminemic tissue edema and increased risk of pressure ulcers. The nurse should assess the patient's prealbumin and albumin values and electrolyte panel. Specific nutrients, such as vitamin C and trace minerals, are needed for tissue maintenance and repair.

### Friction and Shear

Mechanical forces also contribute to the development of pressure ulcers. Friction is the resistance to movement that occurs when two surfaces are moved across each other. Shear is created by the interplay of gravitational forces (forces that push the body down) and friction. When shear occurs, tissue layers slide over one another, blood vessels stretch and twist, and the microcirculation of the skin and subcutaneous tissue is disrupted. Evidence of deep tissue damage may be slow to develop and may present through the development of a sinus tract. The sacrum and heels are most susceptible to the effects of shear. Pressure ulcers from friction and shear occur when the patient slides down in bed (Fig. 11-4) or when the patient is positioned or moved improperly (eg, dragged up in bed). Spastic muscles and paralysis increase the patient's vulnerability to pressure ulcers related to friction and shear.

### Increased Moisture

Prolonged contact with moisture from perspiration, urine, feces, or drainage produces maceration (softening) of the skin. The skin reacts to the caustic substances in the excreta or drainage and becomes irritated. Moist, irritated skin is more vulnerable to pressure breakdown. Once the skin breaks, the area is invaded by microorganisms (eg, streptococci, staphylococci, *Pseudomonas aeruginosa*, *Escherichia coli*), and infection occurs. Foul-smelling infectious drainage is present. The lesion may enlarge and allow a continuous loss of serum, which may further deplete the body of essential protein needed for tissue repair and maintenance. The lesion may continue to enlarge and extend deep into the fascia, muscle, and bone, with multiple sinus tracts radiating from the pressure ulcer. With extensive pressure ulcers, life-threatening infections and sepsis may develop, frequently from gram-negative organisms.

### Gerontologic Considerations

In older adults, the skin has diminished epidermal thickness, dermal collagen, and tissue elasticity. The skin is drier as a result of diminished sebaceous and sweat gland activity. Cardiovascular changes result in decreased tissue perfusion. Muscles atrophy, and bone structures become prominent. Diminished sensory perception and reduced ability to reposition oneself contribute to prolonged pressure on the skin. Therefore, older adults are more susceptible to pressure ulcers, which cause pain and suffering and reduce quality of life.

### Nursing Actions Related to Assessment

In assessing patients for potential risk for pressure ulcer development, the nurse assesses the patient's mobility, sensory perception, cognitive abilities, tissue perfusion, nutritional status, friction and shear forces, sources of moisture on the skin, and age. Nursing actions include the following:

- Assess total skin condition at least twice a day.
- Inspect each pressure site for erythema.
- Assess areas of erythema for blanching response.
- Palpate the skin for increased warmth.
- Inspect for dry skin, moist skin, breaks in skin.
- Note drainage and odor.
- Evaluate level of mobility.
- Note safety and assistive devices (eg, restraints, splints).
- Evaluate circulatory status (eg, peripheral pulses, edema).
- Assess neurovascular status.
- Determine presence of incontinence.
- Evaluate nutritional and hydration status.
- Review the patient's record for laboratory studies, including hematocrit, hemoglobin, electrolytes, albumin, transferrin, and creatinine.
- Note present health problems.
- Review current medications.

Scales such as the Braden or Norton scale may be used to facilitate systematic assessment and quantification of a patient's risk for pressure ulcer, although the nurse should recognize that the reliability of these scales is not well established for all patient populations. Chart 11-9 lists risk factors for pressure ulcers. If a pressure area is noted, the nurse notes its size and location and uses a grading system to describe its severity (Chart 11-10).

Generally, a stage I pressure ulcer is an area of nonblanchable erythema, tissue swelling, and congestion. The patient complains of discomfort. The skin temperature is elevated because of the increased vasodilation. The redness progresses to a dusky, cyanotic blue-gray appearance, which is the result of skin capillary occlusion and subcutaneous weakening.

A stage II pressure ulcer is a break in the skin that extends through the epidermis or the dermis. An abrasion, blister, or shallow crater may be seen. Necrosis occurs along with venous sludging and thrombosis and edema with cellular extravasation and infiltration.

A stage III pressure ulcer extends into the subcutaneous tissues or fascia. Clinically, a deep crater with or without undermining of adjacent tissues is noted.

**FIGURE 11-4.** Mechanical forces contribute to pressure ulcer development. As the person slides down or is improperly pulled up in bed, *friction* resists this movement. *Shear* occurs when one layer of tissue slides over another, disrupting microcirculation of skin and subcutaneous tissue.

## CHART 11-9  Risk Factors for Pressure Ulcers

- Prolonged pressure on tissue
- Immobility, compromised mobility
- Loss of protective reflexes, sensory deficit/loss
- Poor skin perfusion, edema
- Malnutrition, hypoproteinemia, anemia, vitamin deficiency
- Friction, shearing forces, trauma
- Incontinence of urine or feces
- Altered skin moisture: excessively dry, excessively moist
- Advanced age, debilitation
- Equipment: casts, traction, restraints

A stage IV pressure ulcer extends into the underlying structures, including the muscle and possibly the bone. The skin lesion may appear insignificant when, in reality, beneath the small surface ulcer is a large undermined area of necrotic tissue.

The appearance of purulent drainage or foul odor suggests an infection. With an extensive pressure ulcer, deep pockets of infection are often present. Drying and crusting of exudate may be present. Infection of a pressure ulcer may advance to osteomyelitis, pyarthrosis (pus formation within a joint cavity), sepsis, and septic shock.

## Nursing Diagnosis

Based on the assessment data, the nursing diagnoses may include the following:

- Risk for impaired skin integrity
- Impaired skin integrity (related to immobility, decreased sensory perception, decreased tissue perfusion, decreased nutritional status, friction and shear forces, excessive moisture, or advanced age)

## Planning and Goals

The major goals may include relief of pressure, improved mobility, improved sensory perception, improved tissue perfusion, improved nutritional status, minimized friction and shear forces, dry surfaces in contact with skin, and healing of pressure ulcer, if present.

## Nursing Interventions

### Relieving Pressure

Frequent changes of position are needed to relieve and redistribute the pressure on the patient's skin and to prevent prolonged reduced blood flow to the skin and subcutaneous tissues. This can be accomplished by teaching the patient to change position or by turning and repositioning the patient. The patient's family members should be taught how to position and turn the patient at home to prevent pressure ulcers. Shifting weight allows the blood to flow into the ischemic areas and helps tissues recover from the effects of pressure. Thus, the patient should be cared for as follows:

- Turned and repositioned at 1- to 2-hour intervals
- Encouraged to shift weight actively every 15 minutes

### Positioning the Patient

The patient should be positioned laterally, prone, and dorsally in sequence unless a position is not tolerated or is contraindicated. The recumbent position is preferred to the semi-Fowler's position because of increased supporting body surface area in this position. In addition to regular turning, there should be small shifts of body weight, such as repositioning of an ankle, elbow, or shoulder. The skin is inspected at each position change and assessed for temperature elevation. If redness or heat is noted or if the patient complains of discomfort, pressure on the area must be relieved.

Another way to relieve pressure over bony prominences is the bridging technique, accomplished through the correct positioning of pillows. Just as a bridge is supported on pillars to allow traffic to move underneath, the body can be supported by pillows to allow for space between bony prominences and the mattress. A pillow or commercial heel protector may be used to support the heels off the bed when the patient is supine. Placing pillows superior and inferior to the sacrum relieves sacral pressure. Supporting the patient in a 30-degree side-lying position avoids pressure on the trochanter. In aging patients, frequent small shifts of body weight may be effective. Placing a small rolled towel or sheepskin under a shoulder or hip allows a return of blood flow to the skin in the area on which the patient is sitting or lying. The towel or sheepskin is moved around the patient's pressure points in a clockwise fashion. A turning schedule can help the family keep track of the patient's turns.

### Using Pressure-Relieving Devices

At times, special equipment and beds may be needed to help relieve the pressure on the skin. This is particularly important for patients who cannot get out of bed and who have risk factors for pressure ulcer development. These devices are designed to provide support for specific body areas or to distribute pressure evenly.

A patient who sits in a wheelchair for prolonged periods should have wheelchair cushions fitted and adjusted on an individualized basis, using pressure measurement techniques as a guide to selection and fitting. The aim is to redistribute pressure away from areas at risk for ulcers, but no cushion can eliminate excessive pressure completely. The patient should be reminded to shift weight frequently and to rise for a few seconds every 15 minutes while sitting in a chair (Fig. 11-5).

## CHART 11-10

### Assessing for Pressure Ulcer Stages

**Stage I**
- Area of erythema
- Erythema does not blanch with pressure
- Skin temperature elevated
- Tissue swollen and congested
- Patient complains of discomfort
- Erythema progresses to dusky blue-gray

**Stage II**
- Skin breaks
- Abrasion, blister, or shallow crater
- Edema persists
- Ulcer drains
- Infection may develop
- Partial-thickness wound

**Stage III**
- Ulcer extends into subcutaneous tissue
- Necrosis and drainage continue
- Infection develops
- Full-thickness wound

**Stage IV**
- Ulcer extends to underlying muscle and bone
- Deep pockets of infection develop
- Necrosis and drainage continue
- Full-thickness wound

From Weber, J. W., & Kelley, J. (2003). *Health assessment in nursing* (2nd ed.). Philadelphia: Lippincott Williams & Wilkins.

Static support devices (such as high-density foam, air, or liquid mattress overlays) distribute pressure evenly by bringing more of the patient's body surface into contact with the supporting surface. Gel-type flotation pads and air-fluidized beds reduce pressure. The weight of a body floating on a fluid system is evenly distributed over the entire supporting surface (according to Pascal's law). Therefore, as the body sinks into the fluid, additional surface becomes available for weight bearing, body weight per unit area is decreased, and there is less pressure on the body parts.

**FIGURE 11-5.** Wheelchair push-up to prevent ischial pressure ulcers. These push-ups should become an automatic routine (every 15 minutes) for the person with paraplegia. The person should stay up, out of contact with the seat for several seconds. The wheels are kept in the locked position during the exercise.

Soft, moisture-absorbing padding is also useful because the softness and resilience of padding provide for more even distribution of pressure and the dissipation and absorption of moisture, along with freedom from wrinkles and friction. Bony prominences may be protected by gel pads, sheepskin padding, or soft foam rubber beneath the sacrum, the trochanters, heels, elbows, scapulae, and back of the head when there is pressure on these sites.

Specialized beds have been designed to prevent pressure on the skin. Air-fluidized beds allow the patient to float. Dynamic support surfaces, such as low air-loss pockets, alternately inflate and deflate sections to change support pressure for very high-risk patients who are critically ill and debilitated and cannot be repositioned to relieve pressure. Oscillating or kinetic beds change pressure by means of rocking movements of the bed that redistribute the patient's weight and stimulate circulation. These beds are frequently used with patients who have injuries due to multiple trauma.

### Improving Mobility

The patient is encouraged to remain active and is ambulated whenever possible. When sitting, the patient is reminded to change positions frequently to redistribute weight. Active and passive exercises increase muscular, skin, and vascular tone. Activity stimulates circulation, which relieves tissue ischemia, the forerunner of pressure ulcers. For patients at risk for pressure ulcers, turning and exercise schedules are essential: repositioning must occur around the clock.

### Improving Sensory Perception

The nurse helps the patient recognize and compensate for altered sensory perception. Depending on the origin of the alteration (eg, decreased level of consciousness, spinal cord lesion), specific interventions are selected. Strategies to improve cognition and sensory perception may include stimulating the patient to increase awareness of self in the environment, encouraging the patient to participate in self-care, or supporting the patient's efforts toward active compensation for loss of sensation (eg, a patient with paraplegia lifting up from the sitting position every 15 minutes). A patient with quadriplegia should be weight-shifted every 30 minutes while sitting in a wheelchair. When decreased sensory perception exists, the patient and caregivers are taught to inspect potential pressure areas visually every morning and evening, using a mirror if necessary, for evidence of pressure ulcer development.

### Improving Tissue Perfusion

Exercise and repositioning improve tissue perfusion. Massage of erythematous areas is avoided because damage to the capillaries and deep tissue may occur.

**Avoid massaging reddened areas, because this may increase the damage to already traumatized skin and tissue.**

In patients who have evidence of compromised peripheral circulation (eg, edema), positioning and elevation of the edematous body part to promote venous return and diminish congestion improve tissue perfusion. In addition, the nurse or family must be alert to environmental factors (eg, wrinkles in sheets, pressure of tubes) that may contribute to pressure on the skin and diminished circulation and remove the source of pressure.

### Improving Nutritional Status

The patient's nutritional status must be adequate and a positive nitrogen balance must be maintained because pressure ulcers develop more quickly and are more resistant to treatment in patients with nutritional disorders. A high-protein diet with protein supplements may be helpful. Iron preparations may be necessary to raise the hemoglobin concentration so that tissue oxygen levels can be maintained within acceptable limits. Ascorbic acid (vitamin C) is necessary for tissue healing. Other nutrients associated with healthy skin include vitamin A, B vitamins, zinc, and sulfur. With balanced nutrition and hydration, the skin can remain healthy and damaged tissues can be repaired (Table 11-2).

To assess the patient's nutritional status in response to therapeutic strategies, the nurse monitors the patient's hemoglobin, prealbumin level, and body weight weekly. Nutritional assessment is described in further detail in Chapter 5.

### Reducing Friction and Shear

Shear occurs when patients are pulled, allowed to slump, or move by digging heels or elbows into the mattress. Raising the head of the bed by even a few centimeters increases the shearing force over the sacral area; therefore, the semireclining position is avoided in patients at risk. Proper positioning with adequate support is also important when the patient is sitting in a chair. Polyester sheepskin pads are thought to reduce shear and friction and may be used with at-risk patients.

**NURSING ALERT**

To avoid shearing forces when repositioning patients, nurses must lift and must avoid dragging patients across a surface.

### Minimizing Irritating Moisture

Continuous moisture on the skin must be prevented by meticulous hygiene measures. Perspiration, urine, stool, and drainage must be removed from the skin promptly. The soiled skin should be washed immediately with mild soap and water and blotted dry with a soft towel. The skin may be lubricated with a bland lotion to keep it soft and pliable. Drying agents and powders are avoided. Topical barrier ointments (eg, petroleum jelly) may be helpful in protecting the skin of patients who are incontinent.

Absorbent pads that wick moisture away from the body should be used to absorb drainage. Patients who are incontinent need to be checked regularly and have their wet incontinence pads and linens changed promptly. Their skin needs to be cleansed and dried promptly.

### Promoting Pressure Ulcer Healing

Regardless of the stage of the pressure ulcer, the pressure on the area must be eliminated, because the ulcer will not heal until all pressure is removed. The patient must not lie or sit on the pressure ulcer, even for a few minutes. Individualized positioning and turning schedules must be written in the plan of nursing care and followed meticulously.

In addition, inadequate nutritional status and fluid and electrolyte abnormalities must be corrected to promote healing. Wounds from which body fluids and protein drain place the patient in a catabolic state and predispose to hypoproteinemia and serious secondary infections. Protein deficiency must be corrected to heal the pressure ulcer. Carbohydrates are necessary to "spare" the protein and to provide an energy source. Vitamin C and trace elements, especially zinc, are necessary for collagen formation and wound healing.

**STAGE I PRESSURE ULCERS**
To permit healing of stage I pressure ulcers, the pressure is removed to allow increased tissue perfusion, nutritional and fluid and electrolyte balance are maintained, friction and shear are reduced, and moisture to the skin is avoided.

| TABLE 11-2 | Nutritional Requirements to Promote Healing of Pressure Ulcers | |
|---|---|---|
| **Nutrient** | **Rationale** | **Recommended Amount** |
| Protein | Tissue repair | 1.25–1.50 g/kg/day |
| Calories | Spare protein | 30–35 calories/kg/day |
| | Restore normal weight | |
| Water | Maintain homeostasis | 1 mL/calorie fed or 30 mL/kg/day |
| Multivitamin | Promote collagen formation | 1 daily |
| Vitamin C | Promote collagen synthesis | 500–1000 mg daily |
| | Support integrity of capillary wall | |
| Zinc sulfate | Cofactor for collagen formation and protein synthesis | 220 mg daily |
| | Normal lymphocyte and phagocyte response | |
| Vitamin A | Stimulate epithelial cells | — |
| | Stimulate immune response | |
| | *Caution:* An excess can cause an excessive inflammatory response that could impair healing | |

### STAGE II PRESSURE ULCERS

Stage II pressure ulcers have broken skin. In addition to measures listed for stage I pressure ulcers, a moist environment, in which migration of epidermal cells over the ulcer surface occurs more rapidly, should be provided to aid wound healing. The ulcer is gently cleansed with sterile saline solution. Use of a heat lamp to dry the open wound is avoided, as is use of antiseptic solutions that damage healthy tissues and delay wound healing. Semipermeable occlusive dressings, hydrocolloid wafers, or wet saline dressings are helpful in providing a moist environment for healing and in minimizing the loss of fluids and proteins from the body.

### STAGE III AND IV PRESSURE ULCERS

Stage III and IV pressure ulcers are characterized by extensive tissue damage. In addition to the measures listed for stage I, these advanced draining, necrotic pressure ulcers must be cleaned (débrided) to create an area that will heal. Necrotic, devitalized tissue favors bacterial growth, delays granulation, and inhibits healing. Wound cleaning and dressing are uncomfortable; therefore, the nurse must prepare the patient for the procedure by explaining what will occur and administering prescribed analgesia.

Débridement may be accomplished by wet-to-damp dressing changes, mechanical flushing of necrotic and infective exudate, application of prescribed enzyme preparations that dissolve necrotic tissue, or surgical dissection. If an eschar covers the ulcer, it is removed surgically to ensure a clean, vitalized wound. Exudate may be absorbed by dressings or special hydrophilic powders, beads, or gels. Cultures of infected pressure ulcers are obtained to guide the selection of antibiotic therapy.

After the pressure ulcer is clean, a topical treatment is prescribed to promote granulation. New granulation tissue must be protected from reinfection, drying, and damage, and care should be taken to prevent pressure and further trauma to the area. Dressings, solutions, and ointments applied to the ulcer should not disrupt the healing process. Multiple agents and protocols are used to treat pressure ulcers, but consistency is an important key to success. Objective evaluation of the pressure ulcer (eg, measurement of the size and depth of the pressure ulcer, inspection for granulation tissue) for response to the treatment protocol must be made every 4 to 6 days. Taking photographs at weekly intervals is a reliable strategy for monitoring the healing process, which may take weeks to months.

Surgical intervention is necessary when the ulcer is extensive, when complications (eg, fistula) exist, and when the ulcer does not respond to treatment. Surgical procedures include débridement, incision and drainage, bone resection, and skin grafting. Osteomyelitis is a common complication of wounds of stage IV depth. See Chapter 68 for more information on osteomyelitis.

### *Preventing Recurrence*

Recurrence of pressure ulcers should be anticipated; therefore, active, preventive intervention and frequent continuing assessments are essential. The patient's tolerance for sitting or lying on the healed pressure area is increased gradually by increasing the time that pressure is allowed on the area in 5- to 15-minute increments. The patient is taught to increase mobility and to follow a regimen of turning, weight-shifting, and repositioning. The patient teaching plan includes strategies to reduce the risk of pressure ulcers and methods to detect, inspect, and minimize pressure areas. Early recognition and intervention are keys to long-term management of potential impaired skin integrity.

## Evaluation

### *Expected Patient Outcomes*

Expected patient outcomes may include:

1. Maintains intact skin
   a. Exhibits no areas of nonblanchable erythema at bony prominences
   b. Avoids massage of bony prominences
   c. Exhibits no breaks in skin
2. Limits pressure on bony prominences
   a. Changes position every 1 to 2 hours
   b. Uses bridging techniques to reduce pressure
   c. Uses special equipment as appropriate
   d. Raises self from seat of wheelchair every 15 minutes
3. Increases mobility
   a. Performs range-of-motion exercises
   b. Adheres to turning schedule
   c. Advances sitting time as tolerated
4. Sensory and cognitive ability improved
   a. Demonstrates improved level of consciousness
   b. Remembers to inspect potential pressure ulcer areas every morning and evening
5. Demonstrates improved tissue perfusion
   a. Exercises to increase circulation
   b. Elevates body parts susceptible to edema
6. Attains and maintains adequate nutritional status
   a. Verbalizes the importance of protein and vitamin C in diet
   b. Eats diet high in protein and vitamin C
   c. Exhibits hemoglobin, electrolyte, prealbumin, transferrin, and creatinine levels at acceptable levels
7. Avoids friction and shear
   a. Avoids semireclining position
   b. Uses sheepskin pad and heel protectors when appropriate
   c. Lifts body instead of sliding across surfaces
8. Maintains clean, dry skin
   a. Avoids prolonged contact with wet or soiled surfaces
   b. Keeps skin clean and dry
   c. Uses lotion to keep skin lubricated

## Nursing Process

### The Patient With Altered Elimination Patterns

Urinary and bowel incontinence or constipation and impaction are problems that often occur in patients with disabilities. Incontinence curtails the person's independence, causing embarrassment and isolation. It occurs in as much as 15% of the community-based elderly population, and nearly 50% of nursing home residents have bowel or bladder incontinence or both. In addition, constipation may be a problem in patients with disabilities. Complete and predictable evacuation of the bowel is the goal. If a bowel routine is not established, the patient may experience abdominal distention; small, frequent oozing of stool; or impaction.

### Assessment

Urinary incontinence may result from multiple causes, including urinary tract infection, detrusor instability, bladder outlet obstruction or incompetence, neurologic impairment, bladder spasm or contracture, and inability to reach the toilet in time. Urinary incontinence can be classified as urge, reflex, stress, functional, or total:

- *Urge incontinence:* involuntary elimination of urine associated with a strong perceived need to void
- *Reflex (neurogenic) incontinence:* associated with a spinal cord lesion that interrupts cerebral control, resulting in no sensory awareness of the need to void
- *Stress incontinence:* associated with weakened perineal muscles that permit leakage of urine when intra-abdominal pressure is increased (eg, with coughing or sneezing)
- *Functional incontinence:* incontinence in patients with intact urinary physiology who experience mobility impairment, environmental barriers, or cognitive problems and cannot reach and use the toilet before soiling themselves
- *Total incontinence:* occurs in patients who cannot control excreta because of physiologic or psychological impairment; management of the excreta is an essential focus of nursing care.

The health history is used to explore bladder and bowel function, symptoms associated with dysfunction, physiologic risk factors for elimination problems, perception of micturition and defecation cues, and functional toileting abilities. Previous and current fluid intake and voiding patterns may be helpful in designing the plan of nursing care. A record of times of voiding and amounts voided is kept for at least 48 hours. In addition, episodes of incontinence and associated activity (eg, coughing, sneezing, lifting), fluid intake time and amount, and medications are recorded. This record is analyzed and used to determine patterns and relationships of incontinence to other activities and factors.

The ability to get to the bathroom, manipulate clothing, and use the toilet are important functional factors that may be related to incontinence. Related cognitive functioning (perception of need to void, verbalization of need to void, and ability to learn to control urination) must also be assessed. In addition, the nurse reviews the results of the diagnostic studies (eg, urinalysis, urodynamic tests, postvoiding residual volumes). Chart 11-11 presents the factors that affect elimination in older adults.

Bowel incontinence and constipation may result from multiple causes, such as diminished or absent sphincter control, cognitive or perceptual impairment, neurogenic factors, diet, and immobility. The origin of the bowel problem must be determined. The nurse assesses the patient's normal bowel patterns, nutritional patterns, use of laxatives, gastrointestinal problems (eg, colitis), bowel sounds, anal reflex and tone, and functional abilities. The character and frequency of bowel movements are recorded and analyzed.

### Nursing Diagnosis

Based on the assessment data, major nursing diagnoses may include the following:

- Impaired bowel elimination
- Impaired urinary elimination

### Planning and Goals

The major goals may include control of urinary incontinence or urinary retention, control of bowel incontinence, and regular elimination patterns.

---

**CHART 11-11**

### Factors That Alter Urinary Elimination Patterns in the Older Adult

- Decreased bladder capacity
- Decreased muscle tone
- Increased residual volumes
- Delayed perception of elimination cues
- Use of medications that alter elimination patterns, such as diuretics (increase volume of urine produced), sedatives (alter bladder sensitivity to cues), and adrenergics or anticholinergics (cause urinary retention)
- Functional immobility
- Sedentary lifestyle

## Nursing Interventions

### Promoting Urinary Continence

After the nature of the urinary incontinence has been identified, a nursing plan of care is developed based on analysis of the assessment data. Various approaches to promote urinary continence have been developed. Most approaches attempt to condition the body to control urination or to minimize the occurrence of unscheduled urination. Selection of the approach depends on the cause and type of the incontinence. For the program to be successful, participation by the patient and a desire to avoid incontinence episodes are crucial; an optimistic attitude with positive feedback for even slight gains is essential for success. Accurate recording of intake and output and of the patient's response to selected strategies is essential for evaluation.

At no time should the fluid intake be restricted to decrease the frequency of urination. Sufficient fluid intake (2,000 to 3,000 mL per day, according to patient needs) must be ensured. To optimize the likelihood of voiding as scheduled, measured amounts of fluids may be administered about 30 minutes before voiding attempts. In addition, most of the fluids should be consumed before evening to minimize the need to void frequently during the night.

The goal of bladder training is to restore the bladder to normal function. Bladder training can be used with cognitively intact patients experiencing urge incontinence. A voiding and toileting schedule is formulated based on analysis of the assessment data. The schedule specifies times for the patient to try to empty the bladder using a bedpan, toilet, or commode. Privacy should be provided during voiding efforts. The interval between voiding times in the early phase of the bladder training period is short (90 to 120 minutes). The patient is encouraged not to void until the specified voiding time. Voiding success and episodes of incontinence are recorded. As the patient's bladder capacity and control increase, the interval is lengthened. Usually, there is a temporal relationship between drinking, eating, exercising, and voiding. Alert patients can participate in recording intake, activity, and voiding and can plan the schedule to achieve maximum continence. Barrier-free access to the toilet and modification of clothing can help patients with functional incontinence achieve self-care in toileting and continence.

Habit training is used to try to keep patients dry by strict adherence to a toileting schedule and may be successful with stress, urge, or functional incontinence. If the patient is confused, caregivers take the patient to the toilet according to the schedule before involuntary voiding occurs. Simple cuing and consistency promote success. Periods of continence and successful voidings are positively reinforced.

Biofeedback is a system through which patients learn consciously to contract urinary sphincters and control voiding cues. Cognitively intact patients who have stress or urge incontinence may gain bladder control through biofeedback.

Pelvic floor exercises (Kegel exercises) strengthen the pubococcygeus muscle. The patient is instructed to tighten the pelvic floor muscles for 4 seconds ten times, and this is repeated four to six times a day. Stopping and starting the stream during urination is recommended to increase control. Daily practice is essential. These exercises are helpful for cognitively intact women who experience stress incontinence.

Suprapubic tapping or stroking of the inner thigh may produce voiding by stimulating the voiding reflex arc in patients with reflex incontinence. However, this method is not always effective, because of detrusor–sphincter dyssynergy. As the bladder reflexively contracts to expel urine, the bladder sphincter reflexively closes, producing a high residual urine volume and an increased incidence of urinary tract infection.

Intermittent self-catheterization is an appropriate alternative for managing reflex incontinence, urinary retention, and overflow incontinence due to an overdistended bladder. The emphasis of patient teaching is on regular emptying of the bladder rather than sterility. Patients with disabilities may reuse and clean catheters with bleach or hydrogen peroxide solutions or soap and water and may use a microwave oven to sterilize catheters. Aseptic intermittent catheterization technique is required in health care institutions because of the potential for bladder infection from resistant organisms. Intermittent self-catheterization may be difficult for patients with limited mobility, dexterity, or vision; however, family members can be taught the procedure.

Indwelling catheters are avoided if at all possible because of the high incidence of urinary tract infections with their use. Short-term use may be needed during treatment of severe skin breakdown due to continued incontinence. Patients with disabilities who cannot perform intermittent self-catheterization may elect to use suprapubic catheters for long-term bladder management. Suprapubic catheters are easier to maintain than indwelling catheters. A daily fluid intake of 3000 mL is encouraged.

External catheters (condom catheters) and leg bags to collect spontaneous voidings are useful for male patients with reflex or total incontinence. The appropriate design and size must be chosen for maximal success, and the patient or caregiver must be taught how to apply the condom catheter and how to provide daily hygiene, including skin inspection. Instruction on emptying the leg bag must also be provided, and modifications can be made for patients with limited hand dexterity.

Incontinence pads (briefs) may be useful at times for patients with stress or total incontinence to protect clothing, but they should be avoided whenever possible. Incontinence pads only manage, rather than solve, the incontinence problem. Also, they have a negative psychological effect on patients, because many people think of the pads as diapers. Every effort should be made to reduce the incidence of incontinence episodes through the other methods that have been described. When incontinence pads are used, they should wick moisture away from the body to minimize contact of moisture and excreta with the skin. Wet incontinence pads must be changed promptly, the skin cleansed, and a moisture

## NURSING RESEARCH PROFILE

### Satisfaction with Urinary Management Following Spinal Cord Injury

Brillhart, B. (2004). Studying the quality of life and life satisfaction among persons with spinal cord injury undergoing urinary management. *Rehabilitation Nursing, 29*(4), 122–126.

#### Purpose
Patients with spinal cord injury (SCI) have needs related to urinary management and the prevention of urinary complications. The purpose of this study was to investigate quality of life and life satisfaction of patients with SCI who require different types of urinary management, including reflex voiding, indwelling catheter, suprapubic catheter, intermittent catheterization, external catheter, or a combination of intermittent catheterization and external catheter.

#### Design
From a nationwide survey of people with SCI, a sample of 230 people were selected to participate in the study. The mean age of the subjects was 44.6 years, and 75 percent of the subjects were male. The Quality of Life Index (QLI) and a Satisfaction with Life Scale (SWLS) were used as assessment tools to measure quality of life in these patients.

#### Findings
Results of the study revealed no significant differences in QLI and SWLS when comparing patients with the different types of urinary management ($p = .945$) and when comparing patients with different levels (cervical 1–4, cervical 5–7, thoracic 1–12, lumbar 1–4) of SCI ($p = .157$). However, the QLI and SWLS scores were significantly higher ($p = .002$, $p = .001$ and $p = .003$, respectively) for subjects who had greater ability to work, were attending school, and who participated in activities. Subjects who had not experienced skin complications related to urinary dysfunction had significantly higher QLI scores than those who had experienced such complications.

#### Nursing Implications
When caring for patients with SCI, nurses should help these patients focus on self-management of their urinary condition and resolution of any problems related to urinary management. Their plans of care should be individualized to promote maximum activity and function and should be flexible to meet their changing needs. Further studies are needed to determine common factors among SCI patients that promote self-care decision making and activities.

---

barrier applied to protect the skin. It is important for the patient's self-esteem to avoid use of the term "diapers."

### Promoting Bowel Continence

The goals of a bowel training program are to develop regular bowel habits and to prevent uninhibited bowel elimination. Regular, complete emptying of the lower bowel results in bowel continence. A bowel-training program takes advantage of the patient's natural reflexes. Regularity, timing, nutrition and fluids, exercise, and correct positioning promote predictable defecation.

The nurse records defecation time, character of stool, nutritional intake, cognitive abilities, and functional self-care toileting abilities for 5 to 7 days. Analysis of this record is helpful when designing a bowel program for patients with fecal incontinence.

Consistency in implementing the plan is essential. A regular time for defecation is established, and attempts at evacuation should be made within 15 minutes of the designated time daily. Natural gastrocolic and duodenocolic reflexes occur about 30 minutes after a meal; therefore, after breakfast is one of the best times to plan for bowel evacuation. However, if the patient had a previously established habit pattern at a different time of day, it should be followed.

The anorectal reflex may be stimulated by a rectal suppository (eg, glycerin) or by mechanical stimulation (eg, digital stimulation with a lubricated gloved finger or anal dilator). Mechanical stimulation should be used only in patients with a disability who have no voluntary motor function and no sensation as a result of injuries above the sacral segments of the spinal cord, such as patients with quadriplegia, high paraplegia, or severe brain injuries. The technique is not effective in patients who do not have an intact sacral reflex arc (eg, those with flaccid paralysis). Mechanical stimulation, suppository insertion, or both should be initiated about 30 minutes before the scheduled bowel elimination time, and the interval between stimulation and defecation is noted for subsequent modification of the bowel program. Once the bowel routine is well established, stimulation with a suppository may not be necessary.

The patient should assume the normal squatting position and be in a private bathroom for defecation if at all possible, although a padded commode chair or bedside toilet is an alternative. An elevated toilet seat is a simple modification that may make use of the toilet easier for the patient with a disability.

Seating time is limited in patients who are at risk for skin breakdown. Bedpans should be avoided. A patient with a disability who cannot sit on a toilet should be positioned on the left side with legs flexed and the head of the bed elevated 30 to 45 degrees to increase intra-abdominal pressure. Protective padding is placed behind the buttocks. When possible, the patient is instructed to bear down and to contract the abdominal muscles. Massaging the abdomen from right to left facilitates movement of feces in the lower tract.

### Preventing Constipation

The record of bowel elimination, character of stool, food and fluid intake, level of activity, bowel sounds, medications, and other assessment data are reviewed to develop the plan of care. Multiple approaches may be used to prevent constipation. The diet should be well balanced and should include adequate intake of high-fiber foods (vegetables, fruits, bran) to prevent hard stools and to stimulate peristalsis. Daily fluid intake should be 2 to 3 L unless contraindicated. Prune juice or fig juice (120 mL) taken 30 minutes before a meal once daily is helpful in some cases when constipation is a problem. Physical activity and exercise are encouraged, as is self-care in toileting. Patients are encouraged to respond to the natural urge to defecate. Privacy during toileting is provided. Stool softeners, bulk-forming agents, mild stimulants, and suppositories may be prescribed to stimulate defecation and to prevent constipation.

## Evaluation

### Expected Patient Outcomes

Expected patient outcomes may include:

1. Demonstrates control of bowel and bladder function
   a. Experiences no episodes of incontinence
   b. Avoids constipation
   c. Achieves independence in toileting
   d. Expresses satisfaction with level of bowel and bladder control
2. Achieves urinary continence
   a. Uses therapeutic approach that is appropriate to type of incontinence
   b. Maintains adequate fluid intake
   c. Washes and dries skin after episodes of incontinence
3. Achieves bowel continence
   a. Participates in bowel program
   b. Verbalizes need for regular time for bowel evacuation
   c. Modifies diet to promote continence
   d. Uses bowel stimulants as prescribed and needed
4. Experiences relief of constipation
   a. Uses high-fiber diet, fluids, and exercise to promote defecation
   b. Responds to urge to defecate

# Disability and Sexuality Issues

An important issue confronting patients with disabilities, and a vital component of self-concept, is sexuality. Sexuality involves not only biologic sexual activity but also one's concept of masculinity or femininity. It affects the way people react to others and are perceived by them, and it is expressed not only by physical intimacy but also by caring and emotional intimacy.

Sexuality problems experienced by patients with disabilities include limited access to information about sexuality, lack of opportunity to form friendships and loving relationships, impaired self-image, and low self-esteem. People with disabilities may have physical and emotional difficulties that interfere with sexual activities. For example, diabetes and spinal cord injury may affect the ability of men to have erections. Patients who have suffered a heart attack or stroke may fear having a life-threatening event (eg, another heart attack or stroke) during sexual activity. Some patients may fear loss of bowel or bladder control during intimate moments. Changes in desire for sex and in the quality of sexual activities can occur for the patient and his or her partner, who may be too involved as a caregiver to have the desire and energy for sexual activities.

Unfortunately, society and some health care providers contribute to these problems by ignoring the patient's sexuality and by viewing people with disabilities as asexual. Health care providers' own discomfort and lack of knowledge related to sexuality issues prevent them from providing patients with disabilities and their partners with interventions that promote healthy intimacy. Nurses caring for people with disabilities must recognize and address sexual issues to promote feelings of self-worth. The nurse should give the patient "permission" to discuss sexuality concerns and show a willingness to listen and help the patient overcome these concerns. The nurse also plays a key role in providing appropriate patient education about how specific disabilities affect sexual function. For example, arthritis produces fatigue and morning stiffness, making planned afternoon sex a better alternative; spinal cord injury impairs erections and ejaculations; and traumatic brain injury may produce an increased or decreased interest in sexual behavior. Classes, books, movies, and support groups are useful tools to help patients learn about sexuality and disability. When open discussion and education about disability and sexuality do not result in the patient achieving his or her sexuality goals, the nurse should refer the patient for ongoing counseling with a sex counselor or therapist. The patient may need training in communication and in social and assertiveness skills to develop desired relationships.

# Fatigue

People with disabilities frequently experience fatigue. Physical and emotional weariness may be caused by discomfort and pain associated with a chronic health problem, deconditioning associated with prolonged periods of bed rest and immobility, impaired motor function requiring excessive expenditure of energy to ambulate, and the frustrations of performing ADLs. Ineffective coping with the disability, unresolved grief, disordered sleep patterns, and depression can also contribute to fatigue. The patient is encouraged to use coping strategies to manage the psychological impact of the disability and pain management techniques to control the associated discomforts (see Chapter 13 for a discussion of pain management). In addition, the nurse can teach the patient to manage fatigue through priority setting and energy-conserving techniques (Chart 11-12).

## Complementary and Alternative Therapies

People with disabilities may seek a variety of different therapies. For some people, therapeutic horseback riding influences the entire body and has a profound effect on all body systems. Instructors are certified through the North American Riding for the Handicapped Association. Pet therapy and canine companion programs have reduced stress and promoted coping for many people with disabilities. Some animals, including simian monkeys, can pick up the phone, retrieve small assistive devices, assist with drinking beverages, or assist with activating emergency calls. The "working" animals provide companionship as well as physical assistance for elderly people and people with disability who may live alone.

Nurses can also encourage people with disabilities to take advantage of community programs. T'ai chi classes improve muscle strength, balance, and coordination and can help to prevent falls in the elderly. People with disabilities, including wheelchair users, can participate in T'ai chi classes for improved balance, coordination, muscle strength and control, and a sense of well-being.

Daily journal writing has helped depressed people and their families overcome many emotionally draining reactions to adverse circumstances. Nurses are instrumental in teaching patients and family members this cost-effective technique. Relaxation exercises can also be taught by the nurse and encouraged in all settings, including the hospital, rehabilitation setting, outpatient areas, and the home.

### CHART 11-12

### Learning to Cope With Disabilities

**Take Control of Your Life**
- Face the reality of your disability.
- Emphasize areas of strength.
- Remain outward looking.
- Seek inventive ways to tackle problems.
- Share concerns and frustrations.
- Maintain and improve general health.
- Plan for recreation.

**Have Well-Defined Goals and Priorities**
- Keep priorities in order; eliminate nonessential activities.
- Plan and pace your activities.

**Organize Your Life**
- Plan each day.
- Organize work.
- Perform tasks in steps.
- Distribute heavy work throughout the day or week.

**Conserve Energy**
- Rest before undertaking difficult tasks.
- Stop the activity before fatigue occurs.
- Continue with an exercise conditioning program to strengthen muscles.

**Control Your Environment**
- Try to be well organized.
- Keep possessions in the same place, so that they can be found with a minimum of effort.
- Store equipment (personal care, crafts, work) in a box or basket.
- Use energy-conservation and work-simplification techniques.
- Keep work within easy reach and in front of you.
- Use adaptive equipment, self-help aids, and labor-saving devices.
- Recruit assistance from others; delegate when necessary.
- Take safety precautions.

## Promoting Home and Community-Based Care

An important goal of rehabilitation is to assist the patient to return to the home environment after learning to manage the disability. A referral system maintains continuity of care when the patient is transferred to the home or to an extended care facility. The plan for discharge is formulated when the patient is first admitted to the hospital, and discharge plans are made with the patient's functional potential in mind.

### Teaching Patients Self-Care

The patient's support system (family, friends) is assessed. The attitudes of family and friends toward the patient, his or her disability, and the return home are important in making a successful transition to home. Not all families can carry out the arduous programs of exercise, physical therapy, and personal care that the patient may need. They may not have the resources or stability to care for family members with a severe disability. Even a stable family may be overwhelmed by the physical, emotional, economic, and energy strains of a disabling condition. Members of the rehabilitation team must not judge the family but rather should provide supportive interventions that help the family to attain its highest level of function.

The family members need to know as much as possible about the patient's condition and care so that they do not fear the patient's return home. The nurse develops methods to help the patient and family cope with problems that may arise. A skill checklist individualized for the patient and family can be developed to make certain that the family is proficient in assisting the patient with certain tasks (Chart 11-13).

### CHART 11-13

## HOME CARE CHECKLIST • Managing the Therapeutic Regimen at Home

| At the completion of the home care instruction, the patient or caregiver will be able to: | Patient | Caregiver |
|---|:---:|:---:|
| • State the impact of disability on physiologic functioning. | ✔ | ✔ |
| • State changes in lifestyle necessary to maintain health. | ✔ | ✔ |
| • State the name, dose, side effects, frequency, and schedule for all medications. | ✔ | ✔ |
| • State how to obtain medical supplies after discharge. | ✔ | ✔ |
| • Identify durable medical equipment needs, proper usage, and maintenance necessary for safe utilization:<br>    [ ] Wheelchair—manual/power     [ ] Bedside toilet<br>    [ ] Cushion     [ ] Crutches<br>    [ ] Grab bars     [ ] Walker<br>    [ ] Sliding board     [ ] Prosthesis<br>    [ ] Mechanical lift     [ ] Orthosis<br>    [ ] Raised padded commode seat     [ ] Specialty bed<br>    [ ] Padded commode wheelchair | ✔ | ✔ |
| • Demonstrate usage of adaptive equipment for activities of daily living:<br>    [ ] Long-handled sponge     [ ] Rocker-knife, spork, weighted utensils<br>    [ ] Reacher     [ ] Special closures for clothing<br>    [ ] Universal cuff     [ ] Other<br>    [ ] Plate mat and guard | ✔ | ✔ |
| • Demonstrate mobility skills:<br>    [ ] Transfers: bed to chair; in and out of toilet and tub; in and out of car<br>    [ ] Negotiate ramps, curbs, stairs<br>    [ ] Assume sitting from supine position<br>    [ ] Turn side to side in bed<br>    [ ] Maneuver wheelchair; manage arm and leg rests; lock brakes<br>    [ ] Ambulate safely using assistive devices<br>    [ ] Perform range-of-motion exercises<br>    [ ] Perform muscle-strengthening exercises | ✔ | ✔ |
| • Demonstrate skin care:<br>    [ ] Inspect bony prominences every morning and evening<br>    [ ] Identify stage I pressure ulcer and actions to take if present<br>    [ ] Change dressings for stage II to IV pressure ulcers<br>    [ ] State dietary requirements to promote healing of pressure ulcers<br>    [ ] Demonstrate pressure relief at prescribed intervals<br>    [ ] State sitting schedule and demonstrate weight lifts in wheelchair<br>    [ ] Demonstrate adherence to bed turning schedule, bed positioning, and use of bridging techniques<br>    [ ] Apply and wear protective boots at prescribed times<br>    [ ] Demonstrate correct wheelchair sitting posture<br>    [ ] Demonstrate techniques to avoid friction and shear in bed<br>    [ ] Demonstrate proper hygiene to maintain skin integrity | ✔ | ✔ |
| • Demonstrate bladder care:<br>    [ ] State schedule for voiding, toileting, and catheterization<br>    [ ] Identify relationship of fluid intake to voiding and catheterization schedule<br>    [ ] State how to perform pelvic floor exercises<br>    [ ] Demonstrate clean self-intermittent catheterization and care of catheterization equipment<br>    [ ] Demonstrate indwelling catheter care<br>    [ ] Demonstrate application of external condom catheter<br>    [ ] Demonstrate application, emptying, and cleaning of urinary drainage bag | ✔ | ✔ |

## CHART 11-13 HOME CARE CHECKLIST • Managing the Therapeutic Regimen at Home, continued

|  | Patient | Caregiver |
|---|---|---|
| [ ] Demonstrate application of incontinence pads and performing perineal hygiene | | |
| [ ] State signs and symptoms of urinary tract infection | | |
| • Demonstrate bowel care | ✔ | ✔ |
|    [ ] State optimum dietary intake to promote evacuation | | |
|    [ ] Identify schedule for optimum bowel evacuation | | |
|    [ ] Demonstrate techniques to increase intra-abdominal pressure; Valsalva maneuver; abdominal massage; leaning forward | | |
|    [ ] Demonstrate techniques to stimulate bowel movements: ingesting warm liquids; digital stimulation; insertion of suppositories | | |
|    [ ] Demonstrate optimum position for bowel evacuation: on toilet with knees higher than hips; left side in bed with knees flexed and head slightly elevated | | |
|    [ ] Identify complications and corrective strategies for bowel retraining: constipation, impaction, diarrhea, hemorrhoids, rectal bleeding, anal tears | | |
| • Identify community resources for peer and family support | ✔ | ✔ |
|    [ ] Identify phone numbers of support groups for people with disabilities | | |
|    [ ] State meeting locations and times | | |
| • Demonstrate how to access transportation | ✔ | ✔ |
|    [ ] Identify locations of wheelchair accessibility for public buses or trains | | |
|    [ ] Identify phone numbers for private wheelchair van | | |
|    [ ] Contact Division of Motor Vehicles for handicapped parking permit | | |
|    [ ] Contact Division of Motor Vehicles for driving test when appropriate | | |
|    [ ] Identify resources for adapting private vehicle with hand controls or wheelchair lift | | |
| • Identify vocational rehabilitation resources | ✔ | ✔ |
|    [ ] State name and phone number of vocational rehabilitation counselor | | |
|    [ ] Identify educational opportunities that may lead to future employment | | |
| • Identify community resources for recreation | ✔ | ✔ |
|    [ ] State local recreation centers that offer programs for people with disabilities | | |
|    [ ] Identify leisure activities that can be pursued in the community | | |
| • Identify the need for health promotion and screening activities | ✔ | ✔ |

## Continuing Care

A home care nurse may visit the patient in the hospital, interview the patient and the family, and review the ADL sheet to learn which activities the patient can perform. This helps ensure that continuity of care is provided and that the patient does not regress, but instead maintains the independence gained while in the hospital or rehabilitation setting. The family may need to purchase, borrow, or improvise needed equipment, such as safety rails, a raised toilet seat or commode, or a tub bench. Ramps may need to be built or doorways widened to allow full access.

Family members are taught how to use equipment and are given a copy of the equipment manufacturer's instruction booklet, the names of resource people, lists of equipment-related supplies, and locations where they may be obtained. A written summary of the care plan is included in family teaching. The patient and family members are reminded about the importance of routine health screening and other health promotion strategies.

A network of support services and communication systems may be required to enhance opportunities for independent living. The nurse uses collaborative, administrative skills to coordinate these activities and to pull together the network of care. The nurse also provides skilled care, initiates additional referrals when indicated, and serves as a patient advocate and counselor when obstacles are encountered. The nurse continues to reinforce prior teaching and helps the patient to set and achieve attainable goals. The degree to which the patient adapts to the home and community environment depends on the confidence and self-esteem developed during the rehabilitation process and on the acceptance, support, and reactions of family members, employers, and community members.

There is a growing trend toward independent living by people with severe disabilities, either alone or in groups that share resources. Preparation for independent living should include training in managing a household and working with personal care attendants as well as training in mobility. The goal is integration into the community—living and working in the community with accessible housing, employment, public buildings, transportation, and recreation.

State rehabilitation administration agencies provide services to assist people with disabilities in obtaining the help they need to engage in gainful employment. These services include diagnostic, medical, and mental health services. Counseling, training, placement, and follow-up services are available to help people with disabilities select and obtain jobs.

If the patient is transferred to an extended care facility, the transition is planned to promote continued progress. Independence gained continues to be supported, and progress is fostered. Adjustment to the extended care facility is promoted through communication. Family members are encouraged to visit, to be involved, and to take the patient home on weekends and holidays if possible.

## Critical Thinking Exercises

1. A 62-year-old man who is recovering from a heart transplant has just been admitted to your nursing unit. He is very weak and deconditioned as a result of years of debilitating heart disease and the recent surgery. In discussing the patient's level of functioning with the physical rehabilitation team, describe the kinds of self-care activities that you would include in your rehabilitation plan for the patient. How does a functional assessment tool help determine the patient's level of functioning?

2. **ebp** A 22-year-old man who sustained a spinal cord injury with resulting paraplegia is being discharged to his home. He will be cared for by family and will continue physical and occupational therapy as an outpatient. Family members are particularly concerned about what they can do to prevent pressure ulcers. Describe the instructions you would give the patient and the family about prevention of pressure ulcers. What is the evidence base that supports the appropriateness of these instructions, and how strong is this evidence? What criteria did you use to determine the strength of the evidence for interventions that assist in the prevention of pressure ulcers?

3. The patient described in the preceding question has had bowel and bladder training. He and his family have been taught to perform intermittent catheterization to manage his reflex urinary incontinence. As the home care nurse for this patient, what assessment parameters would you use to determine the patient's needs relative to bowel and bladder functioning? What aspects of the home care environment would you assess? What instructions would you provide for the patient and his family?

## REFERENCES AND SELECTED READINGS

### BOOKS

Agency for Health Care Policy and Research, Public Health Service, U.S. Department of Health and Human Services. Panel for the Prediction and Prevention of Pressure Ulcers in Adults. (1992). *Pressure ulcers in adults: Prediction and prevention.* Clinical Practice Guideline No. 3. AHCPR Publication No. 92-0050. Rockville, MD: Author.

Agency for Health Care Policy and Research, Public Health Service, U.S. Department of Health and Human Services. (1994). *Treatment of pressure ulcers.* Clinical Practice Guideline Number 15. AHCPR Publication No. 95-0653. Rockville, MD: Author.

Association of Rehabilitation Nurses. (1995). *Twenty-one rehabilitation nursing diagnoses: A guide to interventions and outcomes.* Glenview, IL: Author.

Association of Rehabilitation Nurses. (1996). *Scope and standards of advanced clinical practice in rehabilitation nursing.* Glenview, IL: Author.

Association of Rehabilitation Nurses. (1997). *Advanced practice in rehabilitation nursing: A core curriculum.* Glenview, IL: Author.

Association of Rehabilitation Nurses. (2000). *Standards and scope of rehabilitation nursing practice.* Glenview, IL: Author.

Association of Rehabilitation Nurses. (2000). *The specialty practice of rehabilitation nursing: A core curriculum* (4th ed.). Skokie, IL: Author.

Centers for Disease Control and Prevention (2004). *Key resources on traumatic brain injury (TBI).* Atlanta, GA, June 3, 2004.

Cuddigan, J., Ayello, E. A., & Sussman, C. (2001). *Pressure ulcers in America: Prevalence, incidence & implications for the future.* Reston, VA: National Pressure Ulcer Advisory Panel.

Derstine, J., & Hargrove, S. (2001). *Comprehensive rehabilitation nursing.* St. Louis, MO: W. B. Saunders.

Hess, C. T. (2000). *Nurse's clinical guide to wound care.* Springhouse, PA: Springhouse.

Jans, L., & Stoddard, S. (1999). *Chartbook on women and disability in the United States.* Washington, DC: U.S. National Institute on Disability and Rehabilitation Research.

McCrory, D. C., Pompeii, L. A., & Skeen, M. B. (2004). *Criteria to determine disability related to multiple sclerosis.* (Rep. No. AHRQ Publication No. 04-E019-1). Rockville, MD: Agency for Healthcare Research and Quality.

Morrison, M. (2001). *The prevention and treatment of pressure ulcers.* St. Louis, MO: Mosby.

National Science Database (2004). *Spinal cord injury facts and figures at a glance.* www.spinal-injury.net. Accessed May 4, 2006.

U.S. Census Bureau (2000). *Disability statistics.* Available at www.census.gov

U.S. Department of Health and Human Services (2003). *HHS Fact Sheet. Substance abuse: A national challenge: Prevention, treatment and research at HHS.* Washington, DC: U.S. Government Printing Office.

### JOURNALS

*Asterisks indicate nursing research articles.

Adedokun, A. O., & Wilson, M. M. (2004). Urinary incontinence: Historical, global, and epidemiologic perspectives. *Clinical Geriatric Medicine, 20*(3), 399–407.

Bodenheimer, C. F., Roig, R. L., Worsowicz, G. M., et al. (2004). Geriatric rehabilitation. 5. The societal aspects of disability in the older adult. *Archives of Physical Medicine and Rehabilitation, 85*(7), S23–S26.

Bogey, R. A., Elovic, E. P., Bryant, P. R., et al. (2004). Rehabilitation of movement disorders. *Archives of Physical Medicine and Rehabilitation, 85*(3), S41–S45.

Bogey, R. A., Geis, C. C., Bryant, P. R., et al. (2004). Stroke and neurodegenerative disorders. 3. Stroke: rehabilitation management. *Archives of Physical Medicine and Rehabilitation, 85*(3), S15–S20.

Bolton, L., McNees, P., van Rijswijk, L., et al. (2004). Wound-healing outcomes using standardized assessment and care in clinical practice. *Journal of Wound Ostomy Continence Nursing, 31*(3), 65–71.

Braden, B. J., & Maklebust, J. (2005). Preventing pressure ulcers with the Braden scale. *American Journal of Nursing, 105*(6), 70–72.

Brem, H., & Lyder, C. (2004). Protocol for the successful treatment of pressure ulcers. *American Journal of Surgery, 188*(1A), 9–17.

*Brillhart, B. (2004). Studying the quality of life and life satisfaction among persons with spinal cord injury undergoing urinary management. *Rehabilitation Nursing, 29*(4), 122–126.

Bryant, P. R., Geis, C. C., Moroz, A., et al. (2004). Stroke and neurodegenerative disorders. 4. Neurodegenerative disorders. *Archives of Physical Medicine and Rehabilitation, 85*(3), S21–S33.

Chaudhuri, A., & Behan, P. O. (2004). Fatigue in neurological disorders. *Lancet, 363*(9413), 978–988.

Cullum, N., McInnes, E., Bell-Syer, S. E., et al. (2004). Support surfaces for pressure ulcer prevention. *Cochrane Database System Reviews,* CD001735.

DeGroot, M. H., Phillips, S. J., & Eskes, G. A. (2003). Fatigue associated with stroke and other neurologic conditions: Implications for stroke rehabilitation. *Archives of Physical Medicine and Rehabilitation, 84*(6), 1714–1720.

Dement, J. M., Pompeii, L. A., Ostbye, T., et al. (2004). An integrated comprehensive occupational surveillance system for health care workers. *American Journal of Industrial Medicine, 45*(6), 528–538.

Doloresco, L. (2001). CARF: Symbol of rehabilitation excellence. *SCI Nursing, 18*(11), 165, 172.

Hackett, M. L., Anderson, C. S., & House, A. O. (2004). Interventions for treating depression after stroke. *Cochrane Database System Reviews,* CD003437.

Horrocks, J. A., Hackett, M. L., Anderson, C. S., et al. (2004). Pharmaceutical interventions for emotionalism after stroke. *Stroke, 35*(11), 2610–2611.

Kelly, A., & Dowling, M. (2004). Reducing the likelihood of falls in older people. *Nursing Standard, 18*(5), 33–40.

*Lutz, B. J. (2004). Determinants of discharge destination for stroke patients. *Rehabilitation Nursing, 29*(5), 154–163.

MacKenzie, A. E., & Change, A. M. (2002). Predictors of quality of life following stroke. *Disability and Rehabilitation, 24*(5), 259–265.

Mechanick, J. I. (2004). Practical aspects of nutritional support for wound-healing patients. *American Journal of Surgery, 188,* 52–56.

*Missik, E. (2001). Women and cardiac rehabilitation: Accessibility issues and policy recommendations. *Rehabilitation Nursing, 26*(4), 141–147.

Moroz, A., Bogey, R. A., Bryant, P. R., et al. (2004). Stroke and neurodegenerative disorders. 2. Stroke: Comorbidities and complications. *Archives of Physical Medicine and Rehabilitation, 85*(3), S11–S14.

O'Neill, B. J., Geis, C. C., Bogey, R. A., et al. (2004). Stroke and neurodegenerative disorders. 1. Acute stroke evaluation, management, risks, prevention, and prognosis. *Archives of Physical Medicine and Rehabilitation, 85*(3), S3–S10.

Olkin, R. (2002). Could you hold the door for me? Including disability in diversity. *Cultural Diversity and Ethnic Minority Psychology, 8*(2), 130–137.

Ostaszkiewicz, J., Johnston, L., & Roe, B. (2004). Habit retraining for the management of urinary incontinence in adults. *Cochrane Database System Reviews,* CD002802.

Ostaszkiewicz, J., Johnston, L., & Roe, B. (2004). Timed voiding for the management of urinary incontinence in adults. *Cochrane Database System Reviews,* CD002802.

Palmer, S. & Wegener, S. T. (2003). Rehabilitation psychology. Overview and key concepts. *Maryland Medical Journal, 4*(2), 20–22.

Phillips, E. M., Bodenheimer, C. F., Roig, R. L., et al. (2004). Geriatric rehabilitation. 4. Physical medicine and rehabilitation interventions for common age-related disorders and geriatric syndromes. *Archives of Physical Medicine and Rehabilitation, 85*(5), S18–S22.

Pompeii, L. A. (1998). Inferential and advanced analysis of research data. *AAOHN Journal, 46*(10), 514–516.

Roig, R. L., Worsowicz, G. M., Stewart, D. G., et al. (2004). Geriatric rehabilitation. 3. Physical medicine and rehabilitation interventions for common disabling disorders. *Archives of Physical Medicine and Rehabilitation, 85*(7), S12–S17.

Saunders, D. H., Greig, C. A., Young, A., et al. (2004). Physical fitness training for stroke patients. *Stroke, 35*(9), 2235.

Siegert, R. J., McPherson, K. M., & Taylor, W. J. (2004). Toward a cognitive-affective model of goal-setting in rehabilitation: Is self-regulation theory a key step? *Disability and Rehabilitation, 26*(20), 1175–1183.

Sipski, M. L., Jackson, A. B., Gomez-Marin, O., et al. (2004). Effects of gender on neurologic and functional recovery after spinal cord injury. *Archives of Physical Medicine and Rehabilitation, 85*(11), 1826–1836.

Smeltzer, S. C. (2000). Viewpoint: Double jeopardy. The health care system slights women with disabilities. *American Journal of Nursing, 100*(8), 11.

Sorensen, J. L., Jorgensen, B., & Gottrup, F. (2004). Surgical treatment of pressure ulcers. *American Journal of Surgery, 188*(1A), 42–51.

Stein, J. (2004). Motor recovery strategies after stroke. *Topics in Stroke Rehabilitation, 11*(1), 12–22.

Stewart, D. G., Phillips, E. M., Bodenheimer, C. F., et al. (2004). Geriatric rehabilitation. 2. Physiatric approach to the older adult. *Archives of Physical Medicine and Rehabilitation, 85*(7), S7–11.

Storey, K. (2003). A review of research on natural support interventions in the workplace for people with disabilities. *International Journal of Rehabilitation Research, 26*(8), 79–84.

Tate, D. G., Roller, S., & Riley, B. (2001). Quality of life for women with physical disabilities. *Physical Medicine and Rehabilitation Clinics of North America, 12*(11), 23–37.

Walsh, N. E. (2004). The Walter J. Zeiter lecture. Global initiatives in rehabilitation medicine. *Archives of Physical Medicine and Rehabilitation, 85*(9), 1395–1402.

Worsowicz, G. M., Stewart, D. G., Phillips, E. M., et al. (2004). Geriatric rehabilitation. 1. Social and economic implications of aging. *Archives of Physical Medicine and Rehabilitation, 85*(7), S3–S6.

Zehr, E. P., & Duysens, J. (2004). Regulation of arm and leg movement during human locomotion. *Neuroscientist, 10*(4), 347–361.

## RESOURCES

ABLEDATA, 8401 Colesville Road, Suite 200, Silver Spring, MD 20910; 1-800-227-0216; http://www.abledata.com. Accessed June 6, 2006.

Agency for Healthcare Research and Quality, 2101 East Jefferson Street, Suite 501, Rockville, MD 20852; 1-800-358-9295; http://www.ahrq.gov. Accessed June 6, 2006.

American Society of Addiction Medicine, 4601 North Park Avenue, Arcade Suite 101, Chevy Chase, MD 20815; 1-301-656-3920; http://www.asam.org. Accessed June 6, 2006.

Assistive Technology Industry Association, 526 Davis Street, Suite 217, Evanston, IL 60201; 1-877-687-2842/847-969-1282; http://www.atia.org. Accessed June 6, 2006.

Association of Rehabilitation Nurses, 4700 W. Lake Avenue, Glenview, IL 60025; 1-800-229-7530; fax 1-847-375-4710; http://www.rehabnurse.org. Accessed June 6, 2006.

Canine Companions for Independence, PO Box 446, Santa Rosa, CA 95402; 1-800-572-2275; www.caninecompanions.org. Accessed June 6, 2006.

Council for Disability Rights, 205 West Randolph, Suite 1650, Chicago, IL 60606; 1-312-444-9484; www.disabilityrights.org. Accessed June 6, 2006.

National Center for the Dissemination of Disability Research 2004–2005; 1-800-266-1832; http://www.ncddr.org. Accessed June 6, 2006.

National Center for Health Statistics, Division of Data Services, Hyattsville, MD 20782; 1-301-458-4636; http://www.cdc.gov/nchs. Accessed June 6, 2006.

National Council on Alcoholism and Drug Dependence, Inc., 20 Exchange Place, Suite 2902, New York, NY 10005; 1-212-269-7797; http://www.ncadd.org. Accessed June 6, 2006.

National Council on Disability, 1331 F Street, NW, Suite 1050, Washington, DC 20004; 1-202-272-2004; http://www.ncd.gov. Accessed June 6, 2006.

National Rehabilitation Information Center (NARIC), 1010 Wayne Avenue, Suite 800, Silver Spring, MD 20910; 1-800-346-2742; http://www.naric.com. Accessed June 6, 2006.

Sexuality and Information and Education Council of the U.S. (SIECUS), 130 West 42nd Street, Suite 350, New York, NY 10036; 1-212-819-9770; http://www.siecus.org. Accessed June 6, 2006.

Substance Abuse Resources and Disability Issues, Wright State University School of Medicine, Dayton, OH 45435; 1-937-775-1484; http://www.med.wright.edu. Accessed June 6, 2006.

U.S. Census Bureau, 4700 Silver Hill Road, Suitland, MD 20746; http://www.census.gov. Accessed June 6, 2006.

U.S. Department of Health and Human Services, 200 Independence Avenue SW, Washington, DC 20201; http://www.hhs.gov. Accessed July 6, 2006.

# CHAPTER 12

# Health Care of the Older Adult

## Learning Objectives

*On completion of this chapter, the learner will be able to:*

1. Describe the aging American population based on demographic trends and statistical data.
2. Describe the significance of preventive health care and health promotion for the elderly.
3. Compare and contrast the physiologic aspects of aging in older adults with those of middle-aged adults.
4. Identify the important physical and mental health problems of aging and their effects on the functioning of older people and their families.
5. Specify nursing implications related to medication therapy in older people.
6. Examine the concerns of older people and their families in the home and community, in the acute care setting, and in the long-term care facility.
7. Identify the resources available to allow older adults to receive medical and nursing services in their own homes.
8. Discuss the potential economic effect on health care of the large aging population in America.
9. Identify ethical and legal issues relevant to the care of older people.

Aging, the normal process of time-related change, begins with birth and continues throughout life. Americans are living longer than ever before, and the number of older Americans is growing more rapidly than the rest of the population. This chapter discusses the theories of aging, normal age-related changes, health problems associated with aging, and how nurses can address the health issues of older adults.

## Overview of Aging

### Demographics of Aging

**Life expectancy**, the average number of years that a person can be expected to live, has risen dramatically in the past 100 years. The proportion of Americans 65 years of age and older has tripled in that time (4.1% in 1900 and 12.3% in 2002). By 2030, it is estimated that 20% of Americans will be 65 years of age or older (Fig. 12-1). In 1900, average life expectancy was 47 years, but by 2001 that figure had increased to 77.2 years. According to data from the National Vital Statistics System, in 2001, a Caucasian 65-year-old could be expected to live until the age of 83.2 years and an African-American 65-year-old could be expected to live until the age of 81.4 years (National Center for Health Statistics,

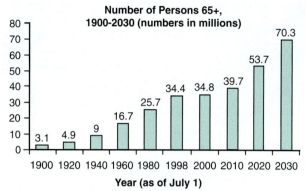

**FIGURE 12-1.** Profile of Americans age 65 and older based on data from the U.S. Bureau of the Census. Data from 1900 to the present is used to predict the millions of Americans aged 65 and older in the year 2030 (www.aoa.gov/aoa/stats/profile/default.htm).

2004). As the older population increases, the number of people who live to a very old age also increases: in 2002, 50,564 people were 100 years of age or older, an increase of 35% from 1990 (Administration on Aging, 2003).

The older population will also become more diverse, reflecting the changing demographics in the United States. Although the older population will increase in all racial and

## Glossary

**advance directive:** a formal, legally endorsed document that provides instructions for care ("living will")

**ageism:** a bias that discriminates, stigmatizes, and disadvantages older people based solely on their chronologic age

**delirium:** an acute, confused state that begins with disorientation but, if not immediately evaluated and treated, can progress to changes in level of consciousness, irreversible brain damage, and sometimes death

**dementia:** broad term for a syndrome characterized by a general decline in higher brain functioning, such as reasoning, with a pattern of eventual decline in ability to perform even basic activities of daily living, such as toileting and eating

**depression:** the most common affective (mood) disorder of old age; results from changes in reuptake of the neurochemical serotonin in response to chronic illness and emotional stresses related to the physical and social changes associated with the aging process

**durable power of attorney:** a formal, legally endorsed document that identifies a proxy decision maker who can make decisions if the signer becomes incapacitated

**elder abuse:** the physical, emotional, or financial harm to an elderly person by one or more of the individual's children, caregivers, or others; includes neglect

**geriatrics:** the study of old age that includes the physiology, pathology, diagnosis, and management of the disorders and diseases of older adults

**gerontologic/geriatric nursing:** the field of nursing that relates to the assessment, nursing diagnosis, planning, implementation, and evaluation of older adults in all environments, including acute, intermediate, and skilled care as well as within the community

**gerontology:** the combined biologic, psychological, and sociologic study of older adults within their environment

**life expectancy:** the average number of years that a person is expected to live

**lifespan:** the maximum number of years an individual can be expected to live in the absence of disease or life-threatening trauma

**orientation:** a person's ability to recognize who and where he or she is in a time continuum; used to evaluate an individual's basic cognitive status

**polypharmacy:** the administration of multiple medications at the same time; common in older persons with several chronic illnesses

**presbycusis:** the decreased ability to hear high-pitched tones that naturally begins in midlife as a result of irreversible inner ear changes

**presbyopia:** the decrease in visual accommodation that occurs with advancing age

**sundowning:** increased confusion at night

**urinary incontinence:** the unplanned loss of urine, which affects up to 50% of community-residing older adults and approximately 75% to 85% of nursing home residents

| TABLE 12-1 | Annual Deaths and Death Rates for the 10 Leading Causes of Death in People 65 Years and Older For Year 2000 | | |
|---|---|---|---|
| Rank | Cause of death | Number | Rate† |
|  | All causes | 1,799,825 | 5,176.4 |
| 1 | Heart diseases | 593,707 | 1,707.2 |
| 2 | Malignant neoplasms, including neoplasms of lymphatic and hematopoietic tissues | 392,966 | 1,128.2 |
| 3 | Cerebrovascular diseases | 148,045 | 425.7 |
| 4 | Chronic obstructive pulmonary diseases and allied conditions | 106,375 | 305.9 |
| 5 | Pneumonia and influenza | 58,557 | 168.4 |
| 6 | Diabetes mellitus | 52,414 | 150.7 |
| 7 | Alzheimer's disease | 48,993 | 140.9 |
| 8 | Nephritis, nephrotic syndrome, and nephrosis | 31,225 | 89.8 |
| 9 | Accidents (unintentional injuries) | 31,061 | 89.8 |
| 10 | Septicemia | 24,796 | 89.3 |
|  | All other causes (residual) | 312,906 | 898.0 |

National Vital Statistics Report, Vol. 50, No. 16, Sept. 16, 2002. Available at: www.cdc.gov/nchs/fastats/pdf/nvbr50_lbtl.pdf

ethnic groups, the rate of growth is projected to be fastest in the Hispanic population, in which it will increase from 2 million in 2000 to 13 million in 2050. By 2028, the older Latino population is expected to outnumber the older African-American population (Older Americans, 2000).

Although most older adults enjoy good health, in national surveys as many as 20% of adults 65 years of age and older report a chronic disability. Chronic disease is the major cause of disability, and between 1980 and 2001, heart disease, cancer, and stroke continued to be the three leading causes of death in people 65 years of age and older in the United States (Table 12-1). In 2002, Alzheimer's disease ranked eighth as a cause of disease and accounted for more than 58,000 deaths (National Center for Health Statistics, 2004).

## Health Status of the Older Adult

The vast majority of deaths (75%) in the United States occur in people 65 years of age and older, and more than half of these are caused by chronic illnesses such as heart disease and cancer. However, improvements in the prevention and early detection and treatment of diseases have had a noticeable impact on the health of people 65 years of age and older. In the past 50 years, there has been a decline in overall deaths (30%) and disability. During the 1990s deaths from heart disease and stroke declined 17.0%. Death from cancer, the second leading cause of death, rose until 1995, when it decreased slightly. Chronic obstructive pulmonary disease, the fourth leading cause of death, has been increasing since 1980, reflecting the effects of smoking.

Diabetes, the sixth leading cause of death, is also identified on death certificates as a contributor to diseases such as heart disease, kidney disease, and stroke (Health, United States, 2003b).

From 1994 to 1996, 72% of older Americans reported their health to be good, very good, or excellent. Men and women reported comparable levels of health status; however, positive health reports declined with advancing age, and a greater number of African-American men and women as well as Hispanic men were less likely to report good health. The proportion of older Americans with a limitation in activities of daily living (ADLs) declined from 6.7% in 1997 to 6.4% in 2001. Similar declines in limitations in instrumental activities of daily living (IADLs) were also reported: 13.7% in 1997 and 12.6% in 2001 (Health, United States, 2003b). These declines in limitations reflect recent trends in health promotion and disease prevention activities, such as improved nutrition, decreased smoking, increased exercise, and early detection and treatment of risk factors such as hypertension and increased serum cholesterol levels.

Many chronic conditions commonly found among older people can be managed, limited, and even prevented. Older people are more likely to maintain good health and functional independence if encouraged to do so and if appropriate community-based support services are available. Nurses are challenged to promote positive lifelong health behaviors among all populations, because the impact of unhealthy behaviors and choices results in many of the chronic diseases seen among the elderly.

## Nursing Care of the Older Adult

**Gerontology**, the scientific study of the aging process, is a multidisciplinary field that draws from the biologic, psychological, and sociologic sciences. Because aging is a normal occurrence, care for the elderly cannot be limited to one discipline but is best provided through a cooperative effort. An interdisciplinary team can combine expertise and resources to provide insight into all aspects of the aging process through comprehensive geriatric assessment and intervention. Nurses collaborate with the team to obtain non-nursing services for patients and provide a holistic approach to care.

**Gerontologic** or **geriatric nursing** is the field of nursing that specializes in the care of the elderly. The *Standards and Scope of Gerontological Nursing Practice* was originally developed in 1969 by the American Nurses Association and was revised in 1976 and again in 1987. The nurse gerontologist can be either a specialist or a generalist offering comprehensive nursing care to older people by combining the basic nursing process of assessment, diagnosis, planning, implementation, and evaluation with a specialized knowledge of aging. Gerontologic nursing is provided in acute care, skilled and assisted living, community, and home settings. Its goals include promoting and maintaining functional status and helping older adults identify and use their strengths to achieve optimal independence.

Nurses who are certified in gerontologic nursing have specialized knowledge of the acute and chronic changes specific to older people. The use of advanced practice nurses (APNs) in long-term care has proved to be very effective; when APNs using current scientific knowledge about clinical problems collaborate with nursing home staff, significantly less deterioration in the overall health issues of patients has been demonstrated (Ryden, Snyder, Gross, et al., 2000).

Nurses who work in all areas of adult medical-surgical nursing encounter elderly patients. They must be knowledgeable about geriatric nursing and skilled in meeting the needs of older patients. It is important that nurses and caregivers who work with older patients understand that aging is not synonymous with disease and that the effects of the aging process alone are not the primary contributors to disability and disease (Fryer, 2001). As research and scientific knowledge increase, it is becoming apparent that aging is a highly complex and varied process.

Functional assessment is a common framework for assessing elderly, dependent people. Age-related changes, as well as additional risk factors such as disease and the effects of medications, can result in functional consequences that have a negative impact on a particular person. However, with nursing interventions that focus on facilitating the highest level of function or quality of life, negative functional consequences can be turned into positive consequences. For example, it is possible to compensate for normal age-related changes in vision by increasing the light for reading or wearing sunglasses to reduce glare. These actions result in increased safety and quality of life (Miller, 2004). Assessing the functional consequences of aging and proposing practical interventions is significant to maintaining and even improving the health of the elderly. The goal is to help older people maintain maximum autonomy and dignity despite physical, social, and psychological losses. Early intervention can prevent further complications and help maximize the quality of life.

## Theories of Aging

Aging has been defined chronologically by the passing of time—subjectively, as in how a person feels, and functionally, as in changes in physical or mental capabilities. Each theory of aging attempts to provide a framework in which to understand aging from different perspectives. Scientists examine the aging process from the biologic and cellular level. Social scientists and psychologists examine the aging process from developmental and experiential models. Each theory is useful to the clinician because a framework and insight into the differences among elderly patients are provided.

### Biologic Theories

It is useful to consider the biologic theories of aging because they help distinguish normal aging from disease. Normal aging is intrinsic aging (from within a person) and refers to those changes caused by the normal aging process that are genetically programmed and essentially universal and irreversible within a species. Universality is the major criterion used to distinguish normal from abnormal aging. Chronologic age is often less predictive of obvious aging characteristics than other factors such as genetics and lifestyle practices.

Many biologic theories of aging are being explored. Much of the current research into biologic aging is at the cellular level. The "wear-and-tear theory" suggests that with use the body, similar to a machine, eventually wears out. The autoimmune theory proposes that over time the body's immune system becomes defective and can no longer recognize and attack foreign invaders. The noticeable changes in the body's collagen that lead to wrinkles as a person ages has led to the "cross-linkage" and "free radical" theories, which suggest that the body accumulates cross-linking compounds or gathers byproducts (free radicals) that eventually impede cell function. It has been suggested that DNA has a genetic "clock" that recognizes a limited **lifespan** or limits cellular reproduction, because cells of older people replicate fewer times than cells of younger people.

### Developmental Theories

Erikson (1963) theorized that a person's life consists of eight stages, each representing a crucial turning point in life stretching from birth to death, with its own developmental conflict to be resolved. According to Erikson, the major developmental task of old age is either to achieve ego integrity or to suffer despair. Achieving ego integrity requires accepting one's lifestyle, believing that one's choices were the best that could be made at a particular time, and being in control of one's life. Despair results when the older person feels dissatisfied and disappointed with his or her life and would live differently if given another chance.

Havighurst (1968) also proposed developmental tasks that occur at certain times in a person's life. The tasks of older people include adjusting to retirement after a lifetime of employment with a possible reduction of income, adjusting to decreases in physical strength and health, adjusting to the death of a spouse, establishing affiliation with one's age group, adapting to new social roles in a flexible way, and establishing satisfactory physical living arrangements.

By combining the concepts of both Erikson and Havighurst, it is possible to identify the following developmental tasks for older adults: (1) maintenance of self-worth, (2) conflict resolution, (3) adjustment to the loss of dominant roles, (4) adjustment to the deaths of significant others, (5) environmental adaptation, and (6) maintenance of optimal levels of wellness. Nurses can facilitate reflection and reminiscence as useful experiences for elderly patients.

### Sociologic Theories

Sociologic theories of aging attempt to predict and explain the social interactions and roles that contribute to successful adjustment to old age in older adults. Older theories include the activity theory, which proposes that life satisfaction in normal aging requires maintaining the active lifestyle of middle age (Havighurst, 1968), and the continuity theory, which proposes that successful adjustment to old age requires continuing life patterns across a lifetime (Atchley, 1989; Neugarten, 1961). Continuity and a connection to the past are maintained through a continuation of well-established habits, values, and interests that are integral to a person's present lifestyle. Other theories suggest that people move through their lives as cohort groups experiencing major life events together, such as war or economic depression, and that these events mold their lives in similar ways. The person-environment fit theory considers the interrelationship between people and their environment (Lawton, 1982). All of these theories provide a framework in which gerontologic nurses can appreciate individual patients within the context of their lives. The theories emphasize the importance of environmental and psychosocial factors in the development and current functioning of the patient.

## Nursing Theory

Miller (2004) has developed the functional consequences theory, which challenges nurses to consider while planning care the effects of normal age-related changes as well as the damage incurred through disease or environmental and behavioral risk factors. Miller suggests that nurses can alter the outcome for patients through nursing interventions that address the consequences of these changes. The functional consequences theory postulates that

> [O]lder adults experience functional consequences because of age-related changes and additional risk factors. Without interventions, many functional consequences are negative; with them, however, functional consequences can be positive. The role of the gerontologic nurse is to identify the factors that cause negative functional consequences and to initiate interventions that will result in positive ones. (p. 59)

According to Miller's theory, normal age-related changes and risk factors may negatively interfere with patient outcomes and actually impair patient activity and quality of life. For example, normal age-related changes in vision may increase sensitivity to glare. Alterations in the environment that reduce glare may enhance patient comfort and safety. In contrast, the development of cataracts, which is not a normal age-related change, also may increase sensitivity to glare. The nurse must differentiate between normal age-related changes that cannot be reversed and risk factors that can be modified. Doing so is useful in designing appropriate nursing interventions that have a positive impact on patient outcomes for the elderly—most importantly, for quality of life.

# Age-Related Changes

The well-being of older people depends on physical, mental, social, economic, and environmental factors. A total assessment includes an evaluation of all major body systems, social and mental status, and the ability of a person to function independently despite having a chronic illness or disability.

## Psychosocial Aspects of Aging

Successful psychological aging is reflected in the ability of older people to adapt to physical, social, and emotional losses and to achieve contentment, serenity, and life satisfaction. Because changes in life patterns are inevitable over a lifetime, older people need resiliency and coping skills when confronting stresses and change. A positive self-image enhances risk taking and participation in new, untested roles.

Although attitudes toward older people differ in ethnic subcultures, a subtle theme of **ageism**—prejudice or discrimination against older people—predominates in our society, and many myths surround aging. Ageism is based on stereotypes, simplified and often untrue beliefs that reinforce society's negative image of older people. Although older people make up an extremely heterogeneous and increasingly a racially and ethnically diverse group, negative stereotypes are attributed to all of them.

Fear of aging and the inability of many to confront their own aging process may trigger ageist beliefs. Retirement and perceived nonproductivity are also responsible for negative feelings, because a younger working person may see an older person as someone who is not contributing to society and who is draining economic resources. Concern about the large numbers of elderly leaving the work force (baby boomers begin to turn age 65 in 2011) is fueling this debate.

Many negative images are so common in society that the elderly themselves often believe and perpetuate them. Only through an understanding of the aging process and respect for each person as an individual can the myths of aging be dispelled. If the elderly are treated with dignity and encouraged to maintain autonomy, the quality of their lives will improve.

## Stress and Coping in the Older Adult

Coping patterns and the ability to adapt to stress develop over the course of a lifetime and remain consistent later in life. Experiencing success in younger adulthood helps a person develop a positive self-image that remains solid through the adversities of old age. A person's abilities to adapt to changes, make decisions, and respond predictably are also determined by past experiences. A flexible, well-functioning person will probably continue as such. However, losses may accumulate within a short period of time and may become overwhelming. The older person will often have fewer choices and diminished resources to deal with stressful events. Common stressors of old age include normal aging changes that impair physical function, activities, and appearance; disabilities from chronic illness; social and environmental losses related to loss of income and decreased ability to perform previous roles and activities; and the deaths of significant others. Many older adults rely strongly on their spiritual beliefs for comfort during stressful times.

## Living Arrangements

More than 95% of the elderly live in the community, and more than 78% own their homes. In 2003, 58.5% of elderly people were living alone. Of the elderly people who live alone in the community, widowed women predominate. In 2003, 71% of men ages 65 to 74 were married compared to 41% of women in the same age group. Among those aged 85 or older, about 50% of the men were married compared to only 13% of the women. This difference in marital status is a result of several factors: women have a longer life expectancy than men do; women tend to marry older men; and women tend to remain widowed, whereas men often remarry (Older Americans 2000, 2005; Administration on Aging, 2004).

Older people often do best in their own environment and can successfully remain at home for many years. Furthermore, the family home and familiar community may have strong emotional significance for them, and this should not be ignored. With advanced age and increasing disability, adjustments to the environment may be required to allow older adults to remain in their own homes or apartments. Additional family support or more formal support such as Meals on Wheels or transportation services may be necessary to compensate for declining function and mobility.

Many elderly people have more-than-adequate financial resources and good health even until very late in life; therefore, they have many housing options. Older people tend to relocate in response to changes in their lives such as retirement or widowhood, a significant deterioration in health, or disability. The type of housing they choose depends on their reason for moving (Hooyman & Kiyak, 2002). For example, there has been a significant increase in the elderly population in the "Sun Belt"—in the states of Florida, California, Texas, and Arizona—as relatively young older adults (60 to 74 years of age) and recent retirees move to warmer climates and retirement communities. With increasing disability and illness, elderly people may move to retirement facilities or assisted living communities that provide some support such as meals, transportation, and housekeeping but allow them to live somewhat independently. If they develop a serious illness or disability and can no longer live independently or semi-independently, they may need to move to a setting where additional support is available. Older people may move in with a relative or to a nursing home or an assisted living setting nearer a child's home. For this reason, while Florida has the largest population of the elderly, it ranks only 24th in the percentage of very old people (Falgoust, 2004).

There are many implications when elderly people choose to remain in their own home. For example, the person tends to be living on a fixed income, which may have been adequate when the person first retired but is no longer sufficient to pay maintenance expenses or taxes and utilities. Creative solutions are available, such as reverse mortgages that lend the older person money via a credit line on his or her mortgage. This is available to elderly people who have little or no mortgage debt and allows them to use the assets of the home to finance daily needs. In addition, house sharing programs with family members or even strangers, although difficult to plan and arrange, can be successful and benefit both the older person and the individual or family sharing the home. Many communities have planned senior housing, much of which may be subsidized for low-income elderly people; some elderly adults who have "downsized" from larger homes and moved into apartment buildings find that they are "aging in place" with other elderly people in similar circumstances.

Sometimes older adults or couples agree to move in with adult children. This can be a rewarding experience as the children, their parents, and the grandchildren interact and share household responsibilities. It can also be stressful, depending on family dynamics. Adult children and their older parents may also choose to pool their financial resources by moving into a house that has an attached "in-law suite." This arrangement provides security for the older adult along with privacy for both families.

Unfortunately, many elderly people and their adult children make housing decisions in times of crisis, such as a serious illness or the death of a spouse. Older people and their families often are unaware of all of the ramifications of shared housing and assuming care for an increasingly dependent person. Families can be helped by anticipatory guidance and long-term planning before a crisis occurs. Older adults should participate in decisions that affect them as much as possible.

## CONTINUING CARE RETIREMENT COMMUNITIES

Continuing care retirement communities (CCRCs), retirement communities that provide three levels of living arrangements and care, are becoming more popular as the first baby boomers enter their retirement years. CCRCs consist of independent single-dwelling houses or apartments for people who can manage all of their day-to-day needs; assisted living apartments for those who need limited assistance with their daily living needs; and skilled nursing services when continuous nursing assistance is required. CCRCs usually contract for a large down payment before the resident moves into the community. This payment gives a person or couple the option to reside in the community from the time of total independence through the need for assisted or skilled nursing care. Decisions about living arrangements and health care can be made before any decline in health status occurs. CCRCs also provide continuity at a time in an older adult's life when many other factors, such as health status, income, and availability of friends and family members, may be changing.

## ASSISTED LIVING FACILITIES

Assisted living facilities are an option when an older person's physical or cognitive changes necessitate at least minimal supervision or assistance. Assisted living allows for a degree of independence while providing minimal nursing assistance (eg, administration of medication and assistance with ADLs or chronic health care needs). Other services, such as laundry, cleaning, and meals, may also be included.

## NURSING HOMES

Skilled nursing facilities offer continuous nursing care. Contrary to the myth of family abandonment and the fear of "ending up in a nursing home," the actual percentage of long-term nursing home residents has declined, from 5.4% in 1985 to 4.5% in 1997 (Older Americans, 2000). However, the actual number of elderly people who reside in nursing homes has risen due to the large increase in the aging population and the multiple uses of nursing homes today for short-term rehabilitation.

Short-term nursing home care is often reimbursed by Medicare if the patient is recovering from an acute illness such as a stroke, myocardial infarction, or cancer and requires skilled nursing care or therapy for recuperation. Usually, if an older adult suffers a major health event and is hospitalized and then goes to a nursing home, Medicare covers the cost of the first 30 to 90 days in a skilled nursing facility if ongoing therapy is needed. The requirement for continued Medicare coverage during this time is documentation of persistent improvement in the condition that requires therapy, most often physical therapy, occupational therapy, respiratory therapy, and cognitive therapy. Some adults choose to have long-term care insurance as a means of paying, at least in part, for the cost of these services should they become necessary. For elderly people who are living in nursing homes and who generally have multiple chronic and debilitating health concerns, costs are primarily paid "out-of-pocket" by the patient. Family members are not responsible for nursing home costs. When a person's financial resources become exhausted as a result of prolonged nursing home care, the patient, the institution, or both may apply for Medicaid reimbursement.

An increasing number of skilled nursing facilities offer subacute care. This area of the facility offers a high level of nursing care that may either prevent the need for a resident to be transferred to a hospital from the nursing home or allow a hospitalized patient to be transferred back to the nursing facility sooner.

## The Role of the Family

Planning for care and understanding the psychosocial issues confronting older people must be accomplished within the context of the family. If dependency needs occur, the spouse often assumes the role of primary caregiver. In the absence of the surviving spouse, an adult child usually assumes caregiver responsibilities and may eventually need help in providing or arranging for care and support. Approximately 81% of elderly people have living children. Of elderly people who live alone, two thirds have at least one child living within 30 minutes of their home, and 62% see at least one adult child weekly (Administration on Aging, 2004).

Two common myths in American society are that adult children and their aged parents are socially alienated and that adult children abandon their parents when health and other dependency problems arise. Extensive research refutes both of these beliefs (Markson, 2003). More than 70% of elderly people receive most of their care from informal caregivers. The family has been and continues to be an important source of support for older people; similarly, older family members provide a great deal of support to younger family members (Fig. 12-2).

Although adult children are not financially responsible for their older parents, social attitudes and cultural values often dictate that adult children should provide services and assume the burden of care if their aged parents cannot care for themselves. In the United States, 70% to 80% of community-based caregiving is provided to the elderly by informal caregivers, predominately by family, friends, and neighbors. This caregiving, which may continue for many years, can become a source of family stress. For prolonged periods, it is not uncommon for caregivers to neglect their own emotional and health needs (Myers, 2003). In addition, because many of the baby boomers (those born between 1946 and 1964) tended to have children later in life, these children face the competing demands of caring for their aging parents while caring for their own dependent children (Spillman, 2001). Furthermore, because of smaller family sizes, future generations of families will have to contend with fewer numbers of siblings to help with parental care issues. If community agencies or adult children cannot provide care, elders are at high risk for institutionalization.

## Physical Aspects of Aging

As previously mentioned, intrinsic aging (from within the person) refers to those changes caused by the normal aging process that are genetically programmed and essentially universal within a species. Universality is the major criterion used to distinguish normal aging from pathologic changes associated with illness. However, people age quite differently and at different rates, so chronologic age is often less predictive of obvious aging characteristics than other factors, such as genetics and lifestyle. For example, extrinsic aging results from influences outside the person. Air pollution and excessive exposure to sunlight are examples of extrinsic factors that may hasten the aging process and that can be eliminated or reduced.

Cellular and extracellular changes of old age cause a change in physical appearance and a decline in function. Measurable changes in shape and body makeup occur. The body's ability to maintain homeostasis becomes increasingly diminished with cellular aging, and organ systems cannot function at full efficiency because of cellular and tissue deficits. Cells become less able to replace themselves, and they accumulate a pigment known as lipofuscin. A degradation of elastin and collagen causes connective tissue to become stiffer and less elastic. All of this results in diminished capacity for organ function and increased vulnerability to disease and stress.

Table 12-2 summarizes the signs and symptoms of age-related changes in the functioning of body systems. More in-depth information about age-related changes can be found in the chapters pertaining to each organ system. Specifics of diseases, medical and surgical management, as well as nursing interventions are also presented in the related chapters.

### Cardiovascular System

Heart disease is the leading cause of death in the elderly. Heart failure is the leading cause of hospitalization among Medicare recipients, and it is also a major cause of morbidity and mortality among the elderly population in the United States. Age-related changes reduce the efficiency of the heart and contribute to decreased compliance of the heart muscle.

**FIGURE 12-2.** Families are an important source of psychosocial and physical support for elderly people and youngsters alike. Caring interaction among grandchildren, grandparents, and other family members typically contributes to the health of all.

## TABLE 12-2    Age-Related Changes in Body Systems and Health Promotion Strategies

| Changes | Subjective and Objective Findings | Health Promotion Strategies |
|---|---|---|
| **Cardiovascular System** | | |
| Decreased cardiac output; diminished ability to respond to stress; heart rate and stroke volume do not increase with maximum demand; slower heart recovery rate; increased blood pressure | Complaints of fatigue with increased activity<br>Increased heart rate recovery time<br>Normal BP ≤140/90 mm Hg | Exercise regularly; pace activities; avoid smoking; eat a low-fat, low-salt diet; participate in stress-reduction activities; check blood pressure regularly; medication compliance; weight control |
| **Respiratory System** | | |
| Increase in residual lung volume; decrease in vital capacity; decreased gas exchange and diffusing capacity; decreased cough efficiency | Fatigue and breathlessness with sustained activity; impaired healing of tissues as a result of decreased oxygenation; difficulty coughing up secretions | Exercise regularly; avoid smoking; take adequate fluids to liquefy secretions; receive yearly influenza immunization; avoid exposure to upper respiratory tract infections |
| **Integumentary System** | | |
| Decreased protection against trauma and sun exposure; decreased protection against temperature extremes; diminished secretion of natural oils and perspiration | Skin appears thin and wrinkled; complaints of injuries, bruises, and sunburn; complaints of intolerance to heat; bone structure is prominent; dry skin | Avoid solar exposure (clothing, sunscreen, stay indoors); dress appropriately for temperature; maintain a safe indoor temperature; shower preferable to tub bath; lubricate skin |
| **Reproductive System**<br>*Female:* Vaginal narrowing and decreased elasticity; decreased vaginal secretions<br>*Male:* Decreased size of penis and testes<br>*Male and Female:* Slower sexual response | *Female:* Painful intercourse; vaginal bleeding following intercourse; vaginal itching and irritation; delayed orgasm<br>*Male:* Delayed erection and achievement of orgasm | May require vaginal estrogen replacement; gynecology/urology follow-up; use a lubricant with intercourse |
| **Musculoskeletal System** | | |
| Loss of bone density; loss of muscle strength and size; degenerated joint cartilage | Height loss; prone to fractures; kyphosis; back pain; loss of strength, flexibility, and endurance; joint pain | Exercise regularly; eat a high-calcium diet; limit phosphorus intake; take calcium and vitamin D supplements as prescribed |
| **Genitourinary System**<br>*Male:* Benign prostatic hyperplasia | Urinary retention; irritative voiding symptoms including frequency, feeling of incomplete bladder emptying, multiple nighttime voidings | Seek referral to urology specialist; have ready access to toilet; wear easily manipulated clothing; drink adequate fluids; avoid bladder irritants (eg, caffeinated beverages, alcohol, artificial sweeteners); pelvic floor muscle exercises, preferably learned via biofeedback; consider urologic workup |
| *Female:* Relaxed perineal muscles, detrusor instability (urge incontinence), urethral dysfunction (stress urinary incontinence) | Urgency/frequency syndrome, decreased "warning time," bathroom mapping; drops of urine lost with cough, laugh, position change | Wear easily manipulated clothing; drink adequate fluids; avoid bladder irritants (eg, caffeinated beverages, alcohol, artificial sweeteners); pelvic floor muscle exercises, preferably learned via biofeedback; consider urologic workup |
| **Gastrointestinal System** | | |
| Decreased salivation; difficulty swallowing food; delayed esophageal and gastric emptying; reduced gastrointestinal motility | Complaints of dry mouth; complaints of fullness, heartburn, and indigestion; constipation, flatulence, and abdominal discomfort | Use ice chips, mouthwash; brush, floss, and massage gums daily; receive regular dental care; eat small, frequent meals; sit up and avoid heavy activity after eating; limit antacids; eat a high-fiber, low-fat diet; limit laxatives; toilet regularly; drink adequate fluids |

*continued >*

### TABLE 12-2  Age-Related Changes in Body Systems and Health Promotion Strategies (Continued)

| Changes | Subjective and Objective Findings | Health Promotion Strategies |
|---|---|---|
| **Nervous System** | | |
| Reduced speed in nerve conduction; increased confusion with physical illness and loss of environmental cues; reduced cerebral circulation (becomes faint, loses balance) | Slower to respond and react; learning takes longer; becomes confused with hospital admission; faintness; frequent falls | Pace teaching; with hospitalization, encourage visitors; enhance sensory stimulation; with sudden confusion, look for cause; encourage slow rising from a resting position |
| **Special Senses** | | |
| *Vision:* Diminished ability to focus on close objects; inability to tolerate glare; difficulty adjusting to changes of light intensity; decreased ability to distinguish colors | Holds objects far away from face; complains of glare; poor night vision; confuses colors | Wear eyeglasses, use sunglasses outdoors; avoid abrupt changes from dark to light; use adequate indoor lighting with area lights and nightlights; use large-print books; use magnifier for reading; avoid night driving; use contrasting colors for color coding; avoid glare of shiny surfaces and direct sunlight |
| *Hearing:* Decreased ability to hear high-frequency sounds | Gives inappropriate responses; asks people to repeat words; strains forward to hear | Recommend a hearing examination; reduce background noise; face person; enunciate clearly; speak with a low-pitched voice; use nonverbal cues |
| *Taste and smell:* Decreased ability to taste and smell | Uses excessive sugar and salt | Encourage use of lemon, spices, herbs |

These changes include sclerosis of the endocardium, fibrosis of the valves, increased myocardial stiffness, decreased muscle fibers, and reduced myocardial strength (Maas et al., 2001). As a result, the heart valves become thicker and stiffer, and the heart muscle and arteries lose their elasticity. Calcium and fat deposits accumulate within arterial walls, and veins become increasingly tortuous.

It is difficult to differentiate between age- and disease-related changes in cardiovascular function because of the significant influence of behavioral factors on cardiovascular health. When cross-cultural studies are conducted, cardiovascular changes that in the past were thought to be age-related do not consistently appear. For example, the higher blood pressure found in older adults in Western societies does not occur in less developed societies and may be a result of different lifestyle behaviors rather than normal age-related changes (Miller, 2004). Under normal circumstances, the cardiovascular system can adapt to the normal age-related changes, and an older person is unaware of any significant decline in cardiovascular performance. However, when challenged, the cardiovascular system of an older person is less efficient under conditions of stress and exercise and when life-sustaining activities are needed.

Careful assessment of older people is necessary because they often present with different symptoms than those seen in younger patients. Older people are more likely to have dyspnea or neurologic symptoms associated with heart disease, and they may experience mental status changes or report vague symptoms such as fatigue, nausea, and syncope. Rather than the typical substernal chest pain associated with myocardial ischemia, older patients may report burning or sharp pain or discomfort in an area of the upper body. Complicating the assessment is the fact that many elderly patients have more than one underlying disease. When a patient complains about symptoms related to digestion and breathing and upper extremity pain, cardiac disease must be considered (Miller, 2004). The absence of chest pain in an older patient is not a good indicator of the absence of heart disease.

Hypotension may be a concern. The risk for orthostatic and postprandial hypotension increases significantly after 75 years of age (Miller, 2004). A patient experiencing hypotension should be counseled to rise slowly (from a lying, to a sitting, to a standing position), to avoid straining when having a bowel movement, and to consider having five or six small meals each day, rather than three, to minimize the hypotension that can occur after a large meal. Extremes in temperature, including hot showers and whirlpool baths, should be avoided.

## Respiratory System

The respiratory system is the one system that seems to be the most able to compensate for the functional changes of aging. In general, healthy, nonsmoking, older adults show very little decline in respiratory function; however, there are substantial individual variations. The age-related changes that do occur are subtle and gradual, and healthy older adults are able to compensate for these changes (Miller, 2004). Diminished respiratory efficiency as well as reduced maximal inspiratory and expiratory force may occur as a result of calcification and weakening of the muscles of the chest wall. The alveoli within the lungs enlarge and become thinner, increasing the amount of anatomic dead space.

Conditions of stress, such as illness, may increase the demand for oxygen and affect the overall function of other systems. Like cardiovascular diseases, respiratory diseases manifest more subtly in older adults than in younger adults and do not necessarily follow the typical pattern of cough, chills, and fever. Older adults may exhibit headache, weakness, lethargy, anorexia, dehydration, and mental status changes (Miller, 2004).

Smoking is the most significant risk factor for respiratory and other diseases. Therefore, a major focus of health promotion activities should be on smoking cessation and avoidance of environmental smoke. Pneumonia and influenza together are the fifth leading cause of death in people older than 65 years of age. Education to promote the use of pneumonia and influenza vaccines is an essential nursing intervention. A pneumococcal vaccine that prevents 85% to 90% of all cases of pneumonia is available, and it is effective in preventing 75% of cases in people older than 65 years of age. Influenza vaccination is less effective in preventing influenza in the elderly than in the younger population, but it reduces influenza-related deaths, hospitalizations, and other complications (Miller, 2004).

Activities that help elderly people maintain adequate respiratory function include regular exercise, appropriate fluid intake, pneumococcal vaccination, yearly influenza immunizations, and avoidance of people who are ill. Hospitalized older adults should be frequently reminded to cough and take deep breaths, particularly postoperatively, because their decreased lung capacity and decreased cough efficiency predispose them to atelectasis and respiratory infections.

## Integumentary System

The functions of the skin include protection, temperature regulation, sensation, and excretion. With aging, changes occur that affect the function and appearance of the skin. There is a decrease of epidermal proliferation, and the dermis becomes thinner. Elastic fibers are reduced in number, and collagen becomes stiffer. Subcutaneous fat diminishes, particularly in the extremities. Decreased numbers of capillaries in the skin result in diminished blood supply. These changes cause a loss of resiliency and wrinkling and sagging of the skin. The skin becomes drier and susceptible to burns, injury, and infection. Hair pigmentation may change, and balding may occur; genetic factors strongly influence these changes. These changes in the integument reduce tolerance to temperature extremes and sun exposure.

Lifestyle practices are likely to have a large impact on skin changes. Therefore, strategies to promote healthy skin function include not smoking, avoiding exposure to the sun, using a sun protection factor (SPF) of 15 or higher, using emollient skin cream containing petrolatum or mineral oil, avoiding hot soaks in the bathtub, and maintaining optimal nutrition and hydration. Older adults should be encouraged to have any suspicious changes in the skin examined, because early detection and treatment of precancerous or cancerous lesions are essential to prevent serious negative consequences.

## Reproductive System

Sexuality is no longer considered pertinent only to the young. However, research about sexuality among the elderly, especially in women, has not been extensive. Ovarian production of estrogen and progesterone ceases with menopause. Changes occurring in the female reproductive system include thinning of the vaginal wall, along with a narrowing in size and a loss of elasticity; decreased vaginal secretions, resulting in vaginal dryness, itching, and decreased acidity; involution (atrophy) of the uterus and ovaries; and decreased pubococcygeal muscle tone, resulting in a relaxed vagina and perineum. Without the use of water-soluble lubricants, these changes may contribute to vaginal bleeding and painful intercourse.

In older men, the penis and testes decrease in size, and levels of androgens diminish. Decreased libido and erectile dysfunction may develop but are more likely to be associated with factors other than age-related changes. These risk factors include cardiovascular disease; neurologic disorders; diabetes; respiratory disease; pain; and medications such as cardiac drugs, vasodilators, antihypertensive agents, and tricyclic antidepressants.

Although there is a less intense response to sexual stimulation and a decline in sexual activity with increasing age, sexual desire does not disappear. Men may experience a decline in sexual function related to health conditions or interference from medications. Women may lose their partner; the absence of a partner is often a primary factor causing lack of sexual activity. Many couples are unaware of the causes of decreased libido or erectile dysfunction and are often reluctant to discuss decreased sexual function, and a thorough assessment is important. There are many methods of improving the quality of sexual interactions, but the assessment and communication require sensitivity and expert knowledge in the field of sexual dysfunction. If sexual dysfunction is present, referral to a gynecologist, urologist, or sex therapist is warranted.

## Genitourinary System

The genitourinary system continues to function adequately in older people, although there is a decrease in kidney mass, primarily because of a loss of nephrons. Changes in kidney function vary widely; about one third of elderly people show no decrease in renal function (Miller, 2004). Therefore, changes in renal function may be a combination of aging and pathologic conditions such as hypertension. The changes most commonly seen include a decreased filtration rate, diminished tubular function with less efficiency in resorbing and concentrating the urine, and a slower restoration of acid–base balance in response to stress. Older adults who take medications may experience serious consequences due to decline in renal function because of impaired absorption, decreased ability to maintain fluid and electrolyte balance, and decreased ability to concentrate urine.

Certain genitourinary disorders are more common in older adults than the general population. Approximately 13 million people in the United States suffer from **urinary incontinence**. About 85% of people with incontinence are women, and this condition is often mistakenly viewed as a normal consequence of aging. It is costly and embarrassing and should be evaluated because in most cases it is reversible or can be treated (Maas et al., 2001) Urinary incontinence is discussed in more detail in Chapter 45. Benign prostatic hyperplasia (enlarged prostate gland), a common finding in older men, causes a gradual increase in urine retention and overflow incontinence. Prostate cancer, a slow-growing cancer, is most often seen in men older than 70 years of age. Kidney and bladder cancers are most frequently seen in people older than 50 years of age. Smoking is known to be a primary factor in these carcinomas.

Adequate consumption of fluids is important to reduce the risk of bladder infections and urinary incontinence.

## Gastrointestinal System

Digestion of food is less influenced by age-related changes than by the risk for poor nutrition. Older people can adjust to the age-related changes but often have more difficulty in purchasing, preparing, and enjoying their meals. The sense of smell diminishes as a result of neurologic changes and environmental factors such as smoking, medications, and vitamin $B_{12}$ deficiencies. The ability to recognize sweet, sour, bitter, or salty foods diminishes over time, altering satisfaction with food. Salivary flow does not decrease in healthy adults, but about 30% of older people may experience a dry mouth as a result of medications and diseases (Miller, 2004). Difficulties with chewing and swallowing are generally associated with disease.

Experts disagree on the extent of gastric changes that occur as a result of normal aging. However, there does appear to be a modest slowing of gastric motility, which results in delayed emptying of stomach contents and early satiation (feeling of fullness). Diminished secretion of gastric acid and pepsin, seemingly the result of pathologic conditions rather than normal aging, reduces the absorption of iron, calcium, and vitamin $B_{12}$. Absorption of nutrients in the small intestine, particularly calcium and vitamin D, appears to diminish with age. The function of the liver, gallbladder, and pancreas is generally maintained, although absorption and tolerance to fat may decrease. The incidence of gallstones and common bile duct stones increases progressively with advancing years.

Difficulty in swallowing, or dysphagia, affects 1 in 17 people, including 6.2 million Americans older than 60 years of age, with 300,000 to 600,000 new cases diagnosed each year. This serious condition can be life-threatening. It is caused by interruption or dysfunction of neural pathways, such as can occur with stroke. It may also result from dysfunction of the striated and smooth muscles of the gastrointestinal tract in as many as 50% of patients with Parkinson's disease and in patients with conditions such as multiple sclerosis, poliomyelitis, and amyotrophic lateral sclerosis (Lou Gehrig's disease). Aspiration of food or fluid is the most serious complication and can occur in the absence of coughing or choking (Galvan, 2001).

Constipation is a common pathologic condition that affects as many as 80% of institutionalized and 45% of community-dwelling elderly people (Miller, 2004). Symptoms of mild constipation are abdominal discomfort and flatulence, and more serious constipation leads to fecal impaction that contributes to diarrhea around the impaction, fecal incontinence, and obstruction. Predisposing factors for constipation include lack of dietary bulk, prolonged use of laxatives, use of some medications, inactivity, insufficient fluid intake, and excessive dietary fat. Ignoring the urge to defecate may also be a contributing factor.

Practices that promote gastrointestinal health include regular tooth brushing and flossing; receiving regular dental care; eating small, frequent meals; avoiding heavy activity after eating; eating a high-fiber, low-fat diet; drinking enough fluids; and avoiding the use of laxatives and antacids. Understanding that there is a direct correlation between loss of smell and taste perception and food intake helps caregivers to intervene to maintain elderly patients' nutritional health.

## Nutritional Health

The social, psychological, and physiologic functions of eating influence the dietary habits of older people. Increasing age alters nutrient requirements; the elderly require fewer calories and a more nutrient-rich, healthy diet in response to alterations in body mass and a more sedentary lifestyle. Recommendations include reducing fat intake while getting enough protein, vitamins, minerals, and dietary fiber for health and disease prevention. Decreased physical activity and a slower metabolic rate reduce the number of calories needed by older adults to maintain an ideal weight. As previously stated, age-related changes that alter pleasure in eating include a decrease in taste and smell. Older people are likely to maintain a taste for sweetness but require more sugar to achieve a sweet flavor. They also may lose the ability to differentiate sour, salty, and bitter tastes. Apathy, immobility, depression, loneliness, poverty, inadequate knowledge, and poor oral health also contribute to suboptimal nutrient intake. Budgetary constraints and physical limitations may interfere with food shopping and meal preparation.

Health promotion includes encouraging a diet that is low in sodium and saturated fats and high in vegetables, fruits, and fish. Education regarding healthy foods versus foods with inadequate nutrients is helpful. Sixty-nine percent of older Americans were considered overweight or obese in 2002, and among those 65 to 74 years of age, the percentage rose from 57% to 73% in just two decades (National Center for Health Statistics, 2004).

Older adults require a variety of foods to maintain healthy nutrition. No more than 20% to 25% of dietary calories should be consumed as fat. Reducing salt intake is also advocated, because sodium reduction has been shown to correct hypertension in some people. Protein intake should be increased in later adulthood to maintain adequate nitrogen equilibrium (Chernoff, 2002). Carbohydrates, a major source of energy, should supply 55% to 60% of the daily calories. Simple sugars should be avoided and complex carbohydrates should be encouraged. Potatoes, whole grains, brown rice, and fruit are sources of minerals, vitamins, and fiber and should be encouraged. Drinking 8 to 10 eight-ounce glasses of water per day is recommended unless contraindicated by a medical condition. A multivitamin each day helps maintain daily nutritional needs. Adults older than 65 years of age should increase their daily calcium intake to 1200 g. In addition, whereas adequate vitamin D can be obtained by 10 to 15 minutes of sun exposure two or three times a week, homebound or institutionalized elderly may need 400 to 800 IU of vitamin D to avoid bone loss (National Osteoporosis Foundation, 2004).

Callen (2004) reports that as many as 50% of surgical patients and 44% of medical patients are malnourished. Furthermore, many people are unaware of dietary deficits. Nurses are in an ideal position to identify nutritional problems among their patients and to work within the patient's own framework of knowledge of his or her health status to improve health behaviors.

## Sleep

Sleep disturbances affect more than 50% of adults 65 years of age or older. The elderly tend to take longer to fall asleep, awaken more easily and frequently, and spend less time in deep sleep. Consequently, they may feel that their sleep is less satisfactory (Miller, 2004). Although older adults require as much sleep as younger people, they may experience variations in their normal sleep–wake cycles, and the lack of quality sleep at night often creates the need for napping during the day. Older people are more likely to awaken because of environmental factors such as noise, pain, or nocturia.

Sleep apnea (a sleep disorder characterized by brief periods in which respirations are absent) increases with age. As many as 24% of those over 65 years of age have been diagnosed with obstructive sleep apnea (Mezey, Fulmer, Abraham, et al., 2002). Sleep apnea is discussed in more detail in Chapter 22.

The nurse is the one caregiver who observes patients while they are sleeping. The nurse can observe problems and also recommend prudent sleep hygiene behaviors such as avoiding use of the bed for activities other than sleeping (or sex), maintaining a consistent bedtime routine, avoiding or limiting daytime napping, limiting alcohol intake to less than three drinks a day, and avoiding caffeine and nicotine after noon.

## Musculoskeletal System

Intact musculoskeletal and neurologic systems are essential for the maintenance of safe mobility and performance of ADLs and IADLs, which allows older adults to remain independent and live in the community. Age-related changes that affect mobility include alterations in bone remodeling, leading to decreased bone density, loss of muscle mass, deterioration of muscle fibers and cell membranes, and degeneration in the function and efficiency of joints. These factors are discussed in detail in Unit 15.

Without exercise, a gradual, progressive decrease in bone mass begins before 40 years of age. The cartilage of joints also progressively deteriorates in middle age. Degenerative joint disease is found in all adults older than 70 years, and weight-bearing joint and back pain is a common complaint. Excessive loss of bone density results in osteoporosis, which leads to potentially life-altering hip and vertebral fractures. Osteoporosis is now considered preventable, but there is concern about the future for today's young people, who are not getting enough exercise and are not consuming adequate calcium and vitamin D, even as children.

The axiom "use it or lose it" is very relevant to the physical capacity of older adults. Nurses play an important role by encouraging older adults to participate in a regular exercise program. The benefits of regular exercise cannot be overstated. Aerobic exercises are the foundation of programs of cardiovascular conditioning, but strength training and flexibility exercises are essential components of an exercise program. *Promoting Exercise and Behavior Change in Older*

---

### NURSING RESEARCH PROFILE

### Nutritional Health in Older Adults

Callen, B. (2004) Understanding nutritional health in older adults: A pilot study. *Journal of Gerontological Nursing, 30*(1), 36–42.

**Purpose**
This study examined the nutritional health of community-dwelling older adults admitted to a hospital for acute care who were identified as being at nutritional risk. This study solicited patients' perceptions of their nutritional health and asked patients how they could improve their nutritional status.

**Design**
This cross-sectional descriptive pilot study used a convenience sample of 10 community-dwelling patients 65 years of age and older who were identified as at nutritional risk by a hospital dietitian. Upon consent, researchers conducted a two-part interview and a nutritional assessment using two tools for comparison. To elicit patients' perception of their nutritional status and recommendations about how to improve their diets, researchers used an open-ended questionnaire.

**Findings**
Although all 10 participants were identified as at nutritional risk, none believed he or she was at risk. Consequently, no participants had suggestions regarding how they could improve their nutritional status. In most cases, the nutritional decline occurred over a long time period, suggesting that if participants had had early nutritional intervention, their state of nutrition could have improved prior to their hospitalization.

**Nursing Implications**
Differences between patients' perceptions of their nutritional health and those identified by the screening tools have important implications for nurses, who are ideally positioned to assess nutritional status. Patients often do not understand the negative effects of their own nutritional practices. It may be necessary to design interventions that are tailored to patients' basic knowledge level and their perceptions of their own nutritional needs.

*Adults* (Burbank & Reibe, 2002) is an excellent reference for designing exercise strategies for the elderly.

Even late in life, it is generally believed that exercise has the benefits of increasing strength, aerobic capacity, and flexibility. One study (Keysor & Jette, 2001) found an 88% increase in strength in older patients who participated in an exercise program compared with those who did not exercise. Even those who are very old benefit from exercise: in an early study, Fiatarone et al. (1990) reported that a group of nursing home residents 90 years of age and older who participated in a high-intensity resistance program showed significant growth in muscle strength and size and in mobility.

## Nervous System

The structure and function of the nervous system change with advanced age, and a reduction in cerebral blood flow accompanies nervous system changes. The loss of nerve cells contributes to a progressive loss of brain mass, and the synthesis and metabolism of the major neurotransmitters are also reduced. Because nerve impulses are conducted more slowly, older people take longer to respond and react. The autonomic nervous system performs less efficiently, and postural hypotension, which causes people to lose consciousness or feel lightheaded when standing up quickly, may occur. Neurologic changes can affect gait and balance, which may interfere with mobility and safety. Nurses advise elderly people to allow a longer time to respond to a stimulus and to move more deliberately. Homeostasis is more difficult to maintain, but in the absence of pathologic changes, older people function adequately and retain their cognitive and intellectual abilities.

This slowed reaction time puts older people at risk for falls and injuries, including driving errors. The per-mile fatality rate for drivers 70 years of age and older is nine times that for drivers 25 to 69 years of age. Elderly people who are driving unsafely should receive a driving fitness evaluation. This is often administered by an occupational therapist in conjunction with a neuropsychologist, who conducts more detailed cognitive testing (Dolinar, McQuillen, & Ranseen, 2001).

Mental function is threatened by physical or emotional stresses. A sudden onset of confusion may be the first symptom of an infection or change in physical condition (eg, pneumonia, urinary tract infection, medication interactions, dehydration).

## Sensory System

People interact with the world through their senses. Sensory losses associated with old age affect all sensory organs, and it can be devastating not to be able to see to read or watch television, hear conversation well enough to communicate, or discriminate taste well enough to enjoy food. In 2002, nearly half of older men and one third of older women reported difficulty hearing without a hearing aid. Sixteen percent of older men and 19% of older women reported difficulty seeing, even with corrective lenses (Older Americans, 2005). An uncompensated alteration in a sensory loss negatively affects the functional ability and quality of life of the older adult.

### SENSORY LOSS VERSUS SENSORY DEPRIVATION

Sensory loss can often be compensated for by assistive devices such as glasses and hearing aids. In contrast, sensory deprivation is the absence of stimuli in the environment or the inability to interpret existing stimuli (perhaps as a result of a sensory loss). Sensory deprivation can lead to boredom, confusion, irritability, disorientation, and anxiety. A decline in sensory input can mimic a decline in cognition that is in fact not present. Meaningful sensory stimulation offered to the older person is often helpful in correcting this problem. One sense can substitute for another in observing and interpreting stimuli. Nurses can enhance sensory stimulation in the environment with colors, pictures, textures, tastes, smells, and sounds. The stimuli are most meaningful if they are interpreted to older people and if the stimuli are changed often. Cognitively impaired people tend to respond well to touch and to familiar music.

### VISION

As new cells form on the outside surface of the lens of the eye, the older central cells accumulate and become yellow, rigid, dense, and cloudy, leaving only the outer portion of the lens elastic enough to change shape (accommodate) and focus at near and far distances. As the lens becomes less flexible, the near point of focus gets farther away. This condition, **presbyopia**, usually begins in the fifth decade of life and requires the person to wear reading glasses to magnify objects. In addition, the yellowing, cloudy lens causes light to scatter and makes the older person sensitive to glare. The ability to discern blue from green decreases. The pupil dilates slowly and less completely because of increased stiffness of the muscles of the iris, so the older person takes more time to adjust when going to and from light and dark settings and needs brighter light for close vision. Pathologic visual conditions are not a part of normal aging, but the incidence of eye disease (most commonly cataracts, glaucoma, diabetic retinopathy, and age-related macular degeneration) increases in older people.

Age-related macular degeneration is the primary cause of vision loss in the elderly. More than 25% of people older than 75 years of age have some signs of this disease, and 6% to 8% have advanced disease associated with severe vision loss. Macular degeneration does not affect peripheral vision, which means that it does not cause blindness. However, it affects central vision, color perception, and fine detail, greatly affecting common visual skills such as reading, driving, and seeing faces. Risk factors include sunlight exposure, cigarette smoking, and heredity, and people with fair skin and blue eyes may be at increased risk. Sunglasses and hats with visors provide some protection, and stopping smoking is paramount in preventing the disease. Although there is no definitive treatment and no cure that restores vision, several treatment options are available, depending on factors such as the location of the abnormal blood vessels. Photodynamic therapy, a "cool laser" therapy, is the mainstay of treatment for the wet type of acute macular degeneration (*Harvard Health Letter*, 2003). The earlier this condition is diagnosed, the greater the chances of preserving sight.

### HEARING

Auditory changes begin to be noticed at about 40 years of age. Environmental factors, such as exposure to noise, medications, and infections, as well as genetics, may contribute to hearing loss as much as age-related changes. **Presbycusis** is a gradual, sensorineural loss that progresses from the loss of the ability to hear high-frequency tones to a generalized loss of hearing. It is attributed to irreversible inner ear changes. Older people often cannot follow conversation because tones of high-frequency consonants (the sounds *f, s, th, ch, sh, b, t, p*) all sound alike. Hearing loss may cause older people to respond inappropriately, misunderstand conversation, and avoid social interaction. This behavior may be erroneously interpreted as confusion. Wax buildup or other correctable problems may also be responsible for hearing difficulties. A properly prescribed and fitted hearing aid may be useful in reducing some types of hearing deficits.

### TASTE AND SMELL

Of the four basic tastes (sweet, sour, salty, and bitter), sweet tastes are particularly dulled in older people. Blunted taste may contribute to the preference for salty, highly seasoned foods, but herbs, onions, garlic, and lemon can be used as substitutes for salt to flavor food.

Changes in the sense of smell are related to cell loss in the nasal passages and in the olfactory bulb in the brain. Environmental factors such as long-term exposure to toxins (eg, dust, pollen, and smoke) contribute to the cellular damage.

## Cognitive Aspects of Aging

Cognition can be affected by many variables, including sensory impairment, physiologic health, environment, and psychosocial influences. Older adults may experience temporary changes in cognitive function when hospitalized or admitted to skilled nursing facilities, rehabilitation centers, or long-term care facilities. These changes are related to differences in the environment or in medical therapy, or to alteration in role performance. In 2002, the proportion of people with moderate to severe memory impairment ranged from approximately 5% among people ages 65 to 69 years to 32% among people 85 years and older (Older Americans, 2005).

### Intelligence

When intelligence test scores from people of all ages are compared, test scores for older adults show a progressive decline beginning in midlife. However, research has shown that environment and health have a considerable influence on scores and that certain types of intelligence (eg, spatial perceptions and retention of nonintellectual information) decline, whereas others (eg, problem-solving ability based on past experiences, verbal comprehension, mathematical ability) do not. Cardiovascular health, a stimulating environment, high levels of education, occupational status, and income all appear to have a positive effect on intelligence scores in later life.

### Learning and Memory

According to Hooyman and Kiyak (2002, p. 271), "significant age-related declines in intelligence, learning, and memory appear not to be inevitable." These authors summarized the major studies on cognitive function in later years and provided the following overview.

Many factors affect the ability of older people to learn and remember and to perform well in testing situations. Older adults who have higher levels of education, good sensory function, good nutrition, and jobs that require complex problem-solving skills continue to demonstrate intelligence, memory, and the capacity for learning. Part of the problem in testing older adults is determining what is actually being tested (eg, speed of response) and whether the test results are indicative of a normal age-related change, a sensory deficit, or poor health. However, age differences continue to emerge even with untimed tests and when the tests are controlled for variations in motor and sensory function. In general, there is a decline in fluid intelligence, the biologically determined intelligence used for flexibility in thinking and problem solving. Crystallized intelligence, that gained through education and lifelong experiences (eg, verbal skills), remains intact. This is termed the classic aging pattern of intelligence. Despite these slight declines, many older people continue to learn and participate in varied educational experiences.

Good health and motivation are important influences on learning. Nurses can support the process by which older adults learn by using the following strategies:

- Supplying mnemonics to enhance recall of related data
- Encouraging ongoing learning
- Linking new information with familiar information
- Using visual, auditory, and other sensory cues
- Encouraging learners to wear prescription glasses and hearing aids
- Providing glare-free lighting
- Providing a quiet, nondistracting environment
- Setting short-term goals with input from the learner
- Keeping teaching periods short
- Pacing learning tasks according to the endurance of the learner
- Encouraging verbal participation by learners
- Reinforcing successful learning in a positive manner

## Pharmacologic Aspects of Aging

Older people use more medications than any other age group. Although they represent only 12.6% of the total population, they use 30% of all prescribed medications and 40% of all over-the-counter medications (Mezey, Fulmer, & Abraham, 2003). Medications improve the health and well-being of older people by relieving pain and discomfort, treating chronic illnesses, and curing infectious processes. However, adverse drug reactions are common because of medication interactions, multiple medication effects, incorrect dosages, and the use of multiple medications (**polypharmacy**). The potential for drug–drug interactions increases with increased drug use; such interactions are responsible for numerous emergency department and physician visits, which cost billions of dollars annually (Delafuente, 2003; Mezey et al., 2003).

Certain types of medications that carry high risks for older patients are often inappropriately prescribed. A study matching explicit criteria for appropriate prescription against a comprehensive drug benefit plan for elderly patients found that significant percentages of patients could be considered to be taking certain medications inappropriately (38% of patients taking antidepressants, 19% taking oral hypoglycemic agents, 18% taking sedative-hypnotics, and 13% taking nonsteroidal anti-inflammatory drugs [NSAIDs]) (Anderson, Beers, & Kerluke, 1997).

Any medication is capable of altering nutritional status, and the nutritional health of the elderly person may already be compromised by a marginal diet or by chronic disease and its treatment. Medications can affect the appetite, cause nausea and vomiting, irritate the stomach, cause constipation or diarrhea, and decrease absorption of nutrients. In addition, these medications may alter electrolyte balance as well as carbohydrate and fat metabolism. For example, antacids cause thiamine deficiency; cathartics diminish absorption; antibiotics and phenytoin (Dilantin) reduce utilization of folic acid; and phenothiazines, estrogens, and corticosteroids increase food intake and cause weight gain.

Combining multiple medications with alcohol, as well as with over-the-counter and herbal medications, complicates the problem. For example, St. John's wort, a common herbal supplement used for mild depression, decreases the anticoagulant effect of warfarin (Coumadin) and interacts with many other medications metabolized in the liver (Lam, 2000).

### Altered Pharmacokinetics

Alterations in absorption, metabolism, distribution, and excretion occur as a result of normal aging and may also result from drug and food interactions. Absorption may be affected by changes in gastric pH and a decrease in gastrointestinal motility. Drug distribution may be altered as a result of decrease in body water and increase in body fat. Normal age-related changes and diseases that alter blood flow, liver and renal function, or cardiac output may affect distribution and metabolism (Mezey et al., 2003) (Table 12-3).

### Nursing Implications

Prescription principles that have been identified for older patients include "start low and go slow" and "keep the medication regimen as simple as possible" (Mezey et al., 2003). A comprehensive assessment that begins with a thorough medication history, including use of alcohol, recreational drugs, and over-the-counter and herbal medications, is essential. It is best to ask the patient or reliable informants to provide all medications for review. Ascertaining the patient's understanding of when and how to take each medication as well as the purpose of each medication allows the nurse to assess the patient's knowledge about and compliance with the medication regimen. The patient's beliefs and concerns about the medications are identified. It is also helpful to know whether patients believe that a given medication is helpful.

Noncompliance leads to significant morbidity and mortality among the elderly. Among people 60 years of age and older, reports of noncompliance with medication regimens range from 26% to 59% (van Eijken, Tsang, Wensing, et al., 2003). The many contributing factors include the number of medications prescribed, the complexity of the regimen, difficulty opening containers, inadequate patient education, financial cost, and the disease or medication interfering with the patient's life. Furthermore, visual and hearing problems may make it difficult to read or to hear directions.

Multifaceted interventions tailored to the individual patient are the most effective strategies in improving compliance (van Eijken et al., 2003). The following steps can help patients manage their medications and improve compliance:

- Explain the purpose, adverse effects, and dosage of each medication.
- Provide the medication schedule in writing.
- Encourage the use of standard containers without safety lids (if there are no children in the household).
- Suggest the use of a multiple-day, multiple-dose medication dispenser to help the patient adhere to the medication schedule (Fig. 12-3).
- Destroy or remove old, unused medications.
- Encourage the patient to inform the primary health care provider about the use of over-the-counter medications and herbal agents, alcohol, and recreational drugs.
- Encourage the patient to keep a list of all medications, including over-the-counter and herbal medications, in his or her purse or wallet to share with the primary care provider at each visit and in case of an emergency.
- Review the medication schedule periodically and update it as necessary.
- Recommend using one supplier for prescriptions; pharmacies frequently track patients and are likely to notice a prescription problem such as duplication or contraindications in the medication regimen.
- If the patient's competence is doubtful, identify a reliable family member or friend who might monitor the patient for compliance.

## Mental Health Problems in the Older Adult

Changes in cognitive ability, excessive forgetfulness, and mood swings are not a part of normal aging. These symptoms should not be dismissed as age-related changes; a thorough assessment may reveal a treatable, reversible physical or mental condition. Changes in mental status may be related to many factors, such as alterations in diet and fluid and electrolyte balance, fever, or low oxygen levels associated with many cardiovascular and pulmonary diseases. Cognitive changes may be reversible when the underlying condition is identified and treated. However, the incidence of dementia and susceptibility to depression and delirium increase with age. Older adults are less likely than younger people to seek treatment for mental health symptoms. Therefore, health professionals must recognize, assess, refer, collaborate, treat, and support older adults who exhibit noticeable changes in intellect or affect.

### Depression

**Depression** is the most common affective or mood disorder of old age. About 15% of older Americans suffer from significant depression (Burke & Laramie, 2004). The incidence of depression is significant among the hospitalized elderly

## TABLE 12-3  Altered Drug Responses in Older People

| Age-Related Changes | Effect of Age-Related Change | Applicable Medications |
|---|---|---|
| **Absorption** | | |
| Reduced gastric acid; increased pH (less acid) | Rate of drug absorption—possibly delayed | Vitamins |
| Reduced gastrointestinal motility; prolonged gastric emptying | Extent of drug absorption—not affected | Calcium |
| **Distribution** | | |
| Decreased albumin sites | Serious alterations in drug binding to plasma proteins (the unbound drug gives the pharmacologic response); highly protein-bound medications have fewer binding sites, leading to increased effects and accelerated metabolism and excretion | Selected highly protein-binding medications:<br>  Oral anticoagulants (warfarin)<br>  Oral hypoglycemic agents (sulfonylureas)<br>  Barbiturates<br>  Calcium channel blockers<br>  Furosemide (Lasix)<br>  Nonsteroidal anti-inflammatory drugs (NSAIDs)<br>  Sulfonamides<br>  Quinidine<br>  Phenytoin (Dilantin) |
| Reduced cardiac output | Decreased perfusion of many bodily organs | |
| Impaired peripheral blood flow | Decreased perfusion | |
| Increased percentage of body fat | Proportion of body fat increases with age, resulting in increased ability to store fat-soluble medications; this causes drug accumulation, prolonged storage, and delayed excretion | Selected fat-soluble medications:<br>  Barbiturates<br>  Diazepam (Valium)<br>  Lidocaine<br>  Phenothiazines (antipsychotics)<br>  Ethanol<br>  Morphine |
| Decreased lean body mass | Decreased body volume allows higher peak levels of medications | |
| **Metabolism** | | |
| Decreased cardiac output and decreased perfusion of the liver | Decreased metabolism and delay of breakdown of medications, resulting in prolonged duration of action, accumulation, and drug toxicity | All medications metabolized by the liver |
| **Excretion** | | |
| Decreased renal blood flow; loss of functioning nephrons; decreased renal efficiency | Decreased rates of elimination and increased duration of action; danger of accumulation and drug toxicity | Selected medications with prolonged action:<br>  Aminoglycoside antibiotics<br>  Cimetidine (Tagamet)<br>  Chlorpropamide (Diabinase)<br>  Digoxin<br>  Lithium<br>  Procainamide |

(12%) and increases to 30% among nursing home residents. Depression among the elderly often follows a major precipitating event or loss but may also be secondary to a medication interaction or an undiagnosed physical condition. Signs of depression include feelings of sadness, fatigue, diminished memory and concentration, feelings of guilt or worthlessness, sleep disturbances, appetite disturbances with excessive weight loss or gain, restlessness, impaired attention span, and suicidal ideation. Depression disrupts quality of life and increases the risk for suicide, especially among elderly Caucasian and Asian-American men (Kennedy-Malone, Fletcher, & Plank, 2004).

Geriatric depression may be confused with dementia. However, the cognitive impairment resulting from depression is a result of apathy rather than decline in brain function. When depression and medical illnesses coexist, as they often

**FIGURE 12-3.** Commercially available, multiple-dose, multiple-day medication dispensers such as this one help older people to follow complex medication regimens safely at home.

do, neglect of the depression can retard physical recovery. Assessing the patient's mental status, including depression, is vital and must not be overlooked (Charts 12-1 and 12-2).

Depression is responsive to treatment but is often overlooked and therefore is undertreated. Initial management involves evaluation of the patient's medication regimen and eliminating or changing any medications that contribute to depression. Furthermore, treatment of underlying medical conditions that may produce depressive symptoms may alleviate the depression. Both antidepressants and short-term psychotherapy, particularly in combination, are effective in treating late-life depression. Newer atypical antidepressants, such as bupropion (Wellbutrin), venlafaxine (Effexor), mirtazapine (Remeron), and nefazodone (Serzone), and selective serotonin reuptake inhibitors, such as paroxetine (Paxil), may be used (Kennedy-Malone et al., 2004). It is recommended that the initial dose of antidepressants be low. The following factors also should be considered: age, coexisting conditions, adverse effects, and prior response to these medications. Tricyclic antidepressants are also clinically effective for depression. However, those with anticholinergic, cardiac, and orthostatic adverse effects, as well as interactions with other medications, should be used with care to avoid medication toxicity. It may take 4 to 6 weeks for symptoms to diminish, and during this period, nurses should offer explanations and encouragement.

### Alcohol and Drug Abuse

Alcohol and drug abuse may be related to depression, and its incidence is significant in the elderly population. In people between 65 and 84 years of age, 35% to 38% of men and 21% to 32% of women have reported drinking moderately (one drink or less a day). Heavy drinking (more than one drink a day) is reportedly between 9% and 10% for men and between 2.2% and 2.6% for women (Breslow, Faden, & Smothers, 2003). Among 565 geriatric veteran inpatients studied, 4% were diagnosed with nonalcoholic substance disorders, 3% had prescription drug use disorders, and 1% had illegal drug use disorders (Widlitz & Marin, 2002).

Alcohol abuse is especially dangerous in older people because of changes in renal and liver function as well as the probability of interactions with prescription medications and the resultant adverse effects. Alcohol- and drug-related problems in older people often remain hidden because many older adults deny their habit when questioned.

---

**CHART 12-1**

## Mini-Mental State Examination

**Maximum Score**

**ORIENTATION**

5    What is the (year) (season) (date) (day) (month)?

5    Where are we (state) (county) (city) (hospital) (floor)?

**REGISTRATION**

3    Name three objects: One second to say each. Then ask the patient all three after you have said them. Give one point for each correct answer. Repeat them until he learns all three. Count trials and record number. Number of trials: _____.

**ATTENTION AND CALCULATION**

5    Begin with 100 and count backwards by 7 (stop after five answers). Alternatively, spell "world" backwards.

**RECALL**

3    Ask for the three objects repeated above. Give one point for each correct answer.

**LANGUAGE**

2    Show a pencil and a watch, and ask subject to name them.

1    Repeat the following: "No 'if's,' 'and's,' or 'but's.'"

3    A three-stage command: "Take a paper in your right hand; fold it in half, and put it on the floor."

1    Read and obey the following: (Show subject the written item.) CLOSE YOUR EYES.

1    Write a sentence.

1    Copy a design (complex polygon as in Bender-Gestalt).

30    **Total score possible**

Reprinted from Folstein, M. F., Folstein, S., & McHugh, P. R. (1975). Mini-mental state: A practical method for grading the cognitive state of patients for the clinician. *Journal of Psychiatric Research, 12*, 189–198. With permission from Pergamon Press Ltd, Headington Hill Hall, Oxford OX3 OBW, UK.

### Delirium

**Delirium**, often called acute confusional state, begins with confusion and progresses to disorientation. Delirium affects an estimated 2.3 million elderly people and accounts for more than 17.5 annual hospital days at a cost of more than $4 billion a year; as many as 10% to 16% of elderly patients are delirious on admission to the hospital (Kennedy-Malone et al., 2004). Delirium is the most frequent complication of

## CHART 12-2

### Geriatric Depression Scale

Choose the best answer for how you felt this past week.

| # | Question | | |
|---|---|---|---|
| *1. | Are you basically satisfied with your life? | YES | NO |
| 2. | Have you dropped many of your activities and interests? | YES | NO |
| 3. | Do you feel that your life is empty? | YES | NO |
| 4. | Do you often get bored? | YES | NO |
| *5. | Are you hopeful about the future? | YES | NO |
| 6. | Are you bothered by thoughts you can't get out of your head? | YES | NO |
| *7. | Are you in good spirits most of the time? | YES | NO |
| 8. | Are you afraid that something bad is going to happen to you? | YES | NO |
| *9. | Do you feel happy most of the time? | YES | NO |
| 10. | Do you often feel helpless? | YES | NO |
| 11. | Do you often get restless and fidgety? | YES | NO |
| 12. | Do you prefer to stay at home, rather than going out and doing new things? | YES | NO |
| 13. | Do you frequently worry about the future? | YES | NO |
| 14. | Do you feel you have more problems with memory than most? | YES | NO |
| *15. | Do you think it is wonderful to be alive now? | YES | NO |
| 16. | Do you often feel downhearted and blue? | YES | NO |
| 17. | Do you feel pretty worthless the way you are now? | YES | NO |
| 18. | Do you worry a lot about the past? | YES | NO |
| *19. | Do you find life very exciting? | YES | NO |
| 20. | Is it hard for you to get started on new projects? | YES | NO |
| *21. | Do you feel full of energy? | YES | NO |
| 22. | Do you feel that your situation is hopeless? | YES | NO |
| 23. | Do you think that most people are better off than you are? | YES | NO |
| 24. | Do you frequently get upset over little things? | YES | NO |
| 25. | Do you frequently feel like crying? | YES | NO |
| 26. | Do you have trouble concentrating? | YES | NO |
| *27. | Do you enjoy getting up in the morning? | YES | NO |
| 28. | Do you prefer to avoid social gatherings? | YES | NO |
| *29. | Is it easy for you to make decisions? | YES | NO |
| *30. | Is your mind as clear as it used to be? | YES | NO |

Score: _____ (Number of "depressed" answers)

**NORMS**

Normal: 5 ± 4
Mildly depressed: 15 ± 6
Very depressed: 23 ± 5

---

* Appropriate (nondepressed) answers = yes; all others = no.

Yesavage, J., et al. (1983). Development and validation of a geriatric screening scale: A preliminary report. *Journal of Psychiatric Research, 17* (1), 37–49. Reprinted with permission from Pergamon Press Ltd., Headington Hill Hall, Oxford OX3 OBW, UK.

---

hospitalization. Patients may experience an altered level of consciousness, ranging from stupor to excessive activity. Thinking is disorganized and the attention span is short. Hallucinations, delusions, fear, anxiety, and paranoia may also be evident.

Delirium occurs secondary to a number of causes, including physical illness, medication or alcohol toxicity, dehydration, fecal impaction, malnutrition, infection, head trauma, lack of environmental cues, and sensory deprivation or overload. Older adults are particularly vulnerable to acute confusion because of their decreased biologic reserve and the large number of medications they may take. Nurses must recognize the grave implications of the acute symptoms and report them immediately. Because of the acute and unexpected onset of symptoms and the unknown underlying cause, delirium is a medical emergency. If the delirium goes unrecognized and the underlying cause is not treated, permanent, irreversible brain damage or death can follow. Attentive clinical assessment is essential, because delirium is sometimes mistaken for dementia; Table 12-4 compares

### TABLE 12-4 Summary of Differences Between Dementia and Delirium

| | Dementia | | Delirium |
|---|---|---|---|
| | **Alzheimer's Disease (AD)** | **Vascular (Multi-Infarct) Dementia** | |
| Etiology | Familial (genetic [chromosomes 14, 19, 21])<br>Sporadic | Cardiovascular (CV) disease<br>Cerebrovascular disease<br>Hypertension | Drug toxicity and interactions; acute disease; trauma; chronic disease exacerbation<br>Fluid and electrolyte disorder |
| Risk factors | Advanced age; genetics | Preexisting CV disease | Preexisting cognitive impairment |
| Occurrence | 50%–60% of dementias | 20% of dementias | 20% of hospitalized older people |
| Onset | Slow | Often abrupt<br>Follows a stroke or transient ischemic attack | Rapid, acute onset<br>A harbinger of acute medical illness |
| Age of onset (yr) | Early onset AD: 30s–65<br>Late onset AD: 65+<br>Most commonly: 85+ | Most commonly 50–70 yr | Any age, but predominantly in older persons |
| Gender | Males and females equally | Predominantly males | Males and females equally |
| Course | Chronic, irreversible; progressive, regular, downhill | Chronic, irreversible<br>Fluctuating, stepwise progression | Acute |
| Duration | 2–20 yr | Variable; years | Lasts 1 day to 1 month |
| Symptom progress | Onset insidious. *Early*—mild and subtle<br>*Middle and late*—intensified<br>Progression to death (infection or malnutrition) | Depends on location of infarct and success of treatment; death due to underlying CV disease | Symptoms are fully reversible with adequate treatment; can progress to chronicity or death if underlying condition is ignored |
| Mood | Early depression (30%) | Labile: mood swings | Variable |
| Speech/language | Speech remains intact until late in disease<br>*Early*—mild anomia (cannot name objects); deficits progress until speech lacks meaning; echoes and repeats words and sounds; mutism. | May have speech deficit/aphasia depending on location of lesion | Fluctuating; often cannot concentrate long enough to speak |
| Physical signs | *Early*—no motor deficits<br>*Middle*—apraxia (70%) (cannot perform purposeful movement)<br>*Late*—Dysarthria (impaired speech)<br>*End stage*—loss of all voluntary activity; positive neurologic signs | According to location of lesion: focal neurologic signs, seizures<br><br>Commonly exhibits motor deficits | Signs and symptoms of underlying disease |
| Orientation | Becomes lost in familiar places (topographic disorientation)<br>Has difficulty drawing three-dimensional objects (visual and spatial disorientation)<br>Disorientation to time, place, and person—with disease progression | | May fluctuate between lucidity and complete disorientation to time, place, and person |
| Memory | Loss is an early sign of dementia; loss of recent memory is soon followed by progressive decline in recent and remote memory | | Impaired recent and remote memory; may fluctuate between lucidity and confusion |
| Personality | Apathy, indifference, irritability<br>*Early disease*—social behavior intact; hides cognitive deficits<br>*Advanced disease*—disengages from activity and relationships; suspicious; paranoid delusions caused by memory loss; aggressive; catastrophic reactions | | Fluctuating; cannot focus attention to converse; alarmed by symptoms (when lucid); hallucinations; paranoid |
| Functional status, activities of daily living | Poor judgment in everyday activities; has progressive decline in ability to handle money, use telephone, function in home and workplace | | Impaired |
| Attention span | Distractable; short attention span | | Highly impaired; cannot maintain or shift attention |

| TABLE 12-4 | Summary of Differences Between Dementia and Delirium (Continued) | | |
|---|---|---|---|
| | **Dementia** | | |
| | Alzheimer's Disease (AD) | Vascular (Multi-Infarct) Dementia | Delirium |
| Psychomotor activity | Wandering, hyperactivity, pacing, restlessness, agitation | | Variable; alternates between high agitation, hyperactivity, restlessness, and lethargy |
| Sleep–wake cycle | Often impaired; wandering and agitation at nighttime | | Takes brief naps throughout day and night |

dementia and delirium. It helps to know an individual patient's mental status prior to hospitalization and whether the changes noted are long term or are abrupt in onset.

In the management of delirium, treatment of the underlying cause is most important, and therapeutic interventions vary depending on the cause. Delirium increases the risk of falls; therefore, management of patient safety and behavioral problems is essential. Because medication interactions and toxicity are often implicated, nonessential medications should be discontinued. Nutritional and fluid intake should be supervised and monitored. The environment should be quiet and calm. To increase function and comfort, the nurse provides familiar environmental cues and encourages family members or friends to touch and talk to the patient. Ongoing mental status assessments using prior mental cognitive status as baseline are helpful in evaluating responses to treatment and to the admission to a hospital or extended-care facility. If the underlying problem is adequately treated, the patient often returns to baseline within several days.

## Dementia

Dementia reportedly affects 3% to 11% of community-residing adults older than 65 years of age and about half of community-residing adults older than 85 years of age. Many of those suffering from dementia who are older than 85 reside in institutional settings. Almost 60% of adults 100 years of age and older demonstrate dementia. Despite this high incidence, clinicians fail to detect dementia in 21% to 72% of patients. For a diagnosis of dementia to be made, at least two domains of function must be altered—memory and at least one of the following: language, perception, visuospatial function, calculation, judgment, abstraction, and problem-solving (Mayo Foundation for Medical Education and Research [Mayo], 2001).

Symptoms of dementia are usually subtle in onset and often progress slowly until they are obvious and devastating. The characteristic changes fall into three general categories—cognitive, functional, and behavioral—and they eventually destroy a person's ability to function. The two most common types of dementia are Alzheimer's disease (AD), which accounts for 50% to 60% of cases, and vascular or multi-infarct dementia, which accounts for 10% to 20% of cases. Other non-Alzheimer dementias include Parkinson's disease, acquired immunodeficiency syndrome (AIDS)-related dementia, and Pick's disease; these types of dementia account for fewer than 15% of cases (National Institute of Neurological Disorders and Stroke, 2006).

### Alzheimer's Disease

AD is a progressive, irreversible, degenerative neurologic disease that begins insidiously and is characterized by gradual losses of cognitive function and disturbances in behavior and affect. Although AD can occur in people as young as 40, it is uncommon before age 65. The prevalence of AD increases dramatically with increasing age, affecting 30% of those 85 and older (Harvard Men's Health Watch, 2002). There are numerous theories about the cause of age-related cognitive decline. Although the greatest risk for AD is increasing age, many environmental, dietary, and inflammatory factors also may affect whether a person suffers from this cognitive disease. AD is a form of dementia, a complex brain disorder caused by a combination of various factors (McDonald, 2002). These factors may include genes, neurotransmitter changes, vascular abnormalities, stress hormones, circadian changes, head trauma, and seizures.

AD can be classified into two types: familial or early-onset AD and sporadic or late-onset AD. Familial AD is rare, accounting for only 5% to 10% of all cases, and is frequently associated with genetic mutations. It occurs in middle-aged adults. If family members have at least one other relative with AD, then there is a familial component, which nonspecifically includes both environmental triggers and genetic determinants. Sporadic AD generally occurs in people older than 65 years of age (Marin, Sewell, & Schlechter, 2002), and it has no obvious pattern of inheritance.

Since 1995, molecular biologists have discovered specific genetic information about the various forms of AD, including genetic differences between early- and late-onset AD. These genetic differences help pinpoint risk factors associated with the disease, although the genetic indicators are not specific enough to be used as reliable diagnostic markers (Mayo, 2001).

**PATHOPHYSIOLOGY**
Specific neuropathologic and biochemical changes are found in patients with AD. These include neurofibrillary tangles (tangled masses of nonfunctioning neurons) and senile or neuritic plaques (deposits of amyloid protein, part of a larger protein called amyloid precursor protein [APP]) in the brain. The neuronal damage occurs primarily in the cerebral cortex and results in decreased brain size. Similar changes are found in the normal brain tissue of older adults, but to a lesser extent. Cells that use the neurotransmitter acetylcholine are those principally affected by AD. Biochemically, the enzyme active in producing acetylcholine, which is specifically involved in memory processing, is decreased.

Several theories are being tested to explain what predisposes people to develop the plaques and neurotangles that can be seen at autopsy in the brains of patients with AD (Mayo, 2001). Scientists continue to increase their understanding of the complex ways in which aging and genetic and nongenetic factors affect and damage brain cells over time, eventually leading to AD. Researchers have recently discovered how amyloid plaques form and cause neuronal death, as well as the possible relationship between various forms of tau protein and impaired function, which leads to neuronal death. (The major role of tau protein is to regulate the assembly and stability of neurons.) Researchers are also beginning to discover the roles of inflammation and oxidative stress and the contribution of brain infarctions to the disease (Iqbal & Grundke-Iqbal, 2004).

## CLINICAL MANIFESTATIONS

In the early stages of AD, forgetfulness and subtle memory loss occur. Patients may experience small difficulties in work or social activities but have adequate cognitive function to hide the loss and function independently. Depression may occur. With further progression of AD, the deficits can no longer be concealed. Forgetfulness is manifested in many daily actions; patients may lose their ability to recognize familiar faces, places, and objects, and they may become lost in a familiar environment. They may repeat the same stories because they forget that they have already told them. Trying to reason with people with AD and using reality **orientation** only increases their anxiety without increasing function. Conversation becomes difficult, and word-finding difficulties occur. The ability to formulate concepts and think abstractly disappears; for example, a patient can interpret a proverb only in concrete terms. Patients are often unable to recognize the consequences of their actions and will therefore exhibit impulsive behavior. For example, on a hot day, a patient may decide to wade in the city fountain fully clothed. Patients have difficulty with everyday activities, such as operating simple appliances and handling money.

Personality changes are also usually evident. Patients may become depressed, suspicious, paranoid, hostile, and even combative. Progression of the disease intensifies the symptoms: speaking skills deteriorate to nonsense syllables, agitation and physical activity increase, and patients may wander at night. Eventually, assistance is needed for most ADLs, including eating and toileting, because dysphagia and incontinence develop. The terminal stage, in which patients are usually immobile and require total care, may last months or years. Occasionally, patients may recognize family members or caregivers. Death occurs as a result of complications such as pneumonia, malnutrition, or dehydration.

## ASSESSMENT AND DIAGNOSTIC FINDINGS

A definitive diagnosis of AD can be made only at autopsy, but an accurate clinical diagnosis can be made in about 90% of cases. The most important goal is to rule out other causes of dementia or reversible causes of confusion, such as other types of dementia, depression, delirium, alcohol or drug abuse, or inappropriate drug dosage or drug toxicity (Marin et al., 2002).

The health history—including medical history, family history, social and cultural history, and medication history—and the physical examination, including functional and mental health status, are essential to the diagnosis of probable AD. Diagnostic tests, including complete blood count, chemistry profile, and vitamin $B_{12}$ and thyroid hormone levels, as well as screening with electroencephalography, computed tomography (CT), magnetic resonance imaging (MRI), and examination of the cerebrospinal fluid may all refute or support a diagnosis of probable AD.

Depression can closely mimic early-stage AD and coexists in many patients. A depression scale is helpful in screening for underlying depression. Tests of cognitive function such as the Mini-Mental State Examination (see Chart 12-1) and the clock-drawing test are useful for screening. CT and MRI scans of the brain are useful for excluding hematoma, brain tumor, stroke, normal-pressure hydrocephalus, and atrophy but are not reliable in making a definitive diagnosis of AD. Infections, physiologic disturbances such as hypothyroidism, Parkinson's disease, and vitamin $B_{12}$ deficiency can cause cognitive impairment that may be misdiagnosed as AD. Biochemical abnormalities can be excluded through examination of the blood and cerebrospinal fluid, but the findings are not sufficiently specific to make the diagnosis. AD is a diagnosis of exclusion, and a diagnosis of probable AD is made when the medical history, physical examination, and laboratory tests have excluded all known causes of other dementias.

## MEDICAL MANAGEMENT

The primary goal in the medical management of AD is to manage the cognitive and behavioral symptoms. There is no cure and no way to slow the progression of the disease. Cholinesterase inhibitors such as donepezil hydrochloride (Aricept), rivastigmine tartrate (Exelon), and galantamine hydrobromide (Reminyl) enhance acetylcholine uptake in the brain, thus maintaining memory skills for a period of time. The drug memantine (Namenda), which is reported to reduce the clinical deterioration in moderate to severe AD, was recently approved for use in the United States (*Mental Health Weekly Digest*, 2004). One clinical trial demonstrated that use of donepezil in combination with memantine increases cognitive function in patients with AD (National Institute of Neurological Disorders and Stroke, 2003). Cognitive ability improves within 6 to 12 months of therapy, but cessation of the medications results in cognitive decline commensurate with disease progression. It is recommended that treatment continue at least through the moderate stage of the illness. Ancillary treatment with an NSAID or vitamin E may be considered; however, research supporting such treatment is limited (Marin et al., 2002).

Behavioral problems such as agitation and psychosis can be managed by behavioral and psychosocial therapies. Associated depression and behavioral problems can also be treated with antidepressants and the newer atypical neuroleptics, which are replacing the typical neuroleptics such as haloperidol (Haldol); the newer drugs have fewer adverse effects. Other atypical neuroleptics include olanzapine (Zyprexa), quetiapine fumarate (Seroquel), and risperidone (Risperdal) (Cohen, 2002).

## NURSING MANAGEMENT

Nursing interventions for dementia are aimed at promoting patient function and independence for as long as possible.

Other important goals include promoting the patient's physical safety, promoting independence in self-care activities, reducing anxiety and agitation, improving communication, providing for socialization and intimacy, promoting adequate nutrition, promoting balanced activity and rest, and supporting and educating family caregivers. Nursing interventions apply to all patients with dementia, regardless of the cause.

**Supporting Cognitive Function.** Because dementia of any type is degenerative and progressive, patients display a decline in cognitive function over time. In the early phase of dementia, minimal cueing and guidance may be all that are needed for the patient to function fairly independently for a number of years. However, as the patient's cognitive ability declines, family members must provide more and more assistance and supervision. A calm, predictable environment helps people with AD interpret their surroundings and activities. Environmental stimuli are limited, and a regular routine is established. A quiet, pleasant manner of speaking, clear and simple explanations, and use of memory aids and cues help minimize confusion and disorientation and give patients a sense of security. Prominently displayed clocks and calendars may enhance orientation to time. Color-coding the doorway may help patients who have difficulty locating their room. Active participation may help patients maintain cognitive, functional, and social interaction abilities for a longer period. Physical activity and communication have also been demonstrated to slow some of the cognitive decline of AD (Tappen, Roach, Applegate, et al., 2000).

**Promoting Physical Safety.** A safe home environment allows the patient to move about as freely as possible and relieves the family of constant worry about safety. To prevent falls and other injuries, all obvious hazards are removed and hand rails are installed. A hazard-free environment allows the patient maximum independence and a sense of autonomy. Adequate lighting, especially in halls, stairs, and bathrooms, is necessary. Nightlights are helpful, particularly if the patient has increased confusion at night (**sundowning**). Driving is prohibited, and smoking is allowed only with supervision. The patient may have a short attention span and be forgetful. Wandering behavior can often be reduced by gentle persuasion or distraction. Restraints should be avoided, because they increase agitation. Doors leading from the house must be secured. Outside the home, all activities must be supervised to protect the patient, and the patient should wear an identification bracelet or neck chain in case he or she becomes separated from the caregiver.

**Promoting Independence in Self-Care Activities.** Pathophysiologic changes in the brain make it difficult for people with AD to maintain physical independence. Patients should be assisted to remain functionally independent for as long as possible. One way to do this is to simplify daily activities by organizing them into short, achievable steps so that the patient experiences a sense of accomplishment. Frequently, occupational therapists can suggest ways to simplify tasks or recommend adaptive equipment. Direct patient supervision is sometimes necessary, but maintaining personal dignity and autonomy is important for people with AD, who should be encouraged to make choices when appropriate and to participate in self-care activities as much as possible.

**Reducing Anxiety and Agitation.** Despite profound cognitive losses, patients are sometimes aware of their diminishing abilities. Patients need constant emotional support that reinforces a positive self-image. When losses of skills occur, goals are adjusted to fit the patient's declining ability.

The environment should be kept familiar and noise-free. Excitement and confusion can be upsetting and may precipitate a combative, agitated state known as a catastrophic reaction (overreaction to excessive stimulation). The patient may respond by screaming, crying, or becoming abusive (physically or verbally); this may be the person's only way of expressing an inability to cope with the environment. When this occurs, it is important to remain calm and unhurried. Forcing the patient to proceed with the activity only increases the agitation. It is better to postpone the activity until later, even to another day. Frequently, the patient quickly forgets what triggered the reaction. Measures such as moving to a familiar environment, listening to music, stroking, rocking, or distraction may quiet the patient. Structuring activity is also helpful. Becoming familiar with a particular patient's predicted responses to certain stressors helps caregivers avoid similar situations.

Many older people with dementia who have progressed to the late stages of the disease typically reside in nursing homes and are predominantly cared for by nurses' aides. Dementia education for caregivers is essential to minimize patient agitation and can be effectively taught by advanced practice nurses.

**Improving Communication.** To promote the patient's interpretation of messages, the nurse should remain unhurried and reduce noises and distractions. Use of clear, easy-to-understand sentences to convey messages is essential, because patients frequently forget the meaning of words or have difficulty organizing and expressing thoughts. In the earlier stages of dementia, lists and simple written instructions that serve as reminders may be helpful. In later stages, the patient may be able to point to an object or use nonverbal language to communicate. Tactile stimuli, such as hugs or hand pats, are usually interpreted as signs of affection, concern, and security.

**Providing for Socialization and Intimacy Needs.** Because socialization with friends can be comforting, visits, letters, and phone calls are encouraged. Visits should be brief and nonstressful; limiting visitors to one or two at a time helps reduce overstimulation. Recreation is important, and people with dementia are encouraged to enjoy simple activities. Realistic goals for activities that provide satisfaction are appropriate. Hobbies and activities such as walking, exercising, and socializing can improve the quality of life. The nonjudgmental friendliness of a pet may provide stimulation, comfort, and contentment. Care of plants or of a pet can also be satisfying and an outlet for energy.

AD does not eliminate the need for intimacy. Patients and their spouses may continue to enjoy sexual activity. Spouses should be encouraged to talk about any sexual concerns, and sexual counseling may be necessary. Simple expressions of love, such as touching and holding, are often meaningful.

**Promoting Adequate Nutrition.** Mealtime can be a pleasant social occasion or a time of upset and distress, and it should be kept simple and calm, without confrontations. Patients prefer familiar foods that look appetizing and taste good. To avoid any "playing" with food, one dish is offered at a time. Food is cut into small pieces to prevent choking. Liquids may be easier to swallow if they are converted to gelatin. Hot food and beverages are served warm, and the temperature of the foods should be checked to prevent burns.

When lack of coordination interferes with self-feeding, adaptive equipment is helpful. Some patients may do well eating with a spoon or with their fingers. If this is the case, an apron or a smock, rather than a bib, is used to protect clothing. As deficits progress, it may be necessary to feed the patient. Forgetfulness, disinterest, dental problems, lack of coordination, overstimulation, and choking may all serve as barriers to good nutrition and hydration.

**Promoting Balanced Activity and Rest.** Many patients with dementia exhibit sleep disturbances, wandering, and behaviors that may be considered inappropriate. These behaviors are most likely to occur when there are unmet underlying physical or psychological needs. Caregivers must identify the needs of patients who are exhibiting these behaviors because further health decline may occur if the source of the problem is not corrected. Adequate sleep and physical exercise are essential. If sleep is interrupted or the patient cannot fall asleep, music, warm milk, or a back rub may help the patient to relax. During the day, patients should be encouraged to participate in exercise because a regular pattern of activity and rest enhances nighttime sleep. Long periods of daytime sleeping are discouraged.

**Supporting Home and Community-Based Care.** The emotional burden on the families of patients with AD is enormous. The physical health of the patient is often very stable, and the mental degeneration is gradual. Family members may cling to the hope that the diagnosis is incorrect and that their relative will improve with greater effort. Family members are faced with numerous difficult decisions (eg, when the patient should stop driving, when to assume responsibility for the patient's financial affairs). Aggression and hostility exhibited by the patient are often misunderstood by families or caregivers, who feel unappreciated, frustrated, and angry. Feelings of guilt, nervousness, and worry contribute to caregiver fatigue, depression, and family dysfunction.

In some cases, caregivers themselves can become so fatigued as a result of the stress of caregiving that self-neglect or neglect or abuse of the patient can occur. This has been documented in home situations as well as in institutions. If neglect or abuse of any kind—including physical, emotional, sexual, or financial abuse—is suspected, the local adult protective services agency must be notified. The role of the nurse is to report the suspected abuse, not to prove it.

The Alzheimer's Disease and Related Disorders Association is a coalition of family members and professionals who share the goals of family support and service, education, research, and advocacy. This national organization has addressed the multiple needs of family caregivers. Family support groups, respite (relief) care, and adult day care may be available through different community resources, such as the Area Agency on Aging or the Alzheimer's Disease and Related Disorders Association, in which concerned volunteers are trained to provide structure to caregiver support groups. Respite care is a commonly provided service in which caregivers can get away from the home for short periods while someone else tends to the needs of the patient.

### Vascular Dementia

Vascular or multi-infarct dementia is associated with hypertension and cardiovascular disease. It is sometimes confused with AD, paranoia, or delirium because of its unpredictable clinical course. Vascular dementia tends to have a more abrupt onset than AD, and it is characterized by an uneven, stepwise downward decline in mental function associated with a vascular incident such as a subclinical stroke. Diagnosis may be even more difficult if a patient has both AD and vascular dementia.

Because vascular dementia is associated with hypertension and cardiovascular disease, risk factors (eg, hypercholesterolemia, history of smoking, diabetes mellitus) are similar. Prevention and management are also similar. Therefore, therapy to decrease blood pressure and lower cholesterol levels may prevent future mini-infarcts. In addition, clinical trials have shown that giving donepezil hydrochloride (Aricept) to patients with vascular dementia enhances cognitive function (*Chemist and Druggist*, 2003).

## Common Health Issues of the Older Adult

To widely varying extents, elderly people tend to acquire multiple problems and illnesses as they age. The decline of physical function leads to a loss of independence and increasing frailty as well as to susceptibility to both acute and chronic health problems, which generally result from several factors rather than from a single cause. When combined with a decrease in host resistance, these factors can lead to illness or injury. Although the problems may develop slowly, the onset of symptoms is often acute. Furthermore, the presenting symptoms may appear in other body systems before becoming apparent in the affected system.

The term "frail" is used to describe elderly people who are at highest risk for adverse health outcomes. According to the most widely accepted definition, people who are frail tend to be 85 or older, suffer from multiple chronic diseases, and have difficulty performing IADLs or ADLs independently. However, there are no standard clinical criteria for frailty.

### Impaired Mobility

The causes of decreased mobility are many and varied. Common causes are Parkinson's disease, diabetic neuropathy, cardiovascular compromise, osteoarthritis, osteoporosis, and sensory deficits. Environmental barriers and iatrogenic factors are also significant. Elderly patients should be encouraged to stay as active as possible to avoid the downward spiral of immobility. During illness, bed rest should be kept to a minimum, because even brief periods of bed rest quickly lead to deconditioning and, consequently, to a wide range of complications. When bed rest cannot be avoided, patients should perform active range-of-motion and strengthening exercises with the unaffected extremities, and nurses or family caregivers should perform passive range-of-motion exercises on the affected extremities. Frequent position changes help offset the hazards of immobility. Both the health care staff and the patient's family can assist in maintaining the current level of mobility (Tappen et al., 2000).

## Dizziness

Older people frequently seek help for dizziness, which presents a particular challenge because there are so many possible internal and external causes. For many, the problem is complicated by an inability to differentiate between true dizziness (a sensation of disorientation in relation to position) and vertigo (a spinning sensation). Other similar sensations include near-syncope and disequilibrium. The causes for these sensations range in severity from minor (eg, buildup of ear wax) to severe (eg, dysfunction of the cerebral cortex, cerebellum, brainstem, proprioceptive receptors, or vestibular system). Even a minor reversible cause, such as ear wax impaction, can result in a loss of balance and a subsequent fall and injury. Because dizziness has many predisposing factors, nurses should seek to identify any potentially treatable factors related to the condition. This preventive strategy may reduce the vulnerability of older people to injury (Tinetti, Williams, & Gill, 2000).

## Falls and Falling

Injuries rank seventh as a cause of death for older people, and falls are the leading cause of injury in the elderly, accounting for 62% of all nonfatal injuries treated in emergency departments in 2001 (Public Health and Aging, 2003). Between 35% and 40% of community-dwelling elderly people and 60% of nursing home residents fall annually, and about half fall multiple times. The incidence of falls rises with increasing age and tends to be highest in those 80 and older.

Although most falls by elderly adults do not result in injury, between 5% and 10% of elderly people who fall sustain serious injury. The most common fracture occurring from falls is hip fracture, which results from both osteoporosis and the situation that provoked the fall. Of the estimated 1% of elderly adults who fall and sustain a hip fracture, 20% to 30% die within 1 year of the fracture (Tideiksaar, 2003). Overall, elderly women who fall sustain a greater degree of injury than elderly men.

Causes of falls are multifactorial. Both extrinsic factors such as changes in the environment or poor lighting and intrinsic factors such as physical illness, neurologic changes, or sensory impairment play a role. Use of many medications, medication interactions, and use of alcohol precipitate falls by causing drowsiness, decreased coordination, and postural hypotension. Falls have physical dangers as well as serious psychological and social consequences. It is not uncommon for an older person who has experienced a fall to become fearful and lose self-confidence (Public Health and Aging, 2003; Tideiksaar, 2003).

Nurses can encourage older adults and their families to make lifestyle and environmental changes to prevent falls. Adequate lighting with minimal glare and shadow can be achieved through the use of small area lamps, indirect lighting, sheer curtains to diffuse direct sunlight, dull rather than shiny surfaces, and nightlights. Sharply contrasting colors can be used to mark the edges of stairs. Grab bars by the bathtub, shower, and toilet are useful. Loose clothing, improperly fitting shoes, scatter rugs, small objects, and pets create hazards and increase the risk for falls. Older adults function best in familiar settings when the arrangement of furniture and objects remains unchanged, if safely possible.

In institutionalized elderly people, physical restraints (lap belts; geriatric chairs; vest, waist, and jacket restraints) and chemical restraints (medications) precipitate many of the injuries they were meant to prevent. Documented injuries and deaths resulting from these restraints include strangulation, vascular and neurologic damage, pressure ulcers, skin tears, fractures, increased confusion, and significant emotional trauma. The time required to supervise restrained patients adequately is better used addressing the unmet need that provoked the behavior that resulted in the use of restraint. Because of the overwhelming negative consequences of restraint use, accrediting agencies of nursing homes and acute care facilities now maintain stringent guidelines concerning their use (Capezuti, Strumpf, Evans, et al., 1999).

## Urinary Incontinence

Urinary incontinence may be acute, occurring during an illness, or it may develop chronically over a period of years. Older patients often do not report this very common problem unless specifically asked. Transient causes may be attributed to *d*elirium and *d*ehydration; *r*estricted mobility and *r*estraints; *i*nflammation, *i*nfection, and *i*mpaction; and *p*harmaceuticals and *p*olyuria (the acronym *drip* may be used to remember them). Once identified, the causative factor can be eliminated. Incontinence may also be a result of neurologic or structural abnormalities. Urinary incontinence has been associated with depression and low self-esteem and may reduce the patient's quality of life by causing restriction in social activities.

The pelvic floor serves as the supporting mechanism or "hammock" for the bladder, uterus, and rectum. It may have become weakened as a result of pregnancy, labor and delivery, prior pelvic surgeries, or activities that required prolonged standing or lifting. Dysfunction of the pelvic floor can be greatly improved with Kegel exercises. Other measures that help prevent episodes of incontinence include having quick access to toilet facilities and wearing clothing that can be unfastened easily.

Patients with incontinence should be urged to seek help from appropriate health care providers, because incontinence can be both emotionally devastating and physically debilitating. Nurses who specialize in behavioral approaches to urinary incontinence management can assist patients to regain full continence or to significantly improve the level of continence. Although medications such as anticholinergics may decrease some of the symptoms of urge incontinence (detrusor instability), the adverse effects of these drugs (dry mouth, slowed gastrointestinal motility, and confusion) may make them inappropriate choices for the elderly. Various surgical procedures are also used to manage urinary incontinence, particularly stress urinary incontinence.

Detrusor hyperactivity with impaired contractility is a type of urge incontinence that is seen predominantly in the elderly population. In this variation of urge incontinence, patients have no warning that they are about to urinate. They often void only a small volume of urine or none at all and then experience a large volume of incontinence after leaving the bathroom. The nursing staff should be familiar with this form of incontinence and should not show disapproval when it occurs. Many patients with dementia suffer from this type of incontinence, because both incontinence and dementia are a result of dysfunction in similar areas of the brain. Prompted, timed voiding can be of assistance in these patients, although clean intermittent catheterization may be necessary because of postvoid residual urine.

## Increased Susceptibility to Infection

Infectious diseases present a significant threat of morbidity and mortality to older people, in part because of the blunted response of host defenses caused by a reduction in both cell-mediated and humoral immunity (see Chapters 50 and 51). Age-related loss of physiologic reserve and chronic illnesses also contribute to increased susceptibility. Pneumonia, urinary tract infections, tuberculosis (TB), gastrointestinal infections, and skin infections are some of the common infections in older people.

The effects of influenza and pneumococcal infections on older people are also significant. An estimated 10% to 20% of Americans have influenza each year; an average of 114,000 are hospitalized with influenza-related complications, and 36,000 die (CDC, 2004). Hospital-acquired pneumonia is responsible for 300,000 deaths annually in the United States, making it the second most common nosocomial infection (after urinary tract infection) and the leading cause of death from hospital-acquired infection. Many of these deaths involve older adults because of their increased vulnerability to infection (Smith-Sims, 2001).

The influenza vaccine is prepared yearly to adjust for the specific immunologic characteristics of the influenza viruses at that time. This inactivated preparation should be administered annually in the fall. The pneumococcal vaccine has 23 type-specific capsular polysaccharides. Protection lasts 4 years or longer, and revaccination is recommended every 5 years. Both of these injections can be received at the same time in separate injection sites. Nurses should urge older people to be vaccinated. All health care providers working with older people or high-risk chronically ill people should also be immunized.

TB affects a significant number of older adults. Case rates for TB are highest among those who are 65 or older, with the exception of people with human immunodeficiency virus (HIV) infection. Nursing home residents account for the majority of the cases of TB in older adults. Much of the infection rate is attributed to reactivation of old infection. Pulmonary TB and extrapulmonary TB often have subtle, nonspecific symptoms. This is of particular concern in nursing homes, because an active case of TB places patients and staff at risk for infection.

The Centers for Disease Control and Prevention (CDC) guidelines suggest that all patients newly admitted to nursing homes have a Mantoux (purified protein derivative [PPD]) test unless there is a history of TB or a previous positive response. All patients whose tests are negative (a positive test is indicated by induration of more than 10 mm at 48 to 72 hours) should have a second test in 1 to 2 weeks. The first PPD serves to boost the suppressed immune response that may occur in older people. Chest x-rays and possibly sputum studies should be used to follow up on PPD-positive responders and converters. For positive converters, a course of preventive therapy for 6 to 9 months with isoniazid (INH) is effective in eliminating active disease. All patients who test negative should be periodically retested (CDC, 2004).

AIDS is no longer only a disease of young people. It is increasingly recognized that AIDS does not spare the older segment of society. According to the CDC, between 1981 and 1989, more than 10% of all AIDS patients nationwide were 50 or older at the time of diagnosis, and about 3% were 60 or older. In that report, male homosexual contact and blood transfusions were the predominant modes of transmission among older patients. Transmission by contaminated blood products has declined in recent years, and the predominant mode of transmission in older people now is by sexual contact. The most common AIDS-indicator disease in older people is *Pneumocystis* pneumonia (PCP). Wasting syndrome and HIV encephalopathy are also common in older HIV-infected people.

## Altered Pain and Febrile Responses

Many altered physical, emotional, and systemic reactions to disease are attributed to age-related changes in older people. Physical indicators of illness that are useful and reliable in young and middle-aged people cannot be relied on for the diagnosis of potential life-threatening problems in older adults. The response to pain in older people may be lessened because of reduced acuity of touch, alterations in neural pathways, and diminished processing of sensory data.

Research has demonstrated that many older adults experiencing a myocardial infarction do not have chest pain. Hiatal hernia or upper gastrointestinal distress is often responsible for chest pain in elderly people. Acute abdominal conditions may go unrecognized in elderly people because of atypical signs and absence of pain.

The baseline body temperature for older people is about 1°F lower than it is for younger people. In the event of illness, therefore, the body temperature of an older person may not be high enough to qualify as a traditionally defined "fever." A temperature of 37.8°C (100°F), in combination with systemic symptoms, may signal infection. A temperature of 38.3°C (101°F) almost certainly indicates a serious infection that needs prompt attention. A blunted fever in the face of an infection often indicates a poor prognosis. Temperatures rarely exceed 39.5°C (103°F). Nurses must be alert to other subtle signs of infection, such as mental confusion, increased respirations, tachycardia, and changed facial appearance and color.

## Altered Emotional Impact

The emotional component of illness in older people may differ from that in younger people. Many elderly people equate good health with the absence of old age and believe "you are as old as you feel." An illness that requires hospitalization or a change in lifestyle is an imminent threat to well-being. Admission to the hospital is often feared and actively avoided. Older people admitted to the hospital are at high risk for disorientation, confusion, change in level of consciousness, and other symptoms of delirium, as well as anxiety and fear. In addition, economic concerns and fear of becoming a burden to families often lead to high anxiety in older people. Nurses must recognize the implications of fear, anxiety, and dependency in elderly patients. They should encourage autonomy and independent decision making. A positive and confident demeanor in nurses and family members promotes a positive mental outlook in elderly patients.

## Altered Systemic Response

In an elderly person, illness has far-reaching repercussions. The decline in organ function that occurs in every system of the aging body eventually depletes the body's ability to respond at full capacity. Illness places new demands on body systems that have little or no reserve to meet the crisis. Homeostasis, the ability of the body to maintain an internal balance of function and chemical composition, is jeopardized. Older people may be unable to respond effectively to an acute illness or, if a chronic health condition is present, they may be unable to sustain appropriate responses over a long period. Furthermore, their ability to respond to definitive treatment is impaired. The altered responses of older adults reinforce the need for nurses to monitor all body system functions closely, being alert to signs of impending systemic complication.

# Other Aspects of Health Care of the Older Adult

## Elder Neglect and Abuse

Older adults who live in communities and institutions are at risk for abuse and neglect, and studies indicate that the prevalence rate is 3% to 5% (about 5 million older Americans). Elder neglect and abuse are believed to be underreported and more widespread than previously thought; one study estimated that 84% of cases are not reported. Both victims and perpetrators are reluctant to report the abuse, and clinicians seemingly are unaware of the frequency of the problems (Levine, 2003).

Neglect is the most common type of abuse, and self-neglect constitutes almost 50% of the caseload of workers in Adult Protective Services. Other forms of abuse are physical, emotional, sexual, and financial abuse. Contributing factors include a family history of violence, mental illness, and drug or alcohol abuse, as well as financial dependency on the older person. In addition, diminished cognitive and physical function or disruptive and abusive behavior on the part of the older person can lead to caregiver strain and emotional exhaustion. Elderly people with disabilities of all types are at increased risk for abuse from family members and paid caregivers (Levine, 2003).

Nurses should be alert to possible **elder abuse** and neglect. During the health history, the elderly person should be asked about abuse during a private portion of the interview. Most states require that care providers, including nurses, report suspected abuse. Preventive action should be taken when caregiver strain is evident, before elder abuse occurs. Early detection and intervention may provide sufficient resources to the family or person at risk to ensure patient safety. Interdisciplinary team members, including the psychologist, social worker, or chaplain, can be enlisted to help the caregiver develop self-awareness, increased insight, and an understanding of the disease or aging process. Community resources also may be useful for both the elderly person and the caregiver (Geldmacher, Heck, & O'Toole, 2001).

## Social Services

Since the 1960s, many programs have been instituted for older Americans, including Medicare, Medicaid, the Older Americans Act, Supplemental Security Income (SSI), Social Security amendments, Section 202 housing, and Title XX social services legislation. These federal programs have dramatically increased health care options and financial support for elderly Americans. The Older Americans Act mandated creation of a federal aging network, resulting in the establishment of the Area Agencies on Aging (AAAs), a national system of social services and network for the elderly. Many community services for the elderly are available through the more than 700 AAAs. Each state has an advisory network that is charged with overseeing statewide planning and advocacy for the elderly throughout the state. Among the services provided by the AAAs are assessment of need, information and referral, case management, transportation, outreach, homemaker services, day care, nutritional education and congregate meals, legal services, respite care, senior centers, and part-time community work. The AAAs target low-income, ethnic minority, rural-living, and frail elders who are at risk for institutionalization; however, the assessment and information services are available to all elderly people (Hooyman & Kiyak, 2002). Similar services such as homemaker, home health aide, and chore services can be obtained at an hourly rate through these agencies or through local community nursing services if the family does not meet the low-income criteria. Informal sources of help, such as family, friends, mail carriers, church members, and neighbors, can all keep an informal watch on community-dwelling senior citizens.

Other community support services are available to help older people outside the home. Senior centers have social and health promotion activities, and some provide a nutritious noontime meal. Adult day care facilities offer daily nursing care and social opportunities for elderly people who cannot be left alone. Adult day care services, although expensive, provide respite and enable family members to carry on daily activities while the older person is at the day care center.

## Health Care Costs of Aging

Health care is a major expenditure for the elderly, especially for those with chronic illness and limited financial resources. The elderly, who make up about 13% of the population, consume more than 33% of health care costs, particularly in the last year of life (Hoover et al., 2002). They occupy about half of the adult hospital beds, use more than two thirds of the available health care services, and spend 3 times as many days in hospitals and 30 times as many days in long-term care facilities than younger people (Miller, 2004). Therefore, whenever nurses work with an adult population, they are likely to encounter a majority of elderly patients.

The two major programs that finance health in the United States are Medicare and Medicaid, both of which are overseen by the Centers for Medicaid and Medicare Services (CMS).

Medicare is funded by the federal government, whereas Medicaid is funded jointly by the federal and state governments to provide health care for the poor. Medicare is the source of payment for acute health care for most older Americans. The services covered under Medicare have changed over the past decade, but principally it covers acute care needs such as inpatient hospitalization, physician care, outpatient care, home health services, and skilled nursing care in a nursing facility. In 2001, Medicare funding covered slightly more than half (54%) of the health care costs for those older than 65 years of age. Medicaid covered 10% of health care costs for older Americans and 46% of nursing home costs. Older Americans paid 15% out of pocket for their health care costs and 48% of their nursing home costs (National Center for Health Statistics, 2004).

In 1996, 1% of Medicare beneficiaries who were 65 or older incurred 13% of health care expenditures in that age group, and the top 5% of beneficiaries with the highest expenditures incurred 37% of all health expenditures (Older Americans, 2003). Medicare pays for only about 55% of all personal health costs, requiring the patient to pay the balance (Liu et al., 2002). For older adults with limited incomes, even with the support of Medicare, paying out-of-pocket expenses can be a hardship that at times they are unable to afford. Despite the recent additional Medicare prescription benefit plan, out-of-pocket expenditures and prescription costs are burdensome.

Use of home care services and skilled nursing home care increases markedly with age (Older Americans, 2003). Eligibility and costs for Medicaid services vary from state to state. As more and more people in the United States become eligible for publicly funded health programs in the future, there are serious concerns about whether sufficient health services will be available.

## Home Health Care

Because of the rapidly growing elderly population and the availability of Medicare funding for acute care, including home care, home health care in the United States rapidly expanded in the 1990s. By the end of the 1990s, home health care had come to represent almost 10% of the total Medicare budget. Home health care, or visiting nursing, is the specialty practice of nursing applied in the home to patients with a wide range of illnesses and chronic conditions. Although people of all ages receive home care, 70% of home care patients are 65 and older (Administration on Aging, 2004). Medicare is a primary payer of home care services.

Home care involves the individual patient, the family, and caregivers. Home care nurses are generally considered skilled generalists who are holistic in their approach to care. In addition to providing skilled nursing care, home care nurses also consider the needs of the family and the impact of the environment and community on the patient situation, and they identify areas for collaboration and referral. Care is episodic (periodic short visits). Home care agencies generally offer several services, including skilled nursing; hospice care; physical, occupational, and speech therapy; and home health aide and homemaker services. Consultation with specialists in nutrition, cardiac, diabetic, and wound care is available. As hospital stays have shortened, the acuity level of home care patients has risen dramatically. "High-tech" therapies such as infusion therapy are frequently available. The primary goal is to promote optimal health and independent function in the home for both patients and their families.

## Hospice Services

Hospice is a program of supportive and palliative services for terminally ill patients and their families that includes physical, psychological, social, and spiritual care. In most cases, patients are not expected to live longer than 6 months. The goal of hospice is to improve the quality of life by focusing on symptom management, pain control, and emotional support. Under Medicare and Medicaid, all needed medical and nursing services are provided to keep patients as pain-free and comfortable as possible. Hospice services may be incorporated into the care of residents in long-term care facilities and include care for end-stage dementia.

Home care and hospice nurses are in a unique position to facilitate discussions about a patient's wishes and goals at the end of life. Too often, discussion regarding end-of-life care is postponed until a crisis occurs, making it difficult or impossible for the patient to be an active participant in the discussion. Home health nurses can assist patients and families by identifying options and initiating conversation about preparing an end-of-life plan. For an in-depth discussion of hospice care, see Chapter 17.

## Aging With a Disability

As the life expectancy of people with all types of physical, cognitive, and mental disabilities has increased, individuals must deal with the normal changes associated with aging in addition to their pre-existing disabilities. There are still large gaps in our understanding of the interaction between disabilities and aging, including how this interaction varies depending on the type and degree of disability and other factors such as socioeconomics and gender. For adults without disabilities, the changes associated with aging may be minor inconveniences. For adults with disorders such as polio, multiple sclerosis, and cerebral palsy, aging may lead to greater disability. In addition, many people with disabilities are greatly concerned and fearful about what will happen to them as they age and whether assistance will be available when they need care.

Minkler and Fadem (2002) support a "new paradigm of disability," which was first suggested by Bleecker (2000). Under this paradigm, a person with a disability should be viewed as someone who needs an accommodation to function rather than as someone who cannot function because of an impairment. Use of this functional approach would encourage public policies that support full participation of all citizens, such as personal assistants and accessible and affordable transportation. Therefore, research and public policy must focus on supports and interventions that allow people with preexisting disabilities who are aging to increase or maintain function within their personal environment as well as in the outside community. Important questions include the following: Who will provide the care? How will it be financed? Qualitative research would be particularly helpful in providing insight into the lives and therefore the needs of older people with disabilities.

Today, children born with intellectual and physical disabilities and those who acquire them early in life are also living into middle and older age. Often, their care has been provided by the family, primarily by the parents. As the parents age and can no longer provide the needed care, they are seeking additional help with the care or long-term care alternatives for their children. However, few services are available at present to support a smooth transition between caregiving by parents and then by others (Bigby, Ozanne, & Gordon, 2002). Again, further research is needed to identify the needs and to guide policy makers who design services and resources for this population of aging adults.

# Ethical and Legal Issues Affecting the Older Adult

Nurses play an important role in supporting and informing patients and families when making treatment decisions. This nursing role becomes even more important in the care of aging patients who are facing serious, life-altering, and possibly end-of-life decisions. There is the potential for loss of rights, victimization, and other serious problems if a patient has made no plans for personal and property management in the event of disability or death. As advocates, nurses can encourage end-of-life decision making and educate older people to prepare advance care planning for future decision making in the event of incapacitation (Plotkin & Roche, 2000).

An **advance directive** is a formal, legally endorsed document that provides instructions for care (living will) or names a proxy decision maker (**durable power of attorney**). It is to be implemented if the signer becomes incapacitated. This written document must be signed by the person and by two witnesses, and a copy should be given to the physician and placed in the medical record. The person must understand that the advance directive is not meant to be used only when certain (or all) types of medical treatment are withheld; rather, it allows for a detailed description of all health care preferences, including full use of all available medical interventions. The health care proxy has the authority to interpret the patient's wishes on the basis of medical circumstances and is not restricted to the decisions or situations stated in the living will, such as whether life-sustaining treatment can be withdrawn or withheld.

When such serious decisions are made, possibilities exist for significant conflict of values among patients, family members, health care providers, and the legal establishment. Autonomy and self-determination are Western concepts, and people from different cultures may view advance directives as a method for denial of care. Elderly people from some cultures may be unwilling to consider the future, or they may wish to protect relatives and not want them to be informed about a serious illness. Nurses can facilitate the decision-making process by being sensitive to the complexity of patients' values and respecting that decision making is a process that occurs over time. Directives must be focused on the wishes of the patient, not those of the family or the designated proxy (Mezey et al., 2003) (Chart 12-3).

---

**CHART 12-3**

### Ethics and Related Issues

**Should an Elderly Person be Allowed to Refuse a Feeding Tube When the Primary Care Practitioner Believes it Would Enhance the Person's Quality of Life?**

**SITUATION**
This patient is an 82-year-old retired office worker who has never married and who has a close relationship with her many nieces and nephews. Until suffering several small strokes following her 80th birthday, she lived independently, drove, and participated in many family and community functions. She appeared to recover from the strokes, and for the next year she continued to drive and engaged in social activities. One year prior to her admission to the nursing home, she suffered another stroke and required a gastric tube for long-term feeding. Gradually, she recovered sufficiently to have the tube removed; however, she continued to experience difficulty swallowing and ate only puddings and ice cream. She was cognitively intact but slowly becoming weaker.

Eight months later, the patient's primary care practitioner recommended reinserting the gastric tube to improve her nutritional status. She refused placement of the gastric tube. The nursing staff and family members disagreed about what should be done about her refusal and can make a case for both positions.

**DILEMMA**
Several ethical issues were relevant to the resolution of the situation. The obligation to respect the patient's autonomy in the decision to refuse gastric feedings affects her nutritional status and may even have put her life at risk. She had had a gastric tube in the past and understood what it is and the purpose of the gastric feedings. The nurses who care for her watched her deteriorate and realized that there was a possible medical solution. However, not all the nurses and family members were in agreement about what to do.

**DISCUSSION**
1. What arguments would you offer *against* reinsertion of the gastric tube?
2. What arguments would you offer *in favor* of reinsertion of the gastric tube?
3. What arguments would you offer *against* and *in favor of* supporting the patient in her decision to refuse the feeding tube?

If no advance arrangement has been made and the older person appears unable to make decisions, anyone can petition the court for a competency hearing. Mezey et al. (2003) report that anecdotally, about 30% of the elderly do not have a relative, friend, or guardian who could make health care decisions for them. If the court rules that an elderly person is incompetent, the judge will appoint a guardian—a third party who is given powers by the court to assume responsibility for making financial or personal decisions for that person.

People with communication difficulties or mild dementia may be viewed as incapable of self-determination. Most people with mild dementia have sufficient cognitive capability to make some, but perhaps not all, decisions. For example, a patient may be able to identify a proxy decision maker yet be unable to select specific treatment options (Mezey et al., 2003). People with mild dementia may be competent to understand the nature and significance of such decisions.

In 1990, the Patient Self-Determination Act (PSDA), a federal law, was enacted to require patient education about advance directives at the time of hospital admission, as well as documentation of this education. Nursing homes are also mandated by PSDA to enhance residents' autonomy by increasing their involvement in health care decision making. A growing body of research indicates that nursing homes implement the PSDA more vigorously than hospitals. However, in both settings, the documentation and placement of advance directives in the medical record and the education of patients about advance directives vary considerably from facility to facility. Processes for fulfilling the requirements of the law are continuously being revised in many facilities to promote compliance. The PSDA provides no guidelines regarding how often the advance directives of nursing home residents should be reviewed. Continuing quality improvement programs that establish guidelines for review are more likely to exist in nursing homes that have ethics committees.

## Critical Thinking Exercises

**1** You recently have accepted a position as staff educator at a local hospital. You have met with a group of newly hired nurses and overheard several of them saying that they hoped they would not be assigned to the skilled nursing facility at the hospital, where many of the patients are elderly. One comment was, "That would be the lowest level of nursing—more like babysitting." You realize you need to plan a program for these new nurses to address their misconceptions about care for the elderly. What would be important for these nurses to learn? What issues would you discuss? What recommendations would you make?

**2** You are a community health nurse assigned to a neighborhood senior center that provides lunch and activities for 50 to 75 seniors a day. You are concerned about the many medications the seniors report taking and would like to provide a "brown bag medication review." To initiate this program, you ask each senior to bring all of the medications he or she takes to the senior center the following week. What information would you also provide to the seniors in preparation for the review to make the review as useful as possible? What health care providers would you ask to participate in this review? During the review, what information would you seek from each senior and what information would you provide?

**3** **ebp** You are a charge nurse in an emergency department when a 75-year-old man with late-stage Alzheimer's disease is admitted with "mental status changes." His vital signs are stable. He is generally pleasant but confused and at times becomes easily agitated. What is the evidence base that indicates how elderly people respond to acute illnesses? What is the strength of the evidence? Based on the evidence-based information that you have found, what assessment parameters would you evaluate? What laboratory and clinical studies would you expect to be ordered? What information would you obtain from the patient's caregiver? What plan of action would you initiate?

## REFERENCES AND SELECTED READINGS

### BOOKS

Administration on Aging (2005). *A profile of older Americans: 2005.* Available at: http://www.aoa.gov/prof/Statistics/profile/2005/2.asp. Accessed May 11, 2006.

Administration on Aging (2004). *A profile of older Americans: 2003.* Available at: http://www.aoa.gov/prof/Statistics/profile/2003/2_pf.asp. Accessed May 11, 2006.

Albert, S. M. (2004). *Public health and aging: An introduction to maximizing function and well-being.* New York: Springer.

Bales, C. W., & Ritchie, C. S. (2003). *Handbook of clinical nutrition and aging.* Totowa, NJ: Humana Press.

Blass, J., Halter, J., Hazzard, W., et al. (2003). *Principles of geriatric medicine and gerontology.* New York: McGraw-Hill.

Beers, M. H. (2004). *Merck manual of health and aging.* Whitehouse Station, NJ: Merck & Co.

Beers, M. H., & Berkow, R. (2000). *Merck manual of geriatrics* (3rd ed.). Whitehouse Station, NJ: Merck & Co.

Burbank, P. M., & Reibe, D. (Eds.). (2002). *Promoting exercise and behavior change in older adults.* New York: Springer.

Burke, M. M., & Laramie, J. A. (2004). *Primary care of the older adult* (2nd ed.). St. Louis: Mosby.

CDC (2004). Key facts about influenza and the influenza vaccine. Available at: http://www.cdc.gov/flu/keyfacts.htm. Accessed May 11, 2006.

Centers for Medicare and Medicaid Services. (2002). *Home health PPS.* Baltimore: Author. Available at: http://www.cms.hhs.gov/HomeHealthPPS. Accessed May 11, 2006.

Division of Tuberculosis Elimination. Available at: http://www.cdc.gov/nchstp/tb/faqs/qa_latenttbinf.htm#Infection3. Accessed May 11, 2003.

Ebersole, P. R., Hess, P., & Luggen, A. S. (2004). *Toward healthy aging: Human needs & nursing response* (6th ed.). Philadelphia: Mosby.

Eliopoulos, C. (2005). *Gerontological nursing* (6th ed.). Philadelphia: Lippincott Williams & Wilkins.

Erikson, E. H. (1963). *Childhood and society* (2nd ed.). New York: W. W. Norton.

Fryer, G. (2001). Normal changes with aging. In M. L. Mass (Ed.), *Nursing care of older adults: Diagnoses, outcomes, & interventions.* Philadelphia: Mosby.

Gallo, J. J., Fulmer, T., Paveza, G. J., et al. (2000). *Handbook of geriatric assessment* (3rd ed.). Gaithersburg, MD: Aspen.

Ham, R. J., & Warshaw G. (2001). *Primary care geriatrics: A case-based approach* (4th ed.). St. Louis: Mosby–Year Book.

Health Services Research on Aging. (2000, January). *Building on biomedical and clinical research. Translating research into practice fact sheet.* (AHRQ Publication No. 00-P012). Rockville, MD: Agency for Healthcare Research and Quality. Available at: http://www.ahrq.gov/research/tripage.htm. Accessed May 11, 2006.

Health, United States (2003a). Chartbook on trends in the health of Americans. National Centers for Health Statistics. Available at: http://www.cdc.gov/nchs/data/hus/hus03cht.pdf. Accessed May 11, 2006.

Health, United States (2003b). Chartbook on trends in the health of Americans. National Centers for Health Statistics. Available at: http://www.cdc.gov/nchs/data/hus/tables/2003/03hus056.pdf. Accessed May 11, 2006.

Hogstel, M. O. (2001). *Gerontology: Nursing care of the older adult.* Albany: Delmar Publishing.

Holmes, D., Teresi, J. A., & Ory, M. (2000). *Special care units: Research and practice in Alzheimer disease,* Vol. 4. New York: Springer.

Hooyman, N. R., & Kiyak, H. A. (2002). *Social gerontology: A multidisciplinary perspective* (6th ed.). Boston: Allyn & Bacon.

Kane, R. L. (2004). *Essentials of clinical geriatrics* (5th ed.). New York: McGraw-Hill.

Kennedy-Malone, L., Fletcher, K. R., & Plank, L. M. (2004). *Management guidelines for nurse practitioners* working with older adults. Philadelphia: F. A. Davis.

Lawton, M. P. (1982). Competence, environmental press, and the adaptation of older people. In M. P. Lawton, P. G., Windley & T. O. Byerts (Eds.), *Aging and the environment: Theoretical approaches.* New York: Springer.

Liu, H., Ginsberg, C. Olin, G., et al. (2002). *Health and health care of the Medicare population: Data from the 1996 Medicare current beneficiary survey.* Rockville, MD: West.

Lueckenotte, A. G. (2000). *Gerontologic nursing* (2nd ed.). St. Louis: Mosby–Year Book.

Maas, M. L., Buckwalter, K. C., Hardy, M. D., et al. (2001). *Nursing care of older adults: Diagnosis, outcomes, & interventions.* St. Louis: Mosby.

Markson, E. W. (2003). *Social gerontology today: An introduction.* Los Angeles: Roxbury Publishing Co.

Mayo Foundation for Medical Education and Research. (2001). *Dementia: Epidemiology.* Available at: http://www.mayo.edu/geriatrics-rst/Dementia.1.html.

Mezey, M., Fulmer, T., Abraham, I., et al. (2002). *Geriatric nursing protocols for best practice* (2nd ed.). New York: Springer.

Mezey, M. D., Berkman, B. J., & Callahan, C. (2000). *The encyclopedia of elder care: The comprehensive resource on geriatric and social care.* New York: Springer.

Miller, C. A. (2004). *Nursing for wellness in older adults: Theory and practice* (4th ed.). Philadelphia: Lippincott Williams & Wilkins.

National Center for Health Statistics (2004). Available at: http://www.cdc.gov/nchs/fastats/pdf/nvbr50_btl.pdf. Accessed May 11, 2006.

National Institute of Neurological Disorders and Stroke (reviewed January 24, 2006). *NINDS Pick's disease information page.* Available at: http://www.ninds.nih.gov/disorders/Niemann/Niemann.htm

National Institute of Neurological Disorders and Stroke (2006). *NINDS Alzheimer disease information page.* Available at: http://www.ninds.nih.gov/health_and_medical/disorders/alzheimersdisease_doc.htm. Accessed May 4, 2006.

National Osteoporosis Foundation (2004). *Prevention, Calcium & Vitamin D.* Available at: http://www.nof.org/prevention/calcium.htm. Accessed May 11, 2006.

Neugarten, B. L. (1961). *Personality in middle and late life.* New York: Atherton Press.

Noelker, L. S., & Harel, Z. (2000). *Linking quality of long term care and quality of life.* New York: Springer.

Older Americans 2000 (2005). *Key indicators of well-being.* Available at: http://www.agingstats.gov/. Accessed May 11, 2006.

Schmidt Luggen, A., Meiner, S. E., & National Gerontological Nursing Association (2000). *NGNA: Core curriculum for gerontological nursing* (2nd ed.). St. Louis: Mosby.

Silin, P. S. (2001). *Nursing homes: The family's journey.* Baltimore: Johns Hopkins University Press.

Strumpf, N. E., Evans, L. K., Wagner, J., et al. (1992). *Reducing restraints: Individualized approaches to behavior. A teaching guide.* Huntingdon Valley, PA: Geriatric Research and Training Center.

## JOURNALS

*Asterisks indicate nursing research articles.*

Adams, W., Atkinson, R., Ganz, S. B., et al. (2000). Alcohol problems in the elderly. *Patient Care for the Nurse Practitioner, 10*(3), 68–89.

Anderson, G. M., Beers, M. H., & Kerluke, K. (1997). Auditing prescription practice using explicit criteria and computerized drug benefit claims data. *Journal of Evaluation in Clinical Practice,* (4)3, 283.

Atchley, R. C. (1989). Continuity theory of normal aging. *Gerontologist, 29*(2), 183–190.

Bigby, C., Ozanne, E., & Gordon, M. (2002). Facilitating transition: Elements of successful case management practice for older parents of adults with intellectual disability. *Journal of Gerontological Social Work, 37*(i3–4), 25.

Bleecker, T. (2000). The new paradigm of disability: Implications for research and policy. *Consumer Choice, 4,* 1, 3.

Breslow, R. A., Faden, V. B., & Smothers, B. (2003). Alcohol consumption by elderly Americans. *Journal of Studies on Alcohol,* (64)6, 884.

*Callen, B. (2004) Understanding nutritional health in older adults: A pilot study. *Journal of Gerontological Nursing, 30*(1), 36.

*Capezuti, E. (2000). Preventing falls and injuries while reducing side rail use. *Annals of Long Term Care, 8*(6), 57–63.

*Capezuti, E., Strumpf, N., Evans, L. K., et al. (1999). Outcomes of nighttime physical restraint removal for severely impaired nursing home residents. *American Journal of Alzheimer Disease, 14*(1), 157–164.

*Capezuti, E., Strumpf, N. E., Evans, L. K., et al. (1998). The relationship between physical restraint removal and falls and injuries among nursing home residents. *Journal of Gerontology, Series A, 53*(1), M47.

*Chemist and Druggist* (Aug. 30, 2003). Donezepil helps vascular dementia, p. 16.

Chernoff, R. (2002). Health promotion for older women: Benefits of nutrition and exercise programs. *Topics in Geriatric Rehabilitation, 1*(18), 59.

Cohen, G. D. (2002). Alzheimer disease: Managing behavioral problems in patients with progressive dementia. *Geriatrics, 2*(57), 53–54.

Delafuente, J. C. (2003). Understanding and preventing drug interactions in elderly patients. *Critical Reviews in Oncology/Hematology, 2*(48), 133.

DiMaria-Ghadili, R. A., & Amello, E. (2005). Nutrition in older adults. *American Journal of Nursing, 105*(3), 40–51.

Dolinar, T. M., McQuillen, A. D., Ranseen, J. D., et al. (2001). Health, safety, and the older driver. *Patient Care, 35*(4), 22–34.

Edwards, N. (2003). Differentiating the three D's: Delirium, dementia, and depression. *MEDSURG Nursing, 12*(6), 347–357.

Falgoust, M. (2004). United States 85 and over population by state. Communication with Mark Falgoust, Statistical Analyst II, PA Department of Health, Aug. 31, 2004.

Fiatarone, M. A., Marks, E. C., Ryan, N. D., et al. (1990). High-intensity strength training in nonagenarians: Effects on skeletal muscle. *Journal of American Medical Association, 263*(8), 3029.

*Forbes, D. A. (2001). Enhancing mastery and sense of coherence: Important determinants of health in older adults. *Geriatric Nursing, 22*(1), 29–32.

*Galvan, T. J. (2001). Dysphagia: Going down and staying down. *American Journal of Nursing, 101*(1), 37–42.

Geldmacher, D. S., Heck, E., & O'Toole, E. (2001). Providing for the caregiver. *Patient Care for the Nurse Practitioner, 4*(2), 36–48.

Goldrick, B. A. (2005). Infection in the older adult. *American Journal of Nursing, 105*(6), 31–34.

*Harvard Health Letter* (2003). The latest on macular degeneration, 28(7).

Harvard Men's Health Watch (June 6, 2002). Lest we forget, II: Alzheimer disease. Issue 11.

Havighurst, R. J. (1968). Personality and patterns of aging. *Gerontologist, 8,* 20–23.

Heidrich, S. M., & Wells, T. J. (2004) Effects of urinary incontinence: Psychological well-being and distress in older community dwelling women. *Journal of Gerontological Nursing, 30*(5), 47–54.

Hoban, S., & Kearney, K. (2000). Elder abuse and neglect: It takes many forms—If you're not looking, you may miss it. *American Journal of Nursing, 100*(1), 49–50.

Hofmann, M. T., & Nahass, D. (2001). Case report: The use of an ethics committee regarding the case of an elderly female with blood loss after hip surgery. *Annals of Long-Term Care, 9*(3), 55–59.

Hoover, D. R., Crystal, S., Kumar, R., et al. (2002). Medical expenditures during the last year of life: Findings from the 1992–1996 Medicare current beneficiary survey. *Health Services Research, 37*(6), 1625–1642.

Iqbal, K., & Grundke-Iqbal, I., (2004). Inhibition of neurofibrillary degeneration: A promising approach to Alzheimer disease and other taupathies. *Current Drug Targets, 5*(6), 495–501.

Keysor, J. J., & Jette, A. M. (2001). Have we over-sold the benefit of late-life exercise? *Journal of Gerontology, Series B, (51)*3, S150.

Kiely, D. K., Simon, S. E., Jones, R. N., et al. (2000). The protective effect of social engagement on mortality in long-term care. *Journal of the American Geriatrics Society, 48*(11), 1367–1372.

Lam, Y. W. F. (2000). Warfarin, St. John's Wort effect on P-450 enzymes. *Psychopharmacology Update, 5*(11), 2.

Levine, J. M. (2003). Elder neglect and abuse: A primer for primary care physicians. *Geriatrics, 58*(10), 37.

Marin, D. B., Sewell, M. C. & Schlechter, A. (2002). Alzheimer disease: Accurate and early diagnosis in the primary care setting. *Geriatrics, 57*(2), 36–40.

McDonald, R. J. (2002). Multiple combinations of co-factors produce variants of age-related cognitive decline: A theory. *Canadian Journal of Experimental Psychology, 56*(3), 221–239.

*Mental Health Weekly Digest* (July 26, 2004). Mechanisms of memantine activity determined. Via NewsRx.com and NewsRx.net, p. 9.

Mezey, M., Mitty, E., & Ramsey, G. (1997). Assessment of decision making capacity: Nurses' role. *Journal of Gerontological Nursing, 23*(3), 28–35.

Miles, S. H., & Irvine, P. (1992). Deaths caused by physical restraints. *Gerontologist, 32*(6), 762–766.

Minkler, M., & Fadem, P. (2002). "Successful aging:" A disability perspective. *Journal of Disability Policy Studies, 12*(4), 229–235.

Myers, J. E. (2003). Coping with caregiver stress: A wellness-oriented, strengths-based approach for family counselors. *Family Journal, 11*(2), 153–161.

*Naylor, M., Brooten, D., Campbell, R., et al. (1999). Comprehensive discharge planning and home follow-up of hospitalized elders. *Journal of American Medical Association, 281*(7), 613–620.

Naylor, M. D., Stephens, C., Bowles, K. H., et al. (2005). Cognitively impaired older adults: From hospital to home. *American Journal of Nursing, 105*(2), 52–61.

*Norlander, L., & McSteen, K. (2000). The kitchen table discussion: A creative way to discuss end-of-life issues. *Home Healthcare Nurse, 18*(8), 532–540.

Nusbaum, N. J. (2000). Issues in home rehabilitative care. *Annals of Long-Term Care, 8*(11), 43–48.

Patient Self-Determination Act (PSDA). (1990). *Omnibus Budget Reconciliation Act.* Title IV, Sec. 4206. *Congressional Record,* 12368, ct 26.

Peterson, J. A. (2001). Osteoporosis overview. *Geriatric Nursing, 22*(5), 17–23.

*Plotkin, K., & Roche, J. (2000). The future of home and hospice care: Linking interventions to outcomes in home health care. *Home Healthcare Nurse, 18*(8), 442–450.

Public health and aging: Non-fatal injuries among older adults treated in hospital emergency departments, United States, 2001. (2003). *Journal of American Medical Association, 290*(20), 2657–2658.

*Resnick, B. (2001). Promoting health in older adults: A four-year analysis. *Journal of the American Academy of Nurse Practitioners, 13*(1), 23–33.

Ruckenstein, M. J. (2001). The dizzy patient: How you can help. *Consultant, 41,* 29–34.

*Ryden, M. B., Snyder, M., Gross, C. R., et al. (2000). Value-added outcomes: The lure of advanced practice nurses in long-term care facilities. *Gerontologist, 40*(6), 654–662.

*Schafer, S. L. (2001). Prescribing for seniors: It's a balancing act. *Journal of American Academy of Nurse Practitioners, 13,* 108–112.

Shugrue, D. T., & Larocque, K. L. (1996). Reducing restraint use in the acute care setting. *Nursing Management, 25*(10), 32H.

Silverstein, M., & Lablotsky, D. L. (1996) Health and social precursors of late life retirement-community migration. *Journal of Gerontology, Series B, (51)*3, S150.

*Smith-Sims, K. (2001). Hospital-acquired pneumonia. *American Journal of Nursing, 101*(1), 24AA–24EE.

Specht, J. K. P. (2005). Myths of incontinence in older adults. *American Journal of Nursing, 105*(6), 58–69.

Spillman, B. (2001). A conversation with Brenda Spillman, Ph.D.: Interface interview. *Long-Term Care Interface, 2,* 27–29.

*Tappen, R., Roach, K., Applegate, E. B., et al. (2000). Effect of a combined walking and conversation intervention on functional mobility of nursing home residents with Alzheimer disease. *Alzheimer Disease and Associated Disorders, 14*(4), 196–201.

Tideiksaar, R. (2003). Best practice approach to fall prevention in community living elders. *Topics in Geriatric Rehabilitation, 19*(3), 199–205.

Tinetti, M. E., Williams, C. S., & Gill, T. M. (2000). Dizziness among older adults: A possible geriatric syndrome. *Annals of Internal Medicine, 132,* 337–344.

Tumolo, J. (2000). Caregivers who hurt: The tragedy of elder abuse. *Advance for Nurse Practitioners, 8*(9), 63–65.

Van Eijken, M., Tsang, S., Wensing, M., et al. (2003). Interventions to improve medication compliance on older patients living in the community: A systematic review of the literature. *Drugs & Aging, 20*(3), 229–240.

Wagner, L. S., & Wagner, T. H. (2003). The effect of age on the use of health and self-care information: Confronting the stereotype. *Gerontologist, 43*(3), 318–324.

Widlitz, M., & Marin, D. B. (2002). Substance in older adults: an overview. *Geriatrics, 57*(12), 29–34.

## RESOURCES

Administration on Aging, 1 Massachusetts Avenue, Suites 4100 & 5100, Washington, DC 20201; 202-619-0724; http://www.aoa.dhhs.gov. Accessed May 13, 2006.

Alzheimer's Disease and Related Disorders Association, Inc., 225 N. Michigan Avenue, 17th floor, Chicago, IL 60601; 800-272-3900; http://www.alz.org. Accessed May 13, 2006.

American Association for Geriatric Psychiatry (AAGP), 7910 Woodmont Ave., Suite 1050, Bethesda, MD 20814; 301-654-7850; http://www.aagpgpa.org. Accessed May 13, 2006.

American Association of Homes and Services for the Aging, 2519 Connecticut Avenue NW, Washington, DC 20008; 1-202-783-2242; http://www.aahsa.org. Accessed May 13, 2006.

American Association of Retired Persons, 601 E Street NW, Washington, DC 20049; 888-687-2277; http://www.aarp.org. Accessed May 13, 2006.

American Federation for Aging Research (AFAR), 70 West 40th Street, 11th Floor, New York, NY 10018; 212-703-9977, 888-582-2327; http://www.afar.org. Accessed May 13, 2006.

American Foundation for the Blind, 15 West 16th Street, New York, NY 10011; 212-620-2000; http://www.afb.org. Accessed May 13, 2006.

American Geriatrics Society, Empire State Building, 350 Fifth Ave, Suite 801, New York, NY 10118; 212-308-1414; http://www.americangeriatrics.org. Accessed May 13, 2006.

Association for Gerontology in Higher Education (AGHE), 1030 15th Street, NW, Suite 240, Washington, DC 20005; 202-289-9806; 202-289-9824 (fax); http://www.aghe.org. Accessed May 13, 2006.

Children of Aging Parents (CAPS), PO Box 167, Richboro, PA 18954; 800-227-7294; http://www.caps4caregivers.org. Accessed May 13, 2006.

Elderhostel, 877-426-8056; http://www.elderhostel.org. Accessed May 13, 2006).

Family Caregiver Alliance (FCA), 690 Market St., San Francisco, CA 94104; 800-445-8106; http://www.caregiver.org. Accessed May 13, 2006.

Gerontological Society of America (GSA), 1030 15th Street NW, Suite 250, Washington, DC 20005; 202-842-1275; http://www.geron.org. Accessed May 13, 2006.

Legal Services for the Elderly, 17th Floor, 130 West 42nd Street, New York, NY 10036; 212-391-0120

National Association of State Units on Aging, 1201 15th Street NW, Suite 350, Washington, DC 20005; 1-202-898-2586; http://www.nasua.org. Accessed May 13, 2006.

National Caucus and Center on Black Aged, Inc., Suite 500, 1424 K Street NW, Washington, DC 20005; 202-637-8400

National Council on the Aging, Inc., 202-479-1200; http://www.ncoa.org. Accessed May 13, 2006.

National Gerontological Nursing Association, 7794 Grow Drive, Pensacola, FL 32514; 800-723-0560; http://www.ngna.org. Accessed May 13, 2006).

Nurse Competence in Aging Initiative; http://www.geronurseonline.org. Accessed May 13, 2006.

Safe Return (program for locating lost patients), Box A-3956, Chicago, IL 60690; 800-572-1122 (to report a lost patient).

# UNIT 3

# Concepts and Challenges in Patient Management

## Case Study
### Applying Concepts from NANDA, NIC, and NOC

**A Patient With Debilitating Pain**

**Mr. Southers** is a 48-year-old man who sustained a back injury in a work-related incident. He reports severe shooting pains in his lower back and both buttocks. Mr. Southers is not a candidate for surgery and has undergone physical therapy with little improvement in his pain. He reports that the pain makes it impossible for him to return to his former job, work around the house, or obtain enjoyment from leisure activities. He has been referred to a pain clinic for management.

 Turn to Appendix C to see a concept map that illustrates the relationships that exist between the nursing diagnoses, interventions, and outcomes for the patient's clinical problems.

## Nursing Classifications and Languages

| NANDA<br>Nursing Diagnoses | NIC<br>Nursing Interventions | NOC<br>Nursing Outcomes<br>Return to functional baseline status, stabilization of, or improvement in: |
|---|---|---|
| **Chronic Pain**—Unpleasant sensory and emotional experience arising from actual or potential tissue damage or described in terms of such damage; sudden or slow onset of any intensity from mild to severe, constant or recurring, without an anticipated or predictable end and a duration of greater than 6 months | **Pain Management**—Alleviation of pain or reduction in pain to a level of comfort that is acceptable to the patient | **Pain Level**—Severity of observed or reported pain |
| **Risk for Powerlessness**—At risk for perceived lack of control over a situation and/or one's ability to significantly affect an outcome | **Medication Management**—Facilitation of safe and effective use of prescribed or over-the-counter medicine | **Comfort Level**—Extent of positive perception of physical and psychological ease |
| | **Simple Relaxation Therapy**—Use of techniques to encourage and elicit relaxation for the purpose of decreasing undesirable signs and symptoms such as pain, muscle tension, or anxiety | **Pain Control**—Personal actions to control pain |
| | **Simple Guided Imagery**—Purposeful use of imagination to achieve relaxation and/or direct attention away from undesirable sensations | **Pain: Disruptive Effects**—Severity of observed or reported disruptive effects of chronic pain on daily functioning |
| | **Emotional Support**—Provision of reassurance, acceptance, and encouragement during times of stress | **Pain: Adverse Psychological Response**—Severity of observed or reported adverse responses to physical pain |
| | **Self-Esteem Enhancement**—Assisting a patient to increase his or her personal judgment of self-worth | |

NANDA International (2005). *Nursing diagnoses: Definitions & classification 2005–2006*. Philadelphia: North American Nursing Diagnosis Association.
Dochterman, J. M. & Bulechek, G. M. (2004). *Nursing interventions classification (NIC)* (4th ed.). St. Louis: Mosby.
Iowa Outcomes Project (2004). In Moorhead, S., Johnson, M. & Maas, M. (2004). *Nursing outcomes classification (NOC)* (3rd ed.). St. Louis: Mosby.
Dochterman, J. M. & Jones, D. A. (2003). *Unifying nursing languages: The harmonization of NANDA, NIC, and NOC*. Washington, D.C.: American Nurses Association.

"Point, click, learn! Visit thePoint for additional resources."

# CHAPTER 13

# Pain Management

## Learning Objectives

*On completion of this chapter, the learner will be able to:*

1. Compare characteristics of acute pain, chronic (persistent) pain, and cancer pain.
2. Describe the negative consequences of pain.
3. Describe the pathophysiology of pain.
4. Describe factors that can alter the perception of pain.
5. Demonstrate appropriate use of pain measurement instruments.
6. Explain the physiologic basis of pain relief interventions.
7. Explain the impact of aging on pain.
8. Discuss when opioid tolerance may be a problem.
9. Identify appropriate pain relief interventions for selected groups of patients.
10. Compare the various types of neurosurgical procedures used to treat intractable pain.
11. Develop a plan to prevent and treat the adverse effects of analgesic agents.
12. Use the nursing process as a framework for the care of patients with pain.

Pain has been defined as an unpleasant sensory and emotional experience associated with actual or potential tissue damage (Merskey & Bogduk, 1994). It is the most common reason for seeking health care. It occurs as the result of many disorders, diagnostic tests, and treatments. It disables and distresses more people than any single disease. Because nurses spend more time with patients in pain than other health care providers do, nurses need to understand the pathophysiology of pain, the physiologic and psychological consequences of acute and chronic (persistent) pain, and the methods used to treat pain. Nurses encounter patients in pain in a variety of settings, including acute care, outpatient, and long-term care settings, as well as in the home. Therefore, they must have the knowledge and skills to assess pain, to implement pain relief strategies, and to evaluate the effectiveness of these strategies, regardless of setting.

## Pain: The Fifth Vital Sign

Pain management is considered such an important part of care that the American Pain Society (2003) refers to pain as "the fifth vital sign" to emphasize its significance and to increase the awareness among health care professionals of the importance of effective pain management. Documentation of pain assessment is now as prominent as documentation of the "traditional" vital signs. Pain assessment and management are also mandated by the Joint Commission on the Accreditation of Healthcare Organizations (JCAHO) (2005).

Identifying pain as the fifth vital sign suggests that the assessment of pain should be as automatic as taking a patient's blood pressure and pulse. The JCAHO (2005) has incorporated pain assessment and management into its standards. JCAHO's standards state that "pain is assessed in all patients" and that "patients have the right to appropriate assessment and management of pain." Most institutions require the nurse to document assessment of the patient's pain in the medical record (Arnstein, 2003).

These standards reflect the importance of pain management. The American Pain Foundation developed the Pain Care Bill of Rights, which addresses the importance of pain management (Chart 13-1). To date, California is the only state to have enacted a Pain Patient's Bill of Rights. In addition, the United States Congress identified 2000 to 2010 as the Decade of Pain Control and Research. In 2003, Congress passed the National Pain Care Policy Act (NPCPA), the first comprehensive and proactive pain care legislation. This Act established a White House Conference on Pain Care to educate the public that pain is a significant health problem. In addition, the NPCPA authorized a National Center for Pain and Palliative Care Research within the National Institutes of Health (headaches.about.com/cs/advocacy/a/npcpa_call.htm; accessed March 12, 2006).

## Glossary

**addiction:** a behavioral pattern of substance use characterized by a compulsion to take the substance (drug or alcohol) primarily to experience its psychic effects

**agonist:** a substance that when combined with the receptor produces the drug effect or desired effect. Endorphins and morphine are agonists on the opioid receptors.

**algogenic:** causing pain

**antagonist:** a substance that blocks or reverses the effects of the agonist by occupying the receptor site without producing the drug effect. Naloxone (Narcan) is an opioid antagonist.

**balanced analgesia:** using more than one form of analgesia concurrently to obtain more pain relief with fewer side effects

**breakthrough pain:** a sudden and temporary increase in pain occurring in a patient being managed with opioid analgesia

**endorphins and enkephalins:** morphine-like substances produced by the body. Primarily found in the central nervous system, they have the potential to reduce pain.

**dependence:** occurs when a patient who has been taking opioids experiences a withdrawal syndrome when the opioids are discontinued; often occurs with opioid tolerance and does not indicate an addiction

**nociception:** activation of sensory transduction in nerves by thermal, mechanical, or chemical energy impinging on specialized nerve endings. The nerves involved convey information about tissue damage to the central nervous system.

**nociceptor:** a receptor preferentially sensitive to a noxious stimulus

**non-nociceptor:** nerve fiber that usually does not transmit pain

**opioid:** a morphine-like compound that produces bodily effects including pain relief, sedation, constipation, and respiratory depression. This term is preferred over narcotic.

**pain:** an unpleasant sensory and emotional experience resulting from actual or potential tissue damage

**pain threshold:** the point at which a stimulus is perceived as painful

**pain tolerance:** the maximum intensity or duration of pain that a person is willing to endure

**patient-controlled analgesia (PCA):** self-administration of analgesic agents by a patient instructed about the procedure

**placebo effect:** analgesia that results from the expectation that a substance will work, not from the actual substance itself

**prostaglandins:** chemical substances that increase the sensitivity of pain receptors by enhancing the pain-provoking effect of bradykinin

**referred pain:** pain perceived as coming from an area different from that in which the pathology is occurring. An example would be the perception of left arm or jaw pain in a person having a myocardial infarction.

**sensitization:** a heightened response seen after exposure to a noxious stimulus. Response to the same stimulus is to feel more pain.

**tolerance:** occurs when a person who has been taking opioids becomes less sensitive to their analgesic properties (and usually side effects). Characterized by the need for increasing doses to maintain the same level of pain relief.

> **CHART 13-1**
>
> ### Pain Care Bill of Rights
>
> Although not always required by law, these are the rights you should expect, and if necessary demand, for your pain care.
>
> As a person with pain, you have the right to
> - Have your report of pain taken seriously and be treated with dignity and respect by doctors, nurses, pharmacists, and other health care professionals.
> - Have your pain thoroughly assessed and promptly treated.
> - Be informed by your health care provider about what may be causing the pain, possible treatments, and the benefits, risks, and cost of each.
> - Participate actively in decisions about how to manage your pain.
> - Have your pain reassessed regularly and your treatment adjusted if your pain has not been eased.
> - Be referred to a pain specialist if your pain persists.
> - Get clear and prompt answers to your questions, take time to make decisions, and refuse a particular type of treatment if you choose.
>
> Courtesy of the American Pain Foundation, 201 N. Charles Street, Suite 710, Baltimore, MD 21201, www.painfoundation.org

The role of primary health care providers is to assess and relieve pain by administering medications and other treatments. Nurses collaborate with other health care professionals while administering most pain relief interventions, evaluating their effectiveness, and serving as patient advocates when the intervention is ineffective. In addition, nurses serve as educators to patients and families, teaching them to manage the pain relief regimen themselves when appropriate.

The definition of pain of the International Association for the Study of Pain identified at the beginning of this chapter encompasses the multidimensional nature of pain (Merskey & Bogduk, 1994). A broad definition of pain is, "whatever the person says it is, existing whenever the experiencing person says it does" (McCaffery & Pasero, 1999). This definition emphasizes the highly subjective nature of pain and pain management. Patients are the best authority on the existence of pain. Therefore, validation of the existence of pain is based on the patient's report that it exists.

Although it is important to believe patients who report pain, it is equally important to be alert to patients who deny pain in situations where pain would be expected. A nurse who suspects pain in a patient who denies it should explore with the patient the reason for suspecting pain, such as the fact that the disorder or procedure is usually painful or that the patient grimaces when moving or avoids movement. It may also be helpful to explore why the patient may be denying that he or she is in pain. Some people deny pain because they fear the treatment that may result if they report or admit pain. Others deny pain for fear of becoming addicted to **opioids** (previously referred to as narcotics) if these medications are prescribed.

## Types of Pain

Pain is categorized according to its duration, location, and etiology. Three basic categories of pain are generally recognized: acute pain, chronic (persistent, nonmalignant) pain, and cancer-related pain. To further clarify pain terminology and treatment, many pain specialists now refer to chronic pain as persistent pain (ie, pain that is not relieved by many different interventions (American Geriatrics Society [AGS] Guidelines, 2002).

### Acute Pain

Usually of recent onset and commonly associated with a specific injury, acute pain indicates that damage or injury has occurred. Pain is significant in that it draws attention to its existence and teaches people to avoid similar potentially painful situations. If no lasting damage occurs and no systemic disease exists, acute pain usually decreases as healing occurs. For purposes of definition, acute pain can be described as lasting from seconds to 6 months. However, the 6-month time frame has been criticized (Brookoff, 2000) as inaccurate, because many acute injuries heal within a few weeks and most heal by 6 weeks. In a situation in which healing is expected in 3 weeks and a patient continues to be in pain, the pain should be considered persistent, and appropriate treatment should be used.

### Chronic Pain

Chronic pain is constant or intermittent pain that persists beyond the expected healing time and that can seldom be attributed to a specific cause or injury. It may have a poorly defined onset, and it is often difficult to treat because the cause or origin may be unclear. Although acute pain may be a useful signal that something is wrong, chronic or persistent pain usually becomes a problem in its own right.

Chronic pain may be defined as pain that lasts for 6 months or longer, although 6 months is an arbitrary period for differentiating between acute and chronic pain. An episode of pain may assume the characteristics of chronic pain before 6 months have elapsed, or some types of pain may remain primarily acute in nature for longer than 6 months. Nevertheless, after 6 months, most pain experiences are accompanied by problems related to the pain itself. Chronic pain serves no useful purpose. If it continues, it may become a patient's primary disorder.

Nurses may come in contact with patients with chronic pain when these patients are admitted to the hospital for treatment or when they are seen out of the hospital for home care. Frequently, nurses are called on in community-based settings to assist patients in managing pain. For more information about common pain syndromes, see Chart 13-2.

## CHART 13-2

### Pain Syndromes and Unusual Severe Pain Problems

**COMPLEX REGIONAL PAIN SYNDROME**
*Complex regional pain syndrome* (CRPS) refers to a group of conditions previously described as causalgia, reflex sympathetic dystrophy (RSD), and other diagnoses. Complex regional pain syndrome describes a variety of painful conditions that often follow an injury. The magnitude and duration of the pain far exceed the expected duration and often result in significant impairment of motor function. There are two categories of CRPS: type I and type II. CRPS type I, the most common type, is characterized by unexplained diffuse burning pain, usually in the periphery of an extremity. RSD is categorized as CRPS type I and occurs after a relatively minor trauma (St. Marie, 2003). Pain is accompanied by weakness, a change in skin color and temperature relative to the other extremity, limited range of motion, hyperesthesia, hypoesthesia, edema, altered hair growth, and sweating.

Pain, which worsens with movement, cutaneous stimulation, or stress, often occurs after surgery or trauma to the extremity but is not limited to the area of surgery or trauma. CRPS type I is usually managed through a pain clinic. Currently, regional sympathetic blockade and regional intravenous (IV) bretylium offer promise for relief. Tricyclic antidepressants may be tried as well.

CRPS type II refers to causalgia. Type II is more likely to develop after trauma with detectable peripheral nerve lesions (Janig, 2001). The pain is characterized as burning and hyperpathia in an extremity after partial injury to a nerve or one of its major branches.

**POSTMASTECTOMY PAIN SYNDROME (PMP)**
*Postmastectomy pain syndrome* (PMP) occurs after mastectomy with node dissection but is not necessarily related to the continuation of disease. Characterized by the sensation of constriction accompanied by a burning, prickling, or numbness in the posterior arm, axilla, or chest wall, PMP is often aggravated by movement of the shoulder, resulting in a frozen shoulder from immobilization (Smith, Bourne, Squair, et al., 1999).

**FIBROMYALGIA (FIBROSITIS)**
*Fibromyalgia,* a chronic pain syndrome characterized by generalized musculoskeletal pain, trigger points, stiffness, fatigability, and sleep disturbances, is aggravated by stress and overexertion. Treatment consists of nonsteroidal anti-inflammatory drugs (NSAIDs), trigger point injections with local anesthetics, tricyclic antidepressants, stress reduction, and regular exercise (Gevirtz, 2004).

**HEMIPLEGIA-ASSOCIATED SHOULDER PAIN**
*Hemiplegia-associated shoulder pain* is a pain syndrome that affects as many as 80% of stroke patients. It may result from stretching of the shoulder joint due to the uncompensated pull of gravity on the impaired arm. It may be preventable with functional electrical stimulation of involved shoulder muscles.

**PAIN ASSOCIATED WITH SICKLE CELL DISEASE**
Pain experienced by patients with sickle cell disease results from venous occlusion caused by the sickle shape of the blood cells, impaired circulation to a muscle or organ, ischemia, and infarction. Acute pain may be managed with IV opioid analgesics administered according to a schedule or by a patient-controlled analgesia (PCA) pump and NSAIDs. Warm soaks and elevating the affected body part may help as well. Meperidine (Demerol) therapy is not recommended in patients with compromised renal function, nor is cold therapy. Patients with sickle cell disease may have a long history of chronic pain. Some issues related to their history include tolerance, possible long-term dependence, racial prejudice, and inadequate pain treatment (Jacob, 2001).

**AIDS-RELATED PAIN**
As AIDS progresses, so do problems that produce increasing amounts of pain, such as neuropathy, esophagitis, headaches, postherpetic pain, and abdominal, back, bone, and joint pain (Marcus, Kerns, Rosenfeld & Breithart, 2000). Pain relief interventions are individualized and may consist of NSAIDs, long-lasting opioids, such as fentanyl patches, and topical lidocaine. Tricyclic antidepressants may provide comfort in neuropathic and postherpetic pain.

**BURN PAIN**
Possibly the most severe pain, burn pain requires accurate assessment by all health care professionals to effectively manage pain. Besides administration of IV opioid analgesic agents, current therapies to relieve or control pain in burn patients include débridement under general anesthesia; anxiety reduction; intervention with PCA devices, such as a handheld nitrous oxide delivery system; and cognitive techniques, particularly hypnosis.

**GUILLAIN-BARRÉ SYNDROME AND PAIN**
A progressive, inflammatory disorder of the peripheral nervous system, Guillain-Barré syndrome is characterized by flaccid paralysis accompanied by paresthesia and pain—muscle pain and severe, unrelenting, burning pain. Complaints of severe pain may be difficult to

*continued >*

## CHART 13-2 Pain Syndromes and Unusual Severe Pain Problems, continued

accept in the face of the characteristic flaccid facial response; therefore, the nurse must be sensitive and learn to disregard nonverbal cues that contradict the verbal report of pain. Treatment interventions include NSAIDs for muscle pain and opioids if NSAIDs are ineffective. Causalgia and neurogenic pain may be relieved by systemic or epidural opioids or, possibly, antiseizure agents or tricyclic antidepressants. To relieve the burning, some patients beg to have windows opened and clothing removed, even in cold weather. This suggests that gentle ice massage may help. Research is needed, however, to test its effectiveness.

### OPIOID TOLERANCE

Opioid tolerance is common among patients treated for chronic pain, especially patients being treated by multiple health care providers. Opioid tolerance should be suspected if a patient (1) complains of significantly more pain than is usually associated with the condition, (2) requires unusually high doses of opioids to achieve pain relief, or (3) experiences an unusually low incidence and severity of side effects from opioids. Cancer patients also often develop a tolerance to opioids, requiring larger and larger doses of medication to obtain pain relief. In such cases, the nurse must recognize the signs of tolerance, seek additional information from the patient or family, and then obtain additional prescriptions for analgesics or an alternative intervention. In patients undergoing surgery, epidural local anesthetic agents provide excellent postoperative analgesia, but the problem of opioid tolerance must be elicited from the patient preoperatively.

A patient recovering from heroin addiction may be seen in an acute pain situation (surgery or trauma). This patient may be undergoing treatment with naltrexone (Trexan), a long-acting form of the opioid antagonist naloxone (Narcan). Both the short-acting naloxone and the long-acting naltrexone act by binding to the opioid receptors, so opioids cannot be effective. If surgery is planned, the naltrexone should be discontinued a few days before the procedure. If a patient receiving naltrexone is in immediate need of pain relief, very high doses of opioids may be necessary. Alternative methods of pain relief (local or regional blockade and NSAIDs) should be incorporated in the pain management plan.

## Cancer-Related Pain

Pain associated with cancer may be acute or chronic. Pain resulting from cancer is so ubiquitous that when cancer patients are asked about possible outcomes, pain is reported to be the most feared outcome (Sutton, Porter & Keefe, 2002). Pain in patients with cancer can be directly associated with the cancer (eg, bony infiltration with tumor cells or nerve compression), a result of cancer treatment (eg, surgery or radiation), or not associated with the cancer (eg, trauma). However, most pain associated with cancer is a direct result of tumor involvement. An approach to cancer pain management is illustrated in Figure 13-1. This three-step approach illustrates the types of analgesic medications used for various levels of pain. A cancer pain algorithm developed as a set of analgesic guiding principles is given in Figure 13-2.

## Pain Classified by Location

The previous discussion of acute and chronic pain is an example of the categorization of pain according to duration. Pain can also be categorized according to location (eg, pelvic pain, headache, chest pain). This type of categorization aids in communication about and treatment of the pain. For example, chest pain suggests angina or a myocardial infarction and indicates the need for diagnostic evaluation and treatment according to cardiac care standards as appropriate.

## Pain Classified by Etiology

Pain can also be categorized according to etiology. Burn pain and postherpetic neuralgia are examples of pain de-

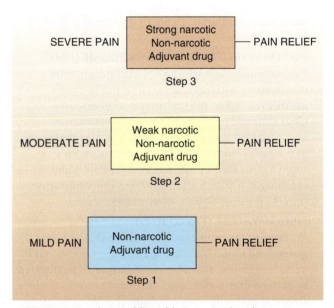

**FIGURE 13-1.** The World Health Organization three-step ladder approach to relieving cancer pain. Analgesic regimens are based on pain reported as ranging from mild to moderate to severe. Various opioid (narcotic) and nonopioid medications may be combined with other medications to control pain.

**FIGURE 13-2.** The cancer pain algorithm (highest-level view) is a decision-tree model for pain treatment that was developed as an interpretation of the AHCPR Guideline for Cancer Pain, 1994. Reproduced with permission from DuPen, A. R., DuPen, S., Hansberry, J., et al. (2000). An educational implementation of a cancer pain algorithm for ambulatory care. *Pain Management Nursing, 1*(4), 118.

scribed in terms of their cause. Clinicians often can predict the course of pain and plan effective treatment using this categorization.

## Harmful Effects of Pain

Regardless of its nature, pattern, or cause, pain that is inadequately treated has harmful effects beyond the suffering it causes. For example, unrelieved pain is associated with sleep alterations. Sleep deprivation affects the pain experience. Kunderman, Kreig, Schreiber, et al. (2004) noted that sleep deprivation produces hyperalgesic changes in which patients report greater pain from the same stimulus when they are sleep deprived. Analgesics may also be less effective if patients experience sleep deprivation.

### Effects of Acute Pain

Unrelieved acute pain can affect the pulmonary, cardiovascular, gastrointestinal, endocrine, and immune systems. The stress response ("neuroendocrine response to stress") that occurs with trauma also occurs with other causes of severe pain. The widespread endocrine, immunologic, and inflammatory changes that occur with stress can have significant negative effects. This is particularly harmful in patients whose health is already compromised by age, illness, or injury.

The stress response generally consists of increased metabolic rate and cardiac output, impaired insulin response, increased production of cortisol, and increased retention of fluids (see Chapter 6 for details about the stress response). The stress response may increase the risk of physiologic disorders (eg, myocardial infarction, pulmonary infection, thromboembolism, prolonged paralytic ileus). Patients with severe pain and associated stress may be unable to take deep breaths and may experience increased fatigue and decreased mobility. Although these effects may be tolerated by young, healthy people, they may hamper recovery in elderly, debilitated, or critically ill people. Effective pain relief may result in faster recovery and improved outcomes.

## Effects of Chronic Pain

Like acute pain, chronic pain also has adverse effects. Suppression of the immune function associated with chronic pain may promote tumor growth. In addition, chronic pain often results in depression and disability. Although health care providers express concern about the large quantities of opioid medications required to relieve chronic pain in some patients, it is safe to use large doses of these medications to control progressive chronic pain. In fact, failure to administer adequate pain relief may be unsafe because of the consequences of unrelieved pain.

Regardless of how patients cope with persistent pain, pain that lasts for an extended period can result in disability. Patients with a number of chronic pain syndromes report depression, anger, and fatigue (Watson & Coyne, 2003; Yezierski, Radison & Vanderah, 2004). Patients may be unable to continue the activities and interpersonal relationships they engaged in before the pain began. Disabilities may range from curtailing participation in physical activities to being unable to take care of personal needs, such as dressing or eating. Nurses should understand the effects of chronic pain on patients and families and should be knowledgeable about pain relief strategies and appropriate resources to assist effectively with pain management.

# Pathophysiology of Pain

The sensory experience of pain depends on the interaction between the nervous system and the environment. The processing of noxious stimuli and the resulting perception of pain involve the peripheral and central nervous systems.

## Pain Transmission

Among the nerve mechanisms and structures involved in the transmission of pain perceptions to and from the area of the brain that interprets pain are nociceptors, or pain receptors, and chemical mediators. **Nociceptors** are receptors that are preferentially sensitive to a noxious stimulus. Nociceptors are also called pain receptors, but the term "nociceptors" is preferred.

### Nociceptors

Nociceptors are free nerve endings in the skin that respond only to intense, potentially damaging stimuli. Such stimuli may be mechanical, thermal, or chemical in nature. The joints, skeletal muscle, fascia, tendons, and cornea also have nociceptors that have the potential to transmit stimuli that produce pain. However, the large internal organs (viscera) do not contain nerve endings that respond only to painful stimuli. Pain originating in these organs results from intense stimulation of receptors that have other purposes. For example, inflammation, stretching, ischemia, dilation, and spasm of the internal organs all cause an intense response in these multipurpose fibers and can cause severe pain.

Nociceptors are part of complex multidirectional pathways. These nerve fibers branch very near their origin in the skin and send fibers to local blood vessels, mast cells, hair follicles, and sweat glands. When these fibers are stimulated, histamine is released from the mast cells, causing vasodilation. Nociceptors respond to high-intensity mechanical, thermal, and chemical stimuli. Some receptors respond to only one type of stimulus, and others, called polymodal nociceptors, respond to all three types. These highly specialized neurons transfer the mechanical, thermal, or chemical stimulus into electrical activity or action potentials (Porth, 2005; Summers, 2000).

The cutaneous fibers located more centrally further branch and communicate with the paravertebral sympathetic chain of the nervous system and with large internal organs. As a result of the connections among these nerve fibers, pain is often accompanied by vasomotor, autonomic, and visceral effects. For example, gastrointestinal peristalsis may decrease or stop in a patient with severe acute pain.

### Peripheral Nervous System

A number of **algogenic** (pain-causing) substances that affect the sensitivity of nociceptors are released into the extracellular tissue as a result of tissue damage. Histamine, bradykinin, acetylcholine, serotonin, and substance P are chemicals that increase the transmission of pain. The transmission of pain is also referred to as **nociception**. **Prostaglandins** are chemical substances that are believed to increase the sensitivity of pain receptors by enhancing the pain-provoking effect of bradykinin. These chemical mediators also cause vasodilation and increased vascular permeability, resulting in redness, warmth, and swelling of the injured area.

Once nociception is initiated, the nociceptive action potentials are transmitted by the peripheral nervous system. The first-order neurons travel from the periphery (skin, cornea, visceral organs) to the spinal cord via the dorsal horn. There are two main types of fibers involved in the transmission of nociception. Smaller, myelinated Aδ (A delta) fibers transmit nociception rapidly, which produces the initial "fast pain." Type C fibers are larger, unmyelinated fibers that transmit what is called "second pain." This type of pain has dull, aching, or burning qualities that last longer than the initial fast pain. The type and concentration of nerve fibers to transmit pain vary by tissue type.

If there is repeated C fiber input, a greater response is noted in dorsal horn neurons, causing the person to perceive more pain. In other words, the same noxious stimulus produces hyperalgesia, and the person reports greater pain than was felt at the first stimulus. For this reason, it is important to treat patients with analgesic agents when they first feel pain. Patients require less medication and experience more effective pain relief if analgesia is administered before they become sensitized to the pain.

Chemicals that reduce or inhibit the transmission or perception of pain include **endorphins** and **enkephalins**. These morphine-like neurotransmitters are endogenous (produced by the body). They are examples of substances that reduce nociceptive transmission when applied to certain nerve fibers. The term "endorphin" is a combination of two words: endogenous and morphine. Endorphins and enkephalins are found in heavy concentrations in the central nervous system (CNS), particularly the spinal and medullary dorsal horn, periaqueductal gray matter, hypothalamus, and amygdala. Morphine and other opioid medications act at receptor sites to suppress the excitation initiated by noxious stimuli. The binding of opioids to receptor sites is responsible for the effects noted after their administration. Each receptor (mu, kappa, delta) responds differently when activated (Porth, 2005). Table 13-1 summarizes the classification and action of opioid receptors.

## Central Nervous System

After tissue injury occurs, nociception (the neurologic transmission of pain impulses) to the spinal cord via the Aδ and C fibers continues. The fibers enter the dorsal horn, which is divided into laminae based on cell type. The laminae II cell type is commonly referred to as the substantia gelatinosa. In the substantia gelatinosa are projections that relay nociception to other parts of the spinal cord (Fig. 13-3).

Nociception continues from the spinal cord to the reticular formation, thalamus, limbic system, and cerebral cortex. Here nociception is localized, and its characteristics become apparent, including the intensity. The involvement of the reticular formation, limbic, and reticular activating systems is responsible for the individual variations in the perception

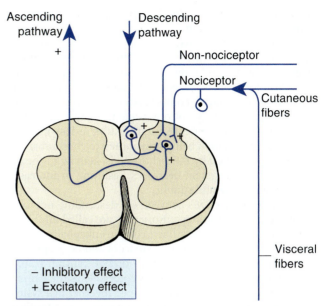

**FIGURE 13-3.** Representative nociception system, showing ascending and descending sensory pathways of the dorsal horn.

of noxious stimuli. People may report the same stimulus differently based on their anxiety, past experiences, and expectations. This is a result of the conscious perception of pain.

For pain to be consciously perceived, neurons in the ascending system must be activated. Activation occurs as a result of input from the nociceptors located in the skin and internal organs. Once activated, the inhibitory interneuronal fibers in the dorsal horn inhibit or turn off the transmission of noxious stimulating information in the ascending pathway.

## Descending Control System

The descending control system is a system of fibers that originate in the lower and midportion of the brain (specifically, in the periaqueductal gray matter) and terminate on the inhibitory interneuronal fibers in the dorsal horn of the spinal cord. This system is probably always somewhat active; it prevents continuous transmission of stimuli as painful, partly through the action of the endorphins.

### TABLE 13-1  Opioid Classification and Action

| Organ Effect | μ | κ | δ |
|---|---|---|---|
| Eye: Pupil | Miosis | Miosis | Mydriasis |
| Lung: Respiratory rate | Stimulation, then depression | No change | Stimulation |
| Heart: Rate | Bradycardia | No change | Tachycardia |
| Body: Temperature | Hypothermia | No change | Unknown |
| Affect | Indifference | Sedation | Dysphoria |
| Gastrointestinal system | Constipation | No effects | Nausea |

μ = mu; κ = kappa; δ = delta

From Willens, J. S. (1994). Pain management in the trauma patient. In V. D. Cardona, P. D. Hurn, P. J. B. Mason, A. M. Scanlon, & S. W. Veise-Berry (Eds.), *Trauma nursing from resuscitation through rehabilitation* (2nd ed., pp 325–362). Philadelphia: W. B. Saunders. With permission of W. B. Saunders. Copyright 1994 by W. B. Saunders.

As nociception occurs, the descending control system is activated to inhibit pain.

Cognitive processes may stimulate endorphin production in the descending control system. The effectiveness of this system is illustrated by the effects of distraction. The distractions of visitors or a favorite TV show may increase activity in the descending control system. Therefore, patients who have visitors may not report pain, because activation of the descending control system results in less noxious or painful information being transmitted to consciousness. Once the distraction by the visitors ends, activity in the descending control system decreases, resulting in increased transmission of painful stimuli.

The interconnections between the descending neuronal system and the ascending sensory tract are called inhibitory interneuronal fibers. These fibers contain enkephalin and are primarily activated through the activity of **non-nociceptor** peripheral fibers (fibers that normally do not transmit painful or noxious stimuli) in the same receptor field as the pain receptor, and descending fibers, grouped together in a system called descending control. The enkephalins and endorphins are thought to inhibit pain impulses by stimulating the inhibitory interneuronal fibers, which in turn reduce the transmission of noxious impulses via the ascending system (Hudspith & Munglani, 2003; Porth, 2005).

The classic gate control theory of pain, described by Melzack and Wall in 1965, was the first to articulate the existence of a pain-modulating system clearly (Melzack, 1996). This theory proposed that stimulation of the skin evokes nervous impulses that are then transmitted by three systems located in the spinal cord. The substantia gelatinosa in the dorsal horn, the dorsal column fibers, and the central transmission cells act to influence nociceptive impulses. The noxious impulses are influenced by a "gating mechanism." Melzack and Wall proposed that stimulation of the large-diameter fibers inhibits the transmission of pain, thus "closing the gate." Conversely, when smaller fibers are stimulated, the gate is opened. The gating mechanism is influenced by nerve impulses that descend from the brain. This theory proposes a specialized system of large-diameter fibers that activate selective cognitive processes via the modulating properties of the spinal gate. Figure 13-4 shows a schematic representation of a gate control system and nociceptive pathways.

The gate control theory was the first theory to suggest that psychological factors play a role in the perception of pain. The theory guided research toward the cognitive-behavioral approaches to pain management. This theory helps explain how interventions such as distraction and music therapy relieve pain.

Melzack (1996) extended the gate control theory after studying phantom limb pain. He proposed that a large, widespread network of neurons exists that consists of loops between the thalamus and cortex and between the cortex and the limbic system. Melzack labeled this network the neuromatrix. As information is processed in the neuromatrix, a characteristic pattern emerges. This pattern, referred to as the neurosignature, is a continuous outflow from the neuromatrix. Ultimately, the neurosignature output, with a constant stream of input and varying patterns, produces the feelings of the whole body with constantly changing qualities.

Melzack (1996) theorized that, in the absence of modulating inputs from the missing limb, the active neuromatrix produces a neurosignature pattern that is perceived as pain. The neuromatrix theory highlights the role of the brain in sustaining the experience of pain. Research to support the theory has been conducted. Andre, Martinet, Paysant, et al. (2001) studied the effects of vestibular caloric stimulation (cold water placed in the ear canal) on people who had an amputation. They noted that vestibular caloric stimulation produced a temporary perception of a normal phantom limb in 16 of 17 of those who previously did not experience phantom limb pain.

## Factors Influencing Pain Response

Several factors, including past experiences with pain, anxiety, culture, age, gender, genetics, and expectations about pain relief, influence a person's experience of pain. These factors may increase or decrease perception of pain, increase or decrease tolerance for pain, and affect responses to pain.

### *Past Experience*

It is tempting to expect that people who have had multiple or prolonged experiences with pain will be less anxious and more tolerant of pain than those who have had little experience with pain. However, this is not true for most people. Often, the more experience a person has had with pain, the more frightened he or she is about subsequent painful events. The person may be less able to tolerate pain; that is, he or she wants relief from pain sooner, before it becomes severe. This reaction is more likely to occur if the person has received inadequate pain relief in the past. A person with repeated pain experiences may have learned to fear the escalation of pain and its inadequate treatment. Once a person experiences severe pain, he or she knows just how severe it can be. Conversely, a person who has never had severe pain may have no fear of such pain.

The way a person responds to pain is a result of many separate painful events during a lifetime. For some, past pain may have been constant and unrelenting, as in chronic pain. Such people may become irritable, withdrawn, and depressed.

The undesirable effects that may result from previous experience point to the need for the nurse to be aware of the patient's past experiences with pain. If pain is relieved promptly and adequately, the person may be less fearful of future pain and better able to tolerate it.

### *Anxiety and Depression*

Although it is commonly believed that anxiety increases pain, this is not necessarily true. Postoperative anxiety is most related to preoperative anxiety and postoperative complications. However, anxiety that is relevant or related to the pain may increase the patient's perception of pain. For example, the patient who was treated 2 years ago for breast cancer and now has hip pain may fear that the pain indicates metastasis. In this case, the anxiety may result in increased pain. Anxiety that is unrelated to the pain may distract the patient and may actually decrease the percep-

**FIGURE 13-4.** A schematic representation of the gate control system and aspects of the nociceptive system. The nervous system is made up of stimulatory and inhibitory fibers. For example, stimulation of the nociceptor results in the transmission of an impulse that will be interpreted as pain. When it is stimulated, it will stimulate transmission at the next fiber junction (represented as +>—). The interneuronal fiber is an inhibitory neuron (–>—). When it is stimulated, it, in turn, inhibits or shuts off transmission at the next junction. So a placebo has a (+) stimulatory effect on the descending control system, which has a stimulatory effect (+) on the interneuronal fiber, which has an inhibitory effect (–) on the ascending control system. A topical anesthetic has an inhibitory effect (–) on nerve transmission at the nociceptor level, and a spinal anesthetic has the same impact (–) on the ascending nociceptive fibers.

tion of pain. For example, a mother who is hospitalized with complications from abdominal surgery and is anxious about her children may perceive less pain as her anxiety about her children increases.

The routine use of antianxiety medications to treat anxiety in patients with pain may prevent patients from reporting pain because of sedation and may impair their ability to take deep breaths, get out of bed, and cooperate with the treatment plan. The most effective way to relieve pain is by directing the treatment at the pain rather than at the anxiety.

Just as anxiety is associated with pain because of concerns and fears about the underlying disease, depression is associated with chronic pain and unrelieved cancer pain. In cases of chronic pain, the incidence of depression is increased (Bair, Robinson, Katon, et al., 2003). Depression is associated with major life changes caused by the limiting effects of persistent pain, specifically unemployment. Unrelieved cancer pain drastically interferes with the patient's quality of life, and relieving the pain may go a long way toward treating the depression.

### Culture

Beliefs about pain and how to respond to it differ from one culture to the next. Early in childhood, people learn from those around them what responses to pain are acceptable or unacceptable. For example, a child may learn that a sports injury is not expected to hurt as much as a comparable injury caused by a motor vehicle crash. The child also learns what stimuli are expected to be painful and what behavioral responses are acceptable. These beliefs vary from one culture to another; therefore, people from different cultures who experience the same intensity of pain may not report it or respond to it in the same ways.

Cultural factors must be taken into account to manage pain effectively. Many studies have examined the cultural aspects of pain. Inconsistent results, methodologic weaknesses or flaws, and failure of many researchers to carefully distinguish ethnicity, culture, and race make it difficult to interpret the findings of many of these studies. Factors that help explain differences in a cultural group include age, gender, education level, and income. In addition, the degree to which patients identify with a culture influences the degree to which they will adopt new health behaviors or rely on traditional health beliefs and practices. Other factors that affect the patient's response to pain include his or her interactions with the health care system and the health care provider (Green et al., 2003; Riley et al., 2002).

The cultural expectations and values of nurses may differ from those of other cultures and may include avoiding exaggerated expressions of pain, such as excessive crying and moaning; seeking immediate relief from pain; and giving complete descriptions of the pain. Whereas patients of one cultural background may moan and complain about pain, refuse pain relief measures that do not cure the cause of the pain, or use adjectives such as "unbearable" in describing the pain, patients of another cultural background may behave in a quiet, stoic manner rather than express the pain loudly. The nurse must react to the person's perception of pain and not to the person's behavior, because the behavior may differ from the nurse's cultural expectations.

Recognizing the values of one's own culture and learning how these values differ from those of other cultures helps avoid evaluating the patient's behavior on the basis of one's own cultural expectations and values. The nurse who recognizes cultural differences has a greater understanding of the patient's pain, is more accurate in assessing pain and behavioral responses to pain, and is more effective at relieving pain.

The main issues to consider when caring for patients of a different culture are

- What does the illness mean to the patient?
- Are there culturally based stigmas related to this illness or pain?
- What is the role of the family in health care decisions?
- Are traditional pain-relief remedies used?
- What is the role of stoicism in the patient's culture?
- Are there culturally determined ways of expressing and communicating pain?
- Does the patient have any fears about the pain?
- Has the patient seen or does the patient want to see a traditional healer?

Regardless of the patient's culture, the nurse should learn about that particular culture and be aware of power and communication issues that affect care outcomes (Watt-Watson, Stevens, Garfinkel, et al., 2001). The nurse should avoid stereotyping the patient by culture and provide individualized care rather than assuming that a patient of a specific culture will exhibit more or less pain. In addition to avoiding stereotyping, health care providers should individualize the amount of medications or therapy according to the information provided by the patient. The nurse should recognize that stereotypes exist and become sensitive to how stereotypes negatively affect care. In turn, patients must be instructed about how and what to communicate about their pain.

## Gerontologic Considerations

Age has long been the focus of research on pain perception and pain tolerance, and again the results have been inconsistent. For example, although some researchers have found that older adults require a higher intensity of noxious stimuli than do younger adults before they report pain (Washington, Gibson & Helme, 2000), others have found no differences in responses of younger and older adults (Edwards & Fillingim, 2000). Other researchers have found that elderly patients (older than 65 years of age) report significantly less pain than younger patients do (Li, Greenwald, Gennis, et al., 2001). Experts in the field of pain management have concluded that if pain perception is diminished in elderly people, it is most likely secondary to a disease process (eg, diabetes) rather than to aging (AGS, 2002). More research is needed in the area of aging and its effects on pain perception to understand what the elderly are experiencing.

Although many elderly people seek health care because of pain, others are reluctant to seek help even when in severe pain because they consider pain to be part of normal aging. Assessment of pain in older adults may be difficult because of the physiologic, psychosocial, and cognitive changes that often accompany aging. Research has revealed that a large number of nursing home residents reported being in pain daily; this pain is often described as excruciating and often persists unrelieved without treatment (Teno, Kabumoto, Wetle, et al., 2004). Unrelieved pain contributes to the problems of depression, sleep disturbances, delayed rehabilitation, malnutrition, and cognitive dysfunction (Miaskowski, 2000).

The way older people respond to pain may differ from the way younger people respond. Because elderly people have a slower metabolism and a greater ratio of body fat to muscle mass than younger people do, small doses of analgesic agents may be sufficient to relieve pain, and these doses may be effective longer. Elderly patients deal with pain according to their lifestyle, personality, and cultural background, as do younger adults. Many elderly people are fearful of addiction and, as a result, do not report that they are in pain or ask for medication to relieve pain. Others fail to seek care because they fear that the pain may indicate serious illness or that pain relief will be associated with a loss of independence.

Elderly patients must receive adequate pain relief after surgery or trauma. When an elderly person becomes confused after surgery or trauma, the confusion is often attributed to medications, which are then discontinued. However, confusion in the elderly may be a result of untreated and unrelieved pain. In some cases, postoperative confusion clears once the pain is relieved. Judgments about pain and the adequacy of treatment should be based on the patient's report of pain and pain relief rather than on age.

## Gender

Researchers have compared pain intensity, pain unpleasantness, and pain-related emotions (depression, anxiety, frustration, fear, and anger) in men and women who were asked to rate their experiences with chronic pain. However, the results of studies of gender in regard to pain levels and response to pain have been inconsistent. A recent study demonstrated that women report significantly greater pain intensity than men in a laboratory setting, but when the level of anxiety and stereotypes about willingness to report pain are taken into account, gender is not a significant predictor of pain. In other studies, women have consistently reported higher pain intensity, pain unpleasantness, frustration, and fear, compared to men (Wise, Price, Myers, et al., 2002). Men and women are thought to be socialized to respond differently and differ in their expectations relative to pain perception. The pharmacokinetics and pharmacodynamics of opioids differ in men and women and have been attributed to hepatic metabolism, where the microsomal enzyme activity differs (Miaskowski, Gear & Levine, 2000).

## Genetics

Genetics factors play a role in the varied responses to nonsteroidal anti-inflammatory drugs (NSAIDs) and opioids seen in patients (Desmeules, Piguet, Ehret, et al., 2004). African Americans reported greater levels of pain than Caucasians for many different types of pain, including migraines, postoperative pain, and myofascial pain. Studying the physiologic responses and clinical pain in combination with subjects with chronic pain, Edwards and colleagues (2001) found that African Americans had higher levels of clinical pain, greater pain-related disability, and less pain tolerance compared with Caucasians. Because African Americans are a genetically mixed population (Collins-Schramm, Phillips, Operario, et al., 2002), these findings may serve as a basis for further study into the potential genetics-based causes of the different responses to analgesics.

The most extensively studied genetics variation in humans is in the metabolism of codeine. Drug metabolism involves genetically controlled enzyme activity for absorption, distribution, inactivation, and excretion. In both experimental and clinical pain, a polymorphism (DNA proteins with variant alleles) in CYP2D6 (encoding cytochrome P450) results both in poor metabolism and poor analgesic efficacy. People who are "poor metabolizers" do not demethylate codeine to morphine; therefore, they do not experience its analgesic effects. See Chapter 9 for further discussion.

## Placebo Effect

A **placebo effect** occurs when a person responds to the medication or other treatment because of an expectation that the treatment will work rather than because it actually does so. Simply receiving a medication or treatment may produce positive effects. The placebo effect results from natural (endogenous) production of endorphins in the descending control system. It is a true physiologic response that can be reversed by naloxone, an opioid antagonist (Wall & Melzack, 1999).

A patient's positive expectations about treatment may increase the effectiveness of a medication or other intervention. Often, the more cues the patient receives about the intervention's effectiveness, the more effective it is. Patients who are told that a medication is expected to relieve pain are more likely to experience pain relief than those who are told that a medication is unlikely to have any effect.

Researchers have shown that different verbal instructions given to patients about therapies affect patient behavior and affect opioid intake significantly. Pollo et al. (2001) studied the effect of information and expectations in patients who had undergone thoracotomy. Patients in three groups were given an intravenous (IV) infusion of normal saline solution and could receive a dose of buprenorphine (Buprenex) on request. The first group was given no information about the analgesic effect of the regimen; the second group was informed that the infusion received could be an analgesic or a placebo; and the third group was told that the infusion was a powerful analgesic. Although subjects in the three groups did not differ in reported level of pain, those in the group told that the infusion was a powerful analgesic used less opioid than patients in the other groups.

Two analyses of multiple published research studies examined the placebo effect in clinical trials and had similar results (Hrobjartsson & Gotzsche, 2001, 2004). Although other clinical conditions were studied, including obesity, asthma, hypertension, insomnia, and anxiety, pain was the only condition in which a placebo effect was demonstrated.

The American Society for Pain Management Nurses (2005) contends that placebos (tablets or injections with no active ingredients) should not be used to assess or manage pain in any patient, regardless of age or diagnosis. Furthermore, the group recommends that all health care institutions have policies in place prohibiting the use of placebos for this purpose. Educational programs should be conducted to educate nurses and other health care providers about effective pain management, and ethics committees should assist in developing and disseminating these policies (Chart 13-3).

---

**CHART 13-3**

### Ethics and Related Issues

**Administration of Placebos**

Because of misperceptions about placebos and the placebo effect, it is important to keep in mind some specific principles and guidelines:

- A placebo effect is not an indication that the person does not have pain; rather, it is a true physiologic response.
- Placebos (tablets or injections with no active ingredients) should never be used to test the person's truthfulness about pain or as the first line of treatment.
- A positive response to a placebo (eg, reduction in pain) should never be interpreted as an indication that the person's pain is not real.
- A patient should never be given a placebo as a substitute for an analgesic medication. Although a placebo can produce analgesia, patients receiving a placebo may report that their pain is relieved or that they feel better simply to avoid disappointing the nurse.

# Nursing Assessment of Pain

The highly subjective nature of pain means that pain assessment and management present challenges for all clinicians. The report of pain is a social transaction; therefore, assessment and management of pain require a good rapport with the person in pain. In assessing a patient with pain, the nurse reviews the patient's description of the pain and other factors that may influence pain (eg, previous experience, anxiety, age), as well as the patient's response to pain relief strategies. Documentation of the pain level as rated on a pain scale becomes part of the patient's medical record, as does the record of the pain relief obtained from interventions.

Pain assessment includes determining what level of pain relief the acutely ill patient believes is needed to recover quickly or improve function, or what level of relief the chronically or terminally ill patient requires to maintain comfort (Chart 13-4). Part of a thorough pain assessment is understanding the patient's expectations and misconceptions about pain (Chart 13-5). People who understand that pain relief not only contributes to comfort but also hastens recovery are more likely to request or self-administer treatment appropriately.

## Characteristics of Pain

The factors to consider in a complete pain assessment are the intensity, timing, location, quality, and personal meaning of pain; aggravating and alleviating factors; and pain behaviors. Pain assessment begins by careful patient observation, noting overall posture and presence or absence of overt pain behaviors. In addition, it is essential to ask the patient to describe, in his or her own words, the specifics of the pain. The words used to describe the pain may point toward the cause. For example, the classic description of chest pain that results from a myocardial infarction includes pressure or squeezing on the chest. A detailed history should follow the initial description of pain.

### Intensity

The intensity of pain ranges from none to mild discomfort to excruciating. There is no correlation between reported intensity and the stimulus that produced it. The reported intensity is influenced by the person's **pain threshold** and **pain tolerance**. Pain threshold is the smallest stimulus for which a person reports pain, and pain tolerance is the maximum amount of pain a person can tolerate. To understand variations, the nurse can ask about the present pain intensity as well as the least and the worst pain intensity. Various scales and surveys are helpful to patients trying to describe pain intensity. Examples of pain scales appear in Figure 13-5.

### Timing

Sometimes the cause of pain can be determined when time aspects are known. Therefore, the nurse inquires about the onset, duration, relationship between time and intensity (eg, at what time is the pain worst), and changes in rhythmic patterns. The patient is asked if the pain began suddenly or increased gradually. Sudden pain that rapidly reaches maximum intensity is indicative of tissue rupture, and immediate intervention is necessary. Pain from ischemia gradually increases and becomes intense over a longer time. The chronic (or persistent) pain of arthritis illustrates the usefulness of determining the relationship between time and intensity, because people with arthritis usually report that pain is worse in the morning.

### Location

The location of pain is best determined by having the patient point to the area of the body involved. Some general assessment forms include drawings of human figures, on which the patient is asked to shade in the area involved. This is especially helpful if the pain radiates (**referred pain**). The shaded figures are helpful in determining the effectiveness of treatment or change in the location of pain over time.

### Quality

The nurse asks the patient to describe the pain in his or her own words without offering clues. For example, the nurse asks the patient to describe what the pain feels like. The nurse must give the patient sufficient time to describe the pain, and the nurse must record all words in the answer. If the patient cannot describe the quality of the pain, the nurse can suggest words such as burning, aching, throbbing, or stabbing. It is important to document the exact words used by the patient to describe the pain and which words were suggested by the nurse conducting the assessment.

### Personal Meaning

Pain means different things to different people; as a result, patients experience pain differently. The meaning of the pain experience helps the clinician understand how the patient is affected and assists in planning treatment. It is important to ask how the pain affects the person's daily life. Some people with pain can continue to work or study, whereas others may be disabled by their pain. The pain may affect family finances. For some patients, the recurrence of pain may mean worsening of disease, such as the spread of cancer.

### Aggravating and Alleviating Factors

The nurse asks the patient what, if anything, makes the pain worse and what makes it better and asks specifically about the relationship between activity and pain. This helps detect factors associated with pain. For example, in a patient with advanced metastatic cancer, pain with coughing may signal spinal cord compression. The nurse ascertains whether environmental factors influence pain, because they may easily be changed to help the patient. For example, making the room warmer may help a patient relax and may decrease the person's pain. Finally, the nurse asks the patient whether the pain is influenced by or affects the quality of sleep or anxiety. Both can significantly affect pain intensity and the quality of life.

Knowledge of alleviating factors assists the nurse in developing a treatment plan. Therefore, it is important to ask about the patient's use of medications (prescribed and over-the-counter [OTC]), including amount and frequency. In addition, the nurse asks if herbal remedies, nonpharmaco-

## CHART 13-4

### Pain at the End of Life

Pain is one of the most feared symptoms at the end of life. Most patients experience pain as a terminal illness progresses. The inadequate treatment of cancer pain has been well documented. In the Study to Understand Prognoses and Preferences for Outcomes and Risks of Treatments (SUPPORT) (1995), investigators noted that nearly 40% of severely chronically ill and older patients who died in hospitals suffered moderate to severe pain in the last 3 days of life. The suffering caused by unrelieved pain touches all aspects of quality of life (activity, appetite, sleep) and can weaken an already fatigued person. Psychologically, unrelieved pain can create anxiety and depression, negatively affect relationships, and promote thoughts of suicide.

The Joint Commission on Accreditation of Health Care Organizations (JCAHO) implemented pain standards in January 2001. These standards present a unique opportunity to improve care for hospitalized patients. Even though hospices and palliative care agencies are not subject to JCAHO review, many patients with chronic illness who are receiving palliative care may be hospitalized at various times. The standards emphasize pain assessment, patient and family education, continuity of care for symptom management, and evaluation of interventions.

Current barriers to pain management include lack of education, lack of access to opioids, fear of addiction, and legislative issues.

### Lack of Education

Strategies to increase knowledge about pain, pain assessment, and pain management in general and at the end of life are needed to ensure that a patient's pain is effectively addressed. Many studies have increased what is known about pain and pain management. However, the information from these studies must be disseminated to health care providers to be translated into evidence-based practice. Health care professionals, including nurses, must remain current about the pharmacokinetics and pharmacodynamics of analgesics and about new technologies to deliver analgesic medications. Continuing education (CE), which can be accessed in many ways, is one option available to improve knowledge about pain and pain management. CE can be provided through conferences, journal articles, and online programs. Chapters of the American Society for Pain Management Nurses provide opportunities for CE about pain assessment and management. National pain organizations list the dates and locations of their CE programs and conferences on the Web sites. Studies are needed to evaluate the effect that educational interventions have on health care providers' knowledge about pain and their ability to manage pain effectively (Gunnarsdottir, Donovan & Ward, 2003).

### ACCESSIBILITY

The lack of access to opioids is another barrier to adequate pain relief. Patients may have difficulty affording medications. Some pharmacists, fearing crime, paperwork, and regulatory oversight, may not stock opioids or may keep limited quantities on hand. Some insurance companies limit the types of medications they will reimburse and the amount and frequency of renewal of analgesics.

### ADDICTION FEARS

The fear of addiction plays a role even at the end of life. Family members may be hesitant to assist the patient in pain management for fear of the social stigma of addiction. This causes needless pain and suffering. Some health care providers continue to have unfounded fears of contributing to a patient's risk for addiction when administering opioids.

### LEGAL BARRIERS

Legislative issues play a role in the inadequate management of pain. Many states are enacting Intractable Pain Statutes. These laws are aimed at reducing physicians' fear of civil or criminal liability or disciplinary action for aggressively managing pain. The tracking system by the Drug Enforcement Agency acts as a deterrent since opioids prescribed by physicians can be tracked. Some physicians fear that prescribing "too many" opioids could be interpreted as treating an addicted patient.

### OTHER ISSUES

Pain management at the end of life differs little from general pain management. Patients still require comprehensive pain assessment and pain management, even though assessment may be hampered by confusion, delirium, or unconsciousness. Caregivers are taught to observe for signs of restlessness or facial expressions as a "proxy" indicator of pain.

Analgesic agents should be titrated to find the most effective dose and the best tolerated route. The nurse and family members should assess the effectiveness of the current pain therapy. If the pain is not relieved, a larger dose of medication may be necessary. If the pain continues, another medication may be needed or the patient should be given a different analgesic. The titration process requires frequent assessment to effectively manage pain. The analgesic agent or treatment should be appropriate for the type of pain. For example,

*continued >*

### CHART 13-4 Pain at the End of Life, continued

neuropathic pain, usually described as burning, tingling, numbness, shooting, stabbing, or electric, requires a different treatment approach than acute pain.

Nonpharmacologic approaches, such as guided imagery and relaxation, can be used to decrease pain and help the patient cope. Careful patient positioning and environmental control are other methods to increase patient comfort.

Respiratory depression should be assessed because over time, the patient's risk for this side effect increases. The rate, depth, and level of consciousness should be monitored to determine whether respiratory depression is occurring and requires treatment. A respiratory rate of 6 per minute or greater is usually adequate. If respiratory depression is suspected, a decrease in the opioid dose may be indicated. Frequent stimulation to encourage deep breathing may be required until the opioid is metabolized. In the last few days of life the patient may become restless, which is an indicator of pain. The need to increase the opioid to provide pain relief and the respiratory effects of opioids are considered in decision making. However, comfort should be a priority in the case of a person who clearly is at the end of life, where cure is no longer the goal.

Side effects from analgesics must be managed as in other painful conditions. Tolerance to constipation is rare. Therefore, a careful bowel regimen involving diet, bowel stimulants, stool softeners, and/or osmotic agents must be instituted. Vigilance in the assessment, management, and treatment of other side effects is similar to that included in previous discussions.

Careful assessment and management of pain at the end of life can make a "good" death possible. Education of health care providers and the family can help patients realize the goal of adequate pain relief throughout the dying process.

---

logic interventions, or alternative therapies have been used with success. This information assists the nurse in determining teaching needs.

### Pain Behaviors

When experiencing pain, people express pain through many different behaviors. These nonverbal and behavioral expressions of pain are not consistent or reliable indicators of the quality or intensity of pain, and they should not be used to determine the presence of or the severity of pain experienced. A patient may grimace, cry, rub the affected area, guard the affected area, or immobilize it. Others may moan, groan, grunt, or sigh. Not all patients exhibit the same behaviors, and there may be different meanings associated with the same behavior.

### CHART 13-5

#### Common Concerns and Misconceptions About Pain and Analgesia

- Complaining about pain will distract my doctor from his primary responsibility—curing my illness.
- Pain is a natural part of aging.
- I don't want to bother the nurse—he/she is busy with other patients.
- Pain medicine can't really control pain.
- People get addicted to pain medicine easily.
- It is easier to put up with pain than with the side effects that come from pain medicine.
- Good patients avoid talking about pain.
- Pain medicine should be saved in case the pain gets worse.
- Pain builds character. It's good for you.
- Patients should expect to have pain; it's part of almost every hospitalization.

Adapted with permission from Gordon, D. B., & Ward, S. E. (1995). Correcting patient misconceptions about pain. *American Journal of Nursing*, 95(7):43–45.

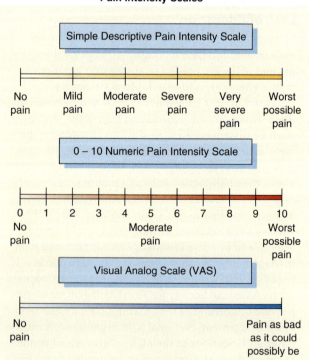

A 10-cm baseline is recommended for each of these scales.

**FIGURE 13-5.** Examples of pain intensity scales.

Sometimes in nonverbal patients, pain behaviors are used as a proxy to assess pain. It is unwise to make judgments and formulate treatment plans based on behaviors that may or may not indicate pain. In unconscious patients, pain should be assumed to be present and treated. All patients have a right to adequate pain management.

Physiologic responses to pain, such as tachycardia, hypertension, tachypnea, pallor, diaphoresis, mydriasis, hypervigilance, and increased muscle tone, are related to stimulation of the autonomic nervous system. These responses are short-lived as the body adapts to the stress. These physiologic signs could be the result of a change in the patient's condition, such as the onset of hypovolemia. Use of physiologic signs to indicate pain is unreliable. Although it is important to observe for any and all pain behaviors, the absence of these behaviors does not indicate an absence of pain.

## Instruments for Assessing the Perception of Pain

Only the patient can accurately describe and assess his or her pain. Clinicians consistently underestimate patients' levels of pain (McCaffery, Ferrell & Pasero, 2000). Therefore, a number of pain assessment tools have been developed to assist in the assessment of the patient's perception of pain (see Fig. 13-5). Such tools may be used to document the need for intervention, to evaluate the effectiveness of the intervention, and to identify the need for alternative or additional interventions if the initial intervention is ineffective in relieving the pain. For a pain assessment tool to be useful, it must require little effort on the part of the patient, be easy to understand and use, be easily scored, and be sensitive to small changes in the characteristic being measured. Figure 13-6 shows a pain assessment pathway that can be used at the time of assessment to direct clinical decisions for pain management.

### Visual Analogue Scales

Visual analogue scales (VAS; see Fig. 13-5) are useful in assessing the intensity of pain. One version of the scale includes a horizontal 10-cm line, with anchors (ends) indicating the extremes of pain. The patient is asked to place a mark indicating where the current pain lies on the line. The left anchor usually represents "none" or "no pain," whereas the right anchor usually represents "severe" or "worst possible pain." To score the results, a ruler is placed along the line, and the distance the patient marked from the left or low end is measured and reported in millimeters or centimeters.

Some patients (eg, children, elderly patients, visually or cognitively impaired patients) may find it difficult to use an unmarked VAS. In those circumstances, ordinal scales, such as a simple descriptive pain intensity scale or a 0-to-10 numeric pain intensity scale, may be used.

## NURSING RESEARCH PROFILE

### Pain Assessment by Nurses Compared With Patients

Puntillo, K., Neighbor, M., O'Neil, N. & Nixon, R. (2004). Accuracy of emergency nurses in assessment of patients' pain. *Pain Management Nursing, 4*(4): 171–175.

#### Purpose
Pain is one of the most common reasons for patients' visits to the emergency department (ED). To manage pain effectively, it must be assessed accurately, treated, and then reassessed to determine treatment efficacy. This study sought to determine if there is a difference between patients' ratings of pain intensity and triage nurses' ratings of patients' pain in the emergency department. The researchers also investigated whether patients' chief complaints influence pain ratings by both nurses and patients.

#### Design
This prospective, descriptive study included a convenience sample of triage nurses, non-triage ED nurses, and patients who presented to a Level 1 trauma center. A horizontal 0-to-10 numeric rating scale was used to measure pain intensity. Research assistants in the triage area asked patients to rate their pain intensity. Nurses who were blinded to the patients' responses were then asked to rate the same patients' pain intensity.

#### Findings
A total of 156 patients and 37 nurses participated in the study. Significant differences ($p = .001$) were found between triage nurses' ratings (mean = $5.1 \pm 2.4$) and patients' ratings (mean = $7.5 \pm 2.2$). Significant differences ($p = .001$) were also found between the non-triage nurses' and patients' intensity ratings. The mean pain intensity scores of non-triage nurses and patients were $4.2 \pm 2.3$ and $7.7 \pm 2.2$, respectively.

To determine what factors may contribute to these discrepancies in ratings, the researchers examined pain intensity ratings between patients and nurses based on patients' chief complaints. The greatest differences in pain intensity ratings occurred in patients with musculoskeletal disorders, abdominal pain, and cellulitis/abscesses. The least differences in pain intensity ratings occurred in patients with headaches, fractures, and radiculopathies.

#### Nursing Implications
The results of this study indicate that nurses continue to underestimate the intensity of patients' pain. Because pain management is based on nurses' assessments of patients' pain intensity, nurses should ask patients to rate their own pain rather than using assessments based on nurses' own assumptions and biases.

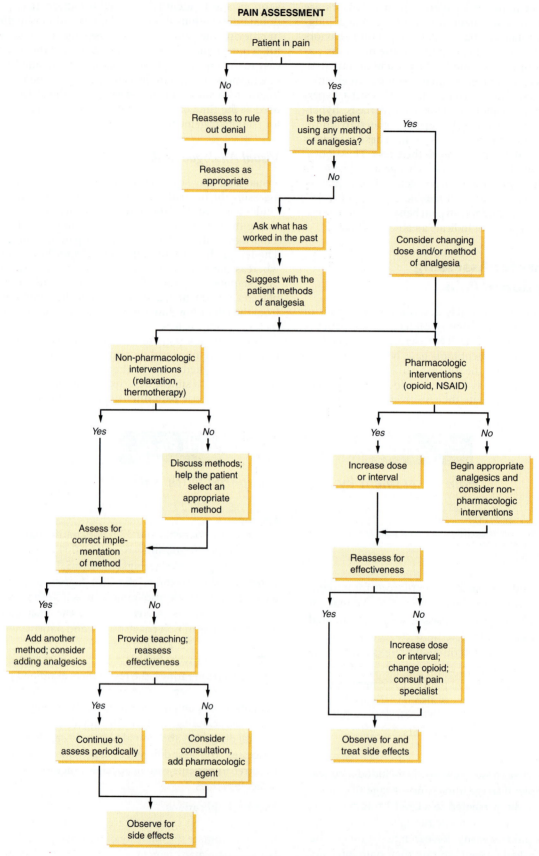

**FIGURE 13-6.** Pain assessment pathway.

## Faces Pain Scale–Revised

This instrument has six faces depicting expressions that range from contented to obvious distress (Fig. 13-7). The patient is asked to point to the face that most closely resembles the intensity of his or her pain. Evidence of reliability and validity of this scale has been established (Hicks, von Baeyer, Spafford, et al., 2001).

## Guidelines for Using Pain Assessment Scales

Using a written scale to assess pain may not be possible if a person is seriously ill, is in severe pain, or has just returned from surgery. In these cases, the nurse can ask the patient, "On a scale of 0 to 10, 0 being no pain and 10 being pain as bad as it can be, how bad is your pain now?" For patients who have difficulty with a 0 to 10 scale, a 0 to 5 scale may be tried. Whichever scale is used, it should be used consistently. Most patients usually can respond without difficulty. Ideally, the nurse teaches the patient how to use the pain scale before the pain occurs (eg, before surgery). The patient's numerical rating is documented and used to assess the effectiveness of pain relief interventions.

If a particular patient does not speak English or cannot clearly communicate information needed to manage pain, an interpreter, translator, or family member familiar with the person's method of communication should be consulted and a method established for pain assessment. Often a chart can be constructed with English words on one side and the foreign language on the other. The patient can then point to the corresponding word to tell the nurse about the pain.

When people with pain are cared for at home by family caregivers or home care nurses, a pain scale may help assess the effectiveness of the interventions if the scale is used before and after the interventions are implemented. The patient and family caregivers can be taught to use a pain assessment scale to assess and manage the patient's pain. Scales that address the location and pattern of pain may be useful in identifying new sources or sites of pain in chronically or terminally ill patients and in monitoring changes in the patient's level of pain. For example, a home care nurse who sees a patient only at intervals may benefit from consulting the patient's or family's written record of the pain scores to evaluate how effective the pain management strategies have been over time.

On occasion, a person will deny having pain when most people in similar circumstances would report significant pain. For example, it is not uncommon for a patient recovering from a total joint replacement to deny feeling "pain," but on further questioning he or she will readily admit to having a "terrible ache, but I wouldn't call it pain." From then on, when evaluating this person's pain, the nurse would use the patient's words rather than the word "pain."

## Guidelines for Assessing Pain in Patients With Disabilities

Alternative forms of communication may be necessary for people with sensory impairments or other disabilities.

- For people who are blind and who know how to read Braille, pain assessment instruments can be obtained in Braille. In addition, there is now computer software that allows written documents to be scanned and converted into Braille. If these programs are not available, agencies that provide services for people who are blind may be able to assist in developing Braille versions.
- For people who are deaf or hard of hearing, outside interpreters (ie, not family members) should be used. Other useful communication strategies may include sign language, written notes, or pictures. When writing notes on a "magic slate" or making written notes, it is necessary to make every effort to guard the patient's privacy and confidentiality.
- For people with disabilities that result in communication impairment, computer-generated speech may be useful.

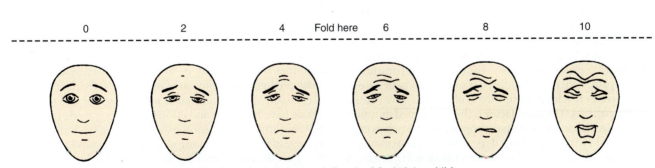

**FIGURE 13-7.** Faces Pain Scale–Revised. This pain scale is especially suited for helping children describe pain. Instructions for using this scale follow: "These faces show how much something can hurt. This face (*point to left-most face*) shows *no pain*. The faces show more and more pain (*point to each from left to right*) up to this one (*point to right-most face*). It shows *very much pain*. Point to the face that shows how much you hurt (right now)." Score the chosen face 0, 2, 4, 6, 8, or 10, counting left to right, so 0 = no pain and 10 = very much pain. Do not use words like "happy" or "sad." This scale is intended to measure how children feel inside, not how their face looks. (From the *Pediatric Pain Sourcebook*. Original copyright © 2001. Used with permission of the International Association for the Study of Pain and the Pain Research Unit, Sydney Children's Hospital, Randwick NSW 2031, Australia.)

# The Nurse's Role in Pain Management

Before discussing what the nurse can do to intervene in the patient's pain, it is necessary to review the role of the nurse in pain management. The nurse helps relieve pain by administering pain-relieving interventions (including both pharmacologic and nonpharmacologic approaches), assessing the effectiveness of those interventions, monitoring for adverse effects, and serving as an advocate for the patient when the prescribed intervention is ineffective in relieving pain. It is important to assess the patient's past medical history and family history for response to analgesics (eg, codeine). It is also critical to assess the patient's ethnic and racial background, because there appears to be a higher frequency of poor drug metabolizers among Caucasian people compared with Asian American and African American people. For example, when assessing a patient's lack of response to codeine, it may be appropriate to consider a genetics cause and obtain a prescription for a different opioid. In addition, the nurse provides education to the patient and family to enable them to manage the prescribed intervention themselves when appropriate.

## Identifying Goals for Pain Management

The information the nurse obtains from the pain assessment is used to identify goals for managing pain. These goals are shared and validated with the patient. For a few patients, the goal may be complete elimination of the pain. However, this expectation may be unrealistic. Other goals may include a decrease in the intensity, duration, or frequency of pain and a decrease in the negative effects of the pain. For example, pain may have a negative effect by interfering with sleep and thereby hampering recovery from an acute illness or decreasing appetite. In such instances, the goals might be to sleep soundly and to take adequate nutrition. Chronic pain may affect the patient's quality of life by interfering with work, interpersonal relationships, or sleep (Call-Schmidt & Richardson, 2003). Therefore, a goal might be to decrease time lost from work, to increase the quality of interpersonal relationships, or to improve the quality of sleep.

To determine the goal, a number of factors are considered. The first factor is the severity of the pain as judged by the patient. The second factor is the anticipated harmful effects of pain. Patients with other serious health issues are at much greater risk for harmful effects of pain than are young, healthy patients. The third factor is the anticipated duration of the pain. In patients with pain from a disease such as cancer, the pain may be prolonged, possibly for the remainder of the patient's life. Therefore, interventions will be needed for some time and should not detract from the patient's quality of life. A different set of interventions is required if the pain is likely to last for only a few days or weeks.

In patients receiving palliative care who had pain when they were conscious, it should be assumed that the pain persists even if the patient cannot communicate. Often family members can be taught what behaviors to look for to assess for pain: a furrowed brow, stiffening of a part of the body, or moaning.

The goals for the patient may be accomplished by pharmacologic or nonpharmacologic means, but most success is achieved with a combination of these methods. In the acute stages of illness, the patient may be unable to participate actively in relief measures, but when sufficient mental and physical energy is present, the patient may learn self-management techniques to relieve the pain. Therefore, as the patient progresses through the stages of recovery, increased patient use of self-management pain relief measures may be a goal.

## Establishing the Nurse–Patient Relationship and Teaching

A positive nurse–patient relationship and teaching are key to managing analgesia in patients with pain, because open communication and patient cooperation are essential to success. A positive nurse–patient relationship characterized by trust is essential. By conveying to the patient the belief that he or she has pain, the nurse often helps reduce the patient's anxiety. Saying to the patient, "I know that you have pain," often eases the patient's mind. Occasionally, a patient who fears that no one believes that he or she has pain feels relieved to know that the nurse can be trusted to believe that the pain exists.

Teaching is equally important, because the patient or family may be responsible for managing the pain at home and preventing or managing side effects. Teaching the patient about pain and strategies to relieve it may reduce pain in the absence of other pain relief measures and may enhance the effectiveness of the pain relief measures used.

The nurse also provides information by explaining how pain can be controlled. For example, the patient should be informed that pain should be reported in the early stages. When the patient waits too long to report pain, **sensitization** may occur, and the pain may be so intense that it is difficult to relieve. The phenomenon of sensitization is important in effective pain management. A heightened response is seen after exposure to a noxious stimulus; as a result, the response to that stimulus is greater, causing the person to feel more pain. When health care providers assess and treat pain before it becomes severe, sensitization is diminished or avoided, and less medication is needed.

## Providing Physical Care

Patients in pain may be unable to participate in the usual activities of daily living or to perform usual self-care and may need assistance to carry out these activities. Patients are usually more comfortable when physical and self-care needs have been met and efforts have been made to ensure as comfortable a position as possible. A fresh gown and change of bed linens, along with efforts to make the person feel refreshed (eg, brushing teeth, combing hair), often increase the level of comfort and improve the effectiveness of the pain relief measures.

In acute, long-term, and home settings, the nurse who provides physical care to patients also has the opportunity to perform complete assessments and to identify problems that may contribute to the patient's discomfort and pain. Appropriate and gentle physical touch during care may be reassuring and comforting. If topical treatments such as fentanyl (an opioid analgesic) patches or intravenous or intraspinal catheters are used, the skin around the patch or catheter should be assessed for integrity during physical care.

## Managing Anxiety Related to Pain

Anxiety may affect the patient's response to pain. A patient who anticipates pain may become increasingly anxious. Teaching the patient about the nature of the impending painful experience and the ways to reduce pain often decreases anxiety; people who experience pain use previously learned strategies to reduce anxiety and pain. Learning about measures to relieve pain may lessen the threat of pain and give the patient a sense of control. The patient's anxiety may be reduced by explanations that point out the degree of pain relief that can be expected from each measure. For example, a patient who is informed that an intervention may not eliminate pain completely is less likely to become anxious when a certain amount of pain persists.

A patient who is anxious about pain may be less tolerant of the pain, which in turn may increase his or her anxiety level. To prevent the pain and anxiety from escalating, the anxiety-producing cycle must be interrupted. Pain relief measures should be used before pain becomes severe. Many patients believe that they should not request pain relief measures until they cannot tolerate the pain, making it difficult for medications to provide relief. It is important to explain to all patients that pain relief or control is more successful if such measures begin before the pain becomes unbearable.

# Pain Management Strategies

Reducing pain to a "tolerable" level was once considered the goal of pain management. However, even patients who have described pain relief as adequate often report disturbed sleep and marked distress because of pain. In view of the harmful effects of pain and inadequate pain management, the goal of tolerable pain has been replaced by the goal of relieving the pain. Pain management strategies include both pharmacologic and nonpharmacologic approaches. These approaches are selected on the basis of the requirements and goals of particular patients. Appropriate analgesic medications are used as prescribed. They are not considered a last resort to be used only when other pain relief measures fail. As previously discussed, any intervention is most successful if it is initiated before pain sensitization occurs, and the greatest success is usually achieved if several interventions are applied simultaneously.

## Pharmacologic Interventions

Pharmacologic management of pain is accomplished in collaboration with physicians, patients, and often families. A physician or nurse practitioner prescribes specific medications for pain or may insert an IV line for administration of analgesic medications. Alternatively, an anesthesiologist or nurse anesthetist may insert an epidural catheter for administration of such analgesic agents. However, it is the nurse who maintains the analgesia, assesses its effectiveness, and reports whether the intervention is ineffective or produces side effects (Table 13-2).

Close collaboration and effective communication among health care providers is necessary. In the home setting, the family often manages the patient's pain and assesses the effectiveness of pharmacologic interventions, and the home care nurse evaluates the adequacy of pain relief strategies and the ability of the family to manage the pain. Home care nurses reinforce teaching and ensure communication among patients, family care providers, physicians, pharmacists, and other health care providers involved in the care of patients.

### Premedication Assessment

Before administering any medication, the nurse should ask the patient about allergies to medications and the nature of any previous allergic responses. True allergic or anaphylactic responses to opioids are rare, but it is not uncommon for patients to report an allergy to one of the opioids. On further questioning, the nurse often learns that the extent of the allergy is "itching" or "nausea and vomiting." These responses are not allergies; rather, they are side effects that can be managed while the patient's pain is relieved. The patient's description of responses or reactions should be documented and reported before medication is administered.

The nurse obtains the patient's medication history (eg, current, usual, or recent use of prescription or OTC medications or herbal agents), along with a history of health disorders. Certain medications or conditions may affect the

**TABLE 13-2　Adverse Interactions of Herbal Substances or Foods With Analgesics**

| Analgesic | Herb or Food | Effect |
|---|---|---|
| NSAIDs | Ginkgo, garlic, ginger, bilberry, dongquai, feverfew, ginseng, turmeric, meadowsweet, willow | Enhanced risk of bleeding |
| Acetaminophen | Ginkgo and possibly some of the above-mentioned herbs | Enhanced risk of bleeding |
|  | Echinacea, kava, willow, meadowsweet | Increased potential for hepatotoxicity and nephrotoxicity |
| Opioids | Valerian, kava, chamomile | Increased central nervous system depression |
|  | Ginseng | Inhibits analgesic effects |
| Alfentanil, fentanyl, sufentanil | Grapefruit juice | Inhibits the cytochrome P450 3A4 enzyme in the liver, blocking metabolism of the drug |

NSAID, nonsteroidal anti-inflammatory drugs.

From Abebe, W. (2002). Herbal medication: Potential for adverse interactions with analgesic drugs. *Journal of Clinical Pharmacologic Therapies, 27*(6), 391–401; and Karch, A. (2004). The grapefruit challenge. *American Journal of Nursing, 104*(12), 33–35.

analgesic medication's effectiveness or its metabolism and excretion. Before administering analgesic agents, the nurse should assess the patient's pain status, including the intensity of current pain, changes in pain intensity after the previous dose of medication, and side effects of the medication.

### Gerontologic Considerations

Physiologic changes in older adults require that analgesic agents be administered with caution. Drug interactions are more likely to occur in older adults because of the higher incidence of chronic illness and the increased use of prescription and OTC medications. Although the elderly population is an extremely heterogeneous group, differences in response to pain or medications by patients over this 40-year span (60 to 100 years) are more likely to be due to chronic illness or other individual factors than to age. Before administering opioid and nonopioid analgesic agents to elderly patients, the nurse should obtain a careful medication history to identify potential drug interactions (see Table 13-2).

Elderly patients are more sensitive to medications and at an increased risk for drug toxicity (American Geriatrics Society [AGS], 2002). Liver, renal, and gastrointestinal functions are decreased in elderly patients, resulting in changes in the absorption and metabolism of medications. In addition, changes in body weight, protein stores, and distribution of body fluid alter the distribution of medications in the body. Consequently, medications are not metabolized as quickly, and blood levels of the medications remain higher for a longer period.

Opioid and nonopioid analgesic medications can be administered to elderly patients but must be used cautiously because of the increased susceptibility to depression of both the nervous and the respiratory systems. Although there is no reason to avoid opioids in patients simply because they are elderly, meperidine should be avoided because its active and neurotoxic metabolite, normeperidine, is more likely to accumulate and cause CNS excitation and seizures. In addition, because of decreased binding of meperidine by plasma proteins, blood concentrations of the medication twice those found in younger patients may occur.

In many cases, the initial dose of analgesic medication prescribed for elderly patients is the same as that for younger patients, or slightly smaller than the normal dose, but because of slowed metabolism and excretion related to aging, the safe interval for subsequent doses may be longer (or prolonged). The AGS (2002) has published clinical practice guidelines for managing persistent pain in elderly patients. As always, the best guide to pain management and administration of analgesic agents in all patients, regardless of age, is what the individual patient says. Elderly patients may obtain more pain relief for a longer time than younger patients do from the same dose. As a result, smaller and less frequent doses of analgesics may be required.

### Approaches for Using Analgesic Agents

Medications are most effective when the dose and interval between doses are individualized to meet the needs of a particular patient. The only safe and effective way to administer analgesic medications is by asking the patient to rate the pain and by observing the response to medications.

### BALANCED ANALGESIA

Pharmacologic interventions are most effective when a multimodal or balanced analgesia approach is used. **Balanced analgesia** refers to the use of more than one form of analgesia concurrently to obtain more pain relief with fewer side effects. The three general categories of analgesic agents are opioids, NSAIDs, and local anesthetics. These agents work by different mechanisms. Using two or three types of agents simultaneously can maximize pain relief while minimizing the potentially toxic effects of any one agent. When one agent is used alone, it usually must be used in a higher dose to be effective. In other words, although it might require 15 mg morphine to relieve a certain pain, it may take only 8 mg morphine plus 30 mg ketorolac (an NSAID) to relieve the same pain.

### PRO RE NATA

In the past, the standard approach was to administer the analgesic *pro re nata* (PRN), or "as needed." The standard practice was for the nurse to wait for the patient to complain of pain and then administer analgesia. As a result, many patients remained in pain because they did not know they needed to ask for medication or waited until the pain became intolerable.

By its very nature, the PRN approach to analgesia leaves patients sedated or in severe pain much of the time. To receive pain relief from an opioid analgesic, the serum level of that opioid must be maintained at a minimum therapeutic level (Fig. 13-8). By the time the patient complains of pain, the serum opioid concentration is below the therapeutic level. From the time the patient requests pain medication until the nurse administers it, the patient's serum levels continue to decrease. The lower the serum opioid level, the more difficult it is to achieve the therapeutic level with the next dose. Using this method, the only way to ensure significant periods of analgesia is to give doses large enough to produce periodic sedation.

### PREVENTIVE APPROACH

Currently, a preventive approach to relieving pain by administering analgesic agents is considered the most effective strategy, because a therapeutic serum level of medication is maintained. With the preventive approach, analgesic agents are administered at set intervals so that the medication acts before the pain becomes severe and before the serum opioid level decreases to a subtherapeutic level.

Administering analgesic medication on a time basis, rather than on the basis of a patient's report of pain, prevents the serum drug level from falling to subtherapeutic levels. For example, a patient takes prescribed morphine or a prescribed NSAID (eg, ibuprofen) every 4 hours rather than waiting until the pain is severe. If the pain is likely to occur around the clock or for a substantial portion of a 24-hour period, a regular around-the-clock schedule of administering analgesia may be indicated. Even if the analgesic is prescribed PRN, it can be administered on a preventive basis before the patient is in severe pain, as long as the prescribed interval between doses is observed. The preventive approach reduces the peaks and troughs in the serum level and provides more pain relief with fewer adverse effects.

Smaller doses of medication are needed with the preventive approach, because the pain does not escalate to a level

**FIGURE 13-8.** Relationship of mode of delivery of analgesia to serum analgesic level. *Top:* intramuscular (IM) and intravenous (IV) patient-controlled analgesia (PCA). *Bottom:* transdermal (TD) and transmucosal (•) delivery.

of severe intensity. Therefore, a preventive approach may result in the administration of less medication over a 24-hour period, helping prevent tolerance to analgesic agents and decreasing the severity of side effects (eg, sedation, constipation). Better pain control can be achieved with a preventive approach, reducing the amount of time patients are in pain.

In using the preventive approach, the nurse assesses the patient for sedation before administering the next dose. The goal is to provide analgesia before the pain becomes severe. It is not safe to medicate the patient with opioids repeatedly if the patient is sedated or not in pain. It may be necessary to decrease the dosage of the opioid analgesic so that the patient receives pain relief with less sedation.

### USE OF "AS NEEDED" RANGE ORDERS FOR OPIOID ANALGESICS

Because of individual variation in patients' needs and responses to analgesics, PRN range doses have been used to relieve pain. Physicians have prescribed opioids with orders that allow the nurse to determine doses of medication to be administered and intervals between doses based on the nurse's assessment of the patient. Because of concern about patient safety with this method of prescribing analgesics, JCAHO established a policy in 2003 requiring specificity (eg, drug name, dose, route) when prescribing medications or a maximal allowable difference between the high and low dose no more than four times the lowest dose. In response, the American Society for Pain Management Nurses and the American Pain Society developed a consensus statement on as-needed range orders for opioids (Gordon et al., 2004). Chart 13-6 provides further information about as-needed range orders for opioids.

### INDIVIDUALIZED DOSAGE

The dosage and the interval between doses should be based on the patient's requirements rather than on an inflexible standard or routine. People metabolize and absorb medications at different rates and experience different levels of pain. Therefore, a certain dose of an opioid medication given at specified intervals may be effective for one patient but ineffective for another.

Because of the fear of promoting addiction or causing respiratory depression, health care providers tend to prescribe and administer inadequate dosages of opioid agents to treat acute pain or persistent pain, particularly in terminally ill patients (Chart 13-7). However, even prolonged administration of opioid agents is associated with an extremely low incidence of addiction (less than 1%). Furthermore, small doses are not necessarily safe doses. For example, some patients receiving a relatively small dose (25 to 50 mg) of meperidine (Demerol) intramuscularly have experienced respiratory depression, whereas other patients have not exhibited any sedation or respiratory depression with very large doses of opioids.

Therefore, the effects of opioid analgesic medications must be monitored, especially when the first dose is given or when the dose is changed or given more frequently. The time, date, patient's pain rating (scale of 0 to 10), analgesic agent, other pain relief measures, side effects, and patient activity are recorded. For example, when the first dose of an analgesic is administered, the nurse should record a pain rating score, blood pressure, and respiratory and pulse rates (all of which are considered "vital signs"). If the pain has not decreased in 30 minutes (sooner if an IV route is used) and the patient is reasonably alert and has a satisfactory respiratory status, blood pressure, and pulse rate, then some change in analgesia is indicated. Although the dose

## CHART 13-6

### Considerations for Writing and Interpreting PRN Range Orders for Opioid Analgesics

- **Reasonable range.** The maximum dose in a range order for an opioid should be at least 2 times, but generally no larger than 4 times, the smallest dose. This range is large enough to provide appropriate options for effective dose titration and small enough to establish a safe dose in a person.
- **Patient's prior drug exposure.** If the patient is opioid naïve, the first dose administered should be the lower dose in the range. If the patient is opioid tolerant or has received a recent dose with inadequate pain relief and tolerable side effects, a dose on the higher end of the range should be administered.
- **Prior response.** Inquire about the patient's response to previous doses. How much relief did prior doses provide, and how long did it last? Did the patient experience side effects?
- **Age.** For very young or elderly patients, "start low and go slow"; begin with a low dose and titrate up slowly and carefully. More frequent reassessments are indicated for more fragile or less resilient patients.
- **Hepatic and renal function.** If the patient has hepatic or renal insufficiency, anticipate a more pronounced peak effect and a longer duration of action.
- **Kinetics.** Know the onset, peak, and duration of action for the specific drug prescribed. Doses of short-acting opioids can be increased at each specified dosing interval, unlike scheduled long-acting opioid formulations.
- **Comorbidities that may affect patient response.** For example, debilitated patients and those with respiratory insufficiency may be at more risk for hypoxia if oversedated.
- **Concomitant administration of other sedating drugs.** If other central nervous system depressants are administered in combination with opioids, the dose of each drug required to achieve the desired effect should be 30% to 50% less than if either drug were administered alone.
- **Combination drugs.** Limit doses of combination drugs (eg, opioids with acetaminophen or an NSAID). Average adults should not receive more than 4000 mg of acetaminophen in 24 hours. Combination drugs may contain as much as 750 mg of acetaminophen per tablet. If substantial upward dose titration is required or anticipated, use opioid-only preparations.

EXAMPLE: An opioid-naïve patient arrives on the unit with the following order: morphine sulfate 2 mg to 6 mg IV every 2 hour PRN for pain.

- Give 2 mg for the first dose. Assess effects after 5 to 15 minutes. If the patient experiences adequate relief, reassess in 1 to 2 hours.
- If the patient experiences no side effects but inadequate relief, give additional 4 mg at time of peak effect from first dose.
- Total dose is 6 mg in a 2-hour period.

NSAID, nonsteroidal anti-inflammatory drug; PRN, "as required."

---

of analgesic medication is safe for this patient, it is ineffective in relieving the pain. Therefore, another dose of medication may be indicated. In such instances, the nurse consults with the physician to determine what further action is warranted.

### PATIENT-CONTROLLED ANALGESIA

Used to manage postoperative pain as well as persistent pain, **patient-controlled analgesia** (PCA) allows patients to control the administration of their own medication within predetermined safety limits. This approach can be used with oral analgesic agents as well as with continuous infusions of opioid analgesic agents by IV, subcutaneous, or epidural routes. PCA can be used in hospitals or in home settings (Pasero & McCaffery, 2005).

The PCA pump permits the patient to self-administer continuous infusions of medication (basal rates) safely and to administer extra medication (bolus doses) with episodes of increased pain or painful activities. A PCA pump is electronically controlled by a timing device. A patient experiencing pain can administer small amounts of medication directly into his or her IV, subcutaneous, or epidural catheter by pressing a button. The pump then delivers a preset amount of medication.

The PCA pump also can be programmed to deliver a constant, background infusion of medication or basal rate and still allow the patient to administer additional bolus doses as needed. The timer can be programmed to prevent additional doses from being administered until a specified time period has elapsed (lock-out time) and until the first dose has had time to exert its maximal effect. Even if the patient pushes the button multiple times in rapid succession, no additional doses are released. If another dose is required at the end of the delay period, the button must be pushed again to receive the dose. Patients who are controlling their own opioid administration usually become sedated and stop pushing the button before any significant respiratory depression occurs. Nevertheless, assessment of respiratory status remains a major nursing role.

To initiate PCA or any analgesia used at home or in the hospital, it is important to avoid playing "catch-up." Pain should be brought under control before PCA starts, often by the use of an initial, larger bolus dose or loading dose. Then, after control is achieved, the pump is programmed to deliver small doses of medication at a time. If a patient with severe pain has a low serum level of opioid analgesic because of an inadequate basal rate, it is difficult to regain control with the small doses available by pump. Before the

### CHART 13-7
### Ethics and Related Issues

#### Inadequate Pain Management

**SITUATION**

When taking over the care of ethnic minority patients at the change of shift from a particular colleague, you usually find these patients to be in a great deal of pain. Your nonsystematic observations have led you to conclude that these patients receive only a small portion of the analgesia prescribed for them. You have heard a nurse colleague state a belief that people of certain ethnic groups have "no pain tolerance" and are "just looking for drugs."

**DILEMMA**

Racial biases are difficult to deal with and change. To confront this nurse may not alter the behavior but will certainly disrupt the working relationships on the unit. It would be easier to look the other way. On the other hand, you believe that the nurse is giving inadequate and unethical care to selected patients and placing them at greater risk for postoperative complications.

**DISCUSSION**

- What information would you need to collect before acting?
- From whom could you seek counsel?
- Are the two aspects of the dilemma equally important?

PCA pump is used, repeated bolus doses of an IV opioid may be administered as prescribed over a short period until the pain is relieved. Then PCA is initiated. If pain control is not achieved with the maximal dose of medication prescribed, further prescriptions are obtained. The goal is to achieve a minimum therapeutic level of analgesia and to allow the patient to maintain that level by using the PCA pump. The patient is instructed not to wait until the pain is severe before pushing the button to obtain a bolus dose. The patient is also reminded not to become so distracted by an activity or visitor that he or she forgets to self-administer a prescribed dose of medication. One potential drawback to distraction is that the patient who is using a PCA pump may not self-administer any analgesia during the time of effective distraction. When distraction ends suddenly (eg, a movie ends, visitors leave), the patient may be left without a therapeutic serum opioid level. When intermittent distraction is used for pain relief, a continuous low-level background infusion of opioid through the PCA pump may be prescribed so that, after the distraction ends, it will not be necessary to try to "catch up."

A continuous infusion plus bolus doses may be effective with cancer patients who require large doses of analgesia and with postsurgical patients. Although this allows more uninterrupted sleep, the risk of sedation increases, especially when the patient has minimal or decreasing pain.

Patients who use PCA achieve better pain relief and often require less pain medication than those who are treated in the standard PRN fashion (Colwell, 2004). Because the patient can maintain a near-constant level of medication, the periods of severe pain and sedation that occur with the traditional PRN regimen are avoided.

If PCA is to be used in the patient's home, the patient and family are taught about the operation of the pump as well as the side effects of the medication and strategies to manage them (Pasero & McCaffery, 2005).

>  **NURSING ALERT**
>
> Family members are cautioned not to push the button for a patient, especially if the patient is asleep, because this overrides some of the safety features of the PCA system.

### Local Anesthetic Agents

Local anesthetics work by blocking nerve conduction when applied directly to the nerve fibers. They can be applied directly to the site of injury (eg, a topical anesthetic spray for sunburn) or directly to nerve fibers by injection or at the time of surgery. They can also be administered through an epidural catheter.

**TOPICAL APPLICATION**

Local anesthetic agents have been successful in reducing the pain associated with thoracic or upper abdominal surgery when injected by the surgeon intercostally. Local anesthetic agents are rapidly absorbed into the bloodstream, resulting in decreased availability at the surgical or injury site and an increased anesthetic level in the blood, increasing the risk of toxicity. Therefore, a vasoconstrictive agent (eg, epinephrine or phenylephrine) is added to the anesthetic agent to decrease its systemic absorption and maintain its concentration at the surgical or injury site.

A topical anesthetic agent known as eutectic mixture or emulsion of local anesthetics, or EMLA cream, has been effective in preventing the pain associated with invasive procedures such as lumbar puncture or the insertion of intravenous lines. To be effective, EMLA must be applied to the site 60 to 90 minutes before the procedure.

A lidocaine 5% (Lidoderm) patch, which has been on the market since 1999, has been shown to be effective in postherpetic neuralgia (Meier, Wasner, Kuntzer, et al., 2003). Currently, this is the only use approved by the U.S. Food and Drug Administration. The patch acts locally by targeting damaged nerves responsible for discharging pain impulses. Because the lidocaine 5% patch does not cause sensory block in the area of application, it has a wide margin of safety. The recommended dose is one to three patches at a time applied for 12 hours daily.

**INTRASPINAL ADMINISTRATION**

Intermittent or continuous administration of local anesthetic agents through an epidural catheter has been used for years to produce anesthesia during surgery. Although the administration of local anesthetic agents in the spinal canal is still largely confined to acute pain, such as postoperative pain and pain associated with labor and delivery, the epidural administration of local anesthetic agents for pain management is increasing.

A local anesthetic agent administered through an epidural catheter is applied directly to the nerve root. The anesthetic agent can be administered continuously in low doses, intermittently on a schedule, or on demand as the patient requires it, and it is often combined with the epidural administration of opioids. Surgical patients treated with this combination experience fewer complications after surgery, ambulate sooner, and have shorter hospital stays than patients who receive standard therapy (Correll, Viscusi, Grunwald, et al., 2001).

## Opioid Analgesic Agents

The goal of administering opioids is to relieve pain and improve quality of life; therefore, the route of administration, dose, and frequency of administration are determined on an individual basis. Factors that are considered in determining the route, dose, and frequency of medication include the characteristics of the pain (eg, its expected duration and severity), the overall status of the patient, the patient's response to analgesic medications, and the patient's report of pain. Opioids can be administered by various routes—oral, IV, subcutaneous, intraspinal, intranasal, rectal, and transdermal. Although the oral route is usually preferred for opioid administration, oral opioids must be given frequently enough and in large enough doses to be effective. Opioid analgesic agents given orally may provide a more consistent serum level than those given intramuscularly.

If the patient is expected to require opioid analgesic agents at home, the clinician should consider the ability of the patient and family to administer opioids as prescribed at the planning stages and should take steps to ensure that the required medications will be available to the patient. Many pharmacies, especially those in smaller rural areas or inner cities, may be reluctant to stock large amounts of opioids. Therefore, arrangements for obtaining these prescription medications must be made ahead of time.

With the administration of opioids by any route, side effects must be considered and anticipated. Clinicians who take steps to minimize the side effects increase the likelihood that the patient will receive adequate pain relief without interrupting therapy to treat the effects.

### RESPIRATORY DEPRESSION AND SEDATION

Respiratory depression is the most serious adverse effect of opioid analgesic agents administered by IV, subcutaneous, or epidural routes. However, it is relatively rare because doses administered through these routes are small, and tolerance to respiratory depressant effects increases if the dose is increased slowly. The risk of respiratory depression increases with age and with the concomitant use of other opioids or other CNS depressants. The risk of respiratory depression also increases when the epidural catheter is placed in the thoracic area and when the intra-abdominal or intrathoracic pressure is increased.

A patient who receives opioids by any route must be assessed frequently for changes in respiratory status. Specific notable changes are shallow respirations and decreasing respiratory rate. Despite the risks associated with their use, IV and epidural opioids are considered safe, with the risks related to epidural administration no greater than those related to IV or other systemic routes of administration. Sedation, which may occur with any method of administering opioids, is likely to occur when opioid doses are increased. However, patients often develop tolerance quickly, so that in a short time they are no longer sedated by the dose that initially caused sedation. Increasing the time between doses or reducing the dose temporarily, as prescribed, usually prevents deep sedation from occurring. Patients at risk for sedation must be monitored closely for changes in respiratory status. Patients are also at risk for problems associated with sedation and immobility. The nurse must initiate strategies to prevent problems such as skin breakdown.

### NAUSEA AND VOMITING

Nausea and vomiting frequently occur with opioid use. Usually these effects occur some hours after the initial injection. Patients, especially postoperative patients, may not think to tell the nurse that they are nauseated, particularly if the nausea is mild. However, a patient receiving opioids should be assessed for nausea and vomiting, which may be triggered by a position change and may be prevented by having the patient change positions slowly. Adequate hydration and the administration of antiemetic agents may also decrease the incidence of nausea. Opioid-induced nausea and vomiting often subside within a few days.

### CONSTIPATION

Constipation, a common side effect of opioid use, may become so severe that the patient is forced to choose between relief of pain and relief of constipation. This situation can occur in patients after surgery and in patients receiving large doses of opioids to treat cancer-related pain. Preventing constipation must be a high priority in all patients receiving opioids. Whenever a patient receives opioids, a bowel regimen should begin at the same time. Tolerance to this side effect does not occur; rather, constipation persists even with long-term use of opioids.

Several strategies may help prevent and treat opioid-related constipation. Mild laxatives and a high intake of fluid and fiber may be effective in managing mild constipation. Unless contraindicated, a mild laxative and a stool softener should be administered on a regular schedule. However, continued severe constipation often requires the use of a stimulating cathartic agent, such as senna derivatives (Senokot) or bisacodyl (Dulcolax). Oral laxatives and stool softeners may prevent constipation. If oral agents fail, rectal suppositories may be used (Plaisance & Ellis, 2002).

### INADEQUATE PAIN RELIEF

One factor commonly associated with ineffective pain relief is an inadequate dose of opioid. This is most likely to occur when the caregiver underestimates the patient's pain or fails to consider differences in absorption and action after a change in the route of administration. Consequently, the patient receives doses that are too small to be effective and, possibly, too infrequent to relieve pain. For example, if opioid delivery is changed from the IV route to the oral route, the oral dose must be approximately three times greater than that given parenterally to provide relief. Because of differences in absorption of orally administered opioids among individuals, patients must be assessed carefully to ensure that the pain is relieved.

Table 13-3 lists opioids and dosages that are equivalent to morphine. It serves only as a guide; the doses listed are

### TABLE 13-3  Selected Opioid Analgesics Commonly Used for Moderate and Severe Pain in Adults

| Name | Starting Dose (milligrams) Moderate Pain | Starting Dose (milligrams) Severe Pain | Comments | Precautions and Contraindications |
|---|---|---|---|---|
| Morphine | — | 30–60 (oral) 10 (parenteral) | Acts as an agonist at specific opioid receptors in the CNS to produce analgesia, euphoria, and sedation. | Use with caution, especially in elderly patients, very ill patients, and those with respiratory impairment. Major risks include respiratory depression, apnea, circulatory depression, and respiratory arrest, shock, and cardiac arrest. Obtain history of hypersensitivity to opioids. Monitor patient closely. If prescribed in correct dose, oral preparations (MS Contin) are effective in treating moderate and severe pain. |
| Codeine | 15–30 (oral) | 60 (oral) up to 360/24 hr | Acts as an agonist at specific opioid receptors in the CNS to produce analgesia, euphoria, and sedation. Is also an antitussive. 10% of people lack the enzyme needed to make codeine active. Codeine may cause more nausea and constipation per unit of analgesia than other mu agonist opioids. | Many preparations of codeine and the other opioids in this table are combinations with nonopioid analgesics. Caution must be used in patients with impaired ventilation, bronchial asthma, increased intracranial pressure, or impaired liver function and in elderly and very ill patients. |
| Oxycodone (OxyContin) | 5 (oral) | 10–20 (oral) | Acts as an agonist at specific opioid receptors in the CNS to produce analgesia, euphoria, and sedation. | Caution must be used in patients with impaired ventilation, bronchial asthma, increased intracranial pressure, or impaired liver function and in elderly and very ill patients. |
| Meperidine (Demerol) | 50 (oral) | 300 (oral) 75 (parenteral) | Acts as an agonist at specific opioid receptors in the CNS to produce analgesia, euphoria, and sedation. Shorter acting than morphine. Meperidine is biotransformed to normeperidine, a toxic metabolite. | Normeperidine, a toxic metabolite of meperidine, accumulates with repetitive dosing, causing CNS excitation. High risk for seizures. Should be avoided in patients with impaired renal function who are receiving MAO inhibitors. Is irritating to tissues with repeated intramuscular injections. Chronic use should be avoided. Should not be used for more than 1 or 2 days. |
| Propoxyphene (Darvon) | 65–130 (oral) | — | Weak analgesic; acts as an agonist at specific opioid receptors in the CNS to produce analgesia, euphoria, and sedation. Many preparations include nonopioid analgesics; biotransformed to potentially toxic metabolite (norpropoxphene). | Accumulation of propoxyphene and toxic metabolites occurs with repetitive dosing. Overdose is complicated by seizures. Propoxyphene is not recommended for older adults or patients with renal impairment. |
| Hydrocodone (Vicodin) | 5–10 (oral) | — | — | Most preparations are combined with nonopioid analgesics. |
| Tramadol (Ultram) | 50–100 (oral) | — | Unique mechanism; analgesia results from the synergy of two mechanisms. Maximum dose is 400 mg/day. | Most common side effects are dizziness, nausea, constipation, and somnolence. Lowers seizure threshold. |

CNS, central nervous system; MAO, monoamine oxidase.

Adapted from American Pain Society. (2003). *Principles of analgesic use in the treatment of acute pain and cancer pain* (5th ed.). Glenview, IL: American Pain Society; and Karch, A. M. (2005). *Lippincott's nursing drug guide.* Philadelphia: Lippincott Williams & Wilkins.

not necessarily the most appropriate doses for all patients. However, the table does give clinicians some idea of equivalency between two different opioids. After administering the first dose of an opioid, clinicians should perform a complete pain assessment to determine the efficacy of that dose. In general, no recalculation needs to be done when changing from one brand of an agent to another brand of the same medication, with the exception of extended-release oral morphine. Currently, three brands of extended-release morphine (MS Contin, Oramorph, Kadian) are commonly used by cancer patients. Although these agents come in the same dosage form and contain the same drug, they are not considered therapeutically equivalent because they use different release mechanisms. Patients who need to change brands should be monitored carefully both for overdose and for inadequate pain relief.

## OTHER EFFECTS OF OPIOIDS

When asked about drug allergies, patients with previous hospital experience (especially for surgery) may report that they are "allergic" to morphine. This report should be thoroughly investigated. Commonly, this "allergy" is described as itching only. Pruritus (itching) is a frequent side effect of opioids administered by any route, but it is not an allergic reaction. It can be relieved by administering prescribed antihistamines. Epidurally administered opioids may also cause urinary retention or pruritus. The patient should be monitored and may require urinary catheterization. Small doses of naloxone may be prescribed to relieve these problems in patients who are receiving epidural opioids for the relief of acute postoperative pain.

A number of factors may influence the safety and effectiveness of opioid administration. Opioid analgesic agents are primarily metabolized by the liver and excreted by the kidney. Therefore, metabolism and excretion of analgesic medications are impaired in patients with liver or kidney disease, increasing the risk of cumulative or toxic effects. In addition, normeperidine, a metabolite of meperidine, may rapidly or unexpectedly accumulate to toxic levels. This is more likely to occur in patients with impaired kidney function and may result in seizures in susceptible patients. Many institutions no longer stock meperidine because of the risks associated with the metabolite normeperidine and because most physicians do not prescribe a high enough dose for it to be effective.

Patients with untreated hypothyroidism are more susceptible to the analgesic effects and side effects of opioids. In contrast, patients with hyperthyroidism may require larger doses for pain relief. Patients with a decreased respiratory reserve from disease or aging may be more susceptible to the depressant effects of opioids and must be carefully monitored for respiratory depression.

Patients who are dehydrated are at increased risk for the hypotensive effects of opioids. Patients who become hypotensive after the administration of an opioid should be kept recumbent and rehydrated unless fluids are contraindicated. Patients who are dehydrated are also more likely to experience nausea and vomiting with opioid use. Rehydration usually relieves these symptoms.

Patients receiving certain other medications, such as monoamine oxidase inhibitors, phenothiazines, or tricyclic antidepressants, may have an exaggerated response to the depressant effects of opioids. Patients taking these medications should receive small doses of opioids and must be monitored closely. Continued pain in these patients indicates that a therapeutic level of the analgesic has not been achieved. Patients must be monitored for sedation even if an analgesic effect has not been obtained.

## TOLERANCE AND ADDICTION

There is no maximum safe dosage of opioids, nor is there any easily identifiable therapeutic serum level. Both the maximal safe dosage and the therapeutic serum level are relative and individual. **Tolerance** (the need for increasing doses of opioids to achieve the same therapeutic effect) develops in almost all patients taking opioids for extended periods. Patients requiring opioids over a long term, especially cancer patients, need increasing doses to relieve pain. After the first few weeks of therapy, their dosing requirements usually level off. Patients who become tolerant to the analgesic effects of large doses of morphine may obtain pain relief by changing to a different opioid. Symptoms of physical dependence may occur when the opioids are discontinued; dependence often occurs with opioid tolerance and does not indicate an addiction. It is an expected physiologic response that will occur in all people exposed to continuous opioid administration (Compton & Athanos, 2003).

> **NURSING ALERT**
>
> Although patients may need increasing levels of opioids, they are not addicted. Physical tolerance usually occurs in the absence of addiction. Tolerance to opioids is common and becomes a problem primarily in terms of delivering or administering the medication (eg, how to administer very large doses of morphine to a patient). On the other hand, addiction is rare and should not be the primary concern of nurses caring for patients in pain.

**Addiction** is a behavioral pattern of substance use characterized by a compulsion to take the substance (drug or alcohol) primarily to experience its psychic effects. Fear that patients will become addicted or dependent on opioids has contributed to inadequate treatment of pain. This fear is commonly expressed by health care providers as well as patients and results from lack of knowledge about the low risk of addiction.

Addiction after therapeutic opioid administration is so negligible that it should not be a consideration when caring for patients in pain. Therefore, patients and health care providers should be dissuaded from withholding opioid analgesics because of concerns about addiction.

When caring for people with a known history of addiction, nurses should consider that each individual person has the right to be treated for pain. The American Society for Pain Management Nurses (2002) developed a position paper on pain management of patients with addictive disease. It stressed education, communication about methods for pain management, and methods to discontinue opioids in this patient population. The opioids should be tapered slowly to prevent withdrawal symptoms (Nichols, 2003).

## Nonsteroidal Anti-inflammatory Drugs

NSAIDs are thought to decrease pain by inhibiting cyclo-oxygenase (COX), the rate-limiting enzyme involved in the production of prostaglandin from traumatized or inflamed tissues. There are two types of COX, COX-1 and COX-2.

COX-1 mediates prostaglandin formation involved in the maintenance of physiologic functions. Some of the physiologic functions of COX-1 include platelet aggregation through the provision of thromboxane precursors and increased gastric mucosal blood flow. This prevents ischemia and promotes mucosal integrity. Inhibition of COX-1 results in gastric ulceration, bleeding, and renal damage.

COX-2 mediates prostaglandin formation that results in symptoms of pain, inflammation, and fever. Therefore, inhibition of COX-2 is desirable. Celecoxib (Celebrex), rofecoxib (Vioxx), and valdecoxib (Bextra) are examples of COX-2 inhibitors. Evidence of increased cardiovascular risk for people taking rofecoxib (Vioxx) for longer than 18 months prompted its manufacturer to withdraw it from the market. The manufacturer noted that there was an increased incidence of cardiovascular events (stroke and myocardial infarction) associated with its use (Shaya & Suwannaprom, 2005). The U.S. Food and Drug Administration then mandated that a warning be added to the label of all COX-2 inhibitors about these risks. The pharmaceutical company that makes valdecoxib (Bextra) withdrew it from the market. Shaya and Suwannaprom (2005) stated that the findings of studies on the cardiovascular effects of COX-2 inhibitors should be interpreted with caution, because if no data were collected about cardiovascular status of patients, researchers cannot conclude that cardiovascular events are or are not related to these medications.

Ibuprofen (Advil, Motrin), another NSAID, blocks both COX-1 and COX-2, is effective in relieving mild to moderate pain, and has a low incidence of adverse effects. Aspirin, the oldest NSAID, also blocks COX-1 as well as COX-2; however, because it causes frequent and severe side effects, aspirin is infrequently used to treat significant acute or persistent pain.

NSAIDs are very helpful in treating arthritic diseases and may be especially powerful in treating cancer-related bone pain. They have been effectively combined with opioids to treat postoperative and other severe pain. The use of NSAIDs in combination with opioids relieves pain more effectively than opioids alone. In such cases, patients may obtain pain relief with decreased doses of opioid and with fewer side effects. In addition, intraoperative administration of NSAIDs reportedly improves postoperative pain control after abdominal hysterectomy surgery (Karamanlioglu, Turan, Memis, et al., 2004). A regimen of a fixed-dose, time-contingent NSAID (eg, every 4 hours) and a separately administered fluctuating dose of opioid may be effective in managing moderate to severe cancer pain. In more severe pain, the opioid dose is also fixed, with an additional fluctuating dose as needed for **breakthrough pain** (a sudden increase in pain despite the administration of pain-relieving medications). These regimens result in better pain relief with fewer opioid-related side effects.

Most patients tolerate NSAIDs well. However, those with impaired kidney function may require a smaller dose and must be monitored closely for side effects. Patients taking NSAIDs bruise easily because the agents have some anticoagulant effect. Furthermore, NSAIDs may displace other medications, such as warfarin (Coumadin), from serum proteins and increase their effects. High doses or prolonged use can irritate the stomach and in some cases result in gastrointestinal bleeding as well. For this reason, monitoring for gastrointestinal bleeding is indicated (Gordon, 2003).

## Tricyclic Antidepressant Agents and Anticonvulsant Medications

Pain of neurologic origin (eg, causalgia, tumor impingement on a nerve, postherpetic neuralgia) is difficult to treat and in general is not responsive to opioid therapy. If these pain syndromes are accompanied by dysesthesia (burning or cutting pain), they may be responsive to a tricyclic antidepressant or an antiseizure agent. When indicated, tricyclic antidepressant agents, such as amitriptyline (Elavil) or imipramine (Tofranil), are prescribed in doses considerably smaller than those generally used for depression. Patients need to know that a therapeutic effect may not occur until they have taken the medication for 3 weeks. Antiseizure medications such as phenytoin (Dilantin) or carbamazepine (Tegretol) also are used in doses lower than those prescribed for seizure disorders. Because a variety of medications can be tried, nurses should be familiar with the possible side effects and should teach patients and families how to recognize these effects.

# Routes of Administration

The route selected for administration of an analgesic agent (Table 13-4) depends on the condition of the individual patient and the desired effect of the medication. Analgesic agents can be administered by parenteral, oral, rectal, transdermal, transmucosal, intraspinal, or epidural routes. Each method of administration has advantages and disadvantages. The route chosen should be based on patient need.

## Parenteral Route

Parenteral administration (intramuscular, IV, or subcutaneous) of the analgesic medication produces effects more rapidly than oral administration does, but these effects are of shorter duration. Parenteral administration may be indicated if the patient is not permitted oral intake or is vomiting.

**TABLE 13-4 Administration Routes for Analgesics**

| Route | Site |
|---|---|
| Parenteral | Intramuscular (IM) |
| | Intravenous (IV) |
| | Subcutaneous (SC) |
| Gastrointestinal | Oral (PO) |
| | Rectal (PR) |
| Transdermal | Skin |
| Transmucosal | Oral mucosa |
| | Intranasal mucosa |
| | Bronchial mucosa |
| Topical | Skin or mucosa |
| Epidural | Epidural space |
| Intraspinal | Spinal canal |

Medication administered by the intramuscular route enters the bloodstream more slowly than medication given IV and is metabolized slowly. The rate of absorption may be erratic; it depends on the site selected and the amount of body fat.

The IV route is an alternative to intramuscular injection for many but not all analgesic medications. The IV route is the preferred parenteral route in most acute care situations because it is much more comfortable for patients. In addition, peak serum levels and pain relief occur more rapidly and more reliably. Because the action of the opioid peaks rapidly (usually within minutes) and it is metabolized quickly, an appropriate IV dose is smaller and is prescribed at shorter intervals than an intramuscular dose.

Intravenous opioids may be administered by intravenous push or slow push (eg, over a 5- to 10-minute period) or by continuous infusion with a pump. Continuous infusion provides a steady level of analgesia and is indicated when pain occurs over a 24-hour period, such as after surgery for the first day or so, or in a patient with prolonged cancer pain who cannot take medication by other routes. The dose of analgesic agent is calculated carefully to relieve pain without producing respiratory depression and other side effects.

The subcutaneous route for infusion of opioid analgesic agents is used for patients with severe pain such as cancer pain. In addition, it is particularly useful for patients with limited intravenous access who cannot take oral medications and for patients who are managing their pain at home. The subcutaneous route is often an effective and convenient way to manage pain, but the dose of opioid that can be infused through this route is limited because of the small volume that can be administered at one time into the subcutaneous tissue.

### Oral Route

Oral administration is preferred over parenteral administration if the patient can take medication by mouth, because it is easy, noninvasive, and not painful. Severe pain can be relieved with oral opioids if the doses are high enough (see Table 13-3). In terminally ill patients with prolonged pain, doses may gradually be increased as the disease progresses and causes more pain or as the patient builds up a tolerance to the medication. If these higher doses are increased gradually, they usually provide additional pain relief without producing respiratory depression or sedation. If the route of administration is changed from a parenteral route to the oral route at a dose that is not equivalent in strength (equianalgesic), the smaller oral dose may result in a withdrawal reaction and recurrence of pain.

### Rectal Route

The rectal route may be indicated in patients who cannot take medications by any other route. The rectal route may also be indicated for patients with bleeding problems, such as hemophilia. The onset of action of opioids administered rectally is unclear but is delayed compared with other routes of administration. Similarly, the duration of action is prolonged.

### Transdermal Route

The transdermal route is used to achieve a consistent opioid serum level through absorption of the medication via the skin. It is most often used in cancer patients at home or in hospice care who take oral sustained-release morphine. The only commercially available transdermal opioids are fentanyl (Duragesic) and buprenorphine (Buprenex), which are marketed as patches consisting of a reservoir containing the medication and a porous membrane.

Fentanyl was the first commercially available transdermal opioid (Chart 13-8). When the fentanyl transdermal system is first applied to the skin, fentanyl, which is fat-soluble, binds to the skin and fat layers. Then it is slowly and systemically absorbed. Therefore, there is a delay in effect while the dermal layer is being saturated. A drug reservoir actually forms in the upper layer of skin. This results in a slowly rising serum level and a slow tapering of the serum level once the patch is removed (see Fig. 13-8). Because it takes 12 to 24 hours for the fentanyl levels to gradually increase from the first patch, the last dose of sustained-release morphine should be administered at the same time the first patch is applied (D'Arcy, 2005a, 2005b; Pasero, 2005). Transdermal fentanyl is associated with slightly less constipation than oral opioids are. Absorption is increased in febrile patients. A heating pad should never be applied to the area where the patch is applied. Transdermal fentanyl is much more expensive than sustained-release morphine, but it is less costly than methods that deliver parenteral opioids.

Buprenorphine, the second transdermal system to be approved, is available in three strengths. It has many of the same advantages as fentanyl and has been shown in limited clinical studies to be associated with a high level of patient adherence and improved quality of life (Bohme, 2002).

---

**CHART 13-8**

### Safe Use of Transdermal Fentanyl

The U.S. Food and Drug Administration issued a public health advisory in 2005 about the use of fentanyl skin patches and warned patients and health care providers about the need for the patches to be used as intended. The advisory also included precautions about safe storage and disposal of fentanyl skin patches:

- Fentanyl skin patches are very strong opioids and should always be prescribed at the lowest dose needed for pain relief. They should be used only for patients with chronic pain that is not well controlled with shorter-acting opioids.
- Patients should be cautioned that a sudden and possibly dangerous rise in the level of fentanyl in their blood can occur with use of alcohol or other medications that affect brain function; an increase in body temperature or exposure to heat; or use of other medicines that affect the metabolism of fentanyl.
- Patients should be informed about signs and symptoms of fentanyl overdose (ie, shallow or difficult breathing; fatigue, extreme sleepiness, or sedation; inability to think, talk, or walk normally; and feeling faint, dizzy, or confused).

Once it is determined that switching from other routes of morphine administration to a transdermal system is appropriate, the correct dosage or strength for the patch must be calculated. If the patient uses an opioid other than morphine, conversion to milligrams of oral morphine is the first step. After determining how many milligrams of morphine (or morphine equivalents) the patient has been using over 24 hours, an initial dose of transdermal fentanyl or buprenorphine is calculated (Skaer, 2004). Patients switched from morphine to transdermal patches of either fentanyl or buprenorphine should be assessed not only for pain and potential side effects but also for dependence, reflected by withdrawal symptoms, which may consist of shivering, a feeling of coldness, sweating, headache, and paresthesia (Gordon & Dahl, 2003). Patients may require short-acting opioids for breakthrough pain before the systemic opioid delivered through the transdermal system reaches a therapeutic level.

**NURSING ALERT**

Conversion tables available for the transdermal systems should be used only to establish the initial dose of the transdermal fentanyl or buprenorphine when patients switch from oral morphine to the transdermal route of delivery (and not vice versa). If these tables are inappropriately used to determine the dosages of oral morphine for patients who have been receiving transdermal fentanyl or buprenorphine, many patients will not achieve satisfactory analgesia and will require an increase in their opioid dose to treat breakthrough pain.

**NURSING ALERT**

If the conversion table or equation is used incorrectly to calculate a morphine dose, there is a risk of overdose. If a patient requires a change from transdermal fentanyl or buprenorphine back to oral or intravenous morphine (as in the case of surgery), the patch should be removed and intravenous morphine administered on an as-needed basis. Before a new patch is applied, the patient should be carefully checked for any older, forgotten patches, which should be removed and discarded. Patches should be replaced every 72 hours.

## Transmucosal Route

People with cancer pain who are being cared for at home may be receiving continuous opioids using sustained-release morphine, hydromorphone, oxycodone, transdermal fentanyl or buprenorphine, or other medications. These patients often experience short episodes of severe pain (eg, after coughing or moving), or they may experience sudden increases in their baseline pain resulting from a change in their condition. These periods, called breakthrough pain, can be well managed with an oral dose of a short-acting transmucosal opioid that has a rapid onset of action. Available transmucosal opioids are fentanyl, buprenorphine, sufentanil, and methadone.

Currently, butorphanol (Stadol) and fentanyl (Duragesic, Sublimaze), sufentanil (Sufenta), and morphine are the only approved transmucosal opioid analgesic agents commercially available in the form of nasal sprays. Butorphanol is a complex medication that simultaneously acts to induce or promote (**agonist**) and inhibit or reverse (**antagonist**) opioid effects. It works like an opioid agonist and an opioid antagonist at the same time. Butorphanol in any form cannot be combined with other opioids (eg, for cancer breakthrough pain), because the antagonist component blocks the action of the opioids the patient is already receiving. The principal use of this agent is for brief, moderate to severe pain, such as migraine headaches.

Intranasal morphine is useful in cancer-related breakthrough pain. When it is given in this form, analgesia is achieved within 5 to 10 minutes, resulting in significant decreases in pain intensity and high patient satisfaction (Fitzgibbon, Morgan, Docketer, et al., 2003).

## Intraspinal and Epidural Routes

Infusion of opioids or local anesthetic agents into the subarachnoid space (intrathecal space or spinal canal) or epidural space has been used for effective control of pain in postoperative patients and those with chronic pain unrelieved by other methods. A catheter is inserted into the subarachnoid or the epidural space at the thoracic or lumbar level for administration of opioid or anesthetic agents (Fig. 13-9). With intrathecal administration, medication infuses directly into the subarachnoid space and cerebrospinal fluid, which surrounds the spinal cord. With epidural administration, medication is deposited in the dura of the spinal canal and diffuses into the subarachnoid space. It is believed that pain relief from intraspinal administration of opioids is based on the existence of opioid receptors in the spinal cord.

Infusion of opioids and local anesthetic agents through an intrathecal or epidural catheter results in pain relief with fewer side effects, including sedation, than with systemic analgesia. Adverse effects associated with intraspinal administration include spinal headache resulting from loss of spinal fluid when the dura is punctured. This is more likely to occur in younger patients (less than 40 years of age). The dura must be punctured with the intrathecal route, and dural puncture may occur inadvertently with the epidural route. If dural puncture inadvertently occurs, spinal fluid seeps out of the spinal canal. The resultant headache is likely to be more severe with an epidural needle because it is larger than a spinal needle, and therefore more spinal fluid escapes.

Respiratory depression generally peaks 6 to 12 hours after epidural opioids are administered, but it can occur earlier or up to 24 hours after the first injection. Depending on the lipophilicity (affinity for body fat) of the opioid injected, the time frame for respiratory depression can be short or long. Morphine is hydrophilic, and the time for

**FIGURE 13-9.** Placement of intraspinal catheters for administration of analgesic medications: (**A**) intrathecal route, (**B**) epidural route.

peak effect is longer than that of fentanyl, which is lipophilic. The patient should be monitored closely for at least 24 hours after the first injection and longer if changes in respiratory status or level of consciousness occur. Opioid antagonist agents such as naloxone must be available for IV use if respiratory depression occurs.

The patient is also observed for urinary retention, pruritus, nausea, vomiting, and dizziness. Precautions must be taken to avoid infection at the catheter site and catheter displacement. Only medications without preservatives should be administered into the subarachnoid or epidural space because of the potential neurotoxic effects of preservatives.

During surgery, intrathecal opioids are used almost exclusively after a spinal anesthetic agent is administered. For patients undergoing large abdominal surgical procedures, especially those at risk for postoperative complications, a combination of a general inhaled anesthetic agent administered before surgery and a local epidural anesthetic agent and epidural opioids administered after surgery results in excellent pain control with fewer postoperative complications.

For patients who have persistent, severe pain that fails to respond to other treatments, or who obtain pain relief only with the risk of serious side effects, medication administered by a long-term intrathecal or epidural catheter may be effective. After the physician tunnels the catheter through the subcutaneous tissue and places the inlet (or port) under the skin, the medication is injected through the skin into the inlet and catheter, which delivers the medication directly into the epidural space. It may be necessary to inject the medication several times a day to maintain an adequate level of pain relief.

For patients who require more frequent doses or continuous infusions of opioid analgesic agents to relieve pain, an implantable infusion device or pump may be used to administer the medication continuously. The medication is administered at a small, constant dose at a preset rate into the epidural or subarachnoid space. The reservoir of the infusion device stores the medication for slow release and needs to be refilled every 1 or 2 months, depending on the patient's needs. This eliminates the need for repeated injections through the skin.

A new delivery method of epidural morphine has been developed that provides effective analgesia for patients who have undergone major surgical procedures. A single-dose extended-release epidural morphine (Depodur) is administered into the epidural space at the lumbar level immediately prior to surgery. The morphine is released slowly from microvesicular liposomes. One dose of 5 to 15 mg is absorbed around the epidural space and systemically. Depodur has been shown to provide up to 48 hours of postoperative analgesia. Although supplemental analgesic agents may be needed, patients who have received Depodur tend to report less intense pain and greater satisfaction with pain relief (Gambling, Hughes, Martin, et al., 2005). Side effects are similar to those of other epidural opioids (ie, nausea, vomiting, pruritus, and hypotension); its use is contraindicated in patients with allergy to morphine, respiratory depression, severe asthma or upper airway obstruction, and circulatory shock.

> **NURSING ALERT**
>
> Epidural catheters inserted for pain control are usually managed by nurses. Baseline information necessary to provide safe and effective pain control includes the level or site of catheter insertion, the medications (eg, local anesthetic agents, opioids) that have been administered, and the medications anticipated in the future. The infusion rate is increased with caution when anesthetic agents are combined with opioids. Sensory deficits can occur, and patients must be assessed frequently. An infusion with a lower concentration of anesthetic agent allows for administration of a greater concentration of opioid with a lower risk of sensory deficits.

### NURSING MANAGEMENT OF SIDE EFFECTS

Headache resulting from spinal fluid loss may be delayed. Therefore, the nurse needs to assess regularly for headache after either type of catheter is placed. If headache develops, the patient should remain flat in bed and should be given large amounts of fluids (provided the medical condition allows), and the physician should be notified. An epidural blood patch may be performed to reduce leakage of spinal fluid.

Cardiovascular effects (hypotension and decreased heart rate) may result from relaxation of the vasculature in the lower extremities. Therefore, the nurse should assess frequently for decreases in blood pressure, pulse rate, and urine output.

Urinary retention and pruritus may develop, and the physician may prescribe small doses of naloxone to combat these effects. The nurse administers these doses in continuous IV infusions that are small enough to reverse the side effects of the opioids without reversing the analgesic effects. Diphenhydramine (Benadryl) may also be used to relieve opioid-related pruritus.

**PROMOTING HOME AND COMMUNITY-BASED CARE**
Patients who receive epidural analgesic agents at home and their families must be taught how to administer the prescribed medication using sterile technique and how to assess for infection. Patients and families also need to learn how to recognize side effects and what to do about them. Respiratory depression is uncommon, but urinary retention may be a problem, and patients and families must be prepared to deal with it if it occurs. Implanted analgesic delivery systems can be safely and confidently used at home only if health care personnel are available for consultation and, possibly, intervention on short notice.

## Nonpharmacologic Interventions

Analgesic medication is the most powerful tool for pain relief that is available, but it is not the only one. Nonpharmacologic nursing activities can assist in pain relief, usually with low risk to the patient. Although such measures are not a substitute for medication, they may be all that is necessary or appropriate to relieve episodes of pain lasting only seconds or minutes. In instances of severe pain that lasts for hours or days, combining nonpharmacologic interventions with medications may be the most effective way to relieve pain. Several of these interventions are used, but the evidence base for many of them is sparse (Rakel & Barr, 2003); further studies of their effectiveness are needed.

### Cutaneous Stimulation and Massage

The gate control theory of pain proposes that stimulation of fibers that transmit nonpainful sensations can block or decrease the transmission of pain impulses. Several nonpharmacologic pain relief strategies, including rubbing the skin and using heat and cold, are based on this theory.

Massage, which is generalized cutaneous stimulation of the body, often concentrates on the back and shoulders. A massage does not specifically stimulate the nonpain receptors in the same receptor field as the pain receptors, but it may have an impact through the descending control system (see previous discussion). Massage also promotes comfort because it produces muscle relaxation (Rakel & Barr, 2003).

### Thermal Therapies

Ice and heat therapies may be effective pain relief strategies in some circumstances; however, their effectiveness and mechanisms of action need further study. Proponents believe that ice and heat stimulate the nonpain receptors in the same receptor field as the injury.

For greatest effect, ice should be placed on the injury site immediately after injury or surgery. Ice therapy after joint surgery can significantly reduce the amount of analgesic medication required. Ice therapy may also relieve pain if applied later. Care must be taken to assess the skin before treatment and to protect the skin from direct application of the ice. Ice should be applied to an area for no longer than 15 to 20 minutes at a time and should be avoided in patients with compromised circulation (Porth, 2005). Long applications of ice may result in frostbite or nerve injury.

Application of heat increases blood flow to an area and contributes to pain reduction by speeding healing. Both dry and moist heat may provide some analgesia, but their mechanisms of action are not well understood.

Both ice and heat therapy must be applied carefully and monitored closely to avoid injuring the skin. Neither therapy should be applied to areas with impaired circulation or used in patients with impaired sensation.

**NURSING ALERT**

Heat should not be applied to a painful area that is the site of acute untreated infection (eg, mastitis, tooth abscess), because it may cause increased pain with increased blood flow to the site.

### Transcutaneous Electrical Nerve Stimulation

Transcutaneous electrical nerve stimulation (TENS) uses a battery-operated unit with electrodes applied to the skin to produce a tingling, vibrating, or buzzing sensation in the area of pain. It has been used in both acute and chronic pain relief and is thought to decrease pain by stimulating the nonpain receptors in the same area as the fibers that transmit the pain. This mechanism is consistent with the gate control theory of pain and explains the effectiveness of cutaneous stimulation when applied in the same area as an injury. For example, when TENS is used in a postoperative patient, the electrodes are placed around the surgical wound. Other possible explanations for the effectiveness of TENS are the placebo effect (the patient expects it to be effective) (Porth, 2005) and release of endorphins and enkephalins (Rakel & Barr, 2003).

### Distraction

Distraction helps relieve both acute and chronic pain (Porth, 2005). Distraction, which involves focusing the patient's attention on something other than the pain, may be the mechanism responsible for other effective cognitive techniques. Distraction is thought to reduce the perception of pain by stimulating the descending control system, resulting in fewer painful stimuli being transmitted to the brain. The effectiveness of distraction depends on the patient's ability to receive and create sensory input other than pain. Distraction techniques may range from simple activities, such as watching TV or listening to music, to highly complex physical and mental exercises. Pain relief generally increases in direct proportion to the patient's active participation, the number of sensory modalities used, and interest in the stimuli. Therefore, the stimulation of sight, sound, and touch is likely to be more effective in reducing pain than is the stimulation of a single sense.

Visits from family and friends are effective in relieving pain. Watching an action-packed movie on a large screen with "Surround Sound" through headphones may be effective (provided the patient finds it acceptable). Others may benefit from games and activities (eg, chess, crossword puzzles) that require concentration. Not all patients obtain pain relief with distraction, especially those in severe pain. Severe pain may prevent patients from concentrating well enough to participate in complex physical or mental activities.

### Relaxation Techniques

Skeletal muscle relaxation is believed to reduce pain by relaxing tense muscles that contribute to the pain. Recent research findings support the use of relaxation in relieving postoperative pain. In a study of pain in patients who had undergone abdominal surgery, Roykulcharoen and Good (2004) reported that fewer participants who used relaxation techniques requested opioids compared with those in the control group. Almost all participants in the relaxation group reported a decrease in pain and an increase in sense of control.

A simple relaxation technique consists of abdominal breathing at a slow, rhythmic rate. The patient may close both eyes and breathe slowly and comfortably. A constant rhythm can be maintained by counting silently and slowly with each inhalation ("in, two, three") and exhalation ("out, two, three"). When teaching this technique, the nurse may count out loud with the patient at first. Slow, rhythmic breathing may also be used as a distraction technique. Relaxation techniques, as well as other noninvasive pain relief measures, may require practice before the patient becomes skilled in using them. Patients who already know a relaxation technique may need to be reminded to use it to reduce or prevent increased pain.

Almost all people with persistent pain can benefit from some method of relaxation. Regular relaxation periods may help combat the fatigue and muscle tension that occur with and increase chronic pain.

### Guided Imagery

Guided imagery is using one's imagination in a special way to achieve a specific positive effect. Guided imagery for relaxation and pain relief may consist of combining slow, rhythmic breathing with a mental image of relaxation and comfort (Antall & Kresevic, 2004). The nurse instructs the patient to close his or her eyes and breathe slowly in and out. With each slowly exhaled breath, the patient imagines muscle tension and discomfort being breathed out, carrying away pain and tension and leaving behind a relaxed and comfortable body. With each inhaled breath, the patient imagines healing energy flowing to the area of discomfort.

If guided imagery is to be effective, it requires a considerable amount of time to explain the technique and time for the patient to practice it. Usually, the patient is asked to practice guided imagery for about 5 minutes, three times a day. Several days of practice may be needed before the intensity of pain is reduced. Many patients begin to experience the relaxing effects of guided imagery the first time they try it. Pain relief can continue for hours after the imagery is used. Patients should be informed that guided imagery may work only for some people. Guided imagery should be used only in combination with all other forms of treatment that have demonstrated effectiveness.

### Hypnosis

Hypnosis, which has been effective in relieving pain or decreasing the amount of analgesic agents required in patients with acute and chronic pain, may promote pain relief in particularly difficult situations (eg, burns). The mechanism by which hypnosis acts is unclear. Its effectiveness depends on the hypnotic susceptibility of the individual (DePascalis, Bellusci, Gallo, et al., 2004). In some cases, hypnosis may be effective in the first session, with effectiveness increasing in additional sessions. In other cases, hypnosis does not work at all. Usually, hypnosis must be induced by specially skilled people (a psychologist or a nurse with specialized training in hypnosis). Some patients may learn to perform self-hypnosis.

### Music Therapy

Music therapy is an inexpensive and effective therapy for the reduction of pain and anxiety. Research has shown that it significantly decreases pain as measured by the short-form McGill questionnaire and VAS in elderly patients with chronic osteoarthritis (McCaffery & Freeman, 2003). The investigators compared the pain of patients who sat quietly for 20 minutes a day for 2 weeks (standard care) to that of similar patients who listened to music 20 minutes daily for the same period. Pain from osteoarthritis was consistently significantly lower in the group who listened to music. Another group of researchers (Nilsson, Rawal & Unosson, 2003) compared two groups of patients undergoing inguinal hernia repair or varicose vein surgery; one group listened to music intraoperatively or postoperatively, and the control group listened to "white" noise. Patients exposed to music reported significantly lower pain intensity at 1 and 2 hours after surgery.

### Alternative Therapies

People suffering chronic, debilitating pain are often desperate. Often they will try anything, recommended by anyone, at any price. Information about an array of potential therapies can be found on the Internet and in the self-help section of many bookstores. Therapies specifically recommended for pain from these sources include, but are not limited to, chelation, therapeutic touch, herbal therapy, reflexology, magnetic therapy, electrotherapy, polarity therapy, acupressure, emu oil, pectin therapy, aromatherapy, homeopathy, and macrobiotic dieting. Many of these "therapies" (with the exception of macrobiotic dieting) are probably not harmful. However, they have yet to be proved effective by the standards used to evaluate the effectiveness of medical and nursing interventions. The National Institutes of Health has established an office to examine the effectiveness of complementary and alternative therapies.

Despite the lack of scientific evidence that these alternative therapies are effective, patients may find any one of them helpful via the placebo response. Problems arise when patients do not find relief but are deprived of conventional therapy because the alternative therapy "should be helping," or when patients abandon conventional therapy for alternative therapy. In addition, few alternative therapies are free. Desperate patients may risk financial ruin seeking alternative therapies that are ineffective.

It is important when caring for patients who are using or considering using untested therapies (often referred to as alternative therapies) not to diminish the patient's hope and the potential placebo response. This must be weighed against the nurse's responsibility to protect the patient from costly and potentially harmful and dangerous therapies that the patient is not in a position to evaluate scientifically.

Nurses should help patients and families understand scientific research and how it differs from anecdotal evidence. Without diminishing the placebo effects that may occur, the nurse encourages the patient to assess the effectiveness of the therapy, continually using standard pain assessment techniques. In addition, the nurse encourages the patient to combine alternative therapies with conventional therapies and to discuss this with their physicians.

# Neurologic and Neurosurgical Approaches to Pain Management

In some situations, especially with long-term and severe intractable pain, usual pharmacologic and nonpharmacologic methods of pain relief are ineffective. In those situations, neurologic and neurosurgical approaches to pain management may be considered. Intractable pain refers to pain that cannot be relieved satisfactorily by the usual approaches, including medications. Such pain often is the result of malignancy (especially of the cervix, bladder, prostate, and lower bowel), but it may occur in other conditions, such as postherpetic neuralgia, trigeminal neuralgia, spinal cord arachnoiditis, and uncontrollable ischemia and other forms of tissue destruction.

Neurologic and neurosurgical methods available for pain relief include (1) stimulation procedures (intermittent electrical stimulation of a tract or center to inhibit the transmission of pain impulses), (2) administration of intraspinal opioids (see previous discussion), and (3) interruption of the tracts conducting the pain impulse from the periphery to cerebral integration centers. Stimulation of nerves with minute amounts of electricity is used if other pharmacologic and nonpharmacologic treatments fail to provide adequate relief. These treatments are reversible. If they need to be discontinued, the nervous system continues to function. However, methods that involve interruption of the tracts are destructive or ablative procedures. They are used only after other methods of pain relief have failed, because their effects are permanent.

## Stimulation Procedures

Electrical stimulation, or neuromodulation, is a method of suppressing pain by applying controlled low-voltage electrical pulses to the different parts of the nervous system. Electrical stimulation is thought to relieve pain by blocking painful stimuli (the gate control theory). This pain-modulating technique is administered by many modes. TENS (discussed earlier) and dorsal spinal cord stimulation are the most common types of electrical stimulation used. There are also brain-stimulating techniques, in which electrodes are implanted in the periventricular area of the posterior third ventricle, allowing the patient to stimulate this area to produce analgesia.

Spinal cord stimulation is a technique used for the relief of persistent, intractable pain, ischemic pain, and pain from angina. A surgically implanted device allows the patient to apply pulsed electrical stimulation to the dorsal aspect of the spinal cord to block pain impulses (Linderoth & Meyerson, 2002). (The largest accumulation of afferent fibers is found in the dorsal column of the spinal cord.) The dorsal column stimulation unit consists of a radiofrequency stimulation transmitter, a transmitter antenna, a radiofrequency receiver, and a stimulation electrode. The battery-powered transmitter and antenna are worn externally; the receiver and electrode are implanted. A laminectomy is performed above the highest level of pain input, and the electrode is placed in the epidural space over the posterior column of the spinal cord. (The placement of the stimulating systems varies.) A subcutaneous pocket is created over the clavicular area or at some other site for placement of the receiver. The two are connected through a subcutaneous tunnel. Careful patient selection is necessary, and not all patients receive total pain relief.

Deep brain stimulation is performed for special pain problems if there is no response to the usual techniques of pain control. Under local anesthesia, electrodes are introduced through a burr hole in the skull and inserted into a selected site in the brain, depending on the location or type of pain. After the effectiveness of stimulation is confirmed, the implanted electrode is connected to a radiofrequency device or pulse-generator system operated by external telemetry. It is used for patients with neuropathic pain that may be caused by damage or injury from a stroke, brain or spinal cord injuries, or phantom limb pain. Use of deep brain stimulation is effective for chronic cluster headaches (Ekbom & Waldenlind, 2004; Leone, 2004).

### Interruption of Pain Pathways

Pain-conducting fibers can be interrupted at any point from their origin to the cerebral cortex. Some part of the nervous system is destroyed, resulting in varying amounts of neurologic deficit and incapacity. In time, pain usually returns as a result of either regeneration of axonal fibers or the development of alternative pain pathways. Destructive procedures used to interrupt the transmission of pain include cordotomy and rhizotomy. These procedures are offered if it is thought that the patient is near the end of life and the procedure will result in an improved quality of life (Linderoth & Meyerson, 2002). Often these procedures can provide pain relief for the duration of the patient's life. The use of other methods to interrupt pain transmission is decreasing, because intraspinal therapies and newer pain management treatments are available.

## CORDOTOMY

Cordotomy is the division of certain tracts of the spinal cord (Fig. 13-10). It may be performed percutaneously, by the open method after laminectomy, or by other techniques. Cordotomy is performed to interrupt the transmission of pain (Hodge & Christensen, 2002). Care must be taken to destroy only the sensation of pain, leaving motor functions intact.

## RHIZOTOMY

Sensory nerve roots are destroyed where they enter the spinal cord. A lesion is made in the dorsal root to destroy neuronal dysfunction and reduce nociceptive input. With the advent of microsurgical techniques, the complications are few, with mild sensory deficits and mild weakness (Fig. 13-11).

### Nursing Interventions

With each of these procedures, the patient is provided with written and verbal instructions about the intervention's expected effect on pain and on possible untoward consequences. The patient is monitored for specific effects of each method of pain intervention, both positive and negative. The specific nursing care of patients who undergo neurologic and neurosurgical procedures for the relief of chronic pain depends on the type of procedure performed, its effectiveness in relieving the pain, and the changes in neurologic function that accompany the procedure. After the procedure, the patient's pain level and neurologic function are assessed. Other nursing interventions that may be indicated include positioning, turning

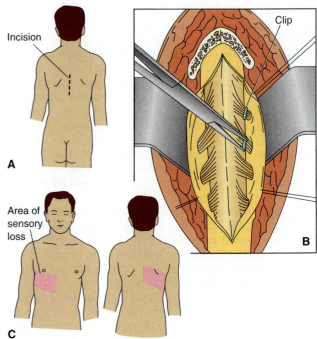

**FIGURE 13-11.** A rhizotomy may be performed surgically, percutaneously, or chemically, depending on a patient's condition and needs. The procedure is usually performed to relieve severe chest pain, for example, from lung cancer. In a surgical rhizotomy (**A**), the spinal roots (**B**) are divided and banded with a clip to form a lesion and produce subsequent loss of sensation (**C**). Adapted with permission from Loeser, J. D. (Ed.) (2000). *Bonica's management of pain* (3rd ed.). Philadelphia: Lippincott Williams & Wilkins.

and skin care, bowel and bladder management, and interventions to promote patient safety. Pain management remains an important aspect of nursing care with each of these procedures.

# Promoting Home and Community-Based Care

In preparing the patient and family to manage pain at home, the patient and family should be taught and guided about what type of pain or discomfort to expect, how long the pain is expected to last, and when the pain indicates a problem that should be reported. People who have experienced pain as a result of injury, illness, a medical procedure, or surgery will probably receive one or more prescriptions for analgesic medication for use at home.

## Teaching Patients Self-Care

The patient and family must understand the purpose of each medication, the appropriate time to use it, the associated side effects, and the strategies that can be used to prevent these problems. The patient and family often need reassurance that pain can be successfully managed at home.

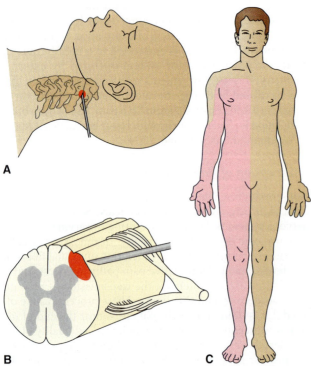

**FIGURE 13-10.** (**A**) Site of percutaneous C1–C2 cordotomy. (**B**) Lesion produced by percutaneous C1–C2 cordotomy. (**C**) Extent of analgesia produced by left C1–C2 percutaneous cordotomy.

Inadequate control of pain at home is a common reason people seek health care or are readmitted to the hospital. When persistent pain exists, anxiety and fear are often intensified at the time the patient is about to return home. The patient and family are instructed about the techniques for assessing pain, using pain assessment tools, and administering medications to relieve pain. These instructions are given verbally and in writing (Chart 13-9).

Opportunities are provided for the patient and family members to practice administering the medication until they are comfortable and confident with the procedure. They are instructed about the risks of respiratory and CNS depression associated with opioids and ways to assess for these complications. If the medications cause other predictable effects, such as constipation, the instructions include measures for preventing and treating the problem, as previously described. Steps are taken to ensure that the needed medications are available from the local pharmacy so that the patient receives the medication when required.

Education for patients and families must stress the need for keeping analgesic agents away from children, who might mistake them for candy. Elderly patients may become lax about this because no children live in the home, but visiting children can be placed at risk. Analgesic agents must also be kept away from other family members who

---

**CHART 13-9**

### Patient Education

**At-Home Pain Management Plan**

**Pain control plan for**
_____

**At home, I will take the following medicines for pain control:**

| Medicine | How to take | How many | How often | Comments |
|---|---|---|---|---|
| _____ | _____ | _____ | _____ | _____ |
| _____ | _____ | _____ | _____ | _____ |
| _____ | _____ | _____ | _____ | _____ |

**Medicines that I may take to help treat side effects:**

| Side effect | Medicine | How to take | How many | How often | Comments |
|---|---|---|---|---|---|
| _____ | _____ | _____ | _____ | _____ | _____ |
| _____ | _____ | _____ | _____ | _____ | _____ |

**Constipation is a very common problem when taking opioid medications. When this occurs, do the following:**
- Increase fluid intake (8 to 10 glasses of fluid).
- Exercise regularly.
- Increase fiber in the diet (bran, fresh fruits, vegetables).
- Use a mild laxative, such as milk of magnesia, if no bowel movement in 3 days.
- Take _____ every day at _____ (time) with a full glass of water.
- Use a glycerin suppository every morning (this may help make a bowel movement less painful).

**Nondrug pain control methods:**
_____
_____

**Additional instructions:**
_____
_____
_____

**Important phone numbers:**
Your doctor _____  Your nurse _____
Your pharmacy _____  Emergencies _____
Call your doctor or nurse immediately if your pain increases or if you have a new pain. Also call your doctor early for refill of pain medicines. Do not let your medicines get below 3 or 4 days' supply.

From Agency for Health Care Policy and Research. (1994). Management of cancer pain. Clinical Practice Guidelines. Rockville, MD: Agency for Health Care Policy and Research, Public Health Service, U.S. Department of Health and Human Services.

**CHART 13-10**

## Plan of Nursing Care: Care of the Patient With Pain

**Nursing Diagnosis:** Pain
**Goal:** Relief of pain or decrease in intensity of pain

| NURSING INTERVENTIONS | RATIONALE | EXPECTED OUTCOMES |
|---|---|---|
| 1. Reassure patient that you know pain is real and will assist him or her in dealing with it. | 1. Fear that pain will not be accepted as real increases tension and anxiety and decreases pain tolerance. | • Reports relief that pain is accepted as real and that he or she will receive assistance in pain relief |
| 2. Use pain assessment scale to identify intensity of pain. | 2. Provides baseline for assessing changes in pain level and evaluating interventions | • Reports lower intensity of pain and discomfort after interventions implemented |
| 3. Assess and record pain and its characteristics: location, quality, frequency, and duration. | 3. Data assist in evaluating pain and pain relief and identifying multiple sources and types of pain. | • Reports less disruption from pain and discomfort after use of intervention |
| 4. Administer balanced analgesics as prescribed to promote optimal pain relief. | 4. Analgesics are more effective if administered early in pain cycle. Simultaneous use of analgesics that work on different portions of the nociceptive system will provide greater pain relief with fewer side effects. | • Uses pain medication as prescribed<br>• Identifies effective pain relief strategies<br>• Demonstrates use of new strategies to relieve pain and reports their effectiveness |
| 5. Readminister pain assessment scale. | 5. Permits assessment of effectiveness of analgesia and identifies need for further action if ineffective | • Experiences minimal side effects of analgesia without interruption to treat side effects<br>• Increases interactions with family and friends |
| 6. Document severity of patient's pain on chart. | 6. Assists in demonstrating need for additional analgesic or alternative approach to pain management | |
| 7. Obtain additional prescriptions as needed. | 7. Inadequate pain relief results in an increased stress response, suffering, and prolonged hospitalizations. | |
| 8. Identify and encourage patient to use strategies that have been successful with previous pain. | 8. Encourages use of pain relief strategies familiar to and accepted by patient | |
| 9. Teach patient additional strategies to relieve pain and discomfort: distraction, relaxation, cutaneous stimulation, etc. | 9. Use of these strategies along with analgesia may produce more effective pain relief. | |
| 10. Instruct patient and family about potential side effects of analgesics and their prevention and management. | 10. Anticipating and preventing side effects enable the patient to continue analgesia without interruption because of side effects. | |

## CHART 13-11

### Expected Patient Outcomes for the Patient With Pain

**Relief of pain,** evidenced when the patient
- Rates pain at a lower intensity (on a scale of 0 to 10) after intervention
- Rates pain at a lower intensity for longer periods

**Correct administration of prescribed analgesic medications,** evidenced when the patient or family
- States correct dose of medication
- Administers correct dose using correct procedure
- Identifies side effects of medication
- Describes actions taken to prevent or correct side effects

**Use of nonpharmacologic pain strategies as recommended,** evidenced when the patient:
- Reports practice of nonpharmacologic strategies
- Describes expected outcomes of nonpharmacologic strategies

**Minimal effects of pain and minimal side effects of interventions,** evidenced when the patient:
- Participates in activities important to recovery (eg, drinking fluids, coughing, ambulating)
- Participates in activities important to self and to family (eg, family activities, interpersonal relationships, parenting, social interaction, recreation, work)
- Reports adequate sleep and absence of fatigue and constipation

---

may take them inadvertently. In addition, analgesic medications should be stored safely in their original containers and clearly labeled. They should be stored out of sight to prevent others from taking them for their own use or diverting them to others.

## Continuing Care

If a patient is to receive parenteral or intraspinal analgesia at home, he or she should be referred to a home care nurse. This nurse will make a home visit to assess the patient, and to determine whether the pain management program is being implemented and the technique for injecting or infusing the analgesic agent is being carried out safely and effectively. If the patient has an implanted infusion pump in place, the nurse examines the condition of the pump or injection site and may refill the reservoir with medication as prescribed or may supervise family members in this procedure. The nurse assesses for any change in the patient's need for analgesic medications, and, in collaboration with the physician, the nurse may assist the patient and family in modifying the medication dose. These efforts enable the patient to obtain adequate pain relief while remaining at home and with family.

As tolerance develops with chronic pain or cancer pain, ever-increasing amounts of opioids are needed. It is important to reassure the patient and family that slowly increasing doses will not increase the risk for respiratory depression and CNS depression, because the patient will become tolerant to these effects also. However, the patient will not become tolerant to the constipating effects of opioids, and increased efforts to prevent constipation will be necessary.

## Evaluating Pain Management Strategies

An important aspect of caring for patients in pain is reassessing the pain after the intervention has been implemented. The measure's effectiveness is based on the patient's assessment of pain, as reflected in pain assessment tools. If the intervention was ineffective, the nurse should consider other measures. If these are ineffective, pain relief goals need to be reassessed in collaboration with the physician. The nurse serves as the patient's advocate in obtaining additional pain relief.

After interventions have had a chance to work, the nurse asks the patient to rate the intensity of pain. The nurse repeats this assessment at appropriate intervals after the intervention and compares the result with the previous rating. These assessments indicate the effectiveness of the pain relief measures and provide a basis for continuing or modifying the plan of care. A plan of nursing care for a patient with pain is given in Chart 13-10. Expected patient outcomes are given in Chart 13-11.

## Critical Thinking Exercises

1. A 65-year-old Hispanic woman is admitted to the hospital with advanced cancer of the left breast with metastasis. She speaks little English, and three of her adult children are with her. Her health history indicates that she initially refused surgery after noticing a lump in her breast, because she believes that the breast is where the soul resides, but finally consented to a left mastectomy. After undergoing surgery, she was transferred from the postanesthesia care unit to a surgical unit. There she is moaning and appears to be writhing in pain. Ten minutes ago, she was given 8 mg of morphine sulfate intravenously. What cultural factors need to be considered in the care of this woman? Identify methods that can be used to communicate with her. How would the nurse assess the patient's pain intensity and the effectiveness of pain management strategies? What level of involvement is appropriate for the family in the assessment and management of her pain? Explain your reasoning.

2. A 27-year-old man is readmitted to a medical center because of severe pain one day after his discharge following an open reduction of his left humerus with internal fixation. He was discharged with a prescription for oxycodone (Percocet), one tablet every 4 hours as needed (total of 20 tablets). He rates his pain intensity as an 11 on a scale of 0 to 10. When the pain escalated at home, he

increased the dose and subsequently ran out of the Percocet. His physician decides to change the analgesic to long-acting morphine in an effort to relieve his pain. How would the nurse determine what prescribed dose of the long-acting morphine to administer? What concerns should the nurse have about the amount of Percocet the patient consumed? What medication should be on hand and what assessments, including laboratory tests, should be performed?

3. A 35-year-old man who is a recovering heroin addict is admitted to the hospital for an emergency appendectomy. During surgery the appendix ruptures, and the patient remains hospitalized for several days for intravenous antibiotics. He tells the nurse that he has been "clean" for the past 3 months. He complains of pain (7 on a 0-to-10 scale) and refuses to use the patient-controlled analgesia that is prescribed for him. He states, "I don't want to get hooked again." Describe how you would address pain relief in this patient, and give the rationale for your actions. How would you address his fears? Who would you consult to help with this patient's pain management?

4. A 76-year-old man with a history of angina and peripheral vascular disease collapses in the street after suffering a massive heart attack and is rushed to a major hospital center. Despite his medical history, he has continued to smoke about one pack of cigarettes a day. He is intubated and placed on a ventilator to provide adequate oxygenation. He is able to report his pain intensity by holding up the number of fingers to correspond to a 0-to-10 rating scale. At first he rates the pain as a 9, but after receiving morphine he rates the pain as a 2. Discuss how morphine works to decrease the intensity of the patient's pain. Identify other interventions, including other medications, that would contribute to decreasing his pain.

5. **ebp** A 48-year-old woman has severe chronic pain secondary to cancer due to metastasis to the bone. She is reluctant to take opioids because she wants to remain alert to enjoy being around her family. Furthermore, she is concerned about having opioids around the house because of the presence of young children in the home. Identify pharmacologic alternatives and nonpharmacologic interventions that might be appropriate. Identify the evidence base and the strength of the evidence for the use of the nonpharmacologic interventions.

## REFERENCES AND SELECTED READINGS

### BOOKS

American Cancer Society. (2001). *American Cancer Society's guide to pain control: Powerful methods to overcome cancer pain.* Atlanta: American Cancer Society.

American Pain Society. (2003). *Principles of analgesic use in the treatment of acute pain and chronic cancer pain* (5th ed.). Skokie, IL: Author.

American Society for Pain Management Nurses. (2002). *Core curriculum for pain management nursing.* Philadelphia: Saunders.

Bonica, J. J. (2000). *The management of pain* (3rd ed.). Philadelphia: Lea & Febiger.

Desmeules, J. A., Piguet, V., Ehret, G. B., et al. (2004). Pharmacogenetics, pharmacokinetics, and analgesia. In Mogil, J. S. (Ed.). *The genetics of pain* (pp. 211–237). Seattle: IASP Press.

Fillingim, R. B. (2000). *Progress in pain research and management: Vol. 17. Sex, gender, and pain.* Seattle: IASP Press.

Freeman, L. W. & Lawlis, G. F. (2001). *Mosby's complementary and alternative medicine: A research-based approach.* St. Louis: Mosby.

Harden, R. N., Baron, R. & Janig, W. (2001). *Progress in pain research and management: Vol. 22. Complex regional pain syndrome.* Seattle: IASP Press.

Hodge, C. J., & Christensen, M. (2002). Anterolateral cordotomy. In K. J. Burchiel (Ed.). *Surgical management of pain.* New York: Thieme.

Hudspith, M. & Munglani, R. (2003). Sites of analgesic action. In Bountra, C., Munglani, R. & Schmidt, W. K. (Eds.). *Pain: Current understanding, emerging therapies, and novel approaches to drug discovery.* New York: Marcel-Dekker.

Janig, W. (2001). CRPS-I and CRPS-II: A strategic view. In Harden, R. N., Baron, R., & Janig, W. (Eds.). *Progress in pain research and management: Vol. 22. Complex regional pain syndrome.* Seattle: IASP Press.

Joint Commission on Accreditation of Healthcare Organizations. (2005). *2005 Hospital accreditation standards.* Oakbrook Terrace, IL: JCAHO.

Kuhn, M. A. (1999). *Complementary therapies for health care providers.* Philadelphia: Lippincott Williams & Wilkins.

Linderoth, B. & Meyerson, B. A. (2002). Spinal cord stimulation: Mechanisms of action. In Burchiel, K. (Ed.). *Surgical management of pain.* New York: Thieme.

MacGregor, A. J. (2004). The heritability of pain in humans. In Mogil, J. S. (Ed.). *Progress in pain research and management: Vol. 28. The genetics of pain.* Seattle: IASP Press.

McCaffery, M. & Pasero, C. (1999). *Pain: Clinical manual* (2nd ed.). St. Louis: Mosby.

Merskey, H. & Bogduk, N. (1994). *Classification of Chronic Pain,* 2nd ed. International Association for the Study of Pain (IASP) Task Force on Taxonomy. Seattle, WA: IASP Press.

Mogil, J. S. (Ed.). (2004). *Progress in pain research and management: Vol. 28. The genetics of pain.* Seattle: IASP Press.

National Institutes of Health. (1995). *Integration of behavioral and relaxation approaches into the treatment of chronic pain and insomnia.* NIH Technology Assessment Statement, Oct. 16–18, 1995. http://consensus.nih.gov/1995/1995BehaviorRelaxPainInsomniata017html.htm. Accessed May 24, 2006.

Porth, C. M. (2005). *Pathophysiology: Concepts of altered health status,* 7th ed. Philadelphia: Lippincott Williams & Wilkins.

Rezai, A. R. & Lozano, A. M. (2002). Deep brain stimulation for chronic pain. In Burchiel, K. J. (Ed.). *Surgical management of pain.* New York: Thieme.

Wall, P. D. & Melzack, R. (Eds.). (1999). *Textbook of pain* (4th ed.). New York: Churchill Livingstone.

### JOURNALS

*Asterisks indicate nursing research articles.

American Geriatrics Society Panel on Persistent Pain in Older Persons. (2002). The management of persistent pain in older persons. *Journal of the American Geriatrics Society, 50*(6S), 205–224.

American Society of Pain Management Nurses. (2005). ASPMN position statement: Use of placebos in pain management. Available at: http://www.aspmn.org/html/Psplacebo.htm. Accessed June 7, 2005. http://www.aspmn.org/Organization/position_papers.htm. Accessed May 22, 2006.

Anderson, R., Saiers, J. H., Abram, S. & Schlicht, C. (2001). Accuracy in equianalgesic dosing: Conversion dilemmas. *Journal of Pain and Symptom Management, 21*(5), 397–406.

Andre, J. M., Martinet, N., Paysant, J., et al. (2001). Temporary phantom limbs evoked by vestibular caloric stimulation in amputees. *Neuropsychiatry Neuropsychology Behavioral Neurology, 14*(3), 190–196.

Antall, G. F. & Kresevic, D. (2004). The use of guided imagery to manage pain in an elderly orthopaedic population. *Orthopaedic Nursing, 23*(5), 335–340.

Arnstein, P. (2003). Comprehensive analysis and management of chronic pain. *Nursing Clinics of North America, 38*(1), 403–417.

Bair, M. J., Robinson, R. L., Katon, W., et al. (2003). Depression and pain comorbidity: A literature review. *Archives of Internal Medicine, 163*(20), 2433–2445.

Bohme, K. (2002). Buprenorphine in a transdermal therapeutic system. A new option. *Clinical Rheumatology, 21* (Suppl.), S13–S16.

Brookoff, D. (2000). Chronic pain: 1. A new disease? *Hospital Practice, 35*(7), 42–59.

California Pain Patients' Bill of Rights. Available at: www.paincare.org/pain_management/advocacy/ca_bill.html (accessed March 12, 2006).

*Call-Schmidt, T. A. & Richardson, S. J. (2003). Prevalence of sleep disturbance and its relationship to pain in adults with chronic pain. *Pain Management Nursing, 4*(3), 124–133.

Collins-Schramm, H. E., Phillips, C. M., Operario, D. J., et al. (2002). Ethnic-difference markers for use in mapping by admixture linkage disequilibrium. *American Journal of Human Genetics, 70*(3), 737–750.

Colwell, C. W. (2004). The use of the pain pump and patient-controlled analgesia in joint reconstruction. *American Journal of Orthopedics, 33*(5S), 10–12.

Compton, P., & Athanos, P. (2003). Chronic pain, substance abuse and addiction. *Nursing Clinics of North America, 38*(1), 525–537.

Correll, D. J., Viscusi, E. R., Grunwald, Z., et al. (2001). Epidural analgesia compared with intravenous morphine patient-controlled analgesia: Postoperative outcome measures after mastectomy with immediate TRAM flap breast reconstruction. *Regional Anesthesia Pain Medicine, 26*(5), 444–449.

Dalton, J. A. & Coyne, P. (2003). Cognitive-behavioral therapy: Tailored to the individual. *Nursing Clinics of North America, 38*(1), 465–476.

D'Arcy, Y. (2005a). What you need to know about fentanyl patches. *Nursing, 35*(8), 73.

D'Arcy, Y. (2005b). Patching together transdermal pain control options. *Nursing, 35*(9), 17

DePascalis, V., Bellusci, A., Gallo, C., et al. (2004). Pain reduction strategies in hypnotic context and hypnosis: ERPs and SCRs during a secondary auditory task. *International Journal of Clinical Experimental Hypnosis, 52*(4), 343–363.

*DuPen, A. R., DuPen, S., Hansberry, J., et al. (2000). An educational implementation of a cancer pain algorithm for ambulatory care. *Pain Management Nursing, 1*(4), 116–128.

*Dysvik, E., Lindstrom, T. C., Eikland, O., et al. (2004). Health-related quality of life and pain beliefs among people suffering from chronic pain. *Pain Management Nursing, 5*(2), 66–74.

Edwards, R., Augustson, E. M., & Fillingim, R. (2000). Sex-specific effects of pain related anxiety on adjustment to chronic pain. *Clinical Journal of Pain, 16*(1), 46–53.

Edwards, R. R., & Fillingim, R. B. (2000). Age-associated differences in responses to noxious stimuli. *Journal of Gerontology Series A: Biological Science and Medical Science, 56*(3), M180–M185.

Ekbom, K. & Waldenlind, E. (2004). Cluster headache: The history of the Cluster Club and a review of clinical research. *Functional Neurology, 19*(2), 73–81.

Fischer, L. M., Schlienger, R. G., Matter, C. M., et al. (2004). Discontinuation of nonsteroidal anti-inflammatory drug therapy and risk of acute myocardial infarction. *Archives of Internal Medicine, 164*(22), 2472–2476.

Fitzgibbon, D., Morgan, D. Dockter, D., et al. (2003). Initial pharmacokinetic, safety and efficacy evaluation of nasal morphine gluconate for breakthrough pain in cancer patients. *Pain, 106*(3), 309–315.

Furlan, A. D., Sandoval, J. A., Mailis-Gagnon, A. et al. (2006). Opioids for chronic noncancer pain: a meta-analysis of effectiveness and side effects. *Canadian Medical Association Journal, 174*(11), 1589–1594.

Gambling, D., Hughes, T., Martin, G., et al. (2005). A comparison of Depodur, a novel, single-dose extended-release epidural morphine, with standard epidural morphine for pain relief after lower abdominal surgery. *Anesthesia & Analgesia, 100*(4), 1065–1074.

Gammaitoni, A. R., Fine, P., Alvarez, N., et al. (2003). Clinical application of opioid equianalgesic data. *Clinical Journal of Pain, 19*(5), 286–297.

Gevirtz, C. (2003). Anesthesia-assisted opiate detoxification. *International Anesthesiology Clinic, 41*(2), 79–93.

Gilron, I., Bailey, J. M., Dongsheng, T., et al. (2005). Morphine, gabapentin, or their combination for neuropathic pain. *New England Journal of Medicine, 352*(13), 1324–1334.

Gordon, D. B. (2003). Nonopioid and adjuvant analgesics in chronic pain management: strategies for effective use. *Nursing Clinics of North America, 38*(1), 447–464.

Gordon, D. & Dahl, J. (2003) Fast facts and concepts #95: Opioid withdrawal. End-of-life/Palliative Education Resource Center. Available at: http://www.eperc.mcw.edu/fastFact/ff_95.htm (accessed March 12, 2006).

Gordon, D. B., Dahl, J., Phillips, P., et al. (2004). The use of "as-needed" range orders for opioid analgesics in the management of acute pain: A consensus statement of the American Society for Pain Management Nurses and the American Pain Society. *Pain Management Nursing, 5*(2), 53–58.

Gordon, D. B. & Ward, S. E. (1995). Correcting patient misconceptions about pain. *American Journal of Nursing, 95*(7), 43–45.

Green, C. R., Anderson, K. O., Baker, T. A., et al. (2003). The unequal burden of pain: Confronting racial and ethnic disparities in pain. *Pain Medicine, 4*(3), 277–294.

Gunnarsdottir, S., Donovan, H. & Ward, S. (2003). Interventions to overcome clinician- and patient-related barriers to pain management. *Nursing Clinics of North America, 38*(1), 419–434.

Holleran, R. S. (2002). The problem of pain in emergency care. *Nursing Clinics of North America, 37*(1), 67–78.

Hicks, C. L., von Baeyer, C. L., Spafford, P. A., et al. (2001). The Faces Pain Scale–Revised: Toward a common metric in pediatric pain measurement. *Pain, 93*(2), 173–183.

*Horgas, A. L. & Dunn, K. (2001). Pain in nursing home residents: Comparison of residents' self-report and nursing assistants' perceptions. Incongruencies exist in resident and caregiver reports of pain; therefore, pain management education is needed to prevent suffering. *Journal of Gerontological Nursing, 27*(3), 44–53.

Hrobjartsson, A. & Gotzsche, P. C. (2001). Is placebo powerless? An analysis of clinical trials comparing placebo with no treatment. *New England Journal of Medicine, 344*(21), 1594–1602.

Hrobjartsson, A. & Gotzsche, P. C. (2004). Is the placebo powerless? Update of a systematic review with 52 new randomized trials comparing placebo with no treatment. *Journal of Internal Medicine, 256*(2), 91–100.

Hunter, M., McDowell, L., Hennessy, R., et al. (2000). An evaluation of the Faces Pain Scale with young children. *Journal of Pain and Symptom Management, 20*(2), 122–129.

Jacob, E. (2001). The pain experience of patients with sickle cell anemia. *Pain Management Nursing, 2*(3), 74–83.

Karamanlioglu, B., Turan, A., Memis, D., et al. (2004). Preoperative oral rofecoxib reduces postoperative pain and tramadol consumption in patients after abdominal hysterectomy. *Anesthesia Analgesia, 98*(4), 1039–1043.

Keefe, F. J., Rumble, M. E., Scipio, C. D., et al. (2004). Psychological aspects of persistent pain: Current state of the science. *Journal of Pain, 5*(4), 195–211.

Kundermann, B., Krieg, J. C., Schreiber, W., et al. (2004). The effect of sleep deprivation on pain. *Pain Research Management, 9*(1), 25–32.

*Lasch, K., Greenhill, K., Wilkes, G., et al. (2002). Why study pain? A qualitative analysis of medical and nursing faculty and students' knowledge of and attitudes to cancer pain management. *Journal of Palliative Medicine, 5*(1), 57–71.

Leone, M. (2004). Chronic cluster headache: New and emerging treatment options. *Current Pain Headache Report, 8*(5), 347–352.

Li, S. F., Greenwald, P. W., Gennis, P., et al. (2001). Effect of age on acute pain perception of a standardized stimulus in the emergency department. *Annals of Emergency Medicine, 38*(6), 644–647.

Marcus, K. S., Kerns, R. D., Rosenfeld, B., et al. (2002). HIV/AIDS-related pain as a chronic pain condition: Implication of a biopsychosocial model for comprehensive assessment and effective management. *Pain Medicine, 1*(3), 260–273.

Mayer, D. M., Torma, L., Byock, I., et al. (2001). Speaking the language of pain. *American Journal of Nursing, 101*(2), 44–49.

McCaffery, M. (2002). What is the role of nondrug methods in the nursing care of patients with acute pain? *Pain Management Nursing, 3*(3), 77–80.

McCaffery, M. (2003). Switching from i.v. to p.o. *American Journal of Nursing, 103*(5), 62–63.

*McCaffery, M., Ferrell, B. R., & Pasero, C. (2000). Nurses' personal opinions about patients' pain and their effect on recorded assessments and titration of opioid doses. *Pain Management Nursing, 1*(3), 79–87.

*McCaffery, R. & Freeman, W. (2003). Effect of music on chronic osteoarthritis pain in older people. *Journal of Advanced Nursing, 44*(5), 517–524.

McCaffery, M., & Pasero, C. (2001). Stigmatizing patients as addicts. *American Journal of Nursing, 101*(5), 77–79.

McCaffery, M., & Pasero, C. (2003). Breakthrough pain. *American Journal of Nursing, 103*(4), 83–84,86.

*McNeill, J. A., Sherwood, G. D., Starck, P. L., et al. (2001). Pain management outcomes for hospitalized Hispanic patients. *Pain Management Nursing, 2*(4), 25–36.

Meier, T., Wasner, G., Kuntzer, T., et al. (2003). Efficacy of lidocaine patch 5% in the treatment of focal peripheral neuropathic pain syndromes: A randomized, double-blind, placebo-controlled study. *Pain, 106*(1–2), 151–158.

Melzack, R. (1996). Gate control theory: On the evolution of pain concepts. *Pain Forum, 5*(1), 128–138.

*Miaskowski, C. (2000). The impact of age on a patient's perception of pain and ways it can be managed. *Pain Management Nursing, 1*(3), S1,S2–S7.

Miaskowski, C. (2004). Psychoeducational interventions for cancer pain serve as a model for behavioral research. *Communicating Nursing Research, 37,* 51,53–71.

Miaskowski, C. (2005). Patient-controlled modalities for acute postoperative pain management. *Journal of Perianesthesia Nursing, 20*(4), 255–267.

*Miaskowski, C., Dodd, M., West, C., et al. (2004). Randomized clinical trial of the effectiveness of a self-care intervention to improve cancer pain management. *Journal of Clinical Oncology, 22*(9), 1713–1720.

Miaskowski, C., Gear, R. W. & Levine, J. D. (2000). Sex-related differences in analgesic responses. In Sex, gender and pain. *Progress in Pain Research and Management, 17,* 209–230.

Nichols, R. (2003). Pain management in patients with addictive disease. *American Journal of Nursing, 103*(3), 87–89.

Nilsson, U., Rawal, N., & Unosson, M. (2003). A comparison of intraoperative or postoperative exposure to music: A controlled trial of the effects on postoperative pain. *Anaesthesia, 58*(7), 699–703.

Panke, J. T. (2002). Difficulties in managing pain at the end of life. *American Journal of Nursing, 102*(7), 26–33.

Pasero, C. (2002a). Subcutaneous opioid infusion. *American Journal of Nursing, 102*(7), 61–62.

Pasero, C. (2002b). The challenge of pain assessment in the PACU. *Journal of Perianesthesia Nursing, 17*(5), 348–350.

Pasero, C. (2003a). Epidural analgesia for postoperative pain. *American Journal of Nursing, 103*(10), 62–64.

Pasero, C. (2003b). Epidural analgesia for postoperative pain: Part 2. *American Journal of Nursing, 103*(11), 43–45.

Pasero, C. (2003c). Lidocaine patch 5%. *American Journal of Nursing, 103*(9),75, 77–78.

Pasero, C. (2003d). Multimodal balanced analgesia in the PACU. *Journal of Perianesthesia Nursing, 18*(4), 265–268.

Pasero, C. (2003e). Pain in the critically ill patient. *Journal of Perianesthesia Nursing, 18*(6), 422–425.

Pasero, C. (2003f). Pain in the emergency department. *American Journal of Nursing, 103*(7), 73–74.

Pasero, C. (2004a). Pain and comfort issues. *Journal of Perianesthesia Nursing, 19*(3), 135–137.

Pasero, C. (2004b). Perineural local anesthetic infusion. *American Journal of Nursing, 104*(7), 89–93.

Pasero, C. (2005). Fentanyl for acute pain management. *Journal of Perianesthesia Nursing, 20*(4), 279–284.

Pasero, C. & McCaffery, M. (2002). Monitoring sedation. *American Journal of Nursing, 102*(2), 67–69.

Pasero, C. & McCaffery, M. (2003). Accountability for pain relief: Use of comfort-function goals. *Journal of Perianesthesia Nursing, 18*(1), 50–52.

Pasero, C. & McCaffery, M. (2004a). Comfort-function goals: A way to establish accountability for pain relief. *American Journal of Nursing, 104*(9), 77–78,81.

Pasero, C. & McCaffery, M. (2004b). Controlled-release oxycodone. *American Journal of Nursing, 104*(1), 30–32.

Pasero, C. & McCaffery, M. (2004c). Safe use of a continuous infusion with i.v. PCA. *Journal of Perianesthesia Nursing, 19*(1), 42–45.

Pasero, C. & McCaffery, M. (2005). Authorized and unauthorized use of PCA pumps. *American Journal of Nursing, 105*(7), 30–31,33.

Pasero, C. & Montgomery, R. (2002). Intravenous fentanyl: Out of the operating room and gaining in popularity. *American Journal of Nursing, 102*(4), 73,75,76.

Perez, R. S. G. M., Kwakkel, G., Zuurmond, W. W. A., et al. (2001). Treatment of reflex sympathetic dystrophy (CRPS type I): A research synthesis of 21 randomized clinical trials. *Journal of Pain and Symptom Management, 21*(6), 511–526.

Perin, M. L. (2000). Corticosteroids for cancer pain. *American Journal of Nursing, 100*(4), 15–16.

Plaisance, L. & Ellis, J. A. (2002). Opioid-induced constipation. *American Journal of Nursing, 102*(3), 72–73.

Pollo, A., Amanzio, M., Arslanina, A., et al. (2001). Response expectancies in placebo analgesia and their clinical relevance. *Pain, 93*(1), 77–84.

*Puntillo, K., Neighbor, M., O'Neil, N., et al. (2004). Accuracy of emergency nurses in assessment of patient's pain. *Pain Management Nursing, 4*(4), 171–175.

*Puntillo, K. A., Stannard, D., Miaskowski, C., et al. (2002). Use of a pain assessment and intervention notation (P.A.I.N.) tool in critical care nursing practice: Nurses' evaluations. *Heart & Lung, 31*(4), 303–314.

Rakel, B., & Barr, J. O. (2003). Physical modalities in chronic pain management. *Nursing Clinics of North America, 38*(1), 477–494.

Rakel, B. & Herr, K. (2004). Assessment and treatment of postoperative pain in older adults. *Journal of Perianesthesia Nursing, 19*(3), 194–208.

Riley, J. L., 3rd, Wade, J. B., Myers, C. D., et al. (2002). Racial/ethnic differences in the experience of chronic pain. *Pain, 100*(3), 291–298.

Robinson, M. E., Wise, E. A., Gagnon, C., et al. (2004). Influences of gender role and anxiety on sex differences in temporal summation of pain. *Journal of Pain, 5*(2), 77–82.

*Roykulcharoen, V., & Good, M. (2004). Systematic relaxation to relieve postoperative pain. *Journal of Advanced Nursing, 48*(2), 140–148.

*Schumacher, K. L., Koresawa, S., West, C., et al. (2002). Putting cancer pain management regimens into practice at home. *Journal of Pain and Symptom Management, 23*(5), 369–382.

Shaya, F. T., & Suwannaprom, P. (2005). Cyclooxygenase-2 inhibitors and cardiovascular risk: How can the evidence guide prescribing decisions? *Topics in Pain Management, 20*(10), 1–7.

Skaer, T. L. (2004). Practice guidelines for transdermal opioids in malignant pain. *Drugs, 64*(23), 2629–2638.

Slaughter, A., Pasero, C., & Manworren, R. (2002). Unacceptable pain levels. *American Journal of Nursing, 102*(5), 75–77.

Smith, W. C., Bourne, D., Squair, J., et al, (1999). A retrospective cohort study of post mastectomy pain syndrome. *Pain, 83*(1), 91–95.

Snyder, M. & Wieland, J. (2003). Complementary and alternative therapies: What is their place in the management of chronic pain? *Nursing Clinics of North America, 38*(1), 495–508.

St. Marie, B. (2003). The complex patient: Interventional treatment and nursing issues. *Nursing Clinics of North America, 38*(1), 539–554.

*Stotts, N. A., Puntillo, K., Morris, A. B., et al. (2004). Wound care pain in hospitalized adult patients. *Heart & Lung, 33*(5), 321–332.

Summers, S. (2000). Evidence-based practice part 1: Pain definitions, pathophysiologic mechanisms and theories. *Journal of Perianesthesia Nursing, 15*(5), 357–365.

The SUPPORT Principal Investigators. (1995). A controlled trial to improve care for seriously ill hospitalized patients. The study to understand prognoses and preferences for outcomes and risks of treatments (SUPPORT). *Journal of American Medical Association, 274*(20), 1591–1598.

Sutton, L. M., Porter, L. S. & Keefe, F. J. (2002). Cancer pain at the end of life: A biopsychosocial perspective. *Pain, 99*(9), 1–2, 5–10.

Teno, J. M., Kabumoto, G., Wetle, T., et al. (2004). Daily pain that was excruciating at some time in the previous week: Prevalence, characteristics, and outcomes in nursing home residents. *Journal of American Geriatrics Society, 52*(5), 762–767.

Vallerand, A. H. (2003). The use of long-acting opioids in chronic pain management. *Nursing Clinics of North America, 38*(1), 435–445.

Walker, B., Shafer, M., Henzi, I., et al. (2002). Efficacy and safety of patient-controlled opioid analgesia for postoperative pain: A quantitative systematic review. *Acta Anaesthesiology Scandinavia, 45*(7), 795–804.

*Wang, H. L. & Keck, J. F. (2004). Foot and hand massage as an intervention for postoperative pain. *Pain Management Nursing, 5*(2), 59–65.

Washington, L. L., Gibson, S. J. & Helme, R. D. (2000). Age-related differences in endogenous analgesic response to repeated cold water immersion in human volunteers. *Pain, 89*(1), 89–96.

Watson, A. C. & Coyne, P. (2003). Recognizing the faces of cancer pain. *Nursing, 33*(4), 32hn1–32hn8. Available at: http://www.nursingworld.com. Accessed May 24, 2006.

*Watt-Watson, J., Chung, F., Chan, V. W., et al. (2004). Pain management following discharge after ambulatory same-day surgery. *Journal of Nursing Management, 12*(3), 153–161.

Watt-Watson, J., Stevens, B., Garfinkel, P., et al. (2001). Relationship between nurses' pain knowledge and pain management outcomes for their postoperative cardiac patients. *Journal of Advanced Nursing, 36*(4), 535–545.

*Watt-Watson, J., Stevens, B., Katz, J., et al. (2004). Impact of preoperative education on pain outcomes after coronary artery bypass graft surgery. *Pain, 109*(1–2), 73–85.

Weiner, D. K. (2004). Pain in nursing home residents: What does it really mean, and how can we help? *Journal of the American Geriatrics Society, 52*(6), 1020–1022.

Westley, C. (2004). Pain: Geriatric self-learning module. *Med Surg Nursing, 13*(6), 399–404.

*Wilkes, G., Lasch, K. E., Lee, J. C., et al. (2003). Evaluation of a cancer pain education module. *Oncology Nursing Forum Online, 30*(6), 1037–1043.

Wise, E. A., Price, D. D., Myers, C. D., et al. (2002). Gender role expectations of pain: Relationship to experimental pain perception. *Pain, 96*(3), 335–342.

Yezierski, R. P., Radson, E. & Vanderah, T. W. (2004). Understanding chronic pain. *Nursing, 34*(4), 22–23.

Zeppetella, G. (2000). An assessment of the safety, efficacy, and acceptability of intranasal fentanyl citrate in the management of breakthrough pain: A pilot study. *Journal of Pain and Symptom Management, 20*(4), 253–258.

## RESOURCES

American Academy of Pain Management, 13947 Mono Way #A, Sonora, CA 95370; 209-533-9744; http://www.aapainmanage.org. Accessed March 12, 2006.

American Chronic Pain Association, P.O. Box 850, Rocklin, CA 95677; 800-533-3231; http://www.theacpa.org. Accessed March 12, 2006.

American Pain Foundation, 201 N. Charles Street, Suite 710, Baltimore, MD 21201; 888-615-7246; http://www.painfoundation.org. Accessed March 3, 2006.

American Pain Society, 4700 W. Lake Street, Glenview, IL 60025; (847) 375-4715; http://www.ampainsoc.org. Accessed March 12, 2006.

American Society for Pain Management Nurses, 7794 Grow Drive, Pensacola, FL 32514; 222-34ASPMN; fax 850-484-8762; http://www.aspmn.org. Accessed March 12, 2006.

National Hospice Organization, Suite 901, 1901 N. Moore St., Arlington, VA 22209; 703-243-5900; http://www.nho.org. Accessed March 12, 2006.

Mendelian Inheritance in Man. A complete listing of inherited genetic conditions. http://www.ncbi.nlm.nih.gov/Omim/mimstats/html. Accessed March 3, 2006.

"Pain Control," a monthly column in *American Journal of Nursing*; http://www.ajnonline.com.

Reflex Sympathetic Dystrophy Syndrome Association, P.O. Box 502, Milford, CN 06460; 203-877-3790 or 877-662-7737; http://www.rsds.org. Accessed March 12, 2006.

# CHAPTER 14

# Fluid and Electrolytes: Balance and Disturbances

## Learning Objectives

*On completion of this chapter, the learner will be able to:*

1. Differentiate between osmosis, diffusion, filtration, and active transport.
2. Describe the role of the kidneys, lungs, and endocrine glands in regulating the body's fluid composition and volume.
3. Identify the effects of aging on fluid and electrolyte regulation.
4. Plan effective care of patients with the following imbalances: fluid volume deficit and fluid volume excess; sodium deficit (hyponatremia) and sodium excess (hypernatremia); potassium deficit (hypokalemia) and potassium excess (hyperkalemia).
5. Describe the cause, clinical manifestations, management, and nursing interventions for the following imbalances: calcium deficit (hypocalcemia) and calcium excess (hypercalcemia); magnesium deficit (hypomagnesemia) and magnesium excess (hypermagnesemia); phosphorus deficit (hypophosphatemia) and phosphorus excess (hyperphosphatemia); chloride deficit (hypochloremia) and chloride excess (hyperchloremia).
6. Explain the roles of the lungs, kidneys, and chemical buffers in maintaining acid–base balance.
7. Compare metabolic acidosis and alkalosis with regard to causes, clinical manifestations, diagnosis, and management.
8. Compare respiratory acidosis and alkalosis with regard to causes, clinical manifestations, diagnosis, and management.
9. Interpret arterial blood gas measurements.
10. Demonstrate a safe and effective procedure of venipuncture.
11. Describe measures used for preventing complications of intravenous therapy.

Fluid and electrolyte balance is a dynamic process that is crucial for life and **homeostasis**. Potential and actual disorders of fluid and electrolyte balance occur in every setting, with every disorder, and with a variety of changes that affect healthy people (eg, increased fluid and sodium loss with strenuous exercise and high environmental temperature, inadequate intake of fluid and electrolytes) as well as those who are ill.

# Fundamental Concepts

Nurses need to understand the physiology of fluid and electrolyte balance and acid–base balance to anticipate, identify, and respond to possible imbalances in each. Nurses also must use effective teaching and communication skills to help prevent and treat various fluid and electrolyte disturbances.

## Amount and Composition of Body Fluids

Approximately 60% of the weight of a typical adult consists of fluid (water and electrolytes). Factors that influence the amount of body fluid are age, gender, and body fat. In general, younger people have a higher percentage of body fluid than older people, and men have proportionately more body fluid than women. People who are obese have less fluid than those who are thin, because fat cells contain little water. The skeleton also has a low water content. Muscle, skin, and blood have the highest amount of water.

Body fluid is located in two fluid compartments: the intracellular space (fluid in the cells) and the extracellular space (fluid outside the cells). Approximately two thirds of body fluid is in the intracellular fluid (ICF) compartment and is located primarily in the skeletal muscle mass. Approximately one third is in the extracellular fluid (ECF) compartment.

The ECF compartment is further divided into the intravascular, interstitial, and transcellular fluid spaces. The intravascular space (the fluid within the blood vessels) contains plasma. Approximately 3 L of the average 6 L of blood volume is made up of plasma. The remaining 3 L is made up of erythrocytes, leukocytes, and thrombocytes. The interstitial space contains the fluid that surrounds the cell and totals about 11 to 12 L in an adult. Lymph is an interstitial fluid. The transcellular space is the smallest division of the ECF compartment and contains approximately 1 L. Examples of transcellular fluids are cerebrospinal, pericardial, synovial, intraocular, and pleural fluids; sweat; and digestive secretions.

Body fluid normally shifts between the two major compartments or spaces in an effort to maintain an equilibrium between the spaces. Loss of fluid from the body can disrupt this equilibrium. Sometimes fluid is not lost from the body but is unavailable for use by either the ICF or ECF. Loss of ECF into a space that does not contribute to equilibrium between the ICF and the ECF is referred to as a third-space fluid shift, or "third spacing" for short.

# Glossary

**acidosis:** an acid–base imbalance characterized by an increase in $H^+$ concentration (decreased blood pH). A low arterial pH due to reduced bicarbonate concentration is called metabolic acidosis; a low arterial pH due to increased $PCO_2$ is respiratory acidosis

**active transport:** physiologic pump that moves fluid from an area of lower concentration to one of higher concentration; active transport requires adenosine triphosphate (ATP) for energy

**alkalosis:** an acid–base imbalance characterized by a reduction in $H^+$ concentration (increased blood pH). A high arterial pH with increased bicarbonate concentration is called metabolic alkalosis; a high arterial pH due to reduced $PCO_2$ is respiratory alkalosis

**diffusion:** the process by which solutes move from an area of higher concentration to one of lower concentration; does not require expenditure of energy

**hemostasis:** a dynamic process that involves the cessation of bleeding from an injured vessel, which requires activity of blood vessels, platelets, coagulation and fibrinolytic systems

**homeostasis:** maintenance of a constant internal equilibrium in a biological system that involves positive and negative feedback mechanisms

**hydrostatic pressure:** the pressure created by the weight of fluid against the wall that contains it. In the body, hydrostatic pressure in blood vessels results from the weight of fluid itself and the force resulting from cardiac contraction

**hypertonic solution:** a solution with an osmolality higher than that of serum

**hypotonic solution:** a solution with an osmolality lower than that of serum

**isotonic solution:** a solution with the same osmolality as serum and other body fluids. Osmolality falls within normal range for serum (280-300 mOsm/kg).

**osmolality:** the number of osmoles (the standard unit of osmotic pressure) per kilogram of solution. Expressed as mOsm/kg. Used more often in clinical practice than the term osmolarity to evaluate serum and urine. In addition to urea and glucose, sodium contributes the largest number of particles to osmolality.

**osmolarity:** the number of osmoles, the standard unit of osmotic pressure per liter of solution. It is expressed as milliosmoles per liter (mOsm/L); describes the concentration of solutes or dissolved particles.

**osmosis:** the process by which fluid moves across a semipermeable membrane from an area of low solute concentration to an area of high solute concentration; the process continues until the solute concentrations are equal on both sides of the membrane.

**tonicity:** the measurement of the osmotic pressure of a solution; another term for osmolality

Early evidence of a third-space fluid shift is a decrease in urine output despite adequate fluid intake. Urine output decreases because fluid shifts out of the intravascular space; the kidneys then receive less blood and attempt to compensate by decreasing urine output. Other signs and symptoms of third spacing that indicate an intravascular fluid volume deficit include increased heart rate, decreased blood pressure, decreased central venous pressure, edema, increased body weight, and imbalances in fluid intake and output (I&O). Third-space shifts occur in ascites, burns, peritonitis, bowel obstruction, and massive bleeding into a joint or body cavity. Fluid shifts may also occur with stress associated with undergoing surgery (van Wissen & Breton, 2004).

## Electrolytes

Electrolytes in body fluids are active chemicals (cations that carry positive charges and anions that carry negative charges). The major cations in body fluid are sodium, potassium, calcium, magnesium, and hydrogen ions. The major anions are chloride, bicarbonate, phosphate, sulfate, and proteinate ions.

These chemicals unite in varying combinations. Therefore, electrolyte concentration in the body is expressed in terms of milliequivalents (mEq) per liter, a measure of chemical activity, rather than in terms of milligrams (mg), a unit of weight. More specifically, a milliequivalent is defined as being equivalent to the electrochemical activity of 1 mg of hydrogen. In a solution, cations and anions are equal in milliequivalents per liter.

Electrolyte concentrations in the ICF differ from those in the ECF, as reflected in Table 14-1. Because special techniques are required to measure electrolyte concentrations in the ICF, it is customary to measure the electrolytes in the most accessible portion of the ECF, namely the plasma.

Sodium ions, which are positively charged, far outnumber the other cations in the ECF. Because sodium concentration affects the overall concentration of the ECF, sodium is important in regulating the volume of body fluid. Retention of sodium is associated with fluid retention, and excessive loss of sodium is usually associated with decreased volume of body fluid.

As shown in Table 14-1, the major electrolytes in the ICF are potassium and phosphate. The ECF has a low concentration of potassium and can tolerate only small changes in potassium concentrations. Therefore, release of large stores of intracellular potassium, typically caused by trauma to the cells and tissues, can be extremely dangerous.

The body expends a great deal of energy maintaining the high extracellular concentration of sodium and the high intracellular concentration of potassium. It does so by means of cell membrane pumps that exchange sodium and potassium ions. Normal movement of fluids through the capillary wall into the tissues depends on **hydrostatic pressure** (the pressure exerted by the fluid on the walls of the blood vessel) at both the arterial and the venous ends of the vessel and the osmotic pressure exerted by the protein of plasma. The direction of fluid movement depends on the differences in these two opposing forces (hydrostatic versus osmotic pressure).

**TABLE 14-1 Approximate Major Electrolyte Content in Body Fluid**

| Electrolytes | mEq/L |
|---|---|
| **Extracellular Fluid (Plasma)** | |
| *Cations* | |
| Sodium (Na) | 142 |
| Potassium (K) | 5 |
| Calcium (Ca$^{++}$) | 5 |
| Magnesium (Mg$^{++}$) | 2 |
| Total cations | 154 |
| *Anions* | |
| Chloride (Cl$^-$) | 103 |
| Bicarbonate (HCO$_3^-$) | 26 |
| Phosphate (HPO$_4^-$) | 2 |
| Sulfate (SO$_4^-$) | 1 |
| Organic acids | 5 |
| Proteinate | 17 |
| Total anions | 154 |
| **Intracellular Fluid** | |
| *Cations* | |
| Potassium (K$^+$) | 150 |
| Magnesium (Mg$^{++}$) | 40 |
| Sodium (Na$^+$) | 10 |
| Total cations | 200 |
| *Anions* | |
| Phosphates and sulfates | 150 |
| Bicarbonate (HCO$_3^-$) | 10 |
| Proteinate | 40 |
| Total anions | 200 |

In addition to electrolytes, the ECF transports other substances, such as enzymes and hormones. It also carries blood components, such as red and white blood cells, throughout the body.

## Regulation of Body Fluid Compartments

### Osmosis and Osmolality

When two different solutions are separated by a membrane that is impermeable to the dissolved substances, fluid shifts through the membrane from the region of low solute concentration to the region of high solute concentration until the solutions are of equal concentration. This diffusion of water caused by a fluid concentration gradient is known as **osmosis** (Fig. 14-1A). The magnitude of this force depends on the number of particles dissolved in the solutions, not on their weights. The number of dissolved particles contained in a unit of fluid determines the osmolality of a solution, which influences the movement of fluid between the fluid compartments. **Tonicity** is the ability of all the solutes to cause an osmotic driving force that promotes water movement from one compartment to another (Porth, 2005). The control of tonicity determines the normal state of cellular hydration and cell size. Sodium, mannitol, glucose, and

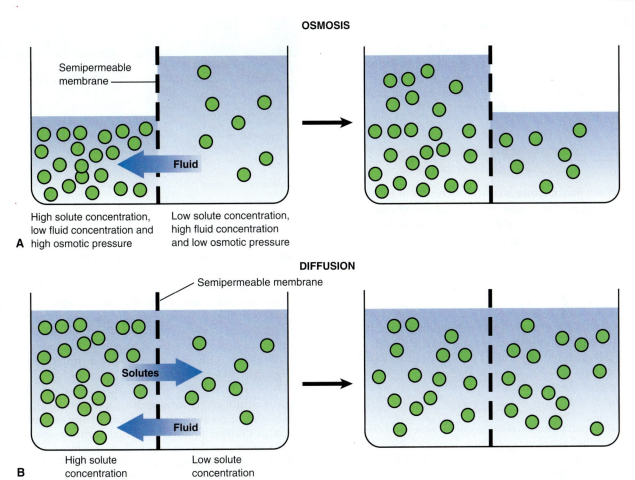

**FIGURE 14-1** (**A**) Osmosis: movement of fluid from an area of lower solute concentration to an area of higher solute concentration with eventual equalization of the solute concentrations. (**B**) Diffusion: movement of solutes from an area of greater concentration to an area of lesser concentration, leading ultimately to equalization of the solute concentrations.

sorbitol are effective osmoles (capable of affecting water movement). Three other terms are associated with osmosis: osmotic pressure, oncotic pressure, and osmotic diuresis.

- Osmotic pressure is the amount of hydrostatic pressure needed to stop the flow of water by osmosis. It is primarily determined by the concentration of solutes.
- Oncotic pressure is the osmotic pressure exerted by proteins (eg, albumin).
- Osmotic diuresis is the increase in urine output caused by the excretion of substances such as glucose, mannitol, or contrast agents in the urine.

## Diffusion

**Diffusion** is the natural tendency of a substance to move from an area of higher concentration to one of lower concentration (see Fig. 14-1B). It occurs through the random movement of ions and molecules (Porth, 2005). Examples of diffusion are the exchange of oxygen and carbon dioxide between the pulmonary capillaries and alveoli and the tendency of sodium to move from the ECF compartment, where the sodium concentration is high, to the ICF, where its concentration is low.

## Filtration

Hydrostatic pressure in the capillaries tends to filter fluid out of the intravascular compartment into the interstitial fluid. Movement of water and solutes occurs from an area of high hydrostatic pressure to an area of low hydrostatic pressure. Filtration allows the kidneys to filter 180 L of plasma per day. Another example of filtration is the passage of water and electrolytes from the arterial capillary bed to the interstitial fluid; in this instance, the hydrostatic pressure is furnished by the pumping action of the heart.

## Sodium–Potassium Pump

As previously stated, the sodium concentration is greater in the ECF than in the ICF, and because of this, sodium tends to enter the cell by diffusion. This tendency is offset by the sodium–potassium pump, which is located in the cell membrane and actively moves sodium from the cell into the ECF. Conversely, the high intracellular potassium concentration is maintained by pumping potassium into the cell. By definition, **active transport** implies that energy must be expended for the movement to occur against a concentration gradient.

## Routes of Gains and Losses

Water and electrolytes are gained in various ways. A healthy person gains fluids by drinking and eating. Fluids may be provided by the parenteral route (intravenously [IV] or subcutaneously) or by means of an enteral feeding tube in the stomach or intestine.

> **NURSING ALERT**
>
> When fluid balance is critical, all routes of gain and all routes of loss must be recorded and all volumes compared. Organs of fluid loss include the kidneys, skin, lungs, and GI tract.

### Kidneys

The usual daily urine volume in the adult is 1 to 2 L. A general rule is that the output is approximately 1 mL of urine per kilogram of body weight per hour (1 mL/kg/h) in all age groups.

### Skin

Sensible perspiration refers to visible water and electrolyte loss through the skin (sweating). The chief solutes in sweat are sodium, chloride, and potassium. Actual sweat losses can vary from 0 to 1000 mL or more every hour, depending on the environmental temperature. Continuous water loss by evaporation (approximately 600 mL/day) occurs through the skin as insensible perspiration, a nonvisible form of water loss. Fever greatly increases insensible water loss through the lungs and the skin, as does loss of the natural skin barrier (eg, through major burns).

### Lungs

The lungs normally eliminate water vapor (insensible loss) at a rate of approximately 400 mL every day. The loss is much greater with increased respiratory rate or depth, or in a dry climate.

### Gastrointestinal Tract

The usual loss through the gastrointestinal (GI) tract is only 100 to 200 mL daily, even though approximately 8 L of fluid circulates through the GI system every 24 hours (called the GI circulation). Because the bulk of fluid is normally reabsorbed in the small intestine, diarrhea and fistulas cause large losses. In healthy people, the daily average intake and output of water are approximately equal (Table 14-2).

## Laboratory Tests for Evaluating Fluid Status

**Osmolality** is the concentration of fluid that affects the movement of water between fluid compartments by osmosis. Osmolality measures the solute concentration per kilogram in blood and urine. It is also a measure of a solution's ability to create osmotic pressure and affect the movement of water. Serum osmolality primarily reflects the concentration of sodium, although blood urea nitrogen (BUN) and glucose also play a major role in determining serum osmolality (Porth, 2005). Urine osmolality is determined by urea, creatinine, and uric acid. When measured with serum osmolality, urine osmolality is the most reliable indicator of urine concentration. Osmolality is reported as milliosmoles per kilogram of water (mOsm/kg).

**Osmolarity**, another term that describes the concentration of solutions, is measured in milliosmoles per liter (mOsm/L). However, the term osmolality is used more often in clinical practice. Normal serum osmolality is 275 to 300 mOsm/kg, and normal urine osmolality is 250 to 900 mOsm/kg. Sodium predominates in ECF osmolality and holds water in this compartment.

Factors that increase and decrease serum and urine osmolality are identified in Chart 14-1. Serum osmolality may be measured directly through laboratory tests or estimated at the bedside by doubling the serum sodium level or by using the following formula:

$$Na^+ \times 2 = \frac{Glucose}{18} + \frac{BUN}{3}$$

= Approximate value of serum osmolality

The calculated value usually is within 10 mOsm of the measured osmolality.

Urine specific gravity measures the kidneys' ability to excrete or conserve water. The specific gravity of urine is compared to the weight of distilled water, which has a specific gravity of 1.000. The normal range of urine specific gravity is 1.010 to 1.025. Urine specific gravity can be measured at the bedside by placing a calibrated hydrometer or urinometer in a cylinder of approximately 20 mL of urine. Specific gravity can also be assessed with a refractometer or dipstick with a reagent for this purpose. Specific gravity varies inversely with urine volume; normally, the larger the volume of urine, the lower the specific gravity. Specific gravity is a less reliable indicator of concentration than urine osmolality; increased glucose or protein in urine can cause a falsely elevated specific gravity. Factors that increase or decrease urine osmolality are the same as those for urine specific gravity.

| TABLE 14-2 | Average Daily Intake and Output in an Adult | | |
|---|---|---|---|
| **Intake (mL)** | | **Output (mL)** | |
| Oral liquids | 1300 | Urine | 1500 |
| Water in food | 1000 | Stool | 200 |
| Water produced by metabolism | 300 | Insensible | |
| | | Lungs | 300 |
| | | Skin | 600 |
| Total gain* | 2600 | Total loss* | 2600 |

*Approximate volumes

## CHART 14-1 Factors Affecting Serum and Urine Osmolality

| FLUID | FACTORS INCREASING OSMOLALITY | FACTORS DECREASING OSMOLALITY |
|---|---|---|
| Serum (275–300 mOsm/kg water) | • Severe dehydration<br>• Free water loss<br>• Diabetes insipidus<br>• Hypernatremia<br>• Hyperglycemia<br>• Stroke or head injury<br>• Renal tubular necrosis<br>• Consumption of methanol or ethylene glycol (antifreeze) | • Fluid volume excess<br>• Syndrome of inappropriate antidiuretic hormone (SIADH)<br>• Renal failure<br>• Diuretic use<br>• Adrenal insufficiency<br>• Hyponatremia<br>• Overhydration<br>• Paraneoplastic syndrome associated with lung cancer |
| Urine (250–900 mOsm/kg water) | • Fluid volume deficit<br>• SIADH<br>• Congestive heart failure<br>• Acidosis | • Fluid volume excess<br>• Diabetes insipidus<br>• Hyponatremia<br>• Aldosteronism<br>• Pyelonephritis |

BUN is made up of urea, which is an end product of the metabolism of protein (from both muscle and dietary intake) by the liver. Amino acid breakdown produces large amounts of ammonia molecules, which are absorbed into the bloodstream. Ammonia molecules are converted to urea and excreted in the urine. The normal BUN is 10 to 20 mg/dL (3.6 to 7.2 mmol/L). The BUN level varies with urine output. Factors that increase BUN include decreased renal function, GI bleeding, dehydration, increased protein intake, fever, and sepsis. Those that decrease BUN include end-stage liver disease, a low-protein diet, starvation, and any condition that results in expanded fluid volume (eg, pregnancy).

Creatinine is the end product of muscle metabolism. It is a better indicator of renal function than BUN because it does not vary with protein intake and metabolic state. The normal serum creatinine is approximately 0.7 to 1.4 mg/dL (62 to 124 mmol/L); however, its concentration depends on lean body mass and varies from person to person. Serum creatinine levels increase when renal function decreases.

Hematocrit measures the volume percentage of red blood cells (erythrocytes) in whole blood and normally ranges from 42% to 52% for males and 35% to 47% for females. Conditions that increase the hematocrit value are dehydration and polycythemia, and those that decrease hematocrit are overhydration and anemia.

Urine sodium values change with sodium intake and the status of fluid volume: as sodium intake increases, excretion increases; as the circulating fluid volume decreases, sodium is conserved. Normal urine sodium levels range from 75 to 200 mEq/24 h (75 to 200 mmol/24 h). A random specimen usually contains more than 40 mEq/L of sodium. Urine sodium levels are used to assess volume status and are useful in the diagnosis of hyponatremia and acute renal failure.

## Homeostatic Mechanisms

The body is equipped with remarkable homeostatic mechanisms to keep the composition and volume of body fluid within narrow limits of normal. Organs involved in homeostasis include the kidneys, lungs, heart, adrenal glands, parathyroid glands, and pituitary gland (Porth, 2005).

### Kidney Functions

Vital to the regulation of fluid and electrolyte balance, the kidneys normally filter 170 L of plasma every day in the adult, while excreting only 1.5 L of urine. They act both autonomously and in response to bloodborne messengers, such as aldosterone and antidiuretic hormone (ADH) (Porth, 2005). Major functions of the kidneys in maintaining normal fluid balance include the following:

- Regulation of ECF volume and osmolality by selective retention and excretion of body fluids
- Regulation of electrolyte levels in the ECF by selective retention of needed substances and excretion of unneeded substances
- Regulation of pH of the ECF by retention of hydrogen ions
- Excretion of metabolic wastes and toxic substances

Given these functions, it is readily apparent that renal failure results in multiple fluid and electrolyte abnormalities. Renal function declines with advanced age, as do muscle mass and daily exogenous creatinine production. Therefore, high-normal and minimally elevated serum creatinine values may indicate substantially reduced renal function in the elderly.

## Heart and Blood Vessel Functions

The pumping action of the heart circulates blood through the kidneys under sufficient pressure to allow for urine formation. Failure of this pumping action interferes with renal perfusion and thus with water and electrolyte regulation.

## Lung Functions

The lungs are also vital in maintaining homeostasis. Through exhalation, the lungs remove approximately 300 mL of water daily in the normal adult. Abnormal conditions, such as hyperpnea (abnormally deep respiration) or continuous coughing, increase this loss; mechanical ventilation with excessive moisture decreases it. The lungs also play a major role in maintaining acid–base balance. Normal aging results in decreased respiratory function, causing increased difficulty in pH regulation in older adults with major illness or trauma.

## Pituitary Functions

The hypothalamus manufactures ADH, which is stored in the posterior pituitary gland and released as needed. ADH is sometimes called the water-conserving hormone because it causes the body to retain water. Functions of ADH include maintaining the osmotic pressure of the cells by controlling the retention or excretion of water by the kidneys and by regulating blood volume (Fig. 14-2).

## Adrenal Functions

Aldosterone, a mineralocorticoid secreted by the zona glomerulosa (outer zone) of the adrenal cortex, has a profound effect on fluid balance. Increased secretion of aldosterone causes sodium retention (and thus water retention) and potassium loss. Conversely, decreased secretion of aldosterone causes sodium and water loss and potassium retention.

Cortisol, another adrenocortical hormone, has only a fraction of the mineralocorticoid potency of aldosterone. However, when secreted in large quantities (or administered as corticosteroid therapy), it can also produce sodium and fluid retention.

## Parathyroid Functions

The parathyroid glands, embedded in the thyroid gland, regulate calcium and phosphate balance by means of parathyroid hormone (PTH). PTH influences bone resorption, calcium absorption from the intestines, and calcium reabsorption from the renal tubules.

## Other Mechanisms

Changes in the volume of the interstitial compartment within the ECF can occur without affecting body function. However, the vascular compartment cannot tolerate change as readily and must be carefully maintained to ensure that tissues receive adequate nutrients.

### BARORECEPTORS

The baroreceptors are small nerve receptors that detect changes in pressure within blood vessels and transmit this information to the central nervous system. They are responsible for monitoring the circulating volume, and they regulate sympathetic and parasympathetic neural activity as well as endocrine activities. They are categorized as either low-pressure or high-pressure baroreceptors. Low-pressure baroreceptors are in the cardiac atria, particularly the left atrium. High-pressure baroreceptors are nerve endings in the aortic arch and the carotid sinus, as well as in the afferent arteriole of the juxtaglomerular apparatus of the nephron.

As arterial pressure decreases, baroreceptors transmit fewer impulses from the carotid sinuses and the aortic arch to the vasomotor center. A decrease in impulses stimulates the sympathetic nervous system and inhibits the parasympathetic nervous system. The outcome is an increase in cardiac rate, conduction, and contractility and an increase in circulating blood volume. Sympathetic stimulation constricts renal arterioles; this increases the release of aldosterone, decreases glomerular filtration, and increases sodium and water reabsorption.

### RENIN–ANGIOTENSIN–ALDOSTERONE SYSTEM

Renin is an enzyme that converts angiotensinogen, an inactive substance formed by the liver, into angiotensin I (Porth, 2005). Renin is released by the juxtaglomerular cells of the kidneys in response to decreased renal perfusion. Angiotensin-converting enzyme (ACE) converts angiotensin I to angiotensin II. Angiotensin II, with its vasoconstrictor properties, increases arterial perfusion pressure and stimulates thirst. As the sympathetic nervous system is stimulated, aldosterone is released in response to an increased release of renin. Aldosterone is a volume regulator and is also released as serum potassium increases, serum sodium decreases, or adrenocorticotropic hormone (ACTH) increases.

### ANTIDIURETIC HORMONE AND THIRST

ADH and the thirst mechanism have important roles in maintaining sodium concentration and oral intake of fluids. Oral intake is controlled by the thirst center located in the hypothalamus (Porth, 2005). As serum concentration or osmolality increases or blood volume decreases, neurons in the hypothalamus are stimulated by intracellular dehydration; thirst then occurs, and the person increases his or her intake of oral fluids. Water excretion is controlled by ADH, aldosterone, and baroreceptors, as mentioned previously. The presence or absence of ADH is the most significant factor in determining whether the urine that is excreted is concentrated or dilute.

### OSMORECEPTORS

Located on the surface of the hypothalamus, osmoreceptors sense changes in sodium concentration. As osmotic pressure increases, the neurons become dehydrated and quickly release impulses to the posterior pituitary, which increases the release of ADH. The ADH then travels in the blood to the kidneys, where it alters permeability to water, causing increased reabsorption of water and decreased urine output. The retained water dilutes the ECF and returns its concentration to normal. Restoration of normal osmotic pressure provides feedback to the osmoreceptors to inhibit further ADH release (see Fig. 14-2).

## Physiology/Pathophysiology

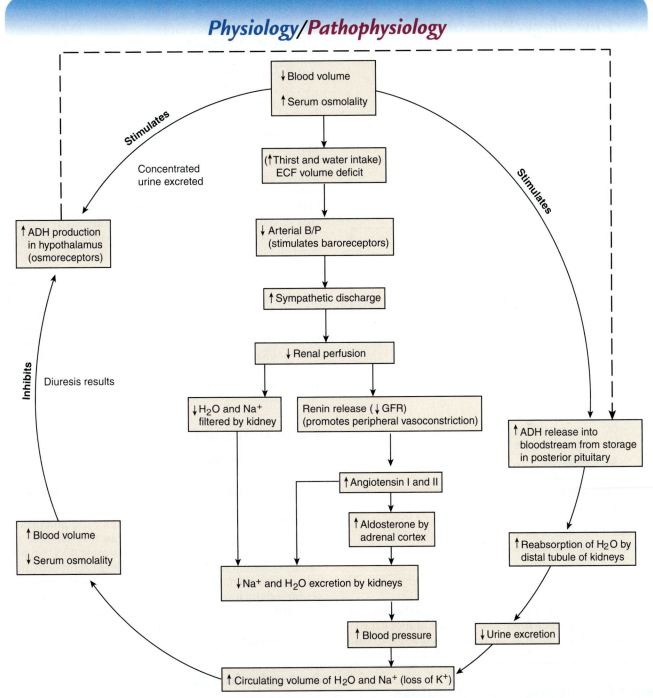

**FIGURE 14-2.** Fluid regulation cycle.

**RELEASE OF ATRIAL NATRIURETIC PEPTIDE**

Atrial natriuretic peptide (ANP), also called atrial natriuretic factor, is a 28-amino-acid peptide that is synthesized, stored, and released by muscle cells of the atria of the heart in response to several factors. These factors include increased atrial pressure, angiotensin II stimulation, endothelin (a powerful vasoconstrictor of vascular smooth muscle peptide released from damaged endothelial cells in the kidneys or other tissues), and sympathetic stimulation (Porth, 2005). In addition, any condition that results in volume expansion (exercise, pregnancy), hypoxia, or increased cardiac filling pressures (eg, high sodium intake, heart failure, chronic renal failure, atrial tachycardia, or use of vasoconstrictor agents such as epinephrine) increases the release of ANP. The action of ANP is the direct opposite of the renin–angiotensin–aldosterone system; ANP decreases blood pressure and volume (Fig. 14-3). The ANP measured in plasma is normally 20 to 77 pg/mL (20 to 77 ng/L). This level increases in acute heart failure, paroxysmal atrial tachycardia, hyperthyroidism, subarachnoid hemorrhage, and small cell lung cancer. The level decreases in chronic heart failure and with the use of medications such as urea

**FIGURE 14-3.** Role of atrial natriuretic peptide (ANP) in maintenance of fluid balance.

(Ureaphil) and prazosin (Minipress). ANP has been shown in studies to improve left ventricular function after left ventricular aneurysm repair by decreasing myocardial fibrosis (Tsuneyoshi, Nishina, Nomoto, et al., 2004).

### Gerontologic Considerations

Normal physiologic changes of aging, including reduced cardiac, renal, and respiratory function and reserve and alterations in the ratio of body fluids to muscle mass, may alter the responses of elderly people to fluid and electrolyte changes and acid–base disturbances. In addition, the frequent use of medications in the older adult can affect renal and cardiac function and fluid balance, thereby increasing the likelihood of fluid and electrolyte disturbances. Routine procedures, such as the vigorous administration of laxatives before colon x-ray studies, may produce a serious fluid volume deficit, necessitating the use of intravenous (IV) fluids to prevent hypotension and other effects of hypovolemia.

Alterations in fluid and electrolyte balance that may produce minor changes in young and middle-aged adults have the potential to produce profound changes in older adults, accompanied by a rapid onset of signs and symptoms. In other elderly patients, the clinical manifestations of fluid and electrolyte disturbances may be subtle or atypical. For example, fluid deficit may cause confusion or cognitive impairment in the elderly person, whereas in the young or middle-aged person the first sign commonly is increased thirst. Rapid infusion of an excessive volume of IV fluids may produce fluid overload and cardiac failure in the elderly patient. These reactions are likely to occur more quickly and with the administration of smaller volumes of fluid than in healthy young and middle-aged adults because of the decreased cardiac reserve and reduced renal function that accompany aging. Dehydration in the elderly is common as a result of decreased reserve capacity of the kidney from the aging process, disease, and use of medications (Suhayda & Walton, 2002).

Increased sensitivity to fluid and electrolyte changes in elderly patients requires careful assessment, with attention to intake and output of fluids from all sources and to changes in daily weight; careful monitoring of side effects and interactions of medications; and prompt reporting and management of disturbances. Additional considerations relating to specific fluid and electrolyte disturbances in older adults are discussed later in this chapter.

## Fluid Volume Disturbances: Hypovolemia

Fluid volume deficit (FVD), or hypovolemia, occurs when loss of ECF volume exceeds the intake of fluid. It occurs when water and electrolytes are lost in the same proportion as they exist in normal body fluids, so that the ratio of serum electrolytes to water remains the same. FVD (hypovolemia) should not be confused with the term dehydration, which refers to loss of water alone, with increased serum sodium levels. FVD may occur alone or in combination with other imbalances. Unless other imbalances are present concurrently, serum electrolyte concentrations remain essentially unchanged.

### Pathophysiology

FVD results from loss of body fluids and occurs more rapidly when coupled with decreased fluid intake. FVD can develop from inadequate intake alone if the decreased intake is prolonged. Causes of FVD include abnormal fluid losses, such as those resulting from vomiting, diarrhea, GI suctioning, and sweating, and decreased intake, as in nausea or inability to gain access to fluids (Heitz & Horne, 2005).

Additional risk factors include diabetes insipidus, adrenal insufficiency, osmotic diuresis, hemorrhage, and coma. Third-space fluid shifts, or the movement of fluid from the vascular system to other body spaces (eg, with edema formation in burns, ascites with liver dysfunction), also cause FVD.

## NURSING RESEARCH PROFILE

### Bowel Cleansing for Colonoscopy

Hayes, A., Buffum, M. & Fuller, D. (2003). Bowel preparation comparison: Flavored versus unflavored colyte. *Gastroenterology Nursing, 26*(3), 106–109.

#### Purpose
Inadequate bowel cleansing prior to colonoscopy often necessitates repeated colon lavage and a second attempt at colonoscopy. Patients who have poorly cleansed bowels often complain about the taste of colon lavage solutions they were required to consume in preparation for colonoscopy. This study was conducted to determine whether flavoring in lavage solutions had an effect on bowel cleansing in preparation for colonoscopy.

#### Design
A randomized clinical trial was conducted with 130 patients, who received either flavored or unflavored lavage solution. The health care staff who assessed the effectiveness of bowel cleansing were blinded to group assignment of patients to the type of lavage solution received. Questionnaires were used to determine patients' opinions about the taste of the solution, the amount consumed, and their willingness to drink the solution again if necessary. A colon preparation rating scale completed by the endoscopist and endoscopy nurse was used to rate the adequacy of bowel cleansing in preparation for the colonoscopy.

#### Findings
Chi square analysis revealed no significant difference in bowel cleansing between the patients who consumed flavored solution and those who consumed unflavored solution. Although both groups reported disliking the flavor of the solution, there was no difference in their adherence to instructions. The authors concluded that taste of the solution did not affect bowel cleansing.

#### Nursing Implications
No differences were detected in the effect of flavoring of colon lavage solution on the adequacy of bowel cleansing in preparation for colonoscopy. Therefore, other factors must be involved. Further research is needed to identify factors that affect adequacy of bowel cleansing with the goals of decreasing the likelihood that patients may have to undergo repeated efforts to cleanse the bowel and increasing the likelihood of successful colonoscopy. Because of the importance of colonoscopy in early detection of colon cancer, efforts are needed to improve the effectiveness of bowel cleansing and to reduce the discomfort and cost associated with ineffective cleansing and potential fluid and electrolyte disturbances associated with repeated doses.

## Clinical Manifestations

FVD can develop rapidly and can be mild, moderate, or severe, depending on the degree of fluid loss. Important characteristics include acute weight loss; decreased skin turgor; oliguria; concentrated urine; postural hypotension; a weak, rapid heart rate; flattened neck veins; increased temperature; decreased central venous pressure; cool, clammy skin related to peripheral vasoconstriction; thirst; anorexia; nausea; lassitude; muscle weakness; and cramps.

## Assessment and Diagnostic Findings

Laboratory data useful in evaluating fluid volume status include BUN and its relation to serum creatinine concentration. A volume-depleted patient has a BUN elevated out of proportion to the serum creatinine (ratio greater than 20:1). The cause of hypovolemia may be determined through the health history and physical examination. The BUN can be elevated because of dehydration or decreased renal perfusion and function. Also, the hematocrit level is greater than normal because the red blood cells become suspended in a decreased plasma volume.

Serum electrolyte changes may also exist. Potassium and sodium levels can be reduced (hypokalemia, hyponatremia) or elevated (hyperkalemia, hypernatremia).

- Hypokalemia occurs with GI and renal losses.
- Hyperkalemia occurs with adrenal insufficiency.
- Hyponatremia occurs with increased thirst and ADH release.
- Hypernatremia results from increased insensible losses and diabetes insipidus.

Urine specific gravity is increased in relation to the kidneys' attempt to conserve water and decreased with diabetes insipidus. Urine osmolality is greater than 450 mOsm/kg, because the kidneys try to compensate by conserving water. Normal values for these tests are listed in Table 14-3.

## Gerontologic Considerations

Elderly patients have special nursing care needs because of their propensity for developing fluid and electrolyte imbalances (Zwicker, 2003). Fluid balance in many elderly patients is often marginal at best because of certain physiologic changes associated with the aging process. Some of these changes include reduction in total body water (associated with increased body fat content and decreased muscle mass); reduction in renal function, resulting in decreased ability to concentrate urine; decreased cardiovascular and respiratory function; and disturbances in hormonal regulatory functions. Although these changes are often viewed as

| TABLE 14-3 | Laboratory Values Used In Evaluating Fluid and Electrolyte Status in Adults | |
|---|---|---|
| Test | Usual Reference Range | SI Units |
| Serum sodium | 135–145 mEq/L | 135–145 mmol/L |
| Serum potassium | 3.5–5.0 mEq/L | 3.5–5.0 mmol/L |
| Total serum calcium | 8.6–10.2 mg/dL | 2.15–2.55 mmol/L |
| Ionized calcium | 4.5–5.0 mg/dL | 1.05–1.30 mmol/L |
| Serum magnesium | 1.3–2.5 mEq/L | 0.65–1.25 mmol/L |
| Serum phosphorus | 2.5–4.5 mg/dL | 0.87–1.45 mmol/L |
| Serum chloride | 97–107 mEq/L | 97–107 mmol/L |
| Carbon dioxide content | 24–32 mEq/L | 24–32 mmol/L |
| Serum osmolality | 275–300 mOsm/kg | 275–300 mmol/kg |
| Blood urea nitrogen (BUN) | 10–20 mg/dL | 3.6–7.2 mmol/L |
| Serum creatinine | 0.7–1.4 mg/dL | 62–124 µmol/L |
| BUN to creatinine ratio | 10:1–20:1 | — |
| Hematocrit | Males: 42–52% | Volume fraction: 0.42–0.52 |
| | Females: 35–47% | Volume fraction: 0.35–0.47 |
| Serum glucose | 60–110 mg/dL | 3.3–6.05 mmol/L |
| Serum albumin | 3.5–5.0 g/dL | 3.5–5.0 g/L |
| Urinary sodium | 75–200 mEq/day | 75–200 mmol/day |
| Urinary potassium (intake-dependent) | 26–123 mEq/day | 26–123 mmol/day |
| Urinary chloride | 110–250 mEq/24 h | 110–250 mmol/24 h |
| Urine specific gravity | 1.003–1.030 | 1.002–1.030 |
| Urine osmolality | 250–900 mOsm/kg | 250–900 mmol/kg |
| Urinary pH | Random: 4.5–8.0 | 4.5–8.0 |
| | Typical urine <5–6 | <5–6 |

a normal part of the aging process, they must be considered when elderly people become ill, because age-related changes predispose people to fluid and electrolyte imbalances. These physiologic changes must be considered during assessment of elderly patients as well as before initiating treatment for fluid and electrolyte imbalances.

Assessment of elderly patients should be modified somewhat from that of younger adults. For example, in an elderly patient, assessment of skin turgor is less valid because the skin has lost some of its elasticity due to the decreased number of papillae and collagen fibers; therefore, other assessment measures (eg, slowness in filling of veins of the hands and feet) become more useful in detecting FVD. In elderly patients, skin turgor is best tested over the forehead or the sternum, because alterations in skin elasticity are less marked in these areas. As in all patients, skin turgor should be monitored serially to detect subtle changes.

The nurse should perform a functional assessment of the ability of the elderly patient to determine fluid and food needs and to obtain adequate intake. For example, is the patient mentally clear? Is the patient able to ambulate and to use both arms and hands to reach fluids and foods? Is the patient able to swallow? All of these questions have a direct bearing on how the patient will be able to meet his or her own need for fluids and foods. During an elderly patient's hospital stay, the nurse provides fluids for the patient if he or she is unable to carry out self-care activities.

Another concern is that some elderly patients deliberately restrict their fluid intake to avoid embarrassing episodes of incontinence. In this situation, the nurse also identifies interventions to deal with the incontinence, such as encouraging the patient to wear protective clothing or devices, to carry a urinal in the car, or to pace fluid intake to allow access to toilet facilities during the day. Elderly people without cardiovascular or renal dysfunction should be reminded to drink adequate fluids, particularly in very warm or humid weather.

## Medical Management

When planning the correction of fluid loss for the patient with FVD, the health care provider considers the usual maintenance requirements of the patient and other factors (eg, fever) that can influence fluid needs. If the deficit is not severe, the oral route is preferred, provided the patient can drink. However, if fluid losses are acute or severe, the IV route is required. Isotonic electrolyte solutions (eg, lactated Ringer's solution, 0.9% sodium chloride) are frequently used to treat the hypotensive patient with FVD because they expand plasma volume. As soon as the patient becomes normotensive, a hypotonic electrolyte solution (eg, 0.45% sodium chloride) is often used to provide both electrolytes and water for renal excretion of metabolic wastes. These and additional fluids are listed in Table 14-4.

Accurate and frequent assessments of I&O, weight, vital signs, central venous pressure, level of consciousness, breath sounds, and skin color should be performed to determine when therapy should be slowed to avoid volume overload. The rate of fluid administration is based on the severity of loss and the patient's hemodynamic response to volume replacement (Suhayda & Walton, 2002).

If the patient with severe FVD is not excreting enough urine and is therefore oliguric, the health care provider needs to determine whether the depressed renal function is caused by reduced renal blood flow secondary to FVD (prerenal azotemia) or, more seriously, by acute tubular necro-

## TABLE 14-4  Selected Water and Electrolyte Solutions

| Solution | Comments |
|---|---|
| **Isotonic Solutions** | |
| 0.9% NaCl (isotonic, also called normal saline [NS]) $Na^+$ 154 mEq/L $Cl^-$ 154 mEq/L (308 mOsm/L) Also available with varying concentrations of dextrose (the most frequently used is a 5% dextrose concentration) | • An isotonic solution that expands the extracellular fluid (ECF) volume, used in hypovolemic states, resuscitative efforts, shock, diabetic ketoacidosis, metabolic alkalosis, hypercalcemia, mild $Na^+$ deficit<br>• Supplies an excess of $Na^+$ and $Cl^-$; can cause fluid volume excess and hyperchloremic acidosis if used in excessive volumes, particularly in patients with compromised renal function, heart failure, or edema<br>• Not desirable as a routine maintenance solution, as it provides only $Na^+$ and $Cl^-$ (and these are provided in excessive amounts)<br>• When mixed with 5% dextrose, the resulting solution becomes hypertonic in relation to plasma and, in addition to the above described electrolytes, provides 170 cal/L<br>• Only solution that may be administered with blood products |
| Lactated Ringer's solution (Hartmann's solution) $Na^+$ 130 mEq/L $K^+$ 4 mEq/L $Ca^{++}$ 3 mEq/L $Cl^-$ 109 mEq/L Lactate (metabolized to bicarbonate) 28 mEq/L (274 mOsm/L) Also available with varying concentrations of dextrose (the most common is 5% dextrose) | • An isotonic solution that contains multiple electrolytes in roughly the same concentration as found in plasma (note that solution is lacking in $Mg^{++}$): provides 9 cal/L<br>• Used in the treatment of hypovolemia, burns, fluid lost as bile or diarrhea, and for acute blood loss replacement<br>• Lactate is rapidly metabolized into $HCO_3^-$ in the body. Lactated Ringer's solution should not be used in lactic acidosis because the ability to convert lactate into $HCO_3^-$ is impaired in this disorder.<br>• Not to be given with a pH > 7.5 because bicarbonate is formed as lactate breaks down, causing alkalosis<br>• Should not be used in renal failure because it contains potassium and can cause hyperkalemia<br>• Similar to plasma |
| 5% dextrose in water ($D_5W$) No electrolytes 50 g of dextrose | • An isotonic solution that supplies 170 cal/L and free water to aid in renal excretion of solutes<br>• Used in treatment of hypernatremia, fluid loss, and dehydration<br>• Should not be used in excessive volumes in the early postoperative period (when antidiuretic hormone secretion is increased due to stress reaction)<br>• Should not be used solely in treatment of fluid volume deficit, because it dilutes plasma electrolyte concentrations<br>• Contraindicated in head injury because it may cause increased intracranial pressure<br>• Should not be used for fluid resuscitation because it can cause hyperglycemia<br>• Should be used with caution in patients with renal or cardiac disease because of risk of fluid overload<br>• Electrolyte-free solutions may cause peripheral circulatory collapse, anuria in patients with sodium deficiency, and increased body fluid loss.<br>• Converts to hypotonic solution as dextrose is metabolized by body. Over time, $D_5W$ without NaCl can cause water intoxication (intracellular fluid volume excess [FVE]) because the solution is hypotonic. |
| **Hypotonic Solutions** | |
| 0.45% NaCl (half-strength saline) $Na^+$ 77 mEq/L $Cl^-$ 77 mEq/L (154 mOsm/L) Also available with varying concentrations of dextrose (the most common is a 5% concentration) | • Provides $Na^+$, $Cl^-$, and free water<br>• Free water is desirable to aid the kidneys in elimination of solute.<br>• Lacking in electrolytes other than $Na^+$ and $Cl^-$<br>• When mixed with 5% dextrose, the solution becomes slightly hypertonic to plasma and in addition to the above-described electrolytes provides 170 cal/L.<br>• Used to treat hypertonic dehydration, $Na^+$ and $Cl^-$ depletion, and gastric fluid loss<br>• Not indicated for third-space fluid shifts or increased intracranial pressure<br>• Administer cautiously, because it can cause fluid shifts from vascular system into cells, resulting in cardiovascular collapse and increased intracranial pressure. |

*continued >*

| TABLE 14-4 | Selected Water and Electrolyte Solutions (Continued) |
|---|---|
| **Solution** | **Comments** |
| **Hypertonic Solutions** | |
| 3% NaCl (hypertonic saline)<br>Na$^+$ 513 mEq/L<br>Cl$^-$ 513 mEq/L<br>(1026 mOsm/L) | • Used to increase ECF volume, decrease cellular swelling<br>• Highly hypertonic solution used only in critical situations to treat hyponatremia<br>• Must be administered slowly and cautiously, because it can cause intravascular volume overload and pulmonary edema<br>• Supplies no calories<br>• Assists in removing intracellular fluid excess |
| 5% NaCL<br>(hypertonic solution)<br>Na$^+$ 855 mEq/L<br>Cl$^-$ 855 mEq/L<br>(1710 mOsm/L) | • Highly hypertonic solution used to treat symptomatic hyponatremia<br>• Administered slowly and cautiously, because it can cause intravascular volume overload and pulmonary edema<br>• Supplies no calories |
| **Colloid Solutions** | |
| Dextran in NS or 5% D$_5$W<br>Available in low-molecular-weight (Dextran 40) and high-molecular-weight (Dextran 70) forms | • Colloid solution used as volume/plasma expander for intravascular part of ECF<br>• Affects clotting by coating platelets and decreasing ability to clot<br>• Remains in circulatory system up to 24 hours<br>• Used to treat hypovolemia in early shock to increase pulse pressure, cardiac output, and arterial blood pressure<br>• Improves microcirculation by decreasing red blood cell aggregation<br>• Contraindicated in hemorrhage, thrombocytopenia, renal disease, and severe dehydration<br>• Not a substitute for blood or blood products |

sis from prolonged FVD. The test used in this situation is referred to as a fluid challenge test. During a fluid challenge test, volumes of fluid are administered at specific rates and intervals while the patient's hemodynamic response to this treatment is monitored (ie, vital signs, breath sounds, sensorium, central venous pressure, urine output).

A typical example of a fluid challenge involves administering 100 to 200 mL of normal saline solution over 15 minutes. The goal is to provide fluids rapidly enough to attain adequate tissue perfusion without compromising the cardiovascular system. The response by a patient with FVD but normal renal function is increased urine output and an increase in blood pressure and central venous pressure.

Shock can occur when the volume of fluid lost exceeds 25% of the intravascular volume, or when fluid loss is rapid. Shock and its causes and treatment are discussed in detail in Chapter 15.

## Nursing Management

To assess for FVD, the nurse monitors and measures fluid I&O at least every 8 hours, and sometimes hourly. As FVD develops, body fluid losses exceed fluid intake. This loss may be in the form of excessive urination (polyuria), diarrhea, vomiting, and so on. Later, after FVD fully develops, the kidneys attempt to conserve needed body fluids, leading to a urine output of less than 30 mL/h in an adult. Urine in this instance is concentrated and represents a healthy renal response. Daily body weights are monitored; an acute loss of 0.5 kg (1 lb) represents a fluid loss of approximately 500 mL. (One liter of fluid weighs approximately 1 kg, or 2.2 lb.)

Vital signs are closely monitored. The nurse observes for a weak, rapid pulse and postural hypotension (ie, a decrease in systolic pressure exceeding 15 mm Hg when the patient moves from a lying to a sitting position). A decrease in body temperature often accompanies FVD, unless there is a concurrent infection.

Skin and tongue turgor is monitored on a regular basis. In a healthy person, pinched skin immediately returns to its normal position when released. This elastic property, referred to as turgor, is partially dependent on interstitial fluid volume. In a person with FVD, the skin flattens more slowly after the pinch is released. In a person with severe FVD, the skin may remain elevated for many seconds. Tissue turgor is best measured by pinching the skin over the sternum, inner aspects of the thighs, or forehead.

**NURSING ALERT**

**The skin turgor test is not as valid in elderly people as in younger people because skin elasticity decreases with age; therefore, other assessment parameters must be considered.**

Evaluating tongue turgor, which is not affected by age, may be more valid than evaluating skin turgor. In a normal person, the tongue has one longitudinal furrow. In the person with FVD, there are additional longitudinal furrows and the tongue is smaller, because of fluid loss. The degree of oral mucous membrane moisture is also assessed; a dry mouth may indicate either FVD or mouth breathing.

Urine concentration is monitored by measuring the urine specific gravity. In a volume-depleted patient, the urine specific gravity should be greater than 1.020, indicating healthy renal conservation of fluid.

Mental function is eventually affected in severe FVD as a result of decreasing cerebral perfusion. Decreased peripheral perfusion can result in cold extremities. In patients with relatively normal cardiopulmonary function, a low central venous pressure is indicative of hypovolemia. Patients with acute cardiopulmonary decompensation require more extensive hemodynamic monitoring of pressures in both sides of the heart to determine if hypovolemia exists.

### Preventing Fluid Volume Deficit

To prevent FVD, the nurse identifies patients at risk and takes measures to minimize fluid losses. For example, if the patient has diarrhea, diarrhea control measures should be implemented and replacement fluids administered. These measures may include administering antidiarrheal medications and small volumes of oral fluids at frequent intervals.

### Correcting Fluid Volume Deficit

When possible, oral fluids are administered to help correct FVD, with consideration given to the patient's likes and dislikes. The type of fluid the patient has lost is also considered, and attempts are made to select fluids most likely to replace the lost electrolytes. If the patient is reluctant to drink because of oral discomfort, the nurse assists with frequent mouth care and provides nonirritating fluids. The patient may be offered small volumes of oral rehydration solutions (eg, Rehydralyte, Elete, Cytomax). These solutions provide fluid, glucose, and electrolytes in concentrations that are easily absorbed. If nausea is present, antiemetics may be needed before oral fluid replacement can be tolerated.

If the patient cannot eat and drink, fluid may need to be administered by an alternative route (enteral or parenteral) until adequate circulating blood volume and renal perfusion are achieved (Suhayda & Walton, 2002). Isotonic fluids are prescribed to increase ECF volume.

## Fluid Volume Disturbances: Hypervolemia

Fluid volume excess (FVE), or hypervolemia, refers to an isotonic expansion of the ECF caused by the abnormal retention of water and sodium in approximately the same proportions in which they normally exist in the ECF. It is always secondary to an increase in the total body sodium content, which, in turn, leads to an increase in total body water. Because there is isotonic retention of body substances, the serum sodium concentration remains essentially normal.

### Pathophysiology

FVE may be related to simple fluid overload or diminished function of the homeostatic mechanisms responsible for regulating fluid balance. Contributing factors can include heart failure, renal failure, and cirrhosis of the liver. Another contributing factor is consumption of excessive amounts of table or other sodium salts. Excessive administration of sodium-containing fluids in a patient with impaired regulatory mechanisms may predispose him or her to a serious FVE as well (Heitz & Horne, 2005).

### Clinical Manifestations

Clinical manifestations of FVE stem from expansion of the ECF and include edema, distended neck veins, and crackles (abnormal lung sounds). Other manifestations include tachycardia; increased blood pressure, pulse pressure, and central venous pressure; increased weight; increased urine output; and shortness of breath and wheezing.

### Assessment and Diagnostic Findings

Laboratory data useful in diagnosing FVE include BUN and hematocrit levels. In FVE, both of these values may be decreased because of plasma dilution. Other causes of abnormalities in these values include low protein intake and anemia. In chronic renal failure, both serum osmolality and the sodium level are decreased due to excessive retention of water. The urine sodium level is increased if the kidneys are attempting to excrete excess volume. Chest x-rays may reveal pulmonary congestion. Hypervolemia occurs when aldosterone is chronically stimulated (ie, cirrhosis, heart failure, and nephrotic syndrome). Therefore, the urine sodium level does not increase in these conditions.

### Medical Management

Management of FVE is directed at the causes. If the fluid excess is related to excessive administration of sodium-containing fluids, discontinuing the infusion may be all that is needed. Symptomatic treatment consists of administering diuretics and restricting fluids and sodium.

### Pharmacologic Therapy

Diuretics are prescribed when dietary restriction of sodium alone is insufficient to reduce edema by inhibiting the reabsorption of sodium and water by the kidneys. The choice of diuretic is based on the severity of the hypervolemic state, the degree of impairment of renal function, and the potency of the diuretic. Thiazide diuretics block sodium reabsorption in the distal tubule, where only 5% to 10% of filtered sodium is reabsorbed. Loop diuretics, such as furosemide (Lasix), bumetanide (Bumex), or torsemide (Demadex), can cause a greater loss of both sodium and water because they block sodium reabsorption in the ascending limb of the loop of Henle, where 20% to 30% of filtered sodium is normally reabsorbed. Generally, thiazide diuretics, such as hydrochlorothiazide (HydroDIURIL) or metolazone (Mykrox, Zaroxolyn), are prescribed for mild to moderate hypervolemia and loop diuretics for severe hypervolemia.

Electrolyte imbalances may result from the effect of the diuretic. Hypokalemia can occur with all diuretics except those that work in the last distal tubule of the nephrons (eg, spironolactone). Potassium supplements can be prescribed to avoid this complication. Hyperkalemia can occur with diuretics that work in the last distal tubule, especially in patients with decreased renal function. Hyponatremia occurs with diuresis due to increased release of ADH secondary to reduction in circulating volume. Decreased magnesium levels occur with administration of loop and thiazide diuretics due to decreased reabsorption and increased excretion of magnesium by the kidney.

Azotemia (increased nitrogen levels in the blood) can occur with FVE when urea and creatinine are not excreted due to decreased perfusion by the kidneys and decreased excretion of wastes. High uric acid levels (hyperuricemia) can also occur from increased reabsorption and decreased excretion of uric acid by the kidneys.

### Hemodialysis

If renal function is so severely impaired that pharmacologic agents cannot act efficiently, other modalities are considered to remove sodium and fluid from the body. Hemodialysis or peritoneal dialysis may be used to remove nitrogenous wastes and control potassium and acid–base balance, and to remove sodium and fluid. Continuous renal replacement therapy may also be required. See Chapter 44 for discussion of these treatment modalities.

### Nutritional Therapy

Treatment of FVE usually involves dietary restriction of sodium. An average daily diet not restricted in sodium contains 6 to 15 g of salt, whereas low-sodium diets can range from a mild restriction to as little as 250 mg of sodium per day, depending on the patient's needs. A mild sodium-restricted diet allows only light salting of food (about half the usual amount) in cooking and at the table, and no addition of salt to commercially prepared foods that are already seasoned. Of course, foods high in sodium must be avoided. It is the sodium salt, sodium chloride, rather than sodium itself that contributes to edema. Therefore, patients are instructed to read food labels carefully to determine salt content.

Because about half of ingested sodium is in the form of seasoning, seasoning substitutes can play a major role in decreasing sodium intake. Lemon juice, onions, and garlic are excellent substitute flavorings, although some patients prefer salt substitutes. Most salt substitutes contain potassium and must therefore be used cautiously by patients taking potassium-sparing diuretics (eg, spironolactone, triamterene, amiloride). They should not be used at all in conditions associated with potassium retention, such as advanced renal disease. Salt substitutes containing ammonium chloride can be harmful to patients with liver damage.

In some communities, the drinking water may contain too much sodium for a sodium-restricted diet. Depending on its source, water may contain as little as 1 mg or more than 1500 mg per quart. Patients may need to use distilled water if the local water supply is very high in sodium. Bottled water can have a sodium content from 0 to 1200 mg/L; therefore, if sodium is restricted, the label must be carefully examined for sodium content before purchasing and drinking bottled water. Also, patients on sodium-restricted diets should be cautioned to avoid water softeners that add sodium to water in exchange for other ions, such as calcium. Protein intake may be increased in patients who are malnourished or who have low serum protein levels in an effort to increase capillary oncotic pressure and pull fluid out of the tissues into vessels for excretion by the kidneys.

## Nursing Management

To assess for FVE, the nurse measures I&O at regular intervals to identify excessive fluid retention. The patient is weighed daily, and acute weight gain is noted. An acute weight gain of 2.2 lb (1 kg) is equivalent to a gain of approximately 1 L of fluid. The nurse also needs to assess breath sounds at regular intervals in at-risk patients, particularly if parenteral fluids are being administered. The nurse monitors the degree of edema in the most dependent parts of the body, such as the feet and ankles in ambulatory patients and the sacral region in patients confined to bed. The degree of pitting edema is assessed, and the extent of peripheral edema is monitored by measuring the circumference of the extremity with a tape marked in millimeters.

### Preventing Fluid Volume Excess

Specific interventions vary somewhat with the underlying condition and the degree of FVE. However, most patients require sodium-restricted diets in some form, and adherence to the prescribed diet is encouraged. Patients are instructed to avoid over-the-counter medications without first checking with a health care provider, because these substances may contain sodium. If fluid retention persists despite adherence to a prescribed diet, hidden sources of sodium, such as the water supply or use of water softeners, should be considered.

### Detecting and Controlling Fluid Volume Excess

It is important to detect FVE before the condition becomes critical. Interventions include promoting rest, restricting sodium intake, monitoring parenteral fluid therapy, and administering appropriate medications.

Regular rest periods may be beneficial, because bed rest favors diuresis of edema fluid. The mechanism is probably related to diminished venous pooling and the subsequent increase in effective circulating blood volume and renal perfusion. Sodium and fluid restriction should be instituted as indicated. Because most patients with FVE require diuretics, the patient's response to these agents is monitored. The rate of parenteral fluids and the patient's response to these fluids are also closely monitored. If dyspnea or orthopnea is present, the patient is placed in a semi-Fowler's position to promote lung expansion. The patient is turned and positioned at regular intervals because edematous tissue is more prone to skin breakdown than normal tissue. Because conditions predisposing to FVE are likely to be chronic, patients are taught to monitor their response to therapy by documenting fluid intake and output and body weight changes. The importance of adhering to the treatment regimen is emphasized.

## Teaching Patients About Edema

Because edema is a common manifestation of FVE, patients need to recognize its symptoms and understand its importance. The nurse gives special attention to edema when teaching the patient with FVE. Edema can occur as a result of increased capillary fluid pressure, decreased capillary oncotic pressure, or increased interstitial oncotic pressure, causing expansion of the interstitial fluid compartment (Porth, 2005). Edema can be localized (eg, in the ankle, as in rheumatoid arthritis) or generalized (as in cardiac and renal failure). Severe generalized edema is called *anasarca*.

Edema occurs when there is a change in the capillary membrane, increasing the formation of interstitial fluid or decreasing the removal of interstitial fluid. Sodium retention is a frequent cause of the increased ECF volume. Burns and infection are examples of conditions associated with increased interstitial fluid volume. Obstruction to lymphatic outflow, a plasma albumin level less than 1.5 to 2 g/dL, or a decrease in plasma oncotic pressure contributes to increased interstitial fluid volume. The kidneys retain sodium and water when there is decreased ECF volume as a result of decreased cardiac output from heart failure. A thorough medication history is necessary to identify any medications that could cause edema, such as nonsteroidal anti-inflammatory drugs (NSAIDs), estrogens, corticosteroids, and antihypertensive agents.

Ascites is a form of edema in which fluid accumulates in the peritoneal cavity; it results from nephrotic syndrome, cirrhosis, and some malignant tumors. The patient commonly reports shortness of breath and a sense of pressure because of pressure on the diaphragm.

Edema usually affects dependent areas. It can be seen in the ankles, sacrum, scrotum, or the periorbital region of the face. Pitting edema is so named because a pit forms after a finger is pressed into edematous tissue. In pulmonary edema, the amount of fluid in the pulmonary interstitium and the alveoli increases. Manifestations include shortness of breath, increased respiratory rate, diaphoresis, and crackles and wheezing on auscultation of the lungs. Decreased hematocrit resulting from hemodilution, arterial blood gas results indicative of respiratory **alkalosis** and hypoxemia, and decreased serum sodium and osmolality from retention of fluid may occur with edema. BUN and creatinine levels increase, urine specific gravity decreases as the kidneys attempt to excrete excess water, and the urine sodium level decreases because of increased aldosterone production.

The goal of treatment is to preserve or restore the circulating intravascular fluid volume. In addition to treating the cause, other treatments may include diuretic therapy, restriction of fluids and sodium, elevation of the extremities, application of elastic compression stockings, paracentesis, dialysis, and continuous renal replacement therapy in cases of renal failure or life-threatening fluid volume overload (See Chapter 44).

# Electrolyte Imbalances

Disturbances in electrolyte balances are common in clinical practice and must be corrected for the patient's health and safety. Table 14-5 summarizes the major fluid and electrolyte imbalances that are described in this chapter. An example of an electrolyte imbalance is an altered sodium balance.

## Sodium Imbalances

Sodium is the most abundant electrolyte in the ECF; its concentration ranges from 135 to 145 mEq/L (135 to 145 mmol/L). Consequently, sodium is the primary determinant of ECF osmolality. Decreased sodium is associated with parallel changes in osmolality. Sodium has a major role in controlling water distribution throughout the body, because it does not easily cross the cell wall membrane and because of its abundance and high concentration in the body. Sodium is regulated by ADH, thirst, and the renin–angiotensin–aldosterone system. It is the primary regulator of ECF volume. A loss or gain of sodium is usually accompanied by a loss or gain of water. Sodium also functions in establishing the electrochemical state necessary for muscle contraction and the transmission of nerve impulses.

Sodium imbalance occurs frequently in clinical practice and can develop under simple or complex circumstances. The two most common sodium imbalances are sodium deficit and sodium excess.

## Sodium Deficit (Hyponatremia)

Hyponatremia refers to a serum sodium level that is below normal (less than 135 mEq/L [135 mmol/L]). Plasma sodium concentration represents the ratio of total body sodium to total body water. A decrease in this ratio can occur because of a low quantity of total body sodium with a lesser reduction in total body water, normal total body sodium content with excess total body water, or an excess of total body sodium with an even greater excess of total body water. However, a hyponatremic state can be superimposed on an existing FVD or FVE.

Sodium may be lost by way of vomiting, diarrhea, fistulas, or sweating, or it may be lost as the result of the use of diuretics, particularly in combination with a low-salt diet. A deficiency of aldosterone, as occurs in adrenal insufficiency, also predisposes to sodium deficiency.

In dilutional hyponatremia (water intoxication), the patient's serum sodium level is diluted by an increase in the ratio of water to sodium. Dilutional hyponatremia, therefore, results from an increased extracellular fluid volume and a normal or increased total body sodium. Predisposing conditions for this type of hyponatremia include syndrome of inappropriate secretion of antidiuretic hormone (SIADH); hyperglycemia; and increased water intake through the administration of electrolyte-poor parenteral fluids, the use of tap-water enemas, or the irrigation of nasogastric tubes with water instead of normal saline solution. Water may be gained abnormally by the excessive parenteral administration of dextrose and water solutions, particularly during periods of stress. It may also be gained by compulsive water drinking (psychogenic polydipsia).

The basic physiologic disturbances in SIADH are excessive ADH activity, with water retention and dilutional hy-

*(text continues on page 318)*

## TABLE 14-5  Major Fluid and Electrolyte Imbalances

| Imbalance | Contributing Factors | Signs/Symptoms and Laboratory Findings |
|---|---|---|
| Fluid volume deficit (hypovolemia) | Loss of water and electrolytes, as in vomiting, diarrhea, fistulas, fever, excess sweating, burns, blood loss, gastrointestinal suction, and third-space fluid shifts; and decreased intake, as in anorexia, nausea, and inability to gain access to fluid. Diabetes insipidus and uncontrolled diabetes mellitus also contribute to a depletion of extracellular fluid volume. | Acute weight loss, decreased skin turgor, oliguria, concentrated urine, weak rapid pulse, capillary filling time prolonged, low CVP, ↓ blood pressure, flattened neck veins, dizziness, weakness, thirst and confusion, ↑ pulse, muscle cramps, sunken eyes<br>*Labs indicate:* ↑ hemoglobin and hematocrit, ↑ serum and urine osmolality and specific gravity, ↓ urine sodium, ↑ BUN and creatinine, ↑ urine specific gravity and osmolality |
| Fluid volume excess (hypervolemia) | Compromised regulatory mechanisms, such as renal failure, heart failure, and cirrhosis; overzealous administration of sodium-containing fluids; and fluid shifts (ie, treatment of burns). Prolonged corticosteroid therapy, severe stress, and hyperaldosteronism augment fluid volume excess. | Acute weight gain, peripheral edema and ascites, distended jugular veins, crackles, and elevated CVP, shortness of breath, ↑ blood pressure, bounding pulse and cough, ↑ respiratory rate<br>*Labs indicate:* ↓ hemoglobin and hematocrit, ↓ serum and urine osmolality, ↓ urine sodium and specific gravity |
| Sodium deficit (hyponatremia) Serum sodium <135 mEq/L | Loss of sodium, as in use of diuretics, loss of GI fluids, renal disease, and adrenal insufficiency. Gain of water, as in excessive administration of $D_5W$ and water supplements for patients receiving hypotonic tube feedings; disease states associated with SIADH such as head trauma and oat-cell lung tumor; medications associated with water retention (oxytocin and certain tranquilizers); and psychogenic polydipsia. Hyperglycemia and heart failure cause a loss of sodium. | Anorexia, nausea and vomiting, headache, lethargy, dizziness, confusion, muscle cramps and weakness, muscular twitching, seizures, papilledema, dry skin, ↑ pulse, ↓ BP, weight gain, edema<br>*Labs indicate:* ↓ serum and urine sodium, ↓ urine specific gravity and osmolality |
| Sodium excess (hypernatremia) Serum sodium >145 mEq/L | Water deprivation in patients unable to drink at will, hypertonic tube feedings without adequate water supplements, diabetes insipidus, heatstroke, hyperventilation, watery diarrhea, burns, and diaphoresis. Excess corticosteroid, sodium bicarbonate, and sodium chloride administration, and salt water near-drowning victims. | Thirst, elevated body temperature, swollen dry tongue and sticky mucous membranes, hallucinations, lethargy, restlessness, irritability, focal or grand mal seizures, pulmonary edema, hyperreflexia, twitching, nausea, vomiting, anorexia, ↑ pulse, and ↑ BP.<br>*Labs indicate.* ↑ serum sodium, ↓ urine sodium, ↑ urine specific gravity and osmolality, ↓ CVP |
| Potassium deficit (hypokalemia) Serum potassium <3.5 mEq/L | Diarrhea, vomiting, gastric suction, corticosteroid administration, hyperaldosteronism, carbenicillin, amphotericin B, bulimia, osmotic diuresis, alkalosis, starvation, diuretics, and digoxin toxicity | Fatigue, anorexia, nausea and vomiting, muscle weakness, polyuria, decreased bowel motility, ventricular asystole or fibrillation, paresthesias, leg cramps, ↓ BP, ileus, abdominal distention, hypoactive reflexes. *ECG:* flattened T waves, prominent U waves, ST depression, prolonged PR interval. |
| Potassium excess (hyperkalemia) Serum potassium >5.0 mEq/L | Pseudohyperkalemia, oliguric renal failure, use of potassium-conserving diuretics in patients with renal insufficiency, metabolic acidosis, Addison's disease, crush injury, burns, stored bank blood transfusions, and rapid IV administration of potassium | Vague muscular weakness, tachycardia → bradycardia, dysrhythmias, flaccid paralysis, paresthesias, intestinal colic, cramps, irritability, anxiety. *ECG:* tall tented T waves, prolonged PR interval and QRS duration, absent P waves, ST depression. |
| Calcium deficit (hypocalcemia) Serum calcium <8.5 mg/dL | Hypoparathyroidism (may follow thyroid surgery or radical neck dissection), malabsorption, pancreatitis, alkalosis, vitamin D deficiency, massive subcutaneous infection, generalized peritonitis, massive transfusion of citrated blood, chronic diarrhea, decreased parathyroid hormone, diuretic phase of renal failure, ↑ $PO_4$, fistulas, burns | Numbness, tingling of fingers, toes, and circumoral region; positive Trousseau's sign and Chvostek's sign; seizures, carpopedal spasms, hyperactive deep tendon reflexes, irritability, bronchospasm, anxiety, impaired clotting time, ↓ prothrombin. *ECG:* prolonged QT interval and lengthened ST.<br>*Labs indicate.* ↓ $Mg^{++}$ |

## TABLE 14-5    Major Fluid and Electrolyte Imbalances (Continued)

| Imbalance | Contributing Factors | Signs/Symptoms and Laboratory Findings |
|---|---|---|
| Calcium excess (hypercalcemia) Serum calcium >10.5 mg/dL | Hyperparathyroidism, malignant neoplastic disease, prolonged immobilization, overuse of calcium supplements, vitamin D excess, oliguric phase of renal failure, acidosis, corticosteroid therapy, thiazide diuretic use, increased parathyroid hormone, and digoxin toxicity | Muscular weakness, constipation, anorexia, nausea and vomiting, polyuria and polydipsia, dehydration, hypoactive deep tendon reflexes, lethargy, deep bone pain, pathologic fractures, flank pain, and calcium stones. *ECG:* shortened ST segment and QT interval, bradycardia, heart blocks. |
| Magnesium deficit (hypomagnesemia) Serum magnesium <1.8 mg/dL | Chronic alcoholism, hyperparathyroidism, hyperaldosteronism, diuretic phase of renal failure, malabsorptive disorders, diabetic ketoacidosis, refeeding after starvation, parenteral nutrition, chronic laxative use, diarrhea, acute myocardial infarction, heart failure, decreased serum K$^+$ and Ca$^{++}$ and certain pharmacologic agents (such as gentamicin, cisplatin, and cyclosporine) | Neuromuscular irritability, positive Trousseau's and Chvostek's signs, insomnia, mood changes, anorexia, vomiting, increased tendon reflexes, and ↑ BP. *ECG:* PVCs, flat or inverted T waves, depressed ST segment, prolonged PR interval and widened QRS |
| Magnesium excess (hypermagnesemia) Serum magnesium >2.7 mg/dL | Oliguric phase of renal failure (particularly when magnesium-containing medications are administered), adrenal insufficiency, excessive IV magnesium administration, DKA, and hypothyroidism | Flushing, hypotension, drowsiness, hypoactive reflexes, depressed respirations, cardiac arrest and coma, diaphoresis. *ECG:* tachycardia → bradycardia, prolonged PR interval and QRS. |
| Phosphorus deficit (hypophosphatemia) Serum phosphorus <2.5 mg/dL | Refeeding after starvation, alcohol withdrawal, diabetic ketoacidosis, respiratory alkalosis, ↓ magnesium, ↓ potassium, hyperparathyroidism, vomiting, diarrhea, hyperventilation, vitamin D deficiency associated with malabsorptive disorders, burns, acid–base disorders, parenteral nutrition, and diuretic and antacid use | Paresthesias, muscle weakness, bone pain and tenderness, chest pain, confusion, cardiomyopathy, respiratory failure, seizures, tissue hypoxia, and increased susceptibility to infection, nystagmus |
| Phosphorus excess (hyperphosphatemia) Serum phosphorus >4.5 mg/dL | Acute and chronic renal failure, excessive intake of phosphorus, vitamin D excess, respiratory acidosis, hypoparathyroidism, volume depletion, leukemia/lymphoma treated with cytotoxic agents, increased tissue breakdown, rhabdomyolysis | Tetany, tachycardia, anorexia, nausea and vomiting, muscle weakness, signs and symptoms of hypocalcemia; hyperactive reflexes; soft tissue calcifications in lungs, heart, kidneys, and cornea |
| Chloride deficit (hypochloremia) Serum chloride <96 mEq/L | Addison's disease, reduced chloride intake or absorption, untreated diabetic ketoacidosis, chronic respiratory acidosis, excessive sweating, vomiting, gastric suction, diarrhea, sodium and potassium deficiency, metabolic alkalosis; loop, osmotic, or thiazide diuretic use; overuse of bicarbonate, rapid removal of ascitic fluid with a high sodium content, intravenous fluids that lack chloride (dextrose and water), draining fistulas and ileostomies, heart failure, cystic fibrosis | Agitation, irritability, tremors, muscle cramps, hyperactive deep tendon reflexes, hypertonicity, tetany, slow shallow respirations, seizures, dysrhythmias, coma *Labs indicate:* ↓ serum chloride, ↓ serum sodium, ↑ pH, ↑ serum bicarbonate, ↑ total carbon dioxide content, ↓ urine chloride level, ↓ serum potassium |
| Chloride excess (hyperchloremia) Serum chloride >108 mEq/L | Excessive sodium chloride infusions with water loss, head injury (sodium retention), hypernatremia, renal failure, corticosteroid use, dehydration, severe diarrhea (loss of bicarbonate), respiratory alkalosis, administration of diuretics, overdose of salicylates, Kayexalate, acetazolamide, phenylbutazone and ammonium chloride use, hyperparathyroidism, metabolic acidosis | Tachypnea, lethargy, weakness, deep rapid respirations, decline in cognitive status, decreased cardiac output, dyspnea, tachycardia, pitting edema, dysrhythmias, coma *Labs indicate:* ↑ serum chloride, ↑ serum potassium and sodium, ↓ serum pH, ↓ serum bicarbonate, normal anion gap, ↑ urinary chloride level |

↑ increased; ↓ decreased; BP, blood pressure; BUN, blood urea nitrogen; CVP, central venous pressure; DKA, diabetic ketoacidosis; GI, gastrointestinal; IV, intravenous; PVCs, premature ventricular contractions; SIADH, syndrome of inappropriate secretion of antidiuretic hormone.

ponatremia, and inappropriate urinary excretion of sodium in the presence of hyponatremia. SIADH can be the result of either sustained secretion of ADH by the hypothalamus or production of an ADH-like substance from a tumor (aberrant ADH production). Conditions associated with SIADH include oat-cell lung tumors; head injuries; endocrine and pulmonary disorders; physical or psychological stress; and the use of medications such as oxytocin, cyclophosphamide, vincristine, thioridazine, and amitriptyline. SIADH is discussed in more detail in Chapter 42.

## Clinical Manifestations

Clinical manifestations of hyponatremia depend on the cause, magnitude, and speed with which the deficit occurs. Poor skin turgor, dry mucosa, headache, decreased saliva production, orthostatic fall in blood pressure, nausea, and abdominal cramping occur. Neurologic changes, including altered mental status, status epilepticus, coma, and obtundation, are probably related to the cellular swelling and cerebral edema associated with hyponatremia. As the extracellular sodium level decreases, the cellular fluid becomes relatively more concentrated and pulls water into the cells (Fig. 14-4). In general, patients with an acute decrease in serum sodium levels have more cerebral edema and higher mortality rates than do those with more slowly developing hyponatremia. Acute decreases in sodium, developing in less than 48 hours, may be associated with brain herniation and compression of midbrain structures. Chronic decreases in sodium, developing over 48 hours or more, can occur in status epilepticus and cerebral pontine myelinolysis.

Features of hyponatremia associated with sodium loss and water gain include anorexia, muscle cramps, and a feeling of exhaustion. The severity of symptoms increases with the degree of hyponatremia and the speed with which it develops. When the serum sodium level decreases to less than 115 mEq/L (115 mmol/L), signs of increasing intracranial pressure, such as lethargy, confusion, muscle twitching, focal weakness, hemiparesis, papilledema, and seizures, may occur.

## Assessment and Diagnostic Findings

Regardless of the cause of hyponatremia, the serum sodium level is less than 135 mEq/L; in SIADH it may be as low as 100 mEq/L (100 mmol/L) or even less. Serum osmolality is also decreased, except in azotemia or ingestion of toxins. When hyponatremia is due primarily to sodium loss, the urinary sodium content is less than 20 mEq/L (20 mmol/L), suggesting increased proximal reabsorption of sodium secondary to ECF volume depletion, and the specific gravity is low (1.002 to 1.004). However, when hyponatremia is due to SIADH, the urinary sodium content is greater than 20 mEq/L, and the urine specific gravity is usually greater than 1.012. Although the patient with SIADH retains water abnormally and therefore gains body weight, there is no peripheral edema; instead, fluid accumulates inside the cells. This phenomenon is sometimes manifested as "fingerprinting" when the finger is pressed over a bony prominence, such as the sternum.

## Medical Management

The key to treating hyponatremia is assessment; this includes assessment of the speed with which hyponatremia occurred, as well as assessment of the patient's actual serum sodium value (Elgart, 2004).

### SODIUM REPLACEMENT

The obvious treatment for hyponatremia is careful administration of sodium by mouth, nasogastric tube, or a parenteral route. For patients who can eat and drink, sodium is easily replaced, because sodium is consumed abundantly in a normal diet. For those who cannot consume sodium, lactated Ringer's solution or isotonic saline (0.9% sodium chloride) solution may be prescribed. Serum sodium must not be increased by more than 12 mEq/L in 24 hours, to avoid neurologic damage due to osmotic demyelination. This condition may occur when the serum sodium concentration is overcorrected (exceeding 140 mEq/L) too rapidly or in the presence of hypoxia or anoxia (Lin, Hsu & Chiu, 2003). It may produce lesions in the pons that cause paraparesis, dysarthria, dysphagia, and coma. The usual daily sodium requirement in adults is approximately 100 mEq, provided there are no abnormal losses. Selected water and electrolyte solutions are described in Table 14-4.

In SIADH, the administration of hypertonic saline solution alone cannot change the plasma sodium concentration. Excess sodium would be excreted rapidly in a highly concentrated urine. With the addition of the diuretic furosemide (Lasix), urine is not concentrated and isotonic urine is excreted to effect a change in water balance. In patients with SIADH, in whom water restriction is difficult, lithium or demeclocycline can antagonize the osmotic effect of ADH on the medullary collecting tubule.

### WATER RESTRICTION

In a patient with normal or excess fluid volume, hyponatremia is treated by restricting fluid to a total of 800 mL

**FIGURE 14-4.** Effect of extracellular sodium level on cell size.

in 24 hours. This is far safer than sodium administration and is usually effective. However, if neurologic symptoms are present, it may be necessary to administer small volumes of a hypertonic sodium solution, such as 3% or 5% sodium chloride. Incorrect use of these fluids is extremely dangerous, because 1 L of 3% sodium chloride solution contains 513 mEq of sodium and 1 L of 5% sodium chloride solution contains 855 mEq of sodium. If edema exists alone, sodium is restricted; if edema and hyponatremia occur together, both sodium and water are restricted.

> **NURSING ALERT**
>
> Highly hypertonic sodium solutions (3% and 5% sodium chloride) should be administered only in intensive care settings under close observation, because only small volumes are needed to elevate the serum sodium concentration from a dangerously low level. These fluids are administered slowly and in small volumes, and the patient is monitored closely for fluid overload. The purpose is to relieve acute manifestations of cerebral edema and to prevent neurologic complications rather than to specifically correct the sodium concentration. Along with the sodium solution, the patient may receive a loop diuretic to prevent ECF volume overload and to increase water excretion.

## Nursing Management

The nurse needs to identify patients at risk of hyponatremia so that they can be monitored. Early detection and treatment of this disorder are necessary to prevent serious consequences. For patients at risk, the nurse monitors fluid I&O as well as daily body weight. It is also necessary to note abnormal losses of sodium or gains of water, as well as GI manifestations such as anorexia, nausea, vomiting, and abdominal cramping. The nurse must be particularly alert for central nervous system changes, such as lethargy, confusion, muscle twitching, and seizures. In general, more severe neurologic signs are associated with very low sodium levels that have fallen rapidly because of fluid overloading. Serum sodium is monitored very closely in patients who are at risk for hyponatremia; when indicated, urine sodium and specific gravity are also monitored.

Hyponatremia is a frequently overlooked cause of confusion in elderly patients, who have an increased risk for hyponatremia because of changes in renal function and subsequent decreased ability to excrete excessive water loads. Administration of medications causing sodium loss or water retention is a predisposing factor.

### DETECTING AND CONTROLLING HYPONATREMIA

For a patient who is experiencing abnormal losses of sodium and can consume a general diet, the nurse encourages foods and fluids with a high sodium content. For example, broth made with one beef cube contains approximately 900 mg of sodium; 8 oz of tomato juice contains approximately 700 mg of sodium. The nurse also needs to be familiar with the sodium content of parenteral fluids (see Table 14-4).

> **NURSING ALERT**
>
> When administering fluids to patients with cardiovascular disease, the nurse assesses for signs of circulatory overload (eg, cough, dyspnea, puffy eyelids, dependent edema, weight gain in 24 hours). The lungs are auscultated for crackles. Extreme care is taken when administering highly hypertonic sodium fluids (eg, 3% or 5% sodium chloride), because these fluids can be lethal if infused carelessly.

For the patient taking lithium, the nurse observes for lithium toxicity, particularly when sodium is lost by an abnormal route. In such instances, supplemental salt and fluid are administered. Because diuretics promote sodium loss, the patient taking lithium is instructed not to use diuretics without close medical supervision. For all patients on lithium therapy, adequate salt intake should be ensured.

Excess water supplements are avoided in patients receiving isotonic or hypotonic enteral feedings, particularly if abnormal sodium loss occurs or water is being abnormally retained (as in SIADH). Actual fluid needs are determined by evaluating fluid I&O, urine specific gravity, and serum sodium levels.

### RETURNING THE SODIUM LEVEL TO NORMAL

If the primary problem is water retention, it is safer to restrict fluid intake than to administer sodium. Administering sodium to a patient with normovolemia or hypervolemia predisposes the patient to fluid volume overload. As stated previously, the nurse must monitor the patient with cardiovascular disease very closely.

In severe hyponatremia, the aim of therapy is to elevate the serum sodium level only enough to alleviate neurologic signs and symptoms. It is generally recommended that the serum sodium concentration be increased to no greater than 125 mEq/L (125 mmol/L) with a hypertonic saline solution.

## Sodium Excess (Hypernatremia)

Hypernatremia is a higher-than-normal serum sodium level (exceeding 145 mEq/L [145 mmol/L]) (Kee, Paulanka & Purnell, 2004). It can be caused by a gain of sodium in excess of water or by a loss of water in excess of sodium. It can occur in patients with normal fluid volume or in those with FVD or FVE. With a water loss, the patient loses more water than sodium; as a result, the serum sodium concentration increases and the increased concentration pulls fluid out of the cell. This is both an extracellular and an intracellular FVD. In sodium excess, the patient ingests or retains more sodium than water.

A common cause of hypernatremia is fluid deprivation in unconscious patients who cannot perceive, respond to, or communicate their thirst (Porth, 2005). Most often affected are very old, very young, and cognitively impaired patients. Administration of hypertonic enteral feedings without adequate water supplements leads to hypernatremia, as does watery diarrhea and greatly increased insensible water loss (eg, hyperventilation, denuding effects of burns).

Diabetes insipidus, a deficiency of ADH from the posterior pituitary gland, leads to hypernatremia if the patient does not experience, or cannot respond to, thirst, or if fluids are excessively restricted. Neurogenic or nephrogenic causes of diabetes insipidus should be considered in the assessment (Olson, Meek & Lynch, 2004).

Less common causes of hypernatremia are heat stroke, near-drowning in sea water (which contains a sodium concentration of approximately 500 mEq/L), and malfunction of either hemodialysis or peritoneal dialysis proportioning systems. IV administration of hypertonic saline or excessive use of sodium bicarbonate also causes hypernatremia (Porth, 2005).

## Clinical Manifestations

The clinical manifestations of hypernatremia are primarily neurologic and are the consequence of increased plasma osmolality caused by an increase in plasma sodium concentration. Water moves out of the cell into the ECF, resulting in cellular dehydration (Rose & Post, 2000). Hypernatremia leads to a relatively concentrated ECF (see Fig. 14-4). Clinically, these changes may be manifested by restlessness and weakness in moderate hypernatremia and by disorientation, delusions, and hallucinations in severe hypernatremia. Dehydration (resulting in hypernatremia) is often overlooked as the primary reason for behavioral changes in elderly patients. If hypernatremia is severe, permanent brain damage can occur (especially in children). Brain damage is apparently due to subarachnoid hemorrhages that result from brain contraction.

A primary characteristic of hypernatremia is thirst. Thirst is such a strong *defender* of serum sodium levels in healthy people that hypernatremia never occurs unless the person is unconscious or does not have access to water. However, ill people may have an impaired thirst mechanism. Other signs include a dry, swollen tongue and sticky mucous membranes. Flushed skin, peripheral and pulmonary edema, postural hypotension, and increased muscle tone and deep tendon reflexes are additional signs and symptoms of hypernatremia. Body temperature may increase mildly, but it returns to normal after the hypernatremia is corrected.

## Assessment and Diagnostic Findings

In hypernatremia, the serum sodium level exceeds 145 mEq/L (145 mmol/L) and the serum osmolality exceeds 300 mOsm/kg (300 mmol/L). The urine specific gravity and urine osmolality are increased as the kidneys attempt to conserve water (provided the water loss is from a route other than the kidneys) (Rose & Post, 2000).

## Medical Management

Treatment of hypernatremia consists of a gradual lowering of the serum sodium level by the infusion of a hypotonic electrolyte solution (eg, 0.3% sodium chloride) or an isotonic nonsaline solution (eg, dextrose 5% in water [$D_5W$]). $D_5W$ is indicated when water needs to be replaced without sodium. Many clinicians consider a hypotonic sodium solution to be safer than $D_5W$ because it allows a gradual reduction in the serum sodium level, thereby decreasing the risk of cerebral edema. It is the solution of choice in severe hyperglycemia with hypernatremia. A rapid reduction in the serum sodium level temporarily decreases the plasma osmolality below that of the fluid in the brain tissue, causing dangerous cerebral edema. Diuretics also may be prescribed to treat the sodium gain.

There is no consensus about the exact rate at which serum sodium levels should be reduced. As a general rule, the serum sodium level is reduced at a rate no faster than 0.5 to 1 mEq/L per hour to allow sufficient time for readjustment through diffusion across fluid compartments. Desmopressin acetate (DDAVP), a synthetic antidiuretic hormone, may be prescribed to treat diabetes insipidus if it is the cause of hypernatremia (Porth, 2005).

## Nursing Management

As in hyponatremia, fluid losses and gains are carefully monitored in patients who are at risk for hypernatremia. The nurse should assess for abnormal losses of water or low water intake and for large gains of sodium, as might occur with ingestion of over-the-counter medications that have a high sodium content (eg, Alka-Seltzer). In addition, the nurse obtains a medication history, because some prescription medications have a high sodium content. The nurse also notes the patient's thirst or elevated body temperature and evaluates it in relation to other clinical signs. The nurse monitors for changes in behavior, such as restlessness, disorientation, and lethargy.

### PREVENTING HYPERNATREMIA

The nurse attempts to prevent hypernatremia by offering fluids at regular intervals, particularly in debilitated or unconscious patients who are unable to perceive or respond to thirst. If fluid intake remains inadequate, the nurse consults with the physician to plan an alternative route for intake, either by enteral feedings or by the parenteral route. If enteral feedings are used, sufficient water should be administered to keep the serum sodium and BUN within normal limits. As a rule, the higher the osmolality of the enteral feeding, the greater the need for water supplementation.

For patients with diabetes insipidus, adequate water intake must be ensured. If the patient is alert and has an intact thirst mechanism, merely providing access to water may be sufficient. If the patient has a decreased level of consciousness or other disability interfering with adequate fluid intake, parenteral fluid replacement may be prescribed. This therapy can be anticipated in patients with neurologic disorders, particularly in the early postoperative period.

### CORRECTING HYPERNATREMIA

When parenteral fluids are necessary for managing hypernatremia, the nurse monitors the patient's response to the fluids by reviewing serial serum sodium levels and by observing for changes in neurologic signs. With a gradual decrease in the serum sodium level, the neurologic signs should improve. As stated in the discussion on management, too-rapid reduction in the serum sodium level renders the plasma temporarily hypo-osmotic to the fluid in the brain tissue, causing movement of fluid into brain cells and dangerous cerebral edema (Hankins, Lonsway-Waldman, Hedrick, et al., 2001).

## Potassium Imbalances

Potassium is the major intracellular electrolyte; in fact, 98% of the body's potassium is inside the cells. The remaining 2% is in the ECF, and it is this 2% that is important in neuromuscular function. Potassium influences both skeletal and cardiac muscle activity. For example, alterations in its concentration change myocardial irritability and rhythm. Under the influence of the sodium–potassium pump and based on the body's needs, potassium is constantly moving in and out of cells. The normal serum potassium concentration ranges from 3.5 to 5.0 mEq/L (3.5 to 5 mmol/L), and even minor variations are significant. Potassium imbalances are commonly associated with various diseases, injuries, medications (diuretics, laxatives, antibiotics), and special treatments, such as parenteral nutrition and chemotherapy (Hogan & Wane, 2003).

To maintain potassium balance, the renal system must function, because 80% of the potassium excreted daily leaves the body by way of the kidneys; the other 20% is lost through the bowel and in sweat. The kidneys are the primary regulators of potassium balance; they accomplish this by adjusting the amount of potassium that is excreted in the urine. As serum potassium levels increase, so does the potassium level in the renal tubular cell. A concentration gradient occurs, favoring the movement of potassium into the renal tubule, with subsequent loss of potassium in the urine. Aldosterone also increases the excretion of potassium by the kidney. Because the kidneys do not conserve potassium as well as they conserve sodium, potassium may still be lost in urine in the presence of a potassium deficit.

## Potassium Deficit (Hypokalemia)

Hypokalemia (below-normal serum potassium concentration) usually indicates an actual deficit in total potassium stores. However, it may occur in patients with normal potassium stores: when alkalosis is present, a temporary shift of serum potassium into the cells occurs (see later discussion).

As previously stated, hypokalemia is a common imbalance, especially with the use of diuretics. GI loss of potassium is probably the most common cause of potassium depletion (Burger, 2004b). Vomiting and gastric suction frequently lead to hypokalemia, partly because potassium is actually lost when gastric fluid is lost, but more so because potassium is lost through the kidneys in association with metabolic alkalosis. Because relatively large amounts of potassium are contained in intestinal fluids, potassium deficit occurs frequently with diarrhea. Intestinal fluid may contain as much potassium as 30 mEq/L. Potassium deficit also occurs from prolonged intestinal suctioning, recent ileostomy, and villous adenoma (a tumor of the intestinal tract characterized by excretion of potassium-rich mucus).

Alterations in acid–base balance have a significant effect on potassium distribution. The mechanism involves shifts of hydrogen and potassium ions between the cells and the ECF. Hypokalemia can cause alkalosis, and in turn alkalosis can cause hypokalemia (Burger, 2004b). For example, hydrogen ions move out of the cells in alkalotic states to help correct the high pH, and potassium ions move in to maintain an electrically neutral state (see later discussion of acid–base balance).

Hyperaldosteronism increases renal potassium wasting and can lead to severe potassium depletion. Primary hyperaldosteronism is seen in patients with adrenal adenomas. Secondary hyperaldosteronism occurs in patients with cirrhosis, nephrotic syndrome, heart failure, or malignant hypertension (Heitz & Horne, 2005).

Potassium-losing diuretics, such as the thiazides (eg, chlorothiazide [Diuril] and polythiazide [Renese]), can induce hypokalemia, particularly when administered in large doses to patients with inadequate potassium intake (Burger, 2004b). Other medications that can lead to hypokalemia include corticosteroids, sodium penicillin, carbenicillin, and amphotericin B.

Because insulin promotes the entry of potassium into skeletal muscle and hepatic cells, patients with persistent insulin hypersecretion may experience hypokalemia, which is often the case in patients receiving high-carbohydrate parenteral fluids (as in parenteral nutrition).

Patients who are unable or unwilling to eat a normal diet for a prolonged period are at risk for hypokalemia. This may occur in debilitated elderly people, patients with alcoholism, and patients with anorexia nervosa. In addition to poor intake, people with bulimia frequently suffer increased potassium loss through self-induced vomiting and laxative and diuretic abuse (Burger, 2004b).

Magnesium depletion causes renal potassium loss and must be corrected first; otherwise, urine loss of potassium will continue. Penicillins may produce renal potassium loss by acting as poorly reabsorbable anions and thereby increasing distal sodium delivery and sodium–potassium loss.

### Clinical Manifestations

Potassium deficiency can result in widespread derangements in physiologic function. Severe hypokalemia can cause death through cardiac or respiratory arrest. Clinical signs rarely develop before the serum potassium level has decreased to less than 3 mEq/L (3 mmol/L) unless the rate of decline has been rapid. Manifestations of hypokalemia include fatigue, anorexia, nausea, vomiting, muscle weakness, leg cramps, decreased bowel motility, paresthesias (numbness and tingling), dysrhythmias, and increased sensitivity to digitalis. If prolonged, hypokalemia can lead to an inability of the kidneys to concentrate urine, causing dilute urine (resulting in polyuria, nocturia) and excessive thirst. Potassium depletion depresses the release of insulin and results in glucose intolerance. Decreased muscle strength and tendon reflexes can be found on physical assessment.

## Assessment and Diagnostic Findings

In hypokalemia, the serum potassium concentration is less than the lower limit of normal. Electrocardiographic (ECG) changes can include flat T waves or inverted T waves or both, suggesting ischemia, and depressed ST segments (Fig. 14-5). An elevated U wave is specific to hypokalemia. Hypokalemia increases sensitivity to digitalis, predisposing the patient to digitalis toxicity at lower digitalis levels.

**FIGURE 14-5.** Effect of potassium on the electrocardiogram (ECG). **(A)** Normal tracing. **(B)** Hypokalemia: serum potassium level below normal. *Left,* flattening of the T wave and the appearance of a U wave. *Right,* further flattening with prominent U wave. **(C)** Hyperkalemia: serum potassium level above normal. *Left,* moderate elevation with wide, flat P wave, wide QRS complex, and peaked T wave. *Right,* ECG changes seen with extreme potassium elevation: widening of QRS complex and absence of P wave.

Metabolic alkalosis is commonly associated with hypokalemia (Burger, 2004b). This is discussed further in the section on acid–base disturbances.

The source of the potassium loss is usually evident from a careful history. However, if the cause of the loss is unclear, a 24-hour urinary potassium excretion test can be performed to distinguish between renal and extrarenal loss. Urinary potassium excretion exceeding 20 mEq/24 h with hypokalemia suggests that renal potassium loss is the cause.

## Medical Management

If hypokalemia cannot be prevented by conventional measures such as increased intake in the daily diet, it is treated with oral or IV replacement therapy (Kee et al., 2004). Potassium loss must be corrected daily; administration of 40 to 80 mEq/day of potassium is adequate in the adult if there are no abnormal losses of potassium.

For patients who are at risk for hypokalemia, a diet containing sufficient potassium should be provided. Dietary intake of potassium in the average adult is 50 to 100 mEq/day. Foods high in potassium include most fruits and vegetables, legumes, whole grains, milk, and meat.

If dietary intake is inadequate for any reason, the physician may prescribe oral or IV potassium supplements (Kee et al., 2004). Many salt substitutes contain 50 to 60 mEq of potassium per teaspoon and may be sufficient to prevent hypokalemia.

> **NURSING ALERT**
>
> Oral potassium supplements can produce small-bowel lesions; therefore, the patient must be assessed for and cautioned about abdominal distention, pain, or GI bleeding.

If oral administration of potassium is not feasible, the IV route is indicated. The IV route is mandatory for patients with severe hypokalemia (eg, serum level of 2 mEq/L). Although potassium chloride is usually used to correct potassium deficits, potassium acetate or potassium phosphate may be prescribed.

## Nursing Management

Because hypokalemia can be life-threatening, the nurse needs to monitor for its early presence in patients who are at risk. Fatigue, anorexia, muscle weakness, decreased bowel motility, paresthesias, and dysrhythmias are signals that warrant assessing the serum potassium concentration. When available, the ECG may provide useful information. For example, patients receiving digitalis who are at risk for potassium deficiency should be monitored closely for signs of digitalis toxicity, because hypokalemia potentiates the action of digitalis. Most physicians prefer to keep the serum potassium level greater than 3.5 mEq/L (3.5 mmol/L) in patients receiving digitalis medications such as digoxin.

### PREVENTING HYPOKALEMIA

Measures are taken to prevent hypokalemia when possible (Kee et al., 2004). Prevention may involve encouraging the patient at risk to eat foods rich in potassium (when the diet allows). Sources of potassium include fruit and fruit juices (bananas, melon, citrus fruit), fresh and frozen vegetables, fresh meats, milk, and processed foods. If the hypokalemia is caused by abuse of laxatives or diuretics, patient education may help alleviate the problem. Part of the health history and assessment should be directed at identifying problems that are amenable to prevention through education. Careful monitoring of fluid intake and output is necessary, because 40 mEq of potassium is lost for every liter of urine output. The ECG is monitored for changes, and arterial blood gas values are checked for elevated bicarbonate and pH levels.

### CORRECTING HYPOKALEMIA
Great care should be exercised when administering potassium, particularly in older adults, who have lower lean body mass and total body potassium levels and therefore lower potassium requirements. In addition, because of the physiologic loss of renal function with advancing years, potassium may be retained more readily in older than in younger people.

### ADMINISTERING INTRAVENOUS POTASSIUM
Potassium should be administered only after adequate urine flow has been established. A decrease in urine volume to less than 20 mL/h for 2 consecutive hours is an indication to stop the potassium infusion until the situation is evaluated. Potassium is primarily excreted by the kidneys; therefore, when oliguria occurs, potassium administration can cause the serum potassium concentration to rise dangerously (Burger, 2004b).

> **NURSING ALERT**
>
> Potassium is *never* administered by IV push or intramuscularly to avoid replacing potassium too quickly. IV potassium must be administered using an infusion pump.

Each health care facility has its own standard of care for the administration of potassium, which should be consulted; however, the maximum concentration of potassium that should be administered on a medical-surgical unit through a peripheral IV line is 20 mEq/100 mL and the rate no faster than 10 to 20 mEq/h. Concentrations of potassium greater than 20 mEq/100 mL should be administered through a central IV catheter using an infusion pump with the patient monitored by ECG. Caution must be used when selecting the correct premixed solution of IV fluid containing potassium chloride as the concentrations range from 10 to 40 mEq/100 mL. IV bags of 1000 mL of fluid containing potassium are also available with 20 to 40 mEq/L. Renal function should be monitored through BUN and creatinine levels and urine output if the patient is receiving potassium replacement (Morton, Fontaine, Hudak et al., 2005).

## Potassium Excess (Hyperkalemia)

Hyperkalemia (greater-than-normal serum potassium concentration) seldom occurs in patients with normal renal function. Like hypokalemia, hyperkalemia is often caused by iatrogenic (treatment-induced) causes. Although hyperkalemia is less common than hypokalemia, it is usually more dangerous, because cardiac arrest is more frequently associated with high serum potassium levels.

Pseudohyperkalemia (a variation of hyperkalemia) has a number of causes. The most common causes are the use of a tight tourniquet around an exercising extremity while drawing a blood sample and hemolysis of the sample before analysis. Other causes include marked leukocytosis (white blood cell count exceeding 200,000) or thrombocytosis (platelet count exceeding 1 million); drawing blood above a site where potassium is infusing; and familial pseudohyperkalemia; in which potassium leaks out of the red blood cells while the blood is awaiting analysis. Failure to be aware of these causes of pseudohyperkalemia can lead to aggressive treatment of a nonexistent hyperkalemia, resulting in serious lowering of serum potassium levels. Therefore, measurements of grossly elevated levels should be verified by retesting.

The major cause of hyperkalemia is decreased renal excretion of potassium (Burger, 2004a). For this reason, significant hyperkalemia is commonly seen in patients with untreated renal failure, particularly those in whom potassium levels increase as a result of infection or excessive intake of potassium in food or medications. In addition, patients with hypoaldosteronism or Addison's disease are at risk for hyperkalemia, because these conditions are characterized by deficient adrenal hormones, leading to sodium loss and potassium retention.

Medications have been identified as a probable contributing factor in more than 60% of hyperkalemic episodes. Medications commonly implicated are potassium chloride, heparin, ACE inhibitors, captopril, NSAIDs, and potassium-sparing diuretics (Palmer, 2004). In most such cases, potassium regulation is compromised by renal insufficiency (Burger, 2004a).

Although a high intake of potassium can cause severe hyperkalemia in patients with impaired renal function, hyperkalemia rarely occurs in people with normal renal function. However, improper use of potassium supplements predisposes all patients to hyperkalemia, especially if salt substitutes are used. Not all patients receiving potassium-losing diuretics require potassium supplements, and patients receiving potassium-conserving diuretics should not receive supplements.

> **NURSING ALERT**
>
> Potassium supplements are extremely dangerous for patients who have impaired renal function and thus decreased ability to excrete potassium. Even more dangerous is the IV administration of potassium to such patients, because serum levels can rise very quickly. Aged (stored) blood should not be administered to patients with impaired renal function, because the serum potassium concentration of stored blood increases as the storage time increases, a result of red blood cell deterioration. It is possible to exceed the renal tolerance of any patient with rapid IV potassium administration, as well as when large amounts of oral potassium supplements are ingested.

In **acidosis**, potassium moves out of the cells and into the ECF. This occurs as hydrogen ions enter the cells, a process that buffers the pH of the ECF (see later discussion). An elevated ECF potassium level should be anticipated when extensive tissue trauma has occurred, as in burns, crushing injuries, or severe infections. Similarly, it can occur with lysis of malignant cells after chemotherapy.

## Clinical Manifestations

The most important consequence of hyperkalemia is its effect on the myocardium. Cardiac effects of elevated serum potassium are usually not significant when the level is less than 7 mEq/L (7 mmol/L), but they are almost always present when the level is 8 mEq/L (8 mmol/L) or greater. As the plasma potassium level rises, disturbances in cardiac conduction occur. The earliest changes, often occurring at a serum potassium level greater than 6 mEq/L (6 mmol/L), are peaked, narrow T waves; ST-segment depression; and a shortened QT interval. If the serum potassium level continues to increase, the PR interval becomes prolonged and is followed by disappearance of the P waves. Finally, there is decomposition and prolongation of the QRS complex (see Fig. 14-5). Ventricular dysrhythmias and cardiac arrest may occur at any point in this progression.

Severe hyperkalemia causes skeletal muscle weakness and even paralysis, related to a depolarization block in muscle. Similarly, ventricular conduction is slowed. Although hyperkalemia has marked effects on the peripheral nervous system, it has little effect on the central nervous system. Rapidly ascending muscular weakness leading to flaccid quadriplegia has been reported in patients with very high serum potassium levels. Paralysis of respiratory and speech muscles can also occur. In addition, GI manifestations, such as nausea, intermittent intestinal colic, and diarrhea, may occur in hyperkalemic patients.

## Assessment and Diagnostic Findings

Serum potassium levels and ECG changes are crucial to the diagnosis of hyperkalemia, as discussed previously. Arterial blood gas analysis may reveal metabolic acidosis; in many cases, hyperkalemia occurs with acidosis (Burger, 2004a).

## Medical Management

An immediate ECG should be obtained to detect changes. Shortened repolarization and peaked T waves are seen initially. To verify results, it is also prudent to obtain a repeat serum potassium level from a vein without an IV infusing a potassium-containing solution.

In nonacute situations, restriction of dietary potassium and potassium-containing medications may suffice. For example, eliminating the use of potassium-containing salt substitutes in a patient who is taking a potassium-conserving diuretic may be all that is needed to deal with mild hyperkalemia.

Prevention of serious hyperkalemia by the administration, either orally or by retention enema, of cation exchange resins (eg, Kayexalate) may be necessary in patients with renal impairment. Cation exchange resins cannot be used if the patient has a paralytic ileus, because intestinal perforation can occur. Kayexalate can bind with other cations in the GI tract and contribute to the development of hypomagnesemia and hypocalcemia; it may also cause sodium retention and fluid overload (Rose & Post, 2000).

### EMERGENCY PHARMACOLOGIC THERAPY

If serum potassium levels are dangerously elevated, it may be necessary to administer IV calcium gluconate. Within minutes after administration, calcium antagonizes the action of hyperkalemia on the heart. Infusion of calcium does not reduce the serum potassium concentration, but it immediately antagonizes the adverse cardiac conduction abnormalities. Calcium chloride and calcium gluconate are not interchangeable: calcium gluconate contains 4.5 mEq of calcium and calcium chloride contains 13.6 mEq of calcium; therefore, caution must be used.

Monitoring the blood pressure is essential to detect hypotension, which may result from the rapid IV administration of calcium gluconate. The ECG should be continuously monitored during administration; the appearance of bradycardia is an indication to stop the infusion. The myocardial protective effects of calcium are transient, lasting about 30 minutes. Extra caution is required if the patient has been "digitalized" (ie, has received accelerated dosages of a digitalis-based cardiac glycoside to reach a desired serum digitalis level rapidly), because parenteral administration of calcium sensitizes the heart to digitalis and may precipitate digitalis toxicity.

IV administration of sodium bicarbonate may be necessary to alkalinize the plasma and cause a temporary shift of potassium into the cells. Also, sodium bicarbonate furnishes sodium to antagonize the cardiac effects of potassium. Effects of this therapy begin within 30 to 60 minutes and may persist for hours; however, they are temporary.

IV administration of regular insulin and a hypertonic dextrose solution causes a temporary shift of potassium into the cells. Glucose and insulin therapy has an onset of action within 30 minutes and lasts for several hours. Loop diuretics, such as furosemide (Lasix), increase excretion of water by inhibiting sodium, potassium, and chloride reabsorption in the ascending loop of Henle and distal renal tubule.

Beta-2 agonists, such as albuterol (Proventil, Ventolin), are highly effective in decreasing potassium but remain controversial, because they can cause tachycardia and chest discomfort (Porth, 2005). Beta-2 agonists also move potassium into the cells and may be used in the absence of ischemic cardiac disease. Administration of these medications is a stopgap measure that only temporarily protects the patient from hyperkalemia. If the hyperkalemic condition is not transient, actual removal of potassium from the body is required; this may be accomplished by using cation exchange resins, peritoneal dialysis, hemodialysis, or other forms of renal replacement therapy.

## Nursing Management

Patients at risk for potassium excess (eg, those with renal failure) should be identified so they can be monitored closely for signs of hyperkalemia. The nurse observes for signs of muscle weakness and dysrhythmias. The presence of paresthesias and GI symptoms such as nausea and intestinal colic are noted. For patients at risk, serum potassium levels are measured periodically (Burger, 2004a).

Because measurements of elevated serum potassium levels may be erroneous, highly abnormal levels should always be verified by repeating the test. To avoid false reports of hyperkalemia, prolonged use of a tourniquet while drawing the blood sample is avoided, and the patient is cautioned not to exercise the extremity immediately before the blood sample is obtained. The blood sample is delivered to the laboratory as soon as possible, because hemolysis of the sample results in a falsely elevated serum potassium level.

### PREVENTING HYPERKALEMIA

Measures are taken to prevent hyperkalemia in patients at risk, when possible, by encouraging the patient to adhere to the prescribed potassium restriction. Potassium-rich foods to be avoided include many fruits and vegetables, legumes, whole-grain breads, meat, milk, eggs, coffee, tea, and cocoa (Dudek, 2006). Conversely, foods with minimal potassium content include butter, margarine, cranberry juice or sauce, ginger ale, gumdrops or jellybeans, hard candy, root beer, sugar, and honey.

### CORRECTING HYPERKALEMIA

As previously stated, it is possible to exceed the tolerance for potassium in any person if it is administered rapidly by the IV route. Therefore, great care should be taken to administer and monitor potassium solutions closely, paying close attention to the solution's concentration and rate of administration. When potassium is added to parenteral solutions, the potassium is mixed with the fluid by inverting the bottle several times. Potassium chloride should never be added to a hanging bottle, because the potassium might be administered as a bolus (potassium chloride is heavy and settles to the bottom of the container).

It is important to caution patients to use salt substitutes sparingly if they are taking other supplementary forms of potassium or potassium-conserving diuretics. Also, potassium-conserving diuretics, such as spironolactone (Aldactone), triamterene (Dyrenium), and amiloride (Midamor); potassium supplements; and salt substitutes should not be administered to patients with renal dysfunction. Most salt substitutes contain approximately 50 to 60 mEq of potassium per teaspoon.

## *Calcium Imbalances*

More than 99% of the body's calcium is located in the skeletal system; calcium is a major component of bones and teeth. About 1% of skeletal calcium is rapidly exchangeable with blood calcium, and the rest is more stable and only slowly exchanged. The small amount of calcium located outside the bone circulates in the serum, partly bound to protein and partly ionized. Calcium plays a major role in transmitting nerve impulses and helps regulate muscle contraction and relaxation, including cardiac muscle. Calcium is instrumental in activating enzymes that stimulate many essential chemical reactions in the body, and it also plays a role in blood coagulation. Because many factors affect calcium regulation, both hypocalcemia and hypercalcemia are relatively common disturbances.

The normal total serum calcium level is 8.6 to 10.2 mg/dL (2.2 to 2.6 mmol/L). Calcium exists in plasma in three forms: ionized, bound, and complexed. About 50% of the serum calcium exists in a physiologically active ionized form that is important for neuromuscular activity and blood coagulation; this is the only physiologically and clinically significant form. The normal ionized serum calcium level is 4.5 to 5.1 mg/dL (1.1 to 1.3 mmol/L). Less than half of the plasma calcium is bound to serum proteins, primarily albumin. The remainder is combined with nonprotein anions: phosphate, citrate, and carbonate.

Calcium is absorbed from foods in the presence of normal gastric acidity and vitamin D. Calcium is excreted primarily in the feces, with the remainder excreted in the urine. The serum calcium level is controlled by PTH and calcitonin. As ionized serum calcium decreases, the parathyroid glands secrete PTH. This, in turn, increases calcium absorption from the GI tract, increases calcium reabsorption from the renal tubule, and releases calcium from the bone. The increase in calcium ion concentration suppresses PTH secretion. When calcium increases excessively, the thyroid gland secretes calcitonin. It briefly inhibits calcium reabsorption from bone and decreases the serum calcium concentration.

## Calcium Deficit (Hypocalcemia)

Hypocalcemia (lower-than-normal serum concentration of calcium) occurs in a variety of clinical situations. A patient may have a total body calcium deficit (as in osteoporosis) but a normal serum calcium level. Elderly people with osteoporosis who spend an increased amount of time in bed have an increased risk for hypocalcemia, because bed rest increases bone resorption.

Several factors can cause hypocalcemia, including primary hypoparathyroidism and surgical hypoparathyroidism. The latter is far more common. Not only is hypocalcemia associated with thyroid and parathyroid surgery, but it can also occur after radical neck dissection and is most likely in the first 24 to 48 hours after surgery. Transient hypocalcemia can occur with massive administration of citrated blood (as in exchange transfusions in newborns or for adults who experience massive hemorrhage and shock), because citrate can combine with ionized calcium and temporarily remove it from the circulation.

Inflammation of the pancreas causes the breakdown of proteins and lipids. It is thought that calcium ions combine with the fatty acids released by lipolysis, forming soaps. As a result of this process, hypocalcemia occurs and is common in pancreatitis. It has also been suggested that hypocalcemia might be related to excessive secretion of glucagon from the inflamed pancreas, which results in increased secretion of calcitonin (a hormone that lowers serum calcium).

Hypocalcemia is common in patients with renal failure, because these patients frequently have elevated serum phosphate levels. Hyperphosphatemia usually causes a reciprocal drop in the serum calcium level. Other causes of hypocalcemia include inadequate vitamin D consumption, magnesium deficiency, medullary thyroid carcinoma, low serum albumin levels, alkalosis, and alcohol abuse. Medications predisposing to hypocalcemia include aluminum-containing antacids, aminoglycosides, caffeine, cisplatin, corticosteroids, mithramycin, phosphates, isoniazid, and loop diuretics.

## Clinical Manifestations

Tetany is the most characteristic manifestation of hypocalcemia and hypomagnesemia. Tetany refers to the entire symptom complex induced by increased neural excitability. These symptoms are caused by spontaneous discharges of both sensory and motor fibers in peripheral nerves. Sensations of tingling may occur in the tips of the fingers, around the mouth, and, less commonly, in the feet. Spasms of the muscles of the extremities and face may occur. Pain may develop as a result of these spasms. These clinical signs indicate tetany and hyperactive deep tendon reflexes.

Trousseau's sign (Fig. 14-6) can be elicited by inflating a blood pressure cuff on the upper arm to about 20 mm Hg above systolic pressure; within 2 to 5 minutes, carpal spasm (an adducted thumb, flexed wrist and metacarpophalangeal joints, extended interphalangeal joints with fingers together) will occur as ischemia of the ulnar nerve develops. Chvostek's sign consists of twitching of muscles supplied by the facial nerve when the nerve is tapped about 2 cm anterior to the earlobe, just below the zygomatic arch.

Seizures may occur because hypocalcemia increases irritability of the central nervous system as well as of the peripheral nerves. Other changes associated with hypocalcemia include mental changes such as depression, impaired memory, confusion, delirium, and even hallucinations. A prolonged QT interval is seen on the ECG due to prolongation of the ST segment, and a form of ventricular tachycardia called torsades de pointes may occur. Respiratory effects with decreasing calcium include dyspnea and laryngospasm. Signs and symptoms of chronic hypocalcemia include hyperactive bowel sounds, dry and brittle hair and nails, and abnormal clotting.

Osteoporosis is associated with prolonged low intake of calcium and represents a total body calcium deficit, even though serum calcium levels are usually normal. This disorder occurs in millions of Americans and is most common in postmenopausal women. It is characterized by loss of bone mass, which causes bones to become porous and brittle and therefore susceptible to fracture. See Chapter 68 for further discussion of osteoporosis.

## Assessment and Diagnostic Findings

When evaluating serum calcium levels, one must consider several other variables, such as the serum albumin level and the arterial pH. Because abnormalities in serum albumin levels may affect interpretation of the serum calcium level, it may be necessary to calculate the corrected serum calcium if the serum albumin level is abnormal. For every decrease in serum albumin of 1 g/dL below 4 g/dL, the total serum calcium level is underestimated by approximately 0.8 mg/dL. The following is a quick method to calculate the corrected serum calcium level:

$$\text{Measured total serum Ca}^{++} \text{ level} (\text{mg/dL}) + 0.8$$
$$\times (4.0 - \text{Measured albumin level } [\text{g/dL}])$$
$$= \text{Corrected total calcium concentration } (\text{mg/dL})$$

An example of the calculations needed to obtain the corrected total serum calcium level is as follows:

A patient's reported serum albumin level is 2.5 g/dL; the reported serum calcium level is 10.5 mg/dL. First, the decrease in serum albumin level from normal (ie, the difference from the normal albumin concentration of 4 g/dL) is calculated: 4 g/dL − 2.5 g/dL = 1.5 g/dL. Next, the following ratio is calculated:

$$0.8 \text{ mg/dL} : 1 \text{ g/dL} = X \text{ mg/dL} : 1.5 \text{ mg/dL}$$
$$X = 0.8 \times 1.5 \text{ mg/dL}$$
$$X = 1.2 \text{ mg/dL calcium}$$

Finally, 1.2 mg/dL is added to 10.5 mg/dL (the reported serum calcium level) to obtain the corrected total serum calcium level: 1.2 mg/dL + 10.5 mg/dL = 11.7 mg/dL

Clinicians often discount a low serum calcium level in the presence of a similarly low serum albumin level. The ionized calcium level is usually normal in patients with reduced total serum calcium levels and concomitant hypoalbuminemia. When the arterial pH increases (alkalosis), more calcium becomes bound to protein. As a result, the ionized portion decreases. Symptoms of hypocalcemia may occur with alkalosis. Acidosis (low pH) has the opposite effect; that is, less calcium is bound to protein and therefore more exists in the ionized form. However, relatively small changes in serum calcium levels occur in these acid–base abnormalities.

Ideally, the ionized level of calcium should be measured in the laboratory. However, in many laboratories, only the total calcium level is reported; therefore, the concentration of the ionized fraction must be estimated by simultaneous measurement of the serum albumin level. PTH levels are decreased in hypoparathyroidism. Magnesium and phosphorus levels need to be assessed to identify possible causes of decreased calcium.

**FIGURE 14-6.** Trousseau's sign. Ischemia-induced carpal spasm can occur with hypocalcemia or hypomagnesemia. Occluding the brachial artery with a blood pressure cuff for 3 minutes can produce carpal spasm that mimics the spasm that occurs with hypocalcemia or hypomagnesemia.

## Medical Management

Acute symptomatic hypocalcemia is life-threatening and requires prompt treatment with IV administration of calcium (Kee et al., 2004). Parenteral calcium salts include calcium gluconate, calcium chloride, and calcium gluceptate. Although calcium chloride produces a significantly higher ionized calcium level than calcium gluconate does, it is not used as often because it is more irritating and can cause sloughing of tissue if it infiltrates. Too-rapid IV administration of calcium can cause cardiac arrest, preceded by bradycardia. IV administration of calcium is particularly dangerous in patients receiving digitalis-derived medications, because calcium ions exert an effect similar to that of digitalis and can cause digitalis toxicity, with adverse cardiac effects. Therefore, calcium should be diluted in $D_5W$ and administered as a slow IV bolus or a slow IV infusion using a volumetric infusion pump. The IV site must be observed often for any evidence of infiltration because of the risk of extravasation and resultant cellulitis or necrosis. A 0.9% sodium chloride solution should not be used with calcium because it increases renal calcium loss. Solutions containing phosphates or bicarbonate should not be used with calcium because they cause precipitation when calcium is added. The nurse must clarify with the physician which calcium salt to administer, because calcium gluconate yields 4.5 mEq of calcium and calcium chloride provides 13.6 mEq of calcium. Calcium can cause postural hypotension; therefore, the patient is kept in bed during IV replacement, and blood pressure is monitored.

Vitamin D therapy may be instituted to increase calcium absorption from the GI tract. Aluminum hydroxide, calcium acetate, or calcium carbonate antacids may be prescribed to decrease elevated phosphorus levels before treating hypocalcemia in the patient with chronic renal failure. Increasing the dietary intake of calcium to at least 1000 to 1500 mg/day in the adult is recommended; calcium-containing foods include milk products; green, leafy vegetables; canned salmon; sardines; and fresh oysters. Hypomagnesemia can also cause tetany; if the tetany responds to IV calcium, then a low magnesium level is considered as a possible cause in chronic renal failure.

## Nursing Management

It is important to observe for hypocalcemia in patients at risk. Seizure precautions are initiated if hypocalcemia is severe. The status of the airway is closely monitored, because laryngeal stridor can occur. Safety precautions are taken, as indicated, if confusion is present.

People who have a high risk for osteoporosis are instructed about the need for adequate dietary calcium intake; it is important to teach the patient what foods are rich in calcium. The nurse must also advise the patient to consider calcium supplements if sufficient calcium is not consumed in the diet. Such supplements should be taken in divided doses with meals. In addition, the value of regular weight-bearing exercise in decreasing bone loss should be emphasized, as well as the effect of medications on calcium balance. For example, alcohol and caffeine in high doses inhibit calcium absorption, and moderate cigarette smoking increases urinary calcium excretion. Additional teaching includes discussion of medications such as alendronate (Fosamax), risedronate (Actonel), raloxifene (Evista), calcitonin, and ibandronate (Boniva), a once-a-month bisphosphonate to reduce the rate of bone loss. Teaching also includes strategies to reduce the risk of falls. The patient is also cautioned to avoid the overuse of laxatives and antacids that contain phosphorus, because their use decreases calcium absorption.

## Calcium Excess (Hypercalcemia)

Hypercalcemia (excess of calcium in the plasma) is a dangerous imbalance when severe; in fact, hypercalcemic crisis has a mortality rate as high as 50% if not treated promptly.

The most common causes of hypercalcemia are malignancies and hyperparathyroidism. Malignant tumors can produce hypercalcemia by a variety of mechanisms (Stewart, 2005). The excessive PTH secretion associated with hyperparathyroidism causes increased release of calcium from the bones and increased intestinal and renal absorption of calcium. Calcifications of soft tissue occur when the calcium–phosphorus product (serum calcium × serum phosphorus) exceeds 70 mg/dL (Rose & Post, 2000).

Bone mineral is lost during immobilization, and sometimes this causes elevation of total (and especially ionized) calcium in the bloodstream. However, symptomatic hypercalcemia from immobilization is rare; when it does occur, it is virtually limited to people with high calcium turnover rates (eg, adolescents during a growth spurt). Most cases of hypercalcemia secondary to immobility occur after severe or multiple fractures or spinal cord injury.

Thiazide diuretics can cause a slight elevation in serum calcium levels because they potentiate the action of PTH on the kidneys, reducing urinary calcium excretion. The milk-alkali syndrome has occurred in patients with peptic ulcer treated previously for a prolonged period with milk and alkaline antacids, particularly calcium carbonate. Vitamin A and D intoxication, as well as the use of lithium, can cause calcium excess. Calcium levels are inversely related to phosphorus levels.

### Clinical Manifestations

As a rule, the symptoms of hypercalcemia are proportional to the degree of elevation of the serum calcium level. Hypercalcemia reduces neuromuscular excitability because it suppresses activity at the myoneural junction. Symptoms such as muscle weakness, incoordination, anorexia, and constipation may be caused by decreased tone in smooth and striated muscle. Cardiac standstill can occur when the serum calcium level is about 18 mg/dL (4.5 mmol/L). The inotropic effect of digitalis is enhanced by calcium; therefore, digitalis toxicity is aggravated by hypercalcemia.

Anorexia, nausea, vomiting, and constipation are common symptoms of hypercalcemia. Dehydration occurs with nausea, vomiting, anorexia, and calcium reabsorption at the proximal renal tubule. Abdominal and bone pain may also be present. Abdominal distention and paralytic ileus may complicate severe hypercalcemic crisis. Excessive urination due to disturbed renal tubular function produced by hypercalcemia may occur. Severe thirst may occur secondary to the polyuria caused by the high solute (calcium) load.

Patients with chronic hypercalcemia may develop symptoms similar to those of peptic ulcer because hypercalcemia increases the secretion of acid and pepsin by the stomach.

Confusion, impaired memory, slurred speech, lethargy, acute psychotic behavior, or coma may occur (Stewart, 2005). The more severe symptoms tend to appear when the serum calcium level is approximately 16 mg/dL (4 mmol/L) or higher. However, some patients become profoundly disturbed with serum calcium levels of only 12 mg/dL (3 mmol/L). These symptoms resolve as serum calcium levels return to normal after treatment.

Hypercalcemic crisis refers to an acute rise in the serum calcium level to 17 mg/dL (4.3 mmol/L) or higher. Severe thirst and polyuria are often present. Other findings may include muscle weakness, intractable nausea, abdominal cramps, obstipation (very severe constipation) or diarrhea, peptic ulcer symptoms, and bone pain. Lethargy, confusion, and coma may also occur. This condition is very dangerous and may result in cardiac arrest.

## Assessment and Diagnostic Findings

The serum calcium level is greater than 10.2 mg/dL (2.6 mmol/L). Cardiovascular changes may include a variety of dysrhythmias (ie, heart blocks) and shortening of the QT interval and ST segment. The PR interval is sometimes prolonged. The double-antibody PTH test may be used to differentiate between primary hyperparathyroidism and malignancy as a cause of hypercalcemia: PTH levels are increased in primary or secondary hyperparathyroidism and suppressed in malignancy. X-rays may reveal the presence of osteoporosis if the patient has hypercalcemia secondary to a malignancy, bone cavitation, or urinary calculi. The Sulkowitch urine test analyzes the amount of calcium in the urine; in hypercalcemia, dense precipitation is observed due to hypercalciuria.

## Medical Management

Therapeutic aims in hypercalcemia include decreasing the serum calcium level and reversing the process causing hypercalcemia. Treating the underlying cause (eg, chemotherapy for a malignancy, partial parathyroidectomy for hyperparathyroidism) is essential.

**PHARMACOLOGIC THERAPY**
General measures include administering fluids to dilute serum calcium and promote its excretion by the kidneys, mobilizing the patient, and restricting dietary calcium intake. IV administration of 0.9% sodium chloride solution temporarily dilutes the serum calcium level and increases urinary calcium excretion by inhibiting tubular reabsorption of calcium. Administering IV phosphate can cause a reciprocal drop in serum calcium. Furosemide (Lasix) is often used in conjunction with administration of a saline solution; in addition to causing diuresis, furosemide increases calcium excretion. Although it is an often-overlooked measure, fluids and medications that contain calcium and dietary sources of calcium should be halted (Stewart, 2005).

Calcitonin can be used to lower the serum calcium level and is particularly useful for patients with heart disease or renal failure who cannot tolerate large sodium loads. Calcitonin reduces bone resorption, increases the depositing of calcium and phosphorus in the bones, and increases urinary excretion of calcium and phosphorus (Karch, 2006). Although several forms are available, calcitonin derived from salmon is commonly used. Skin testing for allergy to salmon calcitonin is necessary before the hormone is administered. Systemic allergic reactions are possible because this hormone is a protein; resistance to the medication may develop later because of antibody formation. Calcitonin is administered by intramuscular injection rather than subcutaneously, because patients with hypercalcemia have poor perfusion of subcutaneous tissue.

For patients with cancer, treatment is directed at controlling the condition by surgery, chemotherapy, or radiation therapy. Corticosteroids may be used to decrease bone turnover and tubular reabsorption for patients with sarcoidosis, myelomas, lymphomas, and leukemias; patients with solid tumors are less responsive. The bisphosphonates inhibit osteoclast activity. Pamidronate (Aredia) is a potent form and is administered intravenously; it causes a transient, mild pyrexia, decreased white blood cell count, and myalgia. Etidronate (Didronel) is another bisphosphonate that is given by IV, but its action is slower. Mithramycin, a cytotoxic antibiotic, inhibits bone resorption and thus lowers the serum calcium level. This agent must be used cautiously because it has significant side effects, including thrombocytopenia, nephrotoxicity, rebound hypercalcemia when discontinued, and hepatotoxicity. Inorganic phosphate salts can be administered orally or by nasogastric tube (in the form of Phospho-Soda or Neutra-Phos), rectally (as retention enemas), or intravenously. IV phosphate therapy is used with extreme caution in the treatment of hypercalcemia, because it can cause severe calcification in various tissues, hypotension, tetany, and acute renal failure.

## Nursing Management

It is important to monitor for hypercalcemia in patients who are at risk. Interventions such as increasing patient mobility and encouraging fluids can help prevent hypercalcemia, or at least minimize its severity. Hospitalized patients who are at risk for hypercalcemia are encouraged to ambulate as soon as possible; outpatients and those cared for in their homes are informed of the importance of frequent ambulation.

When encouraging oral fluids, the nurse considers the patient's likes and dislikes. Fluids containing sodium should be administered unless contraindicated, because sodium favors calcium excretion. Patients are encouraged to drink 3 to 4 quarts of fluid daily. Adequate fiber should be provided in the diet to offset the tendency for constipation. Safety precautions are implemented, as necessary, when mental symptoms of hypercalcemia are present. The patient and family are informed that these mental changes are reversible with treatment. Increased calcium potentiates the effects of digitalis; therefore, the patient is assessed for signs and symptoms of digitalis toxicity. Because ECG changes (premature ventricular contractions, paroxysmal atrial tachycardia, and heart block) can occur, the cardiac rate and rhythm are monitored for any abnormalities.

## Magnesium Imbalances

Magnesium is the most abundant intracellular cation after potassium. It acts as an activator for many intracellular enzyme systems and plays a role in both carbohydrate and protein metabolism. The normal serum magnesium level is 1.3 to 2.3 mEq/L (1.8 to 3.0 mg/dL; 0.8 to 1.2 mmol/L). Approximately one third of serum magnesium is bound to protein; the remaining two thirds exists as free cations—the active component ($Mg^{++}$). Magnesium balance is important in neuromuscular function. Because magnesium acts directly on the myoneural junction, variations in the serum concentration of magnesium affect neuromuscular irritability and contractility. For example, an excess of magnesium diminishes the excitability of the muscle cells, whereas a deficit increases neuromuscular irritability and contractility. Magnesium produces its sedative effect at the neuromuscular junction, probably by inhibiting the release of the neurotransmitter acetylcholine. It also increases the stimulus threshold in nerve fibers.

Magnesium exerts effects on the cardiovascular system, acting peripherally to produce vasodilation. Magnesium is thought to have a direct effect on peripheral arteries and arterioles, which results in a decreased total peripheral resistance. Magnesium is predominantly found in bone and soft tissues. It is primarily eliminated by the kidneys.

## Magnesium Deficit (Hypomagnesemia)

Hypomagnesemia refers to a below-normal serum magnesium concentration (1.3 to 2.3 mEq/L; 1.8 to 3.0 mg/dL; 0.8 to 1.2 mmol/L). Magnesium is similar to calcium in two aspects: (1) it is the ionized fraction of magnesium that is primarily involved in neuromuscular activity and other physiologic processes, and (2) magnesium levels should be evaluated in combination with albumin levels. Low serum albumin levels decrease total magnesium.

Hypomagnesemia is a common yet often overlooked imbalance in acutely and critically ill patients. It may occur with withdrawal from alcohol and administration of tube feedings or parenteral nutrition.

An important route of magnesium loss is the GI tract. Loss of magnesium from the GI tract may occur with nasogastric suction, diarrhea, or fistulas. Because fluid from the lower GI tract has a higher concentration of magnesium (10 to 14 mEq/L) than fluid from the upper tract (1 to 2 mEq/L), losses from diarrhea and intestinal fistulas are more likely to induce magnesium deficit than are those from gastric suction. Although magnesium losses are relatively small in nasogastric suction, hypomagnesemia will occur if losses are prolonged and magnesium is not replaced through IV infusion. Because the distal small bowel is the major site of magnesium absorption, any disruption in small bowel function, as in intestinal resection or inflammatory bowel disease, can lead to hypomagnesemia.

Alcoholism is currently the most common cause of symptomatic hypomagnesemia in the United States. Hypomagnesemia is particularly troublesome during treatment of alcohol withdrawal. Therefore, the serum magnesium level should be measured at least every 2 or 3 days in patients undergoing withdrawal from alcohol. The serum magnesium level may be normal on admission but may decrease as a result of metabolic changes, such as the intracellular shift of magnesium associated with IV glucose administration.

During nutritional replacement, the major cellular electrolytes move from the serum to newly synthesized cells. Therefore, if the enteral or parenteral feeding formula is deficient in magnesium content, serious hypomagnesemia will occur. Because of this, serum magnesium levels should be measured at regular intervals in patients who are receiving parenteral nutrition and enteral feedings, especially those who have undergone a period of starvation. Other causes of hypomagnesemia include the administration of aminoglycosides, cyclosporine, cisplatin, diuretics, digitalis, and amphotericin and the rapid administration of citrated blood, especially to patients with renal or hepatic disease. Magnesium deficiency often occurs in diabetic ketoacidosis, secondary to increased renal excretion during osmotic diuresis and shifting of magnesium into the cells with insulin therapy. Other contributing causes are sepsis, burns, and hypothermia.

### Clinical Manifestations

Clinical manifestations of hypomagnesemia are largely confined to the neuromuscular system. Some of the effects are due directly to the low serum magnesium level; others are due to secondary changes in potassium and calcium metabolism. Symptoms do not usually occur until the serum magnesium level has dropped to less than 1 mEq/L (0.5 mmol/L).

Among the neuromuscular changes are hyperexcitability with muscle weakness, tremors, and athetoid movements (slow, involuntary twisting and writhing). Others include tetany, generalized tonic–clonic or focal seizures, laryngeal stridor, and positive Chvostek's and Trousseau's signs (see earlier discussion), which occur, in part, because of accompanying hypocalcemia.

Magnesium deficiency can disturb the ECG by prolonging the QRS, depressing the ST segment, and predisposing to cardiac dysrhythmias, such as premature ventricular contractions, supraventricular tachycardia, torsades de pointes (a form of ventricular tachycardia), and ventricular fibrillation. Increased susceptibility to digitalis toxicity is associated with low serum magnesium levels. This is important, because patients receiving digoxin are also likely to be receiving diuretic therapy, predisposing them to renal loss of magnesium.

Hypomagnesemia may be accompanied by marked alterations in mood. Apathy, depression, apprehension, and extreme agitation have been noted, as well as ataxia, dizziness, insomnia, and confusion. At times, delirium, auditory or visual hallucinations, and frank psychoses may occur.

### Assessment and Diagnostic Findings

On laboratory analysis, the serum magnesium level is less than 1.3 mEq/L or 1.8 mg/dL (0.75 mmol/L). Hypomagnesemia is frequently associated with hypokalemia and hypocalcemia. About 25% of magnesium is protein-bound, principally to albumin. A decreased serum albumin level can, therefore, reduce the measured total magnesium concentration; however, it does not reduce the ionized plasma magnesium concentration. ECG evaluations reflect magnesium, calcium, and potassium deficiencies, tachydysrhythmias, prolonged PR and QT intervals, widening QRS, ST-segment depression, flattened T waves, and a prominent U wave. Torsades de pointes is associated with a low magnesium level. Premature ventricular contractions, paroxysmal atrial tachycardia, and heart block may also occur. Urine magnesium levels may be helpful in identifying causes of magnesium depletion and are measured after a loading dose of magnesium sulfate is administered. Two newer diagnostic techniques (nuclear magnetic resonance spectroscopy and the ion-selective electrode) are sensitive and direct means of measuring ionized serum magnesium levels.

### Medical Management

Mild magnesium deficiency can be corrected by diet alone. Principal dietary sources of magnesium, which is a component of chlorophyll, are green leafy vegetables, nuts, seeds, legumes, whole grains, and seafood. Magnesium is also plentiful in peanut butter and cocoa.

If necessary, magnesium salts can be administered orally in an oxide or gluconate form to replace continuous excessive losses. Diarrhea is a common complication of excessive ingestion of magnesium. Patients receiving parenteral nutrition require magnesium in the IV solution to prevent hypomagnesemia. Magnesium sulfate must be administered intravenously by an infusion pump and at a rate not to exceed 150 mg/min, or 67 mEq over 8 hours. A bolus dose of magnesium sulfate given too rapidly can produce alterations in cardiac conduction leading to heart block or asystole. Vital signs must be assessed frequently during magnesium administration to detect changes in cardiac rate or rhythm, hypotension, and respiratory distress. Monitoring urine output is essential before, during, and after magnesium administration; the physician is notified if urine volume decreases to less than 100 mL over 4 hours. Calcium gluconate must be readily available to treat hypocalcemic tetany or hypermagnesemia.

Overt symptoms of hypomagnesemia are treated with parenteral administration of magnesium. Magnesium sulfate is the most commonly used magnesium salt. Serial measurements of serum magnesium levels can be used to regulate the dosage.

### Nursing Management

The nurse should be aware of patients who are at risk for hypomagnesemia and observe them for its signs and symptoms. Patients receiving digitalis are monitored closely, because a deficit of magnesium can predispose them to digitalis toxicity. If hypomagnesemia is severe, seizure precautions are implemented. Other safety precautions are instituted, as indicated, if confusion is observed.

Because difficulty in swallowing (dysphagia) may occur in magnesium-depleted patients, the ability to swallow should be tested with water before oral medications or foods are offered. Dysphagia is probably related to the athetoid or choreiform (rapid, involuntary, and irregular jerking) movements associated with magnesium deficit. To determine neuromuscular irritability, the nurse needs to assess and grade deep tendon reflexes (see Chapter 60).

Teaching plays a major role in treating magnesium deficit, particularly that resulting from abuse of diuretic or laxative medications. In such cases, the nurse instructs the patient about the need to consume magnesium-rich foods. For patients experiencing hypomagnesemia from abuse of alcohol, the nurse provides teaching, counseling, support, and possible referral to alcohol abstinence programs or other professional help.

## Magnesium Excess (Hypermagnesemia)

Hypermagnesemia is a rare electrolyte abnormality, because the kidneys are efficient in excreting magnesium. A serum magnesium level can appear falsely elevated if blood specimens are allowed to hemolyze or are drawn from an extremity with a tourniquet that was applied too tightly.

By far the most common cause of hypermagnesemia is renal failure. In fact, most patients with advanced renal failure have at least a slight elevation in serum magnesium levels. This condition is aggravated when such patients receive magnesium to control seizures or inadvertently take one of the many commercial antacids that contain magnesium salts.

Hypermagnesemia can occur in a patient with untreated diabetic ketoacidosis when catabolism causes the release of cellular magnesium that cannot be excreted because of profound fluid volume depletion and resulting oliguria. An excess of magnesium can also result from excessive magnesium administered to treat hypertension of pregnancy or to treat low hypomagnesemia. Increased serum magnesium levels can also occur in adrenocortical insufficiency, Addison's disease, or hypothermia. Excessive use of antacids (eg, Maalox, Riopan, Mylanta); laxatives (Milk of Magnesia); and medications that decrease GI motility, including opioids and anticholinergics, can also increase serum magnesium levels. Decreased elimination of magnesium or its increased absorption due to intestinal hypomotility from any cause can contribute to hypermagnesemia. Lithium intoxication can also cause an increase in serum magnesium levels.

### Clinical Manifestations

Acute elevation of the serum magnesium level depresses the central nervous system as well as the peripheral neuromuscular junction. At mildly increased levels, there is a tendency for lowered blood pressure because of peripheral vasodilation. Nausea, vomiting, weakness, soft tissue calcifications, facial flushing, and sensations of warmth may also occur. At higher magnesium concentrations, lethargy, difficulty speaking (dysarthria), and drowsiness can occur. Deep tendon reflexes are lost, and muscle weakness and paralysis may develop. The respiratory center is depressed when serum magnesium levels exceed 10 mEq/L (5 mmol/L). Coma, atrioventricular heart block, and cardiac arrest can occur when the serum magnesium level is greatly elevated and not treated. High levels of magnesium also result in platelet clumping and delayed thrombin formation (Chernecky & Berger, 2004).

### Assessment and Diagnostic Findings

On laboratory analysis, the serum magnesium level is greater than 2.5 mEq/L or 3.0 mg/dL (1.25 mmol/L). Increased potassium and calcium are present concurrently. As creatinine clearance decreases to less than 3.0 mL/min, the serum magnesium levels increase (Hogan & Wane, 2003). ECG findings may include a prolonged PR interval, tall T waves, a widened QRS, and a prolonged QT interval, as well as an atrioventricular block.

### Medical Management

Hypermagnesemia can be prevented by avoiding the administration of magnesium to patients with renal failure and by carefully monitoring seriously ill patients who are receiving magnesium salts. In patients with severe hypermagnesemia, all parenteral and oral magnesium salts are discontinued. In emergencies, such as respiratory depression or defective cardiac conduction, ventilatory support and IV calcium gluconate are indicated. In addition, hemodialysis with a magnesium-free dialysate can reduce the serum magnesium to a safe level within hours. Administration of loop diuretics (Lasix) and sodium chloride or lactated Ringer's IV solution enhances magnesium excretion in patients with adequate renal function. IV calcium gluconate antagonizes the cardiovascular and neuromuscular effects of magnesium.

### Nursing Management

Patients at risk for hypermagnesemia are identified and assessed. If hypermagnesemia is suspected, the nurse monitors the vital signs, noting hypotension and shallow respirations. The nurse also observes for decreased patellar reflexes and changes in the level of consciousness. Medications that contain magnesium are not administered to patients with renal failure or compromised renal function, and patients with renal failure are cautioned to check with their health care providers before taking over-the-counter medications. Caution is essential when preparing and administering magnesium-containing fluids parenterally, because available parenteral magnesium solutions (eg, 2-mL ampules, 50-mL vials) differ in concentration.

## Phosphorus Imbalances

Phosphorus is a critical constituent of all the body's tissues. It is essential to the function of muscle and red blood cells, the formation of adenosine triphosphate (ATP) and of 2,3-diphosphoglycerate, which facilitates release of oxygen from hemoglobin, and the maintenance of acid–base balance, as well as to the nervous system and the intermediary metabolism of carbohydrate, protein, and fat. It provides structural support to bones and teeth. Phosphorus is the primary anion of the ICF. About 85% of phosphorus is located in bones and teeth, 14% in soft tissue, and less than 1% in the ECF. The normal serum phosphorus level is 2.5 to 4.5 mg/dL (0.8 to 1.45 mmol/L) and may be as high as 6 mg/dL (1.94 mmol/L) in infants and children. Serum phosphorus levels are greater in children presumably because of the high rate of skeletal growth; the levels decrease with age.

## Phosphorus Deficit (Hypophosphatemia)

Hypophosphatemia is a below-normal serum concentration of inorganic phosphorus. Although it often indicates phosphorus deficiency, hypophosphatemia may occur under a variety of circumstances in which total body phosphorus stores are normal. Conversely, phosphorus deficiency is an abnormally low content of phosphorus in lean tissues that may exist in the absence of hypophosphatemia. It can be caused by an intracellular shift of potassium from serum into cells, by increased urinary excretion of potassium, or by decreased intestinal absorption of potassium.

Hypophosphatemia may occur during the administration of calories to patients with severe protein–calorie malnutrition. It is most likely to occur with overzealous intake or administration of simple carbohydrates. This syndrome can be induced in anyone with severe protein–calorie malnutrition (eg, patients with anorexia nervosa or alcoholism, elderly debilitated patients who are unable to eat). As many as 50% of patients hospitalized because of chronic alcoholism have hypophosphatemia.

Marked hypophosphatemia may develop in malnourished patients who receive parenteral nutrition if the phosphorus loss is not adequately corrected. Other causes of hypophosphatemia include pain, heat stroke, prolonged intense hyperventilation, alcohol withdrawal, poor dietary intake, diabetic ketoacidosis, hepatic encephalopathy, and major thermal burns. Low magnesium levels, low potassium levels, and hyperparathyroidism related to increased urinary losses of phosphorus contribute to hypophosphatemia. Loss of phosphorus through the kidneys also occurs with acute volume expansion, osmotic diuresis, use of carbonic anhydrase inhibitors (acetazolamide [Diamox]), and some malignancies. Respiratory alkalosis can cause a decrease in phosphorus because of an intracellular shift of phosphorus, which often stimulates intracellular glycolysis.

Excess phosphorus binding by antacids containing magnesium, calcium, or albumin may decrease the phosphorus available from the diet to an amount lower than required to maintain serum phosphorus balance. The degree of hypophosphatemia depends on the amount of phosphorus in the diet compared to the dose of antacid. Phosphate can occur with chronic diarrhea or through severe potassium restriction. Vitamin D regulates intestinal ion absorption; therefore, a deficiency of vitamin D may cause decreased calcium and phosphorus levels, which may lead to osteomalacia (softened, brittle bones).

### Clinical Manifestations

Most of the signs and symptoms of phosphorus deficiency appear to result from a deficiency of ATP, 2,3-diphosphoglycerate, or both. ATP deficiency impairs cellular energy resources; diphosphoglycerate deficiency impairs oxygen delivery to tissues.

A wide range of neurologic symptoms, such as irritability, fatigue, apprehension, weakness, numbness, paresthesias, dysarthria, dysphagia, diplopia, confusion, seizures, and coma, may occur. Low levels of diphosphoglycerate may reduce the delivery of oxygen to peripheral tissues, resulting in tissue anoxia. Hypoxia then leads to an increase in respiratory rate and respiratory alkalosis, causing phosphorus to move into the cells and potentiating hypophosphatemia. Hemolytic anemia may lead to pale skin and conjunctivae.

It is thought that hypophosphatemia predisposes a person to infection. In laboratory animals, hypophosphatemia is associated with depression of the chemotactic, phagocytic, and bacterial activity of granulocytes.

Muscle damage may develop as the ATP level in the muscle tissue declines. Clinical manifestations are muscle weakness, which may be subtle or profound and may affect any muscle group, muscle pain, and at times acute rhabdomyolysis (disintegration of striated muscle). Weakness of respiratory muscles may greatly impair ventilation. Hypophosphatemia also may predispose a person to insulin resistance and thus hyperglycemia. Chronic loss of phosphorus can cause bruising and bleeding from platelet dysfunction.

### Assessment and Diagnostic Findings

On laboratory analysis, the serum phosphorus level is less than 2.5 mg/dL (0.80 mmol/L) in adults. When reviewing laboratory results, the nurse should keep in mind that glucose or insulin administration causes a slight decrease in the serum phosphorus level. PTH levels are increased in hyperparathyroidism. Serum magnesium may decrease due to increased urinary excretion of magnesium. Alkaline phosphatase is increased with osteoblastic activity. X-rays may show skeletal changes of osteomalacia or rickets.

### Medical Management

Prevention of hypophosphatemia is the goal. In patients at risk for hypophosphatemia, serum phosphate levels should be closely monitored and correction initiated before deficits become severe. Adequate amounts of phosphorus should be added to parenteral solutions, and attention should be paid to the phosphorus levels in enteral feeding solutions.

Severe hypophosphatemia is dangerous and requires prompt attention. Aggressive IV phosphorus correction is usually limited to the patient whose serum phosphorus levels decrease to less than 1 mg/dL (0.3 mmol/L) and whose GI tract is not functioning. Possible dangers of IV administration of phosphorus include tetany from hypocalcemia and calcifications in tissues (blood vessels, heart, lung, kidney, eyes) from hyperphosphatemia. IV preparations of phosphorus are available as sodium or potassium phosphate. The rate of phosphorus administration should not exceed 10 mEq/h, and the site should be carefully monitored because tissue sloughing and necrosis can occur with infiltration. In less acute situations, oral phosphorus replacement is usually adequate.

### Nursing Management

The nurse identifies patients who are at risk for hypophosphatemia and monitors them. Because malnourished patients receiving parenteral nutrition are at risk when calories are introduced too aggressively, preventive measures involve gradually introducing the solution to avoid rapid shifts of phosphorus into the cells.

For patients with documented hypophosphatemia, careful attention is given to preventing infection, because hypophosphatemia may alter the granulocytes. In patients requiring correction of phosphorus losses, the nurse frequently monitors serum phosphorus levels and documents and reports early signs of hypophosphatemia (apprehension, confusion, change in level of consciousness). If the patient experiences mild hypophosphatemia, foods such as milk and milk products, organ meats, nuts, fish, poultry, and whole grains should be encouraged. With moderate hypophosphatemia, supplements such as Neutra-Phos capsules (250 mg phosphorus/capsule) or Fleet's Phospho-Soda (815 mg phosphorus/5 mL) may be prescribed.

## Phosphorus Excess (Hyperphosphatemia)

Hyperphosphatemia is a serum phosphorus level that exceeds normal. Various conditions can lead to this imbalance, but the most common is renal failure. Other causes include increased intake, decreased output, or a shift from the intracellular to extracellular space. Other causes include chemotherapy for neoplastic disease, hypoparathyroidism, metabolic or respiratory acidosis, diabetic ketoacidosis, acute hemolysis, high phosphate intake, profound muscle necrosis, and increased phosphorus absorption. The primary complication of increased phosphorus is metastatic calcification (soft tissue, joints, and arteries), which occurs when the calcium–magnesium product (calcium × magnesium) exceeds 70 mg/dL.

### Clinical Manifestations

An increased serum phosphorus level causes few symptoms. Symptoms that do occur usually result from decreased calcium levels and soft tissue calcifications. The most important short-term consequence is tetany. Because of the reciprocal relationship between phosphorus and calcium, a high serum phosphorus level tends to cause a low serum calcium concentration. Tetany can result, causing tingling sensations in the fingertips and around the mouth. Anorexia, nausea, vomiting, bone and joint pain, muscle weakness, hyperreflexia, and tachycardia may occur.

The major long-term consequence is soft tissue calcification, which occurs mainly in patients with a reduced glomerular filtration rate. High serum levels of inorganic phosphorus promote precipitation of calcium phosphate in nonosseous sites, decreasing urine output, impairing vision, and producing palpitations.

### Assessment and Diagnostic Findings

On laboratory analysis, the serum phosphorus level exceeds 4.5 mg/dL (1.5 mmol/L) in adults. Serum phosphorus levels are normally higher in children, presumably because of the high rate of skeletal growth. The serum calcium level is useful also for diagnosing the primary disorder and assessing the effects of treatments. X-ray studies may show skeletal changes with abnormal bone development. PTH levels are decreased in hypoparathyroidism. BUN and creatinine levels are used to assess renal function. Renal ultrasonography may be indicated as part of the diagnostic assessment for renal failure; bone studies and coronary calcification studies also provide information about the chronicity and prognosis of renal failure.

### Medical Management

When possible, treatment is directed at the underlying disorder. For example, hyperphosphatemia may be related to volume depletion or respiratory or metabolic acidosis. In renal failure, elevated PTH production contributes to a high phosphorus level and bone disease. Measures to decrease the serum phosphate level in these patients include vitamin D preparations, such as calcitriol, which is available in both oral (Rocaltrol) and parenteral (Calcijex, paricalcitol [Zemplar]) forms. IV administration of calcitriol does not increase the serum calcium unless its dose is excessive, thus permitting more aggressive treatment of hyperphosphatemia with calcium-binding antacids (calcium carbonate or calcium citrate), phosphate-binding gels or antacids, restriction of dietary phosphate, forced diuresis with a loop diuretic, volume repletion with saline, and dialysis. Surgery may be indicated for removal of large calcium–phosphorus deposits.

### Nursing Management

The nurse monitors patients at risk for hyperphosphatemia. If a low-phosphorus diet is prescribed, the patient is instructed to avoid phosphorus-rich foods such as hard cheese, cream, nuts, meats, whole-grain cereals, dried fruits, dried vegetables, kidneys, sardines, sweetbreads, and foods made with milk. When appropriate, the nurse instructs the patient to avoid phosphate-containing substances such as laxatives and enemas. The nurse also teaches the patient to recognize the signs of impending hypocalcemia and to monitor for changes in urine output.

## Chloride Imbalances

Chloride, the major anion of the ECF, is found more in interstitial and lymph fluid compartments than in blood. Chloride is also contained in gastric and pancreatic juices, sweat, bile, and saliva. Sodium and chloride in water make up the composition of the ECF and assist in determining osmotic pressure.

The normal serum chloride level is 97 to 107 mEq/L (96 to 106 mmol/L). Inside the cell, the chloride level is 4 mEq/L. The serum level of chloride reflects a change in dilution or concentration of the ECF and does so in direct proportion to the sodium concentration. Serum osmolality parallels chloride levels as well. Aldosterone secretion increases sodium reabsorption, thereby increasing chloride reabsorption. The choroid plexus, where cerebrospinal fluid forms in the brain, depends on sodium and chloride to attract water to form the fluid portion of the cerebrospinal fluid. Bicarbonate has an inverse relationship with chloride. As chloride moves from plasma into the red blood cells (called the chloride shift), bicarbonate moves back into the plasma. Hydrogen ions are formed, which then help release oxygen from hemoglobin. When the level of one of these three electrolytes (sodium, bicarbonate, or chloride) is disturbed, the other two are also affected. Chloride assists in maintaining acid–base balance and works as a buffer in the exchange of oxygen and carbon dioxide in red blood cells. Chloride is primarily obtained from the diet as table salt.

## Chloride Deficit (Hypochloremia)

Chloride control depends on the intake of chloride and the excretion and reabsorption of its ions in the kidneys. Chloride is produced in the stomach, where it combines with hydrogen to form hydrochloric acid. A small amount of chloride is lost in the feces. GI tube drainage and severe vomiting and diarrhea are risk factors for hypochloremia. Administration of chloride-deficient formulas, low sodium intake, decreased serum sodium levels, metabolic alkalosis, prolonged therapy with IV dextrose, diuretic therapy, burns, and fever may also cause hypochloremia. Administration of aldosterone, ACTH, corticosteroids, bicarbonate, or laxatives decreases serum chloride levels as well. As chloride decreases (usually because of volume depletion), sodium and bicarbonate ions are retained by the kidney to balance the loss. Bicarbonate accumulates in the ECF, which raises the pH and leads to hypochloremic metabolic alkalosis.

### Clinical Manifestations

The signs and symptoms of hypochloremia are those of acid–base and electrolyte imbalances. The signs and symptoms of hyponatremia, hypokalemia, and metabolic alkalosis may also be present. Metabolic alkalosis is a disorder that results in a high pH and a high serum bicarbonate level as a result of excess alkali intake or loss of hydrogen ions. With compensation, the partial pressure of carbon dioxide in arterial blood ($PaCO_2$) increases to 50 mm Hg. Hyperexcitability of muscles, tetany, hyperactive deep tendon reflexes, weakness, twitching, and muscle cramps may result. Hypokalemia can cause hypochloremia, resulting in cardiac dysrhythmias. In addition, because low chloride levels parallel low sodium levels, a water excess may occur. Hyponatremia can cause seizures and coma.

### Assessment and Diagnostic Findings

In addition to the chloride level, sodium and potassium levels are also evaluated, because these electrolytes are lost along with chloride. Arterial blood gas analysis identifies the acid–base imbalance, which is usually metabolic alkalosis. The urine chloride level, which is also measured, decreases in hypochloremia.

### Medical Management

Treatment involves correcting the cause of hypochloremia and the contributing electrolyte and acid–base imbalances. Normal saline (0.9% sodium chloride) or half-strength saline (0.45% sodium chloride) solution is administered by IV to replace the chloride. The physician may reevaluate whether the patient receiving a diuretic (loop, osmotic, or thiazide) should discontinue the medications or change to another diuretic.

Foods high in chloride are provided; these include tomato juice, bananas, dates, eggs, cheese, milk, salty broth, canned vegetables, and processed meats. A patient who drinks free water (water without electrolytes) or bottled water excretes large amounts of chloride; therefore, the patient is instructed to avoid this kind of water. Ammonium chloride, an acidifying agent, may be prescribed to treat metabolic alkalosis; the dosage depends on the patient's weight and serum chloride level. This agent is metabolized by the liver, and its effects last for about 3 days. Its use should be avoided in patients with impaired liver or renal function.

### Nursing Management

The nurse monitors the patient's I&O, arterial blood gas values, and serum electrolyte levels, as well as level of consciousness and muscle strength and movement. Changes are reported to the physician promptly. Vital signs are monitored, and respiratory assessment is carried out frequently. The nurse teaches the patient about foods with high chloride content.

## Chloride Excess (Hyperchloremia)

Hyperchloremia exists when the serum level of chloride exceeds 107 mEq/L (107 mmol/L). Hypernatremia, bicarbonate loss, and metabolic acidosis can occur with high chloride levels. Hyperchloremic metabolic acidosis is also known as normal anion gap acidosis (see later discussion). It is usually caused by the loss of bicarbonate ions via the kidney or the GI tract with a corresponding increase in chloride ions. Chloride ions in the form of acidifying salts accumulate and acidosis occurs with a decrease in bicarbonate ions. Head trauma, increased perspiration, excess adrenocortical hormone production, and decreased glomerular filtration can lead to a high serum chloride level.

### Clinical Manifestations

The signs and symptoms of hyperchloremia are the same as those of metabolic acidosis, hypervolemia, and hypernatremia. Tachypnea; weakness; lethargy; deep, rapid respirations; diminished cognitive ability; and hypertension occur. If untreated, hyperchloremia can lead to a decrease in cardiac output, dysrhythmias, and coma. A high chloride level is accompanied by a high sodium level and fluid retention.

### Assessment and Diagnostic Findings

The serum chloride level is 108 mEq/L (108 mmol/L) or greater, the serum sodium level is greater than 145 mEq/L (145 mmol/L), the serum pH is less than 7.35, the serum bicarbonate level is less than 22 mEq/L (22 mmol/L), and there is a normal anion gap of 8 to 12 mEq/L (8 to 12 mmol/L). Urine chloride excretion increases. Increased chloride sweat levels are present in cystic fibrosis, diabetes insipidus, glucose-6-phosphate deficiency, hypothyroidism, malnutrition, and acute renal failure.

Calculation of the serum anion gap is important in analyzing acid–base disorders. The sum of all negatively charged electrolytes (anions) equals the sum of all positively charged electrolytes (cations) with several anions that are not routinely measured leading to an anion gap. It is based primarily on three electrolytes: sodium, chloride, and bicarbonate or serum carbon dioxide ($CO_2$). A low anion gap may be attributed to hypoproteinemia, whereas an elevated anion gap can be due to metabolic acidosis.

### Medical Management

Correcting the underlying cause of hyperchloremia and restoring electrolyte, fluid, and acid–base balance are essential. Hypotonic IV solutions may be given to restore balance. Lactated Ringer's solution may be prescribed to convert lactate to bicarbonate in the liver, which increases the base bicarbonate level and corrects the acidosis. IV sodium bicarbonate may be administered to increase bicarbonate levels, which leads to the renal excretion of chloride ions as bicarbonate and chloride compete for combination with sodium. Diuretics may be administered to eliminate chloride as well. Sodium, chloride, and fluids are restricted.

### Nursing Management

Monitoring vital signs, arterial blood gas values, and I&O is important to assess the patient's status and the effectiveness of treatment. Assessment findings related to respiratory, neurologic, and cardiac systems are documented, and changes discussed with the physician. The nurse teaches the patient about the diet that should be followed to manage hyperchloremia and maintain adequate hydration.

## Acid–Base Disturbances

Acid–base disturbances are commonly encountered in clinical practice. Identification of the specific acid–base imbalance is important in identifying the underlying cause of the disorder and determining appropriate treatment.

Plasma pH is an indicator of hydrogen ion ($H^+$) concentration. Homeostatic mechanisms keep pH within a normal range (7.35 to 7.45). These mechanisms consist of buffer systems, the kidneys, and the lungs. The $H^+$ concentration is extremely important: the greater the concentration, the more acidic the solution and the lower the pH; the lower the $H^+$ concentration, the more alkaline the solution and the higher the pH. The pH range compatible with life (6.8 to 7.8) represents a tenfold difference in $H^+$ concentration in plasma.

Buffer systems prevent major changes in the pH of body fluids by removing or releasing $H^+$; they can act quickly to prevent excessive changes in $H^+$ concentration. Hydrogen ions are buffered by both intracellular and extracellular buffers. The body's major extracellular buffer system is the bicarbonate–carbonic acid buffer system, which is assessed when arterial blood gases are measured. Normally, there are 20 parts of bicarbonate ($HCO_3^-$) to one part of carbonic acid ($H_2CO_3$). If this ratio is altered, the pH will change. It is the ratio of $HCO_3^-$ to $H_2CO_3$ that is important in maintaining pH, not absolute values. $CO_2$ is a potential acid; when dissolved in water, it becomes carbonic acid ($CO_2 + H_2O = H_2CO_3$). Therefore, when $CO_2$ is increased, the carbonic acid content is also increased, and vice versa. If either bicarbonate or carbonic acid is increased or decreased so that the 20:1 ratio is no longer maintained, acid–base imbalance results.

Less important buffer systems in the ECF include the inorganic phosphates and the plasma proteins. Intracellular buffers include proteins, organic and inorganic phosphates, and, in red blood cells, hemoglobin.

The kidneys regulate the bicarbonate level in the ECF; they can regenerate bicarbonate ions as well as reabsorb them from the renal tubular cells. In respiratory acidosis and most cases of metabolic acidosis, the kidneys excrete hydrogen ions and conserve bicarbonate ions to help restore balance. In respiratory and metabolic alkalosis, the kidneys retain hydrogen ions and excrete bicarbonate ions to help restore balance. The kidneys obviously cannot compensate for the metabolic acidosis created by renal failure. Renal compensation for imbalances is relatively slow (a matter of hours or days).

The lungs, under the control of the medulla, control the $CO_2$ and thus the carbonic acid content of the ECF. They do so by adjusting ventilation in response to the amount of $CO_2$ in the blood. A rise in the partial pressure of $CO_2$ in arterial blood ($PaCO_2$) is a powerful stimulant to respiration. Of course, the partial pressure of oxygen in arterial blood ($PaO_2$) also influences respiration. However, its effect is not as marked as that produced by the $PaCO_2$.

In metabolic acidosis, the respiratory rate increases, causing greater elimination of $CO_2$ (to reduce the acid load). In metabolic alkalosis, the respiratory rate decreases, causing $CO_2$ to be retained (to increase the acid load).

## *Acute and Chronic Metabolic Acidosis (Base Bicarbonate Deficit)*

Metabolic acidosis is a clinical disturbance characterized by a low pH (increased $H^+$ concentration) and a low plasma bicarbonate concentration. It can be produced by a gain of hydrogen ion or a loss of bicarbonate (Whittier & Rutecki, 2004). It can be divided clinically into two forms, according to the values of the serum anion gap: high anion gap acidosis and normal anion gap acidosis. The anion gap reflects normally unmeasured anions (phosphates, sulfates, and proteins) in plasma. Measuring the anion gap is essential in analyzing acid–base disorders correctly. The anion gap can be calculated by either one of the following equations:

$$\text{Anion gap} = Na^+ + K^+ - (Cl^- + HCO_3^-)$$

$$\text{Anion gap} = Na^+ - (Cl^- + HCO_3^-)$$

Potassium is often omitted from the equation because of its low level in the plasma; therefore, the second equation is used more often than the first.

The normal value for an anion gap is 8 to 12 mEq/L (8 to 12 mmol/L) without potassium in the equation. If potassium is included in the equation, the normal value for the anion gap is 12 to 16 mEq/L (12 to 16 mmol/L). The unmeasured anions in the serum normally account for less than 16 mEq/L of the anion production. An anion gap greater than 16 mEq (16 mmol/L) suggests excessive accumulation of unmeasured anions. An anion gap occurs because not all electrolytes are measured. More anions are left unmeasured than cations.

Normal anion gap acidosis results from the direct loss of bicarbonate, as in diarrhea, lower intestinal fistulas, ureterostomies, and use of diuretics; early renal insufficiency; excessive administration of chloride; and the administration of parenteral nutrition without bicarbonate or bicarbonate-producing solutes (eg, lactate). Normal anion gap acidosis is also referred to as hyperchloremic acidosis. A reduced or negative anion gap is primarily caused by hypoproteinemia. Disorders that cause a decreased or negative anion gap are rare compared to those related to an increased or high anion gap (Rose & Post, 2000).

High anion gap acidosis results from excessive accumulation of fixed acid. If it is increased to 30 mEq/L (30 mmol/L) or more, then a high anion gap metabolic acidosis is present regardless of what the pH and the $HCO_3^-$ are. High ion gap occurs in ketoacidosis, lactic acidosis, the late phase of salicylate poisoning, uremia, methanol or ethylene glycol toxicity, and ketoacidosis with starvation. The hydrogen is buffered by $HCO_3^-$, causing the bicarbonate concentration to fall. In all of these instances, abnormally high levels of anions flood the system, increasing the anion gap above normal limits.

### Clinical Manifestations

Signs and symptoms of metabolic acidosis vary with the severity of the acidosis. They may include headache, confusion, drowsiness, increased respiratory rate and depth, nausea, and vomiting. Peripheral vasodilation and decreased cardiac output occur when the pH drops to less than 7. Additional physical assessment findings include decreased blood pressure, cold and clammy skin, dysrhythmias, and shock (Whittier & Rutecki, 2004). Chronic metabolic acidosis is usually seen with chronic renal failure. The bicarbonate and pH decrease slowly, and the patient is asymptomatic until the bicarbonate is approximately 15 mEq/L or less.

### Assessment and Diagnostic Findings

Arterial blood gas measurements are valuable in diagnosing metabolic acidosis (Kee et al., 2004). Expected blood gas changes include a low bicarbonate level (less than 22 mEq/L) and a low pH (less than 7.35). The cardinal feature of metabolic acidosis is a decrease in the serum bicarbonate level. Hyperkalemia may accompany metabolic acidosis as a result of the shift of potassium out of the cells. Later, as the acidosis is corrected, potassium moves back into the cells and hypokalemia may occur. Hyperventilation decreases the $CO_2$ level as a compensatory action. As stated previously, calculation of the anion gap is helpful in determining the cause of metabolic acidosis. An ECG detects dysrhythmias caused by the increased potassium.

### Medical Management

Treatment is directed at correcting the metabolic defect (Kee et al., 2004). If the problem results from excessive intake of chloride, treatment is aimed at eliminating the source of the chloride. When necessary, bicarbonate is administered if the pH is less than 7.1 and the serum bicarbonate level is less than 10 mEq/L. Although hyperkalemia occurs with acidosis, hypokalemia may occur with reversal of the acidosis and subsequent movement of potassium back into the cells. Therefore, the serum potassium level is monitored closely, and hypokalemia is corrected as acidosis is reversed.

In chronic metabolic acidosis, low serum calcium levels are treated before the chronic metabolic acidosis is treated, to avoid tetany resulting from an increase in pH and a decrease in ionized calcium. Alkalizing agents may be administered if the serum bicarbonate level is less than 12 mEq/L. Treatment modalities may also include hemodialysis or peritoneal dialysis.

## Acute and Chronic Metabolic Alkalosis (Base Bicarbonate Excess)

Metabolic alkalosis is a clinical disturbance characterized by a high pH (decreased $H^+$ concentration) and a high plasma bicarbonate concentration. It can be produced by a gain of bicarbonate or a loss of $H^+$ (Porth, 2005).

Probably the most common cause of metabolic alkalosis is vomiting or gastric suction with loss of hydrogen and chloride ions. The disorder also occurs in pyloric stenosis, in which only gastric fluid is lost. Gastric fluid has an acid pH (usually 1 to 3), and loss of this highly acidic fluid increases the alkalinity of body fluids. Other situations predisposing to metabolic alkalosis include those associated with loss of potassium, such as diuretic therapy that promotes excretion of potassium (eg, thiazides, furosemide), and excessive adrenocorticoid hormones (as in hyperaldosteronism and Cushing's syndrome).

Hypokalemia produces alkalosis in two ways: (1) the kidneys conserve potassium, and therefore $H^+$ excretion increases; and (2) cellular potassium moves out of the cells into the ECF in an attempt to maintain near-normal serum levels (as potassium ions leave the cells, hydrogen ions must enter to maintain electroneutrality). Excessive alkali ingestion from antacids containing bicarbonate or from use of sodium bicarbonate during cardiopulmonary resuscitation can also cause metabolic alkalosis.

Chronic metabolic alkalosis can occur with long-term diuretic therapy (thiazides or furosemide), villous adenoma, external drainage of gastric fluids, significant potassium depletion, cystic fibrosis, and the chronic ingestion of milk and calcium carbonate.

## Clinical Manifestations

Alkalosis is primarily manifested by symptoms related to decreased calcium ionization, such as tingling of the fingers and toes, dizziness, and hypertonic muscles. The ionized fraction of serum calcium decreases in alkalosis as more calcium combines with serum proteins. Because it is the ionized fraction of calcium that influences neuromuscular activity, symptoms of hypocalcemia are often the predominant symptoms of alkalosis. Respirations are depressed as a compensatory action by the lungs. Atrial tachycardia may occur. As the pH increases to greater than 7.6 and hypokalemia develops, ventricular disturbances may occur. Decreased motility and paralytic ileus may also occur.

Symptoms of chronic metabolic alkalosis are the same as for acute metabolic alkalosis, and as potassium decreases, frequent premature ventricular contractions or U waves are seen on the ECG.

## Assessment and Diagnostic Findings

Evaluation of arterial blood gases reveals a pH greater than 7.45 and a serum bicarbonate concentration greater than 26 mEq/L. The $PaCO_2$ increases as the lungs attempt to compensate for the excess bicarbonate by retaining $CO_2$. This hypoventilation is more pronounced in semiconscious, unconscious, or debilitated patients than in alert patients. The former may develop marked hypoxemia as a result of hypoventilation. Hypokalemia may accompany metabolic alkalosis.

Urine chloride levels may help identify the cause of metabolic alkalosis if the patient's history provides inadequate information. Metabolic alkalosis is the setting in which urine chloride concentration may be a more accurate estimate of volume than the urine sodium concentration. Urine chloride concentrations help to differentiate between vomiting, diuretic therapy, and excessive adrenocorticosteroid secretion as the cause of the metabolic alkalosis. In patients with vomiting or cystic fibrosis, those receiving nutritional repletion, and those receiving diuretic therapy, hypovolemia and hypochloremia produce urine chloride concentrations lower than 25 mEq/L. Signs of hypovolemia are not present, and the urine chloride concentration exceeds 40 mEq/L in patients with mineralocorticoid excess or alkali loading; these patients usually have expanded fluid volume. The urine chloride concentration should be less than 15 mEq/L when decreased chloride levels and hypovolemia occur.

## Medical Management

Treatment of both acute and chronic metabolic alkalosis is aimed at correcting the underlying acid–base disorder (Hogan & Wane, 2003). Because of volume depletion from GI loss, the patient's fluid I&O must be monitored carefully.

Sufficient chloride must be supplied for the kidney to absorb sodium with chloride (allowing the excretion of excess bicarbonate). Treatment also includes restoring normal fluid volume by administering sodium chloride fluids (because continued volume depletion serves to maintain the alkalosis). In patients with hypokalemia, potassium is administered as KCl to replace both $K^+$ and $Cl^-$ losses. $H_2$ receptor antagonists, such as cimetidine (Tagamet), reduce the production of gastric HCl, thereby decreasing the metabolic alkalosis associated with gastric suction. Carbonic anhydrase inhibitors are useful in treating metabolic alkalosis in patients who cannot tolerate rapid volume expansion (eg, patients with heart failure).

## Acute and Chronic Respiratory Acidosis (Carbonic Acid Excess)

Respiratory acidosis is a clinical disorder in which the pH is less than 7.35 and the $PaCO_2$ is greater than 42 mm Hg. It may be either acute or chronic.

Respiratory acidosis is always due to inadequate excretion of $CO_2$ with inadequate ventilation, resulting in elevated plasma $CO_2$ concentrations and, consequently, increased levels of carbonic acid (Morton, Fontaine, Hudak et al., 2005). In addition to an elevated $PaCO_2$, hypoventilation usually causes a decrease in $PaO_2$. Acute respiratory acidosis occurs in emergency situations, such as acute pulmonary edema, aspiration of a foreign object, atelectasis, pneumothorax, overdose of sedatives, sleep apnea syndrome, administration of oxygen to a patient with chronic hypercapnia (excessive $CO_2$ in the blood), severe pneumonia, and acute respiratory distress syndrome. Respiratory acidosis can also occur in diseases that impair respiratory muscles, such as muscular dystrophy, myasthenia gravis, and Guillain-Barré syndrome.

Mechanical ventilation may be associated with hypercapnia if the rate of effective alveolar ventilation is inadequate. Ventilation is fixed, and $CO_2$ may be retained if the rate of $CO_2$ production is increased.

## Clinical Manifestations

Clinical signs in acute and chronic respiratory acidosis vary. Sudden hypercapnia (elevated $PaCO_2$) can cause increased pulse and respiratory rate, increased blood pressure, mental cloudiness, and a feeling of fullness in the head. An elevated $PaCO_2$ causes cerebrovascular vasodilation and increased cerebral blood flow, particularly when it is greater than 60 mm Hg. Ventricular fibrillation may be the first sign of respiratory acidosis in anesthetized patients.

If respiratory acidosis is severe, intracranial pressure may increase, resulting in papilledema and dilated conjunctival blood vessels. Hyperkalemia may result as the hydrogen concentration overwhelms the compensatory mechanisms and $H^+$ moves into cells, causing a shift of potassium out of the cell.

Chronic respiratory acidosis occurs with pulmonary diseases such as chronic emphysema and bronchitis, obstructive sleep apnea, and obesity. As long as the $PaCO_2$ does not exceed the body's ability to compensate, the patient will be asymptomatic. However, if the $PaCO_2$ increases rapidly, cerebral vasodilation will increase the intracranial pressure, and cyanosis and tachypnea will develop. Patients with chronic obstructive pulmonary disease (COPD) who gradually accumulate $CO_2$ over a prolonged period (days to months) may not develop symptoms of hypercapnia because compensatory renal changes have had time to occur.

> **NURSING ALERT**
>
> If the $PaCO_2$ is chronically higher than 50 mm Hg, the respiratory center becomes relatively insensitive to $CO_2$ as a respiratory stimulant, leaving hypoxemia as the major drive for respiration. Oxygen administration may remove the stimulus of hypoxemia, and the patient develops "carbon dioxide narcosis" unless the situation is quickly reversed. Therefore, oxygen is administered only with extreme caution.

## Assessment and Diagnostic Findings

Arterial blood gas analysis reveals a pH lower than 7.35, a $PaCO_2$ greater than 42 mm Hg, and a variation in the bicarbonate level, depending on the duration of the acute respiratory acidosis. When compensation (renal retention of bicarbonate) has fully occurred, the arterial pH may be within the lower limits of normal. Depending on the cause of respiratory acidosis, other diagnostic measures would include monitoring of serum electrolyte levels, chest x-ray for determining any respiratory disease, and a drug screen if an overdose is suspected. An ECG to identify any cardiac involvement as a result of COPD may be indicated as well.

## Medical Management

Treatment is directed at improving ventilation; exact measures vary with the cause of inadequate ventilation (Hogan & Wane, 2003). Pharmacologic agents are used as indicated. For example, bronchodilators help reduce bronchial spasm, antibiotics are used for respiratory infections, and thrombolytics or anticoagulants are used for pulmonary emboli.

Pulmonary hygiene measures are initiated, when necessary, to clear the respiratory tract of mucus and purulent drainage. Adequate hydration (2 to 3 L/day) is indicated to keep the mucous membranes moist and thereby facilitate the removal of secretions. Supplemental oxygen is administered as necessary.

Mechanical ventilation, used appropriately, may improve pulmonary ventilation. Inappropriate mechanical ventilation (eg, increased dead space, insufficient rate or volume settings, high fraction of inspired oxygen [$FiO_2$] with excessive $CO_2$ production) may cause such rapid excretion of $CO_2$ that the kidneys are unable to eliminate excess bicarbonate quickly enough to prevent alkalosis and seizures. For this reason, the elevated $PaCO_2$ must be decreased slowly. Placing the patient in a semi-Fowler's position facilitates expansion of the chest wall. Treatment of chronic respiratory acidosis is the same as for acute respiratory acidosis.

## Acute and Chronic Respiratory Alkalosis (Carbonic Acid Deficit)

Respiratory alkalosis is a clinical condition in which the arterial pH is greater than 7.45 and the $PaCO_2$ is less than 38 mm Hg. As with respiratory acidosis, acute and chronic conditions can occur.

Respiratory alkalosis is always caused by hyperventilation, which causes excessive "blowing off" of $CO_2$ and, hence, a decrease in the plasma carbonic acid concentration. Causes can include extreme anxiety, hypoxemia, the early phase of salicylate intoxication, gram-negative bacteremia, and inappropriate ventilator settings that do not match the patient's requirements.

Chronic respiratory alkalosis results from chronic hypocapnia, and decreased serum bicarbonate levels are the consequence. Chronic hepatic insufficiency and cerebral tumors are predisposing factors.

## Clinical Manifestations

Clinical signs consist of lightheadedness due to vasoconstriction and decreased cerebral blood flow, inability to concentrate, numbness and tingling from decreased calcium ionization, tinnitus, and sometimes loss of consciousness. Cardiac effects of respiratory alkalosis include tachycardia and ventricular and atrial dysrhythmias (Heitz & Horne, 2005).

## Assessment and Diagnostic Findings

Analysis of arterial blood gases assists in the diagnosis of respiratory alkalosis. In the acute state, the pH is elevated above normal as a result of a low $PaCO_2$ and a normal bicarbonate level. (The kidneys cannot alter the bicarbonate level quickly.) In the compensated state, the kidneys have had sufficient time to lower the bicarbonate level to a near-normal level. Evaluation of serum electrolytes is indicated to identify any decrease in potassium as hydrogen is pulled out of the cells in exchange for potassium; decreased calcium, as severe alkalosis inhibits calcium ionization, resulting in carpopedal spasms and tetany; or decreased phosphate due to alkalosis, causing an increased uptake of phosphate by the cells. A toxicology screen should be performed to rule out salicylate intoxication.

Patients with chronic respiratory alkalosis are usually asymptomatic, and the diagnostic evaluation and plan of care are the same as for acute respiratory alkalosis.

## Medical Management

Treatment depends on the underlying cause of respiratory alkalosis. If the cause is anxiety, the patient is instructed to breathe more slowly to allow $CO_2$ to accumulate or to breathe into a closed system (such as a paper bag). A sedative may be required to relieve hyperventilation in very anxious patients. Treatment of other causes of respiratory alkalosis is directed at correcting the underlying problem.

## Mixed Acid–Base Disorders

Patients can simultaneously experience two or more independent acid–base disorders. A normal pH in the presence of changes in the $PaCO_2$ and plasma $HCO_3^-$ concentration immediately suggests a mixed disorder. The only mixed disorder that cannot occur is a mixed respiratory acidosis and alkalosis, because it is impossible to have alveolar hypoventilation and hyperventilation at the same time. An example of a mixed disorder is the simultaneous occurrence of metabolic acidosis and respiratory acidosis during respiratory and cardiac arrest.

## Compensation

Generally, the pulmonary and renal systems compensate for each other to return the pH to normal. In a single acid–base disorder, the system not causing the problem will try to compensate by returning the ratio of bicarbonate to carbonic acid to the normal 20:1. The lungs compensate for metabolic disturbances by changing $CO_2$ excretion. The kidneys compensate for respiratory disturbances by altering bicarbonate retention and $H^+$ secretion.

In respiratory acidosis, excess hydrogen is excreted in the urine in exchange for bicarbonate ions. In respiratory alkalosis, the renal excretion of bicarbonate increases, and hydrogen ions are retained. In metabolic acidosis, the compensatory mechanisms increase the ventilation rate and the renal retention of bicarbonate.

In metabolic alkalosis, the respiratory system compensates by decreasing ventilation to conserve $CO_2$ and increase the $PaCO_2$. Because the lungs respond to acid–base disorders within minutes, compensation for metabolic imbalances occurs faster than compensation for respiratory imbalances. Table 14-6 summarizes compensation effects.

## Blood Gas Analysis

Blood gas analysis is often used to identify the specific acid–base disturbance and the degree of compensation that has occurred. The analysis is usually based on an arterial blood sample, but if an arterial sample cannot be obtained, a mixed venous sample may be used. Results of arterial blood gas analysis provide information about alveolar ventilation, oxygenation, and acid–base balance. It is necessary to evaluate the concentrations of serum electrolytes (sodium, potassium, and chloride) and carbon dioxide along with arterial blood gas data, because they are often the first sign of an acid–base disorder. The health history, physical examination, previous blood gas results, and serum electrolytes should always be part of the assessment used to determine the cause of the acid–base disorder (Porth, 2005). Treatment of the underlying condition usually corrects most acid–base disorders. Table 14-7 compares normal ranges of venous and arterial blood gas values. See also Chart 14-2.

## Parenteral Fluid Therapy

When no other route of administration is available, fluids are administered intravenously in hospitals, outpatient di-

### TABLE 14-6 Acid–Base Disturbances and Compensation

| Disorder | Initial Event | Compensation |
|---|---|---|
| Respiratory acidosis | ↓ pH, ↑ or normal $HCO_3^-$, ↑ $PaCO_2$ | ↑ Renal acid excretion and ↑ serum $HCO_3^-$ |
| Respiratory alkalosis | ↑ pH, ↓ or normal $HCO_3^-$, ↓ $PaCO_2$ | ↓ Renal acid excretion and ↓ serum $HCO_3^-$ |
| Metabolic acidosis | ↓ pH, ↓ $HCO_3^-$, ↓ or normal $PaCO_2$ | Hyperventilation with resulting ↓ PaCO (conserves $HCO_3^-$) |
| Metabolic alkalosis | ↑ pH, ↑ $HCO_3^-$, ↑ or normal $PaCO_2$ | Hypoventilation with resulting ↑ $PaCO_2$ |

| TABLE 14-7 | Normal Values for Arterial and Mixed Venous Blood | |
|---|---|---|
| Parameter | Arterial Blood | Mixed Venous Blood |
| pH | 7.35–7.45 | 7.33–7.41 |
| $PaCO_2$ | 35–45 mm Hg | 41–51 mm Hg |
| $PaO_2$* | 80–100 mm Hg | 35–40 mm Hg |
| $HCO_3^-$ | 22–26 mEq/L | 22–26 mEq/L |
| Base excess/deficit | ± 2 mEq/L | ± 2 mEq/L |
| Oxygen saturation | > 94% | 75% |

*At altitudes of 3,000 feet and higher, the values for oxygen are decreased.

agnostic and surgical settings, clinics, and homes to replace fluids, administer medications, and provide nutrients.

## Purpose

The choice of an IV solution depends on the purpose of its administration. Generally, IV fluids are administered to achieve one or more of the following goals:

- To provide water, electrolytes, and nutrients to meet daily requirements
- To replace water and correct electrolyte deficits
- To administer medications and blood products

IV solutions contain dextrose or electrolytes mixed in various proportions with water. Pure, electrolyte-free water can never be administered IV because it rapidly enters red blood cells and causes them to rupture.

## Types of Intravenous Solutions

Solutions are often categorized as **isotonic**, **hypotonic**, or **hypertonic**, according to whether their total osmolality is the same as, less than, or greater than that of blood (see earlier discussion of osmolality).

Electrolyte solutions are considered isotonic if the total electrolyte content (anions + cations) is approximately 310 mEq/L, hypotonic if the total electrolyte content is less than 250 mEq/L, and hypertonic if the total electrolyte content is greater than 375 mEq/L. The nurse must also consider a solution's osmolality, keeping in mind that the osmolality of plasma is approximately 300 mOsm/L (300 mmol/L). For example, a 10% dextrose solution has an osmolality of approximately 505 mOsm/L.

When administering parenteral fluids, the nurse monitors the patient's response to the fluids, considering the fluid volume, the content of the fluid, and the patient's clinical status.

### Isotonic Fluids

Fluids that are classified as isotonic have a total osmolality close to that of the ECF and do not cause red blood cells to shrink or swell. The composition of these fluids may or may not approximate that of the ECF. Isotonic fluids expand the ECF volume. One liter of isotonic fluid expands the ECF by 1 L; however, it expands the plasma by only 0.25 L because it is a crystalloid fluid and diffuses quickly into the ECF compartment. For the same reason, 3 L of isotonic fluid is needed to replace 1 L of blood loss. Because these fluids expand the intravascular space, patients with hypertension and heart failure should be carefully monitored for signs of fluid overload.

#### $D_5W$

A solution of $D_5W$ has a serum osmolality of 252 mOsm/L. Once administered, the glucose is rapidly metabolized, and this initially isotonic solution then disperses as a hypotonic fluid, one-third extracellular and two-thirds intracellular. It is essential to consider this action of $D_5W$, especially if the patient is at risk for increased intracranial pressure. During fluid resuscitation, this solution should not be used, because it can cause hyperglycemia. Therefore, $D_5W$ is used mainly to supply water and to correct an increased serum osmolality. About 1 L of $D_5W$ provides fewer than 200 kcal and is a minor source of the body's daily caloric requirements.

#### NORMAL SALINE SOLUTION

Normal saline (0.9% sodium chloride) solution has a total osmolality of 308 mOsm/L. Because the osmolality is entirely contributed by electrolytes, the solution remains within the ECF. For this reason, normal saline solution is often used to correct an extracellular volume deficit. Although referred to as "normal," it contains only sodium and chloride and does not actually simulate the ECF. It is used with administration of blood transfusions and to replace large sodium losses, as in burn injuries. It is not used for heart failure, pulmonary edema, renal impairment, or sodium retention. Normal saline does not supply calories.

#### OTHER ISOTONIC SOLUTIONS

Several other solutions contain ions in addition to sodium and chloride and are somewhat similar to the ECF in composition. Lactated Ringer's solution contains potassium and calcium in addition to sodium chloride. It is used to correct dehydration and sodium depletion and replace GI losses. Lactated Ringer's solution contains bicarbonate precursors as well. These solutions are marketed, with slight variations, under various trade names.

### Hypotonic Fluids

One purpose of hypotonic solutions is to replace cellular fluid, because it is hypotonic compared with plasma. Another is to provide free water for excretion of body wastes. At times, hypotonic sodium solutions are used to treat hypernatremia and other hyperosmolar conditions. Half-strength saline (0.45% sodium chloride) solution, with an osmolality of 154 mOsm/L, is frequently used. Multiple-electrolyte solutions are also available. Excessive infusions of hypotonic solutions can lead to intravascular fluid depletion, decreased blood pressure, cellular edema, and cell damage. These solutions exert less osmotic pressure than the ECF.

### Hypertonic Fluids

When normal saline solution or lactated Ringer's solution contains 5% dextrose, the total osmolality exceeds that of the ECF. However, the dextrose is quickly metabolized, and only the isotonic solution remains. Therefore, any effect on the intracellular compartment is temporary.

## CHART 14-2

### Assessing for Arterial Blood Gases

The following steps are recommended to evaluate arterial blood gas values. They are based on the assumption that the average values are:

pH = 7.4
$PaCO_2$ = 40 mm Hg
$HCO_3^-$ = 24 mEq/L

1. *First, note the pH.* It can be high, low, or normal, as follows:

   pH > 7.4 (alkalosis)
   pH < 7.4 (acidosis)
   pH = 7.4 (normal)

   A normal pH may indicate perfectly normal blood gases, *or* it may be an indication of a *compensated* imbalance. A compensated imbalance is one in which the body has been able to correct the pH by either respiratory or metabolic changes (depending on the primary problem). For example, a patient with primary metabolic acidosis starts out with a low bicarbonate level but a normal $CO_2$ level. Soon afterward, the lungs try to compensate for the imbalance by exhaling large amounts of $CO_2$ (hyperventilation). As another example, a patient with primary respiratory acidosis starts out with a high $CO_2$ level; soon afterward, the kidneys attempt to compensate by retaining bicarbonate. If the compensatory mechanism is able to restore the bicarbonate to carbonic acid ratio back to 20:1, full compensation (and thus normal pH) will be achieved.

2. The next step is to determine the primary cause of the disturbance. This is done by evaluating the $PaCO_2$ and $HCO_3^-$ in relation to the pH.

   **Example: pH > 7.4 (alkalosis)**
   a. If the $PaCO_2$ is < 40 mm Hg, the primary disturbance is respiratory alkalosis. (This situation occurs when a patient hyperventilates and "blows off" too much $CO_2$. Recall that $CO_2$ dissolved in water becomes carbonic acid, the acid side of the "carbonic acid–bicarbonate buffer system.")
   b. If the $HCO_3^-$ is >24 mEq/L, the primary disturbance is metabolic alkalosis. (This situation occurs when the body gains too much bicarbonate, an alkaline substance. Bicarbonate is the basic or alkaline side of the "carbonic acid–bicarbonate buffer system.")

   **Example: pH < 7.4 (acidosis)**
   a. If the $PaCO_2$ is >40 mm Hg, the primary disturbance is respiratory acidosis. (This situation occurs when a patient hypoventilates and thus retains too much $CO_2$, an acidic substance.)
   b. If the $HCO_3^-$ is <24 mEq/L, the primary disturbance is metabolic acidosis. (This situation occurs when the body's bicarbonate level drops, either because of direct bicarbonate loss or because of gains of acids such as lactic acid or ketones.)

3. The next step involves determining if compensation has begun. This is done by looking at the value other than the primary disorder. If it is moving in the same direction as the primary value, compensation is underway. Consider the following gases:

   | | pH | $PaCO_2$ | $HCO_3^-$ |
   |---|---|---|---|
   | (1) | 7.2 | 60 mm Hg | 24 mEq/L |
   | (2) | 7.4 | 60 mm Hg | 37 mEq/L |

   The first set (1) indicates acute respiratory acidosis without compensation (the $PaCO_2$ is high, the $HCO_3^-$ is normal). The second set (2) indicates chronic respiratory acidosis. Note that compensation has take place; that is, the $HCO_3^-$ has elevated to an appropriate level to balance the high $PaCO_2$ and produce a normal pH.

4. Two distinct acid–base disturbances may occur simultaneously. These can be identified when the pH does not explain one of the changes.

   **Example: Metabolic and respiratory acidosis**
   a. pH         7.2    decreased acid
   b. $PaCO_2$   52     increased acid
   c. $HCO_3$    13     decreased acid

   This is an example of metabolic and respiratory acidosis.

---

Similarly, with hypotonic multiple-electrolyte solutions containing 5% dextrose, once the dextrose is metabolized, these solutions disperse as hypotonic fluids.

Higher concentrations of dextrose, such as 50% dextrose in water, are administered to help meet caloric requirements. These solutions are strongly hypertonic and must be administered into central veins so that they can be diluted by rapid blood flow.

Saline solutions are also available in osmolar concentrations greater than that of the ECF. These solutions draw water from the ICF to the ECF and cause cells to shrink. If administered rapidly or in large quantity, they may cause an extracellular volume excess and precipitate circulatory overload and dehydration. As a result, these solutions must be administered cautiously and usually only when the serum osmolality has decreased to dangerously low levels. Hypertonic solutions exert an osmotic pressure greater than that of the ECF.

### Other Intravenous Substances

When the patient's GI tract is unable to tolerate food, nutritional requirements are often met using the IV route. Parenteral solutions may include high concentrations of glucose, protein, or fat to meet nutritional requirements (see Chapter 36). The parenteral route may also be used to administer colloids, plasma expanders, and blood products. Examples of blood products include whole blood, packed red blood cells, albumin, and cryoprecipitate; these are discussed in more detail in Chapter 33.

Many medications are also delivered by the IV route, either by infusion or directly into the vein. Because IV medications enter the circulation rapidly, administration by this route is potentially very hazardous. All medications can produce adverse reactions; however, medications administered by the IV route can cause these reactions within 15 minutes after administration, because the medications are delivered directly into the bloodstream. Administration rates and recommended dilutions for individual medications are available in specialized texts pertaining to IV medications and in manufacturers' package inserts; these should be consulted to ensure safe IV administration of medications.

> **! NURSING ALERT**
>
> The nurse must assess the patient for a history of allergic reactions to medications. Although this is important when any medication is to be administered, it is even more important with IV administration, because the medication is delivered directly into the bloodstream.

## Nursing Management of the Patient Receiving Intravenous Therapy

**CONCEPTS in action ANIMATION**

The ability to perform venipuncture to gain access to the venous system for administering fluids and medication is an expected nursing skill in many settings. This responsibility includes selecting the appropriate venipuncture site and type of cannula and being proficient in the technique of vein entry.

### Preparing to Administer Intravenous Therapy

Before performing venipuncture, the nurse carries out hand hygiene, applies gloves, and informs the patient about the procedure. Next, the nurse selects the most appropriate insertion site and type of cannula for a particular patient. Factors influencing these choices include the type of solution to be administered, the expected duration of IV therapy, the patient's general condition, and the availability of veins. The skill of the person initiating the infusion is also an important consideration.

### Choosing an Intravenous Site

Many sites can be used for IV therapy, but ease of access and potential hazards vary. Veins of the extremities are designated as peripheral locations and are ordinarily the only sites used by nurses. Because they are relatively safe and easy to enter, arm veins are most commonly used (Fig. 14-7). The metacarpal, cephalic, basilic, and median veins and their branches are recommended sites because of their size and ease of access. More distal sites should be used first, with more proximal sites used subsequently. Leg veins should rarely, if ever, be used because of the high risk of thromboembolism. Additional sites to avoid include veins distal to a previous IV infiltration or phlebitic area, sclerosed or thrombosed veins, an arm with an arteriovenous shunt or fistula, and an arm affected by edema, infection, blood clot, or skin breakdown. The arm on the side of a mastectomy is avoided because of impaired lymphatic flow.

Central veins commonly used by physicians include the subclavian and internal jugular veins. It is possible to gain access to (or cannulate) these larger vessels even when peripheral sites have collapsed, and they allow for the administration of hyperosmolar solutions. However, the potential hazards are much greater and include inadvertent entry into an artery or the pleural space.

Ideally, both arms and hands are carefully inspected before a specific venipuncture site that does not interfere with

**FIGURE 14-7.** Site selection for peripheral cannulation of veins: anterior (palmar) veins at *left*, posterior (dorsal) veins at *right*. Adapted from Agur, A. M. R., Lee, M. J. & Boileau Grant, M. J. (1999). *Grant's atlas of anatomy* (10th ed.). Philadelphia: Lippincott Williams & Wilkins.

mobility is chosen. For this reason, the antecubital fossa is avoided, except as a last resort. The most distal site of the arm or hand is generally used first, so that subsequent IV access sites can be moved progressively upward. The following factors should be considered when selecting a site for venipuncture:

- Condition of the vein
- Type of fluid or medication to be infused
- Duration of therapy
- Patient's age and size
- Whether the patient is right- or left-handed
- Patient's medical history and current health status
- Skill of the person performing the venipuncture

After applying a tourniquet, the nurse palpates and inspects the vein. The vein should feel firm, elastic, engorged, and round—not hard, flat, or bumpy. Because arteries lie close to veins in the antecubital fossa, the vessel should be palpated for arterial pulsation (even with a tourniquet on), and cannulation of pulsating vessels should be avoided. General guidelines for selecting a cannula include the following:

- Length: 0.75 to 1.25 inches long
- Diameter: narrow diameter of the cannula to occupy minimal space within the vein
- Gauge: 20 to 22 gauge for most IV fluids; a larger gauge for caustic or viscous solutions; 14 to 18 gauge for blood administration and for trauma patients and those undergoing surgery

Hand veins are easiest to cannulate. Cannula tips should not rest in a flexion area (eg, the antecubital fossa), because this could inhibit the IV flow.

## Selecting Venipuncture Devices

Equipment used to gain access to the vasculature includes cannulas, needleless IV delivery systems, and peripherally inserted central catheter or midline catheter access lines.

### CANNULAS

Most peripheral access devices are cannulas. They have an obturator inside a tube that is later removed. "Catheter" and "cannula" are terms that are used interchangeably. The main types of cannula devices available are those referred to as winged infusion sets (butterfly) with a steel needle or as over-the-needle catheters with wings; indwelling plastic cannulas that are inserted over a steel needle; and indwelling plastic cannulas that are inserted through a steel needle. Scalp vein or butterfly needles are short steel needles with plastic wing handles. These are easy to insert, but because they are small and nonpliable, infiltration occurs easily. The use of these needles should be limited to obtaining blood specimens or administering bolus injections or infusions lasting only a few hours, because they increase the risk of vein injury and infiltration. Insertion of an over-the-needle catheter requires the additional step of advancing the catheter into the vein after venipuncture. Because these devices are less likely to cause infiltration, they are frequently preferred over winged infusion sets.

Plastic cannulas inserted through a hollow needle are usually called intracatheters. They are available in long lengths and are well suited for placement in central locations. Because insertion requires threading the cannula through the vein for a relatively long distance, these can be difficult to insert. The most commonly used infusion device is the over-the-needle catheter. A hollow metal stylet is preinserted into the catheter and extends through the distal tip of the catheter to allow puncture of the vessel, in an effort to guide the catheter as the venipuncture is performed. The vein is punctured and a flashback of blood appears in the closed chamber behind the catheter hub. The catheter is threaded through the stylet into the vein and the stylet is then removed. Many safety over-the-needle catheter designs with retracting stylets are available to protect health care workers from needlestick injuries.

Many types of cannulas are available for IV therapy. Some of the variations in these cannulas include the thickness of the cannula wall (affects rate of flow), the sharpness of the insertion needles (determines needle insertion technique), the softening properties of the cannula (influences the length of time the cannula can remain in place), safety features (minimizes risk of needlestick injuries and bloodborne exposure), and the number of lumens (determines the number of solutions that can be infused simultaneously). Cannula systems that help prevent needlesticks and transmission of bloodborne diseases are discussed later in this chapter. Most standard peripheral catheters are composed of some form of plastic. Teflon (polytetrafluoroethylene)–coated catheters have fewer thrombogenic properties and are less inflammatory than those coated with polyurethane or polyvinyl chloride (PVC). Catheters for steel needles can range from 3/8 inch to 1.5 inches in length and can be 27 to 13 gauge in size. Plastic catheters can range in length from 5/8 inch to 2 inches or as long as 12 inches and range in size from 27 to 12 gauge.

To select the ideal product for use, consideration should be given to which product provides the greatest patient satisfaction and offers quality, cost-effective infusion care. All devices should be radiopaque to determine catheter location by x-ray, if necessary. All catheters are thrombogenic and differ only in the incidence of thrombus occurrence. Biocompatibility, another characteristic of a catheter, ensures that inflammation and irritation do not occur. Silicone catheters are the most bioinert catheters available today.

**Needleless Intravenous Delivery Systems.** The federal Needlestick Safety and Prevention Act, which was signed into law in November of 2000, requires needleless systems. In an effort to decrease needlestick injuries and exposure to human immunodeficiency virus (HIV), hepatitis, and other bloodborne pathogens, agencies have implemented needleless IV delivery systems. These systems have built-in protection against needlestick injuries and provide a safe means of using and disposing of an IV administration set (which consists of tubing, an area for inserting the tubing into the container of IV fluid, and an adapter for connecting the tubing to the needle). Numerous companies produce needleless components. IV line connectors allow the simultaneous infusion of IV medications and other intermittent medications (known as a piggyback delivery) without the use of needles (Fig. 14-8). Technology is advancing and moving away from use of the traditional stylet. An

**FIGURE 14-8.** One example of a needleless intravenous access device. The Clearink Access System (Baxter Healthcare Corp., Becton Dickinson Division, Franklin Lakes, NJ) (**A**) is designed to prevent needlesticks and other accidents. After drawing medication into a syringe according to the manufacturer's guidelines and swabbing the Y-site intersection with antiseptic, the nurse can insert the syringe-cannula apparatus into the Y site (**B**) and deliver bolus dose medications. If a blood tube holder (**C**) is attached to the cannula, blood can be withdrawn safely without fear of contact or spills.

example is a self-sheathing stylet that is recessed into a rigid chamber at the hub of the catheter when its insertion is complete. Other designs have placed the stylet at the end of a flexible wire to avoid needlesticks.

Many examples of these devices are on the market. Each institution must evaluate products to determine its own needs based on Occupational Safety and Health Administration (OSHA) guidelines and the institution's policies and procedures.

**Peripherally Inserted Central Catheter or Peripheral-Midline Catheter Access Lines.** Patients who need moderate- to long-term parenteral therapy often receive a peripherally inserted central catheter or a peripheral-midline catheter. These catheters are also used for patients with limited peripheral access (eg, obese or emaciated patients, IV/injection drug users) who require IV antibiotics, blood, and parenteral nutrition. For these devices to be used, the median cephalic, basilic, and cephalic veins must be pliable (not sclerosed or hardened) and not subject to repeated puncture. If these veins are damaged, then central venous access via the subclavian or internal jugular vein, or surgical placement of an implanted port or a vascular access device, must be considered as an alternative. Table 14-8 compares peripherally inserted central and peripheral-midline catheters.

The principles for inserting these lines are much the same as those for inserting peripheral catheters; however, their insertion should be undertaken only by practitioners who are experienced and specially skilled in inserting IV lines.

The physician prescribes the line and the solution to be infused. Insertion of either catheter requires sterile technique. The size of the catheter lumen chosen is based on the type of solution, the patient's body size, and the vein to be used. The patient's consent is obtained before use of these catheters. Use of the dominant arm is recommended as the site for inserting the cannula into the superior vena cava to ensure adequate arm movement, which encourages blood flow and reduces the risk of dependent edema.

## Teaching the Patient

Except in emergency situations, a patient should be prepared in advance for an IV infusion. The venipuncture, the expected length of infusion, and activity restrictions are explained. If the patient requires alternative formats (eg, interpreter, large-print written materials) to understand the procedure, these should be provided. Then the patient should have an opportunity to ask questions and express concerns. For example, some patients believe that they will die if small bubbles in the tubing enter their veins. After acknowledging this fear, the nurse can explain that usually only relatively large volumes of air administered rapidly are dangerous.

| TABLE 14-8 | Comparison of Peripherally Inserted Central and Peripheral-Midline Catheters | |
|---|---|---|
| | **Peripherally Inserted Central Catheter** | **Peripheral-Midline Catheter** |
| Indications | Parenteral nutrition; IV fluid replacement; administration of chemotherapy agents, analgesics, and antibiotics; removal of blood specimens | Parenteral nutrition; IV fluid replacement; administration of analgesics and antibiotics (no solution or medications with a pH <5 or >9 or osmolarity >500 mOsm/L); removal of blood specimens |
| Features | Single- and double-lumen catheters available 40–60 cm long; gauge variable (16–24 gauge) | Single- and double-lumen catheters available (16–24 gauge) 7.5–20 cm in length. Can increase two gauges in size as it softens |
| Material | Radiopaque, polymer (polyurethane), Silastic materials. Flexible. | Silicone, polyurethane, and their derivatives; available impregnated with heparin to ↓ thrombogenicity (radiopaque or clear, with radiopaque strip) |
| Insertion sites | Venipuncture performed in the antecubital fossa, above or below it into the basilic, cephalic, or axillary veins of the dominant arm. The median basilic is the ideal insertion site. | Venipuncture performed 1½ inches above or below the antecubital fossa through the cephalic, basilic, or median cubital vein. |
| Catheter placement | The tip of the catheter lies in the superior vena cava. The catheter is placed via the basilic or cephalic vein at the antecubital fossa. | Between the antecubital area and the head of the clavicle (tip in axilla region). The tip terminates in the proximal portion of the extremity below axilla and proximal to central veins and is advanced 3–10 inches. |
| Insertion method | Through-the-needle technique, with or without a guidewire, breakaway needle with introducer or cannula with introducer (peelaway sheath). (A peripherally inserted central catheter can also be used as a midline catheter.) Insertion can be accomplished at the bedside using sterile technique. Arm to be used should be positioned in abduction to 90-degree angle. Consent is required. Catheter may stay in place for up to 12 months or as long as required without complications. | No separate guidewire or introducer is needed. Stiff catheter is passed using the catheter advancement tab. Insertion can be accomplished at the bedside using sterile technique. Arm to be used should be positioned in abduction to 45-degree angle. Consent is required. Catheter may stay in place for 2–4 weeks. |
| Potential complications | Malposition, pneumothorax, hemothorax, hydrothorax, dysrhythmias, nerve or tendon damage, respiratory distress, catheter embolism, thrombophlebitis, or catheter occlusion. Compared with centrally placed catheters, venipuncture in the antecubital space reduces risk of insertion complications. | Thrombosis, phlebitis, air embolism, infection, vascular perforation, bleeding, catheter transection, occlusion |
| Contraindications | Dermatitis, cellulitis, burns, high fluid volume infusions, rapid bolus injections, hemodialysis, and venous thrombosis. No clamping of this catheter or splinting of the arm permitted. No blood pressure or tourniquets to be used on extremity where peripherally inserted central catheter is inserted. | Dermatitis, cellulitis, burns, high fluid volume infusions, rapid bolus injection, hemodialysis, and venous thrombosis. No blood pressure or tourniquet to be used on extremity where midline catheter is placed. |
| Catheter maintenance | Sterile dressing changes according to agency policy and procedures. Generally, dressing is changed 2 or 3 ×/week or when wet, soiled, or nonocclusive. Line is flushed every 12 hours with 3 mL normal saline followed by heparin 3 mL (100 U/mL) per lumen. | Sterile dressing changes according to policy and procedures. Generally, dressing is changed 2 or 3 ×/week or when wet, soiled, or nonocclusive. Line is flushed after each infusion or every 12 hours with 5–10 mL normal saline followed by 1 mL of heparin (100 U/mL). Catheter must be anchored securely to prevent its dislodgment. |
| Postplacement | Chest x-ray needed to confirm placement of catheter tip. | Chest x-ray to assess placement may be obtained if unable to flush catheter, if no free flow blood return, if difficulty with catheter advancement, or if guidewire difficult to remove or bent on removal. |

| TABLE 14-8 | Comparison of Peripherally Inserted Central and Peripheral-Midline Catheters (Continued) | |
|---|---|---|
| | **Peripherally Inserted Central Catheter** | **Peripheral-Midline Catheter** |
| Assessment | Daily measurement of arm circumference (4″ above insertion site) and length of exposed catheter | Daily measurement of arm circumference (4″ above insertion site) and length of exposed catheter |
| Removal | Catheter should be removed when no longer indicated for use, if contaminated, or if complications occur. | Catheter should be removed when no longer indicated for use, if contaminated, or if complications occur. |
| | Arm is abducted during removal. Patient should be in a dorsal recumbent position with head of bed flat and should perform the Valsalva maneuver while catheter is withdrawn. | Arm is abducted during removal. |
| | Pressure is applied on removal with a sterile dressing and antiseptic ointment to site. Dressing is changed every 24 hours until epithelialization occurs. | Pressure is applied on removal with a sterile dressing and antiseptic ointment to site. Dressing is changed every 24 hours until epithelialization occurs. |
| Advantages | Reduces cost and avoids repeated venipunctures compared with centrally placed catheters. Decreases incidence of catheter-related infections. | Reduces cost and avoids repeated venipunctures compared with centrally placed catheters. Decreases incidence of catheter-related infections. |

## Preparing the Intravenous Site

Before preparing the skin, the nurse should ask the patient whether he or she is allergic to latex or iodine, products commonly used in preparing for IV therapy. Excessive hair at the selected site may be removed by clipping to increase the visibility of the veins and to facilitate insertion of the cannula and adherence of dressings to the IV insertion site. Because infection can be a major complication of IV therapy, the IV device, the fluid, the container, and the tubing must be sterile. The insertion site is scrubbed with a sterile pad soaked in 10% povidone–iodine (Betadine) or chlorhexidine gluconate solution for 30 seconds, working from the center of the area to the periphery and allowing the area to air dry for approximately 2 minutes. The site should not be wiped with 70% alcohol, because the alcohol negates the effect of the disinfecting solution. (Alcohol pledgets are used for 30 seconds instead, only if the patient is allergic to iodine.) The nurse must perform hand hygiene and put on gloves. Gloves (nonsterile, disposable) must be worn during the venipuncture procedure because of the likelihood of coming into contact with the patient's blood.

## Performing Venipuncture

Guidelines and a suggested sequence for venipuncture are presented in Chart 14-3. For veins that are very small or particularly fragile, modifications in the technique may be necessary. Alternative methods can be found in journal articles or in specialized textbooks of IV therapy. Institutional policies and procedures determine whether all nurses must be certified to perform venipuncture. A nurse certified in IV therapy or an IV team can be consulted to assist with initiating IV therapy.

## Maintaining Therapy

Maintaining an existing IV infusion is a nursing responsibility that demands knowledge of the solutions being administered and the principles of flow. In addition, patients must be assessed carefully for both local and systemic complications.

## Factors Affecting Flow

The flow of an IV infusion is governed by the same principles that govern fluid movement in general:

- Flow is directly proportional to the height of the liquid column. Raising the height of the infusion container may improve a sluggish flow.
- Flow is directly proportional to the diameter of the tubing. The clamp on IV tubing regulates the flow by changing the tubing diameter. In addition, the flow is faster through large-gauge rather than small-gauge cannulas.
- Flow is inversely proportional to the length of the tubing. Adding extension tubing to an IV line decreases the flow.
- Flow is inversely proportional to the viscosity of a fluid. Viscous IV solutions, such as blood, require a larger cannula than do water or saline solutions.

## Monitoring Flow

Because so many factors influence gravity flow, a solution does not necessarily continue to run at the speed originally set. Therefore, the nurse monitors IV infusions frequently to make sure that the fluid is flowing at the intended rate. The IV container should be marked with tape to indicate at a glance whether the correct amount has infused. The flow rate is calculated when the solution is originally started and then monitored at least hourly. To calculate the flow rate, the nurse determines the number of drops delivered per milliliter; this varies with equipment and is usually printed on the administration set packaging. A formula that can be used to calculate the drop rate is

$$\text{gtt/mL of infusion set}/60(\text{min in 1 hr}) \times \text{total hourly volume} = \text{gtt/min}$$

## CHART 14-3 Guidelines for Starting an Intravenous Infusion

### NURSING ACTION

**Preparation**
1. Verify prescription for IV therapy, check solution label, and identify patient.
2. Explain procedure to patient.
3. Carry out hand hygiene and put on disposable non-latex gloves.
4. Apply a tourniquet 4–6 inches above the site and identify a suitable vein.
5. Choose site. Use distal veins of hands and arms first.



6. Choose IV cannula or catheter.


7. Connect infusion bag and tubing, and run solution through tubing to displace air; cover end of tubing.
8. Raise bed to comfortable working height and position for patient; adjust lighting. Position patient's arm below heart level to encourage capillary filling. Place protective pad on bed under patient's arm.

**Procedure**
1. Depending on agency policy and procedure, lidocaine 1% (without epinephrine) 0.1–0.2 mL may be injected locally to the IV site or a transdermal analgesic cream (EMLA) may be applied to the site 60 minutes before IV placement or blood withdrawal. Alternatively, topical application of lidocaine (Numby Stuff) via an iontophoretic drug delivery system (iontophoresis) may be used to numb the skin up to a depth of 10 mm; it takes 10 minutes to work. Intradermal injection of bacteriostatic 0.9% sodium chloride may also have a local anesthetic effect.
2. Question the patient carefully about sensitivity to latex; use blood-pressure cuff rather than latex tourniquet if there is possibility of sensitivity.
3. Apply a new tourniquet for each patient or a blood pressure cuff 15 to 20 cm (6–8 in) above injection site. Palpate for a pulse distal to the tourniquet. Ask patient to open and close fist several times or position patient's arm in a dependent position to distend a vein.

### RATIONALE

1. Serious errors can be avoided by careful checking.
2. Knowledge increases patient comfort and cooperation.
3. Asepsis is essential to prevent infection. Use of non-latex gloves prevents exposure of nurse to patient's blood and of patient and nurse to latex.
4. This will distend the veins and allow them to be visualized.
5. Careful site selection will increase likelihood of successful venipuncture and preservation of vein. Using distal sites first preserves sites proximal to the previously cannulated site for subsequent venipunctures. Veins of feet and lower extremity should be avoided due to risk of thrombophlebitis. (In consultation with the physician, the saphenous vein of the ankle or dorsum of the foot may occasionally be used.)
6. Length and gauge of cannula should be appropriate for both site and purpose of infusion. The shortest gauge and length needed to deliver prescribed therapy should be used.
7. Prevents delay; equipment must be ready to connect immediately after successful venipuncture to prevent clotting
8. Proper positioning will increase likelihood of success and provide comfort for patient.



1. Reduces pain locally from procedure and decreases anxiety about pain









2. Reduces risk of allergic reaction

3. The tourniquet distends the vein and makes it easier to enter; it should never be tight enough to occlude arterial flow. If a radial pulse cannot be palpated distal to the tourniquet, it is too tight. A new tourniquet should be used for each patient to prevent the transmission of microorganisms. A blood pressure cuff may be used for elderly patients to avoid

### CHART 14-3  Guidelines for Starting an Intravenous Infusion, continued

| NURSING ACTION | RATIONALE |
|---|---|
| | rupture of the veins. A clenched fist encourages the vein to become round and turgid. Positioning the arm below the level of the patient's heart promotes capillary filling. Warm packs applied for 10–20 min. prior to venipuncture can promote vasodilation. Bedside ultrasound-guided visualization of vein location and assessment of venous pathway and flow using ultrasonic waves may also be used. |
| 4. Ascertain if the patient is allergic to iodine. Prepare site by scrubbing with chlorhexidine gluconate or povidone–iodine swabs for 2–3 min in circular motion, moving outward from injection site. Allow to dry.<br>  a. If the site selected is excessively hairy, clip hair. (Check agency's policy and procedure about this practice.)<br>  b. 70% isopropyl alcohol is an alternative solution that may be used. | 4. Strict asepsis and careful site preparation are essential to prevent infection. |
| 5. With hand not holding the venous access device, steady patient's arm and use finger or thumb to pull skin taut over vessel. | 5. Applying traction to the vein helps to stabilize it. |
| 6. Holding needle bevel up and at 5–25° angle, depending on the depth of the vein, pierce skin to reach but not penetrate vein. | 6. Bevel down technique is necessary for small veins to prevent extravasation. One-step method of catheter insertion directly into vein with immediate thrust through the skin is excellent for large veins but may cause a hematoma if used in small veins. |
| 7. Decrease angle of needle further until nearly parallel with skin, then enter vein either directly above or from the side in one quick motion. | 7. Two-stage procedure decreases chance of thrusting needle through posterior wall of vein as skin is entered. No attempt should be made to reinsert the stylet because of risk of severing or puncturing the catheter. |
| 8. If backflow of blood is visible, straighten angle and advance needle. Additional steps for catheter inserted over needle:<br>  a. Advance needle 0.6 cm (¼–½ in) after successful venipuncture.<br>  b. Hold needle hub, and slide catheter over the needle into the vein. Never reinsert needle into a plastic catheter or pull the catheter back into the needle.<br>  c. Remove needle while pressing lightly on the skin over the catheter tip; hold catheter hub in place. | 8. Backflow may not occur if vein is small; this position decreases chance of puncturing posterior wall of vein.<br>  a. Advancing the needle slightly makes certain the plastic catheter has entered the vein.<br>  b. Reinsertion of the needle or pulling the catheter back can sever the catheter, causing catheter embolism.<br>  c. Slight pressure prevents bleeding before tubing is attached. |
| 9. Release tourniquet and attach infusion tubing; open clamp enough to allow drip. | 9. Infusion must be attached promptly to prevent clotting of blood in cannula. After two unsuccessful attempts at venipuncture, assistance by a more experienced health care provider is recommended to avoid unnecessary trauma to the patient and the possibility of limiting future sites for vascular access. |
| 10. Slip a sterile 2-in × 2-in gauze pad under the catheter hub. | 10. The gauze acts as a sterile field. |
| 11. Anchor needle firmly in place with tape. | 11. A stable needle is less likely to become dislodged or to irritate the vein. |

*continued >*

### CHART 14-3  Guidelines for Starting an Intravenous Infusion, continued

| NURSING ACTION | RATIONALE |
|---|---|
| 12. Cover the insertion site with a transparent dressing, bandage, or sterile gauze; tape in place with nonallergenic tape but do not encircle extremity. | 12. Tape encircling extremity can act as a tourniquet and impede blood flow and infusion of fluid. |
| 13. Tape a small loop of IV tubing onto dressing. | 13. The loop decreases the chance of inadvertent cannula removal if the tubing is pulled. |
| 14. Cover the insertion site with a dressing according to hospital policy and procedure. A gauze or transparent dressing may be used. | 14. Transparent dressings allow assessment of the insertion site for phlebitis, infiltration, and infection without removing the dressing. |
| 15. Label dressing with type and length of cannula, date, time, and initials. | 15. Labeling facilitates assessment and safe discontinuation. |
| 16. A padded, appropriate-length arm board may be applied to an area of flexion (neurovascular checks should be performed frequently). | 16. Secures cannula placement and allows correct flow rate (neurovascular checks assess nerve, muscle, and vascular function to be sure function is not affected by immobilization) |
| 17. Calculate infusion rate and regulate flow of infusion. For hourly IV rate use the following formula: gtt/mL of infusion set/60 (min in hr) × total hourly vol = gtt/min | 17. Infusion must be regulated carefully to prevent overinfusion or underinfusion. Calculation of the IV rate is essential for the safe delivery of fluids. Safe administration requires knowledge of the volume of fluid to be infused, total infusion time, and the calibration of the administration set (found on the IV tubing package; 10, 12, 15, or 60 drops to deliver 1 mL of fluid). |
| 18. Document date and time therapy initiated; type and amount of solution; additives and dosages; flow rate; gauge, length, and type of vascular access device; catheter insertion site; patient response to procedure; and name and title of the health care provider who inserted the catheter. | 18. Documentation is essential to promote continuity of care. |
| 19. Discard needles, stylets, or guidewires into a puncture-resistant needle container that meets OSHA guidelines. | 19. Proper disposal of sharps decreases risk of needlesticks. |

Flushing of a vascular device is performed to ensure patency and to prevent the mixing of incompatible medications or solutions. This procedure should be carried out at established intervals, according to hospital policy and procedure, especially for intermittently used catheters. Most manufacturers and researchers suggest the use of saline for flushing (Hankins et al., 2001). The volume of the flush solution should be at least twice the volume capacity of the catheter. The catheter should be clamped before the syringe is completely empty and withdrawn to prevent reflux of blood into the lumen, which could cause catheter clotting.

A variety of electronic infusion devices are available to assist in IV fluid delivery. These devices allow more accurate administration of fluids and medications than is possible with routine gravity-flow setups. A pump is a positive-pressure device that uses pressure to infuse fluid at a pressure of 10 psi; newer models use a pressure of 5 psi. The pressure exerted by the pump overrides vascular resistance (increased tubing length, low height of the IV container).

Volumetric pumps calculate the volume delivered by measuring the volume in a reservoir that is part of the set and is calibrated in milliliters per hour (mL/h). A controller is an infusion assist device that relies on gravity for infusion; the volume is calibrated in drops (gtt) per minute. A controller uses a drop sensor to monitor the flow. Factors essential for the safe use of pumps include alarms to signify the presence of air in the IV line or an occlusion. The standard for the accurate delivery of fluid or medication via an electronic IV infusion pump is plus or minus 5%. The manufacturer's directions must be read carefully before use of any infusion pump or controller, because there are many variations in available models. Use of these devices does not eliminate the need for the nurse to monitor the infusion and the patient frequently.

### Discontinuing an Infusion

The removal of an IV catheter is associated with two possible dangers: bleeding and catheter embolism. To prevent excessive bleeding, a dry, sterile pressure dressing should be held over the site as the catheter is removed. Firm pressure is applied until hemostasis occurs.

If a plastic IV catheter is severed, the loose fragment can travel to the right ventricle and block blood flow. To detect this complication when the catheter is removed, the nurse compares the expected length of the catheter with its actual length. Plastic catheters should be withdrawn carefully and their length measured to make certain that no fragment has broken off in the vein.

Great care must be exercised when using scissors around the dressing site. If the catheter clearly has been severed, the nurse can attempt to occlude the vein above the site by applying a tourniquet to prevent the catheter from entering the central circulation (until surgical removal is possible). However, as always, it is better to prevent a potentially fatal problem than to deal with it after it has occurred. Fortunately, catheter embolism can be prevented easily by following simple rules:

- Avoid using scissors near the catheter.
- Avoid withdrawing the catheter through the insertion needle.
- Follow the manufacturer's guidelines carefully (eg, cover the needle point with the bevel shield to prevent severance of the catheter).

## Managing Systemic Complications

IV therapy predisposes the patient to numerous hazards, including both local and systemic complications. Systemic complications occur less frequently but are usually more serious than local complications. They include circulatory overload, air embolism, febrile reaction, and infection.

**FLUID OVERLOAD.** Overloading the circulatory system with excessive IV fluids causes increased blood pressure and central venous pressure. Signs and symptoms of fluid overload include moist crackles on auscultation of the lungs, edema, weight gain, dyspnea, and respirations that are shallow and have an increased rate. Possible causes include rapid infusion of an IV solution or hepatic, cardiac, or renal disease. The risk of fluid overload and subsequent pulmonary edema is especially increased in elderly patients with cardiac disease; this is referred to as circulatory overload.

The treatment for circulatory overload is decreasing the IV rate, monitoring vital signs frequently, assessing breath sounds, and placing the patient in a high Fowler's position. The physician is contacted immediately. This complication can be avoided by using an infusion pump for infusions and by carefully monitoring all infusions. Complications of circulatory overload include heart failure and pulmonary edema.

**AIR EMBOLISM.** The risk of air embolism is rare but ever-present. It is most often associated with cannulation of central veins. Manifestations of air embolism include dyspnea and cyanosis; hypotension; weak, rapid pulse; loss of consciousness; and chest, shoulder, and low back pain. Treatment calls for immediately clamping the cannula and replacing a leaking or open infusion system, placing the patient on the left side in the Trendelenburg position, assessing vital signs and breath sounds, and administering oxygen. Air embolism can be prevented by using a Luer-Lok adapter on all lines, filling all tubing completely with solution, and using an air detection alarm on an IV pump. Complications of air embolism include shock and death. The amount of air necessary to induce death in humans is not known; however, the rate of entry is probably as important as the actual volume of air.

**SEPTICEMIA AND OTHER INFECTION.** Pyrogenic substances in either the infusion solution or the IV administration set can induce a febrile reaction and septicemia. Signs and symptoms include an abrupt temperature elevation shortly after the infusion is started, backache, headache, increased pulse and respiratory rate, nausea and vomiting, diarrhea, chills and shaking, and general malaise. In severe septicemia, vascular collapse and septic shock may occur. Causes of septicemia include contamination of the IV product or a break in aseptic technique, especially in immunocompromised patients. Treatment is symptomatic and includes culturing of the IV cannula, tubing, or solution if it is suspect and establishing a new IV site for medication or fluid administration. See Chapter 15 for a discussion of septic shock.

Infection ranges in severity from local involvement of the insertion site to systemic dissemination of organisms through the bloodstream, as in septicemia. Measures to prevent infection are essential at the time the IV line is inserted and throughout the entire infusion. Prevention includes the following:

- Careful hand hygiene before every contact with any part of the infusion system or the patient
- Examining the IV containers for cracks, leaks, or cloudiness, which may indicate a contaminated solution
- Using strict aseptic technique
- Firmly anchoring the IV cannula to prevent to-and-fro motion
- Inspecting the IV site daily and replacing a soiled or wet dressing with a dry sterile dressing. (Antimicrobial agents that should be used for site care include 2% tincture of iodine, 10% povidone–iodine, alcohol, or chlorhexidine gluconate, used alone or in combination.)
- Disinfecting injection/access ports with antimicrobial solution before use
- Removing the IV cannula at the first sign of local inflammation, contamination, or complication
- Replacing the peripheral IV cannula every 48 to 72 hours, or as indicated
- Replacing the IV cannula inserted during emergency conditions (with questionable asepsis) as soon as possible
- Using a 0.2-μm air-eliminating and bacteria/particulate retentive filter with non–lipid-containing solutions that require filtration. The filter can be added to the proximal or distal end of the administration set. If added to the proximal end between the fluid container and the tubing spike, the filter ensures sterility and particulate removal from the infusate container and prevents inadvertent infusion of air. If added to the distal end of the administration set, it filters air particles and contaminants introduced from add-on devices, secondary administration sets, or interruptions to the primary system.
- Replacing the solution bag and administration set in accordance with agency policy and procedure
- Infusing or discarding medication or solution within 24 hours of its addition to an administration set
- Changing primary and secondary continuous administration sets every 72 hours, or immediately if contamination is suspected
- Changing primary intermittent administration sets every 24 hours, or immediately if contamination is suspected

## Managing Local Complications

Local complications of IV therapy include infiltration and extravasation, phlebitis, thrombophlebitis, hematoma, and clotting of the needle.

**INFILTRATION AND EXTRAVASATION.** Infiltration is the unintentional administration of a nonvesicant solution or medication into surrounding tissue. This can occur when the IV cannula dislodges or perforates the wall of the vein. Infiltration is characterized by edema around the insertion site, leakage of IV fluid from the insertion site, discomfort and coolness in the area of infiltration, and a significant decrease in the flow rate. When the solution is particularly irritating, sloughing of tissue may result. Close monitoring of the insertion site is necessary to detect infiltration before it becomes severe.

Infiltration is usually easily recognized if the insertion area is larger than the same site of the opposite extremity; however, it is not always so obvious. A common misconception is that a backflow of blood into the tubing proves that the catheter is properly placed within the vein. However, if the catheter tip has pierced the wall of the vessel, IV fluid will seep into tissues as well as flow into the vein. Although blood return occurs, infiltration has occurred as well. A more reliable means of confirming infiltration is to apply a tourniquet above (or proximal to) the infusion site and tighten it enough to restrict venous flow. If the infusion continues to drip despite the venous obstruction, infiltration is present.

As soon as the nurse notes infiltration, the infusion should be stopped, the IV discontinued, and a sterile dressing applied to the site after careful inspection to determine the extent of infiltration. The infiltration of any amount of blood product, irritant, or vesicant is considered the most severe.

The IV infusion should be started in a new site or proximal to the infiltration if the same extremity must be used again. A warm compress may be applied to the site if small volumes of noncaustic solutions have infiltrated over a long period, or if the solution was isotonic with a normal pH; the affected extremity should be elevated to promote the absorption of fluid. If the infiltration is recent and the solution was hypertonic or had an increased pH, a cold compress may be applied to the area. Infiltration can be detected and treated early by inspecting the site every hour for redness, pain, edema, blood return, coolness at the site, and IV fluid leaking from the IV site. Using the appropriate size and type of cannula for the vein prevents this complication. The Infusion Nursing Standards of Practice state that a standardized infiltration scale should be used to document the infiltration (Alexander, 2000) (Chart 14-4).

Extravasation is similar to infiltration, with an inadvertent administration of vesicant or irritant solution or medication into the surrounding tissue. Medications such as dopamine, calcium preparations, and chemotherapeutic agents can cause pain, burning, and redness at the site. Blistering, inflammation, and necrosis of tissues can occur. The extent of tissue damage is determined by the concentration of the medication, the quantity that extravasated, the location of the infusion site, the tissue response, and the duration of the process of extravasation.

---

**CHART 14-4**

### Assessing for Infiltration

| GRADE | CLINICAL CRITERIA |
|---|---|
| 0 | No clinical symptoms |
| 1 | Skin blanched, edema less than 1 inch in any direction, cool to touch, with or without pain |
| 2 | Skin blanched, edema 1 to 6 inches in any direction, cool to touch, with or without pain |
| 3 | Skin blanched, translucent, gross edema greater than 6 inches in any direction, cool to touch, mild to moderate pain, possible numbness |
| 4 | Skin blanched, translucent, skin tight, leaking, skin discolored, bruised, swollen, gross edema greater than 6 inches in any direction, deep pitting tissue edema, circulatory impairment, moderate to severe pain, infiltration of any amount of blood products, irritant, or vesicant |

---

The infusion must be stopped and the physician notified promptly. The agency's protocol to treat extravasation is initiated; the protocol may specify specific treatments, including antidotes specific to the medication that extravasated, and may indicate whether the IV line should remain in place or be removed before treatment. The protocol often specifies infiltration of the infusion site with an antidote prescribed after assessment by the physician, removal of the cannula; and application of warm compresses to sites of extravasation from vinca alkaloids or cold compresses to sites of extravasation from alkylating and antibiotic vesicants (Hankins et al., 2001). The affected extremity should not be used for further cannula placement. Thorough neurovascular assessments of the affected extremity must be performed frequently.

Reviewing the institution's IV policy and procedures and incompatibility charts and checking with the pharmacist before administering any IV medication, whether given peripherally or centrally, is a prudent way to determine incompatibilities and vesicant potential to prevent extravasation. Careful, frequent monitoring of the IV site, avoiding insertion of IV devices in areas of flexion, securing the IV line, and using the smallest catheter possible that accommodates the vein help minimize the incidence and severity of this complication. In addition, when vesicant medication is administered by IV push, it should be given through a side port of an infusing IV solution to dilute the medication and decrease the severity of tissue damage if extravasation occurs. Extravasation should always be rated as a grade 4 on the infiltration scale.

**PHLEBITIS.** Phlebitis is defined as inflammation of a vein, which can be categorized as chemical, mechanical, or bacterial; however, two or more of these types of irritation often occur simultaneously. Chemical phlebitis can be caused by an irritating medication or solution (increased pH or high osmolality of a solution), rapid infusion rates, and medication incompatibilities. Mechanical phlebitis results from long periods of cannulation, catheters in flexed areas, catheter gauges larger than the vein lumen, and poorly secured catheters. Bacterial phlebitis can develop from poor hand hygiene, lack of aseptic technique, failure to check all equipment before use, and failure to recognize early signs and symptoms of phlebitis. Other factors include poor venipuncture technique, catheter in place for a prolonged period, and failure to adequately secure the catheter. Phlebitis is characterized by a reddened, warm area around the insertion site or along the path of the vein, pain or tenderness at the site or along the vein, and swelling. The incidence of phlebitis increases with the length of time the IV line is in place, the composition of the fluid or medication infused (especially its pH and tonicity), the size and site of the cannula inserted, ineffective filtration, inadequate anchoring of the line, and the introduction of microorganisms at the time of insertion. The Intravenous Nursing Society has identified specific standards for assessing phlebitis (Alexander, 2000); these appear in Chart 14-5. Phlebitis should be graded according to the most severe presenting indication.

Treatment consists of discontinuing the IV and restarting it in another site, and applying a warm, moist compress to the affected site. Phlebitis can be prevented by using aseptic technique during insertion, using the appropriate-size cannula or needle for the vein, considering the composition of fluids and medications when selecting a site, observing the site hourly for any complications, anchoring the cannula or needle well, and changing the IV site according to agency policy and procedures.

**THROMBOPHLEBITIS.** Thrombophlebitis refers to the presence of a clot plus inflammation in the vein. It is evidenced by localized pain, redness, warmth, and swelling around the insertion site or along the path of the vein, immobility of the extremity because of discomfort and swelling, sluggish flow rate, fever, malaise, and leukocytosis.

Treatment includes discontinuing the IV infusion; applying a cold compress first, to decrease the flow of blood and increase platelet aggregation, followed by a warm compress; elevating the extremity; and restarting the line in the opposite extremity. If the patient has signs and symptoms of thrombophlebitis, the IV line should not be flushed (although flushing may be indicated in the absence of phlebitis to ensure cannula patency and to prevent mixing of incompatible medications and solutions). The catheter should be cultured after the skin around the catheter is cleaned with alcohol. If purulent drainage exists, the site is cultured before the skin is cleaned.

Thrombophlebitis can be prevented by avoiding trauma to the vein at the time the IV is inserted, observing the site every hour, and checking medication additives for compatibility.

**HEMATOMA.** Hematoma results when blood leaks into tissues surrounding the IV insertion site. Leakage can result if the opposite vein wall is perforated during venipuncture, the needle slips out of the vein, or insufficient pressure is applied to the site after removal of the needle or cannula. The signs of a hematoma include ecchymosis, immediate swelling at the site, and leakage of blood at the insertion site.

Treatment includes removing the needle or cannula and applying light pressure with a sterile, dry dressing; applying ice for 24 hours to the site to avoid extension of the hematoma; elevating the extremity; assessing the extremity for any circulatory, neurologic, or motor dysfunction; and restarting the line in the other extremity if indicated. A hematoma can be prevented by carefully inserting the needle and by using diligent care with patients who have a bleeding disorder, are taking anticoagulant medication, or have advanced liver disease.

**CLOTTING AND OBSTRUCTION.** Blood clots may form in the IV line as a result of kinked IV tubing, a very slow infusion rate, an empty IV bag, or failure to flush the IV line after intermittent medication or solution administrations. The signs are decreased flow rate and blood backflow into the IV tubing.

If blood clots in the IV line, the infusion must be discontinued and restarted in another site with a new cannula and administration set. The tubing should not be irrigated or milked. Neither the infusion rate nor the solution container should be raised, and the clot should not be aspirated from the tubing. Clotting of the needle or cannula may be prevented by not allowing the IV solution bag to run dry, taping the tubing to prevent kinking and maintain patency, maintaining an adequate flow rate, and flushing the line after intermittent medication or other solution administration. In some cases, a specially trained nurse or physician may inject a thrombolytic agent into the catheter to clear an occlusion resulting from fibrin or clotted blood.

## Promoting Home and Community-Based Care

**TEACHING PATIENTS SELF-CARE.** At times, IV therapy must be administered in the home setting, in which case much of the daily management rests with the patient and

---

### CHART 14-5

### Assessing for Phlebitis

| GRADE | CLINICAL CRITERIA |
|---|---|
| 0 | No clinical symptoms |
| 1 | Erythema at access site with or without pain |
| 2 | Pain at access site<br>Erythema, edema, or both |
| 3 | Pain at access site<br>Erythema, edema, or both<br>Streak formation<br>Palpable venous cord (1 inch or shorter) |
| 4 | Pain at access site with erythema<br>Streak formation<br>Palpable venous cord (longer than 1 inch)<br>Purulent drainage |

Note: If this scale is not being used in an institution, then the description associated with the number can be used to describe the assessment.
From Infusion Nursing Standards of Practice (2000). *Journal of Intravenous Nursing, 23*(6S), S56–S69.

family. Teaching becomes essential to ensure that the patient and family can manage the IV fluid and infusion correctly and avoid complications. Written instructions as well as demonstration and return demonstration help reinforce the key points for all these functions.

**CONTINUING CARE.** Home infusion therapies cover a wide range of treatments, including antibiotic, analgesic, and antineoplastic medications; blood or blood component therapy; and parenteral nutrition. When direct nursing care is necessary, arrangements are made to have an infusion nurse visit the home and administer the IV therapy as prescribed. In addition to implementing and monitoring the IV therapy, the nurse carries out a comprehensive assessment of the patient's condition and continues to teach the patient and family about the skills involved in overseeing the IV therapy setup. Any dietary changes that may be necessary because of fluid or electrolyte imbalances are explained or reinforced during such sessions.

Periodic laboratory testing may be necessary to assess the effects of IV therapy and the patient's progress. Blood specimens may be obtained by a laboratory near the patient's home, or a home visit may be arranged to obtain blood specimens for analysis.

The nurse collaborates with the case manager in assessing the patient, family, and home environment; developing a plan of care in accordance with the patient's treatment plan and level of ability; and arranging for appropriate referral and follow-up if necessary. Any necessary equipment may be provided by the agency or purchased by the patient, depending on the terms of the home care arrangements. Appropriate documentation is necessary to assist in obtaining third-party payment for the service provided.

## Critical Thinking Exercises

**1** A 28-year-old man with a history of diabetes mellitus has an open fracture of the tibia as the result of a motorcycle crash. In the emergency department, his temperature is 103°F. His laboratory test results are as follows: blood glucose, 450 mg/dL; BUN, 35 mg/dL; sodium, 140 mEq/L; potassium, 4.1 mEq/L; pH, 7.1; $PCO_2$, 10 mm Hg; and $HCO_3^-$, 12 mEq/L. His urine ketones are 3+. What fluid and electrolyte or acid–base disorders is the patient experiencing? What IV fluids would you anticipate being prescribed? Give the rationale for their use. What treatments would address the patient's fluid and electrolyte or acid–base disorders?

**2** A 30-year-old woman comes to the emergency department with nausea, confusion, dehydration, and oliguria. Her mother reports that she has been depressed after losing her job as a bank executive. An empty bottle of aspirin was found in her bathroom sink. Her laboratory values are as follows: pH, 7.35; $PaCO_2$, 16 mm Hg; $PaO_2$, 130 mm Hg; and $HCO_3^-$, 15 mEq/L. What acid–base disorder does this patient have? What treatments and relevant nursing actions related to the underlying disorder and its treatment should the nurse anticipate?

**3** A 58-year-old woman is vomiting bright red blood. She is hypotensive. Her pulse rate is 38 bpm, and her pulse is weak and thready. Her arterial blood gases results are as follows: pH, 7.34; $PaCO_2$, 35 mm Hg; $PaO_2$, 69 mm Hg; and $HCO_3^-$, 20 mEq/L. Her hemoglobin is 4 g/dL. How do you interpret the patient's blood gas values? What treatment would you anticipate?

**4** [ebp] A female patient with a developmental delay and cognitive impairment requires frequent and repeated venipunctures and IV infusions for several weeks as part of treatment for osteomyelitis. She becomes very distressed in anticipation of the venipunctures. A nurse on the IV team has suggested the use of the local anesthetic EMLA to decrease her discomfort and distress related to venipuncture. What is the evidence for use of a local anesthetic agent in this case? What criteria would you use to assess the strength of the evidence for the use of the anesthetic? How would you use it in this patient's case?

**5** [ebp] A patient is receiving long-term parenteral fluids to treat recurrent dehydration secondary to GI losses. In an effort to ensure the patency of the IV catheter, the nurse considers irrigating the line with heparin. Do research findings support the use of heparin to keep the IV line open? What is the evidence base to determine whether heparin or saline irrigation is more effective? What are the benefits and risks of irrigation of the IV line with heparin versus saline?

**6** [ebp] A patient who has been receiving IV fluids for more than a week complains of pain and discomfort in the arm in which the fluids are being infused. The nurse assesses the IV insertion site and concludes that the patient has developed phlebitis at the site. The nurse decides to remove the IV catheter and restart the infusion in the patient's other arm. The nurse also applies warm compresses to the site. Identify the evidence that supports the use of warm compresses and evaluate the strength of the evidence. What criteria would you use to determine the strength of the evidence for or against use of warm compresses?

## REFERENCES AND SELECTED READINGS

### BOOKS

Alexander, M. & Corrigan, A. (2004). *Core curriculum for infusion nursing* (4th ed.). Philadelphia: Lippincott Williams & Wilkins.

Baumberger-Henry, M. (2004). *Quick look nursing: Fluid and electrolytes.* Thorofare, NJ: Slack.

Chernecky, C. C. & Berger, B. J. (2004). *Laboratory tests and diagnostic procedures* (3rd ed.). Philadelphia: W. B. Saunders.

Dudek, S. G. (2006). *Nutrition essentials for nursing practice* (5th ed.). Philadelphia: Lippincott Williams & Wilkins.

Hankins, J., Lonsway-Waldman, R., Hedrick, C., et al. (2001). *Infusion therapy in clinical practice* (2nd ed.). Philadelphia: W. B. Saunders.

Heitz, U. & Horne, M. (2005). *Guide to fluid, electrolyte, and acid-base balance* (4th ed.). St. Louis: Mosby.

Hogan, M. & Wane, D. (2003). *Fluids, electrolytes and acid-base balance* (5th ed.). Upper Saddle River, NJ: Pearson Education, Inc. Prentice-Hall.

Holmes, N. H. (2001). *Handbook of pathophysiology*. Philadelphia: Lippincott Williams & Wilkins.

Infusion Nurses Society. (2004). *Policies and procedures for infusion nursing of the older adult*. Norwood, MA: Author.

Infusion Nurses Society. (2006). *Infusion nursing standards of practice*. Norwood, MA: Author.

Karch, A. M. (2006). *Lippincott's nursing drug guide*. Philadelphia: Lippincott Williams & Wilkins.

Kee, J., Paulanka, B. & Purnell, L. (2004). *Handbook of fluids and electrolytes and acid-base imbalances*. Albany, NY: Delmar.

Martin, L. (1999). *All you really need to know how to interpret arterial blood gases* (2nd ed.). Philadelphia: Lippincott Williams & Wilkins.

Metheny, N. M. (2000). *Fluid and electrolyte balance: Nursing considerations* (4th ed.). Philadelphia: Lippincott Williams & Wilkins.

Morton, P. G., Fontaine, D. K., Hudak, C. M., et al. (2005). *Critical care nursing: A holistic approach*. Philadelphia: Lippincott Williams & Wilkins.

Otto, S. E. (2001). *Pocket guide to intravenous therapy* (4th ed.). St. Louis: Mosby.

Porth, C. M. (2005). *Pathophysiology: Concepts of altered health states* (6th ed.). Philadelphia: Lippincott Williams & Wilkins.

Price, S. A., & Wilson, L. M. (2002). *Pathophysiology: Clinical concepts of disease processes* (6th ed.). St. Louis: Mosby–Year Book.

Rose, B. & Post, T. (2000). *Clinical physiology of acid–base disorders* (5th ed.). New York: McGraw-Hill.

Speakman, E. & Weldy, N. J. (2001). *Body fluids and electrolytes: A programmed presentation* (8th ed.). Philadelphia: Elsevier Science Publishers.

Weinstein, S. (2006). *Plumer's principles and practice of intravenous therapy* (8th ed.). Philadelphia: Lippincott Williams & Wilkins.

## JOURNALS

*Asterisks indicate nursing research articles.*

### Fluid and Electrolyte Balances and Imbalances

Allison, S. P., & Lobo, D. N. (2004). Fluid and electrolytes in the elderly. *Current Opinion in Clinical Nutrition and Metabolic Care, 7*(1), 27–33.

American Heart Association. (2005). 2005 guidelines for cardiopulmonary resuscitation and emergency cardiovascular care. *Circulation*. Available at: www.americanheart.org/presenter.jhtml?identifier=3035517 (accessed May 26, 2006).

Burger, C. M. (2004a). Hyperkalemia. *American Journal of Nursing, 104*(10), 66–70.

Burger, C. M. (2004b). Hypokalemia. *American Journal of Nursing, 104*(11), 61–65.

Byrd, R. (2003). Magnesium: Its proven clinical significance. *Southern Medical Journal, 96*(1), 104–105.

Eaton, J. (2003). Detection of hyponatremia in the PACU. *Journal of Perianesthesia Nursing, 18*(6), 392–397.

Elgart, H. N. (2004). Assessment of fluids and electrolytes. *AACN Clinical Issues, 15*(4), 607–621.

*Hayes, A., Buffum, M. & Fuller, D. (2003). Bowel preparation comparison: Flavored versus unflavored colyte. *Gastroenterology Nursing, 26*(3), 106–109.

Inzucchi, S. (2004a). Management of hypercalcemia: Diagnostic work up, therapeutic options for hyperparathyroidism and other common causes. *Postgraduate Medicine, 115*(5), 27–36.

Inzucchi, S. (2004b). Understanding hypercalcemia: Its metabolic basis, signs, and symptoms. *Postgraduate Medicine, 115*(4), 69–70, 73–76.

Lin, S. H., Hsu, Y. J., Chiu, J. S., et al. (2003). Osmotic demyelination syndrome: A potentially avoidable disaster. *Quarterly Journal of Medicine, 96*(12), 935–947.

Lobo, D. N. (2004). Fluid, electrolytes and nutrition: Physiological and clinical aspects. *Proceedings of the Nutrition Society, 63*(3), 453–466.

Luckey, A. E. & Parsa, C. J. (2003). Fluid and electrolytes in the aged. *Archives of Surgery, 138*(10), 1055–1060.

Olson, D. M., Meek, L. G., & Lynch, J. R. (2004). Accurate patient history contributes to differentiating diabetes insipidus: A case study. *Journal of Neuroscience Nursing, 36*(4), 228–230.

Palmer, B. F. (2004). Managing hyperkalemia caused by inhibitors of the rennin-angitensin-aldosterone system. *New England Journal of Medicine, 351*(6), 585–592.

Pirzada, N. A. & Ali, I. I. (2001). Central pontine myelinolysis. *Mayo Clinic Proceedings, 76*(5), 559–562.

Ryland, B. & Thomas, R. (2003). Magnesium: Its proven and potential clinical significance. *Southern Medical Journal, 96*(1), 104.

SAFE Study Investigators. (2004). A comparison of albumin and saline for fluid resuscitation in the intensive care unit. *New England Journal of Medicine, 350*(22), 2247–2256.

Suhayda, R. & Walton, J. C. (2002). Preventing and managing dehydration. *MedSurg Nursing, 11*(6), 267–278.

Stewart, A. F. (2005). Hypercalcemia associated with cancer. *New England Journal of Medicine, 352*(4), 373–379.

Tsuneyoshi, H., Nishina, T., Nomoto, T., et al. (2004). Atrial natriuretic peptide helps prevent late remodeling after left ventricular aneurysm repair. *Circulation, 110*(11 Suppl 1), II174–II179.

van Wissen, L. & Breton, C. (2004). Perioperative influences on fluid distribution. *MedSurg Nursing, 13*(5), 304–311.

Weiss-Guillet, E. M., Takala, J. & Jakob, S. M. (2003). Diagnosis and management of electrolyte emergencies. *Best Practice and Research Clinical Endocrinology and Metabolism, 17*(4), 623–651.

Zwicker, C. D. (2003). The older adult at risk. *Journal of Infusion Nursing, 26*(3), 137–143.

### Acid–Base Balance

Bartlett, D. (2005). Understanding the anion and osmolal gaps laboratory values: What they are and how to use them. *Journal of Emergency Nursing, 31*(1), 109–111.

Herd, A. M. (2005). An approach to complex acid-base problems: Keeping it simple. *Canadian Family Physician, 51*, 226–232.

Kellum, J. A. (2005). Determinants of plasma acid-base balance. *Critical Care Clinics, 21*(2), 329–346.

Kraut, J. A. & Madias, N. E. (2001). Approach to patients with acid-base disorders. *Respiratory Care, 46*(4), 392–403.

Lafrance, J. P., & Leblanc, M. (2005). Metabolic, electrolytes, and nutritional concerns in critical illness. *Critical Care Clinics, 21*(2), 305–327.

Lynes, D. (2003). An introduction to blood gas analysis. *Nursing Times, 99*(11), 54–55.

Whittier, W. L. & Rutecki, G. W. (2004). Primer on clinical acid-base problem solving. *Disease-a-Month, 50*(3), 122–162.

Yucha, C. (2004). Renal regulation of acid-base balance. *Nephrology Nursing Journal, 31*(2), 201–208.

### Intravenous Administration

Alexander, M. (2000). Infusion nursing standards of practice. *Journal of Intravenous Nursing, 23*(6 Suppl), S5–S88.

Anderson, R. N. (2004). Midline catheters. *Journal of Infusion Nursing, 27*(5), 313–321.

*Brown, J. (2003). Using lidocaine for peripheral IV insertions: Patients' preferences and pain experiences. *MedSurg Nursing, 12*(2), 95–100.

*Fetzer, S. J. (2002). Reducing venipuncture and intravenous insertion pain with eutectic mixture of local anesthetic: A meta-analysis. *Nursing Research, 51*(2), 119–124.

Foley, M. (2004). Update on needlestick and sharps injuries: The Needlestick Safety and Prevention Act of 2000. *American Journal of Nursing, 104*(8), 96–97.

Fry, C. & Ahold, D. (2001). Local anesthesia prior to the insertion of peripherally inserted central catheters. *Journal of Infusion Nursing, 24*(6), 404–408.

Gorski, L. A. & Czaplewski, L. M. (2004). Peripherally inserted central catheters and midline catheters for the homecare nurse. *Journal of Infusion Nursing, 27*(6), 399–409.

Haire, W. D. & Herbst, S. (2000). Highlights bulletin: Consensus conference on the use of Alteplase (t-PA) for the management of thrombotic catheter dysfunction. *Journal of Vascular Access Devices, 5*(2), 28–36.

Intravenous Nurses Society. (1997). Position paper: Midline and midclavicular catheters. *Journal of Intravenous Nursing, 20*(4), 175–178.

Intravenous Nurses Society. (1997). Position paper: Peripherally inserted central catheters. *Journal of Intravenous Nursing, 20*(4), 172–174.

Macklin, D. (2003). Phlebitis. *American Journal of Nursing, 103*(2), 55–58.

Macklin, D. (2000). Removing PICC. *American Journal of Nursing, 100*(1), 52–54.

McKnight, S. (2004). Nurse's guide to understanding and treating thrombotic occlusion of central venous access devices. *MedSurg Nursing, 13*(6), 377–382.

O'Grady, N. P., Alexander, M., Dellinger, E. P., et al. (2002). Guidelines for the prevention of intravascular catheter-related infections. Centers for Disease Control and Prevention. *Morbidity and Mortality Weekly Report Recommendations and Reports, 51*(RR-10), 1–29.

Penny-Timmons, E. & Sevedge, S. (2004). Outcome data for peripherally inserted central catheters used in an acute care setting. *Journal of Infusion Nursing, 27*(6), 431–436.

Peter, D. A. & Saxman, C. (2003). Preventing air embolism when removing CVCs: An evidence-based approach to changing practice. *MedSurg Nursing, 12*(4), 223–228.

Shafiee, M. A., Bohn, D., Hoorn, E. J., et al. (2003). How to select optimal maintenance intravenous fluid therapy. *QJM 96*(8), 601–610.

*Snelling, R., Jones, G., Figueredo, A., et al. (2001). Central venous catheters for infusion therapy in gastrointestinal cancer: A comparative study of tunnelled centrally placed catheters and peripherally inserted central catheters. *Journal of Intravenous Nursing, 24*(1), 38–47.

## RESOURCES

Infusion Nurses Society, 220 Norwood Park South, Norwood, MA 02062; 781-440-9408; http://www.ins1.org. Accessed May 25, 2006.

CHAPTER 15

# Shock and Multisystem Failure

## Learning Objectives

*On completion of this chapter, the learner will be able to:*

1. Describe shock and its underlying pathophysiology.
2. Compare clinical findings of the compensatory, progressive, and irreversible stages of shock.
3. Describe organ damage that may occur with shock.
4. Describe similarities and differences in shock due to hypovolemic, cardiogenic, neurogenic, anaphylactic, and septic shock states.
5. Identify medical and nursing management priorities in treating patients in shock.
6. Identify vasoactive medications used in treating shock, and describe nursing implications associated with their use.
7. Discuss the importance of nutritional support in all forms of shock.
8. Discuss the role of nurses in psychosocial support of patients experiencing shock and their families.
9. Discuss multiple organ dysfunction syndrome.

Shock is a life-threatening condition with a variety of underlying causes. It is characterized by inadequate tissue perfusion that, if untreated, results in cell death. The progression of shock is neither linear nor predictable, and shock states, especially septic shock, comprise a current area of aggressive clinical research. Nurses caring for patients with shock and for those at risk for shock must understand the underlying mechanisms of shock and recognize its subtle as well as more obvious signs. Rapid assessment and response are essential to the patient's recovery.

## Shock and Its Significance

**Shock** can best be defined as a condition in which tissue perfusion is inadequate to deliver oxygen and nutrients to support vital organs and cellular function (Hameed, Aird, & Cohn, 2003). Adequate blood flow to the tissues and cells requires the following components: adequate cardiac pump, effective vasculature or circulatory system, and sufficient blood volume. If one component is impaired, perfusion to the tissues is threatened or compromised. Without treatment, inadequate blood flow to the tissues results in poor delivery of oxygen and nutrients to the cells, cellular starvation, cell death, organ dysfunction progressing to organ failure, and eventual death.

Shock affects all body systems. It may develop rapidly or slowly, depending on the underlying cause. During shock, the body struggles to survive, calling on all its homeostatic mechanisms to restore blood flow. Any insult to the body can create a cascade of events resulting in poor tissue perfusion. Therefore, almost any patient with any disease state may be at risk for developing shock.

Nursing care of patients with shock requires ongoing systematic assessment. Many of the interventions required in caring for patients with shock call for close collaboration with other members of the health care team and rapid implementation of physicians' orders. Nurses must anticipate orders, because these orders need to be executed with speed and accuracy.

## Conditions Precipitating Shock

### Classification of Shock

Conventionally, the primary underlying pathophysiologic process and the underlying disorder are used to classify the shock state. Several definitions of shock states are found in the literature. In this chapter, the following shock states will be described:

- **Hypovolemic shock**, which occurs when there is a decrease in the intravascular volume
- **Cardiogenic shock**, which occurs when the heart has an impaired pumping ability; it may be of coronary or noncoronary event origin
- **Septic shock**, which is caused by an infection
- **Neurogenic shock**, which is caused by alterations in vascular smooth muscle tone, caused by either nervous system injury or complications associated with medications such as epidural anesthesia
- **Anaphylactic shock**, which is caused by a hypersensitivity reaction

Shock states that are caused by a loss of vascular tone, including septic, neurogenic, and anaphylactic shock, are discussed later in this chapter as **circulatory shock** (also termed distributive or vasoactive shock). In addition, traumatic shock has been described in the literature (Kellum & Pinsky, 2002).

Regardless of the initial cause of shock, researchers have gradually concluded that certain physiologic responses are common to all types of shock. These physiologic responses are hypoperfusion of the tissues, hypermetabolism, and activation of the inflammatory response. The body responds to shock states by activating the sympathetic nervous system and mounting a hypermetabolic and inflammatory re-

## Glossary

**anaphylactic shock:** circulatory shock state resulting from a severe allergic reaction producing an overwhelming systemic vasodilation and relative hypovolemia

**biochemical mediators:** messenger substances that may be released by a cell to create an action at that site or be carried by the bloodstream to a distant site before being activated; also called cytokines

**cardiogenic shock:** shock state resulting from impairment or failure of the myocardium

**colloids:** intravenous solutions that contain molecules that are too large to pass through capillary membranes

**crystalloids:** electrolyte solutions that move freely between the intravascular compartment and interstitial spaces

**circulatory shock:** shock state resulting from displacement of blood volume creating a relative hypovolemia and inadequate delivery of oxygen to the cells; also called distributive shock

**hypovolemic shock:** shock state resulting from decreased intravascular volume due to fluid loss

**neurogenic shock:** shock state resulting from loss of sympathetic tone causing relative hypovolemia

**septic shock:** circulatory shock state resulting from overwhelming infection causing relative hypovolemia

**shock:** physiologic state in which there is inadequate blood flow to tissues and cells of the body

**systemic inflammatory response syndrome (SIRS):** overwhelming inflammatory response in the absence of infection causing relative hypovolemia and decreased tissue perfusion sponse. A derangement in the compensatory mechanisms to effectively restore physiologic balance is the final pathway of all shock states (Ahrens & Vollman, 2003; Hameed et al., 2003; Kleinpell, 2003). Once shock develops, the patient's survival may have more to do with the body's response than with the initial cause of shock (Kleinpell, 2003). The final common pathway of all forms of shock is inadequate perfusion to the cells that results in cellular hypoxia, end organ damage, and ultimately death.

## Normal Cellular Function

Energy metabolism occurs within the cell, where nutrients are chemically broken down and stored in the form of adenosine triphosphate (ATP). Cells use this stored energy to perform necessary functions, such as active transport, muscle contraction, and biochemical synthesis, as well as specialized cellular functions, such as the conduction of electrical impulses. ATP can be synthesized aerobically (in the presence of oxygen) or anaerobically (in the absence of oxygen). Aerobic metabolism yields far greater amounts of ATP per mole of glucose than does anaerobic metabolism; therefore, it is a more efficient and effective means of producing energy. In addition, anaerobic metabolism results in the accumulation of the toxic end product, lactic acid, which must be removed from the cell and transported to the liver for conversion into glucose and glycogen.

## Pathophysiology

In shock, the cells lack an adequate blood supply and are deprived of oxygen and nutrients; therefore, they must produce energy through anaerobic metabolism. This results in low energy yields from nutrients and an acidotic intracellular environment. Because of these changes, normal cell function ceases (Fig. 15-1). The cell swells and the cell membrane becomes more permeable, allowing electrolytes and fluids to seep out of and into the cell. The sodium–potassium pump becomes impaired; cell structures, primarily the mitochondria, are damaged; and death of the cell results.

Glucose is the primary substrate required for the production of cellular energy in the form of ATP. In stress states, catecholamines, cortisol, glucagons, and inflammatory cytokines and mediators are released, causing hyperglycemia and insulin resistance to mobilize glucose for cellular metabolism. Activation of these substances promotes gluconeogenesis, which is the formation of glucose from noncarbohydrate sources such as proteins and fats. Glycogen that has been stored in the liver is also converted to glucose through glycogenolysis, increasing the amount of glucose in the bloodstream. The net result is hyperglycemia to meet increased metabolic demands.

Continued activation of the stress response by shock states causes a depletion of glycogen stores, resulting in increased proteolysis and eventual organ failure (Baldwin & Morris, 2002; Flynn, 2004). The inability of the body to have enough nutrients and oxygen for normal cellular metabolism causes a buildup of metabolic end products in the cells and interstitial spaces. Cellular metabolism is impaired, and a vicious cycle of negative feedback is initiated.

### Vascular Responses

Oxygen attaches to the hemoglobin molecule in red blood cells, and the blood carries it to body cells. The amount of

**FIGURE 15-1.** Cellular effects of shock. The cell swells and the cell membrane becomes more permeable; fluids and electrolytes seep from and into the cell. Mitochondria and lysosomes are damaged, and the cell dies.

oxygen that is delivered to cells depends both on blood flow to a specific area and on blood oxygen concentration. Blood is continuously recycled through the lungs to be reoxygenated and to eliminate end products of cellular metabolism, such as carbon dioxide. The heart muscle is the pump that propels the freshly oxygenated blood out to the body tissues. This process of circulation is facilitated through an elaborate and dynamic vasculature consisting of arteries, arterioles, capillaries, venules, and veins. The vasculature can dilate or constrict based on central and local regulatory mechanisms. Central regulatory mechanisms stimulate dilation or constriction of the vasculature to maintain an adequate blood pressure (BP). Local regulatory mechanisms, referred to as autoregulation, stimulate vasodilation or vasoconstriction in response to biochemical mediators (cytokines) released by the cell, communicating its need for oxygen and nutrients (Hameed et al., 2003; Kellum & Pinsky, 2002). A biochemical mediator is a substance released by a cell or immune cells such as monocytes and macrophages; the substance triggers an action at a cell site or travels in the bloodstream to a distant site, where it triggers action. Researchers are learning more every day about the physiologic actions of the more than 100 cytokines (Sommers, 2003).

### Blood Pressure Regulation

Three major components of the circulatory system—blood volume, the cardiac pump, and the vasculature—must respond effectively to complex neural, chemical, and hormonal feedback systems to maintain an adequate BP and ultimately perfuse body tissues. BP is regulated through a complex interaction of neural, chemical, and hormonal feedback systems affecting both cardiac output and peripheral resistance. This relationship is expressed in the following equation:

$$\text{Mean arterial BP} = \text{cardiac output} \times \text{peripheral resistance}$$

Cardiac output is determined by stroke volume (the amount of blood ejected at systole) and heart rate. Peripheral resistance is determined by the diameter of the arterioles.

Tissue perfusion and organ perfusion depend on mean arterial pressure (MAP), or the average pressure at which blood moves through the vasculature. MAP must exceed 65 mm Hg for cells to receive the oxygen and nutrients needed to metabolize energy in amounts sufficient to sustain life (Dellinger, Carlet, Masur, et al., 2004). Although true MAP can be calculated only by complex methods, Chart 15-1 displays a convenient formula for clinical use in estimating MAP.

BP is regulated by the baroreceptors (pressure receptors) located in the carotid sinus and aortic arch. These pressure receptors convey impulses to the sympathetic nervous center in the medulla of the brain. When BP drops, catecholamines (epinephrine and norepinephrine) are released from the adrenal medulla. This increases heart rate and vasoconstriction, thus restoring BP. Chemoreceptors, also located in the aortic arch and carotid arteries, regulate BP and respiratory rate using much the same mechanism in response to changes in oxygen and carbon dioxide concentrations in the blood. These primary regulatory mechanisms can respond to changes in BP on a moment-to-moment basis.

The kidneys also play an important role in BP regulation. They regulate BP by releasing renin, an enzyme needed for the conversion of angiotensin I to angiotensin II, a potent vasoconstrictor. This stimulation of the renin–angiotensin mechanism and the resulting vasoconstriction indirectly lead to the release of aldosterone from the adrenal cortex, which promotes the retention of sodium and water. The increased concentration of sodium in the blood then stimulates the release of antidiuretic hormone (ADH) by the pituitary gland. ADH causes the kidneys to retain water further in an effort to raise blood volume and BP. These secondary regulatory mechanisms may take hours or days to respond to changes in BP.

To summarize, adequate blood volume, an effective cardiac pump, and an effective vasculature are necessary to maintain BP and tissue perfusion. When one of the three components of this system begins to fail, the body is able to compensate through increased work by the other two (Fig. 15-2). After compensatory mechanisms can no longer compensate for the failed system, body tissues become inadequately perfused, and shock occurs. Without prompt intervention, shock progresses, resulting in organ dysfunction, organ failure, and death.

---

**CHART 15-1**

### Formula for Estimating Mean Arterial Pressure (MAP)

$$\text{MAP} = \frac{\text{systolic BP} + 2\,(\text{diastolic BP})}{3}$$

Example: patient's BP = 125/75 mm Hg

$$\text{MAP} = \frac{125 + (2 \times 75)}{3}$$

MAP = 92 (rounded to nearest 1/10)

---

## Stages of Shock

Shock is believed to progress along a continuum of stages through which a patient struggles to survive. A convenient way to understand the physiologic responses and subsequent clinical signs and symptoms is to divide the continuum into separate stages: compensatory (stage 1), progressive (stage 2), and irreversible (stage 3). The earlier medical management and nursing interventions can be initiated along this continuum, the greater the patient's chance of survival.

### Compensatory Stage

In the compensatory stage of shock, the BP remains within normal limits. Vasoconstriction, increased heart rate, and increased contractility of the heart contribute to maintain-

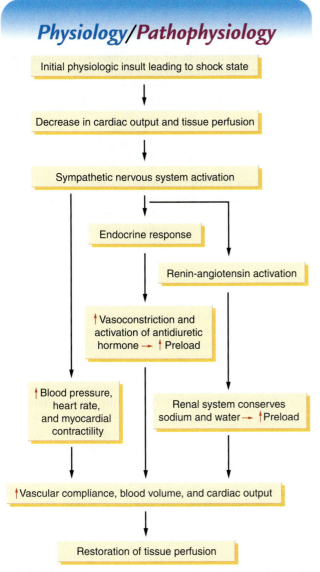

**FIGURE 15-2.** Compensatory mechanisms in shock. Adapted with permission from Jones, K. (1996). Shock. In Clochesy, J. M., Breu, C., Cardin, S., et al. (Eds.). *Critical care nursing* (2nd ed.) Philadelphia: W. B. Saunders.

ing adequate cardiac output. This results from stimulation of the sympathetic nervous system and subsequent release of catecholamines (epinephrine and norepinephrine). Patients display the often-described "fight or flight" response. The body shunts blood from organs such as the skin, kidneys, and gastrointestinal tract to the brain and heart to ensure adequate blood supply to these vital organs. As a result, the skin is cool and clammy, bowel sounds are hypoactive, and urine output decreases in response to the release of aldosterone and ADH.

## Clinical Manifestations

Despite a normal BP, the patient shows numerous clinical signs indicating inadequate organ perfusion (Table 15-1). The result of inadequate perfusion is anaerobic metabolism and a buildup of lactic acid, producing metabolic acidosis. The respiratory rate increases in response to metabolic acidosis. This rapid respiratory rate facilitates removal of excess carbon dioxide but raises the blood pH and often causes a compensatory respiratory alkalosis. The alkalotic state causes mental status changes, such as confusion or combativeness, as well as arteriolar dilation. If treatment begins in this stage of shock, the prognosis for the patient is good.

## Medical Management

Medical treatment is directed toward identifying the cause of the shock, correcting the underlying disorder so that shock does not progress, and supporting those physiologic processes that thus far have responded successfully to the threat. Because compensation cannot be effectively maintained indefinitely, measures such as fluid replacement and medication therapy must be initiated to maintain an adequate BP and reestablish and maintain adequate tissue perfusion.

## Nursing Management

Early intervention along the continuum of shock is the key to improving the patient's prognosis. Therefore, the nurse must assess the patient at risk for shock systematically to recognize the subtle clinical signs of the compensatory stage before the patient's BP drops. Special considerations related

**TABLE 15-1  Clinical Findings in Stages of Shock**

| Finding | Compensatory | Progressive | Irreversible |
|---|---|---|---|
| Blood pressure | Normal | Systolic <80–90 mm Hg | Requires mechanical or pharmacologic support |
| Heart rate | >100 bpm | >150 bpm | Erratic or asystole |
| Respiratory status | >20 breaths/min | Rapid, shallow respirations; crackles | Requires intubation |
| Skin | Cold, clammy | Mottled, petechiae | Jaundice |
| Urinary output | Decreased | 0.5 mL/kg/h | Anuric, requires dialysis |
| Mentation | Confusion | Lethargy | Unconscious |
| Acid-base balance | Respiratory alkalosis | Metabolic acidosis | Profound acidosis |

to recognizing early signs of shock in the elderly patient are given in Chart 15-2.

## Monitoring Tissue Perfusion

In assessing tissue perfusion, the nurse observes for changes in level of consciousness, vital signs (including pulse pressure), urinary output, skin, and laboratory values (base deficit and lactic acid levels). In the compensatory stage of shock, serum sodium and blood glucose levels are elevated in response to the release of aldosterone and catecholamines.

The roles of the nurse at the compensatory stage of shock are to monitor the patient's hemodynamic status and promptly report deviations to the physician, to assist in identifying and treating the underlying disorder by continuous in-depth assessment of the patient, to administer prescribed fluids and medications, and to promote patient safety. Vital signs are key indicators of hemodynamic status; however, BP is an indirect method of monitoring tissue hypoxia. The nurse should report a systolic BP lower than 90 mm Hg or a drop in systolic BP of 40 mm Hg.

Pulse pressure correlates well with stroke volume, or the amount of blood ejected from the heart with systole. Pulse pressure is calculated by subtracting the diastolic measurement from the systolic measurement; the difference is the pulse pressure (Porth, 2005). Normally, the pulse pressure is 30 to 40 mm Hg. Narrowing or decreased pulse pressure is an earlier indicator of shock than a drop in systolic BP. Decreased or narrowing pulse pressure, an early indication of decreased stroke volume, is illustrated in the following example:

Systolic BP − Diastolic BP = Pulse pressure

Normal pulse pressure:

120 mg Hg − 80 mm Hg = 40 mm Hg

Narrowing of pulse pressure:

90 mm Hg − 70 mm Hg = 20 mm Hg

Elevation in the diastolic BP with release of catecholamines and attempts to increase venous return through vasoconstriction is an early compensatory mechanism in response to decreased stroke volume, BP, and overall cardiac output.

**NURSING ALERT**

**By the time BP drops, damage has already been occurring at the cellular and tissue levels. Therefore, the patient at risk for shock must be assessed and monitored closely before the BP falls.**

Several new technologies allow clinicians to detect changes in tissue perfusion before changes in classic signs (BP, heart rate, and urine output) indicate hypoperfusion. These new methods, which sense changes in cellular acidosis caused by the buildup of lactic acid, include sublingual carbon dioxide ($CO_2$) monitoring, gastric tonometry, and central venous or mixed venous blood oxygen saturation ($S\bar{v}O_2$) measurements (Ahrens & Vollman, 2003; Ahrns, 2004; Hameed et al., 2003). $CO_2$ monitoring is referred to as capnography, which measures the exhaled level of $CO_2$ through a device on the exhalation arm of the ventilator. Newer technology allows placement of a probe beneath the tongue to record an estimated $CO_2$. Gastric tonometry is an invasive method in which a nasogastric tube with a $CO_2$-permeable balloon is inserted. The device provides an indirect measurement of the $CO_2$ and pH of intestinal mucosa. Mixed venous blood oxygen saturation can be measured through a central venous ($Sc\bar{v}O_2$) catheter or a pulmonary

---

**CHART 15-2**

### Recognizing Shock in Older Patients

The physiologic changes associated with aging, coupled with pathologic and chronic disease states, place older people at increased risk for developing a state of shock and possibly multiple organ dysfunction syndrome (MODS). Elderly people can recover from shock if it is detected and treated early with aggressive and supportive therapies. Nurses play an essential role in assessing and interpreting subtle changes in older patients' responses to illness.

- Medications such as beta-blocking agents (metoprolol [Lopressor]) used to treat hypertension may mask tachycardia, a primary compensatory mechanism to increase cardiac output, during hypovolemic states.
- The aging immune system may not mount a truly febrile response (temperature more than 40°C or 104°F), but an increasing trend in body temperature should be addressed.
- The heart does not function well in hypoxemic states, and the aging heart may respond to decreased myocardial oxygenation with dysrhythmias that may be misinterpreted as a normal part of the aging process.
- Changes in mentation may be inappropriately misinterpreted as dementia. Older people with a sudden change in mentation should be aggressively treated for the presence of infection and organ hypoperfusion.

artery catheter ($S\bar{v}O_2$) that has a sensor imbedded in the device. The sensor detects changes in saturation of hemoglobin and calculates the venous oxygen saturation.

Although treatments are prescribed and initiated by the physician, the nurse usually implements them, operates and troubleshoots equipment used in treatment, monitors the patient's status during treatment, and assesses the immediate effects of treatment. In addition, the nurse assesses the response of the patient and family to the crisis and its treatment.

### Reducing Anxiety

Patients often become anxious and apprehensive when they face a major threat to health and well-being and are the focus of attention of many health care providers. Providing brief explanations about the diagnostic and treatment procedures, supporting the patient during these procedures, and providing information about their outcomes are usually effective in reducing stress and anxiety and thus promoting the patient's physical and mental well-being. Speaking in a calm, reassuring voice and using gentle touch also help ease the patient's concerns. These actions may provide solace and comfort for critically ill, frightened patients (Benner, 2004).

### Promoting Safety

Another nursing intervention is monitoring potential threats to the patient's safety, because a high anxiety level and altered mental status typically impair judgment. In this stage of shock, patients who were previously cooperative and followed instructions may now disrupt intravenous (IV) lines and catheters and complicate their condition. Therefore, close monitoring and frequent reorientation interventions are essential.

## Progressive Stage

In the second stage of shock, the mechanisms that regulate BP can no longer compensate, and the MAP falls below normal limits. Patients are clinically hypotensive; this is defined as a systolic BP of less than 90 mm Hg or a decrease in systolic BP of 40 mm Hg (Kleinpell, 2003).

## Pathophysiology

Although all organ systems suffer from hypoperfusion at this stage, several events perpetuate the shock syndrome. First, the overworked heart becomes dysfunctional; the body's inability to meet increased oxygen requirements produces ischemia; and biochemical mediators cause myocardial depression (Delling, 2003; Kellum & Pinsky, 2002). This leads to failure of the cardiac pump, even if the underlying cause of the shock is not of cardiac origin. Second, the autoregulatory function of the microcirculation fails in response to the numerous biochemical cytokines and mediators released by the cells, resulting in increased capillary permeability, with areas of arteriolar and venous constriction further compromising cellular perfusion (Ahrens & Vollman, 2003; Ahrns, 2004; Fishel, Are, & Barbul, 2003).

At this stage, the prognosis worsens. The relaxation of precapillary sphincters causes fluid to leak from the capillaries, creating interstitial edema and return of less fluid to the heart. In addition, the inflammatory response to injury is activated, and proinflammatory and anti-inflammatory cytokines and mediators are released, which in turn activate the coagulation system in an effort to reestablish homeostasis (Kleinpell, 2003; Sommers, 2003). The body mobilizes energy stores and increases oxygen consumption to meet the increased metabolic needs of the underperfused tissues and cells.

Even if the underlying cause of the shock is reversed, the sequence of compensatory responses to the decrease in tissue perfusion perpetuates the shock state, and a vicious circle ensues. The cellular reactions that occur during the progressive stage of shock are an active area of clinical research. It is believed that the body's response to shock or lack of response in this stage of shock may be the primary factor determining the patient's survival.

## Assessment and Diagnostic Findings

Chances of survival depend on the patient's general health before the shock state as well as the amount of time it takes to restore tissue perfusion. As shock progresses, organ systems decompensate.

### Respiratory Effects

The lungs, which become compromised early in shock, are affected at this stage. Subsequent decompensation of the lungs increases the likelihood that mechanical ventilation will be needed. Respirations are rapid and shallow. Crackles are heard over the lung fields. Decreased pulmonary blood flow causes arterial oxygen levels to decrease and carbon dioxide levels to increase. Hypoxemia and biochemical mediators cause an intense inflammatory response and pulmonary vasoconstriction, perpetuating the pulmonary capillary hypoperfusion and hypoxemia. The hypoperfused alveoli stop producing surfactant and subsequently collapse. Pulmonary capillaries begin to leak, spilling their contents, thus causing pulmonary edema, diffusion abnormalities (shunting), and additional alveolar collapse. Interstitial inflammation and fibrosis are common as the pulmonary damage progresses (Berry & Pinard, 2003). This condition is sometimes referred to as acute respiratory distress syndrome (ARDS), acute lung injury, shock lung, or noncardiogenic pulmonary edema. Further explanation of ARDS, as well as its nursing management, can be found in Chapter 23.

### Cardiovascular Effects

A lack of adequate blood supply leads to dysrhythmias and ischemia. The heart rate is rapid, sometimes exceeding 150 bpm. The patient may complain of chest pain and even suffer a myocardial infarction. Levels of cardiac enzymes (eg, lactate dehydrogenase [LDH], creatine phosphokinase myocardium and muscle [CPK-MB], cardiac troponin [cTn-I]) increase. In addition, myocardial depression and ventricular dilation may further impair the heart's ability to pump enough blood to the tissues to meet oxygen requirements.

New laboratory markers also can be used to assess the function of the heart. B-type natriuretic peptide (BNP) is one of these markers. BNP is increased when the ventricle is overdistended; therefore, elevations in BNP can be used to assess ventricular function of patients in shock states (Dellinger, 2003; Hachey & Smith, 2003).

### Neurologic Effects

As blood flow to the brain becomes impaired, mental status deteriorates. Changes in mental status occur with decreased cerebral perfusion and hypoxia. Initially, the patient may exhibit a subtle change in behavior or agitation and confusion. Subsequently, lethargy increases, and the patient begins to lose consciousness.

### Renal Effects

When the MAP falls below 70 mm Hg (Huether, 2002), the glomerular filtration rate of the kidneys cannot be maintained, and drastic changes in renal function occur. Acute renal failure (ARF) may develop. ARF is characterized by an increase in blood urea nitrogen (BUN) and serum creatinine levels, fluid and electrolyte shifts, acid–base imbalances, and a loss of the renal-hormonal regulation of BP. Urinary output usually decreases to less than 0.5/mL/kg per hour (or less than 30 mL/h) but may vary depending on the phase of ARF. For further information about ARF, see Chapter 44.

### Hepatic Effects

Decreased blood flow to the liver impairs the ability of liver cells to perform metabolic and phagocytic functions. Consequently, the patient is less able to metabolize medications and metabolic waste products, such as ammonia and lactic acid. Metabolic activities of the liver, including gluconeogenesis and glycogenolysis, are impaired. The patient becomes more susceptible to infection as the liver fails to filter bacteria from the blood. Liver enzymes (aspartate aminotransferase [AST], alanine aminotransferase [ALT], lactate dehydrogenase [LDH]) and bilirubin levels are elevated, and the patient appears jaundiced.

### Gastrointestinal Effects

Gastrointestinal ischemia can cause stress ulcers in the stomach, putting the patient at risk for gastrointestinal bleeding. In the small intestine, the mucosa can become necrotic and slough off, causing bloody diarrhea. Beyond the local effects of impaired perfusion, gastrointestinal ischemia leads to bacterial toxin translocation, in which bacterial toxins enter the bloodstream through the lymph system. In addition to causing infection, bacterial toxins can cause cardiac depression, vasodilation, increased capillary permeability, and an intense inflammatory response with activation of additional biochemical mediators. The net result is interference with healthy cells and their ability to metabolize nutrients (Ceppa, Fuh, & Bulkey, 2003).

### Hematologic Effects

The combination of hypotension, sluggish blood flow, metabolic acidosis, coagulation system imbalance, and generalized hypoxemia can interfere with normal hemostatic mechanisms. In shock states, the inflammatory cytokines activate the clotting cascade, causing deposition of microthrombi in multiple areas of the body and consumption of clotting factors. The alterations of the hematologic system, including imbalance of the clotting cascade, are linked to the overactivation of the inflammatory response of injury (Ahrens & Vollman, 2003). Disseminated intravascular coagulation (DIC) may occur either as a cause or as a complication of shock. In this condition, widespread clotting and bleeding occur simultaneously. Bruises (ecchymoses) and bleeding (petechiae) may appear in the skin. Coagulation times (prothrombin time, partial thromboplastin time) are prolonged. Clotting factors and platelets are consumed and require replacement therapy to achieve hemostasis. Further discussion of DIC appears in Chapter 33.

## Medical Management

Specific medical management in the progressive stage of shock depends on the type of shock and its underlying cause. It is also based on the degree of decompensation in the organ systems. Medical management specific to each type of shock is discussed later in this chapter. Although there are several differences in medical management by type of shock, some medical interventions are common to all types. These include the use of appropriate IV fluids and medications to restore tissue perfusion by the following methods:

- Optimizing intravascular volume
- Supporting the pumping action of the heart
- Improving the competence of the vascular system
- Supporting the respiratory system

Other aspects of management may include early enteral nutritional support, aggressive hyperglycemic control with IV insulin (van den Berghe, Wouters, & Weekers, 2001), and use of antacids, histamine-2 ($H_2$) blockers, or antipeptic agents to reduce the risk of gastrointestinal ulceration and bleeding.

**NURSING ALERT**

Tight glycemic control (blood glucose, 80 to 110 mg/dL) has been shown to reduce morbidity and mortality of acutely ill patients.

## Nursing Management

Nursing care of patients in the progressive stage of shock requires expertise in assessing and understanding shock and the significance of changes in assessment data. Early interventions are essential to the survival of patients in shock; therefore, suspecting that a patient may be in shock and reporting subtle changes in assessment are imperative. Patients in the progressive stage of shock are often cared for in the intensive care setting to facilitate close monitoring (hemodynamic monitoring, electrocardiographic [ECG] monitoring, arterial blood gases, serum electrolyte levels, physical and mental status changes); rapid and frequent administration of various prescribed medications and fluids; and possibly interventions with supportive technologies, such as mechanical ventilation, dialysis, and intra-aortic balloon pump.

Working closely with other members of the health care team, the nurse carefully documents treatments, medications, and fluids that are administered by members of the team, recording the time, dosage or volume, and patient response. In addition, the nurse coordinates both the scheduling of diagnostic procedures that may be carried out at the bedside and the flow of health care personnel involved in care of patients.

### Preventing Complications

If supportive technologies are used, the nurse helps reduce the risk of related complications and monitors the patient for early signs of complications. Monitoring includes evaluating blood levels of medications, observing invasive vascular lines for signs of infection, and checking neurovascular status if arterial lines are inserted, especially in the lower extremities. Simultaneously, the nurse promotes the patient's safety and comfort by ensuring that all procedures, including invasive procedures and arterial and venous punctures, are carried out using correct aseptic techniques and that venous and arterial puncture and infusion sites are maintained with the goal of preventing infection. Nursing interventions that reduce the incidence of ventilator-associated pneumonias must also be implemented. These include frequent oral care, aseptic suction technique, turning, and elevating the head of the bed to prevent aspiration (Rello, Ollendorf, Oster, et al., 2002). Positioning and repositioning of the patient to promote comfort and maintain skin integrity are essential.

### Promoting Rest and Comfort

Efforts are made to minimize the cardiac workload by reducing the patient's physical activity and fear or anxiety. Promoting patient rest and comfort is a priority. To ensure that the patient obtains as much uninterrupted rest as possible, the nurse performs only essential nursing activities. To conserve the patient's energy, the nurse should protect the patient from temperature extremes (excessive warmth or shivering cold), which can increase the metabolic rate and thus the cardiac workload. The patient should not be warmed too quickly, and warming blankets should not be applied, because they can cause vasodilation and a subsequent drop in BP.

### Supporting Family Members

Because patients in shock are the object of intense attention by the health care team, families may be overwhelmed and frightened. Family members may be reluctant to ask questions or seek information for fear that they will be in the way or will interfere with the attention given to the patient. The nurse should make sure that the family is comfortably situated and kept informed about the patient's status. Often, families need advice from the health care team to get some rest; family members are more likely to take this advice if they feel that the patient is being well cared for and that they will be notified of any significant changes in the patient's status. A visit from the hospital chaplain may be comforting and provides some attention to the family while the nurse concentrates on the patient.

## Irreversible Stage

The irreversible (or refractory) stage of shock represents the point along the shock continuum at which organ damage is so severe that the patient does not respond to treatment and cannot survive. Despite treatment, BP remains low. Renal and liver failure, compounded by the release of necrotic tissue toxins, creates an overwhelming metabolic acidosis. Anaerobic metabolism contributes to a worsening lactic acidosis. Reserves of ATP are almost totally depleted, and mechanisms for storing new supplies of energy have been destroyed. Respiratory system failure prevents adequate oxygenation and ventilation despite mechanical ventilatory support, and the cardiovascular system is ineffective in maintaining an adequate MAP for tissue perfusion. Multiple organ dysfunction progressing to complete organ failure has occurred, and death is imminent. Multiple organ dysfunction can occur as a progression along the shock continuum or as a syndrome unto itself and is described in more detail later in this chapter.

## Medical Management

Medical management during the irreversible stage of shock is usually the same as for the progressive stage. Although the patient may have progressed from the progressive to the irreversible stage, the judgment that the shock is irreversible can be made only retrospectively on the basis of the patient's failure to respond to treatment. Strategies that may be experimental (ie, investigational medications, such as antibiotic agents and immunomodulation therapy) may be tried to reduce or reverse the severity of shock.

## Nursing Management

As in the progressive stage of shock, the nurse focuses on carrying out prescribed treatments, monitoring the patient, preventing complications, protecting the patient from injury, and providing comfort. Offering brief explanations to the patient about what is happening is essential even if there is no certainty that the patient hears or understands what is being said. Simple comfort measures, including reassuring touches, should continue to be provided despite the patient's nonresponsiveness to verbal stimuli (Benner, 2004).

As it becomes obvious that the patient is unlikely to survive, the family must be informed about the prognosis and likely outcome. Opportunities should be provided, throughout the patient's care, for the family to see, touch, and talk to the patient. Close family friends or spiritual advisors may be of comfort to the family members in dealing with the inevitable death of their loved one. Whenever possible and appropriate, the patient's family should be approached regarding any living wills, advance directives, or other written or verbal wishes the patient may have shared in the event that he or she became unable to participate in end-of-life decisions. In some cases, ethics committees may assist families and health care teams in making difficult decisions.

During this stage of shock, the family may misinterpret the actions of the health care team. They have been told that nothing has been effective in reversing the shock and that the patient's survival is very unlikely, yet they find physicians and nurses continuing to work feverishly on the patient. Distraught, grieving families may interpret this as a chance for recovery when none exists, and family members may become angry when the patient dies. Conferences with all members of the health care team and the family promote better understanding by the family of the patient's prognosis and the purpose for management measures. During these conferences, it is essential to explain that the equipment and treatments being provided are intended for patient comfort and do not suggest that the patient will recover. Family members should be encouraged to express their wishes concerning the use of life-support measures.

# Overall Management Strategies in Shock

As described previously and in the discussion of types of shock to follow, management in all types and all phases of shock includes the following:

- Fluid replacement to restore intravascular volume
- Vasoactive medications to restore vasomotor tone and improve cardiac function
- Nutritional support to address the metabolic requirements that are often dramatically increased in shock

Therapies described in this section require collaboration among all members of the health care team to ensure that the manifestations of shock are quickly identified and that adequate and timely treatment is instituted to achieve the best outcome possible.

## Fluid Replacement

Fluid replacement is administered in all types of shock. The type of fluids administered and the speed of delivery vary, but fluids are administered to improve cardiac and tissue oxygenation, which in part depends on flow. The fluids administered may include **crystalloids** (electrolyte solutions that move freely between intravascular and interstitial spaces), **colloids** (large-molecule IV solutions), and blood components.

### Crystalloid and Colloid Solutions

The best fluid to treat shock remains controversial. In emergencies, the "best" fluid is often the fluid that is readily available. Fluid resuscitation should be initiated early in shock to maximize intravascular volume. Both crystalloids and colloids, as described later, can be administered to restore intravascular volume. There is no consensus regarding whether crystalloids or colloids should be used; however, with crystalloids, more fluid is necessary to restore intravascular volume (Vincent, 2003). Blood component therapy is used most frequently in hypovolemic shock that is caused by blood loss.

Crystalloids are electrolyte solutions that move freely between the intravascular compartment and the interstitial spaces. Isotonic crystalloid solutions are often selected because they contain the same concentration of electrolytes as the extracellular fluid and therefore can be given without altering the concentrations of electrolytes in the plasma.

Common IV fluids used for resuscitation in hypovolemic shock include 0.9% sodium chloride solution (normal saline) and lactated Ringer's solution (Revell, Greaves, & Porter, 2003). Ringer's lactate is an electrolyte solution containing the lactate ion, which should not be confused with lactic acid. The lactate ion is converted to bicarbonate, which helps buffer the overall acidosis that occurs in shock.

A disadvantage of using isotonic crystalloid solutions is that three parts of the volume are lost to the interstitial compartment for every one part that remains in the intravascular compartment. This occurs in response to mechanisms that store extracellular body fluid. Diffusion of crystalloids into the interstitial space means that more fluid must be administered than the amount lost (Revell et al., 2003; Vincent, 2003).

Care must be taken when rapidly administering isotonic crystalloids to avoid causing excessive edema, particularly pulmonary edema. For this reason, and depending on the cause of the hypovolemia, a hypertonic crystalloid solution, such as 3% sodium chloride, is sometimes administered in hypovolemic shock. Hypertonic solutions produce a large osmotic force that pulls fluid from the intracellular space to the extracellular space to achieve a fluid balance (Ahrns, 2004; Vincent, 2003). The osmotic effect of hypertonic solutions results in fewer fluids being administered to restore intravascular volume. Complications associated with use of hypertonic saline solution include excessive serum osmolality, hypernatremia, hypokalemia, and altered thermoregulation.

Generally, IV colloidal solutions are considered to be plasma proteins, which are molecules that are too large to pass through capillary membranes. Colloids expand intravascular volume by exerting oncotic pressure, thereby pulling fluid into the intravascular space. Colloidal solutions have the same effect as hypertonic solutions in increasing intravascular volume, but less volume of fluid is required than with crystalloids. In addition, colloids have a longer duration of action than crystalloids, because the molecules remain within the intravascular compartment longer.

An albumin solution is commonly used to treat hypovolemic shock. Albumin is a plasma protein; an albumin solution is prepared from human plasma and is heated during production to reduce its potential to transmit disease. The disadvantage of albumin is its high cost. Synthetic colloid preparations, such as hetastarch and dextran solution, are now widely used. However, dextran may interfere with platelet aggregation and therefore is not indicated if hemorrhage is the cause of the hypovolemic shock or if the patient has a coagulation disorder (coagulopathy).

**NURSING ALERT**

With all colloidal solutions, side effects include the rare occurrence of anaphylactic reactions, for which nurses must monitor patients closely.

### Complications of Fluid Administration

Close monitoring of the patient during fluid replacement is necessary to identify side effects and complications. The most common and serious side effects of fluid replacement are cardiovascular overload and pulmonary edema.

The patient receiving fluid replacement must be monitored frequently for adequate urinary output, changes in mental status, skin perfusion, and changes in vital signs. Lung sounds are auscultated frequently to detect signs of fluid accumulation. Adventitious lung sounds, such as crackles, may indicate pulmonary edema.

Often a right atrial pressure line (also known as a central venous pressure [CVP] line) is inserted. In addition to physical assessment, the right atrial pressure value helps in monitoring the patient's response to fluid replacement. A normal right atrial pressure value or CVP is 4 to 12 mm Hg or cm $H_2O$. Several readings are obtained to determine a range, and fluid replacement is continued to achieve a CVP of 8 to 12 mm Hg (Dellinger et al., 2004). With newer technologies, right atrial catheters can be placed that allow the monitoring of intravascular pressures and venous oxygen levels. Assessment of venous oxygenation ($S\bar{v}O_2$, or $Sc\bar{v}O_2$ with a CVP line) is helpful in evaluating the adequacy of intravascular volume (Ahrens & Vollman, 2003; Ahrns, 2004; Kleinpell, 2003). Hemodynamic monitoring with arterial and pulmonary artery lines may be implemented to allow close monitoring of the patient's perfusion and cardiac status as well as response to therapy. For additional information about hemodynamic monitoring, see Chapter 26.

### Vasoactive Medication Therapy

Vasoactive medications are administered in all forms of shock to improve the patient's hemodynamic stability when fluid therapy alone cannot maintain adequate MAP. Specific medications are selected to correct the particular hemodynamic alteration that is impeding cardiac output. Specific vasoactive medications are prescribed for patients in shock because they can support the patient's hemodynamic status. These medications help increase the strength of myocardial contractility, regulate the heart rate, reduce myocardial resistance, and initiate vasoconstriction.

Vasoactive medications are selected for their action on receptors of the sympathetic nervous system. These receptors are known as alpha-adrenergic and beta-adrenergic receptors. Beta-adrenergic receptors are further classified as beta-1 and beta-2 adrenergic receptors. When alpha-adrenergic receptors are stimulated, blood vessels constrict in the cardiorespiratory and gastrointestinal systems, skin, and kidneys. When beta-1 adrenergic receptors are stimulated, heart rate and myocardial contraction increase. When beta-2 adrenergic receptors are stimulated, vasodilation occurs in the heart and skeletal muscles, and the bronchioles relax. The medications used in treating shock consist of various combinations of vasoactive medications to maximize tissue perfusion by stimulating or blocking the alpha- and beta-adrenergic receptors.

When vasoactive medications are administered, vital signs must be monitored frequently (at least every 15 minutes until stable, or more often if indicated). Vasoactive medications should be administered through a central venous line, because infiltration and extravasation of some vasoactive medications can cause tissue necrosis and sloughing. An IV pump or controller should be used to ensure that the medications are delivered safely and accurately.

Individual medication dosages are usually titrated by the nurse, who adjusts drip rates based on the prescribed dose and the patient's response. Dosages are changed to maintain the MAP at a physiologic level that ensures adequate tissue perfusion (usually greater than 65 mm Hg).

**NURSING ALERT**

Vasoactive medications should never be stopped abruptly, because this could cause severe hemodynamic instability, perpetuating the shock state.

Dosages of vasoactive medications should be tapered, and the patient should be weaned from medication with frequent monitoring of BP (every 15 minutes). Table 15-2 presents some of the commonly prescribed vasoactive medications used in treating shock. Occasionally, the patient does not respond as expected to vasoactive medications. A current topic of active research is evaluation of patients' adrenal function. Several recent studies have suggested that critically ill patients should be evaluated for corticosteroid insufficiency, and, if this condition is present, corticosteroid replacement should be initiated (Cooper & Stewart, 2003; Marik & Zaloga, 2003).

### Nutritional Support

Nutritional support is an important aspect of care for patients with shock. Increased metabolic rates during shock increase energy requirements and therefore caloric requirements. Patients in shock may require more than 3000 calories daily.

The release of catecholamines early in the shock continuum causes depletion of glycogen stores in about 8 to 10 hours. Nutritional energy requirements are then met by breaking down lean body mass. In this catabolic process, skeletal muscle mass is broken down even when the patient has large stores of fat or adipose tissue. Loss of skeletal muscle greatly prolongs the patient's recovery time. Parenteral or enteral nutritional support should be initiated as soon as possible, with some form of enteral nutrition always administered. The integrity of the gastrointestinal system depends on direct exposure to nutrients. In addition, glutamine (an essential amino acid during stress) is important in the immunologic function of the gastro-

### TABLE 15-2 — Vasoactive Agents Used in Treating Shock

| Medication | Desired Action in Shock | Disadvantages |
|---|---|---|
| **Sympathomimetics**<br>Amrinone (Inocor)<br>Dobutamine (Dobutrex)<br>Dopamine (Intropin)<br>Epinephrine (Adrenalin)<br>Milrinone (Primacor) | Improve contractility, increase stroke volume, increase cardiac output | Increase oxygen demand of the heart |
| **Vasodilators**<br>Nitroglycerine (Tridil)<br>Nitroprusside (Nipride) | Reduce preload and afterload, reduce oxygen demand of heart | Cause hypotension |
| **Vasoconstrictors**<br>Norepinephrine (Levophed)<br>Phenylephrine (Neo-Synephrine)<br>Vasopressin (Pitressin) | Increase blood pressure by vasoconstriction | Increase afterload, thereby increasing cardiac workload; compromise perfusion to skin, kidneys, lungs, gastrointestinal tract |

intestinal tract, providing a fuel source for lymphocytes and macrophages. Glutamine can be administered through enteral nutrition (DeLegge, 2001; Flynn, 2004).

Stress ulcers occur frequently in acutely ill patients because of the compromised blood supply to the gastrointestinal tract. Therefore, antacids, H$_2$ blockers (eg, famotidine [Pepcid], ranitidine [Zantac]), and proton pump inhibitors (eg, lansoprazole [Prevacid]) are prescribed to prevent ulcer formation by inhibiting gastric acid secretion or increasing gastric pH.

## Hypovolemic Shock

Nurses who care for patients in the different stages of shock must tailor interventions to the type of shock, whether hypovolemic, cardiogenic, or circulatory shock. Hypovolemic shock, the most common type of shock, is characterized by a decreased intravascular volume. Body fluid is contained in the intracellular and extracellular compartments. Intracellular fluid accounts for about two thirds of the total body water. The extracellular body fluid is found in one of two compartments: intravascular (inside blood vessels) or interstitial (surrounding tissues). The volume of interstitial fluid is about three to four times that of intravascular fluid. Hypovolemic shock occurs when there is a reduction in intravascular volume by 15% to 25%, which represents a loss of 750 to 1300 mL of blood in a 70-kg (154-lb) person.

### Pathophysiology

Hypovolemic shock can be caused by external fluid losses, as in traumatic blood loss, or by internal fluid shifts, as in severe dehydration, severe edema, or ascites (Chart 15-3). Intravascular volume can be reduced both by fluid loss and by fluid shifting between the intravascular and interstitial compartments.

The sequence of events in hypovolemic shock begins with a decrease in the intravascular volume. This results in decreased venous return of blood to the heart and subsequent decreased ventricular filling. Decreased ventricular filling results in decreased stroke volume (amount of blood ejected from the heart) and decreased cardiac output. When cardiac output drops, BP drops and tissues cannot be adequately perfused (Fig. 15-3).

### Medical Management

Major goals in the treatment of hypovolemic shock are (1) to restore intravascular volume to reverse the sequence of events leading to inadequate tissue perfusion, (2) to redistribute fluid volume, and (3) to correct the underlying cause of the fluid loss as quickly as possible. Depending on the severity of shock and the patient's condition, it is likely that efforts will be made to address all three goals simultaneously.

#### Treatment of the Underlying Cause

If the patient is hemorrhaging, efforts are made to stop the bleeding. This may involve applying pressure to the bleeding site or surgery to stop internal bleeding. If the cause of the hypovolemia is diarrhea or vomiting, medications to treat diarrhea and vomiting are administered while efforts

### CHART 15-3 — Risk Factors for Hypovolemic Shock

**EXTERNAL: FLUID LOSSES**
- Trauma
- Surgery
- Vomiting
- Diarrhea
- Diuresis
- Diabetes insipidus

**INTERNAL: FLUID SHIFTS**
- Hemorrhage
- Burns
- Ascites
- Peritonitis
- Dehydration

## Physiology/Pathophysiology

**FIGURE 15-3.** Pathophysiologic sequence of events in hypovolemic shock.

are made to identify and treat the cause. In elderly patients, dehydration may be the cause of hypovolemic shock.

### Fluid and Blood Replacement

Beyond reversing the primary cause of the decreased intravascular volume, fluid replacement (also referred to as fluid resuscitation) is of primary concern. At least two large-gauge IV lines are inserted to establish access for fluid administration. Two IV lines allow simultaneous administration of fluid, medications, and blood component therapy if required. Because the goal of the fluid replacement is to restore intravascular volume, it is necessary to administer fluids that will remain in the intravascular compartment, to avoid fluid shifts from the intravascular compartment into the intracellular compartment. Table 15-3 summarizes the fluids commonly used in the treatment of shock.

Lactated Ringer's solution and 0.9% sodium chloride solution are isotonic crystalloid fluids commonly used in hypovolemic shock (Revell et al., 2003; Stern & Bobek, 2001). Large amounts of fluid must be administered to restore intravascular volume, because isotonic crystalloid solutions move freely between the fluid compartments of the body and do not remain in the vascular system.

Colloids (eg, albumin, hetastarch, and dextran) may also be used. Dextran is not indicated if the cause of the hypovolemic shock is hemorrhage, because it interferes with platelet aggregation.

Blood products, which are also colloids, may need to be administered, particularly if the cause of the hypovolemic shock is hemorrhage. However, there is a risk of transmitting bloodborne viruses, as well as scarcity of blood products; therefore, these products are used only if other alternatives are unavailable or blood loss is extensive and rapid. Packed red blood cells are administered to replenish the patient's oxygen-carrying capacity in conjunction with other fluids that will expand volume. Currently, the need for transfusions is based on the patient's oxygenation needs, which are determined by vital signs, blood gas values, and clinical appearance rather than an arbitrary laboratory value. An area of active research is the development of synthetic forms of blood (ie, compounds capable of carrying oxygen in the same way that blood does) as potential alternatives to blood component therapy.

### Redistribution of Fluid

In addition to administering fluids to restore intravascular volume, positioning the patient properly assists fluid redistribution. A modified Trendelenburg position (Fig. 15-4) is recommended in hypovolemic shock. Elevation of the legs promotes the return of venous blood. It is not recom-

| TABLE 15-3 | Fluid Replacement in Shock | |
|---|---|---|
| **Fluids** | **Advantages** | **Disadvantages** |
| **Crystalloids** | | |
| 0.9% sodium chloride (normal saline solution) | Widely available, inexpensive | Requires large volume of infusion; can cause pulmonary edema |
| Lactated Ringer's | Lactate ion helps buffer metabolic acidosis | Requires large volume of infusion; can cause pulmonary edema |
| Hypertonic saline (3%, 5%, 7.5%) | Small volume needed to restore intravascular volume | Danger of hypernatremia |
| **Colloids** | | |
| Albumin (5%, 25%) | Rapidly expands plasma volume | Expensive; requires human donors; limited supply; can cause heart failure |
| Dextran (40, 70) | Synthetic plasma expander | Interferes with platelet aggregation; not recommended for hemorrhagic shock |
| Hetastarch | Synthetic; less expensive than albumin; effect lasts up to 36 h | Prolongs bleeding and clotting times |

**FIGURE 15-4.** Proper positioning (modified Trendelenburg) for the patient who shows signs of shock. The lower extremities are elevated to an angle of about 20 degrees; the knees are straight, the trunk is horizontal, and the head is slightly elevated.

mended that patients be put in a full Trendelenburg position, because this makes breathing difficult.

### Pharmacologic Therapy

If fluid administration fails to reverse hypovolemic shock, then the same medications given in cardiogenic shock are used, because unreversed hypovolemic shock progresses to cardiogenic failure (the vicious circle).

If the underlying cause of the hypovolemia is dehydration, medications are also administered to reverse the cause of the dehydration. For example, insulin is administered if dehydration is secondary to hyperglycemia, desmopressin (DDAVP) is administered for diabetes insipidus, antidiarrheal agents for diarrhea, and antiemetic medications for vomiting.

## Nursing Management

Primary prevention of shock is an essential focus of nursing care. Hypovolemic shock can be prevented in some instances by closely monitoring patients who are at risk for fluid deficits and assisting with fluid replacement before intravascular volume is depleted. In other circumstances, nursing care focuses on assisting with treatment targeted at the cause of the shock and restoring intravascular volume.

General nursing measures include ensuring safe administration of prescribed fluids and medications and documenting their administration and effects. Another important nursing role is monitoring for signs of complications and side effects of treatment and reporting these signs early in treatment.

### Administering Blood and Fluids Safely

Administering blood transfusions safely is a vital nursing role. In emergency situations, it is important to acquire blood specimens quickly, to obtain a baseline complete blood count and to type and cross-match the blood in anticipation of blood transfusions. A patient who receives a transfusion of blood products must be monitored closely for adverse effects (see Chapter 33).

Fluid replacement complications can occur, often when large volumes are administered rapidly. Therefore, the nurse monitors the patient closely for cardiovascular overload and pulmonary edema. The risk of these complications is increased in the elderly and in patients with preexisting cardiac disease. Hemodynamic pressure, vital signs, arterial blood gases, serum lactate levels, hemoglobin and hematocrit levels, and fluid intake and output (I & O) are among the parameters monitored. Temperature should also be monitored closely to ensure that rapid fluid resuscitation does not precipitate hypothermia. IV fluids may need to be warmed during the administration of large volumes. Physical assessment focuses on observing the jugular veins for distention and monitoring jugular venous pressure. Jugular venous pressure is low in hypovolemic shock; it increases with effective treatment and is significantly increased with fluid overload and heart failure. The nurse must monitor cardiac and respiratory status closely and report changes in BP, pulse pressure, heart rate and rhythm, and lung sounds to the physician.

### Implementing Other Measures

Oxygen is administered to increase the amount of oxygen carried by available hemoglobin in the blood. A patient who is confused may feel apprehensive with an oxygen mask or cannula in place, and frequent explanations about the need for the mask may reduce some of the patient's fear and anxiety. Simultaneously, the nurse must direct efforts to the safety and comfort of the patient.

## Cardiogenic Shock

Cardiogenic shock occurs when the heart's ability to contract and to pump blood is impaired and the supply of oxygen is inadequate for the heart and tissues. The causes of cardiogenic shock are known as either coronary or noncoronary. Coronary cardiogenic shock is more common than noncoronary cardiogenic shock and is seen most often in patients with myocardial infarction. Coronary cardiogenic shock occurs when a significant amount of the left ventricular myocardium has been damaged (Hochman, 2003). Patients who experience an anterior wall myocardial infarction are at greatest risk for cardiogenic shock because of the potentially extensive damage to the left ventricle caused by occlusion of the left anterior descending coronary artery. Noncoronary causes of cardiogenic shock are related to conditions that stress the myocardium (eg, severe hypoxemia, acidosis, hypoglycemia, hypocalcemia, and tension pneumothorax) as well as conditions that result in ineffective myocardial function (eg, cardiomyopathies, valvular damage, cardiac tamponade, dysrhythmias).

### Pathophysiology

In cardiogenic shock, cardiac output, which is a function of both stroke volume and heart rate, is compromised. When stroke volume and heart rate decrease or become erratic,

BP falls, and tissue perfusion is compromised. Blood supply for tissues and organs and for the heart muscle itself is inadequate, resulting in impaired tissue perfusion. Because impaired tissue perfusion weakens the heart and impairs its ability to pump blood forward, the ventricle does not fully eject its volume of blood at systole. As a result, fluid accumulates in the lungs. This sequence of events can occur rapidly or over a period of days (Fig. 15-5).

## Clinical Manifestations

Patients in cardiogenic shock may experience the pain of angina and develop dysrhythmias and hemodynamic instability.

## Medical Management

The goals of medical management in cardiogenic shock are (1) to limit further myocardial damage and preserve the healthy myocardium and (2) to improve the cardiac function by increasing cardiac contractility, decreasing ventricular afterload, or both (Hochman, 2003). In general, these goals are achieved by increasing oxygen supply to the heart muscle while reducing oxygen demands.

### Correction of Underlying Causes

As with all forms of shock, the underlying cause of cardiogenic shock must be corrected. It is necessary first to treat the oxygenation needs of the heart muscle to ensure its continued ability to pump blood to other organs. In the case of coronary cardiogenic shock, the patient may require thrombolytic therapy, angioplasty, coronary artery bypass graft surgery, intra-aortic balloon pump therapy, or some combination of these treatments. In the case of noncoronary cardiogenic shock, interventions focus on correcting the underlying cause, such as replacement of a faulty cardiac valve, correction of a dysrhythmia, correction of acidosis and electrolyte disturbances, or treatment of the tension pneumothorax.

**FIGURE 15-5.** Pathophysiologic sequence of events in cardiogenic shock.

### Initiation of First-Line Treatment

First-line treatment of cardiogenic shock involves the following actions:

- Supplying supplemental oxygen
- Controlling chest pain
- Providing selected fluid support
- Administering vasoactive medications
- Controlling heart rate with medication or by implementation of a transthoracic or IV pacemaker
- Implementing mechanical cardiac support (intra-aortic balloon counterpulsation therapy, ventricular assist systems, or extracorporeal cardiopulmonary bypass [CPB])

#### OXYGENATION

In the early stages of shock, supplemental oxygen is administered by nasal cannula at a rate of 2 to 6 L/min to achieve an oxygen saturation exceeding 90%. Monitoring of arterial blood gas values and pulse oximetry values helps determine whether the patient requires a more aggressive method of oxygen delivery.

#### PAIN CONTROL

If a patient experiences chest pain, IV morphine sulfate is administered for pain relief. In addition to relieving pain, morphine dilates the blood vessels. This reduces the workload of the heart by both decreasing the cardiac filling pressure (preload) and reducing the pressure against which the heart muscle has to eject blood (afterload). Morphine also decreases the patient's anxiety.

#### HEMODYNAMIC MONITORING

Hemodynamic monitoring is initiated to assess the patient's response to treatment. In many institutions, this is performed in the intensive care unit (ICU), where an arterial line can be inserted. The arterial line enables accurate and continuous monitoring of BP and provides a port from which to obtain frequent arterial blood samples without having to perform repeated arterial punctures. A multi-lumen pulmonary artery catheter is inserted to allow measurement of the pulmonary artery pressures, myocardial filling pressures, cardiac output, and pulmonary and systemic resistance. For more information, see Chapter 30.

#### LABORATORY MARKER MONITORING

Laboratory markers for ventricular dysfunction (BNP) and cardiac enzyme levels (CPK-MB and cTn-I) are measured, and serial 12-lead ECGs are obtained to assess the degree of myocardial damage.

### Pharmacologic Therapy

Vasoactive medication therapy consists of multiple pharmacologic strategies to restore and maintain adequate cardiac output. In coronary cardiogenic shock, the aims of vasoactive medication therapy are improved cardiac contractility, decreased preload and afterload, and stabilized heart rate and rhythm.

Because improving contractility and decreasing cardiac workload are opposing pharmacologic actions, two types of medications may be administered in combination:

sympathomimetic agents and vasodilators. Sympathomimetic medications increase cardiac output by mimicking the action of the sympathetic nervous system through vasoconstriction, resulting in increased preload, and through increasing myocardial contractility (inotropic action) or increasing the heart rate (chronotropic action). Vasodilators are used to decrease preload and afterload, thus reducing the workload of the heart and the oxygen demand. Medications commonly combined to treat cardiogenic shock include dobutamine, dopamine, and nitroglycerin (see Table 15-2).

### DOBUTAMINE
Dobutamine (Dobutrex) produces inotropic effects by stimulating myocardial beta-receptors, increasing the strength of myocardial activity and improving cardiac output. Myocardial alpha-adrenergic receptors are also stimulated, resulting in decreased pulmonary and systemic vascular resistance (decreased afterload). Dobutamine enhances the strength of cardiac contraction, improving stroke volume ejection and overall cardiac output (Hochman, 2003; Kellum & Pinsky, 2002).

### NITROGLYCERIN
IV nitroglycerin (Tridil) in low doses acts as a venous vasodilator and therefore reduces preload. At higher doses, nitroglycerin causes arterial vasodilation and therefore reduces afterload as well. These actions, in combination with dobutamine, increase cardiac output while minimizing cardiac workload. In addition, vasodilation enhances blood flow to the myocardium, improving oxygen delivery to the weakened heart muscle (Hochman, 2003).

### DOPAMINE
Dopamine (Intropin) is a sympathomimetic agent that has varying vasoactive effects depending on the dosage. It may be used with dobutamine and nitroglycerin to improve tissue perfusion. Low-dose dopamine (0.5 to 3.0 μg/kg/min) is believed to increase renal and mesenteric blood flow, thereby preventing ischemia of these organs, because shock causes blood to be shunted away from the kidneys and the mesentery. However, this dosage does not improve cardiac output. Medium-dose dopamine (4 to 8 μg/kg/min) has sympathomimetic properties, improves contractility (inotropic action), and slightly increases the heart rate (chronotropic action). At this dosage, dopamine may increase cardiac output. High-dose dopamine (8 to 20 μg/kg/min) predominantly causes vasoconstriction, which increases afterload and thus increases cardiac workload. Because this effect is undesirable in patients with cardiogenic shock, dopamine dosages must be carefully titrated. In severe metabolic acidosis, which occurs in the later stages of shock, the effectiveness of dopamine is diminished. To maximize the effectiveness of any vasoactive agent, metabolic acidosis must first be corrected. Physicians often prescribe IV sodium bicarbonate to treat the acidosis (Dellinger et al., 2004).

### OTHER VASOACTIVE MEDICATIONS
Additional vasoactive agents that may be used in managing cardiogenic shock include norepinephrine (Levophed), epinephrine (Adrenalin), milrinone (Primacor), amrinone (Inocor), vasopressin (Pitressin), and phenylephrine (Neo-Synephrine). Each of these medications stimulates different receptors of the sympathetic nervous system. A combination of these medications may be prescribed, depending on the patient's response to treatment. All vasoactive medications have adverse effects, making specific medications more useful than others at different stages of shock. Diuretics such as furosemide (Lasix) may be administered to reduce the workload of the heart by reducing fluid accumulation (see Table 15-2).

### ANTIARRHYTHMIC MEDICATIONS
Multiple factors, such as hypoxemia, electrolyte imbalances, and acid–base imbalances, contribute to serious cardiac dysrhythmias in all patients with shock. In addition, as a compensatory response to decreased cardiac output and BP, the heart rate increases beyond normal limits. This impedes cardiac output further by shortening diastole and thereby decreasing the time for ventricular filling. Consequently, antiarrhythmic medications are required to stabilize the heart rate. For a full discussion of cardiac dysrhythmias as well as commonly prescribed medications, see Chapter 27. General principles regarding the administration of vasoactive medications are discussed later in this chapter.

### FLUID THERAPY
Appropriate fluid administration is also necessary in the treatment of cardiogenic shock. Administration of fluids must be monitored closely to detect signs of fluid overload. Incremental IV fluid boluses are cautiously administered to determine optimal filling pressures for improving cardiac output. A fluid bolus should never be given rapidly, because rapid fluid administration in patients with cardiac failure may result in acute pulmonary edema.

## Mechanical Assistive Devices

If cardiac output does not improve despite supplemental oxygen, vasoactive medications, and fluid boluses, mechanical assistive devices are used temporarily to improve the heart's ability to pump. Intra-aortic balloon counterpulsation is one means of providing temporary circulatory assistance (see Chapter 30). A polyurethane balloon catheter is inserted percutaneously through the common femoral artery and advanced into the descending thoracic aorta. The balloon catheter is connected to a console containing a gas-filled pump. The timing of the balloon inflation is synchronized via ECG with the beginning of diastole, and the balloon deflation occurs just before systole. The goals of intra-aortic balloon counterpulsation include the following (Hollenberg, Ahrens, Annane, et al., 2004):

- Increased stroke volume
- Improved coronary artery perfusion
- Decreased preload
- Decreased cardiac workload
- Decreased myocardial oxygen demand

Other means of mechanical assistance include left and right ventricular assist devices and total temporary artificial hearts. These devices are electrical pumps or pumps driven by air. They assist or replace the ventricular pumping action of the heart. Human heart transplantation may be the only option remaining for a patient who has cardiogenic shock and who cannot be weaned from mechanical assistive devices. (Mechanical assistive devices and heart transplantation are discussed in Chapters 29 and 30.)

Another short-term means of providing cardiac or pulmonary support to the patient in cardiogenic shock is through an extracorporeal device similar to the cardiopulmonary bypass (CPB) system used in open-heart surgery. The CPB system requires systemic anticoagulation; arterial and venous cannulation of the femoral artery and vein; and connection to a centrifugal, oxygenated pump. The catheter tip is advanced into the right atrium. This system lowers left and right ventricular pressures, reducing the workload and oxygen needs of the heart. Complications of CPB include coagulopathies, myocardial ischemia, infection, and thromboembolism. CPB is used only in emergency situations until definitive treatment, such as heart transplantation, can be initiated.

## Nursing Management

### Preventing Cardiogenic Shock

In some circumstances, identifying at-risk patients early, promoting adequate oxygenation of the heart muscle, and decreasing cardiac workload can prevent cardiogenic shock. This can be accomplished by conserving the patient's energy, promptly relieving angina, and administering supplemental oxygen. Often, however, cardiogenic shock cannot be prevented. In such instances, nursing management includes working with other members of the health care team to prevent shock from progressing and to restore adequate cardiac function and tissue perfusion.

### Monitoring Hemodynamic Status

A major role of the nurse is monitoring the patient's hemodynamic and cardiac status. Arterial lines and ECG monitoring equipment must be well maintained and functioning properly. The nurse anticipates the medications, IV fluids, and equipment that might be used and is ready to assist in implementing these measures. Changes in hemodynamic, cardiac, and pulmonary status and laboratory values are documented and reported promptly. In addition, adventitious breath sounds, changes in cardiac rhythm, and other abnormal physical assessment findings are reported immediately.

### Administering Medications and Intravenous Fluids

The nurse plays a critical role in the safe and accurate administration of IV fluids and medications. Fluid overload and pulmonary edema are risks because of ineffective cardiac function and accumulation of blood and fluid in the pulmonary tissues. The nurse documents and records medications and treatments that are administered as well as the patient's response to treatment.

The nurse must be knowledgeable about the desired effects as well as the side effects of medications. For example, it is important to monitor the patient for decreased BP after administering morphine or nitroglycerin. Patients receiving thrombolytic therapy must be monitored for bleeding. Arterial and venous puncture sites must be observed for bleeding, and pressure must be applied at the sites if bleeding occurs. Neurologic assessment is essential after the administration of thrombolytic therapy to assess for the potential complication of cerebral hemorrhage associated with the therapy. IV infusions must be observed closely because tissue necrosis and sloughing may occur if vasopressor medications infiltrate the tissues. Urine output, BUN, and serum creatinine levels are monitored to detect decreased renal function secondary to the effects of cardiogenic shock or its treatment.

### Maintaining Intra-aortic Balloon Counterpulsation

The nurse plays a critical role in caring for the patient receiving intra-aortic balloon counterpulsation (see Chapter 30). The nurse makes ongoing timing adjustments of the balloon pump to maximize its effectiveness by synchronizing it with the cardiac cycle. The patient is at great risk of circulatory compromise to the leg on the side where the catheter for the balloon has been placed; therefore, the nurse must check the neurovascular status of the lower extremities frequently.

### Enhancing Safety and Comfort

Throughout care, the nurse must take an active role in safeguarding the patient, enhancing comfort, and reducing anxiety. This includes administering medication to relieve chest pain, preventing infection at the multiple arterial and venous line insertion sites, protecting the skin, and monitoring respiratory and renal function. Proper positioning of the patient promotes effective breathing without decreasing BP and may also increase patient comfort while reducing anxiety.

Brief explanations about procedures that are being performed and the use of comforting touch often provide reassurance to the patient and family. The family is usually anxious and benefits from opportunities to see and talk to the patient. Explanations of treatments and the patient's responses are often comforting to family members.

## Circulatory Shock

Circulatory shock occurs when blood volume is abnormally displaced in the vasculature (eg, when blood volume pools in peripheral blood vessels). The displacement of blood volume causes a relative hypovolemia because not enough blood returns to the heart, which leads to subsequent inadequate tissue perfusion. The ability of the blood vessels to constrict helps return the blood to the heart. The vascular tone is determined both by central regulatory mechanisms, as in BP regulation, and by local regulatory mechanisms, as in tissue demands for oxygen and nutrients. Therefore, circulatory shock can be caused either by a loss of sympathetic tone or by release of biochemical mediators from cells.

The varied mechanisms leading to the initial vasodilation in circulatory shock further subdivide this classification of shock into three types: (1) **septic shock**, (2) **neurogenic shock**, and (3) **anaphylactic shock**.

The different types of circulatory shock cause variations in the pathophysiologic chain of events and are explained here separately. In all types of circulatory shock, massive arterial and venous dilation allows blood to pool peripherally. Arterial dilation reduces systemic vascular resistance. Initially, cardiac output can be high, both from the reduction in afterload (systemic vascular resistance) and from the heart muscle's increased effort to maintain perfusion despite the incompetent vasculature secondary to arterial dilation. Pooling of blood in the periphery results in decreased venous return. Decreased venous return results in decreased stroke volume and decreased cardiac output. Decreased cardiac output, in turn, causes decreased BP and ultimately decreased tissue perfusion. Figure 15-6 presents the pathophysiologic sequence of events in circulatory shock.

### CHART 15-4

## Risk Factors for Circulatory Shock

**SEPTIC SHOCK**
- Immunosuppression
- Extremes of age (<1 yr and >65 yr)
- Malnourishment
- Chronic illness
- Invasive procedures

**NEUROGENIC SHOCK**
- Spinal cord injury
- Spinal anesthesia
- Depressant action of medications
- Glucose deficiency

**ANAPHYLACTIC SHOCK**
- Penicillin sensitivity
- Transfusion reaction
- Bee sting allergy
- Latex sensitivity
- Severe allergy to some foods or medications

## Septic Shock

Septic shock, the most common type of circulatory shock, is caused by widespread infection (Chart 15-4). Despite the increased sophistication of antibiotic therapy, the incidence of septic shock has continued to rise during the past 60 years. It is the most common cause of death in non-coronary ICUs in the United States; annually, an estimated 215,000 deaths are due to severe sepsis (Aird, 2003). Finding and aggressively treating the source of infection is an important determinant of the clinical outcome.

Nosocomial infections (infections occurring in the hospital) in critically ill patients that may progress to septic shock most frequently originate in the bloodstream, lungs, and urinary tract (in decreasing order of frequency) (Ahrens & Vollman, 2003; Kleinpell, 2003; Sommers, 2003). Other infections include intra-abdominal infections, wound infections, and bacteremia associated with intravascular catheters (Eggimann & Pittet, 2001) and indwelling urinary catheters (urosepsis). Additional risk factors that contribute to the growing incidence of septic shock are increased awareness and identification of the condition; the increased number of immunocompromised patients (due to malnutrition, alcoholism, malignancy, diabetes mellitus, and AIDS); the increased use of invasive procedures and indwelling medical devices; the increased number of resistant microorganisms; and the increasingly older population (Ahrens & Vollman, 2003; Kleinpell, 2003). The incidence of septic shock can be reduced by débriding wounds to remove necrotic tissue; carrying out infection control practices, including the use of meticulous aseptic technique; properly cleaning and maintaining equipment; and using thorough hand-hygiene techniques (Dellinger et al., 2004).

Elderly patients continue to be at particular risk for sepsis because of decreased physiologic reserves and an aging immune system (Kleinpell, 2003; Sommers, 2003). Other patients at risk are those undergoing surgical and other invasive procedures; those with malnutrition or immunosuppression; and those with chronic illness such as diabetes mellitus, hepatitis, chronic renal failure, and immunodeficiency disorders (Kleinpell, 2003).

A significant body of research has been conducted in the past decade in an effort aimed at reducing the morbidity and mortality caused by septic shock. In 1991, the American College of Chest Physicians and the Society of Critical Care Medicine convened a consensus conference to clarify the

### Physiology/Pathophysiology

Precipitating event
↓
Vasodilation
↓
Activation of inflammatory response
↓
Maldistribution of blood volume
↓
Decreased venous return
↓
Decreased cardiac output
↓
Decreased tissue perfusion

**FIGURE 15-6.** Pathophysiologic sequence of events in circulatory shock.

understanding of sepsis and related disorders (Sommers, 2003). In 2002, the Society of Critical Care Medicine further defined the definitions to promote recognition and earlier treatment of patients with sepsis (Chart 15-5). Research efforts continued to define further the physiologic mystery of sepsis progressing to multisystem organ dysfunction and potential treatments. In March 2003, critical care experts and infectious disease experts evaluated the research and provided evidence-based recommendations for the acute management of patients with sepsis and septic shock (Dellinger et al., 2004).

## Pathophysiology

The most common causative microorganisms of septic shock are the gram-negative bacteria. However, there is also an increased incidence of gram-positive bacterial infections. Currently, gram-positive bacteria are responsible for 50% of bacteremic events (Houghton, 2002). Other infectious agents, such as viruses and fungi, also can cause septic shock. However, it is estimated that 20% to 30% of patients with severe sepsis may never have an identifiable site of infection (Sommers, 2003).

When microorganisms invade body tissues, patients exhibit an immune response. This immune response provokes the activation of biochemical cytokines and mediators associated with an inflammatory response and produces a complex cascade of physiologic events that leads to poor tissue perfusion. Increased capillary permeability, which leads to fluid seeping from the capillaries, and vasodilation are two such effects that interrupt the ability of the body to provide adequate perfusion, oxygen, and nutrients to the tissues and cells. In addition, proinflammatory and anti-inflammatory cytokines released during the inflammatory response activate the coagulation system, which begins to form clots in areas where a clot may or may not be needed, further compromising tissue perfusion. The imbalance of the inflammatory response and the clotting and fibrinolysis

---

### CHART 15-5

### Definitions to Promote Recognition and Earlier Treatment of Patients With Sepsis

***Bacteremia:*** the presence of bacteria in the blood
***Infection:*** the presence of microorganisms that trigger an inflammatory response
***Hypotension:*** a systolic blood pressure <90 mm Hg or a drop in systolic blood pressure of >40 mm Hg from the patient's baseline blood pressure
***Sepsis:*** a systemic response to *infection;* may occur after a burn, surgery, or serious illness and is manifested by two or more clinical signs and symptoms:
- Temperature >38°C or <36°C
- Heart rate >90 bpm
- Respiratory rate >30 breaths/min
- PaCO$_2$ <32 mm Hg
- WBC count >12,000 cells/mm$^3$, <4000 cells/mm$^3$, or >10% immature WBC (bands)
- Hyperglycemia and abnormal clotting and bleeding

***PIRO model:*** a method useful in recognizing and trending patients with sepsis
- **P**atient genetic predisposition and response to infection
- **I**nfection
- **R**esponse to infection
- **O**rgan dysfunction associated with infectious response

***Severe sepsis:*** the presence of signs and symptoms of sepsis-related organ dysfunction, hypotension, and/or hypoperfusion; clinical signs and symptoms include those of sepsis as well as
- Lactic acidosis
- Oliguria
- Altered level of consciousness
- Thrombocytopenia
- Alternated level of consciousness

***Septic shock:*** shock associated with sepsis; characterized by symptoms of sepsis plus hypotension and hypoperfusion despite adequate fluid volume replacement

***Systemic inflammatory response syndrome (SIRS):*** a syndrome resulting from a *severe clinical insult* that initiates an overwhelming inflammatory response by the body; clinical signs and symptoms may include
- Temperature >38°C or <36°C (>100.4°F or < 96.8°F)
- Heart rate >90 bpm
- Respiratory rate >30 breaths/min
- PaCO$_2$ <32 mm Hg
- WBC count >12,000 cells/mm$^3$, <4000 cells/mm$^3$, or >10% immature WBC (bands)

***Multiple organ dysfunction syndrome:*** the presence of altered function of one or more organs in an acutely ill patient requiring intervention and support of the organs to achieve physiologic functioning required for homeostasis; clinical signs and symptoms may be
- Cardiovascular: hypotension and hypoperfusion
- Respiratory: hypoxemia, hypercarbia, adventitious breath sounds
- Renal: increased creatinine, decreased urine output
- Hematologic: thrombocytopenia, bleeding
- Metabolic: lactic acidemia, metabolic acidosis
- Neurologic: altered level of consciousness
- Hepatic: elevated liver function tests

Adapted from Sommers, M. S. (2003). The cellular basis of septic shock. *Critical Care Nursing Clinics of North America, 15*(1), 13–26.

cascades are considered critical elements of the devastating physiologic progression that is present in patients with severe sepsis.

Sepsis is an evolving process, with neither clearly definable clinical signs and symptoms nor predictable progression. In the past, septic shock has been described as having two phases, a hyperdynamic and a hypodynamic phase. Although the division into phases may promote understanding of sepsis, its actual progression into severe sepsis and septic shock is not always easy to recognize clinically. Initially, a hyperdynamic response occurs; it is characterized by a high cardiac output with systemic vasodilation. The BP may remain within normal limits, or the patient may be hypotensive but responsive to fluids. The heart rate increases, progressing to tachycardia. Hyperthermia and fever, with warm, flushed skin and bounding pulses, is evident. The respiratory rate is elevated. Urinary output may remain at normal levels or decrease. Gastrointestinal status may be compromised, as evidenced by nausea, vomiting, diarrhea, or decreased bowel sounds. Signs of hypermetabolism include increased serum glucose and insulin resistance. Subtle changes in mental status, such as confusion or agitation, may be present.

As the sepsis progresses, tissues become more underperfused and acidotic, compensation begins to fail, and the patient becomes more hypodynamic. The cardiovascular system also begins to fail, the BP does not respond to vasoactive agents and fluid resuscitation, and signs of end-organ damage are visible (eg, renal failure, pulmonary failure, hepatic failure). As sepsis progresses to septic shock, the BP drops, and the skin becomes cool and pale. Temperature may be normal or below normal. Heart and respiratory rates remain rapid. Urine production no longer occurs, and multiple organ dysfunction progressing to failure develops.

Systemic inflammatory response syndrome (SIRS) presents clinically like sepsis. The only difference between SIRS and sepsis is that there is no identifiable source of infection. SIRS stimulates an overwhelming inflammatory immunologic and hormonal response similar to that seen in septic patients. Any overwhelming insult stimulates SIRS and may progress to sepsis. Therefore, despite an absence of infection, antibiotic agents may still be administered because of the possibility of unrecognized infection. Additional therapies directed to support patients with SIRS are similar to those for sepsis. If the inflammatory process progresses, septic shock may develop.

## Medical Management

Current treatment of septic shock involves identification and elimination of the cause of infection. Specimens of blood, sputum, urine, wound drainage, and tips of invasive catheters are collected for culture using aseptic technique.

Any potential routes of infection must be eliminated. IV lines are removed and reinserted at other body sites. Antibiotic-coated IV central lines may be inserted to decrease the risk of invasive line-related bacteremia in high-risk patients, such as the elderly (Eggimann & Pittet, 2001). If possible, urinary catheters are removed. Any abscesses are drained, and necrotic areas are débrided.

Fluid replacement must be instituted to correct the hypovolemia that results from the incompetent vasculature and the inflammatory response. Crystalloids, colloids, and blood products may be administered to increase intravascular volume.

### Pharmacologic Therapy

If the infecting organism is unknown, broad-spectrum antibiotic agents are started until culture and sensitivity reports are received (Houghton, 2002). A third-generation cephalosporin plus an aminoglycoside may be prescribed initially. This combination works against most gram-negative and some gram-positive organisms. When culture and sensitivity reports become available, the antibiotic agents may be changed to agents that are more specific to the infecting organism and less toxic to the patient.

Research efforts show promise for improving the outcomes of septic shock. Although past treatments focused on destroying the infectious organism, emphasis is now on altering the patient's immune response to the organism as well as modulating the inflammatory and coagulation response to infection. Current research focuses on the development of medications that adjust the effects of biochemical cytokines and mediator responses.

Studies have recently demonstrated that recombinant human activated protein C (rhAPC) reduces mortality in patients with severe sepsis (Ahrens & Vollman, 2003; Angus, Zinde-Zwirble, Clermont, et al., 2003; Kleinpell, 2003). The U.S. Food and Drug Administration has approved its use for treatment of adults with severe sepsis and resulting acute organ dysfunction who are at high risk for death. rhAPC acts as an antithrombotic, anti-inflammatory, and profibrinolytic agent. In sepsis, an imbalance in proinflammatory mediators activates the coagulation cascade and deposits microthrombi that alter tissue perfusion. rhAPC is an anti-inflammatory cytokine that stimulates fibrinolysis, restoring balance in the coagulation–anticoagulation homeostatic process of the body's inflammatory response to injury and infection.

APC, available as drotrecogin alfa (Xigris), has provided a significant breakthrough in the successful pharmacologic treatment of patients with sepsis. However, the medication should be administered as early as possible in the sequence of pathophysiologic events of sepsis. Nurses are critical in the identification of patients in the early stage of sepsis for treatment with drotrecogin alfa (Kleinpell, 2003). The medication is not without side effects, bleeding being the most common serious effect. Stopping the medication reduces the risk of bleeding. The patient should be evaluated with regard to the relative risk of bleeding versus the potential benefit from the medication. Drotrecogin alfa is contraindicated in patients with active internal bleeding, recent hemorrhagic stroke, intracranial surgery, or head injury.

### Nutritional Therapy

Aggressive nutritional supplementation is critical in the management of septic shock, because malnutrition further impairs the patient's resistance to infection. Nutritional supplementation should be initiated within the first 24 hours after ICU admission (DeLegge, 2001), and continuous infusions of insulin should be used to control hyperglycemia (Dellinger et al., 2004). Enteral feedings are preferred to the parenteral route because of the increased risk of iatrogenic infection associated with IV catheters; however, enteral feedings may not be possible if decreased perfusion to the gastrointestinal tract reduces peristalsis and impairs absorption.

## Nursing Management

Nurses caring for patients in any setting must keep in mind the risks of sepsis and the high mortality rate associated with sepsis, severe sepsis, and septic shock. All invasive procedures must be carried out with aseptic technique after careful hand hygiene. In addition, IV lines, arterial and venous puncture sites, surgical incisions, traumatic wounds, urinary catheters, and pressure ulcers must be monitored for signs of infection in all patients. Nurses identify patients who are at particular risk for sepsis and septic shock (ie, elderly and immunosuppressed patients and those with extensive trauma, burns, or diabetes), keeping in mind that these high-risk patients may not develop typical or classic signs of infection and sepsis. For example, confusion may be the first sign of infection and sepsis in elderly patients.

When caring for a patient with septic shock, the nurse collaborates with other members of the health care team to identify the site and source of sepsis and the specific organisms involved. Appropriate specimens for culture and sensitivity are often obtained by the nurse.

Elevated body temperature (hyperthermia) is common with sepsis and raises the patient's metabolic rate and oxygen consumption. Fever is one of the body's natural mechanisms for fighting infections. Therefore, elevated temperatures may not be treated unless they reach dangerous levels (more than 40°C [104°F]) or unless the patient is uncomfortable. Efforts may be made to reduce the temperature by administering acetaminophen or applying a hypothermia blanket. During these therapies, the nurse monitors the patient closely for shivering, which increases oxygen consumption. Efforts to increase comfort are important if the patient experiences fever, chills, or shivering.

The nurse administers prescribed IV fluids and medications, including antibiotic agents and vasoactive medications, to restore vascular volume. Because of decreased perfusion to the kidneys and liver, serum concentrations of antibiotic agents that are normally cleared by these organs may increase and produce toxic effects. Therefore, the nurse monitors blood levels (antibiotic agent, BUN, creatinine, white blood cell count, hemoglobin, hematocrit, platelet levels, coagulation studies) and reports changes to the physician. As with other types of shock, the nurse monitors the patient's hemodynamic status, fluid intake and output, and nutritional status. Daily weights and close monitoring of serum albumin levels help determine the patient's protein requirements.

## Neurogenic Shock

In neurogenic shock, vasodilation occurs as a result of a loss of balance between parasympathetic and sympathetic stimulation. Sympathetic stimulation causes vascular smooth muscle to constrict, and parasympathetic stimulation causes the vascular smooth muscle to relax or dilate. The patient experiences a predominant parasympathetic stimulation that causes vasodilation lasting for an extended period, leading to a relative hypovolemic state. However, blood volume is adequate, because the vasculature is dilated; the blood volume is displaced, producing a hypotensive (low BP) state. The overriding parasympathetic stimulation that occurs with neurogenic shock causes a drastic decrease in the patient's systemic vascular resistance and bradycardia. Inadequate BP results in the insufficient perfusion of tissues and cells that is common to all shock states.

Neurogenic shock can be caused by spinal cord injury, spinal anesthesia, or nervous system damage. It may also result from the depressant action of medications or from lack of glucose (eg, insulin reaction or shock). Neurogenic shock may have a prolonged course (spinal cord injury) or a short one (syncope or fainting). Normally, during states of stress, the sympathetic stimulation causes the BP and heart rate to increase. In neurogenic shock, the sympathetic system is not able to respond to body stressors. Therefore, the clinical characteristics of neurogenic shock are signs of parasympathetic stimulation. It is characterized by dry, warm skin rather than the cool, moist skin seen in hypovolemic shock. Another characteristic is hypotension with bradycardia, rather than the tachycardia that characterizes other forms of shock.

## Medical Management

Treatment of neurogenic shock involves restoring sympathetic tone, either through the stabilization of a spinal cord injury or, in the instance of spinal anesthesia, by positioning the patient properly. Specific treatment depends on cause of the shock. Further discussion of management of patients with a spinal cord injury is presented in Chapter 63. If hypoglycemia (insulin shock) is the cause, glucose is rapidly administered. Hypoglycemia and the insulin reaction are described further in Chapter 41.

## Nursing Management

It is important to elevate and maintain the head of the bed at least 30 degrees to prevent neurogenic shock when a patient receives spinal or epidural anesthesia. Elevation of the head helps prevent the spread of the anesthetic agent up the spinal cord. In suspected spinal cord injury, neurogenic shock may be prevented by carefully immobilizing the patient to prevent further damage to the spinal cord.

Nursing interventions are directed toward supporting cardiovascular and neurologic function until the usually transient episode of neurogenic shock resolves. Applying elastic compression stockings and elevating the foot of the bed may minimize pooling of blood in the legs. Pooled blood increases the risk for thrombus formation. Therefore, the nurse must check the patient daily for any lower-extremity pain, redness, tenderness, and warmth of the calves. If the patient complains of pain and objective assessment of the calf is suspicious, the patient should be evaluated for deep vein thrombosis.

Administration of heparin or low-molecular-weight heparin (Lovenox) as prescribed, application of elastic compression stockings, or use of pneumatic compression of the legs may prevent thrombus formation. Passive range of motion of the immobile extremities helps promote circulation.

A patient who has experienced a spinal cord injury may not report pain caused by internal injuries. Therefore, in the immediate postinjury period, the nurse must monitor the patient closely for signs of internal bleeding that could lead to hypovolemic shock.

# Anaphylactic Shock

Anaphylactic shock occurs rapidly and is life-threatening. Because anaphylactic shock occurs in patients already exposed to an antigen and who have developed antibodies to it, it can often be prevented. Patients with known allergies should understand the consequences of subsequent exposure to the antigen and should wear medical identification that lists their sensitivities. This could prevent inadvertent administration of a medication that would lead to anaphylactic shock. In addition, patients and families need instruction about emergency use of medications for treatment of anaphylaxis.

Anaphylactic shock is caused by a severe allergic reaction when patients who have already produced antibodies to a foreign substance (antigen) develop a systemic antigen–antibody reaction. This process requires that the patient has previously been exposed to the substance. An antigen–antibody reaction provokes mast cells to release potent vasoactive substances, such as histamine or bradykinin, causing widespread vasodilation and capillary permeability.

## Medical Management

Treatment of anaphylactic shock requires removing the causative antigen (eg, discontinuing an antibiotic agent), administering medications that restore vascular tone, and providing emergency support of basic life functions. Epinephrine is given for its vasoconstrictive action. Diphenhydramine (Benadryl) is administered to reverse the effects of histamine, thereby reducing capillary permeability. These medications are given intravenously. Nebulized medications, such as albuterol (Proventil), may be given to reverse histamine-induced bronchospasm.

If cardiac arrest and respiratory arrest are imminent or have occurred, cardiopulmonary resuscitation is performed. Endotracheal intubation or tracheotomy may be necessary to establish an airway. IV lines are inserted to provide access for administering fluids and medications. Anaphylaxis and specific chemical mediators are discussed further in Chapter 53.

## Nursing Management

The nurse has an important role in preventing anaphylactic shock. The nurse must assess all patients for allergies or previous reactions to antigens (eg, medications, blood products, foods, contrast agents, latex) and communicate the existence of these allergies or reactions to others. In addition, the nurse assesses the patient's understanding of previous reactions and steps taken by the patient and family to prevent further exposure to antigens. When new allergies are identified, the nurse advises the patient to wear or carry identification that names the specific allergen or antigen.

When administering any new medication, the nurse observes all patients for allergic reactions. This is especially important with IV medications. Allergy to penicillin is one of the most common causes of anaphylactic shock. Patients who have a penicillin allergy may also develop an allergy to similar medications. For example, they may react to cefazolin sodium (Ancef) because it has a similar antimicrobial action of attaching to the penicillin-binding proteins found on the walls of infectious organisms. Previous adverse drug reactions increase the risk that the patient will develop an undesirable reaction to a new medication. If the patient reports an allergy to a medication, the nurse must be aware of the risks involved in the administration of similar medications.

In the hospital and outpatient diagnostic testing sites, the nurse must identify patients who are at risk for anaphylactic reactions to the contrast agents (radiopaque, dye-like substances that may contain iodine) that are used for diagnostic tests. These include patients with a known allergy to iodine or fish and those who have had previous allergic reactions to contrast agents. This information must be conveyed to the staff at the diagnostic testing site, including x-ray personnel.

The nurse must be knowledgeable about the clinical signs of anaphylaxis, must take immediate action if signs and symptoms occur, and must be prepared to begin cardiopulmonary resuscitation if cardiorespiratory arrest occurs. In addition to monitoring the patient's response to treatment, the nurse assists with intubation if needed, monitors the hemodynamic status, ensures IV access for administration of medications, administers prescribed medications and fluids, and documents treatments and their effects.

Community health and home care nurses who administer medications, including antibiotic agents, in the patient's home or other settings, must be prepared to administer epinephrine subcutaneously or intramuscularly in the event of an anaphylactic reaction.

After recovery from anaphylaxis, the patient and family require an explanation of the event. Furthermore, the nurse provides instruction about avoiding future exposure to antigens and administering emergency medications to treat anaphylaxis (see Chapter 53).

# Multiple Organ Dysfunction Syndrome

Multiple organ dysfunction syndrome (MODS) is altered organ function in acutely ill patients that requires medical intervention to support continued organ function. It is another phase in the progression of shock states. The actual incidence of MODS is difficult to determine, because it develops with acute illnesses that compromise tissue perfusion. In addition, there is a lack of consistent definitions to describe the organ failure that is found in MODS (Vincent et al., 2002). It is estimated that MODS has an associated mortality rate as high as 75% (Schulman, 2003).

## Pathophysiology

MODS can be classified as primary or secondary. Primary MODS is the result of direct tissue insult, which then leads to impaired perfusion or ischemia. Secondary MODS is most often a complication of SIRS and sepsis. However, MODS may be a complication of any form of shock because of inadequate tissue perfusion. As previously described, in shock, all organ systems suffer damage from a lack of adequate perfusion that can result in organ failure. Sequential organ failure has been further observed. The exact triggering mechanism is unknown.

Various causes of MODS have been identified, including dead or injured tissue, infection, and perfusion deficits. However, it is not possible as yet to predict which patients will develop MODS, partly because much of the organ damage occurs at the cellular level and therefore cannot be directly observed or measured. The organ failure usually begins in the lungs and is followed by failure of the liver, gastrointestinal system, and kidneys (Vincent et al., 2002). Advanced age, malnutrition, and coexisting diseases appear to increase the risk of MODS in acutely ill patients.

## Clinical Manifestations

In both primary and secondary MODS, an initial event results in low BP. After treatment for the cause of the decrease in BP, the patient appears to respond.

In primary MODS, which occurs most often when the initiating event is a pulmonary one such as lung injury, the patient experiences respiratory compromise that necessitates intubation. This usually occurs within 72 hours after the initiating event. Respiratory failure leads rapidly to MODS, resulting in a mortality rate of 30% to 75% (Fein & Calalang-Colucci, 2000).

In secondary MODS, which occurs most often in patients with septic shock, the pattern is more insidious and progressively unfolds over about 1 month. Patients also experience respiratory failure and require intubation. They remain hemodynamically stable for about 7 to 14 days. Despite this apparent stability, they exhibit a hypermetabolic state that is characterized by hyperglycemia (elevated blood glucose level), hyperlacticacidemia (excess of lactic acid in the blood), and polyuria (excessive urinary output). The metabolic rate is 1.5 to 2 times the basal metabolic rate. Infection is usually present, and skin breakdown begins. During this stage, there is a severe loss of skeletal muscle mass (autocatabolism). If the hypermetabolic phase can be reversed, the patient may survive with some damage to affected organ systems (DeLegge, 2001). If the hypermetabolic process cannot be halted and cells do not receive adequate oxygen and nutrients, the patient has irreversible organ failure and dies.

If the hypermetabolic phase cannot be reversed, MODS progresses and is characterized by jaundice, hyperbilirubinemia (liver failure), and oliguria progressing to anuria (renal failure) often requiring dialysis. Patients become less hemodynamically stable and begin to require vasoactive medications and fluid support. The onset of organ dysfunction is an ominous prognostic sign; the more organs that fail, the worse the outcome.

## Medical Management

Prevention remains the top priority in managing MODS. Elderly patients are at increased risk for MODS because of the lack of physiologic reserve associated with aging and the natural degenerative process, especially immune compromise (Schulman, 2003; Vincent et al., 2002). Early detection and documentation of initial signs of infection are essential in managing MODS in elderly patients. Subtle changes in mentation and a gradual rise in temperature are early warning signs. Other patients at risk for MODS are those with chronic illness, malnutrition, immunosuppression, or surgical or traumatic wounds.

If preventive measures fail, treatment measures to reverse MODS are aimed at (1) controlling the initiating event, (2) promoting adequate organ perfusion, and (3) providing nutritional support.

## Nursing Management

The general plan of nursing care for patients with MODS is the same as that for patients in septic shock. Primary nursing interventions are aimed at supporting the patient and monitoring organ perfusion until primary organ insults are halted. Providing information and support to family members is a critical role of the nurse. It is important that the health care team address end-of-life decisions to ensure that supportive therapies are congruent with the patient's wishes (see Chapter 17).

### Promoting Communication

Nurses encourage frequent and open communication about treatment modalities and options to ensure that the patient's wishes regarding medical management are met. For patients who survive MODS, it is essential that they be informed about the goals of rehabilitation and expectations for progress toward these goals, because the massive loss of skeletal muscle mass makes rehabilitation a long, slow process. A strong nurse–patient relationship built on effective communication provides needed encouragement during this phase of recovery.

# Promoting Home and Community-Based Care

## Teaching Patients Self-Care

Patients who experience and survive shock may have been unable to get out of bed for an extended period of time and are likely to have a slow, prolonged recovery. The patient and family are instructed about strategies to prevent further episodes of shock by identifying the factors implicated in the initial episode. In addition, the patient and family require instruction about assessments needed to identify the complications that may occur after the patient is discharged from the hospital. Depending on the type of shock and its management, the patient or family may require instruction about treatment modalities such as emergency administration of medications, IV therapy, parenteral nutrition, skin care, exercise, and ambulation. The patient and family are also instructed about the need for gradual increases in ambulation and other activity. The need for adequate nutrition is another crucial aspect of teaching.

## Continuing Care

Because of the physical toll associated with recovery from shock, patients may be cared for in an extended care facility or rehabilitation setting after hospital discharge. Alternatively, a referral may be made for home care. The home care nurse assesses the patient's physical status and monitors recovery. The nurse also assesses the adequacy of treatments that are continued at home and the ability of the patient and family to cope with these treatments. The patient is likely to require close medical supervision until complete recovery occurs. The home care nurse reinforces the importance of continuing medical care and helps the patient and family identify and mobilize community resources.

## Critical Thinking Exercises

**1** You administer an antibiotic to a patient before he goes to surgery. The patient's chart states that he has no known drug allergies. After 15 minutes, the patient complains of anxiety, shortness of breath, and chest discomfort. He is flushed and visibly uncomfortable. What are your nursing priorities in providing care to this patient? What assessment data do you need to obtain to determine if this patient is experiencing cardiogenic or anaphylactic shock? What nursing interventions and medical treatments would you anticipate for cardiogenic shock? In terms of anaphylactic shock, what nursing interventions and medical treatments would you anticipate?

**2** [ebp] An elderly man with a 10-year history of Alzheimer's disease was admitted with sudden, increasing confusion and combative behavior. You know that changes in mental status may be an early sign of sepsis in the elderly. How would you assess this patient for the possibility of sepsis? What risk factors place an older patient at higher risk for sepsis? What is the evidence base for these risk factors? How would you evaluate the strength of the evidence on these risk factors and for strategies to reduce the patient's risks? How would the management of the elderly patient differ from that of a younger patient?

**3** While driving, you witness a car hit a man riding a bicycle. You call 911 and stop to help. The rider of the bicycle has been thrown approximately 25 feet from his bike and appears to be seriously injured. As you approach, you notice that his leg is severely deformed with an open fracture and that he is bleeding profusely. He is unconscious and blood is escaping from under his bike helmet. Describe the type of shock this patient is at greatest risk for developing. What actions would you take at the scene to prevent shock or prevent it from progressing?

**4** A patient who has used a wheelchair for the last 10 years because of a spinal cord injury is burned when her clothing catches fire as she prepares dinner. Her burns are extensive but limited to her upper body. What types of shock are possible in this patient? What therapy directed at prevention or treatment of shock would you anticipate? Describe the rationale for the therapies that you have identified. How would this patient's disability affect management? How would you expect required treatments, in turn, to affect her disability?

## REFERENCES AND SELECTED READINGS

### BOOKS

Baldwin, K. M. & Morris, S. E. (2002). Shock, multiple organ dysfunction syndrome, and burns in adults. In McCance, K. L. & Heuther, S. E. (Eds.). *Pathophysiology: The biologic basis for disease in adults and children* (4th ed.). St. Louis: Mosby.

Huether, S. E. (2002). Alterations of renal and urinary tract function. In McCance, K. L. & Heuther, S. E. (Eds.). *Pathophysiology: The biologic basis for disease in adults and children* (4th ed.). St. Louis: Mosby.

McCance, K. L. & Heuther, S. E. (Eds.). *Pathophysiology: The biologic basis for disease in adults and children* (4th ed.). St. Louis: Mosby.

Morton, P. G., Fontaine, D. K., Hudak, C. M., et al. (2005). *Critical care nursing: A holistic approach.* Philadelphia: Lippincott Williams & Wilkins.

Porth, C. M. (2005). *Pathophysiology: Concepts of altered health states* (7th ed.). Philadelphia: Lippincott Williams & Wilkins.

Stern, S. A. & Bobek, E. M. (2001). Resuscitation: Management of shock. In Ferrera, P. C., Colucciello, S. A., Marx, J. A., et al. (Eds): *Trauma management: An emergency medicine approach.* St. Louis: Mosby.

Vincent, J. L. (2003). Correcting the deficit: Fluids, pressors and RBCs in resuscitation. In Levy, M. M. & Vincent, J. L. (Eds.). *Sepsis: Pathophysiologic insights and current management.* Chicago: Society of Critical Care Medicine.

### JOURNALS

Ahrns, K. S. (2004). Trends in burn resuscitation. *Critical Care Nursing Clinics of North America, 16*(1), 75–98.

Ahrens, T. & Vollman, K. (2003). Severe sepsis management: Are we doing enough? *Critical Care Nurse, 23*(5), S2–S15.

Aird, W. C. (2003). The role of the endothelium in severe sepsis and multiple organ dysfunction syndrome. *Blood, 101*(10), 3765–3777.

Angus, D. C., Linde-Zwirble, W. T., Lidicker, J., et al. (2001). Epidemiology of severe sepsis in the United States: Analysis of incidence, outcome and associated costs of care. *Critical Care Medicine, 29*(7), 1303–1310.

Angus, D. C., Linde-Zwirble, W. T., Clermont, G., et al. (2003). Cost-effectiveness of drotrecogin alfa (activated) in treatment of severe sepsis. *Critical Care Medicine, 31*(1), 1–11.

Benner, P. (2004). Relational ethics of comfort, touch, and solace: Endangered arts? *American Journal of Critical Care, 13*(4), 346–349.

Bernard, G. R., Vincent, J. L., Laterre, R. F., et al. (2001). Efficacy and safety of recombinant human activated protein C for severe sepsis. *New England Journal of Medicine, 344*(10), 699–707.

Berry, B. E. & Pinard, A. E. (2003). Assessing tissue oxygenation. *Critical Care Nurse, 22*(3), 22–42.

Ceppa, E. P., Fuh, C. & Bulkley, G. B. (2003). Mesenteric hemodynamic response to circulatory shock. *Current Opinion in Critical Care, 9*(2), 127–123.

Cooper, M. S. & Stewart, P. M. (2003). Corticosteroid insufficiency in acutely ill patients. *New England Journal of Medicine, 348*(8), 727–734.

Dellinger, R. P. (2003). Cardiovascular management of septic shock. *Critical Care Medicine, 31*(3), 946–955.

Dellinger, R. P., Carlet, J. M., Masur, H., et al. (2004). Surviving Sepsis Campaign guidelines for management of severe sepsis and septic shock. *Critical Care Medicine, 32*(3), 858–873.

DeLegge, M. (2001). Enteral access: The foundation of feeding. *Journal of Parenteral and Enteral Nutrition, 25*(2), S8–S13.

Eggimann, P. & Pittet, D. (2001). Catheter-related infections in intensive care units: An overview with special emphasis on prevention. *Advances in Sepsis, 1*(1), 2–13.

Fein, A. M., & Calalang-Colucci, M. G. (2000). Acute lung injury and acute respiratory distress syndrome in sepsis and septic shock. *Critical Care Clinics, 16*(2), 289–313.

Fishel, R. S., Are, C. & Barbul, A. (2003). Vessel injury and capillary leak. *Critical Care Medicine, 31*(8), S502–S511.

Flynn, M. B. (2004). Nutritional support of the burn-injured patient. *Critical Care Nursing Clinics of North America, 16*(1), 139–144.

Hachey, D. M. & Smith, T. (2003). Use of nesiritide to treat acute decompensated heart failure. *Critical Care Nurse, 23*(1), 53–58.

Hameed, S. M., Aird, W. C., & Cohn, S. M. (2003). Oxygen delivery. *Critical Care Medicine, 31*(12), S658–S667.

Hochman, J. (2003). Cardiogenic shock complicating acute myocardial infarction: Expanding the paradigm. *Circulation, 107*(24), 2998–3002.

Hollenberg, S. M., Ahrens, T. S., Annane, D., et al. (2004). Practice parameters for hemodynamic support of sepsis in adult patients: 2004 update. *Critical Care Medicine, 32*(9), 1928–1949.

Hotchkiss, R. S., & Karl, I. E. (2003). The pathophysiology and treatment of sepsis. *New England Journal of Medicine, 348*(2), 138–149.

Houghton, D. (2002). Antimicrobial resistance in the intensive care unit: Understanding the problem. *AACN Clinical Issues, 13*(2), 410–420.

Kellum, J. A. & Pinsky, M. R. (2002). Use of vasopressor agents in critically ill patients. *Current Opinion in Critical Care, 8*(3), 236–241.

Kleinpell, R. (2003). Advances in treating patients with severe sepsis. *Critical Care Nurse, 23*(3), 16–29.

Marik, P. E. & Zaloga, G. P. (2003). Adrenal insufficiency during septic shock. *Critical Care Medicine, 31*(1), 141–145.

Mikhail, J. (1999). Resuscitation endpoints in trauma. *AACN Clinical Issues, 10*(1), 10–21.

Rello, J., Ollendorf, D. A., Oster, G., et al. (2002). Epidemiology and outcomes of ventilator-associated pneumonia in a large US database. *Chest, 122*(6), 2115–2121.

Revell, M., Greaves, I. & Porter, K. (2003). Endpoints for fluid resuscitation in hemorrhagic shock. *Journal of Trauma, 54*(5), S63–S67.

SAFE Study Investigators. (2005). A comparison of albumin and saline for fluid resuscitation in the intensive care unit. *New England Journal of Medicine, 350*(22), 2247–2256.

Schulman, C. S. (2003). New thoughts on sepsis. *Dimensions in Critical Care Nursing, 22*(1), 20–30.

Sommers, M. S. (2003). The cellular basis of septic shock. *Critical Care Nursing Clinics of North America, 15*(1), 13–26.

Van den Berghe, G., Wouters, P., Weekers, F., et al. (2001). Intensive insulin therapy in critically ill patients. *New England Journal of Medicine, 345*(19), 1359–1367.

Vincent, J. L, Abraham, E., Annane, D., et al. (2002). Reducing mortality in sepsis: New directions. *Critical Care, 6*(3S), S1–S18.

CHAPTER 16

# Oncology: Nursing Management in Cancer Care

## Learning Objectives

*On completion of this chapter, the learner will be able to:*

1. Compare the structure and function of the normal cell and the cancer cell.
2. Differentiate between benign and malignant tumors.
3. Identify agents and factors that have been found to be carcinogenic.
4. Describe the significance of health education and preventive care in decreasing the incidence of cancer.
5. Differentiate among the purposes of surgical procedures used in cancer treatment, diagnosis, prophylaxis, palliation, and reconstruction.
6. Describe the roles of surgery, radiation therapy, chemotherapy, bone marrow transplantation, and other therapies in treating cancer.
7. Describe the special nursing needs of patients receiving chemotherapy.
8. Describe common nursing diagnoses and collaborative problems of patients with cancer.
9. Use the nursing process as a framework for care of patients with cancer.
10. Describe the concept of hospice in providing care for patients with advanced cancer.
11. Discuss the role of the nurse in assessment and management of common oncologic emergencies.

Cancer is not a single disease with a single cause; rather, it is a group of distinct diseases with different causes, manifestations, treatments, and prognoses. Cancer nursing practice covers all age groups and nursing specialties and is carried out in a variety of health care settings, including the home, community, acute care institutions, and rehabilitation centers. The scope, responsibilities, and goals of cancer nursing, also called **oncology** nursing, are as diverse and complex as those of any nursing specialty. Because many people associate cancer with pain and death, nurses need to identify their own reactions to cancer and set realistic goals to meet the challenges inherent in caring for patients with cancer.

In addition, cancer nurses must be prepared to support patients and families through a wide range of physical, emotional, social, cultural, and spiritual crises. Chart 16-1 identifies major areas of responsibility for nurses caring for patients with cancer.

# Epidemiology of Cancer

Although cancer affects people of all ages, most cancers occur in people older than 65 years of age. Overall, the incidence of cancer is higher in men than in women and higher in industrialized sectors and nations.

More than 1.3 million Americans are diagnosed each year with a cancer affecting one of various body sites (Fig. 16-1). Cancer is second only to cardiovascular disease as a leading cause of death in the United States. More than 560,000 Americans die from a malignant process each year. The leading causes of cancer death in the United States, in order of frequency, are lung, prostate, and colorectal cancer in men and lung, breast, and colorectal cancer in women (Jemal, Murray, Ward, et al., 2005).

Relative 5-year survival rates for African Americans compared to whites are lower for cancer at every site. In the United States, cancer mortality in African Americans is

## Glossary

**alopecia:** hair loss
**anaplasia:** cells that lack normal cellular characteristics and differ in shape and organization with respect to their cells of origin; usually, anaplastic cells are malignant
**apoptosis:** programmed cell death
**biologic response modifier (BRM) therapy:** use of agents or treatment methods that can alter the immunologic relationship between the tumor and the host to provide a therapeutic benefit
**biopsy:** a diagnostic procedure to remove a small sample of tissue to be examined microscopically to detect malignant cells
**brachytherapy:** delivery of radiation therapy through internal implants
**cancer:** a disease process whereby cells proliferate abnormally, ignoring growth-regulating signals in the environment surrounding the cells
**carcinogenesis:** process of transforming normal cells into malignant cells
**chemotherapy:** use of medications to kill tumor cells by interfering with cellular functions and reproduction
**control:** containment of the growth of cancer cells
**cure:** prolonged survival and disappearance of all evidence of disease so that the patient has the same life expectancy as anyone else in his or her age group
**cytokines:** substances produced by cells of the immune system to enhance production and functioning of components of the immune system
**dysplasia:** bizarre cell growth resulting in cells that differ in size, shape, or arrangement from other cells of the same type of tissue
**extravasation:** leakage of medication from the veins into the subcutaneous tissues
**grading:** identification of the type of tissue from which the tumor originated and the degree to which the tumor cells retain the functional and structural characteristics of the tissue of origin
**graft-versus-host disease (GVHD):** an immune response initiated by T lymphocytes of donor tissue against the recipient's tissues (skin, gastrointestinal tract, liver); an undesirable response

**graft-versus-disease effect:** the donor cell response against the malignancy; a desirable response
**hyperplasia:** increase in the number of cells of a tissue; most often associated with periods of rapid body growth
**malignant:** having cells or processes that are characteristic of cancer
**metaplasia:** conversion of one type of mature cell into another type of cell
**metastasis:** spread of cancer cells from the primary tumor to distant sites
**myelosuppression:** suppression of the blood cell–producing function of the bone marrow
**nadir:** lowest point of white blood cell depression after therapy that has toxic effects on the bone marrow
**neoplasia:** uncontrolled cell growth that follows no physiologic demand
**neutropenia:** abnormally low absolute neutrophil count
**oncology:** field or study of cancer
**palliation:** relief of symptoms associated with cancer
**radiation therapy:** use of ionizing radiation to interrupt the growth of malignant cells
**stomatitis:** inflammation of the oral tissues, often associated with some chemotherapeutic agents
**staging:** process of determining the size and spread, or metastasis, of a tumor
**targeted therapies:** cancer treatments that seek to minimize the negative effects on healthy tissues by disrupting specific cancer cell functions such as malignant transformation, communication pathways, processes for growth and metastasis, and genetic coding
**thrombocytopenia:** decrease in the number of circulating platelets; associated with the potential for bleeding
**tumor-specific antigen (TSA):** protein on the membrane of cancer cells that distinguishes the malignant cell from a benign cell of the same tissue type
**vesicant:** substance that can cause tissue necrosis and damage, particularly when extravasated
**xerostomia:** dry oral cavity resulting from decreased function of salivary glands

## CHART 16-1

### Responsibilities of the Nurse in Cancer Care

- Support the idea that cancer is a chronic illness that has acute exacerbations rather than one that is synonymous with death and suffering.
- Assess own level of knowledge relative to the pathophysiology of the disease process.
- Make use of current research findings and practices in the care of the patient with cancer and his or her family.
- Identify patients at high risk for cancer.
- Participate in primary and secondary prevention efforts.
- Assess the nursing care needs of the patient with cancer.
- Assess the learning needs, desires, and capabilities of the patient with cancer.
- Identify nursing problems of the patient and the family.
- Assess the social support networks available to the patient.
- Plan appropriate interventions with the patient and the family.
- Assist the patient to identify strengths and limitations.
- Assist the patient to design short-term and long-term goals for care.
- Implement a nursing care plan that interfaces with the medical care regimen and that is consistent with the established goals.
- Collaborate with members of a multidisciplinary team to foster continuity of care.
- Evaluate the goals and resultant outcomes of care with the patient, the family, and members of the multidisciplinary team.
- Reassess and redesign the direction of the care as determined by the evaluation.

### Estimated New Cases*

| Male | Female |
|---|---|
| Prostate (33%) | Breast (32%) |
| Lung and bronchus (13%) | Lung and bronchus (12%) |
| Colon and rectum (10%) | Colon and rectum (11%) |
| Urinary bladder (7%) | Uterine corpus (6%) |
| Melanoma of the skin (5%) | Non-Hodgkin lymphoma (4%) |
| Non-Hodgkin lymphoma (4%) | Melanoma of the skin (4%) |
| Kidney and renal pelvis (3%) | Ovary (3%) |
| Leukemia (3%) | Thyroid (3%) |
| Oral cavity and pharynx (3%) | Urinary bladder (2%) |
| Pancreas (2%) | Pancreas (2%) |
| All sites (100%) | All sites (100%) |

### Estimated Deaths

| Male | Female |
|---|---|
| Lung and bronchus (31%) | Lung and bronchus (27%) |
| Prostate (10%) | Breast (15%) |
| Colon and rectum (10%) | Colon and rectum (10%) |
| Pancreas (5%) | Ovary (6%) |
| Leukemia (4%) | Pancreas (6%) |
| Esophagus (4%) | Leukemia (4%) |
| Liver and intrahepatic bile duct (3%) | Non-Hodgkin lymphoma (3%) |
| Non-Hodgkin lymphoma (3%) | Uterine corpus (3%) |
| Urinary bladder (3%) | Multiple myeloma (2%) |
| Kidney and renal pelvis (3%) | Brain and other nervous system (2%) |
| All sites (100%) | All sites (100%) |

**FIGURE 16-1.** Ten leading types of cancer by gender determined on the bases of estimated new cancer cases and deaths in the United States in 2004. *Excludes basal and squamous cell skin cancers and in situ carcinomas except urinary bladder. Note: Percentages may not total 100 because of rounding. From the American Cancer Society. (2004). Surveillance research, 2004. *CA: A Cancer Journal for Clinicians, 54*[1], 8–29.

higher than in any other racial group. This finding is related to the higher incidence and later stage of diagnosis among African Americans. The increased cancer morbidity and mortality in this group are largely a result of economic factors, education, and access to health care rather than racial characteristics (Ward, Jemal, Cokkinides, et al., 2004).

# Pathophysiology of the Malignant Process

Cancer is a disease process that begins when an abnormal cell is transformed by the genetic mutation of the cellular DNA. This abnormal cell forms a clone and begins to proliferate abnormally, ignoring growth-regulating signals in the environment surrounding the cell. The cells acquire invasive characteristics, and changes occur in surrounding tissues. The cells infiltrate these tissues and gain access to lymph and blood vessels, which carry the cells to other areas of the body. This phenomenon is called **metastasis** (cancer spread to other parts of the body).

## Proliferative Patterns

During the lifespan, various body tissues normally undergo periods of rapid or proliferative growth that must be distinguished from malignant growth activity. Several patterns of cell growth exist: **hyperplasia**, **metaplasia**, **dysplasia**, **anaplasia**, and **neoplasia**.

Cancerous cells are described as **malignant** neoplasms. They demonstrate uncontrolled cell growth that follows no physiologic demand. Benign and malignant growths are classified and named by tissue of origin, as described in Table 16-1. Benign and malignant cells differ in many cellular growth characteristics, including the method and rate of growth, ability to metastasize or spread, general effects, destruction of tissue, and ability to cause death. These differences are summarized in Table 16-2. The degree of anaplasia ultimately determines the malignant potential.

### TABLE 16-1  Names of Selected Benign and Malignant Tumors According to Tissue Types

| Tissue Type | Benign Tumors | Malignant Tumors |
| --- | --- | --- |
| **Epithelial** | | |
| Surface | Papilloma | Squamous cell carcinoma |
| Glandular | Adenoma | Adenocarcinoma |
| **Connective** | | |
| Fibrous | Fibroma | Fibrosarcoma |
| Adipose | Lipoma | Liposarcoma |
| Cartilage | Chondroma | Chondrosarcoma |
| Bone | Osteoma | Osteosarcoma |
| Blood vessels | Hemangioma | Hemangiosarcoma |
| Lymph vessels | Lymphangioma | Lymphangiosarcoma |
| Lymph tissue | | Lymphosarcoma |
| **Muscle** | | |
| Smooth | Leiomyoma | Leiomyosarcoma |
| Striated | Rhabdomyoma | Rhabdomyosarcoma |
| **Neural Tissue** | | |
| Nerve cell | Neuroma | Neuroblastoma |
| Glial tissue | Glioma (benign) | Glioblastoma, astrocytoma, medulloblastoma, oligodendroglioma |
| Nerve sheaths | Neurilemmoma | Neurilemmal sarcoma |
| Meninges | Meningioma | Meningeal sarcoma |
| **Hematologic** | | |
| Granulocytic | | Myelocytic leukemia |
| Erythrocytic | | Erythrocytic leukemia |
| Plasma cells | | Multiple myeloma |
| Lymphocytic | | Lymphocytic leukemia or lymphoma |
| Monocytic | | Monocytic leukemia |
| **Endothelial Tissue** | | |
| Blood vessels | Hemangioma | Hemangiosarcoma |
| Lymph vessels | Lymphangioma | Lymphangiosarcoma |
| Endothelial lining | | Ewing's sarcoma |

Reproduced with permission from Porth, C. M. (2005). *Pathophysiology: Concepts of altered health states* (7th ed.). Philadelphia: Lippincott Williams & Wilkins.

| TABLE 16-2 | Characteristics of Benign and Malignant Neoplasms | |
|---|---|---|
| Characteristics | Benign | Malignant |
| Cell characteristics | Well-differentiated cells that resemble normal cells of the tissue from which the tumor originated | Cells are undifferentiated and often bear little resemblance to the normal cells of the tissue from which they arose |
| Mode of growth | Tumor grows by expansion and does not infiltrate the surrounding tissues; usually encapsulated | Grows at the periphery and sends out processes that infiltrate and destroy the surrounding tissues |
| Rate of growth | Rate of growth is usually slow | Rate of growth is variable and depends on level of differentiation; the more anaplastic the tumor, the faster its growth |
| Metastasis | Does not spread by metastasis | Gains access to the blood and lymphatic channels and metastasizes to other areas of the body |
| General effects | Is usually a localized phenomenon that does not cause generalized effects unless its location interferes with vital functions | Often causes generalized effects, such as anemia, weakness, and weight loss |
| Tissue destruction | Does not usually cause tissue damage unless its location interferes with blood flow | Often causes extensive tissue damage as the tumor outgrows its blood supply or encroaches on blood flow to the area; may also produce substances that cause cell damage |
| Ability to cause death | Does not usually cause death unless its location interferes with vital functions | Usually causes death unless growth can be controlled |

Reproduced with permission from Porth, C. M. (2005). *Pathophysiology: Concepts of altered health states* (7th ed.). Philadelphia: Lippincott Williams & Wilkins.

## Characteristics of Malignant Cells

Despite their individual differences, all cancer cells share some common cellular characteristics in relation to the cell membrane, special proteins, the nuclei, chromosomal abnormalities, and the rate of mitosis and growth. The cell membranes are altered in cancer cells, which affects fluid movement in and out of the cell. The cell membrane of malignant cells also contains proteins called **tumor-specific antigens** (eg, carcinoembryonic antigen [CEA] and prostate-specific antigen [PSA]), which develop as they become less differentiated (mature) over time. These proteins distinguish the malignant cell from a benign cell of the same tissue type. They may be useful in measuring the extent of disease in a person and in tracking the course of illness during treatment or relapse. Malignant cellular membranes also contain less fibronectin, a cellular cement. They are therefore less cohesive and do not adhere to adjacent cells readily.

Typically, nuclei of cancer cells are large and irregularly shaped (pleomorphism). Nucleoli, structures within the nucleus that house ribonucleic acid (RNA), are larger and more numerous in malignant cells, perhaps because of increased RNA synthesis. Chromosomal abnormalities (translocations, deletions, additions) and fragility of chromosomes are commonly found when cancer cells are analyzed.

Mitosis (cell division) occurs more frequently in malignant cells than in normal cells. As the cells grow and divide, more glucose and oxygen are needed. If glucose and oxygen are unavailable, malignant cells use anaerobic metabolic channels to produce energy, which makes the cells less dependent on the availability of a constant oxygen supply.

## Invasion and Metastasis

Malignant disease processes have the ability to allow the spread or transfer of cancerous cells from one organ or body part to another by invasion and metastasis. Patterns of metastasis can be partially explained by circulatory patterns and by specific affinity for certain malignant cells to bind to molecules in specific body tissue.

Invasion, which refers to the growth of the primary tumor into the surrounding host tissues, occurs in several ways. Mechanical pressure exerted by rapidly proliferating neoplasms may force fingerlike projections of tumor cells into surrounding tissue and interstitial spaces. Malignant cells are less adherent and may break off from the primary tumor and invade adjacent structures. Malignant cells are thought to possess or produce specific destructive enzymes (proteinases), such as collagenases (specific to collagen), plasminogen activators (specific to plasma), and lysosomal hydrolyses. These enzymes are thought to destroy surrounding tissue, including the structural tissues of the vascular basement membrane, facilitating invasion of malignant cells. The mechanical pressure of a rapidly growing tumor may enhance this process.

Metastasis is the dissemination or spread of malignant cells from the primary tumor to distant sites by direct spread of tumor cells to body cavities or through lymphatic and blood circulation. Tumors growing in or penetrating body cavities may shed cells or emboli that travel within the body cavity and seed the surfaces of other organs. This can occur in ovarian cancer when malignant cells enter the peritoneal cavity and seed the peritoneal surfaces of such abdominal organs as the liver or pancreas.

## Mechanisms of Metastasis

Lymph and blood are key mechanisms by which cancer cells spread. Angiogenesis, a mechanism by which the tumor cells are ensured a blood supply, is another important process.

### LYMPHATIC SPREAD

Lymphatic spread (the transport of tumor cells through the lymphatic circulation) is the most common mechanism of metastasis. Tumor emboli enter the lymph channels by way of the interstitial fluid, which communicates with lymphatic fluid. Malignant cells also may penetrate lymphatic vessels by invasion. After entering the lymphatic circulation, malignant cells either lodge in the lymph nodes or pass between the lymphatic and venous circulations. Tumors arising in areas of the body with rapid and extensive lymphatic circulation are at high risk for metastasis through lymphatic channels. Breast tumors frequently metastasize in this manner through axillary, clavicular, and thoracic lymph channels.

### HEMATOGENOUS SPREAD

Hematogenous spread is the dissemination of malignant cells via the bloodstream. Hematogenous spread is directly related to the vascularity of the tumor. Few malignant cells can survive the turbulence of arterial circulation, insufficient oxygenation, or destruction by the body's immune system. In addition, the structure of most arteries and arterioles is far too secure to permit malignant invasion. Those malignant cells that do survive this hostile environment are able to attach to endothelium and attract fibrin, platelets, and clotting factors to seal themselves from immune system surveillance. The endothelium retracts, allowing the malignant cells to enter the basement membrane and secrete lysosomal enzymes. These enzymes destroy surrounding body tissues and thereby allow implantation.

### ANGIOGENESIS

Angiogenesis is the growth of new capillaries from the host tissue by the release of growth factors and enzymes such as vascular endothelial growth factor (VEGF). These proteins rapidly stimulate formation of new blood vessels, which helps malignant cells obtain the necessary nutrients and oxygen. It is also through this vascular network that tumor emboli can enter the systemic circulation and travel to distant sites. Large tumor emboli that become trapped in the microcirculation of distant sites may further metastasize to other sites. Therapies that target VEGF or its receptors are being used to treat many cancers effectively.

## Carcinogenesis

Malignant transformation, or **carcinogenesis**, is thought to be at least a three-step cellular process, involving initiation, promotion, and progression.

During *initiation*, initiators (carcinogens), such as chemicals, physical factors, and biologic agents, escape normal enzymatic mechanisms and alter the genetic structure of the cellular DNA. Normally, these alterations are reversed by DNA repair mechanisms, or the changes initiate programmed cellular death (apoptosis). Occasionally, cells escape these protective mechanisms, and permanent cellular mutations occur. These mutations usually are not significant to cells until the second step of carcinogenesis.

During *promotion*, repeated exposure to promoting agents (cocarcinogens) causes the expression of abnormal or mutant genetics information even after long latency periods. Latency periods for the promotion of cellular mutations vary with the type of agent and the dosage of the promoter as well as the innate characteristics of the target cell.

Cellular oncogenes, which exist in all mammalian systems, are responsible for the vital cellular functions of growth and differentiation. Cellular proto-oncogenes act as an "on switch" for cellular growth. Proto-oncogenes are influenced by multiple growth factors that stimulate cell proliferation, such as epidermal growth factor (EGF) and transforming growth factor alpha. Another proto-oncogene that plays an important role in cancer development is the *k-ras (KRAS2)* oncogene located on chromosome 12.

Just as proto-oncogenes "turn on" cellular growth, cancer suppressor genes "turn off," or regulate, unneeded cellular proliferation. When suppressor genes become mutated, rearranged, or amplified or lose their regulatory capabilities, malignant cells are allowed to reproduce. The *p53 (TP53)* gene is a tumor suppressor gene that is frequently mutated in many human cancers. This gene determines whether cells will live or die after their DNA is damaged. Apoptosis is the innate cellular process of programmed cell death. Alterations in *TP53* may decrease apoptotic signals, thus decreasing mutant cell death, giving rise to a survival advantage for mutant cell populations. Mutant *TP53* is associated with a poor prognosis and may be associated with determining response to treatment. Once this genetic expression occurs in cells, the cells begin to produce mutant cell populations that are different from their original cellular ancestors.

During *progression*, the cellular changes formed during initiation and promotion exhibit increased malignant behavior. These cells have a propensity to invade adjacent tissues and to metastasize. Agents that initiate or promote cellular transformation are referred to as carcinogens.

## Etiology

Categories of agents or factors implicated in carcinogenesis include viruses and bacteria, physical agents, chemical agents, genetic or familial factors, dietary factors, and hormonal agents.

### Viruses and Bacteria

Viruses are difficult to evaluate as a cause of human cancers because they are difficult to isolate. However, infectious causes are considered or suspected when specific cancers appear in clusters. Viruses are thought to incorporate themselves in the genetic structure of cells, thus altering future generations of that cell population—perhaps leading to cancer. For example, the Epstein-Barr virus is highly suspect as a cause in Burkitt lymphoma, nasopharyngeal cancers, and some types of non-Hodgkin lymphoma and Hodgkin disease.

Herpes simplex virus type II, cytomegalovirus, and human papillomavirus types 16, 18, 31, and 33 are associated with dysplasia and cancer of the cervix. The hepatitis B and hepatitis C viruses are implicated in cancer of the liver; the human T-cell lymphotropic virus may be a cause of some lymphocytic leukemias and lymphomas; and the human immunodeficiency virus (HIV) is associated with Kaposi's sarcoma. The bacterium *Helicobacter pylori* has been associated with an increased incidence of gastric malignancy, perhaps secondary to inflammation and injury to gastric cells.

## Physical Agents

Physical factors associated with carcinogenesis include exposure to sunlight or radiation, chronic irritation or inflammation, and tobacco use.

Excessive exposure to the ultraviolet rays of the sun, especially in fair-skinned, blue- or green-eyed people, increases the risk of skin cancers. Factors such as clothing styles (sleeveless shirts or shorts); use of sunscreens; occupation; recreational habits; and environmental variables, including humidity, altitude, and latitude, all play a role in the amount of exposure to ultraviolet light.

Exposure to ionizing radiation can occur with repeated diagnostic x-ray procedures or with radiation therapy used to treat disease. Fortunately, improved x-ray equipment appropriately minimizes the risk of extensive radiation exposure. Radiation therapy used in disease treatment and exposure to radioactive materials at nuclear weapon manufacturing sites or nuclear power plants are associated with a higher incidence of leukemias, multiple myeloma, and cancers of the lung, bone, breast, thyroid, and other tissues. Background radiation from the natural decay processes that produce radon has also been associated with lung cancer. Homes with high levels of trapped radon should be ventilated to allow the gas to disperse into the atmosphere.

## Chemical Agents

About 75% of all cancers are thought to be related to the environment. Tobacco smoke, thought to be the single most lethal chemical carcinogen, accounts for at least 30% of cancer deaths (Casciato, 2004). Smoking is strongly associated with cancers of the lung, head and neck, esophagus, pancreas, cervix, and bladder. Tobacco may also act synergistically with other substances, such as alcohol, asbestos, uranium, and viruses, to promote cancer development.

Chewing tobacco is associated with cancers of the oral cavity, which primarily occurs in men younger than 40 years of age. Many chemical substances found in the workplace have proved to be carcinogens or cocarcinogens. The extensive list of suspected chemical substances continues to grow and includes aromatic amines and aniline dyes; pesticides and formaldehydes; arsenic, soot, and tars; asbestos; benzene; betel nut and lime; cadmium; chromium compounds; nickel and zinc ores; wood dust; beryllium compounds; and polyvinyl chloride.

Most hazardous chemicals produce their toxic effects by altering DNA structure in body sites distant from chemical exposure. The liver, lungs, and kidneys are the organ systems most often affected, presumably because of their roles in detoxifying chemicals.

## Genetics and Familial Factors

Almost every cancer type has been shown to run in families. This may be due to genetics, shared environments, cultural or lifestyle factors, or chance alone. Genetic factors play a role in cancer cell development. Abnormal chromosomal patterns and cancer have been associated with extra chromosomes, too few chromosomes, or translocated chromosomes. Specific cancers with underlying genetic abnormalities include Burkitt lymphoma, chronic myelogenous leukemia, meningiomas, acute leukemias, retinoblastomas, Wilms tumor, and skin cancers, including malignant melanoma.

Approximately 5% of cancers of adults display a familial predisposition. The hallmarks of families with a hereditary cancer syndrome include cancer in two or more relatives, cancer in family members younger than 50 years of age, the same type of cancer in several family members, family members with more than one type of cancer, and a rare cancer in one or more family members (Sifri, Gangadharappa & Acheson, 2004). Cancers associated with familial inheritance include retinoblastomas, nephroblastomas, pheochromocytomas, malignant neurofibromatosis, and breast, ovarian, colorectal, stomach, prostate, and lung cancers. In the 1990s, the *BRCA1* and *BRCA2* genes were identified and linked to breast and ovarian cancer syndrome. Mutations in *BRCA1* are associated with an 80 to 90% risk of breast cancer and a 40 to 65% risk of ovarian cancer by 70 years of age (Hutson, 2003).

## Dietary Factors

Dietary factors are also linked to environmental cancers. Dietary substances can be proactive (protective), carcinogenic, or cocarcinogenic. The risk of cancer increases with long-term ingestion of carcinogens or cocarcinogens or chronic absence of protective substances in the diet.

Dietary substances that appear to increase the risk of cancer include fats, alcohol, salt-cured or smoked meats, and nitrate- and nitrite-containing foods. A high caloric dietary intake is also associated with an increased cancer risk. Consumption of high-fiber foods (such as fruits, vegetables, and whole grain cereals) and cruciferous vegetables (such as cabbage, broccoli, cauliflower, Brussels sprouts, and kohlrabi) appears to decrease the risk of cancer. Obesity is associated with endometrial cancer and postmenopausal breast cancers (Casciato, 2004).

## Hormonal Agents

Tumor growth may be promoted by disturbances in hormonal balance, either by the body's own (endogenous) hormone production or by administration of exogenous hormones. Cancers of the breast, prostate, and uterus are thought to depend on endogenous hormonal levels for growth. Diethylstilbestrol (DES) has long been recognized as a cause of vaginal carcinomas. Oral contraceptives and prolonged estrogen replacement therapy are associated with an increased incidence of hepatocellular, endometrial, and breast cancers, but they decrease the risk of ovarian cancer. The combination of estrogen and progesterone appears safer than estrogen alone in decreasing the risk of endometrial cancers; however, the Women's Health Initiative studies support discontinuing hormonal therapy with estrogens and progestins because of the increased risk of breast cancer, coronary heart disease, stroke, and blood clots (National Institutes of Health, 2004).

## GENETICS IN NURSING PRACTICE

### Concepts and Challenges in Management of the Patient with Cancer

Cancer is a genetic disease. Every phase of carcinogenesis is affected by multiple gene mutations. Some of these mutations are inherited (present in germ-line cells), but most (90%) are somatic mutations that are acquired mutations in specific cells. Examples of cancers influenced by genetics include
- Cowden syndrome
- Familial adenomatous polyposis
- Familial melanoma syndrome
- Hereditary breast and ovarian cancer
- Hereditary non-polyposis colon cancer
- Neurofibromatosis type 1
- Retinoblastoma

#### NURSING ASSESSMENTS
#### Family History Assessment
- Obtain information about both maternal and paternal sides of family.
- Obtain cancer history of at least three generations.
- Look for clustering of cancers that occur at young ages, multiple primary cancers in one individual, cancer in paired organs, and two or more close relatives with the same type of cancer suggestive of hereditary cancer syndromes.

#### Patient Assessment
- Physical findings that may predispose the patient to cancer, such as multiple colon polyps, suggestive of a polyposis syndrome
- Skin findings, such as atypical moles, that may be related to familial melanoma syndrome
- Multiple *café au lait* spots, axillary freckling, and two or more neurofibromas associated with neurofibromatosis type 1
- Facial trichilemmomas, mucosal papillomatosis, multinodular thyroid goiter or thyroid adenomas, macrocephaly, fibrocystic breasts and other fibromas or lipomas related to Cowden syndrome

#### MANAGEMENT ISSUES SPECIFIC TO GENETICS
- Assess patient's understanding of genetics factors related to his or her cancer.
- Refer for cancer risk assessment when a hereditary cancer syndrome is suspected so that patient and family can discuss inheritance risk with other family members and availability of genetic testing.
- Offer appropriate genetics information and resources.
- Assess patient's understanding of genetics information.
- Provide support to patients and families with known genetic test results for hereditary cancer syndromes.
- Participate in the management and coordination of risk-reduction measures for those with known gene mutations.

#### GENETICS RESOURCES
American Cancer Society, www.cancer.org—offers general information about cancer and support resources for families

Gene Clinics, www.geneclinics.org—a listing of common genetic disorders with up-to-date clinical summaries, genetic counseling, and testing information

National Organization of Rare Disorders, www.rarediseases.org—a directory of support groups and information for patients and families with rare genetic disorders

National Cancer Institute, www.cancernet.nci.nih.gov—a listing of cancers with clinical summaries and treatment reviews, information on genetic risks for cancer, listing of cancer centers providing genetic cancer risk assessment services

Genetic Alliance, www.geneticalliance.org—a directory of support groups for patients and families with genetic conditions

OMIM: Online Mendelian Inheritance in Man, www.ncbi.nlm.nih.gov/Omim/mimstats.html—a complete listing of known inherited genetic conditions

---

Hormonal changes with reproduction are also associated with cancer incidence. Increased numbers of pregnancies are associated with a decreased incidence of breast, endometrial, and ovarian cancers.

## Role of the Immune System

In humans, malignant cells are capable of developing on a regular basis. However, some evidence indicates that the immune system can detect the development of malignant cells and destroy them before cell growth becomes uncontrolled. When the immune system fails to identify and stop the growth of malignant cells, clinical cancer develops.

Patients who are immunoincompetent have been shown to have an increased incidence of cancer. Organ transplant recipients who receive immunosuppressive therapy to prevent rejection of the transplanted organ have an increased incidence of lymphoma, Kaposi's sarcoma, squamous cell cancer of the skin, and cervical and anogenital cancers. Patients with immunodeficiency diseases, such as acquired immunodeficiency syndrome (AIDS), have an increased incidence of Kaposi's sarcoma, lymphoma, and rectal and head and neck cancers. Some patients who have received alkylating chemotherapeutic agents to treat Hodgkin disease have an increased incidence of secondary malignancies. Autoimmune diseases, such as rheumatoid arthritis and Sjögren syndrome, are associated with increased cancer development. Finally, age-related changes, such as declining organ function, increased incidence of chronic diseases, and diminished immunocompetence, may contribute to an increased incidence of cancer in older people.

### Normal Immune Responses

Normally, an intact immune system has the ability to combat cancer cells in several ways. Usually, the immune system recognizes as foreign certain antigens on the cell membranes of many cancer cells. These antigens, known as tumor-associated antigens (also called tumor cell antigens), are capable of stimulating both cellular and humoral immune responses.

Along with the macrophages, T lymphocytes, the soldiers of the cellular immune response, are responsible for recognizing tumor-associated antigens. When T lymphocytes recognize tumor antigens, other T lymphocytes that are toxic to the tumor cells are stimulated. These lymphocytes proliferate and are released into the circulation. In addition to possessing cytotoxic (cell-killing) properties, T lymphocytes can stimulate other components of the immune system to rid the body of malignant cells.

Certain lymphokines, which are substances produced by lymphocytes, are capable of killing or damaging various types of malignant cells. Other lymphokines can mobilize other cells, such as macrophages, that disrupt cancer cells. Interferon, a substance produced by the body in response to viral infection, also possesses some antitumor properties. Antibodies produced by B lymphocytes, associated with the humoral immune response, also defend the body against malignant cells. These antibodies act either alone or in combination with the complement system or the cellular immune system.

Natural killer (NK) cells are a major component of the body's defense against cancer. NK cells are a subpopulation of lymphocytes that act by directly destroying cancer cells or by producing lymphokines and enzymes that assist in cell destruction.

### Immune System Failure

How is it, then, that malignant cells can survive and proliferate despite the elaborate immune system defense mechanisms? Several theories suggest how tumor cells can evade an apparently intact immune system. If the body fails to recognize the malignant cell as different from "self" (ie, as non-self or foreign), the immune response may not be stimulated. When tumors do not possess tumor-associated antigens that label them as foreign, the immune response is not alerted. The failure of the immune system to respond promptly to the malignant cells allows the tumor to grow too large to be managed by normal immune mechanisms.

Tumor antigens may combine with the antibodies produced by the immune system and hide or disguise themselves from normal immune defense mechanisms. These tumor antigen–antibody complexes can suppress further production of antibodies. Tumors are also capable of changing their appearance or producing substances that impair usual immune responses. These substances not only promote tumor growth but also increase the patient's susceptibility to infection by various pathogenic organisms. As a result of prolonged contact with a tumor antigen, the body may be depleted of the specific lymphocytes and no longer be able to mount an appropriate immune response.

Abnormal concentrations of host suppressor T lymphocytes may play a role in cancer development. Suppressor T lymphocytes normally assist in regulating antibody production and diminishing immune responses when they are no longer required. Low levels of serum antibodies and high levels of suppressor cells have been found in patients with multiple myeloma, a cancer associated with hypogammaglobulinemia (low amounts of serum antibodies). Carcinogens, such as viruses and certain chemicals, including chemotherapeutic agents, may weaken the immune system and ultimately enhance tumor growth.

## Detection and Prevention of Cancer

Nurses and physicians have traditionally been involved with tertiary prevention, the care and rehabilitation of patients after cancer diagnosis and treatment. However, in recent years, the American Cancer Society, the National Cancer Institute, clinicians, and researchers have placed greater emphasis on primary and secondary prevention of cancer. Primary prevention is concerned with reducing the risks of cancer in healthy people. Secondary prevention involves detection and screening to achieve early diagnosis and prompt intervention to halt the cancer process.

### Primary Prevention

By acquiring the knowledge and skills necessary to educate the community about cancer risk, nurses in all settings play a key role in cancer prevention. One way to reduce the risk of cancer is to help patients avoid known carcinogens. Another way involves encouraging patients to make dietary and various lifestyle changes that epidemiologic and laboratory studies show influence the risk for cancer. Nurses can use their teaching and counseling skills to encourage patients to participate in cancer prevention programs and to adopt healthful lifestyles. Several clinical trials have been conducted to identify medications that may help reduce the incidence of certain types of cancer. For example, an important breast cancer prevention study supported by the National Cancer Institute was conducted at multiple medical centers throughout the country. The results of this study indicated that the medication tamoxifen can reduce the incidence of breast cancer by 49% in postmenopausal women identified as being at high risk for breast cancer (Fisher, 1998). Additional trials exploring chemoprevention agents in breast cancer, such as raloxifene, are ongoing (Dunn, Wickerham & Ford, 2005; Goss & Strasser-Weippl, 2004).

### Secondary Prevention

The evolving understanding of the role of genetics in cancer cell development has contributed to prevention and screening efforts. People with specific gene mutations have an increased susceptibility to cancer. For example, people who have the gene for familial adenomatosis polyposis have an increased risk for colon cancer. Women in whom the *BRCA1* and *BRCA2* genes have been identified have an increased risk for breast and ovarian cancer. To provide individualized education and recommendations for continued surveillance and care in high-risk populations, nurses should be familiar with ongoing developments in the field of genetics and cancer (Calzone & Masny, 2004). Many centers across the country are offering innovative cancer risk evaluation programs that provide in-depth screening and follow-up for people who are found to be at high risk for cancer.

Nurses must be aware of factors such as race, cultural influences, access to care, physician–patient relationship, level of education, income, and age, which influence the knowledge, attitudes, and beliefs people have about cancer. These factors also may affect health-promoting behaviors people practice.

Public awareness about health-promoting behaviors can be increased in a variety of ways. Health education and health maintenance programs are sponsored by community organizations such as churches, senior citizen groups, and parent–teacher associations. Although primary prevention programs may focus on the hazards of tobacco use or the importance of nutrition, secondary prevention programs may promote breast and testicular self-examination and Papanicolaou (Pap) tests. Many organizations conduct cancer screening events that focus on cancers with the highest incidence rates or those that have improved survival rates if diagnosed early, such as breast or prostate cancers. These events offer education and examinations such as mammograms, digital rectal examinations, and PSA blood tests for minimal or no cost. These programs are often targeted to people who lack access to health care or cannot afford to participate on their own. In developing these programs, nurses must use strategies that are culturally sensitive to foster participation (Woods, Montgomery & Herring, 2004).

Similarly, nurses in all settings can develop programs that identify risks for patients and families and that incorporate teaching and counseling into all educational efforts, particularly for patients and families with a high incidence of cancer. Nurses support public education campaigns that guide patients and families in taking steps to reduce cancer risks (Chart 16-2). Nurses and physicians can encourage people to comply with detection efforts as suggested by the American Cancer Society (Table 16-3).

## Diagnosis of Cancer and Related Nursing Considerations

A cancer diagnosis is based on assessment for physiologic and functional changes and results of the diagnostic evaluation. Patients with suspected cancer undergo extensive testing to (1) determine the presence of tumor and its extent, (2) identify possible spread (metastasis) of disease or invasion of other body tissues, (3) evaluate the function of involved and uninvolved body systems and organs, and (4) obtain tissue and cells for analysis, including evaluation of tumor stage and grade. The diagnostic evaluation is guided by information

---

### CHART 16-2

### *Health Promotion*

### Reducing Cancer Risk

- Encourage patients to increase consumption of fresh vegetables (especially those of the cabbage family) because studies indicate that roughage and vitamin-rich foods help to prevent certain kinds of cancer.
- Encourage increased fiber intake because high-fiber diets may reduce the risk for certain cancers (eg, breast, prostate, and colon).
- Recommend increased intake of vitamin A, which reduces the risk for esophageal, laryngeal, and lung cancers.
- Recommend increased intake of foods rich in vitamin C, such as citrus fruits and broccoli, which are thought to protect against stomach and esophageal cancers.
- Advise patients to practice weight control because obesity is linked to cancers of the uterus, gallbladder, breast, and colon.
- Advise patients to reduce intake of dietary fat because a high-fat diet increases the risk for breast, colon, and prostate cancers.
- Recommend moderation in consumption of salt-cured, smoked, and nitrate-cured foods; these have been linked to esophageal and gastric cancers.
- Advise patients to stop smoking cigarettes and cigars, which are carcinogens.
- Advise patients to reduce alcohol intake because drinking large amounts of alcohol increases the risk of liver cancer. (*Note:* People who drink heavily and smoke are at greater risk for cancers of the mouth, throat, larynx, and esophagus.)
- Advise patients to avoid overexposure to the sun, wear protective clothing, and use a sunscreen to prevent skin damage from ultraviolet rays that increase the risk of skin cancer.

Adapted from the "Taking Control" program of the American Cancer Society.

| TABLE 16-3 | American Cancer Society Recommendations for Early Detection of Cancer in Asymptomatic, Average Risk People | | | |
|---|---|---|---|---|
| Site | Gender | Age (y) | Evaluation | Frequency |
| Breast | F | 20–39 | Clinical breast examination (CBE) | Every 3 years |
| | | | Self breast examination (SBE) | Every month |
| | | ≥40 | CBE | Every year |
| | | | SBE | Every month |
| | | | Mammogram | Every year |
| Colon/rectum | F/M | ≥50 | Fecal occult blood test and | Every year |
| | | | Flexible sigmoidoscopy or | Every 5 years |
| | | | Colonoscopy or | Every 10 years |
| | | | Double-contrast barium enema | Every 5 years |
| Prostate | M | ≥50 (or 40–45 if at high risk) | Prostate-specific antigen and digital rectal examination | Every year |
| Cervix | F | ≥21 or within 3 y after starting to have intercourse | Papanicolaou (Pap) test* | Every year if regular Pap; every 2 years if liquid Pap test |
| | | | Pelvic examination | Every year |
| Cancer-related checkups | M/F | ≥20–39 | Examination for cancers of the thyroid, testicles, ovaries, lymph nodes, oral cavity, and skin as well as counseling about health practices and risk factors | Every 3 years |
| | | 40+ | Same as for 20–39 | Every year |

*At age 30 after three or more consecutive normal examinations, the Pap test may be performed every 2–3 years at the discretion of the physician; human papillomavirus (HPV) test should be included at that time

Adapted from American Cancer Society (2004). ACS cancer detection guidelines. Available at: www.cancer.org.

obtained through a complete history and physical examination. Knowledge of suspicious symptoms and of the behavior of particular types of cancer assists in determining which diagnostic tests are most appropriate (Table 16-4).

Patients undergoing extensive testing are usually fearful of the procedures and anxious about the possible test results. The nurse can help relieve the patient's fear and anxiety by explaining the tests to be performed, the sensations likely to be experienced, and the patient's role in the test procedures. The nurse encourages the patient and family to voice their fears about the test results, supports the patient and family throughout the test period, and reinforces and clarifies information conveyed by the physician. The nurse also encourages the patient and family to communicate and share their concerns and to discuss their questions and concerns with each other.

## Tumor Staging and Grading

A complete diagnostic evaluation includes identifying the stage and grade of the tumor. This is accomplished before treatment begins to provide baseline data for evaluating outcomes of therapy and to maintain a systematic and consistent approach to ongoing diagnosis and treatment. Treatment options and prognosis are determined on the basis of staging and grading.

**Staging** determines the size of the tumor and the existence of metastasis. Several systems exist for classifying the anatomic extent of disease. The TNM system is frequently used (Green et al., 2002). In this system, "T" refers to the extent of the primary tumor, "N" refers to lymph node involvement, and "M" refers to the extent of metastasis (Chart 16-3). A variety of other staging systems are used to describe the extent of cancers, such as central nervous system (CNS) cancers, hematologic cancers, and malignant melanoma, that are not well described by the TNM system. Staging systems also provide a convenient shorthand notation that condenses lengthy descriptions into manageable terms for comparisons of treatments and prognoses.

**Grading** refers to the classification of the tumor cells. Grading systems seek to define the type of tissue from which the tumor originated and the degree to which the tumor cells retain the functional and histologic characteristics of the tissue of origin. Samples of cells to be used to establish the grade of a tumor may be obtained through cytology (examination of cells from tissue scrapings, body fluids, secretions, or washings), biopsy, or surgical excision.

This information helps the health care team predict the behavior and prognosis of various tumors. The tumor is assigned a numeric value ranging from I to IV. Grade I tumors, also known as well-differentiated tumors, closely resemble the tissue of origin in structure and function. Tumors that do not clearly resemble the tissue of origin in structure or function are described as poorly differentiated or undifferentiated and are assigned grade IV. These tu-

### TABLE 16-4  Diagnostic Aids Used to Detect Cancer

| Test | Description | Diagnostic Uses |
| --- | --- | --- |
| Tumor marker identification | Analysis of substances found in blood or other body fluids that are made by the tumor or by the body in response to the tumor | Breast, colon, lung, ovarian, testicular, prostate cancers |
| Magnetic resonance imaging (MRI) | Use of magnetic fields and radiofrequency signals to create sectioned images of various body structures | Neurologic, pelvic, abdominal, thoracic cancers |
| Computed tomography (CT) | Use of narrow-beam x-ray to scan successive layers of tissue for a cross-sectional view | Neurologic, pelvic, skeletal, abdominal, thoracic cancers |
| Fluoroscopy | Use of x-rays that identify contrasts in body tissue densities; may involve the use of contrast agents | Skeletal, lung, gastrointestinal cancers |
| Ultrasonography (ultrasound) | High-frequency sound waves echoing off body tissues are converted electronically into images; used to assess tissues deep within the body | Abdominal and pelvic cancers |
| Endoscopy | Direct visualization of a body cavity or passageway by insertion of an endoscope into a body cavity or opening; allows tissue biopsy, fluid aspiration, and excision of small tumors; both diagnostic and therapeutic | Bronchial, gastrointestinal cancers |
| Nuclear medicine imaging | Uses intravenous injection or ingestion of radioisotope substances followed by imaging of tissues that have concentrated the radioisotopes | Bone, liver, kidney, spleen, brain, thyroid cancers |
| Positron emission tomography (PET) | Through the use of a tracer; provides black and white or color-coded images of the biologic activity of a particular area, rather than its structure; used in detection of cancer or its response to treatment | Lung, colon, liver, pancreatic, head and neck cancers; Hodgkin and non-Hodgkin lymphoma and melanoma |
| PET fusion | Use of a PET scanner and a CT scanner in one machine to provide an image combining anatomic detail, spatial resolution, and functional metabolic abnormalities | See PET |
| Radioimmunoconjugates | Monoclonal antibodies are labeled with a radioisotope and injected intravenously into the patient; the antibodies that aggregate at the tumor site are visualized with scanners | Colorectal, breast, ovarian, head and neck cancers; lymphoma and melanoma |

mors tend to be more aggressive and less responsive to treatment than well-differentiated tumors.

## Management of Cancer

Treatment options offered to cancer patients should be based on realistic and achievable goals for each specific type of cancer. The range of possible treatment goals may include complete eradication of malignant disease (**cure**), prolonged survival and containment of cancer cell growth (**control**), or relief of symptoms associated with the disease (**palliation**).

The health care team, the patient, and the patient's family must have a clear understanding of the treatment options and goals. Open communication and support are vital as the patient and family periodically reassess treatment plans and goals when complications of therapy develop or disease progresses.

Multiple modalities are commonly used in cancer treatment. A variety of approaches, including surgery, radiation therapy, chemotherapy, and targeted therapies, may be used at various times throughout treatment. Understanding the principles of each and how they interrelate is important in understanding the rationale and goals of treatment.

## Surgery

Surgical removal of the entire cancer remains the ideal and most frequently used treatment method. However, the specific surgical approach may vary for several reasons. Diagnostic surgery is the definitive method of identifying the cellular characteristics that influence all treatment decisions. Surgery may be the primary method of treatment, or it may be prophylactic, palliative, or reconstructive.

### Diagnostic Surgery

Diagnostic surgery, such as a **biopsy**, is usually performed to obtain a tissue sample for analysis of cells suspected to be malignant. In most instances, the biopsy is taken from the actual tumor, but in some situations, it is necessary to biopsy lymph nodes near the suspicious tumor. It is well known that many cancers can metastasize from the primary site to other areas of the body through the lymphatic circulation. Knowing whether adjacent lymph nodes contain tumor cells helps physicians plan for systemic therapies instead of or in addition to surgery, to combat tumor cells that have gone beyond the primary tumor site. The use of injectable dyes and nuclear medicine imaging can help the

> **CHART 16-3**
>
> ## TNM Classification System
>
> T  The extent of the primary tumor
> N  The absence or presence and extent of regional lymph node metastasis
> M  The absence or presence of distant metastasis
>
> The use of numerical subsets of the TNM components indicates the progressive extent of the malignant disease.
>
> **PRIMARY TUMOR (T)**
> Tx  Primary tumor cannot be assessed
> T0  No evidence of primary tumor
> Tis  Carcinoma in situ
> T1, T2, T3, T4  Increasing size and/or local extent of the primary tumor
>
> **REGIONAL LYMPH NODES (N)**
> Nx  Regional lymph nodes cannot be assessed
> N0  No regional lymph node metastasis
> N1, N2, N3  Increasing involvement of regional lymph nodes
>
> **DISTANT METASTASIS (M)**
> Mx  Distant metastasis cannot be assessed
> M0  No distant metastasis
> M1  Distant metastasis
>
> From Green, F., et al. (Eds) (2002). *AJCC cancer staging manual* (6th ed.). New York: Springer-Verlag.

surgeon identify lymph nodes (sentinel nodes) that process lymphatic drainage for the involved area. This procedure has been accepted as the standard of care for melanoma and is rapidly becoming the standard of care for breast cancer. Sentinel node biopsy is still considered investigational for gastrointestinal malignancies and tumors of the vulva (Jakub, Pendas & Reintgen, 2003).

### CHOICE OF BIOPSY METHOD

The choice of biopsy method is based on many factors. Of greatest importance is the type of treatment anticipated if the cancer diagnosis is confirmed. Definitive surgical approaches include excision of the original biopsy site so that any cells disseminated during the biopsy are excised at the time of surgery. Nutrition and hematologic, respiratory, renal, and hepatic function are considered in determining the method of treatment as well. If the biopsy requires general anesthesia and if subsequent surgery is likely, the effects of prolonged anesthesia on the patient are considered.

The patient and family are given the opportunity to discuss the options before definitive plans are made. The nurse, as the patient's advocate, serves as a liaison between the patient and physician to facilitate this process. Time should be set aside to minimize interruptions and distractions. The patient should have time to ask questions and to think through all that has been discussed.

### BIOPSY TYPES

The three most common biopsy methods are the excisional, incisional, and needle methods (Abeloff, Armitage, Niederhuber, et al., 2004).

Excisional biopsy is most frequently used for easily accessible tumors of the skin, breast, upper and lower gastrointestinal tract, and upper respiratory tract. In many cases, the surgeon can remove the entire tumor and surrounding marginal tissues as well. This removal of normal tissue beyond the tumor area decreases the possibility that residual microscopic disease cells may lead to a recurrence of the tumor. This approach not only provides the pathologist, who stages and grades the cells, with the entire tissue specimen but also decreases the chance of seeding the tumor (disseminating cancer cells through surrounding tissues).

Incisional biopsy is performed if the tumor mass is too large to be removed. In this case, a wedge of tissue from the tumor is removed for analysis. The cells of the tissue wedge must be representative of the tumor mass so that the pathologist can provide an accurate diagnosis. If the specimen does not contain representative tissue and cells, negative biopsy results do not guarantee the absence of cancer.

Excisional and incisional approaches are often performed through endoscopy. However, surgical incision may be required to determine the anatomic extent or stage of the tumor. For example, a diagnostic or staging laparotomy (the surgical opening of the abdomen to assess malignant abdominal disease) may be necessary to assess malignancies such as gastric cancer.

Needle biopsies are performed to sample suspicious masses that are easily accessible, such as some growths in the breasts, thyroid, lung, liver, and kidney. Needle biopsies are fast, relatively inexpensive, and easy to perform and usually require only local anesthesia. In general, the patient experiences slight and temporary physical discomfort. In addition, the surrounding tissues are disturbed only minimally, thus decreasing the likelihood of seeding cancer cells. Needle aspiration biopsy involves aspirating tissue fragments through a needle guided into an area suspected of bearing disease. Occasionally, x-ray, computed tomography (CT) scanning, ultrasonography, or magnetic resonance imaging (MRI) is used to help locate the suspicious area and guide the placement of the needle. In some instances, the aspiration biopsy does not yield enough tissue to permit accurate diagnosis. A needle core biopsy uses a specially designed needle to obtain a small core of tissue. Most often, this specimen is sufficient to permit accurate diagnosis.

## Surgery as Primary Treatment

When surgery is the primary approach in treating cancer, the goal is to remove the entire tumor or as much as is feasible (a procedure sometimes called debulking) and any involved surrounding tissue, including regional lymph nodes.

Two common surgical approaches used for treating primary tumors are local and wide excisions. Local excision is warranted when the mass is small. It includes removal of the mass and a small margin of normal tissue that is easily accessible. Wide or radical excisions (en bloc dissections) include removal of the primary tumor, lymph nodes, adjacent involved structures, and surrounding tissues that may be at high risk for tumor spread (Kufe, Pollock, Wechselbaum, et al., 2003). This surgical method can result in disfigurement and altered functioning. However, wide excisions are considered if the tumor can be removed completely and the chances of cure or control are good.

In some situations, video-assisted endoscopic surgery is replacing surgery associated with long incisions and extended recovery periods. In this procedure, an endoscope with intense lighting and an attached multichip minicamera is inserted into the body through a small incision. The surgical instruments are inserted into the surgical field through one or two additional small incisions, each about 3 cm in length. The camera transmits the image of the involved area to a monitor so the surgeon can manipulate the instruments to perform the necessary procedure. Video-assisted endoscopic surgery is now being used for many thoracic and abdominal surgeries.

Salvage surgery is an additional treatment option that uses an extensive surgical approach to treat the local recurrence of a cancer after the use of a less extensive primary approach. A mastectomy to treat recurrent breast cancer after primary lumpectomy and radiation is an example of salvage surgery.

In addition to surgery that uses surgical blades or scalpels to excise the mass and surrounding tissues, several other types of surgical techniques are available. Electrosurgery makes use of electrical current to destroy the tumor cells. Cryosurgery uses liquid nitrogen or a very cold probe to freeze tissue to cause cell destruction. Chemosurgery uses chemicals applied to tissues to facilitate their removal. Laser surgery (light amplification by stimulated emission of radiation) makes use of light and energy aimed at an exact tissue location and depth to vaporize cancer cells. Laser surgery is also referred to as *photocoagulation or photoablation*. Stereotactic radiosurgery is a single and highly precise administration of high-dose radiation therapy used in some types of brain and head and neck cancers. This type of radiation has such a dramatic effect on the target area that the changes are considered to be comparable to more traditional surgical approaches even though no incision is actually made (Law, Mangarin & Kelvin, 2003; Witt, Haas, Marrinan et al., 2003). (Radiation therapy is discussed later in this chapter.)

A multidisciplinary approach to patient care is essential during and after any type of surgery. The effects of surgery on the patient's body image, self-esteem, and functional abilities are addressed. If necessary, a plan for postoperative rehabilitation is made before the surgery is performed.

The growth and dissemination of cancer cells may have produced distant micrometastases by the time the patient seeks treatment. Therefore, attempting to remove wide margins of tissue in the hope of "getting all the cancer cells" may not be feasible. This reality substantiates the need for a coordinated multidisciplinary approach to cancer therapy (Abeloff et al., 2004). Once the surgery has been completed, one or more additional (or adjuvant) modalities may be chosen to increase the likelihood of destroying the remaining cancer cells. However, some cancers that are treated surgically in the very early stages are considered to be curable (eg, skin cancers, testicular cancers).

## Prophylactic Surgery

Prophylactic surgery involves removing nonvital tissues or organs that are likely to develop cancer. The following factors are considered when physicians and patients discuss possible prophylactic surgery:

- Family history and genetic predisposition
- Presence or absence of symptoms
- Potential risks and benefits
- Ability to detect cancer at an early stage
- The patient's acceptance of the postoperative outcome

Colectomy, mastectomy, and oophorectomy are examples of prophylactic surgeries. Recent developments in the ability to identify genetic markers indicative of a predisposition to develop some types of cancer may play a role in decisions concerning prophylactic surgeries. However, what is adequate justification for prophylactic surgery is controversial. For example, several factors are considered when deciding to proceed with a prophylactic mastectomy, including a strong family history of breast cancer; positive *BRCA1* or *BRCA2* findings; an abnormal physical finding on breast examination, such as progressive nodularity and cystic disease; a proven history of breast cancer in the opposite breast; abnormal mammography findings; and abnormal biopsy results.

Because the long-term physiologic and psychological effects are unknown, prophylactic surgery is offered selectively to patients and discussed thoroughly with patients and families. Preoperative teaching and counseling, as well as long-term follow-up, are provided.

## Palliative Surgery

When cure is not possible, the goals of treatment are to make the patient as comfortable as possible and to promote a satisfying and productive life for as long as possible. Whether the period is extremely brief or lengthy, the major goal is a high quality of life—with quality defined by the patient and his or her family. Palliative surgery is performed in an attempt to relieve complications of cancer, such as ulcerations, obstructions, hemorrhage, pain, and malignant effusions (Table 16-5). Honest and informative communication with the patient and family about the goal of surgery is essential to avoid false hope and disappointment.

## Reconstructive Surgery

Reconstructive surgery may follow curative or radical surgery and is carried out in an attempt to improve function or obtain a more desirable cosmetic effect. It may be performed in one operation or in stages. The surgeon who will perform the surgery discusses possible reconstructive surgical options with the patient before the primary surgery is performed. Reconstructive surgery may be indicated for breast, head and neck, and skin cancers.

The nurse must recognize the patient's needs and the impact that altered functioning and altered body image may have on quality of life. It is imperative for the nurse to provide the patient and family with opportunities to discuss these issues. The individual needs of the patient undergoing reconstructive surgery must be accurately assessed and addressed.

## Nursing Management in Cancer Surgery

Patients undergoing surgery for cancer require general perioperative nursing care, as described in Unit 4 of this text,

| TABLE 16-5 | Indications for Palliative Surgical Procedures |
|---|---|
| **Procedure** | **Indications** |
| Pleural drainage tube placement | Pleural effusion |
| Peritoneal drainage tube placement (Tenckoff catheter) | Ascites |
| Abdominal shunt placement (Levine shunt) | Ascites |
| Pericardial drainage tube placement | Pericardial effusion |
| Colostomy or ileostomy | Bowel obstruction |
| Gastrostomy, jejunostomy tube placement | Upper gastrointestinal tract obstruction |
| Biliary stent placement | Biliary obstruction |
| Ureteral stent placement | Ureteral obstruction |
| Nerve block | Pain |
| Cordotomy | Pain |
| Venous access device placement (for administering parenteral analgesics) | Pain |
| Epidural catheter placement (for administering epidural analgesics) | Pain |
| Hormone manipulation (removal of ovaries, testes, adrenals, pituitary) | Tumors that depend on hormones for growth |

along with specific care related to age, organ impairment, nutritional deficits, disorders of coagulation, and altered immunity that may increase the risk of postoperative complications. Combining other treatment methods, such as radiation and chemotherapy, with surgery also contributes to postoperative complications, such as infection, impaired wound healing, altered pulmonary or renal function, and the development of deep vein thrombosis. In these situations, the nurse completes a thorough preoperative assessment for factors that may affect the patient undergoing the surgical procedure.

Patients who are undergoing surgery for the diagnosis or treatment of cancer are often anxious about the surgical procedure, possible findings, postoperative limitations, changes in normal body functions, and prognosis. The patient and family require time and assistance to deal with the possible changes and outcomes resulting from the surgery.

The nurse provides education and emotional support by assessing the needs of the patient and family and by discussing their fears and coping mechanisms with them. The nurse encourages the patient and family to take an active role in decision making when possible. If the patient or family ask about the results of diagnostic testing and surgical procedures, the nurse's response is guided by the information the physician has previously conveyed to the patient and family. The patient and family may also ask the nurse to explain and clarify information that the physician initially provided but that they did not grasp because they were anxious at the time. It is important that the nurse communicate frequently with the physician and other members of the health care team to be certain that the information provided is consistent.

After surgery, the nurse assesses the patient's responses to the surgery and monitors the patient for possible complications, such as infection, bleeding, thrombophlebitis, wound dehiscence, fluid and electrolyte imbalance, and organ dysfunction (Morris & Ward, 2003). The nurse also provides for the patient's comfort. Postoperative teaching addresses wound care, activity, nutrition, and medication information.

Plans for discharge, follow-up and home care, and treatment are initiated as early as possible to ensure continuity of care from hospital to home or from a cancer referral center to the patient's local hospital and health care provider. Patients and families are also encouraged to use community resources such as the American Cancer Society for support and information.

# Radiation Therapy

In **radiation therapy**, ionizing radiation is used to interrupt cellular growth. More than half of patients with cancer receive a form of radiation therapy at some point during treatment. Radiation may be used to cure the cancer, as in Hodgkin disease, testicular seminomas, thyroid carcinomas, localized cancers of the head and neck, and cancers of the uterine cervix. Radiation therapy may also be used to control malignant disease when a tumor cannot be removed surgically or when local nodal metastasis is present, or it can be used prophylactically to prevent leukemic infiltration to the brain or spinal cord.

Palliative radiation therapy is used to relieve the symptoms of metastatic disease, especially when the cancer has spread to brain, bone, or soft tissue, or to treat oncologic emergencies, such as superior vena cava syndrome or spinal cord compression.

Two types of ionizing radiation—electromagnetic rays (x-rays and gamma rays) and particles (electrons [beta particles], protons, neutrons, and alpha particles)—can lead to tissue disruption. The most harmful tissue disruption is the alteration of the DNA molecule within the cells of the tissue. Ionizing radiation breaks the strands of the DNA helix, leading to cell death. Ionizing radiation can also ionize constituents of body fluids, especially water, leading to the formation of free radicals and irreversibly damaging DNA. If the DNA is incapable of repair, the cell may die immediately, or it may initiate cellular suicide (apoptosis), a genetically programmed cell death (Abeloff et al., 2004; Casciato, 2004).

Cells are most vulnerable to the disruptive effects of radiation during DNA synthesis and mitosis (early S, $G_2$, and M phases of the cell cycle). Therefore, those body tissues that undergo frequent cell division are most sensitive to radiation therapy. These tissues include bone marrow, lymphatic tissue, epithelium of the gastrointestinal tract, hair cells, and gonads. Slower-growing tissues and tissues at rest are relatively radioresistant (less sensitive to the effects of radiation). Such tissues include muscle, cartilage, and connective tissues.

A radiosensitive tumor is one that can be destroyed by a dose of radiation that still allows for cell regeneration in the normal tissue. Tumors that are well oxygenated also appear to be more sensitive to radiation. In theory, therefore, radiation therapy may be enhanced if more oxygen can be delivered to tumors. In addition, if the radiation is delivered when most tumor cells are cycling through the cell cycle, the number of cancer cells destroyed (cell kill) is maximal (Abeloff et al., 2004; Casciato, 2004).

Certain chemicals, including chemotherapy agents, act as radiosensitizers and sensitize more hypoxic (oxygen-poor) tumors to the effects of radiation therapy. Radiation is delivered to tumor sites by external or internal means.

### External Radiation

If external radiation therapy is used, one of several delivery methods may be chosen, depending on the depth of the tumor. Depending on the amount of energy they contain, x-rays can be used to destroy cancerous cells at the skin surface or deeper in the body. The higher the energy, the deeper the penetration into the body. Kilovoltage therapy devices deliver the maximal radiation dose to superficial lesions, such as lesions of the skin and breast, whereas linear accelerators and betatron machines produce higher-energy x-rays and deliver their dosage to deeper structures with less harm to the skin and less scattering of radiation within the body tissues. Gamma rays are another form of energy used in radiation therapy. This energy is produced from the spontaneous decay of naturally occurring radioactive elements such as cobalt-60. The gamma rays also deliver this radiation dose beneath the skin surface, sparing skin tissue from adverse effects.

Some centers nationwide treat more hypoxic, radiation-resistant tumors with particle-beam radiation therapy. This type of therapy accelerates subatomic particles (neutrons, photons) through body tissue. This therapy, which is also known as high linear energy transfer radiation, damages target cells as well as other cells in its path (Abeloff et al., 2004; Casciato, 2004).

### Internal Radiation

Internal radiation implantation, or **brachytherapy**, delivers a high dose of radiation to a localized area. The specific radioisotope for implantation is selected on the basis of its half-life, which is the time it takes for half of its radioactivity to decay. This internal radiation can be implanted by means of needles, seeds, beads, or catheters into body cavities (vagina, abdomen, pleura) or interstitial compartments (breast). Brachytherapy may also be administered orally, as with the isotope iodine-131, which is used to treat thyroid carcinomas (Abeloff et al., 2004, Casciato, 2004; Gordils-Perez, Rawlins-Duell & Kelvin, 2003).

Intracavitary radioisotopes are frequently used to treat gynecologic cancers. In these malignancies, the radioisotopes are inserted into specially positioned applicators after the position is verified by x-ray. These radioisotopes remain in place for a prescribed period and then are removed. The patient is maintained on bed rest and log-rolled to prevent displacement of the intracavitary delivery device. An indwelling urinary catheter is inserted to ensure that the bladder remains empty. Low-residue diets and antidiarrheal agents, such as diphenoxylate (Lomotil), are provided to prevent bowel movements during therapy to prevent displacement of the radioisotopes.

Interstitial implants, used in treating such malignancies as prostate, pancreatic, or breast cancer, may be temporary or permanent, depending on the radioisotopes used. These implants usually consist of seeds, needles, wires, or small catheters positioned to provide a local radiation source and are less frequently dislodged. With internal radiation therapy, the farther the tissue is from the radiation source, the lower the dosage. This spares the noncancerous tissue from the radiation dose.

Because patients receiving internal radiation emit radiation while the implant is in place, contacts with the health care team are guided by principles of time, distance, and shielding to minimize exposure of personnel to radiation. Safety precautions used in caring for a patient receiving brachytherapy include assigning the patient to a private room, posting appropriate notices about radiation safety precautions, having staff members wear dosimeter badges, making sure that pregnant staff members are not assigned to the patient's care, prohibiting visits by children or pregnant visitors, limiting visits from others to 30 minutes daily, and seeing that visitors maintain a 6-foot distance from the radiation source. Patients with seed implants may be able to return home; radiation exposure to others is minimal. Information about any precautions, if needed, is provided to the patient and family members to ensure safety.

### Radiation Dosage

The radiation dosage is dependent on the sensitivity of the target tissues to radiation and on the tumor size. The lethal tumor dose is defined as that dose that will eradicate 95% of the tumor yet preserve normal tissue. The total radiation dose is delivered over several weeks to allow healthy tissue to repair and to achieve greater cell kill by exposing more cells to the radiation as they begin active cell division. Repeated radiation treatments over time (fractionated doses) also allow for the periphery of the tumor to be re-oxygenated repeatedly, because tumors shrink from the outside inward. This increases the radiosensitivity of the tumor, thereby increasing tumor cell death (Abeloff et al., 2004; Casciato, 2004).

### Toxicity

Toxicity of radiation therapy is localized to the region being irradiated. Toxicity may be increased if concomitant chemotherapy is administered. Acute local reactions occur when normal cells in the treatment area are also destroyed and cellular death exceeds cellular regeneration. Body tissues most affected are those that normally proliferate rapidly, such as the skin; the epithelial lining of the gastrointestinal tract, including the oral cavity; and the bone marrow. Altered skin integrity is a common effect and can include alopecia (hair loss), erythema, and shedding of skin (desquamation). Reepithelialization occurs after treatments have been completed.

Alterations in oral mucosa secondary to radiation therapy include stomatitis, **xerostomia** (dryness of the mouth), change and loss of taste, and decreased salivation. The entire gastrointestinal mucosa may be involved, and esophageal irritation with chest pain and dysphagia may result. Anorexia, nausea, vomiting, and diarrhea may occur if the stomach or colon is in the irradiated field. Symptoms subside and gastrointestinal reepithelialization occurs after treatments have been completed.

Bone marrow cells proliferate rapidly, and if sites containing bone marrow (e.g., the iliac crest, sternum) are included in the radiation field, anemia, leukopenia (decreased white blood cells [WBCs]), and **thrombocytopenia** (a decrease in platelets) may result. The patient is then at increased risk for infection and bleeding until blood cell counts return to normal. Chronic anemia may occur (Abeloff et al., 2004; Casciato, 2004).

Research to develop cytoprotective agents that can protect normal tissue from radiation damage continues. The most commonly used cytoprotectant is amifostine (Ethyol), which is a scavenger of free radicals that prevents damage to DNA (Wilkes & Barton-Burke, 2004).

Certain systemic side effects are also commonly experienced by patients receiving radiation therapy. These manifestations, which are generalized, include fatigue, malaise, and anorexia. This syndrome may be secondary to substances released when tumor cells break down. The effects are temporary and subside with the cessation of treatment.

Late effects of radiation therapy may also occur in various body tissues. These effects are chronic, usually produce fibrotic changes secondary to a decreased vascular supply, and are irreversible. These late effects can be most severe when they involve vital organs such as the lungs, heart, CNS, and bladder. Toxicities may intensify when radiation is combined with other treatment modalities.

## Nursing Management in Radiation Therapy

Patients receiving radiation therapy and their families often have questions and concerns about its safety. To answer questions and allay fears about the effects of radiation on the tumor and on the patient's normal tissues and organs, the nurses can explain the procedure for delivering radiation and describe the equipment, the duration of the procedure (often minutes only), the possible need for immobilizing the patient during the procedure, and the absence of new sensations, including pain, during the procedure. If a radioactive implant is used, the nurse informs the patient and family about the restrictions placed on visitors and health care personnel and other radiation precautions. The patient also should understand his or her own role before, during, and after the procedure. See Chapter 47 for further discussion of radiation treatment for gynecologic cancers.

### PROTECTING SKIN AND ORAL MUCOSA

The nurse assesses the patient's skin, nutritional status, and general feeling of well-being. The nurse assesses the skin

---

## NURSING RESEARCH PROFILE

### Patients' Need for Information About Cancer Therapy

Skalla, K. A., Bakitas, M., Furstenberg, C. T., et al. (2004). Patients' need for information about cancer therapy. *Oncology Nursing Forum, 31*(2), 313–319.

#### Purpose
Treatment of cancer is a difficult and stressful experience. Research continues to show that patients want information, yet they do not perceive that they are receiving the information they need for successful coping. The purpose of this study was to obtain detailed information about the preferences of patients with cancer and their need for information about side effects of cancer treatment, with the goal of designing an interactive multimedia education program.

#### Design
Data were gathered from focus groups of 51 patients who had undergone chemotherapy, radiation therapy, or combined modality treatment in the past year; the study group included 14 spouses. The questions addressed at each focus group by a trained facilitator were designed to encourage discussion about the nature of the symptoms experienced and patients' informational needs about treatment and management of treatment-related side effects. Each focus group was audiotaped for later discussion and analysis. Participants' comments were reviewed, coded, and organized into categories. A qualitative software program was used to organize data analysis. Categories of themes were developed based on participants' comments.

#### Findings
Results indicated that patients reported that they did not receive the information they wanted or needed to enhance coping. Most patients wanted as much information as possible about treatment and treatment-related side effects. Patients desired individualized, practical information about how the treatments would affect their daily lives, identified as increasingly important because treatment is often being performed on an outpatient basis. Patients reported that it was difficult to absorb and retain information given to them. They often experienced informational overload with traditional teaching methods.

#### Nursing Implications
This study shows that nurses must tailor educational programs to better meet the informational demands of patients with cancer. Interactive multimedia technology (audio, text, graphics, video) offers an innovative approach to patient education that can overcome many educational barriers by allowing patients to control the pace of information. Multimedia technology offers advantages to meet patients' needs, but these tools need to be developed to meet changing educational expectations of patients.

and oral mucosa frequently for changes (particularly if radiation therapy is directed to these areas). The skin is protected from irritation, and the patient is instructed to avoid using ointments, lotions, or powders on the area.

Gentle oral hygiene is essential to remove debris, prevent irritation, and promote healing. If systemic symptoms, such as weakness and fatigue, occur, the patient may need assistance with activities of daily living and personal hygiene. In addition, the nurse offers reassurance by explaining that these symptoms are a result of the treatment and do not represent deterioration or progression of the disease.

### PROTECTING CAREGIVERS

When the patient has a radioactive implant in place, the nurse and other health care providers need to protect themselves as well as the patient from the effects of radiation. Specific instructions are usually provided by the radiation safety officer from the x-ray department. The instructions identify the maximum time that can be spent safely in the patient's room, the shielding equipment to be used, and special precautions and actions to be taken if the implant is dislodged. The nurse should explain the rationale for these precautions to keep the patient from feeling unduly isolated.

## Chemotherapy

In **chemotherapy**, antineoplastic agents are used in an attempt to destroy tumor cells by interfering with cellular functions, including replication. Chemotherapy is used primarily to treat systemic disease rather than localized lesions that are amenable to surgery or radiation. Chemotherapy may be combined with surgery, radiation therapy, or both, to reduce tumor size preoperatively, to destroy any remaining tumor cells postoperatively, or to treat some forms of leukemia. The goals of chemotherapy (cure, control, palliation), must be realistic because they will define the medications to be used and the aggressiveness of the treatment plan.

### Cell Kill and the Cell Cycle

**CONCEPTS in action ANIMATION**

Each time a tumor is exposed to a chemotherapeutic agent, a percentage of tumor cells (20% to 99%, depending on dosage) is destroyed. Repeated doses of chemotherapy are necessary over a prolonged period to achieve regression of the tumor. Eradication of 100% of the tumor is almost impossible. Instead, the goal of treatment is eradication of enough of the tumor so that the remaining tumor cells can be destroyed by the body's immune system.

Actively proliferating cells within a tumor are the most sensitive to chemotherapeutic agents (the ratio of dividing cells to resting cells is referred to as the growth fraction). Nondividing cells capable of future proliferation are the least sensitive to antineoplastic medications and consequently are potentially dangerous. However, the nondividing cells must be destroyed to eradicate a cancer. Repeated cycles of chemotherapy are used to kill more tumor cells by destroying these nondividing cells as they begin active cell division.

Reproduction of both healthy and malignant cells follows the cell cycle pattern (Fig. 16-2). The cell cycle time is the time required for one tissue cell to divide and reproduce two identical daughter cells. The cell cycle of any cell has four distinct phases, each with a vital underlying function:

1. $G_1$ phase—RNA and protein synthesis occur
2. S phase—DNA synthesis occurs
3. $G_2$ phase—premitotic phase; DNA synthesis is complete, mitotic spindle forms
4. Mitosis—cell division occurs

The $G_0$ phase, the resting or dormant phase of cells, can occur after mitosis and during the $G_1$ phase. In the $G_0$ phase are those dangerous cells that are not actively dividing but have the potential for replicating. The administration of certain chemotherapeutic agents (as well as some other forms of therapy) is coordinated with the cell cycle.

### Classification of Chemotherapeutic Agents

Chemotherapeutic agents may be classified by their relationship to the cell cycle. Certain chemotherapeutic agents that are specific to certain phases of the cell cycle are termed cell cycle–specific agents. These agents destroy cells that are actively reproducing by means of the cell cycle; most affect cells in the S phase by interfering with DNA and RNA synthesis. Other agents, such as the vinca or plant alkaloids, are specific to the M phase, where they halt mitotic spindle formation. Chemotherapeutic agents that act independently of the cell cycle phases are termed

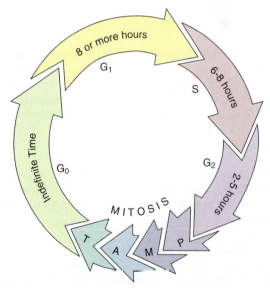

**FIGURE 16-2.** Phases of the cell cycle extend over the interval between the midpoint of mitosis and the subsequent end point in mitosis in a daughter cell. $G_1$ is the postmitotic phase during which ribonucleic acid (RNA) and protein syntheses are increased and cell growth occurs. $G_0$ is the resting, or dormant, phase of the cell cycle. In the S phase, nucleic acids are synthesized and chromosomes are replicated in preparation for cell mitosis. During $G_2$, RNA and protein synthesis occur as in $G_1$. P, prophase; M, metaphase; A, anaphase; T, telophase. From Porth, C. M. (2002). *Pathophysiology: Concepts of altered health states* (6th ed.). Philadelphia: Lippincott Williams & Wilkins.

cell cycle–nonspecific agents. These agents usually have a prolonged effect on cells, leading to cellular damage or death. Many treatment plans combine cell cycle–specific and cell cycle–nonspecific agents to increase the number of vulnerable tumor cells killed during a treatment period (Abeloff et al., 2004; Casciato, 2004; Wilkes & Barton-Burke, 2004).

Chemotherapeutic agents are also classified by chemical group, each with a different mechanism of action. These include the alkylating agents, nitrosoureas, antimetabolites, antitumor antibiotics, plant alkaloids, hormonal agents, and miscellaneous agents. The classification, mechanism of action, common drugs, cell cycle specificity, and common side effects of antineoplastic agents are listed in Table 16-6.

Chemotherapeutic agents from every category may be used to enhance tumor cell kill during therapy by creating multiple cellular lesions. Combined medication therapy relies on agents of differing toxicities and with synergistic actions. Use of combination therapy also prevents the development of drug-resistant mechanisms.

Combining older medications with other agents, such as levamisole, leucovorin, hormones, or interferons, has shown some benefit in combating resistance of cells to chemotherapeutic agents. Newer investigational agents are being studied for effectiveness in resistant tumor lines. For more information about investigational agents, see Chart 16-4.

## Administration of Chemotherapeutic Agents

Chemotherapeutic agents may be administered in the hospital, clinic, or home setting by topical, oral, intravenous, intramuscular, subcutaneous, arterial, intracavitary, and intrathecal routes. The route of administration usually depends on the type of agent; the required dose; and the type, location, and extent of tumor being treated. Guidelines for the administration of chemotherapy have been developed by the Oncology Nursing Society. Patient education is essential to maximize safety if chemotherapy is administered in the home (Chart 16-5).

### DOSAGE
Dosage of antineoplastic agents is based primarily on the patient's total body surface area, previous response to chemotherapy or radiation therapy, and function of major organ systems.

### SPECIAL PROBLEMS: EXTRAVASATION
Special care must be taken whenever intravenous vesicant agents are administered. **Vesicants** are those agents that, if deposited into the subcutaneous tissue (**extravasation**), cause tissue necrosis and damage to underlying tendons, nerves, and blood vessels. Although the complete mechanism of tissue destruction is unclear, it is known that the pH of many antineoplastic drugs is responsible for the severe inflammatory reaction as well as the ability of these drugs to bind to tissue DNA. Sloughing and ulceration of the tissue may be so severe that skin grafting may be necessary. The full extent of tissue damage may take several weeks to become apparent. Medications classified as vesicants include dactinomycin, daunorubicin, doxorubicin (Adriamycin), nitrogen mustard, mitomycin, vinblastine, vincristine, and vindesine.

Only specially trained physicians and nurses should administer vesicants. Careful selection of peripheral veins, skilled venipuncture, and careful administration of medications are essential. Indications of extravasation during administration of vesicant agents include the following:

- Absence of blood return from the intravenous catheter
- Resistance to flow of intravenous fluid
- Swelling, pain, or redness at the site

If extravasation is suspected, the medication administration is stopped immediately, and ice is applied to the site (unless the extravasated vesicant is a vinca alkaloid). The physician may aspirate any infiltrated medication from the tissues and inject a neutralizing solution into the area to reduce tissue damage. Selection of the neutralizing solution depends on the extravasated agent. Examples of neutralizing solutions include sodium thiosulfate, hyaluronidase, and sodium bicarbonate. Recommendations and guidelines for managing vesicant extravasation have been issued by individual medication manufacturers, pharmacies, and the Oncology Nursing Society, and they differ from one medication to the next.

If frequent, prolonged administration of antineoplastic vesicants is anticipated, right atrial Silastic catheters or venous access devices may be inserted to promote safety during medication administration and reduce problems with access to the circulatory system (Figs. 16-3 and 16-4). Complications associated with their use include infection and thrombosis.

### TOXICITY
Toxicity associated with chemotherapy can be acute or chronic. Cells with rapid growth rates (eg, epithelium, bone marrow, hair follicles, sperm) are very susceptible to damage, and various body systems may be affected as well.

**Gastrointestinal System.** Nausea and vomiting are the most common side effects of chemotherapy and may persist for as long as 24–48 hours after its administration. Delayed nausea and vomiting may persist for as long as 1 week after chemotherapy. The vomiting centers in the brain are stimulated by the following mechanisms (Marek, 2003):

- Activation of the receptors found in the chemoreceptor trigger zone (CTZ) of the medulla by serotonin, substance P, and other neurotransmitters such as dopamine
- Stimulation of peripheral autonomic pathways (gastrointestinal tract and pharynx)
- Stimulation of the vestibular pathways (inner ear imbalances, labyrinth input)
- Cognitive stimulation (CNS disease, anticipatory nausea, and vomiting)
- A combination of these factors

Medications that can decrease nausea and vomiting include serotonin blockers, such as ondansetron, granisetron, dolasetron, and palonosetron, which block serotonin receptors of the gastrointestinal tract and CTZ, and dopaminergic blockers, such as metoclopramide (Reglan), which block dopamine receptors of the CTZ. Newer agents include neurokinin-1 receptor antagonists (eg, aprepitant

## TABLE 16-6  Antineoplastic Agents

| Drug Class and Examples | Mechanism of Action | Cell Cycle Specificity | Common Side Effects |
|---|---|---|---|
| **Alkylating Agents** | | | |
| Busulfan, carboplatin, chlorambucil, cisplatin, cyclophosphamide, dacarbazine, hexamethyl melamine, ifosfamide, melphalan, nitrogen mustard, oxaliplatin, thiotepa | Alter DNA structure by misreading DNA code, initiating breaks in the DNA molecule, cross-linking DNA strands | Cell cycle–nonspecific | Bone marrow suppression, nausea, vomiting, cystitis (cyclophosphamide, ifosfamide), stomatitis, alopecia, gonadal suppression, renal toxicity (cisplatin) |
| **Nitrosureas** | | | |
| Carmustine (BCNU), lomustine (CCNU), semustine (methyl CCNU), streptozocin | Similar to the alkylating agents; cross the blood–brain barrier | Cell cycle–nonspecific | Delayed and cumulative myelosuppression, especially thrombocytopenia; nausea, vomiting |
| **Topoisomerase I Inhibitors** | | | |
| Irinotecan, topotecan | Induce breaks in the DNA strand by binding to enzyme topoisomerase I, preventing cells from dividing | Cell cycle–specific (S phase) | Bone marrow suppression, diarrhea, nausea, vomiting, hepatotoxicity |
| **Antimetabolites** | | | |
| 5-Azacytadine, capecitabine (Xeloda), cytarabine, edatrexate fludarabine, 5-fluorouracil (5-FU), FUDR, gemcitabine, hydroxyurea, leustatin, 6-mercaptopurine, methotrexate, pentostatin, 6-thioguanine | Interfere with the biosynthesis of metabolites or nucleic acids necessary for RNA and DNA synthesis | Cell cycle–specific (S phase) | Nausea, vomiting, diarrhea, bone marrow suppression, proctitis, stomatitis, renal toxicity (methotrexate), hepatotoxicity |
| **Antitumor Antibiotics** | | | |
| Bleomycin, dactinomycin, daunorubicin, doxorubicin (Adriamycin), idarubicin, mitomycin, mitoxantrone, plicamycin | Interfere with DNA synthesis by binding DNA; prevent RNA synthesis | Cell cycle–nonspecific | Bone marrow suppression, nausea, vomiting, alopecia, anorexia, cardiac toxicity (daunorubicin, doxorubicin) |
| **Mitotic Spindle Poisons** | | | |
| *Plant alkaloids:* etoposide, teniposide, vinblastine, vincristine (VCR), vindesine, vinorelbine | Arrest metaphase by inhibiting mitotic tubular formation (spindle); inhibit DNA and protein synthesis | Cell cycle–specific (M phase) | Bone marrow suppression (mild with VCR), neuropathies (VCR), stomatitis |
| *Taxanes:* paclitaxel, docetaxel | Arrest metaphase by inhibiting tubulin depolymerization | Cell cycle–specific (M phase) | Bradycardia, hypersensitivity reactions, bone marrow suppression, alopecia, neuropathies |
| **Hormonal Agents** | | | |
| Androgens and antiandrogens, estrogens and antiestrogens, progestins and antiprogestins, aromatase inhibitors, luteinizing hormone–releasing hormone analogues, steroids | Bind to hormone receptor sites that alter cellular growth; block binding of estrogens to receptor sites (antiestrogens); inhibit RNA synthesis; suppress aromatase of P450 system, which decreases estrogen level | Cell cycle–nonspecific | Hypercalcemia, jaundice, increased appetite, masculinization, feminization, sodium and fluid retention, nausea, vomiting, hot flashes, vaginal dryness |
| **Miscellaneous Agents** | | | |
| Asparaginase, procarbazine | Unknown or too complex to categorize | Varies | Anorexia, nausea, vomiting, bone marrow suppression, hepatotoxicity, anaphylaxis, hypotension, altered glucose metabolism |

### CHART 16-4

# PHARMACOLOGY · Investigational Antineoplastic Therapies and Clinical Trials

Evaluation of the effectiveness and toxic potential of promising new modalities for preventing, diagnosing, and treating cancer is accomplished through clinical trials. Before new chemotherapy agents are approved for clinical use, they are subjected to rigorous and lengthy evaluations to identify beneficial effects, adverse effects, and safety.

- *Phase I* clinical trials determine optimal dosing, scheduling, and toxicity.
- *Phase II* trials determine effectiveness with specific tumor types and further define toxicities. Participants in these early trials are most often those who have not responded to standard forms of treatment. Because phase I and II trials may be viewed as last-chance efforts, patients and families are fully informed about the experimental nature of the trial therapies. Although it is hoped that investigational therapy will effectively treat the disease, the purpose of early phase trials is to gather information concerning maximal tolerated doses, adverse effects, and effects of the antineoplastic agents on tumor growth.
- *Phase III* clinical trials establish the effectiveness of new medications or procedures as compared with conventional approaches. Nurses may assist in the recruitment, consent, and education processes for patients who participate. In many cases, nurses are instrumental in monitoring adherence, assisting patients to adhere to the parameters of the trial, and documenting data describing patients' responses. The physical and emotional needs of patients in clinical trials are addressed in much the same way as those of patients who receive standard forms of cancer treatment.
- *Phase IV* testing further investigates medications in terms of new uses, dosing schedule, and toxicities.

[Emend]), which block the activity of substance P, another potent neurotransmitter involved in stimulating nausea and vomiting (Flemm, 2004).

Nausea and vomiting involve multiple pathways; therefore, corticosteroids, phenothiazines, sedatives, and histamines are helpful, especially when used in combination with serotonin blockers to provide improved antiemetic protection. Delayed nausea and vomiting that occur longer than 48 to 72 hours after chemotherapy are troublesome for some patients. To minimize discomfort, some antiemetic medications are necessary for the first week at home after chemotherapy. Relaxation techniques and imagery can also help decrease stimuli contributing to symptoms. Small frequent meals, bland foods, and comfort foods may reduce the frequency or severity of these symptoms.

Although the epithelium that lines the oral cavity quickly renews itself, its rapid rate of proliferation makes it susceptible to the effects of chemotherapy. As a result, stomatitis and anorexia are common. The entire gastrointestinal tract is susceptible to mucositis (inflammation of the mucosal lining), and diarrhea is a common result. Antimetabolites and antitumor antibiotics are the major culprits in mucositis and other gastrointestinal symptoms. Irinotecan is responsible for causing diarrhea, which can be severe in some patients.

**Hematopoietic System.** Most chemotherapeutic agents cause **myelosuppression** (depression of bone marrow

### CHART 16-5

## HOME CARE CHECKLIST · Chemotherapy Administration

| At the completion of the home care instruction, the patient or caregiver will be able to: | Patient | Caregiver |
|---|---|---|
| • Demonstrate how to administer the chemotherapy agent in the home. | ✔ | ✔ |
| • Demonstrate safe disposal of needles, syringes, IV supplies, or unused chemotherapy medications. | ✔ | ✔ |
| • List possible side effects of chemotherapeutic agents. | ✔ | ✔ |
| • List complications of medications necessitating a call to the nurse or physician. | ✔ | ✔ |
| • List complications of medications necessitating a visit to the emergency department. | ✔ | ✔ |
| • List names and telephone numbers of resource personnel involved in care (ie, home care nurse, infusion services, IV vendor, equipment company). | ✔ | ✔ |
| • Explain treatment plan (protocol) and importance of upcoming visits to physician. | ✔ | ✔ |

**FIGURE 16-3.** Right atrial catheter. The right atrial catheter is inserted into the subclavian vein and advanced until its tip lies in the superior vena cava just above the right atrium. The proximal end is then tunneled from the entry site through the subcutaneous tissue of the chest wall and brought out through an exit site on the chest. The Dacron cuff anchors the catheter in place and serves as a barrier to infection.

function), resulting in decreased production of blood cells. Myelosuppression decreases the number of WBCs (leukopenia), red blood cells (RBCs) (anemia), and platelets (thrombocytopenia) and increases the risk of infection and bleeding. Depression of these cells is the usual reason for limiting the dose of the chemotherapeutic agents. Monitoring blood cell counts frequently is essential, because it allows strategies to be implemented to protect patients from infection and injury, particularly while blood cell counts are depressed.

Other agents, called colony-stimulating factors (granulocyte colony-stimulating factor [G-CSF], granulocyte-macrophage colony-stimulating factor [GM-CSF], and erythropoietin [EPO]), can be administered after chemotherapy. G-CSF and GM-CSF stimulate the bone marrow to produce WBCs, especially neutrophils, at an accelerated rate, thus decreasing the duration of neutropenia. The colony-stimulating factors decrease the episodes of infection and the need for antibiotics and allow for more timely cycling of chemotherapy with less need to reduce the dosage. EPO stimulates RBC production, thus decreasing the symptoms of chronic anemia and reducing the need for blood transfusions (Bedell, 2003b; Cappozzo, 2004; Gillespie, 2003).

**Renal System.** Chemotherapeutic agents can damage the kidneys because of their direct effects during excretion and the accumulation of end products after cell lysis. Cisplatin, methotrexate, and mitomycin are particularly toxic to the kidneys. Rapid tumor cell lysis after chemotherapy results in increased urinary excretion of uric acid, which can cause renal damage. In addition, intracellular contents are released into the circulation, resulting in excessive levels of potassium and phosphates (hyperkalemia and hyperphosphatemia) and diminished levels of calcium (hypocalcemia). (See later discussion of tumor lysis syndrome.)

Monitoring blood urea nitrogen (BUN), serum creatinine, creatinine clearance, and serum electrolyte levels is

**FIGURE 16-4.** Implanted vascular access device. (**A**) A schematic diagram of an implanted vascular access device used for administration of medications, fluids, blood products, and nutrition. The self-sealing septum permits repeated puncture by Huber needles without damage or leakage. (**B**) Two Huber needles used to enter the implanted vascular port. The 90-degree needle is used for top-entry ports for continuous infusions.

essential. Adequate hydration, alkalinization of the urine to prevent formation of uric acid crystals, and the use of allopurinol are frequently indicated to prevent these side effects (Richerson, 2004).

**Cardiopulmonary System.** Antitumor antibiotics (daunorubicin and doxorubicin) are known to cause irreversible cumulative cardiac toxicities, especially when total dosage reaches 550 mg/m$^2$. Cardiac ejection fraction (volume of blood ejected from the heart with each beat) and signs of heart failure must be monitored closely. Bleomycin, carmustine (BCNU), and busulfan are known for their cumulative toxic effects on lung function. Pulmonary fibrosis can be a long-term effect of prolonged dosage with these agents. Therefore, patients are monitored closely for changes in pulmonary function, including pulmonary function test results. Total cumulative doses of bleomycin are not to exceed 400 units.

**Reproductive System.** Testicular and ovarian function can be affected by chemotherapeutic agents, resulting in possible sterility. Normal ovulation, early menopause, or permanent sterility may occur. In men, temporary or permanent azoospermia (absence of spermatozoa) may develop. Reproductive cells may be damaged during treatment, resulting in chromosomal abnormalities in offspring. Banking of sperm is recommended for men before treatments are initiated to protect against sterility or any mutagenic damage to sperm.

Patients and their partners need to be informed about potential changes in reproductive function resulting from chemotherapy. They are advised to use reliable methods of birth control while receiving chemotherapy and not to assume that sterility has resulted.

**Neurologic System.** The taxanes and plant alkaloids, especially vincristine, can cause neurologic damage with repeated doses. Peripheral neuropathies, loss of deep tendon reflexes, and paralytic ileus may occur. These side effects are usually reversible and disappear after completion of chemotherapy. Cisplatin is also responsible for peripheral neuropathies, and hearing loss due to damage to the acoustic nerve can also occur (Casciato, 2004; Marrs & Newton, 2003; Wilkes & Barton-Burke, 2004).

**Miscellaneous.** Fatigue is a distressing side effect for most patients that greatly affects quality of life. Fatigue can be debilitating and can last for months after treatment.

## Nursing Management in Chemotherapy

Nurses play an important role in assessing and managing many of the problems experienced by patients undergoing chemotherapy. Chemotherapeutic agents have systemic effects on normal cells as well as malignant ones, which means that these problems are often widespread, affecting many body systems.

### ASSESSING FLUID AND ELECTROLYTE STATUS
Anorexia, nausea, vomiting, altered taste, and diarrhea put patients at risk for nutritional and fluid and electrolyte disturbances. Changes in the mucosa of the gastrointestinal tract may lead to irritation of the oral cavity and intestinal tract, further threatening the patient's nutritional status. Therefore, it is important for the nurse to assess the patient's nutritional and fluid and electrolyte status frequently and to use creative ways to encourage an adequate fluid and dietary intake.

### MODIFYING RISKS FOR INFECTION AND BLEEDING
Suppression of the bone marrow and immune system is an expected consequence of chemotherapy and frequently serves as a guide in determining appropriate chemotherapy dosage. However, this effect also increases the risk of anemia, infection, and bleeding disorders. Nursing assessment and care focus on identifying and modifying factors that would further increase the patient's risk. Aseptic technique and gentle handling are indicated to prevent infection and trauma. Laboratory test results, particularly blood cell counts, are monitored closely. Untoward changes in blood test results and signs of infection and bleeding must be reported promptly. The patient and family members are instructed about measures to prevent these problems at home (see the plan of nursing care for the patient with cancer given in Chart 16-6).

### ADMINISTERING CHEMOTHERAPY
The local effects of the chemotherapeutic agent are also of concern. The patient is observed closely during its administration because of the risk and consequences of extravasation (particularly of vesicant agents, which may produce necrosis if deposited in the subcutaneous tissues). Local difficulties or problems with administration of chemotherapeutic agents are brought to the attention of the physician promptly so that corrective measures can be taken immediately to minimize local tissue damage.

### PROTECTING CAREGIVERS
Nurses involved in handling chemotherapeutic agents may be exposed to low doses of the agents by direct contact, inhalation, or ingestion. Urinalyses of personnel repeatedly exposed to cytotoxic agents have demonstrated mutagenic activity. Although long-term studies of nurses who handle chemotherapeutic agents have not been conducted, it is known that chemotherapeutic agents are associated with secondary formation of cancers and chromosome abnormalities. In addition, nausea, vomiting, dizziness, alopecia, and nasal mucosal ulcerations have been reported in health care personnel who have handled chemotherapeutic agents (Wilkes & Barton-Burke, 2004). The Occupational Safety and Health Administration, Oncology Nursing Society, hospitals, and other health care agencies have developed specific precautions for health care providers involved in the preparation and administration of chemotherapy (Chart 16-7) (Polovich, 2003; Wilkes & Barton-Burke, 2004).

## Bone Marrow Transplantation

Although surgery, radiation therapy, and chemotherapy have resulted in improved survival rates for cancer patients, many cancers that initially respond to therapy recur. This is true of hematologic cancers that affect the bone marrow and solid tumor cancers treated with lower doses of antineoplastics to spare the bone marrow from larger, ablative doses of chemotherapy or radiation therapy. The role of bone marrow transplantation (BMT) for malignant and some nonmalignant diseases continues to grow.

*(text continues on page 415)*

## CHART 16-6 Plan of Nursing Care: The Patient With Cancer

**Nursing Diagnosis:** Risk for infection related to altered immunologic response
**Goal:** Prevention of infection

| NURSING INTERVENTIONS | RATIONALE | EXPECTED OUTCOMES |
|---|---|---|
| 1. Assess patient for evidence of infection:<br>  a. Check vital signs every 4 hours.<br>  b. Monitor WBC count and differential each day.<br>  c. Inspect all sites that may serve as entry ports for pathogens (intravenous sites, wounds, skin folds, bony prominences, perineum, and oral cavity).<br>2. Report fever ≥38.3°C (101°F), chills, diaphoresis, swelling, heat, pain, erythema, exudate on any body surfaces. Also report change in respiratory or mental status, urinary frequency or burning, malaise, myalgias, arthralgias, rash, or diarrhea.<br>3. Obtain cultures and sensitivities as indicated before initiation of antimicrobial treatment (wound exudate, sputum, urine, stool, blood).<br>4. Initiate measures to minimize infection.<br>  a. Discuss with patient and family<br>    (1) Placing patient in private room if absolute WBC count <1,000/mm$^3$<br>    (2) Importance of patient avoiding contact with people who have known or recent infection or recent vaccination<br>  b. Instruct all personnel in careful hand hygiene before and after entering room.<br>  c. Avoid rectal or vaginal procedures (rectal temperatures, examinations, suppositories; vaginal tampons). | 1. Signs and symptoms of infection may be diminished in the immunocompromised host. Prompt recognition of infection and subsequent initiation of therapy will reduce morbidity and mortality associated with infection.<br>2. Early detection of infection facilitates early intervention.<br>3. These tests identify the organism and indicate the most appropriate antimicrobial therapy. Use of inappropriate antibiotics enhances proliferation of additional flora and encourages growth of antibiotic-resistant organisms.<br>4. Exposure to infection is reduced.<br>  a. Preventing contact with pathogens helps prevent infection.<br>  b. Hands are significant source of contamination.<br>  c. Incidence of rectal and perianal abscesses and subsequent systemic infection is high. Manipulation may cause disruption of mem- | • Demonstrates normal temperature and vital signs.<br>• Exhibits absence of signs of inflammation: local edema, erythema, pain, and warmth.<br>• Exhibits normal breath sounds on auscultation.<br>• Takes deep breaths and coughs every 2 hours to prevent respiratory dysfunction and infection.<br>• Exhibits absence of pathologic bacteria on cultures.<br>• Avoids contact with others with infections.<br>• Avoids crowds.<br>• All personnel carry out hand hygiene after each voiding and bowel movement.<br>• Excoriation and trauma of skin are avoided.<br>• Trauma to mucous membranes is avoided (avoidance of rectal thermometers, suppositories, vaginal tampons, perianal trauma).<br>• Uses recommended procedures and techniques if participating in management of invasive lines or catheters.<br>• Uses electric razor.<br>• Is free of skin breakdown and stasis of secretions.<br>• Adheres to dietary and environmental restrictions.<br>• Exhibits no signs of septicemia or septic shock.<br>• Exhibits normal vital signs, cardiac output, and arterial pressures when monitored.<br>• Demonstrates ability to administer colony-stimulating factor. |

*continued >*

## CHART 16-6

### Plan of Nursing Care: The Patient With Cancer (Continued)

| NURSING INTERVENTIONS | RATIONALE | EXPECTED OUTCOMES |
|---|---|---|
| | brane integrity and enhance progression of infection. | |
| d. Use stool softeners to prevent constipation and straining. | d. This minimizes trauma to tissues. | |
| e. Assist patient in practice of meticulous personal hygiene. | e. This prevents skin irritation. | |
| f. Instruct patient to use electric razor. | f. Minimizes skin trauma. | |
| g. Encourage patient to ambulate in room unless contraindicated. | g. Minimizes chance of skin breakdown and stasis of pulmonary secretions. | |
| h. Avoid fresh fruits, raw meat, fish, and vegetables if absolute WBC count <1,000/mm$^3$; remove fresh flowers and potted plants. | h. Fresh fruits and vegetables harbor bacteria not removed by ordinary washing. Flowers and potted plants are sources of organisms. | |
| i. Each day: change water pitcher, denture cleaning fluids, and respiratory equipment containing water. | i. Stagnant water is a source of infection. | |
| 5. Assess intravenous sites every day for evidence of infection: | 5. Nosocomial staphylococcal septicemia is closely associated with intravenous catheters. | |
| a. Change intravenous sites every other day. | a. Incidence of infection is increased when catheter is in place >72 hr. | |
| b. Cleanse skin with povidone-iodine before arterial puncture or venipuncture. | b. Povidone-iodine is effective against many gram-positive and gram-negative pathogens. | |
| c. Change central venous catheter dressings every 48 hours. | c. Allows observation of site and removes source of contamination. | |
| d. Change all solutions and infusion sets every 48 hours. | d. Once introduced into the system, microorganisms are capable of growing in infusion sets despite replacement of container and high flow rates. | |
| 6. Avoid intramuscular injections. | 6. Reduces risk for skin abscesses. | |
| 7. Avoid insertion of urinary catheters; if catheters are necessary, use strict aseptic technique. | 7. Rates of infection greatly increase after urinary catheterization. | |
| 8. Teach patient or family member to administer granulocyte (or granulocyte-macrophage) colony-stimulating factor when prescribed. | 8. Granulocyte colony-stimulating factor decreases the duration of neutropenia and the potential for infection. | |

## CHART 16-6

### Plan of Nursing Care: The Patient With Cancer (Continued)

**Nursing Diagnosis:** Impaired skin integrity: erythematous and wet desquamation reactions to radiation therapy
**Goal:** Maintenance of skin integrity

| NURSING INTERVENTIONS | RATIONALE | EXPECTED OUTCOMES |
|---|---|---|
| 1. In erythematous areas:<br>  a. Avoid the use of soaps, cosmetics, perfumes, powders, lotions and ointments, deodorants.<br>  b. Use only lukewarm water to bathe the area.<br>  c. Avoid rubbing or scratching the area.<br>  d. Avoid shaving the area with a straight-edged razor.<br>  e. Avoid applying hot-water bottles, heating pads, ice, and adhesive tape to the area.<br>  f. Avoid exposing the area to sunlight or cold weather.<br>  g. Avoid tight clothing in the area. Use cotton clothing.<br>  h. Apply vitamin A&D ointment to the area.<br>2. If wet desquamation occurs:<br>  a. Do not disrupt any blisters that have formed.<br>  b. Avoid frequent washing of the area.<br>  c. Report any blistering.<br>  d. Use *prescribed* creams or ointments.<br>  e. If area weeps, apply a thin layer of gauze dressing. | 1. Care to the affected areas must focus on preventing further skin irritation, drying, and damage<br><br><br><br><br><br><br><br><br>g. Allows air circulation to affected area.<br>h. Aids healing.<br>2. Open weeping areas are susceptible to bacterial infection. Care must be taken to prevent introduction of pathogens.<br><br>d. Decreases irritation and inflammation of the area.<br>e. Enhances drying. | • Avoids use of soaps, powders, and other cosmetics on site of radiation therapy.<br>• States rationale for special care of skin.<br>• Exhibits minimal change in skin.<br>• Avoids trauma to affected skin region (avoids shaving, constricting and irritating clothing, extremes of temperature, and use of adhesive tape).<br>• Reports change in skin promptly.<br>• Demonstrates proper care of blistered or open areas.<br>• Exhibits absence of infection of blistered and opened areas. |

**Nursing Diagnosis:** Impaired oral mucous membrane: stomatitis
**Goal:** Maintenance of intact oral mucous membranes

| NURSING INTERVENTIONS | RATIONALE | EXPECTED OUTCOMES |
|---|---|---|
| 1. Assess oral cavity daily.<br>2. Instruct patient to report oral burning, pain, areas of redness, open lesions on the lips, pain associated with swallowing, or decreased tolerance to temperature extremes of food. | 1. Provides baseline for later evaluation.<br>2. Identification of initial stages of stomatitis will facilitate prompt interventions, including modification of treatment as prescribed by physician. | • States rationale for frequent oral assessment and hygiene.<br>• Identifies signs and symptoms of stomatitis to report to nurse or physician.<br>• Participates in recommended oral hygiene regimen.<br>• Avoids mouthwashes with alcohol. |

*continued >*

### CHART 16-6

## Plan of Nursing Care — The Patient With Cancer (Continued)

| NURSING INTERVENTIONS | RATIONALE | EXPECTED OUTCOMES |
|---|---|---|
| 3. Encourage and assist in oral hygiene.<br>**Preventive**<br>  a. Avoid commercial mouthwashes.<br>  b. Brush with soft toothbrush; use non-abrasive toothpaste after meals and bedtime; floss every 24 h unless painful or platelet count falls below 40,000 cu/mm.<br>**Mild stomatitis** (generalized erythema, limited ulcerations, small white patches: *Candida*)<br>  c. Use normal saline mouth rinses every 2 h while awake; every 6 h at night.<br>  d. Use soft toothbrush or toothette.<br>  e. Remove dentures except for meals; be certain dentures fit well.<br>  f. Apply lip lubricant.<br>  g. Avoid foods that are spicy or hard to chew and those with extremes of temperature.<br>**Severe stomatitis** (confluent ulcerations with bleeding and white patches covering more than 25% of oral mucosa)<br>  h. Obtain tissue samples for culture and sensitivity tests of areas of infection.<br>  i. Assess ability to chew and swallow; assess gag reflex.<br>  j. Use oral rinses (may combine in solution saline, anti-*Candida* agent, such as Mycostatin, and topical anesthetic agent as described below) as prescribed or place patient on side and irrigate mouth; have suction available.<br>  k. Remove dentures. | a. Alcohol content of mouthwashes will dry oral tissues and potentiate breakdown.<br>b. Limits trauma and removes debris.<br><br><br>c. Assists in removing debris, thick secretions, and bacteria.<br>d. Minimizes trauma.<br>e. Minimizes friction and discomfort.<br><br>f. Promotes comfort.<br>g. Prevents local trauma.<br><br><br><br>h. Assists in identifying need for anti-microbial therapy.<br>i. Patient may be in danger of aspiration.<br>j. Facilitates cleansing, provides for safety and comfort.<br><br><br><br>k. Prevents trauma from ill-fitting dentures. | • Brushes teeth and mouth with soft toothbrush.<br>• Uses lubricant to keep lips soft and non-irritated.<br>• Avoids hard-to-chew, spicy, and hot foods.<br>• Exhibits clean, intact oral mucosa.<br>• Exhibits no ulcerations or infections of oral cavity.<br>• Exhibits no evidence of bleeding.<br>• Reports absent or decreased oral pain.<br>• Reports no difficulty swallowing.<br>• Exhibits healing (reepithelialization) of oral mucosa within 5 to 7 days (mild stomatitis).<br>• Exhibits healing of oral tissues within 10 to 14 days (severe stomatitis).<br>• Exhibits no bleeding or oral ulceration.<br>• Consumes adequate fluid and food.<br>• Exhibits absence of dehydration and weight loss. |

## CHART 16-6 Plan of Nursing Care: The Patient With Cancer (Continued)

### NURSING INTERVENTIONS | RATIONALE | EXPECTED OUTCOMES

l. Use toothette or gauze soaked with solution for cleansing.
m. Use lip lubricant.
n. Provide liquid or pureed diet.
o. Monitor for dehydration.

l. Limits trauma, promotes comfort.
m. Promotes comfort.
n. Ensures intake of easily digestible foods.
o. Decreased oral intake and ulcerations potentiate fluid deficits.

4. Minimize discomfort.
   a. Consult physician for use of topical anesthetic, such as dyclonine and diphenhydramine, or viscous lidocaine.
   b. Administer systemic analgesics as prescribed.
   c. Perform mouth care as described.

   a. Alleviates pain and increases sense of well-being; promotes participation in oral hygiene and nutritional intake.
   c. Promotes removal of debris, healing, and comfort.

**Nursing Diagnosis:** Impaired tissue integrity: alopecia
**Goal:** Maintenance of tissue integrity; coping with hair loss

### NURSING INTERVENTIONS | RATIONALE | EXPECTED OUTCOMES

1. Discuss potential hair loss and regrowth with patient and family.
2. Explore potential impact of hair loss on self-image, interpersonal relationships, and sexuality.
3. Prevent or minimize hair loss through the following:
   a. Use scalp hypothermia and scalp tourniquets, if appropriate.
   b. Cut long hair before treatment.
   c. Use mild shampoo and conditioner, gently pat dry, and avoid excessive shampooing.
   d. Avoid electric curlers, curling irons, dryers, clips, barrettes, hair sprays, hair dyes, and permanent waves.
   e. Avoid excessive combing or brushing; use wide-toothed comb.

1. Provides information so patient and family can begin to prepare cognitively and emotionally for loss.
2. Facilitates coping.
3. Retains hair as long as possible.
   a. Decreases hair follicle uptake of chemotherapy (not used for patients with leukemia or lymphoma because tumor cells may be present in blood vessels or scalp tissue).
   b–e. Minimizes hair loss due to the weight and manipulation of hair.

- Identifies alopecia as potential side effect of treatment.
- Identifies positive and negative feelings and threats to self-image.
- Verbalizes meaning that hair and possible hair loss have for him or her.
- States rationale for modifications in hair care and treatment.
- Uses mild shampoo and conditioner and shampoos hair only when necessary.
- Avoids hair dryer, curlers, sprays, and other stresses on hair and scalp.
- Wears hat or scarf over hair when exposed to sun.
- Takes steps to deal with possible hair loss before it occurs; purchases wig or hairpiece.
- Maintains hygiene and grooming.
- Interacts and socializes with others.
- States that hair loss and necessity of wig are temporary.

*continued >*

### CHART 16-6 Plan of Nursing Care: The Patient With Cancer (Continued)

| NURSING INTERVENTIONS | RATIONALE | EXPECTED OUTCOMES |
|---|---|---|
| 4. Prevent trauma to scalp.<br>  a. Lubricate scalp with vitamin A&D ointment to decrease itching.<br>  b. Have patient use sunscreen or wear hat when in the sun.<br>5. Suggest ways to assist in coping with hair loss:<br>  a. Purchase wig or hairpiece before hair loss.<br>  b. If hair loss has occurred, take photograph to wig shop to assist in selection.<br>  c. Begin to wear wig before hair loss.<br>  d. Contact the American Cancer Society for donated wigs, or a store that specializes in this product.<br>  e. Wear hat, scarf, or turban.<br>6. Encourage patient to wear own clothes and retain social contacts.<br>7. Explain that hair growth usually begins again once therapy is completed. | 4. Preserves tissue integrity.<br>  a. Assists in maintaining skin integrity.<br>  b. Prevents ultraviolet light exposure.<br>5. Minimizes change in appearance.<br>  a. Wig that closely resembles hair color and style is more easily selected if hair loss has not begun.<br>  b. Facilitates adjustment.<br><br><br><br><br><br>  e. Conceals loss.<br>6. Assists in maintaining personal identity.<br>7. Reassures patient that hair loss is usually temporary. | |

**Nursing Diagnosis:** Imbalanced nutrition, less than body requirements, related to nausea and vomiting
**Goal:** Fewer episodes of nausea and vomiting before, during, and after chemotherapy

| NURSING INTERVENTIONS | RATIONALE | EXPECTED OUTCOMES |
|---|---|---|
| 1. Assess the patient's previous experiences and expectations of nausea and vomiting, including causes and interventions used.<br>2. Adjust diet before and after drug administration according to patient preference and tolerance.<br>3. Prevent unpleasant sights, odors, and sounds in the environment. | 1. Identifies patient concerns, misinformation, potential strategies for intervention. Also gives patient sense of empowerment and control.<br>2. Each patient responds differently to food after chemotherapy. A diet containing foods that relieve the patient's nausea or vomiting is most helpful.<br>3. Unpleasant sensations can stimulate the nausea and vomiting center. | • Identifies previous triggers of nausea and vomiting.<br>• Exhibits decreased apprehension and anxiety.<br>• Identifies previously used successful interventions for nausea and vomiting.<br>• Reports decrease in nausea.<br>• Reports decrease in incidence of vomiting.<br>• Consumes adequate fluid and food when nausea subsides. |

## CHART 16-6

### Plan of Nursing Care: The Patient With Cancer (Continued)

| NURSING INTERVENTIONS | RATIONALE | EXPECTED OUTCOMES |
|---|---|---|
| 4. Use distraction, music therapy, biofeedback, self-hypnosis, relaxation techniques, and guided imagery before, during, and after chemotherapy. | 4. Decreases anxiety, which can contribute to nausea and vomiting. Psychological conditioning may also be decreased. | • Demonstrates use of distraction, relaxation, and imagery when indicated.<br>• Exhibits normal skin turgor and moist mucous membranes.<br>• Reports no additional weight loss. |
| 5. Administer prescribed antiemetics, sedatives, and corticosteroids before chemotherapy and afterward as needed. | 5. Administration of antiemetic regimen before onset of nausea and vomiting limits the adverse experience and facilitates control. Combination drug therapy reduces nausea and vomiting through various triggering mechanisms. | |
| 6. Ensure adequate fluid hydration before, during, and after drug administration; assess intake and output. | 6. Adequate fluid volume dilutes drug levels, decreasing stimulation of vomiting receptors. | |
| 7. Encourage frequent oral hygiene. | 7. Reduces unpleasant taste sensations. | |
| 8. Provide pain relief measures, if necessary. | 8. Increased comfort increases physical tolerance of symptoms. | |
| 9. Assess other causes of nausea and vomiting, such as constipation, gastrointestinal irritation, electrolyte imbalance, radiation therapy, medications, and central nervous system metastasis. | 9. Multiple factors may cause nausea and vomiting. | |

**Nursing Diagnosis:** Imbalanced nutrition: less than body requirements, related to anorexia, cachexia, or malabsorption
**Goal:** Maintenance of nutritional status and of weight within 10% of pretreatment weight

| NURSING INTERVENTIONS | RATIONALE | EXPECTED OUTCOMES |
|---|---|---|
| 1. Teach patient to avoid unpleasant sights, odors, sounds in the environment during mealtime. | 1. Anorexia can be stimulated or increased with noxious stimuli. | • Exhibits weight loss no greater than 10% of pretreatment weight.<br>• Reports decreasing anorexia and increased interest in eating.<br>• Demonstrates normal skin turgor.<br>• Identifies rationale for dietary modifications.<br>• Participates in calorie counts and diet histories.<br>• Uses appropriate relaxation and imagery before meals. |
| 2. Suggest foods that are preferred and well tolerated by the patient, preferably high-calorie and high-protein foods. Respect ethnic and cultural food preferences. | 2. Foods preferred, well tolerated, and high in calories and protein maintain nutritional status during periods of increased metabolic demand. | |
| 3. Encourage adequate fluid intake, but limit fluids at mealtime. | 3. Fluids are necessary to eliminate wastes and prevent dehydration. Increased fluids with meals can lead to early satiety. | |

*continued >*

### CHART 16-6

## Plan of Nursing Care: The Patient With Cancer (Continued)

| NURSING INTERVENTIONS | RATIONALE | EXPECTED OUTCOMES |
|---|---|---|
| 4. Suggest smaller, more frequent meals. | 4. Smaller, more frequent meals are better tolerated because early satiety does not occur. | • Exhibits laboratory and clinical findings indicative of adequate nutritional intake: normal serum protein and transferrin levels; normal serum iron levels; normal hemoglobin, hematocrit, and lymphocyte levels; normal urinary creatinine levels. |
| 5. Promote relaxed, quiet environment during mealtime with increased social interaction as desired. | 5. A quiet environment promotes relaxation. Social interaction at mealtime increases appetite. | • Consumes diet high in required nutrients. |
| 6. If possible, serve wine at mealtime with foods. | 6. Wine often stimulates appetite and adds calories. | • Carries out oral hygiene before meals. |
| 7. Consider cold foods, if desired. | 7. Cold, high-protein foods are often more tolerable and less odorous than hot foods. | • Reports that pain does not interfere with meals. |
| 8. Encourage nutritional supplements and high-protein foods between meals. | 8. Supplements and snacks add protein and calories to meet nutritional requirements. | • Reports decreasing episodes of nausea and vomiting. |
| 9. Encourage frequent oral hygiene. | 9. Oral hygiene stimulates appetite and increases saliva production. | • Participates in increasing levels of activity. |
| 10. Provide pain relief measures. | 10. Pain impairs appetite. | • States rationale for use of tube feedings or parenteral nutrition. |
| 11. Provide control of nausea and vomiting. | 11. Nausea and vomiting increase anorexia. | • Participates in management of tube feedings or parenteral nutrition, if prescribed. |
| 12. Increase activity level as tolerated. | 12. Increased activity promotes appetite. | |
| 13. Decrease anxiety by encouraging verbalization of fears, concerns; use of relaxation techniques; imagery at mealtime. | 13. Relief of anxiety may increase appetite. | |
| 14. Position patient properly at mealtime. | 14. Proper body position and alignment are necessary to aid chewing and swallowing. | |
| 15. For collaborative management, provide enteral tube feedings of commercial liquid diets, elemental diets, or blenderized foods as prescribed. | 15. Tube feedings may be necessary in the severely debilitated patient who has a functioning gastrointestinal system. | |
| 16. Provide parenteral nutrition with lipid supplements as prescribed. | 16. Parenteral nutrition with supplemental fats supplies needed calories and proteins to meet nutritional demands, especially in the nonfunctional gastrointestinal system. | |
| 17. Administer appetite stimulants as prescribed by physician. | 17. Although the mechanism is unclear, medications such as megestrol acetate (Megace) have been noted to improve appetite in patients with cancer and HIV infection. | |

## CHART 16-6

### Plan of Nursing Care
### The Patient With Cancer (Continued)

**Nursing Diagnosis:** Fatigue
**Goal:** Increased activity tolerance and decreased fatigue level

| NURSING INTERVENTIONS | RATIONALE | EXPECTED OUTCOMES |
|---|---|---|
| 1. Encourage several rest periods during the day, especially before and after physical exertion.<br>2. Increase total hours of nighttime sleep.<br>3. Rearrange daily schedule and organize activities to conserve energy expenditure.<br>4. Encourage patient to ask for others' assistance with necessary chores, such as housework, child care, shopping, cooking.<br>5. Encourage reduced job workload, if possible, by reducing number of hours worked per week.<br>6. Encourage adequate protein and calorie intake.<br>7. Encourage use of relaxation techniques, mental imagery.<br>8. Encourage participation in planned exercise programs.<br>9. For collaborative management, administer blood products as prescribed.<br>10. Assess for fluid and electrolyte disturbances.<br>11. Assess for sources of discomfort.<br>12. Provide strategies to facilitate mobility. | 1. During rest, energy is conserved and levels are replenished. Several shorter rest periods may be more beneficial than one longer rest period.<br>2. Sleep helps to restore energy levels.<br>3. Reorganization of activities can reduce energy losses and stressors.<br>4. Conserves energy.<br><br><br><br>5. Reducing workload decreases physical and psychological stress and increases periods of rest and relaxation.<br>6. Protein and calorie depletion decreases activity tolerance.<br>7. Promotion of relaxation and psychological rest decreases physical fatigue.<br>8. Proper exercise programs increase endurance and stamina.<br>9. Lowered hemoglobin and hematocrit predispose patient to fatigue due to decreased oxygen availability.<br>10. May contribute to altered nerve transmission and muscle function.<br>11. Coping with discomfort requires energy expenditure.<br>12. Impaired mobility requires increased energy expenditure. | • Reports decreasing levels of fatigue.<br>• Increases participation in activities gradually.<br>• Rests when fatigued.<br>• Reports restful sleep.<br>• Requests assistance with activities appropriately.<br>• Reports adequate energy to participate in activities important to him or her (eg, visiting with family, hobbies).<br>• Consumes diet with recommended protein and caloric intake.<br>• Uses relaxation exercises and imagery to decrease anxiety and promote rest.<br>• Participates in planned exercise program gradually.<br>• Reports no breathlessness during activities.<br>• Exhibits acceptable hemoglobin and hematocrit levels.<br>• Exhibits normal fluid and electrolyte balance.<br>• Reports decreased discomfort.<br>• Exhibits improved mobility. |

**Nursing Diagnosis:** Chronic pain
**Goal:** Relief of pain and discomfort

| NURSING INTERVENTIONS | RATIONALE | EXPECTED OUTCOMES |
|---|---|---|
| 1. Use pain scale to assess pain and discomfort characteristics: location, quality, frequency, duration, etc. | 1. Provides baseline for assessing changes in pain level and evaluation of interventions. | • Reports decreased level of pain and discomfort on pain scale.<br>• Reports less disruption from pain and discomfort. |

*continued >*

### CHART 16-6

## Plan of Nursing Care — The Patient With Cancer (Continued)

| NURSING INTERVENTIONS | RATIONALE | EXPECTED OUTCOMES |
|---|---|---|
| 2. Assure patient that you know that pain is real and will assist him or her in reducing it.<br>3. Assess other factors contributing to patient's pain: fear, fatigue, anger, etc.<br>4. Administer analgesics to promote optimum pain relief within limits of physician's prescription.<br>5. Assess patient's behavioral responses to pain and pain experience.<br>6. Collaborate with patient, physician, and other health care team members when changes in pain management are necessary.<br>7. Encourage strategies of pain relief that patient has used successfully in previous pain experience.<br>8. Teach patient new strategies to relieve pain and discomfort: distraction, imagery, relaxation, cutaneous stimulation, etc. | 2. Fear that pain will not be considered real increases anxiety and reduces pain tolerance.<br>3. Provides data about factors that decrease patient's ability to tolerate pain and increase pain level.<br>4. Analgesics tend to be more effective when administered early in pain cycle.<br>5. Provides additional information about patient's pain.<br>6. New methods of administering analgesia must be acceptable to patient, physician, and health care team to be effective; patient's participation decreases the sense of powerlessness.<br>7. Encourages success of pain relief strategies accepted by patient and family.<br>8. Increases number of options and strategies available to patient. | • Explains how fatigue, fear, anger, etc., contribute to severity of pain and discomfort.<br>• Accepts analgesia as prescribed.<br>• Exhibits decreased physical and behavioral signs of pain and discomfort in acute pain (no grimacing, crying, moaning; displays interest in surroundings and activities around him).<br>• Takes an active role in administration of analgesia.<br>• Identifies additional effective pain relief strategies.<br>• Uses alternative pain relief strategies appropriately.<br>• Reports effective use of new pain relief strategies and decrease in pain intensity.<br>• Reports that decreased level of pain permits participation in other activities and events. |

**Nursing Diagnosis:** Anticipatory grieving related to loss; altered role functioning
**Goal:** Appropriate progression through grieving process

| NURSING INTERVENTIONS | RATIONALE | EXPECTED OUTCOMES |
|---|---|---|
| 1. Encourage verbalization of fears, concerns, and questions regarding disease, treatment, and future implications.<br>2. Encourage active participation of patient or family in care and treatment decisions.<br>3. Visit family frequently to establish and maintain relationships and physical closeness.<br>4. Encourage ventilation of negative feelings, including projected anger and hostility, within acceptable limits.<br>5. Allow for periods of crying and expression of sadness. | 1. An increased and accurate knowledge base decreases anxiety and dispels misconceptions.<br>2. Active participation maintains patient independence and control.<br>3. Frequent contacts promote trust and security and reduce feelings of fear and isolation.<br>4. This allows for emotional expression without loss of self-esteem.<br>5. These feelings are necessary for separation and detachment to occur. | • The patient and family progress through the phases of grief as evidenced by increased verbalization and expression of grief.<br>• The patient and family identify resources available to aid coping strategies during grieving.<br>• The patient and family use resources and supports appropriately.<br>• The patient and family discuss the future openly with each other.<br>• The patient and family discuss concerns and feelings openly with each other. |

## CHART 16-6

### Plan of Nursing Care: The Patient With Cancer (Continued)

| NURSING INTERVENTIONS | RATIONALE | EXPECTED OUTCOMES |
|---|---|---|
| 6. Involve spiritual advisor as desired by the patient and family. | 6. This facilitates the grief process and spiritual care. | • The patient and family use nonverbal expressions of concern for each other. |
| 7. Advise professional counseling as indicated for patient or family to alleviate pathologic grieving. | 7. This facilitates the grief process. | |
| 8. Allow for progression through the grieving process at the individual pace of the patient and family. | 8. Grief work is variable. Not every person uses every phase of the grief process, and the time spent in dealing with each phase varies with every person. To complete grief work, this variability must be allowed. | |

**Nursing Diagnosis:** Disturbed body image and situational low self-esteem related to changes in appearance, function, and roles
**Goal:** Improved body image and self-esteem

| NURSING INTERVENTIONS | RATIONALE | EXPECTED OUTCOMES |
|---|---|---|
| 1. Assess patient's feelings about body image and level of self-esteem. | 1. Provides baseline assessment for evaluating changes and assessing effectiveness of interventions. | • Identifies concerns of importance.<br>• Takes active role in activities.<br>• Maintains previous role in decision making.<br>• Verbalizes feelings and reactions to losses or threatened losses.<br>• Participates in self-care activities.<br>• Permits others to assist in care when he or she is unable to be independent.<br>• Exhibits interest in appearance and uses aids (cosmetics, scarves, etc.) appropriately.<br>• Participates with others in conversations and social events and activities.<br>• Verbalizes concern about sexual partner and/or significant others.<br>• Explores alternative ways of expressing concern and affection. |
| 2. Identify potential threats to patient's self-esteem (eg, altered appearance, decreased sexual function, hair loss, decreased energy, role changes). Validate concerns with patient. | 2. Anticipates changes and permits patient to identify importance of these areas to him or her. | |
| 3. Encourage continued participation in activities and decision making. | 3. Encourages and permits continued control of events and self. | |
| 4. Encourage patient to verbalize concerns. | 4. Identifying concerns is an important step in coping with them. | |
| 5. Individualize care for the patient. | 5. Prevents or reduces depersonalization and emphasizes patient's self-worth. | |
| 6. Assist patient in self-care when fatigue, lethargy, nausea, vomiting, and other symptoms prevent independence. | 6. Physical well-being improves self-esteem. | |
| 7. Assist patient in selecting and using cosmetics, scarves, hair pieces, and clothing that increase his or her sense of attractiveness. | 7. Promotes positive body image. | |
| 8. Encourage patient and partner to share concerns about altered sexuality and sexual function and to explore alternatives to their usual sexual expression. | 8. Provides opportunity for expressing concern, affection, and acceptance. | |

*continued >*

## CHART 16-6

# Plan of Nursing Care: The Patient With Cancer (Continued)

**Collaborative Problem:** Potential complication: risk for bleeding problems
**Goal:** Prevention of bleeding

### NURSING INTERVENTIONS

1. Assess for potential for bleeding: monitor platelet count.

2. Assess for bleeding:
   a. Petechiae or ecchymosis
   b. Decrease in hemoglobin or hematocrit
   c. Prolonged bleeding from invasive procedures, venipunctures, minor cuts or scratches
   d. Frank or occult blood in any body excretion, emesis, sputum
   e. Bleeding from any body orifice
   f. Altered mental status

3. Instruct patient and family about ways to minimize bleeding:
   a. Use soft toothbrush or toothette for mouth care.
   b. Avoid commercial mouthwashes.
   c. Use electric razor for shaving.
   d. Use emery board for nail care.
   e. Avoid foods that are difficult to chew.

4. Initiate measures to minimize bleeding.
   a. Draw all blood for lab work with one daily venipuncture.
   b. Avoid taking temperature rectally or administering suppositories and enemas.
   c. Avoid intramuscular injections; use smallest needle possible.

### RATIONALE

1. Mild risk: 50,000–100,000/mm³ ($0.05$–$0.1 \times 10^{12}$/L)
   Moderate risk: 20,000–50,000/mm³ ($0.02$–$0.05 \times 10^{12}$/L)
   Severe risk: less than 20,000/mm³ ($0.02 \times 10^{12}$/L)

2. Early detection promotes early intervention.
   a. Indicates injury to microcirculation and larger vessels.
   b–e. Indicates blood loss.




   f. Indicates neurologic involvement.

3. Patient can participate in self-protection.
   a. Prevents trauma to oral tissues.
   b. Contain high alcohol content that will dry oral tissues.
   c. Prevents trauma to skin.
   d. Reduces risk of trauma to nailbeds.
   e. Prevents oral tissue trauma.

4. Preserves circulating blood volume.
   a. Minimizes trauma and blood loss.
   b. Prevents trauma to rectal mucosa.
   c. Prevents intramuscular bleeding.

### EXPECTED OUTCOMES

- Signs and symptoms of bleeding are identified.
- Exhibits no blood in feces, urine, or emesis.
- Exhibits no bleeding of gums or of injection or venipuncture sites.
- Exhibits no ecchymosis (bruising).
- Patient and family identify ways to prevent bleeding.
- Uses recommended measures to reduce risk of bleeding (uses soft toothbrush, shaves with electric razor only).
- Exhibits normal vital signs.
- Reports that environmental hazards have been reduced or removed.
- Consumes adequate fluid.
- Reports absence of constipation.
- Avoids substances interfering with clotting.
- Absence of tissue destruction.
- Exhibits normal mental status and absence of signs of intracranial bleeding.
- Avoids medications that interfere with clotting (eg, aspirin).
- Absence of epistaxis and cerebral bleeding.

## CHART 16-6

### Plan of Nursing Care: The Patient With Cancer (Continued)

| NURSING INTERVENTIONS | RATIONALE | EXPECTED OUTCOMES |
|---|---|---|
| d. Apply direct pressure to injection and venipuncture sites for at least 5 min. | d. Minimizes blood loss. | |
| e. Lubricate lips with petrolatum. | e. Prevents skin from drying. | |
| f. Avoid bladder catheterizations; use smallest catheter if catheterization is necessary. | f. Prevents trauma to urethra. | |
| g. Maintain fluid intake of at least 3 L/24 h unless contraindicated. | g. Hydration helps to prevent skin drying. | |
| h. Use stool softeners or increase bulk in diet. | h. Prevents constipation and straining that may injure rectal tissue. | |
| i. Avoid medications that will interfere with clotting (eg, aspirin). | i. Minimizes risk of bleeding. | |
| j. Recommend use of water-based lubricant before sexual intercourse. | j. Prevents friction and tissue trauma. | |
| 5. When platelet count is less than 20,000/mm³, institute the following: | 5. Platelet count of less than 20,000/mm³ (0.02 × 10¹²/L) is associated with increased risk of spontaneous bleeding. | |
| a. Bed rest with padded side rails | a. Reduces risk of injury | |
| b. Avoidance of strenuous activity | b. Increases intracranial pressure and risk of cerebral hemorrhage. | |
| c. Platelet transfusions as prescribed; administer prescribed diphenhydramine hydrochloride (Benadryl) or hydrocortisone sodium succinate (Solu-Cortef) to prevent reaction to platelet transfusion. | c. Allergic reactions to blood products are associated with antigen–antibody reaction that causes platelet destruction. | |
| d. Supervise activity when out of bed. | d. Reduces risk of falls. | |
| e. Caution against forceful nose blowing. | e. Prevents trauma to nasal mucosa and increased intracranial pressure. | |

The process of obtaining donor cells has evolved over the years. Donor cells can be obtained by the traditional harvesting of large amounts of bone marrow tissue under general anesthesia in the operating room. A second method, referred to as peripheral blood stem cell transplantation (PBSCT), has also gained widespread use. This method of collection uses apheresis of the donor to collect peripheral blood stem cells (PBSCs) for reinfusion. It is a safe and cost-effective means of collection rather than the traditional harvesting of marrow.

Types of BMT based on the source of donor cells include:

- Allogeneic (from a donor other than the patient): either a related donor (ie, family member) or a matched unrelated donor (national bone marrow registry, cord blood registry)

> **CHART 16-7**
>
> ### Safety in Administering Chemotherapy
>
> Safety recommendations from the Occupational Safety and Health Administration (OSHA), Oncology Nursing Society (ONS), hospitals, and other health care agencies for the preparation and handling of antineoplastic agents follow:
>
> - Use a biologic safety cabinet for the preparation of all chemotherapy agents.
> - Wear surgical gloves when handling antineoplastic agents and the excretions of patients who received chemotherapy.
> - Wear disposable, long-sleeved gowns when preparing and administering chemotherapy agents.
> - Use Luer-Lok fittings on all intravenous tubing used to deliver chemotherapy.
> - Dispose of all equipment used in chemotherapy preparation and administration in appropriate, leak-proof, puncture-proof containers.
> - Dispose of all chemotherapy wastes as hazardous materials.
>
> When followed, these precautions greatly minimize the risk of exposure to chemotherapy agents.

- Autologous (from patient)
- Syngeneic (from an identical twin)

Allogeneic BMT, used primarily for disease of the bone marrow, depends on the availability of a human leukocyte antigen–matched donor. This greatly limits the number of possible transplants. An advantage of allogeneic BMT is that the transplanted cells should not be immunologically tolerant of a patient's malignancy and should cause a lethal **graft-versus-disease effect** in the malignant cells. Allogeneic BMT may involve either ablative (high-dose) or nonablative ("mini"-dose) chemotherapy. In ablative allogeneic BMT, the recipient must undergo ablative doses of chemotherapy and possibly total body irradiation to destroy all existing bone marrow and malignant disease. The harvested donor marrow or PBSCs are infused intravenously into the recipients, and they travel to sites in the body where they produce bone marrow and establish themselves. Once engraftment is complete (2 to 4 weeks, sometimes longer), the new bone marrow becomes functional and begins producing RBCs, WBCs, and platelets. In nonablative allogeneic BMT, the chemotherapy doses are lower and are aimed at suppressing the recipient's immune system to allow engraftment of donor bone marrow or PBSCs. The lower doses of chemotherapy create less organ toxicity and thus can be offered to older patients or those with underlying organ dysfunction, for whom high-dose chemotherapy would be prohibitive. After engraftment, it is hoped that the donor cells will create a graft-versus-disease effect (Ezzone, 2004).

Before engraftment, patients are at high risk for infection, sepsis, and bleeding. Side effects of the high-dose chemotherapy and total body irradiation can be acute and chronic. Acute side effects include alopecia, hemorrhagic cystitis, nausea, vomiting, diarrhea, and severe stomatitis. Chronic side effects include sterility, pulmonary dysfunction, cardiac dysfunction, and liver disease.

To prevent **graft-versus-host disease (GVHD)**, patients receive immunosuppressant drugs, such as cyclosporine (Neoral), tacrolimus (FK 506, Prograf), or sirolimus (Rappamune). In allogeneic transplant recipients, GVHD occurs when the T lymphocytes proliferating from the transplanted donor marrow or PBSCs become activated and mount an immune response against the recipient's tissues (skin, gastrointestinal tract, liver). T lymphocytes respond in this manner because they view the recipient's tissue as "foreign," immunologically different from what they recognize as "self" in the donor. GVHD may occur acutely or chronically.

The first 100 days or so after allogeneic BMT are crucial for patients; the immune system and blood-making capacity (hematopoiesis) must recover sufficiently to prevent infection and hemorrhage. Most acute side effects, such as nausea, vomiting, and mucositis, also resolve in the initial 100 days after transplantation. Patients are also at risk for venous occlusive disease (VOD), a vascular injury to the liver caused by high-dose chemotherapy, in the first 30 days or so after BMT. VOD can lead to acute liver failure and death (Ezzone, 2004).

Autologous BMT is considered for patients with disease of the bone marrow who do not have a suitable donor for allogeneic BMT and for patients who have healthy bone marrow but require bone marrow–ablative doses of chemotherapy to cure an aggressive malignancy. Stem cells are collected from the patient and preserved for reinfusion; if necessary, they are treated to kill any malignant cells within the marrow. The patient is then treated with ablative chemotherapy and, possibly, total body irradiation to eradicate any remaining tumor. Stem cells are then reinfused and engraft. Until engraftment occurs in the bone marrow sites of the body, there is a high risk of infection, sepsis, and bleeding. Acute and chronic toxicities from chemotherapy and radiation therapy may be severe. The risk of VOD is also present after autologous transplantation. No immunosuppressant medications are necessary after autologous BMT, because the patient does not receive foreign tissue. A disadvantage of autologous transplantation is the risk that viable tumor cells may remain in the bone marrow despite high-dose chemotherapy (conditioning regimens) (Ezzone, 2004).

Syngeneic transplants use an identical twin as the marrow donor. Syngeneic transplants result in less incidence of GVHD and graft rejection; however, there is also less graft-versus-tumor effect to fight the malignancy. For this reason, even when an identical twin is available for marrow donation, another matched sibling or even an unrelated donor may be the most suitable donor to combat an aggressive malignancy.

## Nursing Management in Bone Marrow Transplantation

Nursing care of patients undergoing BMT is complex and demands a high level of skill. Transplantation nursing can be extremely rewarding yet extremely stressful. The success of BMT is greatly influenced by nursing care throughout the transplantation process.

### IMPLEMENTING PRETRANSPLANTATION CARE

All patients must undergo extensive pretransplantation evaluations to assess the current clinical status of the disease. Nutritional assessments, extensive physical examinations and organ function tests, and psychological evaluations are conducted. Blood work includes assessing past antigen exposure (eg, hepatitis virus, cytomegalovirus, herpes simplex virus, HIV, and syphilis). The patient's social support systems and financial and insurance resources are also evaluated. Informed consent and patient teaching about the procedure and pretransplantation and posttransplantation care are vital.

#### PROVIDING CARE DURING TREATMENT

Skilled nursing care is required during the treatment phase of BMT when high-dose chemotherapy (conditioning regimen) and total body irradiation are administered. The acute toxicities of nausea, diarrhea, mucositis, and hemorrhagic cystitis require close monitoring and constant attention by the nurse.

Nursing management during the bone marrow or stem cell infusions consists of monitoring the patient's vital signs and blood oxygen saturation; assessing for adverse effects, such as fever, chills, shortness of breath, chest pain, cutaneous reactions, nausea, vomiting, hypotension or hypertension, tachycardia, anxiety, and taste changes; and providing ongoing support and patient teaching.

Throughout the period of bone marrow aplasia until engraftment of the new marrow occurs, the patient is at high risk for death from sepsis and bleeding. The patient requires support with blood products and hemopoietic growth factors. Potential infections may be bacterial, viral, fungal, or protozoan in origin. Renal complications arise from the nephrotoxic chemotherapy agents used in the conditioning regimen or those used to treat infection (amphotericin B, aminoglycosides). Tumor lysis syndrome and acute tubular necrosis are also risks after BMT.

GVHD requires skillful nursing assessment to detect early effects on the skin, liver, and gastrointestinal tract. VOD resulting from the conditioning regimens used in BMT can result in fluid retention, jaundice, abdominal pain, ascites, tender and enlarged liver, and encephalopathy. Pulmonary complications, such as pulmonary edema, interstitial pneumonia, and other pneumonias, often complicate the recovery after BMT (Ezonne, 2004).

#### PROVIDING POSTTRANSPLANTATION CARE

**Caring for Recipients.** Ongoing nursing assessment in follow-up visits is essential to detect late effects of therapy after BMT, which occur 100 days or more after the procedure. Late effects include infections (eg, varicella zoster infection), restrictive pulmonary abnormalities, and recurrent pneumonias. Sterility often results. Chronic GVHD involves the skin, liver, intestine, esophagus, eyes, lungs, joints, and vaginal mucosa. Cataracts may also develop after total body irradiation.

Psychosocial assessments by nursing staff must be ongoing. In addition to the stressors affecting patients at each phase of the transplantation experience, marrow donors and family members also have psychosocial needs that must be addressed.

**Caring for Donors.** Like BMT recipients, donors also require nursing care. They commonly experience mood alterations, decreased self-esteem, and guilt from feelings of failure if the transplantation fails. Family members must be educated and supported to reduce anxiety and promote coping during this difficult time. In addition, they must also be assisted to maintain realistic expectations of themselves as well as of the patient. As BMT becomes more prevalent, many moral and ethical issues become apparent, including those related to informed consent, allocation of resources, and quality of life.

## Hyperthermia

Hyperthermia (thermal therapy), the generation of temperatures greater than physiologic fever range (greater than 41.5°C [106.7°F]), has been used for many years to destroy tumors in human cancers. Malignant cells may be more sensitive than normal cells to the harmful effects of high temperatures for several reasons. Malignant cells lack the mechanisms necessary to repair damage caused by elevated temperatures. Most tumor cells lack an adequate blood supply to provide needed oxygen during periods of increased cellular demand, such as during hyperthermia. Cancerous tumors lack blood vessels of adequate size for dissipation of heat. In addition, the body's immune system may be indirectly stimulated when hyperthermia is used.

Hyperthermia is most effective when combined with radiation therapy, chemotherapy, or biologic therapy. Hyperthermia and radiation therapy are thought to work well together because hypoxic tumor cells and cells in the S phase of the cell cycle are more sensitive to heat than radiation; the addition of heat damages tumor cells so that they cannot repair themselves after radiation therapy. Hyperthermia is thought to alter cellular membrane permeability when used with chemotherapy, allowing for an increased uptake of the chemotherapeutic agent. Hyperthermia may enhance the function of immune system cells, such as macrophages and T cells, which are stimulated by many biologic agents.

Heat can be produced by using radiowaves, ultrasound, microwaves, magnetic waves, hot-water baths, or even hot-wax immersions. Hyperthermia may be local or regional, or it may include the whole body. Local or regional hyperthermia may be delivered to a cancerous extremity (for malignant melanoma) by regional perfusion, in which the affected extremity is isolated by a tourniquet and an extracorporeal circulator heats the blood flowing through the affected part. Hyperthermia probes may also be inserted around a tumor in a local area and attached to a heat source during treatment. Chemotherapeutic agents, such as melphalan (Alkeran), may also be heated and instilled into the region's circulating blood. Local or regional hyperthermia may also include infusion of heated solutions into cancerous body organs. Whole-body hyperthermia to treat disseminated disease may be achieved by extracorporeal circulation, immersion of the patient in heated water or paraffin, or enclosure in a heated suit.

Side effects of hyperthermic treatments include skin burns and tissue damage, fatigue, hypotension, peripheral neuropathies, thrombophlebitis, nausea, vomiting, diarrhea, and electrolyte imbalances. Resistance to hyperthermia may develop during the treatment because cells adapt to repeated thermal insult. Research into the effectiveness of hyperthermia, methods of delivery, and side effects is ongoing.

## Nursing Management in Hyperthermia

Although hyperthermia has been used for many years, many patients and their families are unfamiliar with this cancer treatment. Consequently, they need explanations about the procedure, its goals, and its effects. The nurse assesses the patient for adverse effects and acts to reduce the occurrence and severity of adverse effects. Local skin care at the site of the implanted hyperthermic probes is necessary.

## Targeted Therapies

Recent advances in the fields of molecular biology, biochemistry, immunology, and genetics have lead to an improved understanding of cancer development. Traditional therapies such as chemotherapy and radiation are nonspecific, affecting all actively proliferating cells. As a result, both healthy cells and malignant cells are subject to harmful systemic effects of treatment. **Targeted therapies** seek to minimize the negative effects on healthy tissues by disrupting specific cancer cell functions such as malignant transformation, communication pathways, processes for growth and metastasis and genetic coding (Capriotti, 2004; Gemmill & Idell, 2003). Mechanisms of action of targeted therapies include stimulation or augmentation of immune responses through the use of biologic response modifiers, targeting of cancer cell growth factors, promotion of apoptosis (programmed cell death), and genetic manipulation through gene therapy (Gale, 2003; Gemmill & Idell, 2003; Lui, 2003).

### Biologic Response Modifiers

**Biologic response modifier (BRM) therapy** involves the use of naturally occurring or recombinant (reproduced through genetic engineering) agents or treatment methods that can alter the immunologic relationship between the tumor and the cancer patient (host) to provide a therapeutic benefit. Although the mechanisms of action vary with each type of BRM, the goal is to destroy or stop the malignant growth. The basis of BRM treatment lies in the restoration, modification, stimulation, or augmentation of the body's natural immune defenses against cancer (Gemmill & Idell, 2003).

#### NONSPECIFIC BIOLOGIC RESPONSE MODIFIERS

Some of the early investigations of the stimulation of the immune system involved nonspecific agents such as bacille Calmette-Guérin (BCG) and *Corynebacterium parvum*. When injected into the patient, these agents serve as antigens that stimulate an immune response. The hope is that the stimulated immune system will then eradicate malignant cells. Extensive animal and human investigations with BCG have shown promising results, especially in treating localized malignant melanoma. In addition, BCG is considered to be a standard form of treatment for localized bladder cancer. However, use of nonspecific agents in advanced cancer remains limited, and research is continuing in an effort to identify other uses and other agents (Abeloff et al., 2004).

#### MONOCLONAL ANTIBODIES

Monoclonal antibodies (MoAbs), another type of BRM, have become available through technologic advances, enabling investigators to grow and produce targeted antibodies for specific malignant cells. Theoretically, this type of specificity allows MoAbs to destroy the cancer cells and spare normal cells.

The production of MoAbs involves injecting tumor cells that act as antigens into mice (murine models). Antibodies made in response to injected antigens can be found in the spleen of the mouse. Antibody-producing spleen cells are combined with a cancer cell that has the ability to grow indefinitely in culture medium and continue producing more antibodies. The combination of spleen cells and the cancer cells is referred to as a hybridoma. From hybridomas that continue to grow in the culture medium, the desired antibodies are harvested, purified, and prepared for diagnostic or therapeutic use (Fig. 16-5). Recent advances in genetic engineering have led to the production of MoAbs with combinations of mouse and human components (*chimeric MoAbs*) or all-human components (*humanized MoAbs*). MoAbs made with human genes have greater immunologic properties and are less likely to cause allergic reactions (Schmidt & Wood, 2003).

MoAbs are being used as aids in diagnostic evaluation. By attaching radioactive substances to MoAbs, physicians can detect both primary and metastatic tumors through radiologic techniques. This process is referred to as radioimmunodetection. OncoScint (Cytogen Corp., Princeton, NJ) is a U.S. Food and Drug Administration (FDA)–approved MoAb that is used to assist in diagnosing ovarian and colorectal cancers. The use of MoAbs in detecting breast, gastric, and prostate cancers and lymphoma is under investigation. MoAbs are also used in purging residual tumor cells from the bone marrow or peripheral blood of patients who are undergoing BMT or peripheral stem cell rescue after high-dose cytotoxic therapy.

Several MoAbs have been approved for treatment in cancer (Table 16-7). Some of the MoAbs are used alone, whereas others are used in combination with agents that facilitate their antitumor actions. Gemtuzumab ozogamicin (Mylotarg) is a combination of a MoAb and the antitumor antibiotic calicheamicin, which is used for the treatment of a specific type of acute myeloid leukemia (Schmidt & Wood, 2003). Gemtuzumab ozogamicin is an example of immunoconjugate therapy or a "magic bullet" that transports cancer-killing substances to the cancer cells. Ibritumomab-tiuxetan (Zevalin) and tositumomab (Bexxar) are forms of immunoconjugate therapy that combine a monoclonal antibody and a radioactive source for the treatment of specific types of non-Hodgkin lymphoma. The monoclonal antibody delivers the radioactive source to the malignant cells, causing the cells to be destroyed by both radioactivity and normal immune responses (Schmidt & Wood, 2003). Researchers are continuing to explore the development and use of other MoAbs, either alone or in combination with other substances such as radioactive materials, chemotherapeutic agents, toxins, hormones, or other BRMs. Some specific targets for MoAbs under investigation include malignant cell growth factors, cell proteins, and substances that stimulate tumors to develop blood vessels (angiogenesis factors).

#### CYTOKINES

Cytokines, substances produced by cells of the immune system to enhance the production and functioning of com-

**FIGURE 16-5.** Antibody-producing spleen cells are fused with cancer cells. This process produces cells called hybridomas. These cells, which can grow indefinitely in a culture medium, produce antibodies that are harvested, purified, and prepared for diagnostic or treatment purposes.

ponents of the immune system, are also the focus of cancer treatment research (Janeway, Travers, Walport, et al., 2005). Cytokines are grouped into families, such as interferons, interleukins, colony-stimulating factors, and tumor necrosis factors.

**Interferons.** Interferons (IFNs) are examples of cytokines with both antiviral and antitumor properties. When stimulated, all nucleated cells are capable of producing these glycoproteins, which are classified according to their biologic and chemical properties: IFN-α is produced by leukocytes, IFN-β is produced by fibroblasts, and IFN-γ is produced by lymphocytes.

Multiple antitumor effects of IFNs, which have been identified in a variety of malignancies, include antiangiogenesis, direct destruction of tumor cells, inhibition of growth factors, and disruption of the cell cycle (Kufe et al., 2003). IFN-α has been approved by the FDA for treatment of hairy-cell leukemia, Kaposi's sarcoma, chronic myelogenous leuke-

**TABLE 16-7 Food and Drug Administration–Approved Therapeutic Monoclonal Antibodies**

| Monoclonal Antibody | Indication | Target |
|---|---|---|
| Alemtuzumab (Campath) | Chronic lymphocytic leukemia | Marker on cell membrane of lymphocytes, monocytes, and macrophages |
| Bevacizumab (Avastin) | Metastatic colorectal cancer | Vascular endothelial growth factor |
| Cetuximab (Erbitux) | Metastatic colorectal cancer | Epidermal growth factor |
| Gemtuzumab ozogamicin (Mylotarg) | Acute leukemia | Marker on cell membrane of leukemic cells |
| Ibritumomab-tiuxetan (Zevalin) | Non-Hodgkin lymphoma | Marker on cell membrane of lymphocytes |
| Rituximab (Rituxan) | Non-Hodgkin lymphoma | Marker on cell membrane of lymphocytes |
| Tositumomab (Bexxar) | Non-Hodgkin lymphoma | Marker on cell membrane of lymphocytes |
| Trastuzumab (Herceptin) | Breast cancer | Growth factor protein on cell membrane |

mia, high-grade non-Hodgkin lymphoma, renal cell cancer, cutaneous T-cell lymphoma, and melanoma. (IFN-α, IFN-β, and IFN-γ have been approved by the FDA for the treatment of several nonmalignant diseases, such as multiple sclerosis.) IFN is administered by subcutaneous, intramuscular, intravenous, and intracavitary routes. Efforts are underway to establish the effectiveness of IFN in combination with other treatment regimens for treatment of various malignancies.

**Interleukins.** Interleukins (ILs) are a subgroup of cytokines known as lymphokines and monokines because they are primarily produced by lymphocytes and monocytes. About 25 different ILs have been identified (Kufe et al., 2003). They act by signaling and coordinating other cells of the immune system. The FDA has approved IL-2 as a treatment option for renal cell cancer and metastatic melanoma in adults. Originally referred to as T-cell growth factor, IL-2 is known to stimulate the production and activation of several different types of lymphocytes. In addition, IL-2 enhances the production of other types of cytokines and plays a role in influencing both humoral and cell-mediated immunity.

Clinical trials are being conducted on IL-2 as well as other interleukins, such as IL-1, IL-4, IL-10, and IL-12, for their roles in treatment of other cancers. Some early-stage clinical trials are assessing the effects of interleukins in combination with chemotherapy (Breed, 2003; Kufe et al., 2003). In addition, ILs are being investigated as growth factors for treatment of myelosuppression after the use of some forms of chemotherapy.

**Hematopoietic Growth Factors (Colony-Stimulating Factors).** Hematopoietic growth factors, also known as colony-stimulating factors, are hormone-like substances naturally produced by cells within the immune system. Hematopoietic growth factors of different types regulate the production of all cells in the blood, including neutrophils, macrophages, monocytes, RBCs, and platelets. Use of GM-CSF, G-CSF, IL-11, and EPO, all of which are FDA-approved, has contributed significantly to the supportive care of patients with cancer (Bedell, 2003b; Cappozzo, 2004; Mock & Olsen, 2003).

Although these agents do not treat the underlying malignancy, they do target the effects of myelotoxic cancer therapies (ie, those that adversely affect the bone marrow), such as radiation and chemotherapy. Previously, the myelotoxic or bone marrow suppressive effects of chemotherapy had imposed limits on some chemotherapy agents and contributed to the development of life-threatening infections.

GM-CSF is used to treat the **neutropenia** (decreased numbers of neutrophils in the blood) associated with BMT. G-CSF is used to treat neutropenia associated with chemotherapy for solid tumor malignancies. IL-11 is used to prevent severe thrombocytopenia and reduce the need for platelet transfusions after myelosuppressive therapy for nonmyeloid cancers, but its use has been limited because of toxicities such as fatigue, edema, dysrhythmias, and syncope (Capo & Waltzman, 2004). EPO is used to treat anemia in patients with cancer as well as in those with chronic renal disease and in those with HIV infection and zidovudine-induced anemia.

## RETINOIDS
Retinoids are vitamin A derivatives (retinol, all-*trans*-retinoic acid, and 13-*cis*-retinoic acid) that play a role in growth, reproduction, programmed cell death (*apoptosis*), epithelial cell differentiation, and immune function. All-*trans*-retinoic acid (tretinoin) is used in treating acute promyelocytic leukemia, a rare form of leukemia, and cutaneous T-cell lymphoma. Retinoids are being tested for treatment of both hematologic cancers and solid tumors and for prevention of a variety of cancers such as prostate and brain cancers (Galsky & Kelly, 2003; Kristal, 2004).

## CANCER VACCINES
Like viral and bacterial vaccines, cancer vaccines are given to mobilize the body's immune response. Cancer vaccines stimulate the immune system to recognize and attack cancer cells (King, 2004). Cancer vaccines contain either portions of cancer cells alone or portions of cells in combination with other substances (adjuvants) that can augment or boost immune responses. *Autologous* vaccines are made from the patient's own cancer cells, which are obtained during diagnostic biopsy or surgery. The cancer cells are killed and prepared for injection back into the patient. *Allogeneic* vaccines are made from cancer cells that are obtained from other people who have a specific type of cancer. These cancer cells are grown in a laboratory and eventually killed and prepared for injection.

*Prophylactic* vaccines, such as polio vaccine, are given to prevent people from developing a disease. *Therapeutic* vaccines are given to kill existing cancer cells and to provide long-lasting immunity against further cancer development. Multiple clinical trials are being conducted to develop therapeutic vaccines for cancers of the prostate, breast, kidney, and lung, as well as for melanoma, myeloma, and lymphoma (King, 2004). A vaccine that prevents cervical cancer due to two types of human papillomavirus (HPV) is the first to be shown to be effective in prevention of cancer. If widespread use of the vaccine is adopted, it is predicted that the incidence of cervical cancer in vaccinated populations will decrease significantly (National Cancer Institute, 2006).

## NURSING MANAGEMENT IN BIOLOGIC RESPONSE MODIFIER THERAPY
Patients receiving BRM therapy have many of the same needs as cancer patients undergoing other treatment approaches. However, some BRM therapies are still investigational and are considered a last-chance effort by many patients who have not responded to standard treatments. Consequently, it is essential for the nurse to assess the need for education, support, and guidance for both the patient and the family and assist in planning and evaluating patient care.

**Monitoring Therapeutic and Adverse Effects.** The nurse should be familiar with each agent given and its potential effects (Table 16-8). Adverse effects, such as fever, myalgia, nausea, and vomiting, as seen with IFN therapy, may not be life-threatening. However, the nurse must be aware of the impact of these side effects on the patient's quality of life. Other life-threatening adverse effects (eg, capillary leak syndrome, pulmonary edema, hypotension) may occur with IL-2 therapy. The nurse must work closely with the physician to assess and manage potential toxicities of BRM therapy. Because of the investigational nature of many of these agents, the nurse often administers them in a research setting. Accurate observations and careful documentation

## TABLE 16-8  Side Effects of FDA-Approved Biologic Response

| Agent | Selected Side Effects |
|---|---|
| **Monoclonal Antibodies** | |
| Alemtuzumab | Allergic/anaphylactic reactions; fever; chills; rash; hives; itching; sweating; nausea; vomiting; diarrhea; stomatitis; abdominal pain; indigestion; infection; headache; dizziness; muscle pain; insomnia; dyspnea; cough; bronchitis/pneumonitis; pharyngitis; fatigue; skeletal pain; anorexia; weakness; peripheral edema; decreased white blood cell (WBC), platelet, and red blood cell (RBC) counts |
| Bevacizumab | Weakness; abdominal pain; deep vein thrombosis; hypertension; syncope; diarrhea; constipation; decreased WBC count; hemorrhage; gastrointestinal perforation; proteinuria; congestive heart failure |
| Cetuximab | Allergic/anaphylactic reactions; fever; chills; rash; hives; itching; acne-like rash; lung inflammation; sepsis; pulmonary embolus; kidney failure; malaise; weakness; diarrhea; nausea; abdominal pain; vomiting; anorexia; constipation; insomnia |
| Gemtuzumab | Allergic/anaphylactic reactions; fever; chills; weakness; abdominal pain; headache; dyspnea; epistaxis; cough; tachycardia; hemorrhage; local skin reaction; rash; petechiae; peripheral edema; nausea; vomiting; diarrhea; anorexia; stomatitis; constipation; indigestion; dizziness; decreased platelet, WBC and RBC counts; increased bilirubin, potassium, and lactate dehydrogenase (LDH) values |
| Ibritumomab | Decreased platelets, WBC and RBC counts; weakness; chills; abdominal pain; fever; difficulty breathing; nausea and vomiting |
| Rituximab | Allergic/anaphylactic reactions; fever; chills; nausea; headache; abdominal pain; decreased lymphocyte, WBC, platelet, and RBC counts; back pain; night sweats; itching; cough; infection |
| Tositumomab | Allergic/anaphylactic reactions; fever chills, rash, hives, itching; anemia; decreased WBC count; bone marrow impairment; hypothyroidism; infection; nausea; vomiting; abdominal pain; diarrhea; difficulty breathing; headache; weakness; myalgias; arthralgias |
| Trastuzumab | Allergic/anaphylactic reactions; hypotension; fever; chills; heart failure; stroke; diarrhea; infection; rash; nausea; vomiting; anorexia; insomnia; dizziness; headache; chills; back pain; weakness; rhinitis; pharyngitis; cough |
| **Cytokines** | |
| Interferon alfa | Flu-like symptoms (fever, chills, weakness, muscle and joint pain, headaches); fatigue; anorexia; mental status changes; rash; pruritus; hair loss; abdominal pain; nausea; constipation; diarrhea; irritation at the injection site; depression; irritability; insomnia; cough; decreased WBC, RBC, and platelet counts; abnormal liver function values |
| Interleukin-2 | Flu-like symptoms (fever, chills, weakness, muscle and joint pain, headaches); fatigue; anorexia; nausea; vomiting; diarrhea; capillary leak syndrome; edema and fluid retention; hypotension; tachycardia; skin rash; erythema; desquamation; irritation at the injection site; weight gain during therapy due to fluid retention; weight loss after therapy related to anorexia with long-term therapy; decreased WBC, RBC, and platelet counts; abnormal liver function values |
| Filgrastim (granulocyte growth factor) | Bone pain, malaise, fever, fatigue, headache, skin rash, weakness |
| Sargranstim (granulocyte-macrophage growth factor) | Allergic/anaphylactic reaction with first dose; bone pain; fever; fatigue; headache; weakness; chills; skin rash; infection |
| Epoetin alfa (erythrocyte growth factor) | Fever; fatigue; weakness; bone pain; diarrhea; dizziness; nausea; edema; shortness of breath |
| Oprelvekin (platelet growth factor) | Edema; fever; headache; rash; chills; bone pain; fatigue; nausea; vomiting; abdominal pain; constipation; rhinitis; cough; arrhythmia; skin discoloration; bleeding; dehydration; amblyopia; dermatitis |
| **Retinoids** | |
| Retinoic acid | Headache; fever; skin and mucous membrane dryness; bone pain; nausea and vomiting; dyspnea; pleural and pericardial effusions; malaise; chills; bleeding; heart failure; mental status changes; depression; abnormal liver function tests |

are essential components of patient assessment and data collection.

**Promoting Home and Community-Based Care.** The nurse teaches patients self-care and assists in providing for continuing care. Some BRMs, such as IFN, EPO, and G-CSF, can be administered by the patient or family members at home. As needed, the nurse teaches the patient and family how to administer these agents through subcutaneous injections. The nurse also provides instructions about side effects and helps the patient and family identify strategies to manage many of the common side effects of BRM therapy, such as fatigue, anorexia, and flu-like symptoms.

Referral for home care is usually indicated to monitor the patient's responses to treatment and to continue and reinforce patient and family teaching. During home visits, the nurse assesses the patient's and family members' technique in administering medications. The nurse collaborates with physicians, third-party payors, and pharmaceutical companies to help the patient obtain reimbursement for home administration of BRM therapies. The nurse also reminds the patient about the importance of keeping follow-up appointments with the physician and assesses the patient's need for changes in care.

### Gene Therapy

As early as 1914, the somatic mutation theory of cancer suggested that cancer develops as a result of inherited or acquired genetic mutations that lead to a disturbance in the normal chromosomal balance regulating cell growth and reproduction. Technologic advances and information gained through intense study of genetics have helped researchers and clinicians predict, diagnose, and treat cancer. Gene therapy includes approaches that correct genetic defects or manipulate genes to induce tumor cell destruction in the hope of preventing or combating disease.

Three general approaches have been used in the development of gene therapies.

- *Tumor-directed therapy* is introduction of a therapeutic gene (suicide gene) into tumor cells in an attempt to destroy them. This approach is very challenging, because it is difficult to identify which gene would be the most beneficial. In addition, patients with widespread disease would require multiple injections to treat every site of disease.
- *Active immunotherapy* is the administration of genes that will invoke the antitumor responses of the immune system (Lui, 2003).
- *Adoptive immunotherapy* is the administration of genetically altered lymphocytes that are programmed to cause tumor destruction.

Although gene therapy is currently investigational, researchers predict that it will have a profound impact on health care in the 21st century. More than 150 clinical trials in various stages are exploring gene therapy as a treatment for cancer. Tumor-directed gene therapy is being investigated as a treatment for brain, colorectal, and prostate cancers (Lui, 2003); active immunotherapy has been investigated in the treatment of malignant melanoma (Lui, 2003); and adoptive immunotherapy is being explored in the treatment of ovarian, renal, and brain cancers. For more information about investigational therapies, see Chart 16-4.

### Growth Factors

The secretion of growth factors permits cancer cells to avoid apoptosis (normal cell destruction) and grow in an uncontrolled fashion. In addition, growth factors enable cancer cells to develop their own blood supply (angiogenesis), allowing them to continue growing and metastasize to distant sites. Many of the new targeted therapy agents are directed at promoting apoptosis or inhibiting growth factor production and actions (Gemmill & Idell, 2003). Bortezomib (Velcade), which has been approved for the treatment of myeloma, induces cancer cell destruction (Colson, Doss, Swift, et al., 2004). Gefitinib (Iressa), used in the treatment of lung cancer, is an oral agent that targets a specific cancer cell growth factor referred to as epidermal growth factor (Gale, 2003). Many other agents are currently in clinical trials to determine their efficacy in preventing tumor growth and angiogenesis (Gale, 2003).

## Photodynamic Therapy

Photodynamic therapy, or phototherapy, is a cancer treatment that uses photosensitizing agents, such as porfimer (Photofrin). When administered intravenously, these agents are retained in higher concentrations in malignant tissue than in normal tissue. They are then activated by a light source, usually laser light, which penetrates body tissue. The light-activated agent creates activated singlet oxygen molecules that are cytotoxic or harmful to body tissue cells. Because most of the photosensitizing agent has been retained in malignant tissue, a selective cytotoxicity can be achieved with minimal destruction to normal tissues.

Cancers treated with phototherapy include esophageal cancers, lung tumors, and precancerous lesions of the esophagus called Barrett esophagus. The major side effect of therapy is photosensitivity for 4 to 6 weeks after treatment. Patients must protect themselves from direct and indirect sunlight to prevent skin burns. In addition, local reactions are observed in the area treated (Ernst & LoCicero, 2004).

## Unproven and Unconventional Therapies

A diagnosis of cancer evokes many emotions in patients and families, including feelings of fear, frustration, and loss of control. Despite increasing 5-year survival rates with the use of traditional methods of treatment, a significant number of patients use or seriously consider using some form of unconventional treatment. Hopelessness, desperation, unmet needs, lack of factual information, and family or social pressures are major factors that motivate patients to seek unconventional methods of treatment and allow them to fall prey to deceptive practices and quackery.

Unconventional treatments have not demonstrated scientifically—in an objective, reproducible method—the ability to cure or control cancer. In addition to being ineffective, some unconventional treatments may also be harmful to the patient and may cost thousands of dollars. Although research is scant and accuracy of reports may be questionable, it is estimated that as many as 64% of patients with cancer use complementary or alternative methods of treatment (Abeloff et al., 2004).

Caring for patients who choose unconventional methods may place members of the health care team in difficult situations professionally, legally, and ethically. The nurse must keep in mind ethical principles that help guide professional practice, such as autonomy, beneficence, nonmaleficence, and justice.

### Machines and Devices

Electrical gadgets and devices are commonly reputed to cure cancers. Most are operated by people with questionable training who report unrealistic and unlikely success stories. Such machines are often decorated with elaborate lights and dials and produce vibrations or other sensations.

### Drugs and Biologic Agents

Medicinal agents, herbs, proteins (eg, shark cartilage), megavitamins (including vitamin C), immune therapy, vaccines, enzymes, hydrogen peroxide, and sera have been frequent components of fraudulent cancer therapies. These agents have included oral, intravenous, and external medications derived from weeds, flowers, and herbs, as well as from the blood and urine of patients and animals. Many of these agents, especially in megadoses, can be toxic and can have untoward interactions with concomitant medications. Herbs commonly used by people with cancer include echinacea, essiac, ginseng, green tea, pau d'arco, and hoxsey (Montbriand, 2004). Many of these treatments are very costly.

### Metabolic and Dietary Regimens

Metabolic and dietary regimens emphasize the ingestion of only natural substances to purify the body and retard cancerous growth. These regimens include the grape diet; the carrot juice diet; and intake of garlic, onions, various teas, coffee enemas, and raw liver. Laetrile (vitamin B, amygdalin), one of the best-known substances in cancer quackery, was advocated as an agent to kill tumor cells by releasing cyanide, which is especially toxic to malignant cells. The National Cancer Institute, in response to public demand, investigated the effects of laetrile and reported no therapeutic benefits with its use; indeed, many toxic effects (cyanide poisoning, fever, rash, headache, vomiting, diarrhea, and hypotension) were reported. Macrobiotic diets have also been advocated as a cancer treatment to reestablish balance between the major forces in the universe, yin and yang. People who adhere to macrobiotic diets tend to develop vitamin, mineral, and protein deficiencies; experience additional weight loss due to decreased calorie intake; and receive no therapeutic benefits from the diet.

### Mystical and Spiritual Approaches

Traditional Chinese medicine attempts to balance chi forces in order to heal the body. Mystical or spiritual approaches to cancer therapy include such techniques as psychic surgery, faith healing, "laying on of hands," prayer groups, and invocation of mystical universal powers to kill cancerous growths. These techniques are difficult to disclaim because they are based on faith (Abeloff et al., 2004).

### Nursing Management in Unconventional Therapies

The most effective way to protect patients and families from fraudulent therapies and questionable cancer cures is to establish a trusting relationship, provide supportive care, and promote hope. Truthful responses given in a nonjudgmental manner to questions and inquiries about unproven methods of cancer treatments may alleviate the fear and guilt on the part of the patient and family that they are not "doing everything we can" to obtain a cure. The nurse may inform the patient and family of the characteristics common to fraudulent therapies so that they will be informed and cautious when evaluating other forms of "therapy." The nurse also should encourage patients who use unconventional therapies to inform their physicians about such use. This knowledge can help prevent interactions with medications and other therapies that may be prescribed and avoid attributing the side effects of unconventional therapies to prescribed medications.

## Nursing Process

### The Patient With Cancer

The outlook for patients with cancer has greatly improved because of scientific and technologic advances. However, as a result of the underlying disease or various treatment modalities, patients with cancer may experience a variety of secondary problems, such as infection, reduced WBC counts, bleeding, skin problems, nutritional problems, pain, fatigue, and psychological stress.

### Assessment

Regardless of the type of cancer treatment or prognosis, many patients with cancer are susceptible to the following problems and complications. An important role of nurses on oncology teams is to assess patients for these problems and complications.

### Infection

For patients in all stages of cancer, the nurse assesses factors that can promote infection. Infection is the leading cause of death in cancer patients. Factors predisposing patients to infection are summarized in Table 16-9. The nurse monitors laboratory studies to detect early changes in WBC counts. Common sites of infection, such as the pharynx, skin, perianal area, urinary tract, and respiratory tract, are assessed frequently. However, the typical signs of infection

| TABLE 16-9 | Factors Predisposing Cancer Patients to Infection |
|---|---|
| **Factors** | **Underlying Mechanisms** |
| Impaired skin and mucous membrane integrity | Loss of body's first line of defense against invading organisms. |
| Chemotherapy | Many agents cause suppression of bone marrow, resulting in decreased production and function of white blood cells. Chemotherapy agents that cause mucositis impair skin and mucous membrane integrity. Organ damage associated with certain agents may also predispose patients to infection. Organ damage such as pulmonary fibrosis or cardiomyopathy that is associated with certain agents may also predispose patients to infection. |
| Radiation therapy | Radiation involving sites of bone marrow production may result in bone marrow suppression. May also lead to impaired tissue integrity. |
| Biologic response modifiers | Some biologic response modifiers may cause bone marrow suppression and organ dysfunction. |
| Malignancy | Malignant cells may infiltrate the bone marrow and interfere with production of white blood cells and lymphocytes. Hematologic malignancies (leukemias and lymphomas) are associated with impaired function and production of blood cells. |
| Malnutrition | Results in impaired production and function of cells of the immune response. May contribute to impaired skin integrity. |
| Medications | Antibiotics disturb the balance of normal flora, allowing them to become pathogenic. This process occurs most commonly in the gastrointestinal tract. Corticosteroids and nonsteroidal anti-inflammatory drugs (NSAIDs) mask inflammatory responses. |
| Urinary catheter | Creates port and mechanism of entry for organisms. |
| Intravenous catheter | Results in impaired skin integrity and site of entry for organisms. |
| Other invasive procedures (surgery, paracentesis, thoracentesis, drainage tubes, endoscopy, mechanical ventilation) | Create port of entry and possible introduction of exogenous organisms into the system. |
| Contaminated equipment | Environmental objects such as stagnant water in oxygen equipment are associated with growth of microorganisms. |
| Age | Increasing age is associated with declining organ function and decreased production and functioning of the cells of the immune system. |
| Chronic illness | Associated with impaired organ function and altered immune responses. |
| Prolonged hospitalization | Allows increased exposure to nosocomial infection and colonization by new organisms. |

(swelling, redness, drainage, and pain) may not occur in immunosuppressed patients because of a diminished local inflammatory response. Fever may be the only sign of infection. The nurse also monitors the patient for sepsis, particularly if invasive catheters or infusion lines are in place.

WBC function is often impaired in patients with cancer. There are three types of WBCs: neutrophils (granulocytes), basophils, and eosinophils. The neutrophils, totaling 60% to 70% of all the body's WBCs, play a major role in combating infection by engulfing and destroying infective agents in a process called phagocytosis. Both the total WBC count and the concentration of neutrophils are important in determining the patient's ability to fight infection. A decrease in circulating WBCs is referred to as leukopenia. Granulocytopenia is a decrease in neutrophils.

A differential WBC count identifies the relative numbers of WBCs and permits tabulation of polymorphonuclear neutrophils (mature neutrophils, reported as "polys," PMNs, or "segs") and immature forms of neutrophils (reported as bands, metamyelocytes, and "stabs"). These numbers are compiled and reported as the absolute neutrophil count (ANC). The ANC is calculated by the following formula:

$$ANC = \frac{(\text{Total WBC count}) \times [\% \text{ segmented neutrophils} + \% \text{ bands}]}{100}$$

For example, if the total WBC count is 6000 cells/mm$^3$, with segmented neutrophils 25% and bands 25%, the ANC is 3000 cells/mm$^3$.

Neutropenia, an abnormally low ANC, is associated with an increased risk for infection. The risk for infection rises as the ANC decreases and persists. An ANC of less than 1000 cells/mm$^3$ reflects a severe risk of infection. **Nadir** is the lowest ANC after myelosuppressive chemotherapy or radiation therapy. Therapies that suppress bone marrow function are called myelosuppressive. Febrile patients who are neutropenic are assessed for infection through cultures of blood, sputum, urine, stool, catheter, or wounds, if appropriate. In addition, a chest x-ray is often included to assess for pulmonary infections.

## *Bleeding*

The nurse assesses the patient with cancer for factors that may contribute to bleeding. These include bone marrow suppression from radiation, chemotherapy, and other medications that interfere with coagulation and platelet functioning, such as aspirin, dipyridamole (Persantine), heparin, or warfarin (Coumadin). Common bleeding sites include skin and mucous membranes; the intestinal, urinary, and respiratory tracts; and the brain. Gross hemorrhage, as well as blood in the stools, urine, sputum, or vomitus (melena, hematuria, hemoptysis, hematemesis); oozing at injection sites; bruising (ecchymosis); petechiae; and changes in mental status, are monitored and reported.

## *Skin Problems*

The nurse assesses the patient with cancer for any skin problems. Maintaining integrity of skin and tissue poses a problem for patients with cancer because of the effects of chemotherapy, radiation therapy, surgery, and invasive procedures carried out for diagnosis and therapy. As part of the assessment, the nurse identifies which of these predisposing factors are present and assesses the patient for other risk factors, including nutritional deficits, bowel and bladder incontinence, immobility, immunosuppression, multiple skin folds, and changes related to aging. The nurse notes the presence of skin lesions or ulcerations secondary to the tumor. Alterations in tissue integrity throughout the gastrointestinal tract are particularly bothersome to patients. The nurse notes the presence of any lesions of the oral mucous membranes and whether they affect the patient's nutritional status and comfort level.

## *Hair Loss*

The nurse notes the presence of **alopecia** (hair loss), which is another form of tissue disruption common in patients with cancer who receive radiation therapy or chemotherapy. In addition, the nurse assesses the psychological impact of this side effect on the patient and family.

## *Nutritional Concerns*

Assessment of the patient's nutritional status is an important nursing role. Impaired nutritional status may contribute to disease progression, decreased survival, immune incompetence, increased incidence of infection, delayed tissue repair, diminished functional ability, decreased capacity to continue antineoplastic therapy, increased length of hospital stay, and impaired psychosocial functioning. Altered nutritional status, weight loss, and cachexia (muscle wasting, emaciation) may be secondary to decreased protein and caloric intake, metabolic or mechanical effects of the cancer, systemic disease, side effects of the treatment, or the patient's emotional status.

The patient's weight and caloric intake are monitored on a consistent basis. Other information obtained by assessment includes diet history, any episodes of anorexia, changes in appetite, situations and foods that aggravate or relieve anorexia, and medication history. Difficulty in chewing or swallowing is identified, and the presence of nausea, vomiting, or diarrhea is noted.

Clinical and laboratory data useful in assessing nutritional status include anthropometric measurements (triceps skin fold and middle-upper arm circumference), serum protein levels (albumin and transferrin), serum electrolytes, lymphocyte count, skin response to intradermal injection of antigens, hemoglobin levels, hematocrit, urinary creatinine levels, and serum iron levels.

## *Pain*

The nurse assesses the patient with cancer for the source and site of pain. In cancer, pain and discomfort may be related to underlying disease, pressure exerted by the tumor, diagnostic procedures, or the cancer treatment itself. As in any other situation involving pain, cancer pain is affected by both physical and psychosocial influences.

The nurse also assesses those factors that increase the patient's perception of pain, such as fear and apprehension, fatigue, anger, and social isolation. Pain assessment scales (see Chapter 13) are useful for assessing the patient's pain before pain-relieving interventions are instituted and for evaluating the effectiveness of these interventions.

## *Fatigue*

To make an accurate assessment, the nurse must distinguish between acute fatigue, which occurs after an energy-demanding experience, and chronic fatigue, which is often overwhelming, excessive, and not responsive to rest. Acute fatigue serves a protective function, whereas chronic fatigue does not. Chronic fatigue seriously affects quality of life. Fatigue is the most commonly reported side effect in patients who receive chemotherapy and radiation therapy. The nurse assesses for feelings of weariness, weakness, lack of energy, inability to carry out necessary and valued daily functions, lack of motivation, and inability to concentrate. The patient may become less verbal and may appear pale, with relaxed facial musculature. The nurse assesses physiologic and psychological stressors that can contribute to fatigue, including pain, nausea, dyspnea, constipation, fear, and anxiety.

### Psychosocial Status

Nursing assessment also focuses on the patient's psychological and mental status as the patient and family face this life-threatening experience, unpleasant diagnostic tests and treatment modalities, and progression of disease. The nurse assesses the patient's mood and emotional reaction to the results of diagnostic testing and prognosis and looks for evidence that the patient is progressing through the stages of grief and can talk about the diagnosis and prognosis with family members.

### Body Image

The nurse identifies potential threats to the patient's body image and assesses the patient's ability to cope with the many assaults to body image he or she experiences throughout the course of disease and treatment. Entry into the health care system is often accompanied by depersonalization. Threats to self-concept are enormous as the patient faces the realization of illness, disfigurement, possible disability, and death. To accommodate treatments or because of the disease, many patients with cancer are forced to alter their lifestyles. Priorities and values change when body image is threatened. Disfiguring surgery, hair loss, cachexia, skin changes, altered communication patterns, and sexual dysfunction are some of the devastating results of cancer and its treatment that threaten the patients' self-esteem and body image.

## Diagnosis

### Nursing Diagnoses

Based on the assessment data, nursing diagnoses for the patient with cancer may include the following:

- Impaired oral mucous membrane
- Impaired tissue integrity
- Impaired tissue integrity: alopecia
- Impaired tissue integrity: malignant skin lesions
- Imbalanced nutrition, less than body requirements
- Anorexia
- Malabsorption
- Cachexia
- Chronic pain
- Fatigue
- Disturbed body image
- Anticipatory grieving

### Collaborative Problems/ Potential Complications

Based on the assessment data, potential complications include the following:

- Infection and sepsis
- Hemorrhage
- Superior vena cava syndrome (SVCS)
- Spinal cord compression
- Hypercalcemia
- Pericardial effusion
- Disseminated intravascular coagulation (DIC)
- Syndrome of inappropriate secretion of antidiuretic hormone (SIADH)
- Tumor lysis syndrome

See the section on oncologic emergencies for more information.

## Planning and Goal

The major goals for the patient may include management of stomatitis, maintenance of tissue integrity, maintenance of nutrition, relief of pain, relief of fatigue, improved body image, effective progression through the grieving process, and absence of complications.

## Nursing Interventions

Patients with cancer are at risk for various adverse effects of therapy and complications. Nurses in all health care settings, including the home, help patients and families manage these problems.

### Managing Stomatitis

**Mucositis** is a common side effect of radiation and some types of chemotherapy that may lead to inflammation and ulceration of any portion of the gastrointestinal tract from the oral cavity throughout the alimentary canal. One form of mucositis, **stomatitis**, is an inflammatory response of the oral tissues that is characterized by mild redness (erythema) and edema or, if severe, by painful ulcerations, bleeding, and secondary infection. Stomatitis commonly develops 5 to 14 days after patients receive certain chemotherapeutic agents, such as doxorubicin and 5-fluorouracil, and BRMs, such as IL-2 and IFN. As many as 40% of patients receiving chemotherapy experience some degree of stomatitis during treatment. Patients receiving dose-intensive chemotherapy (considerably higher doses than conventional dosing), such as those undergoing BMT, are at increased risk for stomatitis. Stomatitis may also occur after radiation treatments to the head and neck.

As a result of normal everyday wear and tear, the epithelial cells that line the oral cavity undergo rapid turnover and slough off routinely. Until recently, stomatitis was thought to occur because chemotherapy and radiation interfered with this process. Recent molecular studies have improved our understanding of the processes involved. Both chemotherapy and radiation generate chemical substances that lead to the destruction of cells in the mucosa of the epithelium, connective tissue, and blood vessels in the oral cavity (McGuire & Peterson, 2004). This initiates the inflammatory process, leading to further tissue damage. The end result is ulceration and impaired oral tissues. Normal flora of the oral cavity invade the ulcerations and cause additional damage. Poor oral hygiene, existing dental disease, use of other medications that dry mucous membranes, advanced age, smoking, previous cancer treatment, diminished renal function, and impaired nutritional status all contribute to morbidity associated with stomatitis. Radiation-induced xerostomia (dry mouth) associated with decreased function of the salivary glands may contribute to stomatitis in patients who have received radiation to the head and neck.

Myelosuppression (bone marrow depression), resulting from underlying disease or its treatment, predisposes the patient to oral bleeding and infection. Severe pain associated with ulcerated oral tissues can significantly interfere with nutritional intake, speech, and a willingness to maintain oral hygiene. Advanced stomatitis may cause or prolong hospitalizations. In addition, stomatitis may lead to interruptions in chemotherapy and radiation administration or decreases in the intended dosing until the inflammation subsides. Further, it may significantly reduce the patient's quality of life (Garfunkel, 2004).

Although multiple studies on stomatitis have been published, the optimal prevention and treatment approaches have not been identified. Future studies will focus on addressing the cascade of inflammatory events and release of chemical substances that lead to the cellular and tissue destruction underlying stomatitis. At this time, most clinicians agree that good oral hygiene, including brushing, flossing, and rinsing, is necessary to minimize the risk of oral complications associated with cancer therapies. Soft-bristled toothbrushes and nonabrasive toothpaste prevent or reduce trauma to the oral mucosa. Oral swabs with spongelike applicators may be used in place of a toothbrush for painful oral tissues. Flossing may be performed unless it causes pain or unless platelet levels are less than 40,000/mm$^3$ (0.04 × 10$^{12}$/L). Oral rinses with saline solution or tap water may be necessary for patients who cannot tolerate toothbrushing. Products that irritate oral tissues or impair healing, such as alcohol-based mouth rinses, are avoided. Foods that are difficult to chew or are hot or spicy are avoided to minimize further trauma. The patient's lips are lubricated to keep them from becoming dry and cracked. Topical anti-inflammatory and anesthetic agents may be prescribed to promote healing and minimize discomfort. Products that coat or protect oral mucosa are used to promote comfort and prevent further trauma. Patients who experience severe pain and discomfort with stomatitis require systemic analgesics.

Adequate fluid and food intake is encouraged. In some instances, parenteral hydration and nutrition are necessary. Topical or systemic antifungal and antibiotic medications are prescribed to treat local or systemic infections.

Palifermin (Kepivance), a synthetic form of human keratinocyte growth factor, is an intravenous medication approved in 2005 by the FDA for treatment of mucositis in patients with cancer who are undergoing chemotherapy and radiation prior to BMT. Palifermin appears to promote more rapid replacement of cells in the mouth and gastrointestinal tract (Spielberger, Stiff, Bensinger, et al., 2004). It has not yet been tested in other patients with cancer. Careful timing of administration and monitoring are essential for maximum effectiveness and to detect adverse effects.

### Maintaining Tissue Integrity

Some of the most frequently encountered disturbances of tissue integrity, in addition to stomatitis, include skin and tissue reactions to radiation therapy, alopecia, and metastatic skin lesions. Patients with skin and tissue reactions to radiation therapy require careful skin care to prevent further skin irritation, drying, and damage. The skin over the affected area is handled gently; rubbing and use of hot or cold water, soaps, powders, lotions, and cosmetics are avoided. Patients may avoid tissue injury by wearing loose-fitting clothes and avoiding clothes that constrict, irritate, or rub the affected area. If blistering occurs, care is taken not to disrupt the blisters, thus reducing the risk of introducing bacteria. Moisture- and vapor-permeable dressings, such as hydrocolloids and hydrogels, are helpful in promoting healing and reducing pain. Aseptic wound care is indicated to minimize the risk for infection and sepsis. Topical antibiotics, such as 1% silver sulfadiazine cream (Silvadene), may be prescribed for use on areas of moist desquamation (painful, red, moist skin).

### Helping Patients Cope With Alopecia

The temporary or permanent thinning or complete loss of hair is a potential adverse effect of various radiation therapies and chemotherapeutic agents. The extent of alopecia depends on the dose and duration of therapy. These treatments cause alopecia by damaging stem cells and hair follicles. As a result, the hair is brittle and may fall out or break off at the surface of the scalp. Loss of other body hair is less frequent. Hair loss usually begins 2 to 3 weeks after the initiation of treatment; regrowth begins within 8 weeks after the last treatment. Some patients who undergo radiation to the head may sustain permanent hair loss. Many health care providers view hair loss as a minor problem when compared with the potentially life-threatening consequences of cancer. However, for many patients, hair loss is a major assault on body image, resulting in depression, anxiety, anger, rejection, and isolation. To patients and families, hair loss can serve as a constant reminder of the challenges cancer places on their coping abilities, interpersonal relationships, and sexuality.

The nurse provides information about alopecia and supports the patient and family in coping with disturbing effects of therapy, such as hair loss and changes in body image. The patient is encouraged to acquire a wig or hairpiece before hair loss occurs so that the replacement matches the patient's own hair.

Use of attractive scarves and hats may make the patient feel less conspicuous. The nurse can refer the patient to supportive programs, such as "Look Good, Feel Better," offered by the American Cancer Society. Knowledge that hair usually begins to regrow after therapy is completed may comfort some patients, although the color and texture of the new hair may be different.

## Managing Malignant Skin Lesions

Skin lesions may occur with local extension of the tumor or embolization of the tumor into the epithelium and its surrounding lymph and blood vessels. Secondary growth of cancer cells into the skin may result in redness (erythematous areas), or it may progress to wounds involving tissue necrosis and infection. The most extensive lesions tend to disintegrate and are purulent and malodorous. In addition, these lesions are a source of considerable pain and discomfort. Although this type of lesion is most often associated with breast cancer and head and neck cancers, it can also occur with lymphoma, leukemia, melanoma, and cancers of the lung, uterus, kidney, colon, and bladder. The development of severe skin lesions is usually associated with a poor prognosis for extended survival.

Ulcerating skin lesions usually indicate widely disseminated disease that is unlikely to be eradicated. Managing these lesions becomes a nursing priority. Nursing care includes carefully assessing and cleansing the skin, reducing superficial bacteria, controlling bleeding, reducing odor, protecting the skin from further trauma, and relieving pain. The patient and family require assistance and guidance to care for these skin lesions at home. Referral for home care is indicated.

## Promoting Nutrition

Most patients with cancer experience some weight loss during their illness. Anorexia, malabsorption, and cachexia are examples of nutritional problems that commonly occur in patients with cancer; special attention is needed to prevent weight loss and promote nutrition.

### ANOREXIA

Among the many causes of anorexia in patients with cancer are alterations in taste, manifested by increased salty, sour, and metallic taste sensations, and altered responses to sweet and bitter flavors; these changes lead to decreased appetite, decreased nutritional intake, and protein–calorie malnutrition. Taste alterations may result from mineral (eg, zinc) deficiencies, increases in circulating amino acids and cellular metabolites, or the administration of chemotherapeutic agents. Patients undergoing radiation therapy to the head and neck may experience "mouth blindness," which is a severe impairment of taste.

Alterations in the sense of smell also alter taste; this is a common experience of patients with head and neck cancers. Anorexia may occur because people feel full after eating only a small amount of food. This sense of fullness occurs secondary to a decrease in digestive enzymes, abnormalities in the metabolism of glucose and triglycerides, and prolonged stimulation of gastric volume receptors, which convey the feeling of being full. Psychological distress (eg, fear, pain, depression, and isolation) throughout illness may also have a negative impact on appetite. Patients may develop an aversion to food because of nausea and vomiting after treatment.

### MALABSORPTION

Many patients with cancer are unable to absorb nutrients from the gastrointestinal system as a result of tumor activity and cancer treatment. Tumors can affect the gastrointestinal activity in several ways. They may impair enzyme production or produce fistulas. They secrete hormones and enzymes, such as gastrin; this leads to increased gastrointestinal irritation, peptic ulcer disease, and decreased fat digestion. They also interfere with protein digestion.

Chemotherapy and radiation can irritate and damage mucosal cells of the bowel, inhibiting absorption. Radiation therapy can cause sclerosis of the blood vessels in the bowel and fibrotic changes in the gastrointestinal tissue. Surgical intervention may change peristaltic patterns, alter gastrointestinal secretions, and reduce the absorptive surfaces of the gastrointestinal mucosa, all leading to malabsorption.

### CACHEXIA

Cachexia is common in patients with cancer, especially in advanced disease. Cancer cachexia is related to inadequate nutritional intake along with increasing metabolic demand, increased energy expenditure due to anaerobic metabolism of the tumor, impaired glucose metabolism, competition of the tumor cells for nutrients, altered lipid metabolism, and a suppressed appetite. In addition, current literature suggests that cachexia in cancer may be related to a cytokine-induced inflammatory response (Holder, 2003; MacDonald, 2003). Cachexia is characterized by loss of body weight, adipose tissue, visceral protein, and skeletal muscle. Patients with cachexia complain of loss of appetite, early satiety, and fatigue. As a result of protein losses, they often have anemia and peripheral edema.

### GENERAL NUTRITIONAL CONSIDERATIONS

Whenever possible, every effort is used to maintain adequate nutrition through the oral route. Food should be prepared in ways that make it appealing. Unpleasant smells and unappetizing-looking foods are avoided. Family members are included in the plan of care to encourage adequate food intake. The patient's preferences, as well as physiologic and metabolic requirements, are considered when selecting foods. Small, frequent meals are provided, with supplements between meals. Patients often tolerate larger amounts of food earlier in the day rather than later, so meals can be planned accordingly. To avoid early satiety, the patient should avoid drinking fluids while eating. Oral hygiene before mealtime often makes meals more pleasant. It is important to assess and manage pain, nausea, and other symptoms that may interfere with nutrition. Medications such as corticosteroids or progestational agents such as megestrol acetate have been used successfully as appetite stimulants. Prokinetic agents such as metoclopramide are used to increase gastric emptying in patients with early satiety and delayed gastric emptying. A variety of other agents and approaches are currently being investigated as supportive care for patients with anorexia and cachexia (MacDonald, 2003).

If adequate nutrition cannot be maintained by oral intake, nutritional support via the enteral route may be necessary. Short-term nutritional supplementation may be provided through a nasogastric tube. However, if nutritional support is needed for longer than several weeks, a gastrostomy or jejunostomy tube may be inserted. The patient and family are taught to administer enteral nutrition in the home.

If malabsorption is a problem, enzyme and vitamin replacement may be instituted. Additional strategies include changing the feeding schedule, using simple diets, and relieving diarrhea. If malabsorption is severe, parenteral nutrition may be necessary. Parenteral nutrition can be administered in several ways: by a long-term venous access device (eg, right atrial catheter), by an implanted venous port, or by a peripherally inserted central catheter (PICC) (Fig. 16-6). The nurse teaches the patient and family to care for venous access devices and to administer parenteral nutrition. Home care nurses may assist with or supervise parenteral nutrition administration in the home.

Interventions to reduce cachexia usually do not prolong survival or improve nutritional status significantly. Further study is needed to assess the effects of nutritional intervention on disease status and the patient's quality of life (MacDonald, 2003). Before invasive nutritional strategies are instituted, the nurse should assess the patient carefully and discuss options with the patient and family. Creative dietary therapies, enteral (tube) feedings, or parenteral nutrition may be necessary to ensure adequate nutrition. Nursing care is also directed toward preventing trauma, infection, and other complications that increase metabolic demands.

### Relieving Pain

Of all patients with progressive cancer, it is estimated that at least 80% experience pain (Saunders & Booth, 2003). Although the pain may be acute, it is more frequently characterized as chronic. (For more information on cancer-related pain, see Chapter 13.) As in other situations involving pain, the experience of cancer pain is influenced by both physical and psychosocial factors.

Cancer can cause pain in various ways (Table 16-10). Pain is also associated with various cancer treatments. Acute pain is linked with trauma from surgery. Occasionally, chronic pain syndromes, such as postsurgical neuropathies (pain related to nerve tissue injury), occur. Some chemotherapeutic agents cause tissue necrosis, peripheral neuropathies, and stomatitis—all potential sources of pain—whereas radiation therapy can cause pain secondary to skin or organ inflammation. Cancer patients may have other sources of pain, such as arthritis or migraine headaches, that are unrelated to the underlying cancer or its treatment.

In today's society, most people expect pain to disappear or resolve quickly, and in fact it usually does. Although it is controllable, cancer pain is commonly irreversible and not quickly resolved. For many patients, pain is a signal that the tumor is growing and that death is approaching. As patients anticipate the pain and their anxiety increases, pain perception heightens, producing fear and further pain. Chronic cancer pain, then, can be best described as a cycle progressing from pain to anxiety to fear and back to pain.

Pain tolerance, the point past which pain can no longer be tolerated, varies among people. Pain tolerance is decreased by fatigue, anxiety, fear of death, anger, powerlessness, social isolation, changes in role identity, loss of independence, and past experiences. Adequate rest and sleep, diversion, mood elevation, empathy, and medications such as antidepressants, antianxiety agents, and analgesics enhance tolerance to pain.

Inadequate pain management is most often the result of misconceptions and insufficient knowledge about pain assessment and pharmacologic interventions on the part of patients, families, and health care providers. Successful management of cancer pain is based on thorough and objective pain assessment that examines physical, psychosocial, environmental, and spiritual factors. A multidisciplinary team approach is essential to determine optimal management of the patient's pain. Unlike instances of chronic nonmalignant pain, systemic analgesics play a central role in managing cancer pain.

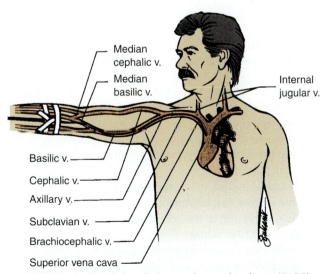

**FIGURE 16-6.** A peripherally inserted central catheter (PICC) is advanced through the cephalic or basilic vein to the axillary, subclavian, or brachiocephalic vein or the superior vena cava.

### TABLE 16-10   Examples of Sources of Cancer Pain

| Source | Descriptions | Underlying Cancer |
|---|---|---|
| Bone metastasis | Throbbing, aching | Breast, prostate, myeloma |
| Nerve compression, infiltration | Burning, sharp, tingling | Breast, prostate, lymphoma |
| Lymphatic or venous obstruction | Dull, aching, tightness | Lymphoma, breast, Kaposi's sarcoma |
| Ischemia | Sharp, throbbing | Kaposi's sarcoma |
| Organ obstruction | Dull, crampy, gnawing | Colon, gastric |
| Organ infiltration | Distention, crampy | Liver, pancreatic |
| Skin inflammation, ulceration, infection, necrosis | Burning, sharp | Breast, head and neck, Kaposi's sarcoma |

The World Health Organization (Hough & Portenoy, 2004) advocates a three-step approach to treat cancer pain (see Chapter 13). Analgesics are administered based on the patient's level of pain. Nonopioid analgesics (eg, acetaminophen) are used for mild pain; weak opioid analgesics (eg, codeine) are used for moderate pain; and strong opioid analgesics (eg, morphine) are used for severe pain. If the pain escalates, the strength of the analgesic medication is increased until the pain is controlled. Adjuvant medications are also administered to enhance the effectiveness of analgesics and to manage other symptoms that may contribute to the pain experience. Examples of adjuvant medications include antiemetics, antidepressants, anxiolytics, antiseizure agents, stimulants, local anesthetics, radiopharmaceuticals (radioactive agents that may be used to treat painful bone tumors), and corticosteroids.

Preventing and reducing pain help to decrease anxiety and break the pain cycle. This can be accomplished best by administering analgesics on a regularly scheduled basis as prescribed (the preventive approach to pain management), with additional analgesics administered for breakthrough pain as needed and as prescribed.

Various pharmacologic and nonpharmacologic approaches offer the best methods of managing cancer pain. No reasonable approaches, even those that may be invasive, should be overlooked because of a poor or terminal prognosis. The nurse helps the patient and family take an active role in managing pain. The nurse provides education and support to correct fears and misconceptions about opioid use. Inadequate pain control leads to suffering, anxiety, fear, immobility, isolation, and depression. Improving the patient's quality of life is as important as preventing a painful death.

### Decreasing Fatigue

In recent years, fatigue has been recognized as one of the most significant and frequent symptoms experienced by patients receiving cancer therapy. The nurse helps the patient and family understand that fatigue is usually an expected and temporary side effect of the cancer process and of many treatments used. Fatigue also stems from the stress of coping with cancer. It does not always signify that the cancer is advancing or that the treatment is failing. Potential sources of fatigue are summarized in Chart 16-8.

Nursing strategies are implemented to minimize fatigue or help the patient cope with existing fatigue. Helping the patient identify sources of fatigue aids in selecting appropriate and individualized interventions. Ways to conserve energy are developed to help the patient plan daily activities. Alternating periods of rest and activity are beneficial. Regular, light exercise may decrease fatigue and facilitate coping, whereas lack of physical activity and "too much rest" can actually contribute to deconditioning and associated fatigue.

The patient is encouraged to maintain as normal a lifestyle as possible by continuing with activities that he or she values and enjoys. Prioritizing necessary and valued activities can help the patient plan for each day. The patient and family are encouraged to plan to reallocate responsibilities, such as attending to child care, cleaning, and preparing meals. Patients who are employed full-time may need to reduce the number of hours worked each day or week. The nurse

### CHART 16-8

### Sources of Fatigue in Cancer Patients

- Pain, pruritus
- Imbalanced nutrition related to anorexia, nausea, vomiting, cachexia
- Electrolyte imbalance related to vomiting, diarrhea
- Ineffective protection related to neutropenia, thrombocytopenia, anemia
- Impaired tissue integrity related to stomatitis, mucositis
- Impaired physical mobility related to neurologic impairments, surgery, bone metastasis, pain, and analgesic use
- Uncertainty and deficient knowledge related to disease process, treatment
- Anxiety related to fear, diagnosis, role changes, uncertainty of future
- Ineffective breathing patterns related to cough, shortness of breath, and dyspnea
- Disturbed sleep pattern related to cancer therapies, anxiety, and pain

helps the patient and family cope with these changing roles and responsibilities.

The nurse also addresses factors that contribute to fatigue and implements pharmacologic and nonpharmacologic strategies to manage pain. The nurse provides nutrition counseling to patients who are not eating enough calories or protein. Small, frequent meals require less energy for digestion. The nurse monitors the patient for deficiencies in serum hemoglobin and hematocrit and administers blood products or EPO as prescribed. In addition, the nurse monitors the patient for alterations in oxygenation and electrolyte balances. Physical therapy and assistive devices are beneficial for patients with impaired mobility.

### Improving Body Image and Self-Esteem

A positive approach is essential when caring for patients with altered body image. To help the patient retain control and positive self-esteem, it is important to encourage independence and continued participation in self-care and decision making. The patient is assisted to assume those tasks and participate in those activities that are personally of most value. Any negative feelings that the patient has or threats to body image should be identified and discussed. The nurse serves as a listener and counselor to both the patient and the family. Referral to a support group can provide the patient with additional assistance in coping with the changes resulting from cancer or its treatment. In many cases, cosmetologists can provide ideas about hair or wig styling, makeup, and the use of scarves and turbans to help with body image concerns.

Patients who experience alterations in sexuality and sexual function are encouraged to discuss concerns openly with their partners. Alternative forms of sexual expression are explored with patients and their partners to promote positive self-worth and acceptance. Nurses who identify serious physiologic, psychological, or communication difficulties related to sexuality or sexual function are in a key position to help patients and partners seek further counseling if necessary.

### Assisting in the Grieving Process

A cancer diagnosis need not indicate a fatal outcome. Many forms of cancer are curable; others may be cured if treated early. Despite these facts, many patients and their families view cancer as a fatal disease that is inevitably accompanied by pain, suffering, debility, and emaciation. Grieving is a normal response to these fears and to the losses anticipated or experienced by patients with cancer. These may include loss of health, normal sensations, body image, social interaction, sexuality, and intimacy. Patients, families, and friends may grieve for the loss of quality time to spend with others, the loss of future and unfulfilled plans, and the loss of control over the patient's body and emotional reactions.

Patients and their families who have just been informed of a cancer diagnosis frequently respond with shock, numbness, and disbelief. It is often during this stage that the patient and family are called on to make important initial decisions about treatment. They require the support of physicians, nurses, and all members of the health care team to make these decisions. The nurse plays an important role in answering any questions the patient and family have and clarifying information provided by physicians.

In addition to assessing the response of the patient and family to the diagnosis and planned treatment, the nurse helps to clarify and present the patient's and family's questions and concerns, identify available resources and support people (eg, spiritual advisor, counselor), and communicate their concerns with each other. Support groups for patients and families are available through hospitals and various community organizations. These groups provide direct assistance, advice, and emotional support.

As the patient and family progress through the grieving process, they may express anger, frustration, and depression. During this time, the nurse encourages the patient and family members to verbalize their feelings in an atmosphere of trust and support. The nurse continues to assess the patient's and family members' reactions and provides assistance and support as the patient and family confront and learn to deal with new problems.

If the patient enters the terminal phase of disease, the nurse may realize that the patient and family members are at different stages of grief. In such cases, the nurse helps the patient and family to acknowledge and cope with their reactions and feelings. The nurse also helps the patient and family to explore preferences for issues related to end-of-life care, such as withdrawal of active disease treatment, desire for the use of life-support measures, and symptom management. Support, which can be as simple as holding a patient's hand or just being with a patient at home or at the bedside, often contributes to peace of mind. After the death of a patient with cancer, maintaining contact with surviving family members may help them work through their feelings of loss and grief. See Chapter 17 for further discussion of end-of-life issues.

### Monitoring and Managing Potential Complications

Despite advances in cancer care, infection remains a common problem for patients with cancer. Defense against infection is compromised in many different ways. The integrity of the skin and mucous membranes, the body's first line of defense, is challenged by multiple invasive diagnostic and therapeutic procedures, by adverse effects of radiation and chemotherapy, and by the detrimental effects of immobility.

Impaired nutrition resulting from anorexia, nausea, vomiting, diarrhea, and the underlying disease alters the body's ability to combat invading organisms. Medications such as antibiotics disturb the balance of normal flora, allowing the overgrowth of pathogenic organisms. Other medications can also alter the immune response (see Chapter 50). Cancer itself may be immunosuppressive. Cancers such as leukemia and lymphoma are often associated with defects in cellular and humoral immunity. Advanced cancer can lead to obstruction by the tumor of the hollow viscera (eg, intestines), blood vessels, and lymphatic vessels, creating a favorable environment for proliferation of pathogenic organisms. In some patients, tumor cells infiltrate bone marrow and prevent normal production of WBCs. However, most often, a decrease in WBCs is a result of bone marrow suppression after chemotherapy or radiation therapy.

The use of the hematopoietic growth factors, also called colony-stimulating factors (see previous discussion), has reduced the severity and duration of neutropenia associated with myelosuppressive chemotherapy and radiation therapy. The administration of these factors assists in reducing the risk for infection and, possibly, in maintaining treatment schedules, drug dosages, treatment effectiveness, and quality of life.

### INFECTION

Gram-positive bacteria (*Streptococcus* and *Staphylococcus* species) and gram-negative organisms (*Escherichia coli, Klebsiella pneumoniae,* and *Pseudomonas aeruginosa*) are the most frequently isolated causes of infection. Fungal organisms, such as *Candida albicans,* also contribute to the incidence of serious infection. Viral infections in immunocompromised patients are caused mostly by herpesviruses and respiratory viruses.

Fever is probably the most important sign of infection in immunocompromised patients. Although fever may be related to a variety of noninfectious conditions, including the underlying cancer, any temperature of 38.3°C (101°F) or higher is reported and dealt with promptly.

Antibiotics may be prescribed to treat infections after cultures of wound drainage, exudate, sputum, urine, stool, or blood are obtained. Patients with neutropenia are treated with broad-spectrum antibiotics before the infecting organism is identified because of the high incidence of mortality associated with untreated infection. Broad-spectrum antibiotic coverage or empiric therapy most often includes a combination of medications to defend the body against the major pathogenic organisms. It is important for the nurse to administer these medications promptly according to the prescribed schedule to achieve adequate blood levels of the medications.

Strict asepsis is essential when handling IV lines, catheters, and other invasive equipment. Exposure of the patient to others with active infections and to crowds is avoided. Patients with profound immunosuppression, such as BMT recipients, may need to be placed in a protective environment where the room and its contents are sterilized and the air is filtered. These patients may also receive low-bacteria diets, avoiding fresh fruits and vegetables. Hand hygiene and appropriate general hygiene are necessary to reduce exposure to potentially harmful bacteria and to eliminate environmental contaminants. Invasive procedures, such as injections, vaginal or rectal examinations, rectal temperatures, and surgery, are avoided. The patient is encouraged to cough and to perform deep-breathing exercises frequently to prevent atelectasis and other respiratory problems. Prophylactic antimicrobial therapy may be used for patients who are expected to be profoundly immunosuppressed and at risk for certain infections. The nurse teaches the patient and family to recognize signs and symptoms of infection to report, perform effective hand hygiene, use antipyretics, maintain skin integrity, and administer hematopoietic growth factors when indicated.

### SEPTIC SHOCK

The nurse assesses the patient frequently for infection and inflammation throughout the course of the disease. Septicemia and septic shock are life-threatening complications that must be prevented or detected and treated promptly. Patients with signs and symptoms of impending sepsis and septic shock require immediate hospitalization and aggressive treatment.

Signs and symptoms of septic shock (see Chapter 15) include altered mental status, either subnormal or elevated temperature, cool and clammy skin, decreased urine output, hypotension, dysrhythmias, electrolyte imbalances, and abnormal arterial blood gas values. Patients and family members are instructed about signs of septicemia, methods for preventing infection, and actions to take if infection or septicemia occurs.

Septic shock is most often associated with overwhelming gram-negative bacterial infections. In a patient with shock, the nurse monitors blood pressure, pulse rate, respirations, and temperature every 15 to 30 minutes. Neurologic assessments are carried out to detect changes in orientation and responsiveness. Fluid and electrolyte status is monitored by measuring fluid intake and output and serum electrolytes. Arterial blood gas values and pulse oximetry are monitored to determine tissue oxygenation. Nurses administer IV fluids, blood products, and vasopressors as prescribed to maintain blood pressure and tissue perfusion, as well as broad-spectrum antibiotics, which may be prescribed to combat the underlying infection (see Chapter 15). Supplemental oxygen is often necessary.

### BLEEDING AND HEMORRHAGE

Platelets are essential for normal blood clotting and coagulation (hemostasis). Thrombocytopenia, a decrease in the circulating platelet count, is the most common cause of bleeding in patients with cancer and is usually defined as a platelet count of less than 100,000/mm³ ($0.1 \times 10^{12}$/L). When the platelet count decreases to between 20,000 and 50,000/mm³ (0.02 to $0.05 \times 10^{12}$/L), the risk of bleeding increases. Platelet counts lower than 20,000/mm³ ($0.02 \times 10^{12}$/L) are associated with an increased risk for spontaneous bleeding, for which patients require a platelet transfusion.

Thrombocytopenia often results from bone marrow depression after certain types of chemotherapy and radiation therapy. Tumor infiltration of the bone marrow can also impair the normal production of platelets. In some cases, platelet destruction is associated with an enlarged spleen (hypersplenism) and abnormal antibody function, which occur with leukemia and lymphoma.

In addition to monitoring laboratory values, the nurse continues to assess the patient for bleeding. The nurse also takes steps to prevent trauma and minimize the risk of bleeding by encouraging the patient to use a soft, not stiff, toothbrush and an electric, not straight-edged, razor. In addition, the nurse avoids unnecessary invasive procedures (eg, rectal temperatures, intramuscular injections, catheterization) and helps the patient and family identify and remove environmental hazards that may lead to falls or other trauma. Soft foods, increased fluid intake, and stool softeners, if prescribed, may be indicated to reduce trauma to the gastrointestinal tract. The joints and extremities are handled and moved gently to minimize the risk of spontaneous bleeding. In limited circumstances, the nurse may administer IL-11, which has been approved by the FDA to prevent severe thrombocytopenia and to reduce the need for platelet transfusions after myelosuppressive chemotherapy in patients with nonmyeloid malignancies (Abehoff et al., 2003). In some instances, the nurse teaches the patient or family members to administer IL-11 in the home.

Hemorrhage may be related to various underlying abnormalities, such as thrombocytopenia and coagulation disorders. These clinical situations are often associated with the cancer itself or with the adverse effects of cancer treatments. Sites of hemorrhage may include the gastrointestinal, respiratory, and genitourinary tracts and the brain. When a hospitalized patient experiences bleeding, the nurse monitors blood pressure and pulse and respiratory rates every 15 to 30 minutes.

Serum hemoglobin and hematocrit are monitored carefully for changes indicating blood loss. The nurse tests all urine, stool, and emesis for occult blood. Neurologic assessments are performed to detect changes in orientation and behavior. The nurse administers fluids and blood products as prescribed to replace any losses. Vasopressor agents may be prescribed to maintain blood pressure and ensure tissue oxygenation. Supplemental oxygen may be necessary.

## Promoting Home and Community-Based Care

### TEACHING PATIENTS SELF-CARE

Patients with cancer usually return home from acute care facilities or receive treatment in the home or outpatient area rather than acute care facilities. The shift from the acute care setting also shifts the responsibility for care to the patient and family. As a result, family members and friends must assume increased involvement in patient care, which requires teaching that enables them to provide care. Teaching initially focuses on providing information needed by the patient and family to address the most immediate care needs likely to be encountered at home.

Side effects of treatments and changes in the patient's status that should be reported are reviewed verbally and reinforced with written information. Strategies to deal with side effects of treatment are discussed with the patient and family. Other learning needs are identified based on the priorities conveyed by the patient and family as well as on the complexity of care provided in the home.

Technologic advances allow home administration of chemotherapy, parenteral nutrition, blood products, parenteral antibiotics, and parenteral analgesics, as well as management of symptoms and care of vascular access devices. Although home care nurses provide care and support for patients receiving this advanced technical care, patients and families need instruction and ongoing support that allow them to feel comfortable and proficient in managing these treatments at home. Follow-up visits and telephone calls from the nurse are often reassuring and increase the patient's and family's comfort in dealing with complex and new aspects of care. Continued contact facilitates evaluation of the patient's progress and assessment of the ongoing needs of the patient and family.

### CONTINUING CARE

Referral for home care is often indicated for patients with cancer. The responsibilities of the home care nurse include assessing the home environment, suggesting modifications in the home or in care to help the patient and family address the patient's physical needs, providing physical care, and assessing the psychological and emotional impact of the illness on the patient and family.

Assessing changes in the patient's physical status and reporting relevant changes to the physician help ensure that appropriate and timely modifications in therapy are made. The home care nurse also assesses the adequacy of pain management and the effectiveness of other strategies to prevent or manage the side effects of treatment modalities.

It is necessary to assess the patient's and family's understanding of the treatment plan and management strategies and to reinforce previous teaching. The nurse often facilitates coordination of patient care by maintaining close communication with all involved health care providers. The nurse may make referrals and coordinate available community resources (eg, local office of the American Cancer Society, home aides, church groups, parish nurses, support groups) to assist patients and caregivers.

## Evaluation

### Expected Patient Outcomes

For specific patient outcomes, see the plan of nursing care (Chart 16-6). Expected patient outcomes may include the following:

1. Maintains integrity of oral mucous membranes
2. Maintains adequate tissue integrity
3. Maintains adequate nutritional status
4. Achieves relief of pain and discomfort
5. Demonstrates increased activity tolerance and decreased fatigue
6. Exhibits improved body image and self-esteem
7. Progresses through the grieving process
8. Experiences no complications, such as infection, or sepsis, and no episodes of bleeding or hemorrhage

# Cancer Rehabilitation

Many patients with cancer, including those who receive primary surgical treatment and adjuvant chemotherapy or radiation therapy, return to work and their usual activities of daily living. These patients may encounter a variety of problems, including changes in their functional abilities and in the attitudes of employers, coworkers, and family members who still view cancer as a terminal, debilitating disease.

Nurses play an important role in the rehabilitation of patients with cancer. Both the patient and family are included as part of any rehabilitation effort, because cancer affects not only the patient but also the family members. In addition, with the shift away from inpatient care, many families are caring for patients at home. To maximize beneficial outcomes, evaluation of the patient's needs related to cancer rehabilitation begins early in cancer treatment (Table 16-11). Depending on the patient's functional abilities, the nurse works with the multidisciplinary health care team to encourage the patient to participate in some form of exercise program to facilitate activity tolerance and quality of life (Young-McCaughan, Mays, Arzola et al., 2003).

Assessment for body image changes as a result of disfiguring treatments is necessary to facilitate the patient's adjustment to changes in appearance or functional abilities. The nurse can refer the patient and family to a variety of support groups sponsored by the American Cancer Society, such as those for people who have had laryngectomies or mastectomies. The nurse also collaborates with physical, occupational, and enterostomal therapists (wound care specialists) in improving the patient's abilities in the use of prosthetic and assistive devices and in altering the home environment as needed.

Patients often experience distress (eg, pain, nausea) related to the underlying cancer or treatments. These symptoms may interfere with work and quality of life. The nurse assesses for these problems and helps the patient identify strategies for coping with them. For patients with gastrointestinal disturbances after chemotherapy, altering work hours or receiving treatments in the evenings may prove helpful. Collaboration with physicians and pharmacists is helpful in identifying appropriate interventions.

The nurse collaborates with the dietitian to help the patient plan meals that will be acceptable and meet nutritional requirements. The nurse is also involved in the ongoing assessment of the patient to detect any long-term consequences of cancer treatment.

Although the Americans With Disabilities Act of 1990 was intended to protect patients with disabling disorders against discrimination, recovering cancer patients have reported instances of unfair practices and discrimination in the workplace. Some employers do not understand that different kinds of cancers have different prognoses and different effects on functional ability. As a result, employers may hesitate to hire or continue to employ people with cancer, especially if ongoing treatment regimens require adjustments in work schedules. Employers, coworkers, and families may continue to view the person as "sick" despite

**TABLE 16-11 Assessing Patient Needs for Cancer Rehabilitation**

| Area of Need | Factors to Assess |
|---|---|
| **Functional** | |
| Activities of daily living | Mobility |
| | Cognitive impairment |
| | Sensory impairments |
| | Communication barriers |
| | Preexisting disabilities |
| **Physiologic** | |
| Nutrition | Need for enteral or parenteral nutrition |
| Elimination | Alterations in bowel and bladder function |
| Symptoms related to disease or treatment | Pain |
| | Nausea, vomiting, diarrhea |
| | Dyspnea, fatigue |
| | Skin impairment, alopecia |
| **Psychosocial Resources** | |
| Family | Availability of caregiver, home physical environment |
| Community | Availability of private transportation; affordability of transportation |
| Personal | Availability of public transportation; affordability of transportation |
| | Availability and access to community organizations for assistance and support |
| | Spiritual concerns |
| | Family relationships |
| | Body image |
| | Coping abilities |
| | Sexuality |
| Financial | Job security for patient and family members |
| | Need for vocational training |

# NURSING RESEARCH PROFILE

## Effects of Exercise in Cancer Rehabilitation

Young-McCaughan, S., Mays, M. Z., Arozola, S. M., et al. (2003). Change in exercise tolerance, activity and sleep patterns, and quality of life in patients with cancer participating in a structured exercise program. *Oncology Nursing Forum, 30*(3), 441–452.

### Purpose
Multiple studies have shown that physical activity in patients with cancer can lead to improvements in functional capacity, levels of fatigue, and quality of life. The purpose of this study was to investigate the feasibility of an exercise intervention program modeled to improve selected physical and psychological parameters of health in patients with cancer. Changes in exercise tolerance, activity, sleep patterns, and quality of life were assessed. In addition, the authors examined whether certain demographic, cancer-related, treatment-related, physical, and psychological variables either encouraged or prevented patients with cancer from participating in the rehabilitation program.

### Design
The Roy Adaptation Model was used as the conceptual framework for this prospective, repeated-measures study. Subjects were recruited from oncology clinics at two major military medical centers in the southwestern United States. To be eligible for the study, participants had to have a biopsy-proven cancer diagnosis within the previous 2 years, be at least 18 years of age, speak and read English, and have a statement from the primary care physician or medical oncologist that participation in the exercise program was not contraindicated. Patients with bone or joint destruction that could have been aggravated by the exercise and patients with severe cognitive impairment were excluded from participation. Of the 323 patients who were approached about the study, 62 (19%) consented to participate.

Patients participated in a 12-week exercise program that included classes on exercise, nutrition, stress management, cancer therapies, drug reviews, sleep, spiritual health, quality of life, and health evaluation and assessment. Exercise tolerance was measured before and after participation in the program by assessing the maximal oxygen uptake. This value was converted into metabolic equivalents (METs), which reflect exercise capacity. Activity and sleep patterns were collected from a wrist-worn actigraph that measured movement in three dimensions. This information was collected at baseline and during weeks 4, 8, and 12 of the study. Quality of life was measured using the Cancer Rehabilitation Evaluation System–Short Form (CARES-SF) at the same four time points.

### Findings
Analysis of data revealed a significant improvement in METs among subjects who completed the exercise program, reflecting improvements in exercise capacity ($p < .001$). In addition, there was a significant improvement in both duration and intensity of exercise between baseline and week 12 testing ($p < .001$). For subjects who completed the exercise program, there was a significant improvement in self-report of energy ($p = .004$), although there was no reported significant change in activity level or percentage of napping. Despite a lack of significant improvement in objective measures of sleep during the course of the rehabilitation program, the subjects' self-reports of difficulty sleeping did show significant improvement ($p = .03$). Analysis of quality-of-life data revealed significant improvement for global scores ($p = .03$), as well as for physical ($p = .002$) and psychological ($p = .09$) subscales.

The authors reported that patients who had completed their cancer treatment were more likely to complete the exercise program than those still in active treatment ($p = .001$). Subjects with early-stage cancer had higher completion rates than those with late stages of cancer ($p = .003$). Some patients reported that the structured program enhanced their return to normal routines.

### Nursing Implications
The findings of this study demonstrate that patients with various types and stages of cancer can benefit from exercise using a cardiac rehabilitation model. Improvements in exercise tolerance, activity, sleep patterns and quality of life are possible for this population. In addition, exercise facilitates both physical and psychological adaptation. Patients with cancer may have limitations based on personal and lifestyle factors and their disease and responses to treatment; however, nurses can collaborate with the multidisciplinary team to assess these limitations and offer individualized cancer rehabilitation through structured exercise programs.

ongoing recovery or completion of treatment. Attitudes of coworkers can be a problem when the patient has a communication impairment, as may occur in some head and neck cancers. Patients may benefit from vocational rehabilitation services of the American Cancer Society or other agencies.

Nurses can participate in efforts to educate employers and the public in general to ensure that the rights of patients with cancer are maintained. Whenever possible, the nurse assists the patient and family to resume preexisting roles. Psychologists and clergy or spiritual advisors are consulted to assist with psychosocial and spiritual concerns. Rehabilitation shifts the focus from what has been lost to what can be done with existing strengths and abilities. In that spirit, the nurse encourages the patient to regain the highest level of function and independence possible.

## Gerontologic Considerations

As a result of an increased life expectancy and an increased risk of cancer with age, nurses are providing cancer-related care for growing numbers of elderly patients. More than 58% of all cancers occur in people older than 65 years of age, and about two thirds of all cancer deaths occur in people 65 years of age and older. Nursing care of this population addresses special needs, including physical, psychosocial, and financial concerns.

Oncology nurses working with the elderly population must understand the normal physiologic changes that occur with aging. These changes include decreased skin elasticity; decreased skeletal mass, structure, and strength; decreased organ function and structure; impaired immune system mechanisms; alterations in neurologic and sensory functions; and altered drug absorption, distribution, metabolism, and elimination. These changes ultimately influence the ability of elderly patients to tolerate cancer treatment. In addition, many elderly patients have other chronic diseases and associated treatments that may limit tolerance to cancer treatments (Table 16-12).

Potential chemotherapy-related toxicities, such as renal impairment, myelosuppression, fatigue, and cardiomyopathy, may increase as a result of declining organ function and diminished physiologic reserves. The recovery of normal tissues after radiation therapy may be delayed, and older patients may experience more severe adverse effects, such as mucositis, nausea and vomiting, and myelosuppression. Because of decreased tissue healing capacity and declining pulmonary and cardiovascular functioning, older patients are slower to recover from surgery. Elderly patients are also at increased risk for complications such as atelectasis, pneumonia, and wound infections.

Access to cancer care for elderly patients may be limited by discriminatory or fatalistic attitudes of health care providers, caregivers, and patients themselves. Issues such as the gradual loss of supportive resources, declining health

### TABLE 16-12 Age-Related Changes and Their Effects on Patients with Cancer

| Age-Related Changes | Implications |
|---|---|
| Impaired immune system | Use special precautions to avoid infection; monitor for atypical signs and symptoms of infection. |
| Altered drug absorption, distribution, metabolism, and elimination | Mandates careful calculation of chemotherapy and frequent assessment for drug response and side effects; dose adjustments may be necessary. |
| Increased prevalence of other chronic diseases | Monitor for effect of cancer or its treatment on patient's other chronic diseases; monitor patient's tolerance for cancer treatment; monitor for interactions with medications used to treat chronic diseases. |
| Diminished renal, respiratory, and cardiac reserve | Be proactive in prevention of decreased renal function, atelectasis, pneumonia, and cardiovascular compromise; monitor for side effects of cancer treatment. |
| Decreased skin and tissue integrity; reduction in body mass; delayed healing | Prevent pressure ulcers secondary to immobility; monitor skin and mucous membranes for changes related to radiation or chemotherapy; monitor nutritional status. |
| Decreased musculoskeletal strength | Prevent falls; assess support for performing activities of daily living in home setting; encourage safe use of assistive mobility devices |
| Decreased neurosensory functioning: loss of vision, hearing, and distal extremity tactile senses | Provide teaching and instructions modified for patient's hearing and vision changes; provide instruction concerning safety and skin care for distal extremities; assess home for safety. |
| Altered social and economic resources | Assess for financial concerns, living conditions, and resources for support |
| Potential changes in cognitive and emotional capacity | Provide teaching and support modified for patient's level of functioning and safety |

or loss of a spouse, and unavailability of relatives or friends may result in limited access to care and unmet needs for assistance with activities of daily living. In addition, the economic impact of health care may be difficult for those living on fixed incomes.

Nurses must be aware of the special needs of the aging population. Cancer prevention, detection, and screening efforts are directed toward the elderly as well as the younger population. Nurses carefully monitor elderly patients receiving cancer treatments for signs and symptoms of adverse effects. In addition, elderly patients are instructed to report all symptoms to the physician. It is not uncommon for elderly patients to delay reporting symptoms, attributing them to "old age." Many elderly people do not want to report illness for fear of losing their independence or financial security. Sensory losses (eg, hearing and visual losses) and memory deficits are considered when planning patient education, because they may affect the patient's ability to process and retain information. In such cases, the nurse acts as a patient advocate, encouraging independence and identifying resources for support when indicated.

## Care of the Patient With Advanced Cancer

Patients with advanced cancer are likely to experience many of the problems previously described, but all to a greater degree. Symptoms of gastrointestinal disturbances, nutritional problems, weight loss, and cachexia make patients more susceptible to skin breakdown, fluid and electrolyte problems, and infection.

Although not all cancer patients experience pain, those who do commonly fear that it will not be adequately treated. Although treatment at this stage of illness is likely to be palliative rather than curative, prevention and appropriate management of problems can improve the patient's quality of life considerably. For example, use of analgesia at set intervals rather than on an "as needed" basis usually breaks the cycle of tension and anxiety associated with waiting until pain becomes so severe that pain relief is inadequate once the analgesic is given. Working with the patient and family as well as with other health care providers on a pain-management program based on the patient's requirements frequently increases the patient's comfort and sense of control. In addition, the dose of opioid analgesic required is often reduced as pain becomes more manageable and other medications (eg, sedatives, tranquilizers, muscle relaxants) are added to assist in relieving pain.

If the patient is a candidate for radiation therapy or surgical intervention to relieve severe pain, the consequences of these procedures (eg, percutaneous nerve block, cordotomy) are explained to the patient and family. Measures are taken to prevent complications resulting from altered sensation, immobility, and changes in bowel and bladder function.

With the appearance of each new symptom, patients may experience dread and fear that the disease is progressing. However, one cannot assume that all symptoms are related to the cancer. The new symptoms and problems are evaluated and treated aggressively if possible to increase the patient's comfort and improve quality of life.

Weakness, immobility, fatigue, and inactivity typically occur in the advanced stages of cancer as a result of the tumor, treatment, inadequate nutritional intake, or shortness of breath. The nurse works with the patient to set realistic goals and to provide rest balanced with planned activities and exercise. Other measures include helping the patient identify energy-conserving methods for accomplishing tasks and promoting activities that the patient values most.

Efforts are made throughout the course of the disease to provide the patient with as much control and independence as desired but with assurance that support and assistance are available when needed. In addition, health care teams work with the patient and family to ascertain and comply with the patient's wishes about treatment methods and care as the terminal phase of illness and death approach.

## Hospice

For many years, society was unable to cope appropriately with patients in the most advanced stages of cancer, and patients died in acute care settings rather than at home or in facilities designed to meet their needs. The needs of patients with terminal illnesses are best met by a comprehensive multidisciplinary program that focuses on quality of life, palliation of symptoms, and provision of psychosocial and spiritual support for patients and families when cure and control of the disease are no longer possible. The concept of hospice, which originated in Great Britain, best addresses these needs. Most important, the focus of care is on the family, not just the patient. Hospice care can be provided in several settings: free-standing, hospital-based, and community or home-based settings.

Because of the high costs associated with maintaining free-standing hospices, care is often delivered through coordination of services provided by hospitals and the community. Although physicians, social workers, clergy, dietitians, pharmacists, physical therapists, and volunteers are involved in patient care, nurses are most often the coordinators of all hospice activities. It is essential that home care and hospice nurses possess advanced skills in assessing and managing pain, nutrition, dyspnea, bowel dysfunction, and skin impairments.

In addition, hospice programs facilitate clear communication among family members and health care providers. Most patients and families are informed of the prognosis and are encouraged to participate in decisions regarding pursuing or terminating cancer treatment. Through collaboration with other support disciplines, the nurse helps the patient and family cope with changes in role identity, family structure, grief, and loss. Hospice nurses are actively involved in bereavement counseling. In many instances, family support for survivors continues for about 1 year. See Chapter 17 for detailed discussion of end-of-life care.

## Oncologic Emergencies

For information about these emergencies, see Table 16-13.

*(text continues on page 442)*

# TABLE 16-13  Oncologic Emergencies: Manifestations and Management

| Emergency | Clinical Manifestations and Diagnostic Findings | Management |
|---|---|---|
| **Superior Vena Cava Syndrome (SVCS)**<br><br>Compression or invasion of the superior vena cava by tumor, enlarged lymph nodes, intraluminal thrombus that obstructs venous circulation, or drainage of the head, neck, arms, and thorax. Typically associated with lung cancer, SVCS can also occur with breast cancer, Kaposi's sarcoma, thymoma, lymphoma and mediastinal metastases (Flounders, 2003a). If untreated, SVCS may lead to cerebral anoxia (because not enough oxygen reaches the brain), laryngeal edema, bronchial obstruction, and death. | *Clinical*<br>Gradually or suddenly impaired venous drainage giving rise to<br>• Progressive shortness of breath (dyspnea), cough, hoarseness, chest pain, and facial swelling<br>• Edema of the neck, arms, hands, and thorax and reported sensation of skin tightness and difficulty swallowing<br>• Possibly engorged and distended jugular, temporal, and arm veins<br>• Dilated thoracic vessels causing prominent venous patterns on the chest wall<br>• Increased intracranial pressure, associated visual disturbances, headache, and altered mental status<br><br>*Diagnostic*<br>Diagnosis is confirmed by<br>• Clinical findings<br>• Chest x-ray<br>• Thoracic computed tomography (CT) scan<br>• Thoracic magnetic resonance imaging (MRI)<br>Intraluminal thrombosis is identified by venogram. | *Medical*<br>• Radiation therapy to shrink tumor size and relieve symptoms<br>• Chemotherapy for chemosensitive cancers (eg, lymphoma, small cell lung cancer) or when the mediastinum has been irradiated to maximum tolerance (Flounders, 2003a)<br>• Anticoagulant or thrombolytic therapy for intraluminal thrombosis<br>• Surgery (less common), such as vena cava bypass graft (synthetic or autologous), to redirect blood flow around the obstruction<br>• Supportive measures such as oxygen therapy, corticosteroids, and diuretics<br><br>*Nursing*<br>• Identify patients at risk for SVCS.<br>• Monitor and report clinical manifestations of SVCS.<br>• Monitor cardiopulmonary and neurologic status.<br>• Avoid upper extremity venipuncture and blood pressure measurement (Flounders, 2003a).<br>• Facilitate breathing by positioning the patient properly. This helps to promote comfort and reduce anxiety produced by difficulty breathing resulting from progressive edema.<br>• Promote energy conservation to minimize shortness of breath.<br>• Monitor the patient's fluid volume status and administer fluids cautiously to minimize edema.<br>• Assess for thoracic radiation-related problems such as dysphagia (difficulty swallowing) and esophagitis.<br>• Monitor for chemotherapy-related problems, such as myelosuppression.<br>• Provide postoperative care as appropriate. |
| **Spinal Cord Compression**<br><br>Potentially leading to permanent neurologic impairment and associated morbidity and mortality, compression of the cord and its nerve roots may result from tumor, lymphomas, intervertebral collapse, or interruption of blood supply to the nerve tissues (Flounders, 2003a).<br>The prognosis depends on the severity and rapidity of onset. About 60% of compressions occur at the thoracic level, 30% in the lumbosacral level, and 10% in the cervical region (Abrahm, 2004). Metastatic cancers (breast, lung, kidney, prostate, myeloma, lymphoma) and related bone erosion are associated with spinal cord compression (Flounders, 2003a). | *Clinical*<br>• Local inflammation, edema, venous stasis, and impaired blood supply to nervous tissues<br>• Local or radicular back or neck pain along the dermatomal areas innervated by the affected nerve root (Flounders, 2003a) (eg, thoracic radicular pain extends in a band around the chest or abdomen)<br>• Pain exacerbated by movement, supine recumbent position, coughing, sneezing, or the Valsalva maneuver<br>• Neurologic dysfunction, and related motor and sensory deficits (numbness, tingling, feelings of coldness in the affected area, inability to detect vibration, loss of positional sense) | *Medical*<br>• Radiation therapy to reduce tumor size to halt progression and corticosteroid therapy to decrease inflammation and swelling at the compression site<br>• Surgery if symptoms progress despite radiation therapy or if vertebral fracture leads to additional nerve damage; surgery is also an option when the tumor is not radiosensitive or is located in an area that was previously irradiated (Flounders, 2003a).<br>• Chemotherapy as adjuvant to radiation therapy for patients with lymphoma or small cell lung cancer<br>• *Note:* Despite treatment, patients with poor neurologic function before treatment are less likely to regain complete motor and sensory function; patients who develop complete paralysis usually do not regain all neurologic function (Abrahm, 2004). |

| TABLE 16-13 | Oncologic Emergencies: Manifestations and Management (Continued) | |
|---|---|---|
| Emergency | Clinical Manifestations and Diagnostic Findings | Management |
| | • Motor loss ranging from subtle weakness to flaccid paralysis<br>• Bladder and/or bowel dysfunction depending on level of compression (above S2, overflow incontinence; from S3 to S5, flaccid sphincter tone and bowel incontinence)<br>**Diagnostic**<br>• Percussion tenderness at the level of compression<br>• Abnormal reflexes<br>• Sensory and motor abnormalities<br>• MRI, myelogram, spinal cord x-rays, bone scans, and CT scan | **Nursing**<br>• Perform ongoing assessment of neurologic function to identify existing and progressing dysfunction.<br>• Control pain with pharmacologic and non-pharmacologic measures.<br>• Prevent complications of immobility resulting from pain and decreased function (eg, skin breakdown, urinary stasis, thrombophlebitis, decreased clearance of pulmonary secretions).<br>• Maintain muscle tone by assisting with range-of-motion exercises in collaboration with physical and occupational therapists.<br>• Institute intermittent urinary catheterization and bowel training programs for patients with bladder or bowel dysfunction.<br>• Provide encouragement and support to patient and family coping with pain and altered functioning, lifestyle, roles, and independence. |
| **Hypercalcemia**<br>In patients with cancer, hypercalcemia is a potentially life-threatening metabolic abnormality resulting when the calcium released from the bones is more than the kidneys can excrete or the bones can reabsorb. It may result from<br>• Bone destruction by tumor cells and subsequent release of calcium<br>• Production of prostaglandins and osteoclast-activating factor, which stimulate bone breakdown and calcium release (Shuey, 2004)<br>• Tumors that produce parathyroid-like substances that promote calcium release (Shuey, 2004)<br>• Excessive use of vitamins and minerals and conditions unrelated to cancer, such as dehydration, renal impairment, primary hyperparathyroidism, thyrotoxicosis, thiazide diuretics, and hormone therapy | **Clinical**<br>Fatigue, weakness, confusion, decreased level of responsiveness, hyporeflexia, nausea, vomiting, constipation, polyuria (excessive urination), polydipsia (excessive thirst), dehydration, and dysrhythmias (Shuey & Brant, 2004)<br>**Diagnostic**<br>Serum calcium level exceeding 11 mg/dL (2.74 mmol/L) | **Medical**<br>See Chapter 14.<br>**Nursing**<br>• Identify patients at risk for hypercalcemia and assess for signs and symptoms of hypercalcemia.<br>• Educate patient and family; prevention and early detection can prevent fatality.<br>• Teach at-risk patients to recognize and report signs and symptoms of hypercalcemia.<br>• Encourage patients to consume 2–3 L of fluid daily unless contraindicated by existing renal or cardiac disease.<br>• Explain the use of dietary and pharmacologic interventions such as stool softeners and laxatives for constipation.<br>• Advise patients to maintain nutritional intake without restricting normal calcium intake.<br>• Discuss antiemetic therapy if nausea and vomiting occur.<br>• Promote mobility by emphasizing its importance in preventing demineralization and breakdown of bones (Shuey & Brant, 2004). |
| **Pericardial Effusion and Cardiac Tamponade**<br>Cardiac tamponade is an accumulation of fluid in the pericardial space. The accumulation compresses the heart and thereby impedes expansion of | **Clinical**<br>• Neck vein distention during inspiration (Kussmaul's sign)<br>• Pulsus paradoxus (systolic blood pressure decrease exceeding 10 mm Hg during inspiration; pulse gets stronger on expiration) | **Medical**<br>• Pericardiocentesis (the aspiration or withdrawal of pericardial fluid by a large-bore needle inserted into the pericardial space). In malignant effusions, pericardiocentesis provides only temporary relief; fluid usually reaccumulates. Windows or openings in the pericardium can be created surgically as a palliative |

*continued >*

## TABLE 16-13    Oncologic Emergencies: Manifestations and Management (Continued)

| Emergency | Clinical Manifestations and Diagnostic Findings | Management |
|---|---|---|
| the ventricles and cardiac filling during diastole. As ventricular volume and cardiac output fall, the heart pump fails, and circulatory collapse develops.<br>With gradual onset, fluid accumulates gradually, and the outer layer of the pericardial space stretches to compensate for rising pressure. Large amounts of fluid accumulate before symptoms of heart failure occur. With rapid onset, pressures rise too quickly for the pericardial space to compensate.<br>Cancerous tumors, particularly from adjacent thoracic tumors (lung, esophagus, breast cancers), and cancer treatment are the most common causes of cardiac tamponade. Radiation therapy of 4000 cGy or more to the mediastinal area has also been implicated in pericardial fibrosis, pericarditis, and resultant cardiac tamponade. Untreated pericardial effusion and cardiac tamponade lead to circulatory collapse and cardiac arrest (Flounders, 2003a). | • Distant heart sounds, rubs and gallops, cardiac dullness<br>• Compensatory tachycardia (heart beats faster to compensate for decreased cardiac output)<br>• Increased venous and vascular pressures<br><br>*Diagnostic*<br>• Electrocardiography (ECG) helps diagnose pericardial effusion<br>• In small effusion, chest x-rays show small amounts of fluid in the pericardium; in large effusions, x-ray films disclose "water-bottle" heart (obliteration of vessel contour and cardiac chambers)<br>• CT scans help diagnose pleural effusions and evaluate effect of treatment<br>• Narrow pulse pressure<br>• Shortness of breath and tachypnea<br>• Weakness, chest pain, orthopnea, anxiety, diaphoresis, lethargy, and altered consciousness from decreased cerebral perfusion (Flounders, 2003a; Casciato, 2004) | measure to drain fluid into the pleural space. Catheters may also be placed in the pericardial space and sclerosing agents (such as tetracycline, talc, bleomycin, 5-fluorouracil, or thiotepa) injected to prevent fluid from reaccumulating.<br>• Radiation therapy or antineoplastic agents, depending on how sensitive the primary tumor is to these treatments. In mild effusions, prednisone and diuretic medications may be prescribed and the patient's status carefully monitored.<br><br>*Nursing*<br>• Monitor vital signs and oxygen saturation frequently.<br>• Assess for pulsus paradoxus.<br>• Monitor ECG tracings.<br>• Assess heart and lung sounds, neck vein filling, level of consciousness, respiratory status, and skin color and temperature.<br>• Monitor and record intake and output.<br>• Review laboratory findings (eg, arterial blood gas and electrolyte levels).<br>• Elevate the head of the patient's bed to ease breathing.<br>• Minimize patient's physical activity to reduce oxygen requirements; administer supplemental oxygen as prescribed.<br>• Provide frequent oral hygiene.<br>• Reposition and encourage the patient to cough and take deep breaths every 2 h.<br>• As needed, maintain patent IV access, reorient the patient, and provide supportive measures and appropriate patient instruction (Flounders, 2003a; Casciato, 2004). |
| **Disseminated Intravascular Coagulation (DIC, also called consumption coagulopathy)**<br>Complex disorder of coagulation or fibrinolysis (destruction of clots), which results in thrombosis or bleeding. DIC is most commonly associated with hematologic cancers (leukemia); cancer of prostate, gastrointestinal (GI) tract, and lungs; chemotherapy (methotrexate, prednisone, l-asparaginase, vincristine, and 6-mercaptopurine); and disease processes such as sepsis, hepatic failure, and anaphylaxis.<br>Blood clots form when normal coagulation mechanisms are triggered. Once activated, the clotting cascade continues to consume clotting factors and | *Clinical*<br>*Chronic DIC:* Few or no observable symptoms or easy bruising, prolonged bleeding from venipuncture and injection sites, bleeding of the gums, and slow GI bleeding<br>*Acute DIC:* life-threatening hemorrhage and infarction; clinical symptoms of this syndrome are varied and depend on the organ system involved in thrombus and infarction or bleeding episodes<br><br>*Diagnostic*<br>• Prolonged prothrombin time (PT or protime)<br>• Prolonged partial thromboplastin time (PTT)<br>• Prolonged thrombin time (TT)<br>• Decreased fibrinogen level<br>• Decreased platelet level<br>• Decrease in clotting factors | *Medical*<br>• Chemotherapy, biologic response modifier therapy, radiation therapy, or surgery is used to treat the underlying cancer.<br>• Antibiotic therapy is used for sepsis.<br>• Anticoagulants, such as heparin or antithrombin III, decrease the stimulation of the coagulation pathways.<br>• Transfusion of fresh-frozen plasma or cryoprecipitates (which contain clotting factors and fibrinogen), packed red blood cells, and platelets may be used as replacement therapy to prevent or control bleeding.<br>• Although controversial, antifibrinolytic agents such as aminocaproic acid (Amicar), which is associated with increased thrombus formation, may be used.<br><br>*Nursing*<br>• Monitor vital signs.<br>• Measure and document intake and output.<br>• Assess skin color and temperature; lung, heart, and bowel sounds; level of consciousness, headache, visual disturbances, chest pain, decreased urine output, and abdominal tenderness.<br>• Inspect all body orifices, tube insertion sites, incisions, and bodily excretions for bleeding. |

| TABLE 16-13 | Oncologic Emergencies: Manifestations and Management (Continued) | |
|---|---|---|
| **Emergency** | **Clinical Manifestations and Diagnostic Findings** | **Management** |
| platelets faster than the body can replace them. Clots are deposited in the microvasculature, placing the patient at great risk for impaired circulation, tissue hypoxia, and necrosis. In addition, fibrinolysis occurs, breaking down clots and increasing the circulating levels of anticoagulant substances, thereby placing the patient at risk for hemorrhage (Casciato, 2004). | • Decreased hemoglobin<br>• Decreased hematocrit<br>• Elevated fibrin split products<br>• Positive protamine sulfate precipitation test (thrombin activation test) (Krimmel, 2003) | • Review laboratory test results.<br>• Minimize physical activity to decrease injury risks and oxygen requirements.<br>• Prevent bleeding; apply pressure to all venipuncture sites, and avoid nonessential invasive procedures; provide electric rather than straight-edged razors; avoid tape on the skin and advise gentle but adequate oral hygiene.<br>• Assist the patient to turn, cough, and take deep breaths every 2 h.<br>• Reorient the patient, if needed; maintain a safe environment; and provide appropriate patient education and supportive measures. |
| **Syndrome of Inappropriate Secretion of Antidiuretic Hormone (SIADH)**<br>The continuous, uncontrolled release of antidiuretic hormone (ADH), produced by tumor cells or by the abnormal stimulation of the hypothalamic–pituitary network, leads to increased extracellular fluid volume, water intoxication, hyponatremia, and increased excretion of urinary sodium. As fluid volume increases, stretch receptors in the right atrium respond by releasing a second hormone, atrial natriuretic factor (ANF). The release of ANF causes increased renal excretion of sodium, which worsens hyponatremia.<br>The most common cause of SIADH is cancer, especially small cell cancers of the lung. Antineoplastics—vincristine, vinblastine, cisplatin, and cyclophosphamide—and morphine also stimulate ADH secretion, which promotes conservation and reabsorption of water by the kidneys. As more fluid is absorbed, the circulatory volume increases, ANF is released, and sodium is actively excreted by the kidneys in compensation (Flounders, 2003a; Casciato, 2004). | *Clinical*<br>*Serum sodium levels lower than 120 mEq/L (120 mmol/L):* symptoms of hyponatremia including personality changes, irritability, nausea, anorexia, vomiting, weight gain, fatigue, muscular pain (myalgia), headache, lethargy, and confusion (Langfeldt & Cooley, 2003).<br>*Serum sodium levels lower than 110 mEq/L (110 mmol/L):* seizure, abnormal reflexes, papilledema, coma, and death. Edema is rare.<br>*Diagnostic*<br>• Decreased serum sodium level<br>• Increased urine osmolality<br>• Increased urinary sodium level<br>• Decreased blood urea nitrogen (BUN), creatinine, and serum albumin levels secondary to dilution<br>• Abnormal water load test results | *Medical*<br>Fluid intake range limited to 500–1000 mL/day to increase the serum sodium level and decrease fluid overload. If water restriction alone is not effective in correcting or controlling serum sodium levels, demeclocycline is often prescribed to interfere with the antidiuretic action of ADH and ANF. If neurologic symptoms are severe, parenteral sodium replacement and diuretic therapy are indicated. Electrolyte levels are monitored carefully to detect secondary magnesium, potassium, and calcium imbalances. After the symptoms of SIADH are controlled, the underlying cancer is treated. If water excess continues despite treatment, pharmacologic intervention (urea and furosemide) may be indicated (Flounders, 2003a; Casciato, 2004).<br>*Nursing*<br>• Maintain intake and output measurements.<br>• Assess level of consciousness, lung and heart sounds, vital signs, daily weight, and urine specific gravity; also assess for nausea, vomiting, anorexia, edema, fatigue, and lethargy.<br>• Monitor laboratory test results, including serum electrolyte levels, osmolality, and BUN, creatinine, and urinary sodium levels.<br>• Minimize the patient's activity; provide appropriate oral hygiene; maintain environmental safety; and restrict fluid intake if necessary.<br>• Reorient the patient and provide instruction and encouragement as needed (Langfeldt & Cooley, 2003). |

*continued >*

## TABLE 16-13     Oncologic Emergencies: Manifestations and Management (Continued)

| Emergency | Clinical Manifestations and Diagnostic Findings | Management |
|---|---|---|
| **Tumor Lysis Syndrome**<br><br>Potentially fatal complication associated with radiation- or chemotherapy-induced cell destruction of large or rapidly growing cancers such as leukemia, lymphoma, and small cell lung cancer (Cope, 2004). The release of intracellular contents from the tumor cells leads to electrolyte imbalances—hyperkalemia, hypocalcemia, hyperphosphatemia, and hyperuricemia—because the kidneys can no longer excrete large volumes of the released intracellular metabolites. | *Clinical*<br>Clinical manifestations depend on the extent of metabolic abnormalities.<br>• Neurologic: fatigue, weakness, memory loss, altered mental status, muscle cramps, tetany, paresthesias (numbness and tingling), seizures<br>• Cardiac: elevated blood pressure, shortened QT complexes, widened QRS waves, dysrhythmias, cardiac arrest<br>• GI: anorexia, nausea, vomiting, abdominal cramps, diarrhea<br>• Renal: flank pain, oliguria, anuria, renal failure, acidic urine pH<br><br>*Diagnostic*<br>Electrolyte imbalances identified by laboratory test results (Casciato, 2004) | *Medical*<br>• To prevent renal failure and restore electrolyte balance, aggressive fluid hydration is initiated 48 hours before and after the initiation of cytotoxic therapy to increase urine volume and eliminate uric acid and electrolytes. Urine is alkalinized by adding sodium bicarbonate to IV fluid to maintain a urine pH of 7 or higher; this prevents renal failure secondary to uric acid precipitation in the kidneys.<br>• Diuretic therapy, with a carbonic anhydrase inhibitor or acetazolamide, to alkalinize the urine<br>• Allopurinol therapy to inhibit the conversion of nucleic acids to uric acid (Cope, 2004)<br>• Administration of a cation-exchange resin, such as sodium polystyrene sulfonate (Kayexalate) to treat hyperkalemia by binding and eliminating potassium through the bowel<br>• Administration of hypertonic dextrose and regular insulin temporarily shifts potassium into cells and lowers serum potassium levels.<br>• Administration of phosphate-binding gels, such as aluminum hydroxide, to treat hyperphosphatemia by promoting phosphate excretion in the feces.<br>• Hemodialysis when patients are unresponsive to the standard approaches for managing uric acid and electrolyte abnormalities (Casciato, 2004)<br><br>*Nursing*<br>• Identify at-risk patients, including those in whom tumor lysis syndrome may develop up to 1 week after therapy has been completed.<br>• Institute essential preventive measures (eg, fluid hydration, allopurinol).<br>• Assess patient for signs and symptoms of electrolyte imbalances.<br>• Assess urine pH to confirm alkalization.<br>• Monitor serum electrolyte and uric acid levels for evidence of fluid volume overload secondary to aggressive hydration.<br>• Instruct patients to report symptoms indicating electrolyte disturbances. |

## Critical Thinking Exercises

**1** **[ebp]** Your patient has been receiving high doses of chemotherapy to treat leukemia. She reports that she wants to stop the chemotherapy because of the oral ulcerations and pain that have developed since she started on the chemotherapy. What would your response be to her? What evidence-based nursing interventions would you implement to relieve the ulcers and her pain? What is the evidence for the interventions you identified? How strong is that evidence, and what criteria did you use to assess the strength of that evidence?

**2** A 74-year-old patient with prostate cancer and metastasis to the bone is to begin a continuous subcutaneous infusion of analgesia through an ambulatory infusion pump to relieve his severe pain. The patient's wife is afraid that he will become addicted, and his adult children state that his pain remains unrelieved. As a home care nurse, what assessments would be of highest priority to you during your initial visit to this patient? What nursing interventions and teaching would be indicated in this situation? How would you modify your interventions if the patient is receiving fentanyl by transdermal patch and still reporting severe pain?

**3** A 45-year-old woman of Ashkenazi Jewish descent has presented to the cancer center for treatment of advanced breast cancer. Her evaluation revealed that she is positive for the *BRCA1* gene. In reviewing her family history, you note that her mother and older sister (who are both deceased) had metastatic breast cancer. You also note that she has two younger sisters. What information about the *BRCA1* gene will guide you as you plan to assess the screening needs for this woman, her sisters, and her children? What type of referral would be appropriate for this woman and her family?

4. Your 68-year-old patient with lung cancer has been admitted for emergent radiation therapy for the diagnosis of superior vena cava syndrome. Describe the underlying pathology that can lead to the signs and symptoms of superior vena cava syndrome. What patient monitoring will be essential during this patient's course of care? Describe the medical and nursing management strategies that will be used for this patient.

5. A patient with colon cancer who has undergone a successful resection of her bowel has been referred to the medical oncologist for participation in an adjuvant therapy clinical trial involving investigational chemotherapy. After the physician reviews the trial and consent form with the patient, she leaves the room for the patient to consider enrollment into the trial. The patient tells you that she is afraid of being a "guinea pig." Describe the role and the importance of clinical trials in oncology care. What would you tell the patient regarding safeguards that are in place to protect patients who participate in human research. How would you support this patient in her decision-making process regarding participation in a clinical trial?

## REFERENCES AND SELECTED READINGS

### BOOKS

Abeloff, M. D., Armitage, J. D., Niederhuber, J. E., et al. (Eds). (2004). *Clinical oncology* (3rd ed.). Philadelphia: Elsevier/Churchill Livingstone.

Boik, J. (1995). *Cancer and natural medicine: A textbook of basic science and clinical research.* Princeton, MN: Oregon Medical Press.

Casciato, D. A. (Ed.). (2004). *Manual of clinical oncology* (5th ed.). Philadelphia: Lippincott Williams & Wilkins.

Ellis, L. E., Curley, S. A. & Tanabe, K. K. (Eds.) (2004). *Radiofrequency ablation for cancer: Current indications, techniques and outcomes.* New York: Springer Verlag.

Ezzone, S. (Ed.) (2004). *Hematopoietic stem cell transplantation: A manual for nursing practice.* Pittsburgh: Oncology Nursing Society.

Govindan, R. (Ed.) (2002). *The Washington manual of oncology.* Philadelphia: Lippincott Williams & Wilkins.

Green, F., Page, D. L., Fleming, I. D., et al. (Eds.). (2002). *AJCC cancer staging manual* (6th ed.). New York: Springer-Verlag.

Higginson, I. J., Hearn, J. & Addington-Hall, J. (2003). Epidemiology of cancer pain. In Sykes, N., Fallon, M. T. & Patt, R. B. (Eds.) *Cancer pain.* New York: Oxford University Press.

Hough, S. W. & Kanner, R. M. (2004). Cancer pain syndromes. In Warfield, C. A. & Bajwa, Z. H. (Eds.) *Principles and practice of pain medicine* (2nd ed.). New York: McGraw-Hill.

Hough, S. W. & Portenoy, R. K. (2004). Medical management of cancer pain. In Warfield, C. A. & Bajwa, Z. H. (Eds.) *Principles and practice of pain medicine* (2nd ed.). New York: McGraw-Hill.

Janeway, C. A., Travers, P., Walport, M., et al. (2005). *Immunobiology: The immune system in health and disease* (6th ed.). New York: Garland Science.

Kufe, D. W., Pollock, R. E., Wechselbaum, R. R., et al. (Eds.) (2003). *Cancer medicine* (6th ed.). Hamilton, Ontario: B. C. Decker.

Lenhard, R. E., Osteen, R. T., & Gansler, T. (Eds.). (2001). *Clinical oncology.* Atlanta: American Cancer Society.

Morris, D. & Ward, K. (2003). Perioperative nursing. In Booker, C. & Nicol, M. J. (Eds.). *Nursing adults: The practice of caring.* Edinburgh: Mosby/Elsevier.

Overcash, J. & Balducci, L. (Eds.). (2003). *The older cancer patient.* New York: Springer.

Pazdur, R., Coia, L. R., Hoskins, H. S., et al. (Eds.). (2003). *Cancer management: A multidisciplinary approach* (7th ed.). New York: The Oncology Group.

Polovich, M. (Ed.). (2003). *Safe handling of hazardous drugs.* Pittsburgh: Oncology Nursing Society.

Ratain, M. J., Tempero, M., & Skosey, C. (2001). *Outline of oncology therapeutics.* Philadelphia: Saunders.

Richerson, M. T. (2004). Electrolyte imbalances. In Yarbro, C. H., Frogge, M. H., & Goodman, M. (Eds.). *Cancer symptom management* (3rd ed.). Boston: Jones and Bartlett.

Saunders, M. & Booth, S. (2003). Cancer pain therapy. In Munglani, C. R. & Schmidt, W. R. (Eds.). *Pain: Current understanding, emerging therapies and novel approaches to drug discovery.* New York: Marcel Dekker.

Vogel, W. H., Wilson, M. A. & Melvin, M. S. (2004). *Advanced practice oncology and palliative care guidelines.* Philadelphia: Lippincott Williams & Wilkins.

Wilkes, G. M. & Barton-Burke, M. (Eds.). (2004). *2004 oncology nursing handbook.* Sudbury, Massachusetts: Jones & Bartlett.

Yarbro, C. H., Frogge, M. H., & Goodman, M. (Eds.). (2004). *Cancer symptom management* (3rd ed.). Boston: Jones & Bartlett.

## JOURNALS

*Asterisks indicate nursing research articles.

### General

American Cancer Society. (2004a). ACS cancer detection guidelines. Available at: www.cancer.org (accessed March 5, 2006).

American Cancer Society. (2004b). Surgery. Available at: www.cancer.org (accessed March 12, 2006).

Anonymous. (2003). Clinical trials in supportive care: Cancer cachexia and anorexia. *Journal of Supportive Oncology,* 1(4), 294–295.

Berger, A. (2003). Treating fatigue in cancer patients. *The Oncologist,* 8(Suppl 1), 10–14.

Braccia, D. P. & Hoffernan, N. (2003). Surgical and ablative modalities for the treatment of colorectal cancer with liver metastasis. *Clinical Journal of Oncology Nursing,* 7(2), 178–184.

Brown, J. K., Byers, T., Doyle, C., et al. (2003). Nutrition and physical activity during and after cancer treatment: An American Cancer Society guide for informed choices. *CA: A Cancer Journal for Clinicians,* 53(5), 268–291.

Bruce, S. D. (2004). Radiation-induced xerostomia: How dry is your patient? *Clinical Journal of Oncology Nursing,* 8(1), 61–67.

Calzone, K. A. & Masny, A. (2004). Genetics and oncology nursing. *Seminars in Oncology Nursing,* 20(3), 178–185.

Coyne, P. (2003). When the Word Health Organization analgesic therapies ladder fails: The role of invasive analgesic therapies. *Oncology Nursing Forum,* 30(5), 777–783.

Dunn, B. N. K., Wickerham, D. L. & Ford, L. G. (2005). Prevention of hormone-related cancers: Breast cancer. *Journal of Clinical Oncology,* 23(2), 357–367.

Ernst, A., Feller-Kopman, D., Becker, H. D., et al. (2004). Central airway obstruction. *American Journal of Respiratory and Critical Care Medicine,* 169(12), 1278–1297.

Fisher, J. P. (1998). Tamoxifen for prevention of breast cancer: Report of the National Surgical Adjuvant Breast and Bowel Project P-1 study. *Journal of National Cancer Institute, 90*(18), 1371–1388.

Garfunkel, A. A. (2004). Oral mucositis: The search for a solution. *New England Journal of Medicine, 351*(25), 2649–2651.

Gillespie, T. W. (2003). Anemia in cancer. *Cancer Nursing, 26*(2), 119–128.

Goodwin, J. A. & Coleman, E. A. (2003). Exploring measures of functional dependence in the older adult with cancer. *MedSurg Nursing, 12*(6), 359–365.

Gordils-Perez, J., Rawlins-Duell, R. & Kelvin, J. F. (2003). Advances in radiation treatment of patients with breast cancer. *Clinical Journal of Oncology Nursing, 7*(6), 629–636.

Goss, P. E., & Strasser-Weippl, K. (2004). Prevention strategies with aromatase inhibitors. *Clinical Cancer Research, 10*(1 Pt 2), 372S–379S.

Haughney, A. (2004). Nausea and vomiting in end-stage cancer. *American Journal of Nursing, 104*(11), 40–48.

Holder, H. (2003). Nursing management of nutrition in cancer and palliative care. *British Journal of Nursing, 12*(11), 667–668,670, 672–674.

Hood, L. E. (2003). Chemotherapy in the elderly: Supportive measures for chemotherapy induced myelotoxicity. *Clinical Journal of Oncology Nursing, 7*(2), 185–190.

Hutson, S. P. (2003). Attitudes and psychological impact of genetic testing, genetic counseling, and breast cancer risk assessment among women at increased risk. *Oncology Nursing Forum, 30*(2), 241–246.

Jakub, J. W., Pendas, S. & Reintgen, D. S. (2003). Current status of sentinel lymph node mapping and biopsy: Facts and controversies. *The Oncologist, 8*(1), 59–68.

Jemal, A., Murray, T., Ward, E., et al. (2005). Cancer statistics. *CA Cancer Journal for Clinicians, 55*(1), 10–30.

Jemal, A., Tiwari, R. C., Murray, T., et al. (2004). Cancer statistics, 2004. *CA Cancer Journal for Clinicians, 54*(1), 8–29.

Law, E., Mangarin, E. & Kelvin, J. F. (2003). Nursing management of patients receiving stereotactic radiosurgery. *Clinical Journal of Oncology Nursing, 7*(4), 387–392.

Leather, A., Bushell, L. & Gillespie, L. (2003, November). The provision of nutritional support for people with cancer. *Nursing Times, 99*(46), 18–24,53–55.

Leon, T. G. & Pase, M. (2004). Essential oncology facts for the float nurse. *MedSurg Nursing, 13*(3), 165–171.

Lobrano, M. B. & Singha, P. (2003). Positron emission tomography in oncology. *Clinical Journal of Oncology Nursing, 7*(4), 379–385.

MacDonald, N. (2003). Is there evidence for earlier intervention in cancer-associated weight loss? *Journal of Supportive Oncology, 1*(4), 279–286.

McGuire, D. B. & Peterson, D. E. (eds.) (2004). Mucositis. *Seminars in Oncology Nursing, 20*(1), 1–68.

Mahon, S. M. (2003). Patient education regarding cancer screening guidelines. *Clinical Journal of Oncology Nursing, 7*(5), 581–585.

Marrs, J. & Newton, S. (2003). Updating your peripheral neuropathy "know-how." *Clinical Journal of Oncology Nursing, 7*(3), 299–303.

Mock, V. (2003). Clinical excellence through evidence-based practice: Fatigue management as a model. *Oncology Nursing Forum, 30*(5), 787–795.

Mock, V. & Olsen, M. (2003). Current management of fatigue and anemia in patients with cancer. *Seminars in Oncology Nursing, 19*(4 Suppl 2), 36–41.

Montbriand, M. J. (1999). Past and present herbs used to treat cancer: Medicine, magic, or poison? *Oncology Nursing Forum, 26*(1), 49–59.

Montbriand, M. (2004). Herbs or natural products that decrease cancer growth (part one of four). *Oncology Nursing Forum, 31*(4), E75–E90.

National Cancer Institute. (2006). Vaccine protects against virus linked to half of all cervical cancers. Available at: http://www.cancer.gov/clinicaltrials/results/cervical-cancer-vaccine1102 (accessed May 25, 2006).

Sadler, G. R., Wasserman, L., Fullerton, J. T., et al. (2004). Supporting patients through genetic screening for cancer risk. *MedSurg Nursing, 13*(4), 233–246.

*Schreier, A. M. & Williams, S. A. (2004). Anxiety and quality of life of women who receive radiation or chemotherapy for breast cancer. *Oncology Nursing Forum, 31*(1), 127–130.

Shelton, B. K. (2003). Evidence-based care for the neutropenic patient with leukemia. *Seminars in Oncology Nursing, 19*(2), 133–141.

Sifri, R., Gangadharappa, S., & Acheson, L. S. (2004). Identifying and testing for hereditary susceptibility to common cancers. *CA Cancer Journal for Clinicians, 54*(6), 309–326.

*Skalla, K. A., Bakitas, M., Furstenberg, C. T., et al. (2004). Patients' need for information about cancer therapy. *Oncology Nursing Forum, 31*(2), 313–319.

Sparber, A., Bauer, L., Curt, G., et al. (2000). Use of complementary medicine by adult patients participating in cancer clinical trials. *Oncology Nursing Forum, 27*(4), 623–630.

Sterman, E, Gauker, S. & Krieger, J. (2003). A comprehensive approach to improving cancer pain management and patient satisfaction. *Oncology Nursing Forum, 30*(5), 857–864.

Stiff, P. J., Erder, H., Bensinger, W. I., et al. (2006). Reliability and validity of a patient self-administered daily questionnaire to assess impact of oral mucositis (OM) on pain and daily functioning in patients undergoing autologous hematopoietic stem cell transplantation (HSCT). *Bone Marrow Transplant, 37*(4), 393–401.

*Thome, B., Dykes, A. K., Gunnars, B., et al. (2003). The experiences of older people living with cancer. *Cancer Nursing, 26*(2), 85–96.

Vickers, A. (2004). Alternative cancer cures: "Unproven" or "disproven"? *CA Cancer Journal for Clinicians, 54*(2), 110–118.

Ward, E., Jemal, A., Cokkinides, V., et al. (2004). Cancer disparities by race/ethnicity and socioeconomic status. *CA Cancer Journal for Clinicians, 544*(2), 78–93.

Whiteside, T. L. (2003). Immune responses to malignancies. *Journal of Allergy and Clinical Immunology, 111*(2 Suppl), S677–S686.

Wickline, M. M. (2004). Prevention and treatment of acute radiation dermatitis: A literature review. *Oncology Nursing Forum, 31*(2), 237–244.

Wohlschlaeger, A. (2004). Prevention and treatment of mucositis: A guide for nurses. *Journal of Pediatric Oncology Nursing, 21*(5), 281–287.

*Woods, D. V., Montgomery, S. B., & Herring, R. P. (2004). Recruiting Black/African American men for research on prostate cancer prevention. *Cancer, 100*(5), 1017–1025.

*Young-McCaughan, S., Mays, M. Z., Arzola, S. M., et al. (2003). Change in exercise tolerance, activity and sleep patterns, and quality of life in patients with cancer participating in a structured exercise program. *Oncology Nursing Forum, 30*(3), 441–452.

## Bone Marrow Transplantation

DeMeyer, D. H. (2003). Hematopoietic cell transplantation in the treatment of leukemia. *Seminars in Oncology Nursing, 19*(2), 118–132.

Hacker, E. D. (2003). Quantitative measurement of quality of life in adult patients undergoing bone marrow transplant or peripheral blood stem cell transplant: A decade in review. *Oncology Nursing Forum, 30*(4), 613–629.

Latchford, T. & Shelton, B. K. (2004). Respiratory syncytial virus in blood and marrow transplant recipients. *Clinical Journal of Oncology Nursing, 7*(4), 418–422.

Moore, S. L. (2003). Bronchiolitis obliterans organizing pneumonia: A late complication of stem cell transplantation. *Clinical Journal of Oncology Nursing, 7*(6), 659–662.

Tierney, D. K. (2004). Sexuality following hematopoietic cell transplantation. *Clinical Journal of Oncology Nursing, 8*(1), 43–47.

West, F. & Mitchell, S. A. (2004). Evidence-based guidelines for the management of neutropenia following outpatient hematopoietic stem cell transplantation. *Clinical Journal of Oncology Nursing, 8*(6), 601–613.

## Carcinogenesis and Risk Factors

Likes, W. M. & Itano, J. (2003). Human papillomavirus and cervical cancer: Not just a sexually transmitted disease. *Clinical Journal of Oncology Nursing, 7*(3), 271–276.

National Institutes of Health, NIH News. (2004). WHI study finds no heart disease benefit, increased stroke risk with estrogen alone. Available at: http://www.nhlbi.nih.gov/new/press/04-04-13.htm (accessed March 15, 2006).

Tsao, A. S., Kim, E. S. & Hong, W. K. (2004). Chemoprevention of cancer. *CA Cancer Journal for Clinicians, 54*(3), 150–180.

## Chemotherapy

Capriotti, T. (2002). Gleevec: Zeroing in on cancer. *MedSurg Nursing*, 11(6), 301–304.

Bedell, C. M. (2003a). A changing paradigm for cancer treatment: The advent of new oral chemotherapy agents. *Clinical Journal of Oncology Nursing*, 7(6 Suppl), 5–9.

Birner, A. (2003). Pharmacology of oral chemotherapy agents. *Clinical Journal of Oncology Nursing*, 7(6 Suppl), 11–19.

Flemm, L. A. (2004). Aprepitant for chemotherapy-induced nausea and vomiting. *Clinical Journal of Oncology Nursing*, 8(3), 303–306.

Green, J. M. & Hacker, E. D. (2004). Chemotherapy in the geriatric population. *Clinical Journal of Oncology Nursing*, 8(6), 591–597.

Griffin, E. (2003). Safety considerations and safe handling of oral chemotherapy agents. *Clinical Journal of Oncology Nursing*, 7(6 Suppl), 25–29.

Harris, D. J. & Knobf, M. T. (2004). Assessing and managing chemotherapy-induced mucositis pain. *Clinical Journal of Oncology Nursing*, 8(6), 622–628.

Marek, C. (2003). Antiemetic therapy in patients receiving cancer chemotherapy. *Oncology Nursing Forum*, 30(2), 259–269.

Rittenberg, C. N. (2004). The next generation of chemotherapy-induced nausea and vomiting prevention and control: A new 5-HT3 antagonist arrives. *Clinical Journal of Oncology Nursing*, 8(3), 307–308.

Sadler, G. R., Stoudt, A., Fullerton, J. T., et al. (2003). Managing the oral sequelae of cancer therapy. *MedSurg Nursing*, 12(1), 28–36.

Sorich, J., Taubes, B., Wagner, A., et al. (2004). Oxaliplatin: Practical guidelines for administration. *Clinical Journal of Oncology Nursing*, 8(3), 251–256.

Spielberger, R., Stiff, P., Bensinger, W. et al. (2004). Palifermin for oral mucositis after intensive therapy for hematologic cancers. *New England Journal of Medicine*, 351(25), 2590–2598.

## Oncologic Emergencies

Abrahm, J. L. (2004). Assessment and treatment of patients with spinal cord compression. *Journal of Supportive Oncology*, 2(5), 377–401.

Cantril, C. A. & Haylock, P. J. (2004). Tumor lysis syndrome. *American Journal of Nursing*, 104(4), 49–52.

Cope, D. (2004). Tumor lysis syndrome. *Clinical Journal of Oncology Nursing*, 8(4), 415–416.

Flounders, J. A. (2003a). Cardiovascular emergencies: Pericardial effusion and cardiac tamponade. *Oncology Nursing Forum*, 30(2), E48–E55.

Flounders, J. A. (2003b). Superior vena cava syndrome. [Online exclusive.] *Oncology Nursing Forum*, 30(4), E84–E90.

Flounders, J. A. (2003c). Syndrome of inappropriate antidiuretic hormone. *Oncology Nursing Forum*, 30(3), E63–E68.

Flounders, J. A. & Ott, B. B. (2003). Oncologic emergency modules: Spinal cord compression. [Online exclusive.] *Oncology Nursing Forum*, 30(1), E17–E23.

Krimmel, T. (2003). Disseminated intravascular coagulation. *Clinical Journal of Oncology Nursing*, 7(4), 479.

Langfeldt, L. A. & Cooley, M. E. (2003). Syndrome of inappropriate antidiuretic hormone secretion in malignancy: Review and implications for nursing management. *Clinical Journal of Oncology Nursing*, 7(4), 425–430.

Shuey, K. M. (2004). Hypercalcemia of malignancy: Part I. *Clinical Journal of Oncology Nursing*, 8(2), 209–210.

Shuey, K. M. & Brant, J., M. (2004). Hypercalcemia of malignancy: Part II. *Clinical Journal of Oncology Nursing*, 8(3), 321–323.

Viale, P. H. & Yamamoto, D. S. (2003). Biphosphonates: Expanded roles in the treatment of patients with cancer. *Clinical Journal of Oncology Nursing*, 7(4), 393–401.

## Radiation Therapy

Abel, L., Dafoe-Lambie, J., Butler, W. M., et al. (2003). Treatment outcomes and quality-of-life issues for patients treated with prostate brachytherapy. *Clinical Journal of Oncology Nursing*, 7(1), 48–54.

Estes, J. M. & Clapp, K. J. (2004). Radioimmunotherapy with tositumomab and iodine-131 tositumomab for low-grade non-Hodgkin lymphoma: Nursing implications. *Oncology Nursing Forum*, 31(6), 1119–1126.

Hogle, W. P., Quinn, A. E., & Heron, D. E. (2003). Advances in brachytherapy: New approaches to target breast cancer. *Clinical Journal of Oncology Nursing*, 7(3), 324–328.

Iwamoto, R. R., & Maher, K. E. (2001). Radiation therapy for prostate cancer. *Seminars in Oncology Nursing*, 17(2), 90–100.

Stajduhar, K. I., Neithercut, J., Chu, E., et al. (2000). Thyroid cancer patients' experiences of receiving iodine-131 therapy. *Oncology Nursing Forum*, 27(8), 1213–1218.

Wickline, M. M. (2004). Prevention and treatment of acute radiation dermatitis: A literature review. *Oncology Nursing Forum*, 31(2), 237–244.

Witt, M. E., Haas, M., Marrinan, M. A., et al. (2003). Understanding stereotactic radiosurgery for intracranial tumors; seed implants for prostate cancer; and intravascular brachytherapy for cardiac restenosis. *Cancer Nursing*, 26(6), 494–502.

## Targeted Therapies

Bedell, C. M. (2003b). Pegfilgrastin for chemotherapy-induced neutropenia. *Clinical Journal of Oncology Nursing*, 7(1), 55–58.

Breed, C. D. (2003). Diagnosis, treatment and nursing care of patients with chronic leukemia. *Seminars in Oncology Nursing*, 19(3), 109–117.

Capo, G. & Waltzman, R. (2004). Managing hematologic toxicities. *Journal of Supportive Oncology*, 2(1), 65–77.

Cappozzo, C. (2004). Optimal use of granulocyte-colony stimulating factor in patients with cancer who are at risk for chemotherapy-induced neutropenia. *Oncology Nursing Forum*, 31(3), 569–574.

Capriotti, T. (2004). New oncology strategy: Molecular targeting of cancer cells. *MedSurg Nursing*, 13(3), 191–195.

Colson, K., Doss, D. S., Swift, R., et al. (2004). Bortezomib, a newly approved proteasome inhibitor for the treatment of multiple myeloma: Nursing implications. *Clinical Journal of Oncology Nursing*, 8(5), 473–480.

Gale, D. M. (2003). Molecular targets in cancer therapy. *Seminars in Oncology Nursing*, 19(2), 193–205.

Galsky, M. & Kelly, W. K. (2003). The development of differentiation agents for the treatment of prostate cancer. *Seminars in Oncology*, 30(5), 689–697.

Gemmill, R. & Idell, C. S. (2003). Biological advances for new treatment approaches. *Seminars in Oncology Nursing*, 19(2), 162–168.

King, S. E. (2004). Therapeutic cancer vaccines: An emerging treatment option. *Clinical Journal of Oncology Nursing*, 8(3), 271–278.

Kristal, A. R. (2004). Vitamin A, retinoids and carotenoids as chemoprevention agents for prostate cancer. *Journal of Urology*, 17(2, part 2 of 2), S54–S58.

Krozely, P. (2004). Epidermal growth factor receptor tyrosine kinase inhibitors: Evolving role of the treatment of solid tumors. *Clinical Journal of Oncology Nursing*, 8(2), 163–168.

Lui, K. (2003). Breakthroughs in cancer gene therapy. *Seminars in Oncology Nursing*, 19(2), 217–226.

Schmidt, K. V. & Wood, B. A. (2003). Trends in cancer therapy: Role of monoclonal antibodies. *Seminars in Oncology Nursing*, 19(2), 169–179.

Stull, D. M. (2003). Targeted therapies for treatment of leukemia. *Seminars in Oncology Nursing*, 19(2), 90–97.

Yarbro, C. H. (Ed.). (2004). Yttrium 90 ibritumamab tiuxetan (Zevalin) radioimmunotherapy for B-cell non-Hodgkin's lymphoma. *Seminars in Oncology Nursing*, 20(1 Suppl 1), 1–25.

## RESOURCES

## PROFESSIONAL ORGANIZATIONS

American Society of Clinical Oncology (ASCO), 1900 Duke Street, Suite 200, Alexandria, VA 22314; 703-299-0150, fax 703-299-1044; http://www.asco.org. Accessed March 15, 2006.

National Comprehensive Cancer Network, 500 Old York Road, Suite 250, Jenkintown, PA 9046; 215-690-0360, fax 215-728-3877, 888-909-NCCN, 888-909-6226; http://www.nccn.org. Accessed March 15, 2006.

Oncology Nursing Society (ONS), 125 Enterprise Drive, RIDC Part West, Pittsburgh, PA 15275-1214; 866-257-4ONS, fax 877-369-5497; http://www.ons.org. Accessed March 15, 2006.

## PATIENT/FAMILY SUPPORT AND EDUCATION

American Brain Tumor Association, 2720 River Road, Des Plaines, IL 60018; 800-886-2282, fax 847-827-9918, Patient line: 800-886-2282; http://www.abta.org. Accessed March 15, 2006.

American Cancer Society. ACS), 800-ACS-2345 (check your local directory for the unit of division nearest you); http://www.cancer.org. Accessed March 15, 2006.

Cancer Care, Inc., National Office, 275 Seventh Ave., New York, NY 10001; Services: 212-302-2400, 800-813-HOPE (×4673); http://www.cancercare.org. Accessed March 15, 2006.

Make Today Count, 1235 East Cherokee Street, Springfield, MO 85804; 407-885-3324 or 800-432-2273.

The National Cancer Institute, Building, 31, Room 10A31, 31 Center Drive, MSC 2580, Bethesda, MD 20892-2580; (800)-4-CANCER; http://www.nci.nih.gov. Accessed March 15, 2006.

National Coalition for Cancer Survivorship, 1010 Wayne Avenue, Suite 770, Silver Spring, MD 20910-5600; 301-650-9127 or 877-NCCS-YES (877-622-7937); fax: 301-565-9670; http://www.canceradvocacy.org. Accessed March 15, 2006.

The National Hospice and Palliative Care Organization, 1700 Diagonal Road, Suite 300, Alexandria, VA 22314; 703-837-1500; http://www.nhpco.org. Accessed March 15, 2006.

Oncolink, the University of Pennsylvania Cancer Center, 3400 Spruce St., Philadelphia, PA 19104; http://www.oncolink.upenn.edu. Accessed March 15, 2006.

The Wellness Community, 919 18th Street NW, Suite 54, Washington, DC 2006, 202-659-9709, fax 202-659-9801, 888-793-WELL; http://www.wellness-community.org. Accessed March 15, 2006.

# CHAPTER 17

# End-of-Life Care

## Learning Objectives

*On completion of this chapter, the learner will be able to:*

1. Discuss the historical, legal, and sociocultural perspectives of palliative and end-of-life care in the United States.
2. Define palliative care.
3. Compare and contrast the settings where palliative care and end-of-life care are provided.
4. Describe the principles and components of hospice care.
5. Identify barriers to improving care at the end of life.
6. Reflect on personal experience with and attitudes toward death and dying.
7. Apply skills for communicating with terminally ill patients and their families.
8. Provide culturally and spiritually sensitive care to terminally ill patients and their families.
9. Implement nursing measures to manage physiologic responses to terminal illness.
10. Support actively dying patients and their families.
11. Identify components of uncomplicated grief and mourning and implement nursing measures to support patients and families.

## Nursing and End-of-Life Care

One of the most difficult realities nurses face is that, despite their very best efforts, some of their patients die. Although nurses cannot change this fact, they can have a significant and lasting effect on the way in which patients live until they die, the manner in which the death occurs, and the enduring memories of that death for the families. Nursing has a long history of holistic, person- and family-centered care. Indeed, the definition of nursing offered by the American Nurses Association (ANA) highlights nursing's commitment to the diagnosis and treatment of human responses to illness (ANA, 2003). There is perhaps no setting or circumstance in which nursing care—that is, attention to human responses—is more important than in caring for dying patients.

Knowledge about end-of-life decisions and principles of care is essential to supporting patients during decision making and in end-of-life closure in ways that recognize patients' unique responses to illness and that support their values and goals. Education, clinical practice, and research concerning end-of-life care are evolving, and the need to prepare nurses and other health care professionals to care for the dying has emerged as a priority. At no time in nursing's history has there been a greater opportunity to bring research, education, and practice together to change the culture of dying, bringing much-needed improvement to care that is relevant across practice settings, age groups, cultural backgrounds, and illnesses. The National Institute for Nursing Research has taken the lead in coordinating research related to end-of-life care within the National Institutes of Health and has included end-of-life care in its strategic plan for the 21st century (see Resources).

## The Context of Death and Dying in America

In the past three to four decades, there has been a surge of interest in the care of the dying, with an emphasis on the settings in which death occurs, the technologies used to sustain life, and the challenges of trying to improve end-of-life care. The focus on care of the dying has been motivated by the aging of the population, the prevalence of and publicity surrounding life-threatening illnesses such as cancer and acquired immunodeficiency syndrome (AIDS), and the efforts of health care providers to build a continuum of service that spans the lifetime from birth until death (Jennings, Ryndes, D'Onofrio, et al., 2003). Although there are more opportunities than ever before to allow peaceful death, the knowledge and technologies available to health care providers have made the process of dying anything but peaceful. According to Callahan (1993), Americans view death as what happens when medicine fails, and this attitude often places the study of death and improvement of the dying process outside the focus of modern medicine and health care. Numerous initiatives aimed at improving end-of-life care have been launched in recent years, spurred by a widespread call for substantive change in the way Americans deal with death.

The Palliative Care Task Force of the Last Acts Campaign (Last Acts, 1997) identified the following as precepts or principles underlying a more comprehensive and humane approach to care of the dying:

- Respecting patients' goals, preferences, and choices
- Attending to the medical, emotional, social, and spiritual needs of dying people

## Glossary

**assisted suicide:** use of pharmacologic agents to hasten the death of a terminally ill patient; illegal in most states

**autonomy:** self-determination; in the health care context, the right of the individual to make choices about the use and discontinuation of medical treatment

**bereavement:** period during which mourning for a loss takes place

**euthanasia:** Greek for "good death;" has evolved to mean the intentional killing by act or omission of a dependent human being for his or her alleged benefit

**grief:** the personal feelings that accompany an anticipated or actual loss

**hospice:** a coordinated program of interdisciplinary care and services provided primarily in the home to terminally ill patients and their families

**interdisciplinary collaboration:** communication and cooperation among members of diverse health care disciplines jointly to plan, implement, and evaluate care

**Medicare Hospice Benefit:** a Medicare entitlement that provides for comprehensive, interdisciplinary palliative care and services for eligible beneficiaries who have a terminal illness and a life expectancy of less than 6 months

**mourning:** individual, family, group, and cultural expressions of grief and associated behaviors

**palliative care:** comprehensive care for patients whose disease is not responsive to cure; care also extends to patients' families

**palliative sedation:** use of pharmacologic agents, at the request of the terminally ill patient, to induce sedation when symptoms have not responded to other management measures. The purpose is not to hasten the patient's death but to relieve intractable symptoms.

**spirituality:** personal belief systems that focus on a search for meaning and purpose in life, intangible elements that impart meaning and vitality to life, and a connectedness to a higher or transcendent dimension

**terminal illness:** progressive, irreversible illness that despite cure-focused medical treatment will result in the patient's death

- Using strengths of interdisciplinary resources
- Acknowledging and addressing caregiver concerns
- Building mechanisms and systems of support

## Technology and End-of-Life Care

In the last century, chronic, degenerative diseases replaced communicable diseases as the major causes of death. Although technologic advances in health care have extended and improved the quality of life for many people, the ability of technologies to prolong life beyond the point that some people would consider meaningful has raised troubling ethical issues. In particular, the use of technology to sustain life has raised perplexing issues with regard to quality of life, prolongation of dying, adequacy of pain relief and symptom management, and allocation of scarce resources. The major ethical question that has emerged concerning the use of technology to extend life is this: Because medical professionals can prolong life through a particular intervention, does it necessarily follow that they must do so? In the latter half of the 20th century, a "technologic imperative" practice pattern among health care professionals emerged, along with an expectation among patients and families that every available means to extend life must be tried.

Decisions to apply every available technology to extend life have contributed to the shift in the place of death from the home to the hospital or extended care facility. In the earlier part of the 20th century, most deaths occurred at home. Because of this, most families had direct experience with death, providing care to family members at the end of life, and mourning for the loss of loved ones. As the place of death shifted to hospitals, families became increasingly distanced from the death experience. By the early 1970s, when hospice care was just beginning in this country, technology had become the expected companion of the critically and terminally ill (Waller & Caroline, 2000). The implications of technologic intervention at the end of life continue to be profound, affecting a societal view of death that influences how clinicians care for the dying, how family and friends participate in care, how patients and families understand and choose among end-of-life care options, how families prepare for **terminal illness** and death, and how they heal after the death of a loved one.

## Sociocultural Context

Although each person experiences terminal illness uniquely, such illness is also shaped substantially by the social and cultural contexts in which it occurs. In the United States, life-threatening illness, life-sustaining treatment decisions, dying, and death occur in a social environment in which illness is largely considered a foe and battles are either lost or won (Benoliel, 1993). A care/cure dichotomy has emerged, in which health care providers may view cure as the ultimate good and care as second best, a good only when cure is no longer possible. In such a model of health or medical care, alleviating suffering is not as valued as curing disease, and patients who cannot be cured feel distanced from the health care team, concluding that, when treatment has failed, they too have failed. Patients and families who have internalized the socially constructed meaning of care as second-best may fear that any shift from curative goals in the direction of comfort-focused care will result in no care or lower-quality care, and that the clinicians on whom they have come to rely will abandon them if they withdraw from the battle for cure.

The reduction of patients to their diseases is exemplified in the frequently relayed message in late-stage illness that "nothing more can be done." This all-too-frequently used statement communicates the belief of many clinicians that there is nothing of value to offer patients who are beyond cure. In a care-focused perspective, mind, body, and spirit are inextricable, and treating the body without attending to the other components is considered inadequate to evoke true healing. This expanded notion of healing as care, along with and beyond cure, implies that healing can take place throughout life and outside the boundaries of contemporary medicine. In this expanded definition, there continue to be opportunities for physical, spiritual, emotional, and social healing, even as body systems begin to fail at the end of life.

### *Clinicians' Attitudes Toward Death*

Clinicians' attitudes toward the terminally ill and dying remain the greatest barrier to improving care at the end of life. Kübler-Ross illuminated the concerns of the seriously ill and dying in her seminal work, *On Death and Dying*, published in 1969. At that time, it was common for patients to be kept uninformed about life-threatening diagnoses, particularly cancer, and for physicians and nurses to avoid open discussion of death and dying with their patients (Krisman-Scott, 2000). Kübler-Ross taught the health care community that having open discussion about life and death issues did not harm patients, and that the patients in fact welcomed such openness. She was plainly critical of what she called "a new but depersonalized science in the service of prolonging life rather than diminishing human suffering" (Kübler-Ross, 1969). She taught the health care community that healing could not take place in a conspiracy of silence, and that as clinicians break the silence and enter the patient's world, they too can be healed by their struggles and strengths. Her work revealed that, given adequate time and some help in working through the process, patients could reach a stage of acceptance in which they were neither angry nor depressed about their fate (Kübler-Ross, 1969).

Clinicians' reluctance to discuss disease and death openly with patients stems from their own anxieties about death as well as misconceptions about what and how much patients want to know about their illnesses. In an early study of care of the dying in hospital settings, sociologists Glaser and Strauss (1965) discovered that health care professionals in hospital settings avoided direct communication about dying in hopes that the patient would discover it on his or her own. They identified four "awareness contexts," described as the patient's, physician's, family's, and other health care professionals' awareness of the patient's status and their recognition of each other's awareness (Glaser & Strauss, 1965):

1. *Closed awareness:* The patient is unaware of his or her terminal state, whereas others are aware. Closed awareness may be characterized as a conspiracy between the family and health care professionals to guard the "secret," fearing that the patient not be able to cope with full disclosure about his or her status, and the patient's

acceptance of others' accounts of his or her "future biography" as long as the others give him or her no reason to be suspicious.
2. *Suspected awareness:* The patient suspects what others know and attempts to find out details about his or her condition. Suspected awareness may be triggered by inconsistencies in the family's and the clinician's communication and behavior, discrepancies between clinicians' accounts of the seriousness of the patient's illness, or a decline in the patient's condition or other environmental cues.
3. *Mutual pretense awareness:* The patient, the family, and the health care professionals are aware that the patient is dying but all pretend otherwise.
4. *Open awareness:* The patient, the family, and the health care professionals are aware that the patient is dying and openly acknowledge that reality.

Glaser and Strauss (1965) also identified a pattern of clinician behavior in which those clinicians who feared or were uncomfortable discussing death developed and substituted "personal mythologies" for appraisals of what level of disclosure patients actually wanted. For example, clinicians avoided direct communication with patients about the seriousness of their illness based on their beliefs that (1) patients already knew the truth or would ask if they wanted to know, or (2) patients would subsequently lose all hope, give up, or be psychologically harmed by disclosure.

Glaser and Strauss' findings were published more than 40 years ago, yet their observations remain valid today. Although a growing number of health care providers are becoming comfortable with assessing patients' and families' information needs and disclosing honest information about the seriousness of illness, many still avoid the topic of death in hopes that the patient will ask or find out on his or her own. Despite progress on many health care fronts, those who work with dying patients have identified the persistence of a "conspiracy of silence" about dying (Stanley, 2000, p. 34).

## Patient and Family Denial

Denial on the part of the patient and family about the seriousness of terminal illness also has been cited as a barrier to discussion about end-of-life treatment options. Kübler-Ross (1969) was one of the first to examine patient denial and expose it as a useful coping mechanism that enables the patient to gain temporary emotional distance from something that is too painful to contemplate fully. Patients who are characterized as being in denial may be using that strategy to preserve important interpersonal relationships, to protect others from the emotional effects of their illness, or to protect themselves because of fears of abandonment.

Connor (1992) studied a small group of terminally ill cancer patients who were characterized by their use of denial as a coping mechanism. Participants in the experimental group were questioned in structured interviews about their perceptions of the most difficult aspects of having cancer and those actions that they or others take that make these difficulties easier or more difficult to bear. They were offered psychosocial intervention that consisted largely of therapeutic communication followed by a postintervention assessment of their use of denial as a defense mechanism. The use of denial by patients in a control group was also assessed, but these patients did not receive the psychosocial intervention. The researcher concluded that terminally ill patients using denial respond favorably to sensitive psychosocial intervention, as indicated by decreased scores on an instrument to measure denial. However, Connor acknowledged the need for additional research to gauge the timing of such interventions according to some measure of patient readiness.

In a more recent study, researchers reported that, although the majority of a sample of 200 patients with advanced cancer were completely aware of their medical prognosis in their final weeks of life, 26.5% were either unaware or only partially aware (Chochinov, Tataryn, Wilson, et al., 2000). Depression was almost three times greater in patients who were unaware of their prognosis. The researchers concluded that patients with underlying psychological or emotional distress are more likely to deny their prognosis. Similarly, Chow and colleagues (2001) reported that many patients surveyed about their understanding of palliative radiation therapy for advanced cancer believed that their disease was curable, that the radiation therapy would cure their cancer, or that the therapy would prolong their lives. Importantly, most also reported that they were unfamiliar with the concept of radiation therapy, were not given information, or were not satisfied with the information their physicians had provided. Clearly, further research is needed to examine the complex interactions between patients' misconceptions about advanced illness, their underlying psychological states, and clinicians' persistent lack of explanations of treatment expectations and prognosis.

The question of how to communicate with patients in a way that acknowledges where they are on the continuum of acceptance, while providing them with unambiguous information, remains a challenge. Zerwekh (1994) analyzed stories from 32 hospice nurses and concluded that nurses in a hospice setting were adept at interventions deemed important in care of the dying, namely truth telling and encouraging patient **autonomy** (Chart 17-1). Although Zerwekh acknowledged that each person views "truth" differently, she observed that hospice nurses deliberately spoke about sensitive matters that were usually avoided and gave patients and families truthful representations of their status when patients were in transition from curative to palliative care. Timing of sensitive questions takes experience, but speaking the truth can be a relief to patients and families, enhancing their autonomy by making way for truly informed consent as the basis for decision making (Pitorak, 2003a).

## Assisted Suicide

The assisted suicide debate has aimed a spotlight on the adequacy and quality of end-of-life care in the United States. **Assisted suicide** refers to providing another person the means to end his or her own life. Physician-assisted suicide involves the prescription by a physician of a lethal dose of medication for the purpose of ending someone's life (not to be confused with the ethically and legally supported practice of withholding or withdrawing medical treatment in accordance with the wishes of the terminally ill person).

## CHART 17-1

### Dying Person's Bill of Rights

- I have the right to be treated as a living human being until I die.
- I have the right to maintain a sense of hopefulness, however changing its focus may be.
- I have the right to be cared for by those who can maintain a sense of hopefulness, however changing this may be.
- I have the right to express my feelings and emotions and my approaching death in my own way.
- I have the right to participate in decisions concerning my care.
- I have the right to expect continuing medical and nursing attention, even though "cure" goals must be changed to "comfort" goals.
- I have the right not to die alone.
- I have the right to be free from pain.
- I have the right to have my questions answered honestly.
- I have the right not to be deceived.
- I have the right to have help from and for my family in accepting my death.
- I have the right to die in peace and dignity.
- I have the right to retain my individuality and not be judged by my decisions, which may be contrary to the beliefs of others.
- I have the right to discuss and enlarge my religious and/or spiritual experiences, regardless of what they mean to others.
- I have the right to expect that the sanctity of the human body will be respected after death.
- I have the right to be cared for by caring, sensitive, knowledgeable people who will attempt to understand my needs and will be able to gain some satisfaction in helping me face my death.

Although the preference to take one's own life instead of awaiting death has been evident through the ages, these recent efforts to legalize assisted suicide underscore the need for changes in the ways people with terminal illnesses are cared for and treated at the end of their lives. This is further emphasized by the efforts of groups such as the Hemlock Society to have physician-assisted suicide legalized and the Hemlock Society's publication of information describing methods for ending one's own life when such assistance from a physician is not available.

Although assisted suicide is expressly prohibited under statutory or common law in all states but Oregon, the calls for legalized assisted suicide have highlighted inadequacies in the care of the dying. In 1990, Dr. Jack Kevorkian, a retired pathologist, assisted a 54-year-old woman with early Alzheimer's disease to end her life using a device that allowed her to control the infusion of a lethal dose of potassium chloride. In 1999, after 130 deaths and nine trials, Kevorkian was convicted on second-degree murder charges in the death of a 52-year-old man with amyotrophic lateral sclerosis and received a 10- to 25-year prison sentence.

Meanwhile, public support for physician-assisted suicide has resulted in a number of state ballot initiatives. In 1994, Oregon voters approved the Oregon Death With Dignity Act, the first—and to date, only—such legislative initiative to pass. This law provides for access to physician-assisted suicide by terminally ill patients under very controlled circumstances. After numerous challenges, a majority of Oregonians voted against an attempted repeal, and the law was enacted in 1997. The most recent challenges to the law, both unsuccessful, were the 1999 federal Pain Relief Promotion Act, a bill designed to derail the implementation of the Oregon law by prohibiting the use of federally controlled substances for physician-assisted suicide, and a 2001 directive from the U.S. Attorney General to the Drug Enforcement Agency to track and prosecute physicians who prescribe under the Oregon law. Oregon subsequently filed a lawsuit in 2001, and a U.S. district court issued a temporary restraining order against Attorney General Ashcroft's ruling. In 2002, the Death with Dignity Act was upheld in U.S. district court and Attorney General Ashcroft filed an appeal. The appeal was denied. After several additional requests by the Attorney General and denials, the U.S. Supreme Court affirmed the lower court's decision on January 6, 2006, allowing the Death with Dignity Act to remain in effect (Oregon Department of Human Services, 2006). Since 1997, the number of Oregonians who have self-administered physician-prescribed lethal medication has remained small, growing from 15 persons in 1999 to 42 persons in 2003, then decreasing to 37 in 2004 and 38 in 2005 (Oregon Department of Human Services, 2006).

Although Oregon is currently the only state with a statute legalizing physician-assisted suicide, it is likely that the issue will be pursued in the courts and through ballot measures in other states. Proponents of physician-assisted suicide argue that terminally ill people should have a legally sanctioned right to make independent decisions about the value of their lives and the timing and circumstances of their deaths, and its opponents argue for greater access to symptom management and psychosocial support for people approaching the end of life. Numerous ethical and legal issues have been raised, including voluntariness and authenticity of requests in relation to the mental competence and decision-making capacity of patients who request physician-assisted suicide, the existence of underlying untreated clinical depression or other suffering, and issues of overt or perceived coercion. Assisted suicide is opposed by nursing and medical organizations as a violation of the ethical traditions of nursing and medicine (Chart 17-2). The ANA Position Statement on Assisted Suicide acknowledges the complexity of the assisted suicide debate but clearly states that nursing participation in assisted suicide is a violation of the Code for Nurses. The ANA Position Statement further stresses the important role of the nurse in supporting effective symptom management, contributing to the creation of environments for care that honor the patient's and family's wishes, and ascertaining and addressing their concerns and fears (ANA, 1994).

### CHART 17-2

### Ethics and Related Issues

#### "What If a Patient Asks You to Help Him End His Life?"

**SITUATION**

You are a hospice nurse visiting a coworker's patients. A 72-year-old man with end-stage congestive heart failure and dyspnea at rest has two-pillow orthopnea while receiving continuous oxygen at 4 L/min by nasal cannula. When compared to the findings reported in your colleague's notes from previous visits, the patient's condition appears to be declining. After you have completed your physical examination, you sit in a chair next to the patient's bed and ask him how he feels he is doing. He sighs and tells you that he thinks he is "getting close to the end" and will "soon be ready for that pill." When you inquire about the pill, the patient says that "John [the name of the usual hospice nurse] knows and is going to help, so don't worry." At this point, the patient says that he is tired and does not want to talk any more today.

**DILEMMA**

The patient's autonomy conflicts with the nurse's obligation to respect and protect human life, to promote comfort and relieve suffering, and to "do no harm."

**DISCUSSION**

1. What should your follow-up consist of?
2. Should you discuss the patient's request with his wife before you end the visit that day? Discuss the moral basis for your decision.
3. What is the position of the American Nurses Association (ANA) on assisted suicide, and how does the ANA position relate to your understanding of your moral obligation?
4. How should you follow up with John?
5. With another student, role play your discussion with John.
6. What would you do next if John will not discuss the patient's request with you?
7. Who are the other stakeholders in this situation, and what is your ethical responsibility to each?

## Settings for End-of-Life Care: Palliative Care Programs and Hospice

### Palliative Care

As concerns have grown about the poor quality of life patients experience during progressive illness, broadening of the concept of palliative care beyond the hospice has begun to take hold in health care settings across the country. **Palliative care** is an approach to care for the seriously ill that has long been a part of cancer care. Both palliative care and hospice care have been recognized as important bridges between a medical bias in the direction of cure-oriented treatment and the needs of the terminally ill patients and their families for comprehensive care in the final years, months, or weeks of life (Hallenbeck, 2003). Advocates for improved care for the dying have stated that acceptance, management, and understanding of death should become fully integrated concepts in mainstream health care. Increasingly, palliative care is being offered to patients with noncancer chronic illnesses, where comprehensive symptom management and psychosocial and spiritual support can enhance the patient's and family's quality of life.

Although hospice care is considered by many to be the "gold standard" for palliative care, the term **hospice** is generally associated with palliative care that is delivered at home or in special facilities to patients who are approaching the end of life. Palliative care is conceptually broader than hospice care, and is defined as the active, total care of patients whose disease is not responsive to treatment (World Health Organization, 1990). When palliative care coexists with disease-oriented treatment, patients and their families benefit from more comprehensive management of the illness experience (Abrahm, 2000).

Palliative care emphasizes management of psychological, social, and spiritual problems in addition to control of pain and other physical symptoms. As the definition suggests, palliative care is not care that begins when cure-focused treatment ends. The goal of palliative care is to improve the patient's and family's quality of life, and many aspects of this type of comprehensive, comfort-focused approach to care are applicable earlier in the process of life-threatening disease, in conjunction with cure-focused treatment. However, definitions of palliative care, the services that are part of it, and the clinicians who provide it are evolving steadily.

Some would argue that palliative care is no different from comprehensive nursing, medical, social, and spiritual care and that patients should not have to be labeled as "dying" to receive person-focused care and symptom management. In addition to a focus on the multiple dimensions of the illness experience for both patients and their families, palliative care emphasizes the interdisciplinary collaboration that is necessary to bring about the desired outcomes for patients and their families. **Interdisciplinary collaboration** is distinguished from multidisciplinary practice in that the former is based on communication and cooperation among the various disciplines, each member of the team contributing to a single integrated care plan that addresses the needs of the patient and family. Multidisciplinary care refers to participation of clinicians with varied backgrounds and skill sets but without coordination and integration.

### *Palliative Care at the End of Life*

As previously discussed, palliative care is broadly conceptualized as comprehensive, person- and family-centered care when disease is not responsive to treatment. The broadening of the concept of palliative care actually followed the development of hospice services in the United States. Hospice care

## NURSING RESEARCH PROFILE

### Nurses' Responses to Their Patients' Requests for Assisted Dying

Schwarz, J. K. (2003). Understanding and responding to patients' requests for assistance in dying. *Journal of Nursing Scholarship, 35*(4), 377–384.

#### Purpose
Nurses have reported increasing numbers of requests from patients or their family members for assistance in dying. Little is known about how nurses have interpreted and responded to such requests. This study explored how nurses understand the meaning of being asked by people competent to make decisions for assistance in dying and how they determine what their response will be.

#### Design
The researcher used interpretive phenomenology to structure and carry out this qualitative study. The research question that guided the study was, "What is the nature of the experience of being asked to help someone die?" Participating nurses self-identified having had an experience when a competent patient asked them for help to die. Participants practiced in settings that included hospice ($n = 4$), with AIDS patients ($n = 3$), in critical care ($n = 2$), and with patients who had spinal cord injuries ($n = 1$). Nine of the 10 participants were interviewed in their homes, one was interviewed by telephone, and all but one received a follow-up interview to react to the researcher's analysis of the data. The researcher began each initial interview by asking the participant to tell her "about a time when a patient asked you for help in dying." As the researcher coded and re-coded interview transcripts, themes and subthemes were identified in the participants' stories.

#### Findings
The researcher identified four major themes: (1) being open to hear and hearing, (2) interpreting and responding to the meaning, (3) responding to persistent requests for assistance in dying, and (4) reflections. Nurses experienced considerable difficulty in dealing with requests. Few directly agreed or refused to participate in assisting patients to die. Instead, they responded by providing supportive end-of-life care and remaining present during difficult times. Participants described "unspoken understandings and covert agreements with family members and collusion with physician colleagues." The participants struggled with identifying a "reliable moral line" for providing palliative interventions that might intentionally or inadvertently hasten death.

#### Nursing Implications
Nurses who care for patients at the end of life witness considerable suffering among the patients and family members for whom they care. Often, they practice in settings in which they are isolated from immediate support from colleagues, such as in home hospice care. Nurses need time with supportive colleagues to reflect on their feelings about morally problematic situations and to determine an ethically and emotionally satisfactory resolution.

---

is in fact palliative care. The difference is that hospice care is associated with the end of life, and although it focuses on quality of life, hospice care by necessity usually includes realistic emotional, social, spiritual, and financial preparation for death. In the mid-1970s, when hospice care was introduced in the United States, it was more broadly conceived as care that addressed the entire person—physical, social, emotional, and spiritual—and was available to patients earlier in the process of life-threatening illness. After hospice care was recognized as a distinct program of services under Medicare in the early 1980s, organizations providing hospice care were able to receive Medicare reimbursement if they could demonstrate that the hospice program met the Medicare "conditions of participation," or regulations, for hospice providers.

Medicare reimbursement resulted in new rules for hospices, and it also defined when Medicare beneficiaries were able to use their **Medicare Hospice Benefit.** In most programs, the Medicare definitions for patient eligibility are used to guide all enrollment decisions. According to Medicare, the patient who wishes to use his or her Medicare Hospice Benefit must be certified by a physician as terminally ill, with a life expectancy of 6 months or less if the disease follows its natural course. Thus, hospice has come to be defined as care provided to terminally ill persons and their families in the last 6 months of the patient's life. Because of additional Medicare rules concerning completion of all cure-focused medical treatment before the Medicare Hospice Benefit may be accessed, many patients delay enrollment in hospice programs until very close to the end of life. Hospice programs are reaching out to patients with very advanced illness and seeking ways to provide them with hospice services while they are completing courses of treatment that many programs previously defined as "life-prolonging," such as certain types of chemotherapy.

The reasons for late referral to hospice and underuse of hospice services are complex. They include values and attitudes of health care providers, inadequate dissemination of existing knowledge about pain and symptom management, health care providers' difficulties in effectively communicating with terminally ill patients, insufficient attention to palliative care concepts in health care providers' education and training, and confusion about eligibility criteria for hospice services.

Hospices provide care for approximately 29% of patients who are eligible (National Hospice and Palliative Care Organization [NHPCO], 2003). For the most part, the remainder of terminally ill patients die in hospitals and long-term care facilities. It is clear that better care for the dying is urgently needed in hospitals, long-term care facilities, home care agencies, and outpatient settings. At the same time, many chronic diseases do not have a predictable "end stage" that fits hospice eligibility criteria, meaning that many patients die after a long, slow, and often painful decline, without the benefit of the coordinated palliative care that is unique to hospice programs. The palliative approach to care could benefit many more patients if it were available across care settings and earlier in the disease process. In an attempt to make this valuable approach to care more widely available, palliative care programs are being developed in other settings for patients who are either not eligible for hospice or who are "not ready" to enroll in a formal hospice program. As yet, there is no dedicated reimbursement to providers for palliative care services when they are delivered outside the hospice setting, making the sustainability of such programs challenging.

### Palliative Care in the Hospital Setting

Since the advent of diagnosis-related groups (DRGs) as the basis for prospective payment for hospital services in the 1980s, hospitals have a financial incentive to transfer patients with terminal illnesses who are no longer in need of acute care to other settings, such as long-term care facilities and home, to receive care (Field & Cassel, 1997). Despite the economic and human costs associated with death in the hospital setting, as many as 50% of all deaths occur in acute care settings (Hogan, Lynn, Gabel, et al., 2000). The landmark Study to Understand Prognoses and Preferences for Outcomes and Risks of Treatments (SUPPORT Principal Investigators, 1995) documented troubling deficiencies in the care of the dying in hospital settings:

- Many patients received unwanted care at the end of life.
- Clinicians were not aware of patient preferences for life-sustaining treatment, even when preferences were documented in the clinical record.
- Pain was often poorly controlled at the end of life.
- Efforts to enhance communication were ineffective.

It is clear that many patients will continue to opt for hospital care or will by default find themselves in hospital settings at the end of life. Increasingly, hospitals are conducting system-wide assessments of end-of-life care practices and outcomes and are developing innovative models for delivering high-quality, person-centered care to patients approaching the end of life. Hospitals cite considerable financial barriers to providing high-quality palliative care in acute care settings (Cassel, Ludden & Moon, 2000). Public policy changes have been called for that would provide reimbursement to hospitals for care delivered via designated hospital-wide palliative care beds, clustered palliative care units, or palliative care consultation services in acute care settings.

### Palliative Care in Long-Term Care Facilities

Although the total number of nursing home residents declined between 1985 and 1999, the number of residents older than 65 years of age has been increasing due to aging of the population (Federal Interagency Forum on Aging-Related Statistics, 2004). As a result, the likely place of death for a growing number of Americans after age 65 will be the long-term care facility. As many as one third of all Medicare beneficiaries who die in any given year spend all or part of their last year of life in a long-term care facility (Hogan et al., 2000). The trend favoring care of dying patients in long-term care facilities will continue as the population ages and as managed care payers pressure health care providers to minimize costs (Field & Cassel, 1997).

Yet residents of long-term care facilities typically have poor access to high-quality palliative care. Regulations that govern how care in these facilities is organized and reimbursed tend to emphasize restorative measures and serve as a disincentive to palliative care (Zerzan, Stearns & Hanson, 2000). Since 1986, home hospice programs have been permitted to enroll long-term care facility residents in hospice programs and to provide interdisciplinary services to residents who qualify for hospice care. However, The Office of the Inspector General (1997), an oversight arm of the federal government, has questioned whether such services are an unnecessary duplication of services already provided by long-term care facility staff. At the same time, long-term care facilities of all types are under increasing public pressure to improve care of the dying and are beginning to develop palliative care units or services; contract with home hospice programs to provide hospice care in the facilities; and educate staff, residents, and their families about pain and symptom management and end-of-life care.

## Hospice Care

Hospice in the United States is not a place, but a concept of care in which the end of life is viewed as a developmental stage. The root of the word hospice is *hospes,* meaning "host." Historically, hospice referred to a shelter or way station for weary travelers on a pilgrimage. In the years that followed Kübler-Ross's groundbreaking work, the concept of hospice care as an alternative to depersonalized death in institutions began as a grassroots movement. Her work, and the development of the concept of hospice in England by Dr. Cicely Saunders, resulted in recognition of gaps in the existing system of care for the terminally ill (Amenta, 1986). Hospice care began in response to "noticeable gaps . . . (1) between treating the disease and treating the person, (2) between technological research and psychosocial support, and (3) between the general denial of the fact of death in our society and the acceptance of death by those who face it" (Wentzel, 1981, p. 11). According to Saunders, who founded the world-renowned St. Christopher's Hospice in London, the principles underlying hospice are as follows:

- Death must be accepted.
- The patient's total care is best managed by an interdisciplinary team whose members communicate regularly with each other.

- Pain and other symptoms of terminal illness must be managed.
- The patient and family should be viewed as a single unit of care.
- Home care of the dying is necessary.
- Bereavement care must be provided to family members.
- Research and education should be ongoing.

## Hospice Care in the United States

Although the concept dates to ancient times, hospice as a way of caring for those at the end of life did not emerge in the United States until the 1960s (Hospice Association of America, 2002). The hospice movement in the United States is based on the belief that meaningful living is achievable during terminal illness and that it is best supported in the home, free from technologic interventions to prolong physiologic dying. After the first hospice in the United States was founded in 1974 in Connecticut, the concept quickly spread, and the number of hospice programs in the United States increased dramatically. In the years between 1984 and 1996, after the creation of the Medicare Hospice Benefit, there was a 73-fold increase in the number of hospices participating in Medicare (Hospice Association of America, 2002). By 2003, there were 3300 hospice programs in operation, serving almost 1 million patients (NHPCO, 2003).

Despite more than 30 years of existence in the United States, hospice remains an option for end-of-life care that has not been fully integrated into mainstream health care. Although hospice care is available to people with any life-limiting condition, it has primarily been used by patients with advanced cancer, in which the disease staging and trajectory lend themselves to more reliable prediction about the end of life (Boling & Lynn, 1998; Christakis & Lamont, 2000). Many reasons have been suggested to explain the reluctance of physicians to refer patients to hospice and the reluctance of patients to accept this form of care. These include the difficulties in making a terminal prognosis, the strong association of hospice with death, advances in "curative" treatment options in late-stage illness, and financial pressures on health care providers that may cause them to retain rather than refer hospice-eligible patients. The result is that patients who could benefit from the comprehensive, interdisciplinary support offered by hospice programs frequently do not enter hospice care until their final days (or hours) of life (Christakis & Lamont, 2000).

Hospice is a coordinated program of interdisciplinary services provided by professional caregivers and trained volunteers to patients with serious, progressive illnesses that are not responsive to cure. In hospice settings, the patient and family make up the unit of care. The goal of hospice care is to enable the patient to remain at home, surrounded by the people and objects that have been important to him or her throughout life. Hospice care does not seek to hasten death, nor does it encourage the prolongation of life through artificial means. Hospice care hinges on the competent patient's full or "open" awareness of dying; it embraces a realism about death and helps patients and families understand the dying process so that they can live each moment as fully as possible.

Although most hospice care is provided in the patient's own home, some hospice programs have developed inpatient facilities or residences where terminally ill patients without family support and those who desire inpatient care may receive hospice services.

Eligibility criteria for hospice vary depending on the hospice program, but generally patients must have a progressive, irreversible illness and limited life expectancy and must have opted for palliative care rather than cure-focused treatment. Although hospices have historically served cancer patients, patients with any life-limiting illness are eligible.

## Medicare Hospice Benefit

In 1983, the Medicare Hospice Benefit was implemented to cover hospice care for Medicare beneficiaries. State Medical Assistance (Medicaid) also provides coverage for hospice care, as do most commercial insurers. Federal reimbursement for hospice care ushered in a new era in hospice, in which program standards developed and published by the federal government codified what had formerly been a grassroots, loosely organized, and somewhat undefined ideal for care at the end of life. To receive Medicare dollars for hospice services, programs are required to comply with conditions of participation promulgated by the Centers for Medicare and Medicaid Services. In many aspects, Medicare standards have come to largely define hospice philosophy and services.

Eligibility criteria for hospice coverage under the Medicare Hospice Benefit are presented in Chart 17-3. Federal rules for hospices require that patients' eligibility be reviewed

### CHART 17-3

### Eligibility Criteria for Hospice Care

**GENERAL**
- Serious, progressive illness
- Limited life expectancy
- Informed choice of palliative care over cure-focused treatment

**HOSPICE-SPECIFIC**
- Presence of a family member or other caregiver continuously in the home when the patient is no longer able to safely care for him/herself (some hospices have created special services within their programs for patients who live alone, but this varies widely)

**MEDICARE AND MEDICAID HOSPICE BENEFITS**
- Medicare Part A; Medical Assistance eligibility
- Waiver of traditional Medicare/Medicaid benefits for the terminal illness
- Life expectancy of 6 months or less
- Physician certification of terminal illness
- Care must be provided by a Medicare-certified hospice program

periodically. There is no limit to the length of time that eligible patients may continue to receive hospice care. Patients who live longer than 6 months under hospice care are not discharged if their physician and the hospice medical director continue to certify that the patient is terminally ill with a life expectancy of 6 months or less, assuming that the disease continues its expected course. The hospice certification and review process and the open-ended benefit structure are intended to address the difficulty physicians face in predicting how long a patient will live, so that patients are not restricted to a lifetime limit on the number of hospice days they may receive.

To use hospice benefits under Medicare or Medicaid, patients must meet eligibility criteria and "elect" to use the hospice benefit in place of traditional Medicare or Medicaid benefits for the terminal illness. Once a patient elects the benefit, the Medicare-certified hospice program assumes responsibility for providing and paying for the care and treatment related to the underlying illness for which hospice care was elected. The Medicare-certified hospice is paid a predetermined dollar amount for each day of hospice care each patient receives. Four levels of hospice care are covered under Medicare and Medicaid hospice benefits:

- *Routine home care:* All services provided are included in the daily rate to the hospice.
- *Inpatient respite care:* A 5-day inpatient stay, provided on an occasional basis to relieve the family caregivers.
- *Continuous care:* Continuous nursing care is provided in the home for management of a medical crisis. Care reverts to the routine home care level after the crisis is resolved. (For example, seizure activity develops, and a nurse is placed in the home continuously to monitor the patient and administer medications. After 72 hours, the seizure activity is under control, the family has been instructed how to care for the patient, and the continuous nursing care is stopped.)
- *General inpatient care:* Inpatient stay for symptom management that cannot be provided in the home. This is not subject to the guidelines for a standard hospital inpatient stay.

Most hospice care is provided at the "routine home care" level and includes the services depicted in Chart 17-4. According to federal guidelines, hospices may provide no more than 20% of the aggregate annual patient days at the inpatient level. Patients may "revoke" their hospice benefits at any time, resuming traditional coverage under Medicare or Medicaid for the terminal illness. They may also reelect to use their hospice benefits at a later time after reassessment for eligibility according to these criteria.

The Medicare Act of 2003 included new provisions for the coverage of hospice services. Effective January 1, 2004, the cost of a consultation visit with the hospice medical director or physicians employed by a hospice are now covered by Medicare. The consultation visit can be provided for pain and symptom management or for counseling regarding end-of-life care options and advance care planning. This provision allows hospice programs to extend their expertise to patients who are terminally ill but have not yet enrolled in a hospice program.

### CHART 17-4

#### Home Hospice Services Covered Under the Medicare / Medicaid Hospice Benefit Routine Home Care Level

- Nursing care provided by or under the supervision of a registered nurse, available 24 hours a day
- Medical social services
- Physician's services
- Counseling services, including dietary counseling
- Home health aide/homemaker
- Physical/occupational/speech therapists
- Volunteers
- Bereavement follow-up (for up to 13 months after the death of the patient)
- Medical supplies for the palliation of the terminal illness
- Medical equipment for the palliation of the terminal illness
- Medications for the palliation of the terminal illness

## Nursing Care of Terminally Ill Patients

Many patients suffer unnecessarily when they do not receive adequate attention for the symptoms accompanying serious illness. Careful evaluation of the patient should include not only the physical problems but also the psychosocial and spiritual dimensions of the patient's and family's experience of serious illness. This approach contributes to a more comprehensive understanding of how the patient's and family's life has been affected by illness and leads to nursing care that addresses the needs in every dimension.

### Psychosocial Issues

Nurses are responsible for educating patients about the possibilities and probabilities inherent in their illness and their life with the illness, and for supporting them as they conduct life review, values clarification, treatment decision making, and end-of-life closure. The only way to do this effectively is to try to appreciate and understand the illness from the patient's perspective.

Kübler-Ross's (1969) work revealed that patients in the final stages of life can and will talk openly about their experiences, exposing as a myth the view that patients are harmed by honest discussion with their caregivers about death. Despite the continued reluctance of health care providers to engage in open discussion about end-of-life issues, studies have confirmed that patients want information about their illness and end-of-life choices and that they are not harmed by open discussion about death (Bailey, 2003).

At the same time, nurses should be both culturally aware and sensitive in their approaches to communication with patients and families about death. Attitudes toward open disclosure about terminal illness vary widely among different cultures, and direct communication with patients about such matters may be viewed as harmful (Blackhall, Murphy, Frank, et al., 1995). To provide effective patient- and family-centered care at the end of life, nurses must be willing to set aside their own assumptions and attitudes so that they can discover what type and amount of disclosure is most meaningful to each patient and family within their unique belief systems.

The social and legal evolution of advance directive documents represents some progress in people's willingness to both contemplate and communicate their wishes surrounding the end of life (Chart 17-5). Now legally sanctioned in every state and federally sanctioned through the Patient Self-Determination Act of 1990, advance directives are written documents that allow competent people to document their preferences regarding the use or nonuse of medical treatment at the end of life, specify their preferred setting for care, and communicate other valuable insights into their values and beliefs. The addition of a proxy directive (the appointment and authorization of another person to make medical decisions on behalf of the person who created the advance directive when he or she can no longer speak for himself or herself) is an important addition to the "living will" or medical directive that specifies the signer's preferences. Although these documents are widely available from health care providers, community organizations, bookstores, and the Internet, their underuse reflects society's continued discomfort with openly confronting the subject of death. Furthermore, the existence of a properly executed advance directive does not reduce the complexity of end-of-life decisions. The advance directive should not be considered a substitute for ongoing communication among the health care provider, patient, and family as the end of life approaches (Wenger & Rosenfeld, 2001).

## Communication

As previously discussed, remarkable strides have been made in the ability to prolong life, but attention to care for the dying lags behind. On one level, this comes as no surprise. Each of us will eventually face death, and most would agree that one's own demise is a subject he or she would prefer not to contemplate. Indeed, Glaser and Strauss (1965) noted that unwillingness in our culture to talk about the process of dying is tied to our discomfort with the notion of particular deaths—those of our patients and our own—rather than death in the abstract. Finucane (2002) observed that our struggle to stay alive is a prerequisite to being human. Confronting death in our patients uncovers our own deeply rooted fears.

To develop a level of comfort and expertise in communicating with seriously and terminally ill patients and their families, nurses and other clinicians should first consider their own experiences with and values concerning illness and death. Reflection, reading, and talking with family members, friends, and colleagues can help nurses examine beliefs about death and dying. Talking with people from different cultural backgrounds can help nurses view personally held beliefs through a different lens and can help nurses become sensitive to death-related beliefs and practices in other cultures. Discussion with nursing and non-nursing colleagues can also be useful; it may reveal the values shared by many health care professionals and identify diversity in the values of patients in their care. Values clarification and personal death awareness exercises can provide a starting point for self-discovery and discussion.

### Skills for Communicating With the Seriously Ill

Nurses need to develop skill and comfort in assessing patients' and families' responses to serious illness and planning interventions that will support their values and choices throughout the continuum of care. Patients and families need ongoing assistance: telling a patient something once is not teaching, and hearing the patient's words is not the same as active listening. Throughout the course of a serious illness, patients and their families encounter complicated treatment decisions, bad news about disease progression, and recurring emotional responses. In addition to the time of initial diagnosis, lack of response to the treatment course, decisions to continue or withdraw particular interventions, and decisions about hospice care are examples of critical points on the treatment continuum that demand patience, empathy, and honesty from nurses. Discussing sensitive issues such as serious illness, hopes for survival, and fears associated with death is never easy. However, the art of therapeutic communication can be

---

**CHART 17-5**

### Methods of Stating End-of-Life Preferences

**Advance directives**—written documents that allow the individual of sound mind to document preferences regarding end-of-life care that should be followed when the signer is terminally ill and unable to verbally communicate his/her wishes. The documents are generally completed in advance of serious illness, but may be completed after a diagnosis of serious illness if the signer is still of sound mind. The most common types are the durable power of attorney for health care and the living will.

**Durable power of attorney for health care**—a legal document through which the signer appoints and authorizes another individual to make medical decisions on his/her behalf when he/she is no longer able to speak for him/herself. This is also known as a health care power of attorney or a proxy directive.

**Living will**—a type of advance directive in which the individual documents treatment preferences. It provides instructions for care in the event that the signer is terminally ill and not able to communicate his/her wishes directly and often is accompanied by a durable power of attorney for health care. This is also known as a medical directive or treatment directive.

Information about the advance care planning and state-specific advance directive documents and instructions are available at www.caringinfo.org.

learned and, like other skills, must be practiced to gain expertise. Similar to other skills, communication should be practiced in a "safe" setting, such as a classroom or clinical skills laboratory with other students or clinicians.

Although communication with each patient and family should be tailored to their particular level of understanding and values concerning disclosure, general guidelines for nurses include the following (Addington, 1991):

- Deliver and interpret the technical information necessary for making decisions without hiding behind medical terminology.
- Realize that the best time for the patient to talk may be when it is least convenient for you.
- Being fully present during any opportunity for communication is often the most helpful form of communication.
- Allow the patient and family to set the agenda regarding the depth of the conversation.

## Nursing Interventions When Patients and Families Receive Bad News

Communicating about a life-threatening diagnosis or about disease progression is best accomplished by the interdisciplinary team in any setting: a physician, nurse, and social worker should be present whenever possible to provide information, facilitate discussion, and address concerns. Most importantly, the presence of the team conveys caring and respect for the patient and family. If the patient wishes to have family present for the discussion, arrangements should be made to have the discussion at a time that is best for everyone (Griffie, Nelson-Marten, & Muchka, 2004). Creating the right setting is particularly important. A quiet area with a minimum of disturbances should be used. All clinicians present should turn off beepers, cell phones, and other communication devices for the duration of the meeting and should allow sufficient time for the patient and family to absorb and respond to the news. Finally, the space in which the meeting takes place should be conducive to seating all participants at eye level. It is difficult enough for the patient and family to be the recipients of bad news without having an array of clinicians standing uncomfortably over them at the foot of the patient's bed.

After the initial discussion of a life-threatening illness or progression of a disease, the patient and family have many questions and may need to be reminded of factual information. Coping with news about a serious diagnosis or poor prognosis is an ongoing process. The nurse should be sensitive to these ongoing needs and may need to repeat previously provided information or simply be present while the patient and family react emotionally. The most important intervention the nurse can provide is listening empathetically. Seriously ill patients and their families need time and support to cope with the changes brought about by serious illness and the prospect of impending death. The nurse who is able to sit comfortably with another's suffering, time and time again, without judgment and without the need to solve the patient's and family's problems, provides an intervention that is a gift beyond measure. Keys to effective listening include the following:

- Resist the impulse to fill the "empty space" in communication with talk.
- Allow the patient and family sufficient time to reflect and respond after asking a question.
- Prompt gently: "Do you need more time to think about this?"
- Avoid distractions (noise, interruptions).
- Avoid the impulse to give advice.
- Avoid canned responses: "I know just how you feel."
- Ask questions.
- Assess understanding—your own and the patient's—by restating, summarizing, and reviewing.

## Responding With Sensitivity to Difficult Questions

Patients often direct questions or concerns to nurses before they have been able to fully discuss the details of their diagnosis and prognosis with their physicians or the entire health care team. Using open-ended questions allows the nurse to elicit the patient's and family's concerns, explore misconceptions and needs for information, and form the basis for collaboration with physicians and other team members.

In one case, a seriously ill patient may ask the nurse, "Am I dying?" The nurse should avoid making unhelpful responses that dismiss the patient's real concerns or defer the issue to another care provider. Nursing assessment and intervention are always possible, even when a need for further discussion with a physician is clearly indicated. Whenever possible, discussions in response to a patient's concerns should occur when the patient expresses a need, although that may be the least convenient time for the nurse. Creating an uninterrupted space of just 5 minutes can do much to identify the source of the concern, allay anxieties, and plan for follow-up.

In another case, in response to the question, "Am I dying?," the nurse could establish eye contact and follow with a statement acknowledging the patient's fears ("This must be very difficult for you") and an open-ended statement or question ("Tell me more about what is on your mind."). The nurse then needs to listen intently, ask additional questions for clarification, and provide reassurance only when it is realistic. In this example, the nurse might quickly ascertain that the patient's question emanates from a need for specific information—about diagnosis and prognosis from the physician, about the physiology of the dying process from the nurse, or perhaps about financial implications for the family from the social worker. The chaplain may also be called to talk with the patient about existential concerns.

As a member of the interdisciplinary team caring for the patient at the end of life, the nurse plays an important role in facilitating the team's understanding of the patient's values and preferences, family dynamics concerning decision making, and the patient's and family's response to treatment and changing health status. Many dilemmas in patient care at the end of life are related to poor communication between team members and the patient and family, as well as to failure of team members to communicate with each other effectively. Regardless of the care setting, the nurse can ensure a proactive approach to the psychosocial care of the patient and family. Periodic, structured assessments provide an opportunity for all parties to consider their priorities and plan for an uncertain future. The nurses can help the patient and family clarify their values and preferences concerning end-of-life care by using a structured approach. Sufficient time must be devoted to each step, so that the patient and family have time to process new information, formulate questions, and consider their options. Nurses may need to plan several meetings to accomplish the four steps described in Table 17-1.

## Providing Culturally Sensitive Care at the End of Life

Although death, grief, and mourning are universally accepted aspects of living, values, expectations, and practices during serious illness, as death approaches, and after death are culturally bound and expressed. Health care providers may share very similar values concerning end-of-life care and may find that they are inadequately prepared to assess for and implement care plans that support culturally diverse perspectives. Historical mistrust of the health care system and unequal access to even basic medical care may underlie the beliefs and attitudes among ethnically diverse populations (West & Levi, 2004). In addition, lack of education or knowledge about end-of-life care treatment options and language barriers influence decisions among many socioeconomically disadvantaged groups.

Much of the formal structure concerning health care decisions in the United States is rooted in the Western notions of autonomy, truth telling, and the acceptability of withdrawing or withholding life-prolonging medical treatment

### TABLE 17-1  Discussing End-of-Life Care

| Steps | Actions |
|---|---|
| 1. Initiate discussion | • Establish a supportive relationship with patient and family<br>  • State the purposes of the patient/family–health care team conference:<br>    • To ensure that the plan of care is consistent with patient and family values and preferences<br>    • To find out how best to support this patient and family<br>    • Inquire if the patient or family have questions or concerns that they want to express<br>• Elicit values and preferences concerning<br>  • Patient and family decision-making roles<br>    • How have major decisions been made in the past?<br>    • How have treatment/care decisions been made during the course of the illness?<br>    • Has the patient appointed a surrogate?<br>      • Formal (Durable Power of Attorney)<br>      • Informal<br>    • How does the patient/family want decisions to be structured from this point on?<br>  • Setting for receiving care at the end of life<br>    • Home<br>    • Home with hospice care<br>    • Assisted living or long-term care with/without hospice<br>    • Disposition when unable to care for self independently (plan for how and where the patient prefers to receive care when he/she can no longer live independently)<br>  • Family involvement in care provision |
| 2. Clarify understanding of the medical treatment plan and prognosis | • Identify what the patient and family understand<br>• Identify gaps in knowledge, need for consultation with other members of the health care team<br>• Use simple, everyday language |
| 3. Identify end-of-life priorities | • Facilitate open discussion about priorities<br>  • "What is most important to you now?"<br>  • "How can (I/we) best help you to meet your goals?"<br>• Allow sufficient time for emotional response |
| 4. Contribute to the interdisciplinary care plan | • Provide guidance and/or referral for understanding medical options<br>• Make recommendations for referrals to other disciplines or services (eg, spiritual care, support groups, community resources)<br>• Identify need for patient/family teaching<br>• Develop a plan for follow-up:<br>  • Schedule (frequency, time, place)<br>  • Participants<br>  • Tasks/assignments<br>  • Communication that needs to occur before the next meeting<br>  • Family member responsible for coordination |

Adapted with permission from Balaban, R. B. (2000). A physician's guide to talking about end-of-life care. *Journal of General Internal Medicine, 15*(3), 195–200. Oxford: Blackwell Science Ltd.

at the end of life. In many cultures, however, interdependence is valued over autonomy, leading to communication styles that favor relinquishment of decision making to family members or to perceived authority figures, such as physicians (Crawley, Marshall, Lo, et al., 2002). In addition, there is variation in preference regarding the use of life-prolonging medical treatments such as cardiopulmonary resuscitation and artificially provided nutrition and hydration at the end of life; some groups are less likely to agree with withholding or withdrawing such life supports from the patient with a terminal illness (Caralis, Davis, Wright et al., 1993).

The nurse's role is to assess the values, preferences, and practices of every patient, regardless of ethnicity, socioeconomic status, or background. The nurse can share knowledge about a patient's and family's cultural beliefs and practices with the health care team and facilitate the adaptation of the care plan to accommodate these practices. For example, a nurse may find that a male patient prefers to have his eldest son make all of his care decisions. Institutional practices and laws governing informed consent are also rooted in the Western notion of autonomous decision making and informed consent. If a patient wishes to defer decisions to his son, the nurse can work with the team to negotiate informed consent, respecting the patient's right not to participate in decision making and honoring his family's cultural practices (Kagawa-Singer & Blackhall, 2001).

The nurse should assess and document the patient's and family's specific beliefs, preferences, and practices regarding end-of-life care, preparation for death, and after-death rituals. Chart 17-6 identifies topics that the nurse should cover and questions that the nurse may use to elicit the information.

### CHART 17-6

## Assessing End-of-Life Care Beliefs, Preferences, and Practices

**Disclosure/truth telling:** "Tell me how you/your family talk about very sensitive or serious matters."
- Content: "Are there any topics that you or your family are uncomfortable discussing?"
- Person responsible for disclosure: "Is there one person in the family who assumes responsibility for obtaining and sharing information?"
- Disclosure practices regarding children: "What kind of information may be shared with children in your family, and who is responsible for communicating with the children?"
- Sharing of information within the family or community group: "What kind/how much information should be shared with your immediate family? Your extended family? Others in the community (for example, members of a religious community)?"

**Decision-making style:** "How are decisions made in your family? Who would you like to be involved in decisions about your treatment or care?"
- Individual
- Family-centered
- Family elder or patriarch/matriarch
- Deference to authority (such as the physician)

**Symptom management:** "How would you like us to help you to manage the physical effects of your illness?"
- Acceptability of medications used for symptom relief
- Beliefs regarding expression of pain and other symptoms
- Degree of symptom management desired

**Life-sustaining treatment expectations:** "Have you thought about what type of medical treatment you or your loved one would want as the end of life is nearing? Do you have an advance directive (living will and/or durable power of attorney)?"
- Nutrition/hydration at the end of life
- Cardiopulmonary resuscitation
- Ventilator
- Dialysis
- Antibiotics
- Medications to treat infection

**Desired location of dying:** "Do you have a preference about being at home or in some other location when you die?"
- Desired role for family members in providing care: "Who do you want to be involved in caring for you at the end of life?"
- Gender-specific prohibitions: "Are you uncomfortable having either males or females provide your care or your loved one's personal care?"

**Spiritual/religious practices and rituals:** "Is there anything that we should know about your spiritual or religious beliefs about death? Are there any practices that you would like us to observe as death is nearing?"

**Care of the body after the death:** "Is there anything that we should know about how a body/your body should be treated after death?"

**Expression of grief:** "What types of losses have you and your family experienced? How do you and your family express grief?"

**Funeral and burial practices:** "Are there any rituals or practices associated with funerals or burial that are especially important to you?"

**Mourning practices:** "How have you and your family carried on after a loss in the past? Are their particular behaviors or practices that are expected or required?"

The nurse must use judgment and discretion about the timing and setting for eliciting this information. Some patients may wish to have a family member speak for them or may be unable to provide information because of advanced illness. The nurse should give the patient and family a context for the discussion, such as, "It is very important to us to provide care that addresses your needs and the needs of your family. We want to honor and support your wishes, and want you to feel free to tell us how we are doing, and what we could do to better meet your needs. I'd like to ask you some questions; what you tell me will help me to understand and support what is most important to you at this time. You don't need to answer anything that makes you uncomfortable. Is it all right to ask some questions?" The assessment of end-of-life beliefs, preferences, and practices probably should be carried out in short segments over a period of time (for example, across multiple days of an inpatient hospital stay or in conjunction with multiple patient visits to an outpatient setting). The discomfort of novice nurses with asking questions and discussing this type of sensitive content can be reduced by prior practice in a classroom or clinical skills laboratory, observation of interviews conducted by experienced nurses, and partnering with experienced nurses during the first few assessments.

## Goal Setting in Palliative Care at the End of Life

As treatment goals begin to shift in the direction of comfort care over aggressive disease-focused treatment, symptom relief and patient/family-defined quality of life assume greater prominence in treatment decision making. Patients, families, and clinicians may all be accustomed to an almost automatic tendency to pursue exhaustive diagnostic testing to locate and treat the source of patients' illnesses or symptoms. Each decision to withdraw treatment or discontinue diagnostic testing is an extremely emotional one for the patient and family. They may fear that the support from health care providers on which they have come to rely will be withdrawn along with the treatment.

Throughout the course of the illness, and especially as the patient's functional status and symptoms indicate approaching death, the clinician should help the patient and family weigh the benefits of continued diagnostic testing and disease-focused medical treatment against the burdens of those activities. The patient and family may be extremely reluctant to forego monitoring that has become routine throughout the illness (eg, blood testing, x-rays) but that may contribute little to a primary focus on comfort. Likewise, health care providers from other disciplines may have difficulty discontinuing such diagnostic testing or medical treatment.

Specifically, the nurse should collaborate with other members of the interdisciplinary team to share assessment findings and develop a coordinated plan of care (Fig. 17-1). In addition, the nurse should help the patient and family clarify their goals, expected outcomes, and values as they consider treatment options (Chart 17-7). The nurse should work with interdisciplinary colleagues to ensure that the patient and family are referred for continuing psychosocial support, symptom management, and assistance with other care-related challenges (eg, arrangements for home care or hospice support, referrals for financial assistance).

## Spiritual Care

Attention to the spiritual component of the illness experienced by the patient and family is not new within the context of nursing care, yet many nurses lack the comfort or skills to assess and intervene in this dimension. **Spirituality** contains features of religiosity, but the two concepts are not interchangeable (Highfield, 2000). Spirituality involves the "search for meaning and purpose in life and relatedness to a transcendent dimension" (Hermann, 2001). For most people, contemplating one's own death raises many issues, such as the meaning of existence, the purpose of suffering, and the existence of an afterlife. In a national survey on spiritual beliefs and the dying process conducted by Gallup for the Nathan Cummings Foundation and the Fetzer Institute in 1996 (George H. Gallup International Institute, 1997), respondents' greatest worries about death included the following:

- The medical matter of greatest worry was the possibility of being vegetable-like for some period of time (73%).
- The emotional matter of greatest worry was not having the chance to say goodbye to someone (73%) or the possibility of having great physical pain before death (67%).
- The practical matter of greatest worry was how family or loved ones will be cared for (65%) or thinking that death will be a cause of inconvenience and stress for those who love them (64%).
- The spiritual matter of greatest worry was not being forgiven by God (56%) or dying when removed or cut off from God or a higher power (51%).

The spiritual assessment is a key component of comprehensive nursing assessment for terminally ill patients and their families. Although the nursing assessment should include religious affiliation, spiritual assessment is conceptually much broader than religion and therefore is relevant regardless of a patient's expression of religious preference or affiliation. In addition to assessment of the role of religious faith and practices, important religious rituals, and connection to a religious community, the nurse should further explore

- The harmony or discord between the patient's and the family's beliefs
- Other sources of meaning, hope, and comfort
- The presence or absence of a sense of peace of mind and purpose in life
- Spiritually or religiously based beliefs about illness, medical treatment, and care of the sick

Maugans (1996) created the useful mnemonic "SPIRIT" to assist health care professionals to include spiritual assessment in their practice:

- **S**piritual belief system
- **P**ersonal spirituality
- **I**ntegration and involvement with others in a spiritual community

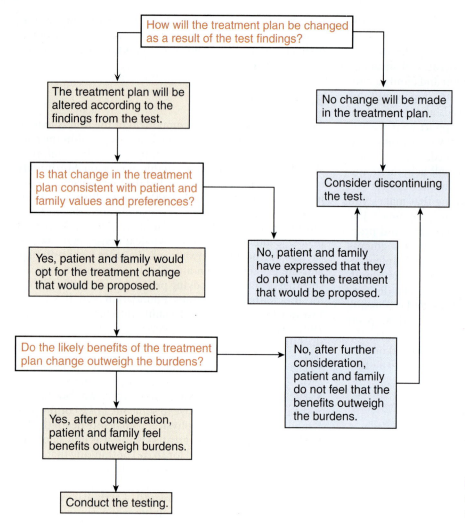

FIGURE 17-1. An algorithm for decision making about diagnostic testing at the end of life.

- *R*itualized practices and restrictions
- *I*mplications for medical care
- *T*erminal events planning

## Hope

Kübler-Ross maintained that hope persists across every stage of terminal illness, noting that "even the most accepting, the most realistic patients left the possibility open for some cure, for the discovery of a new drug, or the 'last-minute success in a research project' " (1969, p 139). Viktor Frankl (1984), a survivor of the Holocaust, described a human capacity for optimism that can be maintained in spite of the possibility or even the certainty of pain and death. In terminal illness, hope represents the patient's imagined future, forming the basis of a positive, accepting attitude and providing the patient's life with meaning, direction, and optimism (O'Gorman, 2002). When hope is viewed in this way, it is not limited to cure of the disease; instead, it focuses on what is achievable in the time remaining. Many patients find hope in working on important relationships and creating legacies. Terminally ill patients can be extremely resilient, reconceptualizing hope repeatedly as they approach the end of life.

The concept of hope has been delineated and studied by numerous nurse researchers, and its presence has been related to concepts such as spirituality, quality of life, and transcendence. Morse and Doberneck (1995) defined hope as a multidimensional construct that provides comfort as one endures life threats and personal challenges. These authors identified seven universal components of hope from their study of patients who had survived serious illness:

- Realistic initial assessment of the threat
- Envisioning alternatives and setting goals
- Bracing for negative outcomes
- Realistic assessment of resources
- Solicitation of mutually supportive relationships
- Continuous evaluation for signs reinforcing the goals
- Determination to endure

Nurses can support the patient and family by using effective listening and communication skills and encouraging realistic hope that is specific to the patient's and family's needs for information, expectations for the future, and values and preferences concerning the end of life. It is important for the nurse to engage in self-reflection and to identify his or her own biases and fears concerning illness, life, and death. As the nurse becomes more skilled in working with seriously ill patients, he or she can become less determined to "fix" and more willing to listen; more comfortable with silence, grief, anger, and sadness; and more fully present with patients and their families.

## CHART 17-7

### Assessing the Patient and Family Perspective: Goal Setting in Palliative Care

Patient and family

- **Awareness of diagnosis, illness stage, and prognosis:** "Tell me your understanding of your illness right now."
- **Values:** "Tell me what is most important to you as you are thinking about the treatment options available to you/your loved one."
- **Preferences:** "You've said that being comfortable and pain-free is most important to you right now. Where would you like to receive care (home, hospital, long-term care facility, doctor's office), and how can I help?"
- **Expected/desired outcomes:** "What are your hopes and expectations for this (diagnostic test [eg, CT scan] or treatment)?"
- **Benefits and burdens:** "Is there a point at which you would say that the testing or treatment is outweighed by the burdens it is causing you (eg, getting from home to the hospital, pain, nausea, fatigue, interference with other important activities)?"

---

tient's report of the pain and its effect, and the importance of systematic assessment of pain. Similarly, symptoms such as dyspnea, nausea, weakness, and anxiety should also be carefully and systematically assessed and managed. Questions that guide the assessment of symptoms are listed in Chart 17-8.

The patient's goals should guide symptom management. Medical interventions may be aimed at treating the underlying causes of the symptoms or reducing the impact of symptoms. For example, a medical intervention such as thoracentesis (an invasive procedure in which fluid is drained from the pleural space) may be performed to temporarily relieve dyspnea in a patient with pleural effusion secondary to lung cancer. Pharmacologic and nonpharmacologic methods for symptom management may be used in combination with medical interventions to modify the physiologic causes of symptoms. In addition, pharmacologic management with low-dose oral morphine is very effective in relieving dyspnea, and guided relaxation may reduce the anxiety associated with the sensation of breathlessness. As is true with pain, the principles of pharmacologic symptom management are use of the smallest dose of the medication to achieve the desired effect, avoidance of polypharmacy, anticipation and management of medical side effects, and creation of a therapeutic regimen that is acceptable to the patient based on his or her goals for maximizing quality of life.

The patient's goals take precedence over the clinicians' goals to relieve all symptoms at all costs. Although clinicians may believe that symptoms must be completely relieved whenever possible, the patient might choose instead to decrease symptoms to a tolerable level rather than to relieve them completely if the side effects of medications are unacceptable to him or her. This often allows the patient to have greater independence, mobility, and alertness, and to

Nursing interventions for enabling and supporting hope include the following:

- Listening attentively
- Encouraging sharing of feelings
- Providing accurate information
- Encouraging and supporting the patient's control over his or her circumstances, choices, and environment whenever possible
- Assisting patients to explore ways for finding meaning in their lives
- Encouraging realistic goals
- Facilitating effective communication within families
- Making referrals for psychosocial and spiritual counseling
- Assisting with the development of supports in the home or community when none exist

## Managing Physiologic Responses to Terminal Illness

Patients approaching the end of life experience many of the same symptoms, regardless of their underlying disease processes. Symptoms in terminal illness may be caused by the disease, either directly (eg, dyspnea due to chronic obstructive lung disease) or indirectly (eg, nausea and vomiting related to pressure in the gastric area); by the treatment for the disease; or by a coexisting disorder that is unrelated to the disease. Chapter 13 presents assessment principles for pain that include identifying the effect of the pain on the patient's life, the importance of believing the pa-

## CHART 17-8

### Assessing Symptoms Associated With Terminal Illness

- How is this symptom affecting the patient's life?
- What is the meaning of the symptom to the patient? To the family?
- How does the symptom affect physical functioning, mobility, comfort, sleep, nutritional status, elimination, activity level, and relationships with others?
- What makes the symptom better?
- What makes it worse?
- Is it worse at any particular time of the day?
- What are the patient's expectations and goals for managing the symptom? The family's?
- How is the patient coping with the symptom?
- What is the economic effect of the symptom and its management?

Adapted from Jacox, A., Carr, D. B., & Payne, R. (1994). *Management of cancer pain*. Rockville, MD: AHCPR.

## NURSING RESEARCH PROFILE

### Assessing Symptoms at the End of Life

McMillan, S. C. & Moody, L. E. (2003). Hospice patient and caregiver congruence in reporting patients' symptom intensity. *Cancer Nursing, 26*(2), 113–118.

#### Purpose
Increasingly, care is provided to patients with advanced illness in their homes, where family members assume responsibility for myriad complex tasks that nurses and others previously performed when the patients were hospitalized. Family members frequently administer medications to a very ill loved one and often must assess the ill family member's symptoms before giving a dose of a medication. This study assessed how well primary caregivers (family members) report the symptom intensity of a family member with cancer.

#### Design
The subjects in this study were participants in a larger, National Institutes of Health–funded clinical trial that examined symptom management and quality of life. Patients had been admitted to hospice within the previous 48 hours and had one of three symptoms (pain, dyspnea, or constipation). Patients were excluded if they were cognitively unable to respond or were close to death. More than 260 patients and their caregivers completed demographic questionnaires, numeric rating scales for pain and dyspnea (providing a rating of 0 to 10 to describe the intensity of a symptom), and the Constipation Assessment Scale. Patients and caregivers completed the instruments independently. The researchers used paired $t$ tests to test for significant differences in patient and caregiver mean ratings for each symptom and Pearson correlations to examine the relationship between scores of patients and caregivers.

#### Findings
For each symptom, caregivers reported higher intensity than did the patients ($p = .000$). Patient and caregiver scores were weakly to moderately correlated ($r = .399$ to $.512$; $p < .000$), which accounted for 16% to 26% of the variance in responses.

#### Nursing Implications
The findings of this study suggest that family members overestimate the intensity of pain, dyspnea, and constipation compared to the patients. Hospice nurses frequently rely on family members' assessments of symptoms, which, according to this study, are generally unreliable. Whenever possible, patients' self-reports should guide treatment. However, patients' declining conditions in combination with other factors, such as language barriers, often require that family members assess and report symptoms. There is a need for better teaching of family members to enable them to accomplish this task more accurately.

---

devote attention to issues he or she considers of higher priority and greater importance.

Anticipating and planning interventions for symptoms that have not yet occurred is a cornerstone of end-of-life care. Both patients and family members cope more effectively with new symptoms and exacerbations of existing symptoms when they know what to expect and how to manage it. Hospice programs typically provide "emergency kits" containing ready-to-administer doses of a variety of medications that are useful to treat symptoms in advanced illness. For example, a kit might contain small doses of oral morphine liquid for pain or shortness of breath, a benzodiazepine for restlessness, and an acetaminophen suppository for fever. Family members can be instructed to administer a prescribed dose from the emergency kit, often avoiding prolonged suffering for the patient as well as rehospitalization for symptom management.

### Pain

Numerous studies have shown that patients with advanced illness, particularly cancer, experience considerable pain (Field & Cassel, 1997; Jacox, Carr, & Payne, 1994). Pain is a significant symptom for many cancer patients throughout their treatment and disease course; it results from both the disease and the modalities used to treat it. It is estimated that this is true in as many as 70% of patients with advanced cancer (Jacox et al., 1994; World Health Organization, 1990). Pain and suffering are among the most feared consequences of cancer (Waller & Caroline, 2000). Although the means to relieve pain have existed for many years, the continued, pervasive undertreatment of pain has been well documented (American Pain Society, 2003). Poorly managed pain affects the psychological, emotional, social, and financial well-being of patients. Despite studies demonstrating the negative effects of inadequate pain management, practice has been slow to change (Spross, 1992).

Patients who are taking an established regimen of analgesics should continue to receive those medications as they approach the end of life. Inability to communicate pain should not be equated with the absence of pain. Although most pain can be managed effectively using the oral route, as the end of life nears, patients may be less able to swallow oral medications due to somnolence or nausea. Patients who have been receiving opioids should continue to receive equianalgesic doses via rectal or sublingual routes. Concentrated morphine solution can be very effectively delivered by the sublingual route, because the small liquid volume is well tolerated even if swallowing is not possible. As long as the patient continues to receive opioids, a regimen to combat constipation must be implemented. If the patient cannot swallow laxatives or stool softeners, rectal suppositories or enemas may be necessary.

The nurse should teach the family about continuation of comfort measures as the patient approaches the end of life, how to administer analgesics via alternative routes, and how to assess for pain when the patient cannot verbally report pain intensity. Because the analgesics administered orally or rectally are short-acting, typically scheduled as frequently as every 3 to 4 hours around the clock, there is always a strong possibility that a patient approaching the end of life will die in close proximity to the time of analgesic administration. If the patient is at home, family members administering analgesics should be prepared for this possibility. They need reassurance that they did not "cause" the death of the patient by administering a dose of analgesic medication (see Chart 13-4 in Chapter 13).

## Dyspnea

Dyspnea is an uncomfortable awareness of breathing that is common in patients approaching the end of life (Brant, 1998). Dyspnea is a highly subjective symptom that often is not associated with visible signs of distress, such as tachypnea, diaphoresis, or cyanosis. Patients with primary lung tumors, lung metastases, pleural effusion, or restrictive lung disease may experience significant dyspnea. Although the underlying cause of the dyspnea can be identified and treated in some cases, the burdens of additional diagnostic evaluation and treatment aimed at the physiologic problem may outweigh the benefits. The treatment of dyspnea varies depending on the patient's general physical condition and imminence of death. For example, a blood transfusion may provide temporary symptom relief for a patient with anemia earlier in the disease process; however, as the patient approaches the end of life, the benefits are typically short-lived or absent.

### NURSING ASSESSMENT AND INTERVENTION

As with assessment and management of pain, reports of dyspnea by patients must be believed. As is true for physical pain, what dyspnea means to an individual patient may increase his or her suffering. For example, the patient may interpret increasing dyspnea as a sign that death is approaching. For some patients, sensations of breathlessness may invoke frightening images of drowning or suffocation, and the resulting cycle of fear and anxiety may increase the sensation of breathlessness. Therefore, the nurse should conduct a careful assessment of the psychosocial and spiritual components of the dyspnea. Physical assessment parameters include

- Symptom intensity, distress, and interference with activities (scale of 0 to 10)
- Auscultation of lung sounds
- Assessment of fluid balance
- Measurement of dependent edema (circumference of lower extremities)
- Measurement of abdominal girth
- Temperature
- Skin color
- Sputum quantity and character
- Cough

To determine the intensity of dyspnea and its interference with daily activities, the patient can be asked to report the severity of the dyspnea using a scale of 0 to 10, where 0 is no dyspnea and 10 is the worst imaginable dyspnea. The patient's baseline rating before treatment and subsequent measurements taken during exacerbation of the symptom, periodically during treatment, and whenever the treatment plan changes provide ongoing objective evidence for the efficacy of the treatment plan. In addition, physical assessment findings may assist in locating the source of the dyspnea and selecting nursing interventions to relieve the symptom. The components of the assessment change as the patient's condition changes. For example, when the patient who has been on daily weights can no longer get out of bed, the goal of comfort may outweigh the benefit of continued weights. Like other symptoms at the end of life, dyspnea can be managed effectively in the absence of assessment and diagnostic data (ie, arterial blood gases) that are standard when a patient's illness or symptom is reversible.

Nursing management of dyspnea at the end of life is directed toward administering medical treatment for the underlying pathology, monitoring the patient's response to treatment, helping the patient and family manage anxiety (which exacerbates dyspnea), altering the perception of the symptom, and conserving energy (Chart 17-9). Pharmacologic intervention is aimed at modifying lung physiology and improving performance as well as altering the perception of the symptom. Bronchodilators and corticosteroids are examples of medications used to treat underlying obstructive pathology, thereby improving overall lung function. Low doses of opioids are very effective in relieving dyspnea, although the mechanism of relief is not entirely clear. Although dyspnea in terminal illness is typically not associated with diminished blood oxygen saturation, low-flow oxygen often provides psychological comfort to both patients and families, particularly in the home setting.

As previously mentioned, dyspnea may be exacerbated by anxiety, and anxiety may trigger episodes of dyspnea, setting off a respiratory crisis in which the patient and family may panic. For patients receiving care at home, patient and family instruction should include anticipation and management of crisis situations and a clearly communicated emergency plan. The patient and family should be instructed about medication administration, condition changes that should be reported to the physician and nurse, and strategies for coping with diminished reserves and increasing symptomatology as the disease progresses. The patient and family need reassurance that the symptom can be effectively managed at home without the need for activation of the emergency medical services or hospitalization and that a nurse will be available at all times via telephone or to make a visit.

## Nutrition and Hydration at the End of Life

### ANOREXIA

Anorexia and cachexia are common problems in the seriously ill. The profound changes in the patient's appearance and the concomitant lack of interest in the socially important rituals of mealtime are particularly disturbing to families. The approach to the problem varies depending on the patient's stage of illness, level of disability associated with the illness, and desires. The anorexia–cachexia syndrome is characterized by disturbances in carbohydrate, protein,

> **CHART 17-9**
>
> ## Palliative Nursing Interventions for Dyspnea
>
> **DECREASE ANXIETY**
> - Administer prescribed anxiolytic medications as indicated for anxiety or panic associated with dyspnea.
> - Assist with relaxation techniques, guided imagery.
> - Provide patient with a means to call for assistance (call bell/light within reach in a hospital or long-term care facility; handheld bell or other device for home).
>
> **TREAT UNDERLYING PATHOLOGY**
> - Administer prescribed bronchodilators and corticosteroids (obstructive pathology).
> - Administer blood products, erythropoietin as prescribed (typically not beneficial in advanced disease).
> - Administer prescribed diuretics and monitor fluid balance.
>
> **ALTER PERCEPTION OF BREATHLESSNESS**
> - Administer prescribed oxygen therapy via nasal cannula, if tolerated; masks may not be well tolerated.
> - Administer prescribed low-dose opioids via oral route (morphine sulfate is used most commonly).
> - Provide air movement in the patient's environment with a portable fan.
>
> **REDUCE RESPIRATORY DEMAND**
> - Teach patient and family to implement energy conservation measures.
> - Place needed equipment, supplies, and nourishment within reach.
> - For home or hospice care, offer bedside commode, electric bed (with head that elevates).

and fat metabolism; endocrine dysfunction; and anemia. The syndrome results in severe asthenia (loss of energy).

Although causes of anorexia may be controlled for a period of time, progressive anorexia is an expected and natural part of the dying process. Anorexia may be related to or exacerbated by situational variables (eg, the ability to have meals with the family versus eating alone in the "sick room"), progression of the disease, treatment for the disease, or psychological distress. The patient and family should be instructed in strategies to manage the variables associated with anorexia (Table 17-2).

**Use of Pharmacologic Agents to Stimulate Appetite.** A number of pharmacologic agents are commonly used to stimulate appetite in anorectic patients. Commonly used medications for appetite stimulation include dexamethasone (Decadron), megestrol acetate (Megace), and dronabinol (Marinol). Although several of these agents may result in temporary weight gain, their use is not associated with an increase in lean body mass in the terminally ill patient. Therapy should be tapered or discontinued after 4 to 8 weeks if there is no response (Wrede-Seaman, 1999).

Dexamethasone initially increases appetite and may provide short-term weight gain in some patients. However, therapy may need to be discontinued in patients with a longer life expectancy, because after 3 to 4 weeks corticosteroids interfere with the synthesis of muscle protein.

Megestrol acetate produces temporary weight gain of primarily fatty tissue, with little effect on protein balance. Because of the time required to see any effect from this agent, therapy should not be initiated if life expectancy is less than 30 days.

Dronabinol is a psychoactive compound found in cannabis that may be helpful in reducing nausea and vomiting, appetite loss, pain, and anxiety, thereby improving food and fluid intake in some patients. However, dronabinol is not as effective as the other agents for appetite stimulation in most patients.

### CACHEXIA

Cachexia refers to severe muscle wasting and weight loss associated with illness. Although anorexia may exacerbate cachexia, it is not the primary cause. Cachexia is associated with changes in metabolism that include hypertriglyceridemia, lipolysis, and accelerated protein turnover, leading to depletion of fat and protein stores (Inui, 2002). However, the pathophysiology of cachexia in terminal illness is not well understood. In terminal illness, the severity of tissue wasting is greater than would be expected from reduced food intake alone, and typically increasing appetite or food intake does not reverse cachexia in the terminally ill.

Anorexia and cachexia differ from starvation (simple food deprivation) in several important ways. Appetite is lost early in the process, the body becomes catabolic in a dysfunctional way, and supplementation by gastric feeding (tube feeding) or parenteral nutrition in advanced disease does not replenish lean body mass that has been lost. At one time it was believed that cancer patients with rapidly growing tumors developed cachexia because the tumor created an excessive nutritional demand and diverted nutrients from the rest of the body. Research links cytokines produced by the body in response to a tumor to a complex inflammatory-immune response present in patients whose tumors have metastasized, leading to anorexia, weight loss, and altered metabolism. An increase in cytokines occurs not only in cancer but also in AIDS and many other chronic diseases (Inui, 2002).

### ARTIFICIAL NUTRITION AND HYDRATION

Along with breathing, eating and drinking are essential to survival throughout life. Near the end of life, the body's nutritional needs change, and the desire for food and fluid may diminish. People may no longer be able to use, eliminate, or store nutrients and fluids adequately. Eating and sharing meals are important social activities in families and communities, and food preparation and enjoyment are linked to happy memories, strong emotions, and hopes for survival. For patients with serious illness, food preparation and mealtimes often become battlegrounds in which well-meaning family members argue, plead, and cajole to encourage ill people to eat. It is not unusual for seriously ill patients to lose their appetites entirely, to develop strong aversions for foods they have enjoyed in the past, or to crave a particular food to the exclusion of all other foods.

Although nutritional supplementation may be an important part of the treatment plan in early or chronic illness, unintended weight loss and dehydration are expected sequelae of progressive illness. As illness progresses, patients, families, and clinicians may believe that, without artificial nutrition and hydration, terminally ill patients will "starve," causing

## TABLE 17-2  Measures for Managing Anorexia

| Nursing Interventions | Patient and Family Teaching Tips |
|---|---|
| Initiate measures to ensure adequate dietary intake without adding stress to the patient at mealtimes. | Reduce the focus on "balanced" meals; offer the same food as often as the patient desires it. |
| Assess the impact of medications (eg, chemotherapy, antiretrovirals) or other therapies (radiation therapy, dialysis) that are being used to treat the underlying illness. | Increase the nutritional value of meals. For example, add dry milk powder to milk, and use this fortified milk to prepare cream soups, milkshakes, and gravies. |
| Administer and monitor effects of prescribed treatment for nausea, vomiting, and delayed gastric emptying. | |
| Encourage patient to eat when effects of medications have subsided. | Allow and encourage the patient to eat when hungry, regardless of usual meal times. |
| Assess and modify environment to eliminate unpleasant odors and other factors that cause nausea, vomiting, and anorexia. | Eliminate or reduce noxious cooking odors, pet odors, or other odors that may precipitate nausea, vomiting, or anorexia. |
| Remove items that may reduce appetite (soiled tissues, bedpans, emesis basins, clutter). | Keep patient's environment clean, uncluttered, and comfortable. |
| Assess and manage anxiety and depression to the extent possible. | Make mealtime a shared experience away from the "sick" room whenever possible. |
| | Reduce stress at mealtimes. |
| | Avoid confrontations about the amount of food consumed. |
| | Reduce or eliminate routine weighing of the patient. |
| Position to enhance gastric emptying. | Encourage patient to eat in a sitting position; elevate the head of the patient's bed. |
| | Plan meals (food selection and portion size) that the patient desires. |
| | Provide small frequent meals if they are easier for patient to eat. |
| Assess for constipation and/or intestinal obstruction. | Ensure that patient and family understand that prevention of constipation is essential, even when the patient's intake is minimal. |
| Prevent and manage constipation on an ongoing basis, even when the patient's intake is minimal. | Encourage adequate fluid intake, dietary fiber, and use of bowel program to prevent constipation. |
| Provide frequent mouth care, particularly following nourishment. | Assist the patient to rinse after every meal. Avoid mouthwashes that contain alcohol or glycerine, which dry mucous membranes. |
| Ensure that dentures fit properly. | Weight loss may cause dentures to loosen and cause irritation. Remove them to inspect the gums and to provide oral care. |
| Administer and monitor effects of topical and systemic treatment for oropharyngeal pain. | The patient's comfort may be enhanced if medications for pain relief given on an as-needed basis for breakthrough pain are administered before mealtimes. |

profound suffering and hastened death. However, starvation should not be viewed as the failure to implant tubes for nutritional supplementation or hydration of terminally ill patients with irreversible progression of disease. Studies have demonstrated that terminally ill patients who were hydrated had neither improved biochemical parameters nor improved states of consciousness (Waller, Hershkowitz & Adunsky, 1994). Similarly, survival was not increased when terminally ill patients with advanced dementia received enteral feeding (Meier, Ahronheim, Morris, et al., 2001). Furthermore, in patients who are close to death, there are beneficial effects to withholding or withdrawing artificial nutrition and hydration, such as decreased urine output and incontinence, decreased gastric fluids and emesis, decreased pulmonary secretions and respiratory distress, decreased edema, and decreased discomfort from pressure associated with accumulated fluids in the tissues (Zerwekh, 1987).

As the patient approaches the end of life, the family and health care providers should offer the patient what he or she prefers and can most easily tolerate. The nurse should instruct the family how to separate feeding from caring, demonstrating love, sharing, and caring by being with the loved one in other ways. Preoccupation with appetite, feeding, and weight loss diverts energy and time that the patient and family could use in other meaningful activities. The following are tips to promote nutrition for terminally ill patients:

- Offer small portions of favorite foods.
- Do not be overly concerned about a "balanced" diet.
- Cool foods may be better tolerated than hot foods.
- Offer cheese, eggs, peanut butter, mild fish, chicken, or turkey. Meat (especially beef) may taste bitter and unpleasant.
- Add milkshakes, "Instant Breakfast" drinks, or other liquid supplements.
- Add dry milk powder to milkshakes and cream soups to increase protein and calorie content.
- Place nutritious foods at the bedside (fruit juices, milkshakes in insulated drink containers with straws).
- Schedule meals when family members can be present to provide company and stimulation.
- Avoid arguments at mealtime.
- Help the patient to maintain a schedule of oral care. Rinse the mouth after each meal or snack. Avoid mouthwashes

that contain alcohol. Use a soft toothbrush. Treat oral ulcers or lesions. Make sure dentures fit well.
- Treat pain and other symptoms.
- Offer ice chips made from frozen fruit juices.
- Allow the patient to refuse foods and fluids.

### Delirium

Many patients remain alert, arousable, and able to communicate until very close to death. Others sleep for long intervals and awaken only intermittently, with eventual somnolence until death. Delirium refers to concurrent disturbances in level of consciousness, psychomotor behavior, memory, thinking, attention, and sleep–wake cycle (Lawlor, Gagnon, Mancini, et al., 2000). In some patients, a period of agitated delirium precedes death, sometimes causing families to be hopeful that suddenly active patients may be getting better. Confusion may be related to underlying, treatable conditions such as medication side effects or interactions, pain or discomfort, hypoxia or dyspnea, or a full bladder or impacted stool. In patients with cancer, confusion may be secondary to brain metastases. Delirium may also be related to metabolic changes, infection, and organ failure.

Patients with delirium may become hypoactive or hyperactive, restless, irritable, and fearful. Sleep deprivation and hallucinations may occur. If treatment of the underlying factors contributing to these symptoms brings no relief, a combination of pharmacologic intervention with neuroleptics or benzodiazepines may be effective in decreasing distressing symptoms. Haloperidol (Haldol) may reduce hallucinations and agitation. Benzodiazepines (eg, lorazepam [Ativan]) can reduce anxiety but do not clear the sensorium and may contribute to worsening cognitive impairment if used alone.

Nursing interventions are aimed at identifying the underlying causes of delirium; acknowledging the family's distress over its occurrence; reassuring family members about what is normal; teaching family members how to interact with and ensure safety for the patient with delirium; and monitoring the effects of medications used to treat severe agitation, paranoia, and fear. Confusion may mask the patient's unmet spiritual needs and fears about dying. Spiritual intervention, music therapy, gentle massage, and therapeutic touch may provide some relief. Reduction of environmental stimuli, avoidance of harsh lighting or very dim lighting (which may produce disturbing shadows), presence of familiar faces, and gentle reorientation and reassurance are also helpful.

### Depression

Clinical depression should not be accepted as an inevitable consequence of dying, nor should it be confused with sadness and anticipatory grieving, which are normal reactions to the losses associated with impending death. Emotional and spiritual support and control of disturbing physical symptoms are appropriate interventions for situational depression associated with terminal illness. Researchers have linked the psychological sequelae of cancer pain to suicidal thought and, less frequently, to carrying out a planned suicide (Ripamonti, Filiberti, Totis, et al., 1999). Cancer patients with advanced disease are especially vulnerable to delirium, depression, suicidal ideation, and severe anxiety. Higher levels of debilitation predict higher levels of pain and depressive symptoms, and the presence of pain doubles the likelihood of developing major psychiatric complications of illness (Roth & Breitbart, 1996). Patients and their families must be given space and time to experience sadness and to grieve, but patients should not have to endure untreated depression at the end of their lives. An effective combined approach to clinical depression includes relief of physical symptoms, attention to emotional and spiritual distress, and pharmacologic intervention with psychostimulants, selective serotonin reuptake inhibitors, and tricyclic antidepressants (Block, 2000).

## Palliative Sedation at the End of Life

Effective control of symptoms can be achieved under most conditions, but some patients may experience distressing, intractable symptoms. Although **palliative sedation** remains controversial, it is offered in some settings to patients who are close to death or who have symptoms that do not respond to conventional pharmacologic and nonpharmacologic approaches, resulting in unrelieved suffering. Palliative sedation is distinguished from **euthanasia** or physician-assisted suicide in that the intent of palliative sedation is to relieve symptoms, not to hasten death. Palliative sedation is most commonly used when the patient exhibits intractable pain, dyspnea, seizures, or delirium, and it is generally considered appropriate in only the most difficult situations. Before implementing palliative sedation, the health care team should assess for the presence of underlying and treatable causes of suffering, such as depression or spiritual pain. Finally, the patient and family should be fully informed about the use of this treatment and alternatives.

Palliative sedation is accomplished through infusion of a benzodiazepine or barbiturate in doses adequate to induce sleep and eliminate signs of discomfort (Quill & Byock, 2000). Nurses act as collaborating members of the interdisciplinary health care team, providing emotional support to patients and families, facilitating clarification of values and preferences, and providing comfort-focused physical care. Once sedation has been induced, the nurse should continue to comfort the patient, monitor the physiologic effects of the sedation, support the family during the final hours or days of their loved one's life, and ensure communication within the health care team and between the team and family.

# Nursing Care of Patients Who Are Close to Death

Providing care to patients who are close to death and being present at the time of death can be one of the most rewarding experiences a nurse can have. Patients and their families are understandably fearful of the unknown, and the approach of death may prompt new concerns or cause previous fears or issues to resurface. It has often been said that as we age and as we approach death, we do not become different people, just more like ourselves. Family members who have always had difficulty communicating or who are part of families in which there are old resentments and hurts may experience heightened difficulty as their loved ones near death. In contrast, the time at the end of life can also afford opportunities to resolve old hurts and learn new ways of being a family. Regardless of the setting, skilled practitioners can make the dying patient comfortable, make space for their loved ones to remain present when they wish, and can give family members the opportunity to experience growth and healing. Likewise, regardless of setting, the patient and family may be less apprehensive near the time of death if they know what to expect and how to respond.

## Expected Physiologic Changes

As death approaches and organ systems begin to fail, observable, expected changes in the body take place. Nursing care measures aimed at patient comfort should be continued: pain medications (administered rectally or sublingually), turning, mouth care, eye care, positioning to facilitate draining of secretions, and measures to protect the skin from urine or feces (if the patient is incontinent) should be continued. The nurse should consult with the physician about discontinuing measures that no longer contribute to patient comfort, such as drawing blood, administering tube feedings, suctioning (in most cases), and invasive monitoring. The nurse should prepare the family for the normal, expected changes that accompany the period immediately preceding death. Although the exact time of death cannot be predicted, it is often possible to identify when the patient is very close to death. Hospice programs frequently provide written information for families so they know what to expect and what to do as death nears (Chart 17-10).

If family members have been prepared for the time of death, they are less likely to panic and are better able to be with their loved ones in a meaningful way. Noisy, gurgling breathing or moaning is generally most distressing to family members. In most cases, the sounds of breathing at the end of life are related to oropharyngeal relaxation and diminished awareness. Family members may have difficulty believing that the patient is not in pain or that the patient's breathing could not be improved by suctioning secretions. Patient positioning and family reassurance are the most helpful responses to these symptoms.

When death is imminent, patients may become increasingly somnolent and unable to clear sputum or oral secretions, which may lead to further impairment of breathing from pooled or dried and crusted secretions. The sound ("terminal bubbling") and appearance of the secretions are often more distressing to family members than is the presence of the secretions to the patient. Family distress over the changes in the patient's condition may be eased by supportive nursing care. Continuation of comfort-focused interventions and reassurance that the patient is not in any distress can do much to ease family concerns. Gentle mouth care with a moistened swab or very soft toothbrush helps maintain the integrity of the patient's mucous membranes. In addition, gentle oral suctioning, positioning to enhance drainage of secretions, and sublingual or transdermal administration of anticholinergic drugs (Table 17-3) reduces the production of secretions and provides comfort to the patient and support to the family. Deeper suctioning may cause significant discomfort to the dying patient and is rarely of any benefit, because secretions reaccumulate rapidly.

## The Death Vigil

Although every death is unique, it is often possible for experienced clinicians to assess that the patient is "actively" or imminently dying and to prepare the family in the final days or hours leading to death. As death nears, the patient may withdraw, sleep for longer intervals, or become somnolent.

Family members should be encouraged to be with the patient, to speak and reassure the patient of their presence, to stroke or touch the patient, or to lie alongside the patient (even in the hospital or long-term care facility) if the family members are comfortable with this degree of closeness and can do so without causing discomfort to the patient.

The family may have gone to great lengths to ensure that their loved one will not die alone. However, despite the best intentions and efforts of the family and clinicians, the patient may die at a time when no one is present. In any setting, it is unrealistic for family members to be at the patient's bedside 24 hours a day, and it is not unusual for a patient to die when family members have stepped away from the bedside just briefly. Experienced hospice clinicians have observed and reported that some patients appear to "wait" until family members are away from the bedside to die, perhaps to spare their loved ones the pain of being present at the time of death. Nurses can reassure family members throughout the death vigil by being present intermittently or continuously, modeling behaviors (such as touching and speaking to the patient), providing encouragement in relation to family caregiving, providing reassurance about normal physiologic changes, and encouraging family rest breaks. If a patient dies while family members are away from the bedside, they may express feelings of guilt and profound grief and may need emotional support.

## After-Death Care

The time of death is generally preceded by a period of gradual diminishment of bodily functions in which increasing intervals between respirations, a weakened and irregular pulse, diminishing blood pressure, and skin color changes or mottling may occur. For patients who have received adequate management of symptoms and for families who have received adequate preparation and support, the actual time of death is commonly peaceful and occurs without struggle. Nurses may or may not be present at the time of a patient's death. In many states, nurses may be authorized to make the pronouncement of death and sign the death certificate. The determination of death is made through a physical examination that includes auscultation for the absence of breathing and heart sounds. Home care or hospice programs in which nurses make the time-of-death visit and pronouncement of death have polices and procedures to guide the nurse's actions during this visit. Immediately on cessation of vital functions, the body begins to change. It becomes dusky or bluish, waxen-appearing, and cool; blood darkens and pools in dependent areas of the body (eg, the back and sacrum if the body is in a supine position); and urine and stool may be evacuated.

Immediately after death, family members should be allowed and encouraged to spend time with the deceased. Normal responses of family members at the time of death vary widely and range from quiet expressions of grief to overt expressions that include wailing and prostration. The family's desire for privacy during their time with the deceased should be honored. Family members may wish to independently manage or assist with care of the body after death. If the death occurs in a long-term care facility, nurses follow the facility's procedure for preparation of the body and transportation to the facility's morgue. However, the needs of families to remain with the deceased, to wait until other family

## CHART 17-10

### Patient Education

### Signs of Approaching Death

**The person will show less interest in eating and drinking.** For many patients, refusal of food is an indication that they are ready to die. Fluid intake may be limited to that which will keep their mouths from feeling too dry.
- What you can do: Offer, but do not force, fluids and medication. Sometimes, pain or other symptoms that have required medication in the past may no longer be present. For most patients, pain medications will still be needed, and can be provided by concentrated oral solutions placed under the tongue or by rectal suppository.

**Urinary output may decrease in amount and frequency.**
- What you can do: No response is needed unless the patient expresses a desire to urinate and cannot. Call the hospice nurse for advice if you are not sure.

**As the body weakens, the patient will sleep more and begin to detach from the environment.** He or she may refuse your attempts to provide comfort.
- What you can do: Allow your loved one to sleep. You may wish to sit with him or her, play soft music, or hold hands. Your loved one's withdrawal is normal and is not a rejection of your love.

**Mental confusion may become apparent,** as less oxygen is available to supply the brain. The patient may report strange dreams or visions.
- What you can do: As he or she awakens from sleep, remind him or her of the day and time, where he or she is, and who is present. This is best done in a casual, conversational way.

**Vision and hearing may become somewhat impaired, and speech may be difficult to understand.**
- What you can do: Speak clearly but no more loudly than necessary. Keep the room as light as the patient wishes, even at night. Carry on all conversations as if they can be heard, because hearing may be the last of the senses to cease functioning.
- Many patients are able to talk until minutes before death and are reassured by the exchange of a few words with a loved one.

**Secretions may collect in the back of the throat and rattle or gurgle as the patient breathes though the mouth.** He or she may try to cough, and his or her mouth may become dry and encrusted with secretions.
- What you can do: if the patient is trying to cough up secretions and is experiencing choking or vomiting, call the hospice nurse for assistance.
- Secretions may drain from the mouth if you place the patient on his/her side and provide support with pillows.
- Cleansing the mouth with moistened mouth swabs will help to relieve the dryness that occurs with mouth breathing.
- Offer water in small amounts to keep the mouth moist. A straw with one finger placed over the end can be used to transfer sips of water to the patient's mouth.

**Breathing may become irregular with periods of no breathing (apnea).** The patient may be working very hard to breathe and may make a moaning sound with each breath. As the time of death nears, the breathing remains irregular and may become more shallow and mechanical.
- What you can do: Raising the head of the bed may help the patient to breathe more easily. The moaning sound does not mean that the patient is in pain or other distress; it is the sound of air passing over very relaxed vocal cords.

**As the oxygen supply to the brain decreases, the patient may become restless.** It is not unusual to pull at the bed linens, to have visual hallucinations, or even to try to get out of bed at this point.
- What you can do: Reassure the patient in a calm voice that you are there. Prevent him or her from falling by trying to get out of bed. Soft music or a back rub may be soothing.

**The patient may feel hot one moment and cold the next as the body loses its ability to control the temperature.** As circulation slows, the arms and legs may become cool and bluish. The underside of the body may darken. It may be difficult to feel a pulse at the wrist.
- What you can do: Provide and remove blankets as needed. Avoid using electric blankets, which may cause burns because the patient cannot tell you if he or she is too warm.
- Sponge the patient's head with a cool cloth if this provides comfort.

**Loss of bladder and bowel control may occur around the time of death.**
- What you can do: Protect the mattress with waterproof padding and change the padding as needed to keep the patient comfortable.

**As people approach death, many times they report seeing gardens, libraries, or family or friends who have died.** They may ask you to pack their bags and find tickets or a passport. Sometimes they may become insistent and attempt to do these chores themselves. They may try getting out of bed (even if they have been confined to bed for a long time) so that they can "leave."
- What you can do: Reassure the patient that it is all right; he or she can "go" without getting out of bed. Stay close, share stories, and be present.

---
Used with permission from the Family Home Hospice of the Visiting Nurse Association of Greater Philadelphia.

### TABLE 17-3 Pharmacologic Management of Excess Oral/Respiratory Secretions When Death is Imminent

| Medication | Dose |
|---|---|
| Atropine sulfate drops 1% | 1 or 2 drops 1% oral/sublingual q4–6h prn or around the clock (ATC) up to 12 drops/d |
| Atropine injection | 0.4–0.6 mg intravenous/subcutaneous/intramuscular q4–6h prn or ATC (if oral therapy is ineffective) |
| Glycopyrrolate (Robinul) | 1–2 mg oral/rectal/sublingual TID prn or ATC (maximum dose 6 mg/d) |
| Hyoscyamine (Levsin) | 0.125–0.25 mg oral/sublingual q4–6h prn or ATC (maximum dose 1.5 mg/d) |
| Scopolamine (Transderm Scop) | 1–3 patches q3d (maximum dose 3 patches every 72 h) |

Reprinted with permission from ExcelleRx, Inc. (2004). *Hospice pharmacia pharmaceutical care tool kit* (6th ed.). Philadelphia: Author.

members arrive before the body is moved, and to perform after-death rituals should be honored. When an expected death occurs in the home setting, the funeral director often transports the body directly to the funeral home.

## Grief, Mourning, and Bereavement

A wide range of feelings and behaviors are normal, adaptive, and healthy reactions to the loss of a loved one. **Grief** refers to the personal feelings that accompany an anticipated or actual loss. **Mourning** refers to individual, family, group, and cultural expressions of grief and associated behaviors. **Bereavement** refers to the period of time during which mourning takes place. Both grief reactions and mourning behaviors change over time as people learn to live with the loss. Although the pain of the loss may be tempered by the passage of time, loss is an ongoing developmental process, and time does not heal the bereaved individual completely (Silverman, 2002). That is, the bereaved do not get over a loss entirely, nor do they return to who they were before the loss. Rather, they develop a new sense of who they are and where they fit in a world that has changed dramatically and permanently.

### Anticipatory Grief and Mourning

Denial, sadness, anger, fear, and anxiety are normal grief reactions in people with life-threatening illness and those close to them. Kübler-Ross (1969) described five common emotional reactions to dying that are applicable to the experience of any loss (Table 17-4). Although the stages that Kübler-Ross described are useful in understanding the overall experience of the dying process, they have been misinterpreted as following a linear, expected trajectory. Not every patient or family member experiences every stage; many patients never reach a stage of acceptance, and patients and families fluctuate on a sometimes daily basis in their emotional responses. Furthermore, although impending loss stresses the patient, people who are close to him or her, and the functioning of the family unit, awareness of dying also provides a unique opportunity for family members to reminisce, resolve relationships, plan for the future, and say goodbye.

Individual and family coping with the anticipation of death is complicated by the varied and conflicting trajectories that grief and mourning may assume in families. For example, although the patient may be experiencing sadness while contemplating role changes that have been brought about by the illness, the patient's spouse or partner may be expressing or suppressing feelings of anger about the current changes in role and impending loss of the relationship. Others in the family may be engaged in denial (eg, "Dad will get better; he just needs to eat more"), fear ("Who will take care of us?" or "Will I get sick too?"), or profound sadness and withdrawal. Although each of these behaviors is normal, tension may arise when one or more family members perceive that others are less caring, too emotional, or too detached.

The nurse should assess the characteristics of the family system and intervene in a manner that supports and enhances the cohesion of the family unit. Parameters for assessing the family facing life-threatening illness are identified in Chart 17-11. The nurse can patiently suggest that family members talk about their feelings and understand them in the broader context of anticipatory grief and mourning. Acknowledging and expressing feelings, continuing to interact with the patient in meaningful ways, and planning for the time of death and bereavement are adaptive family behaviors. Professional support provided by grief counselors, whether in the community, at a local hospital, in the long-term care facility, or associated with a hospice program, can help both the patient and the family sort out and acknowledge feelings and make the end of life as meaningful as possible.

### Grief and Mourning After Death

When a loved one dies, the family members enter a new phase of grief and mourning as they begin to accept the loss, feel the pain of permanent separation, and prepare to live a life without the deceased. Even if the loved one died after a long illness, preparatory grief experienced during the terminal illness does not preclude the grief and mourning that follow the death. With a death after a long or difficult illness, family members may experience conflicting feelings of relief that the loved one's suffering has ended, compounded by guilt and grief related to unresolved issues or the circumstances of death. Grief work may be especially difficult if a patient's death was painful, prolonged, accompanied by unwanted interventions, or unattended. Families who had no preparation or support during the period of imminence and death may have a more difficult time finding a place for the painful memories.

Although some family members may experience prolonged or complicated mourning, most grief reactions fall within a "normal" range. The feelings are often profound, but bereaved people eventually reconcile the loss and find a way to reengage with their lives. Grief and mourning are affected by several factors, including individual characteristics, coping skills, and experiences with illness and death; the nature of the relationship to the deceased; factors surrounding the illness and the death; family dynamics; social support;

| TABLE 17-4 | Kübler-Ross's Five Stages of Dying |
|---|---|
| Stage | Nursing Implications |
| **Denial:** "This cannot be true." Feelings of isolation. May search for another health care professional who will give a more favorable opinion. May seek unproven therapies. | Denial can be an adaptive response, providing a buffer after bad news. It allows time to mobilize defenses but can be maladaptive when it prevents the patient or family from seeking help or when denial behaviors cause more pain or distress than the illness or interfere with everyday functions. Nurses should assess the patient's and family's coping style, information needs, and understanding of the illness and treatment to establish a basis for empathetic listening, education, and emotional support. Rather than confronting the patient with information he or she is not ready to hear, the nurse can encourage him or her to share fears and concerns. Open-ended questions or statements such as "Tell me more about how you are coping with this new information about your illness" can provide a springboard for expression of concerns. |
| **Anger:** "Why me?" Feelings of rage, resentment or envy directed at God, health care professionals, family, others. | Anger can be very isolating, and loved ones or clinicians may withdraw. Nurses should allow the patient and family to express anger, treating them with understanding, respect, and knowledge that the root of the anger is grief over impending loss. |
| **Bargaining:** "I just want to see my grandchild's birth, then I'll be ready. . . ." Patient and/or family plead for more time to reach an important goal. Promises are sometimes made with God. | Terminally ill patients are sometimes able to outlive prognoses and achieve some future goal. Nurses should be patient, allow expression of feelings, and support realistic and positive hope. |
| **Depression:** "I just don't know how my kids are going to get along after I'm gone." Sadness, grief, mourning for impending losses. | Normal and adaptive response. Clinical depression should be assessed and treated when present. Nurses should encourage the patient and family to fully express their sadness. Insincere reassurance or encouragement of unrealistic hopes should be avoided. |
| **Acceptance:** "I've lived a good life, and I have no regrets." Patient and/or family are neither angry nor depressed. | The patient may withdraw as his or her circle of interest diminishes. The family may feel rejected by the patient. Nurses need to support the family's expression of emotions and encourage them to continue to be present for the patient. |

and cultural expectations and norms. Uncomplicated grief and mourning are characterized by emotional feelings of sadness, anger, guilt, and numbness; physical sensations such as hollowness in the stomach and tightness in the chest, weakness, and lack of energy; cognitions that include preoccupation with the loss and a sense of the deceased as still present; and behaviors such as crying, visiting places that are reminders of the deceased, social withdrawal, and restless overactivity (Worden, 1991).

After-death rituals, including preparation of the body, funeral practices, and burial rituals, are socially and culturally significant ways in which family members begin to accept the reality and finality of death. Preplanning of funerals is becoming increasingly common, and hospice professionals in particular help the family make plans for death, often involving the patient, who may wish to play an active role. Preplanning of the funeral relieves the family of the burden of making decisions in the intensely emotional period after a death.

In general, the period of mourning is an adaptive response to loss during which mourners come to accept the loss as real and permanent, acknowledge and experience the painful emotions that accompany the loss, experience life without the deceased, overcome impediments to adjustment, and find a new way of living in a world without the loved one. Particularly immediately after the death, mourners begin to recognize the reality and permanence of the loss by talking about the deceased and telling and retelling the story of the illness and death. Societal norms in the United States are frequently at odds with the normal grieving processes of people; time excused from work obligations is typically measured in days and mourners are often expected to get over the loss quickly and get on with life.

In reality, the work of grief and mourning takes time, and avoiding grief work after the death often leads to long-term adjustment difficulties. According to Rando (2000), mourning for a loss involves the "undoing" of psychosocial ties that bind mourners to the deceased, personal adaptation to the loss, and learning to live in the world without the deceased. Six key processes of mourning allow people to accommodate to the loss in a healthy way (Rando, 2000):

1. Recognition of the loss
2. Reaction to the separation, and experiencing and expressing the pain of the loss
3. Recollection and reexperiencing the deceased, the relationship, and the associated feelings
4. Relinquishing old attachments to the deceased
5. Readjustment to adapt to the new world without forgetting the old
6. Reinvestment

Similarly, Worden (1991) described four tasks of mourning:

1. Acceptance of the reality of the loss
2. Working through the pain of grief
3. Adjusting to the environment in which the deceased is gone

lost a parent, widows, widowers, and gay men and lesbians who have lost a life partner are some examples of specialized support groups available in many communities. Nursing interventions for those experiencing grief and mourning are identified in Chart 17-12.

### Complicated Grief and Mourning

Complicated grief and mourning are characterized by prolonged feelings of sadness and feelings of general worthlessness or hopelessness that persist long after the death, prolonged symptoms that interfere with activities of daily living (anorexia, insomnia, fatigue, panic), or self-destructive behaviors such as alcohol or substance abuse and suicidal ideation or attempts. Complicated grief and mourning require professional assessment and can be treated with pharmacologic and psychological interventions.

## Coping With Death and Dying: Professional Caregiver Issues

Whether practicing in the trauma center, intensive care unit or other acute care setting, home care, hospice, long-term care, or the many locations where patients and their families

---

### CHART 17-11

### Assessing for Anticipatory Mourning in the Family Facing Life-Threatening Illness

**FAMILY CONSTELLATION**
- Identify the members who constitute the patient's family. Who is important to the patient?
- Identify roles and relationships among the family members.
  - Who is the primary caregiver?
  - By what authority is this person the primary caregiver?

**COHESION AND BOUNDARIES**
- How autonomous/interdependent are family members?
  - Degree of involvement with each other as individuals and as a family
  - Degree of bonding between family members
  - Degree of "teamwork" in the family
  - Degree of reliance on individual family members for specific tasks/roles
- How do family members differ in
  - Personality?
  - World view?
  - Priorities?
- What are the implicit and explicit expectations or "rules" for behavior within the family?

**FLEXIBILITY AND ADAPTABILITY**
- What is the family's ability to integrate new information?
- How does the family manage change?
- How able are the family members to assume new roles and responsibilities?

**COMMUNICATION**
- What is the style of communication in the family, in terms of
  - Openness?
  - Directness?
  - Clarity?
- What are the constraints on communication?
- What topics are avoided?

---

### CHART 17-12

### Nursing Interventions for Grief and Mourning

**SUPPORT THE EXPRESSION OF FEELINGS.**
- Encourage the telling of the story using open-ended statements or questions (eg, "Tell me about your husband").
- Assist the mourner to find an outlet for his or her feelings: talking, attending a support group, keeping a journal, finding a safe outlet for angry feelings (writing letters that will not be mailed, physical activity)
- Assess emotional affect and reinforce the normalcy of feelings.
- Assess for guilt and regrets.
  - Are you especially troubled by a certain memory or thought?
  - How do you manage those memories?

**ASSESS FOR THE PRESENCE OF SOCIAL SUPPORT.**
- Do you have someone to whom you can talk about your husband?
- May I help you to find someone you can talk to?

**ASSESS COPING SKILLS.**
- How are you managing day to day?
- Have you experienced other losses? How did you manage those?
- Are there things you are having trouble doing?
- Do you have/need help with specific tasks?

**ASSESS FOR SIGNS OF COMPLICATED GRIEF AND MOURNING AND OFFER PROFESSIONAL REFERRAL.**

---

4. Emotional "relocation" of the deceased to move on with life

Although many people complete the work of mourning with the informal support of families and friends, many find that talking with others who have had a similar experience, such as in formal support groups, normalizes the feelings and experiences and provides a framework for learning new skills to cope with the loss and create a new life. Hospitals, hospices, religious organizations, and other community organizations often sponsor bereavement support groups. Groups for parents who have lost a child, children who have receive ambulatory services, the nurse is closely involved with complex and emotionally laden issues surrounding loss of life. To be most effective and satisfied with the care he or she provides, the nurse should attend to his or her own emotional responses to the losses he or she witnesses every day. Well before the nurse exhibits symptoms of stress or burnout, he or she should acknowledge the difficulty of coping with others' pain on a daily basis and put healthy practices in place that guard against emotional exhaustion. In hospice settings, where death, grief, and loss are expected outcomes of patient care, interdisciplinary colleagues rely on each other for support, using meeting time to express frustration, sadness, anger, and other emotions; to learn coping skills from each other; and to speak about how they were affected by the lives of those patients who have died since the last meeting. In many settings, staff members organize or attend memorial services to support families and other caregivers, who find comfort in joining each other to remember and celebrate the lives of patients. Finally, healthy personal habits, including diet, exercise, stress reduction activities (eg, dance, yoga, tai chi, meditation), and sleep, help guard against the detrimental effects of stress.

## Critical Thinking Exercises

**1** You are conducting your first home care visit to an 88-year-old man who has been hospitalized three times in the last 4 months with acute shortness of breath related to chronic obstructive pulmonary disease. Your assessment reveals that his respiratory rate is 24 breaths per minute, his nail beds and oropharynx are dusky, and he is using accessory muscles to breathe. He is very weak, has a poor appetite, and is able to move from bed to chair only with assistance. He tells you that when he has extreme difficulty breathing, his wife becomes very frightened, causing him to become very anxious as well. His wife, who is also 88 years of age, has heart failure and diabetes. She walks with a walker, and although she tries to take care of her husband, it is becoming increasingly difficult for her to do so. The couple have been married for almost 70 years and are very devoted to each other. What additional assessments would you conduct? What strategies would you implement to (1) relieve the patient's symptoms and discomfort, (2) assist his wife in management of his care, and (3) prepare both of them for his inevitable death?

**2** A 55-year-old married mother of three adult children has been referred for hospice care. During your initial visit to the patient's home, you assess that she is experiencing severe pain in her ribs and pelvis (she reports a score of 8 on a 0-to-10 pain intensity scale). In addition, she reports that she is unable to sleep. Her physician has prescribed morphine for her pain, but you assess that she has used very few doses of the morphine. Her husband tells you privately that he has discouraged her use of the medicine because it has made her very sleepy and nauseated in the past. The interdisciplinary team is meeting to discuss the patient's treatment plan. What additional assessment data are needed to determine the wishes and expectations of the patient as well as the husband? What are the team's options for intervention? What are the pros and cons of each option?

**3** You have been assigned to care for a 44-year-old married man who is in the end stages of AIDS. He was discharged home from the hospital yesterday and is being admitted to the local visiting nurse association's home palliative care program. When you ask him about his religion and beliefs as part of the spiritual assessment that is performed at the time of admission, he says to you, "I know that God is punishing me." How should you respond to his comment? Explain your rationale. What additional questions would you include in your spiritual assessment? Why? Discuss your plan for follow-up.

**4** **ebp** Transcutaneous electrical stimulation (TENS) is prescribed for one of your patients in an effort to relieve his severe bone pain. You are responsible for teaching the patient and his wife how to use the TENS unit. What is the evidence for the effectiveness of TENS in relieving pain? How would you evaluate the strength of the evidence? What are the implications for practice based on the evidence for its effectiveness?

## REFERENCES AND SELECTED READINGS

### BOOKS

Abrahm, J. L. (2000). *A physician's guide to pain and symptom management in cancer patients.* Baltimore, MD: Johns Hopkins University Press.

Addington, T. G. (1991). *Communication and cancer.* Hershey, PA: Central Pennsylvania Oncology Group.

Amenta, M. O. & Bohnet, N. L. (1986). *Nursing care of the terminally ill.* New York: Little Brown.

American Nurses Association. (1994). Position statement on assisted suicide [online]. Available at: www.nursingworld.org/readroom/position/ethics/etsuic.htm (accessed March 31, 2006).

American Nurses Association. (2003). *Nursing's social policy statement.* Washington, DC: Author.

American Pain Society. (2003). *Principles of analgesic use in the treatment of acute pain and cancer pain* (5th ed.). Glenview, IL: Author.

Bailey, F. A. (2003). *The palliative response.* Birmingham, AL: Menasha Ridge.

Barnard, D., Towers, A., Boston, P. & Lambrinidou, Y. (2000). *Crossing over: Narratives of palliative care.* New York: Oxford.

Bennahum, D. A. (1996). The historical development of hospice and palliative care. In Sheehan, D. C. & Forman, W. B. (Eds.), *Hospice and palliative care: Concepts and practice.* Boston: Jones & Bartlett.

Byock, I. (1997). *Dying well: The prospect for growth at the end of life.* New York: Riverhead.

Callahan, D. (1993b). *The troubled dream of life.* New York: Simon & Schuster.

Doyle, D., Hanks, G. W. C., & MacDonald, N. (Eds.). (1998). *Oxford textbook of palliative medicine* (2nd ed.). New York: Oxford.

ExcelleRx, Inc. (2003). *Hospice pharmacia pharmaceutical care tool kit* (5th ed.). Philadelphia: Author.

Family Home Hospice of the Visiting Nurse Association of Greater Philadelphia. (1999). *Signs of approaching death.* Philadelphia: Author.

Federal Interagency Forum on Aging-Related Statistics. (2004). *Older Americans 2004: Key indicators of well-being.* Washington, DC: United States Government Printing Office.

Ferrell, B. R. & Coyle, N. (Eds.). (2001). *Textbook of palliative nursing.* New York: Oxford.

Field, M. J. & Cassel, C. K. (Eds.). (1997). *Approaching death: Improving care at the end of life.* Washington, DC: National Academy Press.

Frankl, V. E. (1984). *Man's search for meaning.* New York: Washington Square.

George H. Gallup International Institute. (1997). *Spiritual beliefs and the dying process.* Princeton, NJ: Author.

Glaser, B. G. & Strauss, A. (1965). *Awareness of dying.* Chicago: Aldine.

Hallenbeck, J. L. (2003). *Palliative care perspectives.* New York: Oxford.

Hogan, C., Lynn, J., Gabel, J., et al. (2000). *Medicare beneficiaries' costs and use of care in the last year of life.* Washington, DC: MedPAC.

Hospice Association of America. (2002). *Hospice facts and statistics.* Washington, DC: Author.

Jacox, A., Carr, D. B. & Payne, R. (1994). *Management of cancer pain.* Clinical practice guideline No. 9 (AHCPR Publication No. 94-0592). Washington, DC: Agency for Health Care Policy and Research, United States Department of Health and Human Services, Public Health Service.

Jennings, B., Ryndes, T., D'Onofrio, C. & Baily, M. A. (2003). *Access to hospice care: Expanding boundaries; overcoming barriers.* Hastings Center Report Supplement: S3.

Kübler-Ross, E. (1969). *On death and dying.* New York: MacMillan.

Lesparre, M. & Matherlee, K. (1998). *Delivering and financing care at the end of life.* Issue Brief (No. 711). Washington, DC: The George Washington University.

Lynn, J., Schuster, J. L. & Kabcenell, A. (2000). *Improving care for the end of life: A sourcebook for health care managers and clinicians.* New York: Oxford.

Matzo, M. L. & Sherman, D. W. (Eds.). (2001). *Palliative care nursing: Quality care to the end of life.* New York: Springer.

McSkimming, S. A., Super, A., Driever, M. J., et al. (1997). *Living and healing during life-threatening illness.* Portland, OR: Supportive Care of the Dying.

National Hospice and Palliative Care Organization. (2003). *Hospice facts and figures.* Alexandria, VA: Author.

Occupational Home Economics Education Series. (1977). Attitudes toward death. In *Care and independent living services for the aging* (Section III-A22). Washington, DC: U.S. Government Printing Office.

Office of the Inspector General, Department of Health and Human Services. (1997). *Hospice patients in nursing homes.* DHHS Publication No. OEI-05-95-00250. Washington, DC: U.S. Government Printing Office.

Plata-Salaman, C. (1997). Symptoms in terminal illness: A research workshop. Cachexia or wasting: Basic perspective [online]. Available at: ninr.nih.gov/ninr/wnew/symptoms_in_terminal_illness.html (accessed March 31, 2006).

Rando, T. A. (2000). Promoting healthy anticipatory mourning in intimates of the life-threatened or dying person. In Rando, T. A. (Ed.). *Clinical dimensions of anticipatory mourning.* Champaign, IL: Research Press.

Saunders, C. & Kastenbaum, R. (Eds.). (1997). *Hospice care on the international scene.* New York: Springer.

Smith, S. A. (2000). *Hospice concepts: A guide to palliative care in terminal illness.* Champaign, IL: Research Press.

Tilly, J. & Wiener, J. (2001). *Medicaid and end-of-life care.* Washington, DC: Last Acts.

Waller, A., & Caroline, N. A. (2000). *Handbook of palliative care in cancer* (2nd ed.). Boston: Butterworth-Heinemann.

Wentzel, K. B. (1981). *To those who need it most, hospice means hope.* Boston: Charles River.

World Health Organization. (1990). *Cancer pain relief and palliative care: Report of a WHO expert committee.* Technical Report Series, 804, 1–75. Geneva: World Health Organization.

Worden, J. W. (1991). *Grief counseling and grief therapy.* New York: Springer.

Wrede-Seaman, L. (1999). *Symptom management algorithms: A handbook for palliative care.* Yakima, WA: Intellicard.

## JOURNALS

*An asterisk indicates a nursing research article.

Ameling, A., & Povilonis, M. (2002). Spirituality, meaning, mental health, and nursing. *Journal of Psychosocial Nursing and Mental Health Services,* 39(4), 14–20.

Balaban, R. B. (2000). A physician's guide to talking about end-of-life care. *Journal of General Internal Medicine,* 15(3), 195–200.

Benoliel, J. Q. (1993). The moral context of oncology nursing. *Oncology Nursing Forum Supplement,* 20(10), 5–12.

Blackhall, L. J., Murphy, S. T., Frank, G., et al. (1995). Ethnicity and attitudes toward patient autonomy. *Journal of the American Medical Association,* 274(10), 820–825.

Block, S. D. (2000). Assessing and managing depression in the terminally ill patient. *Annals of Internal Medicine,* 132(3), 209–218.

Bolling, A. & Lynn, J. (1998). Hospice: Current practice, future possibilities. *Hospice Journal,* 13(1–2), 29–32.

Brant, J. M. (1998). The art of palliative care: Living with hope, dying with dignity. *Oncology Nursing Forum,* 25(96), 995–1004.

Brinson, S. V. & Brunk, Q. (2000). Hospice family caregivers: An experience in coping. *The Hospice Journal,* 15(3), 1–12.

Buchanan, J., Borland, R., Cosolo, W., et al. (1996). Patients' beliefs about cancer management. *Supportive Care in Cancer,* 4(2), 110–117.

Callahan, D. (1993a). Pursuing a peaceful death. *Hastings Center Report,* 23(4), 33–38.

Campbell, M. L. & Field, B. E. (1991). Management of the patient with do not resuscitate status: Compassion and cost containment. *Heart and Lung,* 20(4), 345–348.

Caralis, P. V., Davis, B., Wright, K., et al (1993). The influence of ethnicity and race on attitudes toward advance directives, life-prolonging treatments and euthanasia. *Journal of Clinical Ethics,* 4(2), 155–165.

Cassel, C. K., Ludden, J. M., & Moon, G. M. (2000). Perceptions of barriers to high-quality palliative care in hospitals. *Health Affairs,* 19(5), 166–172.

Chochinov, H. M., Tataryn, D. J., Wilson, K. G., et al. (2000). Prognostic awareness and the terminally ill. *Psychosomatics,* 41(6), 500–504.

Chow, E., Anderson, L., Wong, R., et al. (2001). Patients with advanced cancer: A survey of the understanding of their illness and expectations from palliative radiotherapy for symptomatic metastases. *Clinical Oncology,* 13(3), 204–208.

Christakis, N. A. & Lamont, E. B. (2000). Extent and determinants of error in doctors' prognoses in terminally ill patients: Prospective cohort study. *British Medical Journal,* 320(7233), 469–473.

Connor, S. R. (1992). Denial in terminal illness: To intervene or not to intervene. *Hospice Journal,* 8(4), 1–15.

Cook, D., Rocker, G., Marshall, J., et al. (2003). Withdrawal of mechanical ventilation in anticipation of death in the intensive care unit. *New England Journal of Medicine,* 349(12), 1123–1132.

Crawley, L. M., Marshall, P. A., Lo, B. & Koenig, B. A. (2002). Strategies for culturally effective end-of-life care. *Annals of Internal Medicine,* 136(9), 673–679.

Crawley, L., Payne, R., Bolden, J., et al. (2000). Palliative and end-of-life care in the African American community. *Journal of the American Medical Association,* 284(19), 2518–2521.

Dahlin, C. (2004). Oral complications at the end of life. *American Journal of Nursing,* 104(7), 40–47.

Department of Human Services, Office of Disease Prevention and Epidemiology. (March 6, 2006). Eighth annual report on Oregon's Death with Dignity Act. Available at: http://egov.oregon.gov/DHS/ph/pas/docs/year8.pdf (accessed May 24, 2006).

Egan, K. A. & Arnold, R. L. (2003). Grief and bereavement care. *American Journal of Nursing,* 103(9), 42–52.

Ersek, M., Kagawa-Singer, M., Barnes, D., et al. (1998). Multicultural considerations in the use of advance directives. *Oncology Nursing Forum,* 25(10), 1683–1690.

Ferrell, B. R. & Coyle, N. (2002). An overview of palliative nursing care. *American Journal of Nursing,* 102(5), 26–31.

Ferrell, B., Virani, R., Grant, M., et al. (2000). Beyond the Supreme Court decision: Nursing perspectives on end-of-life care. *Oncology Nursing Forum,* 27(3), 445–455.

Fetters, M. D., Churchill, L. & Danis, M. (2001). Conflict resolution at the end of life. *Critical Care Medicine, 29*(5), 921–925.

Finucane, T. (2002). Care of patients nearing death: Another view. *Journal of the American Geriatrics Society, 50*(3), 551–553.

Ganzini, L., Goy, E. R., Miller, L., et al. (2003). Nurses' experiences with hospice patients who refuse foods and fluids to hasten death. *New England Journal of Medicine, 349*(4), 359–365.

Gbrich, C. (2001). The emotions and coping strategies of caregivers of family members with a terminal cancer. *Journal of Palliative Care, 17*(1), 30–36.

Grady, P. A. (1999). Improving care at the end of life: Research issues. *Journal of Hospice and Palliative Nursing, 1*(94), 151–155.

Griffie, J., Nelson-Marten, P. & Muchka, S. (2004). Acknowledging the "Elephant": Communication in palliative care. *American Journal of Nursing, 104* (1), 48–57.

Helm, A. (1984). Debating euthanasia: An international perspective. *Journal of Gerontological Nursing, 10*(11), 20–24.

Hermann, C. P. (2001). Spiritual needs of dying patients: A qualitative study. *Oncology Nursing Forum, 28*(91), 67.

Hermann, C. & Looney, S. (2001). The effectiveness of symptom management in hospice patients during the last seven days of life. *Journal of Hospice and Palliative Nursing, 3*(3), 88–96.

Highfield, M. E. F. (2000). Providing spiritual care to patients with cancer. *Clinical Journal of Oncology Nursing, 4*(3), 115–120.

Inui, A. (2002). Cancer anorexia-cachexia syndrome: Current issues in research and management. *CA: A Cancer Journal for Clinicians, 52*(2), 72–91.

*Jezuit, D. L. (2000). Suffering of critical care nurses with end-of-life decisions. *MedSurg Nursing, 9*(3), 145–152.

Kagawa-Singer, M., & Blackhall, L. J. (2001). Negotiating cross-cultural issues at the end of life. *Journal of the American Medical Association, 286*(23), 2993–3001.

*Kirchhoff, K. T., Spuhler, V., Walker, L., et al. (2000). Intensive care nurses' experiences with end-of-life care. *American Journal of Critical Care 9*(1), 36–42.

Krisman-Scott, M. A. (2000). An historical analysis of disclosure of terminal status. *Journal of Nursing Scholarship, 32*(1), 47–52.

LaDuke, S. (2001). Terminal dyspnea and palliative care. *American Journal of Nursing 101*(11), 26–31.

Lawlor, P. G., Gagnon, B., Mancini, I. L., et al. (2000). Occurrence, causes, and outcome of delirium in patients with advanced cancer. *Archives of Internal Medicine, 160*(6), 786–794.

Mazanec, P. & Tyler, M. K. (2003). Cultural considerations in end-of-life care. *American Journal of Nursing, 103*(3), 50–58.

Maugans, T. A. (1996). The SPIRITual history. *Archives of Family Medicine, 5*(1), 11–16.

Means to a Better End: A Report on Dying in America Today. (2002). Available at: http://www.rwjf.org/files/publications/other/meansbetterend.pdf (accessed May 24, 2006).

Meier, D. E., Ahronheim, J. C., Morris, J., et al. (2001). High short-term mortality in hospitalized patients with advanced dementia: lack of benefit of tube feeding. *Archives of Internal Medicine, 161*(4), 594–599.

Morrison, R. S. & Meier, D. E. (2004). Palliative care. *New England Journal of Medicine, 350*(25), 2582–2590.

Morrison, R. S., Siu, A. L., Leipzig, R. M., et al. (2000). The hard task of improving care at the end of life. *Archives of Internal Medicine, 160*(6), 743–747.

Morse, J. M. (2000). On comfort and comforting. *American Journal of Nursing, 100*(9), 34–37.

Morse, J. M. & Doberneck, B. (1995). Delineating the concept of hope. *Image: Journal of Nursing Scholarship, 27*, 283–291.

National Institute of Nursing Research (NINR). Mission statement. Available at: ninr.nih.gov/ninr/research/diversity/mission.html (accessed March 31, 2006).

O'Gorman, M. L. (2002). Spiritual care at the end of life. *Critical Care Nursing Clinics of North America, 14*(2), 171–176.

Oregon Department of Human Services. (2004). Physician assisted suicide: Oregon's death with dignity act [online]. Available at: www.ohd.hr.state.or.us/chs/pas/pas.cfm (accessed March 31, 2006).

Paice, J. (2002). Managing psychological conditions in palliative care. *American Journal of Nursing, 102*(11), 36–42.

Patrick, D. L., Engelberg, R. A., & Curtis, J. R. (2001). Evaluating the quality of dying and death. *Journal of Pain and Symptom Management, 22*(3), 717–726.

Pitorak, E. F. (2003a). Care at the time of death. *American Journal of Nursing, 103*(7), 42–51.

Pitorak, E. F. (2003b). Respecting the dying patient's rights. *Home Healthcare Nurse, 21*(12), 833–836.

Post-White, J., Ceronsky, C., Kreitzer, M. J., et al. (1996). Hope, spirituality, sense of coherence, and quality of life in patients with cancer. *Oncology Nursing Forum, 23*(10), 1571–1579.

Quill, T. E., & Byock, I. R. (2000). Responding to intractable terminal suffering: The role of terminal sedation and voluntary refusal of foods and fluids. *Annals of Internal Medicine, 132*(5), 408–414.

Raudonis, B. M. (1992). Ethical considerations in qualitative research with hospice patients. *Qualitative Health Research, 2*(2), 238–249.

Ripamonti, C., Filiberti, A., Totis, A., et al. (1999). Suicide among patients with cancer cared for at home by palliative care teams. *Lancet, 354*(9193), 1877–1878.

Ross, H. M. (2001). Islamic tradition at the end of life. *MedSurg Nursing, 10*(2), 83–87.

Roth, A. J., & Breitbart, W. (1996). Psychiatric emergencies in terminally ill cancer patients. *Hematology/Oncology Clinics of North America, 10*(1), 235–258.

Rushton, C. H. (2004). Ethics and palliative care in pediatrics. *American Journal of Nursing, 104*(4), 54–63.

Sheehan, D. K. & Schirm, V. (2003) End-of-life care of older adults. *American Journal of Nursing, 103*(11), 48–58.

Silverman, P. R. (2002). Living with grief, rebuilding a world. *Journal of Palliative Medicine, 5*(3), 449–454.

Song, M. K. (2004). Effects of end-of-life discussions on patients' affective outcomes. *Nursing Outlook, 52*(3), 118–125.

Sorenson, B. F. (1991). Euthanasia: The "good death"? *Surgical Neurology, 35*, 827–830.

Spross, J. A. (1992). Cancer pain relief: An international perspective. *Oncology Nursing Forum, 19*(7), 5–19.

Stanley, K. J. (2000). Silence is not golden: Conversations with the dying. *Clinical Journal of Oncology Nursing, 4*(1), 34–40.

Steinhauser, K. E., Christakis, N. A., Clipp, E. C., et al. (2004). Family perspectives on end-of-life care at the last place of care. *Journal of the American Medical Association, 291*(1), 88–93.

SUPPORT Principal Investigators. (1995). A controlled trial to improve care for seriously ill hospitalized patients. *Journal of the American Medical Association, 274*(20), 1591–1598.

Teno, J. M., Fisher, E. S., Hamel, M. B., et al. (2002). Medical care inconsistent with patients' treatment goals: Association with 1-year Medicare resource use and survival. *Journal of American Geriatrics Society, 50*(3), 496–500.

Tilden, V. P. (2000). Policy perspectives: Advance directives. *American Journal of Nursing, 100*(12), 49–51.

Tolle, S. W., Tilden, V. P., Rosenfeld, A. G., et al. (2000). Family reports of barriers to optimal care of the dying. *Nursing Research, 49*(6), 310–317.

Tulsky, J. A. (2001). Preparing for the end of life: Preferences of patients, families, physicians and other care providers. *Journal of Pain and Symptom Management, 22*(3), 727–737.

Virani, R. & Sofer, D. (2003). Improving the quality of end-of-life care. *American Journal of Nursing, 103*(5), 52–60.

Virmani, J., Schneiderman, L. J. & Kaplan, R. M. (1994). Relationship of advance directives to physician-patient communication. *Archives of Internal Medicine, 154*(8), 909–913.

Waller, A., Hershkowitz, M. & Adunsky, A. (1994). The effects of intravenous fluid infusion on blood and urine parameters of hydration and on state of consciousness in terminally ill patients. *American Journal of Hospice and Palliative Care, 11*(6), 26–29.

Weissman, D. E. (2004). Decision making at a time of crisis near the end of life. *Journal of the American Medical Association, 292*(14), 1738–1743.

Wenger, N. S. & Rosenfeld, K. (2001). Quality indicators for end-of-life care in vulnerable elders. *Annals of Internal Medicine, 135*(8), 677–685.

Wenrich, M. D., Curtis, J. R., Shannon, S. E., et al. (2001). Communicating with dying patients within the spectrum of medical care from terminal diagnosis to death. *Archives of Internal Medicine, 161*(6), 868–874.

West, S. K. & Levi, L. (2004). Culturally appropriate end-of-life care for the Black American. *Home Healthcare Nurse, 22*(3), 164–168.

Yedidia, M. J. & MacGregor, B. (2001). Confronting the prospect of dying: Reports of terminally ill patients. *Journal of Pain and Symptom Management, 22*(4), 807–819.

Zerwekh, J. V. (1987). Should fluid and nutrition support be withheld from terminally ill patients? *American Journal of Hospice and Palliative Care, 4*(4), 37–38.

Zerwekh, J. (1994). The truth tellers: How hospice nurses help patients confront death. *American Journal of Nursing, 94*(2), 31–34.

Zerwekh, J. V. (1997). Do dying patients really need IV fluids? *American Journal of Nursing, 97*(3), 26–30.

Zerzan, J., Stearns, S. & Hanson, L. (2000). Access to palliative care and hospice in nursing homes. *Journal of the American Medical Association, 284*(19), 2489–2493.

## RESOURCES

American Academy of Hospice and Palliative Medicine, 4700 West Lake Avenue, Glenview, IL 60025; 847-375-4712; http://www.aahpm.org/. Accessed March 31, 2006.

Americans for Better Care of the Dying (ABCD), 4125 Albemarle Street NW, Suite 210, Washington, DC 20016; (202) 895-9485, http://www.abcdcaring.org/. Accessed March 31, 2006.

Association for Death Education and Counseling (ADEC), 342 North Main Street West Hartford, CT 06117; 860-586-7503; fax 860-586-7550; http://www.adec.org/. Accessed March 31, 2006.

American Hospice Foundation, 2120 L Street NW, Suite 200, Washington, DC 20037; 202-223-0204; fax 202-223-0208; e-mail: ahf@msn.com; http://www.americanhospice.org/. Accessed March 31, 2006.

Caring Connections, a program of the National Hospice and Palliative Care Organization, 1700 Diagonal Road, Suite 625, Alexandria, VA 22314; http://www.caringinfo.org. Accessed May 24, 2006.

Center to Improve Care of the Dying (at George Washington University); offices located at the RAND Corporation, 1200 South Hayes Street, Arlington, VA 22202; 703-413-1100; http://www.gwu.edu/~cicd/. Accessed March 31, 2006.

Children's Hospice International, 2202 Mount Vernon Avenue, Suite 3C, Alexandria, VA 22301; 800-24-CHILD; http://www.chionline.org. Accessed March 31, 2006.

Compassion in Dying, 6312 SW Capital Highway, Suite 415, Portland, OR 97201; 503-221-9556; http://www.compassionindying.org/. Accessed March 31, 2006.

Department of Pain Medicine and Palliative Care at Beth Israel Medical Center, 1st Avenue at 16th Street, 12 Baird Hall, New York, NY 10003; 212-844-1472; http://www.stoppain.org. Accessed March 31, 2006.

End-of-Life Nursing Education Consortium; http://www.aacn.nche.edu/elnec/. Accessed March 31, 2006.

Growthhouse, Inc. (provides information and referral services for agencies working with death and dying issues), San Francisco, CA; 415-863-3045; http://www.growthhouse.org. Accessed March 31, 2006.

HMS Center for Palliative Care (Harvard Medical School), Massachusetts General Hospital, Founders House 606, 55 Fruit Street, Boston, MA 02114; 617-724-9509; http://www.hms.harvard.edu/cdi/pallcare/. Accessed March 31, 2006.

Hospice and Palliative Nurses Association (HPNA), Penn Center West One, Suite 229, Pittsburgh, PA 15276; 412-787-9301; http://www.hpna.org. Accessed March 31, 2006.

Hospice Association of America, National Association for Home Care, 228 Seventh Street SE, Washington, DC 20003; 202-547-7424; http://www.hospiceamerica.org/. Accessed March 31, 2006.

Hospice Education Institute, 190 Westbrook Road, Essex, CT 06426; 800-331-1620; http://www.hospiceworld.org/. Accessed March 31, 2006.

Hospice Foundation of America, 2001 S St. NW #300, Washington, DC 20009; 800-854-3402; http://www.hospicefoundation.org. Accessed March 31, 2006.

Hospice Net; http://www.hospicenet.org/index.html. Accessed March 31, 2006.

Hospice Web (links to other resources); http://www.hospiceweb.com/links.htm. Accessed March 31, 2006.

Last Acts Partnership, 1620 Eye Street NW, Suite 202, Washington, DC 20006; 800-989-WILL; http://www.caringinfo.org. Accessed March 31, 2006.

National Consensus Project for Quality Palliative Care (National Guidelines); http://www.nationalconsensusproject.org. Accessed March 31, 2006.

National Hospice and Palliative Care Organization, National Hospice Foundation, 1700 Diagonal Rd, Suite 625, Alexandria, VA 22314; 703-837-1500; http://www.nhpco.org. Accessed March 31, 2006.

National Prison Hospice Association, P.O. Box 4623, Boulder, CO 80306-4623; 303-447-8051; fax 303-447-8055; http://www.npha.org. Accessed March 31, 2006.

Palliative Care Nursing; http://www.palliativecarenursing.net/index.html. Accessed March 31, 2006.

Partnership for Caring: America's Voices for the Dying, National Office, 1620 Eye Street NW, Suite 202, Washington, DC 20006; 202-296-8071; http://www.partnershipforcaring.org. Accessed March 31, 2006.

Population-based Palliative Care Research Network, University of Colorado Health Sciences Center, 4200 East 9th Avenue, Denver, CO 80262; 866-372-9417; http://www.uchsc.edu/popcrn/. Accessed March 31, 2006.

Project on Death in America, Open Society Institute, 400 West 59th Street, New York, NY 10019; 212-548-0150; http://www.soros.org/initiatives/pdia. Accessed March 31, 2006.

Promoting Excellence in End-of-Life Care, The Practical Ethics Center, The University of Montana, 1000 East Beckwith Avenue, Missoula, MT 59812; 406-243-6601; fax 406-243-6633; http://www.promotingexcellence.org. Accessed March 31, 2006.

Supportive Care of the Dying: A Coalition for Compassionate Care; for more information, contact Sylvia McSkimming, PhD, RN, Executive Director, c/o Providence Health System, 4805 NE Glisan Street, 2E07, Portland, OR 97213; 503-215-5053; http://www.careofdying.org. Accessed March 31, 2006.

The Center to Advance Palliative Care at The Mount Sinai School of Medicine, 1255 5th Avenue, Suite C-2, New York, NY, 10029; main line: 212-201-2670; http://www.capcmssm.org. Accessed March 31, 2006.

Toolkit of Instruments to Measure End-of-life Care (TIME; Dr. Joan Teno at Brown University); http://www.chcr.brown.edu/pcoc/toolkit.htm. Accessed March 31, 2006.

Veterans Administration Hospice and Palliative Care Initiative, Office on Academic Affiliations, Department of Veterans Affairs; http://www.va.gov/oaa/flp/. Accessed March 31, 2006.

# UNIT 4

# Perioperative Concepts and Nursing Management

## Case Study
### Applying Concepts from NANDA, NIC, and NOC

**A Patient Recovering From Abdominal Surgery**

**Mr. Dickson,** a 60-year-old smoker, was admitted to the surgical unit 5 hours ago after colon resection for cancer. He is groggy but easily arousable. He can move all extremities with equal strength, but feels better lying still. In the last 4 hours, 125 mL of greenish material has drained from his nasogastric tube, which is connected to low intermittent suction. His abdomen is mildly distended; bowel sounds are absent. The large abdominal dressing has a reconstitutable bulb drain with 30 mL of serosanguineous drainage; the dressing's minimal visible drainage has not increased in several hours. A peripheral IV of D5W ½NS with 20 mEq of KCl is infusing at 125 mL/h. Mr. Dickson has voided 600 mL of clear urine. Vital signs are: Temp 97°F; HR 82, B/P 112/70; Resp 12 and shallow. Lung auscultation reveals scattered crackles throughout and a weak cough. After a 50-mg morphine injection, Mr. Dickson rates his pain at 3 (down from 7). He is reluctant to use his incentive spirometer for fear of more pain.

 Turn to Appendix C to see a concept map that illustrates the relationships that exist between the nursing diagnoses, interventions, and outcomes for the patient's clinical problems.

## Nursing Classifications and Languages

| NANDA<br>Nursing Diagnoses | NIC<br>Nursing Interventions | NOC<br>Nursing Outcomes<br>Return to functional baseline status, stabilization of, or improvement in: |
|---|---|---|
| **Risk for Impaired Gas Exchange**—At risk for excess or deficit in oxygenation and/or carbon dioxide elimination at the alveolar-capillary membrane | **Respiratory Monitoring**—Collection and analysis of patient data to ensure airway patency and adequate gas exchange | **Anxiety Control**—Personal actions to eliminate or reduce feelings of apprehension and tension from an unidentifiable source |
| **Risk for Ineffective Airway Clearance**—At risk for inability to clear secretions or obstructions from the respiratory tract to maintain a clear airway | **Cough Enhancement**—Promotion of deep inhalation by the patient with subsequent generation of high intrathoracic pressures and compression of underlying lung parenchyma for the forceful expulsion of air | **Respiratory Status: Gas Exchange**—The alveolar exchange of $O_2$ and $CO_2$ to maintain arterial blood gas concentrations |
| **Acute Pain**—Unpleasant sensory and emotional experience arising from actual or potential tissue damage or described in terms of such damage | **Pain Management**—Alleviation of pain or reduction in pain to a level of comfort that is acceptable to the patient | **Pain Level**—Severity of observed or reported pain |
| **Impaired Physical Mobility**—Limitation in independent, purposeful physical movement of the body or of one or more extremities | **Teaching: Prescribed Activity/Exercise**—Preparing a patient to achieve and/or maintain a prescribed level of activity | **Mobility**—Ability to move purposefully in own environment independently with or without assistive device |

NANDA International (2005). *Nursing diagnoses: Definitions & classification 2005–2006.* Philadelphia: North American Nursing Diagnosis Association.
Dochterman, J. M. & Bulechek, G. M. (2004). *Nursing interventions classification (NIC)* (4th ed.). St. Louis: Mosby.
Iowa Outcomes Project (2004). In Moorhead, S., Johnson, M. & Maas, M. (2004). *Nursing outcomes classification (NOC)* (3rd ed.). St. Louis: Mosby.
Dochterman, J. M. & Jones, D. A. (2003). *Unifying nursing languages: The harmonization of NANDA, NIC, and NOC.* Washington, D.C.: American Nurses Association.

"Point, click, learn! Visit thePoint for additional resources."

# CHAPTER 18

# Preoperative Nursing Management

## Learning Objectives

*On completion of this chapter, the learner will be able to:*

1. Define the three phases of perioperative nursing.
2. Describe a comprehensive preoperative assessment to identify surgical risk factors.
3. Identify health factors that affect patients preoperatively.
4. Identify legal and ethical considerations related to informed consent.
5. Describe preoperative nursing measures that decrease the risk for infection and other postoperative complications.
6. Describe the immediate preoperative preparation of the patient.
7. Develop a preoperative teaching plan designed to promote the patient's recovery from anesthesia and surgery, thus preventing postoperative complications.

Surgery, whether elective or emergent, is a stressful, complex event. Today, as a result of advances in surgical techniques and instrumentation as well as in anesthesia, many surgical procedures that were once performed in an inpatient setting now take place in ambulatory or outpatient settings. Approximately 60% of elective surgeries are now performed in an ambulatory or outpatient setting; this number is expected to continue to increase over the next decade (Conner, 2004). In the past, the patient scheduled for elective surgery was admitted to the hospital at least one day before surgery for evaluation and preparation; these activities are now completed before the patient is admitted to the hospital. Today, many patients arrive at the hospital on the morning of surgery and go home after recovering from the anesthesia in the postanesthesia care unit (PACU). Often, surgical patients who require hospital stays are trauma patients, acutely ill patients, patients undergoing major surgery, patients who require emergency surgery, and patients with a concurrent medical disorder. As a result, the acuity and complexity of surgical patients and procedures have increased in the inpatient setting. Although each setting (ambulatory, outpatient, or inpatient) offers its own unique advantages for the delivery of patient care, they all require a comprehensive preoperative nursing assessment and nursing interventions to prepare the patient and family before surgery.

Today's technology has led to more complex procedures, more complicated microsurgical and laser technology, more sophisticated bypass equipment, increased use of laparoscopic surgery, and more sensitive monitoring devices. Surgery today can involve the transplantation of multiple human organs, the implantation of mechanical devices, the reattachment of body parts, and the use of robots and minimally invasive procedures in the operating room (OR) (Lotan, Cadeddu & Gettman, 2004; Robinson & Stiegmann, 2004). Advances in anesthesia have kept pace with these surgical technologies. More sophisticated monitoring and new pharmacologic agents, such as short-acting anesthetics and more effective antiemetics, have improved postoperative pain management, reduced postoperative nausea and vomiting, and shortened procedure and recovery times.

Concurrent with technologic advances have been changes in the delivery of and payment for health care. Pressure to reduce hospital stays and contain costs has resulted in diagnostic **preadmission testing (PAT)** and preoperative preparation before admission to the hospital. Many facilities have a presurgical services department to facilitate PAT and to initiate the nursing assessment process, which focuses on patient demographics, health history, and other information pertinent to the surgical procedure (Halaszynski, Juda & Silverman, 2004). The increasing use of **ambulatory**, same-day, or short-stay surgery, means that patients leave the hospital sooner, which increases the need for teaching, discharge planning, preparation for self-care, and referral for home care and rehabilitation services. Competent care of ambulatory, same-day, or short-stay surgical patients requires a sound knowledge of all aspects of perioperative and perianesthesia nursing.

# Perioperative and Perianesthesia Nursing

The special field known as perioperative and perianesthesia nursing includes a wide variety of nursing functions associated with the patient's surgical experience during the perioperative period. **Perioperative** and perianesthesia nursing addresses the nursing roles relevant to the three phases of the surgical experience: preoperative, intraoperative, and postoperative. Each phase begins and ends at a particular point in the sequence of events that constitutes the surgical experience, and each includes a wide range of activities the nurse performs using the nursing process and based on the standards of practice (American Society of PeriAnesthesia Nurses, 2002). Chart 18-1 presents nursing activities characteristic of the three perioperative phases of care.

## Preoperative Phase

The **preoperative phase** begins when the decision to proceed with surgical intervention is made and ends with the transfer of the patient onto the OR table. The scope of nursing activities during this time involves establishing a baseline evaluation of the patient before surgery by carrying out a preoperative interview (which includes a physical

## Glossary

**ambulatory surgery:** includes outpatient (same-day) surgery that does not require an overnight hospital stay or short stay, with admission to an inpatient hospital setting for less than 24 hours

**informed consent:** the patient's autonomous decision about whether to undergo a surgical procedure; based on the nature of the condition, the treatment options, and the risks and benefits involved

**intraoperative phase:** period of time from when the patient is transferred to the operating room table to when he or she is admitted to the postanesthesia care unit (PACU)

**perioperative phase:** period of time that constitutes the surgical experience; includes the preoperative, intraoperative, and postoperative phases of nursing care

**postoperative phase:** period of time that begins with the admission of the patient to the PACU and ends after a follow-up evaluation in the clinical setting or home

**preadmission testing (PAT):** diagnostic testing performed before admission to the hospital

**preoperative phase:** period of time from when the decision for surgical intervention is made to when the patient is transferred to the operating room table

## CHART 18-1

### Examples of Nursing Activities in the Perioperative Phases of Care

**PREOPERATIVE PHASE**

*Preadmission Testing*
1. Initiates initial preoperative assessment
2. Initiates teaching appropriate to patient's needs
3. Involves family in interview
4. Verifies completion of preoperative testing
5. Verifies understanding of surgeon-specific preoperative orders (eg, bowel preparation, preoperative shower)
6. Assesses patient's need for postoperative transportation and care

*Admission to Surgical Center or Unit*
1. Completes preoperative assessment
2. Assesses for risks for postoperative complications
3. Reports unexpected findings or any deviations from normal
4. Verifies that operative consent has been signed
5. Coordinates patient teaching with other nursing staff
6. Reinforces previous teaching
7. Explains phases in perioperative period and expectations
8. Answers patient's and family's questions
9. Develops a plan of care

*In the Holding Area*
1. Assesses patient's status, baseline pain and nutritional status
2. Reviews chart
3. Identifies patient
4. Verifies surgical site and marks site per institutional policy
5. Establishes intravenous line
6. Administers medications if prescribed
7. Takes measures to ensure patient's comfort
8. Provides psychological support
9. Communicates patient's emotional status to other appropriate members of the health care team

**INTRAOPERATIVE PHASE**

*Maintenance of Safety*
1. Maintains aseptic, controlled environment
2. Effectively manages human resources, equipment, and supplies for individualized patient care
3. Transfers patient to operating room bed or table
4. Positions the patient
    a. Functional alignment
    b. Exposure of surgical site
5. Applies grounding device to patient
6. Ensures that the sponge, needle, and instrument counts are correct
7. Completes intraoperative documentation

*Physiologic Monitoring*
1. Calculates effects on patient of excessive fluid loss or gain
2. Distinguishes normal from abnormal cardiopulmonary data
3. Reports changes in patient's vital signs
4. Institutes measures to promote normothermia

*Psychological Support (Before Induction and When Patient Is Conscious)*
1. Provides emotional support to patient
2. Stands near or touches patient during procedures and induction
3. Continues to assess patient's emotional status

**POSTOPERATIVE PHASE**

*Transfer of Patient to Postanesthesia Care Unit*
1. Communicates intraoperative information
    a. Identifies patient by name
    b. States type of surgery performed
    c. Identifies type of anesthetic used
    d. Reports patient's response to surgical procedure and anesthesia
    e. Describes intraoperative factors (eg, insertion of drains or catheters; administration of blood, analgesic agents, or other medications during surgery; occurrence of unexpected events)
    f. Describes physical limitations
    g. Reports patient's preoperative level of consciousness
    h. Communicates necessary equipment needs
    i. Communicates presence of family and/or significant others

*Postoperative Assessment Recovery Area*
1. Determines patient's immediate response to surgical intervention
2. Monitors patient's physiologic status
3. Assesses patient's pain level and administers appropriate pain relief measures
4. Maintains patient's safety (airway, circulation, prevention of injury)
5. Administers medications, fluid, and blood component therapy, if prescribed
6. Provides oral fluids if prescribed for ambulatory surgery patient
7. Assesses patient's readiness for transfer to in-hospital unit or for discharge home based on institutional policy (eg, Alderete score, see Chapter 20)

### CHART 18-1 Examples of Nursing Activities in the Perioperative Phases of Care, continued

**Surgical Unit**
1. Continues close monitoring of patient's physical and psychological response to surgical intervention
2. Assesses patient's pain level and administers appropriate pain relief measures
3. Provides teaching to patient during immediate recovery period
4. Assists patient in recovery and preparation for discharge home
5. Determines patient's psychological status
6. Assists with discharge planning

**Home or Clinic**
1. Provides follow-up care during office or clinic visit or by telephone contact
2. Reinforces previous teaching and answers patient's and family's questions about surgery and follow-up care
3. Assesses patient's response to surgery and anesthesia and their effects on body image and function
4. Determines family's perception of surgery and its outcome

---

and emotional assessment, previous anesthetic and medical history, and identification of known allergies or genetics issues that may affect the surgical outcome), ensuring that necessary tests have been or will be performed in PAT, arranging appropriate consultations, and providing education about recovery from anesthesia and postoperative care (Garcia-Miguel, Serrano-Aguilar & Lopez-Bastida, 2003).

On the day of surgery, patient teaching is reviewed, the patient's identity and the surgical site are verified, informed consent is confirmed, and an intravenous (IV) infusion is started. If the patient is going home the same day, the availability of safe transport and the presence of an accompanying responsible adult are verified. Depending on when the preadmission evaluation and testing were done, nursing activities on the day of surgery include preoperative patient assessment and addressing questions the patient or family may have.

## Intraoperative Phase

The **intraoperative phase** begins when the patient is transferred onto the OR table and ends with admission to the

---

### NURSING RESEARCH PROFILE

### The Effect of Preoperative Teaching on Outcomes

Oetker-Black, S. L., Jones, S., Estok, P., et al. (2003). Preoperative teaching and hysterectomy outcomes. *AORN Journal, 77*(6), 1215–1231.

**Purpose**
This study used a theoretical model of self-efficacy to determine whether an efficacy-enhancing teaching protocol was effective in improving immediate postoperative behaviors and selected short- and long-term health outcomes in women who underwent abdominal hysterectomy.

**Design**
A sample of 108 women admitted to a 486-bed teaching hospital in the Midwest for total abdominal hysterectomy was obtained by convenience sampling. Data collectors used the operating room schedule to identify potential participants based on predetermined criteria (eg, age, able to read English, alert and oriented). Those willing to participate in the 6-month study were randomly assigned to one of the study groups and received either the usual care protocol or the efficacy-enhancing teaching protocol. The efficacy-enhancing group received enhanced preoperative teaching. Sessions stressed the importance of early ambulation, included a detailed demonstration of the effective way to get out of bed, and required that participants demonstrate how to get out of bed.

**Findings**
There were no significant differences found between groups except in ambulation. Patients who received the efficacy-enhancing teaching ambulated significantly longer than those in the usual care group (330 seconds compared to a mean of 56 seconds).

**Nursing Implications**
The most common postoperative complications of hysterectomy or any major abdominal surgery are atelectasis, pneumonia, paralytic ileus, and deep vein thrombosis. Studies have previously shown that postoperative ambulation decreases or prevents all these complications. By incorporating enhanced preoperative patient instruction with return demonstrations, perioperative nurses can improve patients' postoperative ambulation.

PACU. In this phase, the scope of nursing activities includes providing for the patient's safety, maintaining an aseptic environment, ensuring proper function of equipment, providing the surgeon with specific instruments and supplies for the surgical field, and completing appropriate documentation. Nursing activities may include providing emotional support by holding the patient's hand during induction of general anesthesia; assisting in positioning the patient on the OR table using appropriate principles of body alignment; or acting as scrub nurse, circulating nurse, or registered nurse first assistant (RNFA).

## Postoperative Phase

The **postoperative phase** begins with the admission of the patient to the PACU and ends with a follow-up evaluation in the clinical setting or home. The scope of nursing care covers a wide range of activities including maintaining the patient's airway, monitoring vital signs, assessing the effects of the anesthetic agents, assessing the patient for complications, and providing comfort and pain relief. Nursing activities also focus on promoting the patient's recovery and initiating the teaching, follow-up care, and referrals essential for recovery and rehabilitation after discharge. Each phase is reviewed in more detail in this chapter and in the other chapters in this unit.

A conceptual model of patient care, published by the Association of PeriOperative Registered Nurses, formerly known as the Association of Operating Room Nurses (still abbreviated AORN), helps delineate the relationships between various components of nursing practice and patient outcomes. The Perioperative Nursing Data Set (PNDS) categorizes the practice of perioperative nursing practice into four domains: safety, physiologic responses, behavioral responses, and health care systems (Fig. 18-1). The first three domains reflect phenomena of concern to perioperative nurses and are composed of nursing diagnoses, interventions, and outcomes. The fourth domain, the health care system, consists of structural data elements and focuses on clinical processes and outcomes. The model is used to depict the relationship of nursing process components to the achievement of optimal patient outcomes (Kleinbeck, 2004).

## Surgical Classifications

Surgery may be performed for various reasons. A surgical procedure may be diagnostic (eg, biopsy, exploratory laparotomy), curative (eg, excision of a tumor or an inflamed appendix), or reparative (eg, multiple wound repair). It may be reconstructive or cosmetic (eg, mammoplasty or a face-lift) or palliative (eg, to relieve pain or correct a problem—for instance, a gastrostomy tube may be inserted to compensate for the inability to swallow food). Surgery may also be classified according to the degree of urgency involved: emergent, urgent, required, elective, and optional (Table 18-1).

## Preparation for Surgery

### Informed Consent

Voluntary and written **informed consent** from the patient is necessary before nonemergent surgery can be performed. A written consent protects the patient from unsanctioned surgery and protects the surgeon from claims of an unauthorized operation. In the best interests of all parties concerned, sound medical, ethical, and legal principles are followed (Aiken, 2004). The nurse may ask the patient to sign the form and may witness the patient's signature. It is the physician's responsibility to provide appropriate information. Chart 18-2 lists the criteria for a valid informed consent (Bernat, 2004; Schroeter, 2003).

Many ethical principles are integral to informed consent (see Chapter 3). Before the patient signs the consent form, the surgeon must provide a clear and simple explanation of what the surgery will entail. The surgeon must also inform the patient of the benefits, alternatives, possible risks, complications, disfigurement, disability, and removal of body parts as well as what to expect in the early and late postoperative periods. If the patient requests additional information, the nurse notifies the physician. The nurse ascertains that the consent form has been signed before administering psychoactive premedication, because a consent may not be valid if it is obtained while the patient is under the influence of medications that can affect judgment and decision-making capacity. Informed consent is necessary in the following circumstances:

- Invasive procedures, such as a surgical incision, a biopsy, a cystoscopy, or paracentesis
- Procedures requiring sedation and/or anesthesia (see Chapter 19 for a discussion of anesthesia)
- A nonsurgical procedure, such as an arteriography, that carries more than slight risk to the patient
- Procedures involving radiation

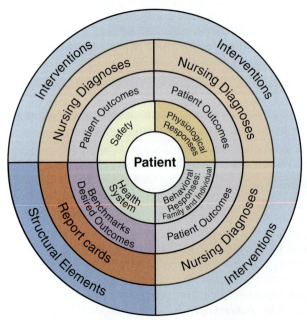

**FIGURE 18-1.** Perioperative patient-focused model. © With permission from Association of PeriOperative Registered Nurses, Inc., Denver, CO.

## TABLE 18-1  Categories of Surgery Based on Urgency

| Classification | Indications for Surgery | Examples |
|---|---|---|
| I. Emergent—Patient requires immediate attention; disorder may be life-threatening | Without delay | Severe bleeding<br>Bladder or intestinal obstruction<br>Fractured skull<br>Gunshot or stab wounds<br>Extensive burns |
| II. Urgent—Patient requires prompt attention | Within 24–30 h | Acute gallbladder infection<br>Kidney or ureteral stones |
| III. Required—Patient needs to have surgery | Plan within a few weeks or months | Prostatic hyperplasia without bladder obstruction<br>Thyroid disorders<br>Cataracts |
| IV. Elective—Patient should have surgery | Failure to have surgery not catastrophic | Repair of scars<br>Simple hernia<br>Vaginal repair |
| V. Optional—Decision rests with patient | Personal preference | Cosmetic surgery |

The patient personally signs the consent if he or she is of legal age and is mentally capable. If the patient is a minor, is neurologically incapacitated, or is incompetent, permission must be obtained from a surrogate, who most often is a responsible family member (preferably next of kin) or legal guardian (Bernat, 2004). An emancipated minor (married or independently earning his or her own living) may sign his or her own consent form. State regulations and agency policy must be followed. In an emergency, it may be necessary for the surgeon to operate as a lifesaving measure without the patient's informed consent. However, every effort must be made to contact the patient's family. In such a situation, contact can be made by telephone, fax, or other electronic means.

If the patient has doubts and has not had the opportunity to investigate alternative treatments, a second opinion may be requested. No patient should be urged or coerced to give informed consent. Refusing to undergo a surgical procedure is a person's legal right and privilege. However, such information must be documented and relayed to the surgeon so that other arrangements can be made. For example, additional explanations may be provided to the patient and family, or the surgery may be rescheduled.

The consent process can be improved by providing audiovisual materials to supplement discussion, by ensuring that the wording of the consent form is understandable, and by using other strategies and resources as needed to help the patient understand its content. It may be necessary to have the consent available in multiple languages or have a trained medical interpreter available. Alternative formats of communication (eg, Braille, large print, sign interpreter) may be needed if the patient is elderly or has a disability (Saufl, 2004).

### CHART 18-2

### Criteria for Valid Informed Consent

**VOLUNTARY CONSENT**
Valid consent must be freely given, without coercion.

**INCOMPETENT PATIENT**
Legal definition: individual who is *not* autonomous and cannot give or withhold consent (eg, individuals who are cognitively impaired, mentally ill, or neurologically incapacitated)

**INFORMED SUBJECT**
Informed consent should be in writing. It should contain the following:
- Explanation of procedure and its risks
- Description of benefits and alternatives
- An offer to answer questions about procedure
- Instructions that the patient may withdraw consent
- A statement informing the patient if the protocol differs from customary procedure

**PATIENT ABLE TO COMPREHEND**
Information must be written and delivered in language understandable to the patient. Questions must be answered to facilitate comprehension if material is confusing.

**NURSING ALERT**

The signed consent form is placed in a prominent place on the patient's chart and accompanies the patient to the OR.

## Assessment of Health Factors That Affect Patients Preoperatively

The goal in the preoperative period is for the patient to have as many positive health factors as possible. Many risk factors may lead to complications (Chart 18-3). Every attempt is made to stabilize those conditions that otherwise

## CHART 18-3

### Risk Factors for Surgical Complications

- Hypovolemia
- Dehydration or electrolyte imbalance
- Nutritional deficits
- Extremes of age (very young, very old)
- Extremes of weight (emaciation, obesity)
- Infection and sepsis
- Toxic conditions
- Immunologic abnormalities
- Pulmonary disease
  - Obstructive disease
  - Restrictive disorder
  - Respiratory infection
- Renal or urinary tract disease
  - Decreased renal function
  - Urinary tract infection
  - Obstruction
- Pregnancy
  - Diminished maternal physiologic reserve
- Cardiovascular disease
  - Coronary artery disease or previous myocardial infarction
  - Cardiac failure
  - Dysrhythmias
  - Hypertension
  - Prosthetic heart valve
  - Thromboembolism
  - Hemorrhagic disorders
  - Cerebrovascular disease
- Endocrine dysfunction
  - Diabetes mellitus
  - Adrenal disorders
  - Thyroid malfunction
- Hepatic disease
  - Cirrhosis
  - Hepatitis
- Preexisting mental or physical disability

hinder recovery. When negative factors dominate, the risks of surgery and postoperative complications increase.

Before any surgical treatment is initiated, a health history is obtained, a physical examination is performed during which vital signs are noted, and a database is established for future comparisons. During the physical examination, many factors that have the potential to affect the patient undergoing surgery are considered (Bickley & Szilagyi, 2003). Health care providers should be alert for signs of abuse, which can occur at all ages and to men and women from all socioeconomic, ethnic, and cultural groups (Fuller, 2003). Findings need to be reported accordingly (see Chapter 5 for further discussion of signs of abuse). Blood tests, x-rays, and other diagnostic tests are prescribed when indicated by information obtained from the history and physical examination.

### Nutritional and Fluid Status

Optimal nutrition is an essential factor in promoting healing and resisting infection and other surgical complications. Assessment of a patient's nutritional status identifies factors that can affect the patient's surgical course, such as obesity, undernutrition, weight loss, malnutrition, deficiencies in specific nutrients, metabolic abnormalities, and the effects of medications on nutrition. Nutritional needs may be determined by measurement of body mass index and waist circumference (U.S. Department of Health and Human Services, 2005). See Chapter 5 for further discussion of nutritional assessment.

Any nutritional deficiency, such as malnutrition, should be corrected before surgery to provide adequate protein for tissue repair. The nutrients needed for wound healing are summarized in Table 18-2.

Dehydration, hypovolemia, and electrolyte imbalances can lead to significant problems in patients with comorbid medical conditions or in patients who are elderly. The severity of fluid and electrolyte imbalances is often difficult to determine. Mild volume deficits may be treated during surgery; however, additional time may be needed to correct pronounced fluid and electrolyte deficits to promote the best possible preoperative condition.

### Drug or Alcohol Use

People who abuse drugs or alcohol frequently deny or attempt to hide it. In such situations, the nurse who is obtaining the patient's health history needs to ask frank questions with patience, care, and a nonjudgmental attitude. See Chapter 5 for an assessment of alcohol and drug use.

Because acutely intoxicated people are susceptible to injury, surgery is postponed if possible. If emergency surgery is required, local, spinal, or regional block anesthesia is used for minor surgery. Otherwise, to prevent vomiting and potential aspiration, a nasogastric tube is inserted before general anesthesia is administered.

The person with a history of chronic alcoholism often suffers from malnutrition and other systemic problems that increase surgical risk. Alcohol withdrawal syndrome or delirium tremens may be anticipated between 48 and 72 hours after alcohol withdrawal (Schofield, 2004) and is associated with a significant mortality rate when it occurs postoperatively.

### Respiratory Status

The goal for surgical patients is optimal respiratory function. The patient is taught breathing exercises and the use of an incentive spirometer if indicated. Because adequate ventilation is potentially compromised during all phases of surgical treatment, surgery is usually postponed if the patient has a respiratory infection. Patients with underlying respiratory disease (eg, asthma, chronic obstructive pulmonary disease) are assessed carefully for current threats to their pulmonary status. Patients also need to be assessed for comorbid conditions such as human immunodeficiency virus (HIV) in-

| TABLE 18-2 | Nutrients Important for Wound Healing | |
|---|---|---|
| Nutrient | Rationale for Increased Need | Possible Deficiency Outcome |
| Protein | To allow collagen deposition and wound healing to occur | Collagen deposition leading to impaired/delayed wound healing<br>Decreased skin and wound strength<br>Increased wound infection rates |
| Arginine (amino acid) | To provide necessary substrate for collagen synthesis and nitric oxide (crucial for wound healing) at wound site<br>To increase wound strength and collagen deposition<br>To stimulate T-cell response<br>Associated with a variety of essential reactions of intermediary metabolism | Impaired wound healing |
| Carbohydrates and fats | Primary source of energy in the body and consequently in the wound healing process<br>To meet the demand for increased essential fatty acids needed for cellular function after an injury<br>To spare protein<br>To restore normal weight | Signs and symptoms of protein deficiency due to use of protein to meet energy requirements<br>Extensive weight loss |
| Water | To replace fluid lost through vomiting, hemorrhage, exudates, fever, drainage, diuresis<br>To maintain homeostasis | Signs, symptoms, and complications of dehydration, such as poor skin turgor, dry mucous membranes, oliguria, anuria, weight loss, increased pulse rate, decreased central venous pressure |
| Vitamin C | Important for capillary formation, tissue synthesis, and wound healing through collagen formation<br>Needed for antibody formation | Impaired/delayed wound healing related to impaired collagen formation and increased capillary fragility and permeability<br>Increased risk of infection related to decreased antibodies |
| Vitamin B complex | Indirect role in wound healing through their influence on host resistance | Decreased enzymes available for energy metabolism |
| Vitamin A | Increases inflammatory response in wounds, reduces anti-inflammatory effects of corticosteroids on wound healing | Impaired/delayed wound healing related to decreased collagen synthesis; impaired immune function<br>Increased risk of infection |
| Vitamin K | Important for normal blood clotting<br>Impaired intestinal synthesis associated with the use of antibiotics | Prolonged prothrombin time<br>Hematomas contributing to impaired healing and predisposition to wound infections |
| Magnesium | Essential cofactor for many enzymes that are involved in the process of protein synthesis and wound repair | Impaired/delayed wound healing (impaired collagen production) |
| Copper | Required cofactor in the development of connective tissue | Impaired wound healing |
| Zinc | Involved DNA synthesis, protein synthesis, cellular proliferation needed for wound healing<br>Essential to immune function | Impaired immune response |

Table prepared and updated using information from Williams, I. & Barbul, A. (2003). Nutrition and wound healing. *Surgical Clinics of North America* 83(3), 571–596.

fection and Parkinson's disease, which may affect respiratory function (Galvez-Jimenez & Lang, 2004; Gotta, 2004).

Patients who smoke are urged to stop 4 to 8 weeks before surgery to significantly reduce pulmonary and wound healing complications, although many patients do not do so. These patients should be counseled to stop smoking at least 24 hours before surgery (Coleman, Cheater & Murphy, 2004).

## Cardiovascular Status

The goal in preparing any patient for surgery is to ensure a well-functioning cardiovascular system to meet the oxygen, fluid, and nutritional needs of the perioperative period. If the patient has uncontrolled hypertension, surgery may be postponed until the blood pressure is under control. At times, surgical treatment can be modified to meet the cardiac tolerance of the patient. For example, in a patient with obstruction of the descending colon and coronary artery disease, a temporary simple colostomy may be performed rather than a more extensive colon resection that would require a prolonged period of anesthesia.

## Hepatic and Renal Function

The presurgical goal is optimal function of the liver and urinary systems so that medications, anesthetic agents, body wastes, and toxins are adequately processed and removed from the body.

The liver is important in the biotransformation of anesthetic compounds. Therefore, any disorder of the liver has an effect on how anesthetic agents are metabolized. Because acute liver disease is associated with high surgical mortality (Wiklund, 2004), preoperative improvement in liver function is a goal. Careful assessment may include various liver function tests (see Chapter 39).

Because the kidneys are involved in excreting anesthetic medications and their metabolites and because acid–base status and metabolism are also important considerations in anesthesia administration, surgery is contraindicated if a patient has acute nephritis, acute renal insufficiency with oliguria or anuria, or other acute renal problems. The exception is surgery that is performed as a lifesaving measure or that is necessary to improve urinary function, as in the case of an obstructive uropathy.

## Endocrine Function

The patient with diabetes who is undergoing surgery is at risk for hypoglycemia and hyperglycemia. Hypoglycemia may develop during anesthesia or postoperatively from inadequate carbohydrates or excessive administration of insulin. Hyperglycemia, which can increase the risk for surgical wound infection, may result from the stress of surgery, which can trigger increased levels of catecholamine (Lorenz, Lorenz & Cody, 2005). Other risks are acidosis and glucosuria. Although the surgical risk in the patient with controlled diabetes is no greater than in the patient without diabetes, the goal is to maintain the blood glucose level at or below 200 mg/dL (Lorenz et al., 2005). Frequent monitoring of blood glucose levels is important before, during, and after surgery (see Chapter 41 for discussion of the patient with diabetes undergoing surgery).

Patients who have received corticosteroids are at risk of adrenal insufficiency. Therefore, the use of corticosteroids for any purpose during the preceding year must be reported to the anesthesiologist, anesthetist (usually a nurse anesthetist), and surgeon. The patient is monitored for signs of adrenal insufficiency.

Patients with uncontrolled thyroid disorders are at risk for thyrotoxicosis (with hyperthyroid disorders) or respiratory failure (with hypothyroid disorders). Therefore, the patient is assessed for a history of these disorders.

## Immune Function

An important function of the preoperative assessment is to determine the presence of allergies. It is especially important to identify and document any sensitivity to medications and past adverse reactions to these agents. The patient is asked to identify any substances that precipitated previous allergic reactions, including medications, blood transfusions, contrast agents, latex, and food products, and to describe the signs and symptoms produced by these substances. A sample latex allergy screening questionnaire is shown in Figure 18-2.

Immunosuppression is common with corticosteroid therapy, renal transplantation, radiation therapy, chemotherapy, and disorders affecting the immune system, such as AIDS and leukemia. The mildest symptoms or slightest temperature elevation must be investigated. Because patients who are immunosuppressed are highly susceptible to infection, great care is taken to ensure strict asepsis.

## Previous Medication Use

A medication history is obtained from each patient because of the possible effects of medications on the patient's perioperative course, including the possibility of drug interactions. Any medication the patient is using or has used in the past is documented, including over-the-counter (OTC) preparations and herbal agents and the frequency with which they are used. Potent medications have an effect on physiologic functions; interactions of such medications with anesthetic agents can cause serious problems, such as arterial hypotension and circulatory collapse.

The potential effects of prior medication therapy are evaluated by the anesthesiologist or anesthetist, who considers the length of time the patient has used the medication, the physical condition of the patient, and the nature of the proposed surgery. Medications that cause particular concern are listed in Table 18-3.

In addition, many patients take self-prescribed or OTC medications. Aspirin is a common OTC medication that inhibits platelet aggregation; therefore, it is prudent to stop aspirin at least 7 to 10 days before surgery if possible, especially for surgeries in which excess bleeding would cause significant complications, such as brain or spinal cord surgeries (Bohan & Glass-Macenka, 2004; Mercado & Petty, 2003). Because of the effects of aspirin or other OTC medications and possible interactions with prescribed medications and anesthetic agents, it is important to ask a patient about their use. The information is noted in the patient's chart and conveyed to the anesthesiologist, anesthetist and surgeon.

The use of herbal medications is widespread among patients; approximately 15 million Americans report using these substances (Heyneman, 2003; MacKichan & Ruthman, 2004). The most commonly used herbal medications are echinacea, ephedra, garlic (*Allium sativum*), ginkgo biloba, ginseng, kava kava (*Piper methysticum*), St. John's wort (*Hypericum perforatum*), licorice (*Glycyrriza glabra*), and valerian (*Valeriana officinalis*). However, many patients fail to report using herbal medicines to their health care providers. Because of the potential effects of herbal medications on coagulation and potentially lethal interactions with other medications, the nurse must ask surgical patients specifically about the use of these agents, document their use, and inform the surgical team and anesthesiologist or anesthetist. Currently, it is recommended that the use of herbal

| Ask the patient the following questions. Check "Yes" or "No" in the box. | YES | NO |
|---|---|---|
| 1. Has a doctor ever told you that you are allergic to latex? | | |
| 2. Do you have on-the-job exposure to latex? | | |
| 3. Were you born with problems involving your spinal cord? | | |
| 4. Have you ever had allergies, asthma, hay fever, eczema or problems with rashes? | | |
| 5. Have you ever had respiratory distress, rapid heart rate or swelling? | | |
| 6. Have you ever had swelling, itching, hives or other symptoms after contact with a balloon? | | |
| 7. Have you ever had swelling, itching, hives or other symptoms after a dental examination or procedure? | | |
| 8. Have you ever had swelling, itching, hives or other symptoms following a vaginal or rectal examination or after contact with a diaphragm or condom? | | |
| 9. Have you ever had swelling, itching, hives or other symptoms during or within one hour after wearing rubber gloves? | | |
| 10. Have you ever had a rash on your hands that lasted longer than one week? | | |
| 11. Have you ever had swelling, itching, hives, runny nose, eye irritation, wheezing, or asthma after contact with any latex or rubber product? | | |
| 12. Have you ever had swelling, itching, hives or other symptoms after being examined by someone wearing rubber or latex gloves? | | |
| 13. Are you allergic to bananas, avocados, kiwi or chestnuts? | | |
| 14. Have you ever had an unexplained anaphylactic episode? | | |

Pre-op RN Signature: _____

Patient Name: _____

Procedure: _____

Scheduled Date / Time: _____

Surgeon: _____

**FIGURE 18-2.** Example of a latex allergy assessment form. Courtesy of Inova Fairfax Hospital, Falls Church, VA.

products be discontinued 2 to 3 weeks before surgery (MacKichan & Ruthman, 2004).

**NURSING ALERT**

Because of possible adverse interactions, the nurse must assess and document the patient's use of prescription medications, OTC medications (especially aspirin), and herbal agents. The nurse must clearly communicate this information to the anesthesiologist or anesthetist.

## Psychosocial Factors

All patients have some type of emotional reaction before any surgical procedure, be it obvious or hidden, normal or abnormal. For example, preoperative anxiety may be an anticipatory response to an experience the patient views as a threat to his or her customary role in life, body integrity, or life itself. Psychological distress directly influences body functioning. Therefore, it is imperative to identify any anxiety the patient is experiencing (Defazio-Quinn & Schick, 2004).

Most patients who are about to undergo surgery have fears, including fear of the unknown, of death, of anesthesia, of pain, or of cancer. Concerns about loss of work time, loss of job, increased responsibilities or burden on family

## TABLE 18-3 Examples of Medications With the Potential to Affect the Surgical Experience

| Agent (Generic and Trade Example) | Effect of Interaction With Anesthetics |
|---|---|
| **Corticosteroids**<br>Prednisone (Deltasone) | Cardiovascular collapse can occur if discontinued suddenly. Therefore, a bolus of corticosteroid may be administered intravenously immediately before and after surgery. |
| **Diuretics**<br>Hydrochlorothiazide (HydroDIURIL) | During anesthesia, may cause excessive respiratory depression resulting from an associated electrolyte imbalance |
| **Phenothiazines**<br>Chlorpromazine (Thorazine) | May increase the hypotensive action of anesthetics |
| **Tranquilizers**<br>Diazepam (Valium) | May cause anxiety, tension, and even seizures if withdrawn suddenly |
| **Insulin** | Interaction between anesthetics and insulin must be considered when a patient with diabetes is undergoing surgery. Intravenous insulin may need to be administered to keep the blood glucose within the normal range. |
| **Antibiotics**<br>Erythromycin (Ery-Tab) | When combined with a curariform muscle relaxant, nerve transmission is interrupted and apnea from respiratory paralysis may result. |
| **Anticoagulants**<br>Warfarin (Coumadin) | Can increase the risk of bleeding during the intraoperative and postoperative periods; should be discontinued in anticipation of elective surgery. The surgeon will determine how long before the elective surgery the patient should stop taking an anticoagulant, depending on the type of planned procedure and the medical condition of the patient. |
| **Antiseizure Medications** | Intravenous administration of medication may be needed to keep the patient seizure-free in the intraoperative and postoperative periods. |
| **Monoamine Oxidase (MAO) Inhibitors**<br>Phenelzine sulfate (Nardil) | May increase the hypotensive action of anesthetics |
| **Thyroid Hormone**<br>Levothyroxine sodium (Levothyroid) | Intravenous administration may be needed during the postoperative period to maintain thyroid levels. |

members, and the threat of permanent incapacity further contribute to the emotional strain created by the prospect of surgery. Less obvious concerns may occur because of previous experiences with the health care system and people the patient has known with the same condition.

People express fear in different ways. For example, some patients may repeatedly ask many questions, even though answers were given previously. Others may withdraw, deliberately avoiding communication, perhaps by reading, watching television, or talking about trivialities. Consequently, the nurse must be empathetic, listen well, and provide information that helps alleviate concerns.

An important outcome of the psychosocial assessment is the determination of the extent and role of the patient's support network. The value and reliability of all available support systems are assessed. Other information, such as usual level of functioning and typical daily activities, may assist in the patient's care and rehabilitation plans. Assessing the patient's readiness to learn and determining the best approach to maximize comprehension provides the basis for preoperative patient education.

### Spiritual and Cultural Beliefs

Spiritual beliefs play an important role in how people cope with fear and anxiety. Regardless of the patient's religious affiliation, spiritual beliefs can be as therapeutic as medication. Every attempt must be made to help the patient obtain the spiritual support that he or she requests. Faith has great sustaining power. Therefore, the beliefs of each patient should be respected and supported. Some nurses avoid the subject of a clergy visit lest the suggestion alarm the patient. Asking whether the patient's spiritual advisor knows about the impending surgery is a caring, nonthreatening approach.

Showing respect for a patient's cultural values and beliefs facilitates rapport and trust. Some areas of assessment include identifying the ethnic group to which the patient relates and the customs and beliefs the patient holds about illness and health care providers. For example, patients from some cultural groups are unaccustomed to expressing feelings openly. Nurses need to consider this pattern of communication when assessing pain. As a sign of respect, people from some cultural groups may not make direct eye contact with others (Flowers, 2004). The nurse should know that this lack of eye contact is not avoidance or a lack of interest.

Perhaps the most valuable skill at the nurse's disposal is listening carefully to the patient, especially when obtaining the history. Invaluable information and insights may be gained through effective communication and interviewing skills. An unhurried, understanding, and caring nurse promotes confidence on the part of the patient.

## Special Situations

In the preoperative period, attention needs to be paid to patients with special situations.

### Patients Undergoing Ambulatory Surgery

The brief time the patient and family spend in the ambulatory setting is an important factor in the preoperative period. The nurse must quickly and comprehensively assess and anticipate the patient's needs and at the same time begin planning for discharge and follow-up home care.

The nurse needs to be sure that the patient and family understand that the patient will first go to the preoperative holding area before going to the OR for the surgical procedure and then will spend some time in the PACU before being discharged home with the family later that day. Other preoperative teaching content should also be verified and reinforced as needed (see later discussion). The nurse should ensure that any plans for follow-up home care are in place if needed.

### Gerontologic Considerations

Preoperative pain assessment and teaching are important in the elderly patient. The older person undergoing surgery may have a combination of chronic illnesses and health issues in addition to the specific one for which surgery is indicated. Elderly people frequently do not report symptoms, perhaps because they fear a serious illness may be diagnosed or because they accept such symptoms as part of the aging process. Subtle clues alert the nurse to underlying problems. Research indicates that key predictors of perioperative complications in the elderly are the patient's preoperative condition and level of functioning (John & Sieber, 2004).

Health care staff must remember that the hazards of surgery for the aged are proportional to the number and severity of coexisting health problems and the nature and duration of the operative procedure. The underlying principle that guides the preoperative assessment, surgical care, and postoperative care is that the aged patient has less physiologic reserve (the ability of an organ to return to normal after a disturbance in its equilibrium) than a younger patient does. Cardiac reserves are lower, renal and hepatic functions are depressed, and gastrointestinal activity is likely to be reduced. Dehydration, constipation, and malnutrition may be evident. Sensory limitations, such as impaired vision or hearing and reduced tactile sensitivity, are often the reasons for falls and burns (Defazio-Quinn & Schick, 2004). Therefore, the nurse must be alert to maintaining a safe environment. Arthritis is common in older people and may affect mobility, making it difficult for the patient to turn from one side to the other or ambulate without discomfort. Protective measures include adequate padding for tender areas, moving the patient slowly, protecting bony prominences from prolonged pressure, and providing gentle massage to promote circulation.

The condition of the mouth is important to assess. Dental caries, dentures, and partial plates are particularly significant to the anesthesiologist or anesthetist, because decayed teeth or dental prostheses may become dislodged during intubation and occlude the airway.

As the body ages, its ability to perspire decreases. Because decreased perspiration leads to dry, itchy skin that becomes fragile and is easily abraded, precautions are taken when moving an elderly person. Decreased subcutaneous fat makes older people more susceptible to temperature changes. A lightweight cotton blanket is an appropriate cover when an elderly patient is moved to and from the OR.

Most elderly people have experienced personal illnesses and possibly life-threatening illnesses of friends and family. Such experiences may result in fears about the surgery and about the future. Providing an opportunity to express these fears enables the patient to gain some peace of mind.

Because the elderly patient may have greater risks during the perioperative period, the following factors are critical: (1) skillful preoperative assessment and treatment, (2) skillful anesthesia and surgery, and (3) meticulous and competent postoperative and postanesthesia management. In addition, the nurse should incorporate pain management information and pain communication skills when teaching the elderly patient how to obtain greater postoperative pain relief.

### Patients Who Are Obese

Like age, obesity increases the risk and severity of complications associated with surgery. During surgery, fatty tissues are especially susceptible to infection. In addition, obesity increases technical and mechanical problems related to surgery. Therefore, dehiscence (wound separation) and wound infections are more common. Moreover, the obese patient may be more difficult to care for because of the added weight. The patient tends to have shallow respirations when supine, which increases the risk of hypoventilation and postoperative pulmonary complications. It has been estimated that for each 30 pounds of excess weight, about 25 additional miles of blood vessels are needed, and this places increased demands on the heart. As the incidence of obesity continues to grow, nurses will be called on to be part of multidisciplinary teams that will develop and implement clinical plans for patients who are obese (Charlebois & Wilmothe, 2004).

## Patients With Disabilities

Special considerations for patients with mental or physical disabilities include the need for appropriate assistive devices, modifications in preoperative teaching, and additional assistance with and attention to positioning or transferring. Assistive devices include hearing aids, eyeglasses, braces, prostheses, and other devices. People who are hearing-impaired may need a sign interpreter or some alternative communication system perioperatively. If the patient relies on signing or speech (lip) reading and his or her eyeglasses or contact lenses are removed or the health care staff wear surgical masks, an alternative method of communication will be needed. These needs must be identified in the preoperative evaluation and clearly communicated to personnel. Specific strategies for accommodating the patient's needs must be identified in advance. Ensuring the security of assistive devices is important, because these devices are expensive and are likely to be lost.

Most patients are directed to move from the stretcher to the OR table and back again. In addition to being unable to see or hear instructions, the patient with a disability may be unable to move without special devices or a great deal of assistance. The patient with a disability that affects body position (eg, cerebral palsy, postpolio syndrome, other neuromuscular disorders) may need special positioning during surgery to prevent pain and injury. Moreover, these patients may be unable to sense whether their extremities are positioned incorrectly.

Patients with respiratory problems related to a disability (eg, multiple sclerosis, muscular dystrophy) may experience difficulties unless the problems are made known to the anesthesiologist or anesthetist and adjustments are made. These factors need to be clearly identified in the preoperative period and communicated to the appropriate personnel.

## Patients Undergoing Emergency Surgery

Emergency surgeries are unplanned and occur with little time for preparation for the patient or the perioperative team. The unpredictable nature of trauma and emergency surgery poses unique challenges to the nurse throughout the perioperative period. In addition, research suggests that older patients undergoing urgent or emergent coronary artery bypass grafting surgery are at higher risk for prolonged mechanical ventilation compared with those undergoing a planned surgery (Bezanson, Weaver, Kinney, et al., 2004).

All of the previously discussed factors that affect patients preparing to undergo surgery apply to these patients, usually in a very condensed time frame. The only preoperative assessment may take place at the same time as resuscitation in the emergency department. For the unconscious patient, informed consent and essential information, such as pertinent past medical history and allergies, need to be obtained from a family member, if one is available. A quick visual survey of the patient is essential to identify all sites of injury if the emergency surgery is due to trauma (see Chapter 71 for more information). The patient, who may have undergone a very frightening experience, may need extra support and explanation of the surgery.

# Preoperative Nursing Interventions

## Preoperative Teaching

Nurses have long recognized the value of preoperative instruction (Rothrock, 2003). Each patient is taught as an individual, with consideration for any unique concerns or learning needs. Multiple teaching strategies should be used (eg, verbal, written, return demonstration), depending on the patient's needs and abilities (Saufl, 2004). Preoperative teaching is initiated as soon as possible. It should start in the physician's office or at the time of PAT and continue until the patient arrives in the OR.

### When and What to Teach

Ideally, instruction is spaced over a period of time to allow the patient to assimilate information and ask questions as they arise. Frequently, teaching sessions are combined with various preparation procedures to allow for an easy and timely flow of information. The nurse should guide the patient through the experience and allow ample time for questions. For some patients, overly detailed descriptions increase anxiety; the nurse should be sensitive to this and provide less detail.

Teaching should go beyond descriptions of the procedure and should include explanations of the sensations the patient will experience. For example, telling the patient only that preoperative medication will cause relaxation before the operation is not as effective as also noting that the medication may result in lightheadedness and drowsiness. Knowing what to expect will help the patient anticipate these reactions and thus attain a higher degree of relaxation than might otherwise be expected. In addition, preoperative teaching includes instruction in breathing and leg exercises used to prevent postoperative complications such as pneumonia and deep vein thrombosis. These exercises may be performed in the hospital or at home (Chart 18-4).

The ideal timing for preoperative teaching is not on the day of surgery but during the preadmission visit, when diagnostic tests are performed. At this time, the nurse or resource person answers questions and provides important patient teaching. During this visit, the patient can meet and ask questions of the perioperative nurse, view audiovisual resources, receive written materials, and be given the telephone number to call as questions arise closer to the date of surgery. Most institutions provide written instructions (designed to be copied and given to patients) about many types of surgery. Patients who are elderly or have impaired vision may need a large-print version of written instructions (Saufl, 2004).

### Deep-Breathing, Coughing, and Incentive Spirometry

One goal of preoperative nursing care is to teach the patient how to promote optimal lung expansion and consequent blood oxygenation after anesthesia. The patient assumes a sitting position to enhance lung expansion. The nurse then demonstrates how to take a deep, slow breath and how to

## GENETICS IN NURSING PRACTICE
### Perioperative Nursing

Nurses who are caring for patients undergoing surgery need to take various genetic considerations into account when assessing patients throughout the perioperative experience. For example, surgical outcomes may be altered by genetic conditions that may cause complications with anesthesia, including the following:
- Malignant hyperthermia
- Central core disease (CCD)
- Duchenne muscular dystrophy
- Hyperkalemic periodic paralysis
- King-Denborough Syndrome

### NURSING ASSESSMENTS
#### Preoperative Family History Assessment
- Obtain a thorough assessment of personal and family history, inquiring about prior problems with surgery or anesthesia with specific attention to complications such as fever, rigidity, dark urine, and unexpected reactions.
- Inquire about any history of musculoskeletal complaints, history of heat intolerance, fevers of unknown origin, or unusual drug reaction.
- Assess for family history of any sudden or unexplained death, especially during participation in athletic events.

#### Patient Assessment
- Assess for subclinical muscle weakness.
- Assess for other physical features suggestive of an underlying genetic condition, such as contractures, kyphoscoliosis, and pterygium with progressive weakness.

#### Management Issues Specific to Genetics
- Inquire whether DNA mutation or other genetic testing has been performed on an affected family member.
- If indicated, refer for further genetic counseling and evaluation so that family members can discuss inheritance, risk to other family members, availability of diagnostic/genetic testing.
- Offer appropriate genetics information and resources.
- Assess patient's understanding of genetics information.
- Provide support to families with newly diagnosed malignant hyperthermia.
- Participate in management and coordination of care of patients with genetic conditions and individuals predisposed to develop or pass on a genetic condition.

### GENETICS RESOURCES FOR NURSES AND THEIR PATIENTS ON THE WEB

Genetic Alliance, www.geneticalliance.org—a directory of support groups for patients and families with genetic conditions

Gene Clinics, www.geneclinics.org—a listing of common genetic disorders with up-to-date clinical summaries, genetic counseling and testing information

International Council of Nurses, www.icn.ch/matters_genetics.htm—ICN's statement re: genetics and nursing.

National Organization of Rare Disorders, www.rarediseases.org—a directory of support groups and information for patients and families with rare genetic disorders

OMIM: Online Mendelian Inheritance in Man, www.ncbi.nlm.nih.gov/entrez/query.fcgi?db-OMIM—a complete listing of inherited genetic conditions

---

exhale slowly. After practicing deep breathing several times, the patient is instructed to breathe deeply, exhale through the mouth, take a short breath, and cough from deep in the lungs (see Chart 18-4). The nurse also demonstrates how to use an incentive spirometer, a device that provides measurement and feedback related to breathing effectiveness (see Chapter 25). In addition to enhancing respiration, these exercises may help the patient relax.

If a thoracic or abdominal incision is anticipated, the nurse demonstrates how to splint the incision to minimize pressure and control pain. The patient should put the palms of both hands together, interlacing the fingers snugly. Placing the hands across the incisional site acts as an effective splint when coughing. In addition, the patient is informed that medications are available to relieve pain and should be taken regularly for pain relief so that effective deep-breathing and coughing exercises can be performed. The goal in promoting coughing is to mobilize secretions so that they can be removed. Deep breathing before coughing stimulates the cough reflex. If the patient does not cough effectively, atelectasis (collapse of the alveoli), pneumonia, or other lung complications may occur.

### Mobility and Active Body Movement

The goals of promoting mobility postoperatively are to improve circulation, prevent venous stasis, and promote optimal respiratory function.

The nurse explains the rationale for frequent position changes after surgery and then shows the patient how to

### CHART 18-4

## Patient Education

### Preoperative Instructions to Prevent Postoperative Complications

**DIAPHRAGMATIC BREATHING**

Diaphragmatic breathing refers to a flattening of the dome of the diaphragm during inspiration, with resultant enlargement of the upper abdomen as air rushes in. During expiration, the abdominal muscles contract.

1. Practice in the same position you would assume in bed after surgery: a semi-Fowler's position, propped in bed with the back and shoulders well supported with pillows.
2. With your hands in a loose-fist position, allow the hands to rest lightly on the front of the lower ribs, with your fingertips against lower chest to feel the movement.

Diaphragmatic breathing

3. Breathe out gently and fully as the ribs sink down and inward toward midline.
4. Then take a deep breath through your nose and mouth, letting the abdomen rise as the lungs fill with air.
5. Hold this breath for a count of five.
6. Exhale and let out *all* the air through your nose and mouth.
7. Repeat this exercise 15 times with a short rest after each group of five.
8. Practice this twice a day preoperatively.

**COUGHING**

1. Lean forward slightly from a sitting position in bed, interlace your fingers together, and place your hands across the incisional site to act as a splintlike support when coughing.

Splinting when coughing

2. Breathe with the diaphragm as described under "Diaphragmatic Breathing."
3. With your mouth slightly open, breathe in fully.
4. "Hack" out sharply for three short breaths.
5. Then, keeping your mouth open, take in a quick deep breath and immediately give a strong cough once or twice. This helps clear secretions from your chest. It may cause some discomfort but will not harm your incision.

**LEG EXERCISES**

1. Lie in a semi-Fowler's position and perform the following simple exercises to improve circulation.
2. Bend your knee and raise your foot—hold it a few seconds, then extend the leg and lower it to the bed.

Leg exercises

3. Do this five times with one leg, then repeat with the other leg.
4. Then trace circles with the feet by bending them down, in toward each other, up, and then out.
5. Repeat these movements five times.

Foot exercises

**TURNING TO THE SIDE**

1. Turn on your side with the uppermost leg flexed most and supported on a pillow.
2. Grasp the side rail as an aid to maneuver to the side.
3. Practice diaphragmatic breathing and coughing while on your side.

**GETTING OUT OF BED**

1. Turn on your side.
2. Push yourself up with one hand as you swing your legs out of bed.

turn from side to side and how to assume the lateral position without causing pain or disrupting IV lines, drainage tubes, or other equipment. Any special position the patient needs to maintain after surgery (eg, adduction or elevation of an extremity) is discussed, as is the importance of maintaining as much mobility as possible despite restrictions. Reviewing the process before surgery is helpful, because the patient may be too uncomfortable or drowsy after surgery to absorb new information.

Exercise of the extremities includes extension and flexion of the knee and hip joints (similar to bicycle riding while lying on the side). The foot is rotated as though tracing the largest possible circle with the great toe (see Chart 18-4). The elbow and shoulder are also put through their range of motion. At first, the patient is assisted and reminded to perform these exercises. Later, the patient is encouraged to do them independently. Muscle tone is maintained so that ambulation will be easier.

The nurse should remember to use proper body mechanics and to instruct the patient to do the same. Whenever the patient is positioned, his or her body needs to be properly aligned.

### Pain Management

A pain assessment should include differentiation between acute and chronic pain. Research suggests that, in older adults, teaching pain communication skills and pain management before surgery may result in greater pain relief during the early postoperative period (McDonald & Molony, 2004). A pain intensity scale should be introduced and explained to the patient to promote more effective postoperative pain management. Chapter 13 contains several examples of pain scales. Preoperative patient teaching also needs to include the difference between acute and chronic pain, so that the patient is prepared to differentiate acute postoperative pain from a chronic condition such as back pain (Nair & Podichetty, 2004).

Postoperatively, medications are administered to relieve pain and maintain comfort without increasing the risk of inadequate air exchange. The patient is instructed to take the medication as frequently as prescribed during the initial postoperative period for pain relief. Anticipated methods of administration of analgesic agents for inpatients include patient-controlled analgesia (PCA), epidural catheter bolus or infusion, or patient-controlled epidural analgesia (PCEA). A patient who is expected to go home will likely receive oral analgesic agents. These methods are discussed with the patient before surgery, and the patient's interest and willingness to use them are assessed.

### Cognitive Coping Strategies

Cognitive strategies may be useful for relieving tension, overcoming anxiety, decreasing fear, and achieving relaxation. Examples of such strategies include the following:

- *Imagery:* The patient concentrates on a pleasant experience or restful scene.
- *Distraction:* The patient thinks of an enjoyable story or recites a favorite poem or song.
- *Optimistic self-recitation:* The patient recites optimistic thoughts ("I know all will go well").

### Instruction for Patients Undergoing Ambulatory Surgery

Preoperative education for the same-day or ambulatory surgical patient comprises all the material presented earlier in this chapter as well as collaborative planning with the patient and family for discharge and follow-up home care. The major difference in outpatient preoperative education is the teaching environment.

Preoperative teaching content may be presented in a group class, on a videotape, at PAT, or by telephone in conjunction with the preoperative interview. In addition to answering questions and describing what to expect, the nurse tells the patient when and where to report, what to bring (insurance card, list of medications and allergies), what to leave at home (jewelry, watch, medications, contact lenses), and what to wear (loose-fitting, comfortable clothes; flat shoes). The nurse in the surgeon's office may initiate teaching before the perioperative telephone contact.

During the final preoperative telephone call, teaching is completed or reinforced as needed, and last-minute instructions are given. The patient is reminded not to eat or drink as directed.

## Preoperative Psychosocial Interventions

### Reducing Preoperative Anxiety

Cognitive strategies useful for reducing anxiety were addressed previously in this chapter. In addition to these strategies, music therapy is an easy-to-administer, inexpensive, noninvasive intervention that can reduce anxiety in the perioperative patient.

The general preoperative teaching addressed earlier in this section also helps decrease anxiety in many patients. Knowing ahead of time about the possible need for a ventilator, drainage tubes, or other types of equipment helps decrease anxiety in the postoperative period.

### Decreasing Fear

During the preoperative assessment, the nurse should assist the patient to identify coping strategies that he or she has previously used to decrease fear. The patient benefits from knowing when family and friends will be able to visit after surgery and that a spiritual advisor will be available if desired.

### Respecting Cultural, Spiritual, and Religious Beliefs

Psychosocial interventions include identifying and showing respect for cultural, spiritual, and religious beliefs. In some cultures, for example, people are stoic in regard to pain, whereas in others they are more expressive. These responses should be recognized as normal for those patients and families and should be respected by perioperative personnel (Flowers, 2004). If patients decline blood transfusions for religious reasons (Jehovah's Witnesses), this information needs to be clearly identified in the preoperative period, documented, and communicated to the appropriate personnel.

## General Preoperative Nursing Interventions

### Maintaining Patient Safety

Protecting patients from injury is one of the major roles of the perioperative nurse. Adherence to AORN recommended practices, the Joint Commission on Accreditation of Healthcare Organizations (JCAHO) recommendations, and national safety goals is crucial (Murphy, 2004). Seven main JCAHO patient safety goals apply throughout the perioperative period (Chart 18-5). These apply to hospitals as well as to ambulatory surgery centers and office-based surgery facilities (JCAHO, 2004).

### Managing Nutrition and Fluids

The major purpose of withholding food and fluid before surgery is to prevent aspiration. Until recently, fluid and food were restricted preoperatively overnight and often longer. However, the American Society of Anesthesiologists reviewed this practice and has made new recommendations for people undergoing elective surgery who are otherwise healthy. Studies show that lengthy restriction of fluid and food is unnecessary in patients who do not have a compromised airway, coexisting disease, or disorders that affect gastric emptying or fluid volume (eg, pregnancy, obesity, diabetes, gastroesophageal reflux, enteral tube feeding, ileus, bowel obstruction) (Brady, Kinn & Stewart, 2004). Specific recommendations depend on the age of the patient and the type of food eaten. For example, adults may be advised to fast for 8 hours after eating fatty food and 4 hours after ingesting milk products. Most patients are currently allowed clear liquids up to 2 hours before an elective procedure (Brady et al., 2004).

### Preparing the Bowel

Enemas are not commonly prescribed preoperatively unless the patient is undergoing abdominal or pelvic surgery. In this case, a cleansing enema or laxative may be prescribed the evening before surgery and may be repeated the morning of surgery. The goals of this preparation are to allow satisfactory visualization of the surgical site and to prevent trauma to the intestine or contamination of the peritoneum by feces. Unless the condition of the patient presents some contraindication, the toilet or bedside commode, rather than the bedpan, is used for evacuating the enema if the patient is hospitalized during this time. In addition, antibiotics may be prescribed to reduce intestinal flora.

### Preparing the Skin

The goal of preoperative skin preparation is to decrease bacteria without injuring the skin. If the surgery is not performed as an emergency, the patient may be instructed to use a soap containing a detergent-germicide to cleanse the skin area for several days before surgery to reduce the number of skin organisms; this preparation may be carried out at home.

Generally, hair is not removed preoperatively unless the hair at or around the incision site is likely to interfere with the operation. If hair must be removed, electric clippers are used for safe hair removal immediately before the operation.

## Immediate Preoperative Nursing Interventions

The patient changes into a hospital gown that is left untied and open in the back. The patient with long hair may braid it, remove hairpins, and cover the head completely with a disposable paper cap.

The mouth is inspected, and dentures or plates are removed. If left in the mouth, these items could easily fall to the back of the throat during induction of anesthesia and cause respiratory obstruction.

Jewelry is not worn to the OR; wedding rings and jewelry of body piercings should be removed to prevent injury (Armstrong, 2004; Larkin, 2004). If a patient objects to removing a ring, some institutions allow the ring to be securely fastened to the finger with tape. All articles of value, including assistive devices, dentures, glasses, and prosthetic devices, are given to family members or are labeled clearly with the patient's name and stored in a safe and secure place according to the institution's policy.

All patients (except those with urologic disorders) should void immediately before going to the OR to promote continence during low abdominal surgery and to make abdominal organs more accessible. Urinary catheterization is performed in the OR as necessary.

### Administering Preanesthetic Medication

The use of preanesthetic medication is minimal with ambulatory or outpatient surgery. If prescribed, it is usually administered in the preoperative holding area. If a preanesthetic medication is administered, the patient is kept in bed with the side rails raised, because the medication can cause lightheadedness or drowsiness. During this time, the nurse observes the patient for any untoward reaction to the medications. The immediate surroundings are kept quiet to promote relaxation.

---

**CHART 18-5**

### Seven Primary National Patient Safety Goals for 2005

- Improve the accuracy of patient identification
- Improve effectiveness of communication among caregivers
- Improve safety of using medications
- Improve safety of using infusion pumps
- Reduce the risk of health care–associated infections
- Accurately and completely reconcile medications across continuum of care
- Reduce the risk of surgical fires

From Joint Commission on Accreditation of Healthcare Organizations (JCAHO). (2004). JCAHO issues 2005 Patient Safety Goals. *OR Manager, 20*(9), 5–8.

Often, surgery is delayed or OR schedules are changed, and it becomes impossible to request that a medication be given at a specific time. In these situations, the preoperative medication is prescribed "on call to OR." The nurse can have the medication ready to administer as soon as a call is received from the OR staff. It usually takes 15 to 20 minutes to prepare the patient for the OR. If the nurse gives the medication before attending to the other details of preoperative preparation, the patient will have at least partial benefit from the preoperative medication and will have a smoother anesthetic and operative course.

## Maintaining the Preoperative Record

Preoperative checklists contain critical elements that must be checked and verified preoperatively (Rothrock, 2003). The nurse completes the preoperative checklist (Fig. 18-3). The nurse also completes the verification form preoperatively, and others provide verification (Fig. 18-4).

The completed chart (with the preoperative checklist and verification form) accompanies the patient to the OR with the surgical consent form attached, along with all laboratory reports and nurses' records. Any unusual last-minute observations that may have a bearing on anesthesia or surgery are noted prominently at the front of the chart.

## Transporting the Patient to the Presurgical Area

The patient is transferred to the holding area or presurgical suite in a bed or on a stretcher about 30 to 60 minutes before the anesthetic is to be given. The stretcher should be as comfortable as possible, with a sufficient number of blankets to prevent chilling in an air-conditioned room. A small head pillow is usually provided.

The patient is taken to the preoperative holding area, greeted by name, and positioned comfortably on the

---

1. Patient's name: _____ Date: _____ Height: _____ Weight: _____
   Identification band present: _____
2. Informed consent signed: _____ Special permits signed: _____
3. Surgical site: _____ (Ex: Sterilization)
4. History & physical examination report present: _____ Date: _____
5. Laboratory records present: _____
   CBC: _____ Hgb: _____ Urinalysis: _____ Hct: _____

6. Item — Present — Removed
   a. Natural teeth
      Dentures; upper, lower, partial
      Bridge, fixed; crown
   b. Contact lenses
   c. Other prostheses—type: _____
   d. Jewelry:
      Wedding band (taped/tied)
      Rings
      Earrings: pierced, clip-on
      Neck chains
      Any other body piercings
   e. Make-up
      Nail polish
7. Clothing
   a. Clean patient gown
   b. Cap
   c. Sanitary pad, etc.
8. Family instructed where to wait? _____
9. Valuables secured? _____
10. Blood available? _____ Ordered? _____ Where? _____
11. Preanesthetic medication given: _____
    Type: _____ Time: _____
12. Voided: _____ Amount: _____ Time: _____ Catheter: _____
    Mouth care given: _____
13. Vital signs: Temperature: _____ Pulse: _____ Resp: _____ Blood Pressure: _____
14. Special problems/precautions: (Allergies, deafness, etc.): _____
15. Area of skin preparation: _____
16. _____ Date: _____ Time: _____
    Signature: Nurse releasing patient

**FIGURE 18-3.** Example of a preoperative checklist.

# Operative/Invasive Procedure Checklist

Procedure Date: ___/___/___

## VERIFICATION #1

Location  ☐ SDA/SPU  ☐ Inpatient Room  ☐ Other

Operative/Invasive Procedure  ☐ Stated By Patient
☐ N/A _____  ☐ Other _____  Relationship to Patient _____

| **Procedure on Left Side of Body** (complete form on Left Side) | **All Other Procedures** (complete form in center) (including non-lateral and bilateral) | **Procedure on Right Side of Body** (complete form on Right Side) |
|---|---|---|
| Consent Completed and In Chart ☐ Yes ☐ No Comments | Consent Completed and In Chart ☐ Yes ☐ No Comments | Consent Completed and In Chart ☐ Yes ☐ No Comments |
| Correct Patient Verification ☐ Name ☐ DOB | Correct Patient Verification ☐ Name ☐ DOB | Correct Patient Verification ☐ Name ☐ DOB |
| Staff Signature/Title | Staff Signature/Title | Staff Signature/Title |

## VERIFICATION #2 (Day of Procedure)

Location  ☐ Holding  ☐ ED  ☐ Radiology  ☐ Critical Care Bedside  ☐ CVIR  ☐ Procedure Room
☐ Endoscopy  ☐ Invasive Cardiology  ☐ Labor/Delivery  ☐ Bronchoscopy  ☐ Other

Operative/Invasive Procedure (as stated by patient)
☐ N/A _____

| **Procedure on Left Side of Body** (complete form on Left Side) | **All Other Procedures** (complete form in center) (including non-lateral and bilateral) | **Procedure on Right Side of Body** (complete form on Right Side) |
|---|---|---|
| Consent Completed and In Chart ☐ Yes ☐ No Comments | Consent Completed and In Chart ☐ Yes ☐ No Comments | Consent Completed and In Chart ☐ Yes ☐ No Comments |
| Correct Patient Verification ☐ Name ☐ DOB | Correct Patient Verification ☐ Name ☐ DOB | Correct Patient Verification ☐ Name ☐ DOB |
| Physician Marking Site | Physician Marking Site | Physician Marking Site |
| Site Marked  ☐ Yes ☐ No ☐ N/A | Site Marked  ☐ Yes ☐ No ☐ N/A | Site Marked  ☐ Yes ☐ No ☐ N/A |
| Site Verified By Patient ☐ Yes ☐ No ☐ N/A | Site Verified By Patient ☐ Yes ☐ No ☐ N/A | Site Verified By Patient ☐ Yes ☐ No ☐ N/A |
| Staff Signature/Title | Staff Signature/Title | Staff Signature/Title |

## VERIFICATION #3 (Immediately Prior to Procedure)

Operative/Invasive Procedure (as stated by patient)
☐ N/A _____

| **Procedure on Left Side of Body** (complete form on Left Side) | **All Other Procedures** (complete form in center) (including non-lateral and bilateral) | **Procedure on Right Side of Body** (complete form on Right Side) |
|---|---|---|
| **Verification Correct Patient/Procedure/Site/Mark visible/Consent read aloud** ☐ Yes ☐ No Comments | **Verification Correct Patient/Procedure/Site/Mark visible/Consent read aloud** ☐ Yes ☐ No Comments | **Verification Correct Patient/Procedure/Site/Mark visible/Consent read aloud** ☐ Yes ☐ No Comments |
| Available in room: | Available in room: | Available in room: |
| Special Equipment ☐ Yes ☐ No Comments | Special Equipment ☐ Yes ☐ No Comments | Special Equipment ☐ Yes ☐ No Comments |
| Implants ☐ Yes ☐ No | Implants ☐ Yes ☐ No | Implants ☐ Yes ☐ No |
| Date/Time | Date/Time | Date/Time |
| Physician Name | Physician Name | Physician Name |
| Anesthesia Name | Anesthesia Name | Anesthesia Name |
| Nurse/Tech Name | Nurse/Tech Name | Nurse/Tech Name |
| Nurse/Tech Name | Nurse/Tech Name | Nurse/Tech Name |

**FIGURE 18-4.** Example of a verification form.

stretcher or bed. The surrounding area should be kept quiet if the preoperative medication is to have maximal effect. Unpleasant sounds or conversation should be avoided, because a sedated patient who overhears them might misinterpret them.

Patient safety in the preoperative area is a priority. Use of a process to verify patient identification, the surgical procedure, and the surgical site is imperative to maximize patient safety (see Fig. 18-4). This allows for prompt intervention if any discrepancies are identified.

**NURSING ALERT**

It is imperative that the entire perioperative team participate in verifying the correct patient identity, surgical procedure, and surgical site before proceeding to the OR.

### Attending to Family Needs

Most hospitals and ambulatory surgery centers have a waiting room where family members and significant others can wait while the patient is undergoing surgery. This room may be equipped with comfortable chairs, television, telephones, and facilities for light refreshment. Volunteers may remain with the family, offer them coffee, and keep them informed of the patient's progress. After surgery, the surgeon may meet the family in the waiting room and discuss the outcome.

The family and significant others should never judge the seriousness of an operation by the length of time the patient is in the OR. A patient may be in surgery much longer than the actual operating time for several reasons:

- Patients are routinely transported well in advance of the actual operating time.
- The anesthesiologist or anesthetist often makes additional preparations that may take 30 to 60 minutes.
- The surgeon may take longer than expected with the preceding case, which delays the start of the next surgical procedure.

After surgery, the patient is taken to the PACU to ensure safe emergence from anesthesia. Family members and significant others waiting to see the patient after surgery should be informed that the patient may have certain equipment or devices (eg, IV lines, indwelling urinary catheter, nasogastric tube, oxygen lines, monitoring equipment, blood transfusion lines) in place when he or she returns from surgery. When the patient returns to the room, the nurse provides explanations regarding the frequent postoperative observations that will be made. However, it is the responsibility of the surgeon, not the nurse, to relay the surgical findings and the prognosis, even when the findings are favorable.

## Expected Patient Outcomes

Expected patient outcomes in the preoperative phase of care are summarized in Chart 18-6.

---

**CHART 18-6**

### Expected Patient Outcomes in the Preoperative Phase of Care

**Relief of anxiety,** evidenced when the patient
- Discusses with the anesthesiologist, anesthetist, or nurse anesthetist concerns related to types of anesthesia and induction
- Verbalizes an understanding of the preanesthetic medication and general anesthesia
- Discusses last-minute concerns with the nurse or physician
- Discusses financial concerns with the social worker, when appropriate
- Requests visit with spiritual advisor when appropriate
- Relaxes quietly after being visited by health care team members

**Decreased fear,** evidenced when the patient
- Discusses fears with health care professionals or a spiritual advisor, or both
- Verbalizes an understanding of any expected bodily changes, including expected duration of bodily changes

**Understanding of the surgical intervention,** evidenced when the patient
- Participates in preoperative preparation
- Demonstrates and describes exercises he or she is expected to perform postoperatively
- Reviews information about postoperative care
- Accepts preanesthetic medication, if prescribed
- Remains in bed once premedicated
- Relaxes during transportation to the OR or unit
- States rationale for use of side rails
- Discusses postoperative expectations

**No evidence of preoperative complications**

## Critical Thinking Exercises

1. A morbidly obese man is scheduled for surgery on his right foot. The patient is noticeably favoring his left foot. What preoperative assessments are indicated? What nursing interventions are warranted?

2. **ebp** A male patient is scheduled for major surgery and asks how long before the surgery he will be without food and fluids. What resources would you use to identify the current fasting guidelines? What is the evidence base for the patient's being NPO after midnight as opposed to a 2-hour fast before surgery? Identify the criteria used to evaluate the strength of the evidence for this practice.

3. **ebp** Two patients are admitted to the same-day surgery unit for knee replacement surgery. What resources would you use to identify current safety practices during the perioperative period? Identify the evidence for and the criteria used to evaluate the strength of the evidence for the safety practices identified for these patients.

## REFERENCES AND SELECTED READINGS

### BOOKS

Aiken, T. D. (2004). *Legal, ethical, and political issues in nursing* (2nd ed.). Philadelphia: F. A. Davis.

American Society of PeriAnesthesia Nurses. (2002). *Standards of perianesthesia nursing practice*. Thorofare, NJ: ASPAN.

Bickley, L. S. & Szilagyi, P. G. (2003). *Bates' guide to physical examination and history taking* (8th ed.). Philadelphia: Lippincott Williams & Wilkins.

Clancy, J., McVicar, A. J. & Baird, N. (2002). *Perioperative practice: Fundamentals of homeostasis*. New York: Routledge.

Conner, R. (2004). *Ambulatory surgery principles and practices* (3rd ed.). Denver: AORN, Inc.

Defazio-Quinn, D. & Schick, L. (Eds). (2004). *Nursing core curriculum: Preoperative, phase I and phase II PACU nursing*. Philadelphia: W. B. Saunders.

Dudek, S. G. (2006). *Nutrition essentials for nursing practice* (5th ed.). Philadelphia: Lippincott Williams & Wilkins.

Kleinbeck, S. V. M. (2004). *Perioperative Nursing Data Set at work: Policies, procedures and pathways*. Denver: AORN, Inc.

Melnyk, B. M. & Fineout-Overholt, E. (2005). *Evidence-based practice in nursing and healthcare: A guide to best practices*. Philadelphia: Lippincott Williams & Wilkins.

Miller, R. D. (2005) *Miller's anesthesia* (6th ed.). New York: Elsevier/Churchill Livingstone.

Murray, M. J., Coursin, D. B., Pearl, R. G., et al. (2002). *Critical care medicine: Perioperative management* (2nd ed.). Philadelphia: Lippincott Williams & Wilkins.

National Institutes of Health, National Heart, Lung and Blood Institute, North American Association for the Study of Obesity. (2000). *The practical guide: Identification, evaluation, and treatment of overweight and obesity in adults*. NIH Publication Number 00-4084. Bethesda, MD: National Institutes of Health.

Phillips, N. (2004). *Berry and Kohn's operating room technique* (10th ed.). St. Louis: Mosby.

Rothrock, J. C. (Ed.). (2003). *Alexander's care of the patient in surgery* (12th ed.). St. Louis: Mosby.

U.S. Department of Health and Human Services, U. S. Department of Agriculture. (2005). *Dietary guidelines for Americans 2005*. Available at: www.healthierus.gov/dietaryguidelines (accessed May 7, 2006).

Weber, J. & Kelley, J. (2006). *Health assessment in nursing* (3rd ed.). Philadelphia: Lippincott Williams & Wilkins.

Worthington, P. H. (2004). *Practical aspects of nutritional support*. Philadelphia: W. B. Saunders.

## JOURNALS

*An asterisk indicates a nursing research article.

### Perioperative

Armstrong, M. L. (2004). Caring for the patient with piercings. *RN, 67*(6), 46–53.

Bernat, J. L. (2004). Ethical issues in the perioperative management of neurologic patients. *Neurologic Clinics of North America, 22*(1), 457–471.

*Bezanson, J. L., Weaver, M., Kinney, M. R., et al. (2004). Presurgical risk factors for late extubation in Medicare recipients after cardiac surgery. *Nursing Research, 53*(1), 46–52.

Bohan, E. & Glass-Macenka, D. (2004). Surgical management of patients with primary brain tumors. *Seminars in Oncology Nursing, 29*(4), 240–252.

Coleman, T., Cheater, R. & Murphy, E. (2004). Qualitative study investigation the process of giving anti-smoking advice in general practice. *Patient Education and Counseling, 52*(2), 159–163.

Flowers, D. L. (2004). Culturally competent nursing care: A challenge for the 21st century. *Critical Care Nurse, 24*(4), 48–52.

Fuller, T. (2003). Elder abuse and neglect assessment. *Journal of Gerontological Nursing, 29*(1), 8–9.

Galvez-Jimenez, N. & Lang, A. E. (2004). The perioperative management of Parkinson's disease revisited. *Neurologic Clinics of North America, 22*(2), 367–377.

Gotta, A. W. (2004). Anesthetic management of the patient with HIV infection. *Current Reviews for Nurse Anesthetists, 27*(11), 117–128.

John, A. D. & Sieber, F. E. (2004). Age associated issues: Geriatrics. *Anesthesiology Clinic of North America, 22*(1), 45–58.

Joint Commission on Accreditation of Healthcare Organizations (JCAHO). (2004). JCAHO issues 2005 patient safety goals. *OR Manager, 20*(9), 5–8.

Lorenz, R. A., Lorenz, R. M. & Cody, J. E. (2005). Home study program: Perioperative blood glucose control during adult coronary artery bypass surgery. *AORN Journal, 81*(1), 126–150.

Lotan, Y., Cadeddu, J. A. & Gettman, M. T. (2004). The new economics of radical prostatectomy: Cost comparison of open, laparoscopic and robot assisted techniques. *Journal of Urology, 172*(4 Pt. 1), 1431–1435.

Matin, S. F., Abreu, S., Ramani, A., et al. (2003). Evaluation of age and comorbidity as risk factors after laparoscopic urological surgery. *Journal of Urology, 170*(4 Pt. 1), 1115–1120.

*McDonald, D. D. & Molony, S. L. (2004). Postoperative pain communication skills for older adults. *Western Journal of Nursing Research, 26*(8), 836–852.

Mercado, D. L. & Petty, B. G. (2003). Perioperative medication management. *Medical Clinics of North America, 87*(1), 41–57.

Pass, S. & Simpson, R. (2004). Discontinuation and reinstitution of medications during the perioperative period. *American Journal of Health-System Pharmacists, 61*(6), 899–912.

Robinson, T. N. & Stiegmann, G. V. (2004). Minimally invasive surgery. *Endoscopy, 36*(1), 48–51.

Saufl, N. M. (2004). Preparing the older adult for surgery and anesthesia. *Journal of Perianesthesia Nursing, 19*(6), 372–377.

Schofield, C. (2004). How do I care for a patient with alcohol withdrawal syndrome? *Nursing, 34*(8), 25.

Ziegeler, S., Tsusaki, B. & Charles, C. (2003). Influence of genotype on perioperative risk and outcome. *Anesthesiology, 99*(1), 212–219.

## Preoperative Assessment

Barkhordarian, S. & Dardik, A. (2004). Preoperative assessment and management to prevent complications during high-risk vascular surgery. *Critical Care Medicine, 32*(4 Suppl.), S174–S185.

Brady, M., Kinn, S. & Stuart, P. (2004). Preoperative fasting for adults to prevent perioperative complications. *Cochrane Library (Oxford) (4),* CD004423.

Bray, A. (2006). Preoperative nursing assessment of the surgical patient. *Nursing Clinics of North America, 41*(2), 135–150.

Charlebois, D. & Wilmothe, D. (2004). Critical care of patients with obesity. *Critical Care Nurse, 24*(4), 19–29.

DeFazio-Quinn, D. M. (2006). How religion, language and ethnicity impact perioperative nursing care. *Nursing Clinics of North America, 41*(2), 231–248.

Garcia-Miguel, F. J., Serrano-Aguilar, P. G. & Lopez-Bastida, J. (2003). Preoperative assessment. *Lancet, 362*(9397), 1749–1757.

Halaszynski, T. M., Juda, R. & Silverman, D. G. (2004). Optimizing postoperative outcomes with efficient preoperative assessment and management. *Critical Care Medicine, 32*(4), S76–S86.

Heyneman, C. (2003). Pharmacology. Preoperative considerations: Which herbal products should be discontinued before surgery? *Critical Care Nurse, 23*(2), 116–123.

Larkin, B. G. (2004). Home Study Program: The ins and outs of body piercing. *AORN Journal, 79*(2), 333–341.

MacKichan, C. & Ruthman, J. (2004). Herbal product use and perioperative patients. *AORN Journal, 79*(5), 947–959.

Mamaril, M. E. (2006). Nursing considerations in the geriatric surgical patient: The perioperative continuum of care. *Nursing Clinics of North America, 41*(2), 313–328.

Murphy, E. K. (2004). OR nursing law. Protecting patients from potential injuries. *AORN Journal, 79*(5), 1013–1016.

Nair, S. & Podichetty, V. K. (2004). The preoperative and postoperative assessment and care of patients with back pain. *Neurologic Clinics of North America, 22*(2), 441–456.

*Oetker-Black, S. L., Jones, S., Estok, P., et al. (2003). Preoperative teaching and hysterectomy outcomes. *AORN Journal, 77*(6), 1215–1231.

Pofahl, W. E. & Pories, W. J. (2003). Current status and future directions of geriatric general surgery. *Journal of American Geriatric Society, 51*(7 Suppl.), S351–S354.

Romanoski, S. (2006). Management of the special needs of the pregnant surgical patient. *Nursing Clinics of North America, 41*(2), 299–311.

Schroeter, K. (2003). Q & A: Informed consent. *Surgical Services Management, 9*(6), 52–54.

Wiklund, R. A. (2004). Preoperative preparation of patients with advanced liver disease. *Critical Care Medicine, 32*(4), S106–S115.

Williams, J. Z. & Barbul, A. (2003) Nutrition and wound healing. *Surgical Clinics of North America, 83*(3), 571–596.

## RESOURCES

American Academy of Ambulatory Care Nursing, East Holly Ave., Box 56, Pitman, NJ, 08071; 856-256-2350, 800-AMB-NURS; http://www.aaacn.org. Accessed March 31, 2006.

American Society of PeriAnesthesia Nurses, 10 Melrose Ave., Suite 110, Cherry Hill, NJ 08003; toll-free 877-9696; fax 856-616-9621; http://www.aspan.org. Accessed March 31, 2006.

Association of Perioperative Registered Nurses, Inc., 2170 S. Parker Rd., Suite 300, Denver, CO 80231; 856-616-9600 or -9601; toll-free 1-877-737-9696; http://www.aorn.org. Accessed March 31, 2006.

Joint Commission on Accreditation of Healthcare Organizations, One Renaissance Blvd., Oakbrook Terrace, IL 60181; 630-792-5000; fax 630-792-5005; http://www.jcaho.org. Accessed March 31, 2006.

# CHAPTER 19

# Intraoperative Nursing Management

## Learning Objectives

*On completion of this chapter, the learner will be able to:*

1. Describe the interdisciplinary approach to the care of the patient during surgery.
2. Describe the principles of surgical asepsis.
3. Describe the roles of the surgical team members during the intraoperative phase of care.
4. Identify adverse effects of surgery and anesthesia.
5. Identify the surgical risk factors related to age-specific populations and nursing interventions to reduce those risks.
6. Compare various types of anesthesia with regard to uses, advantages, disadvantages, and nursing responsibilities.
7. Identify the use of the nursing process for optimizing patient outcomes during the intraoperative period.
8. Describe the role of the nurse in ensuring patient safety during the intraoperative period.

The intraoperative experience has undergone many changes that make it safer and less disturbing to patients. However, even with these advances, anesthesia and surgery place the patient at risk for several complications or adverse events. Consciousness or full awareness, mobility, protective biologic functions, and personal control are totally or partially relinquished by the patient when entering the operating room (OR). Staff from the departments of anesthesia, nursing, and surgery work collaboratively to implement professional standards of care, to control iatrogenic and individual risks, to prevent complications, and to promote high-quality patient outcomes.

## The Surgical Team

The surgical team consists of the patient, the **anesthesiologist** or **anesthetist**, the surgeon, nurses, and the surgical technologists. The anesthesiologist or anesthetist (usually a nurse anesthetist) administers the **anesthetic** agent and monitors the patient's physical status throughout the surgery. The surgeon and assistants scrub and perform the surgery. The person in the scrub role, either a nurse or a surgical technologist, provides sterile instruments and supplies to the surgeon during the procedure. The circulating nurse coordinates the care of the patient in the OR. Care provided by the circulating nurse includes assisting with patient positioning, preparing the patient's skin for surgery, managing surgical specimens, and documenting intraoperative events.

## The Patient

As the patient enters the OR, he or she may feel either relaxed and prepared or fearful and highly stressed. These feelings depend to a large extent on the amount and timing of preoperative sedation and the patient's level of fear and anxiety. Fears about loss of control, the unknown, pain, death, changes in body structure or function, and disruption of lifestyle all may contribute to generalized anxiety. These fears can increase the amount of anesthetic needed, the level of postoperative pain, and overall recovery time.

The patient is also subject to several risks. Infection, failure of the surgery to relieve symptoms, temporary or permanent complications related to the procedure or the anesthetic, and death are uncommon but potential outcomes of the surgical experience (Chart 19-1). In addition to fears and risks, the patient undergoing sedation and anesthesia temporarily loses both cognitive function and biologic self-protective mechanisms. Loss of pain sense, reflexes, and ability to communicate subjects the intraoperative patient to possible injury.

### Gerontologic Considerations

Elderly patients face higher risks from anesthesia and surgery than younger adult patients do (Rothrock, 2003). Statistically, perioperative risk increases with each decade after 60 years of age, often because of the increased incidence of coexisting disease. Key predictors of perioperative complications in the elderly are the patient's preoperative condition and level of function (John & Sieber, 2004). Modifications tailored to the biologic changes of later life and the application of research findings can reduce the risks (Pofahl & Pories, 2003).

Biologic variations of particular importance include age-related cardiovascular and pulmonary changes. The aging heart and blood vessels have decreased ability to respond to stress. Reduced cardiac output and limited cardiac reserve make the elderly patient vulnerable to changes in circulating volume and blood oxygen levels. Excessive or rapid administration of intravenous (IV) solutions can cause pulmonary edema. A sudden or prolonged decline in blood

## Glossary

**anesthesia:** a state of narcosis, analgesia, relaxation, and loss of reflexes

**anesthesiologist:** physician trained to deliver anesthesia and to monitor the patient's condition during surgery

**anesthetic:** the substance, such as a chemical or gas, used to induce anesthesia

**anesthetist:** health care professional, such as a nurse anesthetist, who is trained to deliver anesthesia and to monitor the patient's condition during surgery

**circulating nurse (or circulator):** registered nurse who coordinates and documents patient care in the operating room

**moderate sedation:** use of sedation to depress the level of consciousness without altering the patient's ability to maintain a patent airway and to respond to physical stimuli and verbal commands, previously referred to as conscious sedation

**monitored anesthesia care (MAC):** moderate sedation administered by an anesthesiologist or anesthetist

**restricted zone:** area in the operating room where scrub attire and surgical masks are required; includes operating room and sterile core areas

**scrub role:** registered nurse, licensed practical nurse, or surgical technologist who scrubs and dons sterile surgical attire, prepares instruments and supplies, and hands instruments to the surgeon during the procedure

**semirestricted zone:** area in the operating room where scrub attire is required; may include areas where surgical instruments are processed

**surgical asepsis:** absence of microorganisms in the surgical environment to reduce the risk for infection

**unrestricted zone:** area in the operating room that interfaces with other departments; includes patient reception area and holding area

> **CHART 19-1**
>
> ### Potential Adverse Effects of Surgery and Anesthesia
>
> Anesthesia and surgery disrupt all major body systems. Although most patients can compensate for surgical trauma and the effects of anesthesia, all patients are at risk during the operative procedure. These risks include the following:
> - Allergic reactions
> - Cardiac dysrhythmia from electrolyte imbalance or adverse effect of anesthetic agents
> - Myocardial depression, bradycardia, and circulatory collapse
> - Central nervous system agitation, seizures, and respiratory arrest
> - Oversedation or undersedation
> - Agitation or disorientation, especially in elderly patients
> - Hypoxemia or hypercarbia from hypoventilation and inadequate respiratory support during anesthesia
> - Laryngeal trauma, oral trauma, and broken teeth from difficult intubation
> - Hypothermia from cool operating room temperatures, exposure of body cavities, and impaired thermoregulation secondary to anesthetic agents
> - Hypotension from blood loss or adverse effect of anesthesia
> - Infection
> - Thrombosis from compression of blood vessels or stasis
> - Malignant hyperthermia secondary to adverse effect of anesthesia
> - Nerve damage, skin breakdown from prolonged or inappropriate positioning
> - Electrical shock or burns
> - Laser burns
> - Drug toxicity, faulty equipment, and human error

pressure may lead to cerebral ischemia, thrombosis, embolism, infarction, and anoxia. Reduced gas exchange can result in cerebral hypoxia.

The elderly patient needs fewer and smaller amounts of anesthetic agents to produce anesthesia and eliminates the anesthetic agent over a longer period of time, compared with a younger patient (Yellen, 2003). With increasing age, there is a decrease in the percentage of lean body tissue and a steady increase in fatty tissue (from 20 to 90 years of age). Anesthetic agents that have an affinity for fatty tissue concentrate in body fat and the brain. Lower doses of anesthetic agents are appropriate in an elderly patient if the patient is malnourished and has low plasma protein levels (Williams & Barbul, 2003). With decreased plasma proteins, more of the anesthetic agent remains free or unbound, and the result is more potent action.

In addition, body tissues of the older adult are made up predominantly of water, and those tissues with a rich blood supply, such as skeletal muscle, liver, and kidneys, shrink. Reduced liver size decreases the rate at which the liver can inactivate many anesthetic agents, and decreased kidney function slows the elimination of waste products and anesthetics. Other factors that affect the elderly surgical patient in the intraoperative period include the following:

- Impaired ability to increase metabolic rate and impaired thermoregulatory mechanisms increase susceptibility to hypothermia.
- Bone loss (25% in women, 12% in men) necessitates careful manipulation and positioning during surgery.
- Reduced ability to adjust rapidly to emotional and physical stress influences surgical outcomes and requires meticulous observation of vital functions.

As expected, mortality is higher with emergency surgery (commonly required for traumatic injuries) than with elective surgery, making continuous and careful monitoring and prompt intervention especially important for older surgical patients (Pofahl & Pories, 2003).

## Nursing Care

Throughout surgery, nursing responsibilities include providing for the safety and well-being of the patient, coordinating the OR personnel, and performing scrub and circulating activities. Because the patient's emotional state remains a concern, the care begun by preoperative nurses is continued by the intraoperative nursing staff, who provide the patient with information and reassurance. The nurse supports coping strategies and reinforces the patient's ability to influence outcomes by encouraging his or her active participation in the plan of care.

As patient advocates, intraoperative nurses monitor factors that can cause injury, such as patient position, equipment malfunction, and environmental hazards, and they protect the patient's dignity and interests while the patient is anesthetized. Additional responsibilities include maintaining surgical standards of care and identifying and minimizing risks and complications.

## The Circulating Nurse

The **circulating nurse** (also known as the **circulator**) is preferably a registered nurse (RN). In 20 states in the United States, the circulator is required by law to be an RN (Phillips, 2004). He or she manages the OR and protects the patient's safety and health by monitoring the activities of the surgical team, checking the OR conditions, and continually assessing the patient for signs of injury and implementing appropriate interventions. Main responsibilities include verifying consent; coordinating the team; and ensuring cleanliness, proper temperature, humidity, lighting, safe function of equipment, and the availability of supplies and materials. The circulating nurse monitors aseptic practices to avoid breaks in technique while coordinating the movement of related personnel (medical, x-ray, and laboratory), as well as implementing fire safety precautions. The circulating nurse also monitors the patient and documents specific activities throughout the operation to ensure the patient's safety and well-being.

In addition, the circulating nurse is responsible for ensuring that the second verification of the surgical procedure and site takes place and is documented (see Fig. 18-4 in Chapter 18). In some institutions, this is referred to as a "surgical or preprocedure pause" or "time-out" that takes place among the surgical team prior to incision. Every member of the surgical team verifies the patient's name, procedure, and surgical site using objective documentation and data before beginning the surgery, as mandated by the Joint Commission on Accreditation of Healthcare Organizations (JCAHO). Proper patient identification is one of the seven 2005 National Patient Safety Goals identified by JCAHO (2005) (see Chart 18-5 in Chapter 18).

## The Scrub Role

Activities of the **scrub role** include performing a surgical hand scrub; setting up the sterile tables; preparing sutures, ligatures, and special equipment (eg, laparoscope); and assisting the surgeon and the surgical assistants during the procedure by anticipating the instruments and supplies that will be required, such as sponges, drains, and other equipment. As the surgical incision is closed, the scrub person and the circulator count all needles, sponges, and instruments to be sure they are accounted for and not retained as a foreign body in the patient (Gawande, Studdert, Orav, et al., 2003). Standards call for all sponges to be visible on x-ray and for sponge counts to take place at the beginning of surgery and twice at the end. Tissue specimens obtained during surgery are labeled by the scrub person and sent to the laboratory by the circulator.

## The Surgeon

The surgeon performs the surgical procedure and heads the surgical team. He or she is a licensed physician (MD), osteopath (DO), oral surgeon (DDS or DMD), or podiatrist (DPM) who is specially trained and qualified. Qualifications may include certification by a specialty board, adherence to JCAHO standards, and adherence to hospital standards and admitting practices and procedures (Phillips, 2004).

## The Registered Nurse First Assistant

The registered nurse first assistant (RNFA) is another member of the OR team. Although the scope of practice of the RNFA depends on each state's nurse practice act, the RNFA practices under the direct supervision of the surgeon. RNFA responsibilities may include handling tissue, providing exposure at the operative field, suturing, and maintaining hemostasis (Rothrock, 2003). The role requires a thorough understanding of anatomy and physiology, tissue handling, and the principles of **surgical asepsis**. The RNFA must be aware of the objectives of the surgery, must have the knowledge and ability to anticipate needs and to work as a skilled member of a team, and must be able to handle any emergency situation in the OR.

## The Anesthesiologist and Anesthetist

An **anesthesiologist** is a physician specifically trained in the art and science of anesthesiology. An **anesthetist** is a qualified health care professional who administers anesthetics. Most anesthetists are nurses who have graduated from an accredited nurse anesthesia program and have passed examinations sponsored by the American Association of Nurse Anesthetists to become a certified registered nurse anesthetist (CRNA). The anesthesiologist or anesthetist assesses the patient before surgery, selects the anesthesia, administers it, intubates the patient if necessary, manages any technical problems related to the administration of the anesthetic agent, and supervises the patient's condition throughout the surgical procedure. Before the patient enters the OR, often at preadmission testing, the anesthesiologist or anesthetist visits the patient to supply information and answer questions. The type of anesthetic to be administered, previous reactions to anesthetics, and known anatomic abnormalities that would make airway management difficult are among the topics discussed.

The anesthesiologist or anesthetist uses the American Society of Anesthesiologists (ASA) Physical Status Classification System to determine the patient's status (Chart 19-2). If a patient has a classification of P2, P3, or P4, he or she has a systemic disease that may or may not be related to the cause of surgery. If a patient with a classification of P1, P2, P3, P4, or P5 requires emergency surgery, an E is added to the physical status designation (eg, P1E, P2E). P6 refers to a patient who is brain dead and is undergoing surgery as an organ donor. The abbreviations ASA1 through ASA6 are often used interchangeably with P1 to P6 to designate physical status (Phillips, 2004).

When the patient arrives in the OR, the anesthesiologist or anesthetist reassesses the patient's physical condition immediately prior to initiating anesthesia. The anesthetic is administered, and the patient's airway is maintained through either an endotracheal tube or a laryngeal mask airway (LMA). During surgery, the anesthesiologist or anesthetist monitors the patient's blood pressure, pulse, and respirations as well as the electrocardiogram (ECG), blood oxygen saturation level, tidal volume, blood gas levels, blood pH, alveolar gas concentrations, and body temperature. Monitoring by electroencephalography is sometimes required. Levels of anesthetics in the body can also be determined; a mass spectrometer can provide instant readouts of critical concentration levels on display terminals. This information helps personnel assess the patient's ability to breathe unassisted or the need for mechanical assistance if ventilation is poor and the patient is not breathing well independently.

## The Surgical Environment

The surgical environment is known for its stark appearance and cool temperature. The surgical suite is behind double doors, and access is limited to authorized personnel. External precautions include adhering to principles of surgical asepsis; strict control of the OR environment is required, including traffic pattern restrictions. Policies governing this environment address such issues as the health of the staff; the cleanliness of the

### CHART 19-2

## American Society of Anesthesiologists Physical Status Classification System

Anesthetists and anesthesiologists use the American Society of Anesthesiologists Physical (P) Status Classification System to describe the patient's general status and identify potential risks during surgery. There are six classes of physical status.

- **P1.** A normal healthy patient
  *Example:* No systemic abnormality, localized infection without fever, benign tumor, hernia
- **P2.** A patient with mild systemic disease, without functional limitations
  *Example:* Well-controlled hypertension, well-controlled diabetes mellitus, chronic bronchitis, obesity, age over 80 years
- **P3.** A patient with severe systemic disease associated with functional limitations
  *Example:* Severe disease, compensated heart failure, myocardial infarction more than 6 months ago, angina pectoris, severe dysrhythmia, cirrhosis, poorly controlled diabetes or hypertension, ileus
- **P4.** A patient with an incapacitating systemic disease that is a constant threat to life
  *Example:* Severe heart failure, myocardial infarction less than 6 months ago, severe respiratory failure, advanced liver or renal failure
- **P5.** A moribund patient who is not expected to survive for 24 hours with or without operation
  *Example:* Unconscious patient with traumatic head injury and agonal respirations
- **P6.** Patient is brain dead and is being prepared as an organ donor

Adapted from American Society of Anesthesiologists. (1997). *Manual for anesthesia departments.* Park Ridge, IL: Author.

---

rooms; the sterility of equipment and surfaces; processes for scrubbing, gowning, and gloving; and OR attire.

To provide the best possible conditions for surgery, the OR is situated in a location that is central to all supporting services (eg, pathology, x-ray, laboratory). The OR has special air filtration devices to screen out contaminating particles, dust, and pollutants.

All seven of the JCAHO's 2005 National Patient Safety Goals pertain to the perioperative areas (see Chart 18-5 in Chapter 18), but the one that has the most direct relevance to the OR is the reduction of the risk of surgical fires. The surgical team must be educated about how to control heat sources, manage fuels, and minimize oxygen concentration under drapes (Salmon, 2004). Surgical drapes provide an opportunity for oxygen to concentrate; a stray spark could more easily ignite a fire. This occurs most commonly in ambulatory surgery settings (JCAHO, 2005). To further improve safety, electrical hazards, emergency exit clearances, and storage of equipment and anesthetic gases are monitored periodically by official agencies, such as the state department of health and JCAHO.

To help decrease microbes, the surgical area is divided into three zones: the **unrestricted zone**, where street clothes are allowed; the **semirestricted zone**, where attire consists of scrub clothes and caps; and the **restricted zone**, where scrub clothes, shoe covers, caps, and masks are worn. The surgeons and other surgical team members wear additional sterile clothing and protective devices during the operation.

The Association of PeriOperative Registered Nurses, formerly known as the Association of Operating Room Nurses (still abbreviated as AORN), recommends specific practices for personnel wearing surgical attire to promote a high level of cleanliness in a particular practice setting (AORN, 2004b). OR attire includes close-fitting cotton dresses, pantsuits, jumpsuits, and gowns. Knitted cuffs on sleeves and pant legs prevent organisms shed from the perineum, legs, and arms from being released into the immediate surroundings. Shirts and waist drawstrings should be tucked inside the pants to prevent accidental contact with sterile areas and to contain skin shedding. Wet or soiled garments should be changed.

Masks are worn at all times in the restricted zone of the OR. High-filtration masks decrease the risk of postoperative wound infection by containing and filtering microorganisms from the oropharynx and nasopharynx. Masks should fit tightly; should cover the nose and mouth completely; and should not interfere with breathing, speech, or vision. Masks must be adjusted to prevent venting from the sides. Disposable masks have a filtration efficiency exceeding 95%. Masks are changed between patients and should not be worn outside the surgical department. The mask must be either on or off; it must not be allowed to hang around the neck.

Headgear should completely cover the hair (head and neckline, including beard) so that single strands of hair, bobby pins, clips, and particles of dandruff or dust do not fall on the sterile field.

Shoes should be comfortable and supportive. Shoe covers are worn when it is reasonably anticipated that spills or splashes will occur. If worn, the covers should be changed whenever they become wet, torn, or soiled (Rothrock, 2003).

Barriers such as scrub attire and masks do not entirely protect the patient from microorganisms. Upper respiratory tract infections, sore throats, and skin infections in staff and patients are sources of pathogens and must be reported.

Because artificial fingernails harbor microorganisms and can cause nosocomial infections, a ban on artificial nails by OR personnel is supported by the Centers for Disease Control and Prevention (CDC), AORN, and the Association of Professionals in Infection Control. Short, natural fingernails are encouraged (Gupta, Della-Latta, Todd, et al., 2004).

## Principles of Surgical Asepsis

Surgical asepsis prevents the contamination of surgical wounds. The patient's natural skin flora or a previously existing infection may cause postoperative wound infection. Rigorous adherence to the principles of surgical asepsis by OR personnel is basic to preventing surgical site infections.

All surgical supplies, instruments, needles, sutures, dressings, gloves, covers, and solutions that may come in contact with the surgical wound or exposed tissues must be sterilized before use (Rothrock, 2003). Traditionally, the surgeon, surgical assistants, and nurses prepared themselves by scrubbing their hands and arms with antiseptic soap and water, but this traditional practice is being challenged by research investigating the optimal length of time to scrub and the best preparation to use. In some institutions, an alcohol-based product or scrubless soap is used to prepare for surgery (Paulson, 2004; Rothrock, 2003).

Surgical team members wear long-sleeved, sterile gowns and gloves. Head and hair are covered with a cap, and a mask is worn over the nose and mouth to minimize the possibility that bacteria from the upper respiratory tract will enter the wound. During surgery, only personnel who have scrubbed, gloved, and gowned touch sterilized objects. Nonscrubbed personnel refrain from touching or contaminating anything sterile.

An area of the patient's skin considerably larger than that requiring exposure during the surgery is meticulously cleansed, and an antiseptic solution is applied (Phillips, 2004). If hair needs to be removed, this is done immediately before the procedure to minimize the risk of wound infection (Beyea, 2003). The remainder of the patient's body is covered with sterile drapes.

### Environmental Controls

In addition to the protocols described previously, surgical asepsis requires meticulous cleaning and maintenance of the OR environment. Floors and horizontal surfaces are cleaned frequently with detergent, soap, and water or a detergent germicide. Sterilizing equipment is inspected regularly to ensure optimal operation and performance.

All equipment that comes into direct contact with the patient must be sterile. Sterilized linens, drapes, and solutions are used. Instruments are cleaned and sterilized in a unit near the OR. Individually wrapped sterile items are used when additional individual items are needed.

Airborne bacteria are a concern. To decrease the amount of bacteria in the air, standard OR ventilation provides 15 air exchanges per hour, at least 3 of which are fresh air (Phillips, 2004). A temperature of 20° to 24°C (68° to 73°F), humidity between 30% to 60%, and positive pressure relative to adjacent areas are maintained. Staff members shed skin scales, resulting in about 1000 bacteria-carrying particles (or colony-forming units [CFUs]) per cubic foot per minute. With the standard air exchanges, air counts of bacteria are reduced to 50 to 150 CFUs per cubic foot per minute. Systems with high-efficiency particulate air (HEPA) filters are needed to remove particles larger than 0.3 μm (Rothrock, 2003). Unnecessary personnel and physical movement may be restricted to minimize bacteria in the air and achieve an OR infection rate no greater than 3% to 5% in clean, infection-prone surgery.

Some ORs have laminar airflow units. These units provide 400 to 500 air exchanges per hour (Phillips, 2004). When used appropriately, laminar airflow units result in fewer than 10 CFUs per cubic foot per minute during surgery. The goal for a laminar airflow–equipped OR is an infection rate of less than 1%. An OR equipped with this unit is frequently used for total joint replacement or organ transplant surgery.

Despite these precautions, wound contamination may occur during surgery but may only become apparent days or weeks later in the form of a surgical site infection that results in a longer hospital stay (Pryor, Fahey, Lien, et al., 2004). Constant surveillance and conscientious technique in carrying out aseptic practices are necessary to reduce the risk of contamination and infection.

### Basic Guidelines for Maintaining Surgical Asepsis

All practitioners involved in the intraoperative phase have a responsibility to provide and maintain a safe environment. Adherence to aseptic practice is part of this responsibility. The basic principles of aseptic technique follow:

- All materials in contact with the surgical wound or used within the sterile field must be sterile. Sterile surfaces or articles may touch other sterile surfaces or articles and remain sterile; contact with unsterile objects at any point renders a sterile area contaminated.
- Gowns of the surgical team are considered sterile in front from the chest to the level of the sterile field. The sleeves are also considered sterile from 2 inches above the elbow to the stockinette cuff.
- Sterile drapes are used to create a sterile field. Only the top surface of a draped table is considered sterile. During draping of a table or patient, the sterile drape is held well above the surface to be covered and is positioned from front to back.
- Items are dispensed to a sterile field by methods that preserve the sterility of the items and the integrity of the sterile field. After a sterile package is opened, the edges are considered unsterile. Sterile supplies, including solutions, are delivered to a sterile field or handed to a scrubbed person in such a way that the sterility of the object or fluid remains intact.
- The movements of the surgical team are from sterile to sterile areas and from unsterile to unsterile areas. Scrubbed persons and sterile items contact only sterile areas; circulating nurses and unsterile items contact only unsterile areas.
- Movement around a sterile field must not cause contamination of the field. Sterile areas must be kept in view during movement around the area. At least a 1-foot distance from the sterile field must be maintained to prevent inadvertent contamination.
- Whenever a sterile barrier is breached, the area must be considered contaminated. A tear or puncture of the drape permitting access to an unsterile surface underneath renders the area unsterile. Such a drape must be replaced.
- Every sterile field is constantly monitored and maintained. Items of doubtful sterility are considered unsterile. Sterile fields are prepared as close as possible to the time of use.
- The routine administration of hyperoxia (high levels of oxygen) is *not* recommended to reduce surgical site infections. In a study of 165 patients undergoing general surgery, the rate of surgical site infection was higher in patients who received 80% oxygen during surgery than in those who received 35% oxygen (Pryor et al., 2004).

## Health Hazards Associated With the Surgical Environment

Safety issues in the OR include exposure to blood and body fluids; hazards associated with laser beams; and exposure to latex and adhesive substances, radiation, and toxic agents (Hammarsten, Hammarsten & Jemsby, 2003). Internal monitoring of the OR includes the analysis of surface swipe samples and air samples for infectious and toxic agents. In addition, policies and procedures for minimizing exposure to body fluids and reducing the dangers associated with lasers and radiation have been established.

An additional hazard is the unintentional leaving of an object in a person during a surgical procedure. The risk that foreign objects may be left in a person increases in the following situations: when the procedure is performed on an emergency basis, when there is an unplanned change in the procedure, and when the patient has a high body mass index. Complications from foreign bodies left after a surgical procedure include small bowel fistulas, obstruction, visceral perforation, and death (Gawande et al., 2003).

### Laser Risks

The AORN has recommended practices for laser safety (Phillips, 2004). While lasers are in use, warning signs must be clearly posted to alert personnel. Safety precautions are implemented to reduce the possibility of exposing the eyes and skin to laser beams, to prevent inhalation of the laser plume (smoke and particulate matter), and to protect the patient and personnel from fire and electrical hazards. Several types of lasers are available for clinical use; perioperative personnel should be familiar with the unique features, specific operation, and safety measures for each type of laser used in the practice setting.

Nurses and other intraoperative personnel working with lasers must have a thorough eye examination before participating in procedures involving lasers. All personnel wear special protective goggles, specific to the type of laser used in the procedure (Andersen, 2004).

Whether protection is needed to avoid the laser plume and the effects of its inhalation is controversial. Smoke evacuators are used in some procedures to remove the laser plume from the operative field. In recent years, this technology has been used to protect the surgical team from the potential hazards associated with the generalized smoke plume generated by standard electrocautery units.

### Exposure to Blood and Body Fluids

OR attire has changed dramatically since the advent of acquired immunodeficiency syndrome (AIDS). Double-gloving is routine in trauma and other types of surgery where sharp bone fragments are present. In addition to the routine scrub suit and double gloves, some surgical personnel wear rubber boots, a waterproof apron, and sleeve protectors. Goggles, or a wrap-around face shield, are worn to protect against splashing when the surgical wound is irrigated or when bone drilling is performed. In hospitals where numerous total joint procedures are performed, a complete bubble mask may be used. This mask provides full-barrier protection from bone fragments and splashes.

Ventilation is accomplished through an accompanying hood with a separate air-filtration system.

### Latex Allergy

The AORN has recommended standards of care for the patient with latex allergy (AORN, 2004a). These recommendations include early identification of patients with latex allergies, preparation of a latex allergy supply cart, and maintenance of latex allergy precautions throughout the perioperative period. Because of the increased number of patients with latex allergies, many latex-free products are now available. For safety, manufacturers and hospital material managers need to take responsibility for identifying the latex content in items used by patients and health care personnel. (See Chapters 18 and 53 for assessment for latex allergy.)

**NURSING ALERT**

It is the responsibility of all nurses, and particularly perianesthesia and perioperative nurses, to be aware of latex allergies, necessary precautions, and products that are latex-free. Hospital staff are also at risk for development of a latex allergy secondary to repeated exposure to latex products.

## The Surgical Experience

During the surgical procedure, the patient will need sedation, anesthesia, or some combination of these.

### Types of Anesthesia and Sedation

Anesthesia today is very safe; it is estimated that the number of anesthesia-related deaths is as low as 1 in 200,000 to 300,000 cases (Pine, Holt, & Lou, 2003). For the patient, the anesthesia experience consists of having an IV line inserted, if it was not inserted earlier; receiving a sedating agent prior to induction with an anesthetic agent; losing consciousness; being intubated, if indicated; and then receiving a combination of anesthetic agents. Typically the experience is a smooth one, and the patient has no recall of the events. The main types of anesthesia are general anesthesia, regional anesthesia, moderate sedation, monitored anesthesia care, and local anesthesia.

### General Anesthesia

**Anesthesia** is a state of narcosis (severe central nervous system depression produced by pharmacologic agents), analgesia, relaxation, and reflex loss. Patients under general anesthesia are not arousable, not even to painful stimuli. They lose the ability to maintain ventilatory function and require assistance in maintaining a patent airway. Cardiovascular function may be impaired as well.

In 2004, JCAHO issued an alert regarding the phenomenon of patients being partially awake while under general

## NURSING RESEARCH PROFILE

### Preoperative Skin Testing of Materials Used in Surgical Procedures

Hammarsten, R., Hammarsten, J. & Jemsby, P. (2003). Preoperative skin testing of materials used in surgical procedures. *AORN Journal*, 77(4), 762–771.

**Purpose**

Postoperative skin complications due to allergic or toxic effects of adhesive substances increase health care costs and cause patient discomfort. The purpose of the study was to investigate the incidence of skin reactions with the application of different materials.

**Design**

Study participants included 101 consecutive patients with a history of atopic or contact eczema, allergy, or asthma as indicated by their medical history. The day before surgery, 10 patches containing different adhesive materials that the patient could potentially be exposed to in the operating room were placed on the right forearm or ring finger for 6 hours. The patches were removed and then evaluated for no reaction, redness, itching, rash, and blisters 30 minutes later. The statistical analysis of differences in skin reactions among the various tested patches was performed via chi-square analysis.

**Findings**

From 3% to 50% of the participants showed skin reactions after the preoperative skin test. Surgical drapes with tape caused a skin reaction 50% of the time. Skin reactions included redness, itching, rash, or blisters.

**Nursing Implications**

It is the nurse's responsibility to be the patient advocate during surgery; therefore, it is important to reduce the potential for harm or patient suffering, or even disruption in wound healing. For some time, adhesives have been known to be a source of allergy. Nurses need to be alert to adhesive materials that cause reactions and be instrumental in removing these materials from the OR.

---

anesthesia (referred to as anesthesia awareness). Patients at greatest risk of anesthesia awareness are cardiac, obstetric, and major trauma patients. The entire surgical team must be aware of this phenomenon and help prevent or manage it (JCAHO, 2004).

General anesthesia consists of four stages, each associated with specific clinical manifestations (Rothrock, 2003):

- *Stage I: beginning anesthesia.* As the patient breathes in the anesthetic mixture, warmth, dizziness, and a feeling of detachment may be experienced. The patient may have a ringing, roaring, or buzzing in the ears and, although still conscious, may sense an inability to move the extremities easily. During this stage, noises are exaggerated; even low voices or minor sounds seem loud and unreal. For this reason, unnecessary noises and motions are avoided when anesthesia begins.
- *Stage II: excitement.* The excitement stage, characterized variously by struggling, shouting, talking, singing, laughing, or crying, is often avoided if the anesthetic is administered smoothly and quickly. The pupils dilate, but they contract if exposed to light; the pulse rate is rapid, and respirations may be irregular. Because of the possibility of uncontrolled movements of the patient during this stage, the anesthesiologist or anesthetist must always be assisted by someone ready to help restrain the patient. A strap may be in place across the patient's thighs, and the hands may be secured to an armboard. The patient should not be touched except for purposes of restraint, but restraints should not be applied over the operative site. Manipulation increases circulation to the operative site and thereby increases the potential for bleeding.
- *Stage III: surgical anesthesia.* Surgical anesthesia is reached by continued administration of the anesthetic vapor or gas. The patient is unconscious and lies quietly on the table. The pupils are small but contract when exposed to light. Respirations are regular, the pulse rate and volume are normal, and the skin is pink or slightly flushed. With proper administration of the anesthetic, this stage may be maintained for hours in one of several planes, ranging from light (1) to deep (4), depending on the depth of anesthesia needed.
- *Stage IV: medullary depression.* This stage is reached when too much anesthesia has been administered. Respirations become shallow, the pulse is weak and thready, and the pupils become widely dilated and no longer contract when exposed to light. Cyanosis develops and, without prompt intervention, death rapidly follows. If this stage develops, the anesthetic is discontinued immediately and respiratory and circulatory support is initiated to prevent death. Stimulants, although rarely used, may be administered; narcotic antagonists can be used if the overdosage is due to opioids.

When opioid agents (narcotics) and neuromuscular blockers (relaxants) are administered, several of the stages are absent. During smooth administration of an anesthetic, there is no sharp division between stages I, II, and III, and there is no stage IV. The patient passes gradually from one stage to another, and it is through close observation of the signs exhibited by the patient that an anesthesiologist or anesthetist controls the situation. The responses of the pupils, the blood pressure, and the respiratory and cardiac rates are among the most reliable guides to the patient's condition.

Anesthetic agents used in general anesthesia are inhaled or administered by IV. Anesthetics produce anesthesia because they are delivered to the brain at a high partial pressure that enables them to cross the blood–brain barrier.

Relatively large amounts of anesthetic must be administered during induction and the early maintenance phases because the anesthetic is recirculated and deposited in body tissues. As these sites become saturated, smaller amounts of the anesthetic agent are required to maintain anesthesia because equilibrium or near equilibrium has been achieved between brain, blood, and other tissues.

Any condition that diminishes peripheral blood flow, such as vasoconstriction or shock, may reduce the amount of anesthetic required. Conversely, when peripheral blood flow is unusually high, as in a muscularly active or apprehensive patient, induction is slower, and greater quantities of anesthetic are required because the brain receives a smaller quantity of anesthetic.

### INHALATION

Inhaled anesthetic agents include volatile liquid agents and gases. Volatile liquid anesthetics produce anesthesia when their vapors are inhaled. Commonly used inhalation agents are included in Table 19-1. All are administered with oxygen and usually with nitrous oxide as well.

Gas anesthetics are administered by inhalation and are always combined with oxygen. Nitrous oxide is the most commonly used gas anesthetic agent. When inhaled, the anesthetics enter the blood through the pulmonary capillaries and act on cerebral centers to produce loss of consciousness and sensation. When anesthetic administration is discontinued, the vapor or gas is eliminated through the lungs.

The vapor from inhalation anesthetics can be administered to the patient by several methods. The inhalation anesthetic may be administered through an LMA (Fig. 19-1A), a flexible tube with an inflatable silicone ring and cuff that can be inserted into the larynx. The endotracheal technique for administering anesthetics consists of introducing a soft rubber or plastic endotracheal tube into the trachea, usually by means of a laryngoscope. The endotracheal tube may be inserted through either the nose (see Fig. 19-1B) or mouth

### TABLE 19-1 Inhalation Anesthetic Agents

| Agent | Administration | Advantages | Disadvantages | Implications/Considerations |
|---|---|---|---|---|
| **Volatile Liquids** | | | | |
| Halothane (Fluothane) | Inhalation; special vaporizer | Not explosive or flammable; Induction rapid and smooth; Useful in almost every type of surgery; Low incidence of postoperative nausea and vomiting | Requires skillful administration to prevent overdosage; May cause liver damage; May produce hypotension; Requires special vaporizer for administration | In addition to observation of pulse and respiration postoperatively, blood pressure must be monitored frequently. |
| Enflurane (Ethrane) | Inhalation | Rapid induction and recovery; Potent analgesic; Not explosive or flammable | Respiratory depression may develop rapidly, along with ECG abnormalities. Not compatible with epinephrine | Observe for possible respiratory depression. Administration with epinephrine may cause ventricular fibrillation. |
| Isoflurane (Forane) | Inhalation | Rapid induction and recovery; Muscle relaxants are markedly potentiated. | A profound respiratory depressant | Respirations must be monitored closely and supported when necessary. |
| Sevoflurane (Ultrane) | Inhalation | Rapid induction and excretion; minimal side effects | Coughing and laryngospasm; trigger for malignant hyperthermia | Monitor for malignant hyperthermia. |
| Desflurane (Suprane) | Inhalation | Rapid induction and emergence; rare organ toxicity | Respiratory irritation; trigger for malignant hyperthermia | Monitor for malignant hyperthermia, dysrhythmias. |
| **Gases** | | | | |
| Nitrous oxide ($N_2O$) | Inhalation (semi-closed method) | Induction and recovery rapid; Nonflammable; Useful with oxygen for short procedures; Useful with other agents for all types of surgery | Poor relaxant; Weak anesthetic; May produce hypoxia | Most useful in conjunction with other agents with longer action. Monitor for chest pain, hypertension, and stroke. |
| Oxygen ($O_2$) | Inhalation | Can increase $O_2$ available to tissues | High concentrations are hazardous | Increased fire risk when used with lasers |

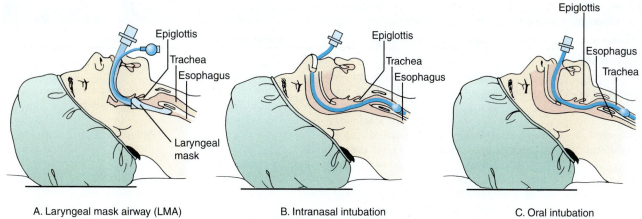

**FIGURE 19-1.** Anesthetic delivery methods: (**A**) laryngeal mask airway (LMA), (**B**) nasal endotracheal catheter (in position with cuff inflated), and (**C**) oral endotracheal intubation (tube is in position with cuff inflated).

(see Fig. 19-1C). When in place, the tube seals off the lungs from the esophagus so that, if the patient vomits, stomach contents do not enter the lungs.

### INTRAVENOUS ADMINISTRATION

General anesthesia can also be produced by the IV administration of various substances, such as barbiturates, benzodiazepines, nonbarbiturate hypnotics, dissociative agents, and opioid agents. Table 19-2 lists commonly used IV anesthetic and analgesic agents, including IV medications used as muscle relaxants in the intraoperative period. These medications may be administered to induce (initiate) or maintain anesthesia. Although they are often used in combination with inhalation anesthetics, they may be used alone. They may also be used to produce moderate sedation, as discussed later in this chapter.

An advantage of IV anesthesia is that the onset of anesthesia is pleasant; there is none of the buzzing, roaring, or dizziness known to follow administration of an inhalation anesthetic. For this reason, induction of anesthesia usually begins with an IV agent and is often preferred by patients who have experienced various methods. The duration of action is brief, and the patient awakens with little nausea or vomiting.

The IV anesthetic agents are nonexplosive, require little equipment, and are easy to administer. The low incidence of postoperative nausea and vomiting makes the method useful in eye surgery, because in this setting vomiting would increase intraocular pressure and endanger vision in the operated eye. IV anesthesia is useful for short procedures but is used less often for the longer procedures of abdominal surgery. It is not indicated for children who have small veins or for those who require intubation because of their susceptibility to respiratory obstruction.

A disadvantage of an IV anesthetic such as thiopental (Pentothal) is its powerful respiratory depressant effect. It must be administered by a skilled anesthesiologist or anesthetist and only when some method of oxygen administration is available immediately in case of difficulty. Sneezing, coughing, and laryngospasm are sometimes noted with its use.

IV neuromuscular blockers (muscle relaxants) block the transmission of nerve impulses at the neuromuscular junction of skeletal muscles. Muscle relaxants are used to relax muscles in abdominal and thoracic surgery, relax eye muscles in certain types of eye surgery, facilitate endotracheal intubation, treat laryngospasm, and assist in mechanical ventilation.

## Regional Anesthesia

Regional anesthesia is a form of local anesthesia in which an anesthetic agent is injected around nerves so that the area supplied by these nerves is anesthetized. The effect depends on the type of nerve involved. Motor fibers are the largest fibers and have the thickest myelin sheath. Sympathetic fibers are the smallest and have a minimal covering. Sensory fibers are intermediate. A local anesthetic blocks motor nerves least readily and sympathetic nerves most readily. An anesthetic cannot be regarded as having worn off until all three systems (motor, sensory, and autonomic) are no longer affected.

The patient receiving regional anesthesia is awake and aware of his or her surroundings unless medications are given to produce mild sedation or to relieve anxiety. The nurse must avoid careless conversation, unnecessary noise, and unpleasant odors; these may be noticed by the patient in the OR and may contribute to a negative response to the surgical experience. A quiet environment is therapeutic. The diagnosis must not be stated aloud if the patient is not to know it at this time.

### EPIDURAL ANESTHESIA

Epidural anesthesia, a commonly used conduction block, is achieved by injecting a local anesthetic into the epidural space that surrounds the dura mater of the spinal cord (Fig. 19-2). (In contrast, spinal anesthesia involves injection through the dura mater into the subarachnoid space surrounding the spinal cord.) Epidural anesthesia blocks sensory, motor, and autonomic functions; it differs from spinal anesthesia by the site of the injection and the amount of anesthetic agent used. Epidural doses are much higher

## TABLE 19-2 Commonly Used Intravenous Medications

| Medication | Common Usage | Advantages | Disadvantages | Comments |
|---|---|---|---|---|
| **Opioid Analgesics** | | | | |
| Morphine sulfate (MS) | Perioperative pain; premedication | Inexpensive; duration of action 4 to 5 hours; euphoria; good cardiovascular stability | Nausea and vomiting; histamine release; postural ↓ BP and ↓ SVR | Used intrathecally and epidurally for postoperative pain; elimination half-life 3 hours |
| Alfentanil (Alfenta) | Surgical analgesia in ambulatory patients | Duration of action 0.5 hour; used as bolus or infusion | | Potency: 750 µg = 10 mg morphine sulfate; elimination half-life 1.6 hours |
| Fentanyl (Sublimaze) | Surgical analgesia: epidural infusion for postoperative analgesia; add to SAB | Good cardiovascular stability; duration of action 0.5 hour | | Most commonly used opioid; potency: 100 µg = 10 mg morphine sulfate; elimination half-life 3.6 hours |
| Remifentanil (Ultiva) | IV infusion for surgical analgesia; small boluses for brief, intense pain | Easily titratable; metabolized by blood and tissue esterases; very short duration; good cardiovascular stability | New; expensive; requires mixing; may cause muscle rigidity | Potency: 25 µg = 10 mg morphine sulfate; 20 to 30 times potency of alfentanil; elimination half-life 3 to 10 min |
| Sufentanil (Sufenta) | Surgical analgesia | Good cardiovascular stability; duration of action 0.5 hour; prolonged analgesia | Prolonged respiratory depression | Potency: 15 µg = 10 mg morphine sulfate; elimination half-life 2.7 hours |
| **Depolarizing Muscle Relaxants** | | | | |
| Succinylcholine (Anectine, Quelicin) | Intubation; short cases | Rapid onset; short duration | Requires refrigeration; may cause fasciculations, postoperative myalgias, and dysrhythmias; ↑ serum K+ with burns, tissue trauma, paralysis, and muscle diseases; slight histamine release | Prolonged muscle relaxation with serum cholinesterase deficiency and certain antibiotics; trigger agent for malignant hyperthermia |
| **Nondepolarizing Muscle Relaxants—Intermediate Onset and Duration** | | | | |
| Atracurium (Tracrium) | Intubation; maintenance of relaxation | No significant cardiovascular or cumulative effects; good with renal failure | Requires refrigeration; slight histamine release | Breakdown by Hofman elimination (non-enzymatic degradation) and ester hydrolysis |
| Cisatracurium (Nimbex) | Intubation; maintenance of relaxation | Similar to atracurium | No histamine release | Similar to atracurium |
| Mivacurium (Mivacron) | Intubation; maintenance of relaxation | Short acting; rapid metabolism by plasma cholinesterase; used as bolus or infusion | Expensive in longer cases | New; rarely need to reverse; prolonged effect with plasma cholinesterase deficiency |
| Rocuronium (Zemuron) | Intubation; maintenance of relaxation | Rapid onset (dose-dependent); elimination via kidney and liver | Vagolytic; may ↑ HR | Duration similar to atracurium and vecuronium |
| Vecuronium (Norcuron) | Intubation; maintenance of relaxation | No significant cardiovascular or cumulative effects; no histamine release | Requires mixing | Mostly eliminated in bile, some in urine |

## TABLE 19-2 Commonly Used Intravenous Medications (Continued)

| Medication | Common Usage | Advantages | Disadvantages | Comments |
|---|---|---|---|---|
| **Nondepolarizing Muscle Relaxants—Longer Onset and Duration** | | | | |
| d-Tubocurarine | Maintenance of relaxation | | May cause histamine release and transient ganglionic blockade | Mostly used for pretreatment with succinylcholine |
| Metocurine (Metubine) | Maintenance of relaxation | Good cardiovascular stability | Slight histamine release | Large bolus may cause ↓ BP |
| Pancuronium (Pavulon) | Maintenance of relaxation | | May cause ↑ HR and ↑ BP | Mostly renal elimination |
| **Intravenous Anesthetics** | | | | |
| Etomidate (Amidate) | Induction | Good cardiovascular stability; fast, smooth induction and recovery | May cause pain with injection and myotonic movements | |
| Diazepam (Valium, Dizac) | Amnesia; hypnotic; preoperative medication | Good sedation | Prolonged duration | Residual effects for 20 to 90 hr; increased effect with alcohol |
| Ketamine (Ketalar) | Induction, occasional maintenance (IV or IM) | Short acting; patient maintains airway; good in small children and burn patients | Large doses may cause hallucinations and respiratory depression | Need darkened, quiet room for recovery; often used in trauma cases |
| Midazolam (Versed) | Hypnotic; anxiolytic; sedation; often used as adjunct to induction | Excellent amnesia; water-soluble (no pain with IV injection); short-acting | Slower induction than thiopental | Often used for amnesia with insertion of invasive monitors or regional anesthesia |
| Propofol (Diprivan) | Induction and maintenance; sedation with regional anesthesia or MAC | Rapid onset; awakening in 4 to 8 min | May cause pain when injected | Short elimination half-life (34–64 min) |
| Sodium methohexital (Brevital) | Induction | Ultrashort-acting barbiturate | May cause hiccups | Can be given rectally |
| Thiopental sodium (Pentothal) | Induction | Induction | May cause laryngospasm; can be given rectally | Large doses may cause apnea and cardiovascular depression |

BP, blood pressure; HR, heart rate; IM, intramuscular; IV, intravenous; MAC, monitored anesthesia care; PO, oral; SAB, subarachnoid block; SVR, stroke volume ratio.

Adapted with permission from Table 7-2, "Commonly Used Anesthetic Drugs," pp. 232–234 in Rothrock, J. C. (2003). *Alexander's care of the patient in surgery* (12th ed.). St. Louis: Mosby.

---

because the epidural anesthetic does not make direct contact with the spinal cord or nerve roots.

An advantage of epidural anesthesia is the absence of headache that occasionally results from spinal anesthesia. A disadvantage is the greater technical challenge of introducing the anesthetic into the epidural rather than the subarachnoid space. If inadvertent puncture of the dura occurs during epidural anesthesia and the anesthetic travels toward the head, high spinal anesthesia can result; this can produce severe hypotension and respiratory depression and arrest. Treatment of these complications includes airway support, IV fluids, and use of vasopressors.

## SPINAL ANESTHESIA

Spinal anesthesia is an extensive conduction nerve block that is produced when a local anesthetic is introduced into the subarachnoid space at the lumbar level, usually between L4 and L5 (see Fig. 19-2). It produces anesthesia of the lower extremities, perineum, and lower abdomen. For the lumbar puncture procedure, the patient usually lies on the side in a knee–chest position. Sterile technique is used as a spinal puncture is made and the medication is injected through the needle. As soon as the injection has been made, the patient is positioned on his or her back. If a relatively high level of block is sought, the head and shoulders are lowered.

The spread of the anesthetic agent and the level of anesthesia depend on the amount of fluid injected, the speed with which it is injected, the positioning of the patient after the injection, and the specific gravity of the agent. If the specific gravity is greater than that of cerebrospinal fluid (CSF), the agent moves to the dependent position of the

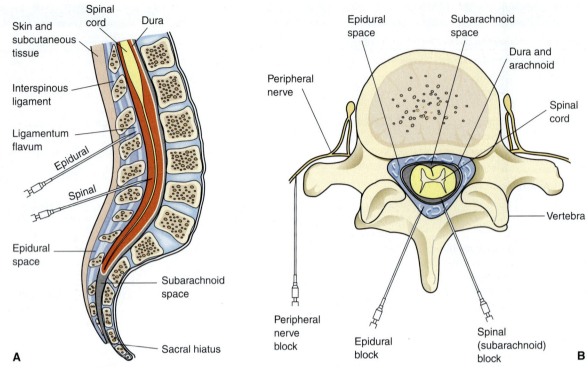

**FIGURE 19-2.** (A) Injection sites for spinal and epidural anesthesia. (B) Cross-section of injection sites for peripheral nerve, epidural, and spinal blocks.

subarachnoid space. If the specific gravity is less than that of CSF, the anesthetic moves away from the dependent position. The anesthesiologist or anesthetist controls the spread of the agent. Table 19-3 contains types of regional anesthesia agents.

A few minutes after induction of a spinal anesthetic, anesthesia and paralysis affect the toes and perineum and then gradually the legs and abdomen. If the anesthetic reaches the upper thoracic and cervical spinal cord in high concentrations, a temporary partial or complete respiratory paralysis results. Paralysis of the respiratory muscles is managed by mechanical ventilation until the effects of the anesthetic on the cranial and thoracic nerves have worn off.

Nausea, vomiting, and pain may occur during surgery when spinal anesthesia is used. As a rule, these reactions result from manipulation of various structures, particularly

### TABLE 19-3 Selected Regional and Local Anesthetic Agents

| Agent | Administration | Advantages | Disadvantages | Implications/Considerations |
|---|---|---|---|---|
| Lidocaine (Xylocaine) | Epidural, spinal, peripheral intravenous anesthesia, and local infiltration | Rapid<br>Longer duration of action (compared with procaine)<br>Free from local irritative effect | Occasional idiosyncrasy | Useful topically for cystoscopy<br>Observe for untoward reactions—drowsiness, depressed respiration, seizures |
| Bupivacaine (Marcaine, Sensoricaine) | Epidural, spinal, peripheral intravenous anesthesia, and local infiltration | Duration is 2–3 times longer than lidocaine | Use cautiously in patients with known drug allergies or sensitivities. | A period of analgesia persists after return of sensation; therefore, need for strong analgesics is reduced.<br>Greater potency and longer action than lidocaine |
| Tetracaine (Pontocaine) | Topical, infiltration, and nerve block | Long acting, produces good relaxation | Occasional allergic reaction | More than 10 times as potent as procaine (Novocaine) |
| Procaine (Novocaine) | Local infiltration | | Occasional allergic reaction | Commonly used in oral or dental surgery |

those within the abdominal cavity. The simultaneous IV administration of a weak solution of thiopental and inhalation of nitrous oxide may prevent such reactions.

Headache may be an after-effect of spinal anesthesia. Several factors are related to the incidence of headache: the size of the spinal needle used, the leakage of fluid from the subarachnoid space through the puncture site, and the patient's hydration status. Measures that increase cerebrospinal pressure are helpful in relieving headache. These include maintaining a quiet environment, keeping the patient lying flat, and keeping the patient well hydrated.

In continuous spinal anesthesia, the tip of a plastic catheter remains in the subarachnoid space during the surgical procedure so that more anesthetic may be injected as needed. This technique allows greater control of the dosage, but there is greater potential for postanesthetic headache because of the large-gauge needle used.

### LOCAL CONDUCTION BLOCKS
Examples of common local conduction blocks are:

- Brachial plexus block, which produces anesthesia of the arm
- Paravertebral anesthesia, which produces anesthesia of the nerves supplying the chest, abdominal wall, and extremities
- Transsacral (caudal) block, which produces anesthesia of the perineum and, occasionally, the lower abdomen

## Moderate Sedation/Analgesia

Moderate sedation (or moderate analgesia), previously referred to as conscious sedation, is a form of anesthesia that involves the IV administration of sedatives and/or analgesic medications to reduce patient anxiety and control pain during diagnostic or therapeutic procedures. It is being used increasingly for specific short-term surgical procedures in hospitals and ambulatory care centers (Rothrock, 2003). The goal is to depress a patient's level of consciousness to a moderate level to enable surgical, diagnostic, or therapeutic procedures to be performed while ensuring the patient's comfort during and cooperation with the procedures. With moderate sedation, the patient is able to maintain a patent airway, retain protective airway reflexes, and respond to verbal and physical stimuli (Morton, Fontaine, Hudak et al., 2005).

Moderate sedation can be administered by an anesthesiologist, anesthetist, or other specially trained and credentialed physician or nurse. The patient receiving moderate sedation is never left alone and is closely monitored by a physician or nurse who is knowledgeable and skilled in detecting dysrhythmias, administering oxygen, and performing resuscitation. The continual assessment of the patient's vital signs, level of consciousness, and cardiac and respiratory function is an essential component of moderate sedation. Pulse oximetry, ECG monitor, and frequent measurement of vital signs are used to monitor the patient. The regulations for use and administration of moderate sedation differ from state to state, and its administration is addressed by standards issued by JCAHO and by institutional policies and nursing specialty organizations, including the Association of PeriAnesthesia Nurses (2004).

## Monitored Anesthesia Care

Monitored anesthesia care (MAC), also referred to as monitored sedation, is administered by an anesthesiologist or anesthetist. Although similar to moderate sedation, the health care provider who administers MAC, usually an anesthesiologist or anesthetist, must be prepared and qualified to convert to general anesthesia if necessary. The skills of an anesthesiologist or anesthetist may be necessary to manage the effects of a level of deeper sedation to return the patient to the appropriate level of sedation (Morton et al., 2005; American Society of Anesthesiologists, 2004). MAC may be used for healthy patients undergoing relatively minor surgical procedures and for some critically ill patients who may be unable to tolerate anesthesia without extensive invasive monitoring and pharmacologic support (Rothrock, 2003). Moderate sedation and monitored anesthesia care are compared in Table 19-4.

## Local Anesthesia

Infiltration anesthesia is the injection of a solution containing the local anesthetic into the tissues at the planned incision site. Often it is combined with a local regional block by injecting the nerves immediately supplying the area. Advantages of local anesthesia are as follows:

- It is simple, economical, and nonexplosive.
- Equipment needed is minimal.
- Postoperative recovery is brief.
- Undesirable effects of general anesthesia are avoided.
- It is ideal for short and superficial surgical procedures.

Local anesthesia is often administered in combination with epinephrine. Epinephrine constricts blood vessels, which prevents rapid absorption of the anesthetic agent

### TABLE 19-4 Comparison of Moderate Sedation and Monitored Anesthesia Care

| | Moderate Sedation | Monitored Anesthesia Care (MAC) |
|---|---|---|
| Responsiveness | Purposeful response to repeated or painful verbal or tactile stimulation | Purposeful response after stimulation |
| Airway | No intervention required | Intervention may be required |
| Spontaneous ventilation | Adequate | May be inadequate |
| Cardiovascular function | Usually maintained | Usually maintained |

From Morton, P. G., Fontaine, D. K., Hudak, C. M. & Gallo, B. M. (2005). *Critical care nursing: A holistic approach* (8th ed.). Philadelphia: Lippincott Williams & Wilkins, p. 179.

and thus prolongs its local action. Rapid absorption of the anesthetic agent into the bloodstream, which could cause seizures, is also prevented. Agents that can be used as local anesthetic agents are listed in Table 19-3; some of the same agents used in regional anesthesia are used as local anesthetics.

Local anesthesia is the preferred method of choice in any surgical procedure in which it can be used. However, contraindications include high preoperative levels of anxiety, because surgery with local anesthesia may increase anxiety. A patient who requests general anesthesia rarely does well under local anesthesia. For some surgical procedures, local anesthesia is impractical because of the number of injections and the amount of anesthetic that would be required (eg, breast reconstruction).

The skin is prepared as for any surgical procedure, and a small-gauge needle is used to inject a modest amount of the anesthetic into the skin layers. This produces blanching or a wheal. Additional anesthetic is then injected into the skin until an area the length of the proposed incision is anesthetized. A larger, longer needle then is used to infiltrate deeper tissues with the anesthetic. The action of the agent is almost immediate, so surgery may begin as soon as the injection is complete. Anesthesia lasts 45 minutes to 3 hours, depending on the anesthetic and the use of epinephrine.

# Potential Intraoperative Complications

The surgical patient is subject to several risks. Potential intraoperative complications include nausea and vomiting, anaphylaxis, hypoxia, hypothermia, malignant hyperthermia, and disseminated intravascular coagulopathy (DIC). The National Surgical Care Improvement Project (SCIP) set a national goal of a 25% reduction in surgical complications by 2010. Targeted areas include surgical site infections, as well as cardiac, respiratory, and venous thromboembolic complications. A SCIP committee has been formed to develop a quality improvement framework to improve both patient safety and the quality of surgical services nationwide (SCIP, 2005).

## Nausea and Vomiting

Nausea and vomiting, or regurgitation, may affect patients during the intraoperative period. If gagging occurs, the patient is turned to the side, the head of the table is lowered, and a basin is provided to collect the vomitus. Suction is used to remove saliva and vomited gastric contents. The advent of new anesthetics has reduced the incidence; however, there is no single way to prevent nausea and vomiting. An interdisciplinary approach involving the surgeon, anesthesiologist or anesthetist, and nurse is best.

In some cases, the anesthesiologist or anesthetist administers antiemetics preoperatively or intraoperatively to counteract possible aspiration. If the patient aspirates vomitus, an asthma-like attack with severe bronchial spasms and wheezing is triggered. Pneumonitis and pulmonary edema can subsequently develop, leading to extreme hypoxia. Increasing medical attention is being paid to silent regurgitation of gastric contents (not related to preoperative fasting times), which occurs more frequently than previously realized. The volume and acidity of the aspirate determine the extent of damage to the lungs. Patients may be given Bicitra, a clear, nonparticulate antacid to increase gastric fluid pH or a histamine-2 ($H_2$) receptor antagonist such as cimetidine (Tagamet), ranitidine (Zantac), or famotidine (Pepcid) to decrease gastric acid production (Rothrock, 2003).

## Anaphylaxis

Any time the patient comes into contact with a foreign substance, there is the potential for an anaphylactic reaction. Because medications are the most common cause of anaphylaxis, intraoperative nurses must be aware of the type and method of anesthesia used as well as the specific agents. An anaphylactic reaction can occur in response to many medications, latex, or other substances. The reaction may be immediate or delayed. Anaphylaxis is a life-threatening acute allergic reaction. See Chapters 15 and 53 for more details about the signs, symptoms, and treatment of anaphylaxis.

Fibrin sealants are used in a variety of surgical procedures, and cyanoacrylate tissue adhesives are used to close wounds without the use of sutures. These sealants have been implicated in allergic reactions and anaphylaxis (Phillips, 2004). Although these reactions are rare, the nurse must be alert to the possibility and observe the patient for changes in vital signs and symptoms of anaphylaxis when these products are used.

## Hypoxia and Other Respiratory Complications

Inadequate ventilation, occlusion of the airway, inadvertent intubation of the esophagus, and hypoxia are significant potential complications associated with general anesthesia. Many factors can contribute to inadequate ventilation. Respiratory depression caused by anesthetic agents, aspiration of respiratory tract secretions or vomitus, and the patient's position on the operating table can compromise the exchange of gases. Anatomic variation can make the trachea difficult to visualize and result in the artificial airway's being inserted into the esophagus rather than into the trachea. In addition to these dangers, asphyxia caused by foreign bodies in the mouth, spasm of the vocal cords, relaxation of the tongue, or aspiration of vomitus, saliva, or blood can occur. Brain damage from hypoxia occurs within minutes; therefore, vigilant monitoring of the patient's oxygenation status is a primary function of the anesthesiologist or anesthetist and the circulating nurse. Peripheral perfusion is checked frequently, and pulse oximetry values are monitored continuously.

## Hypothermia

During anesthesia, the patient's temperature may fall. Glucose metabolism is reduced, and, as a result, metabolic acidosis may develop. This condition is called hypothermia and is indicated by a core body temperature that is lower than normal (36.6°C [98.0°F] or less). Inadvertent hypothermia may occur as a result of a low temperature in the OR, infusion of cold fluids, inhalation of cold gases, open body wounds or cavities, decreased muscle activity, advanced age, or the pharmaceutical agents used (eg, vasodilators, phenothiazines, general anesthetics). Hypothermia may also be intentionally induced in selected surgical procedures (eg, cardiac surgeries requiring cardiopulmonary bypass) to reduce the patient's metabolic rate and energy demands (Seifert, 2002).

Preventing unintentional hypothermia is a major objective. If hypothermia occurs, the goal of intervention is to minimize or reverse the physiologic process. If hypothermia is intentional, the goal is safe return to normal body temperature. Environmental temperature in the OR can temporarily be set at 25° to 26.6°C (78° to 80°F). IV and irrigating fluids are warmed to 37°C (98.6°F). Wet gowns and drapes are removed promptly and replaced with dry materials, because wet linens promote heat loss. Whatever methods are used to rewarm the patient, warming must be accomplished gradually, not rapidly. Conscientious monitoring of core temperature, urinary output, ECG, blood pressure, arterial blood gas levels, and serum electrolyte levels is required.

## Malignant Hyperthermia

Malignant hyperthermia is a rare inherited muscle disorder that is chemically induced by anesthetic agents (Rothrock, 2003). At one time, mortality rates exceeded 80%. Since the introduction of dantrolene sodium in 1979, the development of genetics testing, and early detection and treatment with specific protocols, fatalities have been reduced to approximately 10% (McCarthy, 2004). However, identification of patients at risk for malignant hyperthermia is imperative. Susceptible people include those with strong and bulky muscles, a history of muscle cramps or muscle weakness and unexplained temperature elevation, and an unexplained death of a family member during surgery that was accompanied by a febrile response (Litman & Rosenberg, 2005).

### Pathophysiology

During anesthesia, potent agents such as inhalation anesthetics (halothane, enflurane) and muscle relaxants (succinylcholine) may trigger the symptoms of malignant hyperthermia (Rothrock, 2003). Stress and some medications, such as sympathomimetics (epinephrine), theophylline, aminophylline, anticholinergics (atropine), and cardiac glycosides (digitalis), can induce or intensify such a reaction.

The pathophysiology is related to a hypermetabolic condition in skeletal muscle cells that involves altered mechanisms of calcium function at the cellular level. This disruption of calcium causes clinical symptoms of hypermetabolism, which in turn increases muscle contraction (rigidity) and causes hyperthermia and subsequent damage to the central nervous system.

### Clinical Manifestations

The initial symptoms of malignant hyperthermia are related to cardiovascular and musculoskeletal activity. Tachycardia (heart rate greater than 150 bpm) is often the earliest sign. In addition to the tachycardia, sympathetic nervous stimulation leads to ventricular dysrhythmia, hypotension, decreased cardiac output, oliguria, and, later, cardiac arrest. With the abnormal transport of calcium, rigidity or tetanus-like movements occur, often in the jaw. The rise in temperature is actually a late sign that develops rapidly; body temperature can increase 1° to 2°C (2° to 4°F) every 5 minutes (Rothrock, 2003). The core body temperature can reach or exceed 42°C (104°F) in a very short time and must be properly monitored and recorded during surgery (McCarthy, 2004).

### Medical Management

Recognizing symptoms early and discontinuing anesthesia promptly are imperative. Goals of treatment are to decrease metabolism, reverse metabolic and respiratory acidosis, correct dysrhythmias, decrease body temperature, provide oxygen and nutrition to tissues, and correct electrolyte imbalance. The Malignant Hyperthermia Association of the United States (MHAUS) publishes a treatment protocol that should be posted in the OR and be readily available on a malignant hyperthermia cart.

As soon as the diagnosis is made, anesthesia and surgery are halted and the patient is hyperventilated with 100% oxygen. Dantrolene sodium (Dantrium), a skeletal muscle relaxant, and sodium bicarbonate are administered immediately (McCarthy, 2004). Continued monitoring of all parameters is necessary to evaluate the patient's status. Although malignant hyperthermia usually manifests about 10 to 20 minutes after induction of anesthesia, it can also occur during the first 24 hours after surgery.

### Nursing Management

Although malignant hyperthermia is uncommon, the nurse must identify patients at risk, recognize the signs and symptoms, have the appropriate medication and equipment available, and be knowledgeable about the protocol to follow. This preparation may be lifesaving for the patient.

## Disseminated Intravascular Coagulation

Disseminated intravascular coagulation (also referred to as coagulopathy [DIC]) is a life-threatening condition that is characterized by thrombus formation in the microcirculation and depletion of select coagulation proteins, causing hemorrhaging. The exact cause is unknown, but predisposing factors include many conditions that may occur with emergency surgery, such as massive trauma, head injury, massive transfusion, liver or kidney involvement, embolic events, and shock. The signs and symptoms, nursing assessment, and treatment of DIC are discussed in Chapter 33.

## Nursing Process

### The Patient During Surgery

The Perioperative Nursing Data Set (PNDS) is a helpful model used by nurses in the intraoperative phase of care (see Fig. 18-1 in Chapter 18). Phenomena of concern to intraoperative nurses are nursing diagnoses, interventions, and outcomes that surgical patients and their families experience. Additional areas of concern include collaborative problems and expected goals.

### Assessment

Nursing assessment of the intraoperative patient involves obtaining data from the patient and the patient's record to identify variables that can affect care and serve as guidelines for developing an individualized plan of patient care. The intraoperative nurse uses the focused preoperative nursing assessment documented on the patient record. This includes assessment of physiologic status (eg, health–illness level, level of consciousness), psychosocial status (eg, anxiety level, verbal communication problems, coping mechanisms), physical status (eg, surgical site, skin condition, and effectiveness of preparation; immobile joints), and ethical concerns (Chart 19-3).

### Diagnosis

#### Nursing Diagnoses

Based on the assessment data, some major nursing diagnoses may include the following:

- Anxiety related to expressed concerns due to surgery or OR environment
- Risk for perioperative positioning injury related to positioning in the OR
- Risk for injury related to anesthesia and surgery
- Disturbed sensory perception (global) related to general anesthesia or sedation

#### Collaborative Problems/ Potential Complications

Based on the assessment data, potential complications may include the following:

- Nausea and vomiting
- Anaphylaxis
- Hypoxia
- Unintentional hypothermia
- Malignant hyperthermia
- DIC
- Infection

### CHART 19-3
### Ethics and Related Issues

#### To Resuscitate or Not?
**SITUATION**
Your ambulatory care center has developed a policy, authorized through the medical staff, that allows for patients to have a do-not-resuscitate order (DNR) in place during a surgical procedure. This policy follows the American Society of Anesthesiologists guidelines for DNR in the OR. You are preparing a patient for surgery, and the anesthesiologist who will be administering the anesthetic writes an order for the DNR to be rescinded during surgery. The physician is refusing to talk to the patient concerning the DNR.

**PROBLEM**
The patient believes his/her wishes will be followed with regard to resuscitation in the event of a cardiac arrest and the physician does not believe he can administer anesthesia if the DNR is in place.

**DISCUSSION**
- What are the rights of the patient with regard to advance directives?
- What can you do to advocate for the patient?
- Should you contact the ethics committee of the hospital?
- How do you contact the ethics committee?

### Planning and Goals

Goals for care of the patient during surgery include reducing anxiety, preventing positioning injuries, maintaining safety, maintaining the patient's dignity, and avoiding complications.

### Nursing Interventions

#### Reducing Anxiety

The OR environment can seem cold, stark, and frightening to the patient, who may be feeling isolated and apprehensive. Introducing yourself, addressing the patient by name warmly and frequently, verifying details, providing explanations, and encouraging and answering questions provide a sense of professionalism and friendliness that can help the patient feel secure. When discussing what the patient can expect in surgery, the nurse uses basic communication skills, such as touch and eye contact, to reduce anxiety.

Attention to physical comfort (warm blankets, position changes) helps the patient feel more comfortable. Telling the patient who else will be present in the OR, how long the procedure is expected to take, and other details helps the patient prepare for the experience and gain a sense of control.

### Preventing Intraoperative Positioning Injury

The patient's position on the operating table depends on the surgical procedure to be performed as well as on the patient's physical condition (Fig. 19-3). The potential for transient discomfort or permanent injury is present, because many positions are awkward. Hyperextending joints, compressing arteries, or pressing on nerves and bony prominences usually results in discomfort simply because the position must be sustained for a long period of time (Rothrock, 2003). Factors to consider include the following:

- The patient should be in as comfortable a position as possible, whether conscious or unconscious.
- The operative field must be adequately exposed.
- An awkward position, undue pressure on a body part, or use of stirrups or traction should not obstruct the vascular supply.
- Respiration should not be impeded by pressure of arms on the chest or by a gown that constricts the neck or chest.
- Nerves must be protected from undue pressure. Improper positioning of the arms, hands, legs, or feet can cause serious injury or paralysis. Shoulder braces must be well padded to prevent irreparable nerve injury, especially when the Trendelenburg position is necessary.
- Precautions for patient safety must be observed, particularly with thin, elderly, or obese patients and those with a physical deformity.
- The patient may need light restraint before induction in case of excitement.

The usual position for surgery, called the dorsal recumbent position, is flat on the back. One arm is positioned at the side of the table, with the hand placed palm down; the other is carefully positioned on an

A Patient in position on the operating table for a laparotomy. Note the strap above the knees.

B Patient in Trendelenburg position on operating table. Note padded shoulder braces in place. Be sure that brace does not press on brachial plexus.

C Patient in lithotomy position. Note that the hips extend over the edge of the table.

D Patient lies on unaffected side for kidney surgery. Table is spread apart to provide space between the lower ribs and the pelvis. The upper leg is extended; the lower leg is flexed at the knee and the hip joints; a pillow is placed between the legs.

**FIGURE 19-3.** Positions on the operating table. Captions call attention to safety and comfort features. All surgical patients wear caps to cover the hair completely.

armboard to facilitate IV infusion of fluids, blood, or medications. This position is used for most abdominal surgeries except for surgery of the gallbladder or pelvis (see Fig. 19-3A).

The Trendelenburg position usually is used for surgery on the lower abdomen and pelvis to obtain good exposure by displacing the intestines into the upper abdomen. In this position, the head and body are lowered. The patient is held in position by padded shoulder braces (see Fig. 19-3B).

The lithotomy position is used for nearly all perineal, rectal, and vaginal surgical procedures (see Fig. 19-3C). The patient is positioned on the back with the legs and thighs flexed. The position is maintained by placing the feet in stirrups.

The Sims' or lateral position is used for renal surgery. The patient is placed on the nonoperative side with an air pillow 12.5 to 15 cm (5 to 6 inches) thick under the loin, or on a table with a kidney or back lift (see Fig. 19-3D).

Other procedures, such as neurosurgery or abdominothoracic surgery, may require unique positioning and supplemental apparatus, depending on the operative approach (Bohan & Glass-Macenka, 2004).

### Protecting the Patient From Injury

A variety of activities are used to address the diverse patient safety issues that arise in the OR. The nurse protects the patient from injury by providing a safe environment. Verifying information, checking the chart for completeness, and maintaining surgical asepsis and an optimal environment are critical nursing responsibilities. Verifying that all required documentation is completed is one of the first functions of the intraoperative nurse. The patient is identified, and the planned surgical procedure, correct surgical site, and type of anesthesia are verified. It is important to review the patient's record for the following:

- Correct informed surgical consent, with patient's signature
- Completed records for health history and physical examination
- Results of diagnostic studies
- Allergies (including latex)

In addition to checking that all necessary patient data are complete, the perioperative nurse obtains the necessary equipment specific to the procedure. The need for nonroutine medications, blood components, instruments, and other equipment and supplies is assessed, and the readiness of the room, completeness of physical setup, and completeness of instrument, suture, and dressing setups are determined. Any aspects of the OR environment that may negatively affect the patient are identified. These include physical features, such as room temperature and humidity; electrical hazards; potential contaminants (dust, blood, and discharge on floor or surfaces, uncovered hair, faulty attire of personnel, jewelry worn by personnel); and unnecessary traffic. The circulating nurse also sets up and maintains suction equipment in working order, sets up invasive monitoring equipment, assists with insertion of vascular access and monitoring devices (arterial, Swan-Ganz, central venous pressure, IV lines), and initiates appropriate physical comfort measures for the patient.

Preventing physical injury includes using safety straps and side rails and not leaving the sedated patient unattended. Transferring the patient from the stretcher to the OR table requires safe transferring practices. Other safety measures include properly positioning the grounding pad under the patient to prevent electrical burns and shock, removing excess antiseptic solution from the patient's skin, and promptly and completely draping exposed areas after the sterile field has been created to decrease the risk for hypothermia.

Nursing measures to prevent injury from excessive blood loss include blood conservation using equipment such as a cell-saver (a device for recirculating the patient's own blood cells) and administration of blood products (Phillips, 2004). Few patients undergoing an elective procedure require blood transfusion, but those undergoing higher-risk procedures (such as orthopedic or cardiac surgeries) may require an intraoperative transfusion. The circulating nurse anticipates this need, checks that blood has been cross-matched and held in reserve, and is prepared to administer blood.

### Serving as Patient Advocate

Because the patient undergoing general anesthesia or moderate sedation experiences temporary sensory/perceptual alteration or loss, he or she has an increased need for protection and advocacy. Patient advocacy in the OR entails maintaining the patient's physical and emotional comfort, privacy, rights, and dignity. Patients, whether conscious or unconscious, should not be subjected to excess noise, inappropriate conversation, or, most of all, derogatory comments. As surprising as this sounds, banter in the OR occasionally includes jokes about the patient's physical appearance, job, personal history, and so forth. Cases have been reported in which seemingly deeply anesthetized patients recalled the entire surgical experience, including disparaging personal remarks made by OR personnel. As an advocate, the nurse never engages in this conversation and discourages others from doing so. Other advocacy activities include minimizing the clinical, dehumanizing aspects of being a surgical patient by making sure the patient is treated as a person, respecting cultural and spiritual values, providing physical privacy, and maintaining confidentiality.

### Monitoring and Managing Potential Complications

It is the responsibility of the surgeon and the anesthesiologist or anesthetist to monitor and manage complications. However, intraoperative nurses also play an important role. Being alert to and reporting changes in vital signs and symptoms of nausea and vomiting, anaphylaxis, hypoxia, hypothermia, malignant hyperthermia, or DIC and assisting with their management are important nursing functions. Each of these complications was discussed earlier. Maintaining asepsis and preventing infection are responsibilities of all members of the surgical team (Phillips, 2004; Rothrock, 2003).

## Evaluation

### Expected Patient Outcomes

Expected patient outcomes may include the following:

1. Exhibits low level of anxiety while awake during the intraoperative phase of care
2. Remains free of perioperative positioning injury
3. Experiences no unexpected threats to safety
4. Has dignity preserved throughout OR experience
5. Is free of complications (nausea and vomiting, anaphylaxis, hypoxia, hypothermia, malignant hyperthermia, or DIC) or experiences successful management of adverse effects of surgery and anesthesia should they occur.

## Critical Thinking Exercises

1. An 80-year-old patient with Parkinson's disease is scheduled for surgery to replace a fractured hip. Identify the considerations and associated responsibilities of the OR nurse for safe intraoperative care of this patient.

2. **ebp** A patient has a large open lower-extremity wound caused by a motorcycle accident and is undergoing emergency surgery. What resources would you use to identify the current guidelines for surgical asepsis? What is the evidence base for current patient and environmental surgical asepsis practices? Identify the criteria used to evaluate the strength of the evidence for these practices.

3. A patient develops a temperature of 38°C (100°F) and becomes tachycardic halfway through an abdominal surgery. Five minutes later, the patient's temperature is 42°C (104°F). Describe the protocol you would follow and the medication you would administer for this condition.

4. **ebp** A patient with an infected wound is undergoing an incision and drainage in the OR. Develop an evidence-based plan of care that will reduce the risk of contamination and infection.

## REFERENCES AND SELECTED READINGS

### BOOKS

American Society of Anesthesiologists. (2004). *Distinguishing monitored anesthesia care ("MAC") from moderate sedation/analgesia (conscious sedation).* http://www.asahq.org/publicationsAndServices/standards/35.pdf (accessed May 30, 2006).

American Society of PeriAnesthesia Nurses. (2002). *Standards of perianesthesia nursing practice.* Thorofare, NJ: ASPAN.

AORN standards, recommended practice, and guidelines (2004b). Denver: AORN, Inc.

Clancy, J., McVicar, A. J. & Baird, N. (2002). *Perioperative practice: Fundamentals of homeostasis.* New York: Routledge.

Conner, R. (2004). *Ambulatory surgery principles and practices* (3rd ed.). Denver: AORN, Inc.

Defazio-Quinn, D. & Schick, L. (Eds.). (2004). *Nursing core curriculum-preoperative, phase I and phase II PACU nursing.* Philadelphia: W. B. Saunders.

Joint Commission on Accreditation of Healthcare Organizations (JCAHO). (2004). Sentinel alert: Patient alert under anesthesia. http://www.jcaho.org (accessed March 31, 2006).

Kleinbeck, S. V. M. (2004). *Perioperative nursing data set at work: Policies, procedures and pathways.* Denver: AORN, Inc.

Miller, R. D. (2005). *Miller's anesthesia* (6th ed.). Philadelphia: Elsevier.

Morton, P. G., Fontaine, D. K., Hudak, C. M., et al. (2005). *Critical care nursing: A holistic approach* (8th ed.). Philadelphia: Lippincott Williams & Wilkins.

Murray, M. J., Coursin, D. B., Pearl, R. G., et al. (2002). *Critical care medicine: Perioperative management* (2nd ed.). Philadelphia: Lippincott Williams & Wilkins.

NANDA International. (2005). *NANDA: Nursing diagnoses: Definitions and classification.* Philadelphia: NANDA International.

Phillips, N. (2004). *Berry and Kohn's operating room technique* (10th ed.). St. Louis: Mosby.

Rothrock, J. C. (Ed.). (2003). *Alexander's care of the patient in surgery* (12th ed.). St. Louis: Mosby.

Seifert, P. C. (2002). *Cardiac surgery: Perioperative patient care.* St Louis: Mosby.

Surgical Care Improvement Project (SCIP). (2005). Available at: http://www.medqic.org/scip/scip_contact.html. Accessed May 7, 2006.

Tighe, S. M. (2003). *Instrumentation for the operating room: A photographic manual.* St. Louis: Mosby.

### JOURNALS

*Asterisks indicate nursing research articles.

Andersen, K. (2004). Safe use of lasers in the operating room, *AORN Journal, 79*(1), 171–188.

AORN. (2004a). AORN latex guideline. *AORN Journal, 79*(3), 653–672.

Beyea, S. (2003). Keeping patients safe from infection. *AORN Journal, 78*(1), 133–140.

Bohan, E. & Glass-Macenka, D. (2004). Surgical management of patients with primary brain tumors. *Seminars in Oncology Nursing, 29*(4), 240–252.

DeFazio-Quinn, D. M. (2006). How religion, language and ethnicity impact perioperative nursing care. *Nursing Clinics of North America, 41*(2), 231–248.

Gawande, A. A., Studdert, D. M., Orav, E. J., et al. (2003). Risk for retained instruments and sponges after surgery. *New England Journal of Medicine, 348*(3), 229–235.

Gotta, A. W. (2004). Anesthetic management of the patient with HIV infection. *Current Reviews for Nurse Anesthetists, 27*(11), 117–128.

Gupta, A., Della-Latta, P., Todd, B., et al. (2004) Outbreak of extended-spectrum beta-lactamase-producing *Klebsiella pneumoniae* in a neonatal intensive care unit linked to artificial nails. *Infection Control and Hospital Epidemiology, 25*(3), 210–215.

*Hammarsten, R., Hammarsten, J. & Jemsby, P. (2003). Preoperative skin testing of materials used in surgical procedures. *AORN Journal, 77*(4), 762–771.

Houck, P. M. (2006). Comparison of operating room lasers: Uses, hazards, guidelines. *Nursing Clinics of North America, 41*(2), 193–218.

John, A. D. & Sieber, F. E. (2004). Age associated issues: Geriatrics. *Anesthesiology Clinic of North America, 22*(1), 45–58.

Joint Commission on Accreditation of Healthcare Organizations (JCAHO). (2005). JCAHO issues 2005 patient safety goals. *OR Manager, 20*(9), 5–8.

Litman, R. S. & Rosenberg H. (2005). Malignant hyperthermia: Update on susceptibility testing. *Journal of American Medical Association, 293*(23), 2918–2924.

McCarthy, E. (2004). Malignant hyperthermia. *AACN Clinical Issues, 15*(2), 231–237.

O'Connell, M. P. (2006). Positioning impact on the surgical patient. *Nursing Clinics of North America, 41*(2), 173–192.

Owens, T. M (2006). Bariatric surgery risks, benefits, and care of the morbidly obese. *Nursing Clinics of North America, 41*(2), 249–263.

Paulson, D. (2004). Hand scrub products-performance requirements. *AORN Journal, 80*(2), 225–234.

Pine, M., Holt, K. D. & Lou, Y. (2003). Surgical mortality and type of anesthesia provider. *AANA Journal, 71*(2), 109–116.

Pofahl, W. & Pories, W. (2003). Current status and future directions of geriatric general surgery. *Journal of American Geriatric Society, 51*(7), S351–S354.

Pryor, K. O., Fahey, T. J., Lien, C. A., et al. (2004). Surgical site infection and the routine use of perioperative hyperoxia in a general surgical population: A randomized controlled trial. *Journal of American Medical Association, 291*(1), 79–87.

Salmon, L. (2004). Fire in the OR: Prevention and preparedness. *AORN Journal, 80*(1), 41–54.

Saufl, N. M. (2004). Preparing the older adult for surgery and anesthesia. *Journal of PeriAnesthesia Nursing, 19*(6), 372–377.

Wadlund, D. L. (2006). Prevention, recognition, and management of nursing complications in the intraoperative and postoperative surgical patient. *Nursing Clinics of North America, 41*(2), 151–171.

Wadlund, D. L. (2006). Laparoscopy: Risks, benefits and complications. *Nursing Clinics of North America, 41*(2), 219–229.

Williams, J. & Barbul, A. (2003). Nutrition and wound healing. *Surgical Clinics of America, 83*(3), 571–596.

*Yellen, E. (2003). The influence of nurse-sensitive variables. *AORN Journal, 78*(5), 783–793.

## RESOURCES

American Latex Allergy Association; toll-free 888-972-5378; fax 262-677-2808; http://www.latexallergyresources.org. Accessed March 31, 2006.

American Society of Anesthesiologists, 520 N. Northwest Highway, Park Ridge, IL, 60068; 847-825-2286; http://www.asahq.org. Accessed March 31, 2006.

American Society of PeriAnesthesia Nurses, 10 Melrose Ave., Suite 110, Cherry Hill, NJ 08003; toll-free 877-9696; fax 856-616-9621; http://www.aspan.org. Accessed March 31, 2006.

Association of PeriOperative Registered Nurses, Inc., 2170 S. Parker Rd., Suite 300, Denver, CO 80231; 800-755-2676; http://www.aorn.org. Accessed March 31, 2006.

Centers for Disease Control and Prevention, National Center for Injury Prevention and Control, Mailstop K65, 4770 Buford Highway NE, Atlanta, GA 30341; 770-488-1506; http://www.cdc.gov/nipc/. Accessed March 31, 2006.

Joint Commission on Accreditation Healthcare Organizations (JCAHO), 1 Renaissance Blvd., Oakbrook Terrace, IL; 877-223-6866; http://www.jcaho.org. Accessed March 31, 2006.

Malignant Hyperthermia Association of the United States (MHAUS), 39 East State Street, P.O. Box 1069, Sherburne, NY 13460; 607-674-7901; http://www.mhaus.org. Accessed March 31, 2006.

National SCIP Partnership, Oklahoma Foundation for Medical Quality, 14000 Quail Springs Parkway, Suite 400, Oklahoma City, OK 73134; 405-840-2891 ext. 278; http://www.medqic.org/scip. Accessed May 7, 2006.

# CHAPTER 20

# Postoperative Nursing Management

## Learning Objectives

*On completion of this chapter, the learner will be able to:*

1. Describe the responsibilities of the postanesthesia care unit nurse in the prevention of immediate postoperative complications.
2. Compare postoperative care of the ambulatory surgery patient with that of the hospitalized surgery patient.
3. Identify common postoperative problems and their management.
4. Describe the gerontologic considerations related to postoperative management.
5. Describe variables that affect wound healing.
6. Demonstrate postoperative dressing techniques.
7. Identify assessment parameters appropriate for the early detection of postoperative complications.

The postoperative period extends from the time the patient leaves the operating room (OR) until the last follow-up visit with the surgeon. This may be as short as 1 week or as long as several months. During the postoperative period, nursing care focuses on reestablishing the patient's physiologic equilibrium, alleviating pain, preventing complications, and teaching the patient self-care. Careful assessment and immediate intervention assist the patient in returning to optimal function quickly, safely, and as comfortably as possible. Ongoing care in the community through home care, clinic visits, office visits, or telephone follow-up facilitates an uncomplicated recovery.

## The Postanesthesia Care Unit

The **postanesthesia care unit (PACU)**, also called the recovery room or postanesthesia recovery room, is located adjacent to the operating rooms suite (Phillips, 2004). Patients still under anesthesia or recovering from anesthesia are placed in this unit for easy access to experienced, highly skilled nurses, anesthesiologists or anesthetists, surgeons, advanced hemodynamic and pulmonary monitoring and support, special equipment, and medications.

The PACU is kept quiet, clean, and free of unnecessary equipment. This area is painted in soft, pleasing colors and has indirect lighting. The PACU should also be well ventilated. These features benefit the patient by helping to decrease anxiety and promote comfort. The PACU bed provides easy access to the patient, is safe and easily movable, can readily be positioned to facilitate use of measures to counteract shock and other complications, and has features that facilitate care, such as intravenous (IV) poles, side rails and wheel brakes.

## Phases of Postanesthesia Care

Postanesthesia care in some hospitals and ambulatory surgical centers is divided into three phases (Phillips, 2004). In the **phase I PACU**, used during the immediate recovery phase, intensive nursing care is provided. In the **phase II PACU**, the patient is prepared for self-care or care in the hospital or an extended care setting. In **phase III PACU**, the patient is prepared for discharge. Recliners rather than stretchers or beds are standard in many phase III units, which may also be referred to as step-down, sit-up, or progressive care units. Patients may remain in a PACU unit for as long as 4 to 6 hours, depending on the type of surgery and any preexisting conditions. In facilities without separate phase I, II, and III units, the patient remains in the PACU and may be discharged home directly from this unit.

All PACU nurses have special skills, including strong assessment skills. The PACU nurse provides frequent (every 15 minutes) monitoring of the patient's pulse, electrocardiogram, respiratory rate, blood pressure, and pulse oximeter value (blood oxygen level). In some cases, the end-tidal carbon dioxide ($ETCO_2$) level is monitored as well. The patient's airway may become obstructed because of the latent effects of recent anesthesia, and the PACU nurse must be prepared to assist in reintubation and in handling other emergencies that may occur. Nurses in the phase II and III PACUs must also possess excellent patient teaching skills.

## Admitting the Patient to the PACU

Transferring the postoperative patient from the OR to the PACU is the responsibility of the anesthesiologist or anesthetist. During transport from the OR to the PACU, the anesthesia provider remains at the head of the stretcher (to maintain the airway), and a surgical team member remains at the opposite end. Transporting the patient involves special consideration of the incision site, potential vascular changes, and exposure. The surgical incision is considered every time the postoperative patient is moved; many wounds are closed under considerable tension, and every effort is made to prevent further strain on the incision. The patient is positioned so that he or she is not lying on and obstructing drains or drainage tubes. Serious orthostatic hypotension may occur when a patient is moved too quickly from one position to another (eg, from a lithotomy position to a horizontal position or from a lateral to a supine position), so the patient must be moved slowly and carefully. As soon as the patient is placed on the stretcher or bed, the soiled gown is removed and replaced with a dry gown. The patient

## Glossary

**dehiscence:** partial or complete separation of wound edges
**evisceration:** protrusion of organs through the surgical incision
**first-intention healing:** method of healing in which wound edges are surgically approximated and integumentary continuity is restored without granulation
**Phase I PACU:** area designated for care of surgical patients immediately after surgery and for patients whose condition warrants close monitoring
**Phase II PACU:** area designated for care of surgical patients who have been transferred from a phase I PACU because their condition no longer requires the close monitoring provided in a phase I PACU

**Phase III PACU:** setting in which the patient is cared for in the immediate postoperative period and then prepared for discharge from the facility
**postanesthesia care unit (PACU):** area where postoperative patients are monitored as they recover from anesthesia; formerly referred to as the recovery room or postanesthesia recovery room
**second-intention healing:** method of healing in which wound edges are not surgically approximated and integumentary continuity is restored by the process known as granulation
**third-intention healing:** method of healing in which surgical approximation of wound edges is delayed and integumentary continuity is restored by apposing areas of granulation

is covered with lightweight blankets and warmed. Three side rails may be raised to prevent falls.

The nurse who admits the patient to the PACU reviews essential information with the anesthesiologist or anesthetist (Chart 20-1) (Defazio-Quinn & Schick, 2004; Morton, Fontaine, Hudak, et al., 2005).

## Nursing Management in the PACU

The nursing management objectives for the patient in the PACU are to provide care until the patient has recovered from the effects of anesthesia (eg, until resumption of motor and sensory functions), is oriented, has stable vital signs, and shows no evidence of hemorrhage or other complications.

### Assessing the Patient

Frequent, skilled assessments of the blood oxygen saturation level, pulse rate and regularity, depth and nature of respirations, skin color, level of consciousness, and ability to respond to commands are the cornerstones of nursing care in the PACU. The nurse performs a baseline assessment, then checks the surgical site for drainage or hemorrhage and makes sure that all drainage tubes and monitoring lines are connected and functioning. The nurse checks any IV fluids or medications currently infusing and verifies dosage and rate.

After the initial assessment, the patient's vital signs and general physical status are assessed at least every 15 minutes (Defazio-Quinn & Schick, 2004). Patency of the airway and respiratory function are always evaluated first, followed by assessment of cardiovascular function, the condition of the surgical site, and function of the central nervous system. The nurse must be aware of any pertinent information from the patient's history that may be significant (eg, patient is deaf or hard of hearing, has a history of seizures, has diabetes, is allergic to certain medications or to latex).

### Maintaining a Patent Airway

The primary objective in the immediate postoperative period is to maintain pulmonary ventilation and thus prevent hypoxemia (reduced oxygen in the blood) and hypercapnia (excess carbon dioxide in the blood). Both can occur if the airway is obstructed and ventilation is reduced (hypoventilation). Besides checking the physician's orders for and administering supplemental oxygen, the nurse assesses respiratory rate and depth, ease of respirations, oxygen saturation, and breath sounds.

Patients who have experienced prolonged anesthesia usually are unconscious, with all muscles relaxed. This relaxation extends to the muscles of the pharynx. When the patient lies on his or her back, the lower jaw and the tongue fall backward and the air passages become obstructed (Fig. 20-1A). This is called hypopharyngeal obstruction. Signs of occlusion include choking; noisy and irregular respirations; decreased oxygen saturation scores; and within minutes, a blue, dusky color (cyanosis) of the skin. Because movement of the thorax and the diaphragm does not necessarily indicate that the patient is breathing, the nurse needs to place the palm of the hand at the patient's nose and mouth to feel the exhaled breath.

> **NURSING ALERT**
>
> The treatment of hypopharyngeal obstruction involves tilting the head back and pushing forward on the angle of the lower jaw, as if to push the lower teeth in front of the upper teeth (see Fig. 20-1B,C). This maneuver pulls the tongue forward and opens the air passages.

The anesthesiologist or anesthetist may leave a hard rubber or plastic airway in the patient's mouth (Fig. 20-2) to maintain a patent airway. Such a device should not be removed until signs such as gagging indicate that reflex action is returning. Alternatively, the patient may enter the PACU with an endotracheal tube still in place and may require continued mechanical ventilation. The nurse assists in initiating the use of the ventilator and in the weaning and extubation processes. Some patients, particularly those who have had extensive or lengthy surgical procedures, may be transferred from the OR directly to the intensive care unit (ICU) or from the PACU to the ICU while still intubated and receiving mechanical ventilation.

Respiratory difficulty can also result from excessive secretion of mucus or aspiration of vomitus. Turning the patient to one side allows the collected fluid to escape from the side of the mouth (Defazio-Quinn & Schick, 2004). If the teeth are clenched, the mouth may be opened manually but cautiously with a padded tongue depressor. The head of the bed is elevated 15 to 30 degrees unless contraindicated, and

---

**CHART 20-1**

### Anesthesia Provider-to-Nurse Report: Information to Convey

- Name of patient
- Surgical procedure
- Anesthetic options (agents and reversal agents used)
- Estimated blood loss/fluid loss
- Fluid/blood replacement
- Vital signs—significant problems
- Complications encountered (anesthetic or surgical)
- Preoperative condition (eg, diabetes, hypertension, allergies)
- Considerations for immediate postoperative period (pain management, reversals, ventilator settings)
- Language barrier

Ideally, the anesthesia provider should not leave the patient until the nurse is satisfied with the patient's airway and immediate condition.

From Morton, P. G., Fontaine D. K., Hudak, C. M., et al. (2005). *Critical care nursing: A holistic approach* (8th ed.). Philadelphia: Lippincott Williams & Wilkins.

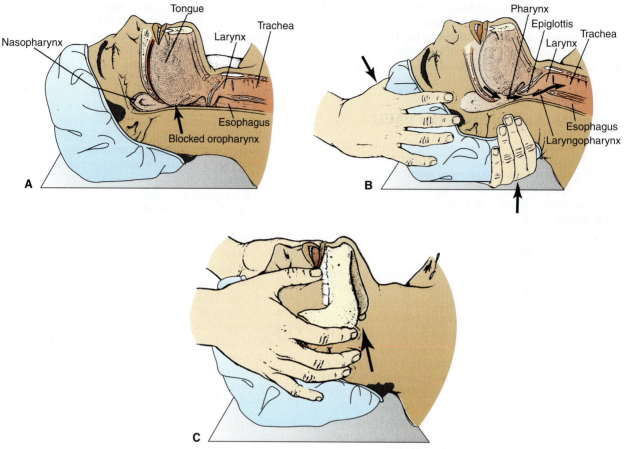

**FIGURE 20-1.** (**A**) A hypopharyngeal obstruction occurs when neck flexion permits the chin to drop toward the chest; obstruction almost always occurs when the head is in the midposition. (**B**) Tilting the head back to stretch the anterior neck structure lifts the base of the tongue off the posterior pharyngeal wall. The direction of the *arrows* indicates the pressure of the hands. (**C**) Opening the mouth is necessary to correct valvelike obstruction of the nasal passage during expiration, which occurs in about 30% of unconscious patients. Open the patient's mouth (separate lips and teeth) and move the lower jaw forward so that the lower teeth are in front of the upper teeth. To regain backward tilt of the neck, lift with both hands at the ascending rami of the mandible.

**FIGURE 20-2.** Use of an airway to maintain a patent airway after anesthesia. The airway passes over the base of the tongue and permits air to pass into the pharynx in the region of the epiglottis. Patients often leave the operating room with an airway in place. The airway should remain in place until the patient recovers sufficiently to breathe normally. As the patient regains consciousness, the airway usually causes irritation and should be removed.

the patient is closely monitored to maintain the airway as well as to minimize the risk of aspiration. If vomiting occurs, the patient is turned to the side to prevent aspiration and the vomitus is collected in the emesis basin. Mucus or vomitus obstructing the pharynx or the trachea is suctioned with a pharyngeal suction tip or a nasal catheter introduced into the nasopharynx or oropharynx. The catheter can be passed into the nasopharynx or oropharynx safely to a distance of 15 to 20 cm (6 to 8 inches). Caution is necessary in suctioning the throat of a patient who has had a tonsillectomy or other oral or laryngeal surgery because of risk of bleeding and discomfort.

## Maintaining Cardiovascular Stability

To monitor cardiovascular stability, the nurse assesses the patient's mental status; vital signs; cardiac rhythm; skin temperature, color, and moisture; and urine output. Central venous pressure, pulmonary artery pressure, and arterial lines are monitored if the patient's condition requires such assessment. The nurse also assesses the patency of all IV

## NURSING RESEARCH PROFILE

### Risk Factors for Extended Mechanical Ventilation Following Surgery

Bezanson, J. L., Weaver, M., Kinney, M., et al. (2004). Presurgical risk factors for late extubation in Medicare recipients after cardiac surgery. *Nursing Research, 53*(1), 46–52.

#### Purpose
The number of Medicare recipients undergoing coronary artery bypass grafting surgery (CABG) is increasing. This study developed and validated a model using selected presurgical patient characteristics to assess the probability of prolonged mechanical ventilation after CABG in Medicare recipients.

#### Design
A retrospective nonexperimental design was used to study 548 Medicare recipients (all 65 years of age or older) who had undergone a CABG. An existing database for the year 1998 was used to assess risks for prolonged mechanical ventilation. 74% of the sample were male, 92% were Caucasian, and the mean age was 72.8 years (SD = 4.99). Logistic regression modeling was used to identify predictors of late extubation.

#### Findings
Based on the time of extubation, the sample was divided into two groups. Group 1, early extubation ($n = 205$), had a mechanical ventilation time of 5 hours or less. Group 2, late extubation ($n = 343$), had a mechanical ventilation time of more than 5 hours. Predictors of late extubation were found to include (1) age 80 years or older, (2) female gender (OR = 1.76, $P = .011$), (3) hypertension (OR = 1.60, $P = .18$), and (4) urgent or emergent preoperative clinical status (OR = 3.04, $P = .002$).

#### Nursing Implications
A better understanding of predictors of prolonged mechanical ventilation may provide information for nurses to optimize the preoperative health status of elderly patients. During preoperative assessments, nurses should note the presence of predictors of prolonged mechanical ventilation and communicate these to the intraoperative and postoperative health care providers.

---

lines. The primary cardiovascular complications seen in the PACU include hypotension and shock, hemorrhage, hypertension, and dysrhythmias.

### HYPOTENSION AND SHOCK
Hypotension can result from blood loss, hypoventilation, position changes, pooling of blood in the extremities, or side effects of medications and anesthetics. The most common cause is loss of circulating volume through blood and plasma loss. If the amount of blood loss exceeds 500 mL (especially if the loss is rapid), replacement is usually indicated.

Shock, one of the most serious postoperative complications, can result from hypovolemia and decreased intravascular volume. The types of shock are classified as hypovolemic, cardiogenic, neurogenic, anaphylactic, and septic shock. The classic signs of hypovolemic shock (the most common type of shock) are

- Pallor
- Cool, moist skin
- Rapid breathing
- Cyanosis of the lips, gums, and tongue
- Rapid, weak, thready pulse
- Narrowing pulse pressure
- Low blood pressure
- Concentrated urine

See Chapter 15 for a detailed discussion of shock.

Hypovolemic shock can be avoided largely by the timely administration of IV fluids, blood, blood products, and medications that elevate blood pressure. Volume replacement is the primary intervention for shock (Defazio-Quinn & Schick, 2004). An infusion of lactated Ringer's solution, 0.9% sodium chloride solution, colloids, or blood component therapy is initiated (see Table 15-2 in Chapter 15). Oxygen is administered by nasal cannula, face mask, or mechanical ventilation. If fluid administration fails to reverse hypovolemic shock, then various cardiac, vasodilator, and corticosteroid medications may be prescribed to improve cardiac function and reduce peripheral vascular resistance. The patient is placed flat in bed with the legs elevated. Respiratory rate, pulse rate, blood pressure, blood oxygen concentration, urinary output, level of consciousness, central venous pressure, pulmonary artery pressure, pulmonary capillary wedge pressure, and cardiac output are monitored to provide information on the patient's respiratory and cardiovascular status. Vital signs are monitored continuously until the patient's condition has stabilized.

Other factors can contribute to hemodynamic instability, and the PACU nurse implements multiple measures to manage these factors. Pain is controlled by making the patient as comfortable as possible and by using opioids judiciously. The patient is kept warm while avoiding overheating to prevent cutaneous vessels from dilating and depriving vital organs of blood. Exposure is avoided, and normothermia is maintained to prevent vasodilation.

### HEMORRHAGE
Hemorrhage is an uncommon yet serious complication of surgery that can result in death. It can present insidiously or emergently at any time in the immediate postoperative period or up to several days after surgery (Table 20-1). When blood loss is extreme, the patient is apprehensive, restless,

| TABLE 20-1 | Classifications of Hemorrhage |
|---|---|
| **Classification** | **Defining Characteristic** |
| **Time Frame** | |
| Primary | Hemorrhage occurs at the time of surgery. |
| Intermediary | Hemorrhage occurs during the first few hours after surgery when the rise of blood pressure to its normal level dislodges insecure clots from untied vessels. |
| Secondary | Hemorrhage may occur some time after surgery if a suture slips because a blood vessel was not securely tied, became infected, or was eroded by a drainage tube. |
| **Type of Vessel** | |
| Capillary | Hemorrhage is characterized by a slow, general ooze. |
| Venous | Darkly colored blood bubbles out quickly. |
| Arterial | Blood is bright red and appears in spurts with each heartbeat. |
| **Visibility** | |
| Evident | Hemorrhage is on the surface and can be seen. |
| Concealed | Hemorrhage is in a body cavity and cannot be seen. |

and thirsty; the skin is cold, moist, and pale. The pulse rate increases, the temperature falls, and respirations are rapid and deep, often of the gasping type spoken of as "air hunger." If hemorrhage progresses untreated, cardiac output decreases, arterial and venous blood pressure and hemoglobin level fall rapidly, the lips and the conjunctivae become pale, spots appear before the eyes, a ringing is heard in the ears, and the patient grows weaker but remains conscious until near death (Defazio-Quinn & Schick, 2004).

Transfusing blood or blood products and determining the cause of hemorrhage are the initial therapeutic measures. The surgical site and incision should always be inspected for bleeding. If bleeding is evident, a sterile gauze pad and a pressure dressing are applied, and the site of the bleeding is elevated to heart level if possible. The patient is placed in the shock position (flat on back; legs elevated at a 20-degree angle; knees kept straight). If hemorrhage is suspected but cannot be visualized, the patient may be taken back to the OR for emergency exploration of the surgical site.

If hemorrhage is suspected, the nurse should be aware of any special considerations related to blood loss replacement. Certain patients may decline blood transfusions for religious or cultural reasons and may identify this request on their advance directives or living will.

### HYPERTENSION AND DYSRHYTHMIAS

Hypertension is common in the immediate postoperative period secondary to sympathetic nervous system stimulation from pain, hypoxia, or bladder distention. Dysrhythmias are associated with electrolyte imbalance, altered respiratory function, pain, hypothermia, stress, and anesthetic agents. Both hypertension and dysrhythmias are managed by treating the underlying causes.

### Relieving Pain and Anxiety

Opioid analgesics are administered judiciously and often by IV in the PACU (Rothrock, 2003). IV opioids provide immediate pain relief and are short-acting, thus minimizing the potential for drug interactions or prolonged respiratory depression while anesthetics are still active in the patient's system. The PACU nurse monitors the patient's physiologic status, manages pain, and provides psychological support in an effort to relive the patient's fears and concerns. The nurse checks the medical record for special needs and concerns of the patient. When the patient's condition permits, a close member of the family may visit in the PACU for a few moments. This often decreases the family's anxiety and makes the patient feel more secure.

### Controlling Nausea and Vomiting

Nausea and vomiting are common issues in the PACU. The nurse should intervene at the patient's first report of nausea to control the problem rather than wait for it to progress to vomiting.

Many medications are available to control nausea and vomiting without oversedating the patient; they are commonly administered during surgery as well as in the PACU. Medications such as metoclopramide (Reglan), prochlorperazine (Compazine), promethazine (Phenergan), dimenhydrinate (Dramamine), hydroxyzine (Vistaril, Atarax) and scopolamine (Transderm-Scop) are commonly prescribed (Rothrock, 2003). Although it is costly, ondansetron (Zofran) is frequently used as an effective antiemetic with few side effects.

A panel of anesthesiologists has reviewed the literature and developed guidelines for the treatment of postoperative nausea and vomiting (PONV). The panel concluded that it was important to evaluate the patient's level of risk for PONV. Based on the risk level, the panel recommended a range of treatments, from no prophylactic antiemetics (for low-risk patients) to double and triple antiemetic combinations for patients at high risk for PONV. The panel identified high-risk patients as females, nonsmokers, those with a history of PONV or motion sickness, and patients undergoing surgical procedures lasting longer than 2 hours (Gan, Meyer, Apfel, et al., 2003).

> **NURSING ALERT**
>
> At the slightest indication of nausea, the patient is turned completely to one side to promote mouth drainage and prevent aspiration of vomitus, which can cause asphyxiation and death.

### Gerontologic Considerations

The elderly patient, like all other patients, is transferred from the OR table to the bed or stretcher slowly and gently. The effects of this action on blood pressure and ventilation are monitored. Special attention is given to keeping the patient warm, because elderly patients are more susceptible to hypothermia. The patient's position is changed frequently to stimulate respirations and to promote circulation and comfort.

Immediate postoperative care for the elderly patient is the same as for any surgical patient, but additional support is given if cardiovascular, pulmonary, or renal function is impaired. With careful monitoring, it is possible to detect cardiopulmonary deficits before signs and symptoms are apparent. The elderly patient has less physiologic reserve, and physiologic responses to stress are diminished or slowed. These changes reinforce the need for close monitoring and prompt treatment of hypotension, shock, and hemorrhage. Because of monitoring and improved individualized preoperative preparation, many older adults tolerate surgery well and have an uneventful recovery. Treating postoperative pain in the elderly patient requires an understanding of the normal changes associated with aging and the impact of aging on metabolism of medications (Barnett, 2003).

Postoperative confusion and delirium affect as many as 51% of older patients (Cofer, 2005; Saufl, 2004). Acute confusion may be caused by pain, analgesic agents, hypotension, fever, hypoglycemia, fluid loss, fecal impaction, urinary retention, or anemia (Cofer, 2005). Providing adequate hydration; reorienting the patient to the environment; and reassessing the doses of sedatives, anesthetics, and analgesics may reduce the risk for confusion. Hypoxia can present as confusion and restlessness, as can blood loss and electrolyte imbalances. Exclusion of all other causes of confusion must precede the assumption that confusion is related to age, circumstances, and medications.

## Determining Readiness for Discharge from the PACU

A patient remains in the PACU until fully recovered from the anesthetic agent. Indicators of recovery include stable blood pressure, adequate respiratory function, adequate oxygen saturation level compared with baseline, and spontaneous movement or movement on command. Ordinarily, the following measures are used to determine the patient's readiness for discharge from the PACU (Defazio-Quinn & Schick, 2004):

- Stable vital signs
- Orientation to person, place, events, and time
- Uncompromised pulmonary function
- Pulse oximetry readings indicating adequate blood oxygen saturation
- Urine output at least 30 mL/hour
- Nausea and vomiting absent or under control
- Minimal pain

Many hospitals use a scoring system (eg, Aldrete score) to determine the patient's general condition and readiness for transfer from the PACU. Throughout the recovery period, the patient's physical signs are observed and evaluated by means of a scoring system based on a set of objective criteria (Aldrete & Wright, 1992). This evaluation guide allows an objective assessment of the patient's condition in the PACU (Fig. 20-3). The patient is assessed at regular intervals (eg, every 15 minutes), and a total score is calculated and recorded on the assessment record. Patients with a score of less than 7 must remain in the PACU until their condition improves or be transferred to an intensive care area, depending on their preoperative baseline score.

The patient is discharged from the phase I PACU by the anesthesiologist or anesthetist to the critical care unit, the medical-surgical unit, the phase II PACU, or home with a responsible family member. In some hospitals and ambulatory care centers, patients are discharged to a phase III PACU, where they are prepared for discharge.

## Preparing the Postoperative Patient for Direct Discharge

Because approximately 60% of elective surgeries are now performed in ambulatory or outpatient settings, the majority of patients are discharged directly home from the PACU (Conner, 2004). Patients being discharged directly to home require verbal and written instructions and information about follow-up care.

### Promoting Home and Community-Based Care

To ensure patient safety and recovery, expert patient teaching and discharge planning are necessary when a patient undergoes same-day or ambulatory surgery. Because anesthetics cloud memory for concurrent events, verbal and written instructions should be given to both the patient and the adult who will be accompanying the patient home. Alternative formats (eg, large print, Braille) of instructions or use of a sign interpreter may be required to ensure patient and family understanding. A translator may be required if the patient and family members do not understand English.

**TEACHING PATIENTS SELF-CARE**
The patient and caregiver (eg, family member or friend) are informed about expected outcomes and immediate postoperative changes anticipated. Written instructions about wound care, activity and dietary recommendations, medications, and follow-up visits to the same-day surgery unit or the surgeon are provided. Written instructions (designed to be copied and given to patients) about postoperative care after many types of surgery are usually provided. The patient's caregiver at home is provided with verbal and written instructions about what to look for and about the actions to take if complications occur. Prescriptions are given to the patient. The nurse's or surgeon's telephone number is provided, and the patient and caregiver are encouraged to call with questions and to schedule follow-up appointments (Chart 20-2).

Although recovery time varies depending on the type and extent of surgery and the patient's overall condition, instructions usually advise limited activity for 24 to 48 hours. During this time, the patient should not drive a vehicle, drink alcoholic beverages, or perform tasks that require energy or skill. Fluids may be consumed as desired, and smaller-than-normal amounts may be eaten at mealtime. Patients are cautioned not to make important decisions at this time, because the medications, anesthesia, and surgery may affect their decision-making ability.

## Post Anesthesia Care Unit
### MODIFIED ALDRETE SCORE

Patient: _____     Final score: _____

Room: _____     Surgeon: _____

Date: _____     PACU nurse: _____

| Area of Assessment | Point Score | Upon Admission | After 15 min | After 30 min | After 45 min | After 60 min |
|---|---|---|---|---|---|---|
| **Activity** (Able to move spontaneously or on command) | | | | | | |
| • Ability to move all extremities | 2 | | | | | |
| • Ability to move 2 extremities | 1 | | | | | |
| • Unable to control any extremity | 0 | | | | | |
| **Respiration** | | | | | | |
| • Ability to breathe deeply and cough | 2 | | | | | |
| • Limited respiratory effort (dyspnea or splinting) | 1 | | | | | |
| • No spontaneous effort | 0 | | | | | |
| **Circulation** | | | | | | |
| • BP ± 20% of preanesthetic level | 2 | | | | | |
| • BP ± 20%–49% of preanesthetic level | 1 | | | | | |
| • BP ± 50% of preanesthetic level | 0 | | | | | |
| **Consciousness** | | | | | | |
| • Fully awake | 2 | | | | | |
| • Arousable on calling | 1 | | | | | |
| • Not responding | 0 | | | | | |
| **O₂ Saturation** | | | | | | |
| • Able to maintain $O_2$ sat >92% on room air | 2 | | | | | |
| • Needs $O_2$ inhalation to maintain $O_2$ sat >90% | 1 | | | | | |
| • $O_2$ sat <90% even with $O_2$ supplement | 0 | | | | | |
| Totals: | | | | | | |

Required for discharge from Post Anesthesia Care Unit: 7–8 points

Time of release _____     Signature of nurse _____

**FIGURE 20-3.** Post anesthesia care unit record; Modified Aldrete Score. ($O_2$ sat = oxygen saturation; BP = blood pressure.) Modified from Aldrete, A., & Wright, A. (1992). Revised Aldrete score for discharge. *Anesthesiology News, 18*(1), 17.

## CONTINUING CARE

Although most patients who undergo ambulatory surgery recover quickly and without complications, some patients require referral for home care. These may be elderly or frail patients, those who live alone, and patients with other health care problems or disabilities that might interfere with self-care or resumption of usual activities. The home care nurse assesses the patient's physical status (eg, respiratory and cardiovascular status, adequacy of pain management, the surgical incision) and the patient's and family's ability to adhere to the recommendations given at the time of discharge. Previous teaching is reinforced as needed. The home care nurse may change surgical dressings, monitor the patency of a drainage system, or administer medications. The patient is assessed for any surgical complications. The patient and family are reminded about the importance of keeping follow-

## CHART 20-2

### HOME CARE CHECKLIST • Discharge After Surgery

| At the completion of the home care instruction, the patient or caregiver will be able to: | Patient | Caregiver |
|---|:---:|:---:|
| Name the procedure that was performed and identify any permanent changes in anatomic structure or function. | ✓ | ✓ |
| Describe ongoing postoperative therapeutic regimen, including medications, diet, activities to perform, (eg, walking and breathing exercises) and to avoid (eg, driving a car; contact sports), adjuvant therapies, dressing changes and wound care, and any other treatments. | ✓ | ✓ |
| Describe signs and symptoms of complications. | ✓ | ✓ |
| State time and date of follow-up appointments. | ✓ | ✓ |
| Identify interventions and strategies to use in adapting to any permanent changes in structure or function. | ✓ | ✓ |
| Relate how to reach health care provider with questions or complications. | ✓ | ✓ |
| State understanding of community resources and referrals (if any). | ✓ | ✓ |
| Describe pertinent health promotion activities (eg, weight reduction, smoking cessation, stress management). | ✓ | ✓ |

up appointments with the surgeon. Follow-up phone calls from the nurse or surgeon may also be used to assess the patient's progress and to answer any questions.

## The Hospitalized Postoperative Patient

The majority of surgeries are now performed in ambulatory care centers, and surgical patients who require hospital stays are trauma patients, acutely ill patients, patients undergoing major surgery, patients who require emergency surgery, and patients with a concurrent medical disorder. Seriously ill patients and those who have undergone major cardiovascular, pulmonary, or neurologic surgery may be admitted to specialized ICUs for close monitoring and advanced interventions and support. The care required by these patients in the immediate postoperative period is discussed in specific chapters. Patients admitted to the clinical unit for postoperative care have multiple needs and stay for a short period of time. Postoperative care for those surgical patients returning to the general medical-surgical unit is discussed later.

## Receiving the Patient in the Clinical Unit

The patient's room is readied by assembling the necessary equipment and supplies: IV pole, drainage receptacle holder, suction equipment, oxygen, emesis basin, tissues, disposable pads, blankets, and postoperative documentation forms. When the call comes to the unit about the patient's transfer from the PACU, the need for any additional items is communicated. The PACU nurse reports data about the patient to the receiving nurse. The report includes relevant demographic data, medical diagnosis, procedure performed, comorbid conditions, allergies, unexpected intraoperative events, estimated blood loss, types and amounts of fluids received, medications administered for pain, types of IV fluids or medications infused, whether the patient has voided, and information that the patient and family have received about the patient's condition. Usually the surgeon speaks to the family after surgery and relates the general condition of the patient. The receiving nurse reviews the postoperative orders, admits the patient to the unit, performs an initial assessment, and attends to the patient's immediate needs (Chart 20-3).

## Nursing Management After Surgery

During the first 24 hours after surgery, nursing care of the hospitalized patient on the general medical-surgical unit involves continuing to help the patient recover from the effects of anesthesia, frequently assessing the patient's physiologic status, monitoring for complications, managing pain, and implementing measures designed to achieve the long-range goals of independence with self-care, successful management of the therapeutic regimen, discharge to home, and full recovery. In the initial hours after admission to the clinical unit, adequate ventilation, hemodynamic stability, incisional pain, surgical site integrity, nausea and vomiting, neurologic status, and spontaneous voiding are primary concerns. The pulse rate, blood pressure, and respiration rate are recorded at least every 15 minutes for the first hour and every 30 minutes for the next 2 hours (Defazio-Quinn & Schick, 2004). Thereafter, they are measured less frequently if they remain stable. The temperature is monitored every 4 hours for the first 24 hours.

Patients usually begin to return to their usual state of health several hours after surgery or after waking up the next morning. Although pain may still be intense, many patients

### CHART 20-3 — Guidelines for Immediate Postoperative Nursing Interventions

| NURSING INTERVENTIONS | RATIONALE |
|---|---|
| 1. Assess breathing and administer supplemental oxygen, if prescribed. | 1. Assessment provides a baseline and helps identify signs and symptoms of respiratory distress early. |
| 2. Monitor vital signs and note skin warmth, moisture, and color. | 2. A careful baseline assessment helps identify signs and symptoms of shock early. |
| 3. Assess the surgical site and wound drainage systems. Connect all drainage tubes to gravity or suction as indicated and monitor closed drainage systems. | 3. Assessment provides a baseline and helps identify signs and symptoms of hemorrhage early. |
| 4. Assess level of consciousness, orientation, and ability to move extremities. | 4. These parameters provide a baseline and help identify signs and symptoms of neurologic complications. |
| 5. Assess pain level, pain characteristics (location, quality) and timing, type, and route of administration of last dose of analgesic. | 5. Assessment provides a baseline of current pain level and for assessment of effectiveness of pain management strategies. |
| 6. Administer analgesics as prescribed and assess their effectiveness in relieving pain. | 6. Administration of analgesics helps decrease pain. |
| 7. Place the call light, emesis basin, ice chips (if allowed), and bedpan or urinal within reach. | 7. Attending to these needs provides for comfort and safety. |
| 8. Position the patient to enhance comfort, safety, and lung expansion. | 8. This promotes safety and reduces risk of postoperative complications. |
| 9. Assess IV sites for patency and infusions for correct rate and solution. | 9. Assessing IV sites and infusions helps detect phlebitis and prevents errors in rate and solution type. |
| 10. Assess urine output in closed drainage system or the patient's urge to void and bladder distention. | 10. Assessment provides a baseline and helps identify signs of urinary retention. |
| 11. Reinforce the need to begin deep-breathing and leg exercises. | 11. These activities help to prevent complications. |
| 12. Provide information to the patient and family. | 12. Patient teaching helps to decrease the patient's and family's anxiety. |

feel more alert, less nauseous, and less anxious. They have begun their breathing and leg exercises, and many will have dangled their legs over the edge of the bed, stood, and ambulated a few feet or been assisted out of bed to the chair at least once. Many will have tolerated a light meal and had IV fluids discontinued. The focus of care shifts from intense physiologic management and symptomatic relief of the adverse effects of anesthesia to regaining independence with self-care and preparing for discharge. Despite these gains, the postoperative patient is still at risk for complications. Atelectasis, pneumonia, deep vein thrombosis, pulmonary embolism, bleeding, constipation, paralytic ileus, and wound infection are ongoing threats for the postoperative patient (Fig. 20-4).

## ◀◀▶▶ Nursing Process

### The Hospitalized Patient Recovering From Surgery

Nursing care of the hospitalized patient recovering from surgery takes place in a compressed time frame, with much of the healing and recovery occurring after the patient is discharged to home or to a rehabilitation center. The Perioperative Nursing Data Set (PNDS) is a helpful model used by nurses in the postoperative phase of care (see Figure 18-1 in Chapter 18). Phenomena of concern to nurses on the clinical unit in the postoperative phase of care include nursing diagnoses, interventions, and outcomes for patients and their families. Additional areas of concern include collaborative problems and expected goals.

### Assessment

Assessment of the hospitalized postoperative patient includes monitoring vital signs and completing a review of the systems on arrival of the patient to the clinical unit (see Chart 20-3) and at regular intervals thereafter.

Respiratory status is important, because pulmonary complications are among the most frequent and serious problems encountered by the surgical patient. The nurse observes for airway patency, watching for laryngeal edema (Letizia, O'Leary & Vodvarka, 2003). The quality of respirations, including depth, rate, and sound, are assessed regularly. Chest auscultation verifies that breath sounds are normal (or abnormal) bilaterally, and the findings are documented as a

**FIGURE 20-4.** The postoperative patient is subject to a number of potential complications.

baseline for later comparisons. Often, because of the effects of analgesic and anesthetic medications, respirations are slow. Shallow and rapid respirations may be caused by pain, constricting dressings, gastric dilation, abdominal distention, or obesity. Noisy breathing may be due to obstruction by secretions or the tongue.

The nurse assesses the patient's pain level using a verbal or visual analogue scale and assesses the characteristics of the pain. The patient's appearance, pulse, respirations, blood pressure, skin color (adequate or cyanotic), and skin temperature (cold and clammy, warm and moist, or warm and dry) are clues to cardiovascular function. When the patient arrives in the clinical unit, the surgical site is observed for bleeding, type and integrity of dressings, and drains.

The nurse also assesses the patient's mental status and level of consciousness, speech, and orientation and compares them with the preoperative baseline. Although a change in mental status or postoperative restlessness may be related to anxiety, pain, or medications, it may also be a symptom of oxygen deficit or hemorrhage. These serious causes must be investigated and excluded before other causes are pursued.

General discomfort resulting from lying in one position on the operating table, the surgeon's handling of tissues, the body's reaction to anesthesia, and anxiety are also common causes of restlessness. These discomforts may be relieved by administering the prescribed analgesics, changing the patient's position frequently, and assessing and alleviating the cause of anxiety. If tight, drainage-soaked bandages are causing discomfort, reinforcing or changing the dressing completely as prescribed by the physician may make the patient more comfortable. The bladder is assessed for distention, because urinary retention can also cause restlessness.

## Diagnosis

### Nursing Diagnoses

Based on the assessment data, major nursing diagnoses may include the following:

- Risk for ineffective airway clearance related to depressed respiratory function, pain, and bed rest
- Acute pain related to surgical incision
- Decreased cardiac output related to shock or hemorrhage
- Risk for activity intolerance related to generalized weakness secondary to surgery
- Impaired skin integrity related to surgical incision and drains
- Ineffective thermoregulation related to surgical environment and anesthetic agents
- Risk for imbalanced nutrition, less than body requirements related to decreased intake and increased need for nutrients secondary to surgery
- Risk for constipation related to effects of medications, surgery, dietary change, and immobility
- Risk for urinary retention related to anesthetic agents
- Risk for injury related to surgical procedure/ positioning or anesthetic agents

- Anxiety related to surgical procedure
- Risk for ineffective management of therapeutic regimen related to wound care, dietary restrictions, activity recommendations, medications, follow-up care, or signs and symptoms of complications

## Collaborative Problems/Potential Complications

Based on the assessment data, potential complications may include the following:

- Pulmonary infection/hypoxia
- Deep vein thrombosis
- Hematoma/hemorrhage
- Infection
- Pulmonary embolism
- Wound dehiscence or evisceration

## Planning and Goals

The major goals for the patient include optimal respiratory function, relief of pain, optimal cardiovascular function, increased activity tolerance, unimpaired wound healing, maintenance of body temperature, and maintenance of nutritional balance. Further goals include resumption of usual pattern of bowel and bladder elimination, identification of any perioperative positioning injury, acquisition of sufficient knowledge to manage self-care after discharge, and absence of complications.

## Nursing Interventions

### Preventing Respiratory Complications

Respiratory depressive effects of opioid medications, decreased lung expansion secondary to pain, and decreased mobility combine to put the patient at risk for common respiratory complications, particularly atelectasis (alveolar collapse; incomplete expansion of the lung), pneumonia, and hypoxemia (Rothrock, 2003). Atelectasis remains a risk for the patient who is not moving well or ambulating or who is not performing deep-breathing and coughing exercises or using an incentive spirometer. Signs and symptoms include decreased breath sounds over the affected area, crackles, and cough. Pneumonia is characterized by chills and fever, tachycardia, and tachypnea. Cough may or may not be present and may or may not be productive. Hypostatic pulmonary congestion, caused by a weakened cardiovascular system that permits stagnation of secretions at lung bases, may develop; this condition occurs most frequently in elderly patients who are not mobilized effectively. The symptoms are often vague, with perhaps a slight elevation of temperature, pulse, and respiratory rate, as well as a cough. Physical examination reveals dullness and crackles at the base of the lungs. If the condition progresses, the outcome may be fatal.

The types of hypoxemia that can affect postoperative patients are subacute and episodic. Subacute hypoxemia is a constant low level of oxygen saturation, although breathing appears normal. Episodic hypoxemia develops suddenly, and the patient may be at risk for cerebral dysfunction, myocardial ischemia, and cardiac arrest. Risk for hypoxemia is present in patients who have undergone major surgery (particularly abdominal), are obese, or have preexisting pulmonary problems. Hypoxemia can be detected by pulse oximetry, which measures blood oxygen saturation. Factors that may affect the accuracy of pulse oximetry readings include cold extremities, tremors, atrial fibrillation, acrylic nails, and black or blue nail polish (these colors interfere with the functioning of the pulse oximeter; other colors do not).

Preventive measures and timely recognition of signs and symptoms help avert pulmonary complications. Strategies to prevent respiratory complications include use of an incentive spirometer and deep-breathing and coughing exercises. Crackles indicate static pulmonary secretions that need to be mobilized by coughing and deep-breathing exercises. When a mucus plug obstructs one of the bronchi entirely, the pulmonary tissue beyond the plug collapses, and massive atelectasis results.

To clear secretions and prevent pneumonia, the nurse encourages the patient to turn frequently and take deep breaths at least every 2 hours. Coughing is also encouraged to dislodge mucus plugs. These pulmonary exercises should begin as soon as the patient arrives on the clinical unit and continue until the patient is discharged. Even if he or she is not fully awake from anesthesia, the patient can be asked to take several deep breaths. This helps expel residual anesthetic agents, mobilize secretions, and prevent alveolar collapse (atelectasis). Careful splinting of abdominal or thoracic incision sites helps the patient overcome the fear that the exertion of coughing might open the incision. Analgesic agents are administered to permit more effective coughing, and oxygen is administered as prescribed to prevent or relieve hypoxia. To encourage lung expansion, the patient is encouraged to yawn or take sustained maximal inspirations to create a negative intrathoracic pressure of −40 mm Hg and expand lung volume to total capacity. Chest physical therapy may be prescribed if indicated.

Coughing is contraindicated in patients who have head injuries or who have undergone intracranial surgery (because of the risk for increasing intracranial pressure), as well as in patients who have undergone eye surgery (because of the risk for increasing intraocular pressure) or plastic surgery (because of the risk for increasing tension on delicate tissues). In patients with an abdominal or thoracic incision, the nurse teaches the patient how to splint the incision while coughing.

Most postoperative patients, especially the elderly and those with an abdominal or thoracic incision, are given an incentive spirometer and instructed in its use. A common recommendation for use of the incentive spirometer is 10 deep breaths every hour while awake. Refer to Chapter 25 for additional discussion of incentive spirometry and other respiratory modalities.

Early ambulation increases metabolism and pulmonary aeration and, in general, improves all body functions. The patient is encouraged to be out of bed as soon as possible (ie, on the day of surgery, or no later than the first postoperative day). This practice is especially valuable in preventing pulmonary complications in older patients.

## Relieving Pain

Most patients experience some pain after a surgical procedure. Many factors (motivational, affective, cognitive, and emotional) influence the pain experience. The degree and severity of postoperative pain and the patient's tolerance for pain depend on the incision site, the nature of the surgical procedure, the extent of surgical trauma, the type of anesthetic agent, and how the agent was administered. The preoperative preparation received by the patient (including information about what to expect, reassurance, psychological support, and teaching specific communication techniques related to pain) is a significant factor in decreasing anxiety, apprehension, and even the amount of postoperative pain (McDonald & Molony, 2004; Nair & Podichetty, 2004).

The reasons for controlling pain are compelling. There is a well-known correlation between frequency of complications and intensity of pain (Barnett, 2003; Milgrom, Brooks, Qi, et al. 2004). Intense pain stimulates the stress response, which adversely affects the cardiac and immune systems. When pain impulses are transmitted, both muscle tension and local vasoconstriction increase. The ischemia in the affected area causes further stimulation of pain receptors. When these impulses travel centrally, sympathetic activity is compounded, which increases myocardial demand and oxygen consumption. Research suggests that outcomes are improved and complications prevented with good pain control in the postoperative period (Barnett & Ochroch, 2004). Cardiovascular insufficiency occurs three times more frequently, and the incidence of infection is five times greater, in people with poor postoperative pain control (Moline, 2001). The hypothalamic stress response is also responsible for an increase in blood viscosity and platelet aggregation; this can lead to phlebothrombosis and pulmonary embolism.

Often the physician has prescribed different medications or dosages to cover various levels of pain. The nurse discusses these options with the patient to determine the best medication. Then the nurse assesses the effectiveness of the medication periodically, beginning 30 minutes after administration, or sooner if the medication is being delivered by patient-controlled analgesia (PCA).

### OPIOID ANALGESICS

About one third of patients report severe pain, one third moderate pain, and one third little or no pain. This does not mean that the patients in the last group have no pain; rather, they appear to activate psychodynamic mechanisms that impair the registering of pain ("gate closing" theory and nociceptive transmission). See Chapter 13 for a more detailed discussion of pain, the factors influencing the pain experience, and use of pain relief strategies.

Opioid analgesics are commonly prescribed for pain and immediate postoperative restlessness. A preventive approach, rather than an "as needed" (PRN) approach, is more effective in relieving pain. With a preventive approach, the medication is administered at prescribed intervals rather than when the pain becomes severe or unbearable. Many patients (and some health care providers) are overly concerned about the risk of drug addiction in the postoperative patient. However, this risk is negligible with the use of opioid medications for short-term pain control.

The postoperative level of opiate analgesia required also depends on whether the patient is a smoker or nonsmoker. Patients who smoke require greater amounts of opioids in the first 48 hours after cardiac surgery (Creekmore, Lugo & Weiland, 2004).

### PATIENT-CONTROLLED ANALGESIA

Given the negative impact of pain on recovery, nurses need to think "pain prevention" rather than sporadic pain control and should encourage the use of PCA. Patients recover more quickly when adequate pain relief measures are used, and PCA permits patients to administer their own pain medication when needed (Defazio-Quinn & Schick, 2004). The amount of medication delivered by the IV or epidural route and the time span during which the opioid medication is released are controlled by the PCA device. Self-administration promotes patient participation in care, eliminates delayed administration of analgesics, and maintains a therapeutic drug level.

Most patients are candidates for PCA. The two requirements for PCA are an understanding of the need to self-dose and the physical ability to self-dose. On sensing pain, the patient activates the medication-delivering pump with a handheld button. PCA enables the patient to move, turn, cough, and take deep breaths with less pain, thus reducing postoperative pulmonary complications.

### EPIDURAL INFUSIONS AND INTRAPLEURAL ANESTHESIA

For thoracic, orthopedic, obstetric, and major abdominal surgery, certain opioid analgesics may be administered by epidural or intrathecal infusion (Defazio-Quinn & Schick, 2004). Epidural infusions provide better postoperative analgesia compared with parenteral opioids (Block, Liu, Rowlingson, et al., 2003; Pasero, 2003). Epidural infusions are used with caution in chest procedures because the analgesic may ascend along the spinal cord and affect respiration. Intrapleural anesthesia involves the administration of local anesthetic by a catheter between the parietal and visceral pleura. It provides sensory anesthesia without affecting motor function to the intercostal muscles. This anesthesia allows more effective coughing and deep breathing in conditions such as cholecystectomy, renal surgery, and rib fractures in which pain in the thoracic region would interfere with these exercises.

A local opioid or a combination anesthetic (opioid plus local anesthetic agent) is used in the epidural infusion. Other local anesthetic methods may be used to provide analgesia and anesthesia. Intrapleural anesthesia has fewer adverse effects than systemic or spinal opioids and is associated with a lowered incidence of urinary retention, vomiting, and pruritus when compared with thoracic epidural opioids (Moline, 2001).

### OTHER PAIN RELIEF MEASURES

For pain that is difficult to control, a subcutaneous pain management system may be used. This is a silicone catheter that is inserted at the site of the affected area. The catheter is attached to a pump that delivers a continuous amount of local anesthetic at a specific amount determined and prescribed by the physician (Fig. 20-5).

Complete absence of pain in the area of the surgical incision may not occur for a few weeks, depending on the site and nature of the surgery, but the intensity of postoperative pain gradually subsides on subsequent days. However, pain control continues to be an important concern for the patient and the nurse. Effective pain management allows the patient to participate in care, perform deep-breathing and leg exercises, and tolerate activity. As stated previously, poor pain control contributes to postoperative complications and increased length of stay. The nurse continues to assess the pain level, the effectiveness of analgesic agents, and factors that influence pain tolerance (eg, energy level, stress level, cultural background, meaning of pain to the patient). The nurse explains that taking an analgesic agent before the pain becomes intense is more effective and offers medication to the patient at intervals rather than waiting for the patient to request it.

Nonpharmacologic pain relief measures, such as imagery, music, relaxation, massage, application of heat or cold (if prescribed), and distraction, can be used to supplement medications (Ikonomidou, Rehnstrom, Naesh, et al., 2004; McRee, Noble & Pasvogel, 2003; Taylor, Galper, Taylor, et al., 2003). Changing the patient's position, using distraction, applying cool washcloths to the face, and rubbing the back with a soothing lotion may be useful in relieving general discomfort temporarily, promoting relaxation, and rendering medication more effective when it is administered.

### Promoting Cardiac Output

If signs and symptoms of shock or hemorrhage occur, treatment and nursing care are implemented as described in the discussion of care in the PACU.

> **NURSING ALERT**
>
> **A systolic blood pressure of less than 90 mm Hg is usually considered reportable at once. However, the patient's preoperative or baseline blood pressure is used to make informed postoperative comparisons. A previously stable blood pressure that shows a downward trend of 5 mm Hg at each 15-minute reading should also be reported.**

Although most patients do not hemorrhage or go into shock, changes in circulating volume, the stress of surgery, and the effects of medications and preoperative preparations all affect cardiovascular function. IV fluid replacement is standard for up to 24 hours after surgery or until the patient is stable and tolerating oral fluids. Close monitoring is indicated to detect and correct conditions such as fluid volume deficit, altered tissue perfusion, and decreased cardiac output, all of which can increase the patient's discomfort, place him or her at risk of complications, and prolong the hospital stay. Some patients are at risk of fluid volume excess secondary to existing cardiovascular or renal disease, advanced age, or the release of adrenocorticotropic hormone and antidiuretic hormone as a result of the stress of surgery (Defazio-Quinn & Schick, 2004). Consequently, fluid replacement must be carefully managed, and intake and output records must be accurate.

**FIGURE 20-5.** Subcutaneous pain management system consists of a pump, filter, and catheter that delivers a specific amount of prescribed local anesthetic at the rate determined by the physician. Used with permission from I-Flow Corporation, Lake Forest, CA.

Nursing management includes assessing the patency of the IV lines and ensuring that the correct fluids are administered at the prescribed rate. Intake and output, including emesis and output from wound drainage systems, are recorded separately and totaled to determine fluid balance. If the patient has an indwelling urinary catheter, hourly outputs are monitored and rates of less than 30 mL/hour are reported; if the patient is voiding, an output of less than 240 mL per 8-hour shift is reported. Electrolyte levels and hemoglobin and hematocrit levels are monitored. Decreased hemoglobin and hematocrit levels can indicate blood loss or dilution of circulating volume by IV fluids. If dilution is contributing to the decreased levels, the hemoglobin and hematocrit will rise as the stress response abates and fluids are mobilized and excreted.

Venous stasis from dehydration, immobility, and pressure on leg veins during surgery put the patient at risk for deep vein thrombosis. Leg exercises and frequent position changes are initiated early in the postoperative period to stimulate circulation. Patients should avoid positions that compromise venous return, such as raising the bed's knee gatch, placing a pillow under the knees, sitting for long periods, and dangling the legs with pressure at the back of the knees. Venous return is promoted by elastic compression stockings and early ambulation. Early ambulation has a significant effect on recovery and the prevention of complications and can begin, in many instances, on the evening of surgery. Postoperative activity orders are checked before the patient is assisted to get out of bed. Sitting up at the edge of the bed for a few minutes may be all that the patient who has undergone a major surgical procedure can tolerate at first.

### Encouraging Activity

Most surgical patients are encouraged to be out of bed as soon as possible. Early ambulation reduces the incidence of postoperative complications, such as atelectasis, hypostatic pneumonia, gastrointestinal discomfort, and circulatory problems (Oetker-Black, Jones, Estok, et al., 2003; Rothrock, 2003). Ambulation increases ventilation and reduces the stasis of bronchial secretions in the lungs. It also reduces postoperative abdominal distention by increasing gastrointestinal tract and abdominal wall tone and stimulating peristalsis. Early ambulation prevents stasis of blood by increasing the rate of circulation in the extremities; as a result, thrombophlebitis or phlebothrombosis occurs less frequently. Pain is often decreased when early ambulation is possible, and the hospital stay is shorter and less costly, a further advantage to the patient and the hospital.

Despite the advantages of early ambulation, patients may be reluctant to get out of bed on the evening of surgery. Reminding them of the importance of early mobility in preventing complications may help patients overcome their fears. When a patient gets out of bed for the first time, orthostatic hypotension, also called postural hypotension, is a concern. Orthostatic hypotension is an abnormal drop in blood pressure that occurs as the patient changes from a supine to a standing position. It is common after surgery because of changes in circulating blood volume and bed rest. Signs and symptoms include a decrease of 20 mm Hg in systolic blood pressure or 10 mm Hg in diastolic blood pressure, weakness, dizziness, and fainting. Older adults are at increased risk for orthostatic hypotension secondary to age-related changes in vascular tone. To detect orthostatic hypotension, the nurse assesses the patient's blood pressure first in the supine position, after the patient sits up, again after the patient stands, and 2 to 3 minutes later. Gradual position change gives the circulatory system time to adjust. If the patient becomes dizzy, he or she should be returned to the supine position, and getting out of bed should be delayed for several hours.

To assist the postoperative patient in getting out of bed for the first time after surgery, the nurse

1. Helps the patient move gradually from the lying position to the sitting position by raising the head of the bed and encourages the patient to splint the incision when applicable.
2. Positions the patient completely upright (sitting) and turned so that both legs are hanging over the edge of the bed.
3. Helps the patient stand beside the bed.

After becoming accustomed to the upright position, the patient may start to walk. The nurse should be at the patient's side to give physical support and encouragement. Care must be taken not to tire the patient; the extent of the first few periods of ambulation varies with the type of surgical procedure and the patient's physical condition and age.

Whether or not the patient can ambulate early in the postoperative period, bed exercises are encouraged to improve circulation. Bed exercises consist of the following:

- Arm exercises (full range of motion, with specific attention to abduction and external rotation of the shoulder)
- Hand and finger exercises
- Foot exercises to prevent deep vein thrombosis, foot drop, and toe deformities and to aid in maintaining good circulation
- Leg flexion and leg-lifting exercises to prepare the patient for ambulation
- Abdominal and gluteal contraction exercises

Hampered by pain, dressings, IV lines, or drains, many patients cannot engage in activity without assistance. Prolonged inactivity may lead to pressure ulcers, deep vein thrombosis, atelectasis, or hypostatic pneumonia. Helping the patient increase his or her activity level on the first postoperative day is an important nursing function. One way to increase the patient's activity is to have the patient perform as much routine hygiene care as possible. Setting up the patient to bathe with a bedside wash basin or, if possible, assisting the patient to the bathroom to sit in a chair at the sink not only gets the patient moving but helps restore a sense of self-control and prepares the patient for discharge.

To be safely discharged to home, patients need to be able to ambulate a functional distance (eg, length of the house or apartment), get in and out of bed unassisted, and be independent with toileting. Patients can be asked to perform as much as they can and then to call for assistance. The patient and the nurse can collaborate on a schedule for progressive activity that includes ambulating in the room and hallway and sitting out of bed in the chair. Assessing the patient's vital signs before, during, and after a scheduled activity helps the nurse and patient determine the rate of progression. By providing physical support, the nurse maintains the patient's safety; by communicating a positive attitude about the patient's ability to perform the activity, the nurse promotes the patient's confidence. The nurse should make sure the patient continues to perform bed exercises, wears pneumatic compression or thigh-high elastic compression stockings when in bed, and rests as needed. If the patient has had orthopedic surgery of the lower extremities or will require a mobility aid (ie, walker, crutches) at home, a physical therapist may be involved the first time the patient gets out of bed to teach him or her to ambulate safely or to use the mobility aid correctly.

### Promoting Wound Healing

**CONCEPTS in action ANIMATION**

Ongoing assessment of the surgical site involves inspection for approximation of wound edges, integrity of sutures or staples, redness, discoloration, warmth, swelling, unusual tenderness, or drainage. The area around the wound should also be inspected for a reaction to tape or trauma from tight bandages.

Nursing interventions to promote wound healing also include management of surgical drains and dressings. Wound drains are tubes that exit the peri-incisional area, either into a portable wound suction device (closed) or into the dressings (open). The principle involved is to allow the escape of blood and serous fluids that could otherwise serve as a culture medium for bacteria. In portable wound suction, the use of gentle, constant suction enhances drainage of these fluids and collapses the skin flaps against the underlying tissue, thus removing "dead space." Types of wound drains include the Penrose, Hemovac, and Jackson-Pratt drains (Fig. 20-6). Output from wound drainage systems and all new drainage is recorded. The amount of bloody drainage on the surgical dressing is assessed frequently. Spots of drainage on the dressings are outlined with a pen, and the date and time of the outline are recorded on the dressing so that increased drainage can be easily seen. A certain amount of bloody drainage in a wound drainage system or on the dressing is expected, but excessive amounts should be reported to the surgeon. Increasing amounts of fresh blood on the dressing should be reported immediately. Some wounds are irrigated heavily before closure in the OR, and open drains exiting the wound may be embedded in the dressings. These wounds may drain large amounts of blood-tinged fluid that saturate the dressing. The dressing can be reinforced with sterile gauze bandages; the time at which they were reinforced should be documented. If drainage continues, the surgeon should be notified so that the dressing can be changed. Multiple similar drains are numbered or otherwise labeled (eg, left lower quadrant, left upper quadrant) so that output measurements can be reliably and consistently recorded.

Surgical wound healing occurs in three phases: the inflammatory, proliferative, and maturation phases (Table 20-2) (Hogan, 2004). Wounds also heal by different mechanisms, depending on the condition of the wound. These mechanisms are first-, second-, and third-intention wound healing (Fig. 20-7) (Rothrock, 2003). With shorter hospital stays, much of the healing takes place at home, and both the hospital and home care nurse should be informed about the principles of wound healing.

#### FIRST-INTENTION HEALING
Wounds made aseptically with a minimum of tissue destruction that are properly closed heal with little tissue reaction by first intention (primary union). When wounds heal by **first-intention healing**, gran-

**FIGURE 20-6.** Types of surgical drains: (**A**) Penrose, (**B**) Jackson-Pratt, (**C**) Hemovac.

### TABLE 20-2 Phases of Wound Healing

| Phase | Duration | Events |
|---|---|---|
| Inflammatory (also called lag or exudative phase) | 1–4 days | Blood clot forms<br>Wound becomes edematous<br>Debris of damaged tissue and blood clot are phagocytosed |
| Proliferative (also called fibroblastic or connective tissue phase) | 5–20 days | Collagen produced<br>Granulation tissue forms<br>Wound tensile strength increases |
| Maturation (also called differentiation, resorptive, remodeling, or plateau phase) | 21 days to months or even years | Fibroblasts leave wound<br>Tensile strength increases<br>Collagen fibers reorganize and tighten to reduce scar size |

ulation tissue is not visible and scar formation is minimal. Postoperatively, many of these wounds are covered with a dry sterile dressing. If a cyanoacrylate tissue adhesive (Liquiband) was used to close the incision without sutures, a dressing is contraindicated.

### SECOND-INTENTION HEALING

**Second-intention healing** (granulation) occurs in infected wounds (abscess) or in wounds in which the edges have not been approximated. When an abscess is incised, it collapses partly, but the dead and the dying cells forming its walls are still being released

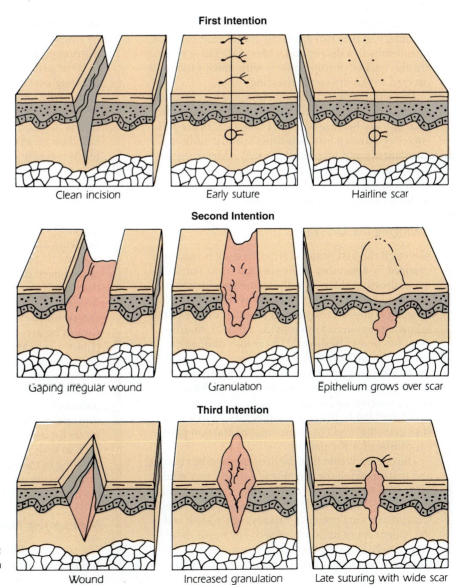

**FIGURE 20-7.** Types of wound healing: first-intention healing, second-intention healing, and third-intention healing.

into the cavity. For this reason, drainage tubes or gauze packing is inserted into the abscess pocket to allow drainage to escape easily. Gradually, the necrotic material disintegrates and escapes, and the abscess cavity fills with a red, soft, sensitive tissue that bleeds easily. This tissue is composed of minute, thin-walled capillaries and buds that later form connective tissue. These buds, called granulations, enlarge until they fill the area left by the destroyed tissue (see Fig. 20-7). The cells surrounding the capillaries change their round shape to become long, thin, and intertwined to form a scar (cicatrix). Healing is complete when skin cells (epithelium) grow over these granulations. This method of repair is called healing by granulation, and it takes place whenever pus is formed or when loss of tissue has occurred for any reason. When the postoperative wound is to be allowed to heal by secondary intention, it is usually packed with saline-moistened sterile dressings and covered with a dry sterile dressing.

### THIRD-INTENTION HEALING

**Third-intention healing** (secondary suture) is used for deep wounds that either have not been sutured early or break down and are resutured later, thus bringing together two apposing granulation surfaces. This results in a deeper and wider scar. These wounds are also packed postoperatively with moist gauze and covered with a dry sterile dressing.

As a wound heals, many factors, such as adequate nutrition, cleanliness, rest, and position, determine how quickly healing occurs. These factors are influenced by nursing interventions. Specific nursing assessments and interventions that address these factors and help promote wound healing are presented in Table 20-3. Other nursing interventions include assessment and care of the wound.

## Changing the Dressing

Although the first postoperative dressing is usually changed by a member of the surgical team, subsequent dressing changes in the immediate postoperative period are usually performed by the nurse. A dressing is applied to a wound for one or more of the following reasons: (1) to provide a proper environment for wound healing; (2) to absorb drainage; (3) to splint or immobilize the wound; (4) to protect the wound and new epithelial tissue from mechanical injury; (5) to protect the wound from bacterial contamination and from soiling by feces, vomitus, and urine; (6) to promote hemostasis, as in a pressure dressing; and (7) to provide mental and physical comfort for the patient.

The patient is told that the dressing is to be changed and that changing the dressing is a simple procedure associated with little discomfort. The dressing change is performed at a suitable time (eg, not at mealtimes or when visitors are present). Privacy is provided, and the patient is not unduly exposed. The nurse should avoid referring to the incision as a scar, because the term may have negative connotations for the patient.

> **NURSING ALERT**
>
> If disruption of a wound occurs, the patient is placed in low Fowler's position and instructed to lie quietly. These actions minimize protrusion of body tissues. The protruding coils of intestine are covered with sterile dressings moistened with sterile saline solution, and the surgeon is notified at once.

Assurance is given that the incision will shrink as it heals and that the redness will fade.

The nurse carries out hand hygiene before and after the dressing change and wears disposable gloves for the dressing change itself. The tape or adhesive portion of the dressing is removed by pulling it parallel with the skin surface and in the direction of hair growth, rather than at right angles. Alcohol wipes or nonirritating solvents aid in removing adhesive painlessly and quickly. The old dressing is removed and then deposited in a container designated for disposal of biomedical waste. In accordance with standard precautions, dressings are never touched by ungloved hands because of the danger of transmitting pathogenic organisms.

If the patient is sensitive to adhesive tape, the dressing may be held in place with hypoallergenic tape. Many tapes are porous to permit ventilation and prevent skin maceration. The correct way to apply tape is to place the tape at the center of the dressing and then press the tape down on both sides, applying tension evenly away from the midline. The incorrect way to apply tape—to fix one end of the tape to the skin and to pull it tight over the dressing—often wrinkles and pulls the skin in the process. The resulting continuous and forceful traction produces a shearing effect, causing the epidermal layer to slip sideways and become separated from the deeper dermal layers. Some wounds become edematous after having been dressed, causing considerable tension on the tape. If the tape is not flexible, the stretching bandage will also cause a shear injury to the skin. This can result in denuded areas or large blisters and should be avoided. An elastic adhesive bandage (Elastoplast, Microfoam-3M) may be used to hold dressings in place over mobile areas, such as the neck or the extremities, or where pressure is required.

While changing the dressing, the nurse has an opportunity to teach the patient how to care for the incision and change the dressings at home. The nurse observes for indicators of the patient's readiness to learn, such as looking at the incision, expressing interest, or assisting in the dressing change. Information on self-care activities and possible signs of infection is summarized in Chart 20-4.

## Maintaining Normal Body Temperature

The patient is still at risk for malignant hyperthermia and hypothermia in the postoperative period. Efforts

## TABLE 20-3 Factors Affecting Wound Healing

| Factors | Rationale | Nursing Interventions |
|---|---|---|
| Age of patient | The older the patient, the less resilient the tissues. | Handle all tissues gently. |
| Handling of tissues | Rough handling causes injury and delayed healing. | Handle tissues carefully and evenly. |
| Hemorrhage | Accumulation of blood creates dead spaces as well as dead cells that must be removed. The area becomes a growth medium for organisms. | Monitor vital signs. Observe incision site for evidence of bleeding and infection. |
| Hypovolemia | Insufficient blood volume leads to vasoconstriction and reduced oxygen and nutrients available for wound healing. | Monitor for volume deficit (circulatory impairment). Correct by fluid replacement as prescribed. |
| Local factors | | |
|   Edema | Reduces blood supply by exerting increased interstitial pressure on vessels | Elevate part; apply cool compresses. |
|   Inadequate dressing technique | | |
|     Too small | Permits bacterial invasion and contamination | Follow guidelines for proper dressing technique. |
|     Too tight | Reduces blood supply carrying nutrients and oxygen | |
| Nutritional deficits | Protein–calorie depletion may occur. Insulin secretion may be inhibited, causing blood glucose to rise. | Correct deficits; this may require parenteral nutritional therapy. Monitor blood glucose levels. Administer vitamin supplements as prescribed. |
| Foreign bodies | Foreign bodies retard healing. | Keep wounds free of dressing threads and talcum powder from gloves. |
| Oxygen deficit (tissue oxygenation insufficient) | Insufficient oxygen may be due to inadequate lung and cardiovascular function as well as localized vasoconstriction. | Encourage deep breathing, turning, controlled coughing. |
| Drainage accumulation | Accumulated secretions hamper healing process. | Monitor closed drainage systems for proper functioning. Institute measures to remove accumulated secretions. |
| Medications | | |
|   Corticosteroids | May mask presence of infection by impairing normal inflammatory response | Be aware of action and effect of medications patient is receiving. |
|   Anticoagulants | May cause hemorrhage | |
|   Broad-spectrum and specific antibiotics | Effective if administered immediately before surgery for specific pathology or bacterial contamination. If administered after wound is closed, ineffective because of intravascular coagulation. | |
| Patient overactivity | Prevents approximation of wound edges. Resting favors healing. | Use measures to keep wound edges approximated: taping, bandaging, splints. Encourage rest. |
| Systemic disorders<br>  Hemorrhagic shock<br>  Acidosis<br>  Hypoxia<br>  Renal failure<br>  Hepatic disease<br>  Sepsis | These depress cell functions that directly affect wound healing. | Be familiar with the nature of the specific disorder. Administer prescribed treatment. Cultures may be indicated to determine appropriate antibiotic. |
| Immunosuppressed state | Patient is more vulnerable to bacterial and viral invasion; defense mechanisms are impaired. | Provide maximum protection to prevent infection. Restrict visitors with colds; institute mandatory hand hygiene by all staff. |
| Wound stressors<br>  Vomiting<br>  Valsalva maneuver<br>  Heavy coughing<br>  Straining | Produce tension on wounds, particularly of the torso. | Encourage frequent turning and ambulation and administer antiemetic medications as prescribed. Assist patient in splinting incision. |

## CHART 20-4

### Patient Education

### Wound Care Instructions

**UNTIL SUTURES ARE REMOVED**
1. Keep the wound dry and clean.
   - If there is no dressing, ask your nurse or physician if you can bathe or shower.
   - If a dressing or splint is in place, do not remove it unless it is wet or soiled.
   - If wet or soiled, change dressing yourself if you have been taught to do so; otherwise, call your nurse or physician for guidance.
   - If you have been taught, instruction might be as follows:
     - Cleanse area *gently* with sterile normal saline once or twice daily.
     - Cover with a sterile Telfa pad or gauze square large enough to cover wound.
     - Apply hypoallergenic tape (Dermacel or paper). Adhesive is not recommended because it is difficult to remove without possible injury to the incisional site.
2. Immediately report any of these signs of infection:
   - Redness, marked swelling exceeding ½ inch (2.5 cm) from incision site; tenderness; or increased warmth around wound
   - Red streaks in skin near wound
   - Pus or discharge, foul odor
   - Chills or temperature higher than 37.7°C (100°F)
3. If soreness or pain causes discomfort, apply a dry cool pack (containing ice or cold water) or take prescribed acetaminophen tablets (2) every 4–6 hours. Avoid using aspirin without direction or instruction because bleeding can occur with its use.
4. Swelling after surgery is common. To help reduce swelling, elevate the affected part to the level of the heart.
   - Hand or arm
     - Sleep—elevate arm on pillow at side
     - Sitting—place arm on pillow on adjacent table
     - Standing—rest affected hand on opposite shoulder; support elbow with unaffected hand
   - Leg or foot
     - Sitting—place a pillow on a facing chair; provide support underneath the knee
     - Lying—place a pillow under affected leg

**AFTER SUTURES ARE REMOVED**

Although the wound appears to be healed when sutures are removed, it is still tender and will continue to heal and strengthen for several weeks.
1. Follow recommendations of physician or nurse regarding extent of activity.
2. Keep suture line clean; do not rub vigorously; pat dry. Wound edges may look red and may be slightly raised. This is normal.
3. If the site continues to be red, thick, and painful to pressure after 8 weeks, consult the health care provider. (This may be due to excessive collagen formation and should be checked.)

---

are made to identify malignant hyperthermia and to treat it early and promptly (McCarthy, 2004; Rothrock, 2003). (See the discussion of malignant hyperthermia in Chapter 19.)

Patients who have been anesthetized are susceptible to chills and drafts. Attention to hypothermia management, begun in the intraoperative period, extends into the postoperative period to prevent significant nitrogen loss and catabolism. Signs of hypothermia are reported to the physician. The room is maintained at a comfortable temperature, and blankets are provided to prevent chilling. Treatment includes oxygen administration, adequate hydration, and proper nutrition. The patient is also monitored for cardiac dysrhythmias. The risk of hypothermia is greater in the elderly and in patients who were in the cool OR environment for a prolonged period.

### Managing Gastrointestinal Function and Resuming Nutrition

Gastrointestinal discomfort (nausea, vomiting, hiccups) and resumption of oral intake are issues for both the patient and the nurse. Nausea and vomiting are common after anesthesia (Rothrock, 2003). They are more common in women, in obese people (fat cells act as reservoirs for the anesthetic), in patients prone to motion sickness, and in patients who have undergone lengthy surgical procedures. Other causes of postoperative vomiting include an accumulation of fluid in the stomach, inflation of the stomach, and the ingestion of food and fluid before peristalsis resumes.

If vomiting is likely because of the nature of surgery, a nasogastric tube is inserted preoperatively and remains in place throughout the surgery and the immediate postoperative period. A nasogastric tube also may be inserted before surgery if postoperative distention is anticipated. In addition, a nasogastric tube may be inserted if a patient who has food in the stomach requires emergency surgery.

Hiccups, produced by intermittent spasms of the diaphragm secondary to irritation of the phrenic nerve, can occur after surgery. The irritation may be direct, such as from stimulation of the nerve by a distended stomach, subdiaphragmatic abscess, or abdominal distention; indirect, such as from toxemia or uremia that stimulates the nerve; or reflexive, such as irritation from a drainage tube or obstruction of the intestines. Usually these occurrences are mild, transitory attacks that cease spontaneously. If hiccups persist, they may produce considerable distress and serious effects such as vomiting, exhaustion, and wound dehiscence. The physician may prescribe phenothiazine medications (e.g., Thorazine) for intractable hiccups (Zunderman & Doyle, 2006).

Once nausea and vomiting have subsided and the patient is fully awake and alert, the sooner he or she can tolerate a usual diet, the more quickly normal gastrointestinal function will resume. Taking food by mouth stimulates digestive juices and promotes gastric function and intestinal peristalsis. The return to normal dietary intake should proceed at a pace set by the patient. Of course, the nature of the surgery and the type of anesthesia directly affect the rate at which normal gastric activity resumes. Liquids are typically the first substances desired and tolerated by the patient after surgery. Water, juice, and tea may be given in increasing amounts. Cool fluids are tolerated more easily than those that are ice cold or hot. Soft foods (gelatin, custard, milk, and creamed soups) are added gradually after clear fluids have been tolerated. As soon as the patient tolerates soft foods well, solid food may be given.

Assessment and management of gastrointestinal function are important after surgery because the gastrointestinal tract is subject to uncomfortable or potentially life-threatening complications. Any postoperative patient may suffer from distention. Postoperative distention of the abdomen results from the accumulation of gas in the intestinal tract. Manipulation of the abdominal organs during surgery may produce a loss of normal peristalsis for 24 to 48 hours, depending on the type and extent of surgery. Even though nothing is given by mouth, swallowed air and gastrointestinal secretions enter the stomach and intestines; if not propelled by peristalsis, they collect in the intestines, producing distention and causing the patient to complain of fullness or pain in the abdomen. Most often, the gas collects in the colon. Abdominal distention is further increased by immobility, anesthetic agents, and the use of opioid medications.

After major abdominal surgery, distention may be avoided by having the patient turn frequently, exercise, and ambulate as early as possible. This also alleviates distention produced by swallowing air, which is common in anxious patients. A nasogastric tube inserted before surgery may remain in place until full peristaltic activity (indicated by the passage of flatus) has resumed. The nurse can determine when peristaltic bowel sounds return by listening to the abdomen with a stethoscope. Bowel sounds are documented so that diet progression can occur.

Paralytic ileus and intestinal obstruction are potential postoperative complications that occur more frequently in patients undergoing intestinal or abdominal surgery. Refer to Chapter 37 for discussion of treatment.

### Promoting Bowel Function

Constipation is common after surgery and can range from a minor to a serious complication. Decreased mobility, decreased oral intake, and opioid analgesics contribute to difficulty having a bowel movement. In addition, irritation and trauma to the bowel during surgery may inhibit intestinal movement for several days. The combined effect of early ambulation, improved dietary intake, and a stool softener (if prescribed) promotes bowel elimination. Until the patient reports return of normal bowel function, the nurse should assess the abdomen for distention and the presence and frequency of bowel sounds. If the abdomen is not distended and bowel sounds are normal, and if the patient does not have a bowel movement by the second or third postoperative day, the physician should be notified so that a laxative can be given that evening.

### Managing Voiding

Urinary retention after surgery can occur for various reasons. Anesthetics, anticholinergic agents, and opioids interfere with the perception of bladder fullness and the urge to void and inhibit the ability to initiate voiding and completely empty the bladder. Abdominal, pelvic, and hip surgery may increase the likelihood of retention secondary to pain. In addition, some patients find it difficult to use the bedpan or urinal in the recumbent position.

Bladder distention and the urge to void should be assessed at the time of the patient's arrival on the unit and frequently thereafter. The patient is expected to void within 8 hours after surgery (this includes time spent in the PACU). If the patient has an urge to void and cannot, or if the bladder is distended and no urge is felt or the patient cannot void, catheterization is not delayed solely on the basis of the 8-hour time frame. All methods to encourage the patient to void should be tried (eg, letting water run, applying heat to the perineum). The bedpan should be warm; a cold bedpan causes discomfort and automatic tightening of muscles (including the urethral sphincter). If the patient cannot void on a bedpan, it may be possible to use a commode rather than resorting to catheterization. Male patients are often permitted to sit up or stand beside the bed to use the urinal, but safeguards should be taken to prevent the patient from falling or fainting due to loss of coordination from medications or orthostatic hypotension. If the patient cannot void in the specified time frame, the patient is catheterized and the catheter is removed after the bladder has emptied. Straight intermittent catheterization is preferred over indwelling catheterization, because the risk of infection is increased with an indwelling catheter.

Even if the patient voids, the bladder may not necessarily be empty. The nurse notes the amount of urine voided and palpates the suprapubic area for distention or tenderness. A portable ultrasound device may also be used to assess residual volume. Intermittent catheterization may be prescribed every 4 to 6 hours until the patient can void spontaneously and the postvoid residual is less than 100 mL.

### Maintaining a Safe Environment

During the immediate postoperative period, the patient recovering from anesthesia should have three side rails up, and the bed should be in the low position. The nurse assesses the patient's level of consciousness and orientation and determines whether the patient needs his or her eyeglasses or hearing aid, because impaired vision, inability to hear postoperative instructions, or inability to communicate verbally places the patient at risk for injury. All objects the patient may need should be within reach, especially the call light. Any immediate postoperative orders concerning special positioning, equipment, or interventions should be implemented as soon as possible. The patient is instructed to ask for assistance with any activity. Although restraints are occasionally necessary for the disoriented patient, they should be avoided if at all possible. Agency policy on the use of restraints must be consulted and followed.

Any surgical procedure has the potential for injury due to disrupted neurovascular integrity resulting from prolonged awkward positioning in the OR, manipulation of tissues, inadvertent severing of nerves, or tight bandages. Any orthopedic surgery or surgery involving the extremities carries a risk of peripheral nerve damage. Vascular surgeries, such as replacing sections of diseased peripheral arteries or inserting an arteriovenous graft, put the patient at risk for thrombus formation at the surgical site and subsequent ischemia of tissues distal to the thrombus. Assessment includes having the patient move the hand or foot distal to the surgical site through a full range of motion, assessing all surfaces for intact sensation, and assessing peripheral pulses (Rothrock, 2003).

### Providing Emotional Support to the Patient and Family

Although patients and families are undoubtedly relieved that surgery is over, anxiety levels may remain high in the immediate postoperative period. Many factors contribute to this anxiety: pain, being in an unfamiliar environment, inability to control one's circumstances or care for oneself, fear of the long-term effects of surgery, fear of complications, fatigue, spiritual distress, altered role responsibilities, ineffective coping, and altered body image are all potential reactions to the surgical experience. The nurse helps the patient and family work through their anxieties by providing reassurance and information and by spending time listening to and addressing their concerns. The nurse describes hospital routines and what to expect in the ensuing hours and days until discharge and explains the purpose of nursing assessments and interventions. Informing patients when they will be able to drink fluids or eat, when they will be getting out of bed, and when tubes and drains will be removed helps them gain a sense of control and participation in recovery and engages them in the plan of care. Acknowledging family members' concerns and accepting and encouraging their participation in the patient's care assists them in feeling that they are helping their loved one. The nurse can modify the environment to enhance rest and relaxation by providing privacy, reducing noise, adjusting lighting, providing enough seating for family members, and encouraging a supportive atmosphere.

### Managing Potential Complications

**DEEP VEIN THROMBOSIS**

Deep vein thrombosis and other complications, such as pulmonary embolism, are serious potential complications of surgery (Chart 20-5) (Defazio-Quinn & Schick, 2004). The stress response that is initiated by

---

**CHART 20-5**

### Risk Factors for Postoperative Complications

**DEEP VEIN THROMBOSIS**

- Orthopedic patients having hip surgery, knee reconstruction, and other lower extremity surgery
- Urologic patients having transurethral prostatectomy and older patients having urologic surgery
- General surgical patients older than 40 years of age, those who are obese, those with a malignancy, those who have had prior deep vein thrombosis or pulmonary embolism, and those undergoing extensive, complicated surgical procedures
- Gynecologic (and obstetric) patients older than 40 years of age with added risk factors (varicose veins, previous venous thrombosis, infection, malignancy, obesity)
- Neurosurgical patients, similar to other surgical high-risk groups (in patients with stroke, for instance, the risk of deep vein thrombosis in the paralyzed leg is as high as 75%)

**PULMONARY COMPLICATIONS**

- Type of surgery—greater incidence after all forms of abdominal surgery when compared with peripheral surgery
- Location of incision—the closer the incision to the diaphragm, the higher the incidence of pulmonary complications
- Preoperative respiratory problems
- Age—greater risk after age 40 than before age 40
- Sepsis
- Obesity—weight greater than 110% of ideal body weight
- Prolonged bed rest
- Duration of surgical procedure—more than 3 hours
- Aspiration
- Dehydration
- Malnutrition
- Hypotension and shock
- Immunosuppression

surgery inhibits the fibrinolytic system, resulting in blood hypercoagulability. Dehydration, low cardiac output, blood pooling in the extremities, and bed rest add to the risk of thrombosis formation. Although all postoperative patients are at some risk, factors such as a history of thrombosis, malignancy, trauma, obesity, indwelling venous catheters, and hormone (eg, estrogen) use increase the risk (Farray, Carman & Fernandez, 2004). The first symptom of deep vein thrombosis may be a pain or cramp in the calf. Initial pain and tenderness may be followed by a painful swelling of the entire leg, often accompanied by a fever, chills, and diaphoresis.

Prophylactic treatment for postoperative patients at risk is common practice. Low-dose heparin may be prescribed and administered subcutaneously until the patient is ambulatory (Roper, Gress, Diringer, et al., 2004). Low-molecular-weight heparin and low-dose warfarin are other anticoagulants that may be used. External pneumatic compression and thigh-high elastic compression stockings can be used alone or in combination with low-dose heparin.

The benefits of early ambulation and hourly leg exercises in preventing deep vein thrombosis cannot be overemphasized, and these activities are recommended for all patients, regardless of their risk. It is important to avoid the use of blanket rolls, pillow rolls, or any form of elevation that can constrict vessels under the knees. Even prolonged "dangling" (having the patient sit on the edge of the bed with legs hanging over the side) can be dangerous and is not recommended in susceptible patients because pressure under the knees can impede circulation. Adequate hydration is also encouraged; the patient can be offered juices and water throughout the day to avoid dehydration. Refer to Chapter 30 for a complete discussion of deep vein thrombosis and to Chapter 23 for discussion of pulmonary embolus.

### HEMATOMA

At times, concealed bleeding occurs beneath the skin at the surgical site. This hemorrhage usually stops spontaneously but results in clot (hematoma) formation within the wound. If the clot is small, it will be absorbed and need not be treated. If the clot is large, the wound usually bulges somewhat, and healing will be delayed unless the clot is removed. After several sutures are removed by the physician, the clot is evacuated and the wound is packed lightly with gauze. Healing occurs usually by granulation, or a secondary closure may be performed.

### INFECTION (WOUND SEPSIS)

The creation of a surgical wound disrupts the integrity of the skin and its protective function. Exposure of deep body tissues to pathogens in the environment places the patient at risk for infection of the surgical site, a potentially life-threatening complication. Surgical site infection increases hospital length of stay, costs of care, and risk of further complications. In postoperative patients, surgical site infection is the most common nosocomial infection, with 67% of these infections occurring within the incision and 33% occurring in an organ or space around the surgical site. The administration of supplemental oxygen during colorectal resection and for 2 hours postoperatively has been shown to reduce the incidence of postoperative infection (Hopf, Hunt & Rosen, 2004).

Multiple factors place the patient at risk of wound infection. One risk factor relates to the type of wound. Surgical wounds are classified according to the degree of contamination. Table 20-4 defines the

### TABLE 20-4 Wound Classification and Associated Surgical Site Infection Risk

| Surgical Category | Determinants of Category | Expected Risk of Postsurgical Infection (%) |
|---|---|---|
| Clean | Nontraumatic site<br>Uninfected site<br>No inflammation<br>No break in aseptic technique<br>No entry into respiratory, alimentary, genitourinary, or oropharyngeal tracts | 1–3 |
| Clean-contaminated | Entry into respiratory, alimentary, genitourinary or oropharyngeal tracts without unusual contamination<br>Appendectomy<br>Minor break in aseptic technique<br>Mechanical drainage | 3–7 |
| Contaminated | Open, newly experienced traumatic wounds<br>Gross spillage from gastrointestinal tract<br>Major break in aseptic technique<br>Entry into genitourinary or biliary tract when urine or bile is infected | 7–16 |
| Dirty | Traumatic wound with delayed repair, devitalized tissue, foreign bodies, or fecal contamination<br>Acute inflammation and purulent drainage encountered during procedure | 16–29 |

terms used to describe surgical wounds and gives the expected rate of wound infection per category. Other risk factors include both patient-related factors and those associated with the surgical procedure. Patient-related factors include age, nutritional status, diabetes, smoking, obesity, remote infections, endogenous mucosal microorganisms, altered immune response, length of preoperative stay, and severity of illness (Defazio-Quinn & Schick, 2004; Worley, 2004). Factors related to the surgical procedure include the method of preoperative skin preparation, surgical attire of the team, method of sterile draping, duration of surgery, antimicrobial prophylaxis, aseptic technique, factors related to surgical technique, drains or foreign material, OR ventilation, length of procedure, and exogenous microorganisms. Efforts to prevent wound infection are directed at reducing these risks. Preoperative and intraoperative risks and interventions are discussed in Chapters 18 and 19. Although the conditions for surgical site infection and serious contamination of the wound occur in the preoperative and intraoperative time frames, postoperative care of the wound centers on assessing the wound, preventing contamination and infection before wound edges have sealed, and enhancing healing.

Wound infection may not be evident until at least postoperative day 5. Most patients are discharged before that time, and more than half of wound infections are diagnosed after discharge, highlighting the importance of patient education regarding wound care. Risk factors for wound sepsis include wound contamination, foreign body, faulty suturing technique, devitalized tissue, hematoma, debilitation, dehydration, malnutrition, anemia, advanced age, extreme obesity, shock, length of preoperative hospitalization, duration of surgical procedure, and associated disorders (eg, diabetes mellitus, immunosuppression). Signs and symptoms of wound infection include increased pulse rate and temperature; an elevated white blood cell count; wound swelling, warmth, tenderness, or discharge; and incisional pain. Local signs may be absent if the infection is deep. *Staphylococcus aureus* accounts for many postoperative wound infections. Other infections may result from *Escherichia coli, Proteus vulgaris, Aerobacter aerogenes, Pseudomonas aeruginosa,* and other organisms. Although they are rare, beta-hemolytic streptococcal or clostridial infections can be rapid and deadly. If wound infection due to beta-hemolytic streptococcus or clostridium occurs, strict infection control practices are needed to prevent the spread of infection to others. Intensive medical and nursing care is essential if the patient is to survive.

When a wound infection is diagnosed in a surgical incision, the surgeon may remove one or more sutures or staples and, using aseptic precautions, separate the wound edges with a pair of blunt scissors or a hemostat. Once the incision is opened, a drain is inserted. If the infection is deep, an incision and drainage procedure may be necessary. Antimicrobial therapy and a wound care regimen are also initiated.

## WOUND DEHISCENCE AND EVISCERATION

Wound **dehiscence** (disruption of surgical incision or wound) and **evisceration** (protrusion of wound contents) are serious surgical complications (Fig. 20-8). Dehiscence and evisceration are especially serious when they involve abdominal incisions or wounds. These complications result from sutures giving way, from infection, or, more frequently, from marked distention or strenuous cough. They may also occur because of increasing age, poor nutritional status, or pulmonary or cardiovascular disease in patients undergoing abdominal surgery.

When the wound edges separate slowly, the intestines may protrude gradually or not at all, and the earliest sign may be a gush of bloody (serosanguineous) peritoneal fluid from the wound. When a wound ruptures suddenly, coils of intestine may push out of the abdomen. The patient may report that "something gave way." The evisceration causes pain and may be associated with vomiting.

An abdominal binder, properly applied, is an excellent prophylactic measure against an evisceration and often is used along with the primary dressing, especially in patients with weak or pendulous abdominal walls or when rupture of a wound has occurred.

### *Gerontologic Considerations*

Elderly patients recover more slowly, have longer hospital stays, and are at greater risk for development of postoperative complications. Delirium, pneumonia, decline in functional ability, exacerbation

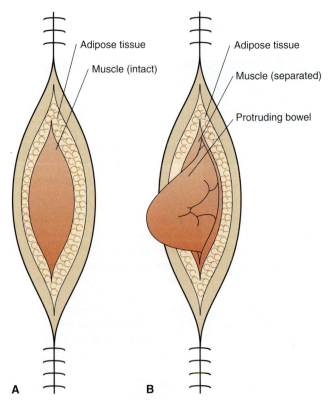

**FIGURE 20-8.** (**A**) Wound dehiscence; (**B**) wound evisceration.

of comorbid conditions, pressure ulcers, decreased oral intake, gastrointestinal disturbance, and falls are all threats to recovery in the older adult (Saufl, 2004). Expert nursing care can help the older adult avoid these complications or minimize their effects.

Postoperative delirium, characterized by confusion, perceptual and cognitive deficits, altered attention levels, disturbed sleep patterns, and impaired psychomotor skills, is a significant problem for older adults. Causes of delirium are multifactorial (Chart 20-6). Skilled and frequent assessment of mental status and of all physiologic factors influencing mental status helps the nurse plan care, because delirium may be the initial or only early indicator of infection, fluid and electrolyte imbalance, or deterioration of respiratory or hemodynamic status in the elderly patient. Factors that determine whether a patient is at risk for delirium include age, history of alcohol abuse, preoperative cognitive function, physical function, serum chemistries, and type of surgery.

Recognizing postoperative delirium and identifying and treating its underlying cause are the goals of care. Postoperative delirium is sometimes mistaken for preexisting dementia or is attributed to age. In addition to monitoring and managing identifiable causes, the nurse implements supportive interventions. Keeping the patient in a well-lit room and close to the nurses' station can help with sensory deprivation. At the same time, distracting and unfamiliar noises should be minimized. Because pain can contribute to postoperative delirium, adequate pain control is essential. The nurse collaborates with the physician or geriatric nurse specialist and the patient to achieve pain relief without oversedation (Barnett, 2003).

The patient is reoriented as often as necessary, and staff should introduce themselves each time they come in contact with the patient. Engaging the patient in conversation and care activities and placing a clock and calendar nearby may improve cognitive function. Physical activity should not be neglected while the patient is confused, because physical deterioration can worsen delirium and place the patient at increased risk for other complications. Restraints should be avoided, because they can also worsen confusion. If possible, a family member or staff member is asked to stay with the patient instead. Haloperidol (Haldol) or lorazepam (Ativan) may be administered during episodes of acute confusion, but these medications should be discontinued as soon as possible to avoid side effects.

Other problems confronting the elderly postoperative patient, such as pneumonia, altered bowel function, deep vein thrombosis, weakness, and functional decline, often can be prevented by early and progressive ambulation. Ambulation means walking, not just getting out of bed and sitting in a chair. Prolonged sitting positions that promote venous stasis in the lower extremities should be avoided. Assistance with ambulation may be required to keep the patient from bumping into objects and falling. A physical therapy referral may be indicated to promote safe, regular exercise for the older adult.

Urinary incontinence can be prevented by providing easy access to the call bell and the commode and by prompting voiding. Early ambulation and familiarity with the room help the patient to become self-sufficient sooner.

Optimal nutritional status is important for wound healing, return of normal bowel function, and fluid and electrolyte balance. The nurse and patient can consult with the dietitian to plan appealing, high-protein meals that provide sufficient fiber, calories, and vitamins. Nutritional supplements, such as Ensure or Sustacal, may be recommended. Multivitamins, iron, and vitamin C supplements aid in tissue healing, formation of new red blood cells, and overall nutritional status and are commonly prescribed postoperatively.

In addition to monitoring and managing physiologic recovery of the older adult, the nurse identifies and addresses psychosocial needs. The older adult may require much encouragement and support to resume activities, and the pace may be slow. Sensory deficits may require frequent repetition of instructions, and decreased physiologic reserve may necessitate frequent rest periods. The older adult may require extensive discharge planning to coordinate both professional and family care providers, and the nurse, social

### CHART 20-6

### Causes of Postoperative Delirium

- Acid–base disturbances
- Age greater than 80 years
- Fluid and electrolyte imbalance
- Dehydration
- History of dementia-like symptoms
- Hypoxia
- Hypercarbia
- Infection (urinary tract, wound, respiratory)
- Medications (anticholinergics, benzodiazepines, central nervous system depressants)
- Unrelieved pain
- Blood loss
- Decreased cardiac output
- Cerebral hypoxia
- Heart failure
- Acute myocardial infarction
- Hypothermia or hyperthermia
- Unfamiliar surroundings and sensory deprivation
- Emergent surgery
- Alcohol withdrawal
- Urinary retention
- Fecal impaction
- Polypharmacy
- Presence of multiple diseases
- Sensory impairments
- High stress or anxiety levels

worker, or nurse case manager may institute the plan for continuing care.

### Promoting Home and Community-Based Care

**TEACHING PATIENTS SELF-CARE**

Patients have always required detailed discharge instructions to become proficient in special self-care needs after surgery; however, dramatically reduced hospital lengths of stay during the past decade have greatly increased the amount of information needed while reducing the amount of time in which to provide it. Although needs are specific to individual patients and the procedures they have undergone, general patient education needs for postoperative care have been identified (see Chart 20-2).

**CONTINUING CARE**

Continuing care provided by community-based services is frequently necessary after surgery. Older patients, patients who live alone, patients without family support, and patients with preexisting chronic illness or disabilities are often in greatest need. Planning for discharge involves arranging for necessary services early in the acute care hospitalization. Wound care, drain management, catheter care, infusion therapy, and physical or occupational therapy are some of the needs addressed by community-based health care providers. The home care nurse coordinates these activities and services.

During home care visits, the nurse assesses the patient for postoperative complications; the nurse also assesses the surgical incision, respiratory and cardiovascular status, adequacy of pain management, fluid and nutritional status, and the patient's progress in returning to preoperative status. The nurse assesses the patient's and family's ability to manage dressing changes and drainage systems and other devices and to administer prescribed medications. The nurse may change dressings or catheters if needed. The nurse determines whether any additional services are needed and assists the patient and family to arrange for them. Previous teaching is reinforced, and the patient is reminded to keep follow-up appointments. The patient and family are instructed about signs and symptoms to be reported to the surgeon. In addition, the nurse provides information about how to obtain needed supplies and suggests resources or support groups the patient may want to contact. In many settings, postoperative telephone calls are made to answer questions, assess recovery, and reassure patients and families.

### Evaluation

#### Expected Patient Outcomes

Expected patient outcomes may include the following:

1. Maintains optimal respiratory function
    a. Performs deep-breathing exercises
    b. Displays clear breath sounds
    c. Uses incentive spirometer as prescribed
    d. Splints incisional site when coughing to reduce pain
2. Indicates that pain is decreased in intensity
3. Increases activity as prescribed
    a. Alternates periods of rest and activity
    b. Progressively increases ambulation
    c. Resumes normal activities within prescribed time frame
    d. Performs activities related to self-care
4. Wound heals without complication
5. Maintains body temperature within normal limits
6. Resumes oral intake
    a. Reports absence of nausea and vomiting
    b. Eats at least 75% of usual diet
    c. Is free of abdominal distress and gas pains
    d. Exhibits normal bowel sounds
7. Reports resumption of usual bowel elimination pattern
8. Resumes usual voiding pattern
9. Is free of injury
10. Exhibits decreased anxiety
11. Acquires knowledge and skills necessary to manage therapeutic regimen
12. Experiences no complications

## Critical Thinking Exercises

**1** A 35-year-old woman who has had a right-sided mastectomy for cancer is admitted to the phase II PACU. Identify what information is essential to obtain during report from the OR, describe the Aldrete scoring system, and explain how you will know when the patient is ready to be discharged from the PACU.

**2** A frail 75-year-old man, who was brought in to the emergency department last night, has undergone an appendectomy. How would you direct your assessment to identify the factors that might affect his recovery? How would you prioritize his care needs, and what complications would you anticipate? Create a nursing care plan for this patient that addresses discharge to home in the next 24 hours.

**3** [ebp] An obese woman is admitted to the PACU after knee surgery, and she is complaining of nausea. What resources would you use to identify the current guidelines for treatment of PONV? What is the evidence base for PONV management practices? Identify the criteria used to evaluate the strength of the evidence for these practices.

**4** [ebp] A 45-year-old patient who is a smoker is admitted to the postoperative nursing unit after abdominal surgery and is complaining of severe pain. Develop an evidence-based plan of care for this patient, addressing priorities from admission to the unit until discharge to home.

# REFERENCES AND SELECTED READINGS

## BOOKS

American Society of PeriAnesthesia Nurses. (2002). *Standards of perianesthesia nursing practice.* Thorofare, NJ: ASPAN.

Clancy, J., McVicar, A. J. & Baird, N. (2002). *Perioperative practice: Fundamentals of homeostasis.* New York: Routledge.

Conner, R. (2004). *Ambulatory surgery principles and practices* (3rd ed.). Denver: AORN.

Defazio-Quinn, D. & Schick, L. (Eds.). (2004). *Nursing core curriculum: Preoperative, phase I and phase II PACU nursing.* Philadelphia: W. B. Saunders.

Dudek, S. G. (2006). *Nutrition essentials for nursing practice* (5th ed.). Philadelphia: Lippincott Williams & Wilkins.

Kost, M. (2004). *Moderate sedations/analgesia: Core competencies for practice.* Philadelphia: W. B. Saunders.

Miller, R. D. (2005) *Miller's anesthesia* (6th ed.). Philadelphia: Elsevier.

Morton, P. G., Fontaine, D. K., Hudak, C. M., et al. (2005). *Critical care nursing: A holistic approach* (8th ed.). Philadelphia: Lippincott Williams & Wilkins.

Murray, M. J., Coursin, D. B., Pearl, R. G., et al. (2002). *Critical care medicine: Perioperative management* (2nd ed.). Philadelphia: Lippincott Williams & Wilkins.

Phillips, N. (2004). *Berry and Kohn's operating room technique* (10th ed.). St. Louis: Mosby.

Roper, A. H., Gress, D., Diringer, M. N., et al. (2004). *Neurological and neurosurgical intensive care* (4th ed.). Philadelphia: Lippincott Williams & Wilkins.

Rothrock, J. C. (Ed.). (2003). *Alexander's care of the patient in surgery* (12th ed.). St. Louis: Mosby.

Seifert, P. C. (2002). *Cardiac surgery: Perioperative patient care.* St Louis: Mosby.

Zonderman, J. & Doyle, R. (2006). *Springhouse nurse's drug guide 2006.* Philadelphia: Lippincott Williams & Wilkins.

## JOURNALS

*Asterisks indicate nursing research articles.

Aldrete, A. & Wright, A. (1992). Revised Aldrete score for discharge. *Anesthesiology News, 18*(1), 17.

Barnett, R. & Ochroch, E. (2004). Epidural analgesia: Management and outcomes. *Annals of Long-Term Care, 11*(11), 33–38.

Barnett, S. (2003). Acute pain in the elderly surgical patient. *Clinical Geriatrics, 11*(9), 30–35.

*Bezanson, J. L., Weaver, M., Kinney, M., et al. (2004). Presurgical risk factors for late extubation in Medicare recipients after cardiac surgery. *Nursing Research, 53*(1), 46–52.

Block, B. M., Liu, S. S., Rowlingson, A. J., et al. (2003). Efficacy of postoperative epidural analgesia. *Journal of the American Medical Association, 290*(18), 2455–2463.

Cofer, M. J. (2005). Unwelcome companion to older patients: Postoperative delirium. *Nursing, 35*(1), 32hn1–32hn3.

Creekmore, F., Lugo, R. A., & Weiland, K. J. (2004). Postoperative opiate analgesic requirements of smokers and nonsmokers. *Annals of Pharmacotherapy, 38*(4), 949–953.

DeFazio-Quinn, D. M. (2006). How religion, language and ethnicity impact perioperative nursing care. *Nursing Clinics of North America, 41*(2), 231–248.

Farray, D., Carman, T. L. & Fernandez, B. B. (2004). The treatment and prevention of deep vein thrombosis in the preoperative management of patients who have neurologic diseases. *Neurologic Clinics of North America, 22*(2), 423–439.

Gan, T., Meyer, T., Apfel, C., et al. (2003). Consensus guidelines for managing postoperative nausea and vomiting. *Anesthesia and Analgesia, 97*(1), 62–71.

Happ, M. B., Roesch, T. & Kagan, S. (2004). Communication needs, methods and perceived voice quality following head and neck surgery: A literature review. *Cancer Nursing, 27*(1), 1–9.

Hogan, S. L. (2004). How to help wounds heal. *RN, 67*(8), 26–31.

Holmes, C. L. & Walley, K. R. (2003). The evaluation and management of shock. *Clinics in Chest Medicine, 24*(4), 775–789.

Hopf, H., Hunt, T. & Rosen, N. (2004). Supplemental oxygen and risk of surgical site infection. *Journal of the American Medical Association, 291*(1), 79–87.

*Ikonomidou, E., Rehnstrom, A., Naesh, O., et al. (2004). Effect of music on vital signs and postoperative pain. *AORN Journal, 80*(2), 269–278.

Letizia, M., O'Leary, J. & Vodvarka, J. (2003). Laryngeal edema: Perioperative nursing considerations. *MedSurg Nursing, 12*(2), 111–115.

McCarthy, E. (2004). Malignant hyperthermia. *AACN Clinical Issues, 15*(2), 231–237.

*McDonald, D. D. & Molony, S. L. (2004). Postoperative pain communication skills for older adults. *Western Journal of Nursing Research, 25*(8), 836–852.

*McRee, L., Noble, S. & Pasvogel, A. (2003). Using massage and music therapy to improve postoperative outcomes. *AORN Journal, 78*(3), 433–447.

Milgrom, L. B., Brooks, J. A., Qi, R., et al. (2004). Pain levels experienced with activities after cardiac surgery. *American Journal of Critical Care, 13*(2), 116–125.

Moline, B. M. (2001). Pain management in the ambulatory surgical population. *Journal of Perianesthesia Nursing, 16*(6), 388–398.

Nair, S. & Podichetty, V. K. (2004). The preoperative and postoperative assessment and care of patients with back pain. *Neurologic Clinics of North America, 22*(2), 441–456.

*Oetker-Black, S. L., Jones, S., Estok, P., et al. (2003). Preoperative teaching and hysterectomy outcomes. *AORN Journal, 77*(6), 1215–1231.

Pasero, C. (2003). Epidural analgesia for postoperative pain. *American Journal of Nursing, 103*(10), 62–65.

Saufl, N. M. (2004). Preparing the older adult for surgery and anesthesia. *Journal of Perianesthesia Nursing, 19*(6), 372–377.

Taylor, A., Galper, D., Taylor, P., et al. (2003). Effects of adjunctive Swedish massage and vibration therapy on short-term postoperative outcomes: A randomized, controlled trial. *Journal of Alternative and Complementary Medicine, 9*(1), 77–89.

Wadlund, D. L. (2006). Prevention, recognition, and management of nursing complications in the intraoperative and postoperative surgical patient. *Nursing Clinics of North America, 41*(2), 151–171.

Worley, C. (2004). "Why won't this wound heal?" Factors affecting wound healing. *Dermatology Nursing, 16*(4), 360–362.

*Yellen, E. (2003). The influence of nurse-sensitive variables on patient satisfaction. *AORN Journal, 78*(5), 783–793.

*Zalon, M. L. (2004). Correlates of recovery among older adults after major abdominal surgery. *Nursing Research, 53*(2), 99–106.

## RESOURCES

American Academy of Ambulatory Care Nursing, East Holly Ave., Box 56, Pitman, NJ, 08071; 856-256-2350 or 800-AMB-NURS; http://www.aacn.org. Accessed March 31, 2006.

American Society of PeriAnesthesia Nurses, 10 Melrose Ave., Suite 110, Cherry Hill, NJ 08003; 856-616-9600 or -9601; toll-free 877-737-9696; fax 856-616-9621; http://www.aspan.org. Accessed March 31, 2006.

Association of PeriOperative Registered Nurses, Inc., 2170 S. Parker Road, Suite 300, Denver, CO 80231; 800-755-2676 or 303-755-6304; http://www.aorn.org. Accessed March 31, 2006.

Centers for Disease Control and Prevention, Surgical Site Infection Guideline, Division of Healthcare Quality Promotion, National Center for Infectious Diseases, Atlanta, GA 30333; 404-639-3534 or 800-311-3435; http://www.cdc.gov/ncidod/dhqp/gl_surgicalsite.html. Accessed March 31, 2006.

Malignant Hyperthermia Association of the United States (MHAUS), 39 East State Street, P.O. Box 1069, Sherburne, NY 13460; 607-674-7901; http://www.mhaus.org. Accessed March 31, 2006.

# UNIT 5

# Gas Exchange and Respiratory Function

## Case Study
### Applying Concepts from NANDA, NIC, and NOC

**A Patient With Impaired Cough Reflex**

**Mrs. Lewis,** age 77 years, is admitted to the hospital for left lower lobe pneumonia. Her vital signs are: Temp 100.6°F; HR 90 and regular; B/P: 142/74; Resp 28. She has a weak cough, diminished breath sounds over the lower left lung field, and coarse rhonchi over the midtracheal area. She can expectorate some sputum, which is thick and grayish-green. She has a history of stroke. Secondary to the stroke she has impaired gag and cough reflexes and mild weakness of her left side. She is allowed food and fluids because she can swallow safely if she uses the chin-tuck maneuver.

 Turn to Appendix C to see a concept map that illustrates the relationships that exist between the nursing diagnoses, interventions, and outcomes for the patient's clinical problems.

## Nursing Classifications and Languages

| NANDA<br>Nursing Diagnoses | NIC<br>Nursing Interventions | NOC<br>Nursing Outcomes<br>Return to functional baseline status, stabilization of, or improvement in: |
|---|---|---|
| **Ineffective Airway Clearance**—Inability to clear secretions or obstructions from the respiratory tract to maintain a clear airway | **Respiratory Monitoring**—Collection and analysis of patient data to ensure airway patency and adequate gas exchange | **Respiratory Status: Airway Patency**—Extent to which the tracheobronchial passages remain open |
| **Impaired Gas Exchange**—Excess or deficit in oxygenation and/or carbon dioxide elimination at the alveolar-capillary membrane | **Airway Management**—Facilitation of patency of air passages | **Respiratory Status: Gas Exchange**—The alveolar exchange of $O_2$ and $CO_2$ to maintain arterial blood gas concentrations |
| **Ineffective Breathing Pattern**—Inspiration and/or expiration that does not provide adequate ventilation | **Cough Enhancement**—Promotion of deep inhalation by the patient with subsequent generation of high intrathoracic pressures and compression of underlying lung parenchyma for the forceful expulsion of air | **Respiratory Status: Ventilation**—Movement of air in and out of the lungs |
| **Risk for Aspiration**—At risk for entry of gastrointestinal secretions, oropharyngeal secretions, solids, or fluids into tracheobronchial passages | **Airway Suctioning**—Removal of airway secretions by inserting a suction catheter into the patient's oral airway and/or trachea | |
| | **Aspiration Precautions**—Prevention or minimization of risk factors in the patient at risk for aspiration | |

NANDA International (2005). *Nursing diagnoses: Definitions & classification 2005–2006.* Philadelphia: North American Nursing Diagnosis Association.
Dochterman, J. M. & Bulechek, G. M. (2004). *Nursing interventions classification (NIC)* (4th ed.). St. Louis: Mosby.
Iowa Outcomes Project (2004). In Moorhead, S., Johnson, M. & Maas, M. (2004). *Nursing outcomes classification (NOC)* (3rd ed.). St. Louis: Mosby.
Dochterman, J. M. & Jones, D. A. (2003). *Unifying nursing languages: The harmonization of NANDA, NIC, and NOC.* Washington, D.C.: American Nurses Association.

"Point, click, learn! Visit thePoint for additional resources."

# CHAPTER 21

# Assessment of Respiratory Function

## Learning Objectives

*On completion of this chapter, the learner will be able to:*

1. Describe the structures and functions of the upper and lower respiratory tracts.
2. Describe ventilation, perfusion, diffusion, shunting, and the relationship of pulmonary circulation to these processes.
3. Discriminate between normal and abnormal breath sounds.
4. Use assessment parameters appropriate for determining the characteristics and severity of the major symptoms of respiratory dysfunction.
5. Identify the nursing implications of the various procedures used for diagnostic evaluation of respiratory function.

Disorders of the respiratory system are common and are encountered by nurses in every setting from the community to the intensive care unit. To assess the respiratory system, the nurse must be skilled at differentiating between normal and abnormal assessment findings. Expert assessment skills must be developed and used when caring for patients with acute and chronic respiratory problems. In addition, an understanding of respiratory function and the significance of abnormal diagnostic test results is essential.

# Anatomic and Physiologic Overview

The respiratory system is composed of the upper and lower respiratory tracts. Together, the two tracts are responsible for **ventilation** (movement of air in and out of the airways). The upper tract, known as the upper airway, warms and filters inspired air so that the lower respiratory tract (the lungs) can accomplish gas exchange. Gas exchange involves delivering oxygen to the tissues through the bloodstream and expelling waste gases, such as carbon dioxide, during expiration. The respiratory system works in concert with the cardiovascular system; the respiratory system is responsible for ventilation and diffusion, and the cardiovascular system is responsible for perfusion (Farquhar & Fantasia, 2005).

## Anatomy of the Upper Respiratory Tract

Upper airway structures consist of the nose, sinuses and nasal passages, pharynx, tonsils and adenoids, larynx, and trachea.

### Nose

The nose is composed of an external and an internal portion. The external portion protrudes from the face and is supported by the nasal bones and cartilage. The anterior nares (nostrils) are the external openings of the nasal cavities.

The internal portion of the nose is a hollow cavity separated into the right and left nasal cavities by a narrow vertical divider, the septum. Each nasal cavity is divided into three passageways by the projection of the turbinates (also called conchae) from the lateral walls. The nasal cavities are lined with highly vascular ciliated mucous membranes called the nasal mucosa. Mucus, secreted continuously by goblet cells, covers the surface of the nasal mucosa and is moved back to the nasopharynx by the action of the **cilia** (fine hairs).

The nose serves as a passageway for air to pass to and from the lungs. It filters impurities and humidifies and warms the air as it is inhaled. It is responsible for olfaction (smell) because the olfactory receptors are located in the nasal mucosa. This function diminishes with age.

### Paranasal Sinuses

The paranasal sinuses include four pairs of bony cavities that are lined with nasal mucosa and ciliated pseudostratified columnar epithelium. These air spaces are connected by a series of ducts that drain into the nasal cavity. The sinuses are named by their location: frontal, ethmoidal, sphenoidal, and maxillary (Fig. 21-1). A prominent function of the sinuses is to serve as a resonating chamber in speech. The sinuses are a common site of infection.

### Turbinate Bones (Conchae)

The turbinate bones are also called conchae (the name suggested by their shell-like appearance). Because of their curves, these bones increase the mucous membrane surface of the nasal passages and slightly obstruct the air flowing through them (Fig. 21-2).

Air entering the nostrils is deflected upward to the roof of the nose, and it follows a circuitous route before it reaches the nasopharynx. It comes into contact with a large surface of moist, warm mucous membrane that traps practically all the dust and organisms in the inhaled air. The air is moistened, warmed to body temperature, and brought into contact with sensitive nerves. Some of these nerves detect odors; others provoke sneezing to expel irritating dust.

## Glossary

**bronchoscopy:** direct examination of larynx, trachea, and bronchi using an endoscope

**cilia:** short hairs that provide a constant whipping motion that serves to propel mucus and foreign substances away from the lung toward the larynx

**crackles:** soft, high-pitched, discontinuous popping sounds during inspiration caused by delayed reopening of the airways

**diffusion:** exchange of gas molecules from areas of high concentration to areas of low concentration

**dyspnea:** labored breathing or shortness of breath

**hemoptysis:** expectoration of blood from the respiratory tract

**hypoxemia:** decrease in arterial oxygen tension in the blood

**hypoxia:** decrease in oxygen supply to the tissues and cells

**orthopnea:** inability to breathe easily except in an upright position

**physiologic dead space:** portion of the tracheobronchial tree that does not participate in gas exchange

**pulmonary perfusion:** blood flow through the pulmonary vasculature

**respiration:** gas exchange between atmospheric air and the blood and between the blood and cells of the body

**ventilation:** movement of air in and out of airways

**wheezes:** continuous musical sounds associated with airway narrowing or partial obstruction

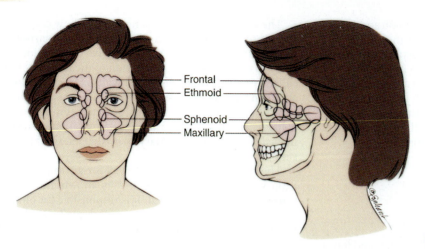

**FIGURE 21-1.** The paranasal sinuses.

## Pharynx, Tonsils, and Adenoids

The pharynx, or throat, is a tubelike structure that connects the nasal and oral cavities to the larynx. It is divided into three regions: nasal, oral, and laryngeal. The nasopharynx is located posterior to the nose and above the soft palate. The oropharynx houses the faucial, or palatine, tonsils. The laryngopharynx extends from the hyoid bone to the cricoid cartilage. The epiglottis forms the entrance to the larynx.

The adenoids, or pharyngeal tonsils, are located in the roof of the nasopharynx. The tonsils, the adenoids, and other lymphoid tissue encircle the throat. These structures are important links in the chain of lymph nodes guarding the body from invasion by organisms entering the nose and the throat. The pharynx functions as a passageway for the respiratory and digestive tracts.

## Larynx

The larynx, or voice organ, is a cartilaginous epithelium-lined structure that connects the pharynx and the trachea. The major function of the larynx is vocalization. It also protects the lower airway from foreign substances and facilitates coughing. It is frequently referred to as the voice box and consists of the following:

- Epiglottis—a valve flap of cartilage that covers the opening to the larynx during swallowing
- Glottis—the opening between the vocal cords in the larynx
- Thyroid cartilage—the largest of the cartilage structures; part of it forms the Adam's apple
- Cricoid cartilage—the only complete cartilaginous ring in the larynx (located below the thyroid cartilage)
- Arytenoid cartilages—used in vocal cord movement with the thyroid cartilage
- Vocal cords—ligaments controlled by muscular movements that produce sounds; located in the lumen of the larynx

## Trachea

The trachea, or windpipe, is composed of smooth muscle with C-shaped rings of cartilage at regular intervals. The cartilaginous rings are incomplete on the posterior surface and give firmness to the wall of the trachea, preventing it from collapsing. The trachea serves as the passage between the larynx and the bronchi.

## Anatomy of the Lower Respiratory Tract

The lower respiratory tract consists of the lungs, which contain the bronchial and alveolar structures needed for gas exchange.

**FIGURE 21-2.** Cross-section of nasal cavity.

## Lungs

The lungs are paired elastic structures enclosed in the thoracic cage, which is an airtight chamber with distensible walls (Fig. 21-3). Ventilation requires movement of the walls of the thoracic cage and of its floor, the diaphragm. The effect of these movements is alternately to increase and decrease the capacity of the chest. When the capacity of the chest is increased, air enters through the trachea (inspiration) because of the lowered pressure within and inflates the lungs. When the chest wall and diaphragm return to their previous positions (expiration), the lungs recoil and force the air out through the bronchi and trachea. Inspiration occurs during the first third of the respiratory cycle, expiration during the latter two thirds. The inspiratory phase of respiration normally requires energy; the expiratory phase is normally passive requiring very little energy. In respiratory diseases, such as chronic obstructive pulmonary disease (COPD), expiration requires energy.

### PLEURA

The lungs and wall of the thorax are lined with a serous membrane called the pleura. The visceral pleura covers the lungs; the parietal pleura lines the thorax. The visceral and parietal pleura and the small amount of pleural fluid between these two membranes serve to lubricate the thorax and lungs and permit smooth motion of the lungs within the thoracic cavity with each breath.

### MEDIASTINUM

The mediastinum is in the middle of the thorax, between the pleural sacs that contain the two lungs. It extends from the sternum to the vertebral column and contains all the thoracic tissue outside the lungs.

### LOBES

Each lung is divided into lobes. The left lung consists of an upper and lower lobe, whereas the right lung has an upper, middle, and lower lobe (Fig. 21-4). Each lobe is further

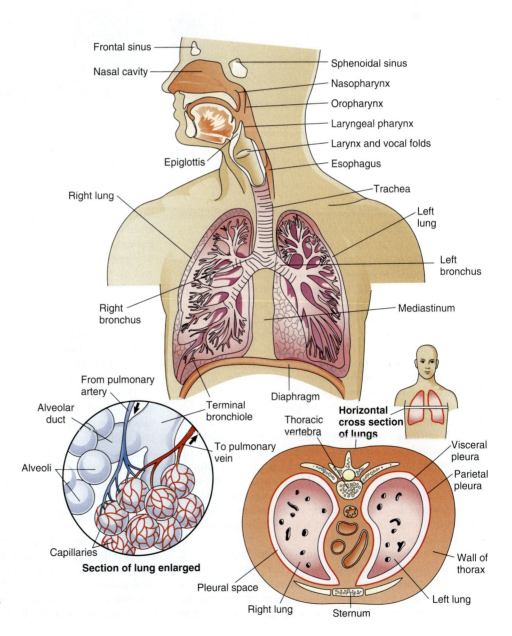

**FIGURE 21-3.** The respiratory system; upper respiratory structures and the structures of the thorax (*top*); alveoli and a horizontal cross section of the lungs (*bottom*).

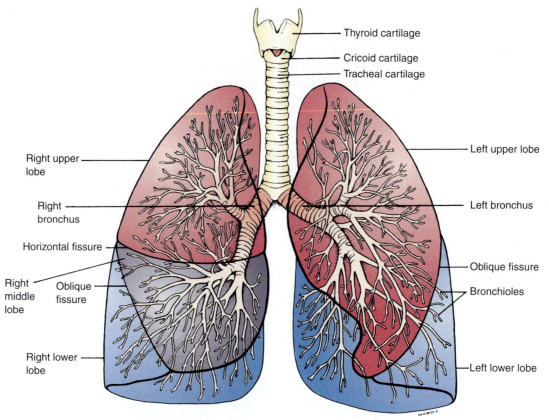

**FIGURE 21-4.** Anterior view of the lungs. The lungs consist of five lobes. The right lung has three lobes (upper, middle, lower); the left has two (upper and lower). The lobes are further subdivided by fissures. The bronchial tree, another lung structure, inflates with air to fill the lobes.

subdivided into two to five segments separated by fissures, which are extensions of the pleura.

### BRONCHI AND BRONCHIOLES

There are several divisions of the bronchi within each lobe of the lung. First are the lobar bronchi (three in the right lung and two in the left lung). Lobar bronchi divide into segmental bronchi (10 on the right and 8 on the left), which are the structures identified when choosing the most effective postural drainage position for a given patient. Segmental bronchi then divide into subsegmental bronchi. These bronchi are surrounded by connective tissue that contains arteries, lymphatics, and nerves.

The subsegmental bronchi then branch into bronchioles, which have no cartilage in their walls. Their patency depends entirely on the elastic recoil of the surrounding smooth muscle and on the alveolar pressure. The bronchioles contain submucosal glands, which produce mucus that covers the inside lining of the airways. The bronchi and bronchioles are lined also with cells that have surfaces covered with cilia. These cilia create a constant whipping motion that propels mucus and foreign substances away from the lungs toward the larynx.

The bronchioles then branch into terminal bronchioles, which do not have mucus glands or cilia. Terminal bronchioles then become respiratory bronchioles, which are considered to be the transitional passageways between the conducting airways and the gas exchange airways. Up to this point, the conducting airways contain about 150 mL of air in the tracheobronchial tree that does not participate in gas exchange. This is known as **physiologic dead space**. The respiratory bronchioles then lead into alveolar ducts and alveolar sacs and then alveoli. Oxygen and carbon dioxide exchange takes place in the alveoli.

### ALVEOLI

The lung is made up of about 300 million alveoli, which are arranged in clusters of 15 to 20. These alveoli are so numerous that if their surfaces were united to form one sheet, it would cover 70 square meters—the size of a tennis court.

There are three types of alveolar cells. Type I alveolar cells are epithelial cells that form the alveolar walls. Type II alveolar cells are metabolically active. These cells secrete surfactant, a phospholipid that lines the inner surface and prevents alveolar collapse. Type III alveolar cell macrophages are large phagocytic cells that ingest foreign matter (eg, mucus, bacteria) and act as an important defense mechanism.

## Function of the Respiratory System

The cells of the body derive the energy they need from the oxidation of carbohydrates, fats, and proteins. As with any type of combustion, this process requires oxygen. Certain vital tissues, such as those of the brain and the heart, cannot survive for long without a continuous supply of oxygen. However, as a result of oxidation in the body tissues, carbon dioxide is produced and must be removed from the cells to prevent the buildup of acid waste products. The respiratory system performs this function by facilitating life-sustaining processes such as oxygen transport, respiration and ventilation, and gas exchange.

## Oxygen Transport

Oxygen is supplied to, and carbon dioxide is removed from, cells by way of the circulating blood. Cells are in close contact with capillaries, the thin walls of which permit easy passage or exchange of oxygen and carbon dioxide. Oxygen diffuses from the capillary through the capillary wall to the interstitial fluid. At this point, it diffuses through the membrane of tissue cells, where it is used by mitochondria for cellular respiration. The movement of carbon dioxide occurs by diffusion in the opposite direction—from cell to blood.

## Respiration

After these tissue capillary exchanges, blood enters the systemic veins (where it is called venous blood) and travels to the pulmonary circulation. The oxygen concentration in blood within the capillaries of the lungs is lower than in the lungs' air sacs (alveoli). Because of this concentration gradient, oxygen diffuses from the alveoli to the blood. Carbon dioxide, which has a higher concentration in the blood than in the alveoli, diffuses from the blood into the alveoli. Movement of air in and out of the airways (ventilation) continually replenishes the oxygen and removes the carbon dioxide from the airways and lungs. This whole process of gas exchange between the atmospheric air and the blood and between the blood and cells of the body is called **respiration**.

## Ventilation

During inspiration, air flows from the environment into the trachea, bronchi, bronchioles, and alveoli. During expiration, alveolar gas travels the same route in reverse.

Physical factors that govern air flow in and out of the lungs are collectively referred to as the mechanics of ventilation and include air pressure variances, resistance to air flow, and lung compliance.

### AIR PRESSURE VARIANCES

Air flows from a region of higher pressure to a region of lower pressure. During inspiration, movement of the diaphragm and other muscles of respiration enlarges the thoracic cavity and thereby lowers the pressure inside the thorax to a level below that of atmospheric pressure. As a result, air is drawn through the trachea and bronchi into the alveoli. During expiration, the diaphragm relaxes and the lungs recoil, resulting in a decrease in the size of the thoracic cavity. The alveolar pressure then exceeds atmospheric pressure, and air flows from the lungs into the atmosphere.

### AIRWAY RESISTANCE

Resistance is determined chiefly by the radius or size of the airway through which the air is flowing. Any process that changes the bronchial diameter or width affects airway resistance and alters the rate of air flow for a given pressure gradient during respiration (Chart 21-1). With increased resistance, greater-than-normal respiratory effort is required to achieve normal levels of ventilation.

> **CHART 21-1**
> ### Causes of Increased Airway Resistance
>
> Common phenomena that may alter bronchial diameter, which affects airway resistance, include the following:
> - Contraction of bronchial smooth muscle—as in asthma
> - Thickening of bronchial mucosa—as in chronic bronchitis
> - Obstruction of the airway—by mucus, a tumor, or a foreign body
> - Loss of lung elasticity—as in emphysema, which is characterized by connective tissue encircling the airways, thereby keeping them open during both inspiration and expiration

### COMPLIANCE

The pressure gradient between the thoracic cavity and the atmosphere causes air to flow in and out of the lungs. When pressure changes occur in the normal lung, there is a proportional change in the lung volume. A measure of the elasticity, expandability, and distensibility of the lungs and thoracic structures is called compliance. Factors that determine lung compliance are the surface tension of the alveoli (normally low with the presence of surfactant) and the connective tissue (ie, collagen and elastin) of the lungs.

Compliance is determined by examining the volume–pressure relationship in the lungs and the thorax. Compliance is normal (1.0 L/cm $H_2O$) if the lungs and thorax easily stretch and distend when pressure is applied. High or increased compliance occurs if the lungs have lost their elasticity and the thorax is overdistended (ie, in emphysema). Low or decreased compliance occurs if the lungs and thorax are "stiff." Conditions associated with decreased compliance include pneumothorax, hemothorax, pleural effusion, pulmonary edema, atelectasis, pulmonary fibrosis, and acute respiratory distress syndrome (ARDS), all of which are discussed in later chapters in this unit. Measurement of compliance is one method used to assess the progression and improvement in patients with ARDS. Lungs with decreased compliance require greater-than-normal energy expenditure by the patient to achieve normal levels of ventilation. Compliance is usually measured under static conditions.

## Lung Volumes and Capacities

Lung function, which reflects the mechanics of ventilation, is viewed in terms of lung volumes and lung capacities. Lung volumes are categorized as tidal volume, inspiratory reserve volume, expiratory reserve volume, and residual volume. Lung capacity is evaluated in terms of vital capacity, inspiratory capacity, functional residual capacity, and total lung capacity. These terms are described in Table 21-1.

## Diffusion and Perfusion

**Diffusion** is the process by which oxygen and carbon dioxide are exchanged at the air–blood interface. The alveolar–

### TABLE 21-1  Lung Volumes and Lung Capacities

| Term | Symbol | Description | Normal Value* | Significance |
|---|---|---|---|---|
| **Lung Volumes** | | | | |
| Tidal volume | VT or TV | The volume of air inhaled and exhaled with each breath | 500 mL or 5–10 mL/kg | The tidal volume may not vary, even with severe disease. |
| Inspiratory reserve volume | IRV | The maximum volume of air that can be inhaled after a normal inhalation | 3000 mL | |
| Expiratory reserve volume | ERV | The maximum volume of air that can be exhaled forcibly after a normal exhalation | 1100 mL | Expiratory reserve volume is decreased with restrictive conditions, such as obesity, ascites, pregnancy. |
| Residual volume | RV | The volume of air remaining in the lungs after a maximum exhalation | 1200 mL | Residual volume may be increased with obstructive disease. |
| **Lung Capacities** | | | | |
| Vital capacity | VC | The maximum volume of air exhaled from the point of maximum inspiration VC = TV + IRV + ERV | 4600 mL | A decrease in vital capacity may be found in neuromuscular disease, generalized fatigue, atelectasis, pulmonary edema, and COPD. |
| Inspiratory capacity | IC | The maximum volume of air inhaled after normal expiration IC = TV + IRV | 3500 mL | A decrease in inspiratory capacity may indicate restrictive disease. |
| Functional residual capacity | FRC | The volume of air remaining in the lungs after a normal expiration FRV = ERV + RV | 2300 mL | Functional residual capacity may be increased with COPD and decreased in ARDS. |
| Total lung capacity | TLC | The volume of air in the lungs after a maximum inspiration TLC = TV + IRV + ERV + RV | 5800 mL | Total lung capacity may be decreased with restrictive disease (atelectasis, pneumonia) and increased in COPD. |

*Values for healthy men; women are 20–25% less.
ARDS, acute respiratory distress syndrome; COPD, chronic obstructed pulmonary disease.

capillary membrane is ideal for diffusion because of its thinness and large surface area. In the normal healthy adult, oxygen and carbon dioxide travel across the alveolar–capillary membrane without difficulty as a result of differences in gas concentrations in the alveoli and capillaries.

**Pulmonary perfusion** is the actual blood flow through the pulmonary circulation. The blood is pumped into the lungs by the right ventricle through the pulmonary artery. The pulmonary artery divides into the right and left branches to supply both lungs. These two branches divide further to supply all parts of each lung. Normally about 2% of the blood pumped by the right ventricle does not perfuse the alveolar capillaries. This shunted blood drains into the left side of the heart without participating in alveolar gas exchange.

The pulmonary circulation is considered a low-pressure system because the systolic blood pressure in the pulmonary artery is 20 to 30 mm Hg and the diastolic pressure is 5 to 15 mm Hg. Because of these low pressures, the pulmonary vasculature normally can vary its capacity to accommodate the blood flow it receives. However, when a person is in an upright position, the pulmonary artery pressure is not great enough to supply blood to the apex of the lung against the force of gravity. Thus, when a person is upright, the lung may be considered to be divided into three sections: an upper part with poor blood supply, a lower part with maximal blood supply, and a section between the two with an intermediate supply of blood. When a person lying down turns to one side, more blood passes to the dependent lung.

Perfusion also is influenced by alveolar pressure. The pulmonary capillaries are sandwiched between adjacent alveoli. If the alveolar pressure is sufficiently high, the capillaries are squeezed. Depending on the pressure, some capillaries completely collapse, whereas others narrow.

Pulmonary artery pressure, gravity, and alveolar pressure determine the patterns of perfusion. In lung disease these factors vary, and the perfusion of the lung may become very abnormal.

## Ventilation and Perfusion Balance and Imbalance

Ventilation is the flow of gas in and out of the lungs, and perfusion is the filling of the pulmonary capillaries with blood. Adequate gas exchange depends on an adequate ventilation–perfusion ($\dot{V}/\dot{Q}$) ratio. In different areas of the lung, the $\dot{V}/\dot{Q}$ ratio varies. Alterations in perfusion may occur with a change in the pulmonary artery pressure, alveolar pressure, or gravity. Airway blockages, local changes in compliance, and gravity may alter ventilation.

$\dot{V}/\dot{Q}$ imbalance occurs as a result of inadequate ventilation, inadequate perfusion, or both. There are four possible $\dot{V}/\dot{Q}$ states in the lung: normal $\dot{V}/\dot{Q}$ ratio, low $\dot{V}/\dot{Q}$ ratio (shunt), high $\dot{V}/\dot{Q}$ ratio (dead space), and absence of ventilation and perfusion (silent unit) (Chart 21-2). $\dot{V}/\dot{Q}$ imbalance causes shunting of blood, resulting in **hypoxia** (low level of cellular oxygen). Shunting appears to be the main cause of hypoxia after thoracic or abdominal surgery and most types of respiratory failure. Severe hypoxia results when the amount of shunting exceeds 20%. Supplemental oxygen may eliminate hypoxia, depending on the type of $\dot{V}/\dot{Q}$ imbalance.

## Gas Exchange

**CONCEPTS in action ANIMATION**

The air we breathe is a gaseous mixture consisting mainly of nitrogen (78.62%) and oxygen (20.84%), with traces of carbon dioxide (0.04%), water vapor (0.05%), helium, and argon. The atmospheric pressure at sea level is about 760 mm Hg. Partial pressure is the pressure exerted by

---

### CHART 21-2

### Ventilation-Perfusion Ratios

**NORMAL RATIO (A)**
In the healthy lung, a given amount of blood passes an alveolus and is matched with an equal amount of gas (**A**). The ratio is 1:1 (ventilation matches perfusion).

**LOW VENTILATION–PERFUSION RATIO: SHUNTS (B)**
Low ventilation–perfusion states may be called shunt-producing disorders. When perfusion exceeds ventilation, a shunt exists (**B**). Blood bypasses the alveoli without gas exchange occurring. This is seen with obstruction of the distal airways, such as with pneumonia, atelectasis, tumor, or a mucus plug.

**HIGH VENTILATION–PERFUSION RATIO: DEAD SPACE (C)**
When ventilation exceeds perfusion, dead space results (**C**). The alveoli do not have an adequate blood supply for gas exchange to occur. This is characteristic of a variety of disorders, including pulmonary emboli, pulmonary infarction, and cardiogenic shock.

**SILENT UNIT (D)**
In the absence of ventilation and perfusion or with limited ventilation and perfusion, a condition known as a silent unit occurs (**D**). This is seen with pneumothorax and severe acute respiratory distress syndrome.

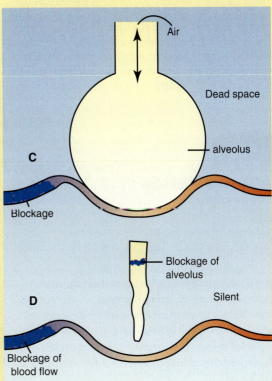

each type of gas in a mixture of gases. The partial pressure of a gas is proportional to the concentration of that gas in the mixture. The total pressure exerted by the gaseous mixture is equal to the sum of the partial pressures.

## PARTIAL PRESSURE OF GASES

Based on these facts, the partial pressures of nitrogen and oxygen can be calculated. The partial pressure of nitrogen is 79% of 760 (0.79 × 760), or 600 mm Hg; that of oxygen is 21% of 760 (0.21 × 760), or 160 mm Hg. Chart 21-3 identifies and defines terms and abbreviations related to partial pressure of gases.

Once the air enters the trachea, it becomes fully saturated with water vapor, which displaces some of the gases so that the air pressure within the lung remains equal to the air pressure outside (760 mm Hg). Water vapor exerts a pressure of 47 mm Hg when it fully saturates a mixture of gases at the body temperature of 37°C (98.6°F). Nitrogen and oxygen are responsible for the remaining 713 mm Hg (760–47) pressure. Once this mixture enters the alveoli, it is further diluted by carbon dioxide. In the alveoli, the water vapor continues to exert a pressure of 47 mm Hg. The remaining 713 mm Hg pressure is now exerted as follows: nitrogen, 569 mm Hg (74.9%); oxygen, 104 mm Hg (13.6%); and carbon dioxide, 40 mm Hg (5.3%).

## PARTIAL PRESSURE IN GAS EXCHANGE

When a gas is exposed to a liquid, the gas dissolves in the liquid until an equilibrium is reached. The dissolved gas also exerts a partial pressure. At equilibrium, the partial pressure of the gas in the liquid is the same as the partial pressure of the gas in the gaseous mixture. Oxygenation of venous blood in the lung illustrates this point. In the lung, venous blood and alveolar oxygen are separated by a very thin alveolar membrane. Oxygen diffuses across this membrane to dissolve in the blood until the partial pressure of oxygen in the blood is the same as that in the alveoli (104 Hg). However, because carbon dioxide is a byproduct of oxidation in the cells, venous blood contains carbon dioxide at a higher partial pressure than that in the alveolar gas. In the lung, carbon dioxide diffuses out of venous blood into the alveolar gas. At equilibrium, the partial pressure of carbon dioxide in the blood and in alveolar gas is the same (40 mm Hg). The changes in partial pressure are shown in Figure 21-5.

## EFFECTS OF PRESSURE ON OXYGEN TRANSPORT

**CONCEPTS** in action **ANIMATION**

Oxygen and carbon dioxide are transported simultaneously dissolved in blood or combined with some of the elements of blood. Oxygen is carried in the blood in two forms: first as physically dissolved oxygen in the plasma, and second in combination with the hemoglobin of the red blood cells. Each 100 mL of normal arterial blood carries 0.3 mL of oxygen physically dissolved in the plasma and 20 mL of oxygen in combination with hemoglobin. Large amounts of oxygen can be transported in the blood because oxygen combines easily with hemoglobin to form oxyhemoglobin:

$$O_2 + Hgb \leftrightarrow HgbO_2$$

The volume of oxygen physically dissolved in the plasma varies directly with the partial pressure of oxygen in the arteries ($PaO_2$). The higher the $PaO_2$, the greater the amount of oxygen dissolved. For example, at a $PaO_2$ of 10 mm Hg, 0.03 mL of oxygen is dissolved in 100 mL of plasma. At 20 mm Hg, twice this amount is dissolved in plasma, and at 100 mm Hg, 10 times this amount is dissolved. Therefore, the amount of dissolved oxygen is directly proportional to the partial pressure, regardless of how high the oxygen pressure becomes.

The amount of oxygen that combines with hemoglobin also depends on $PaO_2$, but only up to a $PaO_2$ of about 150 mm Hg. When the $PaO_2$ is 150 mm Hg, hemoglobin is 100% saturated and does not combine with any additional oxygen. When hemoglobin is 100% saturated, 1 g of hemoglobin combines with 1.34 mL of oxygen. Therefore, in a person with 14 g/dL of hemoglobin, each 100 mL of blood contains about 19 mL of oxygen associated with hemoglobin. If the $PaO_2$ is less than 150 mm Hg, the percentage of hemoglobin saturated with oxygen decreases. For example, at a $PaO_2$ of 100 mm Hg (normal value), saturation is 97%; at a $PaO_2$ of 40 mm Hg, saturation is 70%.

## OXYHEMOGLOBIN DISSOCIATION CURVE

The oxyhemoglobin dissociation curve (Chart 21-4) shows the relationship between the partial pressure of oxygen ($PaO_2$) and the percentage of saturation of oxygen ($SaO_2$). The percentage of saturation can be affected by the following factors: carbon dioxide, hydrogen ion concentration, temperature, and 2,3-diphosphoglycerate. An increase in these factors shifts the curve to the right, so that more oxygen is released to the tissues at the same $PaO_2$. A decrease in these factors causes the curve to shift to the left, making the bond between oxygen and hemoglobin stronger, so that less oxygen is given up to the tissues at the same $PaO_2$. The unusual shape of the oxyhemoglobin dissociation curve is a distinct advantage to the patient for two reasons:

1. If the $PaO_2$ decreases from 100 to 80 mm Hg as a result of lung disease or heart disease, the hemoglobin of the arterial blood remains almost maximally saturated (94%), and the tissues do not suffer from hypoxia.

---

### CHART 21-3

### Partial Pressure Symbols

P = pressure
$PO_2$ = partial pressure of oxygen
$PCO_2$ = partial pressure of carbon dioxide
$PAO_2$ = partial pressure of alveolar oxygen
$PACO_2$ = partial pressure of alveolar carbon dioxide
$PaO_2$ = partial pressure of arterial oxygen
$PaCO_2$ = partial pressure of arterial carbon dioxide
$P\bar{v}O_2$ = partial pressure of venous oxygen
$P\bar{v}CO_2$ = partial pressure of venous carbon dioxide
$P_{50}$ = partial pressure of oxygen when the hemoglobin is 50% saturated

**FIGURE 21-5.** Changes occur in the partial pressure of gases during respiration. These values vary as a result of the exchange of oxygen and carbon dioxide and the changes that occur in their partial pressures as venous blood flows through the lungs.

## CHART 21-4

### Oxyhemoglobin Dissociation Curve

The oxyhemoglobin dissociation curve is marked to show three oxygen levels:
1. Normal levels—$PaO_2$ above 70 mm Hg
2. Relatively safe levels—$PaO_2$ 45 to 70 mm Hg
3. Dangerous levels—$PaO_2$ below 40 mm Hg

The normal (middle) curve (N) shows that 75% saturation occurs at a $PaO_2$ of 40 mm Hg. If the curve shifts to the right (R), the same saturation (75%) occurs at the higher $PaO_2$ of 57 mm Hg. If the curve shifts to the left (L), 75% saturation occurs at a $PaO_2$ of 25 mm Hg.

2. When the arterial blood passes into tissue capillaries and is exposed to the tissue tension of oxygen (about 40 mm Hg), hemoglobin gives up large quantities of oxygen for use by the tissues.

With a normal value for $PaO_2$ of 80 to 100 mm Hg (95% to 98% saturation), there is a 15% margin of excess oxygen available to the tissues. With a normal hemoglobin level of 15 mg/dL and a $PaO_2$ level of 40 mm Hg (oxygen saturation 75%), there is adequate oxygen available for the tissues but no reserve for physiologic stresses that increase tissue oxygen demand. When a serious incident occurs (eg, bronchospasm, aspiration, hypotension, or cardiac dysrhythmias) that reduces the intake of oxygen from the lungs, tissue hypoxia results.

An important consideration in the transport of oxygen is cardiac output, which determines the amount of oxygen delivered to the body and which affects lung and tissue perfusion. If the cardiac output is normal (5 L/min), the amount of oxygen delivered to the body per minute is normal. If cardiac output falls, the amount of oxygen delivered to the tissues also falls. Under normal conditions, most of the oxygen delivered to the body is not used. In fact, only 250 mL of oxygen is used per minute. Under normal conditions, this is approximately 25% of available oxygen. The rest of the oxygen returns to the right side of the heart, and the $PaO_2$ of venous blood drops from 80 to 100 mm Hg to about 40 mm Hg.

### Carbon Dioxide Transport

At the same time that oxygen diffuses from the blood into the tissues, carbon dioxide diffuses in the opposite direction (ie, from tissue cells to blood) and is transported to the lungs for excretion. The amount of carbon dioxide in transit is one of the major determinants of the acid–base balance of the body. Normally, only 6% of the venous carbon dioxide is removed, and enough remains in the arterial blood to exert a pressure of 40 mm Hg. Most of the carbon dioxide (90%) enters the red blood cells; the small portion (5%) that remains dissolved in the plasma ($PCO_2$) is the critical factor that determines carbon dioxide movement in or out of the blood.

In summary, the many processes involved in respiratory gas transport do not occur in intermittent stages; rather, they are rapid, simultaneous, and continuous.

## Neurologic Control of Ventilation

Resting respiration is the result of cyclic excitation of the respiratory muscles by the phrenic nerve. The rhythm of breathing is controlled by respiratory centers in the brain. The inspiratory and expiratory centers in the medulla oblongata and pons control the rate and depth of ventilation to meet the body's metabolic demands.

The apneustic center in the lower pons stimulates the inspiratory medullary center to promote deep, prolonged inspirations. The pneumotaxic center in the upper pons is thought to control the pattern of respirations.

Several groups of receptor sites assist in the brain's control of respiratory function. The central chemoreceptors are located in the medulla and respond to chemical changes in the cerebrospinal fluid, which result from chemical changes in the blood. These receptors respond to an increase or decrease in the pH and convey a message to the lungs to change the depth and then the rate of ventilation to correct the imbalance. The peripheral chemoreceptors are located in the aortic arch and the carotid arteries and respond first to changes in $PaO_2$, then to $PaCO_2$ and pH. The Hering–Breuer reflex is activated by stretch receptors in the alveoli. When the lungs are distended, inspiration is inhibited; as a result, the lungs do not become overdistended. In addition, proprioceptors in the muscles and joints respond to body movements, such as exercise, causing an increase in ventilation. Thus, range-of-motion exercises in an immobile patient stimulate breathing. Baroreceptors, also located in the aortic and carotid bodies, respond to an increase or decrease in arterial blood pressure and cause reflex hypoventilation or hyperventilation.

### Gerontologic Considerations

A gradual decline in respiratory function begins in early to middle adulthood and affects the structure and function of the respiratory system. The vital capacity of the lungs and strength of the respiratory muscles peak between 20 and 25 years of age and decrease thereafter. With aging (40 years and older), changes occur in the alveoli that reduce the surface area available for the exchange of oxygen and carbon dioxide. At approximately 50 years of age, the alveoli begin to lose elasticity. A decrease in vital capacity occurs with loss of chest wall mobility, which restricts the tidal flow of air. The amount of respiratory dead space increases with age. These changes result in a decreased diffusion capacity for oxygen with increasing age, producing lower oxygen levels in the arterial circulation. Elderly people have a decreased ability to rapidly move air in and out of the lungs.

Gerontologic changes in the respiratory system are summarized in Table 21-2. Despite these changes, in the absence of chronic pulmonary disease, elderly people are

**TABLE 21-2 Age-Related Changes in the Respiratory System**

| | Structural Changes | Functional Changes | History and Physical Findings |
|---|---|---|---|
| Defense mechanisms (respiratory and nonrespiratory) | ↓ Number of cilia and ↓ mucus<br>↓ Cough and gag reflex<br>Loss of surface area of the capillary membrane<br>Lack of a uniform or consistent ventilation and/or blood flow | ↓ Protection against foreign particles<br>↓ Protection against aspiration<br>↓ Antibody response to antigens<br>↓ Response to hypoxia and hypercapnia (chemoreceptors) | ↓ Cough reflex and mucus<br>↑ Infection rate<br>History of respiratory infections, COPD, pneumonia.<br>Risk factors: smoking, environmental exposure, TB exposure |
| Lung | ↓ Size of airway<br>↑ Diameter of alveolar ducts<br>↑ Collagen of alveolar walls<br>↑ Thickness of alveolar membranes<br>↓ Elasticity of alveolar sacs | ↑ Airway resistance<br>↑ Pulmonary compliance<br>↓ Expiratory flow rate<br>↓ Oxygen diffusion capacity<br>↑ Dead space<br>Premature closure of airways<br>↑ Air trapping<br>↓ Expiratory flow rates<br>Ventilation–perfusion mismatch<br>↓ Exercise capacity<br>↑ Anteroposterior (AP) diameter | Unchanged total lung capacity (TLC)<br>↑ Residual volume (RV)<br>↓ Inspiratory reserve volume (IRV)<br>↓ Expiratory reserve volume (ERV)<br>↓ Forced vital capacity (FVC) and vital capacity (VC)<br>↑ Functional residual capacity (FRC)<br>↓ $PaO_2$<br>↑ $CO_2$ |
| Chest wall and muscles | Calcification of intercostal cartilages<br>Arthritis of costovertebral joints<br>↓ Continuity of diaphragm<br>Osteoporotic changes<br>↓ Muscle mass<br>Muscle atrophy | ↑ Rigidity and stiffness of thoracic cage<br>↓ Respiratory muscle strength<br>↑ Work of breathing<br>↓ Capacity for exercise<br>↓ Peripheral chemosensitivity<br>↑ Risk for inspiratory muscle fatigue | Kyphosis, barrel chest<br>Skeletal changes<br>↑ AP diameter<br>Shortness of breath<br>↑ Abdominal and diaphragmatic breathing<br>↓ Maximum expiratory flow rates |

able to carry out activities of daily living, but they may have decreased tolerance for and require additional rest after prolonged or vigorous activity.

# Assessment

## Health History

The health history focuses on the physical and functional problems of the patient and the effects of these problems on the patient, including his or her ability to carry out activities of daily living. The reason the patient is seeking health care often is related to one of the following: **dyspnea** (shortness of breath), pain, accumulation of mucus, wheezing, **hemoptysis** (blood spit up from the respiratory tract), edema of the ankles and feet, cough, and general fatigue and weakness. If the patient is experiencing severe dyspnea, the nurse may need to modify or abbreviate the questions asked and the timing of the health history to avoid increasing the patient's breathlessness and anxiety.

In addition to identifying the chief reason why the patient is seeking health care, the nurse tries to determine when the health problem or symptom started, how long it lasted, if it was relieved at any time, and how relief was obtained. The nurse obtains information about precipitating factors, duration, severity, and associated factors or symptoms and also assesses for risk factors and genetics factors that may contribute to the patient's lung condition (Chart 21-5).

The nurse assesses the impact of signs and symptoms on the patient's ability to perform activities of daily living and to participate in usual work and family activities. In addition, psychosocial factors that may affect the patient are explored (Chart 21-6). These factors include anxiety, role changes, family relationships, financial problems, employment status, and the strategies the patient uses to cope with them.

Many respiratory diseases are chronic and progressively debilitating and disabling. Therefore, ongoing assessment of the patient's physical abilities, psychosocial supports, and quality of life is needed to plan appropriate interventions. It is important that the patient with a respiratory disorder understand the condition and be familiar with necessary self-care interventions. The nurse evaluates these factors over time and provides education as needed.

The major signs and symptoms of respiratory disease are dyspnea, cough, sputum production, chest pain, wheezing, clubbing of the fingers, hemoptysis, and cyanosis. These clinical manifestations are related to the duration and severity of the disease.

### Dyspnea

Dyspnea (difficult or labored breathing, breathlessness, shortness of breath) is a symptom common to many pulmonary and cardiac disorders, particularly when there is decreased lung compliance or increased airway resistance. The right ventricle of the heart is affected ultimately by lung disease because it must pump blood through the lungs against greater resistance. It may also be associated with neurologic or neuromuscular disorders (ie, myasthenia gravis, Guillain-Barré syndrome, muscular dystrophy) that affect respiratory function. Dyspnea can also occur after physical exercise in people without disease (Porth, 2005). It is also common at the end of life in patients with a variety of disorders.

**CLINICAL SIGNIFICANCE**

In general, acute diseases of the lungs produce a more severe grade of dyspnea than do chronic diseases. Sudden dyspnea in a healthy person may indicate pneumothorax (air in the pleural cavity), acute respiratory obstruction, or ARDS. In immobilized patients, sudden dyspnea may denote pulmonary embolism. **Orthopnea** (inability to breathe easily except in an upright position) may be found in patients with heart disease and occasionally in patients with COPD; dyspnea with an expiratory wheeze occurs with COPD. Noisy breathing may result from a narrowing of the airway or localized obstruction of a major bronchus by a tumor or foreign body. The presence of both inspiratory and expiratory wheezing usually signifies asthma if the patient does not have heart failure. Because dyspnea can occur with other disorders (eg, cardiac disease, anaphylactic reactions, severe anemia), these disorders also need to be considered when obtaining the patient's health history (Zoorob & Campbell, 2003).

The circumstance that produces the dyspnea must be determined. Therefore, it is important to ask the patient the following questions:

1. How much exertion triggers shortness of breath?
2. Is there an associated cough?
3. Is the shortness of breath related to other symptoms?
4. Was the onset of shortness of breath sudden or gradual?
5. At what time of day or night does the shortness of breath occur?
6. Is the shortness of breath worse when the patient is flat in bed?
7. Does the shortness of breath occur at rest? With exercise? Running? Climbing stairs?
8. Is the shortness of breath worse while walking? If so, when walking how far? How fast?

Other issues that are important in assessment of dyspnea include the following: the patient's rating of the intensity of breathlessness, the effort required to breathe, and the severity of the breathlessness or dyspnea. Patients use a variety of terms and phrases to describe breathlessness, and the nurse needs to clarify what terms are most familiar to the patient and what these terms mean (Bailey, 2004; de Souza Caroci & Lareau, 2004; Michaels & Meek, 2004). Several scales are available to assess the severity of dyspnea,

### CHART 21-5

### Risk Factors for Respiratory Disease

- Smoking (the single most important contributor to lung disease)
- Exposure to secondhand smoke
- Personal or family history of lung disease
- Genetic make-up
- Allergens and environmental pollutants
- Recreational and occupational exposure

## GENETICS IN NURSING PRACTICE
### Genetic Influences

Various conditions that affect gas exchange and respiratory function are influenced by genetics factors, including:
- Asthma
- Chronic obstructive pulmonary disease
- Cystic fibrosis
- Alpha-1 antitrypsin deficiency

### NURSING ASSESSMENTS
**Family History Assessment**
- Assess family history for other family members with histories of respiratory impairment.
- Assess family history for individuals with early-onset chronic pulmonary disease, family history of hepatic disease in infants (clinical symptoms of alpha-1 antitrypsin deficiency).
- Inquire about family history of genetic cystic fibrosis.

### PATIENT ASSESSMENT
- Assess for symptoms such as changes in respiratory status associated with asthma (eg, wheezing, hyperresponsiveness, mucosal edema, and mucus production).
- Assess for multisystem effects characteristic of cystic fibrosis (eg, productive cough, wheezing, obstructive airways disease, gastrointestinal problems including pancreatic insufficiency, clubbing of the fingers).

### MANAGEMENT ISSUES SPECIFIC TO GENETICS
- Inquire whether DNA mutation or other genetic testing has been performed on affected family members.
- Refer for further genetics counseling and evaluation so that family members can discuss inheritance, risk to other family members, availability of genetics testing and gene-based interventions.
- Offer appropriate genetics information and resources.
- Assess patient's understanding of genetics information.
- Provide support to families with newly diagnosed genetic-related respiratory disorders.
- Participate in management and coordination of care of patients with genetic conditions, individuals predisposed to develop or pass on a genetic condition.

### GENETIC RESOURCES
American Lung Association, www.lungusa.org
Cystic Fibrosis Foundation, www.cff.org
Genetic Alliance, www.geneticalliance.org—a directory of support groups for patients and families with genetic conditions
Gene Clinics, www.geneclinics.org—a listing of common genetic disorders with clinical summaries, genetics counseling and testing information
National Organization of Rare Disorders, www.rarediseases.org—a directory of support groups and information for patients and families with rare genetic disorders
OMIM: Online Mendelian Inheritance in Man, www.ncbi.nlm.nih.gov/cntrez/query.fcgi?db=OMIM—a complete listing of inherited genetic conditions

---

including visual analog scales that can be used to assess changes in its severity over time (Leidy, Rennard, Schmier, et al., 2003; Porth, 2005).

### RELIEF MEASURES
The management of dyspnea is aimed at identifying and correcting its cause. Relief of the symptom sometimes is achieved by placing the patient at rest with the head elevated (high Fowler's position) and, in severe cases, by administering oxygen. Strategies that enable patients with chronic or persistent dyspnea to decrease or prevent breathlessness and to cope with it can lead to improved quality of life (Hately, Laurence, Scott, et al. 2003).

## Cough

Although cough is a reflex that protects the lungs from the accumulation of secretions or the inhalation of foreign bodies, it can also be a symptom of a number of disorders of the pulmonary system or it can be suppressed in other disorders. The cough reflex may be impaired by weakness or paralysis of the respiratory muscles, prolonged inactivity, the presence of a nasogastric tube, or depressed function of the medullary centers in the brain (eg, anesthesia, brain disorders) (Ebihara, Saito, Kanda, et al., 2003; Porth, 2005).

Cough results from irritation of the mucous membranes anywhere in the respiratory tract. The stimulus that produces a cough may arise from an infectious process or from an airborne irritant, such as smoke, smog, dust, or a gas. A persistent and frequent cough can be exhausting and cause pain. Cough may indicate serious pulmonary disease, but it may be caused by a variety of other problems as well, including cardiac disease, medications (eg, amiodarone, angiotensin-converting enzyme [ACE] inhibitors), smoking, and gastroesophageal reflux disease (Ott, Khoor, Leventhal, et al. 2003; Poe & Kallay, 2003).

### CLINICAL SIGNIFICANCE
To help determine the cause of the cough, the nurse describes the cough: dry, hacking, brassy, wheezing, loose, or severe. A dry, irritative cough is characteristic of an upper respiratory tract infection of viral origin, or it may

## CHART 21-6

### Assessing for Psychosocial Factors Related to Pulmonary Disease and Respiratory Function

- What strategies does the patient use to cope with the signs and symptoms and challenges associated with pulmonary disease?
- What effect has the pulmonary disease had on the patient's quality of life, goals, role within the family, and occupation?
- What changes has the pulmonary disease had on the patient's family and relationships with family members?
- Does the patient exhibit depression, anxiety, anger, hostility, dependency, withdrawal, isolation, avoidance, noncompliance, acceptance, or denial?
- What support systems does the patient use to cope with the illness?
- Are resources (relatives, friends, or community groups) available? Do the patient and family use them effectively?

---

be a side effect of ACE inhibitor therapy. Laryngotracheitis causes an irritative, high-pitched cough. Tracheal lesions produce a brassy cough. A severe or changing cough may indicate bronchogenic carcinoma. Pleuritic chest pain that accompanies coughing may indicate pleural or chest wall (musculoskeletal) involvement.

The time of coughing is also noted. Coughing at night may herald the onset of left-sided heart failure or bronchial asthma. A cough in the morning with sputum production may indicate bronchitis. A cough that worsens when the patient is supine suggests postnasal drip (sinusitis). Coughing after food intake may indicate aspiration of material into the tracheobronchial tree. A cough of recent onset is usually from an acute infection.

A persistent cough may affect a patient's quality of life and may produce embarrassment, exhaustion, inability to sleep, and pain. Therefore, the effect of a chronic cough on the patient and the patient's view about the significance of the cough and its effect on his or her life should also be obtained during the health history (French, Fletcher & Irwin, 2004).

### RELIEF MEASURES

Cough suppressants must be used with caution, because they may relieve the cough but do not address the cause of the cough. If used inappropriately, they may prevent the patient from clearing mucus from the airways and result in a delay in seeking indicated health care. If the cause of the cough has been investigated and addressed but the cough persists, cough suppressants may be prescribed. If the cough is a result of irritation, smoking cessation strategies are indicated. Drinking warm beverages may relieve cough caused by throat irritation.

The American College of Chest Physicians (ACCP) issued guidelines for the assessment and management of acute cough (a cough that lasts for less than 3 weeks), subacute cough (a cough that lasts 3 to 8 weeks), and chronic cough (a cough that lasts for more than 8 weeks) (Irwin, Baumann, Bolser, et al., 2006). The guidelines recommend use of first-generation antihistamines with a decongestant for treatment of acute cough or upper airway cough syndrome secondary to rhinosinus disease (previously referred to as postnasal drip syndrome) instead of over-the-counter cough expectorants or suppressants (ie, cough syrups and cough drops). The guidelines contain a number of algorithms for use in evaluating different patterns of cough and identifying appropriate treatment strategies (Irwin et al., 2006).

### Sputum Production

A patient who coughs long enough almost invariably produces sputum. Violent coughing causes bronchial spasm, obstruction, and further irritation of the bronchi and may result in syncope (fainting). A severe, repeated, or uncontrolled cough that is nonproductive is exhausting and potentially harmful. Sputum production is the reaction of the lungs to any constantly recurring irritant. It also may be associated with a nasal discharge.

### CLINICAL SIGNIFICANCE

The nature of the sputum is indicative of the causal condition. A profuse amount of purulent sputum (thick and yellow, green, or rust-colored) or a change in color of the sputum is a common sign of a bacterial infection. Thin, mucoid sputum frequently results from viral bronchitis. A gradual increase of sputum over time may indicate the presence of chronic bronchitis or bronchiectasis. Pink-tinged mucoid sputum suggests a lung tumor. Profuse, frothy, pink material, often welling up into the throat, may indicate pulmonary edema. Foul-smelling sputum and bad breath point to the presence of a lung abscess, bronchiectasis, or an infection caused by fusospirochetal or other anaerobic organisms.

### RELIEF MEASURES

If the sputum is too thick for the patient to expectorate, it is necessary to decrease its viscosity by increasing its water content through adequate hydration (drinking water) and inhalation of aerosolized solutions, which may be delivered by any type of nebulizer. Strategies to help the patient cough productively are discussed later in this chapter.

Smoking is contraindicated with excessive sputum production because it interferes with ciliary action, increases bronchial secretions, causes inflammation and hyperplasia of the mucous membranes, and reduces production of surfactant. Thus, smoking impairs bronchial drainage. When a person stops smoking, sputum volume decreases and resistance to bronchial infections increases.

The patient's appetite may decrease because of the odor of the sputum or the taste it leaves in the mouth. The nurse encourages adequate oral hygiene and wise selection of food, measures that stimulate the appetite. In addition, the nurse encourages the patient and family to remove sputum cups, emesis basins, and soiled tissues before mealtime. Encouraging the patient to drink citrus juices at the beginning of the meal may increase the palatability of the rest of

## NURSING RESEARCH PROFILE

### Patients' Descriptions of Respiratory Symptoms

Michaels, C. & Meek, P. M. (2004). The language of breathing among individuals with chronic obstructive pulmonary disease. *Heart and Lung, 33*(6), 390–400.

### Purpose
The words patients use to describe pulmonary symptoms and changes in their symptoms to their health care providers may determine whether further assessment and treatment are performed. Difficulty with breathing can include effort required to breathe and the distress associated with impaired breathing. The purpose of this study was to examine the everyday language used by people with moderate to severe chronic obstructive pulmonary disease (COPD) to describe the effort of breathing and the distress associated with breathlessness.

### Design
A longitudinal study was conducted using descriptive naturalistic research methods. The convenience sample included 15 people with a clinical diagnosis of COPD, moderate to severe pulmonary impairment based on results of pulmonary function tests, and no history of an exacerbation of COPD in the 3 months before enrollment in the study. Study participants were asked to perform each of the following tasks:

- From a list of 20 terms used in other studies, select the word or phrase that most accurately describes their breathing each day for 28 consecutive days.
- Complete a daily description and rating of breathing intensity for 28 days using a visual analogue scale (VAS) for breathing distress and another VAS for breathing effort.
- Describe the experience of breathing intensity during the previous 24 hours and record their breathing at the same time each day.
- Record physical sensations, associated emotions, or details they believed pertinent to the study.

Participants were visited at home weekly for 4 weeks. At each home visit, the daily logs and VAS scores for the previous week were reviewed. Terminology used was analyzed using qualitative data analysis techniques, and mean VAS scores on breathing effort and breathing distress were calculated.

### Findings
Data were available from 11 of 15 participants who were originally recruited into the study. The mean VAS score (on a scale ranging from 0 = no distress or no effort to 100 = greatest distress or greatest effort possible) was 28.4 (SD ± 18.5) for breathing distress and 31.3 (SD ± 18.2) for breathing effort. Ten participants reported at least one episode of breathing distress or effort greater than 20 mm above their baseline VAS scores. In 30 instances, breathing distress and/or effort exceeded individual means by greater than 20 mm, representing 1% of the total days reviewed. Distress and effort both increased 50% of the time. In the remaining instances, distress was increased above effort 8 times, and effort was increased above distress 7 times. Descriptors that were frequently identified included "hard to breathe," "difficulty breathing," and "out of breath." Other terms that were often reported were "short of breath," "tightness," and "breathless." Occasionally, participants used more than one term or phrase to describe their breathing each day. The use of more intense wording or phrases to describe breathing difficulty tended to be associated with VAS scores indicating more breathing effort and greater breathing distress.

Typically, the highest VAS scores reported for distress and effort occurred on the same day, although there were inconsistencies. For example, "no problem" was used to describe breathing on days with high breathing distress and effort scores when participants had ceased all physical activity to minimize respiratory distress.

### Nursing Implications
This study provides some insight into the everyday language used by people with moderate to severe COPD to describe their breathing effort and breathing distress. In a natural setting (ie, patients' homes), factors other than altered breathing may contribute to wording used by patients to describe their breathing. Participants used some of the words or phrases identified in previous research conducted in laboratory settings, added other words or phrases, and described the range of intensity of breathing difficulty. It is important that health care professionals understand the nuances of a patient's descriptions of changes in breathing, because the patient's language is essential for communication about problems that necessitate self-care and those that require professional treatment. To detect significant breathing changes, it is essential that nurses and other clinicians be sensitive to the various words and phrases patients use in describing their breathing difficulties and clarify terms used by patients.

## NURSING RESEARCH PROFILE

### Dyspnea-Anxiety-Dyspnea Cycle in Patients With Chronic Obstructive Pulmonary Disease

Bailey, P. H. (2004). The dyspnea-anxiety-dyspnea cycle—COPD patients' stories of breathlessness: "It's scary when you can't breathe." *Qualitative Health Research, 14*(6), 760–778.

#### Purpose
Dyspnea, or the sensation of breathlessness, is a major subjective symptom of chronic obstructive pulmonary disease (COPD) that is invisible to others because it is subjective. The purpose of this study was to explore the affective component of dyspnea, specifically anxiety, as described by patients and family caregivers, associated with acute exacerbations of COPD characterized by severe dyspnea.

#### Design
The researcher used qualitative research methods to gain insight into the meaning and experience of severe dyspnea associated with acute exacerbations of COPD. Ten patients with advanced COPD and at least two previous hospital admissions for acute exacerbations of COPD and 15 of their family caregivers participated in in-depth interviews about their experiences. Narrative analysis of the transcriptions of the interviews was used to examine the data.

#### Findings
Patients with COPD and their caregivers identified and described a close relationship between acute dyspnea and patients' physical and emotional functioning. Stories about the experiences of acute dyspnea and the relationship between dyspnea and patients' emotional function, labeled Emotional Vulnerability Stories by the researcher, revealed that patients were often unable to cope emotionally with everyday experiences (eg, having a heated discussion with others, becoming excited about an event) because of intractable breathlessness. Normal emotional responses to everyday events often produced an increase in patients' feelings of breathlessness. Patients who were emotionally disabled because of increased breathlessness were unable to participate in normal physical or emotional activities because doing so increased the likelihood of even greater breathlessness.

#### Nursing Implications
The findings of this study demonstrate the complex and often circular relationship between dyspnea and emotional functioning in patients with severe COPD. Other researchers have described a cycle of anxiety-breathlessness-anxiety, in which patients' emotional reactions to being dyspneic have further increased their sense of breathlessness and have led to greater anxiety. However, the findings of this study suggest a cycle of dyspnea–anxiety–dyspnea in which anxiety is not the underlying cause of acute episodes of dyspnea. Patients who can control or suppress their emotional reactions can decrease the severity of their dyspnea. Thus, when they feel anxious, their anxiety is not a cause of dyspnea; rather, their acute episodes of anxiety may be indicators of increasing breathlessness. This study suggests that nurses and other health care providers should consider anxiety as a sign of increasing dyspnea rather than as a cause of the breathlessness in patients with COPD who are in acute respiratory distress.

---

the meal, because these juices cleanse the palate of the sputum taste.

## Chest Pain

Chest pain or discomfort may be associated with pulmonary or cardiac disease. Chest pain associated with pulmonary conditions may be sharp, stabbing, and intermittent, or it may be dull, aching, and persistent. The pain usually is felt on the side where the pathologic process is located, but it may be referred elsewhere—for example, to the neck, back, or abdomen.

#### CLINICAL SIGNIFICANCE
Chest pain may occur with pneumonia, pulmonary embolism with lung infarction, and pleurisy. It also may be a late symptom of bronchogenic carcinoma. In carcinoma, the pain may be dull and persistent because the cancer has invaded the chest wall, mediastinum, or spine.

Lung disease does not always cause thoracic pain, because the lungs and the visceral pleura lack sensory nerves and are insensitive to pain stimuli. However, the parietal pleura has a rich supply of sensory nerves that are stimulated by inflammation and stretching of the membrane. Pleuritic pain from irritation of the parietal pleura is sharp and seems to "catch" on inspiration; patients often describe it as "like the stabbing of a knife." Patients are more comfortable when they lie on the affected side, because this splints the chest wall, limits expansion and contraction of the lung, and reduces the friction between the injured or diseased pleurae on that side. Pain associated with cough may be reduced manually by splinting the rib cage.

The nurse assesses the quality, intensity, and radiation of pain and identifies and explores precipitating factors and their relationship to the patient's position. In addition, it is important to assess the relationship of pain to the inspiratory and expiratory phases of respiration.

#### RELIEF MEASURES
Analgesic medications may be effective in relieving chest pain, but care must be taken not to depress the respiratory center or a productive cough, if present. Nonsteroidal anti-

inflammatory drugs (NSAIDs) achieve this goal and therefore are used for pleuritic pain. A regional anesthetic block may be performed to relieve extreme pain.

### Wheezing

Wheezing is often the major finding in a patient with bronchoconstriction or airway narrowing. It is heard with or without a stethoscope, depending on its location. Wheezing is a high-pitched, musical sound heard mainly on expiration.

Oral or inhalant bronchodilator medications reverse wheezing in most instances.

### Clubbing of the Fingers

Clubbing of the fingers is a sign of lung disease that is found in patients with chronic hypoxic conditions, chronic lung infections, or malignancies of the lung (Bickley & Szilagyi, 2003). This finding may be manifested initially as sponginess of the nail bed and loss of the nail bed angle (Fig. 21-6).

### Hemoptysis

Hemoptysis (expectoration of blood from the respiratory tract) is a symptom of both pulmonary and cardiac disorders. The onset of hemoptysis is usually sudden, and it may be intermittent or continuous. Signs, which vary from blood-stained sputum to a large, sudden hemorrhage, always merit investigation. The most common causes are

- Pulmonary infection
- Carcinoma of the lung
- Abnormalities of the heart or blood vessels
- Pulmonary artery or vein abnormalities
- Pulmonary embolus and infarction

Diagnostic evaluation to determine the cause includes several studies: chest x-ray, chest angiography, and bronchoscopy. A careful history and physical examination are necessary to diagnose the underlying disease, irrespective of whether the bleeding involved a very small amount of blood in the sputum or a massive hemorrhage. The amount of blood produced is not always proportional to the seriousness of the cause.

First, it is important to determine the source of the bleeding—the gums, nasopharynx, lungs, or stomach. The nurse may be the only witness to the episode. When documenting the bleeding episode, the nurse considers the following points:

- Bloody sputum from the nose or the nasopharynx is usually preceded by considerable sniffing, with blood possibly appearing in the nose.
- Blood from the lung is usually bright red, frothy, and mixed with sputum. Initial symptoms include a tickling sensation in the throat, a salty taste, a burning or bubbling sensation in the chest, and perhaps chest pain, in which case the patient tends to splint the bleeding side. The term "hemoptysis" is reserved for the coughing up of blood arising from a pulmonary hemorrhage. This blood has an alkaline pH (greater than 7.0).
- If the hemorrhage is in the stomach, the blood is vomited (hematemesis) rather than coughed up. Blood that has been in contact with gastric juice is sometimes so dark that it is referred to as "coffee grounds." This blood has an acid pH (less than 7.0).

### Cyanosis

Cyanosis, a bluish coloring of the skin, is a very late indicator of hypoxia. The presence or absence of cyanosis is determined by the amount of unoxygenated hemoglobin in the blood. Cyanosis appears when there is at least 5 g/dL of unoxygenated hemoglobin. A patient with a hemoglobin level of 15 g/dL does not demonstrate cyanosis until 5 g/dL of that hemoglobin becomes unoxygenated, reducing the effective circulating hemoglobin to two thirds of the normal level.

A patient with anemia rarely manifests cyanosis, and a patient with polycythemia may appear cyanotic even if adequately oxygenated. Therefore, cyanosis is *not* a reliable sign of hypoxia.

Assessment of cyanosis is affected by room lighting, the patient's skin color, and the distance of the blood vessels from the surface of the skin. In the presence of a pulmonary condition, central cyanosis is assessed by observing the color of the tongue and lips. This indicates a decrease in oxygen tension in the blood. Peripheral cyanosis results from decreased blood flow to a certain area of the body, as in vasoconstriction of the nail beds or earlobes from exposure to cold, and does not necessarily indicate a central systemic problem.

## Physical Assessment of the Upper Respiratory Structures

For a routine examination of the upper airway, only a simple light source, such as a penlight, is necessary. A more thorough examination requires the use of a nasal speculum.

### Nose and Sinuses

The nurse inspects the external nose for lesions, asymmetry, or inflammation and then asks the patient to tilt the head backward. Gently pushing the tip of the nose upward,

**FIGURE 21-6.** Clubbed finger. In clubbing, the distal phalanx of each finger is rounded and bulbous. The nail plate is more convex, and the angle between the plate and the proximal nail fold increases to 180 degrees or more. The proximal nail fold, when palpated, feels spongy or floating. Among the many causes are chronic hypoxia and lung cancer.

the nurse examines the internal structures of the nose, inspecting the mucosa for color, swelling, exudate, or bleeding. The nasal mucosa is normally redder than the oral mucosa. It may appear swollen and hyperemic if the patient has a common cold, but in allergic rhinitis the mucosa appears pale and swollen.

Next the nurse inspects the septum for deviation, perforation, or bleeding. Most people have a slight degree of septal deviation, but actual displacement of the cartilage into either the right or left side of the nose may produce nasal obstruction. Such deviation usually causes no symptoms.

While the head is still tilted back, the nurse inspects the inferior and middle turbinates. In chronic rhinitis, nasal polyps may develop between the inferior and middle turbinates; they are distinguished by their gray appearance. Unlike the turbinates, they are gelatinous and freely movable.

Next the nurse may palpate the frontal and maxillary sinuses for tenderness (Fig. 21-7). Using the thumbs, the nurse applies gentle pressure in an upward fashion at the supraorbital ridges (frontal sinuses) and in the cheek area adjacent to the nose (maxillary sinuses). Tenderness in either area suggests inflammation. The frontal and maxillary sinuses can be inspected by transillumination (passing a strong light through a bony area, such as the sinuses, to inspect the cavity; Fig. 21-8). If the light fails to penetrate, the cavity likely contains fluid or pus.

### Pharynx and Mouth

After the nasal inspection, the nurse assesses the mouth and pharynx, instructing the patient to open the mouth wide and take a deep breath. Usually this flattens the posterior tongue and briefly allows a full view of the anterior and posterior pillars, tonsils, uvula, and posterior pharynx (Fig. 21-9). The nurse inspects these structures for color, symmetry, and evidence of exudate, ulceration, or enlargement. If a tongue blade is needed to depress the tongue to visualize the pharynx, it is pressed firmly beyond the midpoint of the tongue to avoid a gagging response.

### Trachea

Next the position and mobility of the trachea are noted by direct palpation. This is performed by placing the thumb and index finger of one hand on either side of the trachea just above the sternal notch. The trachea is highly sensitive, and palpating too firmly may trigger a coughing or gagging response. The trachea is normally in the midline as it enters the thoracic inlet behind the sternum, but it may be deviated by masses in the neck or mediastinum. Pleural or pulmonary disorders, such as a pneumothorax, may also displace the trachea.

## Physical Assessment of the Lower Respiratory Structures and Breathing

### Thorax

Inspection of the thorax provides information about the musculoskeletal structure, the patient's nutritional status, and the respiratory system. The nurse observes the skin over the thorax for color and turgor and for evidence of loss of subcutaneous tissue. It is important to note asymmetry, if present. In recording or reporting the findings, anatomic landmarks are used as points of reference (Chart 21-7).

#### CHEST CONFIGURATION

Normally, the ratio of the anteroposterior diameter to the lateral diameter is 1:2. However, there are four main deformities of the chest associated with respiratory disease that alter this relationship: barrel chest, funnel chest (pectus excavatum), pigeon chest (pectus carinatum), and kyphoscoliosis.

**Barrel Chest.** Barrel chest occurs as a result of overinflation of the lungs. There is an increase in the anteroposterior diameter of the thorax. In a patient with emphysema, the ribs are more widely spaced and the intercostal spaces tend

**FIGURE 21-7.** Technique for palpating the frontal sinuses at left and the maxillary sinuses at right. From Weber, J. & Kelley, J. (2003). *Health assessment in nursing* (2nd ed.). Philadelphia: Lippincott Williams & Wilkins.

**FIGURE 21-8.** At left, the nurse positions the light source for transillumination of the frontal sinus. At right, the nurse shields the patient's brow and shines the light. In normal conditions (a darkened room), the light should shine through the tissues and appear as a reddish glow (above the nurse's hand) over the sinus. From Weber, J. & Kelley, J. (2003). *Health assessment in nursing* (2nd ed.). Philadelphia: Lippincott Williams & Wilkins.

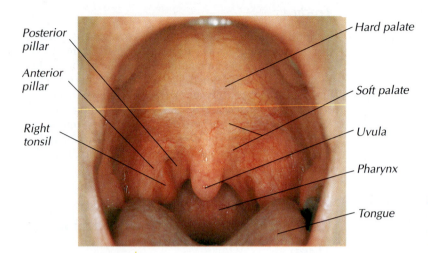

**FIGURE 21-9.** The pharynx and other oral structures—pillars, tonsils, uvula, hard and soft palates, posterior pharynx, and tongue—are easily seen when the mouth is open.

to bulge on expiration. The appearance of the patient with advanced emphysema is thus quite characteristic and often allows the observer to detect its presence easily, even from a distance.

**Funnel Chest (Pectus Excavatum).** Funnel chest occurs when there is a depression in the lower portion of the sternum. This may compress the heart and great vessels, resulting in murmurs. Funnel chest may occur with rickets or Marfan's syndrome.

**Pigeon Chest (Pectus Carinatum).** A pigeon chest occurs as a result of displacement of the sternum. There is an increase in the anteroposterior diameter. This may occur with rickets, Marfan's syndrome, or severe kyphoscoliosis.

**Kyphoscoliosis.** A kyphoscoliosis is characterized by elevation of the scapula and a corresponding S-shaped spine. This deformity limits lung expansion within the thorax. It may occur with osteoporosis and other skeletal disorders that affect the thorax.

### BREATHING PATTERNS AND RESPIRATORY RATES

Observing the rate and depth of respiration is a simple but important aspect of assessment (Finesilver, 2003). The normal adult who is resting comfortably takes 12 to 18 breaths per minute. Except for occasional sighs, respirations are regular in depth and rhythm. This normal pattern is described as eupnea.

Bradypnea, or slow breathing, is associated with increased intracranial pressure, brain injury, and drug overdose. Tachypnea, or rapid breathing, is commonly seen in patients with pneumonia, pulmonary edema, metabolic acidosis, septicemia, severe pain, or rib fracture. Shallow, irregular breathing is referred to as hypoventilation.

Hyperpnea is an increase in depth of respirations. Hyperventilation is an increase in both rate and depth that results in a decreased arterial $PaCO_2$ level. With rapid breathing, inspiration and expiration are nearly equal in duration. Hyperventilation that is marked by an increase in rate and depth, associated with severe acidosis of diabetic or renal origin, is called Kussmaul's respiration.

Apnea describes varying periods of cessation of breathing. If sustained, apnea is life-threatening.

Cheyne-Stokes respiration is characterized by alternating episodes of apnea (cessation of breathing) and periods of deep breathing. Deep respirations become increasingly shallow, followed by apnea that may last approximately 20 seconds. The cycle repeats after each apneic period. The duration of the period of apnea may vary and may progressively lengthen; therefore, it is timed and reported. Cheyne-Stokes respiration is usually associated with heart failure and damage to the respiratory center (drug-induced, tumor, trauma).

Biot's respirations, or cluster breathing, are cycles of breaths that vary in depth and have varying periods of apnea. Biot's respirations are seen with some central nervous system disorders.

Certain patterns of respiration are characteristic of specific disease states. Respiratory rhythms and their deviation from normal are important observations that the nurse reports and documents. The rate and depth of various patterns of respiration are presented in Table 21-3.

In thin people, it is quite normal to note a slight retraction of the intercostal spaces during quiet breathing. Bulging of the intercostal spaces during expiration implies obstruction of expiratory airflow, as in emphysema. Marked retraction on inspiration, particularly if asymmetric, implies blockage of a branch of the respiratory tree. Asymmetric bulging of the intercostal spaces, on one side or the other, is created by an increase in pressure within the hemithorax. This may be a result of air trapped under pressure within the pleural cavity, where it is not normally present (pneumothorax), or the pressure of fluid within the pleural space (pleural effusion).

## Thoracic Palpation

The nurse palpates the thorax for tenderness, masses, lesions, respiratory excursion, and vocal fremitus. If the patient has reported an area of pain or if lesions are apparent, the nurse performs direct palpation with the fingertips (for skin lesions and subcutaneous masses) or with the ball of the hand (for deeper masses or generalized flank or rib discomfort).

### RESPIRATORY EXCURSION

Respiratory excursion is an estimation of thoracic expansion and may disclose significant information about thoracic movement during breathing. The nurse assesses the patient for range and symmetry of excursion. The

### CHART 21-7

## Locating Thoracic Landmarks

With respect to the thorax, location is defined both horizontally and vertically. With respect to the lungs, location is defined by lobe.

### HORIZONTAL REFERENCE POINTS

Horizontally, thoracic locations are identified according to their proximity to the rib or the intercostal space under the examiner's fingers. On the anterior surface, identification of a specific rib is facilitated by first locating the angle of Louis. This is where the manubrium joins the body of the sternum in the midline. The second rib joins the sternum at this prominent landmark.

Other ribs may be identified by counting down from the second rib. The intercostal spaces are referred to in terms of the rib immediately above the intercostal space; for example, the fifth intercostal space is directly below the fifth rib.

Locating ribs on the posterior surface of the thorax is more difficult. The first step is to identify the spinous process. This is accomplished by finding the seventh cervical vertebra (*vertebra prominens*), which is the most prominent spinous process. When the neck is slightly flexed, the seventh cervical spinous process stands out. Other vertebrae are then identified by counting downward.

### VERTICAL REFERENCE POINTS

Several imaginary lines are used as vertical referents or landmarks to identify the location of thoracic findings. The *midsternal line* passes through the center of the sternum. The *midclavicular line* is an imaginary line that descends from the middle of the clavicle. The *point of maximal impulse* of the heart normally lies along this line on the left thorax.

When the arm is abducted from the body at 90°, imaginary vertical lines may be drawn from the anterior axillary fold, from the middle of the axilla, and from the posterior axillary fold. These lines are called, respectively, the *anterior axillary line*, the *midaxillary line*, and the *posterior axillary line*. A line drawn vertically through the superior and inferior poles of the scapula is called the *scapular line*, and a line drawn down the center of the vertebral column is called the *vertebral line*. Using these landmarks, for example, the examiner communicates findings by referring to an area of dullness extending from the vertebral to the scapular line between the seventh and tenth ribs on the right.

### LOBES OF THE LUNGS

The lobes of the lung may be mapped on the surface of the chest wall in the following manner. The line between the upper and lower lobes on the left begins at the fourth thoracic spinous process posteriorly, proceeds around to cross the fifth rib in the midaxillary line, and meets the sixth rib at the sternum. This line on the right divides the right middle lobe from the right lower lobe. The line dividing the right upper lobe from the middle lobe is an incomplete one that begins at the fifth rib in the midaxillary line, where it intersects the line between the upper and lower lobes and traverses horizontally to the sternum. Thus, the upper lobes are dominant on the anterior surface of the thorax and the lower lobes are dominant on the posterior surface. There is no presentation of the right middle lobe on the posterior surface of the chest.

| TABLE 21-3 | Rates and Depths of Respiration | |
|---|---|---|
| | Definition | Graphic Representation |
| Eupnea | Normal, breathing at 12–18 breaths/minute | |
| Bradypnea | Slower than normal rate (<10 breaths/minute), with normal depth and regular rhythm | |
| Tachypnea | Rapid, shallow breathing >24 breaths/minute | |
| Hypoventilation | Shallow, irregular breathing | |
| Hyperventilation | Increased rate and depth of breathing (called Kussmaul's respiration if caused by diabetic ketoacidosis) | |
| Apnea | Period of cessation of breathing. Time duration varies; apnea may occur briefly during other breathing disorders, such as with sleep apnea. Life threatening if sustained. | |
| Cheyne-Stokes | Regular cycle where the rate and depth of breathing increase, then decrease until apnea (usually about 20 seconds) occurs. | |
| Biot's respiration | Periods of normal breathing (3–4 breaths) followed by a varying period of apnea (usually 10–60 seconds). | |

patient is instructed to inhale deeply while the movement of the nurse's thumbs (placed along the costal margin on the anterior chest wall) during inspiration and expiration is observed. This movement is normally symmetric (Bickley & Szilagyi, 2003).

Posterior assessment is performed by placing the thumbs adjacent to the spinal column at the level of the tenth rib (Fig. 21-10). The hands lightly grasp the lateral rib cage. Sliding the thumbs medially about 2.5 cm (1 inch) raises a small skinfold between the thumbs. The patient is instructed to take a full inspiration and to exhale fully. The nurse observes for normal flattening of the skinfold and feels the symmetric movement of the thorax.

Decreased chest excursion may be caused by chronic fibrotic disease. Asymmetric excursion may be due to splinting secondary to pleurisy, fractured ribs, trauma, or unilateral bronchial obstruction (Bickley & Szilagyi, 2003).

## TACTILE FREMITUS

Sound generated by the larynx travels distally along the bronchial tree to set the chest wall in resonant motion. This is especially true of consonant sounds. The detection of the resulting vibration on the chest wall by touch is called tactile fremitus.

Normal fremitus is widely varied. It is influenced by the thickness of the chest wall, especially if that thickness is muscular. However, the increase in subcutaneous tissue associated with obesity may also affect fremitus. Lower-pitched sounds travel better through the normal lung and produce greater vibration of the chest wall. Therefore, fremitus is more pronounced in men than in women because of the deeper male voice. Normally, fremitus is most pronounced where the large bronchi are closest to the chest wall and least palpable over the distant lung fields. Therefore, it is most palpable in the upper thorax, anteriorly and posteriorly.

The patient is asked to repeat "ninety-nine" or "one, two, three," or "eee, eee, eee" as the nurse's hands move down

**FIGURE 21-10.** Method for assessing posterior respiratory excursion. Place both hands posteriorly at the level of T9 or T10. Slide hands medially to pinch a small amount of skin between your thumbs. Observe for symmetry as the patient exhales fully following a deep inspiration.

the patient's thorax. The vibrations are detected with the palmar surfaces of the fingers and hands, or the ulnar aspect of the extended hands, on the thorax. The hand or hands are moved in sequence down the thorax. Corresponding areas of the thorax are compared (Fig. 21-11). Bony areas are not tested.

Air does not conduct sound well, but a solid substance such as tissue does, provided that it has elasticity and is not compressed. Therefore, an increase in solid tissue per unit volume of lung enhances fremitus, and an increase in air per unit volume of lung impedes sound. Patients with emphysema, which results in the rupture of alveoli and trapping of air, exhibit almost no tactile fremitus. A patient with consolidation of a lobe of the lung from pneumonia has increased tactile fremitus over that lobe. Air in the pleural space does not conduct sound (Bickley & Szilagyi, 2003).

## Thoracic Percussion

Percussion sets the chest wall and underlying structures in motion, producing audible and tactile vibrations. The nurse uses percussion to determine whether underlying tissues are filled with air, fluid, or solid material (Finesilver, 2003). Percussion also is used to estimate the size and location of certain structures within the thorax (eg, diaphragm, heart, liver).

Percussion usually begins with the posterior thorax. Ideally, the patient is in a sitting position with the head flexed forward and the arms crossed on the lap. This position separates the scapulae widely and exposes more lung area for assessment. The nurse percusses across each shoulder top, locating the 5-cm width of resonance overlying the lung apices (Fig. 21-12). Then the nurse proceeds down the posterior thorax, percussing symmetric areas at intervals of 5 to 6 cm (2 to 2.5 inches). The middle finger is positioned parallel to the ribs in the intercostal space; the finger is placed firmly against the chest wall before it is struck with the middle finger of the opposite hand. Bony structures (scapulae or ribs) are not percussed.

Percussion over the anterior chest is performed with the patient in an upright position with shoulders arched backward and arms at the side. The nurse begins in the supraclavicular area and proceeds downward, from one intercostal space to the next. In the female patient, it may be necessary to displace the breasts for an adequate examination. Dullness noted to the left of the sternum between the third and fifth intercostal spaces is a normal finding, because that is the location of the heart. Similarly, there is a normal span of liver dullness in the right thorax, from the fifth intercostal space to the right costal margin at the midclavicular line (Bickley & Szilagyi, 2003).

The anterior and lateral thorax is examined with the patient in a supine position. If the patient cannot sit up, percussion of the posterior thorax is performed with the patient positioned on the side.

Dullness over the lung occurs when air-filled lung tissue is replaced by fluid or solid tissue. Table 21-4 reviews percussion sounds and their characteristics.

### DIAPHRAGMATIC EXCURSION

The normal resonance of the lung stops at the diaphragm. The position of the diaphragm is different during inspiration and expiration.

To assess the position and motion of the diaphragm, the nurse instructs the patient to take a deep breath and hold it while the maximal descent of the diaphragm is percussed. The point at which the percussion note at the midscapular line changes from resonance to dullness is marked with a pen. The patient is then instructed to exhale fully and hold it while the nurse again percusses downward to the dullness

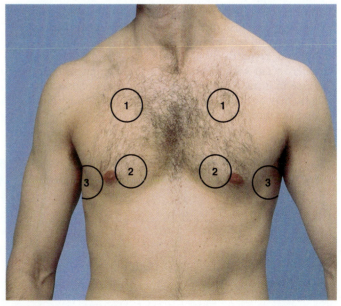

**FIGURE 21-11.** When palpating for tactile fremitus (*left*), the nurse places the ball or ulnar surface of the hands on the chest area being assessed. The palpation sequence is at *right*. From Bickley, L. S. & Szilagyi, P. G. (2003). *Bates' guide to physical examination and history taking* (8th ed.). Philadelphia: Lippincott Williams & Wilkins.

**FIGURE 21-12.** Percussion of the posterior thorax. With the patient in a sitting position, symmetric areas of the lungs are percussed at 5-cm intervals. This progression starts at the apex of each lung and concludes with percussion of each lateral chest wall.

of the diaphragm. This point is also marked. The distance between the two markings indicates the range of motion of the diaphragm.

Maximal excursion of the diaphragm may be as much as 8 to 10 cm (3 to 4 inches) in healthy, tall young men, but for most people it is usually 5 to 7 cm (2 to 2.75 inches). Normally, the diaphragm is about 2 cm (0.75 inches) higher on the right because of the position of the heart and the liver above and below the left and right segments of the diaphragm, respectively. Decreased diaphragmatic excursion may occur with pleural effusion and emphysema. An increase in intra-abdominal pressure, as in pregnancy or ascites, may account for a diaphragm that is positioned high in the thorax (Bickley & Szilagyi, 2003).

## Thoracic Auscultation

Auscultation is useful in assessing the flow of air through the bronchial tree and in evaluating the presence of fluid or solid obstruction in the lung. The nurse auscultates for normal breath sounds, adventitious sounds, and voice sounds (Finesilver, 2003).

Examination includes auscultation of the anterior, posterior, and lateral thorax and is performed as follows. The nurse places the diaphragm of the stethoscope firmly against the chest wall as the patient breathes slowly and deeply through the mouth. Corresponding areas of the chest are auscultated in a systematic fashion from the apices to the bases and along midaxillary lines. The sequence of auscultation and the positioning of the patient are similar to those used for percussion. It often is necessary to listen to two full inspirations and expirations at each anatomic location for valid interpretation of the sound heard. Repeated deep breaths may result in symptoms of hyperventilation (eg, lightheadedness); this is avoided by having the patient rest and breathe normally periodically during the examination.

### BREATH SOUNDS

Normal breath sounds are distinguished by their location over a specific area of the lung and are identified as vesicular, bronchovesicular, and bronchial (tubular) breath sounds (Table 21-5).

The location, quality, and intensity of breath sounds are determined during auscultation. When airflow is decreased by bronchial obstruction (atelectasis) or when fluid (pleural effusion) or tissue (obesity) separates the air passages from the stethoscope, breath sounds are diminished or absent. For example, the breath sounds of the patient with emphysema are faint or often completely inaudible. When they are heard, the expiratory phase is prolonged. Bronchial and bronchovesicular sounds that are audible anywhere except over the main bronchus in the lungs signify pathology, usually indicating consolidation in the lung (eg, pneumonia, heart failure). This finding requires further evaluation.

### ADVENTITIOUS SOUNDS

An abnormal condition that affects the bronchial tree and alveoli may produce adventitious (additional) sounds. Adventitious sounds are divided into two categories: dis-

| TABLE 21-4 | Characteristics of Percussion Sounds | | | | |
|---|---|---|---|---|---|
| Sound | Relative Intensity | Relative Pitch | Relative Duration | Location Example | Examples |
| Flatness | Soft | High | Short | Thigh | Large pleural effusion |
| Dullness | Medium | Medium | Medium | Liver | Lobar pneumonia |
| Resonance | Loud | Low | Long | Normal lung | Simple chronic bronchitis |
| Hyperresonance | Very loud | Lower | Longer | None normally | Emphysema, pneumothorax |
| Tympany | Loud | High* | —* | Gastric air bubble or puffed-out cheek | Large pneumothorax |

*Distinguished mainly by its musical timbre.

### TABLE 21-5 Breath Sounds

| | Duration of Sounds | Intensity of Expiratory Sound | Pitch of Expiratory Sound | Locations Where Heard Normally |
|---|---|---|---|---|
| Vesicular* | Inspiratory sounds last longer than expiratory ones | Soft | Relatively low | Entire lung field except over the upper sternum and between the scapulae |
| Broncho-vesicular | Inspiratory and expiratory sounds are about equal | Intermediate | Intermediate | Often in the 1st and 2nd interspaces anteriorly and between the scapulae (over the main bronchus) |
| Bronchial | Expiratory sounds last longer than inspiratory ones | Loud | Relatively high | Over the manubrium, if heard at all |
| Tracheal | Inspiratory and expiratory sounds are about equal | Very loud | Relatively high | Over the trachea in the neck |

*The thickness of the bars indicates intensity of breath sounds; the steeper their incline, the higher the pitch of the sounds.

crete, noncontinuous sounds (crackles) and continuous musical sounds (wheezes). The duration of the sound is the important distinction to make in identifying the sound as noncontinuous or continuous.

**Crackles** (formerly referred to as rales) are discrete, noncontinuous sounds that result from delayed reopening of deflated airways. Crackles may or may not be cleared by coughing. They reflect underlying inflammation or congestion and are often present in such conditions as pneumonia, bronchitis, heart failure, bronchiectasis, and pulmonary fibrosis. Crackles are usually heard on inspiration, but they may also be heard on expiration.

Pleural friction rubs are specific examples of crackles (Table 21-6). Friction rubs result from inflammation of the

### TABLE 21-6 Abnormal (Adventitious) Breath Sounds

| Breath Sound | Description | Etiology |
|---|---|---|
| **Crackles** | | |
| Crackles in general | Soft, high-pitched, discontinuous popping sounds that occur during inspiration | Secondary to fluid in the airways or alveoli or to opening of collapsed alveoli |
| Coarse crackles | Discontinuous popping sounds heard in early inspiration; harsh, moist sound originating in the large bronchi | Associated with obstructive pulmonary disease |
| Fine crackles | Discontinuous popping sounds heard in late inspiration; sounds like hair rubbing together; originates in the alveoli | Associated with interstitial pneumonia, restrictive pulmonary disease (eg, fibrosis). Fine crackles in early inspiration are associated with bronchitis or pneumonia. |
| **Wheezes** | | |
| Sonorous wheezes (rhonchi) | Deep, low-pitched rumbling sounds heard primarily during expiration; caused by air moving through narrowed tracheobronchial passages | Secretions or tumor |
| Sibilant wheezes | Continuous, musical, high-pitched, whistle-like sounds heard during inspiration and expiration caused by air passing through narrowed or partially obstructed airways; may clear with coughing | Bronchospasm, asthma, and buildup of secretions |
| **Friction rubs** | | |
| Pleural friction rub | Harsh, crackling sound, like two pieces of leather being rubbed together. Heard during inspiration alone or during both inspiration and expiration. May subside when patient holds breath. Coughing will not clear sound. | Secondary to inflammation and loss of lubricating pleural fluid |

pleural surfaces that induces a crackling, grating sound usually heard in inspiration and expiration. The sound can be enhanced by applying pressure to the chest wall with the diaphragm of the stethoscope. The sound is imitated by rubbing the thumb and index finger together near the ear. A friction rub is best heard over the lower lateral anterior surface of the thorax.

**Wheezes** are associated with bronchial wall oscillation and changes in airway diameter. Like crackles, wheezes are usually heard on expiration but may be heard on inspiration. They are commonly heard in patients with asthma, chronic bronchitis, or bronchiectasis.

### VOICE SOUNDS

The sound heard through the stethoscope as the patient speaks is known as vocal resonance. The vibrations produced in the larynx are transmitted to the chest wall as they pass through the bronchi and alveolar tissue. During the process, the sounds are diminished in intensity and altered so that syllables are not distinguishable. Voice sounds are usually assessed by having the patient repeat "ninety-nine" or "eee" while the nurse listens with the stethoscope in corresponding areas of the chest from the apices to the bases.

Bronchophony describes vocal resonance that is more intense and clearer than normal. Egophony describes voice sounds that are distorted. It is best appreciated by having the patient repeat the letter E. The distortion produced by consolidation transforms the sound into a clearly heard A rather than E. Bronchophony and egophony have precisely the same significance as bronchial breathing with an increase in tactile fremitus. When an abnormality is detected, it should be evident using more than one assessment method. A change in tactile fremitus is more subtle and can be missed, but bronchial breathing and bronchophony can be noted loudly and clearly.

Whispered pectoriloquy is a very subtle finding, which is heard only in the presence of rather dense consolidation of the lungs. Transmission of high-frequency components of sound is so enhanced by the consolidated tissue that even whispered words are heard, a circumstance not noted in normal physiology. The significance is the same as that of bronchophony (Bickley & Szilagyi, 2003). The physical findings for the most common respiratory diseases are summarized in Table 21-7.

## Assessment of Respiratory Function in the Acutely or Critically Ill Patient

Assessment of respiratory status is essential for the well-being of the patient who is acutely or critically ill. Often, such a patient is intubated and receiving mechanical ventilation. This requires that the nurse have expertise in physical assessment, be skilled in monitoring techniques, and be knowledgeable about possible ventilator-induced lung injury (Winters & Munro, 2004). The nurse reviews the patient's health history, including the history of disorders affecting lung function, signs and symptoms, and exposure to medications and other agents that can affect respiratory status. The nurse also observes the patient's respiratory status to analyze and interpret a variety of clinical findings and laboratory test results. Checking the ventilator settings to make sure that they are set as prescribed and that alarms are always in the "on" position, the nurse must assess for patient–ventilator synchrony as well as for agitation, restlessness, and other signs of respiratory distress (nasal flaring, excessive use of intercostals and accessory muscles, uncoordinated movement of the chest and abdomen, and a report by the patient of shortness of breath). The nurse must note changes in the patient's vital signs and evidence of hemodynamic instability and report them to the physician, because they may indicate that the mechanical ventilation is ineffective or that the patient's status has deteriorated. It is necessary to assess the position of the patient to be certain that the head of the bed is elevated to prevent aspiration, especially if the patient is receiving enteral feedings. In addition, the patient's mental status should be assessed and compared to previous status. Lethargy and somnolence may be signs of increasing carbon dioxide levels and should not be considered insignificant, even if the patient is receiving sedation or analgesic agents (Johnson, 2004).

### TABLE 21-7  Assessment Findings in Common Respiratory Disorders

| Disorder | Tactile Fremitus | Percussion | Auscultation |
| --- | --- | --- | --- |
| Consolidation (eg, pneumonia) | Increased | Dull | Bronchial breath sounds, crackles, bronchophony, egophony, whispered pectoriloquy |
| Bronchitis | Normal | Resonant | Normal to decreased breath sounds, wheezes |
| Emphysema | Decreased | Hyperresonant | Decreased intensity of breath sounds, usually with prolonged expiration |
| Asthma (severe attack) | Normal to decreased | Resonant to hyperresonant | Wheezes |
| Pulmonary edema | Normal | Resonant | Crackles at lung bases, possibly wheezes |
| Pleural effusion | Absent | Dull to flat | Decreased to absent breath sounds, bronchial breath sounds and bronchophony, egophony, and whispered pectoriloquy above the effusion over the area of compressed lung |
| Pneumothorax | Decreased | Hyperresonant | Absent breath sounds |
| Atelectasis | Absent | Flat | Decreased to absent breath sounds |

Chest auscultation, percussion, and palpation are essential parts of the evaluation of the critically ill patient with or without mechanical ventilation. Assessment of the anterior and posterior lung fields is part of the nurse's routine evaluation. If the patient is recumbent, it is essential to turn the patient to assess all lung fields so that dependent areas can be assessed for breath sounds, including the presence of normal breath sounds and adventitious sounds. Failure to examine the dependent areas of the lungs can result in missing the findings associated with disorders such as atelectasis or pleural effusion. Percussion is performed to assess for pleural effusion; if pleural effusion is present, the affected lung fields are dull to percussion and breath sounds are absent. A pleural friction rub may also be present (Winters & Munro, 2004).

Tests of the patient's respiratory status are easily performed at the bedside by measuring the respiratory rate (see earlier discussion), tidal volume, minute ventilation, vital capacity, inspiratory force, and compliance. These tests are particularly important for patients who are at risk for pulmonary complications, including those who have undergone chest or abdominal surgery, have had prolonged anesthesia, have preexisting pulmonary disease, or are elderly. These tests are also used routinely for mechanically ventilated patients.

The patient whose chest expansion is limited by external restrictions such as obesity or abdominal distention and who cannot breathe deeply because of postoperative pain or sedation will inhale and exhale a low volume of air (referred to as low tidal volumes). Prolonged hypoventilation at low tidal volumes can produce alveolar collapse (atelectasis). The amount of air remaining in the lungs after a normal expiration (functional residual capacity) decreases, the ability of the lungs to expand (compliance) is reduced, and the patient must breathe faster to maintain the same degree of tissue oxygenation. These events can be exaggerated in patients who have preexisting pulmonary diseases and in elderly patients whose airways are less compliant, because the small airways may collapse during expiration. More details of the assessment of the patient with lung disease, including arterial blood gas (ABG) analysis, are described in subsequent chapters in this unit and in Chapter 14.

> **NURSING ALERT**
> One should not rely only on visual inspection of the rate and depth of a patient's respiratory excursions to determine the adequacy of ventilation. Respiratory excursions may appear normal or exaggerated due to an increased work of breathing, but the patient may actually be moving only enough air to ventilate the dead space. If there is any question regarding adequacy of ventilation, auscultation or pulse oximetry (or both) should be used for additional assessment of respiratory status.

## Tidal Volume

The volume of each breath is referred to as the tidal volume (see Table 21-1 to review lung capacities and volumes). A spirometer is an instrument that can be used at the bedside to measure volumes. If the patient is breathing through an endotracheal tube or tracheostomy, the spirometer is directly attached to it and the exhaled volume is obtained from the reading on the gauge. In other patients, the spirometer is attached to a face mask or a mouthpiece positioned so that it is airtight, and the exhaled volume is measured.

The tidal volume may vary from breath to breath. To ensure that the measurement is reliable, it is important to measure the volumes of several breaths and to note the range of tidal volumes, together with the average tidal volume.

## Minute Ventilation

Respiratory rates and tidal volume alone are unreliable indicators of adequate ventilation, because both can vary widely from breath to breath. However, together the tidal volume and respiratory rate are important because the minute ventilation, which is useful in detecting respiratory failure, can be determined from them. Minute ventilation is the volume of air expired per minute. It is equal to the product of the tidal volume in liters multiplied by the respiratory rate or frequency. In practice, the minute ventilation is not calculated but is measured directly using a spirometer.

Minute ventilation may be decreased by a variety of conditions that result in hypoventilation. When the minute ventilation falls, alveolar ventilation in the lungs also decreases, and the $PaCO_2$ increases. Risk factors for hypoventilation are listed in Chart 21-8.

## Vital Capacity

Vital capacity is measured by having the patient take in a maximal breath and exhale fully through a spirometer. The normal value depends on the patient's age, gender, body build, and weight.

---

**CHART 21-8**

### Risk Factors for Hypoventilation

- Limited neurologic impulses transmitted from the brain to the respiratory muscles, as in spinal cord trauma, cerebrovascular accidents, tumors, myasthenia gravis, Guillain-Barré syndrome, polio, and drug overdose
- Depressed respiratory centers in the medulla, as with anesthesia, sedation, and drug overdose
- Limited thoracic movement (kyphoscoliosis), limited lung movement (pleural effusion, pneumothorax), or reduced functional lung tissue (chronic pulmonary diseases, severe pulmonary edema)

> **NURSING ALERT**
>
> Most patients can generate a vital capacity twice the volume they normally breathe in and out (tidal volume). If the vital capacity is less than 10 mL/kg, the patient will be unable to sustain spontaneous ventilation and will require respiratory assistance.

When the vital capacity is exhaled at a maximal flow rate, the forced vital capacity is measured. Most patients can exhale at least 80% of their vital capacity in 1 second (forced expiratory volume in 1 second, or $FEV_1$) and almost all of it in 3 seconds ($FEV_3$). A reduction in $FEV_1$ suggests abnormal pulmonary air flow. If the patient's $FEV_1$ and forced vital capacity are proportionately reduced, maximal lung expansion is restricted in some way. If the reduction in $FEV_1$ greatly exceeds the reduction in forced vital capacity, the patient may have some degree of airway obstruction.

### Inspiratory Force

Inspiratory force evaluates the effort the patient is making during inspiration. It does not require patient cooperation and therefore is a useful measurement in the unconscious patient. The equipment needed for this measurement includes a manometer that measures negative pressure and adapters that are connected to an anesthesia mask or a cuffed endotracheal tube. The manometer is attached and the airway is completely occluded for 10 to 20 seconds while the inspiratory efforts of the patient are registered on the manometer. The normal inspiratory pressure is about 100 cm $H_2O$. If the negative pressure registered after 15 seconds of occluding the airway is less than about 25 cm $H_2O$, mechanical ventilation is usually required because the patient lacks sufficient muscle strength for deep breathing or effective coughing.

## Diagnostic Evaluation

A wide range of diagnostic studies, described on the following pages, may be performed in patients with respiratory conditions.

### Pulmonary Function Tests

Pulmonary function tests (PFTs) are routinely used in patients with chronic respiratory disorders. They are performed to assess respiratory function and to determine the extent of dysfunction. Such tests include measurements of lung volumes, ventilatory function, and the mechanics of breathing, diffusion, and gas exchange (Table 21-8).

PFTs are useful in monitoring the course of a patient with an established respiratory disease and assessing the response to therapy (Conner & Meng, 2003). They are useful as screening tests in potentially hazardous industries, such as coal mining and those that involve exposure to asbestos and other noxious fumes, dusts, or gases. They are used to screen patients who are scheduled for thoracic and upper abdominal surgery (Beckles, Spiro, Colice, et al., 2003; Wang, 2004) and symptomatic patients with a history suggesting high risk. In addition, PFTs may be used for evaluation of respiratory symptoms and disability for insurance or legal purposes (Porth, 2005) and to diagnose occupational respiratory disease (Anees, 2003).

PFTs generally are performed by a technician using a spirometer that has a volume-collecting device attached to a recorder that demonstrates volume and time simultaneously. A number of tests are carried out, because no single measurement provides a complete picture of pulmonary function. The most frequently used PFTs are described in Table 21-8. Technology is available that allows for more complex assessment of pulmonary function. Methods include exercise tidal flow–volume loops, negative expiratory pressure, nitric oxide, and forced oscillation. These assessment methods

### TABLE 21-8 Pulmonary Function Tests

| Term Used | Symbol | Description | Remarks |
|---|---|---|---|
| Forced vital capacity | FVC | Vital capacity performed with a maximally forced expiratory effort | Forced vital capacity is often reduced in COPD because of air trapping. |
| Forced expiratory volume (qualified by subscript indicating the time interval in seconds) | $FEV_t$ (usually $FEV_1$) | Volume of air exhaled in the specified time during the performance of forced vital capacity; $FEV_1$ is volume exhaled in 1 second | A valuable clue to the severity of the expiratory airway obstruction |
| Ratio of timed forced expiratory volume to forced vital capacity | $FEV_t/FVC\%$, usually $FEV_1/FVC\%$ | $FEV_t$ expressed as a percentage of the forced vital capacity | Another way of expressing the presence or absence of airway obstruction |
| Forced expiratory flow | $FEF_{200-1200}$ | Mean forced expiratory flow between 200 and 1200 mL of the FVC | An indicator of large airway obstruction |
| Forced midexpiratory flow | $FEF_{25-75\%}$ | Mean forced expiratory flow during the middle half of the FVC | Slowed in small airway obstruction |
| Forced end expiratory flow | $FEF_{75-85\%}$ | Mean forced expiratory flow during the terminal portion of the FVC | Slowed in obstruction of smallest airways |
| Maximal voluntary ventilation | MVV | Volume of air expired in a specified period (12 seconds) during repetitive maximal effort | An important factor in exercise tolerance |

allow for detailed evaluation of expiratory flow limitations and airway inflammation (Conner & Meng, 2003).

PFT results are interpreted on the basis of the degree of deviation from normal, taking into consideration the patient's height, weight, age, and gender. Because there is a wide range of normal values, PFTs may not detect early localized changes. The patient with respiratory symptoms (dyspnea, wheezing, cough, sputum production) usually undergoes a complete diagnostic evaluation, even if the results of PFTs are "normal." Trends of results provide information about disease progression as well as the patient's response to therapy (Conner & Meng, 2003).

Patients with respiratory disorders may be taught how to measure their peak flow rate (which reflects maximal expiratory flow) at home using a spirometer (Ramirez, 2003). This allows them to monitor the progress of therapy, to alter medications and other interventions as needed based on caregiver guidelines, and to notify the health care provider if there is inadequate response to their own interventions. Home care teaching instructions are described in Chapter 24, which discusses asthma.

## Arterial Blood Gas Studies

Measurements of blood pH and of arterial oxygen and carbon dioxide tensions are obtained when managing patients with respiratory problems and adjusting oxygen therapy as needed. The arterial oxygen tension ($PaO_2$) indicates the degree of oxygenation of the blood, and the arterial carbon dioxide tension ($PaCO_2$) indicates the adequacy of alveolar ventilation. ABG studies aid in assessing the ability of the lungs to provide adequate oxygen and remove carbon dioxide and the ability of the kidneys to reabsorb or excrete bicarbonate ions to maintain normal body pH. Serial ABG analysis also is a sensitive indicator of whether the lung has been damaged after chest trauma. ABG levels are obtained through an arterial puncture at the radial, brachial, or femoral artery or through an indwelling arterial catheter. ABG levels are discussed in detail in Chapter 14.

Patients whose ABG levels are monitored repeatedly with blood obtained from arterial punctures should receive an explanation of the purpose of the procedure. It has been reported that patients often experience considerable pain with repeated ABG levels yet are often unaware of the purpose of the puncture and the fact that the ABG results could make a major difference in their treatment (Crawford, 2004).

## Pulse Oximetry

Pulse oximetry is a noninvasive method of continuously monitoring the oxygen saturation of hemoglobin ($SaO_2$). When oxygen saturation is measured with pulse oximetry, it is referred to as $SpO_2$ (Johnson, 2004; Woodrow, 2004). Although pulse oximetry does not replace ABG measurement, it is an effective tool to monitor for subtle or sudden changes in oxygen saturation. It is used in all settings where oxygen saturation monitoring is needed, such as the home, clinics, ambulatory surgical settings, and hospitals.

A probe or sensor is attached to the fingertip (Fig. 21-13), forehead, earlobe, or bridge of the nose. The sensor detects changes in oxygen saturation levels by monitoring light

**FIGURE 21-13.** Measuring blood oxygenation with pulse oximetry reduces the need for invasive procedures, such as drawing blood for analysis of oxygen levels. After the pulse oximeter sensor slips easily over a patient's finger, the oxygen saturation level appears on the monitor. The oximeter is portable and ideal for home use. Courtesy of Novametrix Medical Systems, Inc.

signals generated by the oximeter and reflected by blood pulsing through the tissue at the probe. Normal $SpO_2$ values are 95% to 100%. Values less than 85% indicate that the tissues are not receiving enough oxygen, and further evaluation is needed. $SpO_2$ values obtained by pulse oximetry are unreliable in cardiac arrest and shock, if dyes (ie, methylene blue) or vasoconstrictor medications have been used, or if the patient has severe anemia or a high carbon monoxide level. Furthermore, they are not reliable detectors of hypoventilation if the patient is receiving supplemental oxygen (Fu, Downs, Schweiger, et al., 2004).

## Cultures

Throat cultures may be performed to identify organisms responsible for pharyngitis. Throat culture may also assist in identifying organisms responsible for infection of the lower respiratory tract. Nasal swabs also may be performed for the same purpose.

## Sputum Studies

Sputum is obtained for analysis to identify pathogenic organisms and to determine whether malignant cells are present. It also may be used to assess for hypersensitivity states (in which there is an increase in eosinophils). Periodic sputum examinations may be necessary for patients receiving antibiotics, corticosteroids, and immunosuppressive medications for prolonged periods, because these agents are associated with opportunistic infections. In general, sputum cultures are used in diagnosis, for drug sensitivity testing, and to guide treatment.

Expectoration is the usual method for collecting a sputum specimen. The patient is instructed to clear the nose and throat and rinse the mouth to decrease contamination of the sputum. After taking a few deep breaths, the patient coughs (rather than spits), using the diaphragm, and expectorates into a sterile container.

If the sputum cannot be raised spontaneously, the patient often can be induced to cough deeply by breathing an irritating aerosol of supersaturated saline, propylene glycol, or some other agent delivered with an ultrasonic nebulizer. Other methods of collecting sputum specimens include endotracheal aspiration, bronchoscopic removal, bronchial brushing, transtracheal aspiration, and gastric aspiration—usually for tuberculosis organisms (see Chapter 23). Generally, the deepest specimens (those from the base of the lungs) are obtained in the early morning after they have accumulated overnight.

The specimen is delivered to the laboratory within 2 hours by the patient or nurse. Allowing the specimen to stand for several hours in a warm room results in the overgrowth of contaminant organisms and may make it difficult to identify the pathogenic organisms (especially *Mycobacterium tuberculosis*). The home care nurse may assist patients who need help obtaining the sample or who cannot deliver the specimen to the laboratory in a timely fashion.

## Imaging Studies

Imaging studies, including x-rays, computed tomography (CT), magnetic resonance imaging (MRI), contrast studies, and radioisotope diagnostic scans may be part of any diagnostic workup, ranging from a determination of the extent of infection in sinusitis to tumor growth in cancer.

### Chest X-Ray

Normal pulmonary tissue is radiolucent; therefore, densities produced by fluid, tumors, foreign bodies, and other pathologic conditions can be detected by x-ray examination. A chest x-ray may reveal an extensive pathologic process in the lungs in the absence of symptoms. The routine chest x-ray consists of two views—the posteroanterior projection and the lateral projection. Chest x-rays are usually taken after full inspiration (a deep breath), because the lungs are best visualized when they are well aerated. Also, the diaphragm is at its lowest level and the largest expanse of lung is visible. If taken on expiration, x-ray films may accentuate an otherwise unnoticed pneumothorax or obstruction of a major artery.

### Computed Tomography

CT is an imaging method in which the lungs are scanned in successive layers by a narrow-beam x-ray. The images produced provide a cross-sectional view of the chest. Whereas a chest x-ray shows major contrasts between body densities such as bone, soft tissue, and air, CT can distinguish fine tissue density. CT may be used to define pulmonary nodules and small tumors adjacent to pleural surfaces that are not visible on routine chest x-rays and to demonstrate mediastinal abnormalities and hilar adenopathy, which are difficult to visualize with other techniques. Contrast agents are useful when evaluating the mediastinum and its contents.

### Magnetic Resonance Imaging

MRI is similar to CT except that magnetic fields and radiofrequency signals are used instead of a narrow-beam x-ray. MRI yields a much more detailed diagnostic image than CT. MRI is used to characterize pulmonary nodules, to help stage bronchogenic carcinoma (assessment of chest wall invasion), and to evaluate inflammatory activity in interstitial lung disease, acute pulmonary embolism, and chronic thrombolytic pulmonary hypertension.

### Fluoroscopic Studies

Fluoroscopy is used to assist with invasive procedures, such as a chest needle biopsy or transbronchial biopsy, that are performed to identify lesions. It also may be used to study the movement of the chest wall, mediastinum, heart, and diaphragm; to detect diaphragm paralysis; and to locate lung masses.

### Pulmonary Angiography

Pulmonary angiography is most commonly used to investigate thromboembolic disease of the lungs, such as pulmonary emboli, and congenital abnormalities of the pulmonary vascular tree. It involves the rapid injection of a radiopaque agent into the vasculature of the lungs for radiographic study of the pulmonary vessels. It can be performed by injecting the radiopaque agent into a vein in one or both arms (simultaneously) or into the femoral vein, with a needle or catheter. The agent also can be injected into a catheter that has been inserted in the main pulmonary artery or its branches or into the great veins proximal to the pulmonary artery.

### Radioisotope Diagnostic Procedures (Lung Scans)

Several types of lung scans—V/Q scan, gallium scan, and positron emission tomography (PET)—are used to assess normal lung functioning, pulmonary vascular supply, and gas exchange.

A V/Q lung scan is performed by injecting a radioactive agent into a peripheral vein and then obtaining a scan of the chest to detect radiation. The isotope particles pass through the right side of the heart and are distributed into the lungs in proportion to the regional blood flow, making it possible to trace and measure blood perfusion through the lung. This procedure is used clinically to measure the integrity of the pulmonary vessels relative to blood flow and to evaluate blood flow abnormalities, as seen in pulmonary emboli. The imaging time is 20 to 40 minutes, during which the patient lies under the camera with a mask fitted over the nose and mouth. This is followed by the ventilation component of the scan. The patient takes a deep breath of a mixture of oxygen and radioactive gas, which diffuses throughout the lungs. A scan is performed to detect ventilation abnormalities in patients who have regional differences in ventilation. It may be helpful in the diagnosis of bronchitis, asthma, inflammatory fibrosis, pneumonia, emphysema, and lung cancer. Ventilation without perfusion is seen with pulmonary emboli.

A gallium scan is a radioisotope lung scan used to detect inflammatory conditions, abscesses, adhesions, and the presence, location, and size of tumors. It is used to stage bronchogenic cancer and document tumor regression after chemotherapy or radiation. Gallium is injected intravenously, and scans are taken at intervals (eg, 6, 24, and 48 hours) to evaluate gallium uptake by the pulmonary tissues.

PET is a radioisotope study with advanced diagnostic capabilities that is used to evaluate lung nodules for malignancy. PET can detect and display metabolic changes in tissue, distinguish normal tissue from diseased tissue (such as in cancer), differentiate viable from dead or dying tissue, show regional blood flow, and determine the distribution and fate of medications in the body. PET is more accurate in detecting malignancies than CT and has equivalent accuracy in detecting malignant nodules when compared with invasive procedures such as thoracoscopy.

## Endoscopic Procedures

### Bronchoscopy

**Bronchoscopy** is the direct inspection and examination of the larynx, trachea, and bronchi through either a flexible fiberoptic bronchoscope or a rigid bronchoscope (Fig. 21-14). The fiberoptic scope is used more frequently in current practice.

The purposes of diagnostic bronchoscopy are: (1) to examine tissues or collect secretions, (2) to determine the location and extent of the pathologic process and to obtain a tissue sample for diagnosis (by biting or cutting forceps, curettage, or brush biopsy), (3) to determine whether a tumor can be resected surgically, and (4) to diagnose bleeding sites (source of hemoptysis).

Therapeutic bronchoscopy is used to (1) remove foreign bodies from the tracheobronchial tree, (2) remove secretions obstructing the tracheobronchial tree when the patient cannot clear them, (3) treat postoperative atelectasis, and (4) destroy and excise lesions. It has also been used to insert stents to relieve airway obstruction that is caused by tumors or miscellaneous benign conditions or that occurs as a complication of lung transplantation (Saad, Murthy, Krizmanich, et al., 2003).

The fiberoptic bronchoscope is a thin, flexible bronchoscope that can be directed into the segmental bronchi. Because of its small size, its flexibility, and its excellent optical system, it allows increased visualization of the peripheral airways and is ideal for diagnosing pulmonary lesions. Fiberoptic bronchoscopy allows biopsy of previously inaccessible tumors and can be performed at the bedside. It also can be performed through endotracheal or tracheostomy tubes of patients on ventilators. Cytologic examinations can be performed without surgical intervention.

The rigid bronchoscope is a hollow metal tube with a light at its end. It is used mainly for removing foreign substances, investigating the source of massive hemoptysis, or performing endobronchial surgical procedures. Rigid bronchoscopy is performed in the operating room, not at the bedside.

Possible complications of bronchoscopy include a reaction to the local anesthetic, infection, aspiration, bronchospasm, **hypoxemia** (low blood oxygen level), pneumothorax, bleeding, and perforation.

#### NURSING INTERVENTIONS

Before the procedure, a signed consent form is obtained from the patient. Food and fluids are withheld for 6 hours before the test to reduce the risk of aspiration when the cough reflex is blocked by anesthesia. The nurse explains the procedure to the patient to reduce fear and decrease anxiety and administers preoperative medications (usually atropine and a sedative or opioid) as prescribed to inhibit vagal stimulation (thereby guarding against bradycardia, dysrhythmias, and hypotension), suppress the cough reflex, sedate the patient, and relieve anxiety.

> **NURSING ALERT**
>
> Sedation given to patients with respiratory insufficiency may precipitate respiratory arrest.

The patient must remove dentures and other oral prostheses. The examination is usually performed under local anesthesia or moderate sedation, but general anesthesia may be used for rigid bronchoscopy. A topical anesthetic such as lidocaine (Xylocaine) may be sprayed on the pharynx or

Fiberoptic bronchoscopy

Rigid bronchoscopy

**FIGURE 21-14.** Endoscopic bronchoscopy permits visualization of bronchial structures. The bronchoscope is advanced into bronchial structures orally. Bronchoscopy permits the clinician not only to diagnose but also to treat various lung problems.

dropped on the epiglottis and vocal cords and into the trachea to suppress the cough reflex and minimize discomfort. Sedatives or opioids are administered intravenously as prescribed to provide moderate sedation.

After the procedure, it is important that the patient takes nothing by mouth until the cough reflex returns, because the preoperative sedation and local anesthesia impair the protective laryngeal reflex and swallowing for several hours. Once the patient demonstrates a cough reflex, the nurse may offer ice chips and eventually fluids. In the elderly patient, the nurse assesses for confusion and lethargy, which may be due to the large doses of lidocaine administered during the procedure. The nurse also monitors the patient's respiratory status and observes for hypoxia, hypotension, tachycardia, dysrhythmias, hemoptysis, and dyspnea. Any abnormality is reported promptly. The patient is not discharged from the recovery area until adequate cough reflex and respiratory status are present. The nurse instructs the patient and family caregivers to report any shortness of breath or bleeding immediately.

### Thoracoscopy

Thoracoscopy is a diagnostic procedure in which the pleural cavity is examined with an endoscope (Fig. 21-15). Small incisions are made into the pleural cavity in an intercostal space; the location of the incision depends on the clinical and diagnostic findings. After any fluid present in the pleural cavity is aspirated, the fiberoptic mediastinoscope is inserted into the pleural cavity, and its surface is inspected through the instrument. After the procedure, a chest tube may be inserted, and the pleural cavity is drained by negative-pressure water-seal drainage.

Thoracoscopy is primarily indicated in the diagnostic evaluation of pleural effusions, pleural disease, and tumor staging. Biopsies of the lesions can be performed under visualization for diagnosis.

Thoracoscopic procedures have expanded with the availability of video monitoring, which permits improved visualization of the lung. Video-assisted thoracoscopy may be used in the diagnosis and treatment of empyema, pleural effusion, and other respiratory disorders (Luh, Chou, Wang, et al., 2005). Such procedures also have been used with the carbon dioxide laser in the removal of pulmonary blebs and bullae and in the treatment of spontaneous pneumothorax. Lasers have also been used in the excision of peripheral pulmonary nodules. Although the laser does not replace the need for thoracotomy in the treatment of some lung cancers, its use continues to expand, because it is less invasive than open surgical procedures and hospitalization and recovery are shorter.

**NURSING INTERVENTIONS**
Follow-up care in the health care facility and at home involves monitoring the patient for shortness of breath (which might indicate a pneumothorax) and minor activity restrictions, which vary depending on the intensity of the procedure. If a chest tube was inserted during the procedure, monitoring of the chest drainage system and chest tube insertion site is essential (see Chapter 25).

### Thoracentesis

A thin layer of pleural fluid normally remains in the pleural space. An accumulation of pleural fluid may occur with some disorders. A sample of this fluid can be obtained by thoracentesis (aspiration of pleural fluid for diagnostic or therapeutic purposes). It is important to position the patient as shown in Chart 21-9. When thoracentesis is performed under ultrasound guidance, it has a lower rate of complications than when it is performed without ultrasound guidance (Jones, Moyers, Rogers, et al., 2003; Mayo, Goltz, Tafreshi, et al., 2004).

A needle biopsy of the pleura may be performed at the same time. Studies of pleural fluid include Gram stain culture and sensitivity, acid-fast staining and culture, differential cell count, cytology, pH, specific gravity, total protein, and lactic dehydrogenase.

### Biopsy

Biopsy, the excision of a small amount of tissue, may be performed to permit examination of cells from the pharynx, larynx, and nasal passages. Local, topical, moderate sedation, or general anesthesia may be administered, depending on the site and the procedure.

### Pleural Biopsy

Pleural biopsy is accomplished by needle biopsy of the pleura or by pleuroscopy, a visual exploration through a fiberoptic

**FIGURE 21-15.** Endoscopic thoracoscopy. Like bronchoscopy, thoracoscopy uses fiberoptic instruments and video cameras for visualizing thoracic structures. Unlike bronchoscopy, thoracoscopy usually requires the surgeon to make a small incision before inserting the endoscope. A combined diagnostic–treatment procedure, thoracoscopy includes excising tissue for biopsy.

## CHART 21-9  Guidelines for Assisting the Patient Undergoing Thoracentesis

A thoracentesis (aspiration of fluid or air from the pleural space) is performed on patients with various clinical problems. A diagnostic or therapeutic procedure, thoracentesis may be used for
- Removal of fluid and air from the pleural cavity
- Aspiration of pleural fluid for analysis
- Pleural biopsy
- Instillation of medication into the pleural space

The responsibilities of the nurse and rationale for the nursing actions are summarized below.

### NURSING ACTIVITIES

1. Ascertain in advance that a chest x-ray has been ordered and completed and the consent form has been signed.

2. Assess the patient for allergy to the local anesthetic to be used.

3. Administer sedation if prescribed

4. Inform the patient about the nature of the procedure and
    a. The importance of remaining immobile
    b. Pressure sensations to be experienced
    c. That minimal discomfort is anticipated after the procedure

5. Position the patient comfortably with adequate supports. If possible, place the patient upright or in one of the following positions:
    a. Sitting on the edge of the bed with the feet supported and arms and head on a padded over-the-bed table

### RATIONALE

1. Posteroanterior and lateral chest x-ray films are used to localize fluid and air in the pleural cavity and to aid in determining the puncture site. When fluid is loculated (isolated in a pocket of pleural fluid), ultrasound scans are performed to help select the best site for needle aspiration.

2. If the patient is allergic to the initially prescribed anesthetic, assessment findings provide an opportunity to use a safer anesthetic.

3. Sedation enables the patient to cooperate with the procedure and promotes relaxation

4. An explanation helps to orient the patient to the procedure, assists the patient to mobilize resources, and provides an opportunity to ask questions and verbalize anxiety.

5. The upright position facilitates the removal of fluid that usually localizes at the base of the thorax. A position of comfort helps the patient to relax.

Pleural effusion

*continued >*

## CHART 21-9 Guidelines for Assisting the Patient Undergoing Thoracentesis, continued

| NURSING ACTIVITIES | RATIONALE |
|---|---|
|    b. Straddling a chair with arms and head resting on the back of the chair<br>   c. Lying on the unaffected side with the head of the bed elevated 30 to 45 degrees if unable to assume a sitting position | |
| 6. Support and reassure the patient during the procedure.<br>   a. Prepare the patient for the cold sensation of skin germicide solution and for a pressure sensation from infiltration of local anesthetic agent.<br>   b. Encourage the patient to refrain from coughing. | 6. Sudden and unexpected movement, such as coughing, by the patient can traumatize the visceral pleura and lung. |
| 7. Expose the entire chest. The site for aspiration is visualized by chest x-ray and percussion. If fluid is in the pleural cavity, the thoracentesis site is determined by the chest x-ray, ultrasound scanning, and physical findings, with attention to the site of maximal dullness on percussion. | 7. If air is in the pleural cavity, the thoracentesis site is usually in the second or third intercostal space in the midclavicular line because air rises in the thorax. |
| 8. The procedure is performed under aseptic conditions. After the skin is cleansed, the physician uses a small-caliber needle to inject a local anesthetic slowly into the intercostal space. | 8. An intradermal wheal is raised slowly; rapid injection causes pain. The parietal pleura is very sensitive and should be well infiltrated with anesthetic before the physician passes the thoracentesis needle through it. |
| 9. The physician advances the thoracentesis needle with the syringe attached. When the pleural space is reached, suction may be applied with the syringe.<br>   a. A 20-mL syringe with a three-way stopcock is attached to the needle (one end of the adapter is attached to the needle and the other to the tubing leading to a receptacle that receives the fluid being aspirated).<br>   b. If a considerable quantity of fluid is removed, the needle is held in place on the chest wall with a small hemostat. | 9. Use of thoracentesis needle allows proper insertion.<br><br>   a. When a large quantity of fluid is withdrawn, a three-way stopcock serves to keep air from entering the pleural cavity.<br><br><br><br>   b. The hemostat steadies the needle on the chest wall. Sudden pleuritic chest pain or shoulder pain may indicate that the needle point is irritating the visceral or the diaphragmatic pleura. |
| 10. After the needle is withdrawn, pressure is applied over the puncture site and a small, airtight, sterile dressing is fixed in place. | 10. Pressure helps to stop bleeding, and the airtight dressing protects the site and prevents air from entering the pleural cavity. |
| 11. Advise the patient that he or she will be on bed rest and a chest x-ray will be obtained after thoracentesis. | 11. A chest x-ray verifies that there is no pneumothorax. |
| 12. Record the total amount of fluid withdrawn from the procedure and document the nature of the fluid, its color, and its viscosity. If indicated, prepare samples of fluid for laboratory evaluation. A specimen container with formalin may be needed for a pleural biopsy. | 12. The fluid may be clear, serous, bloody, purulent, etc. |
| 13. Monitor the patient at intervals for increasing respiratory rate; asymmetry in respiratory movement; faintness; vertigo; tightness in chest; uncontrollable cough; blood-tinged, frothy mucus; a rapid pulse; and signs of hypoxemia. | 13. Pneumothorax, tension pneumothorax, subcutaneous emphysema, and pyrogenic infection are complications of a thoracentesis. Pulmonary edema or cardiac distress can occur after a sudden shift in mediastinal contents when large amounts of fluid are aspirated. |

bronchoscope inserted into the pleural space. Pleural biopsy is performed when there is pleural exudate of undetermined origin or when there is a need to culture or stain the tissue to identify tuberculosis or fungi.

## Lung Biopsy Procedures

If the chest x-ray findings are inconclusive or show pulmonary density (indicating an infiltrate or lesion), biopsy may be performed to obtain lung tissue for examination to identify the nature of the lesion. Several nonsurgical lung biopsy techniques are used because they yield accurate information with low morbidity: (1) transcatheter bronchial brushing, (2) transbronchial lung biopsy, and (3) percutaneous (through-the-skin) needle biopsy.

In transcatheter bronchial brushing, a fiberoptic bronchoscope is introduced into the bronchus under fluoroscopy. A small brush attached to the end of a flexible wire is inserted through the bronchoscope. Under direct visualization, the area under suspicion is brushed back and forth, causing cells to slough off and adhere to the brush. The catheter port of the bronchoscope may be used to irrigate the lung tissue with saline solution to secure material for additional studies. The brush is removed from the bronchoscope and a slide is made for examination under the microscope. The brush may be cut off and sent to the pathology laboratory for analysis.

This procedure is useful for cytologic evaluations of lung lesions and for the identification of pathogenic organisms (eg, *Nocardia, Aspergillus, Pneumocystis carinii*). It is especially useful in the immunologically compromised patient.

Another method of bronchial brushing involves the introduction of the catheter through the transcricothyroid membrane by needle puncture. After this procedure, the patient is instructed to hold a finger or thumb over the puncture site while coughing to prevent air from leaking into the surrounding tissues.

In transbronchial lung biopsy, biting or cutting forceps are introduced by a fiberoptic bronchoscope. A biopsy is indicated when a lung lesion is suspected and the results of routine sputum samples and bronchoscopic washings are negative.

In percutaneous needle biopsy, a cutting needle or a spinal-type needle is used to obtain a tissue specimen for histologic study. Analgesia may be administered before the procedure. The skin over the biopsy site is cleansed and anesthetized, and a small incision is made. The biopsy needle is inserted through the incision into the pleura with the patient holding the breath in midexpiration. Using fluoroscopic monitoring, the surgeon guides the needle into the periphery of the lesion and obtains a tissue sample from the mass. Possible complications include pneumothorax, pulmonary hemorrhage, and empyema.

### NURSING INTERVENTIONS

After the procedure, recovery and home care are similar to those for bronchoscopy and thoracoscopy. Nursing care involves monitoring the patient for shortness of breath, bleeding, and infection. In preparation for discharge, the patient and family are instructed to report pain, shortness of breath, visible bleeding, redness of the biopsy site, or purulent drainage (pus) to the health care provider immediately. Patients who have undergone biopsy are often anxious because of the need for the biopsy and the potential findings; the nurse must consider this in providing postbiopsy care and teaching.

## Lymph Node Biopsy

The scalene lymph nodes are enmeshed in the deep cervical pad of fat overlying the scalenus anterior muscle. They drain the lungs and mediastinum and may show histologic changes from intrathoracic disease. If these nodes are palpable on physical examination, a scalene node biopsy may be performed. A biopsy of these nodes may be performed to detect spread of pulmonary disease to the lymph nodes and to establish a diagnosis or prognosis in such diseases as Hodgkin disease, sarcoidosis, fungal disease, tuberculosis, and carcinoma.

Mediastinoscopy is the endoscopic examination of the mediastinum for exploration and biopsy of mediastinal lymph nodes that drain the lungs; this examination does not require a thoracotomy. Biopsy is usually performed through a suprasternal incision. Mediastinoscopy is carried out to detect mediastinal involvement of pulmonary malignancy and to obtain tissue for diagnostic studies of other conditions (eg, sarcoidosis).

An anterior mediastinotomy is thought to provide better exposure and diagnostic possibilities than a mediastinoscopy. An incision is made in the area of the second or third costal cartilage. The mediastinum is explored, and biopsies are performed on any lymph nodes found. Chest tube drainage is required after the procedure. Mediastinotomy is particularly valuable to determine whether a pulmonary lesion is resectable.

### NURSING INTERVENTIONS

Postprocedure care focuses on providing adequate oxygenation, monitoring for bleeding, and providing pain relief. The patient may be discharged a few hours after the chest drainage system is removed. The nurse should instruct the patient and family about monitoring for changes in respiratory status, taking into consideration the impact of anxiety about the potential findings of the biopsy on their ability to remember those instructions.

## Critical Thinking Exercises

**1** A man with a long history of smoking (60 pack-years) is scheduled for surgery to remove a nonfunctioning kidney. In preparation for surgery, he is scheduled for PFTs, which he refuses to have because he says his breathing has nothing to do with his kidney problem or his scheduled kidney surgery. How would you respond to his statement? What impact does his 60-pack-year history of cigarette smoking have on your preoperative, intraoperative, and postoperative assessment?

**2** When obtaining a health history from a 55-year-old patient who is seeking health care because of a persistent cough and extreme fatigue, you note that she is able to speak only in short sentences before having to stop to catch her breath. What specific information about signs and symptoms would you obtain during the health history? How would you modify your physical examination based on your observations? What initial laboratory tests would you anticipate will be ordered for this patient?

**3** A patient who has cancer of the lung has undergone a thoracentesis for removal of pleural fluid in an effort to relieve his shortness of breath. Soon after the procedure is completed, the patient reports that his shortness of breath has increased rather than decreased. Based on your knowledge of risks associated with thoracentesis, what assessment data would you obtain from this patient and report to the physician? What additional nursing measures are warranted for the patient at this time? How would you respond if the patient had been discharged an hour after the thoracentesis and provided this information to you by telephone from home?

**4** [ebp] A woman reports that she has had a cough with sputum production in the morning for the past 2 weeks. She says that she is a smoker and has a 20-pack-year history of smoking. Her primary health care provider explains to her why smoking is contraindicated with cough and sputum production and explains the importance of smoking cessation. As the nurse in the clinic, your role is to discuss smoking cessation techniques with her and to identify a plan that is likely to be successful for her. Describe the specific smoking cessation strategies that you will discuss with this patient. Identify the evidence base that supports the use of the smoking cessation strategies selected. What is the strength of the evidence, and what criteria will you use to evaluate the effectiveness of various smoking cessation strategies?

## REFERENCES AND SELECTED READINGS

## BOOKS

Bickley, L. S. & Szilagyi, P. G. (2003). *Bates' guide to physical examination and history taking* (8th ed.). Philadelphia: Lippincott Williams & Wilkins.

Levitzky, M. G. (2003). *Pulmonary physiology* (6th ed.). New York: McGraw-Hill Medical.

Morton, P. G., Fontaine, D. K., Hudak, C. M., et al. (2005). *Critical care nursing: A holistic approach* (8th ed.). Philadelphia: Lippincott Williams & Wilkins.

Porth, C. M. (2005). *Pathophysiology: Concepts of altered health states* (7th ed.). Philadelphia: Lippincott Williams & Wilkins.

Sole, M. L., Klein, D. G., & Moseley, M. J. (2005). *Introduction to critical care nursing* (4th ed.). St. Louis: Elsevier Saunders.

Stanley, M., Blair, K. A. & Beare, P. G. (2005). *Gerontological nursing: Promoting successful aging with older adults* (3rd ed.). Philadelphia: F. A. Davis.

Urden, L. D., Stacy, K. M. & Lough, M. E. (2002). *Thelan's critical care nursing: Diagnosis and management* (4th ed.). St. Louis: Mosby.

Weber, J. & Kelley, J. (2003). *Health assessment in nursing* (2nd ed.). Philadelphia: Lippincott Williams & Wilkins.

West, J. B. (2004). *Respiratory physiology* (7th ed.). Philadelphia: Lippincott Williams & Wilkins.

Wilkins, R. L., Sheldon, R. L. & Krider, S. J. (2005). *Clinical assessment in respiratory care* (5th ed.). St. Louis: Elsevier Mosby.

## JOURNALS

*Asterisks indicate nursing research articles.

Anees, W. (2003). Use of pulmonary function tests in the diagnosis of occupational asthma. *Annals of Allergy, Asthma, and Immunology, 90*(5 Suppl. 2), 47–51.

Ayers, D. M. M. & Lappin, J. S. (2004). Act fast when your patient has dyspnea. *Nursing, 34*(7), 36–42.

Bahhady, I. J. & Unterborn, J. (2003a). Pulmonary function tests: An update. *Consultant, 43*(7), 813–818,820.

Bahhady, I. J. & Unterborn, J. (2003b). What pulmonary function tests can and cannot tell you: Results help assess disease severity in ILD and COPD. *Journal of Respiratory Diseases, 24*(4), 170–176.

*Bailey, P. H. (2004). The dyspnea-anxiety-dyspnea cycle—COPD patients' stories of breathlessness: "It's scary when you can't breathe." *Qualitative Health Research, 14*(6), 760–778.

Beckles, M. A., Spiro, S. G., Colice, G. L., et al. (2003). The physiologic evaluation of patients with lung cancer being considered for resectional surgery. *Chest, 123*(1 Suppl.), 105S–114S.

Bledsoe, B. E., Porter, R. S., & Cherry, R. A. (2005). 25 Physical examination pearls: Important tips to help you polish your hands-on patient assessment skills. *JEMS: Journal of Emergency Medical Services, 30*(3), 58–60, 62–63, 64–74.

Boyle, A. H. & Waters, H. F. (2000). Issues in respiratory nursing. Focus on prevention: Recommendations of the National Lung Health Education Program. *Heart and Lung, 29*(6), 446–449.

Burki, N. (2003). Evaluating dyspnea: A practical guide. *Journal of Respiratory Diseases, 24*(1), 10–15.

*Chernecky, C., Sarna, L., Waller, J. L., et al. (2004). Assessing coughing and wheezing in lung cancer: A pilot study. *Oncology Nursing Forum, 31*(6), 1095–1101.

Conklin B. (2005). B-type natriuretic peptide: A new measurement to distinguish cardiac from pulmonary causes of acute dyspnea. *Journal of Emergency Nursing, 31*(1), 73–75,117–123.

Conner, B. & Meng, A. (2003). Pulmonary function testing in asthma: Nursing applications. *Nursing Clinics of North America, 38*(4), 571–583.

Considine, J. (2005). The role of nurses in preventing adverse events related to respiratory dysfunction: Literature review. *Journal of Advanced Nursing, 49*(6), 624–633.

Crawford, A. (2004). Respiratory nursing. An audit of the patient's experience of arterial blood gas testing. *British Journal of Nursing, 13*(9), 529–532.

Davis, M. & Holliday, J. Jr. (2005). Differentiating causes of respiratory distress. *Emergency Medical Services, 34*(1), 72–73.

*de Souza Caroci, A. D. S. & Lareau, S. C. (2004). Descriptors of dyspnea by patients with chronic obstructive pulmonary disease versus congestive heart failure. *Heart and Lung, 33*(2), 102–110.

Ebihara, S., Saito, H., Kanda, A., et al. (2003). Impaired efficacy of cough in patients with Parkinson disease. *Chest, 124*(3), 1009–1015.

Farquhar, S. L. & Fantasia, L. (2005). Pulmonary anatomy and physiology and the effects of COPD. *Home Healthcare Nurse, 23*(3), 167–176.

Finesilver, C. (2003). Pulmonary assessment: What you need to know. *Progress in Cardiovascular Nursing, 18*(2), 83–92.

French, C. T., Fletcher, K. E. & Irwin, R. S. (2004). Gender differences in health-related quality of life in patients complaining of chronic cough. *Chest, 125*(2), 482–488.

Fu, E. S., Downs, J. B., Schweiger, J. W., et al. (2004). Supplemental oxygen impairs detection of hypoventilation by pulse oximetry. *Chest, 126*(5), 1552–1558.

Garrett, K., Laurer, K., & Christopher, B. (2004). The effects of obesity on the cardiopulmonary system: Implications for critical care nursing. *Progress in Cardiovascular Nursing, 19*(4), 155–161.

Hardie, J. A., Vollmer, W. M., Buist, A. S., et al. (2004). Reference values for arterial blood gases in the elderly. *Chest, 125*(6), 2053–2060.

Hately, J., Laurence, V., Scott, A., et al. (2003). Breathlessness clinics within specialist palliative care settings can improve the quality of life and functional capacity of patients with lung cancer. *Palliative Medicine, 17*(5), 410–417.

Irwin, R. S., Baumann, M. H., Bolser, D. C., et al. (2006). Diagnosis and management of cough: Executive summary. ACCP evidence-based clinical practice guidelines. *Chest, 129*(1 Suppl.), 1S–23S.

Johnson, K. L. (2004). Diagnostic measures to evaluate oxygenation in critically ill adults: Implications and limitations. *AACN Clinical Issues: Advanced Practice in Acute and Critical Care, 15*(4), 506–524, 640–642.

Jones, P. W., Moyers, J. P., Rogers, J. T., et al. (2003). Ultrasound-guided thoracentesis: Is it a safer method? *Chest, 123*(2), 418–423.

Karnani, N. G., Reisfield, G. M. & Wilson, G. R. (2005). Evaluation of chronic dyspnea. *American Family Physician, 71*(8), 1529–1538, 1473–1475, 1612.

Leidy, N. K., Rennard, S. I., Schmier, J., et al. (2003). The Breathlessness, Cough, and Sputum Scale: The development of empirically based guidelines for interpretation. *Chest, 124*(6), 2182–2191.

Lim, K. G. & Morgenthaler, T. I. (2005). Defining obstruction or restriction remains the goal: Pulmonary function tests. Part 1: Applying the basics. *Journal of Respiratory Diseases, 26*(1), 26–30,32.

Luh, S. P., Chou, M. C., Wang, L. S., et al. (2005). Video-assisted thoracoscopic surgery in the treatment of complicated parapneumonic effusions or empyemas: Outcome of 234 patients. *Chest, 127*(4), 1427–1432.

Lung, C. L. & Lung, M. L. (2003). General principles of asthma management: Symptom monitoring. *Nursing Clinics of North America, 38*(4), 585–596.

Mahler, D. A., Fierro-Carrion, G., & Baird, J. C. (2003). Evaluation of dyspnea in the elderly. *Clinics in Geriatric Medicine, 19*(1), 19–33.

Mayo, P. H., Goltz, H. R., Tafreshi, M., et al. (2004). Safety of ultrasound-guided thoracentesis in patients receiving mechanical ventilation. *Chest, 125*(3), 1059–1067.

*Meek, P. M., Lareau, S. C., & Hu, J. (2003). Are self-reports of breathing effort and breathing distress stable and valid measures among persons with asthma, persons with COPD, and healthy persons? *Heart and Lung, 32*(5), 335–346.

Mehta, M. (2003). Assessing respiratory status: Learn how to evaluate your patient's lungs through sight, sound, and touch. *Nursing, 33*(2), 54–56.

Meng, A. & McConnell, S. (2003). Symptom perception and respiratory sensation: Clinical applications. *Nursing Clinics of North America, 38*(4), 737–748.

*Michaels, C. & Meek, P. M. (2004). The language of breathing among individuals with chronic obstructive pulmonary disease. *Heart and Lung, 33*(6), 390–400.

*Moody, L. E., Webb, M., Cheung, R., et al. (2004). A focus group for caregivers of hospice patients with severe dyspnea. *American Journal of Hospice and Palliative Care, 21*(2), 121–130, 160.

Noppen, M., Poppe, K., D'Haese, J., et al. (2004). Interventional bronchoscopy for treatment of tracheal obstruction secondary to benign or malignant thyroid disease. *Chest, 125*(2), 723–730.

*Nguyen, H. Q., Carrieri-Kuhlman, V., Rankin, S. H., et al. (2005). Is Internet-based support for dyspnea self-management in patients with chronic obstructive pulmonary disease possible? Results of a pilot study. *Heart and Lung, 34*(1), 51–62.

Ott, M. C., Khoor, A., Leventhal, J. P., et al. (2003). Pulmonary toxicity in patients receiving low-dose amiodarone. *Chest, 123*(2), 646–651.

Pezzoli, L., Giardini, G., Consonni, S., et al. (2003). Quality of spirometric performance in older people. *Age and Ageing, 21*(1), 43–46.

Poe, R. H. & Kallay, M. C. (2003). Chronic cough and gastroesophageal reflux disease: Experience with specific therapy for diagnosis and treatment. *Chest, 123*(3), 679–684.

Prigmore, S. (2005). Respiratory care: Assessment and nursing care of the patient with dyspnoea. *Nursing Times, 101*(4), 50–53.

Ramirez, E. G. (2003). Management of asthma emergencies. *Nursing Clinics of North America, 38*(4), 713–724.

Saad, C. P., Murthy, S., Krizmanich, G., et al. (2003). Bronchoscopy. Self-expandable metallic airway stents and flexible bronchoscopy: Long-term outcomes analysis. *Chest, 124*(5), 1993–1999.

Simpson, H. (2004). Respiratory nursing. Interpretation of arterial blood gases: A clinical guide for nurses. *British Journal of Nursing, 13*(9), 522–528.

Smetana, G. W. (2003). Preoperative pulmonary assessment of the older adult. *Clinics in Geriatric Medicine, 19*(1), 35–55.

Vrijhoef, H. J. M., Diederiks, J. P. M., Wesseling, G. J., et al. (2003). Undiagnosed patients and patients at risk for COPD in primary health care: Early detection with the support of non-physicians. *Journal of Clinical Nursing, 12*(3), 366–373.

Wang, J. S. (2004). Pulmonary function tests in preoperative pulmonary evaluation. *Respiratory Medicine, 98*(7), 598–605.

Winters, A. C. & Munro, N. (2004). Assessment of the mechanically ventilated patient: An advanced practice approach. *AACN Clinical Issues: Advanced Practice in Acute and Critical Care, 15*(4), 525–533.

Woodrow, P. (2004). Arterial blood gas analysis. *Nursing Standard, 18*(21), 45–52.

*Wu, H., Wu, S., Lin, J., et al. (2004). Effectiveness of acupressure in improving dyspnoea in chronic obstructive pulmonary disease. *Journal of Advanced Nursing, 45*(3), 252–259.

Zeleznik, J. (2003). Normative aging of the respiratory system. *Clinics in Geriatric Medicine, 19*(1), 1–18.

Zoorob, R. J. & Campbell, J. S. (2003). Acute dyspnea in the office. *American Family Physician, 68*(9), 1803–1810.

## RESOURCES

American Association for Respiratory Care, 11030 Ables Lane, Dallas, TX 75229; 972-243-2272; http://www.aarc.org. Accessed March 31, 2006.

American Lung Association, 1740 Broadway, New York, NY 10019; 212-315-8700 or 800-LUNG USA; http://www.lungusa.org. Accessed March 31, 2006.

National Heart, Lung, and Blood Institute/National Institutes of Health, Rockville Pike, Bldg. 31, Bethesda, MD 20892; 301-496-5166; http://www.nhlbi.nih.gov/index.htm. Accessed March 31, 2006.

National Lung Health Education Program; http://www.nlhep.org. Accessed March 31, 2006. Has easy-to-read teaching resources for patients.

# CHAPTER 22

# Management of Patients With Upper Respiratory Tract Disorders

## Learning Objectives

*On completion of this chapter, the learner will be able to:*

1. Describe nursing management of patients with upper airway disorders.
2. Compare and contrast the upper respiratory tract infections with regard to cause, incidence, clinical manifestations, management, and the significance of preventive health care.
3. Use the nursing process as a framework for care of patients with upper airway infection.
4. Describe nursing management of the patient with epistaxis.
5. Use the nursing process as a framework for care of patients undergoing laryngectomy.

Many upper airway disorders are relatively minor, and their effects are limited to mild and temporary discomfort and inconvenience for the patient. Others, however, are acute, severe, and life-threatening and may require permanent alterations in breathing and speaking. Therefore, the nurse must have expert assessment skills, an understanding of the wide variety of disorders that may affect the upper airway, and an awareness of the impact of these alterations on patients. Because many of the disorders are treated outside the hospital or at home by patients themselves, patient teaching is an important aspect of nursing care. When caring for patients with acute, life-threatening disorders, the nurse needs highly developed assessment and clinical management skills, along with a focus on rehabilitation needs.

## Upper Airway Infections

Upper airway infections are the most common cause of illness and affect most people on occasion. Some infections are acute, with symptoms that last several days; others are chronic, with symptoms that last a long time or recur. Patients with these conditions seldom require hospitalization. However, nurses working in community settings or long-term care facilities may encounter patients who have these infections. Therefore, it is important for the nurse to recognize the signs and symptoms and to provide appropriate care.

Infections of the upper airway are also known as upper respiratory tract infections (URIs). They occur when microorganisms such as viruses and bacteria are inhaled. URIs are the most common reason for seeking health care and for absences from school and work throughout the year. There are many causative organisms, and people are susceptible throughout life.

URIs affect the nasal cavity; ethmoidal air cells; and frontal, maxillary, and sphenoid sinuses, as well as the larynx and trachea. About 90% of upper respiratory disorders stem from a viral infection of the upper respiratory passages and subsequent mucous membrane inflammation. Although patients with these conditions rarely require hospitalization, the nurse can influence patient outcomes in community settings and in long-term facilities through patient teaching and use of resources when warranted.

Special considerations with regard to URIs in the elderly are summarized in Chart 22-1.

## Rhinitis

**Rhinitis** is a group of disorders characterized by inflammation and irritation of the mucous membranes of the nose. It may be acute or chronic, nonallergic or allergic. It is estimated that 20% of the population of the United States has allergic rhinitis (Bush, 2004). Allergic rhinitis is further classified as seasonal or perennial rhinitis. Seasonal rhinitis occurs during pollen seasons, and perennial rhinitis occurs throughout the year. Allergies, including allergic rhinitis, affect more than 40 million people in the United States yearly (National Institute of Allergy and Infectious Diseases, 2005). Allergic disorders are described in detail in Chapter 53.

### Pathophysiology

Nonallergic rhinitis may be caused by a variety of factors, including environmental factors such as changes in temperature or humidity, odors, or foods; infection; age; systemic disease; drugs (eg, cocaine), over-the-counter (OTC) and prescribed nasal decongestants, and other medications; and the presence of a foreign body. The most common cause of nonallergic rhinitis is the common cold. Drug-induced rhinitis is associated with use of antihypertensive agents and oral contraceptives and chronic use of nasal decongestants. Other causes of rhinitis are identified in Table 22-1. Figure 22-1 shows the pathologic processes involved in rhinitis and sinusitis.

## Glossary

**alaryngeal communication:** alternative modes of speaking that do not involve the normal larynx; used by patients whose larynx has been surgically removed

**aphonia:** impaired ability to use one's voice due to disease or injury to the larynx

**apnea:** cessation of breathing

**dysphagia:** difficulties in swallowing

**epistaxis:** hemorrhage from the nose due to rupture of tiny, distended vessels in the mucous membrane of any area of the nose

**herpes simplex:** cold sore (cutaneous viral infection with painful vesicles and erosions on the tongue, palate, gingiva, buccal membranes, or lips)

**laryngitis:** inflammation of the larynx; may be caused by voice abuse, exposure to irritants, or infectious organisms

**laryngectomy:** removal of all or part of the larynx and surrounding structures

**nuchal rigidity:** stiffness of the neck or inability to bend the neck

**pharyngitis:** inflammation of the throat; usually viral or bacterial in origin

**rhinitis:** inflammation of the mucous membranes of the nose; may be infectious, allergic, or inflammatory in origin

**rhinorrhea:** drainage of a large amount of fluid from the nose

**sinusitis:** inflammation of the sinuses; may be acute or chronic; may be viral, bacterial, or fungal in origin

**submucosal resection:** surgical procedure to correct nasal obstruction due to deviated septum; also called septoplasty

**tonsillitis:** inflammation of the tonsils, usually due to an acute infection

**xerostomia:** dryness of the mouth from a variety of causes

## CHART 22-1

### Upper Respiratory Tract Disorders in the Elderly

- Upper respiratory infections in the elderly may have more serious consequences if patients have concurrent medical problems that compromise their respiratory or immune status.
- Antihistamines to treat upper respiratory disorders must be used cautiously in the elderly because of their side effects and potential interactions with other medications.
- Sinusitis in the elderly is often preceded by nasal packing for treatment of epistaxis.
- Laryngitis in the elderly is common and most frequently occurs secondary to gastroesophageal reflux disease (GERD). The elderly are more likely to have impaired esophageal peristalsis and a weaker esophageal sphincter. Treatment measures include sleeping with the head of the bed elevated and the use of medications such as $H_2$-receptor blockers (eg, famotidine [Pepcid], ranitidine [Zantac]) or proton pump inhibitors (omeprazole [Prilosec]).

## Physiology/Pathophysiology

A. Rhinitis

B. Sinusitis

**FIGURE 22-1.** Pathophysiologic processes in rhinitis and sinusitis. Although pathophysiologic processes are similar in rhinitis and sinusitis, they affect different structures. In rhinitis (**A**), the mucous membranes lining the nasal passages become inflamed, congested, and edematous. The swollen nasal conchae block the sinus openings, and mucus is discharged from the nostrils. Sinusitis (**B**) is also marked by inflammation and congestion, with thickened mucous secretions filling the sinus cavities and occluding the openings.

### TABLE 22-1  Causes of Rhinitis

| Category | Causes |
| --- | --- |
| Vasomotor | Idiopathic |
|  | Abuse of nasal decongestants (rhinitis medicamentosa) |
|  | Psychological stimulation (anger, sexual arousal) |
|  | Irritants (smoke, air pollution, exhaust fumes, cocaine) |
| Mechanical | Tumor |
|  | Deviated septum |
|  | Crusting |
|  | Hypertrophied turbinates |
|  | Foreign body |
|  | Cerebrospinal fluid leak |
| Chronic inflammatory | Polyps (in cystic fibrosis) |
|  | Sarcoidosis |
|  | Wegener's granulomatosis |
|  | Midline granuloma |
| Infectious | Acute viral infection |
|  | Acute or chronic sinusitis |
|  | Rare nasal infections (syphilis, tuberculosis) |
| Hormonal | Pregnancy |
|  | Use of oral contraceptives |
|  | Hypothyroidism |

Adapted from Carr, M. M. Differential diagnosis of rhinitis. Available at: icarus.med.utoronto.ca/carr/manual/ddxrhinitis.html (accessed March 31, 2006).

## Clinical Manifestations

The signs and symptoms of nonallergic rhinitis include **rhinorrhea** (excessive nasal drainage, runny nose); nasal congestion; nasal discharge (purulent with bacterial rhinitis); sneezing; and pruritus of the nose, roof of the mouth, throat, eyes, and ears. Headache may occur, particularly if sinusitis is also present. Nonallergic rhinitis can occur throughout the year.

## Medical Management

The management of rhinitis depends on the cause, which may be identified through the history and physical examination. The examiner asks the patient about recent symptoms as well as possible exposure to allergens in the home, environment, or workplace. If viral rhinitis is the cause, medications are given to relieve the symptoms. In allergic rhinitis, tests may be performed to identify possible allergens. Depending on the severity of the allergy, desensitizing immunizations and corticosteroids may be required (see Chapter 53 for more details). If symptoms suggest a bacterial infection, an antimicrobial agent will be used (see later discussion of sinusitis). Patients with nasal septal deformities or nasal polyps may be referred to an ear, nose, and throat specialist.

### Pharmacologic Therapy

Medication therapy for allergic and nonallergic rhinitis focuses on symptom relief. Antihistamines are administered for sneezing, pruritus, and rhinorrhea. Examples of first-generation antihistamines include diphenhydramine (Benadryl), chlorpheniramine (Chlor-Trimeton), and brompheniramine. Newer, second-generation antihistamines used to treat rhinitis include loratadine (Alavert, Claritin), fexofenadine (Allegra), and cetirizine (Zyrtec). Dimetapp (brompheniramine/pseudoephedrine) is an example of a combination antihistamine. Oral decongestant agents are used for nasal obstruction. Another medication used in the treatment of rhinitis is cromolyn (Nasalcrom), which inhibits the release of histamine and other chemicals. Use of saline nasal spray can act as a mild decongestant and can liquefy mucus to prevent crusting. Two inhalations of intranasal ipratropium (Atrovent) can be administered in each nostril 2 to 3 times per day for symptomatic relief of rhinorrhea. In addition, intranasal corticosteroids may be used for severe congestion, and ophthalmic agents are used to relieve irritation, itching, and redness of the eyes. The choice of medications depends on the symptoms, adverse reactions, adherence factors, risk of drug interactions, and cost to the patient.

## Nursing Management

### Teaching Patients Self-Care

The nurse instructs the patient with allergic rhinitis to avoid or reduce exposure to allergens and irritants, such as dusts, molds, animals, fumes, odors, powders, sprays, and tobacco smoke. Patient education is essential when assisting the patient in the use of OTC medications. To prevent possible drug interactions, the nurse teaches the patient to read drug labels before taking any OTC medication.

The nurse instructs the patient about the importance of controlling the environment at home and at work. Saline nasal or aerosol sprays may be helpful in soothing mucous membranes, softening crusted secretions, and removing irritants. The nurse instructs the patient in the proper technique for administering nasal medications. To achieve maximal relief, the patient is instructed to blow the nose before applying any medication into the nasal cavity. In addition, the patient is taught to keep the head upright; spray quickly and firmly into each nostril away from the nasal septum, and wait at least 1 minute before administering the second spray. The container should be cleaned after each use.

In the case of infectious rhinitis, the nurse reviews hand hygiene technique with the patient as a measure to prevent transmission of organisms. This is especially important for infected people who are in contact with vulnerable populations such as the very young, the elderly, or people who are immunosuppressed (eg, patients with HIV infection, those taking immunosuppressive medications). The nurse teaches methods to treat symptoms of viral rhinitis. In the elderly and other high-risk populations, the nurse reviews the value of receiving an influenza vaccination each year to achieve immunity before the beginning of the "flu season."

## Viral Rhinitis (Common Cold)

Viral rhinitis is the most frequent viral infection in the general population. The term "common cold" often is used when referring to a URI that is self-limited and caused by a virus. The term "cold" refers to an afebrile, infectious, acute inflammation of the mucous membranes of the nasal cavity characterized by nasal congestion, rhinorrhea, sneezing, sore throat, and general malaise. More broadly, the term refers to an acute URI, whereas terms such as "rhinitis," "pharyngitis," and "laryngitis" distinguish the sites of the symptoms. It is also used when the causative virus is influenza ("the flu"). Colds are highly contagious, because virus is shed for about 2 days before the symptoms appear and during the first part of the symptomatic phase.

Adults in the United States average two to three colds each year (American Lung Association, 2005). Adult women are more susceptible than adult men. In the United States, colds are more frequent during the late fall and winter seasons. The incidence of viral rhinitis follows a specific pattern during the year, depending on the causative agent (Fig. 22-2). Even though viral rhinitis can occur at any time of the year, three time periods account for the epidemics in the United States:

- In September, just after the opening of school
- In late January
- Toward the end of April

Colds are believed to be caused by as many as 200 different viruses. Rhinoviruses are the most likely causative organisms and are believed to cause more than 40% of colds. Other viruses implicated in the common cold include coronaviruses, adenovirus, respiratory syncytial virus (RSV), influenza virus, and parainfluenza virus. Each virus may have multiple strains. Because of this diversity, development of a vaccine is almost impossible. Immunity after recovery is variable and depends on many factors, including a person's natural host resistance and the specific virus that caused the cold. Despite popular belief, cold temperatures and exposure to cold rainy weather do not increase the incidence or severity of the common cold.

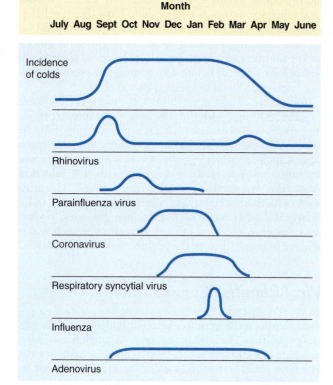

**FIGURE 22-2.** Schematic diagram incidence of viral rhinitis (common cold) in the United States and the frequency of the causative agents. Redrawn from Goldman, L. & Bennett, J. C. (Eds.) (2000). *Cecil textbook of medicine* (21st ed., Vol. 2). Philadelphia: W. B. Saunders, p. 1791.

## Clinical Manifestations

Signs and symptoms of viral rhinitis are nasal congestion, rhinorrhea and nasal discharge, sneezing, tearing watery eyes, "scratchy" or sore throat, general malaise, low-grade fever, chills, and often headache and muscle aches. As the illness progresses, cough usually appears. In some people, the virus exacerbates **herpes simplex,** commonly called a "cold sore" (Chart 22-2).

The symptoms of viral rhinitis may last from 1 to 2 weeks. If there is significant fever or more severe systemic respiratory symptoms, it is no longer considered viral rhinitis but one of the other acute URIs. Allergic conditions can also affect the nose, mimicking the symptoms of a cold.

## Medical Management

Management consists of symptomatic therapy. Some measures include providing adequate fluid intake, encouraging rest, preventing chilling, and using expectorants as needed. Warm salt-water gargles soothe the sore throat, and nonsteroidal anti-inflammatory agents (NSAIDs), such as aspirin or ibuprofen, relieve the aches, pains, and fever in adults. Antihistamines are used to relieve sneezing, rhinorrhea, and nasal congestion. Topical (nasal) decongestant agents may relieve nasal congestion; however, if they are overused they

### CHART 22-2

## Colds and Cold Sores (Herpes Simplex Virus HSV-1)

Herpes labialis is an infection that is caused by the herpes simplex virus. It is characterized by an eruption of small, painful blisters on the skin of the lips, mouth, gums, tongue, or the skin around the mouth. The blisters are commonly referred to as "cold sores" or "fever blisters." Once the person is infected with this virus, it can lie latent in the cells for a period of time. The incubation period is about 2 to 12 days. It is activated by overexposure to sunlight or wind, colds, influenza and similar infections, heavy alcohol use, and physical or emotional stress.

Herpes labialis is extremely common and is caused by the herpes simplex virus type 1. (Herpes type 2 virus causes genital herpes.) Most Americans are infected with the type 1 virus by 20 years of age. Herpes labialis is extremely contagious and can be spread through contaminated razors, towels, and dishes. Oral/genital contact can spread oral herpes to the genitals (and vice versa). People with active herpetic lesions should avoid oral sex. It is extremely important for patients to understand that the virus can be transmitted by asymptomatic people.

Early symptoms of herpes labialis include burning, itching and increased sensitivity or tingling sensation. These symptoms occur about 2 days before the appearance of lesions. The lesions appear as small blisters (vesicles) that are filled with clear, yellowish fluid. They are raised, red, and painful and can break and ooze. Eventually yellow crusts slough to reveal pink, healing skin.

The lesions will eventually subside (10 to 14 days). Medications used in the management of herpes labialis include acyclovir (Zovirax) and valacyclovir (Valtrex), which help to minimize the symptoms and the duration or length of flare-up. Other medications used for analgesia include acetaminophen with codeine and other milder forms of opioids. Topical anesthetics such as xylocaine or over-the-counter medications such as Herpecin-L or docosanol [Abreva] can help in the control of discomfort.

may create a rebound congestion that can be worse than the original symptoms. Some research suggests that zinc lozenges may reduce the duration of cold symptoms if taken within the first 24 hours of onset (Marshall, 2006). Amantadine (Symmetrel) or rimantadine (Flumadine) may be prescribed prophylactically to decrease the signs and symptoms as well. Antimicrobial agents (antibiotics) should not be used, because they do not affect the virus or reduce the incidence of bacterial complications.

Most patients treat the common cold with OTC medications that produce moderate clinical benefits. OTC medications provide symptomatic relief along with other measures to improve well-being through the course of the illness. Other treatment measures include adequate fluid intake, adequate rest, and warm salt-water gargles to soothe the sore throat. Acetaminophen or NSAIDs such as ibuprofen can relieve generalized aches, pains, and fevers. Antihistamines and decongestants can be used to treat sneezing and congestion. Topical nasal decongestants can be used with caution. Topical therapy delivers medication directly to the nasal mucosa, but its overuse can produce rhinitis medicamentosa or rebound rhinitis.

## Nursing Management

### Teaching Patients Self-Care

Most viruses can be transmitted in several ways: direct contact with infected secretions; inhalation of large particles from others' coughing or sneezing; or inhalation of small particles (aerosol) that may be suspended in the air for up to an hour. The nurse teaches the patient how to break the chain of infection. Handwashing remains the most effective measure to prevent transmission of organisms. The nurse teaches methods to treat symptoms of the common cold and preventive measures (Chart 22-3) and provides both verbal and written information to assist the patient in the prevention and management of URIs.

> **NURSING ALERT**
>
> Due to the risk of gastrointestinal bleeding, aspirin, ibuprofen, and naproxen should be avoided by persons who are not eating well, have a history of peptic ulcer or related disorder, have aspirin-sensitive asthma, or have renal dysfunction.
>
> Patients who have high blood pressure, diabetes, or thyroid disease, and those who are pregnant should check with their physician before using a decongestant.
>
> Patients should avoid use of zinc and dextromethorphan (Benylin) if pregnancy is possible.
>
> Patients taking monoamine oxidase (MAO) inhibitors (eg, phenelzine sulfate [Nardil], tranylcypromine [Parnate]) should not use dextromethorphan [Robitussin].

## Acute Sinusitis

The sinuses, mucus-lined cavities filled with air, normally drain into the nose and are involved in many URIs. If their openings into the nasal passages are clear, the infections resolve promptly. However, if their drainage is obstructed by a deviated septum or by hypertrophied turbinates, spurs, or nasal polyps or tumors, sinus infection may persist as a smoldering (persistent) secondary infection or progress to an acute suppurative process (causing purulent discharge). **Sinusitis** (inflammation of the sinuses) affects 14% to 16% of the population and accounts for billions of dollars in direct health care costs (Shashy, Moore & Weaver, 2004). Some people are more prone to sinusitis because of their occupations. For example, continuous exposure to environmental hazards such as paint, sawdust, and chemicals may result in chronic inflammation of the nasal passages.

## Pathophysiology

Acute sinusitis is an infection of the mucous membranes that line the paranasal sinuses. Five subtypes of sinusitis have been identified: acute, subacute, chronic, allergic, and hyperplastic sinusitis. Acute sinusitis refers to rapid-onset infection in one or more of the paranasal sinuses that resolves with treatment, whereas subacute sinusitis is persistent purulent nasal discharge despite therapy with symptoms lasting less than 3 months. Chronic sinusitis occurs with episodes of prolonged inflammation and with repeated or inadequate treatment of acute infections. Irreversible damage to the mucosa may occur. Symptoms last for longer than 3 months. Sinusitis often follows a URI or cold, such as an unresolved viral or bacterial infection, or an exacerbation of allergic rhinitis. Nasal congestion, caused by inflammation, edema, and transudation of fluid secondary to URI, leads to obstruction of the sinus cavities (see Fig. 22-1). This provides an excellent medium for bacterial growth. Other conditions that can block the normal flow of sinus secretions include abnormal structures of the nose, enlarged adenoids, diving and swimming, tooth infection, trauma to the nose, tumors, and the pressure of foreign objects. Bacterial organisms account for more than 60% of the cases of acute sinusitis. *Streptococcus pneumonia*, *Haemophilus influenzae*, and *Moraxella catarrhalis* are the most common organisms associated with sinusitis. Less common organisms include *Chlamydia pneumoniae*, *Streptococcus pyogenes*, viruses, and fungi (*Aspergillus fumigatus*). Fungal infections occur most often in immunosuppressed patients. Pathogens in chronic or subacute sinusitis are likely to be polymicrobial, involving anaerobic bacteria (Uphold & Graham, 2003).

## Clinical Manifestations

Symptoms of sinusitis vary among people and are dependent on the age of the person. Most infections in adults involve the maxillary and anterior ethmoidal sinuses. Symptoms may include facial pain or pressure over the affected sinus area, nasal obstruction, fatigue, purulent nasal discharge, fever, headache, ear pain and a sense of fullness, dental pain, decreased sense of smell, sore throat, early morning

**CHART 22-3**

## HOME CARE CHECKLIST • Preventing and Managing Upper Respiratory Infections

| At the completion of home care instructions, the patient and significant other will be able to: | Patient | Caregiver |
|---|:---:|:---:|
| **Prevention** | | |
| • Identify strategies to prevent infection and, if infected, to prevent the spread of infection to others. | | |
|    • Perform hand hygiene often | ✔ | ✔ |
|    • Use disposable tissues | ✔ | |
|    • Cover mouth when coughing or sneezing | ✔ | |
|    • Avoid crowds during the flu season | ✔ | |
|    • Avoid people with infections | ✔ | |
|    • Obtain annual influenza vaccination (especially if patient is elderly or has a chronic illness or disability) | ✔ | |
| • Practice good health habits | | |
|    • Eat a nutritious diet | ✔ | |
|    • Get adequate sleep, rest, and exercise | ✔ | |
|    • Avoid the use of tobacco in all forms | ✔ | |
|    • Avoid secondhand smoke | ✔ | |
|    • Increase the humidity in the home (especially in the winter) | ✔ | ✔ |
|    • Avoid irritants (dust, chemicals) to include exposure to animals | ✔ | ✔ |
|    • Use central air conditioning with microstatic air filters | ✔ | ✔ |
| **Management** | | |
| • Describe strategies to relieve symptoms of upper respiratory infection | | |
|    • Increase fluid intake. Warm fluids (eg, chicken soup) are especially soothing for irritated throats. | ✔ | ✔ |
|    • Elevate head of bed. | ✔ | ✔ |
|    • Gargle with salt water frequently for sore throat (1/4 teaspoon of salt dissolved in eight ounces warm water) | ✔ | |
|    • Use throat lozenge for sore throat or cough. | ✔ | |
|    • Use saline nose drops/sprays (1/4 teaspoon salt dissolved in eight ounces warm water; use dropper, or purchase prepared saline drops) | ✔ | |
| • Recognize signs and symptoms of infection and state when to contact health care provider | | |
|    • If symptoms worsen after 3 to 5 days; new symptoms develop or symptoms do not improve after 14 days. | ✔ | ✔ |
|    • If the following signs or symptoms occur, obtain immediate health care: | | |
|       • Upper respiratory distress (stridor, drooling, inability to swallow) | ✔ | ✔ |
|       • Lower respiratory distress (moderate to severe dyspnea) | ✔ | ✔ |
|       • Severe headache ("worst ever," rigid neck, altered mental state, focal neurologic symptoms) | ✔ | |

periorbital edema, and cough that worsens when the patient is supine. Acute sinusitis can be difficult to differentiate from a URI or allergic rhinitis. The presence of fewer than two symptoms rules out acute bacterial sinusitis, and four or more symptoms suggest acute bacterial sinusitis (DeAlleaume, Parker & Reider, 2003).

## Assessment and Diagnostic Findings

A careful history and physical examination are performed. The head and neck, particularly the nose, ears, teeth, sinuses, pharynx, and chest, are examined. There may be tenderness to palpation over the infected sinus area. The sinuses are percussed using the index finger, tapping lightly to determine whether the patient experiences pain. The affected area is also transilluminated; with sinusitis, there is a decrease in the transmission of light (see Chapter 21). Diagnostic tests are not indicated for sinusitis with a typical presentation or for the first episode of acute sinusitis. Sinus x-rays and computed tomography (CT) scans may be obtained for patients with frontal headaches, in refractory cases, if complications are suspected, or when the diagnosis is unclear (Reider, Nashelsky & Neher, 2003; Uphold & Graham, 2003). To confirm the diagnosis of maxillary and frontal sinusitis and identify the pathogen, sinus aspirates may be obtained. Flexible endoscopic culture techniques have been used for this purpose as well as swabbing of the sinuses.

## Complications

If untreated, acute sinusitis may lead to severe and occasionally life-threatening complications such as meningitis, brain abscess, ischemic brain infarction, and osteomyelitis. Other complications of sinusitis, although uncommon, include severe orbital cellulitis, subperiosteal abscess, cavernous sinus thrombosis, and meningitis. Brain abscesses occur by direct spread and can be life-threatening. Frontal epidural abscesses are usually quiescent and can be detected by CT scan.

## Medical Management

The goals of treatment of acute sinusitis are to treat the infection, shrink the nasal mucosa, and relieve pain. Because of growing concern about the inappropriate use of antibiotics for viral URIs and the resulting resistance that has occurred, careful consideration must be given to the potential pathogen before antimicrobial agents are prescribed.

Antibiotic therapy is used to eradicate the infecting organism. First-line antibiotics include amoxicillin, ampicillin, trimethoprim/sulfamethoxazole (Bactrin, Septra), and erythromycin. Second-line antibiotic therapy includes cephalosporins such as cefuroxime axetil (Ceftin) and cefprozil (Cefzil) and amoxicillin clavulanate (Augmentin). Newer and more expensive antibiotics such as macrolides (clarithromycin [Biaxin], azithromycin [Zithromax]) and quinolones such as levofloxacin (Levaquin) can be used if the patient has a severe allergy to penicillin. Studies suggest that most patients will improve spontaneously, and antibiotics should be reserved for those with prolonged symptoms (Lindbaek, 2004). However, deep-seated bacterial sinusitis can be a serious infection that requires antibiotic treatment for 2 to 3 weeks. A narrow-spectrum antibiotic such as amoxicillin is often a good initial choice (Jackson, 2003).

Treatment of acute sinusitis typically involves nasal decongestants (pseudoephedrine hydrochloride [Sudafed]). Decongestants or nasal saline spray can improve patency of the ostiomeatal unit and improve drainage of the sinuses. Topical decongestants are used only in adults and should not be used for longer than 3 or 4 days. Oral decongestants must be used cautiously in patients with hypertension. OTC antihistamines, including diphenhydramine (Benadryl) and antihistamines (cetirizine, fexofenadine) are used if an allergic component is suspected.

Heated mist and saline irrigation also may be effective for opening blocked passages. If the patient continues to have symptoms after 7 to 10 days, the sinuses may need to be irrigated and hospitalization may be required.

## Nursing Management

### Teaching Patients Self-Care

Patient teaching is an important aspect of nursing care for the patient with acute sinusitis. The nurse instructs the patient about symptoms of complications that require immediate follow-up. Referral to a physician is indicated if periorbital edema and severe pain on palpation occur. The nurse instructs the patient about methods to promote drainage of the sinuses, including humidification of the air in the home and use of steam inhalation and warm compresses to relieve pressure. The patient is advised to avoid swimming, diving, and air travel during the acute infection. Patients using tobacco are instructed to immediately stop smoking or using any form of tobacco. The nurse also teaches the patient about the side effects of nasal sprays and about rebound congestion. In the case of rebound congestion, the body's receptors have become dependent on the decongestant sprays to keep the nasal passages open. Once the decongestant is discontinued, the nasal passages close and congestion results. Patients with recurrent sinusitis should be instructed to begin decongestants at the first sign of sinusitis. This will promote drainage and decrease the risk of bacterial infection.

The nurse stresses the importance of following the recommended antibiotic regimen, because a consistent blood level of the medication is critical to treat the infection. The nurse teaches the patient the early signs of a sinus infection and recommends preventive measures such as following healthy practices and avoiding contact with people who have URIs (see Chart 22-3).

The nurse explains to the patient that fever, severe headache, and **nuchal rigidity** (stiffness of the neck/inability to bend the neck) are signs of potential complications. Patients with chronic symptoms of sinusitis who do not have marked improvement in 4 weeks with continuous medical treatment may be candidates for aspiration of the sinus or sinus surgery.

## Chronic Sinusitis

Chronic sinusitis is one of the most common illnesses in the United States, reportedly affecting up to 16% of the population. It affects more than 32 million persons each year and ranks fifth in frequency of antibiotic use associated with treatment. It is considered a common disease worldwide. The data on the incidence, however, rely largely on patients' self report and can lead to inaccuracies and likely overestimation (Shashy et al., 2004). Chronic sinusitis is a result of prolonged inflammation or repeated or inadequately treated acute sinus infections. People with symptoms lasting longer than 3 months are usually classified as having chronic sinusitis.

## Pathophysiology

Mechanical obstruction in the ostia of the frontal, maxillary, and anterior ethmoid sinuses (known collectively as the ostiomeatal complex) is the usual cause of chronic sinusitis. Obstruction prevents adequate drainage to the nasal passages. Blockage that persists longer than 3 weeks in an adult may occur because of infection, allergy, or structural abnormalities. This results in stagnant secretions, an ideal medium for growth of bacteria. The organisms that cause chronic sinusitis are the same as those implicated in acute sinusitis. Immunocompromised patients, however, are at increased risk for development of fungal sinusitis. Fungal sinusitis in immunocompromised patients can be divided into three categories: (1) fungus ball, (2) chronic erosive (noninvasive) sinusitis, and (3) allergic fungal sinusitis. *A. fumigatus* is the most common organism associated with fungal sinusitis.

## Clinical Manifestations

Clinical manifestations of chronic sinusitis include impaired mucociliary clearance and ventilation, cough (because the thick discharge constantly drips backward into the nasopharynx), chronic hoarseness, chronic headaches in the periorbital area, and facial pain. As a result of chronic nasal congestion, the patient is usually required to breathe through the mouth. Snoring, sore throat, and, in some situations, adenoidal hypertrophy may also occur. Periorbital edema and facial pain are common. These symptoms are generally most pronounced on awakening in the morning. Fatigue and nasal congestion are also common. Many patients experience a decrease in smell and taste and a sense of fullness in the ears.

## Assessment and Diagnostic Findings

The health assessment focuses on onset and duration of symptoms. It addresses the quantity and quality of nasal discharge and cough, the presence of pain, factors that relieve or aggravate the pain, and allergies. It is essential to obtain any history of comorbid conditions, including asthma, and history of tobacco use. A history of fever, fatigue, previous episodes and treatments, and previous response to therapies is also obtained. The physical assessment includes vital signs and examination of the eyes, nasal mucosa, ears, throat, mouth, and pharynx for signs of erythema and exudates. The nose is inspected for septal deviation and polyps and the eyes for periorbital edema. Pain on examination of the teeth and tapping them with a tongue blade suggests tooth infection. The frontal and maxillary sinuses are palpated, and the patient is asked whether this produces tenderness.

Diagnostic tests may include CT scan or magnetic resonance imaging (if fungal sinusitis is suspected) of the sinuses to rule out other local or systemic disorders, such as tumor, fistula, and allergy. Nasal endoscopy may be indicated to rule out underlying diseases such as tumors and sinus mycetomas (fungus balls). The fungus ball is usually a brown or greenish-black material with the consistency of peanut butter or cottage cheese.

## Complications

Complications of chronic sinusitis, although uncommon, include severe orbital cellulitis, subperiosteal abscess, cavernous sinus thrombosis, meningitis, encephalitis, and ischemic infarction.

## Medical Management

Medical management of chronic sinusitis is almost the same as for acute sinusitis. The antimicrobial agents of choice include amoxicillin clavulanate (Augmentin) or ampicillin (Ampicin). Clarithromycin (Biaxin) and third-generation cephalosporins such as cefuroxime axetil (Ceftin), cefpodoxime (Vantin), and cefprozil (Cefzil) have also been effective. Macrolides (eg, clarithromycin [Biaxin]) increase mucociliary clearance and improve sinusitis symptoms and are known to decrease nasal secretions and polyp size associated with chronic sinusitis. In addition to their antimicrobial activity, the macrolides' immunomodulatory properties may be effective in chronic inflammation (Gotfried, 2004). Levofloxacin (Levaquin), a quinolone, may also be used. The course of treatment may be 3 to 4 weeks. As with acute sinusitis, decongestant agents, antihistamines, saline sprays, and heated mist may also provide some symptom relief.

The use of intranasal nebulized medications is emerging as a treatment of chronic sinusitis. Specially formulated medication compounds delivered by nebulizer are an innovative and advanced approach to treating acute and chronic sinusitis. The role of leukotriene inhibitors in patients with paranasal sinus disease is also under study. This class of medications blocks the binding of leukotrienes (inflammatory mediators) to receptors and in a number of studies has demonstrated a role in inhibiting nasal symptoms in asthmatic patients (Chung & Adcock, 2004; Singh, 2004). As a result, studies are ongoing to determine the role of these agents in patients with chronic sinusitis and their role in endoscopic surgical treatment. Endoscopic sinus surgery has evolved over the past 20 years as an accepted treatment for people with chronic sinusitis refractory to medical management (Colclasure, Gross & Kountakis, 2004).

## Surgical Management

If standard medical therapy fails and symptoms persist, surgery, usually endoscopic, may be indicated to correct structural deformities that obstruct the ostia (openings) of the sinuses. Minimally invasive surgical procedures are used, reducing postoperative discomfort and producing significant improvement in the patient's quality of life. Excising and cauterizing nasal polyps, correcting a deviated septum, incising and draining the sinuses, aerating the sinuses, and removing tumors are some of the specific procedures performed. If sinusitis is caused by a fungal infection, surgery is required to excise the fungus ball and necrotic tissue and drain the sinuses. Antimicrobial agents are administered before and after surgery. Some patients with severe chronic sinusitis obtain relief only by moving to a dry climate.

## Nursing Management

Because the patient usually performs care measures for sinusitis at home, nursing management consists mainly of patient teaching.

### Teaching Patients Self-Care

Many people with sinus infections tend to blow their nose frequently and with force to clear their nasal passages. Doing so, however, often increases the symptoms. Therefore, the patient is instructed to blow the nose gently and to use tissue to remove the nasal drainage. Increasing the environmental humidity (eg, steam bath, hot shower, vaporizer), increasing fluid intake, applying local heat (hot wet packs), and elevating the head of the bed promote drainage of the sinuses. The nurse also instructs the patient about the importance of following the medication regimen. Instructions on the early signs of a sinus infection are provided, and preventive measures are reviewed. The nurse instructs the patient about signs and symptoms that require follow-up and provides these instructions in writing.

# Acute Pharyngitis

Acute **pharyngitis** is a sudden inflammation of the pharynx that is more common in patients younger than 25 years of age (particularly between 5 and 15 years). It is most common in adolescents and young adults. It occurs less frequently in the elderly. The primary symptom is a sore throat.

## Pathophysiology

Most cases of acute pharyngitis are caused by viral infection. Responsible viruses include the adenovirus, influenza virus, Epstein-Barr virus and herpes simplex virus. Bacterial organisms known to cause pharyngitis include group A beta-hemolytic streptococci, *Neisseria gonorrhoeae*, *H. influenzae* type B, and *Mycoplasma*. When group A beta-hemolytic streptococcus, the most common bacterial organism, causes acute pharyngitis, the condition is known as strep throat (Wald & Fischer, 2004). The body responds by triggering an inflammatory response in the pharynx. This results in pain, fever, vasodilation, edema, and tissue damage, manifested by redness and swelling in the tonsillar pillars, uvula, and soft palate. A creamy exudate may be present in the tonsillar pillars (Fig. 22-3).

Uncomplicated viral infections usually subside promptly, within 3 to 10 days after the onset. However, pharyngitis caused by more virulent bacteria, such as group A beta-hemolytic streptococci, is a more severe illness. If left untreated, the complications can be severe and life-threatening. Complications include sinusitis, otitis media, peritonsillar abscess, mastoiditis, and cervical adenitis. In rare cases, the infection may lead to bacteremia, pneumonia, meningitis, rheumatic fever, or nephritis.

## Clinical Manifestations

The signs and symptoms of acute pharyngitis include a fiery-red pharyngeal membrane and tonsils, lymphoid follicles that are swollen and flecked with white-purple exudate, enlarged and tender cervical lymph nodes, and no cough. Fever, malaise, and sore throat also may be present. Occasionally patients with group A beta-hemolytic streptococcal pharyngitis exhibit vomiting, anorexia, and a scarlatina-form rash with urticaria.

## Assessment and Diagnostic Findings

Diagnosis of group A streptococcal pharyngitis must be made by laboratory testing rather than by clinical findings alone. Rapid strep test (RST) and strep culture (sometimes referred to as STCX) require proper collection technique, because improper collection reduces the accuracy of the test. RST must be performed according to the manufacturer's guidelines. When the test is performed correctly, the swabs touch both the tonsillar pillars and the posterior pharyngeal wall; the tongue should not be included. If the RST result is negative, a second culture should be performed. Treatment is usually delayed until the culture results are available (Armengol, Schlager & Hendley, 2004; Neuner,

**FIGURE 22-3.** Pharyngitis—inflammation without exudate. **(A)** Redness and vascularity of the pillars and uvula are mild to moderate. **(B)** Redness is diffuse and intense. Each patient would probably complain of a sore throat. From Bickley, L. S. & Szilagyi, P. G. (2003). *Bates' guide to physical examination and history taking* (8th ed.). Philadelphia: Lippincott Williams & Wilkins.

Hamel, Phillips et al., 2003). In most communities, preliminary culture reports are available in 24 hours. Rapid screenings include the latex agglutination (LA) antigen test and solid-phase enzyme immunoassays (ELISA), optical immunoassay (OIA), and streptolysin titers. Nasal swabs and blood cultures may also be necessary to identify the organism.

## Medical Management

Viral pharyngitis is treated with supportive measures, because antibiotics will have no effect on the organism. Bacterial pharyngitis is treated with a variety of antimicrobial agents.

### Pharmacologic Therapy

If a bacterial cause is suggested or demonstrated, penicillin is usually the treatment of choice. For patients who are allergic to penicillin or have organisms that are resistant to erythromycin (one fifth of group A beta-hemolytic streptococci and most *Staphylococcus aureus* organisms are resistant to penicillin and erythromycin), cephalosporins and macrolides (clarithromycin and azithromycin) may be used. Antibiotics are administered for at least 10 days to eradicate the infection from the oropharynx.

Severe sore throats can also be relieved by analgesic medications, as prescribed. For example, aspirin or acetaminophen (Tylenol) can be taken at 3- to 6-hour intervals; if required, acetaminophen with codeine can be taken three or four times daily. Antitussive medication, in the form of codeine, dextromethorphan (Robitussin DM), or hydrocodone bitartrate (Hycodan), may be required to control the persistent and painful cough that often accompanies acute pharyngitis.

### Nutritional Therapy

A liquid or soft diet is provided during the acute stage of the disease, depending on the patient's appetite and the degree of discomfort that occurs with swallowing. Cool beverages, warm liquids, and flavored frozen desserts such as popsicles are often soothing. Occasionally, the throat is so sore that liquids cannot be taken in adequate amounts by mouth. In severe situations, IV fluids may be needed. Otherwise, the patient is encouraged to drink as much fluid as possible (at least 2 to 3 L per day).

## Nursing Management

Nursing care for patients with viral pharyngitis focuses on symptomatic management. For patients who demonstrate signs of strep throat and have a history of rheumatic fever, who appear toxic, who have clinical scarlet fever, or who have symptoms suggesting peritonsillar abscess, nursing care focuses on prompt initiation and correct administration of prescribed antibiotic therapy. The nurse instructs the patient about signs and symptoms that warrant prompt contact with the physician. These include dyspnea, drooling, inability to swallow, and inability to fully open the mouth.

The nurse instructs the patient to stay in bed during the febrile stage of illness and to rest frequently once up and about. Used tissues should be disposed of properly to prevent the spread of infection. The nurse (or the patient or family member, if the patient is not hospitalized) should examine the skin once or twice daily for possible rash, because acute pharyngitis may precede some other communicable diseases (eg, rubella).

Depending on the severity of the lesion and the degree of pain, warm saline gargles or throat irrigations are used. The benefits of this treatment depend on the degree of heat that is applied. The nurse teaches the patient about these procedures and about the recommended temperature of the solution: high enough to be effective and as warm as the patient can tolerate, usually 105°F to 110°F (40.6°C to 43.3°C). Irrigating the throat properly is an effective means of reducing spasm in the pharyngeal muscles and relieving soreness of the throat.

An ice collar also can relieve severe sore throats. Mouth care may add greatly to the patient's comfort and prevent the development of fissures (cracking) of the lips and oral inflammation when bacterial infection is present. The nurse instructs the patient to resume activity gradually and to delay returning to work or school until after 24 hours of antibiotic therapy. A full course of antibiotic therapy is indicated in patients with group A beta-hemolytic streptococcal infection because of the potential complications such as nephritis and rheumatic fever, which may have their onset 2 or 3 weeks after the pharyngitis has subsided. The nurse instructs the patient and family about the importance of taking the full course of therapy and informs them about the symptoms to watch for that may indicate complications.

# Chronic Pharyngitis

Chronic pharyngitis is a persistent inflammation of the pharynx. It is common in adults who work or live in dusty surroundings, use their voice to excess, suffer from chronic cough, or habitually use alcohol and tobacco.

There are three types of chronic pharyngitis:

- Hypertrophic: characterized by general thickening and congestion of the pharyngeal mucous membrane
- Atrophic: probably a late stage of the first type (the membrane is thin, whitish, glistening, and at times wrinkled)
- Chronic granular ("clergyman's sore throat"), characterized by numerous swollen lymph follicles on the pharyngeal wall.

## Clinical Manifestations

Patients with chronic pharyngitis complain of a constant sense of irritation or fullness in the throat, mucus that collects in the throat and can be expelled by coughing, and difficulty swallowing. This is often associated with intermittent postnasal drip that causes minor irritation and inflammation of the pharynx. A sore throat that is worse with swallowing in the absence of pharyngitis suggests the possibility of thyroiditis, and patients with this symptom are referred for evaluation for possible thyroiditis.

## Medical Management

Treatment of chronic pharyngitis is based on relieving symptoms, avoiding exposure to irritants, and correcting any upper respiratory, pulmonary, or cardiac condition that might be responsible for a chronic cough.

Nasal congestion may be relieved by short-term use of nasal sprays or medications containing ephedrine sulfate (Kondon's Nasal) or phenylephrine hydrochloride (Neo-Synephrine). For a patient with a history of allergy, one of the antihistamine decongestant medications, such as Drixoral or Dimetapp, is prescribed orally every 4 to 6 hours. Aspirin or acetaminophen is recommended for its anti-inflammatory and analgesic properties.

## Nursing Management

### Teaching Patients Self-Care

To prevent the infection from spreading, the nurse instructs the patient to avoid contact with others until the fever subsides. The nurse recommends avoidance of alcohol, tobacco, secondhand smoke, and exposure to cold or to environmental or occupational pollutants. The patient may minimize exposure to pollutants by wearing a disposable facemask. The nurse encourages the patient to drink plenty of fluids. Gargling with warm saline solution may relieve throat discomfort. Lozenges will keep the throat moistened.

## Tonsillitis and Adenoiditis

The tonsils are composed of lymphatic tissue and are situated on each side of the oropharynx. The faucial or palatine tonsils and lingual tonsils are located behind the pillars of fauces and tongue, respectively. They frequently serve as the site of acute infection (**tonsillitis**). Acute tonsillitis can be confused with pharyngitis. Chronic tonsillitis is less common and may be mistaken for other disorders such as allergy, asthma, and sinusitis.

The adenoids or pharyngeal tonsils consist of lymphatic tissue near the center of the posterior wall of the nasopharynx. Infection of the adenoids frequently accompanies acute tonsillitis. Group A beta-hemolytic streptococcus is the most common organism associated with tonsillitis and adenoiditis. Often thought of as a childhood disorder, tonsillitis can also occur in adults.

## Clinical Manifestations

The symptoms of tonsillitis include sore throat, fever, snoring, and difficulty swallowing. Enlarged adenoids may cause mouth-breathing, earache, draining ears, frequent head colds, bronchitis, foul-smelling breath, voice impairment, and noisy respiration. Unusually enlarged adenoids fill the space behind the posterior nares, making it difficult for the air to travel from the nose to the throat and resulting in nasal obstruction. Infection can extend to the middle ears by way of the auditory (eustachian) tubes and may result in acute otitis media, which can lead to spontaneous rupture of the tympanic membranes (eardrums) and further extension of the infection into the mastoid cells, causing acute mastoiditis. The infection also may reside in the middle ear as a chronic, low-grade, smoldering process that eventually may cause permanent deafness.

## Assessment and Diagnostic Findings

A thorough physical examination is performed, and a careful history is obtained to rule out related or systemic conditions. The tonsillar site is cultured to determine the presence of bacterial infection. In adenoiditis, if recurrent episodes of suppurative otitis media result in hearing loss, the patient should be given a comprehensive audiometric examination (see Chapter 59).

## Medical Management

Tonsillitis is treated through the use of supportive measures that include increased fluid intake, analgesics, salt-water gargles, and rest. Bacterial infections are treated with penicillin as first-line therapy. Viral tonsillitis is not effectively treated by antibiotic therapy.

Tonsillectomy or adenoidectomy is indicated if the patient has had repeated episodes of tonsillitis despite antibiotic therapy; hypertrophy of the tonsils and adenoids that could cause obstruction and obstructive sleep apnea; repeated attacks of purulent otitis media; suspected hearing loss due to serous otitis media that has occurred in association with enlarged tonsils and adenoids; and in some other conditions, such as an exacerbation of asthma or rheumatic fever. Surgery is also indicated if the patient has developed a peritonsillar abscess that occludes the pharynx, making swallowing difficult and endangering the patency of the airway (particularly during sleep). Enlargement of the tonsils is rarely an indication for their removal; most children normally have large tonsils, which decrease in size with age. Despite the continuing debate over the effectiveness of tonsillectomy, it is a common surgical procedure in the United States (Discolo, Darrow & Koltai, 2003). Appropriate antibiotic therapy is initiated for patients undergoing tonsillectomy or adenoidectomy. The most common antimicrobial agent is oral penicillin, which is prescribed for 7 to 10 days. Amoxicillin and erythromycin are alternatives. Indications for adenoidectomy include chronic nasal airway obstruction, chronic rhinorrhea, obstruction of the eustachian tube with related ear infections, and abnormal speech.

## Nursing Management

### Providing Postoperative Care

Continuous nursing observation is required in the immediate postoperative and recovery periods because of the significant risk of hemorrhage. In the immediate postoperative period, the most comfortable position is prone with the head turned to the side to allow drainage from the mouth and pharynx. The nurse must not remove the oral airway until the patient's gag and swallowing reflexes have returned. The nurse applies an ice collar to the neck, and a basin and tissues are provided for the expectoration of blood and mucus.

Symptoms of postoperative complications include fever, throat pain, ear pain, and bleeding. Pain is effectively controlled with analgesic medications. Bleeding may be bright red if the patient expectorates blood before swallowing it. If the patient swallows the blood, it becomes brown because of the action of the acidic gastric juice. Hemorrhage is a potential complication after tonsillectomy and adenoidectomy. Risk factors associated with post-tonsillectomy hemorrhage include male gender, age older than 70 years, infectious mononucleosis, and history of recurrent tonsillitis (Windfuhr & Chen, 2003). Postoperative hemorrhage rates are not significantly different with tonsillectomy by electrodissection versus sharp dissection (Leinbach, Markwell, Colliver, et al., 2003).

If the patient vomits large amounts of dark blood or bright-red blood at frequent intervals, or if the pulse rate and temperature rise and the patient is restless, the nurse notifies the surgeon immediately. The nurse should have the following items ready for examination of the surgical site for bleeding: a light, a mirror, gauze, curved hemostats, and a waste basin.

Occasionally, suture or ligation of the bleeding vessel is required. In such cases, the patient is taken to the operating room and given general anesthesia. After ligation, continuous nursing observation and postoperative care are required, as in the initial postoperative period. If there is no bleeding, water and ice chips may be given to the patient as soon as desired. The patient is instructed to refrain from too much talking and coughing, because these activities can produce throat pain.

### Teaching Patients Self-Care

Tonsillectomy and adenoidectomy are usually performed as outpatient surgery with a short length of stay. Because the patient will be sent home soon after surgery, the patient and family must understand the signs and symptoms of hemorrhage. Hemorrhage usually occurs in the first 12 to 24 hours; however, the risk is present for up to 18 days after the procedure (Windfuhr & Chen, 2003). The patient is instructed to report frank red bleeding to the physician.

Alkaline mouthwashes and warm saline solutions are useful in coping with the thick mucus and halitosis that may be present after surgery. The nurse should explain to the patient that a sore throat, stiff neck, and vomiting may occur in the first 24 hours. A liquid or semiliquid diet is given for several days. Sherbet and gelatin are acceptable foods. The patient should avoid spicy, hot, acidic, or rough foods. Milk and milk products (ice cream and yogurt) may be restricted because they make removal of mucus more difficult for some patients. The patient is informed that halitosis and some minor ear pain may occur for the first few days. The nurse instructs the patient to avoid vigorous tooth brushing or gargling, because these activities can cause bleeding.

## Peritonsillar Abscess

Peritonsillar abscess is a collection of purulent exudate between the tonsillar capsule and the surrounding tissues, including the soft palate. It may develop after an acute tonsillar infection that progresses to a local cellulitis and abscess. Beta-hemolytic streptococcus is the usual organism responsible for peritonsillar abscesses (Brook, 2004). In more severe cases, the infection can spread over the palate and to the neck and chest. Edema can cause airway obstruction, which can become life-threatening and is a medical emergency. Peritonsillar abscess is an uncommon infection in older adults. However, the possibility of a peritonsillar abscess as well as pharyngeal space abscess should be considered in afebrile, nontoxic patients older than 50 years of age who have complaints of new-onset sore throat and **dysphagia** (difficulty swallowing) lasting several days (Franzese & Isaacson, 2003).

### Clinical Manifestations

The person with a peritonsillar abscess appears acutely ill. The patient often has fever, trismus (inability to open the mouth), and drooling. Local symptoms include a raspy voice, odynophagia (a severe sensation of burning, squeezing pain while swallowing), dysphagia, and otalgia (pain in the ear). The patient may also demonstrate tender and enlarged cervical lymph nodes. On physical examination, the patient shows signs of marked swelling of the soft palate, often occluding almost half of the opening from the mouth into the pharynx; unilateral tonsillar hypertrophy; and dehydration. The patient may also present with erythema of the skin of the chest.

### Assessment and Diagnostic Findings

Emergency room physicians are often required to make the diagnosis of peritonsillar abscess and to decide whether aspiration, an invasive procedure, should be carried out based on the patient's clinical picture. Intraoral ultrasound is used in the management of peritonsillar abscess to assist in distinguishing between peritonsillar cellulitis (inflammation) and abscess. This diagnostic tool also helps to provide ultrasound needle guidance during peritonsillar abscess drainage, avoiding the multiple attempts to aspirate the abscess that often occur with a blind approach (Blaivas, Theodoro & Duggal, 2003). The aspirated material is sent for culture and Gram stain. A CT scan may be performed if it is not possible to aspirate the abscess or to confirm the diagnosis before surgical intervention.

### Medical Management

Studies have evaluated the best treatment for peritonsillar abscess, including use of corticosteroids, permucosal aspiration with a fine needle versus incision and drainage, and tonsillectomy (Johnson, Stewart & Wright, 2003). Rarely, the patient with a peritonsillar abscess may present with acute airway obstruction and require immediate airway management. Procedures may include intubation, cricothyroidotomy, or tracheotomy. Antibiotics (usually penicillin) are extremely effective in controlling the infection in peritonsillar abscess. If antibiotics are prescribed early in the course of the disease, the abscess may resolve without needing to be incised. Patients with signs of toxicity or complications require hospitalization for IV antibiotics, imaging studies, observation, and proper airway management.

## Surgical Management

If pharmacologic treatment is delayed or ineffective, the abscess must be evacuated as soon as possible. Untreated abscesses can rupture spontaneously into the pharynx and cause catastrophic aspiration and death (Brook, 2004). Fine needle aspiration of purulent material (pus) has traditionally been the treatment of choice once the diagnosis has been made. Evidence suggests that these treatment methods (ie, aspiration, incision and drainage) are equally effective, with low rates of recurrence of peritonsillar abscess (Johnson et al., 2003). The mucous membrane over the swelling is first sprayed with a topical anesthetic and then injected with a local anesthetic. Single or repeated needle aspirations are performed to decompress the abscess. Alternatively, the abscess may be incised and drained. These procedures are performed best with the patient in the sitting position to make it easier to expectorate the pus and blood that accumulate in the pharynx. Almost immediate relief is experienced. In a small number of cases, needle aspiration is unsuccessful, so incision and drainage therapy will be used with later tonsillectomy. Approximately 30% of patients with peritonsillar abscess have indications for tonsillectomy (Tierney, McPhee & Papadakis, 2005).

If the patient requires intubation, cricothyroidotomy, or tracheotomy to treat airway obstruction, the nurse assists with the procedure and provides support to the patient before, during, and after the procedure. The nurse also assists with the needle aspiration when indicated.

Considerable relief may be obtained by the use of topical anesthetic agents and throat irrigations or the frequent use of mouthwashes or gargles, using saline or alkaline solutions at a temperature of 105°F to 110°F (40.6°C to 43.3°C). Gentle gargling after the procedure with a cool normal saline gargle may relieve discomfort. The patient must be upright and clearly expectorate forward. The nurse instructs the patient to gargle *gently* at intervals of 1 or 2 hours for 24 to 36 hours. Liquids that are cool or at room temperature are usually well tolerated. Adequate fluids must be provided to treat dehydration and prevent its recurrence.

## Laryngitis

**Laryngitis**, an inflammation of the larynx, often occurs as a result of voice abuse or exposure to dust, chemicals, smoke, and other pollutants, or as part of a URI. It also may be caused by isolated infection involving only the vocal cords.

Laryngitis is very often caused by the same pathogens that cause the common cold and pharyngitis; the most common cause is a virus and laryngitis is often associated with allergic rhinitis or pharyngitis. Bacterial invasion may be secondary. The onset of infection may be associated with exposure to sudden temperature changes, dietary deficiencies, malnutrition, or an immunosuppressed state. Viral laryngitis is common in the winter and is easily transmitted to others.

### Clinical Manifestations

Signs of acute laryngitis include hoarseness or **aphonia** (complete loss of voice) and severe cough. Chronic laryngitis is marked by persistent hoarseness. Laryngitis may be a complication of URIs. Other signs of acute laryngitis include sudden onset made worse by cold dry wind. The throat feels worse in the morning and improves when the patient is indoors in a warmer climate. At times the patient presents with a dry cough and a dry, sore throat that worsens in the evening hours. If allergies are present, the uvula will be visibly edematous. Many patients also complain of a "tickle" in the throat that is made worse by cold air or cold liquids. Chronic laryngitis is marked by persistent hoarseness. Laryngitis may be a complication of a URI.

### Medical Management

Management of acute laryngitis includes resting the voice, avoiding irritants (including smoking), resting, and inhaling cool steam or an aerosol. If the laryngitis is part of a more extensive respiratory infection caused by a bacterial organism or if it is severe, appropriate antibacterial therapy is instituted. The majority of patients recover with conservative treatment; however, laryngitis tends to be more severe in elderly patients and may be complicated by pneumonia.

For chronic laryngitis, the treatment includes resting the voice, eliminating any primary respiratory tract infection, eliminating smoking, and avoiding secondhand smoke. Topical corticosteroids, such as beclomethasone dipropionate (Vanceril), may also be given by inhalation. These preparations have few systemic or long-lasting effects and may reduce local inflammatory reactions.

### Nursing Management

The nurse instructs the patient to rest the voice and to maintain a well-humidified environment. If laryngeal secretions are present during acute episodes, expectorant agents are suggested, along with a daily fluid intake of 2 to 3 L to thin secretions. In cases involving infection, the nurse informs the patient that the symptoms of laryngitis often extend a week to 10 days after completion of antibiotic therapy. The nurse also informs the patient of signs and symptoms that require contacting the health care provider. These signs and symptoms include loss of voice with sore throat that makes swallowing saliva difficult, hemoptysis, and noisy respirations. Continued hoarseness after voice rest or laryngitis that persists for longer than 5 days should be reported because of the possibility of malignancy.

## ◄◄▼►► Nursing Process

### The Patient With Upper Airway Infection

#### Assessment

A health history may reveal signs and symptoms of headache, sore throat, pain around the eyes and on either side of the nose, difficulty in swallowing, cough, hoarseness, fever, stuffiness, and generalized discomfort and fatigue. Determining when the symptoms began, what precipitated them, what if anything relieves them, and what aggravates them is part of the assessment. The nurse should also determine any history of allergy or the existence of a concomitant illness. Inspection may reveal swelling, lesions, or asymmetry of the nose as well as bleeding or discharge. The nurse inspects the nasal mucosa for abnormal findings such as increased redness, swelling, exudate, and nasal polyps, which may develop in chronic rhinitis. The nurse palpates the frontal and maxillary sinuses for tenderness, which suggests inflammation, and then inspects the throat by having the patient open the mouth wide and take a deep breath. The tonsils and pharynx are inspected for abnormal findings such as redness, asymmetry, or evidence of drainage, ulceration, or enlargement. The nurse also palpates the trachea to determine the midline position in the neck and to detect any masses or deformities. The neck lymph nodes are palpated for enlargement and tenderness.

## Diagnosis

### Nursing Diagnoses

Based on the assessment data, the patient's major nursing diagnoses may include the following:

- Ineffective airway clearance related to excessive mucus production secondary to retained secretions and inflammation
- Acute pain related to upper airway irritation secondary to an infection
- Impaired verbal communication related to physiologic changes and upper airway irritation secondary to infection or swelling
- Deficient fluid volume related to decreased fluid intake and increased fluid loss secondary to diaphoresis associated with a fever
- Deficient knowledge regarding prevention of URIs, treatment regimen, surgical procedure, or postoperative care

### Collaborative Problems/ Potential Complications

Based on assessment data, potential complications include

- Sepsis
- Meningitis
- Peritonsillar abscess
- Otitis media
- Sinusitis

## Planning and Goals

The major goals for the patient may include maintenance of a patent airway, relief of pain, maintenance of effective means of communication, normal hydration, knowledge of how to prevent upper airway infections, and absence of complications.

### Nursing Interventions

#### Maintaining a Patent Airway

An accumulation of secretions can block the airway in patients with an upper airway infection. As a result, changes in the respiratory pattern occur, and the work of breathing increases to compensate for the blockage. The nurse can implement several measures to loosen thick secretions or to keep the secretions moist so that they can be easily expectorated. Increasing fluid intake helps thin the mucus. Use of room vaporizers or steam inhalation also loosens secretions and reduces inflammation of the mucous membranes. To enhance drainage from the sinuses, the nurse instructs the patient about the best position to assume; this depends on the location of the infection or inflammation. For example, drainage for sinusitis or rhinitis is achieved in the upright position. In some conditions, topical or systemic medications, when prescribed, help to relieve nasal or throat congestion.

#### Promoting Comfort

URIs usually produce localized discomfort. In sinusitis, pain may occur in the area of the sinuses, or a general headache may be produced. In pharyngitis, laryngitis, or tonsillitis, a sore throat occurs. The nurse encourages the patient to take analgesics, such as acetaminophen with codeine, as prescribed, to relieve this discomfort. A pain intensity rating scale (see Chapter 13) may be used to assess effectiveness of pain relief measures. Other helpful measures include topical anesthetic agents for symptomatic relief of herpes simplex blisters (see Chart 22-2) and sore throats, hot packs to relieve the congestion of sinusitis and promote drainage, and warm-water gargles or irrigations to relieve the pain of a sore throat. The nurse encourages rest to relieve the generalized discomfort and fever that accompany many upper airway conditions (especially rhinitis, pharyngitis, and laryngitis). The nurse instructs the patient in general hygiene techniques to prevent the spread of infection. For postoperative care after tonsillectomy and adenoidectomy, an ice collar may reduce swelling and decrease bleeding.

#### Promoting Communication

Upper airway infections may result in hoarseness or loss of speech. The nurse instructs the patient to refrain from speaking as much as possible and, if possible, to communicate in writing instead. Additional strain on the vocal cords may delay full return of the voice. The nurse encourages the patient and family to use alternative forms of communication, such as a memo pad and a bell to signal for assistance when needed.

### Encouraging Fluid Intake

In upper airway infections, the work of breathing and the respiratory rate increase as inflammation and secretions develop. This, in turn, may increase insensible fluid loss. Fever further increases the metabolic rate, diaphoresis, and fluid loss.

Sore throat, malaise, and fever may interfere with a patient's willingness to eat and drink. The nurse provides a list of easily ingested foods to increase caloric intake during the acute phase of illness. These include soups, pudding, yogurt, cottage cheese, high protein drinks, and popsicles. The nurse encourages the patient to drink 2 to 3 L of fluid per day during the acute stage of airway infection, unless contraindicated, to thin the secretions and promote drainage. Liquids (hot or cold) may be soothing, depending on the disorder.

### Promoting Home and Community-Based Care

#### TEACHING PATIENTS SELF-CARE

Prevention of most upper airway infections is difficult because of the many potential causes. But because most URIs are transmitted by hand-to-hand contact, the nurse teaches the patient and family techniques to minimize the spread of infection to others, including frequent handwashing. Other preventive strategies are identified in Chart 22-3. The nurse advises the patient to avoid exposure to people who are at risk for serious illness if respiratory infection is transmitted. Those at risk include elderly adults, immunosuppressed people, and those with chronic health problems.

The nurse teaches patients and their families strategies to relieve symptoms of URIs. These include increasing the humidity level, encouraging adequate fluid intake, getting adequate rest, using warm-water gargles or irrigations and topical anesthetic agents to relieve sore throat, and applying hot packs to relieve congestion. The nurse reinforces the need to complete the treatment regimen, particularly when antibiotics are prescribed.

#### CONTINUING CARE

Referral for home care is rare. However, it may be indicated for people whose health status was compromised before the onset of the respiratory infection and for those who cannot manage self-care without assistance. In such circumstances, the home care nurse assesses the patient's respiratory status and progress in recovery. The nurse may advise elderly patients and those who would be at increased risk from a respiratory infection to consider an annual influenza vaccine. A follow-up appointment with the primary care provider may be indicated for patients with compromised health status to ensure that the respiratory infection has resolved.

### Monitoring and Managing Potential Complications

Although major complications of URIs are rare, the nurse must be aware of them and assess the patient for them. Because most patients with URIs are managed at home, patients and their families must be instructed to monitor for signs and symptoms and to seek immediate medical care if the patient's condition does not improve or if the patient's physical status appears to be worsening.

Sepsis and meningitis may occur in patients with compromised immune status or in those with an overwhelming bacterial infection. The patient with a URI and family members are instructed to seek medical care if the patient's condition fails to improve within several days after the onset of symptoms, if unusual symptoms develop, or if the patient's condition deteriorates. They are instructed about signs and symptoms that require further attention: persistent or high fever, increasing shortness of breath, confusion, and increasing weakness and malaise. The patient with sepsis requires expert care to treat the infection, stabilize vital signs, and prevent or treat septicemia and shock. Deterioration of the patient's condition necessitates intensive care measures (eg, hemodynamic monitoring and administration of vasoactive medications, IV fluids, nutritional support, corticosteroids) to monitor the patient's status and to support the patient's vital signs. High doses of antibiotics may be administered to treat the causative organism. The nurse's role is to monitor the patient's vital signs, hemodynamic status, and laboratory values, administer needed treatment, alleviate the patient's physical discomfort, and provide explanations, teaching, and emotional support to the patient and family.

Peritonsillar abscess may develop after an acute infection of the tonsils. The patient requires treatment to drain the abscess and receives antibiotics for infection and topical anesthetic agents and throat irrigations to relieve pain and sore throat. Follow-up is necessary to ensure that the abscess resolves; tonsillectomy may be required. The nurse assists the patient in administering throat irrigations and instructs the patient and family about the importance of adhering to the prescribed treatment regimen and recommended follow-up appointments.

Otitis media and sinusitis may develop with URI. The patient and family are instructed about the signs and symptoms of otitis media and sinusitis and about the importance of follow-up with the primary health care practitioner to ensure adequate evaluation and treatment of these conditions.

### Evaluation

#### Expected Patient Outcomes

Expected patient outcomes may include the following:

1. Maintains a patent airway by managing secretions
   a. Reports decreased congestion
   b. Assumes best position to facilitate drainage of secretions
   c. Uses self-care measures appropriately and consistently to manage secretions during the acute phase of illness

2. Reports relief of pain and discomfort using pain intensity scale
    a. Uses comfort measures: analgesics, hot packs, gargles, rest
    b. Demonstrates adequate oral hygiene
3. Demonstrates ability to communicate needs, wants, level of comfort
4. Maintains adequate fluid and nutrition intake
5. Utilizes strategies to prevent upper airway infections and allergic reactions
    a. Demonstrates hand hygiene technique
    b. Identifies the value of the influenza vaccine
6. Demonstrates an adequate level of knowledge and performs self-care adequately
7. Becomes free of signs and symptoms of infection
    a. Exhibits normal vital signs (temperature, pulse, respiratory rate)
    b. Absence of purulent drainage
    c. Free of pain in ears, sinuses, and throat
    d. Absence of signs of inflammation
8. Absence of complications
    a. No signs of sepsis: fever, hypotension, deterioration of cognitive status
    b. Vital signs and hemodynamic status normal
    c. No evidence of neurologic involvement
    d. No signs of development of peritonsillar abscess
    e. Resolution of URI without development of otitis media or sinusitis

# Obstruction and Trauma of the Upper Respiratory Airway

## Obstruction During Sleep

A variety of respiratory disorders are associated with sleep, the most common being sleep apnea syndrome. Chronic loss of sleep, along with untreated sleep disorders, affects the health and quality of life of 70 million people in the United States. Health care costs for sleep disorders average $15 billion annually plus $50 billion in lost productivity (Lamberg, 2004). Sleep apnea syndrome is defined as cessation of breathing (**apnea**) during sleep usually caused by repetitive upper airway obstruction. It interferes with the person's ability to obtain adequate rest and ultimately can affect memory, learning, and decision making.

Various definitions of obstructive sleep apnea (OSA)—also referred to as obstructive sleep apnea/hypopnea syndrome (OSAHS)—exist, leading to overestimation of the prevalence of this syndrome. More research is needed to accurately estimate the number of people with sleep apnea syndrome (Stradling & Davis, 2004). It is currently estimated that 12 million Americans each year suffer from chronic sleep disorders, including sleep apnea. Sleep apnea is more prevalent in men, especially those who are older and overweight. However, patients who are not obese should also be evaluated for OSA, because it is not always associated with obesity. Cigarette smoking has also been identified as another possible risk factor, although more studies on this topic are needed (Young, Skatrud & Peppard, 2004).

## Pathophysiology

Sleep apnea is classified into three types:

- Obstructive—lack of air flow due to pharyngeal occlusion
- Central—simultaneous cessation of both air flow and respiratory movements
- Mixed—a combination of central and obstructive apnea within one apneic episode

The most common type of sleep apnea syndrome, OSA, will be presented here. The obstruction may be caused by mechanical factors such as a reduced diameter of the upper airway or dynamic changes in the upper airway during sleep. The tone of the muscles of the upper airway is reduced during sleep. These sleep-related changes may predispose the patient to upper airway collapse when small amounts of negative pressure are generated during inspiration.

## Clinical Manifestations

OSA is characterized by frequent and loud snoring with breathing cessation for 10 seconds or longer, for at least five episodes per hour, followed by awakening abruptly with a loud snort as the blood oxygen level drops. Patients with sleep apnea may experience anywhere from five apneic episodes per hour to several hundred per night. Signs and symptoms of OSA are given in (Chart 22-4).

OSA may be associated with obesity and with other conditions that reduce pharyngeal muscle tone (eg, neuromuscular disease, sedative/hypnotic medications, acute ingestion of alcohol). The diagnosis of sleep apnea is based on clinical features plus polysomnographic findings (sleep study), in which the patient's cardiopulmonary status, eye

---

**CHART 22-4**

### Assessing for Obstructive Sleep Apnea (OSA)

Be alert for the following signs and symptoms:
- Excessive daytime sleepiness
- Frequent nocturnal awakening
- Insomnia
- Loud snoring
- Morning headaches
- Intellectual deterioration
- Personality changes, irritability
- Impotence
- Systemic hypertension
- Dysrhythmias
- Pulmonary hypertension, cor pulmonale
- Polycythemia
- Enuresis

movements, and muscle activity are monitored during an episode of sleep (Merritt & Berger, 2004).

The patient with OSA is at high risk for coronary artery disease, cerebrovascular disease, and premature death (von Känel & Dimsdale, 2003). Repetitive apneic events result in hypoxia and hypercapnia, which triggers a sympathetic response. As a consequence, patients have a high prevalence of hypertension and an increased risk of myocardial infarction and stroke. In patients with underlying cardiovascular disease, the nocturnal hypoxemia may predispose to dysrhythmias.

## Medical Management

Patients usually seek medical treatment because their sleeping partners express concern or because they experience excessive sleepiness at inappropriate times or settings (eg, while driving a car). A variety of treatments are used. In mild cases, the patient is advised to avoid sleeping on the back, avoid alcohol and medications that depress the upper airway, and lose weight. In more severe cases involving hypoxemia with severe carbon dioxide retention (hypercapnia), the treatment includes continuous positive airway pressure (CPAP) or bilevel positive airway pressure (BiPAP) therapy with supplemental oxygen via nasal cannula. These treatment methods are described in Chapter 25. CPAP is used to prevent airway collapse, whereas BiPAP makes breathing easier and results in a lower average airway pressure.

Surgical procedures (eg, uvulopalatopharyngoplasty) may be performed to correct the obstruction. As a last resort, a tracheostomy is performed to bypass the obstruction if the potential for respiratory failure or life-threatening dysrhythmias exists. The tracheostomy is unplugged only during sleep. Although this is an effective treatment, it is used in a limited number of patients because of its associated physical disfigurement (Thatcher & Maisel, 2003).

### Pharmacologic Therapy

Although medications are not generally recommended for OSA, some preliminary data suggest that modafinil (Provigil) may help reduce daytime sleepiness (Boutrel & Koob, 2004). Protriptyline (Triptil) given at bedtime may increase the respiratory drive and improve upper airway muscle tone. Medroxyprogesterone acetate (Provera) and acetazolamide (Diamox) have been recommended for sleep apnea associated with chronic alveolar hypoventilation, but their benefits have not been well established. The patient must understand that these medications are not a substitute for CPAP or BiPAP. Administration of low-flow nasal oxygen at night can help relieve hypoxemia in some patients but has little effect on the frequency or severity of apnea. Clinical trials are needed to assess the effectiveness of these treatment approaches.

## Nursing Management

The patient with OSA may not recognize the potential consequences of the disorder. Therefore, the nurse explains the disorder in terms that are understandable to the patient and relates symptoms (daytime sleepiness) to the underlying disorder. The nurse also instructs the patient and family about treatments, including the correct and safe use of CPAP, BiPAP, and oxygen therapy, if prescribed.

## Epistaxis (Nosebleed)

**Epistaxis**, a hemorrhage from the nose, is caused by the rupture of tiny, distended vessels in the mucous membrane of any area of the nose. Rarely does epistaxis originate in the densely vascular tissue over the turbinates. Most commonly, the site is the anterior septum, where three major blood vessels enter the nasal cavity: (1) the anterior ethmoidal artery on the forward part of the roof (Kiesselbach's plexus), (2) the sphenopalatine artery in the posterosuperior region, and (3) the internal maxillary branches (the plexus of veins located at the back of the lateral wall under the inferior turbinate).

A variety of causes are associated with epistaxis (Chart 22-5).

## Medical Management

Management of epistaxis depends on its cause and the location of the bleeding site. A nasal speculum, penlight, or headlight may be used to determine the site of bleeding in the nasal cavity. Most nosebleeds originate from the anterior portion of the nose. Initial treatment may include applying direct pressure. The patient sits upright with the head tilted forward to prevent swallowing and aspiration of blood and is directed to pinch the soft outer portion of the nose against the midline septum for 5 or 10 minutes continuously. If this measure is unsuccessful, additional treatment is indicated. In anterior nosebleeds, the area may be treated with a silver nitrate applicator and Gelfoam, or by electrocautery.

Topical vasoconstrictors, such as adrenaline (1:1,000), cocaine (0.5%), and phenylephrine may be prescribed.

### CHART 22-5 — Risk Factors for Epistaxis

- Local infections (vestibulitis, rhinitis, sinusitis)
- Systemic infections (scarlet fever, malaria)
- Drying of nasal mucous membranes
- Nasal inhalation of illicit drugs (eg, cocaine)
- Trauma (digital trauma as in picking the nose; blunt trauma; fracture; forceful nose blowing)
- Arteriosclerosis
- Hypertension
- Tumor (sinus or nasopharynx)
- Thrombocytopenia
- Use of aspirin
- Liver disease
- Redu-Osler-Weber syndrome (hereditary hemorrhagic telangiectasia)

Cotton pledgets soaked in a vasoconstricting solution (ie, epinephrine, ephedrine, cocaine) may be inserted into the nose to reduce the blood flow and improve the examiner's view of the bleeding site. Alternatively, a cotton tampon may be used to try to stop the bleeding. Suction may be used to remove excess blood and clots from the field of inspection. The search for the bleeding site should shift from the anteroinferior quadrant to the anterosuperior, then to the posterosuperior, and finally to the posteroinferior area. The field is kept clear by using suction and by shifting the cotton tampon. Only about 60% of the total nasal cavity can actually be seen, however.

If the origin of the bleeding cannot be identified, the nose may be packed with gauze impregnated with petrolatum jelly or antibiotic ointment; a topical anesthetic spray and decongestant agent may be used before the gauze packing is inserted, or a balloon-inflated catheter may be used (Fig. 22-4). Alternatively, a compressed nasal sponge may be used. Once the sponge becomes saturated with blood or is moistened with a small amount of saline, it will expand and produce tamponade to halt the bleeding. The packing may remain in place for 48 hours or up to 5 or 6 days if necessary to control bleeding. Antibiotics may be prescribed because of the risk of iatrogenic sinusitis and toxic shock syndrome.

## Nursing Management

The nurse monitors the patient's vital signs, assists in the control of bleeding, and provides tissues and an emesis basin to allow the patient to expectorate any excess blood. It is common for patients to be anxious in response to a nosebleed. Blood loss on clothing and handkerchiefs can be frightening, and the nasal examination and treatment are uncomfortable. Assuring the patient in a calm, efficient manner that bleeding can be controlled can help reduce anxiety. The nurse continuously assesses the patient's airway and breathing as well as vital signs. On rare occasions, a patient with significant hemorrhage requires IV infusions of crystalloid solutions (normal saline) as well as cardiac and pulse oximetry monitoring.

### Teaching Patients Self-Care

Discharge teaching includes reviewing ways to prevent epistaxis: avoiding forceful nose blowing, straining, high altitudes, and nasal trauma (including nose picking). Adequate humidification may prevent drying of the nasal passages. The nurse instructs the patient how to apply direct pressure to the nose with the thumb and the index finger for 15 minutes in the case of a recurrent nosebleed. If recurrent bleeding cannot be stopped, the patient is instructed to seek additional medical attention.

## Nasal Obstruction

The passage of air through the nostrils is frequently obstructed by a deviation of the nasal septum, hypertrophy of the turbinate bones, or the pressure of nasal polyps, which are grapelike swellings that arise from the mucous membrane of the sinuses, especially the ethmoids. Chronic nasal congestion seriously affects the patient throughout the day as well as during sleep. It forces the patient to breath through the mouth, thus producing dryness of the oral mucosa and associated problems including persistent dry, cracked lips. Patients with chronic nasal congestion often suffer from sleep deprivation due to difficulty maintaining an adequate airway while lying flat and during sleep.

Persistent nasal obstruction also may lead to chronic infection of the nose and result in frequent episodes of nasopharyngitis. Frequently, the infection extends to the nasal sinuses. When sinusitis develops and the drainage from these cavities is obstructed by deformity or swelling within the nose, pain is experienced in the region of the affected sinus.

## Medical Management

The treatment of nasal obstruction requires the removal of the obstruction, followed by measures to treat whatever chronic infection exists. In many patients an underlying allergy also requires treatment. Measures to reduce or alleviate nasal obstruction include nonsurgical as well as surgical techniques. Commonly used medications include fluticasone propionate aqueous nasal spray (Flonase) and montelukast (Singulair). Additional medications may include antibiotics for the treatment of underlying infection or antihistamines for management of allergies. Hypertrophied turbinates may be treated by applying an astringent agent to shrink them.

A more aggressive approach in treating nasal obstruction caused by turbinate hypertrophy involves surgical reduction of the hypertrophy. Available surgical procedures include turbinectomy, laser cautery, electrocautery, cryotherapy, submucosal resection, and submucosal resection

**FIGURE 22-4.** Packing to control bleeding from the posterior nose. (**A**) Catheter is inserted and packing is attached. (**B**) Packing is drawn into position as the catheter is removed. (**C**) Strip is tied over a bolster to hold the packing in place with an anterior pack installed "accordion pleat" style. (**D**) Alternative method, using a balloon catheter instead of gauze packing.

with lateral displacement (Passali, Passali, Damiani, et al., 2003). During **submucosal resection** to treat a deviated septum, the surgeon makes an incision into the mucous membrane and, after raising it from the bone, removes the deviated bone and cartilage with bone forceps. The mucosa then is allowed to fall back in place and is held there by tight packing. Generally, the packing is soaked in liquid petrolatum so that it can be removed easily after 24 to 36 hours. At times endoscopic surgery is also indicated to drain the nasal sinuses. The specific procedure performed depends on the type of nasal obstruction found. Nasal polyps are removed by clipping them at their base with a wire snare. Usually, these surgical procedures are performed under local anesthesia.

## Nursing Management

Most of these procedures are performed on an outpatient basis. The nurse explains the procedure after the physician provides the initial instruction. Postoperatively, the nurse elevates the head of the bed to promote drainage and to alleviate discomfort from edema. Frequent oral hygiene is encouraged to overcome dryness caused by breathing through the mouth. Before discharge from the outpatient or same-day surgical unit, the patient is instructed to avoid blowing the nose with force during the postoperative recovery period. The patient is also instructed about the signs and symptoms of bleeding and infection and when to contact the physician. The patient is provided with written postoperative instructions including emergency phone numbers.

## Fractures of the Nose

The location of the nose makes it susceptible to injury. Nasal fracture is the most common facial fracture and the most common fracture in the body. Fractures of the nose usually result from a direct assault. Nasal fractures may affect the ascending process of the maxilla and the septum. The torn mucous membrane results in a nosebleed. In a series of complications, the patient could ultimately experience a hematoma, infection, abscess, and avascular/septic necrosis. However, as a rule, serious consequences usually do not occur.

## Clinical Manifestations

The signs and symptoms of a nasal fracture are pain, bleeding from the nose externally and internally into the pharynx, swelling of the soft tissues adjacent to the nose, periorbital ecchymosis, nasal obstruction, and deformity. The patient's nose may have an asymmetric appearance that may not be obvious until the edema subsides.

## Assessment and Diagnostic Findings

The nose is examined internally to rule out the possibility that the injury may be complicated by a fracture of the nasal septum and a submucosal septal hematoma. Because of the swelling and bleeding that occur with a nasal fracture, an accurate diagnosis can be made only after the swelling subsides.

Clear fluid draining from either nostril suggests a fracture of the cribriform plate with leakage of cerebrospinal fluid. Because cerebrospinal fluid contains glucose, it can readily be differentiated from nasal mucus by means of a dipstick (Dextrostix). Usually, careful inspection or palpation discloses any deviations of the bone or disruptions of the nasal cartilages. An x-ray may reveal displacement of the fractured bones and may help rule out extension of the fracture into the skull.

## Medical Management

The nose is assessed for symmetry either before swelling has occurred or after it has subsided. A nasal fracture very often produces bleeding from the nasal passage. As a rule, bleeding is controlled with the use of packing. Cold compresses are used to prevent or reduce edema. For the patient who has sustained enough trauma to break the nose or any facial bone, the emergency medical team must consider the possibility of a cervical spine fracture. Therefore, it is essential to ensure a patent airway and to rule out a cervical spine fracture. Uncomplicated nasal fractures may be treated initially with antibiotics, analgesic agents, and a decongestant nasal spray.

Treatment of nasal fractures is aimed at restoring nasal function and returning the aesthetic appearance of the nose to baseline. The patient is referred to a specialist, usually 3 to 5 days after the injury, to evaluate the need to realign the bones. Although improved outcomes are obtained when reduction of the fracture is performed during the first 3 hours after the injury, this is often not possible because of the edema. If immediate reduction of the fracture is not possible, it is performed within 3 to 7 days. Timing is important when treating nasal fractures because a delay in treatment longer than 7 to 10 days may result in significant bone healing, which ultimately may require surgical intervention that includes rhinoplasty to reshape the external appearance of the nose. A septorhinoplasty is performed when the nasal septum needs to be repaired. In patients who develop a septal hematoma, the physician will drain the hematoma through a small incision. A septal hematoma that is not drained can lead to permanent deformity of the nose.

## Nursing Management

Immediately after the fracture, the nurse applies ice and encourages the patient to keep the head elevated. The nurse instructs the patient to apply ice packs to the nose for 20 minutes four times each day to decrease swelling. The patient who experiences bleeding from the nose (epistaxis) is usually frightened and anxious and needs reassurance. The packing inserted to stop the bleeding may be uncomfortable and unpleasant, and obstruction of the nasal passages by the packing forces the patient to breathe through the mouth. This in turn causes the oral mucous membranes to become dry. Mouth rinses help to moisten the mucous membranes and to reduce the odor and taste of dried blood in the oropharynx and nasopharynx. Use of analgesic agents such as acetaminophen or NSAIDs such as ibuprofen or naproxen is encouraged. For people younger than 20 years of age, aspirin is avoided because of the risk of Reye's syndrome. When removing the cotton pledgets, the nurse carefully inspects the mucosa for lacerations or a septal hematoma. The nurse reminds the patient to avoid sports activities for 6 weeks.

## Laryngeal Obstruction

Obstruction of the larynx because of edema is a serious, often fatal, condition. The larynx is a stiff box that will not stretch. It contains a narrow space between the vocal cords (glottis), through which air must pass. Swelling of the laryngeal mucous membranes may close off the opening tightly, leading to life-threatening hypoxia or suffocation. Edema of the glottis occurs rarely in patients with acute laryngitis, occasionally in patients with urticaria, and more frequently in patients with severe inflammation of the throat, as in scarlet fever. It is an occasional but usually preventable cause of death in severe anaphylaxis (angioneurotic edema).

Hereditary angioedema (HAE) is also characterized by episodes of life-threatening laryngeal edema. Laryngeal edema in people with HAE can occur at any age, although young adults are at greatest risk. Risk factors for laryngeal obstruction are given in Table 22-2.

Foreign bodies frequently are aspirated into the pharynx, the larynx, or the trachea and cause a twofold problem. First, they obstruct the air passages and cause difficulty in breathing, which may lead to asphyxia; later, they may be drawn farther down, entering the bronchi or a bronchial branch and causing symptoms of irritation, such as a croupy cough, expectoration of blood or mucus, or labored breathing. The physical signs and x-ray findings confirm the diagnosis.

### TABLE 22-2 Risk Factors for Laryngeal Obstruction

| Precipitating Event | Mechanism of Obstruction |
|---|---|
| History of allergies; exposure to medications, latex, foods (tree nuts [eg, walnuts, pecans]), bee stings | Anaphylaxis |
| Foreign body | Inhalation/ingestion of meat or other food items, coin, chewing gum, balloon fragments, drug packets (ingested to avoid arrest) |
| Heavy alcohol consumption; heavy tobacco use | Obstruction from tumor |
| Family history of airway problems | Suggests angioedema (type I hypersensitivity reaction) |
| Use of angiotensin-converting enzyme (ACE) inhibitors | Increased risk for angioedema of the mucous membranes |
| Recent throat pain or recent fever | Infectious process |
| History of surgery or previous tracheostomy | Possible subglottic stenosis |

## Clinical Manifestations

The patient's clinical presentation and x-ray findings confirm the diagnosis of laryngeal obstruction. The patient may demonstrate lowered oxygen saturation; however, a normal oxygen saturation should not be interpreted as a sign that the obstruction is not significant. Use of accessory muscles to maximize airflow may occur and is often manifested by retractions in the neck or abdomen during inspirations. Patients who demonstrate these symptoms are at an immediate risk of collapse, and respiratory support (ie, mechanical ventilation or positive-pressure ventilation) is considered.

## Assessment and Diagnostic Findings

A thorough history can be very useful to the health care team in diagnosing and treating the patient with a laryngeal obstruction. However, emergency measures to secure the patient's airway should not be delayed to obtain a history or perform tests. If possible, the nurse obtains a history from the patient or family about heavy alcohol or tobacco consumption, current medications, family history of airway problems, recent infections, pain or fever, dental pain or poor dentition, and any previous surgeries or trauma.

## Medical Management

Medical management is based on the initial evaluation of the patient and the need to ensure a patent airway. If the airway is obstructed by a foreign body and signs of asphyxia are apparent, immediate treatment is necessary. Frequently, if the foreign body has lodged in the pharynx and can be visualized, the finger can dislodge it. If the obstruction is in the larynx or the trachea, the clinician or other rescuer tries the subdiaphragmatic abdominal thrust maneuver (Chart 22-6). If all efforts are unsuccessful, an immediate tracheotomy is necessary (see Chapter 25 for further discussion). If the obstruction is caused by edema resulting from an allergic reaction, treatment may include administration of subcutaneous epinephrine and a corticosteroid (see Chapter 53). Ice may be applied to the neck in an effort to reduce edema. Continuous pulse oximetry is essential in the patient who has experienced acute upper airway obstruction.

## Cancer of the Larynx

Cancer of the larynx is a malignant tumor in and around the larynx (voice box). Squamous cell carcinoma is the most common form of cancer of the larynx (95%). Adenocarcinoma or sarcoma of the larynx is diagnosed less often. More than 10,000 new cases of cancer of the larynx occur annually. Cancer of the larynx occurs more frequently in men than in women, and it is most common in people between the ages of 50 and 70 years. The incidence of laryngeal cancer continues to decline, but the incidence in women versus men continues to increase. The disease is also about 50% more common among African Americans than among Caucasian Americans.

Carcinogens that have been associated with laryngeal cancer include tobacco (smoke, smokeless) and alcohol

## CHART 22-6

### Performing the Abdominal Thrust Maneuver

To assist a patient or other person who is choking on a foreign object, the nurse performs the abdominal thrust maneuver (sometimes called the Heimlich maneuver) according to guidelines set forth by the American Heart Association. (*Note:* Hands crossed at the neck is the universal sign for choking.)

1. Stand behind the person who is choking.
2. Place both arms around the person's waist.
3. Make a fist with one hand with the thumb outside the fist.
4. Place thumb side of fist against the person's abdomen above the navel and below the xiphoid process.
5. Grasp fist with other hand.
6. Quickly and forcefully exert pressure against the person's diaphragm, pressing upward with quick, firm thrusts.
7. Apply thrusts 6 to 10 times until the obstruction is cleared.
8. The pressure from the thrusts should lift the diaphragm, force air into the lungs, and create an artificial cough powerful enough to expel the aspirated object.

and their combined effects, as well as exposure to asbestos, mustard gas, wood dust, cement dust, tar products, leather, and metals (Dietz, Ramroth, Urban, et al., 2004). Other contributing factors include straining the voice, chronic laryngitis, nutritional deficiencies (riboflavin), and family predisposition (Chart 22-7).

Laryngeal cancer can be classified into three categories: supraglottic (false vocal cords), glottic (true vocal cords), and subglottic (downward extension of disease from the vocal cords) (National Cancer Institute, 2003). Two thirds of laryngeal cancers are in the glottic area. Supraglottic cancers account for approximately one third of the cases, subglottic tumors for fewer than 1%. Glottic tumors seldom spread if found early, because of the limited lymph vessels found in the vocal cords.

Approximately 25% to 50% of patients with laryngeal cancer present with involved lymph nodes. Metastatic disease from the true vocal cords is very rare, because they are devoid of lymph nodes. The prognosis for patients who have small laryngeal cancers without evidence of spread to the lymph nodes is about 75% to 95%. Recurrence occurs usually within the first 2 to 3 years after diagnosis. The presence of disease after 5 years is very often secondary to a new primary malignancy (National Cancer Institute, 2003).

## Clinical Manifestations

Hoarseness of more than 2 weeks' duration occurs in the patient with cancer in the glottic area, because the tumor impedes the action of the vocal cords during speech. The

## CHART 22-7

### Risk Factors for Laryngeal Cancer

**CARCINOGENS**
- Tobacco (smoke, smokeless)
- Combined effects of alcohol and tobacco
- Asbestos
- Secondhand smoke
- Paint fumes
- Wood dust
- Cement dust
- Chemicals
- Tar products
- Mustard gas
- Leather and metals

**OTHER FACTORS**
- Straining the voice
- Chronic laryngitis
- Nutritional deficiencies (riboflavin)
- History of alcohol abuse
- Familial predisposition
- Age (higher incidence after 60 years of age)
- Gender (more common in men)
- Race (more prevalent in African Americans)
- Weakened immune system

voice may sound harsh, raspy, and lower in pitch. Affected voice sounds are not early signs of subglottic or supraglottic cancer. The patient may complain of a persistent cough or sore throat and pain and burning in the throat, especially when consuming hot liquids or citrus juices. A lump may be felt in the neck. Later symptoms include dysphagia, dyspnea (difficulty breathing), unilateral nasal obstruction or discharge, persistent hoarseness, persistent ulceration, and foul breath. Cervical lymph adenopathy, unintentional weight loss, a general debilitated state, and pain radiating to the ear may occur with metastasis.

## Assessment and Diagnostic Findings

An initial assessment includes a complete history and physical examination of the head and neck. This includes identification of risk factors, family history, and any underlying medical conditions. An indirect laryngoscopy, using a flexible endoscope, is initially performed in the otolaryngologist's office to visually evaluate the pharynx, larynx, and possible tumor. Mobility of the vocal cords is assessed; if normal movement is limited, the growth may affect muscle, other tissue, and even the airway. The neck and the thyroid gland are palpated for enlarged lymph nodes (Timon, Toner & Conlon, 2003).

If a tumor of the larynx is suspected on an initial examination, a direct laryngoscopic examination is performed under local or general anesthesia to evaluate all areas of the larynx. In some cases, intraoperative examination obtained by direct microscopic visualization and palpation of the vocal folds may yield a more accurate diagnosis. Samples of the suspicious tissue are obtained for histologic evaluation. The tumor may involve any of the three areas of the larynx and may vary in appearance. Additionally, tumor markers (p53 and cyclin D1) obtained through analysis of biopsy tissue provide information about the prognosis of patients with laryngeal epidermoid carcinomas (Vielba, Bilbao, Ispizua, et al., 2003).

The stage of the tumor serves as a basis for the therapeutic regimen. The TNM classification system, developed by the American Joint Committee on Cancer (AJCC), is used to classify head and neck tumors. The classification of the tumor is used to determine treatment modalities. The presence of metastatic disease in lymph nodes is the foremost prognostic indicator (Timon et al., 2003). Because many of these lesions are submucosal, obtaining tissue for biopsy may require an incision made with microlaryngeal techniques or with the use of a $CO_2$ laser to transect the mucosa and reach the tumor.

CT and magnetic resonance imaging (MRI) are used to assess regional adenopathy and soft tissue and to help stage and determine the extent of a tumor. MRI is also helpful in post-treatment follow-up to detect a recurrence. Positron emission tomography (PET) scanning may also be used to detect recurrence of a laryngeal tumor after treatment.

## Medical Management

Treatment of laryngeal cancer depends on the staging of the tumor, which includes the location, size, and histology of the tumor and the presence and extent of cervical lymph node involvement. Treatment options include surgery, radiation therapy, and chemotherapy. The prognosis depends on a variety of factors: tumor stage, the patient's gender and age, and pathologic features of the tumor, including the grade and depth of infiltration. The treatment plan also depends on whether this is an initial diagnosis or a recurrence.

Patients with early-stage disease (stage I or II) can be treated with either radiation therapy or surgery. Survival with radiation alone is 80% to 90% for patients with stage I disease and 70% to 80% for patients with stage II disease. Surgery alone can be used; however, voice preservation is better with radiation alone than with partial laryngectomy (American Cancer Society, 2005). Patients with stage III or IV or advanced tumors require a combined treatment modality approach consisting of either surgery and irradiation, radiation therapy and chemotherapy, or all three treatment regimens. Because of the advanced nature of the disease, surgery often requires the complete removal of the larynx. Patients with advanced laryngeal cancer have longer disease-free survival when treated with chemotherapy along with radiotherapy rather than with radiotherapy alone (Forastiere, Goepfert, Maor, et al., 2003).

Treatment with hyperfractionated accelerated irradiation and concomitant cisplatin has also been effective against locally advanced laryngeal carcinomas. In hyperfractionated radiotherapy, the patient receives a radiation treatment twice daily for a prescribed period of time (DeVita, Hellman & Rosenberg, 2005).

Surgery and radiation therapy are both effective methods in the early stages of cancer of the larynx. Chemotherapy traditionally has been used for recurrence or metastatic disease. It has also been used more recently in conjunction with radiation therapy, to avoid a total laryngectomy, or preoperatively, to shrink a tumor before surgery.

The highest risk of laryngeal cancer recurrence is in the first 2 to 3 years. Combined treatment for patients with stage III cancers yields a survival rate of 30% to 50% at 3 years. The survival rate decreases to 20% to 30% at 5 years. Patients with resectable stage IV disease treated with combined therapy have a 5-year survival rate of 15% to 25% (American Cancer Society, 2005).

Before treatment, a complete dental examination is performed to rule out any oral disease. Any dental problems are resolved, if possible, before surgery and radiotherapy. If surgery is to be performed, a multidisciplinary team evaluates the needs of the patient and family to develop a successful plan of care (Harrison, Dale, Haverman, et al., 2003; Marques & Dib, 2004).

### *Surgical Management*

Surgical management depends largely on the stage of the disease. The overall goals for the patient include minimizing the effects of surgery on speech, swallowing, and breathing while maximizing the cure of the cancer. Complete removal of the larynx (total **laryngectomy**) can provide the desired cure, but it also leaves the patient with significant loss of the natural voice and the need to breathe through an opening (stoma) created in the lower neck. Advances in surgical techniques for treating laryngeal cancer may minimize the cosmetic and functional deficits previously seen with total laryngectomy. Partial laryngectomy is often used for smaller cancers of the larynx. Several different curative procedures are available that can offer voice-sparing results for the patient who has an early laryngeal carcinoma while achieving a positive cure rate. Some microlaryngeal surgery can be performed endoscopically. The $CO_2$ laser can be used for the treatment of many laryngeal tumors, with the exception of large vascular tumors.

Some less extensive procedures are used to treat dysplasia, hyperkeratosis, and leukoplakia. Complete stripping of the cord is often the curative treatment for this classification of lesions. Stripping of the cord involves removal of the mucosa of the edge of the cord. It is performed with use of an operating microscope. Early vocal cord lesions are initially treated with radiation therapy. An excision of the vocal cord (cordectomy) is usually performed via transoral laser. This procedure is used for confined lesions involving the middle third of the vocal cord. The probability of poor voice quality is related to the extent of tissue removed. High-volume, bilateral, advanced lesions in patients who either refuse laryngectomy or are unable to tolerate surgery may be treated with radiation therapy, with a cure rate of 10% to 20%. Patients with a fixed cord but minimal total tumor bulk may be treated with radiation therapy. Chemotherapy is often considered, and the patients are informed that the need for a subsequent total laryngectomy will be based on clinical suspicion of disease recurrence (ie, in the absence of a biopsy).

Several different types of laryngectomy (surgical removal of part or all of the larynx and surrounding structures) are considered for patients with more extensive involvement:

- Partial laryngectomy
- Supraglottic laryngectomy
- Hemilaryngectomy
- Total laryngectomy
- Other surgical procedures

**PARTIAL LARYNGECTOMY.** A partial laryngectomy (laryngofissure–thyrotomy) is recommended in the early stages of cancer in the glottic area when only one vocal cord is involved. The surgery is associated with a very high cure rate. It may also be performed for recurrence when high-dose radiation has failed. A portion of the larynx is removed, along with one vocal cord and the tumor; all other structures remain. The airway remains intact, and the patient is expected to have no difficulty swallowing. The voice quality may change, or the patient may sound hoarse.

**SUPRAGLOTTIC LARYNGECTOMY.** This is a voice-sparing operation that can be tailored to the supraglottic lesion. It is used for lesions that involve the epiglottis, a single arytenoid cartilage, the aryepiglottic fold, and false vocal cords. A neck dissection of one or both sides may also be performed. Postoperative irradiation is indicated based on the pathologic findings from the surgery. A supraglottic laryngectomy is indicated in the management of early (stage I) supraglottic and stage II lesions. The hyoid bone, glottis, and false cords are removed. The true vocal cords, cricoid cartilage, and trachea remain intact. A tracheostomy tube (see Chapter 25) is left in the trachea until the glottic airway is established. It is usually removed after a few days, and the stoma is allowed to close.

Nutrition is provided through enteral feedings until there is healing, followed by a semisolid diet. Postoperatively, the patient may experience some difficulty swallowing for the first 2 weeks. Aspiration is a potential complication, because the patient must learn a new method of swallowing (supraglottic swallowing). The chief advantage of this surgical procedure is that it preserves the voice, even though the quality of the voice may change. Speech therapy is required before and after surgery. The major problem is the high risk for recurrence of the cancer; therefore, patients are selected carefully. For patients with early disease, the surgeon may consider an endoscopic supraglottic laryngectomy with postoperative radiation therapy (Davis, Kriskovich, Galloway, et al., 2004).

**HEMILARYNGECTOMY.** A hemilaryngectomy is performed when the tumor extends beyond the vocal cord but is less than 1 cm in size and is limited to the subglottic area. It may be used in stage I glottic lesions. In this procedure, the thyroid cartilage of the larynx is split in the midline of the neck, and the portion of the vocal cord (one true cord and one false cord) is removed with the tumor. The arytenoid cartilage and half of the thyroid are removed. The patient will have a tracheostomy tube and nasogastric tube in place for a number of days after the surgery. The patient is at risk for aspiration postoperatively. Some change may occur in the voice quality. The voice may be rough, raspy, and hoarse and have limited projection. The airway and swallowing remain intact. Usually, this procedure is reserved for patients with lesions that involve only one cord. Extension of the lesion to the epiglottis, false cord, or intra-arytenoid areas is a contraindication to a hemilaryngectomy.

**TOTAL LARYNGECTOMY.** A total laryngectomy is performed in most advanced stage IV laryngeal cancers, when the tumor extends beyond the vocal cords, or for cancer that recurs or persists after radiation therapy. In a total laryngectomy, the laryngeal structures are removed, including the hyoid bone, epiglottis, cricoid cartilage, and two or three rings of the trachea. The tongue, pharyngeal walls, and trachea are preserved. A total laryngectomy results in permanent loss of the voice and a change in the airway, requiring a permanent tracheostomy (Fig. 22-5). Patients who have this procedure require alternatives to normal speech; these may include a prosthetic device such as the Singer-Blom valve to speak without aspirating.

Although this procedure can be performed with or without neck dissection, many surgeons recommend that a radical neck dissection be performed on the same side as the lesion even if no lymph nodes are palpable, because metastasis to the cervical lymph nodes is common. Surgery is more difficult when the lesion involves the midline structures or both vocal cords. With or without neck dissection, a total laryngectomy requires a permanent tracheal stoma, because the larynx that provides the protective sphincter is no longer present. The tracheal stoma prevents the aspiration of food and fluid into the lower respiratory tract. The patient will have no voice but will have normal swallowing. A total laryngectomy changes the manner in which airflow is used for breathing and speaking, as depicted in Figure 22-5. Complications that may occur include a salivary leak, wound infection from the development of a pharyngocutaneous fistula, stomal stenosis, and dysphagia secondary to pharyngeal and cervical esophageal stricture.

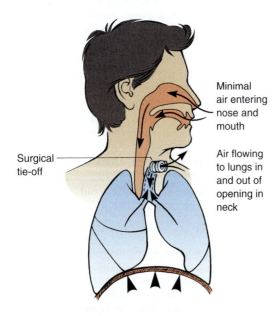

**FIGURE 22-5.** Total laryngectomy produces a change in airflow for breathing and speaking. **(A)** Normal airflow. **(B)** Airflow after total laryngectomy.

In some cases, the patient may be a candidate for a near-total laryngectomy (NTL). In this situation, the patient would be a candidate for chemotherapy and radiotherapy regimens postoperatively. Voice preservation can be achieved in most cases. NTL enhances speech rehabilitation options for the patient by adding a physiologic, nonprosthetic tissue technique (ie, the myomucosal shunt) that provides a prosthesis-free method for rehabilitating the voice (Kasperbauer & Thomas, 2004).

**OTHER SURGICAL APPROACHES.** Other surgical procedures include the supracricoid laryngectomy, which was initially developed in the late 1950s as an alternative to total laryngectomy but was not widely adopted in the United States until 30 years later. Two types of this procedure exist; they differ in the extent of resection and reconstruction. Both procedures are alternatives to the total laryngectomy and have been used to preserve or restore speech in patients with more advanced larynx cancers (Shiotani, Araki, Moro, et al., 2004).

In the supracricoid partial laryngectomy (SCPL), the true and false cords, both paraglottic spaces, and the thyroid cartilage are resected. The reconstruction requires suturing of the cricoid to the hyoid and the epiglottis. The procedure is thus termed cricohyoidoepiglottopexy (CHEP).

The second procedure involves the resection of both true and false cords, both paraglottic spaces, the entire preepiglottic space, the epiglottis, and the entire thyroid cartilage. The reconstruction is extensive and requires suturing of the cricoid to the hyoid. The procedure is therefore termed cricohyoidopexy (CHP).

## Radiation Therapy

The goal of radiation therapy is to eradicate the cancer and preserve the function of the larynx. The decision to use radiation therapy is based on several factors, including the staging of the tumor (usually used for stage I and stage II tumors as a standard treatment option) and the patient's overall health status, lifestyle (including occupation), and personal preference. Excellent results have been achieved with radiation therapy in patients with early-stage (stage I or II) glottic tumors when only one vocal cord is involved and there is normal mobility (ie, with phonation), as well as in small supraglottic lesions. One of the benefits of radiation therapy is that patients retain a near-normal voice. A few may develop chondritis (inflammation of the cartilage) or stenosis; a small number may later require laryngectomy.

Radiation therapy may also be used preoperatively to reduce the tumor size. Radiation therapy is combined with surgery in advanced laryngeal cancer (stages III and IV) as adjunctive therapy to surgery or chemotherapy and as a palliative measure. A variety of clinical trials have combined chemotherapy and radiation therapy in the treatment of advanced laryngeal tumors.

Advances in research and treatment of these tumors with surgery, chemotherapy, and radiation therapy have improved outcomes and decreased the incidence of post-treatment morbidities (DeVita et al., 2005). Radiation therapy combined with chemotherapy may be an alternative to a total laryngectomy.

Complications from radiation therapy are a result of external radiation to the head and neck area, which may also include the parotid gland, which is responsible for mucus production. Symptoms may include acute mucositis, ulceration of the mucous membranes, pain, **xerostomia** (dry mouth), loss of taste, dysphasia, fatigue, and skin reactions. Later complications may include laryngeal necrosis, edema, and fibrosis.

## Speech Therapy

The patient who undergoes a laryngectomy faces potentially complex and frustrating communication problems. These are related to alterations in communication methods, perceived voice quality, and perceptions of quality of life related to communication, disfigurement, and socialization (Happ, Roesch & Kagan, 2004). Often, communication needs and voice quality of patients are ignored during the hospital stay. To minimize anxiety and frustration on the part of the patient and family, the loss or alteration of speech is discussed with the patient and family before surgery, and the speech therapist conducts a preoperative evaluation. During this time, the nurse discusses with the patient and family methods of communication that will be available in the immediate postoperative period. These include writing, lip speaking, and communication or word boards. A system of communication is established with the patient, family, nurse, and physician and is implemented consistently after surgery.

In addition, a long-term postoperative communication plan for **alaryngeal communication** is developed. The three most common techniques of alaryngeal communication are esophageal speech, artificial larynx (electrolarynx), and tracheoesophageal puncture. Training in these techniques begins once medical clearance is obtained from the physician.

**ESOPHAGEAL SPEECH.** Esophageal speech was the primary method of alaryngeal speech taught to patients until the 1980s. The patient needs the ability to compress air into the esophagus and expel it, setting off a vibration of the pharyngeal esophageal segment. The technique can be taught once the patient begins oral feedings, approximately 1 week after surgery. First, the patient learns to belch and is reminded to do so an hour after eating. Then the technique is practiced repeatedly. Later, this conscious belching action is transformed into simple explosions of air

## NURSING RESEARCH PROFILE

### Communication Needs after Head and Neck Surgery

Happ, M. B., Roesch, T. & Kagan, S. H. (2004). Communication needs, methods, and perceived voice quality following head and neck surgery: A literature review. *Cancer Nursing, 27*(1), 1–9.

#### Purpose
Limited data on the topic of communication immediately after surgery for treatment of head and neck cancer stimulated this review. The authors conducted a review and critique of research and related medical, nursing, and psychological literature on in-hospital postoperative communication with adult patients with head and neck cancer.

#### Design
The authors conducted a comprehensive literature review of available research to address the communication needs, methods, or perceived voice quality of patients with head and neck cancer during the postoperative period. A combined computerized and hand search of the medical, psychological and nursing literature was evaluated through MEDLINE, Cancerlit, and CINHL, as well as a review of health and psychosocial instruments. The search included the following terms: head and neck cancer, head and neck surgery, head and neck surgery complications, and nonverbal communication. Due to the significant lack of in-hospital research, the authors expanded their search to include the first 12 months after surgery. Ten published research articles and one clinical case report were used in the analysis.

#### Findings
The review and synthesis of the articles included in this review addressed the communication needs, communication methods, and perceptions of voice quality of patients with head and neck cancer in the postoperative period. Three major themes emerged from the small body of research; these themes included (1) information needs, (2) communication methods and perceived voice quality, and (3) quality-of-life perceptions related to communication, disfigurement and socialization.

The patients and family members addressed in the studies reported the need for more information about the consequences of head and neck surgery, specifically the loss of speech and the alternative communication methods available to them. The patients' experiences of being voiceless immediately after surgery were largely ignored during their hospital stays. The emotional and social changes associated with loss of voice and the lack of congruence between actual voice quality and expected voice quality were significant issues for patients in the studies. The effect of surgery, disfigurement, and loss of socialization on perceived quality of life was addressed in several studies. The authors reported that disfigurement and perceptions of disfigurement are factors that influence social interaction and quality of life after head and neck cancer surgery.

#### Nursing Implications
The results of this critical review and synthesis of articles revealed that health care personnel, including nurses, need to address the physical, emotional and social changes resulting from surgery to treat head and neck cancer. Educational needs and preparation for postoperative communication impairment remain largely unaddressed in caring for the patient with head and neck cancer. Strategies to address patients' and families' educational, emotional, and communication needs are needed and should be subjected to research studies to determine best practices.

from the esophagus for speech purposes. The speech therapist continues to work with the patient to make speech intelligible and as close to normal as possible. Because it takes a long time to become proficient, the success rate is low.

**ELECTRIC LARYNX.** If esophageal speech is not successful, or until the patient masters the technique, an electric larynx may be used for communication. This battery-powered apparatus projects sound into the oral cavity. When the mouth forms words (articulated), the sounds from the electric larynx become audible words. The voice that is produced sounds mechanical, and some words may be difficult to understand. The advantage is that the patient is able to communicate with relative ease while working to become proficient at either esophageal or tracheoesophageal puncture speech.

**TRACHEOESOPHAGEAL PUNCTURE.** The third technique of alaryngeal speech is tracheoesophageal puncture (Fig. 22-6). This technique has become the most widely used because the speech associated with it most resembles normal speech (the sound produced is a combination of esophageal speech and voice), and it is easily learned. A valve is placed in the tracheal stoma to divert air into the esophagus and out the mouth. Once the puncture is surgically created and has healed, a voice prosthesis (Singer–Blom) is fitted over the puncture site. A speech therapist teaches the patient how to produce sounds. Moving the tongue and lips to form the sound into words produces speech as before. To prevent airway obstruction, the prosthesis is removed and cleaned when mucus builds up.

The success of these various approaches to preserve or restore speech varies. In one study that evaluated the effectiveness of these methods, the electric larynx was used more often than the other methods of speaking, and tracheoesophageal speech was preferred over esophageal speech. (DeVita et al., 2005).

**FIGURE 22-6.** Schematic representation of tracheoesophageal puncture speech (TEP). Air travels from the lung through a puncture in the posterior wall of the trachea into the esophagus and out the mouth. A voice prosthesis is fitted over the puncture site.

## Nursing Process

# The Patient Undergoing Laryngectomy

## Assessment

The nurse obtains a health history and assesses the patient's physical, psychosocial, and spiritual domains. The health history addresses the following symptoms: hoarseness, sore throat, dyspnea, dysphagia, and pain or burning in the throat. The physical assessment includes a thorough head and neck examination with an emphasis on the patient's airway. In addition, the neck is palpated for swelling or adenopathy.

The nurse also assesses the patient's general state of nutrition, including height and weight and body mass index and reviews laboratory values that assist in determining the patient's nutritional status (albumin, protein, glucose, and electrolyte levels). If treatment includes surgery, the nurse must know the nature of the surgery to plan appropriate care. If the patient is expected to have no voice as a result of the surgical procedure, a preoperative evaluation by the speech therapist is essential. The patient's ability to hear, see, read, and write is assessed. Visual impairment and functional illiteracy may create additional problems with communication and may require creative approaches to ensure that the patient is able to communicate any needs. Because alcohol abuse is a risk factor for cancer of the larynx, it is essential to assess the patient's pattern of alcohol intake. Patients who are accustomed to daily consumption of alcohol are at risk for alcohol withdrawal syndrome (delirium tremens) when alcohol intake is stopped suddenly.

In addition, the nurse determines the psychological readiness of the patient and family. The thought of having cancer is frightening to most people. Fear is compounded by the possibility of permanent voice loss and, in some cases, some degree of disfigurement (Chart 22-8). The nurse evaluates the patient's and family's knowledge of the planned surgical procedure and expected postoperative course, and assesses the patient's and family's coping methods and support systems. The nurse assesses the patient's spirituality needs based on the patient's individual preferences, beliefs, and culture.

## Diagnosis

### Nursing Diagnoses

Based on all the assessment data, major nursing diagnoses may include the following:

## CHART 22-8

### Ethics and Related Issues

**SITUATION**

A 60-year-old singer was diagnosed with cancer of the larynx 6 years ago. He was treated successfully with radiation therapy, resulting in an altered voice quality. Recently, he has complained of shortness of breath and difficulty swallowing. In the past few months, he also has noticed a marked change in his voice and physical condition, yet has not sought health care.

After a complete physical examination and an extensive diagnostic workup and biopsy, it is determined that the cancer has recurred. His health care provider recommends surgery (a total laryngectomy) and chemotherapy as the best options. The patient states that he is not willing to "lose my voice and my livelihood" but instead will "take my chances." He has also expressed concern about his quality of life after surgery. His family has approached you about trying to convince him to have surgery.

**DILEMMA**

The patient's right to refuse treatment conflicts with the family's wishes and recommendation from his health care provider.

**DISCUSSION**

1. Is the patient making a decision based upon all pertinent information concerning his health status, treatment, options, risk/benefits, and long-term prognosis?
2. What arguments can be made to support the patient's decision to forego treatment?
3. What arguments can be made to question the patient's decision to forego treatment?

---

- Deficient knowledge about the surgical procedure and postoperative course
- Anxiety and depression related to the diagnosis of cancer and impending surgery
- Ineffective airway clearance related to excess mucus production secondary to surgical alterations in the airway
- Impaired verbal communication related to anatomic deficit secondary to removal of the larynx and to edema
- Imbalanced nutrition: less than body requirements, related to inability to ingest food secondary to swallowing difficulties
- Disturbed body image and low self-esteem secondary to major neck surgery, change in appearance, and altered structure and function
- Self-care deficit related to pain, weakness, fatigue, musculoskeletal impairment related to surgical procedure and postoperative course

### Collaborative Problems/Potential Complications

Based on assessment data, potential complications that may develop include the following:

- Respiratory distress (hypoxia, airway obstruction, tracheal edema)
- Hemorrhage
- Infection
- Wound breakdown
- Aspiration

## Planning and Goals

The major goals for the patient may include attainment of an adequate level of knowledge, reduction in anxiety, maintenance of a patent airway (patient is able to handle own secretions), effective use of alternative means of communication, attainment of optimal levels of nutrition and hydration, improvement in body image and self-esteem, improved self-care management, and absence of complications.

## Nursing Interventions

### Teaching the Patient Preoperatively

The diagnosis of laryngeal cancer often produces misconceptions and fears. Many people assume that loss of speech and disfigurement are inevitable with this condition. Once the physician explains the diagnosis and discusses treatment options with the patient and family, the nurse clarifies any misconceptions by identifying the location of the larynx, its function, the nature of the planned surgical procedure, and its effect on speech. Informational materials (written and audiovisual) about the surgery are given to the patient and family for review and reinforcement. If a complete laryngectomy is planned, the patient must understand that the natural voice will be lost, but that special training can provide a means for communicating. The patient needs to know that until this training is started, communication will be possible by using the call light, by writing, or by using a special communication board. The nurse answers questions about the nature of the surgery and reinforces the physician's explanation that the patient will lose the ability to vocalize, but that a rehabilitation program is available. The patient's ability to sing, laugh, and whistle will be lost. The interdisciplinary team conducts an initial assessment of the patient and family. The team might include the nurse, physician, speech therapist, respiratory therapist, clinical nurse specialist, social worker, dietitian, and home care nurse. The services of a spiritual advisor are made available to the patient and family, as appropriate.

The nurse also reviews equipment and treatments for postoperative care with the patient and family, teaches important coughing and deep-breathing exercises, and assists the patient to perform return demonstrations. The nurse clarifies the patient's role in the postoperative and rehabilitation periods.

### Reducing Anxiety and Depression

Because surgery of the larynx is performed most commonly for a malignant tumor, the patient may have many questions: Will the surgeon be able to remove all of the tumor? Is it cancer? Will I die? Will I choke? Will I suffocate? Will I ever speak again? What will I look like? Because of these and other questions, the psychological preparation of the patient is as important as the physical preparation.

Any patient undergoing surgery may have many fears. In laryngeal surgery, these fears may relate to the diagnosis of cancer and the possibility of permanent loss of the voice and disfigurement. The nurse provides the patient and family with opportunities to ask questions, verbalize feelings, and discuss perceptions. The nurse should address any questions and misconceptions the patient and family have. During the preoperative or postoperative period, a visit from someone who has had a laryngectomy may reassure the patient that people are available to assist and that rehabilitation is possible.

In the immediate postoperative period, the nurse attempts to spend time with the patient that is uninterrupted and focused on building trust and reducing the patient's anxiety. Active listening provides an environment that promotes open communication and allows the patient to verbalize feelings. Clear instructions and explanations are given to the patient and family in a calm, reassuring manner before and during each contact with the patient. The nurse listens attentively, encourages the patient, and identifies and reduces environmental stressors. The nurse seeks to learn from the patient what activities promote feelings of comfort and assists the patient in such activities (eg, listening to music, reading). The nurse remains with the patient during episodes of severe anxiety and includes the patient in decision making. The nurse also supports the family by allowing extra visiting periods if indicated. Relaxation techniques such as guided imagery and meditation are often helpful to the patient.

### Maintaining a Patent Airway

The nurse promotes a patent airway by positioning the patient in the semi-Fowler's or Fowler's position after recovery from anesthesia. This position decreases surgical edema and promotes lung expansion. Observing the patient for restlessness, labored breathing, apprehension, and increased pulse rate helps to identify possible respiratory or circulatory problems. The nurse assesses the patient's lung sounds and reports changes that may indicate impending complications. Medications that depress respiration, particularly opioids, should be used cautiously. However, adequate use of analgesic medications is essential for pain relief, because postoperative pain can result in shallow breathing and an ineffective cough. As with other surgical patients, the nurse encourages the patient to turn, cough, and take deep breaths. If necessary, suctioning may be performed to remove secretions, but the nurse must avoid disruption of suture lines. The nurse also encourages and assists the patient with early ambulation to prevent atelectasis, pneumonia, and deep vein thrombosis. Pulse oximetry is used to monitor the patient's oxygen saturation level.

If a total laryngectomy was performed, a laryngectomy tube will most likely be in place. In some instances a laryngectomy tube is not used; in others it is used temporarily; and in many it is used permanently. The laryngectomy tube, which is shorter than a tracheostomy tube but has a larger diameter, is the patient's only airway. The care of this tube is the same as for a tracheostomy tube (see Chapter 25). The nurse changes the inner cannula of the tube every 8 hours if it is disposable. Although nondisposable tubes are used infrequently, if one is used, the nurse cleans the inner cannula every 8 hours. If a tracheostomy tube without an inner cannula is used, humidification and suctioning of this tube is essential to prevent formation of mucous plugs. The nurse must suction both sides of the T-tube to relieve the obstruction (Shores, Hacking & Triana, 2004). This prevents obstruction of the airway due to copious secretions. The nurse should also maintain secure tracheostomy ties to prevent tube dislodgement.

The nurse cleans the stoma daily with saline solution or another prescribed solution. If a non–oil-based antibiotic ointment is prescribed, the nurse applies it around the stoma and suture line. If crusting appears around the stoma, the nurse removes the crusts with sterile tweezers and applies additional ointment.

Wound drains, inserted during surgery, may be in place to assist in removal of fluid and air from the surgical site. Suction also may be used, but cautiously, to avoid trauma to the surgical site and incision. The nurse observes, measures, and records drainage. When drainage is less than 50 to 60 mL/day, the physician usually removes the drains.

Frequently, the patient coughs up large amounts of mucus through this opening. Because air passes directly into the trachea without being warmed and moistened by the upper respiratory mucosa, the tracheobronchial tree compensates by secreting excessive amounts of mucus. Therefore, the patient will have frequent coughing episodes and may develop a brassy-sounding, mucus-producing cough. The nurse reassures the patient that these problems will diminish in time, as the tracheobronchial mucosa adapts to the altered physiology.

After the patient coughs, the tracheostomy opening must be wiped clean and clear of mucus. A simple gauze dressing, washcloth, or even paper towel (because of its size and absorbency) worn below the tracheostomy may serve as a barrier to protect the clothing from the copious mucus that the patient may initially expel.

One of the most important factors in decreasing cough, mucus production, and crusting around the stoma is adequate humidification of the environment. Mechanical humidifiers and aerosol generators (nebulizers) increase the humidity and are important for the patient's comfort. The laryngectomy tube may be removed when the stoma is well healed, within 3 to 6 weeks after surgery. The nurse teaches the patient how to clean and change the tube (see Chapter 25) and remove secretions.

### Promoting Alternative Communication Methods

Understanding and anticipating the patient's postoperative needs are critical. Alternative means of communication are established preoperatively and must be used consistently by all personnel who come in contact with the patient postoperatively. For example, a call bell or hand bell must be placed within easy reach of the patient. Because a Magic Slate often is used for communication, the nurse documents which hand the patient uses for writing so that the opposite arm can be used for IV infusions. (To ensure the patient's privacy, the nurse discards any old notes used for communication.) If the patient cannot write, a picture-word-phrase board or hand signals can be used.

Writing everything or communicating through gestures can be very time-consuming and frustrating. The patient must be given adequate time to communicate his or her needs. The patient may become impatient and angry when not understood. In addition, other staff members need to be alerted to the problem and also be aware that the patient will be unable to use the intercom system.

Establishing an effective means of communication is usually the ultimate goal in the rehabilitation of the laryngectomy patient. The nurse works with the patient, speech therapist, and family to encourage use of alternative communication methods.

### Promoting Adequate Nutrition and Hydration

Postoperatively, the patient may not be permitted to eat or drink for several days. Alternative sources of nutrition and hydration include IV fluids, enteral feedings through a nasogastric or gastrostomy tube, and parenteral nutrition.

When the patient is ready to start oral feedings, a speech therapist or radiologist may conduct a swallow study (a video fluoroscopy radiology procedure) to evaluate the patient's risk for aspiration. Once the patient is cleared for oral feedings, the nurse explains that thick liquids will be used first, because they are easy to swallow. Different swallowing maneuvers are attempted with various food consistencies. Once the patient is cleared for food intake, the nurse stays with the patient during initial oral feedings and keeps a suction setup at the bedside for needed suctioning. The nurse instructs the patient to avoid sweet foods, which increase salivation and suppress the appetite. Solid foods are introduced as tolerated. The patient is instructed to rinse the mouth with warm water or mouthwash after oral feedings and to brush the teeth frequently.

Because taste and smell are so closely related, taste sensations are altered for a while after surgery because inhaled air passes directly into the trachea, bypassing the nose and the olfactory end organs. In time, however, the patient usually accommodates to this change and olfactory sensation adapts, often with return of interest in eating. The nurse observes the patient for any difficulty swallowing, particularly when eating resumes, and reports its occurrence to the physician.

The patient's weight and laboratory data are monitored to ensure that nutritional and fluid intake are adequate. In addition, skin turgor and vital signs are assessed for signs of decreased fluid volume.

### Promoting Positive Body Image and Self-Esteem

Disfiguring surgery and an altered communication pattern are a threat to a patient's body image and self-esteem. The reaction of family members and friends is a major concern for the patient. The nurse encourages the patient to express feelings about the changes brought about by surgery, particularly feelings related to fear, anger, depression, and isolation. Encouraging use of previous effective coping strategies may be helpful. Referral to a support group, such as Lost Chord or New Voice clubs (through the International Association of Laryngectomees [IAL]) and I Can Cope (through the American Cancer Society), may help the patient and family deal with the changes in their lives.

### Promoting Self-Care Management

A positive approach is important when caring for the patient and includes promotion of self-care activities. The patient and family should begin participating in self-care activities as soon as possible. The nurse assesses the patient's readiness for decision making and encourages the patient to participate actively in performing care. The nurse provides positive reinforcement when the patient makes an effort in self-care. The nurse needs to be a good listener and a support to the family, especially when explaining the tubes, dressings, and drains that are in place postoperatively. Groups such as Lost Chord and New Voice promote and support the rehabilitation of people who have had a laryngectomy by providing an opportunity for exchanging ideas and sharing information.

In addition to its work through support groups, the International Association of Laryngectomees encourages an exchange of ideas and methods for learning and teaching alaryngeal methods of communication. It also works to promote employers' understanding about cancer of the larynx, to enable patients to retain or obtain employment after surgery.

### Monitoring and Managing Potential Complications

The potential complications after laryngectomy include respiratory distress and hypoxia, hemorrhage, infection, wound breakdown, and aspiration.

### RESPIRATORY DISTRESS AND HYPOXIA

The nurse monitors the patient for signs and symptoms of respiratory distress and hypoxia, particularly restlessness, irritation, agitation, confusion, tachypnea, use of accessory muscles, and decreased oxygen saturation on pulse oximetry ($SpO_2$). Any change in respiratory status requires immediate intervention. Hypoxia may cause restlessness and an initial rise in blood pressure; this is followed by hypotension and somnolence. Cyanosis is a late sign of hypoxia. Obstruction needs to be ruled out immediately by suctioning and by having the patient cough and breathe deeply. Hypoxia and airway obstruction, if not immediately treated, are life-threatening.

Other nursing measures include repositioning of the patient to ensure an open airway and administering oxygen as prescribed and used with caution in patients with chronic obstructive pulmonary disease. The nurse should always be prepared for possible intubation and mechanical ventilation. The nurse must be knowledgeable about the hospital's emergency code protocols and skilled in use of emergency equipment. The nurse must remain with the patient at all times during respiratory distress. The emergency call bell and telephone should be used to initiate a code, call for further assistance, and summon the physician immediately if nursing measures do not improve the patient's respiratory status.

### HEMORRHAGE

Bleeding from the drains at the surgical site or with tracheal suctioning may signal the occurrence of hemorrhage. The nurse promptly notifies the surgeon of any active bleeding, which can occur at a variety of sites, including the surgical site, drains, and trachea. Rupture of the carotid artery is especially dangerous. Should this occur, the nurse must apply direct pressure over the artery, summon assistance, and provide emotional support to the patient until the vessel is ligated. The nurse monitors vital signs for changes, particularly increased pulse rate, decreased blood pressure, and rapid deep respirations. Cold, clammy, pale skin may indicate active bleeding. IV fluids and blood components may be administered and other measures implemented to prevent or treat hemorrhagic shock. Management of the patient with shock is discussed in detail in Chapter 15.

### INFECTION

The nurse monitors the patient for signs of postoperative infection. These include an increase in temperature and pulse, a change in the type of wound drainage, and increased areas of redness or tenderness at the surgical site. Other signs include purulent drainage, odor, and increased wound drainage. The nurse monitors the patient's white blood cell (WBC) count; a rise in WBCs may indicate the body's effort to combat infection. In elderly patients, infection can be present without an increase in the patient's WBC count; therefore, the nurse must monitor the patient for more subtle signs. WBCs will be suppressed in the patient with decreased immune function (eg, patients with HIV infection, those receiving chemotherapy or radiation therapy); this predisposes the patient to a severe infection and sepsis. Antimicrobial (antibiotic) medications must be administered as scheduled. All suspicious drainage is cultured, and the patient may be placed in isolation as indicated. Strategies are implemented to minimize the exposure of the patient to microorganisms and their spread to others. The nurse reports any significant change in the patient's status to the surgeon.

### WOUND BREAKDOWN

Wound breakdown caused by infection, poor wound healing, development of a fistula, radiation therapy, or tumor growth can create a life-threatening emergency. The carotid artery, which is close to the stoma, may rupture from erosion if the wound does not heal properly. The nurse observes the stoma area for wound breakdown, hematoma, and bleeding and reports their occurrence to the surgeon. If wound breakdown occurs, the patient must be monitored carefully and identified as being at high risk for carotid hemorrhage.

### ASPIRATION

The patient who has undergone a laryngectomy is at risk for aspiration and aspiration pneumonia due to depressed cough, the sedating effects of anesthetic and analgesic medications, alteration in the airway, impaired swallowing, and the administration of tube feedings. The nurse assesses for the presence of nausea and administers antiemetic medications, as prescribed. The nurse keeps a suction set-up available in the hospital and instructs the family to do so at home for use if needed. Patients receiving tube feedings are positioned with the head of the bed at 30 degrees or higher during feedings and for 30 to 45 minutes after tube feedings. Adding a small amount of food coloring to the tube feedings assists in distinguishing tube feeding aspirate from other secretions from the pulmonary system. When the patient begins oral feeding, the nurse maintains the head of the bed in an upright position for 30 to 45 minutes after each feeding. For patients with a nasogastric or gastrostomy tube, the placement of the tube and residual gastric volume must be checked before each feeding. High amounts of residual volume (greater than 50% of previous intake) indicate delayed gastric emptying; this can lead to reflux and aspiration. Signs or symptoms of aspiration are reported to the physician immediately.

## Promoting Home and Community-Based Care

### TEACHING PATIENTS SELF-CARE

The nurse has an important role in the recovery and rehabilitation of the patient who has had a laryngectomy. In an effort to facilitate the patient's ability to manage self-care, discharge instruction begins as soon as the patient is able to participate. Nursing care and patient teaching in the hospital, outpatient setting, and rehabilitation or long-term care facility must take into consideration the many emotions, physical changes, and lifestyle changes experienced by the patient. In preparing the patient to go home, the nurse assesses the patient's readiness to learn and the level of knowledge about self-care management. The nurse also reassures the patient and family that most self-care management strategies can be mastered. The patient will need to learn a variety of self-care behaviors, including tracheostomy and stoma care, wound care, and oral hygiene. The nurse also instructs the patient about the need for adequate dietary intake, safe hygiene, and recreational activities.

**Tracheostomy and Stoma Care.** The nurse provides specific instructions to the patient and family about what to expect with a tracheostomy and its management. The nurse teaches the patient and caregiver to perform suctioning and emergency measures and tracheostomy and stoma care. The nurse stresses the importance of humidification at home and instructs the family to obtain and set up a humidification system before the patient returns home. In addition, the nurse cautions the patient and family that air-conditioned air may be too cool or too dry, and therefore irritating for the patient with a new laryngectomy. (See Chapter 25 for details about tracheostomy care.)

**Hygiene and Safety Measures.** The nurse instructs the patient and family about safety precautions that are needed because of the changes in structure and function resulting from the surgery. Special precautions are needed in the shower to prevent water from entering the stoma. Wearing a loose-fitting plastic bib over the tracheostomy or simply holding a hand over the opening is effective. Swimming is not recommended, because a person with a laryngectomy can drown without submerging his or her face. Barbers and beauticians need to be alerted so that hair sprays, loose hair, and powder do not get near the stoma, because they can block or irritate the trachea and possibly cause infection. These self-care points are summarized in Chart 22-9.

The nurse teaches the patient and caregiver the signs and symptoms of infection and identifies indications that require contacting the physician after discharge. A discussion regarding cleanliness and infection control behaviors is essential in the education of the patient. The nurse teaches the patient and family to wash their hands before and after caring for the tracheostomy, to use tissue to remove mucus, and to dispose of soiled dressings and equipment properly. If the patient's surgery included cervical lymph node dissection, the nurse teaches the patient exercises for strengthening the shoulder and neck muscles.

### CHART 22-9

## HOME CARE CHECKLIST • The Patient With a Laryngectomy

| At the completion of the home care instruction, the patient or caregiver will be able to: | Patient | Caregiver |
|---|---|---|
| • Demonstrate methods to clear the airway and handle secretions | ✓ | ✓ |
| • Explain the rationale for maintaining adequate humidification with a humidifier or nebulizer | ✓ | ✓ |
| • Demonstrate how to clean the skin around the stoma and how to use ointments and tweezers to remove encrustations | ✓ | ✓ |
| • State the rationale for wearing a loose-fitting protective cloth at the stoma | ✓ | ✓ |
| • Discuss the need to avoid cold air from air conditioning and the environment to prevent irritation of the airway | ✓ | ✓ |
| • Demonstrate safe technique in changing the laryngectomy/tracheostomy tube | ✓ | ✓ |
| • Identify the signs and symptoms of wound infection and state what to do about them | ✓ | ✓ |
| • Describe safety or emergency measures to implement in case of breathing difficulty or bleeding | ✓ | ✓ |
| • State the rationale for wearing or carrying special medical identification and ways to obtain help in an emergency | ✓ | ✓ |
| • Explain the importance of covering the stoma when showering or bathing | ✓ | ✓ |
| • Identify fluid and caloric needs | ✓ | ✓ |
| • Describe mouth care and discuss its importance | ✓ | ✓ |
| • Demonstrate alternative communication methods | ✓ | |
| • Identify support groups and agency resources | ✓ | ✓ |
| • State the need for regular checkups and reporting of any problems immediately | ✓ | ✓ |

Recreation and exercise are important for the patient's well-being and quality of life, and all but very strenuous exercise can be enjoyed safely. Avoidance of strenuous exercise and fatigue is important because the patient will have more difficulty speaking when tired, which can be discouraging. Additional safety points to address include the need for the patient to wear or carry medical identification, such as a bracelet or card, to alert medical personnel to the special requirements for resuscitation should this need arise. If resuscitation is needed, direct mouth-to-stoma ventilation should be performed. For home emergency situations, prerecorded emergency messages for police, the fire department, or other rescue services can be kept near the phone to be used quickly.

The nurse instructs and encourages the patient to perform oral care on a regular basis to prevent halitosis and infection. If the patient is receiving radiation therapy, synthetic saliva may be required because of decreased saliva production. The nurse instructs the patient to drink water or sugar-free liquids throughout the day and to use a humidifier at home. Brushing the teeth or dentures and rinsing the mouth several times a day will assist in maintaining proper oral hygiene.

**CONTINUING CARE**

Referral for home care is an important aspect of postoperative care for the patient who has had a laryngectomy and will assist the patient and family in the transition to the home. The home care nurse assesses the patient's general health status and the ability of the patient and family to care for the stoma and tracheostomy. The nurse assesses the surgical incisions, nutritional and respiratory status, and adequacy of pain management. The nurse assesses for signs and symptoms of complications and the patient's and family's knowledge of signs and symptoms to be reported to the physician. During the home visit, the nurse identifies and addresses other learning needs and concerns of the patient and family, such as adaptation to physical, lifestyle, and functional changes, as well as the patient's progress with learning and using new communication strategies. The nurse assesses the patient's psychological status as well. The home care nurse reinforces previous teaching and provides reassurance and support to the patient and family as needed.

The nurse encourages the person who has had a laryngectomy to have regular physical examinations and to seek advice concerning any problems related to recovery and rehabilitation. The patient is also reminded to participate in health promotion activities and health screening and about the importance of keeping scheduled appointments with the physician, speech therapist, and other health care providers.

## Evaluation

### Expected Patient Outcomes

Expected patient outcomes may include the following:

1. Demonstrates an adequate level of knowledge, verbalizing an understanding of the surgical procedure and performing self-care adequately
2. Demonstrates less anxiety and depression
   a. Expresses a sense of hope
   b. Is aware of available community organizations and agencies such as the Lost Chord and New Voice groups
   c. Participates in support group, such as I Can Cope.
3. Maintains a clear airway and handles own secretions; also demonstrates practical, safe, and correct technique for cleaning and changing the laryngectomy tube
4. Acquires effective communication techniques
   a. Uses assistive devices and strategies for communication (Magic Slate, call bell, picture board, sign language, lip reading, computer aids)
   b. Follows the recommendations of the speech therapist
   c. Demonstrates ability to communicate with new communication strategy
   d. Reports availability of prerecorded messages to summon emergency assistance by telephone
5. Maintains adequate nutrition and adequate fluid intake
6. Exhibits improved body image, self-esteem, and self-concept
   a. Expresses feelings and concerns
   b. Participates in self-care and decision making
   c. Accepts information about support group
7. Adheres to rehabilitation and home care program
   a. Practices recommended speech therapy
   b. Demonstrates proper methods for caring for stoma and laryngectomy or tracheostomy tube (if present)
   c. Verbalizes understanding of symptoms that require medical attention
   d. States safety measures to take in emergencies
   e. Performs oral hygiene as prescribed
8. Absence of complications
   a. Demonstrates a patent airway
   b. No bleeding from surgical site and minimal bleeding from drains; vital signs (blood pressure, temperature, pulse, respiratory rate) normal
   c. No redness, tenderness, or purulent drainage at surgical site
   d. No wound breakdown
   e. Clear breath sounds; oxygen saturation level within acceptable range; chest x-ray clear

## Critical Thinking Exercises

**1** A 49-year-old man presents to the employee health clinic with generalized fatigue and low-grade fever. He reports a history of recently "having a cold" that "lasted 3 weeks." He also states that he is "stuffy all the time." What further information would you request from the patient to obtain a more accurate health history? Is the patient at risk for sinusitis? What are the symptoms of acute and chronic sinusitis? What teaching is warranted for a patient with acute sinusitis? How does teaching for a patient with chronic sinusitis differ?

2. A 75-year-old woman comes to the clinic today with complaints of a persistent runny nose that is producing yellow to greenish drainage. She lives in an assisted-living environment and is accompanied to the clinic by an aide from the facility. The aide reports that the patient has complained of a sore throat and that she "sleeps all the time" and had a fever of 100.6°F early this morning. Discuss your assessment of this patient. You suspect that the patient is at risk for which upper respiratory illnesses? As a community health nurse, what actions would you take to ensure control of the infection at the assisted-living facility?

3. **ebp** A 55-year-old woman is brought to the emergency department by her husband, who tells you that her nose has been bleeding for more than 3 hours. The patient reports that she takes one aspirin a day (325 mg), has a history of atrial fibrillation, and takes medication for hypertension. What immediate action would you take to care for this patient? What are the risk factors for epistaxis in this patient? What medical treatment would you anticipate for her? What nursing measures would you provide for this patient? How would you modify your discharge instructions if the patient lived alone? What strategies would you recommend to the patient and her husband to stop a nosebleed if it occurs again at home? What is the evidence for your recommendations? How will you determine the strength of the evidence on which your recommendations are based?

4. You are caring for a 78-year-old patient on a medical-surgical nursing unit. He has recently been diagnosed with cancer of the larynx and is scheduled for a total laryngectomy in the morning. What patient education is needed before this patient's surgery? Discuss nursing management of the patient's airway in the immediate postoperative period. What critical elements would you include in teaching the patient how to care for his tracheostomy? What community resources would you provide or arrange for this patient once he is discharged? What modifications in teaching and care would be necessary if this man had one-sided weakness secondary to an earlier stroke?

5. A 65-year-old man is referred for home care after a total laryngectomy performed to treat cancer of the larynx. As the home health nurse, you are responsible to provide continued patient education regarding tracheostomy care and gastric tube feedings. The overall plan is for the patient to begin oral feedings; however, both the patient and his wife believe that he is not ready to begin to eat. What are your priorities in terms of assessment of this patient? What are your recommendations to the patient regarding fear, anxiety, communication, and nutrition? What additional medical and support services will the patient need to assist him in his recovery? How would your care differ if this patient lived alone?

# REFERENCES AND SELECTED READINGS

## BOOKS

Abeloff, M., Armitage, J., Niederhuber, J., et al. (2004). *Clinical oncology*. Philadelphia: Churchill Livingstone.

American Cancer Society. (2005). *Cancer facts and figures*. Atlanta: American Cancer Society Inc.

American Lung Association. (2005). *Guidelines for the prevention and treatment of influenza and the common cold*. www.lungusa.org/site/pp.asp?c=dvLUK9O0E&b=23161 (accessed May 30, 2006).

Bickley, L. S. & Szilagyi, P. G. (2003). *Bates' guide to physical examination and history taking* (8th ed.). Philadelphia: Lippincott Williams & Wilkins.

Cameron, J. L. (2004). *Current surgical therapy*. St. Louis: Mosby.

Casciato, D. A. (2004). *Manual of clinical oncology* (5th ed.). Philadelphia: Lippincott Williams & Wilkins.

De Vita, V. T., Hellman, S. & Rosenberg, S. A. (Eds.)(2004). *Cancer: Principles and practice of oncology* (7th ed.). Philadelphia: Lippincott Williams & Wilkins.

Evans, P. R., Montgomery, P. Q. & Gullane, P. J. (2003). *Principles and practice of head and neck oncology*. London: Taylor & Francis Group.

Goldman, L. & Ausiello, D. A. (Eds.)(2003). *Cecil textbook of medicine* (22nd ed.). Philadelphia: Saunders.

Green, F., Balch, C., Flemming, I., et al. (Eds.)(2002). *AJCC cancer staging manual* (6th ed), New York: Springer.

Gulanick, M. & Myers, J. (2003). *Nursing care plans: Nursing diagnosis and intervention* (5th ed.). St. Louis: Mosby.

Kufe, D., Pollock, R., Weichselbaum, R., et al. (2003). *Holland-Frei cancer medicine* (6th ed.). Hamilton, Ontario: B. C. Decker.

Mandell, G. L., Bennett, J. E. & Dolin, R. (Eds.). (2004). *Principles and practice of infectious diseases* (6th ed.). Philadelphia: Churchill Livingstone.

Murray, J. F. & Nadel, J. A. (2005). *Textbook of respiratory medicine* (4th ed.). Philadelphia: Saunders.

National Cancer Institute. (2003). *What you need to know about cancer of the larynx*. NIH Publication No. 02-1568. Washington, DC: U.S. Department of Health and Human Services. http://www.cancer.gov/cancertopics/wyntk/larynx (accessed May 30, 2006).

National Institute of Allergy and Infectious Diseases. (2005). *Allergy statistics*. http://www.niaid.nih.gov/factsheets/allergystat.htm (accessed May 30, 2006).

National Institute of Allergy and Infectious Diseases. (2004). *The common cold*. http://www.niaid.nih.gov/factsheets/cold.htm (accessed May 30, 2006).

Shores, C., Hacking, T. & Triana, R. (2004). Complications of airway management. In Tintinalli, J., Kelan, G. & Stapczynski, S. (Eds.). *Emergency medicine: A comprehensive study guide* (6th ed.). New York: McGraw-Hill.

Tierney, L. M., McPhee, S. J. & Papadakis, M. A. (Eds.). (2005). *Current medical diagnosis and treatment* (44th ed.). New York: McGraw-Hill.

Townsend, C. M., Beauchamp, R. D., Evans, B. M., et al. (Ed.)(2004). *Sabiston textbook of surgery* (17th ed.). Philadelphia: Saunders.

Uphold, C. & Graham, M. (2003). *Clinical guidelines in family practice* (4th ed.). Gainesville: Barmarrae Books.

Yunglinger, J., Busse, W., Bochner, B., et al. (2003). *Allergy: Principles and practice* (6th ed.). St. Louis: Mosby.

## JOURNALS

*Asterisks indicate nursing research articles.

### General

Banerjee, D., Vitiello, M. V. & Grunstein, R. R. (2004). Pharmacology for excessive daytime sleepiness. *Sleep Medicine Reviews, 8*(5), 319–354.

Boutrel, B. & Koob, G. G. (2004). What keeps us awake: The neuropharmacology of stimulants and wakefulness-promoting medications. *Sleep, 27*(6), 1181–1194.

Bush, R. K. (2004). Etiopathogenesis and management of perennial allergic rhinitis: A state-of-the-art review. *Treatments in Respiratory Medicine, 3*(1), 45–57.

Colclasure, J. C., Gross, C. W. & Kountakis, S. E. (2004). Endoscopic sinus surgery in patients older than sixty. *Otolaryngology Head & Neck Surgery, 131*(6), 946–949.

Lamberg, L. (2004). Promoting adequate sleep finds a place on the public health agenda. *Journal of the American Medical Association, 291*(20), 2415–2417.

Leinbach, R. F., Markwell, S. J., Colliver, J. A., et al. (2003). Hot versus cold tonsillectomy: A systematic review of the literature. *Otolaryngology Head & Neck Surgery, 129*(4), 360–364.

Marshall, I. (2006). Zinc for the common cold. *Cochrane Database of Systematic Reviews (2)*, CD001364.

Parmet, S. (2004). Sore throat. *Journal of the American Medical Association, 291*(13), 1664.

Reider, J. M., Nashelsky, J. & Neher, J. (2003). Do imaging studies aid diagnosis of acute sinusitis? *Journal of Family Practice, 52*(7), 565–567.

Windfuhr, J. P. & Chen, Y. S. (2003). Post-tonsillectomy and adenoidectomy hemorrhage in nonselected patients. *Annals of Otology, Rhinology and Laryngology, 112*(1), 63–70.

### Upper Respiratory Infections

Armengol, C. E., Schlager, T. A. & Hendley, J. O. (2004). Sensitivity of a rapid antigen detection test for group A streptococci in a private pediatric office setting: Answering the Red book's request for validation. *Pediatrics, 113*(4), 924–926.

Blaivas, M., Theodoro, D. & Duggal, S. (2003). Ultrasound-guided drainage of peritonsillar abscess by the emergency physician. *American Journal of Emergency Medicine, 21*(2), 155–158.

Brook, I. (2004). Microbiology and management of peritonsillar, retropharyngeal, and parapharyngeal abscesses. *Journal of Oral and Maxillofacial Surgery, 62*(12), 1545–1550.

DeAlleaume, L., Parker, S. & Reider, J. M. (2003). What findings distinguish acute bacterial sinusitis? *Journal of Family Practice, 52*(7), 563–565.

Del Mar, C. B., Glasziou, P. P. & Spinks, A. B. (2004). Antibiotics for sore throat. *Cochrane Database of Systematic Reviews (2)*, CD000023.

Discolo, C. M., Darrow, D. H. & Koltai, P. J. (2003). Infectious indications for tonsillectomy. *Pediatric Clinics of North America, 50*(2), 445–458.

Eiles, W. & Huber, K. (2004). Short-course therapy for acute sinusitis: How long is enough? *Treatments in Respiratory Medicine, 3*(5), 269–277.

Franzese, C. B. & Isaacson, J. E. (2003). Peritonsillar and parapharyngeal space abscess in the older adult. *American Journal of Otolaryngology, 24*(3), 169–173.

Gotfried, M. H. (2004). Macrolides for the treatment of chronic sinusitis, asthma, and COPD. *Chest, 125*(2), 52S–61S.

Jackson, E. A. (2003). Amoxicillin-clavulanate ineffective for suspected acute sinusitis. *Journal of Family Practice, 529*(12), 930, 932.

Johnson, R. F., Stewart, M. G. & Wright, C. C. (2003). An evidence-based review of the treatment of peritonsillar abscess. *Otolaryngology Head & Neck Surgery, 128*(3), 332–343.

Jull, A. (2003). Review: Specific signs and symptoms can help practitioners to diagnose acute purulent sinusitis in general practice. *Evidence-Based Nursing, 6*(1), 24.

Lindbaek, M. (2004). Acute sinusitis: Guide to selection of antibacterial therapy. *Drugs, 64*(8), 805–819.

Neuner, J. M., Hamel, M. B., Phillips, R. S., et al. (2003). Diagnosis and management of adults with pharyngitis a cost effective analysis. *Annals of Internal Medicine, 139*(2), 113–122.

Scheid, D. C. & Hamm, R. M. (2004). Acute bacterial rhinosinusitis in adults: Part I. Evaluation. *American Family Physician, 70*(9), 1685–1692.

Shashy, R. G., Moore, E. J. & Weaver, A. (2004). Prevalence of the chronic sinusitis in Olmsted County, Minnesota. *Archives of Otolaryngology Head & Neck Surgery, 130*(3), 320–323.

Singh, M. (2004). Newer drugs for asthma. *Indian Journal of Pediatrics, 71*(8), 721–727

Wald, E. R. & Fischer, D. R. (2004). Diagnosing and treating strep throat. *Family Practice Management, 11*(2), 20.

Williams, J. W., Jr., Aguilar, C., Cornell, J., et al. (2004). Antibiotics for acute maxillary sinusitis. *Cochrane Database of Systematic Reviews (2)*, CD000243.

### Obstruction and Trauma of the Airway

Chung, K. F. & Adcock, I. M. (2004). Combination therapy of long-acting beta2-adrenoceptor agonists and corticosteroids for asthma. *Treatments in Respiratory Medicine, 3*(5), 279–289.

Letizia, M., O'Leary, J. & Vodvarka, J. (2003). Laryngeal edema: Perioperative nursing considerations. *MedSurg Nursing, 12*(2), 111–115.

Merritt, S. L. (2004). Sleep-disordered breathing and the association with cardiovascular risk. *Progress in Cardiovascular Nursing, 19*(1), 19–27.

Merritt, S. L. & Berger, B. E. (2004). Obstructive sleep apnea-hypopnea syndrome. *American Journal of Nursing, 104*(7), 49–52.

Passali, D., Passali, F. M., Damiani, V., et al. (2003). Treatment of inferior turbinate hypertrophy: A randomized clinical trial. *Annals of Otology, Rhinology & Laryngology, 112*(8), 683–688.

Stradling, J. R. & Davies, R. J. O. (2004). Sleep. 1: Obstructive sleep apnoea/hypopnea syndrome: Definitions, epidemiology, and natural history. *Thorax, 59*(1), 73–78.

Thatcher, G. W. & Maisel, R. H. (2003). The long-term evaluation of tracheostomy in the management of severe obstructive sleep apnea. *Laryngoscope, 113*(2), 201–204.

Von Känel, R. & Dimsdale, J. E. (2003). Hemostatic alterations in patients with obstructive sleep apnea and the implications for cardiovascular disease. *Chest, 124*(5), 1956–1967.

Yantis, M. A. & Neatherlin, J. (2005). Obstructive sleep apnea in neurological patients. *Journal of Neuroscience Nursing, 37*(3), 150–155.

Young, T., Skatrud, J. & Peppard, P. E. (2004). Risk factors for obstructive sleep apnea in adults. *Journal of the American Medical Association, 291*(16), 2013–2016.

### Cancer of the Larynx

Davis, R. K., Kriskovich, M. D., Galloway, E. B., III, et al. (2004). Endoscopic supraglottic laryngectomy with postoperative irradiation. *Annals of Otology, Rhinology, and Laryngology, 113*(2), 132–138.

Dietz, A., Ramroth, H., Urban, T., et al. (2004). Exposure to cement dust, related occupational groups and laryngeal cancer risk: Results of a population based case control study. *International Journal of Cancer, 108*(6), 907–911.

Forastiere, A. A., Goepfert, H., Maor, M., et al. (2003). Concurrent chemotherapy and radiotherapy for organ preservation in advanced laryngeal cancer. *New England Journal of Medicine, 249*(22), 2091.

*Happ, M. B., Roesch, T. & Kagan, S. H. (2004). Communication needs, methods, and perceived voice quality following head and neck surgery: A literature review. *Cancer Nursing, 27*(1), 1–9.

Harrison, J. S., Dale, R. A., Haverman, C. W., et al. (2003). Oral complications in radiation therapy. *General Dentistry, 51*(6), 552–560.

International Association of Laryngectomees, 2004

Kasperbauer, J. L. & Thomas, J. E. (2004). Voice rehabilitation after near-total laryngectomy. *Otolaryngologic Clinics of North America, 37*(3), 655–657.

*Krouse, H. J., Rudy, S. F., Vallerand, A. H., et al. (2004). Impact of tracheostomy or laryngectomy on spousal and caregiver relationships. *ORL Head & Neck Nursing, 22*(1), 10–25.

Marques, M. A. & Dib, L. L. (2004). Peridontal changes in patients undergoing radiotherapy. *Journal of Periodontology, 75*(9), 1178–1187.

*Rodriguez, C. S. & VanCott, M. L. (2005). Speech impairment in the postoperative head and neck and neck cancer patient: Nurses' and patients' perceptions. *Qualitative Health Research, 15*(7), 897–911.

Shiotani, A., Araki, K., Moro, K., et al. (2003). CHEP with the total removal of the arytenoids on the tumor-bearing side. *Journal of the Oto-Rhino-Laryngological Society of Japan, 106*(11), 1100–1103.

Timon, C. V., Toner, M. & Conlon, B. J. (2003). Paratracheal lymph node involvement in advanced cancer of the larynx, hypopharynx, and cervical esophagus. *Laryngoscope, 113*(9), 595–1599.

Vielba, R., Bilbao, J., Ispizua, A. et al. (2003). P53 and cyclin D1 as prognostic factors in squamous cell carcinoma of the larynx. *Laryngoscope, 113*(1), 167–172.

## RESOURCES

American Cancer Society, 1599 Clifton Rd. NE, Atlanta, GA 30329; 404-320-3333 or 800-ACS-2345; http://www.cancer.org. Accessed March 31, 2006.

American Lung Association, 1740 Broadway, New York, NY 10019; 212-315-8700; http://www.lungusa.org. Accessed March 31, 2006.

American Sleep Apnea Association, 1424 K Street NW, Suite 302, Washington, DC 20005; 202-293-3650; http://www.sleepapnea.org. Accessed March 31, 2006.

Differential Diagnosis of Rhinitis; http://icarus.med.utoronto.ca/carr/manual/ddxrhinitis.html. Accessed March 31, 2006; by M. M. Carr, Otolaryngologist, Department of Otolaryngology, Toronto General Hospital, 200 Elizabeth Street, Toronto, Ontario, Canada M5G 2C4, 416-340-3490; fax 416-340-5116.

E-Medicine: Instant Access to the Minds of Medicine. http://www.emedicine.com. Accessed March 31, 2006.

International Association of Laryngectomees, 7400 N. Shadeland Ave., Suite 100, Indianapolis, IN 46250; 317-570-4568; http://www.larynxlink.com. Accessed March 31, 2006.

National Cancer Institute (NCI), Bldg. 31, 31 Center Drive, MSC 2580, Bethesda, MD 20892; http://cancernet.nci.nih.gov. Accessed March 31, 2006.

National Cancer Institute: US National Institutes of Health. http://www.cancer.gov. Accessed March 31, 2006); NCI Public Inquiries, Office 6116, Executive Boulevard Room 3036A, Bethesda, MD 20892, 1-800-422-6237.

National Heart, Lung, and Blood Institute (NHBLI), National Institutes of Health, Bldg. 31, Rm. 4A21, Bethesda, MD 20892; 301-592-8573 or 800-575-9355; http://www.nhlbi.nih.gov. Accessed March 31, 2006.

National Institute of Allergy and Infectious Disease, Building 31, 31 Center Drive MSC 2520, Bethesda, MD 20892; http://www.niaid.nih.gov. Accessed March 31, 2006.

National Sleep Foundation, 1522 K Street NW, Suite 500, Washington, DC 20005; 202-437-3471; fax 202-347-3472; http://www.sleepfoundation.org. Accessed March 31, 2006.

Voice Center at Eastern Virginia Medical School, Department of Otolaryngology, P.O. Box 1980, Norfolk, VA 23507; 757-446-5934, http://www.evms.edu/about/centers.html. Accessed March 31, 2006.

University of Kansas Medical Center—Head and Neck Surgery, 3001 Eaton, Kansas City, KS 66160; 913-588-6719; http://www2.kumc.edu/otolaryngology/. Accessed March 31, 2006.

# CHAPTER 23

# Management of Patients With Chest and Lower Respiratory Tract Disorders

## Learning Objectives

*On completion of this chapter, the learner will be able to:*

1. Identify patients at risk for atelectasis and nursing interventions related to its prevention and management.
2. Compare the various pulmonary infections with regard to causes, clinical manifestations, nursing management, complications, and prevention.
3. Use the nursing process as a framework for care of the patient with pneumonia.
4. Relate pleurisy, pleural effusion, and empyema to pulmonary infection.
5. Describe smoking and air pollution as causes of pulmonary disease.
6. Relate the therapeutic management techniques of acute respiratory distress syndrome to the underlying pathophysiology of the syndrome.
7. Describe risk factors and measures appropriate for prevention and management of pulmonary embolism.
8. Describe preventive measures appropriate for controlling and eliminating occupational lung disease.
9. Discuss the modes of therapy and related nursing management for patients with lung cancer.
10. Describe the complications of chest trauma and their clinical manifestations and nursing management.
11. Describe nursing measures to prevent aspiration.

Conditions affecting the lower respiratory tract range from acute problems to chronic disorders. Many of these disorders are serious and often life-threatening. Patients with lower respiratory tract disorders require care from nurses with astute assessment and clinical management skills who also understand the impact of the particular disorder on the patient's quality of life and ability to carry out usual activities of daily living. Patient and family teaching is an important nursing intervention in the management of all lower respiratory tract disorders.

# Atelectasis

**Atelectasis** refers to closure or collapse of alveoli and often is described in relation to x-ray findings and clinical signs and symptoms. Atelectasis may be acute or chronic and may cover a broad range of pathophysiologic changes, from microatelectasis (which is not detectable on chest x-ray) to macroatelectasis with loss of segmental, lobar, or overall lung volume. The most commonly described atelectasis is acute atelectasis, which occurs frequently in the postoperative setting or in people who are immobilized and have a shallow, monotonous breathing pattern. Excess secretions or mucus plugs may also cause obstruction of airflow and result in atelectasis in an area of the lung. Atelectasis also is observed in patients with a chronic airway obstruction that impedes or blocks air flow to an area of the lung (eg, obstructive atelectasis in the patient with lung cancer that is invading or compressing the airways). This type of atelectasis is more insidious and slower in onset.

## Pathophysiology

Atelectasis may occur in adults as a result of reduced alveolar ventilation or any type of blockage that impedes passage of air to and from the alveoli that normally receive air through the bronchi and network of airways. The trapped alveolar air becomes absorbed into the bloodstream, and no additional air can enter into the alveoli because of the blockage. As a result, the affected portion of the lung becomes airless and the alveoli collapse. This may result from altered

## Glossary

**acute lung injury (ALI):** an umbrella term for hypoxemic, respiratory failure; ARDS is a severe form of ALI

**acute respiratory distress syndrome (ARDS):** nonspecific pulmonary response to a variety of pulmonary and non-pulmonary insults to the lung; characterized by interstitial infiltrates, alveolar hemorrhage, atelectasis, decreased compliance, and refractory hypoxemia

**asbestosis:** diffuse lung fibrosis resulting from exposure to asbestos fibers

**atelectasis:** collapse or airless condition of the alveoli caused by hypoventilation, obstruction to the airways, or compression

**central cyanosis:** bluish discoloration of the skin or mucous membranes due to hemoglobin carrying reduced amounts of oxygen

**consolidation:** lung tissue that has become more solid in nature due to collapse of alveoli or infectious process (pneumonia)

**cor pulmonale:** "heart of the lungs"; enlargement of the right ventricle from hypertrophy or dilation or as a secondary response to disorders that affect the lungs

**empyema:** accumulation of purulent material in the pleural space

**fine-needle aspiration:** insertion of a needle through the chest wall to obtain cells of a mass or tumor; usually performed under fluoroscopy or chest CT guidance

**hemoptysis:** the coughing up of blood from the lower respiratory tract

**hemothorax:** partial or complete collapse of the lung due to blood accumulating in the pleural space; may occur after surgery or trauma

**induration:** an abnormally hard lesion or reaction, as in a positive tuberculin skin test

**nosocomial:** pertaining to or originating from a hospitalization; not present at the time of hospital admission

**open lung biopsy:** biopsy of lung tissue performed through a limited thoracotomy incision

**orthopnea:** shortness of breath when reclining or in the supine position

**pleural effusion:** abnormal accumulation of fluid in the pleural space

**pleural friction rub:** localized grating or creaking sound caused by the rubbing together of inflamed parietal and visceral pleurae

**pleural space:** the area between the parietal and visceral pleurae; a potential space

**pneumothorax:** partial or complete collapse of the lung due to positive pressure in the pleural space

**pulmonary edema:** increase in the amount of extravascular fluid in the lung

**pulmonary embolism:** obstruction of the pulmonary vasculature with an embolus; embolus may be due to blood clot, air bubbles, or fat droplets

**purulent:** consisting of, containing, or discharging pus

**restrictive lung disease:** disease of the lung that causes a decrease in lung volumes

**tension pneumothorax:** pneumothorax characterized by increasing positive pressure in the pleural space with each breath; this is an emergency situation and the positive pressure needs to be decompressed or released immediately

**thoracentesis:** insertion of a needle into the pleural space to remove fluid that has accumulated and decrease pressure on the lung tissue; may also be used diagnostically to identify potential causes of a pleural effusion

**transbronchial:** through the bronchial wall, as in a transbronchial lung biopsy

**ventilation–perfusion ratio:** the ratio between ventilation and perfusion in the lung; matching of ventilation to perfusion optimizes gas exchange breathing patterns, retained secretions, pain, alterations in small airway function, prolonged supine positioning, increased abdominal pressure, reduced lung volumes due to musculoskeletal or neurologic disorders, restrictive defects, and specific surgical procedures (eg, upper abdominal, thoracic, or open heart surgery). Persistent low lung volumes, secretions or a mass obstructing or impeding airflow, and compression of lung tissue may all cause collapse or obstruction of the airways, which leads to atelectasis.

Patients are at high risk for atelectasis postoperatively because of the numerous respiratory changes that may occur. A monotonous, low tidal breathing pattern may cause small airway closure and alveolar collapse. This can result from the effects of anesthesia or analgesic agents, supine positioning, splinting of the chest wall because of pain, or abdominal distention. Postoperative patients may also have secretion retention, airway obstruction, and an impaired cough reflex, or they may be reluctant to cough because of pain. Figure 23-1 shows the pathogenic mechanisms and consequences of acute atelectasis in postoperative patients.

Atelectasis resulting from bronchial obstruction by secretions may occur in postoperative patients, in those with impaired cough mechanisms (eg, musculoskeletal or neurologic disorders), and in debilitated, bedridden patients. Atelectasis may also result from excessive pressure on the lung tissue, which restricts normal lung expansion on inspiration. Such pressure may be produced by fluid accumulating within the pleural space (**pleural effusion**), air in the pleural space (**pneumothorax**), or blood in the pleural space (**hemothorax**). The **pleural space** is the area between the parietal and the visceral pleurae. Pressure may also be produced by a pericardium distended with fluid (pericardial effusion), tumor growth within the thorax, or an elevated diaphragm.

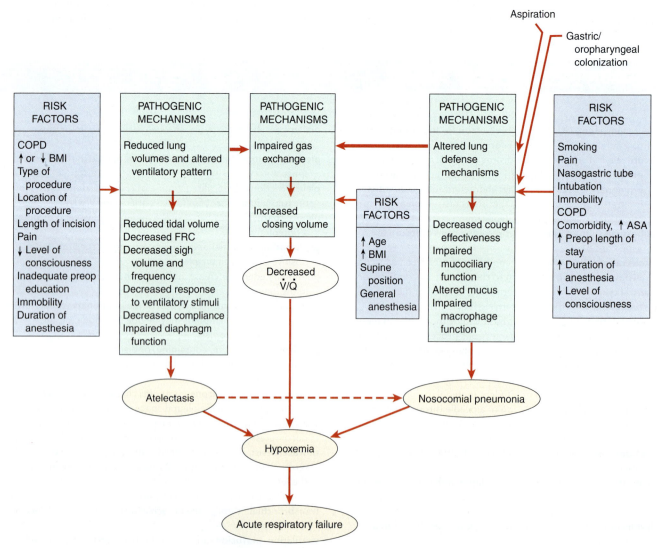

**FIGURE 23-1.** Relationship of risk factors, pathogenic mechanisms, and consequences of acute atelectasis in the postoperative patient. COPD, chronic obstructive pulmonary disease; BMI, body mass index; FRC, functional residual capacity; diaphragm fx, diaphragm function; ASA, American Society of Anesthesiology physical status; V̇/Q̇, ventilation-perfusion ratio. From the work of Jo Ann Brooks-Brunn, DNS, RN, FAAN, FCCP, Indiana University Medical Center, Indianapolis.

## Clinical Manifestations

The development of atelectasis usually is insidious. Signs and symptoms include cough, sputum production, and low-grade fever. Fever is universally cited as a clinical sign of atelectasis, but there are few data to support this. Most likely, the fever that accompanies atelectasis is due to infection or inflammation distal to the obstructed airway.

In acute atelectasis involving a large amount of lung tissue (lobar atelectasis), marked respiratory distress may be observed. In addition to the previously mentioned signs and symptoms, dyspnea, tachycardia, tachypnea, pleural pain, and **central cyanosis** (a bluish skin hue that is a late sign of hypoxemia) may be anticipated. Patients characteristically have difficulty breathing in the supine position and are anxious.

In chronic atelectasis, signs and symptoms are similar to those of acute atelectasis. The chronic nature of the alveolar collapse predisposes patients to infection distal to the obstruction. Therefore, the signs and symptoms of a pulmonary infection also may be present.

## Assessment and Diagnostic Findings

When clinically significant atelectasis develops, it is generally characterized by increased work of breathing and hypoxemia. The patient may demonstrate an increased respiratory rate and appear to labor with breathing. Decreased breath sounds and crackles are heard over the affected area. In addition, chest x-ray findings may reveal patchy infiltrates or consolidated areas. In patients who are confined to bed, atelectasis is usually diagnosed by chest x-ray or identified by physical assessment in the dependent, posterior, basilar areas of the lungs. Depending on the degree of hypoxemia, pulse oximetry ($SpO_2$) may demonstrate a low saturation of hemoglobin with oxygen (less than 90%) or a lower-than-normal partial pressure of arterial oxygen ($PaO_2$).

## Prevention

Nursing measures to prevent atelectasis include frequent turning, early mobilization, and strategies to expand the lungs and to manage secretions. Voluntary deep-breathing maneuvers (at least every 2 hours) assist in preventing and treating atelectasis. The performance of these maneuvers requires the patient to be alert and cooperative. Patient education and reinforcement are key to the success of these interventions. The use of incentive spirometry or voluntary deep breathing enhances lung expansion, decreases the potential for airway closure, and may generate a cough. Secretion management techniques include directed cough, suctioning, aerosol nebulizer treatments followed by chest physical therapy (postural drainage and chest percussion), and bronchoscopy. In some settings, a metered-dose inhaler is used to dispense a bronchodilator rather than an aerosol nebulizer. Chart 23-1 summarizes measures used to prevent atelectasis.

## Management

The goal of treatment is to improve ventilation and remove secretions. Strategies to prevent atelectasis, which include frequent turning, early ambulation, lung volume expansion maneuvers (eg, deep-breathing exercises, incentive spirometry), and coughing, also serve as the first-line measures to minimize or treat atelectasis by improving ventilation. In patients who do not respond to first-line measures or who cannot perform deep-breathing exercises, other treatments such as positive end-expiratory pressure (PEEP; a simple mask and one-way valve system that provides varying amounts of expiratory resistance, usually 5 to 15 cm $H_2O$), continuous or intermittent positive pressure-breathing (IPPB), or bronchoscopy may be used. An older therapy, IPPB continues to be used in some settings to improve lung volume expansion; however, other types of lung volume expansion maneuvers should be tried first in the postoperative setting (Sorenson & Shelledy, 2003). Before initiating more complex, costly, and labor-intensive therapies, nurses should ask several questions:

- Has the patient been given an adequate trial of deep-breathing exercises?
- Has the patient received adequate education, supervision, and coaching to carry out the deep-breathing exercises?
- Have other factors been evaluated that may impair ventilation or prevent a good patient effort (eg, lack of turning, mobilization; excessive pain; excessive sedation)?

If the cause of atelectasis is bronchial obstruction from secretions, the secretions must be removed by coughing or suctioning to allow air to re-enter that portion of the lung. Chest physical therapy (chest percussion and postural drainage) may also be used to mobilize secretions. Nebulizer treatments with a bronchodilator or sodium bicarbonate may be used to assist patients in the expectoration of secretions. If respiratory care measures fail to remove the obstruction, a bronchoscopy is performed. Although bronchoscopy is an excellent measure to acutely remove secretions and increase ventilation, it is imperative for the nurse to assist the patient

---

**CHART 23-1**

### Preventing Atelectasis

- Change patient's position frequently, especially from supine to upright position, to promote ventilation and prevent secretions from accumulating.
- Encourage early mobilization from bed to chair followed by early ambulation.
- Encourage appropriate deep breathing and coughing to mobilize secretions and prevent them from accumulating.
- Teach/reinforce appropriate technique for incentive spirometry.
- Administer prescribed opioids and sedatives judiciously to prevent respiratory depression.
- Perform postural drainage and chest percussion, if indicated.
- Institute suctioning to remove tracheobronchial secretions, if indicated.

with maintaining the patency of the airways after bronchoscopy, using the traditional techniques of deep breathing, coughing, and suctioning. Severe or massive atelectasis may lead to acute respiratory failure, especially in patients with underlying lung disease. Endotracheal intubation and mechanical ventilation may be necessary. Prompt treatment reduces the risk for development of acute respiratory failure, pneumonia, or both.

If the cause of atelectasis is compression of lung tissue, the goal is to decrease the compression. With a large pleural effusion that is compressing lung tissue and causing alveolar collapse, treatment may include **thoracentesis** (removal of the fluid by needle aspiration) or insertion of a chest tube. The measures to increase lung expansion described previously also are used.

Management of chronic atelectasis focuses on removing the cause of the obstruction of the airways or the compression of the lung tissue. For example, bronchoscopy may be used to open an airway obstructed by lung cancer or a nonmalignant lesion, and the procedure may involve cryotherapy or laser therapy. If the atelectasis is a result of obstruction caused by lung cancer, an airway stent or radiation therapy to shrink a tumor may be used to open the airways and provide ventilation to the collapsed area. However, in patients who have experienced chronic, long-term collapse, it may not be possible to reopen the airways and reaerate the area of the lung. In some cases, surgical management may be indicated.

# Respiratory Infections

## Acute Tracheobronchitis

Acute tracheobronchitis, an acute inflammation of the mucous membranes of the trachea and the bronchial tree, often follows infection of the upper respiratory tract. Patients with viral infections have decreased resistance and can readily develop a secondary bacterial infection. Adequate treatment of upper respiratory tract infection is one of the major factors in the prevention of acute bronchitis.

## Pathophysiology

In acute tracheobronchitis, the inflamed mucosa of the bronchi produces mucopurulent sputum, often in response to infection by *Streptococcus pneumoniae, Haemophilus influenzae,* or *Mycoplasma pneumoniae*. In addition, a fungal infection (eg, *Aspergillus*) may also cause tracheobronchitis. A sputum culture is essential to identify the specific causative organism. In addition to infection, inhalation of physical and chemical irritants, gases, or other air contaminants can also cause acute bronchial irritation.

## Clinical Manifestations

Initially, the patient has a dry, irritating cough and expectorates a scanty amount of mucoid sputum. The patient may report sternal soreness from coughing and have fever or chills, night sweats, headache, and general malaise. As the infection progresses, the patient may be short of breath, have noisy inspiration and expiration (inspiratory stridor and expiratory wheeze), and produce **purulent** (pus-filled) sputum. In severe tracheobronchitis, blood-streaked secretions may be expectorated as a result of the irritation of the mucosa of the airways.

## Medical Management

Antibiotic treatment may be indicated depending on the symptoms, sputum purulence, and results of the sputum culture. Antihistamines usually are not prescribed, because they can cause excessive drying and make secretions more difficult to expectorate. Expectorants may be prescribed, although their efficacy is questionable. Fluid intake is increased to thin the viscous and tenacious secretions. Copious, purulent secretions that cannot be cleared by coughing place patients at risk for increasing airway obstruction and the development of more severe lower respiratory tract infections, such as pneumonia. Suctioning and bronchoscopy may be needed to remove secretions. Rarely, endotracheal intubation may be necessary in cases of acute tracheobronchitis leading to acute respiratory failure, such as in patients who are severely debilitated or who have coexisting diseases that also impair the respiratory system.

In most cases, treatment of tracheobronchitis is largely symptomatic. Increasing the vapor pressure (moisture content) in the air reduces airway irritation. Cool vapor therapy or steam inhalations may help relieve laryngeal and tracheal irritation. Moist heat to the chest may relieve the soreness and pain. Mild analgesics or antipyretics may be indicated.

## Nursing Management

Acute tracheobronchitis is usually treated in the home setting. A primary nursing function is to encourage bronchial hygiene, such as increased fluid intake and directed coughing to remove secretions. The nurse encourages and assists the patient to sit up frequently to cough effectively and to prevent retention of mucopurulent sputum. If the patient is taking antibiotics for an underlying infection, it is important to emphasize the need to complete the full course of antibiotics prescribed. Fatigue is a consequence of tracheobronchitis; therefore, the nurse cautions the patient against overexertion, which can induce a relapse or exacerbation of the infection. The patient is advised to rest.

## Pneumonia

Pneumonia is an inflammation of the lung parenchyma caused by various microorganisms, including bacteria, mycobacteria, chlamydiae, mycoplasma, fungi, parasites, and viruses. "Pneumonitis" is a more general term that describes an inflammatory process in the lung tissue that may predispose or place the patient at risk for microbial invasion. Pneumonia is the most common cause of death from infectious diseases in the United States. It accounts for almost 66,000 deaths per year and ranks as the seventh leading cause of death in the United States (Kochanek & Smith, 2004). A costly disorder, pneumonia occurs in both inpatients and outpatients.

## Classification

Several systems are used to classify pneumonias. Classically, pneumonia has been categorized into one of four categories: bacterial or typical, atypical, anaerobic/cavitary, and opportunistic. However, there is overlap in the microorganisms thought to be responsible for typical and atypical pneumonias. A more widely used classification scheme categorizes the major pneumonias as community-acquired pneumonia (CAP), hospital-acquired (nosocomial) pneumonia (HAP), pneumonia in the immunocompromised host, and aspiration pneumonia (Table 23-1). There is overlap in how specific pneumonias are classified, because they may occur in differing settings.

### Community-Acquired Pneumonia

CAP occurs either in the community setting or within the first 48 hours after hospitalization or institutionalization. The need for hospitalization for CAP depends on the severity of the pneumonia. The causative agents for CAP that requires hospitalization are most frequently S. pneumoniae, H. influenzae, Legionella, Pseudomonas aeruginosa, and other gram-negative rods. The specific etiologic agent is identified in about 50% of cases. More than 5.5 million people develop CAP and as many as 1.1 million of these require hospitalization each year. (The absence of a responsible caregiver in the home may be another indication for hospitalization.) In the United States, CAP is the major cause of death from infectious disease (Andrews, Nadjm, Gant, et al., 2003).

Pneumonia caused by S. pneumoniae (pneumococcus) is the most common CAP in people younger than 60 years of age without comorbidity and in those 60 years and older with comorbidity. It is most prevalent during the winter and spring, when upper respiratory tract infections are most frequent. S. pneumoniae is a gram-positive, capsulated, nonmotile coccus that resides naturally in the upper respiratory tract. The organism colonizes the upper respiratory tract and can cause the following types of illnesses: disseminated invasive infections, pneumonia and other lower respiratory tract infections, and upper respiratory tract infections, including otitis media and sinusitis. It may occur as a lobar or bronchopneumonic form in patients of any age and may follow a recent respiratory illness.

Mycoplasma pneumonia, another type of CAP, is caused by M. pneumoniae. Mycoplasma pneumonia occurs most often in older children and young adults and is spread by infected respiratory droplets through person-to-person contact. Patients can be tested for mycoplasma antibodies. The inflammatory infiltrate is primarily interstitial rather than alveolar. It spreads throughout the entire respiratory tract, including the bronchioles, and has the characteristics of a bronchopneumonia. Earache and bullous myringitis are common. Impaired ventilation and diffusion may occur.

H. influenzae is another cause of CAP. This type of pneumonia frequently affects elderly people and those with comorbid illnesses (eg, chronic obstructive pulmonary disease [COPD], alcoholism, diabetes mellitus). The presentation is indistinguishable from that of other forms of bacterial CAP and may be subacute, with cough or low-grade fever for weeks before diagnosis. Chest x-rays may reveal multilobar, patchy bronchopneumonia or areas of **consolidation** (tissue that solidifies as a result of collapsed alveoli or pneumonia).

Viruses are the most common cause of pneumonia in infants and children but are relatively uncommon causes of CAP in adults. In immunocompetent adults, the chief causes of viral pneumonia are influenza viruses types A and B, adenovirus, parainfluenza virus, coronavirus, and varicella-zoster virus. In immunocompromised adults, cytomegalovirus is the most common viral pathogen, followed by herpes simplex virus, adenovirus, and respiratory syncytial virus. The acute stage of a viral respiratory infection occurs within the ciliated cells of the airways. This is followed by infiltration of the tracheobronchial tree. With pneumonia, the inflammatory process extends into the alveolar area, resulting in edema and exudation. The clinical signs and symptoms of a viral pneumonia are often difficult to distinguish from those of a bacterial pneumonia.

### Hospital-Acquired Pneumonia

HAP, also known as **nosocomial** pneumonia, is defined as the onset of pneumonia symptoms more than 48 hours after admission in patients with no evidence of infection at the time of admission. HAP accounts for approximately 15% of hospital-acquired infections but is the most lethal nosocomial infection. It is estimated to occur in 0.5% to 1% of all hospitalized patients and in 15% to 20% of intensive care patients (Centers for Disease Control and Prevention [CDC], 2004d). Ventilator-associated pneumonia can be considered a type of nosocomial pneumonia that is associated with endotracheal intubation and mechanical ventilation. Ventilator-associated pneumonia is defined as bacterial pneumonia that develops in patients with acute respiratory failure who have been receiving mechanical ventilation for at least 48 hours.

HAP occurs when at least one of three conditions exists: host defenses are impaired, an inoculum of organisms reaches the lower respiratory tract and overwhelms the host's defenses, or a highly virulent organism is present. Certain factors may predispose patients to HAP because of impaired host defenses (eg, severe acute or chronic illness), a variety of comorbid conditions, supine positioning and aspiration, coma, malnutrition, prolonged hospitalization, hypotension, and metabolic disorders. Hospitalized patients are also exposed to potential bacteria from other sources (eg, respiratory therapy devices and equipment, transmission of pathogens by the hands of health care personnel). Numerous intervention-related factors also may play a role in the development of HAP (eg, therapeutic agents leading to central nervous system depression with decreased ventilation, impaired removal of secretions, or potential aspiration; prolonged or complicated thoracoabdominal procedures, which may impair mucociliary function and cellular host defenses; endotracheal intubation; prolonged or inappropriate use of antibiotics; use of nasogastric tubes). In addition, immunocompromised patients are at particular risk. HAP is associated with a high mortality rate, in part because of the virulence of the organisms, their resistance to antibiotics, and the patient's underlying disorder.

The common organisms responsible for HAP include the pathogens Enterobacter species, Escherichia coli, H. influenzae,

(text continues on page 633)

## TABLE 23-1 Commonly Encountered Pneumonias

| Type | Organism Responsible | Epidemiology | Clinical Features | Treatment | Comments |
|---|---|---|---|---|---|
| **Community-Acquired Pneumonia** | | | | | |
| Streptococcal pneumonia (pneumococcal) | Streptococcus pneumoniae | Highest occurrence in winter months. Incidence greatest in the elderly and in patients with COPD, heart failure, alcoholism, asplenia, and after influenza. Leading infectious cause of illness worldwide among young children, persons with underlying chronic health conditions, and the elderly. Death occurs in 14% of hospitalized adults with invasive disease. | Abrupt onset, toxic appearance, pleuritic chest pain. Usually involves one or more lobes. Lobar infiltrate common on chest x-ray or bronchopneumonia pattern. Bacteremia in 15% to 25% of all patients. | Penicillins Alternative antibiotic therapy, such as cefotaxime or ceftriaxone; antipseudomonal fluoroquinolones (levofloxacin, gatifloxacin, moxifloxacin). | Complications include shock, pleural effusion, superinfections, pericarditis, and otitis media. |
| Haemophilus influenzae | Haemophilus influenzae | Incidence greatest in alcoholics, the elderly, patients in long-term care facilities and nursing homes, patients with diabetes or COPD, and children <5 years of age. Accounts for 5–20% of community-acquired pneumonias. Mortality rate: 30%. | Frequently insidious onset associated with upper respiratory tract infection 2 to 6 weeks before onset of illness. Fever, chills, productive cough. Usually involves one or more lobes. Bacteremia is common. Infiltrate, occasional bronchopneumonia pattern on chest x-ray. | Ampicillin, third- or fourth-generation cephalosporin, macrolides (azithromycin, clarithromycin), fluoroquinolones | Complications include lung abscess, pleural effusion, meningitis, arthritis, pericarditis, epiglottitis. |
| Legionnaires' disease | Legionella pneumophila | Highest occurrence in summer and fall. May cause disease sporadically or as part of an epidemic. Incidence greatest in middle-aged and older men, smokers, patients with chronic diseases, those receiving immunosuppressive therapy, and those in close proximity to excavation sites. Accounts for 15% of community-acquired pneumonias. Mortality rate: 15–50%. | Flulike symptoms. High fevers, mental confusion, headache, pleuritic pain, myalgias, dyspnea, productive cough, hemoptysis, leukocytosis. Bronchopneumonia, unilateral or bilateral disease, lobar consolidation. | Erythromycin +/− rifampin (in severely compromised patient) or clarithromycin, or a macrolide (azithromycin), or a fluoroquinolone (ofloxacin, levofloxacin, sparfloxacin). | Complications include hypotension, shock, and acute renal failure. |

| TABLE 23-1 | Commonly Encountered Pneumonias (Continued) | | | | |
|---|---|---|---|---|---|
| Type | Organism Responsible | Epidemiology | Clinical Features | Treatment | Comments |
| Mycoplasma pneumoniae | Mycoplasma pneumoniae | Increase in fall and winter. Responsible for epidemics of respiratory illness. Most common type of atypical pneumonia. Accounts for 20% of community-acquired pneumonias. More common in children and young adults. Mortality rate: <0.1%. | Onset is usually insidious. Patients not usually as ill as in other pneumonias. Sore throat, nasal congestion, ear pain, headache, low-grade fever, pleuritic pain, myalgias, diarrhea, erythematous rash, pharyngitis. Interstitial infiltrates on chest x-ray. | Doxycycline, macrolide or fluoroquinolone. | Complications include aseptic meningitis, meningoencephalitis, transverse myelitis, cranial nerve palsies, pericarditis, myocarditis. |
| Viral pneumonia | Influenza viruses types A, B adenovirus, parainfluenza, cytomegalovirus, coronavirus | Incidence greatest in winter months. Epidemics occur every 2 to 3 years. Most common causative organisms in adults. Other organisms in children (eg, cytomegalovirus, respiratory syncytial virus). Accounts for 20% of community-acquired pneumonias. | Patchy infiltrate, small pleural effusion on chest x-ray. In most patients, influenza begins as an acute upper respiratory infection; others have bronchitis, pleurisy, and so on, and still others develop gastrointestinal symptoms. | Type A: amantadine and rimantadine Type A/B: zanamivir, oseltamivir phosphate. Treated symptomatically. Does not respond to treatment with currently available antimicrobials. | Complications include a superimposed bacterial infection, bronchopneumonia. |
| Chlamydial pneumonia (TWAR agent) | Chlamydia pneumoniae | Reported mainly in college students, military recruits, and the elderly. May be a common cause of community-acquired pneumonia or observed in combination with other pathogens. Mortality rate is low because the majority of cases are relatively mild. The elderly with coexistent infections, comorbidities, and reinfections may require hospitalization. | Hoarseness, fever, chills, pharyngitis, rhinitis, nonproductive cough, myalgias, arthralgias. Single infiltrate on chest x-ray; pleural effusion possible. | Tetracycline, erythromycin, macrolide, quinolone. | Complications include reinfection and acute respiratory failure. |

*continued >*

| TABLE 23-1 | Commonly Encountered Pneumonias (Continued) | | | | |
|---|---|---|---|---|---|
| Type | Organism Responsible | Epidemiology | Clinical Features | Treatment | Comments |
| **Hospital-Acquired Pneumonia** | | | | | |
| *Pseudomonas* pneumonia | *Pseudomonas aeruginosa* | Incidence greatest in those with pre-existing lung disease, cancer (particularly leukemia); those with homograft transplants, burns; debilitated persons; and patients receiving antimicrobial therapy and treatments such as tracheostomy, suctioning, and in postoperative settings. Almost always of nosocomial origin. Accounts for 15% of hospital-acquired pneumonias. Mortality rate: 40–60%. | Diffuse consolidation on chest x-ray. Toxic appearance: fever, chills, productive cough, relative bradycardia, leukocytosis. | Aminoglycoside and anti-pseudomonal agents (ticarcillin, piperacillin, mezlocillin, ceftazidine). | Complications include lung cavitation. Has capacity to invade blood vessels, causing hemorrhage and lung infarction. Usually requires hospitalization. |
| Staphylococcal pneumonia | *Staphylococcus aureus* | Incidence greatest in immunocompromised patients, IV drug users, and as a complication of epidemic influenza. Commonly nosocomial in origin. Accounts for 10–30% of hospital-acquired pneumonias. Mortality rate: 25–60%. | Severe hypoxemia, cyanosis, necrotizing infection. Bacteremia is common. | Nafcillin/oxacillin; clindamycin or linezolid; methicillin-resistant: vancomycin or linezolid | Complications include pleural effusion/pneumothorax, lung abscess, empyema, meningitis, endocarditis. Frequently requires hospitalization. Treatment must be vigorous and prolonged because disease tends to destroy lung tissue. |
| *Klebsiella* pneumonia | *Klebsiella pneumoniae* (Friedlander's bacillus-encapsulated gram-negative aerobic bacillus) | Incidence greatest in the elderly; alcoholics; patients with chronic disease, such as diabetes, heart failure, COPD; patients in chronic care facilities and nursing homes. Accounts for 2–5% of community-acquired and 10–30% of hospital-acquired pneumonias. Mortality rate: 40–50%. | Tissue necrosis occurs rapidly. Toxic appearance: fever, cough, sputum production, bronchopneumonia, lung abscess. Lobar consolidation, bronchopneumonia pattern on chest x-ray. | Third- and/or fourth-generation cephalosporins (cefotaxime, ceftriaxone) plus aminoglycoside, antipseudomonal penicillin, monobactam (aztreonam), or quinolone. | Complications include multiple lung abscesses with cyst formation, empyema, pericarditis, pleural effusion. May be fulminating, progressing to fatal outcome. |

| TABLE 23-1 | Commonly Encountered Pneumonias (Continued) | | | | |
|---|---|---|---|---|---|
| Type | Organism Responsible | Epidemiology | Clinical Features | Treatment | Comments |
| **Pneumonia in Immunocompromised Host** | | | | | |
| Pneumocystis pneumonia (PCP) | Pneumocystis jiroveci | Incidence greatest in patients with AIDS and patients receiving immunosuppressive therapy for cancer, organ transplantation, and other disorders. Frequently seen with cytomegalovirus infection. Mortality rate 15–20% in hospitalized patients and fatal if not treated. | Pulmonary infiltrates on chest x-ray. Nonproductive cough, fever, dyspnea. | Trimethoprim/ sulfamethoxazole (TMP-SMZ), dapsone-trimethoprim, pentamidine, primequine plus clindamycin. | Complications include respiratory failure. |
| Fungal pneumonia | Aspergillus fumigatus | Incidence greatest in immunocompromised and neutropenic patients. Mortality rate: 15–20%. | Cough, hemoptysis, infiltrates, fungus ball on chest x-ray. | Flucytosine with amphotericin B in non-neutropenic patients, amphotericin B, itraconazole, ketoconazole. Lobectomy for fungus ball. | Complications include dissemination to brain, myocardium, and/or thyroid gland. |
| Tuberculosis | Mycobacterium tuberculosis | Incidence increased in indigent, immigrant, and prison populations, people with AIDS, and the homeless. Mortality rate <1% (depending on comorbidity) | Weight loss, fever, night sweats, cough, sputum production, hemoptysis, nonspecific infiltrate (lower lobe), hilar node enlargement, pleural effusion on chest x-ray. | Rifampin, ethambutol, INH (isoniazid), pyrazinamide | Complications include reinfection and acute respiratory infection. |

+/− may add depending upon situation; COPD, chronic obstructive pulmonary disease.

*Klebsiella* species, *Proteus*, *Serratia marcescens*, *P. aeruginosa*, methicillin-sensitive or methicillin-resistant *Staphylococcus aureus* (MRSA), and *S. pneumoniae*. Some risk factors for infection are shared, and others are unique to the specific organisms; however, most patients with HAP are colonized with multiple organisms. Pseudomonal pneumonia, which accounts for 15% of cases of HAP, occurs in patients who are debilitated, those with altered mental status, and those with prolonged intubation or with tracheostomy. Staphylococcal pneumonia, which accounts for more than 30% of cases of HAP but less than 10% of cases of CAP, can occur through inhalation of the organism or spread through the hematogenous route. It is often accompanied by bacteremia and positive blood cultures. Its mortality rate is high. Specific strains of staphylococci are resistant to all available antimicrobial agents except vancomycin. Overuse and misuse of antimicrobial agents are major risk factors for the emergence of these resistant pathogens. Because MRSA is highly virulent, steps must be taken to prevent its spread. Patients with MRSA are isolated in a private room, and contact precautions (gown, mask, glove, and antibacterial soap) are used. The number of people in contact with affected patients is minimized, and appropriate precautions must be taken when transporting these patients within or between facilities.

The usual presentation of HAP is a new pulmonary infiltrate on chest x-ray combined with evidence of infection such as fever, respiratory symptoms, purulent sputum, or leukocytosis. Pneumonias from *Klebsiella* or other gram-negative organisms (*E. coli, Proteus, Serratia*) are characterized by destruction of lung structure and alveolar walls, consolidation, and bacteremia. Elderly patients and those with alcoholism, chronic lung disease, or diabetes are at particular risk. Development of a cough or increased cough and sputum production are common presentations, along with low-grade fever and general malaise. In debilitated or dehydrated patients, sputum production may be minimal or absent. Pleural effusion, high fever, and tachycardia are common. Even with treatment, the mortality rate remains high.

### Pneumonia in the Immunocompromised Host

Pneumonia in immunocompromised hosts includes *Pneumocystis* pneumonia (PCP), fungal pneumonias, and *Mycobacterium tuberculosis*. The organism that causes PCP is now known as *Pneumocystis jiroveci* instead of *Pneumocystis carinii*. The acronym PCP still applies because it can be read "*Pneumocystis* pneumonia."

Pneumonia in the immunocompromised host occurs with use of corticosteroids or other immunosuppressive agents, chemotherapy, nutritional depletion, use of broad-spectrum antimicrobial agents, acquired immunodeficiency syndrome (AIDS), genetic immune disorders, and long-term advanced life-support technology (mechanical ventilation). It is seen with increasing frequency because affected patients constitute a growing portion of the population; however, pneumonias that typically occur in immunocompromised people may also occur in immunocompetent people. Patients with compromised immune systems commonly develop pneumonia from organisms of low virulence. In addition, increasing numbers of patients with impaired defenses develop HAP from gram-negative bacilli (*Klebsiella, Pseudomonas, E. coli,* Enterobacteriaceae, *Proteus, Serratia*).

Pneumonia in immunocompromised hosts may be caused by the organisms also observed in CAP or HAP (*S. pneumoniae, S. aureus, H. influenzae, P. aeruginosa, M. tuberculosis*). PCP is rarely observed in immunocompetent hosts and is often an initial AIDS-defining complication. Whether patients are immunocompromised or immunocompetent, the clinical presentation of pneumonia is similar. PCP has a subtle onset, with progressive dyspnea, fever, and a nonproductive cough.

### Aspiration Pneumonia

Aspiration pneumonia refers to the pulmonary consequences resulting from entry of endogenous or exogenous substances into the lower airway. The most common form of aspiration pneumonia is bacterial infection from aspiration of bacteria that normally reside in the upper airways. Aspiration pneumonia may occur in the community or hospital setting. Common pathogens are *S. pneumoniae, H. influenzae,* and *S. aureus*. Substances other than bacteria may be aspirated into the lung, such as gastric contents, exogenous chemical contents, or irritating gases. This type of aspiration or ingestion may impair the lung defenses, cause inflammatory changes, and lead to bacterial growth and a resulting pneumonia. (See later discussion of aspiration.)

## Pathophysiology

Upper airway characteristics normally prevent potentially infectious particles from reaching the sterile lower respiratory tract. Pneumonia arises from normal flora present in patients whose resistance has been altered or from aspiration of flora present in the oropharynx; patients often have an acute or chronic underlying disease that impairs host defenses. Pneumonia may also result from bloodborne organisms that enter the pulmonary circulation and are trapped in the pulmonary capillary bed.

Pneumonia affects both ventilation and diffusion. An inflammatory reaction can occur in the alveoli, producing an exudate that interferes with the diffusion of oxygen and carbon dioxide. White blood cells, mostly neutrophils, also migrate into the alveoli and fill the normally air-containing spaces. Areas of the lung are not adequately ventilated because of secretions and mucosal edema that cause partial occlusion of the bronchi or alveoli, with a resultant decrease in alveolar oxygen tension. Bronchospasm may also occur in patients with reactive airway disease. Because of hypoventilation, a ventilation–perfusion mismatch occurs in the affected area of the lung. Venous blood entering the pulmonary circulation passes through the underventilated area and travels to the left side of the heart poorly oxygenated. The mixing of oxygenated and unoxygenated or poorly oxygenated blood eventually results in arterial hypoxemia.

If a substantial portion of one or more lobes is involved, the disease is referred to as "lobar pneumonia." The term "bronchopneumonia" is used to describe pneumonia that is distributed in a patchy fashion, having originated in one or more localized areas within the bronchi and extending to the adjacent surrounding lung parenchyma. Bronchopneumonia is more common than lobar pneumonia (Fig. 23-2).

### Risk Factors

Being knowledgeable about the factors and circumstances that commonly predispose people to pneumonia helps identify patients at high risk for the disease (Table 23-2).

Increasing numbers of patients who have compromised defenses against infections are susceptible to pneumonia. Some types of pneumonia, such as those caused by viral infections, occur in previously healthy people, often after a viral illness.

**FIGURE 23-2.** Distribution of lung involvement in bronchial and lobar pneumonia. In bronchopneumonia (*left*), patchy areas of consolidation occur. In lobar pneumonia (*right*), an entire lobe is consolidated.

## TABLE 23-2  Risk Factors and Preventive Measures for Pneumonia

| Risk Factor | Preventive Measure |
|---|---|
| Conditions that produce mucus or bronchial obstruction and interfere with normal lung drainage (eg, cancer, cigarette smoking, COPD) | Promote coughing and expectoration of secretions. Encourage smoking cessation. |
| Immunosuppressed patients and those with a low neutrophil count (neutropenic) | Initiate special precautions against infection. |
| Smoking; cigarette smoke disrupts both mucociliary and macrophage activity | Encourage smoking cessation. |
| Prolonged immobility and shallow breathing pattern | Reposition frequently and promote lung expansion exercises and coughing. Initiate suctioning and chest physical therapy if indicated. |
| Depressed cough reflex (due to medications, a debilitated state, or weak respiratory muscles); aspiration of foreign material into the lungs during a period of unconsciousness (head injury, anesthesia, depressed level of consciousness), or abnormal swallowing mechanism | Reposition frequently to prevent aspiration and administer medications judiciously, particularly those that increase risk for aspiration. Perform suctioning and chest physical therapy if indicated. |
| Nothing-by-mouth (NPO) status; placement of nasogastric, orogastric, or endotracheal tube | Promote frequent oral hygiene. Minimize risk for aspiration by checking placement of tube and proper positioning of patient. |
| Supine positioning in patients unable to protect their airway | Elevate head of bed at least 30 degrees. |
| Antibiotic therapy (in very ill people, the oropharynx is likely to be colonized by gram-negative bacteria) | Monitor patients receiving antibiotic therapy for signs and symptoms of pneumonia. |
| Alcohol intoxication (because alcohol suppresses the body's reflexes, may be associated with aspiration, and decreases white cell mobilization and tracheobronchial ciliary motion) | Encourage reduced or moderate alcohol intake (in case of alcohol stupor, position patient to prevent aspiration). |
| General anesthetic, sedative, or opioid preparations that promote respiratory depression, which causes a shallow breathing pattern and predisposes to the pooling of bronchial secretions and potential development of pneumonia | Observe the respiratory rate and depth during recovery from general anesthesia and before giving medications. If respiratory depression is apparent, withhold the medication and contact the physician. |
| Advanced age, because of possible depressed cough and glottic reflexes and nutritional depletion | Promote frequent turning, early ambulation and mobilization, effective coughing, breathing exercises, and nutritious diet. |
| Respiratory therapy with improperly cleaned equipment | Make sure that respiratory equipment is cleaned properly; participate in continuous quality improvement monitoring with the respiratory care department. |
| Transmission of organisms from health care providers | Use strict hand hygiene and gloves. Implement health care provider education. |

Pneumonia occurs in patients with certain underlying disorders such as heart failure, diabetes, alcoholism, COPD, and AIDS. Certain diseases also have been associated with specific pathogens. For example, staphylococcal pneumonia has been noted after epidemics of influenza, and patients with COPD are at increased risk for development of pneumonia caused by pneumococci or *H. influenzae*. In addition, cystic fibrosis is associated with respiratory infection caused by pseudomonal and staphylococcal organisms, and PCP has been associated with AIDS. Pneumonias occurring in hospitalized patients often involve organisms not usually found in CAP, including enteric gram-negative bacilli and *S. aureus*.

The CDC (2004d) has identified four specific strategies for preventing HAP: (1) staff education and involvement in infection prevention, (2) infection and microbiologic surveillance, (3) prevention of transmission of microorganisms, and (4) modifying host risk for infection. The CDC (2003a) has also established guidelines for environmental infection control in health care facilities. Providing anticipatory interventions and preventive care are important nursing measures.

Pneumococcal disease is more prevalent (threefold to fivefold higher) in African American adults as compared with Caucasians. Pneumococcal vaccination has been demonstrated to prevent pneumonia in otherwise healthy populations with an efficiency of 65% to 85% (Niederman & Ahmed, 2003). To reduce or prevent serious complications of CAP in high-risk groups, vaccination against pneumococcal infection is advised for the following:

- People 65 years of age or older
- Immunocompetent people who are at increased risk for illness and death associated with pneumococcal disease because of chronic illness (eg, cardiovascular disease, pulmonary disease, diabetes mellitus, chronic liver disease) or disability
- People with functional or anatomic asplenia
- People living in environments or social settings in which the risk of disease is high
- Immunocompromised people at high risk for infection

The vaccine provides specific prevention against pneumococcal pneumonia and other infections caused by *S. pneumoniae* (otitis media, other upper respiratory tract infections). Vaccines should be avoided during the first trimester of pregnancy.

## Clinical Manifestations

Pneumonia varies in its signs and symptoms depending on the causal organism and the presence of underlying disease. However, it is not possible to diagnose a specific type of pneumonia (CAP, HAP, immunocompromised host, or aspiration) by clinical manifestations alone. The patient with streptococcal (pneumococcal) pneumonia usually has a sudden onset of chills, rapidly rising fever (38.5° to 40.5°C [101° to 105°F]), and pleuritic chest pain that is aggravated by deep breathing and coughing. The patient is severely ill, with marked tachypnea (25 to 45 breaths/min), accompanied by other signs of respiratory distress (eg, shortness of breath, use of accessory muscles in respiration). The pulse is rapid and bounding, and it usually increases about 10 bpm for every degree (Celsius) of temperature elevation. A relative bradycardia for the amount of fever may suggest viral infection, mycoplasma infection, or infection with a *Legionella* organism.

Some patients exhibit an upper respiratory tract infection (nasal congestion, sore throat), and the onset of symptoms of pneumonia is gradual and nonspecific. The predominant symptoms may be headache, low-grade fever, pleuritic pain, myalgia, rash, and pharyngitis. After a few days, mucoid or mucopurulent sputum is expectorated. In severe pneumonia, the cheeks are flushed and the lips and nail beds demonstrate central cyanosis (a late sign of poor oxygenation [hypoxemia]).

The patient may exhibit **orthopnea** (shortness of breath when reclining), preferring to be propped up or sitting in bed leaning forward (orthopneic position) in an effort to achieve adequate gas exchange without coughing or breathing deeply. Appetite is poor, and the patient is diaphoretic and tires easily. Sputum is often purulent; however, this is not a reliable indicator of the etiologic agent. Rusty, blood-tinged sputum may be expectorated with streptococcal (pneumococcal), staphylococcal, and *Klebsiella* pneumonia.

Signs and symptoms of pneumonia may also depend on a patient's underlying condition. Different signs occur in patients with conditions such as cancer, and in those who are undergoing treatment with immunosuppressants, which decrease the resistance to infection. Such patients have fever, crackles, and physical findings that indicate consolidation of lung tissue, including increased tactile fremitus (vocal vibration detected on palpation), percussion dullness, bronchial breath sounds, egophony (when auscultated, the spoken "E" becomes a loud, nasal-sounding "A"), and whispered pectoriloquy (whispered sounds are easily auscultated through the chest wall). These changes occur because sound is transmitted better through solid or dense tissue (consolidation) than through normal air-filled tissue; these sounds are described in Chapter 21.

Purulent sputum or slight changes in respiratory symptoms may be the only sign of pneumonia in patients with COPD. It may be difficult to determine whether an increase in symptoms is an exacerbation of the underlying disease process or an additional infectious process.

## Assessment and Diagnostic Findings

The diagnosis of pneumonia is made by history (particularly of a recent respiratory tract infection), physical examination, chest x-ray, blood culture (bloodstream invasion, called bacteremia, occurs frequently), and sputum examination. The sputum sample is obtained by having patients do the following: (1) rinse the mouth with water to minimize contamination by normal oral flora, (2) breathe deeply several times, (3) cough deeply, and (4) expectorate the raised sputum into a sterile container.

More invasive procedures may be used to collect specimens. Sputum may be obtained by nasotracheal or orotracheal suctioning with a sputum trap or by fiberoptic bronchoscopy (see Chapter 21). Bronchoscopy is often used in patients with acute severe infection, in patients with chronic or refractory infection, in immunocompromised patients when a diagnosis cannot be made from an expectorated or induced specimen, and in mechanically ventilated patients.

## Medical Management

### Pharmacologic Therapy

The treatment of pneumonia includes administration of the appropriate antibiotic as determined by the results of a Gram stain. However, an etiologic agent is not identified in half of CAP cases, and empiric therapy must be initiated. Therapy for CAP is continuing to evolve. Guidelines exist to guide antibiotic choice; however, the resistance patterns, prevalence of etiologic agents, patient risk factors, and costs and availability of newer antibiotic agents must all be considered.

Several organizations have published guidelines and comprehensive reviews of the medical management of CAP (File, Garau, Blasi, et al., 2004; Institute for Clinical Systems Improvement [ICSI], 2003; Mandell, Bartlett, Dowell, et al., 2003). However, guidelines take time to develop, and by the time they are published, they are often out-of-date. In addition, different organizations may publish slightly different recommendations, making treatment decisions even more difficult (File et al., 2004). Guidelines may be classified in terms of risk factors, treatment setting (inpatient versus outpatient), or specific pathogens. Examples of risk factors that may increase the risk of infection with certain types of pathogens appear in Chart 23-2.

Prompt administration (within 4 to 8 hours) of antibiotics in patients in whom CAP is strongly suspected or confirmed is a key treatment measure. For outpatients with CAP who have no cardiopulmonary disease or other modifying factors, treatment should include an oral macrolide (azithromycin [Zithromax] or clarithromycin [Biaxin]), doxycycline (Vibramycin), or a fluoroquinolone (eg, gatifloxacin [Tequin], levofloxacin [Levaquin]) with enhanced activity against *S. pneumoniae* (File et al. 2004; ICSI, 2003). For outpatients with CAP who have cardiopulmonary disease or other modifying factors, treatment should include a beta-lactam agent (oral cefpodoxime [Vantin], cefurox-

## CHART 23-2

### Risk Factors for Pathogenic Lung Infections

**RISK FACTORS FOR INFECTION WITH PENICILLIN-RESISTANT AND DRUG-RESISTANT PNEUMOCOCCI**
- Age over 65 years
- Alcoholism
- Beta-lactam therapy (eg, cephalosporins) in past 3 months
- Immunosuppressive disorders
- Multiple medical comorbidities
- Exposure to a child in a day care facility

**RISK FACTORS FOR INFECTION WITH ENTERIC GRAM-NEGATIVE BACTERIA**
- Residency in a long-term care facility
- Underlying cardiopulmonary disease
- Multiple medical comorbidities
- Recent antibiotic therapy

**RISK FACTORS FOR INFECTION WITH *PSEUDOMONAS AERUGINOSA***
- Structural lung disease (eg, bronchiectasis)
- Corticosteroid therapy
- Broad-spectrum antibiotic therapy (more than 7 days in the past month)
- Malnutrition

---

ime [Zinacef, Ceftin], high-dose amoxicillin or amoxicillin/clavulanate [Augmentin, Clavulin]) plus a macrolide or doxycycline. Also, a beta-lactam agent plus an antipneumococcal fluoroquinolone can be used (File et al., 2004; ICSI, 2003). For older patients with multiple comorbidities, a fluoroquinolone may be preferred. Fluoroquinolones are sometimes reserved for use in higher-risk or drug-intolerant patients to slow the emergence of resistance to this class of antibiotics (File et al., 2004; ICSI, 2003). These are guidelines only; treatment regimens may be modified for individual patients.

For patients with CAP who are hospitalized and do not have cardiopulmonary disease or other significant risk factors, management consists of intravenous (IV) azithromycin or doxycycline plus a beta-lactam agent or mono therapy with an antipneumococcal fluoroquinolone. For inpatients with cardiopulmonary disease or other significant risk factors who are not in the intensive care unit, treatment involves IV ceftriaxone plus azithromycin. For acutely ill patients admitted to the intensive care unit, management includes an IV beta-lactam agent plus either an IV macrolide or fluoroquinolone. In a setting in which MRSA is a potential organism, an IV fluoroquinolone plus vancomycin or linezolid may be administered. For patients at high risk for *P. aeruginosa,* more select antipseudomonal antibiotics are administered by IV.

If specific pathogens responsible for the CAP are identified, more specific agents may be used. Mycoplasma pneumonia is treated with doxycycline or a macrolide. PCP responds best to pentamidine (Pentacarinat, NebuPent) or trimethoprim–sulfamethoxazole (TMP-SMZ [Bactrim, Septra]). Amantadine (Symmetrel) and rimantadine (Flumadine) are effective with influenza type A, and zanamivir and oseltamivir are effective with influenza type A/B. These medications have been shown to reduce the duration of fever and other systemic complications when administered within 24 to 48 hours of the onset of an uncomplicated influenza infection (CDC, 2004e). These medications also reduce the duration and quantity of virus shed in the respiratory secretions. They are most effective when used in combination with influenza vaccine. Ganciclovir (Cytovene, Vitrasert) is used to treat cytomegalovirus in patients who do not have AIDS; cytomegalovirus immunoglobulin may also be used.

HAP has a different etiology from CAP. In suspected HAP or nosocomial pneumonia, empiric treatment is usually initiated with a broad-spectrum IV antibiotic and may be monotherapy or combination therapy. In patients who are mildly to moderately ill with a low risk of *Pseudomonas* infection, the following antibiotics may be used: second-generation cephalosporins (eg, cefuroxime [Ceftin, Zinacef], cefamandole [Mandol]), nonpseudomonal third-generation cephalosporins (ceftriaxone [Rocephin], cefotaxime [Claforan], ampicillin-sulbactam [Unasyn]), fluoroquinolones (eg, ciprofloxacin [Cipro], levofloxacin [Levaquin]), or a carbapenem (meropenem [Merrem]). For combination therapy, any of these may be used with an aminoglycoside.

For patients who are at high risk for *Pseudomonas* infection, an antipseudomonal penicillin plus an aminoglycoside (amikacin [Amikin], gentamicin) or a beta-lactamase inhibitor (ampicillin/sulbactam [Unasyn], ticarcillin/clavulanate [Timentin]) may be used. Other types of combination therapy may also be used, depending on patient characteristics.

For patients with MRSA infection, vancomycin (Vancocin) or linezolid (Zyvox) is used. For patients with methicillin-sensitive *S. aureus,* nafcillin (Unipen), clindamycin (Cleocin), or linezolid (Zyvox) may be used.

Of concern is the rampant rise in respiratory pathogens that are resistant to available antibiotics. Examples include vancomycin-resistant enterococcus (VRE), MRSA, and drug-resistant *S. pneumoniae*. There is a tendency for clinicians to use antibiotics aggressively and inappropriately; they may use broad-spectrum agents when narrow-spectrum agents are more appropriate. Mechanisms to monitor and minimize the inappropriate use of antibiotics are in place. Education of clinicians about the use of evidence-based guidelines in the treatment of respiratory infection is important, and some institutions have implemented algorithms to assist clinicians in making the appropriate choice of antibiotics. Monitoring and surveillance of susceptibility patterns for pathogens are also important.

Usually, therapy with parenteral agents is changed to oral antimicrobial agents when there is evidence of a clinical response and patients are stable and able to tolerate oral medications. The recommended duration of treatment for pneumococcal pneumonia is 72 hours after the patient become afebrile. Patients with most other forms of pneumonia caused by bacterial pathogens are treated for 1 to 2 weeks after they become afebrile. Those with atypical pneumonia (eg, *Legionella*, *M. pneumoniae*) are usually treated for 10 to 21 days.

### Other Therapeutic Regimens

Antibiotics are ineffective in viral upper respiratory tract infections and pneumonia, and their use may be associated with adverse effects. Treatment of viral infections with antibiotics is a major reason for the overuse of these medications in the United States. Antibiotics are indicated with a viral respiratory infection *only* if a secondary bacterial pneumonia, bronchitis, or sinusitis is present. With the exception of the use of antimicrobial therapy, treatment of viral pneumonia is the same as that for bacterial pneumonia.

Treatment of viral pneumonia is primarily supportive. Hydration is a necessary part of therapy, because fever and tachypnea may result in insensible fluid losses. Antipyretics may be used to treat headache and fever; antitussive medications may be used for the associated cough. Warm, moist inhalations are helpful in relieving bronchial irritation. Antihistamines may provide benefit with reduced sneezing and rhinorrhea. Nasal decongestants may also be used to treat symptoms and improve sleep; however, excessive use can cause rebound nasal congestion. Bed rest is prescribed until the infection shows signs of clearing. If the patient is hospitalized, he or she is observed carefully until the clinical condition improves.

If hypoxemia develops, oxygen is administered. Pulse oximetry or arterial blood gas analysis is performed to determine the need for oxygen and to evaluate the effectiveness of the therapy. Arterial blood gases may be used to obtain a baseline measure of the patient's oxygenation and acid–base status; however, pulse oximetry is used to continuously monitor the patient's oxygen saturation and response to therapy. A high concentration of oxygen is contraindicated in the patient with COPD because it may worsen alveolar ventilation by decreasing the patient's ventilatory drive, leading to further respiratory decompensation. More aggressive respiratory support measures include administration of high concentrations of oxygen (fraction of inspired oxygen [$FIO_2$]), endotracheal intubation, and mechanical ventilation. Different modes of mechanical ventilation may be required; see Chapter 25. Figure 23-3 provides an example of a treatment algorithm for patients with suspected CAP.

### Gerontologic Considerations

Pneumonia in elderly patients may occur as a primary diagnosis or as a complication of a chronic disease process. Pulmonary infections in older people frequently are difficult to treat and result in a higher mortality rate than in younger people. General deterioration, weakness, abdominal symptoms, anorexia, confusion, tachycardia, and tachypnea may signal the onset of pneumonia. The diagnosis of pneumonia may be missed because the classic symptoms of cough, chest pain, sputum production, and fever may be absent or masked in elderly patients. Also, the presence of some signs may be misleading. Abnormal breath sounds, for example, may be caused by microatelectasis that occurs as a result of decreased mobility, decreased lung volumes, or other respiratory function changes. It may be necessary to obtain chest x-rays to differentiate chronic heart failure, which is often seen in the elderly, from pneumonia as the cause of clinical signs and symptoms.

Supportive treatment includes hydration (with caution and with frequent assessment because of the risk of fluid overload in the elderly), supplemental oxygen therapy, and assistance with deep breathing, coughing, frequent position changes, and early ambulation. All of these are particularly important in the care of elderly patients with pneumonia. To reduce or prevent serious complications of pneumonia in the elderly, vaccination against pneumococcal and influenza infections is recommended.

## Complications

### Shock and Respiratory Failure

Severe complications of pneumonia include hypotension and shock and respiratory failure (especially with gram-negative bacterial disease in elderly patients). These complications are encountered chiefly in patients who have received no specific treatment or inadequate or delayed treatment. These complications are also encountered when the infecting organism is resistant to therapy, when a co-morbid disease complicates the pneumonia, or when the patient is immunocompromised.

If the patient is seriously ill, aggressive therapy may include hemodynamic and ventilatory support to combat peripheral collapse, maintain arterial blood pressure, and provide adequate oxygenation. A vasopressor agent may be administered by continuous IV infusion and at a rate adjusted in accordance with the pressure response. Corticosteroids may be administered parenterally to combat shock and toxicity in patients who are extremely ill with pneumonia and at apparent risk for death from the infection. Patients may require endotracheal intubation and mechanical ventilation. Heart failure, cardiac dysrhythmias, pericarditis, and myocarditis also are complications of pneumonia that may lead to shock.

### Atelectasis and Pleural Effusion

Atelectasis (from obstruction of a bronchus or small airways by accumulated secretions) may occur at any stage of acute pneumonia. Parapneumonic pleural effusions occur in at least 40% of bacterial pneumonias. A parapneumonic effusion is any pleural effusion associated with bacterial pneumonia, lung abscess, or bronchiectasis. After the pleural effusion is detected on a chest x-ray, a thoracentesis may be performed to remove the fluid. The fluid is sent to the laboratory for analysis. There are three stages of parapneumonic pleural effusions based on pathogenesis: uncomplicated, complicated, and thoracic empyema. An **empyema** occurs when thick, purulent fluid accumulates within the pleural space, often with fibrin development and a loculated (walled-off) area where the infection is located (see later discussion). A chest tube may be inserted to treat pleural infection by establishing proper drainage of the empyema. Sterilization of the empyema cavity requires 4 to 6 weeks of antibiotics. Frequently used antibiotics include clindamycin (Cleocin), meropenem (Merrem), or piperacillin/tazobactam (Zosyn). Sometimes surgical management is required.

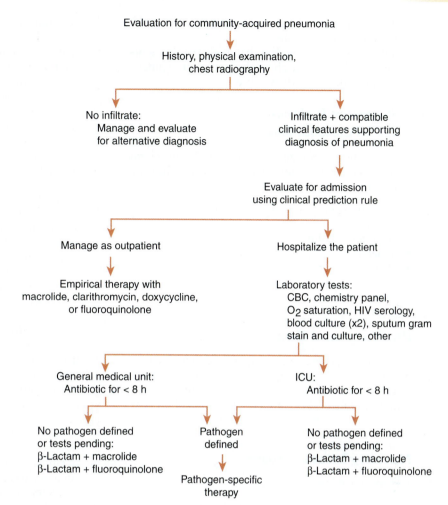

**FIGURE 23-3.** Example of a treatment algorithm for patient with suspected community-acquired pneumonia (CAP). From Bartlett, J. G., Dowell, S. F., Mandell, F. A., et al. (2000). Practice guidelines for the management of community-acquired pneumonia in adults. *Clinical Infectious Diseases, 31*(2), 347–382.

## Superinfection

Superinfection may occur with the administration of very large doses of antibiotics, such as penicillin, or with combinations of antibiotics. Superinfection may also occur in patients who have been receiving numerous courses and types of antibiotics. In such cases, bacteria may become resistant to the antibiotic therapy. If the patient improves and fever decreases after initial antibiotic therapy, but subsequently a rise in temperature occurs with increasing cough and evidence that the pneumonia has spread, a superinfection is likely. Antibiotics are changed appropriately or discontinued entirely in some cases to reevaluate the causative organisms, antibiotic resistance, and sensitivity.

## ◂◂▸▸ Nursing Process

## The Patient With Pneumonia

### Assessment

Nursing assessment is critical in detecting pneumonia. Fever, chills, or night sweats in a patient who also has respiratory symptoms should alert the nurse to the possibility of bacterial pneumonia. Respiratory assessment further identifies the clinical manifestations of pneumonia: pleuritic-type pain, fatigue, tachypnea, use of accessory muscles for breathing, bradycardia or relative bradycardia, coughing, and purulent sputum. The nurse monitors the patient for the following:

- Changes in temperature and pulse
- Amount, odor, and color of secretions
- Frequency and severity of cough
- Degree of tachypnea or shortness of breath
- Changes in physical assessment findings (primarily assessed by inspecting and auscultating the chest)
- Changes in the chest x-ray findings

In addition, it is important to assess elderly patients for unusual behavior, altered mental status, dehydration, excessive fatigue, and concomitant heart failure.

### Diagnosis

#### Nursing Diagnoses

Based on the assessment data, the major nursing diagnoses may include the following:

- Ineffective airway clearance related to copious tracheobronchial secretions
- Activity intolerance related to impaired respiratory function

- Risk for deficient fluid volume related to fever and a rapid respiratory rate
- Imbalanced nutrition: less than body requirements
- Deficient knowledge about the treatment regimen and preventive health measures

### Collaborative Problems/ Potential Complications

Based on the assessment data, collaborative problems or potential complications that may occur include the following:

- Continuing symptoms after initiation of therapy
- Shock
- Respiratory failure
- Atelectasis
- Pleural effusion
- Confusion
- Superinfection

## Planning and Goals

The major goals may include improved airway patency, rest to conserve energy, maintenance of proper fluid volume, maintenance of adequate nutrition, an understanding of the treatment protocol and preventive measures, and absence of complications.

## Nursing Interventions

### Improving Airway Patency

Removing secretions is important, because retained secretions interfere with gas exchange and may slow recovery. The nurse encourages hydration (2 to 3 L/day), because adequate hydration thins and loosens pulmonary secretions. Hydration must be achieved more slowly and with careful monitoring in patients with preexisting conditions, such as heart failure. Humidification may be used to loosen secretions and improve ventilation. A high-humidity face mask (using either compressed air or oxygen) delivers warm, humidified air to the tracheobronchial tree, helps to liquefy secretions, and relieves tracheobronchial irritation. Coughing can be initiated either voluntarily or by reflex. Lung expansion maneuvers, such as deep breathing with an incentive spirometer, may induce a cough. A directed cough may be necessary to improve airway patency. The nurse encourages the patient to perform an effective, directed cough, which includes correct positioning, a deep inspiratory maneuver, glottic closure, contraction of the expiratory muscles against the closed glottis, sudden glottic opening, and an explosive expiration. In some cases, the nurse may assist the patient by placing both hands on the lower rib cage (either anteriorly or posteriorly) to focus the patient on a slow deep breath, and then manually assisting the patient by applying constant, external pressure during the expiratory phase.

Chest physiotherapy (percussion and postural drainage) is important in loosening and mobilizing secretions (see Chapter 25). Indications for chest physiotherapy include sputum retention not responsive to spontaneous or directed cough, a history of pulmonary problems previously treated with chest physiotherapy, continued evidence of retained secretions (decreased or abnormal breath sounds, change in vital signs), abnormal chest x-ray findings consistent with atelectasis or infiltrates, and deterioration in oxygenation. The patient is placed in the proper position to drain the involved lung segments, and then the chest is percussed and vibrated either manually or with a mechanical percussor. Other devices, such as the Flutter device (Axcan Pharma), assist in secretion removal. The nurse may consult the respiratory therapy department for volume-expansion protocols and secretion-management protocols that help direct the respiratory care of the patient and match the patient's needs with appropriate treatment schedules.

After each position change, the nurse encourages the patient to breathe deeply and cough. If the patient is too weak to cough effectively, the nurse may need to remove the mucus by nasotracheal suctioning (see Chapter 25). It may take time for secretions to mobilize and move into the central airways for expectoration. Therefore, it is important for the nurse to monitor the patient for cough and sputum production after the completion of chest physiotherapy.

The nurse also administers and titrates oxygen therapy as prescribed or via protocols. The effectiveness of oxygen therapy is monitored by improvement in clinical signs and symptoms, patient comfort, and adequate oxygenation values as measured by pulse oximetry or arterial blood gas analysis.

### Promoting Rest and Conserving Energy

The nurse encourages the debilitated patient to rest and avoid overexertion and possible exacerbation of symptoms. The patient should assume a comfortable position to promote rest and breathing (eg, semi-Fowler's position) and should change positions frequently to enhance secretion clearance and ventilation and perfusion in the lungs. It is important to instruct outpatients not to overexert themselves and to engage in only moderate activity during the initial phases of treatment.

### Promoting Fluid Intake

The respiratory rate of patients with pneumonia increases because of the increased workload imposed by labored breathing and fever. An increased respiratory rate leads to an increase in insensible fluid loss during exhalation and can lead to dehydration. Therefore, it is important to encourage increased fluid intake (at least 2 L/day), unless contraindicated.

### Maintaining Nutrition

Many patients with shortness of breath and fatigue have a decreased appetite and consume only fluids. Fluids with electrolytes (commercially available drinks, such as Gatorade) may help provide fluid, calories, and electrolytes. Other nutritionally enriched drinks or shakes may be helpful. In addition, IV fluids and nutrients may be administered if necessary.

### Promoting Patients' Knowledge

The patient and family are instructed about the cause of pneumonia, management of symptoms of pneumonia, signs and symptoms that should be reported to the physician or nurse, and the need for follow-up. The patient also needs information about factors (both patient risk factors and external factors) that may have contributed to development of pneumonia and strategies to promote recovery and prevent recurrence. If the patient is hospitalized, he or she is instructed about the purpose and importance of management strategies that have been implemented and about the importance of adhering to them during and after the hospital stay. Explanations should be given simply and in language that the patient can understand. If possible, written instructions and information should be provided, and alternative formats should be provided for patients with hearing or vision loss, if necessary. Because of the severity of symptoms, the patient may require that instructions and explanations be repeated several times.

### Monitoring and Managing Potential Complications

#### CONTINUING SYMPTOMS AFTER INITIATION OF THERAPY

The patient is observed for response to antibiotic therapy; patients usually begin to respond to treatment within 24 to 48 hours after antibiotic therapy is initiated. If the patient started taking antibiotics before evaluation by culture and sensitivity of the causative organisms, antibiotics may need to be changed once the results are available. The patient is monitored for changes in physical status (deterioration of condition or resolution of symptoms) and for persistent recurrent fever, which may be a result of medication allergy (signaled possibly by a rash); medication resistance or slow response (greater than 48 hours) of the susceptible organism to therapy; superinfection; pleural effusion; or pneumonia caused by an unusual organism, such as *P. jiroveci* or *Aspergillus fumigatus*. Failure of the pneumonia to resolve or persistence of symptoms despite changes on the chest x-ray raises the suspicion of other underlying disorders, such as lung cancer. As previously described, lung cancers may invade or compress airways, causing an obstructive atelectasis that may lead to pneumonia.

In addition to monitoring for continuing symptoms of pneumonia, the nurse also monitors for other complications, such as shock and multisystem failure and atelectasis, which may develop during the first few days of antibiotic treatment.

#### SHOCK AND RESPIRATORY FAILURE

The nurse assesses for signs and symptoms of shock and respiratory failure by evaluating the patient's vital signs, pulse oximetry values, and hemodynamic monitoring parameters. The nurse reports signs of deteriorating patient status and assists in administering IV fluids and medications prescribed to combat shock. Intubation and mechanical ventilation may be required if respiratory failure occurs. Shock is described in detail in Chapter 15, and care of the patient receiving mechanical ventilation is described in Chapter 25.

#### ATELECTASIS AND PLEURAL EFFUSION

The patient is assessed for atelectasis, and preventive measures are initiated to prevent its development. If pleural effusion develops and thoracentesis is performed to remove fluid, the nurse assists in the procedure and explains it to the patient. After thoracentesis, the nurse monitors the patient for pneumothorax or recurrence of pleural effusion. If a chest tube needs to be inserted, the nurse monitors the patient's respiratory status (see Chapter 25 for more information on care of patients with chest tubes).

#### SUPERINFECTION

The patient is monitored for manifestations of superinfection (ie, minimal improvement in signs and symptoms, increase in temperature with increasing cough, increasing fremitus and adventitious breath sounds on auscultation of the lungs). These signs are reported, and the nurse assists in implementing therapy to treat superinfection.

#### CONFUSION

A patient with pneumonia is assessed for confusion and other more subtle changes in cognitive status. Confusion and changes in cognitive status resulting from pneumonia are poor prognostic signs. Confusion may be related to hypoxemia, fever, dehydration, sleep deprivation, or developing sepsis. The patient's underlying comorbid conditions may also play a part in the development of confusion. Addressing the underlying factors and ensuring patient safety are important nursing interventions.

### Promoting Home and Community-Based Care

#### TEACHING PATIENTS SELF-CARE

Depending on the severity of the pneumonia, treatment may occur in the hospital or in the outpatient setting. Patient education is crucial regardless of the setting, and the proper administration of antibiotics is important. In some instances, the patient may be initially treated with IV antibiotics as an inpatient and then discharged to continue the IV antibiotics at home. It is important that a seamless system of care be maintained for the patient from hospital to home; this includes communication between the nurses caring for the patient in both settings.

If oral antibiotics are prescribed, it is important to teach the patient about their proper administration and potential side effects. The patient should be instructed about symptoms that require contacting the health care provider: difficulty breathing, worsening cough, recurrent/increasing fever, and medication intolerance.

After the fever subsides, the patient may gradually increase activities. Fatigue and weakness may be prolonged after pneumonia, especially in the elderly. The nurse encourages breathing exercises to promote secretion clearance and volume expansion. A patient who is being treated as an outpatient should be contacted by the health care team or instructed to contact the health care provider 24 to 48 hours after starting therapy. The patient is also instructed to return to the clinic or physician's office for a follow-up chest x-ray and physical examination. Often improvement in chest x-ray findings lags behind improvement in clinical signs and symptoms.

The nurse encourages the patient to stop smoking. Smoking inhibits tracheobronchial ciliary action, which is the first line of defense of the lower respiratory tract. Smoking also irritates the mucous cells of the bronchi and inhibits the function of alveolar macrophage (scavenger) cells. The patient is instructed to avoid stress, fatigue, sudden changes in temperature, and excessive alcohol intake, all of which lower resistance to pneumonia. The nurse reviews with the patient the principles of adequate nutrition and rest, because one episode of pneumonia may make a patient susceptible to recurring respiratory tract infections.

### CONTINUING CARE

A patient who is severely debilitated or who cannot care for himself or herself may require referral for home care. During home visits, the nurse assesses the patient's physical status, monitors for complications, assesses the home environment, and reinforces previ-

---

## NURSING RESEARCH PROFILE

### Tobacco-Related Nursing Interventions

Ratner, P. A., Johnson, J. L., Richardson, C. G., et al. (2004). Efficacy of a smoking-cessation intervention for elective-surgical patients. *Research in Nursing & Health, 27*(3), 148–161.

#### Purpose
Smoking remains a major cause of morbidity and mortality in the United States. The purpose of this study was to evaluate a smoking-cessation intervention for elective surgical patients to determine whether patients could (1) abstain from cigarette use just prior to surgery, (2) sustain abstinence from tobacco in the postoperative period, and (3) maintain long-term 12-month post-surgery abstinence.

#### Design
This randomized, pretest-posttest study targeted patients admitted for presurgical assessment who smoked tobacco. Variables assessed were smoking status, smoking-cessation self-efficacy, smoking stage of change, demographic and personal information, smoking history/nicotine dependence, and psychological state. There were 120 subjects in the control group and 117 in the intervention group. Subjects in the intervention group received the following:

- A 15-minute counseling session in the preoperative assessment clinic, including one-on-one counseling, written information, nicotine replacement therapy, and phone numbers for assistance/information
- Nurse visitation within 24 hours after surgery (or when stable) for provision of reinforcement information regarding smoking cessation
- Telephone contact approximately 1 week later and weekly thereafter
- Final telephone contact to provide educational information at 16 weeks after discharge
- Telephone contact at 6 and 12 months regarding smoking habits

Subjects assigned to the control group received routine care and were seen by the study nurse immediately after surgery and contacted by telephone at 6 and 12 months.

#### Findings
Subjects in the intervention group were more likely to abstain from smoking prior to surgery ($P = .003$) than subjects in the control group and were more likely to abstain from smoking at 6 months after surgery (31.2% versus 20.2%; however, the unadjusted effect of treatment was not statistically significant). There was no significant difference in the abstinence rates at 12 months in subjects in the two groups (18.8% versus 19.2%).

#### Nursing Implications
Nurses have frequent contacts with active smokers in inpatient and outpatient settings. Therefore, nurses could have a tremendous impact on smoking prevention and cessation. This study demonstrates that educating patients prior to surgery may be an excellent strategy to begin the process of smoking cessation. In addition, these results show that continued contact and support with patients may increase the probability of cessation. Nurses need advanced education regarding evidence-based guidelines for smoking cessation techniques. Nurses need to raise the issue of tobacco use with patients, discuss smoking cessation, and provide potential resources that are accessible to patients.

ous teaching. The nurse evaluates the patient's adherence to the therapeutic regimen (ie, taking medications as prescribed, performing breathing exercises, consuming adequate fluid and dietary intake, and avoiding smoking, alcohol, and excessive activity). The nurse stresses to the patient and family the importance of monitoring for complications or exacerbation of the pneumonia. The nurse encourages the patient to obtain an influenza vaccination at the prescribed times, because influenza increases susceptibility to secondary bacterial pneumonia, especially that caused by staphylococci, *H. influenzae,* and *S. pneumoniae* (CDC, 2004e). The nurse also urges the patient to seek medical advice about receiving the vaccine (Pneumovax) against *S. pneumoniae.*

## Evaluation

### Expected Patient Outcomes

Expected patient outcomes may include the following:

1. Demonstrates improved airway patency, as evidenced by adequate oxygenation by pulse oximetry or arterial blood gas analysis, normal temperature, normal breath sounds, and effective coughing
2. Rests and conserves energy by limiting activities and remaining in bed while symptomatic and then slowly increasing activities
3. Maintains adequate hydration, as evidenced by an adequate fluid intake and urine output and normal skin turgor
4. Consumes adequate dietary intake, as evidenced by maintenance or increase in body weight without excess fluid gain
5. States explanation for management strategies
6. Complies with management strategies
7. Exhibits no complications
    a. Exhibits acceptable vital signs, pulse oximetry, and arterial blood gas measurements
    b. Reports productive cough that diminishes over time
    c. Has absence of signs or symptoms of shock, respiratory failure, or pleural effusion
    d. Remains oriented and aware of surroundings
    e. Maintains or increases weight
8. Complies with treatment protocol and prevention strategies

## Severe Acute Respiratory Syndrome

Severe acute respiratory syndrome (SARS) is a viral respiratory illness caused by a coronavirus, called SARS-associated coronavirus (Denison, 2004). SARS was first reported in Asia in February 2003. The illness quickly spread to countries in North America, South America, Europe, and Asia. The World Health Organization (WHO) reported that 8098 people worldwide became sick with SARS during the 2003 outbreak, and 774 died (CDC, 2004c).

The SARS-associated coronavirus is transmitted via respiratory droplets when an infected person coughs or sneezes; the droplets may be deposited on the mucous membranes (mouth, nose, eyes) of a nearby person. The virus may also be spread when a person touches a surface or object contaminated by the droplets and then touches his or her mucous membranes. The SARS virus may be transmitted in other ways, but those methods of transmission are unknown at this time.

The constellation of symptoms characteristic of SARS are a high fever in association with headache, overall discomfort, and body aches. Mild respiratory symptoms may also be present. Approximately 10% to 20% of patients develop diarrhea. After 2 to 7 days, a dry cough may develop, which often includes progressive hypoxemia and subsequent pneumonia. Based on available information, SARS is most likely to be contagious only when symptoms are present; patients are most contagious during the second week of illness. It is recommended that people with SARS limit interactions outside the home until 10 days after the fever is no longer present and respiratory symptoms have improved. At this time, treatment of SARS is the same for a severe community-acquired atypical pneumonia (CDC, 2004c).

Infection control measures designed to limit transmission of SARS are a priority. In health care settings, the general CDC guidelines for infection control in health care facilities should be followed; in addition, specific strategies for SARS should be in place regarding use of negative pressure isolation rooms, personal protective equipment, hand hygiene, environmental cleaning and disinfection techniques, and source control measures to contain patients' secretions (CDC, 2003a; Levy, Baylor, Bernard, et al., 2005).

## Pulmonary Tuberculosis

Tuberculosis (TB) is an infectious disease that primarily affects the lung parenchyma. It also may be transmitted to other parts of the body, including the meninges, kidneys, bones, and lymph nodes. The primary infectious agent, *M. tuberculosis,* is an acid-fast aerobic rod that grows slowly and is sensitive to heat and ultraviolet light. *Mycobacterium bovis* and *Mycobacterium avium* have rarely been associated with the development of a TB infection.

TB is a worldwide public health problem, and mortality and morbidity rates continue to rise. *M. tuberculosis* infects an estimated one third of the world's population and remains the leading cause of death from infectious disease in the world. The World Health Organization estimates that TB is the cause of death for 11% of all patients with AIDS (Corbett, Walt, Walker, et al., 2003). TB is closely associated with poverty, malnutrition, overcrowding, substandard housing, and inadequate health care.

In 1952, anti-TB medications were introduced, and the rate of reported cases of TB in the United States declined an average of 6% each year between 1953 and 1985. It was thought that, by the early part of the 21st century, TB might be eliminated in the United States. However, since 1985 the trend has reversed, and the number of cases has increased. This change has been attributed to several factors, including increased immigration, the human immunodeficiency virus (HIV) epidemic, the emergence of multidrug-resistant strains of TB, increased homelessness, decreased interest and detection by health care providers, and inadequate funding of the United States public health system. Almost 15,000 cases of TB are reported annually to the CDC (2005). Progress toward TB elimination in the United States focuses on programs that provide services to foreign-born persons with latent TB infection, collaborative efforts that reduce the burden of TB globally, and intensified TB control efforts that address higher rates in the population of non-Hispanic blacks born in the United States (CDC, 2003c).

## Transmission and Risk Factors

TB spreads from person to person by airborne transmission. An infected person releases droplet nuclei (usually particles 1 to 5 μm in diameter) through talking, coughing, sneezing, laughing, or singing. Larger droplets settle; smaller droplets remain suspended in the air and are inhaled by a susceptible person. Risk factors for TB are listed in Chart 23-3.

> **CHART 23-3**
>
>
> ### Risk Factors for Tuberculosis
>
> - Close contact with someone who has active TB. Inhalation of airborne nuclei from an infected person is proportional to the amount of time spent in the same air space, the proximity of the person, and the degree of ventilation.
> - Immunocompromised status (eg, those with HIV infection, cancer, transplanted organs, and prolonged high-dose corticosteroid therapy)
> - Substance abuse (IV/injection drug users and alcoholics)
> - Any person without adequate health care (the homeless; impoverished; minorities, particularly children under age 15 y and young adults between ages 15 and 44 y)
> - Preexisting medical conditions or special treatment (eg, diabetes, chronic renal failure, malnourishment, selected malignancies, hemodialysis, transplanted organ, gastrectomy, jejunoileal bypass)
> - Immigration from countries with a high prevalence of TB (southeastern Asia, Africa, Latin America, Caribbean)
> - Institutionalization (eg, long-term care facilities, psychiatric institutions, prisons)
> - Living in overcrowded, substandard housing
> - Being a health care worker performing high-risk activities: administration of aerosolized pentamidine and other medications, sputum induction procedures, bronchoscopy, suctioning, coughing procedures, caring for the immunosuppressed patient, home care with the high-risk population, and administering anesthesia, and related procedures (eg, intubation, suctioning)

Chart 23-4 summarizes the CDC's recommendations for prevention of TB transmission in health care settings.

## Pathophysiology

TB begins when a susceptible person inhales mycobacteria and becomes infected. The bacteria are transmitted through the airways to the alveoli, where they are deposited and begin to multiply. The bacilli also are transported via the lymph system and bloodstream to other parts of the body (kidneys, bones, cerebral cortex) and other areas of the lungs (upper lobes). The body's immune system responds by initiating an inflammatory reaction. Phagocytes (neutrophils and macrophages) engulf many of the bacteria, and TB-specific lymphocytes lyse (destroy) the bacilli and normal tissue. This tissue reaction results in the accumulation of exudate in the alveoli, causing bronchopneumonia. The initial infection usually occurs 2 to 10 weeks after exposure.

Granulomas, new tissue masses of live and dead bacilli, are surrounded by macrophages, which form a protective wall. They are then transformed to a fibrous tissue mass, the central portion of which is called a Ghon tubercle. The material (bacteria and macrophages) becomes necrotic, forming a cheesy mass. This mass may become calcified and form a collagenous scar. At this point, the bacteria become dormant, and there is no further progression of active disease.

After initial exposure and infection, active disease may develop because of a compromised or inadequate immune system response. Active disease also may occur with reinfection and activation of dormant bacteria. In this case, the Ghon tubercle ulcerates, releasing the cheesy material into the bronchi. The bacteria then become airborne, resulting in further spread of the disease. Then the ulcerated tubercle heals and forms scar tissue. This causes the infected lung to become more inflamed, resulting in further development of bronchopneumonia and tubercle formation.

Unless the process is arrested, it spreads slowly downward to the hilum of the lungs and later extends to adjacent lobes. The process may be prolonged and is characterized by long remissions when the disease is arrested, followed by periods of renewed activity. Approximately 10% of people who are initially infected develop active disease. Some people develop reactivation TB (also called adult-type TB). This type of TB results from a breakdown of the host defenses. It most commonly occurs in the lungs, usually in the apical or posterior segments of the upper lobes or the superior segments of the lower lobes.

## Clinical Manifestations

The signs and symptoms of pulmonary TB are insidious. Most patients have a low-grade fever, cough, night sweats, fatigue, and weight loss. The cough may be nonproductive, or mucopurulent sputum may be expectorated. Hemoptysis also may occur. Both the systemic and the pulmonary symptoms are chronic and may have been present for weeks to months. Elderly patients usually present with less pronounced symptoms than younger patients do. Extrapulmonary disease occurs in up to 16% of cases in the United States. In patients with AIDS, extrapulmonary disease is more prevalent.

> **CHART 23-4**
>
> ### CDC Recommendations for Preventing Transmission of Tuberculosis in Health Care Settings
>
> 1. Early identification and treatment of persons with active TB
>    a. Maintain a high index of suspicion for TB to identify cases rapidly.
>    b. Promptly initiate effective multidrug anti-TB therapy based on clinical and drug-resistance surveillance data.
> 2. Prevention of spread of infectious droplet nuclei by source control methods and by reduction of microbial contamination of indoor air
>    a. Initiate acid-fast bacilli (AFB) isolation precautions immediately for all patients who are suspected or confirmed to have active TB and who may be infectious. AFB isolation precautions include use of a private room with negative pressure in relation to surrounding areas and a minimum of six air exchanges per hour. Air from the room should be exhausted directly to the outside. Use of ultraviolet lamps and/or high-efficiency particulate air filters to supplement ventilation may be considered.
>    b. Persons entering the AFB isolation room should use disposable particulate respirators that fit snugly around the face.
>    c. Continue AFB isolation precautions until there is clinical evidence of reduced infectiousness (ie, cough has substantially decreased, and the number of organisms on sequential sputum smears is decreasing). If drug resistance is suspected or confirmed, continue AFB precautions until the sputum smear is negative for AFB.
>    d. Use special precautions during cough-inducing procedures.
> 3. Surveillance for TB transmission
>    a. Maintain surveillance for TB infection among health care workers (HCWs) by routine, periodic tuberculin skin testing. Recommend appropriate preventive therapy for HCWs when indicated.
>    b. Maintain surveillance for TB cases among patients and HCWs.
>    c. Promptly initiate contact investigation procedures among HCWs, patients, and visitors exposed to an untreated, or ineffectively treated, patient with infectious TB for whom appropriate AFB procedures are not in place. Recommend appropriate therapy or preventive therapy for contacts with disease or TB infection without current disease. Therapeutic regimens should be chosen based on the clinical history and local drug-resistance surveillance data.

## Assessment and Diagnostic Findings

A complete history, physical examination, tuberculin skin test, chest x-ray, acid-fast bacillus smear, and sputum culture are used to diagnose TB. If the patient is infected with TB, the chest x-ray usually reveals lesions in the upper lobes, and the acid-fast bacillus smear contains mycobacteria.

### Tuberculin Skin Test

The Mantoux test is used to determine whether a person has been infected with the TB bacillus. The Mantoux test is a standardized procedure and should be performed only by those trained in its administration and reading. Tubercle bacillus extract (tuberculin), purified protein derivative (PPD), is injected into the intradermal layer of the inner aspect of the forearm, approximately 4 inches below the elbow (Fig. 23-4). Intermediate-strength PPD, in a tuberculin syringe with a half-inch 26- or 27-gauge needle, is used. The needle, with the bevel facing up, is inserted beneath the skin. Then 0.1 mL of PPD is injected, creating an elevation in the skin, a wheal or bleb. The site, antigen name, strength, lot number, date, and time of the test are recorded. The test result is read 48 to 72 hours after injection. Tests read after 72 hours tend to underestimate the true size of **induration** (hardening). A delayed localized reaction indicates that the person is sensitive to tuberculin.

A reaction occurs when both induration and erythema (redness) are present. After the area is inspected for induration, it is lightly palpated across the injection site, from the area of normal skin to the margins of the induration. The diameter of the induration (not erythema) is measured in millimeters at its widest part (see Fig. 23-4), and the size of the induration is documented. Erythema without induration is not considered significant.

### Interpretation of Results

The size of the induration determines the significance of the reaction. A reaction of 0 to 4 mm is considered not significant; a reaction of 5 mm or greater may be significant in people who are considered to be at risk. An induration of 10 mm or greater is usually considered significant in people who have normal or mildly impaired immunity. A significant reaction indicates past exposure to *M. tuberculosis* or vaccination with bacille Calmette-Guérin (BCG) vaccine. The BCG vaccine is given to produce a greater resistance to development of TB. It is effective in up to 76% of people who receive it. The BCG vaccine is used in Europe and Latin America but not routinely in the United States.

A reaction of 5 mm or greater is defined as positive in patients who are HIV-positive or have HIV risk factors and are of unknown HIV status; in those who are close contacts

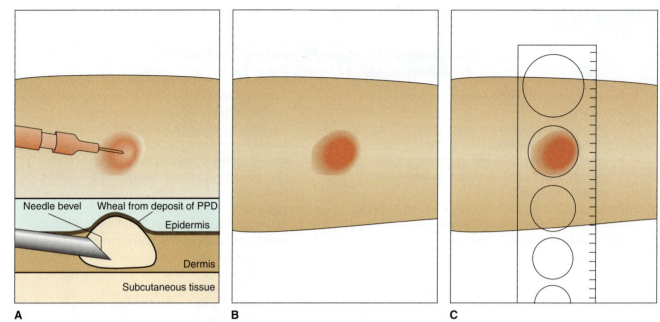

**FIGURE 23-4.** The Mantoux test for tuberculosis. **(A)** Correct technique for inserting the needle involves depositing the PPD subcutaneously with the needle bevel facing upward. **(B)** The reaction to the Mantoux test usually consists of a wheal, a hivelike, firm welt. **(C)** To determine the extent of the reaction, the wheal is measured using a commercially prepared gauge. Interpretation of the Mantoux test is discussed in the text.

of someone with active TB; and in those who have chest x-ray results consistent with TB.

A significant (positive) reaction does not necessarily mean that active disease is present in the body. More than 90% of people who are tuberculin-significant reactors do not develop clinical TB. However, all significant reactors are candidates for active TB. In general, the more intense the reaction, the greater the likelihood of an active infection.

A nonsignificant (negative) skin test does not exclude TB infection or disease, because patients who are immunosuppressed cannot develop an immune response that is adequate to produce a positive skin test. This is referred to as anergy.

### QuantiFERON-TB Gold (QFT-G) Test

In 2005, the U.S. Food and Drug Administration approved a new test for the detection of TB. The QuantiFERON-TB Gold (QFT-G) test is an enzyme-linked immunosorbent assay (ELISA) that detects the release of interferon-gamma by white blood cells when the blood of a patient with TB is incubated with peptides similar to those in *M. tuberculosis*. The results of the QFT-G test are available in less than 24 hours and are not affected by prior vaccination with BCG. The test results are also less influenced than those of TST by previous infection with nontuberculous mycobacteria. The CDC has recommended that the QFT-G be used in place of, rather than in addition to, the TST, although the new test is not yet widely used. Additional studies of the QFT-G test are under way to evaluate the use of this new diagnostic test (CDC, 2005).

### Classification

Data from the history, physical examination, TB test, chest x-ray, and microbiologic studies are used to classify TB into one of five classes. A classification scheme provides public health officials with a systematic way to monitor epidemiology and treatment of the disease (American Thoracic Society, 2000).

- Class 0: no exposure; no infection
- Class 1: exposure; no evidence of infection
- Class 2: latent infection; no disease (eg, positive PPD reaction but no clinical evidence of active TB)
- Class 3: disease; clinically active
- Class 4: disease; not clinically active
- Class 5: suspected disease; diagnosis pending

### Gerontologic Considerations

TB may have atypical manifestations in elderly patients, whose symptoms may include unusual behavior and altered mental status, fever, anorexia, and weight loss. In many elderly patients, the tuberculin skin test produces no reaction (loss of immunologic memory) or delayed reactivity for up to 1 week (recall phenomenon). A second skin test is performed in 1 to 2 weeks.

### Medical Management

Pulmonary TB is treated primarily with chemotherapeutic agents (antituberculosis agents) for 6 to 12 months. A prolonged treatment duration is necessary to ensure eradication of the organisms and to prevent relapse. The continuing (since the 1950s) and increasing resistance of *M. tuberculosis* to TB medications is a worldwide concern and challenge in TB therapy. Several types of drug resistance must be considered when planning effective therapy:

- Primary drug resistance: resistance to one of the first-line antituberculosis agents in people who have not had previous treatment
- Secondary or acquired drug resistance: resistance to one or more antituberculosis agents in patients undergoing therapy
- Multidrug resistance: resistance to two agents, isoniazid (INH) and rifampin. The populations at greatest risk for multidrug resistance are those who are HIV-positive, institutionalized, or homeless.

The increasing prevalence of drug resistance points out the need to begin TB treatment with four or more medications, to ensure completion of therapy, and to develop and evaluate new anti-TB medications.

### Pharmacologic Therapy

In current TB therapy, four first-line medications are used (Table 23-3), INH, rifampin, pyrazinamide, and ethambutol. Combination medications, such as INH and rifampin (Rifamate) or INH, pyrazinamide, and rifampin (Rifater) and medications administered twice a week (eg, rifapentine) are available to help improve patient adherence. Capreomycin, ethionamide, para-aminosalicylate sodium, and cycloserine are second-line medications. Additional potentially effective medications include other aminoglycosides, quinolones, rifabutin, clofazimine, and combinations of medications.

### TABLE 23-3  First-Line Antituberculosis Medications

| Commonly Used Agents | Adult Daily Dosage* | Most Common Side Effects | Drug Interactions† | Remarks* |
|---|---|---|---|---|
| Isoniazid (INH) | 5 mg/kg (300 mg maximum daily) | Peripheral neuritis, hepatic enzyme elevation, hepatitis, hypersensitivity | Phenytoin—synergistic Antabuse Alcohol | Bactericidal. Pyridoxine is used as prophylaxis for neuritis. Monitor AST and ALT. |
| Rifampin (Rifadin) | 10 mg/kg (600 mg maximum daily) | Hepatitis, febrile reaction, purpura (rare), nausea, vomiting | Rifampin increases metabolism of oral contraceptives, quinidine, corticosteroids, coumarin derivatives and methadone, digoxin, oral hypoglycemics; PAS may interfere with absorption of rifampin. | Bactericidal. Orange urine and other body secretions. Discoloring of contact lenses. Monitor AST and ALT. |
| Rifabutin (Mycobutin) | 5 mg/kg (300 mg maximum daily) | | | |
| Rifapentine (Priftin) | 10 mg/kg (600 mg twice weekly) | Hepatotoxicity, thrombocytopenia | Avoid protease inhibitors | Orange-red coloration of body secretions, contact lenses, dentures. Use with caution in elderly or in those with renal disease. |
| Pyrazinamide | 15 to 30 mg/kg (2.0 g maximum daily)* | Hyperuricemia, hepatotoxicity, skin rash, arthralgias, GI distress | | Bactericidal. Monitor uric acid, AST, ALT. |
| Ethambutol (Myambutol) | 15 to 25 mg/kg (no maximum daily dose, but base on lean body wt)* | Optic neuritis (may lead to blindness; very rare at 15 mg/kg), skin rash | | Bacteriostatic. Use with caution with renal disease or when eye testing is not feasible. Monitor visual acuity, color discrimination.‡ |
| Combinations: INH + rifampin (eg, Rifamate) | 150-mg & 300-mg caps (2 caps daily) | | | |

*Check product labeling for detailed information on dose, contraindications, drug interaction, adverse reactions, and monitoring.
† Refer to current literature, particularly on rifampin, because it increases hepatic microenzymes and therefore interacts with many drugs.
‡ Initial examination should be performed at start of treatment.

Recommended treatment guidelines for newly diagnosed cases of pulmonary TB (CDC, 2003b) have two parts: an initial treatment phase and a continuation phase. The initial phase consists of a multiple-medication regimen of INH, rifampin, pyrazinamide, and ethambutol. This initial intensive-treatment regimen is administered daily for 8 weeks, after which options for the continuation phase of treatment include INH and rifampin or INH and rifapentine. The continuation course of treatment lasts for an additional 4 or 7 months. The 4-month period is used for the large majority of patients (CDC, 2003b). The 7-month period is recommended for patients with cavitary pulmonary TB whose sputum culture after the initial 2 months of treatment is positive, for those whose initial phase of treatment did not include pyrazinamide (PZA), and for those being treated once weekly with INH and rifapentine whose sputum culture is positive at the end of the initial phase of treatment. People are considered noninfectious after 2 to 3 weeks of continuous medication therapy. Vitamin B (pyridoxine) is usually administered with INH to prevent INH-associated peripheral neuropathy (see Table 23-3). The total number of doses taken, not simply the duration of treatment, more accurately determines whether a course of therapy has been completed.

INH also may be used as a prophylactic (preventive) measure for people who are at risk for significant disease, including

- Household family members of patients with active disease
- Patients with HIV infection who have a PPD test reaction with 5 mm of induration or more
- Patients with fibrotic lesions suggestive of old TB detected on a chest x-ray and a PPD reaction with 5 mm of induration or more
- Patients whose current PPD test results show a change from former test results, suggesting recent exposure to TB and possible infection (skin test converters)
- Users of IV/injection drugs who have PPD test results with 10 mm of induration or more
- Patients with high-risk comorbid conditions and a PPD result with 10 mm of induration or more

Other candidates for preventive INH therapy are those 35 years or younger who have PPD test results with 10 mm of induration or more and one of the following criteria:

- Foreign-born individuals from countries with a high prevalence of TB
- High-risk, medically underserved populations
- Institutionalized patients

Prophylactic INH treatment involves taking daily doses for 6 to 12 months. Liver enzymes, blood urea nitrogen (BUN), and creatinine levels are monitored monthly. Sputum culture results are monitored for acid-fast bacillus to evaluate the effectiveness of treatment and the patient's adherence to the treatment regimen.

In 1998, the federal Advisory Council for the Elimination of Tuberculosis published recommendations for the development of TB vaccines. The recommendations include a focus on a "postinfection vaccine" to prevent people who are infected with TB from developing active disease. To date, this vaccine has not become clinically available. Recommendations regarding the treatment of latent TB infection were released in 2000 and updated in 2003 and 2005 (CDC, 2003b, 2005a). The 2000 recommendations focused on treating latent infections for a shorter period of time. The CDC released case reports of liver injury associated with the 2-month rifampin-pyrazinamide (RIF-PZA) dosing regimen in August 2001. RIF plus PZA is no longer recommended for treatment of latent tuberculosis infection (CDC, 2003b). Nine months of daily INH remains the preferred treatment, and 4 months of daily RIF is an acceptable alternative.

## ◄◄►► Nursing Process

### The Patient With Tuberculosis

#### Assessment

The nurse performs a complete history and physical examination. Clinical manifestations of fever, anorexia, weight loss, night sweats, fatigue, cough, and sputum production prompt a more thorough assessment of respiratory function—for example, assessing the lungs for consolidation by evaluating breath sounds (diminished, bronchial sounds, crackles), fremitus, egophony, and dullness on percussion. Enlarged, painful lymph nodes may be palpated as well. The nurse also assesses the patient's living arrangements, perceptions and understanding of TB and its treatment, and readiness to learn.

#### Diagnosis

##### Nursing Diagnoses

Based on the assessment data, nursing diagnoses may include the following:

- Ineffective airway clearance related to copious tracheobronchial secretions
- Deficient knowledge about treatment regimen and preventive health measures and related ineffective individual management of the therapeutic regimen (noncompliance)
- Activity intolerance related to fatigue, altered nutritional status, and fever

##### Collaborative Problems/ Potential Complications

Based on the assessment data, collaborative problems or potential complications that may occur include the following:

- Malnutrition
- Adverse side effects of medication therapy: hepatitis, neurologic changes (deafness or neuritis), skin rash, gastrointestinal upset
- Multidrug resistance
- Spread of TB infection (miliary TB)

## Planning and Goals

The major goals include maintenance of a patent airway, increased knowledge about the disease and treatment regimen and adherence to the medication regimen, increased activity tolerance, and absence of complications.

## Nursing Interventions

### Promoting Airway Clearance

Copious secretions obstruct the airways in many patients with TB and interfere with adequate gas exchange. Increasing the fluid intake promotes systemic hydration and serves as an effective expectorant. The nurse instructs the patient about correct positioning to facilitate airway drainage (postural drainage); this is described in Chapter 25.

### Advocating Adherence to Treatment Regimen

The multiple-medication regimen that the patient must follow can be quite complex. Understanding of the medications, schedule, and side effects is important. The patient must understand that TB is a communicable disease and that taking medications is the most effective means of preventing transmission. The major reason treatment fails is that patients do not take their medications regularly and for the prescribed duration. The nurse carefully instructs the patient about important hygiene measures, including mouth care, covering the mouth and nose when coughing and sneezing, proper disposal of tissues, and handwashing. The nurse's positive reinforcement and monitoring of the patient's adherence are important follow-up measures.

### Promoting Activity and Adequate Nutrition

Patients with TB are often debilitated from prolonged chronic illness and impaired nutritional status. The nurse plans a progressive activity schedule that focuses on increasing activity tolerance and muscle strength. Anorexia, weight loss, and malnutrition are common in patients with TB. The patient's willingness to eat may be altered by fatigue from excessive coughing, sputum production, chest pain, generalized debilitated state, or cost, if the patient has few resources. A nutritional plan that allows for small, frequent meals may be required. Liquid nutritional supplements may assist in meeting basic caloric requirements.

### Monitoring and Managing Potential Complications

#### MALNUTRITION

Malnutrition may be a consequence of the patient's lifestyle, lack of knowledge about adequate nutrition and its role in health maintenance, lack of resources, fatigue, or lack of appetite because of coughing and mucus production. To counter the effects of these factors, the nurse collaborates with the dietitian, physician, social worker, family, and patient to identify strategies to ensure an adequate nutritional intake and availability of nutritious food. Identifying facilities (eg, shelters, soup kitchens, Meals on Wheels) that provide meals in the patient's neighborhood may increase the likelihood that the patient with limited resources and energy will have access to a more nutritious intake. High-calorie nutritional supplements may be suggested as a strategy for increasing dietary intake using food products normally found in the home. Purchasing food supplements may be beyond the patient's budget, but dietitians can help develop recipes to increase caloric intake despite minimal resources.

#### SIDE EFFECTS OF MEDICATION THERAPY

It is important to assess medication side effects, because they are often a reason why patients fail to adhere to the prescribed medication regimen. Efforts are made to reduce the side effects and to motivate the patient to take the medications as prescribed.

The nurse instructs the patient to take the medication either on an empty stomach or at least 1 hour before meals, because food interferes with medication absorption (although taking medications on an empty stomach frequently results in gastrointestinal upset). Patients taking INH should avoid foods that contain tyramine and histamine (tuna, aged cheese, red wine, soy sauce, yeast extracts), because eating them while taking INH may result in headache, flushing, hypotension, lightheadedness, palpitations, and diaphoresis.

In addition, rifampin can increase the metabolism of certain other medications, making them less effective. These medications include beta-blockers, oral anticoagulants such as warfarin (Coumadin), digoxin, quinidine, corticosteroids, oral hypoglycemic agents, oral contraceptives, theophylline, and verapamil (Calan, Isoptin). This issue should be discussed with the physician and pharmacist so that medication dosages can be adjusted accordingly. The nurse informs the patient that rifampin may discolor contact lenses and that the patient may want to wear eyeglasses during treatment. The nurse monitors for other side effects of anti-TB medications, including hepatitis, neurologic changes (hearing loss, neuritis), and rash. Liver enzymes, BUN, and serum creatinine levels are monitored to detect changes in liver and kidney function. Sputum culture results are monitored for acid-fast bacilli to evaluate the effectiveness of the treatment regimen and adherence to therapy.

#### MULTIDRUG RESISTANCE

The nurse carefully monitors vital signs and observes for spikes in temperature or changes in the patient's clinical status. Changes in the patient's respiratory status are reported to the primary health care provider. The nurse instructs the patient about the risk of drug resistance if the medication regimen is not strictly and continuously followed.

### SPREAD OF TUBERCULOSIS INFECTION

Spread or dissemination of TB infection to nonpulmonary sites of the body is known as miliary TB. It is the result of invasion of the bloodstream by the tubercle bacillus (Ghon tubercle). Usually it results from late reactivation of a dormant infection in the lung or elsewhere. The origin of the bacilli that enter the bloodstream is either a chronic focus that has ulcerated into a blood vessel or multitudes of miliary tubercles lining the inner surface of the thoracic duct. The organisms migrate from these foci into the bloodstream, are carried throughout the body, and disseminate throughout all tissues, with tiny miliary tubercles developing in the lungs, spleen, liver, kidneys, meninges, and other organs.

The clinical course of miliary TB may vary from an acute, rapidly progressive infection with high fever to a slowly developing process with low-grade fever, anemia, and debilitation. At first, there may be no localizing signs except an enlarged spleen and a reduced number of leukocytes. However, within a few weeks, the chest x-ray reveals small densities scattered diffusely throughout both lung fields; these are the miliary tubercles, which gradually grow.

The possibility of spread to nonpulmonary sites in the body requires careful monitoring for this very serious form of TB. The nurse monitors vital signs and observes for spikes in temperature as well as changes in renal and cognitive function. Few physical signs may be elicited on physical examination of the chest, but at this stage the patient has a severe cough and dyspnea. Treatment of miliary TB is the same as for pulmonary TB.

## Promoting Home and Community-Based Care

### TEACHING PATIENTS SELF-CARE

The nurse plays a vital role in caring for the patient with TB and the family, which includes assessing the patient's ability to continue therapy at home. The nurse instructs the patient and family about infection control procedures, such as proper disposal of tissues, covering the mouth during coughing, and frequent handwashing. Assessment of the patient's adherence to the medication regimen is essential because of the risk of emergence of resistance if the regimen is not followed faithfully. In some cases, when the patient's ability to comply with the medication regimen is in question, referral to an outpatient clinic for daily medication administration may be required. This is referred to as directly observed therapy (DOT).

### CONTINUING CARE

The nurse evaluates the patient's environment, including the home or workplace and social setting, to identify other people who may have been in contact with the patient during the infectious stage. It is important to arrange follow-up screening for any such contacts. The nurse who has contact with a patient in the home, shelter, hospital, clinic, or work setting continues to assess the patient's physical and psychological status and ability to adhere to the prescribed treatment. The nurse also assesses the patient for adverse effects of medications and adherence to the therapeutic regimen (eg, taking medications as prescribed, practicing safe hygiene, consuming a nutritious and adequate diet, and participating in an appropriate level of activity). In addition, the nurse reinforces previous teaching, emphasizes the importance of keeping scheduled appointments with the primary health care provider, and reminds the patient about the importance of other health promotion activities and recommended health screening.

## Evaluation

### Expected Patient Outcomes

Expected patient outcomes may include the following:

1. Maintains a patent airway by managing secretions with hydration, humidification, coughing, and postural drainage
2. Demonstrates an adequate level of knowledge
    a. Lists medications by name and the correct schedule for taking them
    b. Identifies expected side effects of medications
    c. Identifies how and when to contact health care provider
3. Adheres to treatment regimen by taking medications as prescribed and reporting for follow-up screening
4. Participates in preventive measures
    a. Disposes of used tissues properly
    b. Encourages people who are close contacts to undergo testing
    c. Adheres to handwashing or hand hygiene recommendations
5. Maintains activity schedule
6. Exhibits no complications
    a. Maintains adequate weight or gains weight if indicated
    b. Exhibits normal results of tests of liver and kidney function
7. Takes steps to minimize side effects of medications
    a. Takes supplemental vitamins (vitamin B), as prescribed, to minimize peripheral neuropathy
    b. Avoids use of alcohol
    c. Avoids foods containing tyramine and histamine
    d. Has regular physical examinations and blood tests to evaluate liver and kidney function, neuropathy, hearing and visual acuity

# Lung Abscess

A lung abscess is a localized necrotic lesion of the lung parenchyma containing purulent material that collapses and forms a cavity. It is generally caused by aspiration of anaerobic bacteria. In a lung abscess, by definition, the chest x-ray demonstrates a cavity of at least 2 cm. Patients who have impaired cough reflexes and cannot close the glottis, and those with swallowing difficulties, are at risk for aspiration of foreign material and development of a lung abscess. Other at-risk patients include those with central nervous system disorders (eg, seizure, stroke), drug addiction, alcoholism, esophageal disease, or compromised immune function; patients without teeth and those receiving nasogastric tube feedings; and patients with an altered state of consciousness due to anesthesia.

## Pathophysiology

Most lung abscesses are a complication of bacterial pneumonia or are caused by aspiration of oral anaerobes into the lung. Abscesses also may occur secondary to mechanical or functional obstruction of the bronchi by a tumor, foreign body, or bronchial stenosis, or from necrotizing pneumonias, TB, pulmonary embolism (PE), or chest trauma.

Most lung abscesses are found in areas of the lung that may be affected by aspiration. The site of the lung abscess is related to gravity and is determined by position. For patients who are confined to bed, the posterior segment of an upper lobe and the superior segment of the lower lobe are the most common areas in which lung abscess occurs. However, atypical presentations may occur, depending on the position of the patient when the aspiration occurred.

Initially, the cavity in the lung may or may not extend directly into a bronchus. Eventually, the abscess becomes surrounded, or encapsulated, by a wall of fibrous tissue. The necrotic process may extend until it reaches the lumen of a bronchus or the pleural space and establishes communication with the respiratory tract, the pleural cavity, or both. If the bronchus is involved, the purulent contents are expectorated continuously in the form of sputum. If the pleura is involved, an empyema results. A communication or connection between the bronchus and pleura is known as a bronchopleural fistula.

The organisms frequently associated with lung abscesses are *S. aureus, Klebsiella,* and other gram-negative species. However, anaerobic organisms may also be present. The organisms vary depending on the underlying predisposing factors.

## Clinical Manifestations

The clinical manifestations of a lung abscess may vary from a mild productive cough to acute illness. Most patients have a fever and a productive cough with moderate to copious amounts of foul-smelling, sometimes bloody, sputum. The fever and cough may develop insidiously and may have been present for several weeks before diagnosis. Leukocytosis may be present. Pleurisy or dull chest pain, dyspnea, weakness, anorexia, and weight loss are common.

## Assessment and Diagnostic Findings

Physical examination of the chest may reveal dullness on percussion and decreased or absent breath sounds with an intermittent **pleural friction rub** (grating or rubbing sound) on auscultation. Crackles may be present. Confirmation of the diagnosis is made by chest x-ray, sputum culture, and, in some cases, fiberoptic bronchoscopy. The chest x-ray reveals an infiltrate with an air–fluid level. A computed tomography (CT) scan of the chest may be required to provide more detailed pictures of different cross-sectional areas of the lung.

## Prevention

The following measures reduce the risk of lung abscess:

- Appropriate antibiotic therapy before any dental procedures in patients who must have teeth extracted while their gums and teeth are infected
- Adequate dental and oral hygiene, because anaerobic bacteria play a role in the pathogenesis of lung abscess
- Appropriate antimicrobial therapy for patients with pneumonia

## Medical Management

The findings of the history, physical examination, chest x-ray, and sputum culture indicate the type of organism and the treatment required. Adequate drainage of the lung abscess may be achieved through postural drainage and chest physiotherapy. Patients should be assessed for an adequate cough. Some patients require insertion of a percutaneous chest catheter for long-term drainage of the abscess. Therapeutic use of bronchoscopy to drain an abscess is uncommon. A diet high in protein and calories is necessary, because chronic infection is associated with a catabolic state, necessitating increased intake of calories and protein to facilitate healing. Surgical intervention is rare, but pulmonary resection (lobectomy) is performed if massive **hemoptysis** (coughing up of blood) occurs or if there is little or no response to medical management.

### Pharmacologic Therapy

IV antimicrobial therapy depends on the results of the sputum culture and sensitivity and is administered for an extended period. Antibiotics used include clindamycin (Cleocin), meropenem (Merrem), or piperacillin/tazobactam (Zosyn). Large IV doses are usually required, because the antibiotic must penetrate the necrotic tissue and the fluid in the abscess. The IV dose is continued until there is evidence of symptom improvement.

Long-term therapy with oral antibiotics replaces IV therapy after the patient shows signs of improvement (usually 3 to 5 days). Improvement is demonstrated by normal temperature, decreased white blood cell count, and improvement on chest x ray (resolution of surrounding infiltrate, reduction in cavity size, absence of fluid). Oral administration of antibiotic therapy is continued for an additional 4 to 8 weeks. If treatment is stopped too soon, a relapse may occur.

## Nursing Management

The nurse administers antibiotics and IV treatments as prescribed and monitors for adverse effects. Chest physiotherapy is initiated as prescribed to facilitate drainage of the abscess. The nurse teaches the patient to perform deep-breathing and coughing exercises to help expand the lungs.

To ensure proper nutritional intake, the nurse encourages a diet that is high in protein and calories. The nurse also offers emotional support, because the abscess may take a long time to resolve.

### Promoting Home and Community-Based Care

**TEACHING PATIENTS SELF-CARE.** A patient who has had surgery may return home before the wound closes entirely or with a drain or tube in place. In these cases, the patient or caregivers require instruction about how to change the dressings to prevent skin excoriation and odor, how to monitor for signs and symptoms of infection, and how to care for and maintain the drain or tube. The nurse instructs the patient to perform deep-breathing and coughing exercises every 2 hours during the day and shows caregivers how to perform chest percussion and postural drainage to facilitate expectoration of lung secretions.

**CONTINUING CARE.** A patient whose condition requires therapy at home may need referral for home care. During home visits, the nurse assesses the physical condition, nutritional status, and home environment of the patient, as well as the ability of the patient and family to carry out the therapeutic regimen. Patient teaching is reinforced, and nutritional counseling is provided with the goal of attaining and maintaining an optimal state of nutrition. To prevent relapses, the nurse emphasizes the importance of completing the antibiotic regimen and of following suggestions for rest and appropriate activity. If IV antibiotic therapy is to continue at home, the services of home care nurses may be arranged to initiate IV therapy and to evaluate its administration by the patient or family.

Although most outpatient IV therapy is administered in the home setting, the patient may visit a nearby clinic or physician's office for this treatment. In some cases, patients with lung abscess may have ignored their health. Therefore, it is important to use this opportunity to address health promotion strategies and health screening with the patient.

# Pleural Conditions

Pleural conditions are disorders that involve the membranes covering the lungs (visceral pleura) and the surface of the chest wall (parietal pleura) or disorders affecting the pleural space.

## Pleurisy

### Pathophysiology

Pleurisy (pleuritis) refers to inflammation of both layers of the pleurae (parietal and visceral). Pleurisy may develop in conjunction with pneumonia or an upper respiratory tract infection, TB, or collagen disease; after trauma to the chest, pulmonary infarction, or PE; in patients with primary or metastatic cancer; and after thoracotomy. The parietal pleura has nerve endings; the visceral pleura does not. When the inflamed pleural membranes rub together during respiration (intensified on inspiration), the result is severe, sharp, knifelike pain.

### Clinical Manifestations

The key characteristic of pleuritic pain is its relationship to respiratory movement. Taking a deep breath, coughing, or sneezing worsens the pain. Pleuritic pain is limited in distribution rather than diffuse; it usually occurs only on one side. The pain may become minimal or absent when the breath is held. It may be localized or radiate to the shoulder or abdomen. Later, as pleural fluid develops, the pain decreases.

### Assessment and Diagnostic Findings

In the early period, when little fluid has accumulated, a pleural friction rub can be heard with the stethoscope, only to disappear later as more fluid accumulates and separates the inflamed pleural surfaces. Diagnostic tests may include chest x-rays, sputum examinations, thoracentesis to obtain a specimen of pleural fluid for examination, and, less commonly, a pleural biopsy.

### Medical Management

The objectives of treatment are to discover the underlying condition causing the pleurisy and to relieve the pain. As the underlying disease (pneumonia, infection) is treated, the pleuritic inflammation usually resolves. At the same time, it is necessary to monitor for signs and symptoms of pleural effusion, such as shortness of breath, pain, assumption of a position that decreases pain, and decreased chest wall excursion.

Prescribed analgesics and topical applications of heat or cold provide symptomatic relief. Indomethacin (Indocin), a nonsteroidal anti-inflammatory agent, may provide pain relief while allowing the patient to take deep breaths and cough more effectively. If the pain is severe, an intercostal nerve block may be required.

### Nursing Management

Because the patient has considerable pain on inspiration, the nurse offers suggestions to enhance comfort, such as turning frequently onto the affected side to splint the chest wall and reduce the stretching of the pleurae. The nurse also teaches the patient to use the hands or a pillow to splint the rib cage while coughing.

## Pleural Effusion

Pleural effusion, a collection of fluid in the pleural space, is rarely a primary disease process but is usually occurs secondary to other diseases. Normally, the pleural space contains a small amount of fluid (5 to 15 mL), which acts as a lubricant that allows the pleural surfaces to move without friction (Fig. 23-5). Pleural effusion may be a complication of heart failure, TB, pneumonia, pulmonary infections (par-

# CHAPTER 23 • Management of Patients With Chest and Lower Respiratory Tract Disorders

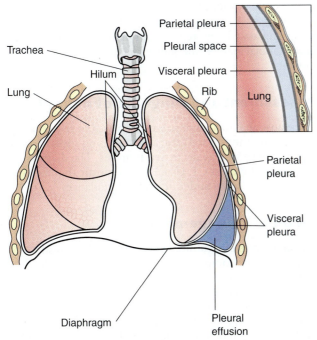

**FIGURE 23-5.** In pleural effusion, an abnormal volume of fluid collects in the pleural space, causing pain and shortness of breath. Pleural effusion is usually secondary to other disease processes.

ticularly viral infections), nephrotic syndrome, connective tissue disease, pulmonary embolus, and neoplastic tumors. The most common malignancy associated with a pleural effusion is bronchogenic carcinoma.

## Pathophysiology

In certain disorders, fluid may accumulate in the pleural space to a point at which it becomes clinically evident. This almost always has pathologic significance. The effusion can be composed of a relatively clear fluid, or it can be bloody or purulent. An effusion of clear fluid may be a transudate or an exudate. A transudate (filtrate of plasma that moves across intact capillary walls) occurs when factors influencing the formation and reabsorption of pleural fluid are altered, usually by imbalances in hydrostatic or oncotic pressures. The finding of a transudative effusion generally implies that the pleural membranes are not diseased. A transudative effusion most commonly results from heart failure. An exudate (extravasation of fluid into tissues or a cavity) usually results from inflammation by bacterial products or tumors involving the pleural surfaces.

## Clinical Manifestations

Usually, the clinical manifestations are caused by the underlying disease. Pneumonia causes fever, chills, and pleuritic chest pain, whereas a malignant effusion may result in dyspnea, difficulty lying flat, and coughing. The severity of symptoms is determined by the size of the effusion, the speed of its formation, and the underlying lung disease. A large pleural effusion causes dyspnea (shortness of breath). A small to moderate pleural effusion causes minimal or no dyspnea.

## Assessment and Diagnostic Findings

Assessment of the area of the pleural effusion reveals decreased or absent breath sounds, decreased fremitus, and a dull, flat sound on percussion. In the case of an extremely large pleural effusion, the assessment reveals a patient in acute respiratory distress. Tracheal deviation away from the affected side may also be apparent.

Physical examination, chest x-ray, chest CT, and thoracentesis confirm the presence of fluid. In some instances, a lateral decubitus x-ray is obtained. For this x-ray, the patient lies on the affected side in a side-lying position. A pleural effusion can be diagnosed because this position allows for the "layering out" of the fluid, and an air–fluid line is visible.

Pleural fluid is analyzed by bacterial culture, Gram stain, acid-fast bacillus stain (for TB), red and white blood cell counts, chemistry studies (glucose, amylase, lactic dehydrogenase, protein), cytologic analysis for malignant cells, and pH. A pleural biopsy also may be performed as a diagnostic tool.

## Medical Management

The objectives of treatment are to discover the underlying cause of the pleural effusion; to prevent reaccumulation of fluid; and to relieve discomfort, dyspnea, and respiratory compromise. Specific treatment is directed at the underlying cause (eg, heart failure, pneumonia, cirrhosis). If the pleural fluid is an exudate, more extensive diagnostic procedures are performed to determine the cause. Treatment for the primary cause is then instituted.

Thoracentesis is performed to remove fluid, to obtain a specimen for analysis, and to relieve dyspnea and respiratory compromise (see Chapter 21). Thoracentesis may be performed under ultrasound guidance. Depending on the size of the pleural effusion, the patient may be treated by removing the fluid during the thoracentesis procedure or by inserting a chest tube connected to a water-seal drainage system or suction to evacuate the pleural space and re-expand the lung.

However, if the underlying cause is a malignancy, the effusion tends to recur within a few days or weeks. Repeated thoracenteses result in pain, depletion of protein and electrolytes, and sometimes pneumothorax. Once the pleural space is adequately drained, a chemical pleurodesis may be performed to obliterate the pleural space and prevent reaccumulation of fluid. Pleurodesis may be performed using either a thoracoscopic approach or a chest tube. A chemically irritating agent (eg., talc) is instilled or aerosolized into the pleural space. With the chest tube approach, after the agent is instilled, the chest tube is clamped for 60 to 90 minutes and the patient is assisted to assume various positions to promote uniform distribution of the agent and to maximize its contact with the pleural surfaces. The tube is unclamped as prescribed, and chest drainage may be continued several days longer to prevent reaccumulation of fluid and to promote the formation of adhesions between the visceral and parietal pleurae.

Other treatments for malignant pleural effusions include surgical pleurectomy, insertion of a small catheter attached to a drainage bottle for outpatient management (Pleurx catheter [Denver Biomedical]), or implantation of a pleuroperitoneal shunt. A pleuroperitoneal shunt consists of two catheters connected by a pump chamber containing two one-way valves. Fluid moves from the pleural space to the pump chamber and then to the peritoneal cavity. The patient manually pumps on the reservoir daily to move fluid from the pleural space to the peritoneal space.

## Nursing Management

The nurse's role in the care of patients with a pleural effusion includes implementing the medical regimen. The nurse prepares and positions the patient for thoracentesis and offers support throughout the procedure. The nurse is responsible for making sure the thoracentesis fluid amount is recorded and sent for appropriate laboratory testing. If a chest tube drainage and water-seal system is used, the nurse is responsible for monitoring the system's function and recording the amount of drainage at prescribed intervals. Nursing care related to the underlying cause of the pleural effusion is specific to the underlying condition. Care of the patient with a chest tube is discussed in Chapter 25.

If a chest tube is inserted for talc instillation, pain management is a priority and the nurse helps the patient assume positions that are the least painful. However, frequent turning and movement are important to facilitate adequate spreading of the talc over the pleural surface. The nurse evaluates the patient's pain level and administers analgesics as prescribed and as needed.

If the patient is to be managed as an outpatient with a pleural catheter for drainage, the nurse is responsible for educating the patient and family regarding management and care of the catheter and drainage system.

## *Empyema*

An empyema is an accumulation of thick, purulent fluid within the pleural space, often with fibrin development and a loculated (walled-off) area where infection is located.

## Pathophysiology

Most empyemas occur as complications of bacterial pneumonia or lung abscess. They also result from penetrating chest trauma, hematogenous infection of the pleural space, nonbacterial infections, and iatrogenic causes (after thoracic surgery or thoracentesis). At first the pleural fluid is thin, with a low leukocyte count, but it frequently progresses to a fibropurulent stage and, finally, to a stage where it encloses the lung within a thick exudative membrane (loculated empyema).

## Clinical Manifestations

The patient is acutely ill and has signs and symptoms similar to those of an acute respiratory infection or pneumonia (fever, night sweats, pleural pain, cough, dyspnea, anorexia, weight loss). If the patient is immunocompromised, the symptoms may be more vague. If the patient has received antimicrobial therapy, the clinical manifestations may be less obvious.

## Assessment and Diagnostic Findings

Chest auscultation demonstrates decreased or absent breath sounds over the affected area, and there is dullness on chest percussion as well as decreased fremitus. The diagnosis is established by chest CT. Usually a diagnostic thoracentesis is performed, often under ultrasound guidance.

## Medical Management

The objectives of treatment are to drain the pleural cavity and to achieve complete expansion of the lung. The fluid is drained, and appropriate antibiotics, in large doses, are prescribed based on the causative organism. Sterilization of the empyema cavity requires 4 to 6 weeks of antibiotics. Drainage of the pleural fluid depends on the stage of the disease and is accomplished by one of the following methods:

- Needle aspiration (thoracentesis) with a thin percutaneous catheter, if the volume is small and the fluid is not too purulent or too thick
- Tube thoracostomy (chest drainage using a large-diameter intercostal tube attached to water-seal drainage [see Chapter 25]) with fibrinolytic agents instilled through the chest tube in patients with loculated or complicated pleural effusions
- Open chest drainage via thoracotomy, including potential rib resection, to remove the thickened pleura, pus, and debris and to remove the underlying diseased pulmonary tissue

With long-standing inflammation, an exudate can form over the lung, trapping it and interfering with its normal expansion. This exudate must be removed surgically (decortication). The drainage tube is left in place until the pus-filled space is obliterated completely. The complete obliteration of the pleural space is monitored by serial chest x-rays, and the patient should be informed that treatment may be long term. Patients are frequently discharged from the hospital with a chest tube in place, with instructions to monitor fluid drainage at home.

## Nursing Management

Resolution of empyema is a prolonged process. The nurse helps the patient cope with the condition and instructs the patient in lung-expanding breathing exercises to restore normal respiratory function. The nurse also provides care specific to the method of drainage of the pleural fluid (eg, needle aspiration, closed chest drainage, rib resection and drainage). When the patient is discharged home with a drainage tube or system in place, the nurse instructs the patient and family on care of the drainage system and drain site, measurement and observation of drainage, signs and symptoms of infection, and how and when to contact the health care provider. (See Nursing Process: The Patient Undergoing Thoracic Surgery in Chapter 25.)

## Pulmonary Edema

**Pulmonary edema** is defined as abnormal accumulation of fluid in the lung tissue, the alveolar space, or both. It is a severe, life-threatening condition.

### Pathophysiology

Pulmonary edema most commonly occurs as a result of increased microvascular pressure from abnormal cardiac function. The backup of blood into the pulmonary vasculature resulting from inadequate left ventricular function causes an increased microvascular pressure, and fluid begins to leak into the interstitial space and the alveoli. Other causes of pulmonary edema are hypervolemia or a sudden increase in the intravascular pressure in the lung. One example occurs in the patient who has undergone pneumonectomy. When one lung has been removed, all the cardiac output goes to the remaining lung. If the patient's fluid status is not monitored closely, pulmonary edema can quickly develop in the postoperative period as the patient's pulmonary vasculature attempts to adapt. This type of pulmonary edema is sometimes termed "flash" pulmonary edema. A second example is called re-expansion pulmonary edema. This may result from a rapid reinflation of the lung after removal of air from a pneumothorax or evacuation of fluid from a large pleural effusion.

### Clinical Manifestations

Increasing respiratory distress, characterized by dyspnea, air hunger, and central cyanosis, is present. Patients are usually very anxious and often agitated. As the fluid leaks into the alveoli and mixes with air, a foam or froth is formed. The patient coughs up (or the nurse suctions out) these foamy, frothy, and often blood-tinged secretions. The patient experiences acute respiratory distress and may become confused or stuporous.

### Assessment and Diagnostic Findings

Auscultation reveals crackles in the lung bases (especially in the posterior bases) that rapidly progress toward the apices of the lungs. These crackles are caused by the movement of air through the alveolar fluid. The chest x-ray reveals increased interstitial markings. The patient may have tachycardia. Pulse oximetry values begin to fall, and arterial blood gas analysis demonstrates worsening hypoxemia.

### Medical Management

Management focuses on correcting the underlying disorder. If the pulmonary edema is cardiac in origin, then improvement in left ventricular function is the goal. Vasodilators, inotropic medications, afterload or preload agents, or contractility medications may be administered. Additional cardiac measures (eg, intra-aortic balloon pump) may be indicated if there is no response. If the problem is fluid overload, diuretics are administered and fluids are restricted. Oxygen is administered to correct the hypoxemia; in some circumstances, intubation and mechanical ventilation are necessary. The patient is extremely anxious, and morphine is prescribed to reduce anxiety and control pain.

### Nursing Management

Nursing management includes assisting with administration of oxygen and intubation and mechanical ventilation if respiratory failure occurs. The nurse also administers medications (eg, morphine, vasodilators, inotropic medications, preload and afterload agents) as prescribed and monitors the patient's responses. Nursing management in pulmonary edema is described in more detail in Chapter 30.

## Acute Respiratory Failure

Respiratory failure is a sudden and life-threatening deterioration of the gas exchange function of the lung. It exists when the exchange of oxygen for carbon dioxide in the lungs cannot keep up with the rate of oxygen consumption and carbon dioxide production by the cells of the body. Acute respiratory failure (ARF) is defined as a decrease in arterial oxygen tension ($PaO_2$) to less than 50 mm Hg (hypoxemia) and an increase in arterial carbon dioxide tension ($PaCO_2$) to greater than 50 mm Hg (hypercapnia), with an arterial pH of less than 7.35.

It is important to distinguish between ARF and chronic respiratory failure. Chronic respiratory failure is defined as a deterioration in the gas exchange function of the lung that has developed insidiously or has persisted for a long period after an episode of ARF. The absence of acute symptoms and the presence of a chronic respiratory acidosis suggest the chronicity of the respiratory failure. Two causes of chronic respiratory failure are COPD (discussed in Chapter 24) and neuromuscular diseases (discussed in Chapter 65). Patients with these disorders develop a tolerance to the gradually worsening hypoxemia and hypercapnia. However, patients with chronic respiratory failure can develop ARF. For example, a patient with COPD may develop an exacerbation or infection that causes additional deterioration of gas exchange. The principles of management of acute versus chronic respiratory failure are different; the following discussion is limited to ARF.

### Pathophysiology

In ARF, the ventilation or perfusion mechanisms in the lung are impaired. Impaired respiratory system mechanisms leading to ARF include

- Alveolar hypoventilation
- Diffusion abnormalities
- Ventilation–perfusion mismatching
- Shunting

Common causes of ARF can be classified into four categories: decreased respiratory drive, dysfunction of the chest wall, dysfunction of the lung parenchyma, and other causes.

### Decreased Respiratory Drive

Decreased respiratory drive may occur with severe brain injury, large lesions of the brainstem (multiple sclerosis), use of sedative medications, and metabolic disorders such as severe hypothyroidism. These disorders impair the response of chemoreceptors in the brain to normal respiratory stimulation.

### Dysfunction of the Chest Wall

The impulses arising in the respiratory center travel through nerves that extend from the brainstem down the spinal cord to receptors in the muscles of respiration. Any disease or disorder of the nerves, spinal cord, muscles, or neuromuscular junction involved in respiration seriously affects ventilation and may ultimately lead to ARF. These include musculoskeletal disorders (muscular dystrophy, polymyositis), neuromuscular junction disorders (myasthenia gravis, poliomyelitis), some peripheral nerve disorders, and spinal cord disorders (amyotrophic lateral sclerosis, Guillain-Barré syndrome, and cervical spinal cord injuries).

### Dysfunction of Lung Parenchyma

Pleural effusion, hemothorax, pneumothorax, and upper airway obstruction are conditions that interfere with ventilation by preventing expansion of the lung. These conditions, which may cause respiratory failure, usually are produced by an underlying lung disease, pleural disease, or trauma and injury. Other diseases and conditions of lung parenchyma that lead to ARF include pneumonia, status asthmaticus, lobar atelectasis, PE, and pulmonary edema.

### Other Causes

In the postoperative period, especially after major thoracic or abdominal surgery, inadequate ventilation and respiratory failure may occur because of several factors. During this period, for example, ARF may be caused by the effects of anesthetic agents, analgesics, and sedatives, which may depress respiration (as described earlier) or enhance the effects of opioids and lead to hypoventilation. Pain may interfere with deep breathing and coughing. A ventilation–perfusion mismatch is the usual cause of respiratory failure after major abdominal, cardiac, or thoracic surgery.

### Clinical Manifestations

Early signs are those associated with impaired oxygenation and may include restlessness, fatigue, headache, dyspnea, air hunger, tachycardia, and increased blood pressure. As the hypoxemia progresses, more obvious signs may be present, including confusion, lethargy, tachycardia, tachypnea, central cyanosis, diaphoresis, and finally respiratory arrest. Physical findings are those of acute respiratory distress, including use of accessory muscles, decreased breath sounds if the patient cannot adequately ventilate, and other findings related specifically to the underlying disease process and cause of ARF.

### Medical Management

The objectives of treatment are to correct the underlying cause and to restore adequate gas exchange in the lung. Intubation and mechanical ventilation may be required to maintain adequate ventilation and oxygenation while the underlying cause is corrected.

### Nursing Management

Nursing management of patients with ARF includes assisting with intubation and maintaining mechanical ventilation (described in Chapter 25). Patients are usually managed in the intensive care unit. The nurse assesses the patient's respiratory status by monitoring the level of responsiveness, arterial blood gases, pulse oximetry, and vital signs. In addition, the nurse assesses the entire respiratory system and implements strategies (eg, turning schedule, mouth care, skin care, range of motion of extremities) to prevent complications. The nurse also assesses the patient's understanding of the management strategies that are used and initiates some form of communication to enable the patient to express concerns and needs to the health care team.

Finally, the nurse addresses the problems that led to the ARF. As the patient's status improves, the nurse assesses the patient's knowledge of the underlying disorder and provides teaching as appropriate to address the disorder.

# Acute Respiratory Distress Syndrome

**Acute respiratory distress syndrome** (ARDS; previously called adult respiratory distress syndrome) is a severe form of **acute lung injury**. This clinical syndrome is characterized by a sudden and progressive pulmonary edema, increasing bilateral infiltrates on chest x-ray, hypoxemia refractory to oxygen supplementation, and reduced lung compliance. These signs occur in the absence of left-sided heart failure. Patients with ARDS usually require mechanical ventilation with a higher-than-normal airway pressure. A wide range of factors are associated with the development of ARDS (Chart 23-5), including direct injury to the lungs (eg, smoke inhalation) or indirect insult to the lungs (eg, shock). ARDS has been associated with a mortality rate as high as 50% to 60%. The major cause of death in ARDS is nonpulmonary multiple-system organ failure, often with sepsis.

## Pathophysiology

ARDS occurs as a result of an inflammatory trigger that initiates the release of cellular and chemical mediators, causing injury to the alveolar capillary membrane. This leads to leakage of fluid into the alveolar interstitial spaces and alterations in the capillary bed.

Severe ventilation–perfusion mismatching occurs in ARDS. Alveoli collapse because of the inflammatory infiltrate, blood, fluid, and surfactant dysfunction. Small air-

## CHART 23-5

### Etiologic Factors Related to Acute Respiratory Distress Syndrome (ARDS)

- Aspiration (gastric secretions, drowning, hydrocarbons)
- Drug ingestion and overdose
- Hematologic disorders (disseminated intravascular coagulopathy [DIC], massive transfusions, cardiopulmonary bypass)
- Prolonged inhalation of high concentrations of oxygen, smoke, or corrosive substances
- Localized infection (bacterial, fungal, viral pneumonia)
- Metabolic disorders (pancreatitis, uremia)
- Shock (any cause)
- Trauma (pulmonary contusion, multiple fractures, head injury)
- Major surgery
- Fat or air embolism
- Systemic sepsis

ways are narrowed because of interstitial fluid and bronchial obstruction. Lung compliance becomes markedly decreased (stiff lungs), and the result is a characteristic decrease in functional residual capacity and severe hypoxemia. The blood returning to the lung for gas exchange is pumped through the nonventilated, nonfunctioning areas of the lung, causing shunting. This means that blood is interfacing with nonfunctioning alveoli and gas exchange is markedly impaired, resulting in severe, refractory hypoxemia. Figure 23-6 shows the sequence of pathophysiologic events leading to ARDS.

## Clinical Manifestations

Clinically, the acute phase of ARDS is marked by a rapid onset of severe dyspnea that usually occurs 12 to 48 hours after the initiating event. A characteristic feature is arterial hypoxemia that does not respond to supplemental oxygen. On chest x-ray, the findings are similar to those seen with cardiogenic pulmonary edema and appear as bilateral infiltrates that quickly worsen. The acute lung injury then progresses to fibrosing alveolitis with persistent, severe hypoxemia. The patient also has increased alveolar dead space (ventilation to alveoli, but poor perfusion) and decreased pulmonary compliance ("stiff lungs," which are difficult to ventilate). Clinically, the patient is thought to be in the recovery phase if the hypoxemia gradually resolves, the chest x-ray improves, and the lungs become more compliant.

## Assessment and Diagnostic Findings

Intercostal retractions and crackles, as the fluid begins to leak into the alveolar interstitial space, are evident on physical examination. A diagnosis of ARDS may be made based on the following criteria: a history of systemic or pulmonary risk factors, acute onset of respiratory distress, bilateral pulmonary infiltrates, clinical absence of left-sided heart failure, and a ratio of $PaO_2$ to fraction of inspired oxygen ($FiO_2$) less than 200 mm Hg (severe refractory hypoxemia).

## Medical Management

The primary focus in the management of ARDS includes identification and treatment of the underlying condition. Aggressive, supportive care must be provided to compensate for the severe respiratory dysfunction. This supportive therapy almost always includes intubation and mechanical

**FIGURE 23-6.** Pathogenesis and pathophysiology of acute respiratory distress syndrome. Adapted from Farzan, S. (1997). *A concise handbook of respiratory diseases* (4th ed.). Stamford, CT: Appleton & Lange.

ventilation. In addition, circulatory support, adequate fluid volume, and nutritional support are important. Supplemental oxygen is used as the patient begins the initial spiral of hypoxemia. As the hypoxemia progresses, intubation and mechanical ventilation are instituted. The concentration of oxygen and ventilator settings and modes are determined by the patient's status. This is monitored by arterial blood gas analysis, pulse oximetry, and bedside pulmonary function testing.

PEEP is a critical part of the treatment of ARDS. PEEP usually improves oxygenation, but it does not influence the natural history of the syndrome. Use of PEEP helps increase functional residual capacity and reverse alveolar collapse by keeping the alveoli open, resulting in improved arterial oxygenation and a reduction in the severity of the ventilation–perfusion imbalance. By using PEEP, a lower $FiO_2$ may be required. The goal is a $PaO_2$ greater than 60 mm Hg or an oxygen saturation level of greater than 90% at the lowest possible $FiO_2$. Evidence suggests that ARDS should be managed with a low tidal volume, pressure-limited approach with low or moderately high PEEP (Kallet, 2004; Young, Manning, Wilson, et al., 2004). PEEP and modes of mechanical ventilation are discussed in Chapter 25.

Systemic hypotension may occur in ARDS as a result of hypovolemia secondary to leakage of fluid into the interstitial spaces and depressed cardiac output from high levels of PEEP therapy. Hypovolemia must be carefully treated without causing further overload. IV crystalloid solutions are administered, with careful monitoring of pulmonary status. Inotropic or vasopressor agents may be required. Pulmonary artery pressure catheters are used to monitor the patient's fluid status and the severe and progressive pulmonary hypertension sometimes observed in ARDS.

## Pharmacologic Therapy

Numerous pharmacologic treatments are under investigation to stop the cascade of events leading to ARDS. These include human recombinant interleukin-1 receptor antagonist, neutrophil inhibitors, pulmonary-specific vasodilators, surfactant replacement therapy, antisepsis agents, antioxidant therapy, and corticosteroids administered late in the course of ARDS.

## Nutritional Therapy

Adequate nutritional support is vital in the treatment of ARDS. Patients with ARDS require 35 to 45 kcal/kg per day to meet caloric requirements. Enteral feeding is the first consideration; however, parenteral nutrition also may be required.

# Nursing Management

## General Measures

A patient with ARDS is critically ill and requires close monitoring in the intensive care unit, because the patient's condition could quickly become life-threatening. Most of the respiratory modalities discussed in Chapter 25 are used in this situation (oxygen administration, nebulizer therapy, chest physiotherapy, endotracheal intubation or tracheostomy, mechanical ventilation, suctioning, bronchoscopy). Frequent assessment of the patient's status is necessary to evaluate the effectiveness of treatment.

In addition to implementing the medical plan of care, the nurse considers other needs of the patient. Positioning is important. The nurse turns the patient frequently to improve ventilation and perfusion in the lungs and enhance secretion drainage. However, the nurse must closely monitor the patient for deterioration in oxygenation with changes in position. Oxygenation in patients with ARDS is sometimes improved in the prone position. This position may be evaluated for improvement in oxygenation and used in special circumstances. Devices and specialty beds are available to assist the nurse in placing the patient in a prone position ("proning") (Powers & Daniels, 2004).

The patient is extremely anxious and agitated because of the increasing hypoxemia and dyspnea. The nurse explains all procedures and provides care in a calm, reassuring manner. It is important to reduce the patient's anxiety, because anxiety increases oxygen expenditure by preventing rest. Rest is essential to limit oxygen consumption and reduce oxygen needs.

## Ventilator Considerations

If the patient is intubated and receiving mechanical ventilation with PEEP, several considerations must be addressed. PEEP, which causes increased end-expiratory pressure, is an unnatural pattern of breathing and feels strange to patients. The patients may be anxious and "fight" the ventilator. Nursing assessment is important to assess for problems with ventilation that may be causing the anxiety reaction: tube blockage by kinking or retained secretions; other acute respiratory problems (eg, pneumothorax, pain); a sudden decrease in the oxygen level; the level of dyspnea; or ventilator malfunction. In some cases, sedation may be required to decrease the patient's oxygen consumption, allow the ventilator to provide full support of ventilation, and decrease the patient's anxiety. Sedatives that may be used are lorazepam (Ativan), midazolam (Versed), dexmedetomidine (Precedex), propofol (Diprivan), and short-acting barbiturates.

If the PEEP level cannot be maintained despite the use of sedatives, neuromuscular blocking agents, such as pancuronium (Pavulon), vecuronium (Norcuron), atracurium (Tracrium), and rocuronium (Zemuron), may be administered to paralyze the patient. This allows the patient to be ventilated more easily. With paralysis, the patient appears to be unconscious; loses motor function; and cannot breathe, talk, or blink independently. However, the patient retains sensation and is awake and able to hear. The nurse must reassure the patient that the paralysis is a result of the medication and is temporary. Paralysis should be used for the shortest possible time and never without adequate sedation and pain management.

Use of paralytic agents has many dangers and side effects. The nurse must be sure the patient does not become disconnected from the ventilator, because respiratory muscles are paralyzed and the patient will be apneic. Consequently, the nurse ensures that the patient is closely monitored, and all ventilator and patient alarms must be on at all times. Eye care is important as well, because the patient cannot blink, increasing the risk of corneal abrasions.

Neuromuscular blockers predispose the patient to deep venous thrombi, muscle atrophy, and skin breakdown. Nursing assessment is essential to minimize the complications related to neuromuscular blockade. The patient may have discomfort or pain but cannot communicate these sensations. Analgesia is usually administered concurrently with neuromuscular blocking agents. The nurse must anticipate the patient's needs regarding pain and comfort. The nurse checks the patient's position to ensure it is comfortable and in normal alignment and talks to, and not about, the patient while in the patient's presence.

In addition, it is important for the nurse to describe the purpose and effects of the paralytic agents to the patient's family. If family members are unaware that these agents have been administered, they may become distressed by the change in the patient's status.

# Pulmonary Arterial Hypertension

Pulmonary arterial hypertension exists when the systolic pulmonary artery pressure exceeds 30 mm Hg or the mean pulmonary artery pressure exceeds 25 mm Hg at rest or 30 mm Hg with activities. These pressures cannot be measured indirectly as can systemic blood pressure; instead, they must be measured during right-sided heart catheterization. In the absence of these measurements, clinical recognition becomes the only indicator for the presence of pulmonary hypertension. However, pulmonary arterial hypertension is a condition that is not clinically evident until late in its progression.

There are two types of pulmonary arterial hypertension: idiopathic (or primary) pulmonary arterial hypertension and pulmonary arterial hypertension due to a known cause (American College of Chest Physicians, 2004). Idiopathic hypertension is an uncommon disease; the incidence is 1 to 2 cases per million persons per year (Eells, 2004). It occurs most often in women 20 to 40 years of age, either sporadically or in patients with a family history, and is usually fatal within 5 years of diagnosis. There are several possible causes, but the exact cause is unknown (Chart 23-6). The clinical presentation may occur with no evidence of pulmonary or cardiac disease or PE.

In contrast, pulmonary arterial hypertension due to a known cause is more common and results from existing cardiac or pulmonary disease. The prognosis depends on the severity of the underlying disorder and the changes in the pulmonary vascular bed. A common cause of pulmonary arterial hypertension is pulmonary artery constriction due to hypoxemia from COPD (cor pulmonale).

## Pathophysiology

Conditions such as collagen vascular disease, congenital heart disease, portal hypertension, and HIV infection increase the risk for pulmonary arterial hypertension in susceptible patients. Vascular injury occurs with endothelial dysfunction and vascular smooth muscle dysfunction, which leads to disease progression (vascular smooth muscle hypertrophy, adventitial and intimal proliferation [thickening of the wall], and advanced vascular lesion formation). Normally, the pulmonary vascular bed can handle the blood volume delivered by the right ventricle. It has a low resistance to blood flow and compensates for increased blood volume by dilation of the vessels in the pulmonary circulation. However, if the pulmonary vascular bed is destroyed or obstructed, as in pulmonary hypertension, the ability to handle whatever flow or volume of blood it receives is impaired, and the increased blood flow then increases the pulmonary artery pressure. As the pulmonary arterial pressure increases, the pulmonary vascular resistance also increases. Both pulmonary artery constriction (as in hypoxemia or hypercapnia) and a reduction of the pulmonary vascular bed (which occurs with pulmonary emboli) result in increased pulmonary vascular resistance and pressure. This increased workload affects right ventricular function. The myocardium ultimately cannot meet the increasing demands imposed on it, leading to right ventricular hypertrophy (enlargement and dilation) and failure.

### CHART 23-6

**Causes of Pulmonary Arterial Hypertension**

**IDIOPATHIC (PRIMARY) ARTERIAL HYPERTENSION AND PULMONARY ARTERIAL HYPERTENSION DUE TO A KNOWN CAUSE**
- Collagen vascular diseases
- Congenital systemic-to-pulmonary shunts
- Portal hypertension
- Altered immune mechanisms (HIV infection)
- Diseases associated with significant venous or capillary involvement
- Chronic thrombotic or embolic disease
- Pulmonary venous hypertension
- Pulmonary vasoconstriction due to hypoxemia
- Chronic obstructive pulmonary disease (COPD), interstitial lung disease, sleep-disordered breathing
- Miscellaneous causes: sarcoidosis, histiocytosis, compression of pulmonary vessels

## Clinical Manifestations

Dyspnea, the main symptom of pulmonary hypertension, occurs at first with exertion and eventually at rest. Substernal chest pain also is common, affecting 25% to 50% of patients. Other signs and symptoms include weakness, fatigue, syncope, occasional hemoptysis, and signs of right-sided heart failure (peripheral edema, ascites, distended neck veins, liver engorgement, crackles, heart murmur).

## Assessment and Diagnostic Findings

Several tests are used to determine whether there is a known cause for the pulmonary hypertension. If the diagnostic tests and thorough evaluation of the patient reveal no known cause, a diagnosis of primary pulmonary hypertension is made. Complete diagnostic evaluation includes a history, physical examination, chest x-ray, pulmonary function studies, electrocardiogram (ECG), echocardiogram, ventilation–perfusion scan, sleep studies, autoantibody tests (to identify diseases of collagen vascular origin), HIV tests, liver function testing, and cardiac catheterization. Pulmonary function studies may be normal or show a slight decrease in vital capacity and lung compliance, with a mild decrease in the diffusing capacity. The $PaO_2$ also is decreased (hypoxemia). The ECG reveals right ventricular hypertrophy, right axis deviation, and tall peaked P waves in inferior leads; tall anterior R waves; and ST-segment depression, T-wave inversion, or both anteriorly. An echocardiogram can assess the progression of the disease and rule out other conditions with similar signs and symptoms. A ventilation–perfusion scan or pulmonary angiography detects defects in pulmonary vasculature, such as pulmonary emboli. Cardiac catheterization of the right side of the heart reveals elevated pulmonary arterial pressure and determines whether there is a vasoactive component to the pulmonary hypertension.

## Medical Management

The goal of treatment is to manage the underlying condition related to pulmonary hypertension of known cause. Most patients with pulmonary hypertension do not have hypoxemia at rest but require supplemental oxygen with exercise. However, patients with severe right ventricular failure, decreased cardiac output, and progressive disease may have resting hypoxemia and require continuous oxygen supplementation. Appropriate oxygen therapy (see Chapter 25) reverses the vasoconstrictive effect and reduces the pulmonary hypertension in a relatively short time.

Bosentan, an endothelin receptor antagonist, causes vasodilation and is prescribed for its antihypertensive effects in patients with pulmonary hypertension (Eells, 2004). Other medications, including diuretics, digoxin, anticoagulant therapy, and calcium-channel blockers (nifedipine [Procardia], diltiazem [Cardizem]) may be prescribed. Because calcium-channel blockers are effective in only a small percentage of patients, other treatment options, including prostacyclin, are often necessary (Humbert, Sitbon & Simonneau, 2004).

Prostaglandin (prostacyclin) relaxes vascular smooth muscle by stimulating the production of cyclic adenosine monophosphate (AMP) and inhibiting the growth of smooth muscle cells. Additionally, it inhibits platelet aggregation. Because of its short-half life in the circulation (ie, 3 minutes), IV prostacyclin (epoprostenol [Flolan]) can be administered only by continuous IV infusion (Humbert et al., 2004). It helps to decrease pulmonary hypertension by reducing pulmonary vascular resistance and pressures and increasing cardiac output. For long-term administration, epoprostenol can be infused with the use of a portable infusion pump connected to a permanent catheter inserted in the subclavian vein. The use of epoprostenol has led to improvement in some patients without lung transplantation, which had previously been the only treatment.

Despite its role in improving function in some patients, epoprostenol is not an ideal treatment because it has significant side effects, is uncomfortable for patients, and is very costly. Continuous subcutaneous infusion of treprostinil (Remodulin), a prostacyclin analogue, was approved for treatment of pulmonary hypertension in 2002 and is an alternative for some patients. Iloprost (Ventavis) is an inhaled, synthetic form of prostacyclin and a powerful vasodilator of the pulmonary arteries. It has been shown to improve patients' overall symptoms and their ability to exercise (walk). Bosentan is an oral endothelin-receptor antagonist; other agents with similar action are under investigation.

Nitric oxide, sildenafil, vasoactive intestinal peptide, and selective serotonin-reuptake inhibitors (SSRIs), and various combinations of these agents are undergoing studies to determine if they have a role in the treatment of patients with pulmonary hypertension (Humbert et al., 2004). Although several treatments for pulmonary arterial hypertension (epoprostenol, treprostinil, and bosentan) are now approved for use in the United States, the long-term effects of many of these therapies are unknown. Lung transplantation remains an option for all eligible patients who have severe disease and symptoms after 3 months of receiving epoprostenol. Atrial septostomy may be considered for selected patients with severe disease (Humbert et al., 2004).

## Nursing Management

The major nursing goal is to identify patients at high risk for pulmonary arterial hypertension, such as those with COPD, pulmonary emboli, congenital heart disease, and mitral valve disease. The nurse also must be alert for signs and symptoms, administer oxygen therapy appropriately, and instruct the patient and family about the use of home oxygen supplementation. In patients treated with prostacyclin (ie, epoprostenol or treprostinil), education about the need for central venous access (epoprostenol), subcutaneous infusion (treprostinil), proper administration and dosing of the medication, pain at the injection site, and potential severe side effects is extremely important. Emotional and psychosocial aspects of this disease must be addressed. Formal and informal support groups for patients and families are extremely valuable (Eells, 2004).

# Pulmonary Heart Disease (Cor Pulmonale)

**Cor pulmonale** is a condition in which the right ventricle of the heart enlarges (with or without right-sided heart failure) as a result of diseases that affect the structure or function of the lung or its vasculature. It is a type of pulmonary arterial hypertension due to a known cause. Any disease affecting the lungs and accompanied by hypoxemia may result in cor pulmonale. The most frequent cause is severe COPD (see Chapter 24), in which changes in the airway and retained secretions reduce alveolar ventilation. Other causes are conditions that restrict or compromise ventilatory function, leading to hypoxemia or acidosis (eg, deformities of the thoracic cage, massive obesity) and conditions that reduce the pulmonary vascular bed (eg, primary idiopathic pulmonary arterial hypertension, pulmonary embolus). Certain disorders of the nervous system, respiratory muscles, chest wall, and pulmonary arterial tree also may be responsible for cor pulmonale.

## Pathophysiology

Pulmonary disease can produce physiologic changes that in time affect the heart and cause the right ventricle to enlarge and eventually fail. Any condition that deprives the lungs of oxygen can cause hypoxemia and hypercapnia, resulting in ventilatory insufficiency. Hypoxemia and hypercapnia cause pulmonary arterial vasoconstriction and possibly reduction of the pulmonary vascular bed, as in emphysema or pulmonary emboli. The result is increased resistance in the pulmonary circulatory system, with a subsequent rise in pulmonary blood pressure (pulmonary hypertension). A mean pulmonary arterial pressure of 45 mm Hg or more may occur in cor pulmonale. Right ventricular hypertrophy may result, followed by right ventricular failure. In short, cor pulmonale results from pulmonary hypertension, which causes the right side of the heart to enlarge because of the increased work required to pump blood against high resistance through the pulmonary vascular system.

## Clinical Manifestations

Symptoms of cor pulmonale are usually related to the underlying lung disease, such as COPD. With right ventricular failure, the patient may develop increasing edema of the feet and legs, distended neck veins, an enlarged palpable liver, pleural effusion, ascites, and heart murmurs. Headache, confusion, and somnolence may occur as a result of increased levels of carbon dioxide (hypercapnia). Patients often complain of increasing shortness of breath, wheezing, cough, and fatigue.

## Medical Management

The objectives of treatment are to improve ventilation and to treat both the underlying lung disease and the manifestations of heart disease. Supplemental oxygen is administered to improve gas exchange and to reduce pulmonary arterial pressure and pulmonary vascular resistance. Improved oxygen transport relieves the pulmonary hypertension that is causing the cor pulmonale.

Continuous, 24-hour oxygen therapy in patients with severe hypoxemia reportedly leads to better survival rates and greater reduction in pulmonary vascular resistance. Substantial improvement may require 4 to 6 weeks of oxygen therapy, usually in the home. Periodic assessment of pulse oximetry and arterial blood gases is necessary to determine the adequacy of alveolar ventilation and to monitor the effectiveness of oxygen therapy.

Chest physical therapy and bronchial hygiene maneuvers as indicated to remove accumulated secretions and the administration of bronchodilators further improve ventilation. Additional measures depend on the patient's condition. If the patient is in respiratory failure, endotracheal intubation and mechanical ventilation may be necessary. If the patient is in heart failure, hypoxemia and hypercapnia must be relieved to improve cardiac function and output. Bed rest, sodium restriction, and diuretic therapy also are instituted judiciously to reduce peripheral edema (ie, to lower pulmonary arterial pressure through a decrease in total blood volume) and the circulatory load on the right side of the heart. Digitalis may be prescribed to relieve pulmonary hypertension if the patient also has left ventricular failure, a supraventricular dysrhythmia, or right ventricular failure that does not respond to other therapy.

ECG monitoring may be indicated because of the high incidence of dysrhythmias in patients with cor pulmonale. Any respiratory infection must be treated promptly to avoid further impaired gas exchange and exacerbations of hypoxemia and pulmonary heart disease. The prognosis depends on whether the pulmonary hypertension is reversible. (See earlier discussion of the management of acute respiratory failure.)

## Nursing Management

Nursing care addresses the underlying disorder leading to cor pulmonale as well as the problems related to pulmonary hyperventilation and right-sided cardiac failure. If intubation and mechanical ventilation are required to manage ARF, the nurse assists with the intubation procedure and maintains mechanical ventilation. The nurse assesses the patient's respiratory and cardiac status and administers medications as prescribed.

During the patient's hospital stay, the nurse instructs the patient about the importance of close self-monitoring (fluid retention, weight gain, edema) and adherence to the therapeutic regimen, especially the 24-hour use of oxygen. It is important to address factors that affect the patient's adherence to the treatment regimen.

### Promoting Home and Community-Based Care

#### TEACHING PATIENTS SELF-CARE
Because cor pulmonale is a chronic disorder, most of the care and monitoring of patients with cor pulmonale is performed by patients and families in the home. If supplemental oxygen is administered, the nurse instructs the patient and family in its safe and correct use. Nutrition counseling is warranted if the patient is on a sodium-restricted diet or is taking diuretics. The nurse teaches the family to monitor for signs and symptoms of right ventricular failure and about emergency interventions and when to call for assistance. Most importantly, the nurse works with the patient to stop smoking.

#### CONTINUING CARE
Referral for home care may be warranted for patients who cannot manage self-care and for those whose physical condition warrants close assessment. During home visits, the home care nurse evaluates the patient's status and the patient's and family members' understanding of the therapeutic regimen and their adherence to it. If oxygen is used in the home, the nurse determines whether it is being administered safely and as prescribed. It is important to assess the patient's progress in stopping smoking and to reinforce the importance of smoking cessation with the patient and family. The nurse identifies strategies to assist with smoking cessation and refers the patient and family to community support groups. In addition, the nurse reminds the patient about the importance of other health promotion and screening practices.

# Pulmonary Embolism

Pulmonary embolism (PE) refers to the obstruction of the pulmonary artery or one of its branches by a thrombus (or thrombi) that originates somewhere in the venous system or in the right side of the heart. It is estimated that more than half a million people develop PE yearly, resulting in more than 50,000 deaths (Goldhaber, 2004). PE is a common disorder and often is associated with trauma, surgery (orthopedic, major abdominal, pelvic, gynecologic), pregnancy, heart failure, age older than 50 years, hypercoagulable states, and prolonged immobility. It also may occur in apparently healthy people. Risk factors for PE are identified in Chart 23-7.

## Pathophysiology

Most commonly, PE is due to a blood clot or thrombus. However, there are other types of emboli: air, fat, amniotic fluid, and septic (from bacterial invasion of the thrombus). Although most thrombi originate in the deep veins of the legs, other sites include the pelvic veins and the right atrium of the heart. Venous thrombosis can result from slowing of blood flow (stasis) secondary to damage to the blood vessel wall (particularly the endothelial lining) or changes in the blood coagulation mechanism. Atrial fibrillation also causes PE. An enlarged right atrium in fibrillation causes blood to stagnate and form clots in this area. These clots are prone to travel into the pulmonary circulation.

When a thrombus completely or partially obstructs a pulmonary artery or its branches, the alveolar dead space is increased. The area, although continuing to be ventilated, receives little or no blood flow. Therefore, gas exchange is impaired or absent in this area. In addition, various substances are released from the clot and surrounding area that cause regional blood vessels and bronchioles to constrict. This results in an increase in pulmonary vascular resistance. This reaction compounds the ventilation–perfusion imbalance.

The hemodynamic consequences are increased pulmonary vascular resistance due to the regional vasoconstriction and reduced size of the pulmonary vascular bed. This results in an increase in pulmonary arterial pressure and, in turn, an increase in right ventricular work to maintain pulmonary blood flow. When the work requirements of the right ventricle exceed its capacity, right ventricular failure occurs, leading to a decrease in cardiac output followed by a decrease in systemic blood pressure and the development of shock.

## Clinical Manifestations

Symptoms depend on the size of the thrombus and the area of the pulmonary artery occluded by the thrombus; they may be nonspecific. Dyspnea is the most frequent symptom; tachypnea (very rapid respiratory rate) is the most frequent sign (Goldhaber, 2004). The duration and intensity of the dyspnea depend on the extent of embolization. Chest pain is common and is usually sudden and pleuritic in origin. It may be substernal and may mimic angina pectoris or a myocardial infarction. Other symptoms include anxiety, fever, tachycardia, apprehension, cough, diaphoresis, hemoptysis, and syncope.

Deep venous thrombosis is closely associated with development of PE. Typically, patients report sudden onset of pain and/or swelling and warmth of the proximal or distal extremity, skin discoloration, and superficial vein distention. The pain is usually relieved with elevation.

A massive PE is best defined by the degree of hemodynamic instability rather than the percentage of pulmonary vasculature occlusion. It is described as an occlusion of the outflow tract of the main pulmonary artery or of the bifurcation of the pulmonary arteries that produces pronounced dyspnea, sudden substernal pain, rapid and weak pulse, shock, syncope, and sudden death. Multiple small emboli can lodge in the terminal pulmonary arterioles, producing multiple small infarctions of the lungs. A pulmonary in-

---

### CHART 23-7

### Risk Factors for Pulmonary Embolus

**VENOUS STASIS (SLOWING OF BLOOD FLOW IN VEINS)**
- Prolonged immobilization (especially postoperative)
- Prolonged periods of sitting/traveling
- Varicose veins
- Spinal cord injury

**HYPERCOAGULABILITY (DUE TO RELEASE OF TISSUE THROMBOPLASTIN AFTER INJURY/SURGERY)**
- Injury
- Tumor (pancreatic, gastrointestinal, genitourinary, breast, lung)
- Increased platelet count (polycythemia, splenectomy)

**VENOUS ENDOTHELIAL DISEASE**
- Thrombophlebitis
- Vascular disease
- Foreign bodies (IV/central venous catheters)

**CERTAIN DISEASE STATES (COMBINATION OF STASIS, COAGULATION ALTERATIONS, AND VENOUS INJURY)**
- Heart disease (especially heart failure)
- Trauma (especially fracture of hip, pelvis, vertebra, lower extremities)
- Postoperative state/postpartum period
- Diabetes mellitus
- Chronic obstructive pulmonary disease (COPD)

**OTHER PREDISPOSING CONDITIONS**
- Advanced age
- Obesity
- Pregnancy
- Oral contraceptive use
- History of previous thrombophlebitis, pulmonary embolism
- Constrictive clothing

farction causes ischemic necrosis of an area of the lung. The clinical picture may mimic that of bronchopneumonia or heart failure. In atypical instances, PE causes few signs and symptoms, whereas in other instances it mimics various other cardiopulmonary disorders.

## Assessment and Diagnostic Findings

Death from PE commonly occurs within 1 hour after the onset of symptoms; therefore, early recognition and diagnosis are priorities. Because the symptoms of PE can vary from few to severe, a diagnostic workup is performed to rule out other diseases. The initial diagnostic workup includes chest x-ray, ECG, peripheral vascular studies, arterial blood gas analysis, and ventilation–perfusion (V̇/Q̇) scan.

The chest x-ray is usually normal but may show infiltrates, atelectasis, elevation of the diaphragm on the affected side, or a pleural effusion. The chest x-ray is most helpful in excluding other possible causes. The ECG usually shows sinus tachycardia, PR-interval depression, and nonspecific T-wave changes. Peripheral vascular studies may include impedance plethysmography, Doppler ultrasonography, or venography (see Chapter 31). Test results confirm or exclude the diagnosis of PE. Arterial blood gas analysis may show hypoxemia and hypocapnia (from tachypnea); however, arterial blood gas measurements may be normal even in the presence of PE.

The V̇/Q̇ scan was once the second choice for diagnosis of a PE (with pulmonary angiogram [discussed below] considered the best diagnostic procedure). It is still used, especially in facilities that do not have access to a spiral CT scanner. The V̇/Q̇ scan is minimally invasive, involving the IV administration of a contrast agent. This scan evaluates different regions of the lung (upper, middle, lower) and allows comparisons of the percentage of ventilation and perfusion in each area. This test has a high sensitivity but can be more cumbersome then a CT scan and is not as accurate as a pulmonary angiogram.

A high suspicion of PE may warrant a spiral computed CT scan of the lung, D-dimer assay (blood test for evidence of blood clots), and pulmonary arteriogram. Spiral CT of the chest may also assist in the diagnosis. Spiral CT scan has recently gained popularity for use in the diagnosis of PE; it is more advanced and quicker than routine tomography. The term "spiral" comes from the shape of the path taken by the x-ray beam during scanning. The examination table advances at a constant rate through the scanner while the x-ray tube rotates continuously around the patient, following a spiral path, thus allowing the gathering of continuous data with no gaps between images. Unlike the traditional CT scan, the spiral CT scan evaluates slices as narrow as 1.0 mm, as compared with 5.0 mm slices obtained by traditional CT scan. This allows for a more accurate visualization of a PE. However, spiral CT has limitations. It cannot be performed at the bedside, so unstable patients must be transported to a CT scanner. In addition, IV infusion of contrast agent is necessary for visualization.

The D-dimer assay is becoming a more commonly used method for evaluating patients with possible PE. Because it is a simple test to perform, involving only a venipuncture, it has been studied as a possible method for ruling out PE; it is not used to make the diagnosis of PE. Emergency departments in particular have used this as a rapid, cost-effective test. D-dimer is a product of fibrin degradation and occurs as a result of fibrin lysis. An increased D-dimer value is usually indicative of a clotting abnormality. When a clot is dislodged, similar elevations of clotting factors should be present in the blood, especially in the case of a large embolus.

Pulmonary angiography is considered the best method to diagnose PE; however, it may not be feasible, cost-effective, or easily performed, especially with critically ill patients. The pulmonary angiogram allows for direct visualization under fluoroscopy of the arterial obstruction and accurate assessment of the perfusion deficit. A catheter is threaded through the vena cava to the right side of the heart to inject dye, similar to a cardiac catheterization, and a specially trained team must be available to perform the procedure.

## Prevention

For patients at risk for PE, the most effective approach for prevention is to prevent deep venous thrombosis. Active leg exercises to avoid venous stasis, early ambulation, and use of elastic compression stockings are general preventive measures. Additional strategies for prevention are listed in Chart 23-8.

Anticoagulant therapy may be prescribed for patients who are older than 40 years of age, whose hemostasis is adequate, and who are undergoing major elective abdominal or thoracic surgery. Low doses of heparin may be administered before surgery to reduce the risk of postoperative deep venous thrombus and PE. Heparin should be administered subcutaneously 2 hours before surgery and continued every 8 to 12 hours until the patient is discharged. Low-dose heparin is thought to enhance the activity of antithrombin III, a major plasma inhibitor of clotting factor X. This regimen is not recommended for patients with an active thrombotic process or for those undergoing major orthopedic surgery, open prostatectomy, or surgery on the eye or brain. Low-molecular-weight heparin (eg, enoxaparin [Lovenox]) is an alternative therapy. It has a longer half-life, enhanced subcutaneous absorption, a reduced incidence of thrombocytopenia, and reduced interaction with platelets, compared with unfractionated heparin (Goldhaber, 2004).

Sequential compression devices (SCDs) are often used to prevent venous stasis through compression and relaxation of the calf muscles, similar to the effect of muscle contraction. SCDs have been proven to effectively reduce the risk of deep venous thrombosis and have been shown to be an effective primary therapy for patients who are unable to receive anticoagulation therapy (Nagahiro, Andou, Aoe, et al., 2004; Ramirez, Pantelis, Gonzalez-Ruiz, et al., 2003). Several types of SCDs, using foot, calf, and thigh-high compression as well as graduated, asymmetric, and circumferential compression, are available. There is little evidence favoring any particular type of compression. Graduated compression involves the sequential movement of air in the sleeve up the leg, followed by relaxation of the sleeve. The advantage of this therapy is the extended duration of compression compared with standard inflation. Asymmetric compression involves inflating only the area on the back of the leg or foot. Circumferential compression involves even compression of the entire leg.

### CHART 23-8

## HOME CARE CHECKLIST • Prevention of Recurrent Pulmonary Embolism

| At the completion of the home care instruction, the patient or caregiver will be able to: | Patient | Caregiver |
|---|---|---|
| • Describe the underlying process leading to pulmonary embolism. | ✔ | ✔ |
| • Describe the need for continued anticoagulant therapy after the initial embolism. | ✔ | ✔ |
| • Name the anticoagulant prescribed and identify dosage and schedule of administration. | ✔ | ✔ |
| • Describe potential side effects of coagulation such as bruising and bleeding and identify ways to prevent bleeding. | ✔ | ✔ |
|   • Avoid the use of sharps (razors, knives, etc.) to prevent cuts; shave with an electric shaver. | | |
|   • Use a toothbrush with soft bristles to prevent gum injury. | | |
|   • Do not take aspirin or antihistamines while taking warfarin sodium (Coumadin). | | |
|   • Always check with health care provider before taking any medicine, including over-the-counter medications. | | |
|   • Avoid laxatives, because they may affect vitamin K absorption. | | |
|   • Report the occurrence of dark, tarry stools to the health care provider immediately. | | |
|   • Wear an identification bracelet or carry a medicine card stating that you are taking anticoagulants. | | |
| • Describe strategies to prevent recurrent deep venous thrombosis and pulmonary emboli: | ✔ | ✔ |
|   • Continue to wear elastic pressure stockings (compression hose) as long as directed. | | |
|   • Avoid sitting with legs crossed or sitting for prolonged periods of time. | | |
|   • When traveling, change position regularly, walk occasionally, and do active exercises of moving the legs and ankles while sitting. | | |
|   • Drink fluids, especially while traveling and in warm weather, to avoid hemoconcentration due to fluid deficit. | | |
| • Describe the signs and symptoms of lower extremity circulatory compromise and potential deep venous thrombosis: calf or leg pain, swelling, pedal edema. | ✔ | ✔ |
| • Describe the signs and symptoms of pulmonary compromise related to recurrent pulmonary embolism. | ✔ | ✔ |
| • Describe how and when to contact the health care provider if symptoms of circulatory compromise or pulmonary compromise are identified. | ✔ | ✔ |

## Medical Management

Because PE is often a medical emergency, emergency management is of primary concern. After emergency measures have been initiated and the patient is stabilized, the treatment goal is to dissolve (lyse) the existing emboli and prevent new ones from forming. Treatment may include a variety of modalities:

- General measures to improve respiratory and vascular status
- Anticoagulation therapy
- Thrombolytic therapy
- Surgical intervention

## Emergency Management

Massive PE is a life-threatening emergency. The immediate objective is to stabilize the cardiopulmonary system. A sudden increase in pulmonary resistance increases the work of the right ventricle, which can cause acute right-sided heart failure with cardiogenic shock. Emergency management consists of the following actions:

- Nasal oxygen is administered immediately to relieve hypoxemia, respiratory distress, and central cyanosis.
- Intravenous infusion lines are inserted to establish routes for medications or fluids that will be needed.
- A perfusion scan, hemodynamic measurements, and arterial blood gas determinations are performed. spiral (helical) CT or pulmonary angiography may be performed.
- Hypotension is treated by a slow infusion of dobutamine (Dobutrex), which has a dilating effect on the pulmonary vessels and bronchi, or dopamine (Intropin).
- The ECG is monitored continuously for dysrhythmias and right ventricular failure, which may occur suddenly.
- Digitalis glycosides, IV diuretics, and antiarrhythmic agents are administered when appropriate.

- Blood is drawn for serum electrolytes, complete blood count, and hematocrit.
- If clinical assessment and arterial blood gas analysis indicate the need, the patient is intubated and placed on a mechanical ventilator.
- If the patient has suffered massive embolism and is hypotensive, an indwelling urinary catheter is inserted to monitor urinary output.
- Small doses of IV morphine or sedatives are administered to relieve patient anxiety, to alleviate chest discomfort, to improve tolerance of the endotracheal tube, and to ease adaptation to the mechanical ventilator.

## General Management

Measures are initiated to improve respiratory and vascular status. Oxygen therapy is administered to correct the hypoxemia, relieve the pulmonary vascular vasoconstriction, and reduce the pulmonary hypertension. Use of elastic compression stockings or intermittent pneumatic leg compression devices reduces venous stasis. These measures compress the superficial veins and increase the velocity of blood in the deep veins by redirecting the blood through the deep veins. Elevating the leg (above the level of the heart) also increases venous flow.

## Pharmacologic Therapy

### ANTICOAGULATION THERAPY

Anticoagulant therapy (heparin, warfarin sodium) has traditionally been the primary method for managing acute deep vein thrombosis and PE (Goldhaber, 2004; Karin, 2003). Heparin is used to prevent recurrence of emboli but has no effect on emboli that are already present. Heparin is generally recommended for all patients who have been diagnosed with PE. Generally, a therapeutic heparin dose is administered as a one-time 5000-unit bolus and a continuous IV infusion is then started to maintain the partial thromboplastin time (PTT) at 1.5 to 2.0 times the normal level.

Heparin administration is associated with several concerns. Because the half-life of heparin is dose dependent, it is difficult and time-consuming to adjust and maintain the IV drip infusion at a therapeutic level; frequent laboratory testing is necessary. With long-term heparin use, there is also the risk of antibody formation and bleeding. Despite the risks, anticoagulation after initial clot formation and dislodgement is necessary because of the high risk for a recurrent thrombus. Therapy may be changed to an oral regimen, such as warfarin (Coumadin), as soon as the patient is able to take oral medications. Heparin must be continued until the international normalized ratio (INR) is within a therapeutic range, typically 2.0 to 2.5. Once the patient starts an oral regimen, it is important that he or she continue to take the same brand of warfarin, because the bioavailability may vary greatly among brands.

High doses of subcutaneous low-molecular-weight heparin or heparinoids may also be used to maintain a therapeutic PTT while oral anticoagulation therapy is being adjusted. Lepirudin (Refludan) and argatroban are alternatives for patients in whom heparin or heparinoids are contraindicated. These agents are direct thrombin inhibitors; therefore, they require less frequent monitoring and dose adjustment. Both medications have contraindications and side effects that the nurse must be aware of before administration. Lepirudin and argatroban are both contraindicated in patients with overt major bleeding and in patients who are hypersensitive to these agents or at high risk for bleeding (eg, recent cerebrovascular accident [CVA, brain attack], anomaly of vessels or organs, recent major surgery, recent puncture of large vessels or organ biopsy). Major side effects are bleeding anywhere in the body and anaphylactic reaction resulting in shock or death. Other side effects include fever, abnormal liver function, and allergic skin reaction. All patients must continue to take some form of anticoagulation for at least 3 to 6 months after the embolic event.

### THROMBOLYTIC THERAPY

Thrombolytic therapy (urokinase, streptokinase, alteplase, anistreplase, reteplase) also may be used in treating PE, particularly for patients who are severely compromised (eg, those who are hypotensive and have significant hypoxemia despite oxygen supplementation). Thrombolytic therapy resolves the thrombi or emboli more quickly and restores more normal hemodynamic functioning of the pulmonary circulation, thereby reducing pulmonary hypertension and improving perfusion, oxygenation, and cardiac output. However, bleeding is a significant side effect. Contraindications to thrombolytic therapy include a CVA within the past 2 months, other active intracranial processes, active bleeding, surgery within 10 days of the thrombotic event, recent labor and delivery, trauma, or severe hypertension. Consequently, thrombolytic agents are advocated only for PE affecting a significant area of blood flow to the lung and causing hemodynamic instability.

Before thrombolytic therapy is started, INR, PTT, hematocrit, and platelet counts are obtained. Heparin is stopped prior to administration of a thrombolytic agent. During therapy, all but essential invasive procedures are avoided because of potential bleeding. If necessary, fresh whole blood, packed red cells, cryoprecipitate, or frozen plasma is administered to replace blood loss and reverse the bleeding tendency. After the thrombolytic infusion is completed (which varies in duration according to the agent used and the condition being treated), anticoagulant therapy is initiated.

## Surgical Management

A surgical embolectomy is rarely performed but may be indicated if the patient has a massive PE or hemodynamic instability or if there are contraindications to thrombolytic therapy. This invasive procedure involves removal of the actual clot and must be performed by a cardiovascular surgical team with the patient on cardiopulmonary bypass. It may be used for patients who fail to improve with thrombolytic therapy, have contraindications to thrombolytic therapy and have had a massive PE, or must have the clot removed to help reduce right-sided heart failure. Although surgical embolectomy ensures removal of the clot, it is not without risk. The procedure has a high intraoperative mortality rate and has typical postoperative complications.

Transvenous catheter embolectomy is a technique in which a vacuum-cupped catheter is introduced transvenously into the affected pulmonary artery. Suction is applied to the end of the embolus, and the embolus is aspirated into the cup. The surgeon maintains suction to hold the embolus within the cup, and the entire catheter is withdrawn through the right side of the heart and out the femoral vein. Catheters are available that pulverize the clot with high-velocity jets of normal saline solution. An inferior vena cava filter is usually inserted at the time of surgery to protect against a recurrence.

Interrupting the inferior vena cava is another surgical technique used when PE recurs or when the patient does not tolerate anticoagulant therapy. This approach prevents dislodged thrombi from being swept into the lungs while allowing adequate blood flow. The preferred approach is the application of Teflon clips to the inferior vena cava to divide the lumen into small channels without occluding caval blood flow. Also, the use of transvenous devices that occlude or filter the blood through the inferior vena cava is a fairly safe way to prevent recurrent PE. One such technique involves insertion of a filter (eg, Greenfield filter) through the internal jugular vein or common femoral vein (Fig. 23-7). This filter is advanced into the inferior vena cava, where it is opened. The perforated umbrella permits the passage of blood but prevents the passage of large thrombi. It is recommended that anticoagulation be continued in patients with a vena cava filter, if there are no contraindications to its use.

## Nursing Management

### Minimizing the Risk of Pulmonary Embolism

A key role of the nurse is to identify the patient at high risk for PE and to minimize the risk of PE in all patients. The nurse must have a high degree of suspicion for PE in all patients, but particularly in those with conditions predisposing to a slowing of venous return (see Chart 23-7).

### Preventing Thrombus Formation

Preventing thrombus formation is a major nursing responsibility. The nurse encourages ambulation and active and passive leg exercises to prevent venous stasis in patients prescribed bed rest. The nurse instructs the patient to move the legs in a "pumping" exercise so that the leg muscles can help increase venous flow. The nurse also advises the patient not to sit or lie in bed for prolonged periods, not to cross the legs, and not to wear constrictive clothing. Legs should not be dangled or feet placed in a dependent position while the patient sits on the edge of the bed; instead, feet should rest on the floor or on a chair. In addition, IV catheters (for parenteral therapy or measurements of central venous pressure) should not be left in place for prolonged periods.

### Assessing Potential for Pulmonary Embolism

All patients are evaluated for risk factors for thrombus formation and pulmonary embolus. The nurse does a careful assessment of the patient's health history, family history, and medication record. On a daily basis, the patient is asked about pain or discomfort in the extremities. In addition, the extremities are evaluated for warmth, redness, and inflammation.

### Monitoring Thrombolytic Therapy

The nurse is responsible for monitoring thrombolytic and anticoagulant therapy. Thrombolytic therapy (streptokinase, urokinase, tissue plasminogen activator) causes lysis of deep vein thrombi and pulmonary emboli, which helps dissolve the clots. During thrombolytic infusion, while the patient remains on bed rest, vital signs are assessed every 2 hours and invasive procedures are avoided. Tests to determine INR or PTT are performed 3 to 4 hours after the thrombolytic infusion is started to confirm that the fibrinolytic systems have been activated. See Chapter 31 for nursing management for the patient receiving anticoagulant or thrombolytic therapy.

**NURSING ALERT**

Because of the prolonged clotting time, only essential arterial punctures or venipunctures are performed, and manual pressure is applied to any puncture site for at least 30 minutes. Pulse oximetry is used to monitor changes in oxygenation. The thrombolytic infusion is discontinued immediately if uncontrolled bleeding occurs.

### Managing Pain

Chest pain, if present, is usually pleuritic rather than cardiac in origin. A semi-Fowler's position provides a more comfortable position for breathing. However, it is important to continue to turn patients frequently and reposition them to improve the **ventilation–perfusion ratio** in the lung. The nurse administers opioid analgesics as prescribed for severe pain.

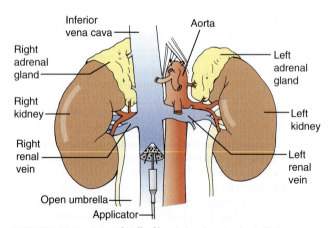

**FIGURE 23-7.** An umbrella filter is in place in the inferior vena cava to prevent pulmonary embolism. The filter (compressed within an applicator catheter) is inserted through an incision in the right internal jugular vein. The applicator is withdrawn when the filter fixes itself to the wall of the inferior vena cava after ejection from the applicator.

### Managing Oxygen Therapy

Careful attention is given to the proper use of oxygen. It is important to ensure that the patient understands the need for continuous oxygen therapy. The nurse assesses the patient frequently for signs of hypoxemia and monitors the pulse oximetry values to evaluate the effectiveness of the oxygen therapy. Deep breathing and incentive spirometry are indicated for all patients to minimize or prevent atelectasis and improve ventilation. Nebulizer therapy or percussion and postural drainage may be used for management of secretions.

### Relieving Anxiety

The nurse encourages the stabilized patient to talk about any fears or concerns related to this frightening episode, answers the patient's and family's questions concisely and accurately, explains the therapy, and describes how to recognize untoward effects early.

### Monitoring for Complications

When caring for a patient who has had PE, the nurse must be alert for the potential complication of cardiogenic shock or right ventricular failure subsequent to the effect of PE on the cardiovascular system. Nursing activities for managing shock are found in Chapter 15.

### Providing Postoperative Nursing Care

The nurse measures the patient's pulmonary arterial pressure and urinary output. The nurse also assesses the insertion site of the arterial catheter for hematoma formation and infection. It is important to maintain the blood pressure at a level that supports perfusion of vital organs. To prevent peripheral venous stasis and edema of the lower extremities, the nurse elevates the foot of the bed and encourages isometric exercises, use of elastic compression stockings, and walking when the patient is permitted out of bed. Sitting is discouraged, because hip flexion compresses the large veins in the legs.

### Promoting Home and Community-Based Care

#### TEACHING PATIENTS SELF-CARE
Before hospital discharge and at follow-up visits to the clinic, the nurse instructs the patient about preventing recurrence and reporting signs and symptoms. Patient instructions, as presented in Chart 23-8, are intended to help prevent recurrences and side effects of treatment.

#### CONTINUING CARE
During follow-up or home care visits, the nurse monitors the patient's adherence to the prescribed management plan and reinforces previous instructions. The nurse also monitors the patient for residual effects of the PE and recovery. The patient is reminded about the importance of keeping follow-up appointments for coagulation tests and appointments with the primary care provider. The nurse also reminds the patient about the importance of participation in health promotion activities (eg, immunizations) and health screening.

## Sarcoidosis

Sarcoidosis is a multisystem, granulomatous disease of unknown etiology. It may involve almost any organ or tissue but most commonly involves the lungs, lymph nodes, liver, spleen, central nervous system, skin, eyes, fingers, and parotid glands. The disease is not gender-specific, but some manifestations are more common in women. Prevalence rates are 10 to 40 cases per 100,000 population. In the United States, the disease is more common in African Americans (36 cases per 100,000) than in Caucasians (11 cases per 100,000), and the disease usually begins in the third or fourth decade of life (Doty & Judson, 2004).

### Pathophysiology

Sarcoidosis is thought to be a hypersensitivity response to one or more agents (bacteria, fungi, virus, chemicals) in people with an inherited or acquired predisposition to the disorder. The hypersensitivity response results in noncaseating granuloma formation due to the release of cytokines and other substances that promote replication of fibroblasts. In the lung, granuloma infiltration and fibrosis may occur, resulting in low lung compliance, impaired diffusing capacity, and reduced lung volumes.

### Clinical Manifestations

Hallmarks of sarcoidosis are its insidious onset and lack of prominent clinical signs or symptoms. The clinical picture depends on the systems affected. The lung is most commonly involved; signs and symptoms may include dyspnea, cough, hemoptysis, and congestion. Generalized symptoms include anorexia, fatigue, and weight loss. Other signs include uveitis, joint pain, fever, and granulomatous lesions of the skin, liver, spleen, kidney, and central nervous system. The granulomas may disappear or gradually convert to fibrous tissue. With multisystem involvement, patients may also have fatigue, fever, anorexia, and weight loss.

### Assessment and Diagnostic Findings

Chest x-rays and CT are used to assess pulmonary adenopathy. These may show hilar adenopathy and disseminated miliary and nodular lesions in the lungs. A mediastinoscopy or **transbronchial** biopsy (in which a tissue specimen is obtained through the bronchial wall) may be used to confirm the diagnosis. In rare cases, an **open lung biopsy** is performed. Diagnosis is confirmed by a biopsy that shows noncaseating granulomas. Pulmonary function test results are abnormal if there is restriction of lung function (reduction in total lung capacity). Arterial blood gas measurements may be normal or may show reduced oxygen levels (hypoxemia) and increased carbon dioxide levels (hypercapnia).

## Medical Management

Many patients undergo remission without specific treatment. Corticosteroids may be beneficial because of their anti-inflammatory effects, which relieve symptoms and improve organ function. They are useful in patients with ocular and myocardial involvement, skin involvement, extensive pulmonary disease that compromises pulmonary function, hepatic involvement, and hypercalcemia. Other cytotoxic and immunosuppressive agents have been used, but without the benefit of controlled clinical trials. There is no single test that monitors the progression or recurrence of sarcoidosis. Multiple tests are used to monitor involved systems.

## Occupational Lung Diseases: Pneumoconioses

Pneumoconiosis refers to a nonneoplastic alteration of the lung resulting from inhalation of mineral or inorganic dust (eg, "dusty lung"). Pneumoconioses are caused by inhalation and deposition of mineral dusts in the lungs, resulting in pulmonary fibrosis and parenchymal changes. Many people with early pneumoconiosis are asymptomatic, but advanced disease often is accompanied by disability and premature death (CDC, 2004b). Between 1968 and 2000, pneumoconiosis was cited as the cause of death of 124,846 people in the United States (CDC, 2004b).

Diseases of the lungs occur in numerous occupations as a result of exposure to several different types of agents. Examples include mineral dusts (asbestos, silica, coal), metal dusts, biological dusts (spores, mycelia, bird droppings), manufactured fibers (glass or ceramic fibers), and toxic fumes (nitrogen dioxide, sulfur dioxide, chlorine, ammonia). The effects of inhaling these materials depend on the composition of the substance, its concentration, its ability to initiate an immune response, its irritating properties, the duration of exposure, and the individual's response or susceptibility to the irritant. Smoking may compound the problem and may increase the risk of lung cancers in people exposed to the mineral asbestos and other potential carcinogens.

Key aspects of any assessment of patients with a potential occupational respiratory history include job and job activities, exposure levels, general hygiene, time frame of exposure, amount of respiratory protection used, and direct versus indirect exposures. Specific information that should be obtained includes the following:

- Exposure to an agent known to cause an occupational disorder
- Length of time from exposure of agent to onset of symptoms
- Congruence of symptoms with those of known exposure-related disorder
- Lack of other more likely explanations of the signs and symptoms

Occupational health nurses serve as employee advocates, making every effort to promote measures to reduce the exposure of workers to industrial products. Resources for occupational health nurses include the United States Department of Labor Occupational Safety and Health Administration (OSHA) as well as state-specific resources. The mission of OSHA is to ensure the safety and health of America's workers by setting and enforcing standards; providing training, outreach, and education; establishing partnerships; and encouraging continual improvement in workplace safety and health. Laws require that the work environment be ventilated properly to remove any noxious agent.

Dust control can prevent many of the pneumoconioses. Dust control includes ventilation, spraying an area with water to control dust, and effective and frequent floor cleaning. Air samples need to be monitored. Toxic substances should be enclosed and placed in restricted areas. Workers must wear or use protective devices (face masks, hoods, industrial respirators) to provide a safe air supply when a toxic element is present. Employees who are at risk should be carefully screened and monitored. There is a risk of developing serious smoking-related illness (cancer) in industries in which there are unsafe levels of certain gases, dusts, fumes, fluids, and other toxic substances. In addition, there is the potential for second-hand exposure. Asbestos and toxic dusts and substances may be transferred to others through the handling of clothing or shoes that have been exposed. Ongoing educational programs should be designed to teach workers to take responsibility for their own health and to stop smoking and receive an influenza vaccination.

Federal "right to know" laws stipulate that employees must be informed about all hazardous and toxic substances in the workplace. Specifically, they must be informed about any hazardous or toxic substances they work with, what effects these substances can have on their health, and the measures they can take to protect themselves. The responsibility for implementing these controls inevitably falls on the federal or state government.

In addition to teaching preventive measures to patients and their families, the nurse assesses patients for a history of exposure to environmental agents (eg, dusts, fibers, fumes) and makes referrals so that pulmonary function can be evaluated and the patient can be treated early in the course of the disease. Patients with occupational lung disease often experience increasing chronic dyspnea, cough, and a prolonged illness culminating in respiratory failure. Strategies to prevent superimposed infection are implemented, and the patient and family are assisted in coping with the increasing disability that accompanies occupational lung disease. Home care referrals are often helpful in identifying measures to decrease the patient's dyspnea, ensure appropriate and safe use of oxygen, and make the patient as comfortable as possible. In addition, referral to a pulmonary rehabilitation program may be considered in some patients.

The most common pneumoconioses are silicosis, asbestosis, and coal worker's pneumoconiosis.

### Silicosis

Silicosis is a chronic fibrotic pulmonary disease caused by inhalation of silica dust (crystalline silicon dioxide particles). Exposure to silica and silicates occurs in almost all mining, quarrying, and tunneling operations. Glass manufacturing, stone-cutting, manufacturing of abrasives and pottery, and foundry work are other occupations with exposure hazards. Finely ground silica, such as that found in soaps, polishes and filters, is extremely dangerous.

## Pathophysiology

When the silica particles, which have fibrogenic properties, are inhaled, nodular lesions are produced throughout the lungs. With the passage of time and further exposure, the nodules enlarge and coalesce. Dense masses form in the upper portion of the lungs, resulting in the loss of pulmonary volume. **Restrictive lung disease** (disease of the lungs that limits their ability to expand fully) and obstructive lung disease from secondary emphysema result. Cavities can form as a result of superimposed TB. Exposure of 15 to 20 years is usually required before the onset of the disease and shortness of breath occurs. Fibrotic destruction of pulmonary tissue can lead to emphysema, pulmonary hypertension, and cor pulmonale.

## Clinical Manifestations

Patients with acute silicosis present with dyspnea, fever, cough, and weight loss, and progression of the disease is rapid. Symptoms are more severe in patients whose disease is complicated by progressive massive fibrosis. More commonly, this disease is a chronic problem with a long latency period. Patients may have slowly progressive symptoms indicative of hypoxemia, severe air-flow obstruction, and right-sided heart failure. Edema may occur because of the cardiac failure.

## Medical Management

There is no specific treatment for silicosis, because the fibrotic process in the lung is irreversible. Supportive therapy is directed at managing complications and preventing infection. Testing is performed to rule out other lung diseases, such as TB, lung cancer, and sarcoidosis. If TB is present, it is aggressively treated. Additional therapy may include oxygen, diuretics, inhaled beta-adrenergic agonists, anticholinergics, and bronchodilator therapy.

# Asbestosis

Asbestosis is a disease characterized by diffuse pulmonary fibrosis from the inhalation of asbestos dust. Current laws restrict the use of asbestos, but many industries used it in the past. Therefore, exposure occurred, and may still occur, in people in numerous occupations, including asbestos mining and manufacturing, shipbuilding, demolition of structures containing asbestos, and roofing. Materials such as shingles, cement, vinyl asbestos tile, fireproof paint and clothing, brake linings, and filters all contained asbestos at one time, and many of these materials are still in existence. Chronic exposure may also occur by washing clothes that have been in contact with asbestos. Additional diseases related to asbestos exposure include lung cancer, mesothelioma, and asbestos-related pleural effusion.

## Pathophysiology

Inhaled asbestos fibers enter the alveoli, where they are surrounded by fibrous tissue. The fibrous tissue eventually obliterates the alveoli. Fibrous changes also affect the pleura, which thickens and develops plaque. The result of these physiologic changes is a restrictive lung disease, with a decrease in lung volume, diminished exchange of oxygen and carbon dioxide, and hypoxemia.

## Clinical Manifestations

The onset of the disease is insidious, and patients have progressive dyspnea, persistent, dry cough, mild to moderate chest pain, anorexia, weight loss, and malaise. Early physical findings include bibasilar fine, end-inspiratory crackles and, in more advanced cases, clubbing of the fingers. As the disease progresses, cor pulmonale and respiratory failure occur. A high proportion of workers who have been exposed to asbestos dust, especially those who smoke or have a history of smoking, die of lung cancer. Malignant mesothelioma, a rare cancer of the pleura or peritoneum that is strongly associated with asbestos exposure, may also occur.

## Medical Management

There is no effective treatment for asbestosis, because the lung damage is permanent and often progressive. Management is directed at controlling infection and treating the lung disease. When oxygen–carbon dioxide exchange becomes severely impaired, continuous oxygen therapy may help improve activity tolerance. The patient must be instructed to avoid additional exposure to asbestos and to stop smoking. A significant contributing cause to mortality in this population is the high incidence of lung carcinoma.

# Coal Worker's Pneumoconiosis

Coal worker's pneumoconiosis ("black lung disease") includes a variety of respiratory diseases found in coal workers who have inhaled coal dust over the years. Coal miners are exposed to dusts that are mixtures of coal, kaolin, mica, and silica.

## Pathophysiology

When coal dust is deposited in the alveoli and respiratory bronchioles, macrophages engulf the particles (by phagocytosis) and transport them to the terminal bronchioles, where they are removed by mucociliary action. In time, the clearance mechanisms cannot handle the excessive dust load, and the macrophages aggregate in the respiratory bronchioles and alveoli. Fibroblasts appear and a network of reticulin is laid down surrounding the dust-laden macrophages. The bronchioles and the alveoli become clogged with coal dust, dying macrophages, and fibroblasts. This leads to the formation of the coal macule, the primary lesion of the disorder. Macules appear as blackish dots on the lungs. Fibrotic lesions develop and, as the macules enlarge, the weakening bronchioles dilate, with subsequent development of localized emphysema. The disease begins in the upper lobes of the lungs but may progress to the lower lobes.

## Clinical Manifestations

The first signs are a chronic cough and sputum production, similar to the signs encountered in chronic bronchitis. As the disease progresses, patients develop dyspnea and cough up large amounts of sputum with varying amounts of black fluid (melanoptysis), particularly if they are smokers. Eventually, cor pulmonale and respiratory failure result. The diagnosis may first be made based on chest x-ray findings and history of exposure.

## Medical Management

Preventing this disease is key, because there is no effective treatment. Instead, treatment focuses on early diagnosis and management of complications. (See Chapter 24 for discussion of emphysema.)

# Chest Tumors

Tumors of the lung may be benign or malignant. A malignant chest tumor can be primary, arising within the lung, chest wall, or mediastinum, or it can be a metastasis from a primary tumor site elsewhere in the body. Metastatic lung tumors occur frequently because the bloodstream transports cancer cells from primary cancers elsewhere in the body to the lungs.

## Lung Cancer (Bronchogenic Carcinoma)

Lung cancer is the leading cancer killer among men and women in the United States. In 2005, there were an estimated 172,500 new cases of cancer of the lung and bronchus (93,000 men and 79,500 women). In the same year, it was estimated that 163,500 would die from this disease (American Cancer Society, 2005). For men, the incidence of lung cancer has remained relatively constant and in women it has begun to plateau after a continuous rise over the past 30 years (American Cancer Society, 2005). Two thirds of the United States population with lung cancer is 65 years of age or older (Hurria & Kris, 2003).

In approximately 70% of patients with lung cancer, the disease has spread to regional lymphatics and other sites by the time of diagnosis. As a result, the long-term survival rate is low.

### Pathophysiology

Between 80% and 90% of lung cancers are caused by inhaled carcinogens, most commonly cigarette smoke (Baldwin, 2003); other carcinogens include radon gas and occupational and environmental agents. Lung cancers arise from a single transformed epithelial cell in the tracheobronchial airways, in which the carcinogen binds to and damages the cell's DNA. This damage results in cellular changes, abnormal cell growth, and eventually a malignant cell. As the damaged DNA is passed on to daughter cells, the DNA undergoes further changes and becomes unstable. With the accumulation of genetic changes, the pulmonary epithelium undergoes malignant transformation from normal epithelium eventually to invasive carcinoma. Evidence indicates that carcinoma tends to arise at sites of previous scarring (TB, fibrosis) in the lung.

### Classification and Staging

For purposes of staging and treatment, most lung cancers are classified into one of two major categories: small cell lung cancer and non–small cell lung cancer. Non–small cell lung cancer is further classified with cell types. Squamous cell cancer is usually more centrally located and arises more commonly in the segmental and subsegmental bronchi. Adenocarcinoma is the most prevalent carcinoma of the lung in both men and women; it occurs peripherally as peripheral masses or nodules and often metastasizes. Large cell carcinoma (also called undifferentiated carcinoma) is a fast-growing tumor that tends to arise peripherally. Bronchoalveolar cell cancer is found in the terminal bronchi and alveoli and is usually slower growing compared with other bronchogenic carcinomas.

Non–small cell lung carcinoma (NSCLC) represents 75% to 80% of tumors; small cell carcinoma represents 15% to 20% of tumors. In NSCLC, the cell types include squamous cell carcinoma (20% to 30%), large cell carcinoma (10%), and adenocarcinoma (30% to 40%), including bronchoalveolar carcinoma. Most small cell carcinomas arise in the major bronchi and spread by infiltration along the bronchial wall. Small cell lung cancer accounts for 20% to 25% of all bronchogenic cancers (Baldwin, 2003).

In addition to classification according to cell type, lung cancers are staged. The stage of the tumor refers to the size of the tumor, its location, whether lymph nodes are involved, and whether the cancer has spread (American Joint Committee on Cancer, 2002). NSCLC is staged as I to IV. Stage I is the earliest stage and has the highest cure rates, whereas stage IV designates metastatic spread. Estimated 5-year survival rates for the stages of NSCLC are as follows: stages IA and IB, 50% to 80%; stage IIA and IIB, 30% to 50%; stage IIIA, 10% to 40%; stage IIIB, 5% to 20%; and stage IV, less than 5% (Baldwin, 2003). Small cell lung cancers are classified as limited or extensive. Diagnostic tools and further information on staging are described in Chapter 16.

### Risk Factors

Various factors have been associated with the development of lung cancer, including tobacco smoke, secondhand (passive) smoke, environmental and occupational exposures, gender, genetics, and dietary deficits. Other factors that have been associated with lung cancer include genetic predisposition and underlying respiratory diseases, such as COPD and TB.

## Tobacco Smoke

Tobacco use is responsible for more than one of every six deaths in the United States from pulmonary and cardiovascular diseases. Smoking is the most important single preventable cause of death and disease in this country. Lung cancer is 10 times more common in cigarette smokers than nonsmokers. Risk is determined by the pack-year history (number of packs of cigarettes used each day, multiplied by the number of years smoked), the age of initiation of smoking, the depth of inhalation, and the tar and nicotine levels in the cigarettes smoked. The younger a person is when he or she starts smoking, the greater the risk of developing lung cancer. The risk of cancer is always higher for former smokers than for people who have never smoked. However, the risk decreases beginning at approximately 5 years after smoking cessation occurs and continues to decrease over time.

## Secondhand Smoke

Passive smoking has been identified as a possible cause of lung cancer in nonsmokers. It is estimated that secondhand smoke causes about 3000 deaths per year (Baldwin, 2003). When compared with unexposed nonsmokers, people who are involuntarily exposed to tobacco smoke in a closed environment (house, automobile, building) have an increased risk of lung cancer.

## Environmental and Occupational Exposure

Various carcinogens have been identified in the atmosphere, including motor vehicle emissions and pollutants from refineries and manufacturing plants. Evidence suggests that the incidence of lung cancer is greater in urban areas as a result of the buildup of pollutants and motor vehicle emissions.

Radon is a colorless, odorless gas found in soil and rocks. For many years it has been associated with uranium mines, but it is now known to seep into homes through ground rock. High levels of radon have been associated with the development of lung cancer, especially when combined with cigarette smoking. Homeowners are advised to have radon levels checked in their houses and to arrange for special venting if the levels are high.

Chronic exposure to industrial carcinogens, such as arsenic, asbestos, mustard gas, chromates, coke oven fumes, nickel, oil, and radiation, has been associated with the development of lung cancer. Laws have been passed to control exposure to these carcinogens in the workplace.

## Genetics

Some familial predisposition to lung cancer seems apparent, because the incidence of lung cancer in close relatives of patients with lung cancer appears to be two to three times that in the general population regardless of smoking status.

## Dietary Factors

Smokers who eat a diet low in fruits and vegetables have an increased risk of developing lung cancer. The actual active agents in a diet rich in fruits and vegetables have yet to be determined. It has been hypothesized that carotenoids, particularly carotene or vitamin A, may be important. Several ongoing trials may help determine whether carotene supplementation has anticancer properties. Other nutrients, including vitamin E, selenium, vitamin C, fat, and retinoids, are also being evaluated regarding their protective role against lung cancer.

## Clinical Manifestations

Often, lung cancer develops insidiously and is asymptomatic until late in its course. The signs and symptoms depend on the location and size of the tumor, the degree of obstruction, and the existence of metastases to regional or distant sites.

The most frequent symptom of lung cancer is cough or change in a chronic cough. People frequently ignore this symptom and attribute it to smoking or a respiratory infection. The cough starts as a dry, persistent cough, without sputum production. When obstruction of airways occurs, the cough may become productive due to infection.

**A cough that changes in character should arouse suspicion of lung cancer.**

Dyspnea occurs in 35% to 50% of patients (Baldwin, 2003). Hemoptysis or blood-tinged sputum may be expectorated. Chest or shoulder pain may indicate chest wall or pleural involvement by a tumor. Pain also is a late manifestation and may be related to metastasis to the bone.

In some patients, a recurring fever is an early symptom in response to a persistent infection in an area of pneumonitis distal to the tumor. In fact, cancer of the lung should be suspected in people with repeated unresolved upper respiratory tract infections. If the tumor spreads to adjacent structures and regional lymph nodes, the patient may present with chest pain and tightness, hoarseness (involving the recurrent laryngeal nerve), dysphagia, head and neck edema, and symptoms of pleural or pericardial effusion. The most common sites of metastases are lymph nodes, bone, brain, contralateral lung, adrenal glands, and liver. Nonspecific symptoms of weakness, anorexia, and weight loss also may be present.

## Assessment and Diagnostic Findings

If pulmonary symptoms occur in heavy smokers, cancer of the lung should always be considered. A chest x-ray is performed to search for pulmonary density, a solitary pulmonary nodule (coin lesion), atelectasis, and infection. CT scans of the chest are used to identify small nodules not easily visualized on the chest x-ray and also to serially examine areas for lymphadenopathy.

Sputum cytology is rarely used to make a diagnosis of lung cancer. Fiberoptic bronchoscopy is more commonly used; it provides a detailed study of the tracheobronchial tree and allows for brushings, washings, and biopsies of suspicious areas. For peripheral lesions not amenable to bronchoscopic biopsy, a transthoracic **fine-needle aspiration** may be performed under CT guidance to aspirate cells from a suspicious area. In some circumstances, an endoscopy with esophageal ultrasound may be used to obtain a transesophageal biopsy of enlarged subcarinal lymph nodes that are not easily accessible by other means.

A variety of scans may be used to assess for metastasis of the cancer. These may include bone scans, abdominal scans, positron emission tomography (PET) scans, and liver ultrasound. CT of the brain, magnetic resonance imaging (MRI), and other neurologic diagnostic procedures are used to detect central nervous system metastases. Mediastinoscopy or mediastinotomy may be used to obtain biopsy samples from lymph nodes in the mediastinum.

If surgery is a potential treatment, the patient is evaluated to determine whether the tumor is resectable and whether the patient can tolerate the physiologic impairment resulting from such surgery. Pulmonary function tests, arterial blood gas analysis, V/Q scans, and exercise testing may all be used as part of the preoperative assessment.

## Medical Management

The objective of management is to provide a cure, if possible. Treatment depends on the cell type, the stage of the disease, and the patient's physiologic status (particularly cardiac and pulmonary status). In general, treatment may involve surgery, radiation therapy, or chemotherapy—or a combination of these. Newer and more specific therapies to modulate the immune system (gene therapy, therapy with defined tumor antigens) are under study and show promise.

### Surgical Management

Surgical resection is the preferred method of treating patients with localized non–small cell tumors, no evidence of metastatic spread, and adequate cardiopulmonary function. If the patient's cardiovascular status, pulmonary function, and functional status are satisfactory, surgery is generally well tolerated. However, coronary artery disease, pulmonary insufficiency, and other comorbidities may contraindicate surgical intervention. The cure rate of surgical resection depends on the type and stage of the cancer. Surgery is primarily used for NSCLCs, because small cell cancer of the lung grows rapidly and metastasizes early and extensively. Lesions of many patients with bronchogenic cancer are inoperable at the time of diagnosis.

Several different types of lung resection may be performed (Chart 23-9). The most common surgical procedure for a small, apparently curable tumor of the lung is lobectomy (removal of a lobe of the lung). In some cases, an entire lung may be removed (pneumonectomy) (see Chapter 25 for further details).

### Radiation Therapy

Radiation therapy may offer cure in a small percentage of patients. It is useful in controlling neoplasms that cannot be surgically resected but are responsive to radiation. Irradiation also may be used to reduce the size of a tumor, to make an inoperable tumor operable, or to relieve the pressure

---

**CHART 23-9**

### Types of Lung Resection

- **Lobectomy:** a single lobe of lung is removed
- **Bilobectomy:** two lobes of the lung are removed
- **Sleeve resection:** cancerous lobe(s) is removed and a segment of the main bronchus is resected
- **Pneumonectomy:** removal of entire lung
- **Segmentectomy:** a segment of the lung is removed*
- **Wedge resection:** removal of a small, pie-shaped area of the segment*
- **Chest wall resection with removal of cancerous lung tissue:** for cancers that have invaded the chest wall

*Not recommended as curative resection for lung cancer.

---

of the tumor on vital structures. It can reduce symptoms of spinal cord metastasis and superior vena caval compression. Also, prophylactic brain irradiation is used in certain patients to treat microscopic metastases to the brain. Radiation therapy may help relieve cough, chest pain, dyspnea, hemoptysis, and bone and liver pain. Relief of symptoms may last from a few weeks to many months and is important in improving the quality of the remaining period of life.

Radiation therapy usually is toxic to normal tissue within the radiation field, and this may lead to complications such as esophagitis, pneumonitis, and radiation lung fibrosis. These may impair ventilatory and diffusion capacity and significantly reduce pulmonary reserve. The patient's nutritional status, psychological outlook, fatigue level, and signs of anemia and infection are monitored throughout the treatment. See Chapter 16 for management of the patient receiving radiation therapy.

### Chemotherapy

Chemotherapy is used to alter tumor growth patterns, to treat distant metastases or small cell cancer of the lung, and as an adjunct to surgery or radiation therapy. Chemotherapy may provide relief, especially of pain, but it does not usually cure the disease or prolong life to any great degree. Chemotherapy is also accompanied by side effects. It is valuable in reducing pressure symptoms of lung cancer and in treating brain, spinal cord, and pericardial metastasis. See Chapter 16 for a discussion of chemotherapy for the patient with cancer.

The choice of agent depends on the growth of the tumor cell and the specific phase of the cell cycle that the medication affects. In combination with surgery, chemotherapy may be administered before surgery (neoadjuvant therapy) or after surgery (adjuvant therapy). Combinations of two or more medications may be more beneficial than single-dose regimens. A variety of agents are used, including platinum analogues (cisplatin and carboplatin) and non–platinum-containing agents—taxanes (paclitaxel, docetaxel), vinca alkaloids (vinblastine and vindesine), doxorubicin, gemcitabine, vinorelbine, irinotecan (CPT-11), etoposide (VP-16), and pemetrexed (Alimta). Recently approved chemotherapeutic agents in oral form are gefitinib (Iressa) and erlotinib (Tarceva), which are epidermal growth factor tyrosine kinase inhibitors. Numerous new agents with cellular targets, including protein kinase C, vascular endothelial growth factor, cyclooxygenase-2, and farnesyl transferase, are being tested for various types of lung cancer.

### Palliative Therapy

Palliative therapy may include radiation therapy to shrink the tumor to provide pain relief, a variety of bronchoscopic interventions to open a narrowed bronchus or airway, and pain management and other comfort measures. Evaluation and referral for hospice care are important in planning for comfortable and dignified end-of-life care for the patient and family.

## Treatment-Related Complications

A variety of complications may occur as a result of treatment for lung cancer. Surgical resection may result in respiratory failure, particularly if the cardiopulmonary system is compromised before surgery. Surgical complications and prolonged mechanical ventilation are potential outcomes. Radiation therapy may result in diminished cardiopulmonary function and other complications, such as pulmonary fibrosis, pericarditis, myelitis, and cor pulmonale. Chemotherapy, particularly in combination with radiation therapy, can cause pneumonitis. Pulmonary toxicity is a potential side effect of chemotherapy.

## Nursing Management

Nursing care of patients with lung cancer is similar to that for other patients with cancer (see Chapter 16) and addresses the physiologic and psychological needs of the patient. The physiologic problems are primarily due to the respiratory manifestations of the disease. Nursing care includes strategies to ensure relief of pain and discomfort and to prevent complications.

### Managing Symptoms

The nurse instructs the patient and family about the potential side effects of the specific treatment and strategies to manage them. Strategies for managing such symptoms as dyspnea, fatigue, nausea and vomiting, and anorexia help the patient and family cope with therapeutic measures.

### Relieving Breathing Problems

Airway clearance techniques are key to maintaining airway patency through the removal of excess secretions. This may be accomplished through deep-breathing exercises, chest physiotherapy, directed cough, suctioning, and in some instances bronchoscopy. Bronchodilator medications may be prescribed to promote bronchial dilation. As the tumor enlarges or spreads, it may compress a bronchus or involve a large area of lung tissue, resulting in an impaired breathing pattern and poor gas exchange. At some stage of the disease, supplemental oxygen will probably be necessary.

Nursing measures focus on decreasing dyspnea by encouraging the patient to assume positions that promote lung expansion and to perform breathing exercises for lung expansion and relaxation. Patient education about energy conservation and airway clearance techniques is also necessary. Many of the techniques used in pulmonary rehabilitation can be applied to patients with lung cancer. Depending on the severity of disease and the patient's wishes, a referral to a pulmonary rehabilitation program may be helpful in managing respiratory symptoms.

### Reducing Fatigue

Fatigue is a devastating symptom that affects quality of life in patients with cancer. It is commonly experienced by patients with lung cancer and may be related to the disease itself, the cancer treatment and complications (eg, anemia), sleep disturbances, pain and discomfort, hypoxemia, poor nutrition, or the psychological ramifications of the disease (eg, anxiety, depression). The nurse is pivotal in thoroughly assessing the patient's level of fatigue, identifying potentially treatable causes, and validating with the patient that fatigue is indeed an important symptom. Educating the patient about energy conservation techniques or referral to physical therapy, occupational therapy, or pulmonary rehabilitation programs may be helpful. In addition, guided exercise has been recently identified as a potential intervention for treating fatigue in cancer patients. This is an important area for research, because few studies have been conducted, and only in select populations of patients with cancer.

### Providing Psychological Support

Another important part of the nursing care of patients with lung cancer is provision of psychological support and identification of potential resources for the patient and family. Often, the nurse must help the patient and family deal with the following:

- The poor prognosis and relatively rapid progression of this disease
- Informed decision making regarding the possible treatment options
- Methods to maintain the patient's quality of life during the course of this disease
- End-of-life treatment options

## Gerontologic Considerations

At the time of diagnosis of lung cancer, most patients are older than 65 years of age and have stage III or IV disease (Hurria & Kris, 2003). Although age is not a significant prognostic factor for overall survival and response to treatment for either NSCLC or small cell lung cancer, older patients have specific needs (Hurria & Kris, 2003). Depending on the comorbidities and functional status of elderly patients, chemotherapy agents, doses, and cycles may need to be adjusted to maintain quality of life. Issues that must be considered in care of elderly patients with lung cancer include functional status, comorbid conditions, nutritional status, cognition, concomitant medications, and psychological

## NURSING RESEARCH PROFILE

### Lung Cancer

Gift, A. G., Stommel, M., Jablonski, A., et al. (2003). A cluster of symptoms over time in patients with lung cancer. *Nursing Research, 52*(6), 393–400.

**Purpose**

Lung cancer is a leading type of cancer diagnosed in both men and women. The purpose of this study was to determine whether the symptom cluster identified at the time of diagnosis remained constant at 3 and 6 months after diagnosis and whether there was a difference in the number or severity of symptoms. Lastly, the ability of number of symptoms and cluster of symptoms to predict survival was explored.

**Design**

An existing data set of 112 patients (58 men and 54 women) with newly diagnosed lung cancer was evaluated. Only patients who survived at least 6 months after diagnosis were included in the analysis. Symptoms were assessed using the Physical Symptom Experience technique, a self-report measure used to assess the occurrence and severity of 37 common symptoms. Symptom clusters were evaluated at the time of diagnosis and 3 and 6 months later. Survival was evaluated at 19 months after diagnosis.

**Findings**

A cluster of seven symptoms (fatigue, weakness, weight loss, appetite loss, nausea, vomiting, altered taste) was identified at diagnosis. Both the mean number and severity of symptoms declined over time. Correlations between severity of vomiting and weight loss at diagnosis, at 3 months, and at 6 months were low; however, fatigue, weakness, poor appetite, altered taste, and nausea were reported more consistently over time. Stage of cancer at diagnosis was the most predictive of the number of cluster symptoms reported, and death occurring 6 to 19 months after diagnosis was predicted by age, stage at diagnosis, and symptom severity at 6 months.

**Nursing Implications**

Symptom management is a major nursing priority in patients with cancer. Many nurses focus on only one symptom; however, multiple symptoms are frequently experienced. These clusters of symptoms most likely have a multiplicative effect on patients and their cancers. These symptoms relate not only to the cancer diagnosis but also to the patient's comorbidities, treatment regimen, or palliative care plan. It is important to identify symptom clusters and symptom distress in patients with cancer and to further develop and evaluate nursing interventions to help patients deal with different symptom clusters.

---

and social support (Barrocas, Purdy, Brady, et al., 2002; Hurria & Kris, 2003).

## Tumors of the Mediastinum

Tumors of the mediastinum include neurogenic tumors, tumors of the thymus, lymphomas, germ cell tumors, cysts, and mesenchymal tumors. These tumors may be malignant or benign. They are usually described in relation to location: anterior, middle, or posterior masses or tumors.

### Clinical Manifestations

Nearly all symptoms of mediastinal tumors result from the pressure of the mass against important intrathoracic organs. Symptoms may include cough, wheezing, dyspnea, anterior chest or neck pain, bulging of the chest wall, heart palpitations, angina, other circulatory disturbances, central cyanosis, superior vena cava syndrome (ie, swelling of the face, neck, and upper extremities), marked distention of the veins of the neck and the chest wall (evidence of the obstruction of large veins of the mediastinum by extravascular compression or intravascular invasion), and dysphagia and weight loss from pressure or invasion into the esophagus.

### Assessment and Diagnostic Findings

Chest x-rays are the major method used initially to diagnose mediastinal tumors and cysts. CT is the standard diagnostic test for assessment of the mediastinum and surrounding structures. MRI, as well as PET, may be used in some circumstances.

### Medical Management

If the tumor is malignant and has infiltrated the surrounding tissue and complete surgical removal is not feasible, radiation therapy, chemotherapy, or both are used.

### Surgical Management

Many mediastinal tumors are benign and operable. The location of the tumor (anterior, middle, or posterior compartment) in the mediastinum dictates the type of incision. The common incision used is a median sternotomy; however, a thoracotomy may be used, depending on the location of the tumor. Additional approaches include a bilateral anterior thoracotomy (clamshell incision) and video-assisted thoracoscopic surgery (see Chapter 25). The care is the same as for any patient undergoing thoracic surgery. Major complications include hemorrhage, injury to the phrenic or recurrent laryngeal nerve, and infection.

# Chest Trauma

Major chest trauma may occur alone or in combination with multiple other injuries. Chest trauma is classified as either blunt or penetrating. Blunt chest trauma results from sudden compression or positive pressure inflicted to the chest wall. Penetrating trauma occurs when a foreign object penetrates the chest wall.

## Blunt Trauma

Blunt thoracic injuries are responsible for approximately 8% of all trauma admissions (Karmy-Jones & Jurkovich, 2004). Although blunt chest trauma is more common than penetrating trauma, it is often difficult to identify the extent of the damage because the symptoms may be generalized and vague. In addition, patients may not seek immediate medical attention, which may complicate the problem.

## Overview
### Pathophysiology

The most common causes of blunt chest trauma are motor vehicle crashes (trauma from steering wheel, seat belt), falls, and bicycle crashes (trauma from handlebars). Mechanisms of blunt chest trauma include acceleration (moving object hitting the chest or patient being thrown into an object), deceleration (sudden decrease in rate of speed or velocity, such as a motor vehicle crash), shearing (stretching forces to areas of the chest causing tears, ruptures, or dissections), and compression (direct blow to the chest, such as a crush injury). Injuries to the chest are often life-threatening and result in one or more of the following pathologic states:

- Hypoxemia from disruption of the airway; injury to the lung parenchyma, rib cage, and respiratory musculature; massive hemorrhage; collapsed lung; and pneumothorax
- Hypovolemia from massive fluid loss from the great vessels, cardiac rupture, or hemothorax
- Cardiac failure from cardiac tamponade, cardiac contusion, or increased intrathoracic pressure

These pathologic states frequently result in impaired ventilation and perfusion leading to ARF, hypovolemic shock, and death.

### Assessment and Diagnostic Findings

Time is critical in treating chest trauma. Therefore, it is essential to assess the patient immediately to determine the following:

- Time elapsed since injury occurred
- Mechanism of injury
- Level of responsiveness
- Specific injuries
- Estimated blood loss
- Recent drug or alcohol use
- Prehospital treatment

Initial assessment of thoracic injuries includes assessment for airway obstruction, tension pneumothorax, open pneumothorax, massive hemothorax, flail chest, and cardiac tamponade. These injuries are life-threatening and require immediate treatment. Secondary assessment includes assessment for simple pneumothorax, hemothorax, pulmonary contusion, traumatic aortic rupture, tracheobronchial disruption, esophageal perforation, traumatic diaphragmatic injury, and penetrating wounds to the mediastinum. Although listed as secondary, these injuries may be life-threatening as well.

The physical examination includes inspection of the airway, thorax, neck veins, and breathing difficulty. Specifics include assessing the rate and depth of breathing for abnormalities such as stridor, cyanosis, nasal flaring, use of accessory muscles, drooling, and overt trauma to the face, mouth, or neck. The chest is assessed for symmetric movement, symmetry of breath sounds, open chest wounds, entrance or exit wounds, impaled objects, tracheal shift, distended neck veins, subcutaneous emphysema, and paradoxical chest wall motion. In addition, the chest wall is assessed for bruising, petechiae, lacerations, and burns. The vital signs and skin color are assessed for signs of shock. The thorax is palpated for tenderness and crepitus, and the position of the trachea is also assessed.

The initial diagnostic workup includes a chest x-ray, CT scan, complete blood count, clotting studies, type and cross-match, electrolytes, oxygen saturation, arterial blood gas analysis, and ECG. The patient is completely undressed to avoid missing additional injuries that may complicate care. Many patients with injuries involving the chest have associated head and abdominal injuries that require attention. Ongoing assessment is essential to monitor the patient's response to treatment and to detect early signs of clinical deterioration.

### Medical Management

The goals of treatment are to evaluate the patient's condition and to initiate aggressive resuscitation. An airway is immediately established with oxygen support and, in some cases, intubation and ventilatory support. Reestablishing fluid volume and negative intrapleural pressure and draining intrapleural fluid and blood are essential.

The potential for massive blood loss and exsanguination with blunt or penetrating chest injuries is high because of injury to the great blood vessels. Many patients die at the scene of the injury or are in shock by the time help arrives. Agitation and irrational and combative behavior are signs of decreased oxygen delivery to the cerebral cortex. Strategies to restore and maintain cardiopulmonary function include ensuring an adequate airway and ventilation; stabilizing and reestablishing chest wall integrity; occluding any opening into the chest (open pneumothorax); and draining or removing any air or fluid from the thorax to relieve pneumothorax, hemothorax, or cardiac tamponade. Hypovolemia and low cardiac output must be corrected. Many of these treatment efforts, along with the control of hemorrhage, are carried out simultaneously at the scene of the injury or in the emergency department. Depending on the success of efforts to control the hemorrhage in the emergency department, the patient may be taken immediately to the operating room. Principles of management are essentially those pertaining to care of the postoperative thoracic patient (see Chapter 25).

## Sternal and Rib Fractures

Sternal fractures are most common in motor vehicle crashes with a direct blow to the sternum via the steering wheel. Rib fractures are the most common type of chest trauma, occurring in more than 60% of patients admitted with blunt chest injury (Karmy-Jones & Jurkovich, 2004). Most rib fractures are benign and are treated conservatively. Fractures of the first three ribs are rare but can result in a high mortality rate because they are associated with laceration of the subclavian artery or vein. The fifth through ninth ribs are the most common sites of fractures. Fractures of the lower ribs are associated with injury to the spleen and liver, which may be lacerated by fragmented sections of the rib.

### Clinical Manifestations

Patients with sternal fractures have anterior chest pain, overlying tenderness, ecchymosis, crepitus, swelling, and possible chest wall deformity. For patients with rib fractures, clinical manifestations are similar: severe pain, point tenderness, and muscle spasm over the area of the fracture that are aggravated by coughing, deep breathing, and movement. The area around the fracture may be bruised. To reduce the pain, the patient splints the chest by breathing in a shallow manner and avoids sighs, deep breaths, coughing, and movement. This reluctance to move or breathe deeply results in diminished ventilation, atelectasis (collapse of unaerated alveoli), pneumonitis, and hypoxemia. Respiratory insufficiency and failure can be the outcomes of such a cycle.

### Assessment and Diagnostic Findings

The patient must be closely evaluated for underlying cardiac injuries. A crackling, grating sound in the thorax (subcutaneous crepitus) may be detected with auscultation. The diagnostic workup may include a chest x-ray, rib films of a specific area, ECG, continuous pulse oximetry, and arterial blood gas analysis.

### Medical Management

Medical management is directed toward relieving pain, avoiding excessive activity, and treating any associated injuries. Surgical fixation is rarely necessary unless fragments are grossly displaced and pose a potential for further injury.

The goals of treatment for rib fractures are to control pain and to detect and treat the injury. Sedation is used to relieve pain and to allow deep breathing and coughing. Care must be taken to avoid oversedation and suppression of respiratory drive. Alternative strategies to relieve pain include an intercostal nerve block and ice over the fracture site. A chest binder may be used as supportive treatment to provide stability to the chest wall and may decrease pain. The patient is instructed to apply the binder snugly enough to provide support, but not to impair respiratory excursion. Usually the pain abates in 5 to 7 days, and discomfort can be relieved with epidural analgesia, patient-controlled analgesia, or nonopioid analgesia. Most rib fractures heal in 3 to 6 weeks. The patient is monitored closely for signs and symptoms of associated injuries.

## Flail Chest

Flail chest is frequently a complication of blunt chest trauma from a steering wheel injury. It usually occurs when three or more adjacent ribs (multiple contiguous ribs) are fractured at two or more sites, resulting in free-floating rib segments. It may also result as a combination fracture of ribs and costal cartilages or sternum. As a result, the chest wall loses stability, causing respiratory impairment and usually severe respiratory distress.

### Pathophysiology

During inspiration, as the chest expands, the detached part of the rib segment (flail segment) moves in a paradoxical manner (pendelluft movement) in that it is pulled inward during inspiration, reducing the amount of air that can be drawn into the lungs. On expiration, because the intrathoracic pressure exceeds atmospheric pressure, the flail segment bulges outward, impairing the patient's ability to exhale. The mediastinum then shifts back to the affected side (Fig. 23-8). This paradoxical action results in increased dead space, a reduction in alveolar ventilation, and decreased compliance. Retained airway secretions and atelectasis frequently accompany flail chest. The patient has hypoxemia, and if gas exchange is greatly compromised, respiratory acidosis develops as a result of carbon dioxide retention. Hypotension, inadequate tissue perfusion, and metabolic acidosis often follow as the paradoxical motion of the mediastinum decreases cardiac output.

### Medical Management

As with rib fracture, treatment of flail chest is usually supportive. Management includes providing ventilatory support, clearing secretions from the lungs, and controlling pain. Specific management depends on the degree of respiratory dysfunction. If only a small segment of the chest is involved, the objectives are to clear the airway through positioning, coughing, deep breathing, and suctioning to aid in the expansion of the lung, and to relieve pain by intercostal nerve blocks, high thoracic epidural blocks, or cautious use of IV opioids.

For mild to moderate flail chest injuries, the underlying pulmonary contusion is treated by monitoring fluid intake and appropriate fluid replacement while relieving chest pain. Pulmonary physiotherapy focusing on lung volume expansion, and secretion management techniques are performed. The patient is closely monitored for further respiratory compromise.

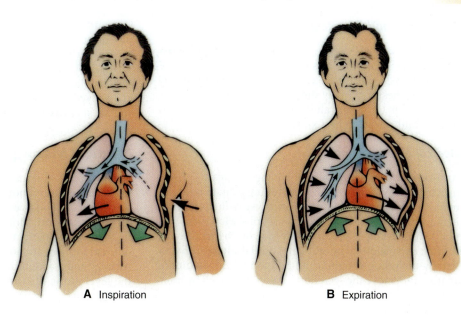

**FIGURE 23-8.** Flail chest is caused by a free-floating segment of rib cage resulting from multiple rib fractures. (**A**) Paradoxical movement on inspiration occurs when the flail rib segment is sucked inward and the mediastinal structures shift to the unaffected side. The amount of air drawn into the affected lung is reduced. (**B**) On expiration, the flail segment bulges outward and the mediastinal structures shift back to the affected side.

**A** Inspiration  **B** Expiration

For severe flail chest injuries, endotracheal intubation and mechanical ventilation are required to provide internal pneumatic stabilization of the flail chest and to correct abnormalities in gas exchange. This helps treat the underlying pulmonary contusion, serves to stabilize the thoracic cage to allow the fractures to heal, and improves alveolar ventilation and intrathoracic volume by decreasing the work of breathing. This treatment modality requires endotracheal intubation and ventilator support. Differing modes of ventilation are used depending on the patient's underlying disease and specific needs.

In rare circumstances, surgery may be required to more quickly stabilize the flail segment. This may be used for patients who are difficult to ventilate or for high-risk patients with underlying lung disease who may be difficult to wean from mechanical ventilation.

Regardless of the type of treatment, the patient is carefully monitored by serial chest x-rays, arterial blood gas analysis, pulse oximetry, and bedside pulmonary function monitoring. Pain management is key to successful treatment. Patient-controlled analgesia, intercostal nerve blocks, epidural analgesia, and intrapleural administration of opioids may be used to relieve or manage thoracic pain.

## Pulmonary Contusion

Pulmonary contusion is a common thoracic injury and is frequently associated with flail chest. It is defined as damage to the lung tissues resulting in hemorrhage and localized edema. It is associated with chest trauma when there is rapid compression and decompression to the chest wall (ie, blunt trauma). Pulmonary contusion represents a spectrum of lung injury characterized by the development of infiltrates and various degrees of respiratory dysfunction and sometimes respiratory failure. It is often cited as the most common potentially life-threatening chest injury; however, mortality is often attributed to other associated injuries (Karmy-Jones & Jurkovich, 2004). A contusion is sustained in 30% to 70% of patients who experience blunt force trauma. Pulmonary contusion may not be evident initially on examination but develops in the posttraumatic period; it may involve a small portion of one lung, a massive section of a lung, one entire lung, or both lungs.

### Pathophysiology

The primary pathologic defect is an abnormal accumulation of fluid in the interstitial and intra-alveolar spaces. It is thought that injury to the lung parenchyma and its capillary network results in a leakage of serum protein and plasma. The leaking serum protein exerts an osmotic pressure that enhances loss of fluid from the capillaries. Blood, edema, and cellular debris (from cellular response to injury) enter the lung and accumulate in the bronchioles and alveoli, where they interfere with gas exchange. An increase in pulmonary vascular resistance and pulmonary artery pressure occurs. The patient has hypoxemia and carbon dioxide retention. Occasionally, a contused lung occurs on the other side of the point of body impact; this is called a contrecoup contusion.

### Clinical Manifestations

Pulmonary contusion may be mild, moderate, or severe. The clinical manifestations vary from decreased breath sounds, tachypnea, tachycardia, chest pain, hypoxemia, and blood-tinged secretions to more severe tachypnea, tachycardia, crackles, frank bleeding, severe hypoxemia (cyanosis), and respiratory acidosis. Changes in sensorium, including increased agitation or combative irrational behavior, may be signs of hypoxemia.

In addition, patients with moderate pulmonary contusion have a large amount of mucus, serum, and frank blood in the tracheobronchial tree; patients often have a constant cough but cannot clear the secretions. Patients with severe pulmonary contusion have the signs and symptoms of ARDS; these may include central cyanosis, agitation, combativeness, and productive cough with frothy, bloody secretions.

### Assessment and Diagnostic Findings

The efficiency of gas exchange is determined by pulse oximetry and arterial blood gas measurements. Pulse oximetry is also used to measure oxygen saturation continuously. The initial chest x-ray may show no changes; changes may not appear for 1 or 2 days after the injury and appear as pulmonary infiltrates on chest x-ray.

### Medical Management

Treatment priorities include maintaining the airway, providing adequate oxygenation, and controlling pain. In mild pulmonary contusion, adequate hydration via IV fluids and oral intake is important to mobilize secretions. However, fluid intake must be closely monitored to avoid hypervolemia. Volume expansion techniques, postural drainage, physiotherapy including coughing, and endotracheal suctioning are used to remove the secretions. Pain is managed by intercostal nerve blocks or by opioids via patient-controlled analgesia or other methods. Usually, antimicrobial therapy is administered because the damaged lung is susceptible to infection. Supplemental oxygen is usually given by mask or cannula for 24 to 36 hours.

In patients with moderate pulmonary contusions, bronchoscopy may be required to remove secretions. Intubation and mechanical ventilation with PEEP (see Chapter 25) may also be necessary to maintain the pressure and keep the lungs inflated. Diuretics may be administered to reduce edema. A nasogastric tube is inserted to relieve gastrointestinal distention.

In patients with severe contusion, who may develop respiratory failure, aggressive treatment with endotracheal intubation and ventilatory support, diuretics, and fluid restriction may be necessary. Colloids and crystalloid solutions may be used to treat hypovolemia.

Antimicrobial medications may be prescribed for the treatment of pulmonary infection. This is a common complication of pulmonary contusion (especially pneumonia in the contused segment), because the fluid and blood that extravasates into the alveolar and interstitial spaces serve as an excellent culture medium.

## Penetrating Trauma: Gunshot and Stab Wounds

Gunshot and stab wounds are the most common causes of penetrating chest trauma. These wounds are classified according to their velocity. Stab wounds are generally considered low-velocity trauma because the weapon destroys a small area around the wound. Knives and switchblades cause most stab wounds. The appearance of the external wound may be very deceptive, because pneumothorax, hemothorax, lung contusion, and cardiac tamponade, along with severe and continuing hemorrhage, can occur from any small wound, even one caused by a small-diameter instrument such as an ice pick.

Gunshot wounds may be classified as low, medium, or high velocity. The factors that determine the velocity and resulting extent of damage include the distance from which the gun was fired, the caliber of the gun, and the construction and size of the bullet. A bullet can cause damage at the site of penetration and along its pathway, and a gunshot wound to the chest can produce a variety of pathophysiologic changes. The bullet may ricochet off bony structures and damage the chest organs and great vessels. If the diaphragm is involved in a gunshot wound or a stab wound, injury to the chest cavity must be considered.

### Medical Management

The objective of immediate management is to restore and maintain cardiopulmonary function. After an adequate airway is ensured and ventilation is established, examination for shock and intrathoracic and intra-abdominal injuries is necessary. The patient is undressed completely so that additional injuries are not missed. There is a high risk for associated intra-abdominal injuries with stab wounds below the level of the fifth anterior intercostal space. Death can result from exsanguinating hemorrhage or intra-abdominal sepsis.

The diagnostic workup includes a chest x-ray, chemistry profile, arterial blood gas analysis, pulse oximetry, and ECG. The patient's blood is typed and cross-matched in case blood transfusion is required. After the status of the peripheral pulses is assessed, a large-bore IV line is inserted. An indwelling catheter is inserted to monitor urinary output. A nasogastric tube is inserted and connected to low suction to prevent aspiration, minimize leakage of abdominal contents, and decompress the gastrointestinal tract.

Shock is treated simultaneously with colloid solutions, crystalloids, or blood, as indicated by the patient's condition. Diagnostic procedures are carried out as dictated by the needs of the patient (eg, CT scans of chest or abdomen, flat plate x-ray of the abdomen, abdominal tap to check for bleeding).

A chest tube is inserted into the pleural space in most patients with penetrating wounds of the chest to achieve rapid and continuing reexpansion of the lungs. The insertion of the chest tube frequently results in a complete evacuation of the blood and air. The chest tube also allows early recognition of continuing intrathoracic bleeding, which would make surgical exploration necessary. If the patient has a penetrating wound of the heart or great vessels, the esophagus, or the tracheobronchial tree, surgical intervention is required.

## Pneumothorax

Pneumothorax occurs when the parietal or visceral pleura is breached and the pleural space is exposed to positive atmospheric pressure. Normally the pressure in the pleural space is negative or subatmospheric; this negative pressure is required to maintain lung inflation. When either pleura is breached, air enters the pleural space, and the lung or a portion of it collapses.

### Types of Pneumothorax

Types of pneumothorax include simple, traumatic, and tension pneumothorax.

### Simple Pneumothorax

A simple, or spontaneous, pneumothorax occurs when air enters the pleural space through a breach of either the parietal or visceral pleura. Most commonly this occurs as air enters the pleural space through the rupture of a bleb or a bronchopleural fistula. A spontaneous pneumothorax may occur in an apparently healthy person in the absence of trauma due to rupture of an air-filled bleb, or blister, on the surface of the lung, allowing air from the airways to enter the pleural cavity. It may be associated with diffuse interstitial lung disease and severe emphysema.

### Traumatic Pneumothorax

A traumatic pneumothorax occurs when air escapes from a laceration in the lung itself and enters the pleural space or enters the pleural space through a wound in the chest wall. It may result from blunt trauma (eg, rib fractures), penetrating chest or abdominal trauma (eg, stab wounds or gunshot wounds), or diaphragmatic tears. Traumatic pneumothorax may occur during invasive thoracic procedures (ie, thoracentesis, transbronchial lung biopsy, insertion of a subclavian line) in which the pleura is inadvertently punctured, or with barotrauma from mechanical ventilation.

A traumatic pneumothorax resulting from major injury to the chest is often accompanied by hemothorax (collection of blood in the pleural space resulting from torn intercostal vessels, lacerations of the great vessels, or lacerations of the lungs). Often both blood and air are found in the chest cavity (hemopneumothorax) after major trauma. Chest surgery can be classified as a traumatic pneumothorax as a result of the entry into the pleural space and the accumulation of air and fluid in the pleural space.

Open pneumothorax is one form of traumatic pneumothorax. It occurs when a wound in the chest wall is large enough to allow air to pass freely in and out of the thoracic cavity with each attempted respiration. Because the rush of air through the wound in the chest wall produces a sucking sound, such injuries are termed sucking chest wounds. In such patients, not only does the lung collapse, but the structures of the mediastinum (heart and great vessels) also shift toward the uninjured side with each inspiration and in the opposite direction with expiration. This is termed mediastinal flutter or swing, and it produces serious circulatory problems.

**Traumatic open pneumothorax calls for emergency interventions. Stopping the flow of air through the opening in the chest wall is a life-saving measure.**

### Tension Pneumothorax

A **tension pneumothorax** occurs when air is drawn into the pleural space from a lacerated lung or through a small opening or wound in the chest wall. It may be a complication of other types of pneumothorax. In contrast to open pneumothorax, the air that enters the chest cavity with each inspiration is trapped; it cannot be expelled during expiration through the air passages or the opening in the chest wall. In effect, a one-way valve or ball valve mechanism occurs where air enters the pleural space but cannot escape. With each breath, tension (positive pressure) is increased within the affected pleural space. This causes the lung to collapse and the heart, the great vessels, and the trachea to shift toward the unaffected side of the chest (mediastinal shift). Both respiration and circulatory function are compromised because of the increased intrathoracic pressure, which decreases venous return to the heart, causing decreased cardiac output and impairment of peripheral circulation. In extreme cases, the pulse may be undetectable—this is known as pulseless electrical activity.

**Relief of tension pneumothorax is considered an emergency measure.**

## Clinical Manifestations

The signs and symptoms associated with pneumothorax depend on its size and cause. Pain is usually sudden and may be pleuritic. The patient may have only minimal respiratory distress with slight chest discomfort and tachypnea with a small simple or uncomplicated pneumothorax. If the pneumothorax is large and the lung collapses totally, acute respiratory distress occurs. The patient is anxious, has dyspnea and air hunger, has increased use of the accessory muscles, and may develop central cyanosis from severe hypoxemia. In assessing the chest for any type of pneumothorax, the nurse assesses tracheal alignment, expansion of the chest, breath sounds and percussion of the chest. In a simple pneumothorax the trachea is midline, expansion of the chest is decreased, breath sounds may be diminished, and percussion of the chest may reveal normal sounds or hyperresonance depending on the size of the pneumothorax.

In a tension pneumothorax, the trachea is shifted away from the affected side, chest expansion may be decreased or fixed in a hyperexpansion state, breath sounds are diminished or absent, and percussion to the affected side is hyperresonant. The clinical picture is one of air hunger, agitation, increasing hypoxemia, central cyanosis, hypotension, tachycardia, and profuse diaphoresis. Figure 23-9 compares open and tension pneumothorax.

## Medical Management

Medical management of pneumothorax depends on its cause and severity. The goal of treatment is to evacuate the air or blood from the pleural space. A small chest tube (28 French) is inserted near the second intercostal space; this space is used because it is the thinnest part of the chest wall, minimizes the danger of contacting the thoracic nerve, and leaves

**FIGURE 23-9.** Open pneumothorax (*top*) and tension pneumothorax (*bottom*). In open pneumothorax, air enters the chest during inspiration and exits during expiration. A slight shift of the affected lung may occur because of a decrease in pressure as air moves out of the chest. In tension pneumothorax, air enters but cannot leave the chest. As the pressure increases, the heart and great vessels are compressed and the mediastinal structures are shifted toward the opposite side of the chest. The trachea is pushed from its normal midline position toward the opposite side of the chest, and the unaffected lung is compressed.

a less visible scar. If a patient also has a hemothorax, a large-diameter chest tube (32 French or greater) is inserted, usually in the fourth or fifth intercostal space at the midaxillary line. The tube is directed posteriorly to drain the fluid and air. Once the chest tube or tubes are inserted and suction is applied (usually to 20 mm Hg suction), effective decompression of the pleural cavity (drainage of blood or air) occurs.

If an excessive amount of blood enters the chest tube in a relatively short period, an autotransfusion may be needed. This technique involves taking the patient's own blood that has been drained from the chest, filtering it, and then transfusing it back into the vascular system.

In such an emergency, anything may be used that is large enough to fill the chest wound—a towel, a handkerchief, or the heel of the hand. If conscious, the patient is instructed to inhale and strain against a closed glottis. This action assists in reexpanding the lung and ejecting the air from the thorax. In the hospital, the opening is plugged by sealing it with gauze impregnated with petrolatum. A pressure dressing is applied. Usually, a chest tube connected to water-seal drainage is inserted to permit air and fluid to drain. Antibiotics usually are prescribed to combat infection from contamination.

The severity of open pneumothorax depends on the amount and rate of thoracic bleeding and the amount of air in the pleural space. The pleural cavity can be decompressed by needle aspiration (thoracentesis) or by chest tube drainage of the blood or air. The lung is then able to re-expand and resume the function of gas exchange. As a rule of thumb, the chest wall is opened surgically (thoracotomy) if more than 1500 mL of blood is aspirated initially by thoracentesis (or is the initial chest tube output) or if chest tube output continues at greater than 200 mL/hour. The urgency with which the blood must be removed is determined by the degree of respiratory compromise. An emergency thoracotomy may also be performed in the emergency department if a cardiovascular injury secondary to chest or penetrating trauma is suspected. The patient with a possible tension pneumothorax should immediately be given a high concentration of supplemental oxygen to treat the hypoxemia, and pulse oximetry should be used to monitor oxygen saturation. In an emergency situation, a tension pneumothorax can be decompressed or quickly converted to a simple pneumothorax by inserting a large-bore needle (14-gauge) at the second intercostal space, midclavicular line on the affected side. This relieves the pressure and vents the positive pressure to the external environment. A chest tube is then inserted and connected to suction to remove the remaining air and fluid, reestablish the negative pressure, and reexpand the lung. If the lung reexpands and air leakage from the lung parenchyma stops, further drainage may be unnecessary. If a prolonged air leak continues despite chest tube drainage to underwater seal, surgery may be necessary to close the leak.

## Cardiac Tamponade

Cardiac tamponade is compression of the heart resulting from fluid or blood within the pericardial sac. It usually is caused by blunt or penetrating trauma to the chest. A penetrating wound of the heart is associated with a high mortality rate. Cardiac tamponade also may follow diagnostic cardiac catheterization, angiographic procedures, and pacemaker insertion, which can produce perforations of the heart and great vessels. Pericardial effusion with fluid compressing the heart also may develop from metastases to the pericardium from malignant tumors of the breast, lung, or mediastinum and may occur with lymphomas and leukemias, renal failure, TB, and high-dose radiation to the chest. Cardiac tamponade is discussed in detail in Chapter 30.

## Subcutaneous Emphysema

No matter what kind of chest trauma a patient has, when the lung or the air passages are injured, air may enter the tissue planes and pass for some distance under the skin (eg, neck, chest). The tissues give a crackling sensation when palpated, and the subcutaneous air produces an alarming appearance as the face, neck, body, and scrotum become misshapen by subcutaneous air. Fortunately, subcutaneous emphysema is of itself usually not a serious complication. The subcutaneous air is spontaneously absorbed if the underlying air leak is treated or stops spontaneously. In severe cases in which there is widespread subcutaneous emphysema, a tracheostomy is indicated if airway patency is threatened.

# Aspiration

Aspiration of stomach contents into the lungs is a serious complication that can cause pneumonia and result in the following clinical picture: tachycardia, dyspnea, central cyanosis, hypertension, hypotension, and finally death. It can occur when the protective airway reflexes are decreased or absent due to a variety of factors (Chart 23-10).

**NURSING ALERT**

When a nonfunctioning nasogastric tube allows the gastric contents to accumulate in the stomach, a condition known as silent aspiration may result. Silent aspiration often occurs unobserved and may be more common than suspected. If untreated, massive inhalation of gastric contents develops in a period of several hours.

## Pathophysiology

The primary factors responsible for death and complications after aspiration of gastric contents are the volume and character of the aspirated gastric contents. For example, a small, localized aspiration from regurgitation can cause pneumonia and acute respiratory distress; a massive aspiration is usually fatal.

A full stomach contains solid particles of food. If these are aspirated, the problem then becomes one of mechanical blockage of the airways and secondary infection. During periods of fasting, the stomach contains acidic gastric juice, which, if aspirated, can be very destructive to the alveoli and capillaries. Fecal contamination (more likely seen in intestinal obstruction) increases the likelihood of death, because the endotoxins produced by intestinal organisms may be absorbed systemically, or the thick proteinaceous material found in the intestinal contents may obstruct the airway, leading to atelectasis and secondary bacterial invasion.

Aspiration pneumonitis may develop from aspiration of substances with a pH of less than 2.5 and a volume of gastric aspirate greater than 0.3 mL per kilogram of body weight (approximately 20 to 25 mL in adults) (Marik, 2001). Aspiration of gastric contents causes a chemical burn of the tracheobronchial tree and pulmonary parenchyma (Marik, 2001). An inflammatory response occurs. This results in the destruction of alveolar–capillary endothelial cells, with a consequent outpouring of protein-rich fluids into the interstitial and intra-alveolar spaces. As a result, surfactant is lost, which in turn causes the airways to close and the alveoli to collapse. Finally, the impaired exchange of oxygen and carbon dioxide causes respiratory failure.

Aspiration pneumonia develops after inhalation of colonized oropharyngeal material. The pathologic process involves an acute inflammatory response to bacteria and bacterial products. Most commonly, the bacteriologic findings include gram-positive cocci, gram-negative rods, and occasionally anaerobic bacteria (Marik, 2001).

## Prevention

Prevention is the primary goal when caring for patients at risk for aspiration. Examples of risk factors for aspiration include decreased level of consciousness, supine positioning, presence of a nasogastric tube, tracheal intubation and mechanical ventilation, bolus or intermittent feeding delivery methods, and advanced age (Metheny, 2002). Evidence confirms that one of the main preventive measures for aspiration is placing at-risk patients in a semirecumbent position (elevation of the head of the bed to a 30- to 45-degree angle) (CDC, 2004d; Keithley & Swanson, 2004).

### Compensating for Absent Reflexes

Aspiration may occur if the patient cannot adequately coordinate protective glottic, laryngeal, and cough reflexes. This hazard is increased if the patient has a distended abdomen, is supine, has the upper extremities immobilized by IV infusions or hand restraints, receives local anesthetics to the oropharyngeal or laryngeal area for diagnostic procedures, has been sedated, or has had long-term intubation.

When vomiting, people can normally protect their airway by sitting up or turning on the side and coordinating breathing, coughing, gag, and glottic reflexes. If these reflexes are active, an oral airway should not be inserted. If an airway is in place, it should be pulled out the moment the patient gags so as not to stimulate the pharyngeal gag reflex and promote vomiting and aspiration. Suctioning of oral secretions with a catheter should be performed with minimal pharyngeal stimulation.

### Assessing Feeding Tube Placement

When a patient is intubated, aspiration may occur even with a nasogastric tube in place and may result in nosocomial pneumonia. Assessment of nasogastric tube placement is

**CHART 23-10**

**Risk Factors for Aspiration**

- Seizure activity
- Decreased level of consciousness from trauma, drug or alcohol intoxication, excessive sedation, or general anesthesia
- Nausea and vomiting in the patient with a decreased level of consciousness
- Stroke
- Swallowing disorders
- Cardiac arrest
- Silent aspiration

key to prevention of aspiration. The best method for determining tube placement is via an x-ray. Other methods have been studied; observation of the aspirate and testing of its pH are the most reliable. Gastric fluid may be grassy green, brown, clear, or colorless. An aspirate from the lungs may be off-white or tan mucus. Pleural fluid is watery and usually straw-colored. Gastric pH values are typically lower (more acidic) than those of the intestinal or respiratory tract. Gastric pH is usually between 1 and 5, whereas intestinal or respiratory pH is 7 or higher. There are differences in assessing tube placement with continuous versus intermittent feedings. For intermittent feedings with small-bore tubes, observation of aspirated contents and pH evaluation should be performed. For continuous feedings, the pH method is not clinically useful because of the infused formula (Metheny, 2002; Metheny & Titler, 2001).

Patients who receive continuous or timed-interval tube feedings must be positioned properly. Patients receiving continuous infusions are given small volumes under low pressure in an upright position, which helps prevent aspiration. Patients receiving tube feedings at timed intervals are maintained in an upright or semirecumbent position (elevation of the head of the bed to a 30- to 45-degree angle) during the feeding and for a minimum of 30 minutes afterward to allow the stomach to empty partially (Keithley & Swanson, 2004). Tube feedings must be given only when it is certain that the feeding tube is positioned correctly in the stomach. Many patients today receive enteral feeding directly into the duodenum through a small-bore flexible feeding tube or surgically implanted tube. Feedings are given slowly and are regulated by a feeding pump. Correct placement is confirmed by chest x-ray.

### Identifying Delayed Stomach Emptying

A full stomach can cause aspiration because of increased intragastric or extragastric pressure. The following clinical situations delay emptying of the stomach and may contribute to aspiration: intestinal obstruction; increased gastric secretions in gastroesophageal reflex disease; increased gastric secretions during anxiety, stress, or pain; and abdominal distention because of ileus, ascites, peritonitis, use of opioids or sedatives, severe illness, or vaginal delivery.

When a feeding tube is present, contents are aspirated, usually every 4 hours, to determine the amount of the last feeding left in the stomach (residual volume). Preliminary evidence in this area suggests that gastric residuals are insensitive and unreliable markers of tolerance to tube feedings. Except in high-risk, selected patients, few data support withholding tube feedings in patients with gastric residuals less than 500 mL (Keithley & Swanson, 2004).

### Managing Effects of Prolonged Intubation

Prolonged endotracheal intubation or tracheostomy can depress the laryngeal and glottic reflexes because of disuse. Patients with prolonged tracheostomies are encouraged to phonate and exercise their laryngeal muscles. For patients who have had long-term intubation or tracheostomies, it may be helpful to have a rehabilitation therapist experienced in speech and swallowing disorders (ie, speech therapist) work with the patient to assess the swallowing reflex.

## Critical Thinking Exercises

**1** **ebp** You are caring for an 82-year-old woman who was recently transferred to the hospital from a nursing home with the diagnosis of presumed nursing home–acquired pneumonia. She has a nasogastric feeding tube in place and is lethargic, dehydrated, and confused. What strategies would you initiate to prevent aspiration? What nursing care interventions would you use to assess for aspiration? What is the evidence base for the interventions that you consider? How will you evaluate the strength of the evidence? What suggestions might you have regarding appropriate devices for long-term enteral feeding in this patient once she is discharged back to the nursing home?

**2** On a surgical unit, you are caring for a 42-year-old woman who underwent a total abdominal hysterectomy and bilateral salpingo-oophorectomy and has developed severe postoperative deep venous thrombosis that resulted in a pulmonary embolism. She is a smoker and is taking multiple medications. She was stable when you started your shift, but she has become increasingly anxious with some shortness of breath in the past hour. What are potential risk factors you might observe or identify in this patient? What assessment strategies would you use to evaluate changes in her respiratory status? What decision process would you use to determine when the physician should be contacted?

**3** You are caring for a patient who experienced blunt chest trauma in a motor vehicle crash. A chest tube has been inserted to treat a simple pneumothorax and hemothorax. The chest drainage system has drained 400 mL of light red fluid during the first 6 hours after insertion. The patient has become increasingly short of breath during the past hour. What physical assessment skills and strategies would you use to determine potential changes in the patient's respiratory condition? What are potential causes of this increasing shortness of breath? What would you do to prepare for an emergency situation in this patient?

**4** **ebp** On a surgical unit, you are caring for a 62-year-old man who has undergone right upper lobectomy for lung cancer. The patient has chronic obstructive pulmonary disease (COPD) and has continued to smoke despite the diagnoses of COPD and lung cancer. What strategies would you use to prevent or minimize pulmonary complications in this patient? What are methods you might use to assess the patient's progress from a respiratory standpoint? What strategies would you consider to encourage the patient to stop smoking? What is the evidence base for the strategies that you consider? How will you evaluate the strength of the evidence?

# REFERENCES AND SELECTED READINGS

## BOOKS

Agency for Healthcare Research and Quality. (2003). *Diagnosis and treatment of deep venous thrombosis and pulmonary embolism*. Rockville, MD: Agency for Healthcare Research and Quality.

Albert, R., Spiro, S. & Jett, J. (2004). *Clinical respiratory medicine* (2nd ed.). St. Louis: Mosby.

American Cancer Society. (2005). *Cancer facts and figures*. Atlanta: American Cancer Society.

American Joint Committee on Cancer (AJCC). (2002). *Cancer staging manual* (6th ed.). New York: Springer-Verlag.

Fossella, F. V., Putnam, J. B. & Komaki, K. (2003). *Lung cancer*. New York: Springer-Verlag.

Haas, M. (2003). *Contemporary issues in lung cancer: A nursing perspective*. Sudbury, MA: Jones and Bartlett.

Pazdur, R., Coia, L. R., Hoskins, W. J., et al. (2003). *Cancer management: A multidisciplinary approach* (7th ed.). New York: The Oncology Group.

Schwartz, A. L. (2004). *Pocket guide to managing cancer fatigue*. Sudbury, MA: Jones and Bartlett.

Tapson, V. F. (2003). *Venous thromboembolism*. Philadelphia: Saunders.

Williams, N. R. & Harrison, J. (2004). *Atlas of occupational health and disease*. Oxford, UK: Oxford University Press.

## JOURNALS

*Asterisks indicate nursing research articles.

### General

American College of Chest Physicians. (2004). Diagnosis and management of pulmonary arterial hypertension: ACCP evidence-based clinical practice guidelines. *Chest, 126*(1 Suppl.), 4S–92S.

American Thoracic Society and European Respiratory Society. (2000). Idiopathic pulmonary fibrosis: Diagnosis and treatment. International consensus statement. *American Journal of Respiratory and Critical Care Medicine, 161*(2), 646–664.

Azoulay, E. (2003). Pleural effusions in the intensive care unit. *Current Opinions in Pulmonary Medicine, 9*(4), 291–297.

Barrocas, A., Purdy, D., Brady, P., et al. (2002). Cancer: Nutritional management for older adults. From *A physician's guide to nutrition in chronic disease management in older adults*. Washington, DC: Nutrition Screening Initiative.

Centers for Disease Control and Prevention. (2004b). Changing patterns of pneumoconiosis mortality United States, 1968–2000. *MMWR Morbidity and Mortality Weekly Report, 53*(28), 627–632.

Davies, R. J. O. & Gleeson, F. V. (2003). Introduction to methods used in the generation of the British Thoracic Society guidelines for the management of pleural diseases. *Thorax, 58*(Suppl. II), ii1–ii7.

Doty, J. D. & Judson, M. A. (2004). Sarcoidosis, part 1: A thorough look at the clinical aspects. *Journal of Respiratory Diseases, 25*(1), 31–36.

Eells, P. L. (2004). Advances in prostacyclin therapy for pulmonary arterial hypertension. *Critical Care Nursing, 24*(2), 42–54.

Goldhaber, S. Z. (2004). Pulmonary embolism. *Lancet, 363*(9417), 1295–1305.

Humbert, M., Sitbon, O. & Simonneau, G. (2004). Drug therapy: Treatment of pulmonary arterial hypertension. *New England Journal of Medicine, 351*(14), 1425–1436.

Kaboli, P., Henderson, M. C., & White, R. H. (2003). DVT prophylaxis and anticoagulation in the surgical patient. *Medical Clinics of North America, 87*(1), 77–110.

Karin, J. (2003). Managing pulmonary embolism. *British Medical Journal, 326*(7403), 1341–1342.

Keithley, J. K., & Swanson, B. (2004). Enteral nutrition: An update on practice recommendations. *MedSurg Nursing, 13*(2), 131–134.

Marik, P. E. (2001). Aspiration pneumonitis and aspiration pneumonia. *New England Journal of Medicine, 344*(9), 665–671.

McClave, S. A., DeMeo, M. T., DeLegge, M. H., et al. (2002). North American summit on aspiration in the critically ill patient: Consensus statement. *Journal of Parenteral and Enteral Nutrition, 26*(6 Suppl), S80–S85.

Metheny, N. A. (2002). Risk factors for aspiration. *Journal of Parenteral and Enteral Nutrition, 26*(Suppl 6), S26–S33.

Metheny, N. A. & Titler, M. G. (2001). Assessing placement of feeding tubes. *American Journal of Nursing, 101*(5), 36–45.

Morris, R. J. & Woodcock, J. P. (2004). Evidence-based compression: prevention of stasis and deep vein thrombosis. *Annals of Surgery, 239*(2), 162–171.

Nagahiro, I., Andou, A., Aoe, M., et al. (2004). Intermittent pneumatic compression is effective in preventing symptomatic pulmonary embolism after thoracic surgery. *Surgery Today, 34*(1), 6–10.

Ramirez, J., Pantelis, V., Gonzalez-Ruiz, C., et al. (2003). Sequential compression devices as prophylaxis for venous thromboembolism in high-risk colorectal surgery patients: Reconsidering American Society of Colorectal Surgeons parameters. *American Surgeon, 69*(11), 941–945.

*Ratner, P. A., Johnson, J. L., Richardson, C. G., et al. (2004). Efficacy of a smoking-cessation intervention for elective-surgical patients. *Research in Nursing and Health, 27*(3), 148–161.

Sorenson, H. M. & Shelledy, D. C. (2003). AARC clinical practice guideline. Intermittent positive pressure breathing—2003 revision and update. *Respiratory Care, 48*(5), 540–546.

Wood, K., & Joffe, A. (2003). Major pulmonary embolism part 3: A practical treatment strategy. *The Journal of Respiratory Diseases, 24*(10), 446–451.

### Acute Respiratory Failure and ARDS

Bernard, G. R., Artigas, A., Brigham, K. L., et al. (1994). Report of the American-European consensus conference on acute respiratory distress syndrome: Definitions, mechanisms, relevant outcomes, and clinical trial coordination. *American Journal of Critical Care Medicine, 9*(1), 72–81.

Kallet, R. H. (2004). Evidence-based management of acute lung injury and acute respiratory distress syndrome. *Respiratory Care, 49*(7), 793–809.

Marini, J. (2004). Advances in the understanding of acute respiratory distress syndrome: Summarizing a decade of progress. *Current Opinion in Critical Care, 10*(4), 265–271.

Powers, J., & Daniels, D. (2004). Turning points: Implementing kinetic therapy in the ICU. *Nursing Management, 35*(Suppl. 3), 2–7.

Young, M. P., Manning, H. L., Wilson, D. L., et al. (2004). Ventilation of patients with acute lung injury and acute respiratory distress syndrome: Has new evidence changed clinical practice? *Critical Care Medicine, 32*(6), 1260–1265.

### Lung Cancer

Baldwin, P. D. (2003). Lung cancer. *Clinical Journal of Oncology Nursing, 7*(6), 699–702.

Centers for Disease Control and Prevention. (2004a). Cancer mortality surveillance—United States, 1990–2000. *MMWR Morbidity and Mortality Weekly Report, 53*(SS03), 1–108.

*Gift, A. G., Stommel, M., Jablonski, A., et al. (2003). A cluster of symptoms over time in patients with lung cancer. *Nursing Research, 52*(6), 393–400.

Gohagan, J., Marcus, P., Fagerstsrom, R., et al. (2004). Baseline findings of a randomized feasibility trial of lung cancer screening with spiral CT scan vs. chest radiograph. *Chest, 126*(1), 114–121.

Hurria, A. & Kris, M. G. (2003). Management of lung cancer in older adults. *CA: A Cancer Journal for Clinicians, 53*(6), 325–341.

Jemal, A., Tiwari, R. C., Murray, T., et al. (2004). Cancer statistics 2004. *CA: A Cancer Journal for Clinicians, 54*(1), 8–29.

Mulshine, J. L. & Sullivan, D. C. (2005). Lung cancer screening. *New England Journal of Medicine, 352*(26), 2714–2719.

Spira, A. & Ettinger, D. S. (2004). Drug therapy: Multidisciplinary management of lung cancer. *New England Journal of Medicine, 350*(4), 379–392.

## *Pulmonary Infections*

Andrews, J., Nadjm, B., Gant, V., et al. (2003). Community acquired pneumonia. *Current Opinion in Pulmonary Medicine, 9*(3), 175–180.

Centers for Disease Control and Prevention. (2003a). Guidelines for environmental infection control in health-care facilities: Recommendations of CDC and the Healthcare Infection Control Practice Advisory Committee (HICPAC). *MMWR Morbidity and Mortality Weekly Report, 52*(RR10).

Centers for Disease Control and Prevention. (2004c). Clinical guidance on the identification and evaluation of possible SARS-CoV disease among persons presenting with community-acquired illness, version 2. January, 2004.

Centers for Disease Control and Prevention. (2004d). Guidelines for preventing health-care–associated pneumonia, 2004. *MMWR Morbidity and Mortality Weekly Report, 53*(RR03), 1–36.

Centers for Disease Control and Prevention. (2004e). Prevention and control of influenza: recommendations of the Advisory Committee on Immunization Practices (ACIP). *MMWR Morbidity and Mortality Weekly Report, 53*(RR-6), 1–40.

Collard, H. R., Saint, S., & Matthay, M. A. (2003). Prevention of ventilator-associated pneumonia: An evidence-based systematic review. *Annals of Internal Medicine, 138*(6), 494–501.

Denison, M. R. (2004). Severe acute respiratory syndrome coronavirus pathogenesis, disease and vaccines: An update. *Pediatric Infectious Disease Journal, 23*(11), S207–S214.

File, T. M., Garau, J., Blasi, F., et al. (2004). Guidelines for empiric antimicrobial prescribing in community-acquired pneumonia. *Chest, 125*(5), 1888–1901.

Frazee, B. W. (2004). Community-acquired pneumonia: Getting down to the basics. *Journal of Respiratory Diseases, 25*(1), 37–44.

Institute for Clinical Systems Improvement (ISCI). (2003). Community acquired pneumonia in adults. Bloomington, MN: Institute for Clinical Systems Improvement.

Kochanek, K. D., & Smith, B. L. (2004). Deaths: Preliminary data for 2002. *National Vital Statistics Reports, 52*(13). Hyattsville, MD: National Center for Heath Statistics.

Levy, M. M., Baylor, M. S., Bernard, G. R., et al. (2005). Clinical issues and research in respiratory failure from severe acute respiratory syndrome. *American Journal of Respiratory and Critical Care Medicine, 171*(5), 518–526.

Mandell, L. A., Bartlett, J. G., Dowell, S. F., et al. (2003). Update of practice guidelines for the management of community-acquired pneumonia in immunocompetent adults. *Clinical Infectious Diseases, 37*(11), 1405–1433.

Niederman, M. S. & Ahmed, Q. A. (2003). Community-acquired pneumonia in elderly patients. *Clinical Geriatric Medicine, 21*(1), 101–120.

Stringer, J. R., Beard, C. B., Miller, R. F., et al. (2002). A new name (*Pneumocystis jiroveci*) for pneumocystis from humans. *Emerging Infectious Diseases, 8*(9), 891–896.

Wilkinson, M. & Woodhead, M. A. (2004). Guidelines for community-acquired pneumonia in the ICU. *Current Opinions in Critical Care, 10*(1), 59–64.

## *Trauma*

Karmy-Jones, R. & Jurkovich, G. J. (2004). Blunt chest trauma. *Current Problems in Surgery, 41*(3), 223–380.

Kulshrestha, P., Munshi, I., & Wait, R. (2004). Profile of chest trauma in a level 1 trauma center. *Journal of Trauma Injury, Infection and Critical Care, 57*(3), 576–581.

Sirmali, M., Turut, H., Topcu, S. et al. (2003). A comprehensive analysis of traumatic rib fractures: Morbidity, mortality and management. *European Journal of Cardio-thoracic Surgery, 24*(2003), 133–138.

Wanek, S. & Mayberry, J. C. (2004). Blunt thoracic trauma: Flail chest, pulmonary contusion and blast injury. *Critical Care Clinics, 20*(1), 71–81.

## *Tuberculosis*

American Thoracic Society. (2000). Diagnostic standards and classification of tuberculosis in adults and children. *American Journal of Respiratory and Critical Care Medicine, 161*(4), 1376–1395.

Centers for Disease Control and Prevention. (2003b). Treatment of tuberculosis. American Thoracic Society, CDC, and Infectious Diseases Society of America. *MMWR Morbidity and Mortality Weekly Report, 52*(RR-11), 1–74.

Centers for Disease Control and Prevention. (2003c). Trends in tuberculosis morbidity—United States, 1992–2002. *MMWR Morbidity and Mortality Weekly Report, 52*(11), 217–222.

Centers for Disease Control and Prevention. (2004f). Trends in tuberculosis—United States, 1998–2003. *MMWR Morbidity and Mortality Weekly Report, 53*(10), 209–214.

Centers for Disease Control and Prevention. (2005a). Treatment options for latent tuberculosis infection. Document 250004. CDC, Atlanta, GA.

Centers for Disease Control and Prevention. (2005b). Guidelines for using the QuantiFERON®-TB Gold Test for detecting *Mycobacterium tuberculosis* infection, United States. *MMWR Morbidity and Mortality Weekly Report, 54*(RR 15), 49–55.

Corbett, E. L., Watt, C. J., Walker, N., et al. (2003). The growing burden of tuberculosis: Global trends and interactions with the HIV epidemic. *Archives of Internal Medicine, 163*(9), 1009–1021.

## RESOURCES

Agency for Healthcare Quality and Research, John M. Eisenberg Bldg, 540 Gaither Road, Rockville, MD 20850; 301-427-1364; http://www.ahrq.gov. Accessed March 31, 2006.

American Association for Respiratory Care, 9425 N. MacArthur Blvd., Suite 100, Irving, TX 75063; 972-243-2272; http://www.aarc.org. Accessed March 31, 2006.

American Cancer Society, 1599 Clifton Road NE, Atlanta, GA 30329; 888-ACS-2345; http://www.cancer.org. Accessed March 31, 2006.

American College of Chest Physicians, 3300 Dundee Road, Northbrook, IL 60062; 847-498-1400; http://www.chestnet.org. Accessed March 31, 2006.

American Lung Association, 61 Broadway 6th Floor, New York, NY 10006; 800-LUNGUSA; http://www.lungusa.org. Accessed March 31, 2006.

American Thoracic Society, 61 Broadway, New York, NY 10006; 212-315-8600; http://www.thoracic.org. Accessed March 31, 2006.

Centers for Disease Control and Prevention, 1600 Clifton Road NE, Atlanta, GA 30333; 800-311-3435; http://www.cdc.gov. Accessed March 31, 2006.

National Cancer Institute, National Institutes of Health, 6116 Executive Blvd, Room 3036A, Bethesda, MD 20892; 800-4-CANCER (Cancer Information Services); http://www.cancer.gov. Accessed March 31, 2006.

National Heart, Lung and Blood Institute, National Institutes of Health, Bldg. 31, 31 Center Drive MSC, Bethesda, MD 20892; 301-592-8573; http://www.nhlbi.nih.gov. Accessed March 31, 2006.

Occupational Safety and Health Administration (OSHA), United States Department of Labor, 200 Constitution Avenue NW., Washington, DC 20210; 800-321-6742; http://www.osha.gov. Accessed March 31, 2006.

Respiratory Nursing Society, c/o NYSNA, 11 Cornell Road, Latham, NY 12110; 518-782-9400 ×286; http://www.respiratorynursingsociety.org. Accessed March 31, 2006.

# CHAPTER 24

# Management of Patients With Chronic Obstructive Pulmonary Disorders

## Learning Objectives

*On completion of this chapter, the learner will be able to:*

1. Describe the pathophysiology of chronic obstructive pulmonary disease (COPD).
2. Discuss the major risk factors for developing COPD and nursing interventions to minimize or prevent these risk factors.
3. Use the nursing process as a framework for care of patients with COPD.
4. Develop a teaching plan for patients with COPD.
5. Describe the pathophysiology of asthma.
6. Discuss the medications used in asthma management.
7. Describe asthma self-management strategies.
8. Describe the pathophysiology of cystic fibrosis.

Chronic pulmonary disorders are a leading cause of morbidity and mortality in the United States. Nurses are involved with patients with chronic pulmonary disease across the spectrum of care, from outpatient and home care to critical care and the hospice setting. Patients with chronic pulmonary disorders need care from nurses who not only have astute assessment and clinical management skills but who also understand how these disorders can affect quality of life. In addition, the nurse's knowledge of palliative and end-of-life care is important for affected patients. Patient and family teaching is an important nursing intervention to enhance self-management in patients with any chronic pulmonary disorder.

# Chronic Obstructive Pulmonary Disease

**Chronic obstructive pulmonary disease (COPD)** is a disease state characterized by airflow limitation that is not fully reversible. This newest definition of COPD, provided by the Global Initiative for Chronic Obstructive Lung Disease (GOLD), is a broad description that better explains this disorder and its signs and symptoms (GOLD, World Health Organization [WHO] & National Heart, Lung and Blood Institute [NHLBI], 2004). Although previous definitions have included emphysema and chronic bronchitis under the umbrella classification of COPD, this was often confusing because most patients with COPD present with overlapping signs and symptoms of these two distinct disease processes.

COPD may include diseases that cause airflow obstruction (eg, emphysema, chronic bronchitis) or any combination of these disorders. Other diseases such as cystic fibrosis, bronchiectasis, and asthma that were previously classified as types of chronic obstructive lung disease are now classified as chronic pulmonary disorders. However, asthma is now considered a separate disorder and is classified as an abnormal airway condition characterized primarily by reversible inflammation. COPD can coexist with asthma. Both of these diseases have the same major symptoms; however, symptoms are generally more variable in asthma than in COPD. This chapter discusses COPD as a disease and describes chronic bronchitis and emphysema as distinct disease states, providing a foundation for understanding the pathophysiology of COPD. Bronchiectasis, asthma, and cystic fibrosis are discussed separately.

Currently, COPD is the fourth leading cause of mortality and the 12th leading cause of disability in the United States; however, by the year 2020 it is estimated that COPD will be the third leading cause of death and the fifth leading cause of disability (Sin, McAlister, Man, et al., 2003). In 2001, chronic pulmonary disorders caused 123,013 deaths in people of all ages, regardless of gender, and the male/female age-adjusted ratio was 1:4 (Arias, Anderson, Hsiang-Ching, et al., 2003). At present, approximately 16 million people in the United States have some form of COPD. The annual cost of COPD is approximately $32.1 billion, including health care expenditures of $18.0 billion and indirect costs of $14.1 billion (American Lung Association, 2004).

People with COPD commonly become symptomatic during the middle adult years, and the incidence of the disease increases with age. Although certain aspects of lung function normally decrease with age—for example, vital capacity and forced expiratory volume in 1 second ($FEV_1$), COPD accentuates and accelerates these physiologic changes.

## Pathophysiology

In COPD, the airflow limitation is both progressive and associated with an abnormal inflammatory response of the lungs to noxious particles or gases. The inflammatory response occurs throughout the airways, parenchyma, and pulmonary vasculature (GOLD, WHO & NHLBI, 2004). Because of the chronic inflammation and the body's attempts to repair it, narrowing occurs in the small peripheral airways. Over time, this injury-and-repair process causes

## Glossary

**air trapping:** incomplete emptying of alveoli during expiration due to loss of lung tissue elasticity (emphysema), bronchospasm (asthma), or airway obstruction

**alpha$_1$-antitrypsin deficiency:** genetic disorder resulting from deficiency of alpha$_1$ antitrypsin, a protective agent for the lung; increases patient's risk for developing panacinar emphysema even in the absence of smoking

**asthma:** a disease with multiple precipitating mechanisms resulting in a common clinical outcome of reversible airflow obstruction; no longer considered a category of COPD

**bronchiectasis:** chronic dilation of a bronchus or bronchi; the dilated airways become saccular and are a medium for chronic infection. No longer considered a category of COPD.

**bronchitis:** a disease of the airways defined as the presence of cough and sputum production for at least a combined total of 3 months in each of 2 consecutive years; a category of COPD

**chronic obstructive pulmonary disease:** disease state characterized by airflow limitation that is not fully reversible; sometimes referred to as chronic airway obstruction or chronic obstructive lung disease

**emphysema:** a disease of the airways characterized by destruction of the walls of overdistended alveoli; a category of COPD

**metered-dose inhaler (MDI):** patient-activated medication canister that provides aerosolized medication that the patient inhales into the lungs

**polycythemia:** increase in the red blood cell concentration in the blood; in COPD, the body attempts to improve oxygen carrying capacity by producing increasing amounts of red blood cells

**spirometry:** pulmonary function tests that measure specific lung volumes (eg, $FEV_1$, FVC) and rates ($FEF_{25-75\%}$); may be measured before and after bronchodilator administration scar tissue formation and narrowing of the airway lumen. Airflow obstruction may also be caused by parenchymal destruction, as is seen with emphysema, a disease of the alveoli or gas exchange units.

In addition to inflammation, processes related to imbalances of proteinases and antiproteinases in the lung may be responsible for airflow limitation. When activated by chronic inflammation, proteinases and other substances may be released, damaging the parenchyma of the lung. The parenchymal changes may occur as a consequence of inflammation or environmental or genetic factors (eg, alpha$_1$-antitrypsin deficiency).

Early in the course of COPD, the inflammatory response causes pulmonary vasculature changes that are characterized by thickening of the vessel wall. These changes may result from (1) exposure to cigarette smoke, (2) use of tobacco products, or (3) the release of inflammatory mediators (GOLD, WHO & NHLBI, 2004).

## Chronic Bronchitis

Chronic **bronchitis**, a disease of the airways, is defined as the presence of cough and sputum production for at least 3 months in each of two consecutive years. In many cases, smoke or other environmental pollutants irritate the airways, resulting in hypersecretion of mucus and inflammation. This constant irritation causes the mucus-secreting glands and goblet cells to increase in number. Ciliary function is reduced, and more mucus is produced. The bronchial walls become thickened, the bronchial lumen narrows, and mucus may plug the airway (Fig. 24-1). Alveoli adjacent to the bronchioles may become damaged and fibrosed, resulting in altered function of the alveolar macrophages. This is significant because the macrophages play an important role in destroying foreign particles, including bacteria. As a result, the patient becomes more susceptible to respiratory infection. A wide range of viral, bacterial, and mycoplasmal infections can produce acute episodes of bronchitis. Exacerbations of chronic bronchitis are most likely to occur during the winter.

## Emphysema

In **emphysema**, impaired gas oxygen and carbon dioxide exchange results from destruction of the walls of overdistended alveoli. "Emphysema" is a pathologic term that describes an abnormal distention of the air spaces beyond the terminal bronchioles, with destruction of the walls of the alveoli. It is the end stage of a process that has progressed slowly for many years. As the walls of the alveoli are destroyed (a process accelerated by recurrent infections), the alveolar surface area in direct contact with the pulmonary capillaries continually decreases, causing an increase in dead space (lung area where no gas exchange can occur) and impaired oxygen diffusion, which leads to hypoxemia. In the later stages of disease, carbon dioxide elimination is impaired, resulting in increased carbon dioxide tension in arterial blood (hypercapnia) and causing respiratory acidosis. As the alveolar walls continue to break down, the pulmonary capillary bed is reduced in size. Consequently, resistance to pulmonary blood flow is increased, forcing the right ventricle to maintain a higher blood pressure in the pulmonary artery. Hypoxemia may further increase pulmonary artery pressures. For this reason, right-sided heart failure (cor pulmonale) is one of the complications of emphysema. Congestion, dependent edema, distended neck veins, or pain in the region of the liver suggests the development of cardiac failure.

**FIGURE 24-1.** Pathophysiology of chronic bronchitis as compared to a normal bronchus. The bronchus in chronic bronchitis is narrowed and has impaired air flow due to multiple mechanisms: inflammation, excess mucus production, and potential smooth muscle constriction (bronchospasm).

There are two main types of emphysema, based on the changes taking place in the lung (Fig. 24-2). Both types may occur in the same patient.

In the panlobular (panacinar) type of emphysema, there is destruction of the respiratory bronchiole, alveolar duct, and alveolus. All air spaces within the lobule are essentially enlarged, but there is little inflammatory disease. A hyperinflated (hyperexpanded) chest (barrel chest on physical examination), marked dyspnea on exertion, and weight loss typically occur. To move air into and out of the lungs, negative pressure is required during inspiration, and an adequate level of positive pressure must be attained and maintained during expiration. The resting position is one of inflation. Instead of being an involuntary passive act, expiration becomes active and requires muscular effort. Patients become increasingly short of breath; the chest becomes rigid, and the ribs are fixed at their joints.

In the centrilobular (centroacinar) form, pathologic changes take place mainly in the center of the secondary lobule, preserving the peripheral portions of the acinus. Frequently, there is a derangement of ventilation–perfusion ratios, producing chronic hypoxemia, hypercapnia, **polycythemia**, and episodes of right-sided heart failure. This leads to central cyanosis and respiratory failure. The patient also develops peripheral edema, which is treated with diuretic therapy.

## Risk Factors

Risk factors for COPD include environmental exposures and host factors (Chart 24-1). The most important risk factor for COPD is cigarette smoking. Other risk factors are pipe, cigar, and other types of tobacco smoking. In addition, passive smoking contributes to respiratory symptoms and COPD (NIH, 2001). Smoking depresses the activity of scavenger cells and affects the respiratory tract's ciliary cleansing mechanism, which keeps breathing passages free of inhaled irritants, bacteria, and other foreign matter. When smoking damages this cleansing mechanism, airflow is obstructed and air becomes trapped behind the obstruction. The alveoli greatly distend, diminishing lung capacity. Smoking also irritates the goblet cells and mucus glands, causing an increased accumulation of mucus, which in turn produces more irritation, infection, and damage to the lung. In addition, carbon monoxide (a byproduct of smoking) combines with hemoglobin to form carboxyhemoglobin. Hemoglobin that is bound by carboxyhemoglobin cannot carry oxygen efficiently.

Other factors that put people at risk for COPD include prolonged and intense exposure to occupational dusts and chemicals, indoor air pollution, and outdoor air pollution. This exposure adds to the total burden of inhaled particles on the lung (GOLD, WHO & NHLBI, 2004).

A host risk factor for COPD is a deficiency of alpha$_1$-antitrypsin, an enzyme inhibitor that protects the lung parenchyma from injury. This deficiency predisposes young people to rapid development of lobular emphysema, even if they do not smoke. **Alpha$_1$-antitrypsin deficiency** is one of the most common genetically linked lethal diseases among Caucasians and affects approximately 1 in every 3000 Americans (approximately 80,000 to 100,000 cases) (American Lung Association, 2005). Genetically susceptible people are sensitive to environmental factors (eg, smoking, air pollution, infectious agents, allergens) and eventually develop chronic obstructive symptoms. Carriers of this genetic defect must be identified so that they can modify environmental risk factors to delay or prevent overt symptoms of disease. Genetics counseling should be offered. Alpha-protease inhibitor replacement therapy, which slows the progression of the disease, is available for patients with this genetic defect and for those with severe disease. However, this intermittent infusion therapy is costly and is required on an ongoing basis.

> ### CHART 24-1
> ### Risk Factors for Chronic Obstructive Pulmonary Disease (COPD)
>
> - Exposure to tobacco smoke accounts for an estimated 80% to 90% of COPD cases
> - Passive smoking
> - Occupational exposure
> - Ambient air pollution
> - Genetic abnormalities, including a deficiency of alpha$_1$-antitrypsin, an enzyme inhibitor that normally counteracts the destruction of lung tissue by certain other enzymes

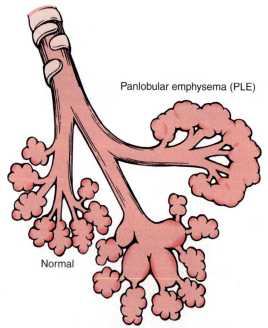

**FIGURE 24-2.** Changes in alveolar structure in centrilobular and panlobular emphysema. In panlobular emphysema, the bronchioles, alveolar ducts, and alveoli are destroyed, and the air spaces within the lobule are enlarged. In centrilobular emphysema, the pathologic changes occur in the lobule, whereas the peripheral portions of the acinus are preserved.

## Clinical Manifestations

COPD is characterized by three primary symptoms: chronic cough, sputum production, and dyspnea on exertion (GOLD, WHO & NHLBI, 2004). These symptoms often worsen over time. Chronic cough and sputum production often precede the development of airflow limitation by many years. However, not all people with cough and sputum production develop COPD. Dyspnea may be severe and often interferes with the patient's activities. Weight loss is common, because dyspnea interferes with eating and the work of breathing is energy-depleting. Often patients cannot participate in even mild exercise because of dyspnea; as COPD progresses, dyspnea occurs even at rest. As the work of breathing increases over time, the accessory muscles are recruited in an effort to breathe. Patients with COPD are at risk for respiratory insufficiency and respiratory infections, which in turn increase the risk of acute and chronic respiratory failure.

In patients with COPD that has a primary emphysematous component, chronic hyperinflation leads to the "barrel chest" thorax configuration. This results from fixation of the ribs in the inspiratory position (due to hyperinflation) and from loss of lung elasticity (Fig. 24-3). Retraction of the supraclavicular fossae occurs on inspiration, causing the shoulders to heave upward (Fig. 24-4). In advanced emphysema, the abdominal muscles also contract on inspiration.

## Assessment and Diagnostic Findings

The nurse should obtain a thorough health history for patients with known or potential COPD. Chart 24-2 lists the key factors to assess. Pulmonary function studies are used to help confirm the diagnosis of COPD, determine disease severity, and monitor disease progression. **Spirometry** is used to evaluate airflow obstruction, which is determined by the ratio of $FEV_1$ to forced vital capacity (FVC). Spirometric results are expressed as an absolute volume and as a percentage of the predicted value using appropriate normal values for gender, age, and height. With obstruction, the patient either has difficulty exhaling or cannot forcibly exhale air from the lungs, reducing the $FEV_1$. Obstructive lung disease is defined as a $FEV_1/FVC$ ratio of less than 70%.

In addition, bronchodilator reversibility testing may be performed to rule out the diagnosis of asthma and to guide initial treatment. With this type of testing, spirometry is first obtained, then the patient is given an inhaled bronchodilator treatment according to a protocol, and finally spirometry is repeated. The patient demonstrates a degree of reversibility if the pulmonary function values improve after administration of the bronchodilator. Even patients who do not show a significant response to a short-acting bronchodilator test may benefit symptomatically from long-term bronchodilator treatment.

Arterial blood gas measurements may also be obtained to assess baseline oxygenation and gas exchange and are especially important in advanced COPD. In addition, a chest x-ray may be obtained to exclude alternative diagnoses. A chest x-ray is seldom diagnostic in COPD unless obvious bullous disease is present. A computed tomography (CT) scan is not routinely obtained in the diagnosis of COPD, but a high-resolution CT scan may help in the differential diagnosis. Lastly, screening for alpha$_1$-antitrypsin deficiency

**FIGURE 24-3.** Characteristics of normal chest wall and chest wall in emphysema. (**A**) The normal chest wall and its cross-section. (**B**) The barrel-shaped chest of emphysema and its cross-section.

**FIGURE 24-4.** Typical posture of a person with chronic obstructive pulmonary disease (COPD)—primarily emphysema. The person tends to lean forward and uses the accessory muscles of respiration to breathe, forcing the shoulder girdle upward and causing the supraclavicular fossae to retract on inspiration.

may be performed for patients younger than 45 years and for those with a strong family history of COPD.

COPD is classified into five stages depending on severity (Table 24-1) (GOLD, WHO & NHLBI, 2004). Factors that determine the clinical course and survival of patients with COPD include history of cigarette smoking, passive smoking exposure, age, rate of decline of $FEV_1$, hypoxemia, pulmonary artery pressure, resting heart rate, weight loss, and reversibility of airflow obstruction.

In diagnosing COPD, several differential diagnoses must be ruled out. The primary differential diagnosis is asthma. Key characteristics of asthma often include onset early in life; variation in daily symptoms and day-to-day occurrence or timing of symptoms; symptoms at night or in the early morning; family history of asthma; potential presence of allergy, rhinitis, or eczema; and a largely reversible airflow obstruction. It may be difficult to differentiate between a patient with COPD and one with chronic asthma. Key parts of differentiation are the patient history and the patient's responsiveness to bronchodilators. Other diseases that must be considered in the differential diagnosis include heart failure, bronchiectasis, tuberculosis, obliterative bronchiolitis, and diffuse panbronchiolitis (GOLD, WHO & NHLBI, 2004).

## Complications

Respiratory insufficiency and failure are major life-threatening complications of COPD. The acuity of the onset

### CHART 24-2

**Assessing Key Factors in the Health History of Patients with COPD**

- Exposure to risk factors—types, intensity, duration
- Past medical history—respiratory diseases/problems, including asthma, allergy, sinusitis, nasal polyps, history of respiratory infections
- Family history of COPD or other chronic respiratory diseases
- Pattern of symptom development
- History of exacerbations or previous hospitalizations for respiratory problems
- Presence of comorbidities
- Appropriateness of current medical treatments
- Impact of the disease on quality of life
- Available social and family support for patient
- Potential for reducing risk factors (eg, smoking cessation)

**TABLE 24-1 Classifications of Chronic Obstructive Pulmonary Disease (COPD) by Severity**

| Stage | Characteristics |
|---|---|
| 0 (at risk) | Normal spirometry |
|  | Chronic symptoms of cough, sputum production |
| I (mild COPD) | $FEV_1/FVC < 70\%$ |
|  | $FEV_1 \geq 80\%$ predicted |
|  | With or without chronic symptoms of cough, sputum production |
| II (moderate COPD) | $FEV_1/FVC < 70\%$ |
|  | $FEV_1$ 50–80% predicted |
|  | With or without chronic symptoms of cough, sputum production |
| III (severe COPD) | $FEV_1/FVC < 70\%$ |
|  | $FEV_1 < 30$–50% predicted |
|  | With or without chronic symptoms |
| IV (very severe COPD) | $FEV_1/FVC < 70\%$ |
|  | $FEV_1 < 30$–50% predicted |
|  | Chronic respiratory failure |

COPD, chronic obstructive pulmonary disease; $FEV_1$, forced expiratory volume in 1 second; FVC, forced vital capacity.

From Global Initiative for Chronic Obstructive Lung Disease (GOLD), World Health Organization (WHO), & National Heart, Lung and Blood Institute (NHLBI). (2004). *Global strategy for the diagnosis, management, and prevention of chronic obstructive pulmonary disease.* Bethesda, MD: National Heart, Lung and Blood Institute.

## NURSING RESEARCH PROFILE

### Fatigue in Patients With COPD

Theander, K. & Unosson, M. (2004). Fatigue in patients with chronic obstructive pulmonary disease. *Journal of Advanced Nursing, 45*(2), 172–177.

**Purpose**
This study described the frequency, duration, and severity of fatigue in patients with COPD. In addition, it compared the impact of perceived fatigue on cognitive, physical, and psychosocial functioning between patients with COPD and control subjects.

**Design**
The convenience sample in this study was made up of 36 patients with COPD (19 women and 17 men) with mean ages of 63 ± 4.6 years and 68 ± 5.3 years, respectively. Using a control group comparison design, two gender- and age-matched controls were randomly assigned for each patient with COPD (control group, n = 88). A total of 36 patients with COPD and 37 controls completed questionnaires that included a demographic form and the Fatigue Impact Scale, which was used to assess perceptions of the impact of functional limitations due to fatigue on cognitive, physical, and psychosocial functioning during the past 4 weeks.

**Findings**
Forty-seven percent of patients with COPD reported fatigue every day during the preceding month compared to 13.5% of the control group ($p < .001$). In evaluation of the duration of fatigue, 52.7% of the patients with COPD reported fatigue more than 6 hours per day versus 18.9% of the controls ($p < .001$). In rating the impact of fatigue, 44.4% of patients with COPD reported fatigue as either the worst or one of the worst symptoms experienced, while 10.8% of the control group did so ($p < .01$). Patients with COPD reported a significantly greater ($p < .001$) impact of fatigue on cognitive, physical, and psychosocial functioning than did members of the control group.

**Nursing Implications**
Fatigue is a common symptom experienced by patients with COPD on a daily basis. Nursing interventions must include assessment of this symptom and the impact of all dimensions of fatigue (cognitive, physical, and psychosocial) on activities of daily living and quality of life. Future studies must focus on specific interventions related to fatigue for the COPD population.

---

and the severity of respiratory failure depend on baseline pulmonary function, pulse oximetry or arterial blood gas values, comorbid conditions, and the severity of other complications of COPD. Respiratory insufficiency and failure may be chronic (with severe COPD) or acute (with severe bronchospasm or pneumonia in a patient with severe COPD). Acute respiratory insufficiency and failure may necessitate ventilatory support until other acute complications, such as infection, can be treated. Management of the patient requiring ventilatory support is discussed in Chapter 25. Other complications of COPD include pneumonia, atelectasis, pneumothorax, and pulmonary arterial hypertension (cor pulmonale).

## Medical Management

### Risk Reduction

Smoking cessation is the only intervention proven to slow the accelerated decline in lung function and the progression of COPD (GOLD, WHO & NHLBI, 2004; Sin et al., 2003). Recent surveys indicate that 22.5% (46.2 million) of all American adults smoke. According to the Centers for Disease Control and Prevention (CDC), 28.5% of all high school students report that they smoke (CDC, 2004). Smoking cessation is difficult to achieve and even more difficult to sustain in the long term. Nurses play a key role in promoting smoking cessation and educating patients about ways to do so. Patients diagnosed with COPD who continue to smoke must be encouraged and assisted to quit. Factors associated with continued smoking vary among patients and may include the strength of the nicotine addiction, continued exposure to smoking-associated stimuli (at work or in social settings), stress, depression, and habit. Continued smoking is also more prevalent among those with low incomes, low levels of education, or psychosocial problems (CDC, 2004).

Because multiple factors are associated with continued smoking, successful cessation often requires multiple strategies. Health care providers should promote cessation by explaining the risks of smoking and personalizing the "at-risk" message to the patient. After giving a strong warning about smoking, health care providers should work with the patient to set a definite "quit date." Referral to a smoking cessation program may be helpful. Follow-up within 3 to 5 days after the "quit date" to review progress and to address any problems is associated with an increased rate of success; this should be repeated as needed. Continued reinforcement with telephone calls or clinic visits is extremely beneficial. Relapses should be analyzed, and the patient and health care provider should jointly identify possible solutions to prevent future backsliding. It is important to emphasize successes rather than failures. First-line pharmacotherapy that reliably increases long-term smoking abstinence rates is nicotine replacement (gum, inhaler, nasal spray, transdermal patch, sublingual tablet, or lozenges). Bupropion SR (Zyban,

Wellbutrin) and nortriptyline (Aventyl) may also increase long-term quit rates. Second-line pharmacotherapy includes the antihypertensive agent clonidine (Catapres); however, its use is limited by its side effects (GOLD, WHO & NHLBI, 2004). Patients with medical contraindications, light smokers (less than 10 cigarettes per day), and pregnant and adolescent smokers are not appropriate candidates for the use of pharmacotherapy.

Smoking cessation can begin in a variety of health care settings—outpatient clinic, pulmonary rehabilitation, community, hospital, and the home. Regardless of the setting, nurses have the opportunity to teach patients about the risks of smoking and the benefits of smoking cessation. Various materials, resources, and programs developed by several organizations (eg, Agency for Healthcare Research and Quality, U.S. Public Health Service, CDC, National Cancer Institute, American Lung Association, American Cancer Society) are available to assist with this effort.

## Pharmacologic Therapy

**BRONCHODILATORS.** Bronchodilators relieve bronchospasm and reduce airway obstruction by allowing increased oxygen distribution throughout the lungs and improving alveolar ventilation. These medications, which are central in the management of COPD (GOLD, WHO & NHLBI, 2004), are delivered through a metered-dose inhaler or other type of inhaler, by nebulization, or via the oral route in pill or liquid form. Bronchodilators are often administered regularly throughout the day as well as on an as-needed basis. They may also be used prophylactically to prevent breathlessness by having the patient use them before participating in or completing an activity, such as eating or walking.

A **metered-dose inhaler** (MDI) is a pressurized device that contains an aerosolized powder of medication. A precise amount of medication is released with each activation of the canister. Patients must be instructed on the correct use of the device. A spacer (holding chamber) may also be used to enhance deposition of the medication in the lung and help the patient coordinate activation of the MDI with inspiration. Spacers come in several designs, but all are attached to the MDI and have a mouthpiece on the opposite end (Fig. 24-5). Once the canister is activated, the spacer holds the aerosol in the chamber until the patient inhales. The patient should take a slow, 3- to 5-second inhalation immediately after activation of the MDI (Expert Panel Report, 1997; NHLBI/WHO, 2001). Other types of inhalers include the discus inhaler (Serevent) and the Aerolizer inhaler (Foradil). Specific package insert information is available on the use of these inhalers.

Several classes of bronchodilators are used, including beta-adrenergic agonists, anticholinergic agents, methylxanthines, and combination agents. These medications may be used in combination to optimize bronchodilation. Some of these medications are short-acting, and others are long-acting. Long-acting bronchodilators are more convenient for patient use. Examples of medications are shown in Table 24-2. Nebulized medications (nebulization of medication via an air compressor) may also be effective in patients who cannot use an MDI properly or who prefer this method of administration.

**CORTICOSTEROIDS.** Inhaled and systemic corticosteroids (oral or intravenous) may also be used in COPD but are used more frequently in asthma. They may improve symptoms, but it has been shown that they do not slow the decline in lung function. A short trial course of oral corticosteroids may be prescribed for patients to determine

**FIGURE 24-5.** (A) Examples of metered-dose inhalers and spacers. (B) A metered-dose inhaler and spacer in use.

## TABLE 24-2  Common Types of Bronchodilator Medications

| Class/Drug | Inhaler* | Nebulizer | Oral | Duration of Action |
|---|---|---|---|---|
| **Beta$_2$-Adrenergic Agonist Agents** | | | | |
| Albuterol (Proventil, Ventolin, Volmax) | X | X | X | Short |
| Bitolterol (Tornalate) | | X | | Long |
| Formoterol (Foradil) | X | | | Long |
| Levalbuterol (Xopenax) | | X | | Medium |
| Metaproterenol (Alupent) | X | X | X | Short |
| Pirbuterol (Maxair) | X | | | Short |
| Salmeterol (Serevent Diskus) | X | | | Long |
| **Anticholinergic Agents** | | | | |
| Ipratropium bromide (Atrovent) | X | | | Short |
| Oxitropium bromide (Oxivent) | X | X | | Medium |
| **Methylxanthines** | | | | |
| Aminophylline (Phyllocontin) | | | X | Variable |
| Theophylline (Slo-bid, Theo-Dur) | | | X | Variable |

Short-acting, 4–6 hours; medium-acting, 6–9 hours; long-acting, 12+ hours.
*Inhaler may include metered-dose inhaler, powdered inhalation with inhaler, or discus.

whether pulmonary function improves and symptoms decrease. Regular treatment with inhaled glucocorticosteroids is appropriate for symptomatic stage III and IV patients and for those with repeated exacerbations of the disease (eg, three episodes in the past 3 years). Long-term treatment with oral corticosteroids is not recommended in COPD and can cause steroid myopathy, leading to muscle weakness, decreased ability to function, and, in advanced disease, respiratory failure (GOLD, WHO & NHLBI, 2004). Examples of corticosteroids in the inhaled form are beclomethasone (Beclo-vent, Vanceril, Qvar), budesonide (Pulmicort Turbuhaler, Pulmicort Respules), flunisolide (AeroBid), fluticasone (Flovent), and triamcinolone (Azmacort).

Medication regimens used to manage COPD are based on disease severity. For stage I (mild) COPD, a short-acting bronchodilator may be prescribed. For stage II or III COPD, a short-acting bronchodilator along with regular treatment of one or more long-acting bronchodilators may be used. For stage III or IV (severe or very severe) COPD, medication therapy includes regular treatment with one or more bronchodilators and inhaled corticosteroids for repeated exacerbations (GOLD, WHO & NHLBI, 2004).

**OTHER MEDICATIONS.** There is little evidence regarding the usefulness of influenza and pneumococcal vaccinations specifically for patients with COPD. However, it has been demonstrated that influenza and pneumococcal vaccinations reduce the incidence of pneumonia, hospitalizations for cardiac conditions, and deaths in the general elderly population (Sin et al., 2003). As a preventive measure, patients should receive a yearly influenza vaccine and the pneumococcal vaccine every 5 to 7 years. In most healthy adults, pneumococcal vaccine titers persist for 5 or more years. Other pharmacologic treatments that may be used in COPD include alpha1-antitrypsin augmentation therapy, antibiotic agents, mucolytic agents, and antitussive agents.

## Management of Exacerbations

An exacerbation of respiratory symptoms requiring medical intervention is an important clinical event in COPD. An exacerbation of COPD is difficult to diagnose, but signs and symptoms may include increased dyspnea, increased sputum production and purulence, respiratory failure, changes in mental status, or worsening blood gas abnormalities. Primary causes of an acute exacerbation include tracheobronchial infection and air pollution. However, the cause of approximately one third of severe exacerbations cannot be identified (GOLD, WHO & NHLBI, 2004). First the primary cause of the exacerbation is identified, if possible, and then specific treatment is administered. Optimization of bronchodilator medications is the first-line therapy and involves identifying the best medication or combinations of medications taken on a regular schedule for a specific patient. Depending on the signs and symptoms, corticosteroids, antibiotic agents, oxygen therapy, and intensive respiratory interventions may also be used. Indications for hospitalization for acute exacerbation of COPD include severe dyspnea that does not respond adequately to initial therapy, confusion or lethargy, respiratory muscle fatigue, paradoxical chest wall movement, peripheral edema, worsening or new onset of central cyanosis, persistent or worsening hypoxemia, and need for noninvasive or invasive assisted mechanical ventilation (GOLD, WHO & NHLBI, 2004). The risk of death from an exacerbation of COPD is closely related to the development of respiratory acidosis, the presence of significant comorbidities, and the need for noninvasive or invasive positive-pressure ventilatory support.

The GOLD, WHO & NHLBI guidelines (2004) provide indications for assessment, hospital admission, and intensive care admission for patients with exacerbation of COPD.

## Oxygen Therapy

Oxygen therapy can be administered as long-term continuous therapy, during exercise, or to prevent acute dyspnea. Supplemental oxygen is effective in prolonging survival of patients with COPD who have a resting partial arterial pressure of oxygen ($PaO_2$) of less than 60 mm Hg at sea level (Sin et al., 2003). Long-term oxygen therapy (more than 15 hours per day) has also been shown to improve quality of life, has a mild beneficial effect on pulmonary arterial pressure, and decreases dyspnea (Sin et al., 2003). Long-term oxygen therapy is usually introduced in stage IV (very severe) COPD, and indications generally include a $PaO_2$ of 55 mm Hg or less or evidence of tissue hypoxia and organ damage such as cor pulmonale, secondary polycythemia, edema from right-sided heart failure, or impaired mental status (GOLD, WHO & NHLBI, 2004). For patients with exercise-induced hypoxemia, oxygen supplementation during exercise may improve performance. However, there is no evidence to support the idea that short bursts of oxygen before or after exercise provide any symptomatic relief (GOLD, WHO & NHLBI, 2004). Patients who are hypoxemic while awake are likely to be so during sleep. Therefore, nighttime oxygen therapy is recommended as well, and the prescription for oxygen therapy is for continuous, 24-hour use. Intermittent oxygen therapy is indicated for patients who desaturate only during exercise or sleep.

For years, the hypoxic drive theory has influenced clinicians. This theory proposed that administering oxygen to patients with COPD could result in apnea, cardiopulmonary arrest, or death as a result of blunting of the hypoxic drive to breathe (Simmons & Simmons, 2004). This theory is now considered obsolete. A small subset of COPD patients with chronic hypercapnia (elevated $PaCO_2$ levels) may be oxygen sensitive; however, the theories of ventilation–perfusion mismatch in the lungs and the Haldane effect are probably more important. The Haldane effect relates to the ability of hemoglobin to carry oxygen and carbon dioxide. When supplemental oxygen is administered, increased oxygen saturation results, and carbon dioxide is unable to be carried by the hemoglobin or is cast off by the hemoglobin. It must be transported in the dissolved form or as bicarbonate. This results in an overall increased load of carbon dioxide in the body. When patients with COPD cannot increase ventilation to adjust for this increased load, increasing hypercapnia occurs (Simmons & Simmons, 2004). Key in the care of patients with COPD on supplemental oxygen is monitoring and assessment. Pulse oximetry is helpful in assessing response to therapy but does not assess $PaCO_2$ levels. Optimal oxygenation of patients is important while monitoring for any possible complications of oxygen supplementation (Simmons & Simmons, 2004).

## Surgical Management

**BULLECTOMY.** A bullectomy is a surgical option for select patients with bullous emphysema. Bullae are enlarged airspaces that do not contribute to ventilation but occupy space in the thorax; these areas may be surgically excised. Many times these bullae compress areas of the lung that do have adequate gas exchange. Bullectomy may help reduce dyspnea and improve lung function. It can be performed thoracoscopically (with a video-assisted thoracoscope) or via a limited thoracotomy incision (see Chapter 25).

**LUNG VOLUME REDUCTION SURGERY.** Treatment options for patients with end-stage COPD (stage IV) with a primary emphysematous component are limited, although lung volume reduction surgery is an option for a selected subset of patients. This subset includes patients with homogenous disease or disease that is focused in one area and not widespread throughout the lungs. Lung volume reduction surgery involves the removal of a portion of the diseased lung parenchyma. This reduces hyperinflation and allows the functional tissue to expand, resulting in improved elastic recoil of the lung and improved chest wall and diaphragmatic mechanics. This type of surgery does not cure the disease or improve life expectancy, but it may decrease dyspnea, improve lung function, and improve the patient's overall quality of life (GOLD, WHO & NHLBI, 2004).

Careful selection of patients for lung volume reduction surgery is essential to decrease morbidity and mortality. The National Emphysema Treatment Trial found that the addition of lung volume reduction surgery to optimal medical management and rehabilitation led to overall improvement in exercise tolerance and survival in a subgroup of patients with predominantly upper lobe disease (National Emphysema Treatment Trial Research Group, 2003).

**LUNG TRANSPLANTATION.** Lung transplantation is a viable alternative for definitive surgical treatment of end-stage emphysema. It has been shown to improve quality of life and functional capacity in a selected group of patients with COPD (GOLD, WHO & NHLBI, 2004). Single-lung transplantation may be considered for patients with end-stage emphysema who have an $FEV_1$ less than 25% of the predicted normal and who have complications such as pulmonary hypertension, marked hypoxemia, and hypercapnia. However, surgery does not appear to significantly improve survival (Sutherland & Cherniack, 2004). Specific criteria exist for referral for lung transplantation. Organs are in short supply, and many patients die while waiting for a transplant.

## Pulmonary Rehabilitation

Pulmonary rehabilitation for patients with COPD is well established and widely accepted as a means to alleviate symptoms and optimize functional status. The primary goals of rehabilitation are to reduce symptoms, improve quality of life, and increase physical and emotional participation in everyday activities (GOLD, WHO & NHLBI, 2004). Pulmonary rehabilitation services are multidisciplinary and include assessment, education, physical reconditioning, skills training, and psychological support. Patients are taught methods to alleviate symptoms. Breathing exercises as well as retraining and exercise programs are used to improve functional status.

Pulmonary rehabilitation may be used therapeutically in other disorders besides COPD, including asthma, cystic fibrosis, lung cancer, interstitial lung disease, thoracic surgery, and lung transplantation. It may be conducted in inpatient, outpatient, or home settings, and the lengths of programs vary. Patients at all stages of COPD may benefit from pulmonary rehabilitation. The minimum length of an effective program is 2 months, and the longer the program continues, the more effective the results (GOLD, WHO &

NHLBI, 2004). Selection of a program depends on the patient's physical, functional, and psychosocial status; insurance coverage; availability of programs; and preference.

## Nursing Management

Nurses play a key role in identifying potential candidates for pulmonary rehabilitation and in facilitating and reinforcing the material learned in the rehabilitation program. Not all patients have access to a formal rehabilitation program. However, nurses can be instrumental in teaching patients and families as well as facilitating specific services, such as respiratory therapy education, physical therapy for exercise and breathing retraining, occupational therapy for conserving energy during activities of daily living, and nutritional counseling.

Numerous educational materials are available to assist nurses in teaching patients with COPD. Potential resources include those of organizations such as the American Lung Association, the American Association of Cardiovascular and Pulmonary Rehabilitation, the American Thoracic Society, the American College of Chest Physicians, and the American Association for Respiratory Therapy.

### Patient Education

Patient education is a major component of pulmonary rehabilitation and includes a broad variety of topics. Depending on the length and setting of the educational program, topics may include normal anatomy and physiology of the lung, pathophysiology and changes with COPD, medications and home oxygen therapy, nutrition, respiratory therapy treatments, symptom alleviation, smoking cessation, sexuality and COPD, coping with chronic disease, communicating with the health care team, and planning for the future (advance directives, living wills, informed decision making about health care alternatives).

**BREATHING EXERCISES.** The breathing pattern of most people with COPD is shallow, rapid, and inefficient; the more severe the disease, the more inefficient the breathing pattern. With practice, this type of upper chest breathing can be changed to diaphragmatic breathing, which reduces the respiratory rate, increases alveolar ventilation, and sometimes helps expel as much air as possible during expiration (see Chapter 25 for technique). Pursed-lip breathing helps slow expiration, prevents collapse of small airways, and helps the patient control the rate and depth of respiration. It also promotes relaxation, enabling the patient to gain control of dyspnea and reduce feelings of panic.

**INSPIRATORY MUSCLE TRAINING.** Once the patient masters diaphragmatic breathing, a program of inspiratory muscle training may be prescribed to help strengthen the muscles used in breathing. This program involves use of a respiratory training device, which is placed in the mouth. The patient is instructed to inhale against a set resistance for a prescribed amount of time every day. As the resistance is gradually increased, the muscles become better conditioned. To be effective, inspiratory muscle training must be intense, and it is not recommended for all patients with COPD.

**ACTIVITY PACING.** People with COPD have decreased exercise tolerance during specific periods of the day, especially in the morning on arising, because bronchial secretions have collected in the lungs during the night while the person was lying down. The patient may have difficulty bathing or dressing and may become fatigued. Activities that require the arms to be supported above the level of the thorax may produce fatigue or respiratory distress but may be tolerated better after the patient has been up and moving around for an hour or more. The nurse can help the patient reduce these limitations by planning self-care activities and determining the best times for bathing, dressing, and other daily activities.

**SELF-CARE ACTIVITIES.** As gas exchange, airway clearance, and the breathing pattern improve, the patient is encouraged to assume increasing participation in self-care activities. The patient is taught to coordinate diaphragmatic breathing with activities such as walking, bathing, bending, or climbing stairs. The patient should bathe, dress, and take short walks, resting as needed to avoid fatigue and excessive dyspnea. Fluids should always be readily available, and the patient should begin to drink fluids without having to be reminded. If secretion management is a problem and some type of postural drainage or airway clearance maneuver is to be performed at home, the nurse or respiratory therapist instructs and supervises the patient before discharge or in an outpatient setting.

**PHYSICAL CONDITIONING.** People with COPD of all stages benefit from exercise training programs, which result in increased exercise tolerance and decreased dyspnea and fatigue (GOLD, WHO & NHLBI, 2004). Physical conditioning techniques include breathing exercises and general exercises intended to conserve energy and increase pulmonary ventilation. There is a close relationship between physical fitness and respiratory fitness (Covey & Larson, 2004). Graded exercises and physical conditioning programs using treadmills, stationary bicycles, and measured level walks can improve symptoms and increase work capacity and exercise tolerance. Any physical activity that can be performed regularly is helpful. Walking aids may be beneficial (GOLD, WHO & NHLBI, 2004). Lightweight portable oxygen systems are available for ambulatory patients who require oxygen therapy during physical activity.

**OXYGEN THERAPY.** Oxygen supplied to the home comes in compressed gas, liquid, or concentrator systems. Portable oxygen systems allow the patient to exercise, work, and travel. To help the patient adhere to the oxygen prescription, the nurse explains the proper flow rate and required number of hours for oxygen use as well as the dangers of arbitrary changes in flow rate or duration of therapy (Simmons & Simmons, 2004). The nurse should caution the patient that smoking with or near oxygen is extremely dangerous. The nurse also reassures the patient that oxygen is not "addictive" and explains the need for regular evaluations of blood oxygenation by pulse oximetry or arterial blood gas analysis.

**NUTRITIONAL THERAPY.** Nutritional assessment and counseling are important aspects in the rehabilitation process for patients with COPD. Weight loss as well as a depletion of muscle mass may be observed in stable patients with COPD, irrespective of the degree of airflow limitation. Weight loss and loss of fat mass are primarily the result of a negative balance between dietary intake and energy expenditure, whereas muscle wasting is a consequence of an impaired balance between protein synthesis and protein breakdown (American Thoracic Society & European Respiratory

Society, 2004). A thorough assessment of caloric needs and counseling about meal planning and supplementation is part of the rehabilitation process. Continual monitoring of weight and interventions as necessary are important parts of the care of patients with COPD.

**COPING MEASURES.** Any factor that interferes with normal breathing quite naturally induces anxiety, depression, and changes in behavior. Many patients find the slightest exertion exhausting, and fatigue is a major symptom of patients with COPD (Theander & Unosson, 2004). Constant shortness of breath and fatigue may make the patient irritable and apprehensive to the point of panic. Restricted activity (and reversal of family roles due to loss of employment), the frustration of having to work to breathe, and the realization that the disease is prolonged and unrelenting may cause the patient to become angry, depressed, and demanding (Andenaes, Kalfoss & Wahl, 2004). Sexual function may be compromised, which also diminishes self-esteem. The nurse should provide education and support to spouses or significant others and families, because the caregiver role in end-stage COPD can be difficult.

# Nursing Process

## The Patient With COPD

### Assessment

Assessment involves obtaining information about current symptoms as well as previous disease manifestations. Chart 24-3 lists sample questions that may be used to obtain a clear history of the disease process. In addition to the history, nurses review the results of available diagnostic tests.

### Diagnosis

#### Nursing Diagnoses

Based on the assessment data, major nursing diagnoses may include the following:

- Impaired gas exchange and airway clearance due to chronic inhalation of toxins
- Impaired gas exchange related to ventilation–perfusion inequality
- Ineffective airway clearance related to bronchoconstriction, increased mucus production, ineffective cough, bronchopulmonary infection, and other complications
- Ineffective breathing pattern related to shortness of breath, mucus, bronchoconstriction, and airway irritants
- Activity intolerance due to fatigue, ineffective breathing patterns, and hypoxemia
- Deficient knowledge of self-care strategies to be performed at home
- Ineffective coping related to reduced socialization, anxiety, depression, lower activity level, and the inability to work

### CHART 24-3

### Assessing Patients With Chronic Obstructive Pulmonary Disease

**HEALTH HISTORY**
- How long has the patient had respiratory difficulty?
- Does exertion increase the dyspnea? What type of exertion?
- What are the limits of the patient's tolerance for exercise?
- At what times during the day does the patient complain most of fatigue and shortness of breath?
- Which eating and sleeping habits have been affected?
- What does the patient know about the disease and his or her condition?
- What is the patient's smoking history (primary and secondary)?
- Is there occupational exposure to smoke or other pollutants?
- What are the triggering events (eg, exertion, strong odors, dust, exposure to animals)?

**PHYSICAL ASSESSMENT**
- What position does the patient assume during the interview?
- What are the pulse and the respiratory rates?
- What is the character of respirations? Even and without effort? Other?
- Can the patient complete a sentence without having to take a breath?
- Does the patient contract the abdominal muscles during inspiration?
- Does the patient use accessory muscles of the shoulders and neck when breathing?
- Does the patient take a long time to exhale (prolonged expiration)?
- Is central cyanosis evident?
- Are the patient's neck veins engorged?
- Does the patient have peripheral edema?
- Is the patient coughing?
- What is the color, amount, and consistency of the sputum?
- Is clubbing of the fingers present?
- What types of breath sounds (ie, clear, diminished or distant, crackles, wheezes) are heard? Describe and document findings and locations.
- What is the status of the patient's sensorium?
- Is there short-term or long-term memory impairment?
- Is there increasing stupor?
- Is the patient apprehensive?

## Collaborative Problems/ Potential Complications

Based on the assessment data, potential complications may include the following:

- Respiratory insufficiency or failure
- Atelectasis
- Pulmonary infection
- Pneumonia
- Pneumothorax
- Pulmonary hypertension

## Planning and Goals

Major patient goals may include smoking cessation, improved gas exchange, airway clearance, improved breathing pattern, improved activity tolerance, maximal self-management, improved coping ability, adherence to the therapeutic program and home care, and absence of complications.

## Nursing Interventions

### Promoting Smoking Cessation

Because smoking has such a detrimental effect on the lungs, the nurse must discuss smoking cessation strategies with the patient. Although the patient may believe that smoking cessation is futile, because it is too late to reverse the damage caused by years of smoking, the nurse should inform the patient that continuing to smoke impairs the mechanisms used to clear the airways and keep them free of irritants. The nurse should educate the patient regarding the hazards of smoking and cessation strategies and provide resources regarding smoking cessation, counseling, and formalized programs available in the community.

### Improving Gas Exchange

Bronchospasm, which occurs in many pulmonary diseases, reduces the caliber of the small bronchi and may cause dyspnea, static secretions, and infection. Bronchospasm can sometimes be detected on auscultation with a stethoscope when wheezing or diminished breath sounds are heard. Increased mucus production, along with decreased mucociliary action, contributes to further reduction in the caliber of the bronchi and results in decreased airflow and decreased gas exchange. This is further aggravated by the loss of lung elasticity that occurs with COPD (GOLD, WHO & NHLBI, 2004). These changes in the airway require that the nurse monitor the patient for dyspnea and hypoxemia. If bronchodilators or corticosteroids are prescribed, the nurse must administer the medications properly and be alert for potential side effects. The relief of bronchospasm is confirmed by measuring improvement in expiratory flow rates and volumes (the force of expiration, how long it takes to exhale, and the amount of air exhaled) as well as by assessing the dyspnea and making sure that it has lessened.

### Achieving Airway Clearance

Diminishing the quantity and viscosity of sputum can clear the airway and improve pulmonary ventilation and gas exchange. All pulmonary irritants should be eliminated or reduced, particularly cigarette smoking, which is the most persistent source of pulmonary irritation. The nurse instructs the patient in directed or controlled coughing, which is more effective and reduces the fatigue associated with undirected forceful coughing. Directed coughing consists of a slow, maximal inspiration followed by breath-holding for several seconds and then two or three coughs. "Huff" coughing may also be effective. The technique consists of one or two forced exhalations ("huffs") from low to medium lung volumes with the glottis open.

Chest physiotherapy with postural drainage, intermittent positive-pressure breathing, increased fluid intake, and bland aerosol mists (with normal saline solution or water) may be useful for some patients with COPD. The use of these measures must be based on the response and tolerance of the particular patient.

### Improving Breathing Patterns

Ineffective breathing patterns and shortness of breath are due to the ineffective respiratory mechanics of the chest wall and lung resulting from **air trapping**, ineffective diaphragmatic movement, airway obstruction, the metabolic cost of breathing, and stress. Inspiratory muscle training and breathing retraining may help improve breathing patterns. Training in diaphragmatic breathing reduces the respiratory rate, increases alveolar ventilation, and sometimes helps expel as much air as possible during expiration. Pursed-lip breathing helps slow expiration, prevent collapse of small airways, and control the rate and depth of respiration. It also promotes relaxation, which allows patients to gain control of dyspnea and reduce feelings of panic.

### Improving Activity Tolerance

Patients with COPD experience progressive activity and exercise intolerance and disability. Education is focused on rehabilitative therapies to promote independence in executing activities of daily living. These may include pacing activities throughout the day or using supportive devices to decrease energy expenditure. The nurse evaluates the patient's activity tolerance and limitations and uses teaching strategies to promote independent activities of daily living. The patient may be a candidate for exercise training to strengthen the muscles of the upper and lower extremities and to improve exercise tolerance and endurance. Use of walking aids may be recommended to improve activity levels and ambulation (GOLD, WHO & NHLBI, 2004). Other health care professionals (rehabilitation therapist, occupational therapist, physical therapist) may be consulted as additional resources.

### Enhancing Self-Care Strategies

In addition to a pulmonary rehabilitation program, the nurse helps the patient manage self-care by emphasizing the importance of setting realistic goals, avoiding temperature extremes, and modifying lifestyle (particularly stopping smoking) as applicable.

**SETTING REALISTIC GOALS**

A major area of teaching is the importance of setting and accepting realistic short-term and long-range goals. If the patient is severely disabled, the objectives of treatment are to preserve current pulmonary function and relieve symptoms as much as possible. If the COPD is mild, the objectives are to increase exercise tolerance and prevent further loss of pulmonary function. It is important to plan and share the goals and expectations of treatment with the patient. Both the patient and the care provider need patience to achieve these goals.

**AVOIDING TEMPERATURE EXTREMES**

The nurse instructs the patient to avoid extremes of heat and cold. Heat increases the body temperature, thereby raising oxygen requirements, and cold tends to promote bronchospasm. Air pollutants such as fumes, smoke, dust, and even talcum, lint, and aerosol sprays may initiate bronchospasm. High altitudes aggravate hypoxemia.

**MODIFYING LIFESTYLES**

A patient with COPD should adopt a lifestyle of moderate activity, ideally in a climate with minimal shifts in temperature and humidity. The patient should avoid emotional disturbances and stressful situations that might trigger a coughing episode as much as possible. The medication regimen can be quite complex; patients receiving aerosol medications by an MDI or other type of inhaler may be particularly challenged. It is crucial to review educational information and to have the patient demonstrate correct MDI use before discharge, during follow-up visits to a caregiver's office or clinic, and during home visits (Chart 24-4).

Smoking cessation goes hand in hand with lifestyle changes, and reinforcement of the patient's efforts is a key nursing activity. Smoking cessation is the single most important therapeutic intervention for patients with COPD. There are many strategies, including prevention, cessation with or without oral or topical patch medications, and behavior modification techniques.

### Enhancing Individual Coping Strategies

COPD and its progression promote a cycle of physical, social, and psychological consequences, all of which are interrelated. The patient experiences depression, altered mood states, social isolation, and altered functional status. The nurse is crucial to identifying this cycle and promoting interventions for improved physical functioning, psychological and emotional stability, and social support. After the initial assessment of the patient, the nurse may provide referrals to health care professionals in these specific areas.

### Monitoring and Managing Potential Complications

The nurse must assess for various complications of COPD, such as life-threatening respiratory insufficiency and failure, as well as respiratory infection and atelectasis, which may increase the risk of respiratory failure. The nurse monitors for cognitive changes (personality and behavioral changes, memory impairment), increasing dyspnea, tachypnea, and tachycardia, which may indicate increasing hypoxemia and impending respiratory failure.

The nurse monitors pulse oximetry values to assess the patient's need for oxygen and administers supplemental oxygen as prescribed. The nurse also instructs the patient about signs and symptoms of respiratory infection that may worsen hypoxemia and reports changes in the patient's physical and cognitive status to the physician. The nurse also assists with the management of developing complications, with possible noninvasive positive-pressure ventilation or intubation, and with mechanical ventilation (see Chapter 25).

Bronchopulmonary infections must be controlled to diminish inflammatory edema and to permit recovery of normal ciliary action. Minor respiratory infections that are of no consequence to people with normal lungs can be life-threatening to people with COPD. The cough associated with bronchial infection introduces a vicious cycle with further trauma and damage to the lungs, progression of symptoms, increased bronchospasm, and increased susceptibility to bronchial infection. Infection compromises lung function and is a common cause of respiratory failure in people with COPD.

In COPD, infection may be accompanied by subtle changes. The nurse instructs the patient to report any signs of infection, such as a fever or change in sputum color, character, consistency, or amount. Any worsening of symptoms (increased tightness of the chest, increased dyspnea and fatigue) also suggests infection and must be reported. Viral infections are hazardous to the patient because they are often followed by infections caused by bacterial organisms, such as *Streptococcus pneumoniae* and *Haemophilus influenzae*.

To prevent infection, the nurse should encourage the patient with COPD to be immunized against influenza and *S. pneumoniae*, because the patient is prone to respiratory infection. It is important to caution the patient to avoid going outdoors if the pollen count is high or if there is significant air pollution, because of the risk of bronchospasm. The patient also should avoid exposure to high outdoor temperatures with high humidity.

Pneumothorax is a potential complication of COPD and can be life-threatening in patients with COPD who have minimal pulmonary reserve. Patients with severe emphysematous changes can develop large bullae, which may rupture and cause a pneumo-

## CHART 24-4

### HOME CARE CHECKLIST • Use of Metered-Dose Inhaler (MDI)

| At the completion of the home care instruction, the patient or caregiver will be able to: | Patient | Caregiver |
|---|---|---|
| • Describe the rationale for using the MDI to administer inhaled medicine. | ✔ | ✔ |
| • Describe how the medication enters the lungs. | ✔ | ✔ |
| • Demonstrate the correct steps in administering medication with an MDI: | | |
|   • Remove the cap and hold the inhaler upright. | ✔ | |
|   • Shake the inhaler. | ✔ | |
|   • Tilt your head back slightly and breathe out slowly. | ✔ | |
|   • Position the inhaler approximately 1–2 inches away from the open mouth, or use a spacer/holding chamber. When using a medicine chamber, place the lips around the mouthpiece. | ✔ | |
|   • Press down on the inhaler to release the medication as you start to breathe in slowly through the mouth. Continue breathing in as the medication is released (press the cartridge down). | ✔ | |

| | | |
|---|---|---|
|   • Breathe in slowly and deeply for 3–5 seconds. | ✔ | |
|   • Hold your breath for 8–10 seconds to allow the medication to reach down into your airways. | ✔ | |
|   • Repeat puffs as directed, allowing 1–2 minutes between puffs. | ✔ | |
|   • Apply the cap to the MDI for storage. | ✔ | |
|   • After inhalation, rinse mouth with water when using a corticosteroid-containing MDI. | ✔ | |
| • Describe how to clean the MDI. | ✔ | ✔ |
| • Describe how to assess the amount of medication remaining in the MDI. | ✔ | ✔ |
| • Describe how and when to contact the health care provider for assessment, and how to obtain a refill of the MDI prescription. | ✔ | ✔ |

Expert Panel Report II. (1997). *Guidelines for the diagnosis and management of asthma*. Bethesda, MD: National Asthma Education and Prevention Program, National Institutes of Health.

---

thorax. Development of a pneumothorax may be spontaneous or related to an activity such as severe coughing or large intrathoracic pressure changes. If a rapid onset of shortness of breath occurs, the nurse should quickly evaluate the patient for potential pneumothorax by assessing the symmetry of chest movement, differences in breath sounds, and pulse oximetry.

Over time, pulmonary hypertension may occur as a result of chronic hypoxemia. The pulmonary arteries respond to hypoxemia by constricting, which results in pulmonary hypertension. The complication may be prevented by maintaining adequate oxygenation through an adequate hemoglobin level, improved ventilation–perfusion of the lungs, or continuous administration of supplemental oxygen (if needed).

## Promoting Home and Community-Based Care

### TEACHING PATIENTS SELF-CARE

Teaching is essential throughout the course of COPD and should be part of the nursing care given to all patients with COPD. The knowledge of patients and family members and their comfort level with this knowledge should be assessed and considered when providing instructions about self-management strategies. In addition to the previously described aspects of patient education, patients and family members must become familiar with the medications prescribed and knowledgeable about potential side effects. Patients and family members need to learn the early signs and symptoms of infection and other complications so that they seek appropriate health care promptly.

### CONTINUING CARE

Referral for home care is important to enable the nurse to assess the patient's home environment and physical and psychological status, to evaluate the patient's adherence to a prescribed regimen, and to assess the patient's ability to cope with changes in lifestyle and physical status. The nurse assesses the patient's and family's understanding of the complications and side effects of medications. Home care visits provide an opportunity to reinforce the information and activities learned in the inpatient or outpatient pulmonary rehabilitation program and to have the patient and family demonstrate correct administration of medications and oxygen, if indicated, and performance of exercises. If the patient does not have access to a formal pulmonary rehabilitation program, it is important to provide the education and breathing retraining necessary to optimize the patient's functional status.

The nurse may direct the patient to community resources such as pulmonary rehabilitation programs and smoking cessation programs to help improve the patient's ability to cope with his or her chronic condition and the therapeutic regimen and to give the patient a sense of worth, hope, and well-being. In addition, the nurse reminds the patient and family about the importance of participating in general health promotion activities and health screening.

It is important to address quality of life and issues surrounding the end of life in patients with end-stage COPD. Patients with COPD have identified lack of information about diagnosis and the disease process, treatment, prognosis, advance care planning, and the dying process as areas of major concern (Curtis, Wenrich, Carline et al., 2002). Areas identified as being of major importance in palliative care for patients with end-stage COPD include symptom management, psychological and emotional needs, spiritual needs, privacy and dignity, equitable care at the end of life, and safety (Blackler, Mooney & Jones, 2004). It is crucial that patients know what to expect as the disease progresses. In addition, they should have information about their role in decisions regarding aggressiveness of care near the end of life and access to specialists who may help them and their families. As the disease course progresses, a holistic assessment of physical and psychological needs should be undertaken at each hospitalization, clinic visit, or home visit. This helps to gauge the patient's assessment of the progression of the disease and its impact on quality of life and guides planning for future interventions and management.

## Evaluation

### Expected Patient Outcomes

Expected patient outcomes may include the following:

1. Demonstrates knowledge of hazards of smoking
   a. Verbalizes willingness/interest to quit smoking
   b. Verbalizes information about smoking, risks of continuing, benefits of quitting, and techniques to optimize cessation efforts
2. Demonstrates improved gas exchange
   a. Shows no signs of restlessness, confusion, or agitation
   b. Has stable pulse oximetry or arterial blood gas values (but not necessarily normal values due to chronic changes in the gas exchange ability of the lungs)
3. Achieves maximal airway clearance
   a. Stops smoking
   b. Avoids noxious substances and extremes of temperature
   c. Maintains adequate hydration
   d. If indicated, performs postural drainage correctly
   e. Knows signs of early infection and is aware of how and when to report them if they occur
   f. Performs controlled coughing without experiencing excessive fatigue
4. Improves breathing pattern
   a. Practices and uses pursed-lip and diaphragmatic breathing
   b. Shows signs of decreased respiratory effort (decreased respiratory rate, less dyspnea)
5. Demonstrates knowledge of strategies to improve activity tolerance and maintain maximum level of self-care
   a. Performs self-care activities within tolerance range
   b. Paces self to avoid fatigue and dyspnea
   c. Uses controlled breathing while performing activities
   d. Uses assistive devices to increase activity tolerance and decrease energy expenditure
6. Demonstrates knowledge of self-care strategies
   a. Participates in determining the therapeutic program
   b. Understands the rationale for activities and medications
   c. Follows the medication plan
   d. Uses bronchodilators and oxygen therapy as prescribed
   e. Stops smoking
   f. Maintains acceptable activity level

## NURSING RESEARCH PROFILE

### Psychological Distress and Quality of Life in Hospitalized Patients With COPD

Andenaes, R., Kalfoss, M. H. & Wahl, A. (2004). Psychological distress and quality of life in hospitalized patients with chronic obstructive pulmonary disease. *Journal of Advanced Nursing, 46*(5), 522–530.

#### Purpose
The purpose of this study was to describe the influence of psychological distress on health status and self-reported quality of life in hospitalized patients with COPD.

#### Design
This longitudinal study evaluated a convenience sample of 92 acutely ill hospitalized patients with COPD. Inclusion criteria included diagnosis of COPD, 45 years of age and older with no other chronic disabling diseases, and ability to communicate in the native language (Norwegian). Participants were evaluated after hospitalization and up to 9 months after discharge. Background and demographic information was collected for each participant. Questionnaires were used to assess health status (St. George's Respiratory Questionnaire), psychological distress (Hopkins Symptom Checklist-25), and quality of life (World Health Organization Quality of Life Abbreviated Questionnaire). Correlational coefficient analysis and multiple linear regression were used to assess relationships between disease factors, psychological distress, and quality-of-life variables.

#### Findings
The majority of the subjects were older (mean age, 69.1 years), lived alone, and had a low educational level. Their physiologic status was poor, with a mean $FEV_1\%$ of 38.9%, indicating severe COPD according to the GOLD classification system. There were significant relationships demonstrated between the St. George's Respiratory Questionnaire Total Impact subscores (measure of social functioning and the psychological disturbances resulting from airways disease) with psychological distress (Hopkins Symptom Checklist-25). Physiologic status as measured by pulmonary function tests was moderately associated with perceived quality of life. Psychological distress was significantly associated with quality of life and accounted for 34% of the total 39% variance explained in the regression model.

#### Nursing Implications
There is a relationship between psychological distress and perceived quality of life, and care of patients with COPD includes planning for interventions related not only to patients' physiologic needs but also their psychological needs. Nursing interventions must focus on helping patients decrease psychological distress to improve perceived quality of life.

---

7. Uses effective coping mechanisms to deal with consequences of disease
    a. Uses self-care strategies to lessen stress associated with disease
    b. Verbalizes resources available to deal with psychological burden of disease
    c. Participates in pulmonary rehabilitation, if appropriate
8. Uses community resources and home-based care
    a. Verbalizes knowledge of community resources (eg, smoking cessation, hospital/community-based support groups)
    b. Participates in pulmonary rehabilitation, if appropriate
    c. Identifies preferences for care as the disease progresses
9. Avoids or reduces complications
    a. Has no evidence of respiratory failure or insufficiency
    b. Maintains adequate pulse oximetry and arterial blood gas values
    c. Shows no signs or symptoms of infection, pneumothorax, or pulmonary hypertension

For more information, see the plan of nursing care for the patient with COPD given in Chart 24-5.

## Bronchiectasis

**Bronchiectasis** is a chronic, irreversible dilation of the bronchi and bronchioles. Under the new definition of COPD, it is considered a separate disease process from COPD (GOLD, WHO & NHLBI, 2004). Bronchiectasis may be caused by a variety of conditions, including

- Airway obstruction
- Diffuse airway injury
- Pulmonary infections and obstruction of the bronchus or complications of long-term pulmonary infections
- Genetic disorders such as cystic fibrosis
- Abnormal host defense (eg, ciliary dyskinesia or humoral immunodeficiency)
- Idiopathic causes

People may be predisposed to bronchiectasis as a result of recurrent respiratory infections in early childhood, measles, influenza, tuberculosis, or immunodeficiency disorders.

*(text continues on page 708)*

### CHART 24-5 Plan of Nursing Care: Care of the Patient With COPD

**Nursing Diagnosis:** Impaired gas exchange and airway clearance due to chronic inhalation of toxins
**Goal:** Improvement in gas exchange

| NURSING INTERVENTIONS | RATIONALE | EXPECTED OUTCOMES |
|---|---|---|
| 1. Evaluate current smoking status, educate regarding smoking cessation, and facilitate efforts to quit.<br>  a. Evaluate current smoking habits of patient and family.<br>  b. Educate regarding hazards of smoking and relationship to COPD.<br>  c. Evaluate previous smoking cessation attempts.<br>  d. Provide educational materials.<br>  e. Refer to a smoking cessation program or resource.<br>2. Evaluate current exposure to occupational toxins or pollutants and indoor/outdoor pollution.<br>  a. Evaluate current exposures to occupational toxins, indoor and outdoor air pollution (eg, smog, toxic fumes, chemicals).<br>  b. Emphasize primary prevention to occupational exposures. This is best achieved by elimination or reduction of exposures in the workplace.<br>  c. Educate regarding types of indoor and outdoor air pollution (eg, biomass fuel burned for cooking and heating in poorly ventilated buildings, outdoor air pollution).<br>  d. Advise patient to monitor public announcements regarding air quality. | 1. Smoking causes permanent damage to the lung and diminishes the lungs' protective mechanisms. Airflow is obstructed, secretions are increased, and lung capacity is reduced. Continued smoking increases morbidity and mortality in COPD and is also a risk factor for lung cancer.<br><br>2. Chronic inhalation of both indoor and outdoor toxins causes damage to the airways and impairs gas exchange. | • Identifies the hazards of cigarette smoking<br>• Identifies resources for smoking cessation<br>• Enrolls in smoking cessation program<br>• Reports success in stopping smoking<br>• Verbalizes types of inhaled toxins<br>• Minimizes or eliminates exposures<br>• Monitors public announcements regarding air quality and minimizes or eliminates exposures during episodes of severe pollution |

**Nursing Diagnosis:** Impaired gas exchange related to ventilation–perfusion inequality
**Goal:** Improvement in gas exchange

| NURSING INTERVENTIONS | RATIONALE | EXPECTED OUTCOMES |
|---|---|---|
| 1. Administer bronchodilators as prescribed:<br>  a. Inhalation is the preferred route. | 1. Bronchodilators dilate the airways. The medication dosage is carefully adjusted for each patient, in accordance with clinical response. | • Verbalizes need for bronchodilators and for taking them as prescribed<br>• Evidences minimal side effects; heart rate near normal, absence of dysrhythmias, normal mentation |

## CHART 24-5 Plan of Nursing Care: Care of the Patient With COPD (Continued)

### NURSING INTERVENTIONS

b. Observe for side effects: tachycardia, dysrhythmias, central nervous system excitation, nausea, and vomiting.
c. Assess for correct technique of metered-dose inhaler (MDI) or other type of administration.
2. Evaluate effectiveness of nebulizer or MDI treatments.
   a. Assess for decreased shortness of breath, decreased wheezing or crackles, loosened secretions, decreased anxiety.
   b. Ensure that treatment is given before meals to avoid nausea and to reduce fatigue that accompanies eating.
3. Instruct and encourage patient in diaphragmatic breathing and effective coughing.

4. Administer oxygen by the method prescribed.
   a. Explain rationale and importance to patient.
   b. Evaluate effectiveness; observe for signs of hypoxemia. Notify physician if restlessness, anxiety, somnolence, cyanosis, or tachycardia is present.
   c. Analyze arterial blood gases and compare with baseline values. When arterial puncture is performed and a blood sample is obtained, hold puncture site for 5 minutes to prevent arterial bleeding and development of ecchymoses.
   d. Initiate pulse oximetry to monitor oxygen saturation.
   e. Explain that no smoking is permitted by patient or visitors while oxygen is in use.

### RATIONALE

2. Combining medication with aerosolized bronchodilators is typically used to control bronchoconstriction in an acute exacerbation. Generally, however, the MDI with spacer is the preferred route (less cost and time to treatment).

3. These techniques improve ventilation by opening airways to facilitate clearing the airways of sputum. Gas exchange is improved and fatigue is minimized.

4. Oxygen will correct the hypoxemia. Careful observation of the liter flow or the percentage administered and its effect on the patient is important. These patients generally require low-flow oxygen rates of 1 to 2 L/min. Monitor and titrate to achieve desired $PaO_2$. Periodic arterial blood gases and pulse oximetry help evaluate adequacy of oxygenation. Smoking may render pulse oximetry inaccurate because the carbon monoxide from cigarette smoke also saturates hemoglobin.

### EXPECTED OUTCOMES

- Reports a decrease in dyspnea
- Shows an improved expiratory flow rate
- Uses and cleans respiratory therapy equipment as applicable
- Demonstrates diaphragmatic breathing and coughing
- Uses oxygen equipment appropriately when indicated
- Evidences improved arterial blood gases or pulse oximetry
- Demonstrates correct technique for use of MDI

*continued >*

### CHART 24-5

## Plan of Nursing Care — Care of the Patient With COPD (Continued)

**Nursing Diagnosis:** Ineffective airway clearance related to bronchoconstriction, increased mucus production, ineffective cough, bronchopulmonary infection, and other complications
**Goal:** Achievement of airway clearance

| NURSING INTERVENTIONS | RATIONALE | EXPECTED OUTCOMES |
|---|---|---|
| 1. Adequately hydrate the patient. | 1. Systemic hydration keeps secretions moist and easier to expectorate. Fluids must be given with caution if right- or left-sided heart failure is present. | • Verbalizes need to drink fluids<br>• Demonstrates diaphragmatic breathing and coughing<br>• Performs postural drainage correctly<br>• Coughing is minimized<br>• Does not smoke<br>• Verbalizes that pollens, fumes, gases, dusts, and extremes of temperature and humidity are irritants to be avoided<br>• Identifies signs of early infection<br>• Is free of infection (no fever, no change in sputum, lessening of dyspnea)<br>• Verbalizes need to notify health care provider at the earliest sign of infection<br>• Verbalizes need to stay away from crowds or people with colds in flu season<br>• Discusses flu and pneumonia vaccines with clinician to help prevent infection |
| 2. Teach and encourage the use of diaphragmatic breathing and coughing techniques. | 2. These techniques help to improve ventilation and mobilize secretions without causing breathlessness and fatigue. | |
| 3. Assist in administering nebulizer or MDI. | 3. This ensures adequate delivery of medication to the airways. | |
| 4. If indicated, perform postural drainage with percussion and vibration in the morning and at night as prescribed. | 4. Uses gravity to help raise secretions so they can be more easily expectorated or suctioned. | |
| 5. Instruct patient to avoid bronchial irritants such as cigarette smoke, aerosols, extremes of temperature, and fumes. | 5. Bronchial irritants cause bronchoconstriction and increased mucus production, which then interfere with airway clearance. | |
| 6. Teach early signs of infection that are to be reported to the clinician immediately:<br>  a. Increased sputum production<br>  b. Change in color of sputum<br>  c. Increased thickness of sputum<br>  d. Increased shortness of breath, tightness in chest, or fatigue<br>  e. Increased coughing<br>  f. Fever or chills | 6. Minor respiratory infections that are of no consequence to the person with normal lungs can produce fatal disturbances in the lungs of the person with emphysema. Early recognition is crucial. | |
| 7. Administer antibiotics as prescribed. | 7. Antibiotics may be prescribed to prevent or treat infection. | |
| 8. Encourage patient to be immunized against influenza and *Streptococcus pneumoniae*. | 8. People with respiratory conditions are prone to respiratory infections and are encouraged to be immunized. | |

**Nursing Diagnosis:** Ineffective breathing pattern related to shortness of breath, mucus, bronchoconstriction, and airway irritants
**Goal:** Improvement in breathing pattern

| NURSING INTERVENTIONS | RATIONALE | EXPECTED OUTCOMES |
|---|---|---|
| 1. Teach patient diaphragmatic and pursed-lip breathing. | 1. Helps patient prolong expiration time and decreases air trapping. With these techniques, patient will breathe more efficiently and effectively. | • Practices pursed-lip and diaphragmatic breathing and uses them when short of breath and with activity |

## CHART 24-5

# Plan of Nursing Care — Care of the Patient With COPD (Continued)

| NURSING INTERVENTIONS | RATIONALE | EXPECTED OUTCOMES |
|---|---|---|
| 2. Encourage alternating activity with rest periods. Allow patient to make some decisions (bath, shaving) about care based on tolerance level. | 2. Pacing activities permits patient to perform activities without excessive distress. | • Shows signs of decreased respiratory effort and paces activities<br>• Uses inspiratory muscle trainer as prescribed |
| 3. Encourage use of an inspiratory muscle trainer if prescribed. | 3. Strengthens and conditions the respiratory muscles. | |

**Nursing Diagnosis:** Self-care deficits related to fatigue secondary to increased work of breathing and insufficient ventilation and oxygenation
**Goal:** Independence in self-care activities

| NURSING INTERVENTIONS | RATIONALE | EXPECTED OUTCOMES |
|---|---|---|
| 1. Teach patient to coordinate diaphragmatic breathing with activity (eg, walking, bending). | 1. This will allow the patient to be more active and to avoid excessive fatigue or dyspnea during activity. | • Uses controlled breathing while bathing, bending, and walking<br>• Paces activities of daily living to alternate with rest periods to reduce fatigue and dyspnea<br>• Describes energy conservation strategies<br>• Performs same self-care activities as before<br>• Performs postural drainage correctly |
| 2. Encourage patient to begin to bathe self, dress self, walk, and drink fluids. Discuss energy conservation measures. | 2. As condition resolves, patient will be able to do more but needs to be encouraged to avoid increasing dependence. | |
| 3. Teach postural drainage if appropriate. | 3. Encourages patient to become involved in own care. Prepares patient to manage at home. | |

**Nursing Diagnosis:** Activity intolerance due to fatigue, hypoxemia, and ineffective breathing patterns
**Goal:** Improvement in activity tolerance

| NURSING INTERVENTIONS | RATIONALE | EXPECTED OUTCOMES |
|---|---|---|
| 1. Support patient in establishing a regular regimen of exercise using treadmill and exercise bicycle, walking, or other appropriate exercises, such as mall walking.<br>  a. Assess the patient's current level of functioning and develop exercise plan based on baseline functional status.<br>  b. Suggest consultation with a physical therapist or pulmonary rehabilitation program to determine an exercise program specific to the patient's capability. Have portable oxygen unit available if oxygen is prescribed for exercise. | 1. Muscles that are deconditioned consume more oxygen and place an additional burden on the lungs. Through regular, graded exercise, these muscle groups become more conditioned, and the patient can do more without getting as short of breath. Graded exercise breaks the cycle of debilitation. | • Performs activities with less shortness of breath<br>• Verbalizes need to exercise daily and demonstrates an exercise plan to be carried out at home<br>• Walks and gradually increases walking time and distance to improve physical condition<br>• Exercises both upper and lower body muscle groups |

*continued >*

## CHART 24-5 Plan of Nursing Care: Care of the Patient With COPD (Continued)

**Nursing Diagnosis:** Ineffective coping related to reduced socialization, anxiety, depression, lower activity level, and the inability to work
**Goal:** Attainment of an optimal level of coping

| NURSING INTERVENTIONS | RATIONALE | EXPECTED OUTCOMES |
|---|---|---|
| 1. Help the patient develop realistic goals. | 1. Developing realistic goals will promote a sense of hope and accomplishment rather than defeat and hopelessness. | • Expresses interest in the future<br>• Participates in the discharge plan<br>• Discusses activities or methods that can be performed to ease shortness of breath<br>• Uses relaxation techniques appropriately<br>• Expresses interest in a pulmonary rehabilitation program |
| 2. Encourage activity to level of symptom tolerance. | 2. Activity reduces tension and decreases degree of dyspnea as patient becomes conditioned. | |
| 3. Teach relaxation technique or provide a relaxation tape for patient. | 3. Relaxation reduces stress, anxiety, and dyspnea and helps patient to cope with disability. | |
| 4. Enroll patient in pulmonary rehabilitation program where available. | 4. Pulmonary rehabilitation programs have been shown to promote a subjective improvement in a patient's status and self-esteem as well as increased exercise tolerance and decreased hospitalizations. | |

**Nursing Diagnosis:** Deficient knowledge about self-management to be performed at home.
**Goal:** Adherence to therapeutic program and home care

| NURSING INTERVENTIONS | RATIONALE | EXPECTED OUTCOMES |
|---|---|---|
| 1. Help patient identify/develop short- and long-term goals.<br>  a. Teach the patient about disease, medications, procedures, and how and when to seek help.<br>  b. Refer patient to pulmonary rehabilitation. | 1. Patient needs to be a partner in developing the plan of care and needs to know what to expect. Teaching about the condition is one of the most important aspects of care; it will prepare the patient to live and cope with the condition and improve quality of life. | • Understands disease and what affects it<br>• Verbalizes the need to preserve existing lung function by adhering to the prescribed program<br>• Understands purposes and proper administration of medications<br>• Stops smoking or enrolls in a smoking cessation program<br>• Identifies when and whom to call for assistance |
| 2. Give strong message to stop smoking. Discuss smoking cessation strategies. Provide information about resource groups (eg, SmokEnders, American Cancer Society, American Lung Association). | 2. Smoking causes permanent damage to the lung and diminishes the lungs' protective mechanisms. Air flow is obstructed and lung capacity is reduced. Smoking increases morbidity and mortality and is also a risk factor for lung cancer. | |

## CHART 24-5 Plan of Nursing Care: Care of the Patient With COPD (Continued)

**Collaborative Problem:** Atelectasis
**Goal:** Absence of atelectasis on x-ray and physical examination

| NURSING INTERVENTIONS | RATIONALE | EXPECTED OUTCOMES |
|---|---|---|
| 1. Monitor respiratory status, including rate and pattern of respirations, breath sounds, signs and symptoms of respiratory distress, and pulse oximetry.<br>2. Instruct in and encourage diaphragmatic breathing and effective coughing techniques.<br>3. Promote use of lung expansion techniques (eg, deep-breathing exercises, incentive spirometry) as prescribed. | 1. A change in respiratory status, including tachypnea, dyspnea, and diminished or absent breath sounds, may indicate atelectasis.<br>2. These techniques improve ventilation and lung expansion and ideally improve gas exchange.<br>3. Deep-breathing exercises and incentive spirometry promote maximal lung expansion. | • Normal (baseline for patient) respiratory rate and pattern<br>• Normal breath sounds for patient<br>• Demonstrates diaphragmatic breathing and effective coughing<br>• Performs deep-breathing exercises, incentive spirometry as prescribed<br>• Pulse oximetry is ≥ 90% |

**Collaborative Problem:** Pneumothorax
**Goal:** Absence of signs and symptoms of pneumothorax

| NURSING INTERVENTIONS | RATIONALE | EXPECTED OUTCOMES |
|---|---|---|
| 1. Monitor respiratory status, including rate and pattern of respirations, symmetry of chest wall movement, breath sounds, signs and symptoms of respiratory distress, and pulse oximetry.<br>2. Assess pulse.<br>3. Assess for chest pain and precipitating factors.<br>4. Palpate for tracheal deviation/shift away from the affected side.<br>5. Monitor pulse oximetry and if indicated arterial blood gases.<br>6. Administer supplemental oxygen therapy, as indicated.<br>7. Administer analgesics, as indicated, for chest pain.<br>8. Assist with chest tube insertion and use pleural drainage system, as prescribed. | 1. Dyspnea, tachypnea, tachycardia, acute pleuritic chest pain, tracheal deviation away from the affected side, absence of breath sounds on the affected side, and decreased tactile fremitus may indicate pneumothorax.<br>2. Tachycardia is associated with pneumothorax and anxiety.<br>3. Pain may accompany pneumothorax.<br>4. Early detection of pneumothorax and prompt intervention will prevent other serious complications.<br>5. Recognition of a deterioration in respiratory function will prevent serious complications.<br>6. Oxygen will correct hypoxemia; administer it with caution.<br>7. Pain interferes with deep breathing, resulting in a decrease in lung expansion.<br>8. Removal of air from the pleural space will reexpand the lung. | • Normal respiratory rate and pattern for patient<br>• Normal breath sounds bilaterally<br>• Normal pulse for patient<br>• Normal tactile fremitus<br>• Absence of pain<br>• Tracheal position is midline<br>• Pulse oximetry ≥ 90%<br>• Maintains normal oxygen saturation and arterial blood gas measurements for patient<br>• Exhibits no hypoxemia and hypercapnia (or returns to baseline values)<br>• Absence of pain<br>• Symmetric chest wall movement<br>• Lung is reexpanded on chest x-ray<br>• Breath sounds are heard on the affected side |

*continued >*

# CHART 24-5

## Plan of Nursing Care: Care of the Patient With COPD (Continued)

**Collaborative Problem:** Respiratory failure
**Goal:** Absence of signs and symptoms of respiratory failure; no evidence of respiratory failure on laboratory tests

| NURSING INTERVENTIONS | RATIONALE | EXPECTED OUTCOMES |
|---|---|---|
| 1. Monitor respiratory status, including rate and pattern of respirations, breath sounds, and signs and symptoms of acute respiratory distress.<br>2. Monitor pulse oximetry and arterial blood gases.<br>3. Administer supplemental oxygen and initiate mechanisms for mechanical ventilation, as prescribed. | 1. Early recognition of a deterioration in respiratory function will avert further complications, such as respiratory failure, severe hypoxemia, and hypercapnia.<br>2. Recognition of changes in oxygenation and acid–base balance will guide in correcting and preventing complications.<br>3. Acute respiratory failure is a medical emergency. Hypoxemia is a hallmark sign. Administration of oxygen therapy and mechanical ventilation (if indicated) are critical to survival. | • Normal respiratory rate and pattern for patient with no acute distress<br>• Recognizes symptoms of hypoxemia and hypercapnia<br>• Maintains normal arterial blood gases/pulse oximetry or returns to baseline values |

**Collaborative Problem:** Pulmonary arterial hypertension
**Goal:** Absence of evidence of pulmonary arterial hypertension on physical examination or laboratory tests

| NURSING INTERVENTIONS | RATIONALE | EXPECTED OUTCOMES |
|---|---|---|
| 1. Monitor respiratory status, including rate and pattern of respirations, breath sounds, pulse oximetry, and signs and symptoms of acute respiratory distress.<br>2. Assess for signs and symptoms of right-sided heart failure, including peripheral edema, ascites, distended neck veins, crackles, and heart murmur.<br>3. Administer oxygen therapy, as prescribed. | 1. Dyspnea is the primary symptom of pulmonary arterial hypertension. Other symptoms include fatigue, angina, near syncope, edema, and palpitations.<br>2. Right-sided heart failure is a common clinical manifestation of pulmonary arterial hypertension due to increased right ventricular workload.<br>3. Continuous oxygen therapy is a major component of management of pulmonary arterial hypertension by preventing hypoxemia and thereby reducing pulmonary vascular constriction (resistance) secondary to hypoxemia. | • Normal respiratory rate and pattern for patient<br>• Exhibits no signs and symptoms of right-sided failure<br>• Maintains baseline pulse oximetry values and arterial blood gases |

## Pathophysiology

The inflammatory process associated with pulmonary infections damages the bronchial wall, causing a loss of its supporting structure and resulting in thick sputum that ultimately obstructs the bronchi. The walls become permanently distended and distorted, impairing mucociliary clearance. The inflammation and infection extend to the peribronchial tissues; in the case of saccular bronchiectasis, each dilated tube virtually amounts to a lung abscess, the exudate of which drains freely through the bronchus. Bronchiectasis is usually localized, affecting a segment or lobe of a lung, most frequently the lower lobes.

The retention of secretions and subsequent obstruction ultimately cause the alveoli distal to the obstruction to collapse (atelectasis). Inflammatory scarring or fibrosis replaces functioning lung tissue. In time, the patient develops respiratory insufficiency with reduced vital capacity, decreased ventilation, and an increased ratio of residual volume to total lung capacity. There is impairment in the matching of ventilation to perfusion (ventilation–perfusion imbalance) and hypoxemia.

## Clinical Manifestations

Characteristic symptoms of bronchiectasis include chronic cough and the production of purulent sputum in copious amounts. Many patients with this disease have hemoptysis. Clubbing of the fingers also is common because of respiratory insufficiency. Patients usually have repeated episodes of pulmonary infection. Even with modern treatment approaches, the average age at death is approximately 55 years.

## Assessment and Diagnostic Findings

Bronchiectasis is not readily diagnosed because the symptoms can be mistaken for those of simple chronic bronchitis. A definite sign is offered by the prolonged history of productive cough, with sputum consistently negative for tubercle bacilli. The diagnosis is established by a CT scan, which demonstrates either the presence or absence of bronchial dilation.

## Medical Management

Treatment objectives are to promote bronchial drainage to clear excessive secretions from the affected portion of the lungs and to prevent or control infection. Postural drainage is part of all treatment plans, because draining of the bronchiectatic areas by gravity reduces the amount of secretions and the degree of infection. Sometimes mucopurulent sputum must be removed by bronchoscopy. Chest physiotherapy, including percussion and postural drainage, is important in the management of secretions.

Smoking cessation is important, because smoking impairs bronchial drainage by paralyzing ciliary action, increasing bronchial secretions, and causing inflammation of the mucous membranes, resulting in hyperplasia of the mucous glands. Infection is controlled with antimicrobial therapy based on the results of sensitivity studies on organisms cultured from sputum. A year-round regimen of antibiotic agents may be prescribed, with different types of antibiotics at intervals. Some clinicians prescribe antibiotic agents throughout the winter or when acute upper respiratory tract infections occur. Patients should be vaccinated against influenza and pneumococcal pneumonia. Bronchodilators, which may be prescribed for patients who also have reactive airway disease, may also assist with secretion management.

Surgical intervention, although used infrequently, may be indicated for patients who continue to expectorate large amounts of sputum and have repeated bouts of pneumonia and hemoptysis despite adherence to treatment regimens. The disease must involve only one or two areas of the lung that can be removed without producing respiratory insufficiency. The goals of surgical treatment are to conserve normal pulmonary tissue and to avoid infectious complications. Diseased tissue is removed, provided that postoperative lung function will be adequate. It may be necessary to remove a segment of a lobe (segmental resection), a lobe (lobectomy), or rarely an entire lung (pneumonectomy). (See Chart 25-16 in Chapter 25 for further information.) Segmental resection is the removal of an anatomic subdivision of a pulmonary lobe. The chief advantage is that only diseased tissue is removed, and healthy lung tissue is conserved.

The surgery is preceded by a period of careful preparation. The objective is to obtain a dry (free of infection) tracheobronchial tree to prevent complications (atelectasis, pneumonia, bronchopleural fistula, and empyema). This is accomplished by postural drainage or, depending on the location, by direct suction through a bronchoscope. A course of antibacterial therapy may be prescribed. After surgery, care is the same as for any patient who has undergone chest surgery (see Chapter 25).

## Nursing Management

Nursing management of patients with bronchiectasis focuses on alleviating symptoms and helping patients clear pulmonary secretions. Patient teaching targets smoking and other factors that increase the production of mucus and hamper its removal. Patients and families are taught to perform postural drainage and to avoid exposure to people with upper respiratory or other infections. If the patient experiences fatigue and dyspnea, he or she is informed about strategies to conserve energy while maintaining as active a lifestyle as possible. The patient is taught about the early signs of respiratory infection and the progression of the disorder, so that appropriate treatment can be implemented promptly. The presence of a large amount of mucus may decrease the patient's appetite and result in an inadequate dietary intake; therefore, the patient's nutritional status is assessed and strategies are implemented to ensure an adequate diet.

# Asthma

**Asthma** is a chronic inflammatory disease of the airways that causes airway hyperresponsiveness, mucosal edema, and mucus production. This inflammation ultimately leads to recurrent episodes of asthma symptoms: cough, chest tightness, wheezing, and dyspnea (Fig. 24-6). In 2001, there were 11.3 million visits to physicians' offices for treatment of asthma and approximately 4300 deaths attributable to asthma. In 2002, 1.9 million hospital emergency department visits were due to asthma. In that same year, 14 million non-institutionalized adults and 6.4 million children were diagnosed with asthma in the United States (CDC, 2004).

Asthma differs from other obstructive lung diseases in that it is largely reversible, either spontaneously or with treatment. Patients with asthma may experience symptom-free periods alternating with acute exacerbations that last from minutes to hours or days. Asthma is the most common

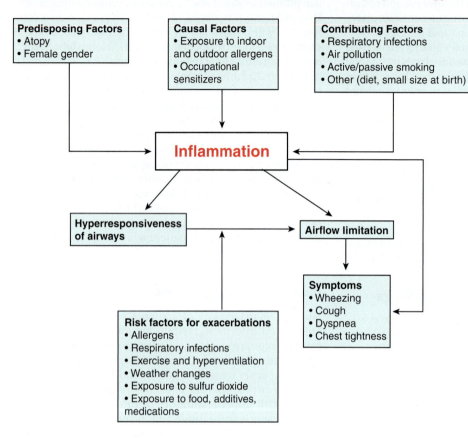

**FIGURE 24-6.** Pathophysiology of asthma. Adapted from materials developed for the Global Initiative for Asthma (GINA): Global Strategy for Asthma Management and Prevention, National Institutes of Health, National Heart, Lung, and Blood Institute (revised 2003).

chronic disease of childhood and can occur at any age. Despite increased knowledge regarding the pathology of asthma and the development of better medications and management plans, the death rate from this disease continues to increase. For most patients, asthma is a disruptive disease, affecting school and work attendance, occupational choices, physical activity, and general quality of life.

Allergy is the strongest predisposing factor for asthma. Chronic exposure to airway irritants or allergens also increases the risk of asthma. Common allergens can be seasonal (grass, tree, and weed pollens) or perennial (eg, mold, dust, roaches, animal dander). Common triggers for asthma symptoms and exacerbations include airway irritants (eg, air pollutants, cold, heat, weather changes, strong odors or perfumes, smoke), exercise, stress or emotional upset, sinusitis with postnasal drip, medications, viral respiratory tract infections, and gastroesophageal reflux. Most people who have asthma are sensitive to a variety of triggers. A person's asthma changes depending on the environment, activities, management practices, and other factors (American Thoracic Society, 2004).

## Pathophysiology

**CONCEPTS** in action **ANIMATION**

The underlying pathology in asthma is reversible and diffuse airway inflammation. The inflammation leads to obstruction due to the following factors: (1) swelling of the membranes that line the airways (mucosal edema), which reduces the airway diameter; (2) contraction of the bronchial smooth muscle that encircles the airways (bronchospasm), which causes further narrowing; and (3) increased mucus production, which diminishes airway size and may entirely plug the bronchi.

The bronchial muscles and mucous glands enlarge; thick, tenacious sputum is produced; and the alveoli hyperinflate. Some patients have airway subbasement membrane fibrosis. This is called airway "remodeling" and occurs in response to chronic inflammation. The fibrotic changes in the airway lead to airway narrowing and potentially irreversible airflow limitation (Expert Panel Report, 2003). Cells that play a key role in the inflammation of asthma are mast cells, neutrophils, eosinophils, and lymphocytes. Mast cells, when activated, release several chemicals called mediators. These chemicals, which include histamine, bradykinin, prostaglandins, and leukotrienes, perpetuate the inflammatory response, causing increased blood flow, vasoconstriction, fluid leak from the vasculature, attraction of white blood cells to the area, and bronchoconstriction (Expert Panel Report, 2003). Regulation of these chemicals is the aim of much of the current research regarding pharmacologic therapy for asthma.

In addition, alpha- and beta$_2$-adrenergic receptors of the sympathetic nervous system located in the bronchi play a role. When the alpha-adrenergic receptors are stimulated, bronchoconstriction occurs. When the beta$_2$-adrenergic receptors are stimulated, bronchodilation occurs. The balance between alpha and beta$_2$-adrenergic receptors is controlled primarily by cyclic adenosine monophosphate (cAMP). Alpha-adrenergic receptor stimulation results in a decrease in cAMP, which leads to an increase of chemical mediators released by the mast cells and bronchoconstriction. Beta$_2$-adrenergic stimulation results in increased levels of cAMP, which inhibits the release of chemical mediators and causes bronchodilation.

## Clinical Manifestations

The three most common symptoms of asthma are cough, dyspnea, and wheezing. In some instances, cough may be the only symptom. An asthma attack often occurs at night or early in the morning, possibly because of circadian variations that influence airway receptor thresholds.

An asthma exacerbation may begin abruptly but most frequently is preceded by increasing symptoms over the previous few days. There is cough, with or without mucus production. At times the mucus is so tightly wedged in the narrowed airway that the patient cannot cough it up. There may be generalized wheezing (the sound of airflow through narrowed airways), first on expiration and then possibly during inspiration as well. Generalized chest tightness and dyspnea occur. Expiration requires effort and becomes prolonged. As the exacerbation progresses, diaphoresis, tachycardia, and a widened pulse pressure may occur along with hypoxemia and central cyanosis (a late sign of poor oxygenation). Although life-threatening and severe hypoxemia can occur in asthma, it is relatively uncommon. The hypoxemia is secondary to a ventilation–perfusion mismatch and readily responds to supplemental oxygenation.

Symptoms of exercise-induced asthma include maximal symptoms during exercise, absence of nocturnal symptoms, and sometimes only a description of a "choking" sensation during exercise.

Asthma is categorized according to symptoms and objective measures of airflow obstruction (Table 24-3) (Expert Panel Report, 2003).

## Assessment and Diagnostic Findings

A complete family, environmental, and occupational history is essential. To establish the diagnosis, the clinician must determine that periodic symptoms of airflow obstruction are present, airflow is at least partially reversible, and other causes have been excluded. A positive family history and environmental factors, including seasonal changes, high pollen counts, mold, pet dander, climate changes (particularly cold air), and air pollution, are primarily associated with asthma. In addition, asthma is associated with a variety of occupation-related chemicals and compounds, including metal salts, wood and vegetable dust, medications (eg, aspirin, antibiotics, piperazine, cimetidine), industrial chemicals and plastics, biologic enzymes (eg, laundry detergents), animal and insect dusts, sera, and secretions. Comorbid conditions that may accompany asthma include gastroesophageal reflux, drug-induced asthma, and allergic bronchopulmonary aspergillosis. Other possible allergic reactions that may accompany asthma include eczema, rashes, and temporary edema.

During acute episodes, sputum and blood tests may disclose eosinophilia (elevated levels of eosinophils). Serum levels of immunoglobulin E may be elevated if allergy is present. Arterial blood gas analysis and pulse oximetry reveal hypoxemia during acute attacks. Initially, hypocapnia and respiratory alkalosis are present. As the patient's condition worsens and he or she becomes more fatigued, the PaCO$_2$ may increase. A normal PaCO$_2$ value may be a signal of impending respiratory failure. Because carbon dioxide is 20 times more diffusible than oxygen, it is rare for PaCO$_2$ to be normal or elevated in a person who is breathing very rapidly. During an exacerbation, the FEV$_1$ and FVC are markedly decreased but improve with bronchodilator administration (demonstrating reversibility). Pulmonary function is usually normal between exacerbations.

The occurrence of a severe, continuous reaction is referred to as status asthmaticus and is considered life-threatening (see later discussion).

## Prevention

Patients with recurrent asthma should undergo tests to identify the substances that precipitate the symptoms. Possible causes are dust, dust mites, roaches, certain types of cloth, pets, horses, detergents, soaps, certain foods, molds, and pollens. If the attacks are seasonal, pollens can be strongly suspected. Patients are instructed to avoid the causative agents whenever possible. Knowledge is the key to quality asthma care. National guidelines are available for the care of patients with asthma. Unfortunately, not all health care providers follow them.

## Complications

Complications of asthma may include status asthmaticus, respiratory failure, pneumonia, and atelectasis. Airway obstruction, particularly during acute asthmatic episodes, often results in hypoxemia, requiring the administration of oxygen and the monitoring of pulse oximetry and arterial blood gases. Fluids are administered, because people with asthma are frequently dehydrated from diaphoresis and insensible fluid loss with hyperventilation.

## Medical Management

Immediate intervention is necessary, because the continuing and progressive dyspnea leads to increased anxiety, aggravating the situation.

### Pharmacologic Therapy

There are two general classes of asthma medications: quick-relief medications for immediate treatment of asthma symptoms and exacerbations (see Table 24-2) and long-acting medications to achieve and maintain control of persistent asthma (Table 24-4). Because the underlying pathology of asthma is inflammation, control of persistent asthma is accomplished primarily with regular use of anti-inflammatory medications. These medications have systemic side effects

# TABLE 24-3. Stepwise Approach for Managing Asthma in Adults and Children Older Than 5 Years of Age: Treatment

| Classify Severity: Clinical Features Before Treatment or Adequate Control | | | Medications Required To Maintain Long-Term Control |
|---|---|---|---|
| | **Symptoms/Day** **Symptoms/Night** | **PEF or FEV₁** **PEF Variability** | **Daily Medications** |
| **Step 4** **Severe Persistent** | Continual Frequent | ≤60% >30% | • Preferred treatment: <br> — High-dose inhaled corticosteroids AND <br> — Long-acting inhaled beta₂-agonists AND, if needed, <br> — Corticosteroid tablets or syrup long term (2 mg/kg/day, generally do not exceed 60 mg per day). (Make repeat attempts to reduce systemic corticosteroids and maintain control with high-dose inhaled corticosteroids.) |
| **Step 3** **Moderate Persistent** | Daily >1 night/week | >60% – <80% >30% | • Preferred treatment: <br> — Low-to-medium dose inhaled corticosteroids and long-acting inhaled beta₂-agonists. <br> • Alternative treatment (listed alphabetically): <br> — Increase inhaled corticosteroids within medium-dose range OR <br> — Low-to-medium dose inhaled corticosteroids and either leukotriene modifier or theophylline. <br> If needed (particularly in patients with recurring severe exacerbations): <br> • Preferred treatment: <br> — Increase inhaled corticosteroids within medium-dose range and add long-acting inhaled beta₂-agonists. <br> • Alternative treatment (listed alphabetically): <br> — Increase inhaled corticosteroids within medium-dose range and add either leukotriene modifier or theophylline. |
| **Step 2** **Mild Persistent** | >2 weeks but < 1x/day >2 nights/month | ≥80% 20–30% | • Preferred treatment: <br> — Low-dose inhaled corticosteroids. <br> • Alternative treatment: (listed alphabetically): cromolyn, leukotriene modifier, nedocromil, OR sustained-release theophylline to serum concentration of 5–15 mcg/mL. |
| **Step 1** **Mild Intermittent** | ≤2 days/week ≤2 nights/month | ≥80% <20% | • No daily medication needed <br> • Severe exacerbations may occur, separated by long periods of normal lung function and no symptoms. A course of systemic corticosteroids is recommended. |
| **Quick Relief** **All Patients** | | | • Short-acting bronchodilator: 2–4 puffs short-acting inhaled beta₂-agonists as needed for symptoms. <br> • Intensity of treatment will depend on severity of exacerbation; up to 3 treatments at 20-minute intervals or a single nebulizer treatment as needed. Course of systemic corticosteroids may be needed. <br> • Use of short-acting beta₂-agonists >2 times a week in intermittent asthma (daily, or increasing use in persistent asthma) may indicate the need to initiate (increase) long-term-control therapy. |

**↓ Step down**

Review treatment every 1 to 6 months: a gradual stepwise reduction in treatment may be possible.

**↑ Step up**

If control is not maintained, consider step up. First, review patient medication technique, adherence, and environmental control.

**Goals of Therapy: Asthma Control**

- Minimal or no chronic symptoms day or night
- Minimal or no exacerbations
- No limitations on activities; no school/work missed
- Maintain (near) normal pulmonary function
- Minimal use of short-acting inhaled beta₂-agonist
- Minimal or no adverse effects from medications

**Note**

- The stepwise approach is meant to assist, not replace, the clinical decision-making required to meet individual patient needs.
- Classify severity: assign patient to most severe step in which any feature occurs (PEF is % of personal best; FEV₁ is % predicted).
- Gain control as quickly as possible (consider a short course of systemic corticosteroids); then step down to the least medication necessary to maintain control.
- Minimize use of short-acting inhaled beta₂-agonists. Overreliance on short-acting inhaled beta₂-agonists (e.g., use of approximately one canister a month even if not using it every day) indicates inadequate control of asthma and the need to initiate or intensify long-term-control therapy.
- Provide education on self-management and controlling environmental factors that make asthma worse (e.g., allergens and irritants).
- Refer to an asthma specialist if there are difficulties controlling asthma or if step 4 care is required. Referral may be considered if step 3 care is required.

From Expert Panel Report (2003). *Guidelines for the diagnosis and management of asthma: Update on selected topics 2002*. NIH Publication No 02-5074. Bethesda, MD: National Institutes of Health, National Heart, Lung and Blood Institute.

### TABLE 24-4  Usual Dosages for Long-Term Asthma Control Medications

| Medication | Dosage Form | Adult Dose |
|---|---|---|
| **Inhaled Corticosteroids** (See Guidelines for the diagnosis and management of asthma: update on selected topics, 2002, for comparative daily dosages for inhaled corticosteroids.) | | |
| **Systemic Corticosteroids** (Applies to all three corticosteroids.) | | |
| Methylprednisolone | 2, 4, 8, 16, 32 mg tablets | • 7.5–60 mg daily in a single dose in a.m. or qod as needed for control |
| Prednisolone | 5 mg tablets, 5 mg/5 mL, 15 mg/5 mL | • Short-course "burst" to achieve control: 40–60 mg per day as single or 2 divided doses for 3–10 days |
| Prednisone | 1, 2.5, 5, 10, 20, 50 mg tablets; 5 mg/mL, 5 mg/5 mL | |
| **Long-Acting Inhaled Beta$_2$-Agonists** (Should not be used for symptom relief or for exacerbations. Use with inhaled corticosteroids.) | | |
| Salmeterol | MDI 21 mcg/puff | 2 puffs q12h |
|  | DPI 50 mcg/blister | 1 blister q12h |
| Formoterol | DPI 12 mcg/single-use capsule | 1 capsule q12h |
| **Combined Medication** | | |
| Fluticasone/Salmeterol | DPI 100, 250, or 500 mcg/50 mcg | 1 inhalation bid; dose depends on severity of asthma |
| **Cromolyn and Nedocromil** | | |
| Cromolyn | MDI 1 mg/puff | 2–4 puffs tid-qid |
|  | Nebulizer 20 mg/ampule | 1 ampule tid-qid |
| Nedocromil | MDI 1.75 mg/puff | 2–4 puffs tid-qid |
| **Leukotriene Modifiers** | | |
| Montelukast | 5 mg chewable tablet, 10 mg tablet | 10 mg qhs |
| Zafirlukast | 10 or 20 mg tablet | 40 mg daily (20 mg tablet bid) |
| Zileuton | 300 or 600 mg tablet | 2,400 mg daily (give tablets qid) |
| **Methylxanthines** (Serum monitoring is important, serum concentration of 5–15 mcg/mL at steady state) | | |
| Theophylline | Liquids, sustained-release tablets, and capsules | Starting dose 10 mg/kg/day up to 300 mg max; usual max 800 mg/day |

DPI, dry powder inhaler; MDI, metered-dose inhaler.

Expert Panel Report (2003). *Guidelines for the diagnosis and management of asthma: Update on selected topics 2002.* NIH Publication No 02-5074. Bethesda, MD: National Institutes of Health, National Heart, Lung and Blood Institute.

when used over the long term. The route of choice for administration of these medications is an MDI or other type of inhaler, because it allows for topical administration. Critical to the success of inhaled therapy is the proper use of the MDI (see Chart 24-4). If patients have difficulty with this procedure, a spacer device may be used. Management of asthma involves a stepwise approach (see Table 24-3) (Expert Panel Report, 2003).

**LONG-ACTING CONTROL MEDICATIONS.** Corticosteroids are the most potent and effective anti-inflammatory medications currently available. They are broadly effective in alleviating symptoms, improving airway function, and decreasing peak flow variability. Initially, an inhaled form is used. A spacer should be used with inhaled corticosteroids, and the patient should rinse his or her mouth after administration to prevent thrush, a common complication associated with use of inhaled corticosteroids. A systemic preparation may be used to gain rapid control of the disease; to manage severe, persistent asthma; to treat moderate to severe exacerbations; to accelerate recovery; and to prevent recurrence. Cromolyn sodium (Intal) and nedocromil (Tilade) are mild to moderate anti-inflammatory agents that are used more commonly in children. They also are effective on a prophylactic basis to prevent exercise-induced asthma or in unavoidable exposure to known triggers. These medications are contraindicated in acute asthma exacerbations.

Long-acting beta$_2$-adrenergic agonists are used with anti-inflammatory medications to control asthma symptoms, particularly those that occur during the night. These agents are also effective in the prevention of exercise-induced asthma. Long-acting beta$_2$-adrenergic agonists are not indicated for immediate relief of symptoms. Theophylline (Slo-bid, Theo-24, Theo-Dur) is a mild to moderate bronchodilator that is usually used in addition to inhaled corticosteroids, mainly for relief of nighttime asthma symptoms.

Leukotriene modifiers (inhibitors), or antileukotrienes, are a new class of medications that include montelukast (Singulair), zafirlukast (Accolate), and zileuton (Zyflo). Leukotrienes, which are synthesized from membrane phospholipids through a cascade of enzymes, are potent bronchoconstrictors that also dilate blood vessels and alter permeability. Leukotriene inhibitors act either by interfering with leukotriene synthesis or by blocking the receptors where leukotrienes exert their action. They may provide an alternative to inhaled corticosteroids for mild persistent asthma, or they may be added to a regimen of inhaled corticosteroids in more severe asthma to attain further control.

**QUICK-RELIEF MEDICATIONS.** Short-acting beta$_2$-adrenergic agonists are the medications of choice for relief of acute symptoms and prevention of exercise-induced asthma (see Table 24-2). They have a rapid onset of action. Anticholinergics (eg, ipratropium bromide [Atrovent]) may have an added benefit in severe exacerbations of asthma, but they are used more frequently in COPD.

### Management of Exacerbations

Asthma exacerbations are best managed by early treatment and education, including the use of written action plans as part of any overall effort to educate patients about self-management techniques, especially those with moderate or severe persistent asthma and those with a history of severe exacerbations (Expert Panel Report, 2003). Quick-acting beta$_2$-adrenergic agonist medications are first used for prompt relief of airflow obstruction. Systemic corticosteroids may be necessary to decrease airway inflammation in patients who fail to respond to inhaled beta-adrenergic medications. In some patients, oxygen supplementation may be required to relieve hypoxemia associated with moderate to severe exacerbations (Expert Panel Report, 2003). In addition, response to treatment may be monitored by serial measurements of lung function.

Evidence from clinical trials suggests that antibiotic therapy, whether administered routinely or when suspicion of bacterial infection is low, is not beneficial for asthma exacerbations (Expert Panel Report, 2003). Antibiotics may be appropriate in the treatment of acute asthma exacerbations in patients with comorbid conditions (eg, fever and purulent sputum, evidence of pneumonia, suspected bacterial sinusitis).

Despite insufficient data supporting or refuting the benefits of using a written asthma action plan as compared to medical management alone, the 2003 Expert Panel Report continues to recommend the use of a written plan to educate patients about self-management (Fig. 24-7). Such a plan gives patients self-management strategies to combat exacerbations and provides instructions about early warning signs of worsening asthma. Patient self-management and early recognition of problems lead to more efficient communication with health care providers about asthma exacerbations (Expert Panel Report, 2003).

### Peak Flow Monitoring

Peak flow meters measure the highest airflow during a forced expiration (Fig. 24-8). Daily peak flow monitoring is recommended for all patients with moderate or severe asthma, because it helps measure asthma severity and, when added to symptom monitoring, indicates the current degree of asthma control. The patient is instructed in the proper technique (Chart 24-6), particularly about giving maximal effort, and peak flows are monitored for 2 or 3 weeks after receipt of optimal asthma therapy. Then the patient's "personal best" value is measured. The green (80% to 100% of personal best), yellow (60% to 80%), and red (less than 60%) zones are determined, and specific actions are delineated for each zone, enabling the patient to monitor and manipulate his or her own therapy after careful instruction (Expert Panel Report, 1997).

The 2003 Expert Panel Report recommends that peak flow monitoring should be considered as an adjunct to asthma management for patients with moderate to severe persistent asthma. Peak flow monitoring plans may enhance communication between the patient and health care providers and may increase the patient's awareness of disease status and control (Expert Panel Report, 2003).

## Nursing Management

The immediate nursing care of patients with asthma depends on the severity of symptoms. The patient may be treated successfully as an outpatient if asthma symptoms are relatively mild or may require hospitalization and intensive care if symptoms are acute and severe. The patient and family are often frightened and anxious because of the patient's dyspnea. Therefore, a calm approach is an important aspect of care. The nurse assesses the patient's respiratory status by monitoring the severity of symptoms, breath sounds, peak flow, pulse oximetry, and vital signs.

The nurse generally performs the following tasks:

- Obtains a history of allergic reactions to medications before administering medications.
- Identifies medications the patient is currently taking.
- Administers medications as prescribed and monitors the patient's responses to those medications. An antibiotic may be prescribed if the patient has an underlying respiratory infection.
- Administers fluids if the patient is dehydrated.

If the patient requires intubation because of acute respiratory failure, the nurse assists with the intubation procedure, continues close monitoring of the patient, and keeps the patient and family informed about procedures.

### Promoting Home and Community-Based Care

**TEACHING PATIENTS SELF-CARE.** A major challenge is to implement basic asthma management principles at the community level. Key issues include education of health care providers, establishment of programs for asthma education (for patients and providers), use of outpatient follow-up care for patients, and a focus on chronic management versus acute episodic care. Nurses are pivotal to achievement of these objectives.

Patient teaching is a critical component of care for patients with asthma. Multiple inhalers, different types of inhalers, antiallergy therapy, antireflux medications, and avoidance measures are essential for long-term control. This complex therapy requires a partnership between the patient and the health care providers to determine the desired outcomes and to formulate a plan to achieve those outcomes. The patient then carries out daily therapy as part of self-care management, with input and guidance by his or her health care providers. Before a partnership can be established, the patient must understand the following:

- The nature of asthma as a chronic inflammatory disease
- The definition of inflammation and bronchoconstriction
- The purpose and action of each medication
- Triggers to avoid, and how to do so
- Proper inhalation technique
- How to perform peak flow monitoring (see Chart 24-6)

# ASTHMA ACTION PLAN FOR _____ Date _____

Doctor's Name _____  
Doctor's Phone Number _____  
Hospital/Emergency Room Phone Number _____

## GREEN ZONE: Doing Well

- No cough, wheeze, chest tightness, or shortness of breath during the day or night
- Can do usual activities

And, if a peak flow meter is used,  
Peak flow: more than _____  
(80% or more of my best peak flow)

My best peak flow is: _____

**Take These Long-Term-Control Medicines Each Day** (include an anti-inflammatory)

| Medicine | How much to take | When to take it |
|---|---|---|
|  |  |  |
|  |  |  |
|  |  |  |
|  |  |  |

Before exercise ☐ 2 or ☐ 4 puffs  5 to 60 minutes before exercise

## YELLOW ZONE: Asthma Is Getting Worse

- Cough, wheeze, chest tightness, or shortness of breath, or
- Waking at night due to asthma, or
- Can do some, but not all, usual activities

-Or-

Peak flow: _____ to _____  
(50% - 80% of my best peak flow)

**FIRST** ➔ **Add: Quick-Relief Medicine – and keep taking your GREEN ZONE medicine**

☐ 2 or ☐ 4 puffs, every 20 minutes for up to 1 hour  
☐ Nebulizer, once  
_____ (short-acting beta₂-agonist)

**SECOND** ➔ **If your symptoms (and peak flow, if used) return to GREEN ZONE after 1 hour of above treatment:**

☐ Take the quick-relief medicine every 4 hours for 1 to 2 days.  
☐ Double the dose of your inhaled steroid for _____ (7-10) days.

-Or-

**If your symptoms (and peak flow, if used) do not return to GREEN ZONE after 1 hour of above treatment:**

☐ Take: _____  ☐ 2 or ☐ 4 puffs or ☐ Nebulizer  
(short-acting beta₂-agonist)

☐ Add: _____ mg. per day  For _____ (3-10) days  
(oral steroid)

☐ Call the doctor ☐ before/ ☐ within _____ hours after taking the oral steroid.

## RED ZONE: Medical Alert!

- Very short of breath, or
- Quick-relief medicines have not helped, or
- Cannot do usual activities, or
- Symptoms are same or get worse after 24 hours in Yellow Zone

-Or-

Peak flow: less than _____  
(50% of my best peak flow)

**Take this medicine:**

☐ _____  ☐ 4 or ☐ 6 puffs or ☐ Nebulizer  
(short-acting beta₂-agonist)

☐ _____  _____ mg.  
(oral steroid)

**Then call your doctor NOW.**  Go to the hospital or call for an ambulance if:
- You are still in the red zone after 15 minutes AND
- You have not reached your doctor.

## DANGER SIGNS

- Trouble walking and talking due to shortness of breath
- Lips or fingernails are blue

➔ ■ Take ☐ 4 or ☐ 6 puffs of your quick-relief medicine AND  
■ Go to the hospital or call for an ambulance (_____) NOW!

**FIGURE 24-7.** Asthma action plan. From *Facts about controlling asthma*, National Asthma Education and Prevention Program, National Heart, Lung, and Blood Institute. NIH Publication No. 97-2339. Bethesda, MD: National Institutes of Health.

**FIGURE 24-8.** Peak flow meters measure the highest volume of air flow during a forced expiration (*left*). Volume is measured in color-coded zones (*right*): the green zone signifies 80% to 100% of personal best; yellow, 60% to 80%; and red, less than 60%. If peak flow falls below the red zone, the patient should take the appropriate actions prescribed by his or her health care provider.

### CHART 24-6

## HOME CARE CHECKLIST • Use of Peak Flow Meter

| At the completion of the home care instruction, the patient or caregiver will be able to: | Patient | Caregiver |
|---|:---:|:---:|
| • Describe the rationale for using a peak flow meter in asthma management. | ✔ | ✔ |
| • Explain how peak flow monitoring is used along with symptoms to determine severity of asthma. | ✔ | ✔ |
| • Demonstrate steps for using the peak flow meter correctly: | ✔ | |
|   • Move the indicator to the bottom of the numbered scale. | ✔ | |
|   • Stand up. | ✔ | |
|   • Take a deep breath and fill the lungs completely. | ✔ | |
|   • Place mouthpiece in mouth and close lips around mouthpiece (do not put tongue inside opening). | ✔ | |
|   • Blow out hard and fast with a single blow. | ✔ | |
|   • Record the number achieved on the indicator. | ✔ | |
| • Repeat steps 1–5 two more times and write the highest number in the asthma diary. | ✔ | |
| • Explain how to determine the "personal best" peak flow reading. | ✔ | ✔ |
| • Describe the significance of the color zones for peak flow monitoring. | ✔ | ✔ |
| • Demonstrate how to clean the peak flow meter. | ✔ | ✔ |
| • Discuss how and when to contact the health care provider about changes or decreases in peak flow values. | ✔ | ✔ |

- How to implement an action plan
- When to seek assistance, and how to do so

An assortment of excellent educational materials is available from the NHLBI and other sources. The nurse should obtain current educational materials for the patient based on the patient's diagnosis, causative factors, educational level, and cultural background. If a patient has a coexisting sensory impairment (ie, vision loss or hearing impairment), materials should be provided in an alternative format.

**CONTINUING CARE.** Nurses who have contact with patients in the hospital, clinic, school, or office use the opportunity to assess the patient's respiratory status and ability to manage self-care to prevent serious exacerbations. Nurses emphasize adherence to the prescribed therapy, preventive measures, and the need to keep follow-up appointments with health care providers. Home visits to assess the home environment for allergens may be indicated for patients with recurrent exacerbations. Nurses refer patients to community support groups. In addition, nurses remind patients and families about the importance of health promotion strategies and recommended health screening.

## Status Asthmaticus

Status asthmaticus is severe and persistent asthma that does not respond to conventional therapy. The attacks can occur with little or no warning and can progress rapidly to asphyxiation. Infection, anxiety, nebulizer abuse, dehydration, increased adrenergic blockage, and nonspecific irritants may contribute to these episodes. An acute episode may be precipitated by hypersensitivity to aspirin.

### Pathophysiology

The basic characteristics of asthma (inflammation of bronchial mucosa, constriction of the bronchiolar smooth muscle, and thickened secretions) decrease the diameter of the bronchi and occur in status asthmaticus. The most common scenario is severe bronchospasm, with mucus plugging leading to asphyxia. A ventilation–perfusion abnormality results in hypoxemia and respiratory alkalosis initially, followed by respiratory acidosis. There is a reduced $PaO_2$ and initial respiratory alkalosis, with a decreased $PaCO_2$ and an increased pH. As status asthmaticus worsens, the $PaCO_2$ increases and the pH decreases, reflecting respiratory acidosis.

### Clinical Manifestations

The clinical manifestations are the same as those seen in severe asthma; signs and symptoms include labored breathing, prolonged exhalation, engorged neck veins, and wheezing. However, the extent of wheezing does not indicate the severity of the attack. As the obstruction worsens, the wheezing may disappear; this is frequently a sign of impending respiratory failure.

### Assessment and Diagnostic Findings

Pulmonary function studies are the most accurate means of assessing acute airway obstruction. Arterial blood gas measurements are obtained if the patient cannot perform pulmonary function maneuvers because of severe obstruction or fatigue, or if the patient does not respond to treatment. Respiratory alkalosis (low $PaCO_2$) is the most common finding in patients with asthma. An increasing $PaCO_2$ (to normal levels or levels indicating respiratory acidosis) frequently is a danger sign indicating impending respiratory failure.

### Medical Management

Close monitoring of the patient and objective reevaluation for response to therapy are key in status asthmaticus. In the emergency setting, the patient is treated initially with a short-acting beta$_2$-adrenergic agonist and subsequently a short course of systemic corticosteroids, especially if the patient does not respond to the short-acting beta$_2$-adrenergic agonist. Corticosteroids are critical in the therapy of status asthmaticus and are used to decrease the intense airway inflammation and swelling. Short-acting inhaled beta$_2$-adrenergic agonists provide the most rapid relief from bronchospasm. An MDI with or without a spacer may be used for nebulization of the drugs. The patient usually requires supplemental oxygen and IV fluids for hydration. Oxygen therapy is initiated to treat dyspnea, central cyanosis, and hypoxemia. High-flow supplemental oxygen is best delivered using a partial or complete non-rebreather mask with the objective of maintaining the $PaO_2$ at a minimum of 92 mm Hg or $O_2$ saturation greater than 95% (Higgins, 2003). Sedative medications are contraindicated. Magnesium sulfate, a calcium antagonist, may be administered to induce smooth muscle relaxation. In trials, magnesium sulfate has improved symptoms of patients with severe asthma who did not respond to other treatments. Magnesium may be beneficial in patients who are prone to hypomagnesemia because of prolonged use of inhaled beta$_2$-adrenergic agonists (Higgins, 2003). In addition, magnesium can relax smooth muscle and hence cause bronchodilation by competing with calcium at calcium-mediated smooth muscle binding sites. Adverse effects of magnesium sulfate may include facial warmth, flushing, tingling, nausea, central nervous system depression, respiratory depression, and hypotension.

If there is no response to repeated treatments, hospitalization is required. Other criteria for hospitalization include poor pulmonary function test results and deteriorating blood gas levels (respiratory acidosis), which may indicate that the patient is tiring and will require mechanical ventilation. Most patients do not need mechanical ventilation, but it is used for patients in respiratory failure, for those who tire and are too fatigued by the attempt to breathe, and for those whose conditions do not respond to initial treatment.

Death from asthma is associated with several risk factors, including the following (Expert Panel Report, 1997):

- Past history of sudden and severe exacerbations
- Prior endotracheal intubation for asthma
- Prior admission to the intensive care unit for an asthma exacerbation
- Two or more hospitalizations for asthma within the past year
- Three or more emergency care visits for asthma in the past year
- Excessive use of short-acting beta-adrenergic inhalers (more than two canisters per month)

- Recent withdrawal from systemic corticosteroids
- Comorbidity of cardiovascular disease or COPD
- Psychiatric disease
- Low socioeconomic status
- Urban residence

## Nursing Management

The main focus of nursing management is to actively assess the airway and the patient's response to treatment. The nurse should be prepared for the next intervention if the patient does not respond to treatment.

The nurse constantly monitors the patient for the first 12 to 24 hours, or until status asthmaticus is under control. The nurse also assesses the patient's skin turgor for signs of dehydration. Fluid intake is essential to combat dehydration, to loosen secretions, and to facilitate expectoration. Nurses administer IV fluids as prescribed, up to 3 to 4 L/day, unless contraindicated. Blood pressure and cardiac rhythm should be monitored continuously during the acute phase and until the patient stabilizes and responds to therapy. The patient's energy needs to be conserved, and his or her room should be quiet and free of respiratory irritants, including flowers, tobacco smoke, perfumes, or odors of cleaning agents. Nonallergenic pillows should be used.

# Cystic Fibrosis

Cystic fibrosis (CF) is the most common fatal autosomal recessive disease among the Caucasian population. A person must inherit a defective copy of the CF gene (one from each parent) to have CF. One in 31 Americans are unknowing carriers of this gene, and approximately 30,000 children and adults in the United States have CF (Cystic Fibrosis Foundation, 2004).

The frequency of CF is 1 in 1900 to 1 in 3700 live births among Caucasian Americans (Aronson & Marquis, 2004). CF is less frequently found among Hispanic, Asian, and African Americans. Although CF was once considered a fatal childhood disease, approximately 37% of people living with the disease are 18 years of age or older. Researchers have documented survival past age 76 years (Aronson & Marquis, 2004).

This multisystem genetic disease is usually diagnosed in infancy or early childhood but may be diagnosed later in life. Respiratory symptoms are frequently the major manifestation of CF when it is diagnosed later in life.

## Pathophysiology

CF is caused by mutations in the CF transmembrane conductance regulator protein, which is a chloride channel found in all exocrine tissues. Chloride transport problems lead to thick, viscous secretions in the lungs, pancreas, liver, intestine, and reproductive tract as well as increased salt content in sweat gland secretions. The CF gene was discovered in 1989 and mapped to a single locus on the long arm of chromosome 7. More than 1000 mutations have been identified on the CF transmembrane conductance regulator gene, thus creating multiple variations in presentation and progression of the disease (Aronson & Marquis, 2004).

The ability to detect the common mutations of this gene allows for routine screening for CF and the detection of carriers of the disease. Genetics counseling is an important part of health care for couples at risk. People who are heterozygous for CF (ie, having one defective gene and one normal gene) do not have the disease but can be carriers and pass the defective gene on to their children. If both parents are carriers, their risk of having a child with CF is 1 in 4 (25%) with each pregnancy. Genetics testing should be offered to adults with a positive family history of CF and to partners of people with CF who are planning a pregnancy or seeking prenatal counseling. Currently, genetics testing for CF is not recommended for the general population.

## Clinical Manifestations

The pulmonary manifestations of CF include a productive cough, wheezing, hyperinflation of the lung fields on chest x-ray, and pulmonary function test results consistent with obstructive disease of the airways. Chronic respiratory inflammation and infection are caused by impaired mucus clearance. Colonization of the airways with pathogenic bacteria usually occurs early in life. *Staphylococcus aureus* and *H. influenzae* are common organisms during early childhood. As the disease progresses, *Pseudomonas aeruginosa* is ultimately isolated from the sputum of most patients. Upper respiratory manifestations of the disease include sinusitis and nasal polyps.

Nonpulmonary clinical manifestations include gastrointestinal problems (eg, pancreatic insufficiency, recurrent abdominal pain, biliary cirrhosis, vitamin deficiencies, recurrent pancreatitis, weight loss), CF-related diabetes, genitourinary problems (male and female infertility), and clubbing of the digits (fingers and toes). (See Chapter 40 for a discussion of pancreatitis.)

## Assessment and Diagnostic Findings

The diagnosis of CF is suspected in patients with typical clinical features of CF, once other diseases have been excluded. Diagnosis is based on an elevated sweat chloride concentration, together with clinical signs and symptoms consistent with the disease. Repeated sweat chloride values of greater than 60 mEq/L distinguish most people with CF from those with other obstructive diseases. The only acceptable procedure for sweat testing is the quantitative pilocarpine iontophoresis sweat test. It should be performed in a laboratory that frequently does this test. A molecular diagnosis or genetics evaluation may also be used in evaluating common genetic mutations of the CF gene.

## Medical Management

Pulmonary problems remain the leading cause of morbidity and mortality in CF and account for death in more than 95% of patients (Aronson & Marquis, 2004). A variety of management techniques are necessary.

Because chronic bacterial infection of the airways occurs in CF, control of infections is essential to treatment. Antibiotic medications are routinely prescribed for acute pulmonary exacerbations of the disease. Depending on the severity of the exacerbation, aerosolized, oral, or IV antibiotic therapy may be used. Antibiotic agents are selected based on the results of a sputum culture and sensitivity. Patients with CF may be infected with bacteria that are resistant to multiple antibiotics and require multiple courses of antibiotic agents over long periods.

Bronchodilators, including beta$_2$-adrenergic agonists and anticholinergics, are frequently administered to treat airway hyperactivity and to reverse bronchospasm.

Airway clearance is a key intervention in the care of patients with CF, and various pulmonary techniques are used to enhance secretion clearance. Examples include manual postural drainage and chest physical therapy, high-frequency chest wall oscillation, autogenic drainage (a combination of breathing techniques at different lung volume levels to move the secretions to where they can be "huff"-coughed out), and other devices that assist in airway clearance, such as masks that generate positive expiratory pressure (PEP masks) and "flutter devices" (devices that provide an oscillatory expiratory pressure pattern with positive expiratory pressure and assist with expectoration of secretions). Inhaled mucolytic agents such as dornase alfa (Pulmozyme) or N-acetylcysteine (Mucomyst) may also be used. These agents help decrease the viscosity of the sputum and promote expectoration of secretions.

To decrease the inflammation and ongoing destruction of the airways, anti-inflammatory agents, including inhaled corticosteroids or systemic therapy, may also be used. Corticosteroids are used in late-stage disease and during severe respiratory exacerbations. Their routine use is not recommended because of unacceptable short-term and long-term side effects (Aronson & Marquis, 2004). Other anti-inflammatory medications have also been studied in CF. Ibuprofen has been studied in younger patients, and some benefit has been demonstrated in reducing the rate of deterioration of pulmonary function in specific groups of patients; however, it is not routinely used to treat CF.

Supplemental oxygen is used to treat the progressive hypoxemia that occurs with CF. It helps correct the hypoxemia and may minimize the complications seen with chronic hypoxemia (pulmonary hypertension).

Lung transplantation is an option for a small, selected population of patients with CF. A double-lung transplantation technique is used because of chronic infection of both lungs in end-stage CF. Because there is a long waiting list for lung transplants, many patients die while waiting for suitable lungs for transplantation.

Gene therapy is a promising approach to management, and clinical trials are underway. It is hoped that techniques will be developed to carry healthy genes to the damaged cells and correct defective CF cells. Efforts are underway to develop innovative methods of delivering therapy to the CF cells of the airways. In addition, clinical trials are focusing on chloride channel therapies and anti-inflammatory therapies for CF (Cystic Fibrosis Foundation, 2004).

## Nursing Management

Nursing is crucial to the interdisciplinary approach required for care of adults with CF. Nursing care includes helping patients manage pulmonary symptoms and prevent complications of CF. Specific nursing measures include strategies that promote removal of pulmonary secretions; chest physiotherapy (including postural drainage, chest percussion, and vibration); and breathing exercises, which are implemented and are taught to the patient and family when the patient is very young. The patient is reminded of the need to reduce risk factors associated with respiratory infections (eg, exposure to crowds or to persons with known infections). In addition, the patient is taught the early signs and symptoms of respiratory infection and disease progression that indicate the need to notify a primary health care provider.

Nurses emphasize the importance of an adequate fluid and dietary intake to promote removal of secretions and to ensure an adequate nutritional status. Because CF is a lifelong disorder, patients often have learned to modify their daily activities to accommodate their symptoms and treatment modalities. However, as the disease progresses, assessment of the home environment may be warranted to identify modifications required to address changes in the patient's needs, increasing dyspnea and fatigue, and non-pulmonary symptoms.

Although gene therapy and double-lung transplantation are promising therapies for CF, they are limited in availability and are largely experimental. As a result, the overall life expectancy of adults with CF is shortened. Despite this, pregnancy is possible in patients with CF. Preconception counseling and evaluation are needed because of high risks associated with pregnancy. Very frequent monitoring is needed throughout pregnancy and delivery in women with CF. End-of-life issues and concerns need to be addressed with the patient when warranted. For the patient whose disease is progressing and who is developing increasing hypoxemia, preferences for end-of-life care should be discussed, documented, and honored (see Chapter 17). Patients and family members require support as they face a shortened life span and an uncertain future.

## Critical Thinking Exercises

1. A 74-year-old man with end-stage COPD has been admitted with impending respiratory failure. He is extremely anxious and short of breath and shows signs of central cyanosis. He is unable to lie flat in bed and is on supplemental oxygen at 2 L/min. What tests or examinations might be appropriate to assess the severity of the patient's respiratory failure and his oxygenation status? What comfort measures would you institute for this patient?

2. **ebp** A 69-year-old farmer with COPD reports that he has been using continuous oxygen for the past 5 years. He reports increasing shortness of breath and asks you to increase his oxygen flow. How do you respond to his request? What is the evidence base for your response? How do you evaluate the strength of the evidence?

3. As a nurse in an outpatient asthma clinic in a tertiary care medical center, you see a 35-year-old Mexican-American mother with asthma. When you inquire about symptom

management and medication history, she provides minimal information and reports that she does not take any medication on a regular basis but has an MDI. In her medical record, you note that use of an MDI on a regular daily schedule has been repeatedly prescribed for her, but she reports that she does not use it except as needed when she is extremely short of breath. Describe the assessment method you would use to evaluate her asthma symptoms and severity. Describe teaching techniques you might use to assess the patient's knowledge of her medications and provide education about the action of the MDI, frequency of use, and correct administration of medication. What methods would you use to monitor use of the MDI and reinforce education about its use?

4 As a nurse in your hospital's community outreach clinic, you are responsible for providing group education and counseling to patients with newly diagnosed asthma. What areas would you address regarding triggers for asthma? How might you have patients assess or change their home and work environments? What resources might you suggest?

5 A 35-year-old woman with CF is admitted to your unit from the emergency room. Her husband accompanies her and states that this is the first time she has been admitted to the hospital for her disease. She cannot lie flat in bed, is extremely short of breath, and is having paroxysms of coughing. The cough is productive of thick, yellow sputum. What is the pathophysiology associated with these findings? What medical and nursing interventions might be used to decrease or alleviate these signs and symptoms? What members of the health care team would you consult to be involved in her care and why?

## REFERENCES AND SELECTED READINGS

### BOOKS

American Lung Association. (2004). *Chronic obstructive pulmonary disease fact sheet.* New York: Author.

Brown, E. S. (Ed.). (2003). *Asthma: Social and psychological factors and psychosomatic syndromes.* New York: Karger.

Cazzola, M. (2004). *Therapeutic strategies in COPD.* London: Taylor & Francis.

Expert Panel Report. (1997). *Guidelines for the diagnosis and management of asthma.* Bethesda, MD: National Asthma Education and Prevention Program, National Institutes of Health.

Expert Panel Report. (2003). *Guidelines for the diagnosis and management of asthma-update on selected topics 2002.* NIH Publication No. 02-5074. Bethesda, MD: National Institutes of Health, National Heart, Lung and Blood Institute.

Global Initiative for Asthma Management and Prevention. (2004). *National Heart, Lung and Blood Institute NHLBI/World Health Organization WHO workshop report, 2004.* NIH Publication No. 02-3659. Bethesda, MD: National Institutes of Health.

Global Initiative for Asthma Management and Prevention. (2001). *Inhaler Charts for Use with GINA Documents.* National Heart, Lung and Blood Institute NHLBI/World Health Organization. Geneva: WHO.

Global Initiative for Chronic Obstructive Lung Disease (GOLD), World Health Organization (WHO) & National Heart, Lung and Blood Institute (NHLBI). (2004). *Global strategy for the diagnosis, management, and prevention of chronic obstructive pulmonary disease.* Bethesda, MD: National Heart, Lung and Blood Institute.

Hansel, T. T. & Barnes, P. (2004). *An atlas of chronic obstructive pulmonary disease: COPD. A resource for reference, teaching and lecturing.* London: Taylor & Francis.

Institute for Clinical Systems Improvement (ICSI). (2003). *Chronic obstructive pulmonary disease.* Bloomington, MN: Author.

National Heart, Lung and Blood Institute & World Health Organization. (2004). *NHLBI/WHO Workshop Report: Global initiative for asthma management and prevention.* NIH Publication No. 02-3659. Bethesda, MD: National Heart, Lung and Blood Institute.

National Institutes of Health. (2001). *Global initiative for chronic obstructive lung disease: Global strategy for the diagnosis, management, and prevention of chronic obstructive pulmonary disease.* NIH Publication No. 2701B. Washington, DC: U.S. Department of Health and Human Services.

Petty, T. L. (2003). *Coping with COPD: Understanding, treating, and living with chronic obstructive pulmonary disease.* New York: St. Martin's Press.

Reid, W. D. (2004). *Clinical management notes and case histories in cardiopulmonary physical therapy.* Thorofare, NJ: Slack.

Ruppel, G. (2003). *Manual of pulmonary function testing.* St. Louis: Mosby.

### JOURNALS

*Asterisks indicate nursing research articles.

#### General

ACCP/AACVPR Pulmonary Rehabilitation Guidelines Panel. (1997). Pulmonary rehabilitation: Joint ACCP/AACVPR evidence-based guidelines. *Chest, 112*(5), 1363–1396.

American Thoracic Society. (1999). Statement on pulmonary rehabilitation. *American Journal of Respiratory and Critical Care Medicine, 159*(5), 1666–1682.

#### Asthma

Adams, R. J., Wilson, D. H., Taylor, A. W., et al. (2004). Psychological factors and asthma quality of life: A population based study. *Thorax, 59*(11), 930–935.

American Thoracic Society. (2004). Guidelines for assessing and managing asthma risk at work, school, and recreation. *American Journal of Respiratory and Critical Care Medicine, 169*(7), 873–881.

Bender, B. G. & Bender S. E. (2005). Patient-identified barriers to asthma treatment adherence: Responses to interviews, focus groups, and questionnaires. *Immunology and Allergy Clinics of North America, 25*(1), 107–130.

Centers for Disease Control and Prevention. (2004). *Fast stats sheet: Asthma.* Atlanta: National Center for Health Statistics.

Gelb, A. F., Schein, A., Nussbaum, E., et al. (2004). Risk factors for near-fatal asthma. *Chest, 126*(4), 1138–1146.

Higgins, J. C. (2003). The "crashing asthmatic." *American Family Physician, 67*(5), 997–1004.

Sin, D. D., Man, J., Sharpe, H., et al. (2004). Pharmacological management to reduce exacerbations in adults with asthma: A systematic review and meta-analysis. *Journal of the American Medical Association, 293*(2), 367–376.

#### Chronic Obstructive Pulmonary Disease

American Lung Association. (2005). Alpha-1 related emphysema. Available at: http://www.lungusa.org. Accessed June 17, 2006.

American Thoracic Society & European Respiratory Society. (2004). *ATS and ERS standards for the diagnosis and management of patients with COPD.* Available at: www.thoracic.org. Accessed April 20, 2006.

Andenaes, R., Kalfoss, M. H. & Wahl, A. (2004). Psychological distress and quality of life in hospitalized patients with chronic obstructive pulmonary disease. *Journal of Advance Nursing, 46*(5), 522–530.

Arias, E., Anderson, R. N., Hsiang-Ching, K., et al. (2003). Deaths: Final data for 2001. *National Vital Statistics Reports, 52*(3), 1–116.

Blackler, L., Mooney, C. & Jones, C. (2004). Palliative care in the management of chronic obstructive pulmonary disease. *British Journal of Nursing, 13*(9), 518–521.

Brenner, M., Hanna, N. M., Mina-Araghi, R., et al. (2004). Innovative approaches to lung volume reduction for emphysema. *Chest, 126*(1), 238–248.

Centers for Disease Control and Prevention. (2004). *Smoking fact sheets.* Atlanta: Office on Smoking and Heath.

Covey, M. K. & Larson, J. L. (2004). Exercise and COPD. *American Journal of Nursing, 104*(5), 40–43.

Curtis, J., Wenrich, M., Carline, J., et al. (2002). Patients' perspectives on physician skill in end-of-life care. Differences between patients with COPD, cancer and AIDS. *Chest, 122*(1), 356–362.

*Meek, P. M. & Lareau, S. C. (2003). Critical outcomes in pulmonary rehabilitation: Assessment and evaluation of dyspnea and fatigue. *Journal of Rehabilitation Research and Development, 50*(5), 13–24.

National Emphysema Treatment Trial Research Group. (2003). A randomized trial comparing lung-volume reduction surgery with medical therapy for severe emphysema. *New England Journal of Medicine, 348*(21), 2059–2073.

Simmons, P. & Simmons, M. (2004). Informed nursing practice: The administration of oxygen to patients with COPD. *MedSurg Nursing, 13*(2), 82–85.

Sin, D., McAlister, F., Man, S. F. P., et al. (2003). Contemporary management of chronic obstructive pulmonary disease: Scientific review. *Journal of the American Medical Association, 290*(7), 2301–2312.

Sutherland, R. E. & Cherniack, R. M. (2004). Management of chronic obstructive pulmonary disease. *New England Journal of Medicine, 350*(26), 2689–2697.

Theander, K. & Unosson, M. (2004). Fatigue in patients with chronic obstructive pulmonary disease. *Journal of Advanced Nursing, 45*(2), 172–177.

## Cystic Fibrosis

Aronson, B. S. & Marquis, M. (2004). Care of the adult with cystic fibrosis. *MedSurg Nursing, 13*(3), 143–154

Cystic Fibrosis Adult Care: Consensus Committee Report. (2004). *Chest, 125*(1 Suppl.), 1S–39S.

Cystic Fibrosis Foundation. (2004). What is cystic fibrosis? Available at: http://www.cff.org/about_cystic_fibrosis. Accessed June 16, 2006.

## RESOURCES

Agency for Healthcare Research and Quality, John M. Eisenberg Bldg, 540 Gaither Road, Rockville, MD 20850; 1-301-427-1364; http://www.ahrq.gov or www.ahcpr.gov. Accessed April 20, 2006.

Alpha-1 Association, 275 West Street, Suite 210, Annapolis, MD 21401; 1-800-521-3025; http://www.alpha1.org. Accessed April 20, 2006.

American Academy of Allergy, Asthma, and Immunology, 611 E. Wells St. Suite 1100, Milwaukee, WI 53202; 414-272-6071; http://www.aaaai.org. Accessed April 20, 2006.

American Association of Cardiovascular and Pulmonary Rehabilitation, 401 North Michigan Ave, Suite 2200, Chicago, IL 60611; 312-321-5146; http://www.aacvpr.org. Accessed April 20, 2006.

American Association for Respiratory Care, 9425 N. MacArthur Blvd., Suite 100, Irving, TX 75063; 1-972-243-2272; http://www.aarc.org. Accessed April 20, 2006.

American College of Chest Physicians, 3300 Dundee Road, Northbrook, IL 60062; 1-847-498-1400; http://www.chestnet.org. Accessed April 20, 2006.

American Lung Association, 61 Broadway 6th Floor, New York, NY 10006; 1-800-LUNGUSA; http://www.lungusa.org. Accessed April 20, 2006.

American Thoracic Society, 61 Broadway, New York, NY 10006; 1-212-315-8600; http://www.thoracic.org. Accessed June 17, 2006.

Centers for Disease Control and Prevention, 1600 Clifton Road, NE, Atlanta, GA 30333; 1-800-311-3435; http://www.cdc.gov. Accessed June 17, 2006.

Cystic Fibrosis Foundation, 6931 Arlington Road, Bethesda, MD 20814; 310-951-4422 or 800-FIGHT-CF; http://www.cff.org. Accessed April 20, 2006.

National Heart, Lung and Blood Institute, National Institutes of Health, Bldg. 31, 31 Center Drive MSC, Bethesda, MD 20892; 1-301-592-8573; http://www.nhlbi.nih.gov. Accessed April 20, 2006.

Respiratory Nursing Society, c/o NYSNA, 11 Cornell Road, Latham, NY 12110; 1-518-782-9400 × 286; http://www.respiratorynursingsociety.org. Accessed April 20, 2006.

U.S. Department of Health and Human Services, Department of Health and Human Services, 200 Independence Avenue, S.W., Washington DC 20201; 202-619-0257; http://www.hhs.gov or http://www.healthfinder.gov. Accessed April 20, 2006.

# CHAPTER 25

# Respiratory Care Modalities

## Learning Objectives

*On completion of this chapter, the learner will be able to:*

1. Describe the nursing management for patients receiving oxygen therapy, intermittent positive-pressure breathing, mini-nebulizer therapy, incentive spirometry, chest physiotherapy, and breathing retraining.
2. Describe the patient education and home care considerations for patients receiving oxygen therapy.
3. Describe the nursing care for a patient with an endotracheal tube and for a patient with a tracheostomy.
4. Demonstrate the procedure of tracheal suctioning.
5. Use the nursing process as a framework for care of patients who are mechanically ventilated.
6. Describe the process of weaning the patient from mechanical ventilation.
7. Describe the significance of preoperative nursing assessment and patient teaching for the patient who is to have thoracic surgery.
8. Explain the principles of chest drainage and the nursing responsibilities related to the care of the patient with a chest drainage system.
9. Describe the patient education and home care considerations for patients who have had thoracic surgery.

Numerous treatment modalities are used when caring for patients with various respiratory conditions. The choice of modality is based on the oxygenation disorder and whether there is a problem with gas ventilation, diffusion, or both. Therapies range from simple and noninvasive (oxygen and nebulizer therapy, chest physiotherapy, breathing retraining) to complex and highly invasive treatments (intubation, mechanical ventilation, surgery). Assessment and management of the patient with respiratory disorders are best accomplished when the approach is multidisciplinary and collaborative.

# Noninvasive Respiratory Therapies

Noninvasive respiratory therapies include oxygen therapy, incentive spirometry, mini-nebulizer therapy, intermittent positive-pressure breathing, and chest physiotherapy.

# Oxygen Therapy

Oxygen therapy is the administration of oxygen at a concentration greater than that found in the environmental atmosphere. At sea level, the concentration of oxygen in room air is 21%. The goal of oxygen therapy is to provide adequate transport of oxygen in the blood while decreasing the work of breathing and reducing stress on the myocardium.

Oxygen transport to the tissues depends on factors such as cardiac output, arterial oxygen content, concentration of hemoglobin, and metabolic requirements. These factors must be kept in mind when oxygen therapy is considered. (Respiratory physiology and oxygen transport are discussed in Chapter 21.)

## Glossary

**airway pressure release ventilation (APRV):** mode of mechanical ventilation that allows unrestricted, spontaneous breaths throughout the ventilatory cycle; produces tidal ventilation by release of airway pressure from an elevated baseline airway pressure to simulate expiration

**assist–control ventilation:** mode of mechanical ventilation in which the patient's breathing pattern may trigger the ventilator to deliver a preset tidal volume; in the absence of spontaneous breathing, the machine delivers a controlled breath at a preset minimum rate and tidal volume

**chest drainage system:** use of a chest tube and closed drainage system to reexpand the lung and to remove excess air, fluid, and blood

**chest percussion:** manually cupping over the chest wall to mobilize secretions by mechanically dislodging viscous or adherent secretions in the lungs

**chest physiotherapy (CPT):** therapy used to remove bronchial secretions, improve ventilation, and increase the efficiency of the respiratory muscles. Types include postural drainage, chest percussion, and vibration.

**continuous positive airway pressure (CPAP):** positive pressure applied throughout the respiratory cycle to a spontaneously breathing patient to promote alveolar and airway stability; may be administered with endotracheal or tracheostomy tube, or by mask

**controlled ventilation:** mode of mechanical ventilation in which the ventilator completely controls the patient's ventilation according to preset tidal volumes and respiratory rate. Because of problems with synchrony, it is rarely used except in paralyzed or anesthetized patients.

**endotracheal intubation:** insertion of a breathing tube through the nose or mouth into the trachea

**fraction of inspired oxygen (FiO$_2$):** concentration of oxygen delivered (1.0 = 100% oxygen)

**hypoxemia:** decrease in arterial oxygen tension in the blood

**hypoxia:** decrease in oxygen supply to the tissues and cells

**incentive spirometry:** method of deep breathing that provides visual feedback to help the patient inhale deeply and slowly and achieve maximum lung inflation

**intermittent mandatory ventilation (IMV):** mode of mechanical ventilation that provides a combination of mechanically assisted breaths and spontaneous breaths

**mechanical ventilator:** a positive- or negative-pressure breathing device that supports ventilation and oxygenation

**pneumothorax:** partial or complete collapse of the lung due to positive pressure in the pleural space

**positive end-expiratory pressure (PEEP):** positive pressure maintained by the ventilator at the end of exhalation (instead of a normal zero pressure) to increase functional residual capacity and open collapsed alveoli; improves oxygenation with lower FiO$_2$

**postural drainage:** positioning the patient to allow drainage from all the lobes of the lungs and airways

**pressure support ventilation (PSV):** mode of mechanical ventilation in which preset positive pressure is delivered with spontaneous breaths to decrease work of breathing

**proportional assist ventilation (PAV):** mode of mechanical ventilation that provides partial ventilatory support in proportion to the patient's inspiratory efforts; decreases the work of breathing

**respiratory weaning:** process of gradual, systematic withdrawal and/or removal of ventilator, breathing tube, and oxygen

**synchronized intermittent mandatory ventilation (SIMV):** mode of mechanical ventilation in which the ventilator allows the patient to breathe spontaneously while providing a preset number of breaths to ensure adequate ventilation; ventilated breaths are synchronized with spontaneous breathing

**thoracotomy:** surgical opening into the chest cavity

**tracheotomy:** surgical opening into the trachea

**tracheostomy tube:** indwelling tube inserted directly into the trachea to assist with ventilation

**vibration:** a type of massage administered by quickly tapping the chest with the fingertips or alternating the fingers in a rhythmic manner, or by using a mechanical device to assist in mobilizing lung secretions

## Indications

A change in the patient's respiratory rate or pattern may be one of the earliest indicators of the need for oxygen therapy. The change in respiratory rate or pattern may result from hypoxemia or hypoxia. **Hypoxemia** (a decrease in the arterial oxygen tension in the blood) is manifested by changes in mental status (progressing through impaired judgment, agitation, disorientation, confusion, lethargy, and coma), dyspnea, increase in blood pressure, changes in heart rate, dysrhythmias, central cyanosis (late sign), diaphoresis, and cool extremities. Hypoxemia usually leads to **hypoxia**, which is a decrease in oxygen supply to the tissues. Hypoxia, if severe enough, can be life-threatening.

The signs and symptoms signaling the need for oxygen may depend on how suddenly this need develops. With rapidly developing hypoxia, changes occur in the central nervous system because the higher neurologic centers are very sensitive to oxygen deprivation. The clinical picture may resemble that of alcohol intoxication, with the patient exhibiting lack of coordination and impaired judgment. Longstanding hypoxia (as seen in chronic obstructive pulmonary disease [COPD] and chronic heart failure) may produce fatigue, drowsiness, apathy, inattentiveness, and delayed reaction time. The need for oxygen is assessed by arterial blood gas analysis and pulse oximetry as well as by clinical evaluation. More information about hypoxia is presented in Chart 25-1.

## Complications

As with other medications, the nurse administers oxygen with caution and carefully assesses its effects on each patient. Oxygen is a medication, and except in emergency situations it is administered only when prescribed by a physician.

In general, patients with respiratory conditions are given oxygen therapy only to increase the arterial oxygen pressure ($PaO_2$) back to the patient's normal baseline, which may vary from 60 to 95 mm Hg. In terms of the oxyhemoglobin dissociation curve (see Chapter 21), the blood at these levels is 80% to 98% saturated with oxygen; higher **fraction of inspired oxygen** (**$FiO_2$**) flow values add no further significant amounts of oxygen to the red blood cells or plasma. Instead of helping, increased amounts of oxygen may produce toxic effects on the lungs and central nervous system or may depress ventilation (see later discussion).

It is important to observe for subtle indicators of inadequate oxygenation when oxygen is administered by any method. Therefore, the nurse assesses the patient frequently for confusion, restlessness progressing to lethargy, diaphoresis, pallor, tachycardia, tachypnea, and hypertension. Intermittent or continuous pulse oximetry is used to monitor oxygen levels.

### Oxygen Toxicity

Oxygen toxicity may occur when too high a concentration of oxygen (greater than 50%) is administered for an extended period (longer than 48 hours). It is caused by overproduction of oxygen free radicals, which are byproducts of cell metabolism. If oxygen toxicity is untreated, these radicals can severely damage or kill cells. Antioxidants such as vitamin E, vitamin C, and beta-carotene may help defend against oxygen free radicals. The dietitian can adjust the patient's diet so that it is rich in antioxidants; supplements are also available for patients who have a decreased appetite or who are unable to eat.

Signs and symptoms of oxygen toxicity include substernal discomfort, paresthesias, dyspnea, restlessness, fatigue, malaise, progressive respiratory difficulty, refractory hypoxemia, alveolar atelectasis, and alveolar infiltrates evident on chest x-rays.

Prevention of oxygen toxicity is achieved by using oxygen only as prescribed. If high concentrations of oxygen are necessary, it is important to minimize the duration of administration and reduce its concentration as soon as possible. Often, **positive end-expiratory pressure (PEEP)** or **continuous positive airway pressure (CPAP)** is used

---

**CHART 25-1**

### Types of Hypoxia

Hypoxia can occur from either severe pulmonary disease (inadequate oxygen supply) or from extrapulmonary disease (inadequate oxygen delivery) affecting gas exchange at the cellular level. The four general types of hypoxia are hypoxemic hypoxia, circulatory hypoxia, anemic hypoxia, and histotoxic hypoxia.

#### HYPOXEMIC HYPOXIA
Hypoxemic hypoxia is a decreased oxygen level in the blood resulting in decreased oxygen diffusion into the tissues. It may be caused by hypoventilation, high altitudes, ventilation–perfusion mismatch (as in pulmonary embolism), shunts in which the alveoli are collapsed and cannot provide oxygen to the blood (commonly caused by atelectasis), and pulmonary diffusion defects. It is corrected by increasing alveolar ventilation or providing supplemental oxygen.

#### CIRCULATORY HYPOXIA
Circulatory hypoxia is hypoxia resulting from inadequate capillary circulation. It may be caused by decreased cardiac output, local vascular obstruction, low-flow states such as shock, or cardiac arrest. Although tissue partial pressure of oxygen ($PO_2$) is reduced, arterial oxygen ($PaO_2$) remains normal. Circulatory hypoxia is corrected by identifying and treating the underlying cause.

#### ANEMIC HYPOXIA
Anemic hypoxia is a result of decreased effective hemoglobin concentration, which causes a decrease in the oxygen-carrying capacity of the blood. It is rarely accompanied by hypoxemia. Carbon monoxide poisoning, because it reduces the oxygen-carrying capacity of hemoglobin, produces similar effects but is not strictly anemic hypoxia because hemoglobin levels may be normal.

#### HISTOTOXIC HYPOXIA
Histotoxic hypoxia occurs when a toxic substance, such as cyanide, interferes with the ability of tissues to use available oxygen.

with oxygen therapy to reverse or prevent microatelectasis, thus allowing a lower percentage of oxygen to be used. The level of PEEP that allows the best oxygenation without hemodynamic compromise is known as "best PEEP."

### Suppression of Ventilation

In many patients with COPD, the stimulus for respiration is a decrease in blood oxygen rather than an elevation in carbon dioxide levels. The administration of a high concentration of oxygen removes the respiratory drive that has been created largely by the patient's chronic low oxygen tension. The resulting decrease in alveolar ventilation can cause a progressive increase in arterial carbon dioxide pressure ($PaCO_2$). This hypoventilation can, in rare cases, lead to acute respiratory failure secondary to carbon dioxide narcosis, acidosis, and death. Oxygen-induced hypoventilation is prevented by administering oxygen at low flow rates (1 to 2 L/min) and by closely monitoring the respiratory rate and the oxygen saturation as measured by pulse oximetry ($SpO_2$).

### Other Complications

Because oxygen supports combustion, there is always a danger of fire when it is used. It is important to post "No Smoking" signs when oxygen is in use. Oxygen therapy equipment is also a potential source of bacterial cross-infection; therefore, the nurse (or respiratory therapist) changes the tubing according to infection control policy and the type of oxygen delivery equipment.

## Methods of Oxygen Administration

Oxygen is dispensed from a cylinder or a piped-in system. A reduction gauge is necessary to reduce the pressure to a working level, and a flow meter regulates the flow of oxygen in liters per minute. When oxygen is used at high flow rates, it should be moistened by passing it through a humidification system to prevent it from drying the mucous membranes of the respiratory tract.

The use of oxygen concentrators is another means of providing varying amounts of oxygen, especially in the home setting. These devices are relatively portable, easy to operate, and cost-effective. However, they require more maintenance than tank or liquid systems and probably cannot deliver oxygen flows in excess of 4 L/min, which provides an $FiO_2$ of about 36%.

Many different oxygen devices are used, and all deliver oxygen if they are used as prescribed and maintained correctly (Table 25-1). The amount of oxygen delivered is expressed as a percentage concentration (eg, 70%). The

**TABLE 25-1  Oxygen Administration Devices**

| Device | Suggested Flow Rate (L/min) | $O_2$ Percentage Setting | Advantages | Disadvantages |
|---|---|---|---|---|
| **Low-Flow Systems** | | | | |
| Cannula | 1–2<br>3–5<br>6 | 23–30<br>30–40<br>42 | Lightweight, comfortable, inexpensive, continuous use with meals and activity | Nasal mucosal drying, variable $FiO_2$ |
| Oropharyngeal catheter | 1–6 | 23–42 | Inexpensive, does not require a tracheostomy | Nasal mucosa irritation; catheter should be changed frequently to alternate nostril |
| Mask, simple | 6–8 | 40–60 | Simple to use, inexpensive | Poor fitting, variable $FiO_2$, must remove to eat |
| Mask, partial rebreather | 8–11 | 50–75 | Moderate $O_2$ concentration | Warm, poorly fitting, must remove to eat |
| Mask, non-rebreather | 12 | 80–100 | High $O_2$ concentration | Poorly fitting |
| **High-Flow Systems** | | | | |
| Transtracheal catheter | ¼–4 | 60–100 | More comfortable, concealed by clothing, less oxygen liters per minute needed than nasal cannula | Requires frequent and regular cleaning, requires surgical intervention |
| Mask, Venturi | 4–6<br>6–8 | 24, 26, 28<br>30, 35, 40 | Provides low levels of supplemental $O_2$<br>Precise $FiO_2$, additional humidity available | Must remove to eat |
| Mask, aerosol | 8–10 | 30–100 | Good humidity, accurate $FiO_2$ | Uncomfortable for some |
| Tracheostomy collar | 8–10 | 30–100 | Good humidity, comfortable, fairly accurate $FiO_2$ | |
| T-piece | 8–10 | 30–100 | Same as tracheostomy collar | Heavy with tubing |
| Face tent | 8–10 | 30–100 | Good humidity, fairly accurate $FiO_2$ | Bulky and cumbersome |
| **Oxygen Conserving Devices** | | | | |
| Pulse dose (or demand) | 10–40 mL/breath | | Deliver $O_2$ only on inspiration, conserve 50% to 75% of $O_2$ used | Must carefully evaluate function individually |

appropriate form of oxygen therapy is best determined by arterial blood gas levels, which indicate the patient's oxygenation status.

Oxygen delivery systems are classified as low-flow or high-flow delivery systems. Low-flow systems contribute partially to the inspired gas the patient breathes, which means that the patient breathes some room air along with the oxygen. These systems do not provide a constant or known concentration of inspired oxygen. The amount of inspired oxygen changes as the patient's breathing changes. Examples of low-flow systems include nasal cannula, oropharyngeal catheter, simple mask, partial-rebreather, and non-rebreather masks. In contrast, high-flow systems provide the total amount of inspired air. A specific percentage of oxygen is delivered independent of the patient's breathing. High-flow systems are indicated for patients who require a constant and precise amount of oxygen. Examples of such systems include transtracheal catheters, Venturi masks, aerosol masks, tracheostomy collars, T-pieces, and face tents.

A nasal cannula is used when the patient requires a low to medium concentration of oxygen for which precise accuracy is not essential. This method is relatively simple and allows the patient to move about in bed, talk, cough, and eat without interrupting oxygen flow. Flow rates in excess of 6 to 8 L/min may lead to swallowing of air or may cause irritation and drying of the nasal and pharyngeal mucosa.

The oropharyngeal catheter is rarely used but may be prescribed for short-term therapy to administer low to moderate concentrations of oxygen. The catheter should be changed every 8 hours, alternating nostrils to prevent nasal irritation and infection.

When oxygen is administered via cannula or catheter, the percentage of oxygen reaching the lungs varies with the depth and rate of respirations, particularly if the nasal mucosa is swollen or if the patient is a mouth breather.

Oxygen masks come in several forms. Each is used for different purposes (Fig. 25-1). *Simple masks* are used to administer low to moderate concentrations of oxygen. The body of the mask itself gathers and stores oxygen between breaths. The patient exhales directly through openings or ports in the body of the mask. If oxygen flow ceases, the patient can draw air in through these openings around the mask edges. Although widely used, these masks cannot be used for controlled oxygen concentrations and must be adjusted for proper fit. They should not press too tightly against the skin, because this can cause a sense of claustrophobia as well as skin breakdown; adjustable elastic bands are provided to ensure comfort and security.

*Partial-rebreathing masks* have a reservoir bag that must remain inflated during both inspiration and expiration. The nurse adjusts the oxygen flow to ensure that the bag does not collapse during inhalation. A high concentration of oxygen can be delivered, because both the mask and the bag serve as reservoirs for oxygen. Oxygen enters the mask through small-bore tubing that connects at the junction of the mask and bag. As the patient inhales, gas is drawn from the mask, from the bag, and potentially from room air through the exhalation ports. As the patient exhales, the first third of the exhalation fills the reservoir bag. This is mainly dead space and does not participate in gas exchange in the lungs. Therefore, it has a high oxygen concentration. The remainder of the exhaled gas is vented through the exhalation ports. The actual percentage of oxygen delivered is influenced by the patient's ventilatory pattern (Kacmarek, Dimas, & Mack, 2005).

*Non-rebreathing masks* are similar in design to partial-rebreathing masks except that they have additional valves. A one-way valve located between the reservoir bag and the base of the mask allows gas from the reservoir bag to enter the mask on inhalation but prevents gas in the mask from flowing back into the reservoir bag during exhalation. One-way valves located at the exhalation ports prevent room air from entering the mask during inhalation. They also allow the patient's exhaled gases to exit the mask on exhalation.

Venturi mask

Nonrebreathing mask

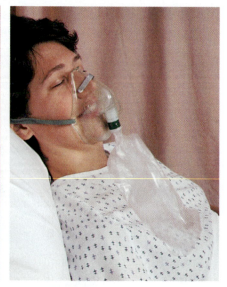
Partial rebreathing mask

**FIGURE 25-1.** Types of oxygen masks used to deliver varying concentrations of oxygen. Photos © Ken Kaspar.

As with the partial-rebreathing mask, it is important to adjust the oxygen flow so that the reservoir bag does not completely collapse on inspiration. In theory, if the non-rebreathing mask fits the patient snugly and both side exhalation ports have one-way valves, it is possible for the patient to receive 100% oxygen, making the non-rebreathing mask a high-flow oxygen system. However, because it is difficult to get an exact fit from the mask on every patient, and some non-rebreathing masks have only one one-way exhalation valve, it is almost impossible to ensure 100% oxygen delivery, making it a low-flow oxygen system.

The *Venturi mask* is the most reliable and accurate method for delivering precise concentrations of oxygen through noninvasive means. The mask is constructed in a way that allows a constant flow of room air blended with a fixed flow of oxygen. It is used primarily for patients with COPD because it can accurately provide appropriate levels of supplemental oxygen, thus avoiding the risk of suppressing the hypoxic drive.

The Venturi mask uses the Bernoulli principle of air entrainment (trapping the air like a vacuum), which provides a high air flow with controlled oxygen enrichment. For each liter of oxygen that passes through a jet orifice, a fixed proportion of room air is entrained. A precise volume of oxygen can be delivered by varying the size of the jet orifice and adjusting the flow of oxygen. Excess gas leaves the mask through the two exhalation ports, carrying with it the exhaled carbon dioxide. This method allows a constant oxygen concentration to be inhaled regardless of the depth or rate of respiration.

The mask should fit snugly enough to prevent oxygen from flowing into the patient's eyes. The nurse checks the patient's skin for irritation. It is necessary to remove the mask so that the patient can eat, drink, and take medications, at which time supplemental oxygen is provided through a nasal cannula.

The *transtracheal oxygen catheter* is inserted directly into the trachea and is indicated for patients with chronic oxygen therapy needs. These catheters are more comfortable, less dependent on breathing patterns, and less obvious than other oxygen delivery methods. Because no oxygen is lost into the surrounding environment, the patient achieves adequate oxygenation at lower rates, making this method less expensive and more efficient.

The *T-piece* connects to the endotracheal tube and is useful in weaning patients from mechanical ventilation (Fig. 25-2).

Other oxygen devices include *aerosol masks, tracheostomy collars,* and *face tents,* all of which are used with aerosol devices (nebulizers) that can be adjusted for oxygen concentrations from 27% to 100% (0.27 to 1.00). If the gas mixture flow falls below patient demand, room air is pulled in, diluting the concentration. The aerosol mist must be available for the patient during the entire inspiratory phase.

Although most oxygen therapy is administered as continuous flow oxygen, new methods of oxygen conservation are coming into use. The *demand oxygen delivery system* (DODS) interrupts the flow of oxygen during exhalation, when it is otherwise mostly wasted. Several versions of the DODS are being evaluated for their effectiveness. Studies show that DODS models conserve oxygen and maintain oxygen saturations better than continuous-flow oxygen systems when the respiratory rate increases (Langenhof & Fichter, 2005).

*Hyperbaric oxygen therapy* is the administration of oxygen at pressures greater than 1 atmosphere. As a result, the amount of oxygen dissolved in plasma is increased, which increases oxygen levels in the tissues.

**FIGURE 25-2.** T-pieces and tracheostomy collars are devices used when weaning patients from mechanical ventilation.

During therapy, the patient is placed in a small (single patient use) or large (multiple patient use) cylinder chamber. Hyperbaric oxygen therapy is used to treat conditions such as air embolism, carbon monoxide poisoning, gangrene, tissue necrosis, and hemorrhage.

Other, more controversial, uses for this therapy include treatment for multiple sclerosis (Bennett & Heard, 2004; Moon, 2002), diabetic foot ulcers (Broussard, 2003;. Roeckl-Wiedmann, Bennett & Kranke, 2005), closed head trauma (Bennett, Trytko, & Jonker, 2004; McDonagh, Helfand, Carson et al., 2004), and acute myocardial infarction (Dekleva, Neskovic, Vlahovic, et al., 2004; Sharifi, Fares, Abdel-Karim, et al., 2004). Potential side effects include ear trauma, central nervous system disorders, and oxygen toxicity.

## Gerontologic Considerations

The respiratory system changes throughout the aging process, and it is important for nurses to be aware of these changes when assessing patients who are receiving oxygen therapy. As the respiratory muscles weaken and the large bronchi and alveoli become enlarged, the available surface area of the lungs decreases, resulting in reduced ventilation and respiratory gas exchange. The number of functional cilia is also reduced, decreasing ciliary action and the cough reflex. As a result of osteoporosis and calcification of the costal cartilages, chest wall compliance is decreased. Patients may display increased chest rigidity and respiratory rate and decreased $PaO_2$ and lung expansion. Nurses should be aware that the older adult is at risk for aspiration and infection related to these changes. In addition, patient education regarding adequate nutrition is essential, because appropriate dietary intake can help diminish the excess buildup of carbon dioxide and maintain optimal respiratory functioning.

## Nursing Management

### Promoting Home and Community-Based Care

**TEACHING PATIENTS SELF-CARE**

At times oxygen must be administered to the patient at home. The nurse instructs the patient or family in the methods for administering oxygen safely and informs the patient and family that oxygen is available in gas, liquid, and concentrated forms. The gas and liquid forms come in portable devices so that the patient can leave home while receiving oxygen therapy. Humidity must be provided while oxygen is used (except with portable devices) to counteract the dry, irritating effects of compressed oxygen on the airway (Chart 25-2).

**CONTINUING CARE**

Home visits by a home health nurse or respiratory therapist may be arranged based on the patient's status and needs. It is important to assess the patient's home envi-

---

**CHART 25-2**

### HOME CARE CHECKLIST • Oxygen Therapy

| At the completion of the home care instruction, the patient or caregiver will be able to: | Patient | Caregiver |
|---|:---:|:---:|
| • State proper care of and administration of oxygen to patient | | |
|   • State physician's prescription for oxygen and the manner in which it is to be used | ✓ | ✓ |
|   • Indicate when a humidifier should be used | ✓ | ✓ |
|   • Identify signs and symptoms indicating the need for change in oxygen therapy | ✓ | ✓ |
|   • Describe precautions and safety measures to be used when oxygen is in use | ✓ | ✓ |
|   • Know **NOT** to smoke while using oxygen | ✓ | ✓ |
|   • Post "No smoking—oxygen in use" signs on doors | ✓ | ✓ |
|   • Notify local fire department and electric company of oxygen use in home | ✓ | ✓ |
|   • Keep oxygen tank at least 15 feet away from matches, candles, gas stove, or other source of flame | ✓ | ✓ |
|   • Keep oxygen tank 5 feet away from TV, radio, and other appliances | ✓ | ✓ |
|   • Keep oxygen tank out of direct sunlight | ✓ | ✓ |
|   • When traveling in automobile, place oxygen tank on floor behind front seat | ✓ | ✓ |
|   • If traveling by airplane, notify air carrier of need for oxygen at least 2 weeks in advance | ✓ | ✓ |
|   • State how and when to place an order for more oxygen | ✓ | ✓ |
|   • Describe a diet that meets energy demands | ✓ | ✓ |
| • Maintain equipment properly | | |
|   • Demonstrate correct adjustment of prescribed flow rate | ✓ | ✓ |
|   • Describe how to clean and when to replace oxygen tubing | ✓ | ✓ |
|   • Identify when a portable oxygen delivery device should be used | ✓ | ✓ |
|   • Demonstrate safe and appropriate use of portable oxygen delivery device | ✓ | ✓ |
|   • Identify causes of malfunction of equipment and when to call for replacement of equipment | ✓ | ✓ |
|   • Describe the importance of determining that all electrical outlets are working properly | ✓ | ✓ |

ronment, the patient's physical and psychological status, and the need for further teaching. The nurse reinforces the teaching points on how to use oxygen safely and effectively, including fire safety tips. To maintain a consistent quality of care and to maximize the patient's financial reimbursement for home oxygen therapy, the nurse ensures that the physician's prescription includes the diagnosis, the prescribed oxygen flow, and conditions for use (eg, continuous use, nighttime use only). Because oxygen is a medication, the nurse reminds the patient receiving long-term oxygen therapy and the family about the importance of keeping follow-up appointments with the physician. The patient is instructed to see the physician every 6 months or more often, if indicated. Arterial blood gas measurements and laboratory tests are repeated annually, or more often if the patient's condition changes.

## Incentive Spirometry (Sustained Maximal Inspiration)

**Incentive spirometry** is a method of deep breathing that provides visual feedback to encourage the patient to inhale slowly and deeply to maximize lung inflation and prevent or reduce atelectasis. Ideally, the patient assumes a sitting or semi-Fowler's position to enhance diaphragmatic excursion (Chart 25-3). However, this procedure may be performed with the patient in any position.

Incentive spirometers are available in two types: volume or flow. In the volume type, the tidal volume of the spirometer is set according to the manufacturer's instructions. The purpose of the device is to ensure that the volume of air inhaled is increased gradually as the patient takes deeper and deeper breaths. The patient takes a deep breath through the mouthpiece, pauses at peak lung inflation, and then relaxes and exhales. Taking several normal breaths before attempting another with the incentive spirometer helps avoid fatigue. The volume is periodically increased as tolerated.

A flow spirometer has the same purpose as a volume spirometer, but the volume is not preset. The spirometer contains a number of movable balls that are pushed up by the force of the breath and held suspended in the air while the patient inhales. The amount of air inhaled and the flow of the air are estimated by how long and how high the balls are suspended.

### Indications

Incentive spirometry is used after surgery, especially thoracic and abdominal surgery, to promote the expansion of the alveoli and to prevent or treat atelectasis.

### CHART 25-3

#### Assisting the Patient to Perform Incentive Spirometry

- Explain the reason and objective for the therapy: the inspired air helps to inflate the lungs. The ball or weight in the spirometer will rise in response to the intensity of the intake of air. The higher the ball rises, the deeper the breath.
- Assess the patient's level of pain and administer pain medication if prescribed.
- Position the patient in semi-Fowler's position or in an upright position (although any position is acceptable).
- Demonstrate how to use diaphragmatic breathing.
- Instruct the patient to place the mouthpiece of the spirometer firmly in the mouth, to breathe air in (inspire), and to hold the breath at the end of inspiration for about 3 seconds. The patient then exhales slowly.
- Encourage the patient to perform the procedure approximately 10 times in succession, repeating the 10 breaths with the spirometer each hour during waking hours.
- Set a reasonable volume and repetition goal (to provide encouragement and give the patient a sense of accomplishment).
- Encourage coughing during and after each session.

© B. Proud

- Assist the patient to splint the incision when coughing postoperatively.
- Place the spirometer within easy reach of the patient.
- For the postoperative patient, begin the therapy immediately. (If the patient begins to hypoventilate, atelectasis can start to develop within an hour.)
- Record how effectively the patient performs the therapy and the number of breaths achieved with the spirometer every 2 hours.

## Nursing Management

Nursing management of the patient using incentive spirometry includes placing the patient in the proper position, teaching the technique for using the incentive spirometer, setting realistic goals for the patient, and recording the results of the therapy.

## Mini-Nebulizer Therapy

The mini-nebulizer is a handheld apparatus that disperses a moisturizing agent or medication, such as a bronchodilator or mucolytic agent, into microscopic particles and delivers it to the lungs as the patient inhales. The mini-nebulizer is usually air-driven by means of a compressor through connecting tubing. In some instances, the nebulizer is oxygen-driven rather than air-driven. To be effective, a visible mist must be available for the patient to inhale.

### Indications

The indications for use of a mini-nebulizer include difficulty in clearing respiratory secretions, reduced vital capacity with ineffective deep breathing and coughing, and unsuccessful trials of simpler and less costly methods for clearing secretions, delivering aerosol, or expanding the lungs. The patient must be able to generate a deep breath. Diaphragmatic breathing (Chart 25-4) is a helpful technique to prepare for proper use of the mini-nebulizer. Mini-nebulizers are frequently used for patients with COPD to dispense inhaled medications, and they are commonly used at home on a long-term basis.

### Nursing Management

#### Promoting Home and Community-Based Care

**TEACHING PATIENTS SELF-CARE**
The nurse instructs the patient to breathe through the mouth, taking slow, deep breaths, and then to hold the breath for a few seconds at the end of inspiration to increase intrapleural pressure and reopen collapsed alveoli, thereby increasing functional residual capacity. The nurse encourages the patient to cough and to monitor the effectiveness of the therapy. The nurse instructs the patient and family about the purpose of the treatment, equipment setup, medication additive, and proper cleaning and storage of the equipment.

## Intermittent Positive-Pressure Breathing

Intermittent positive-pressure breathing (IPPB) is an older form of assisted or controlled respiration in which compressed gas is delivered under positive pressure into a person's airways until a preset pressure is reached. Passive exhalation is allowed through a valve.

### CHART 25-4 — Patient Education

### Breathing Exercises

**GENERAL INSTRUCTIONS**
- Breathe slowly and rhythmically to exhale completely and empty the lungs completely.
- Inhale through the nose to filter, humidify, and warm the air before it enters the lungs.
- If you feel out of breath, breathe more slowly by prolonging the exhalation time.
- Keep the air moist with a humidifier.

**DIAPHRAGMATIC BREATHING**
Goal: To use and strengthen the diaphragm during breathing
- Place one hand on the abdomen (just below the ribs) and the other hand on the middle of the chest to increase the awareness of the position of the diaphragm and its function in breathing.
- Breathe in slowly and deeply through the nose, letting the abdomen protrude as far as possible.
- Breathe out through pursed lips while tightening (contracting) the abdominal muscles.
- Press firmly inward and upward on the abdomen while breathing out.
- Repeat for 1 minute; follow with a rest period of 2 minutes.
- Gradually increase duration up to 5 minutes, several times a day (before meals and at bedtime).

**PURSED-LIP BREATHING**
Goal: To prolong exhalation and increase airway pressure during expiration, thus reducing the amount of trapped air and the amount of airway resistance.
- Inhale through the nose while slowly counting to 3—the amount of time needed to say "Smell a rose."
- Exhale slowly and evenly against pursed lips while tightening the abdominal muscles. (Pursing the lips increases intratracheal pressure; exhaling through the mouth offers less resistance to expired air.)
- Count to 7 slowly while prolonging expiration through pursed lips—the length of time to say "Blow out the candle."
- While sitting in a chair:
  Fold arms over the abdomen.
  Inhale through the nose while counting to 3 slowly.
  Bend forward and exhale slowly through pursed lips while counting to 7 slowly.
- While walking:
  Inhale while walking two steps.
  Exhale through pursed lips while walking four or five steps.

## Indications

IPPB is indicated for patients who need to increase lung expansion. Although it has been used to administer aerosolized medications, spontaneous inhalation of medications using a metered-dose inhaler or a nebulizer is equally effective (Kacmarek et al., 2005).

## Complications

IPPB therapy is used rarely today because of its inherent hazards, which include pneumothorax, mucosal drying, increased intracranial pressure (ICP), hemoptysis, gastric distention, vomiting with possible aspiration, psychological dependency (especially with long-term use, as in patients with COPD), hyperventilation, excessive oxygen administration, and cardiovascular problems.

# Chest Physiotherapy

Chest physiotherapy (CPT) includes **postural drainage**, **chest percussion** and **vibration**, and breathing retraining. In addition, teaching the patient effective coughing technique is an important part of CPT. The goals of CPT are to remove bronchial secretions, improve ventilation, and increase the efficiency of the respiratory muscles.

## Postural Drainage (Segmented Bronchial Drainage)

Postural drainage uses specific positions that allow the force of gravity to assist in the removal of bronchial secretions. The secretions drain from the affected bronchioles into the bronchi and trachea and are removed by coughing or suctioning. Postural drainage is used to prevent or relieve bronchial obstruction caused by accumulation of secretions.

Because the patient usually sits in an upright position, secretions are likely to accumulate in the lower parts of the lungs. With postural drainage, different positions (Fig. 25-3) are used so that the force of gravity helps move secretions from the smaller bronchial airways to the main bronchi and trachea. The secretions then are removed by coughing. The nurse instructs the patient to inhale bronchodilators and mucolytic agents, if prescribed, before postural drainage, because these medications improve drainage of the bronchial tree.

Postural drainage exercises can be directed at any of the segments of the lungs. The lower and middle lobe bronchi drain more effectively when the head is down, the upper lobe bronchi drain more effectively when the head is up. Frequently, five positions are used, one for drainage of each lobe: head down, prone, right and left lateral, and sitting upright.

### Nursing Management

The nurse should be aware of the patient's diagnosis as well as the lung lobes or segments involved, the cardiac status, and any structural deformities of the chest wall and spine. Auscultating the chest before and after the procedure helps identify the areas needing drainage and assess the effectiveness of treatment. The nurse teaches family members who will be assisting the patient at home to evaluate breath sounds before and after treatment. The nurse explores strategies that will enable the patient to assume the indicated positions at home. This may require the creative use of objects readily available at home, such as pillows, cushions, or cardboard boxes.

Postural drainage is usually performed two to four times daily, before meals (to prevent nausea, vomiting, and aspiration) and at bedtime. Prescribed bronchodilators, water, or saline may be nebulized and inhaled before postural drainage to dilate the bronchioles, reduce bronchospasm, decrease the thickness of mucus and sputum, and combat edema of the bronchial walls. The recommended sequence starts with positions to drain the lower lobes, followed by positions to drain the upper lobes.

The nurse makes the patient as comfortable as possible in each position and provides an emesis basin, sputum cup, and paper tissues. The nurse instructs the patient to remain in each position for 10 to 15 minutes and to breathe in slowly through the nose and out slowly through pursed lips to help keep the airways open so that secretions can drain while in each position. If a position cannot be tolerated, the nurse helps the patient assume a modified position. When the patient changes position, the nurse explains how to cough and remove secretions (Chart 25-5).

If the patient cannot cough, the nurse may need to suction the secretions mechanically. It also may be necessary to use chest percussion and vibration or a high-frequency chest wall oscillation (HFCWO) vest to loosen bronchial secretions and mucus plugs that adhere to the bronchioles and bronchi and to propel sputum in the direction of gravity drainage (see later discussion). If suctioning is required at home, the nurse instructs caregivers in safe suctioning technique and care of the suctioning equipment.

After the procedure, the nurse notes the amount, color, viscosity, and character of the expelled sputum. It is important to evaluate the patient's skin color and pulse the first few times the procedure is performed. It may be necessary to administer oxygen during postural drainage.

If the sputum is foul-smelling, it is important to perform postural drainage in a room away from other patients or family members. (Deodorizers may be used to counteract the odor, but aerosol sprays can cause bronchospasm and irritation; therefore, they should be used sparingly and with caution.) After the procedure, the patient may find it refreshing to brush the teeth and use a mouthwash before resting.

## Chest Percussion and Vibration

Thick secretions that are difficult to cough up may be loosened by tapping (percussing) and vibrating the chest or through use of an HFCWO vest. Chest percussion and vibration help dislodge mucus adhering to the bronchioles and bronchi.

Percussion is carried out by cupping the hands and lightly striking the chest wall in a rhythmic fashion over the lung segment to be drained. The wrists are alternately flexed and extended so that the chest is cupped or clapped in a painless manner (Fig. 25-4). A soft cloth or towel may be placed over the segment of the chest that is being cupped to prevent skin irritation and redness from direct contact.

**FIGURE 25-3.** Postural drainage positions and the areas of lung drained by each position.

## CHART 25-5

### Effective Coughing Technique

1. The patient assumes a sitting position and bends slightly forward. This upright position permits a stronger cough.
2. The patient's knees and hips are flexed to promote relaxation and reduce the strain on the abdominal muscles while coughing.
3. The patient inhales slowly through the nose and exhales through pursed lips several times.
4. The patient should cough twice during each exhalation while contracting (pulling in) the abdomen sharply with each cough.
5. The patient splints the incisional area, if any, with firm hand pressure or supports it with a pillow or rolled blanket while coughing (see Fig. 25-12). (The nurse can initially demonstrate this by using the patient's hands.)

An inflatable HFCWO vest (Fig. 25-5) may be used to provide chest therapy. The vest uses air pulses to compress the chest wall 8 to 18 times/second, causing secretions to detach from the airway wall, enabling the patient to expel them by coughing. Vest therapy is considered more effective than manual percussion because it is more gentle and acts on all lobes of the lung simultaneously (Oermann, Sockrider, Giles, et al., 2001).

A scheduled program of coughing and clearing sputum, together with hydration, reduces the amount of sputum in most patients. The number of times the percussion and coughing cycle is repeated depends on the patient's tolerance and clinical response. It is important to evaluate breath sounds before and after the procedures.

To increase the effectiveness of coughing, a flutter valve is sometimes used, especially by people who have cystic fibrosis. The flutter valve looks like a pipe but has a cap covering the bowl, which contains a steel ball. When the patient exhales actively into the valve, movement of the ball causes pressure oscillations, thereby decreasing mucus viscosity, allowing it to move within the airways and be coughed out.

### Nursing Management

When performing CPT, the nurse ensures that the patient is comfortable, is not wearing restrictive clothing, and has not just eaten. The uppermost areas of the lung are treated first. The nurse gives medication for pain, as prescribed, before percussion and vibration and splints any incision and provides pillows for support as needed. The positions are varied, but focus is placed on the affected areas. On completion of the treatment, the nurse assists the patient to assume a comfortable position.

If an HFCWO vest is being used, the patient may assume whatever position is most comfortable and may even continue to perform light activity during therapy within the length of the compressed air hose. It is not necessary for the patient to assume specific positions for the vest to be effective.

The nurse must stop treatment if any of the following occur: increased pain, increased shortness of breath, weakness, lightheadedness, or hemoptysis. Therapy is indicated

Percussion, alternating with vibration, is performed for 3 to 5 minutes for each position. The patient uses diaphragmatic breathing during this procedure to promote relaxation (see later discussion). As a precaution, percussion over chest drainage tubes, the sternum, spine, liver, kidneys, spleen, or breasts (in women) is avoided. Percussion is performed cautiously in the elderly because of their increased incidence of osteoporosis and risk of rib fracture.

Vibration is the technique of applying manual compression and tremor to the chest wall during the exhalation phase of respiration (see Fig. 25-4). This helps increase the velocity of the air expired from the small airways, thus freeing the mucus. After three or four vibrations, the patient is encouraged to cough, using the abdominal muscles. (Contracting the abdominal muscles increases the effectiveness of the cough.)

**FIGURE 25-4.** Percussion and vibration. (**A**) Proper hand position for percussion. (**B**) Proper technique for vibration. The wrists and elbows remain stiff; the vibrating motion is produced by the shoulder muscles. (**C**) Proper hand position for vibration.

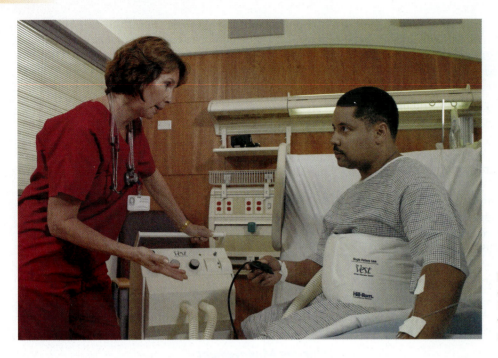

**FIGURE 25-5.** High-frequency chest wall oscillation vest. © 2005 Hill-Rom Services, Inc. Reprinted with permission—all rights reserved.

until the patient has normal respirations, can mobilize secretions, and has normal breath sounds, and until the chest x-ray findings are normal.

**PROMOTING HOME AND COMMUNITY-BASED CARE**

**Teaching Patients Self-Care.** CPT is frequently indicated at home for patients with COPD, bronchiectasis, or cystic fibrosis. The techniques are the same as described previously, but gravity drainage is achieved by placing the hips over a box, a stack of magazines, or pillows (unless a hospital bed is available). The nurse instructs the patient and family in the positions and techniques of percussion and vibration so that therapy can be continued in the home. In addition, the nurse instructs the patient to maintain an adequate fluid intake and air humidity to prevent secretions from becoming thick and tenacious. It also is important to teach the patient to recognize early signs of infection, such as fever and a change in the color or character of sputum. Resting 5 to 10 minutes in each postural drainage position before CPT maximizes the amount of secretions obtained.

**Continuing Care.** CPT may be carried out during visits by a home care nurse. The nurse also assesses the patient's physical status, understanding of the treatment plan, and compliance with recommended therapy, as well as the effectiveness of therapy. It is important to reinforce patient and family teaching during these visits. The nurse reports to the patient's physician any deterioration in the patient's physical status or inability to clear secretions.

## Breathing Retraining

Breathing retraining consists of exercises and breathing practices that are designed to achieve more efficient and controlled ventilation and to decrease the work of breathing. Breathing retraining is especially indicated in patients with COPD and dyspnea. These exercises promote maximal alveolar inflation and muscle relaxation; relieve anxiety; eliminate ineffective, uncoordinated patterns of respiratory muscle activity; slow the respiratory rate; and decrease the work of breathing. Slow, relaxed, and rhythmic breathing also helps to control the anxiety that occurs with dyspnea. Specific breathing exercises include diaphragmatic and pursed-lip breathing (see Chart 25-4).

The goal of diaphragmatic breathing is to use and strengthen the diaphragm during breathing. Diaphragmatic breathing can become automatic with sufficient practice and concentration. Pursed-lip breathing, which improves oxygen transport, helps induce a slow, deep breathing pattern and assists the patient to control breathing, even during periods of stress. This type of breathing helps prevent airway collapse secondary to loss of lung elasticity in emphysema. The goal of pursed-lip breathing is to train the expiratory muscles to prolong exhalation and increase airway pressure during expiration, thus lessening the amount of airway trapping and resistance. The nurse instructs the patient in diaphragmatic breathing and pursed-lip breathing, as described earlier in Chart 25-4. Breathing exercises may be practiced in several positions, because air distribution and pulmonary circulation vary with the position of the chest.

Many patients require additional oxygen, using a low-flow method, while performing breathing exercises. Emphysema-like changes in the lung occur as part of the natural aging process of the lung; therefore, breathing exercises are appropriate for all elderly patients who are hospitalized and for elderly patients in any setting who are sedentary, even without primary lung disease.

### Nursing Management

**PROMOTING HOME AND COMMUNITY-BASED CARE**

**Teaching Patients Self-Care.** The nurse instructs the patient to breathe slowly and rhythmically in a relaxed manner and to exhale completely to empty the lungs. The patient is instructed to always inhale through the nose because this filters, humidifies, and warms the air. If short of breath, the patient should concentrate on breathing slowly and rhythmically. To avoid initiating a cycle of increasing shortness of breath and panic, it is often helpful to instruct the patient to concentrate on prolonging the length of exhalation rather than merely slowing the rate of breathing. Minimizing the amount of dust or particles in the air and providing adequate humidification may also make it easier for the patient to breathe. Strategies to decrease dust or particles in the air include removing drapes and upholstered furniture, using air filters, and washing floors, dusting, and vacuuming frequently.

The nurse instructs the patient that an adequate dietary intake promotes gas exchange and increases energy levels. It is important to provide adequate nutrition without overfeeding the patient. The nurse teaches the patient to consume small, frequent meals and snacks. Having ready-prepared meals and favorite foods available helps encourage nutrient consumption. Gas-producing foods such as beans, legumes, broccoli, cabbage, and Brussels sprouts should be avoided to prevent gastric distress. Because many of these patients lack the energy to eat, they should be taught to rest before and after meals to conserve energy.

# Airway Management

Adequate ventilation is dependent on free movement of air through the upper and lower airways. In many disorders, the airway becomes narrowed or blocked as a result of disease, bronchoconstriction (narrowing of airway by contraction of muscle fibers), a foreign body, or secretions. Maintaining a patent (open) airway is achieved through meticulous airway management, whether in an emergency situation such as airway obstruction or in long-term management, as in caring for a patient with an endotracheal or a tracheostomy tube.

## Emergency Management of Upper Airway Obstruction

Upper airway obstruction has a variety of causes. Acute upper airway obstruction may be caused by food particles, vomitus, blood clots, or any other particle that enters and obstructs the larynx or trachea. It also may occur from enlargement of tissue in the wall of the airway, as in epiglottitis, obstructive sleep apnea, laryngeal edema, laryngeal carcinoma, or peritonsillar abscess, or from thick secretions. Pressure on the walls of the airway, as occurs in retrosternal goiter, enlarged mediastinal lymph nodes, hematoma around the upper airway, and thoracic aneurysm, also may result in upper airway obstruction.

The patient with an altered level of consciousness from any cause is at risk for upper airway obstruction because of loss of the protective reflexes (cough and swallowing) and loss of the tone of the pharyngeal muscles, which causes the tongue to fall back and block the airway.

The nurse makes the following rapid observations to assess for signs and symptoms of upper airway obstruction:

- Inspection: Is the patient conscious? Is there any inspiratory effort? Does the chest rise symmetrically? Is there use or retraction of accessory muscles? What is the skin color? Are there any obvious signs of deformity or obstruction (trauma, food, teeth, vomitus)? Is the trachea midline?
- Palpation: Do both sides of the chest rise equally with inspiration? Are there any specific areas of tenderness, fracture, or subcutaneous emphysema (crepitus)?
- Auscultation: Is there any audible air movement, stridor (inspiratory sound), or wheezing (expiratory sound)? Are breath sounds present over the lower trachea and bilaterally in all lobes?

As soon as an upper airway obstruction is identified, the nurse takes emergency measures (Chart 25-6). (See Chapter 71 for more details on managing a foreign body airway obstruction, or see Chapter 22.)

## Endotracheal Intubation

**Endotracheal intubation** involves passing an endotracheal tube through the mouth or nose into the trachea (Fig. 25-6). Intubation provides a patent airway when the patient is having respiratory distress that cannot be treated with simpler methods. It is the method of choice in emergency care. Endotracheal intubation is a means of providing an airway for patients who cannot maintain an adequate airway on their own (eg, comatose patients, patients with upper airway obstruction), for patients needing mechanical ventilation, and for suctioning secretions from the pulmonary tree.

An endotracheal tube usually is passed with the aid of a laryngoscope by specifically trained medical, nursing, or respiratory therapy personnel (see Chapter 71). Once the tube is inserted, a cuff is inflated to prevent air from leaking around the outer part of the tube, to minimize the possibility of subsequent aspiration, and to prevent movement of the tube.

The nurse should be aware that complications could occur from pressure exerted by the cuff on the tracheal wall. Cuff pressures should be checked with a calibrated aneroid manometer device every 6 to 8 hours to maintain cuff pressure between 15 and 20 mm Hg (Morton, Fontaine, Hudak, et al., 2005). High cuff pressure can cause tracheal bleeding, ischemia, and pressure necrosis, whereas low cuff pressure can increase the risk for aspiration pneumonia. Routine deflation of the cuff is not recommended because of the increased risk for aspiration and hypoxia. The cuff is deflated before the endotracheal tube is removed. Tracheobronchial secretions are suctioned through the tube. Warmed, humidified oxygen should always be introduced through the tube, whether the patient is breathing spontaneously or is receiving ventilatory support. Endotracheal intubation may be used for no longer than 3 weeks, by which time a tracheostomy must be considered to decrease irritation of and trauma to the tracheal lining, to reduce the incidence of vocal cord paralysis (secondary to laryngeal nerve damage), and to decrease the work of breathing. Chart 25-7 discusses the nursing care of the patient with an endotracheal tube.

Endotracheal and tracheostomy tubes have several disadvantages. The tubes cause discomfort. The cough reflex is depressed because closure of the glottis is hindered.

**CHART 25-6**

## Clearing an Upper Airway Obstruction

### CLEARING THE AIRWAY
- Hyperextend the patient's neck by placing one hand on the forehead and placing the fingers of the other hand underneath the jaw and lifting upward and forward. This action pulls the tongue away from the back of the pharynx.

Opening the airway.

- Assess the patient by observing the chest and listening and feeling for the movement of air.
- Use a cross-finger technique to open the mouth and observe for obvious obstructions such as secretions, blood clots, or food particles.
- If no passage of air is detected, apply five quick sharp abdominal thrusts just below the xiphoid process to expel the obstruction. Repeat this procedure until the obstruction is expelled.
- After the obstruction is expelled, roll the patient as a unit onto the side for recovery.
- When the obstruction is relieved, if the patient can breathe spontaneously but not cough, swallow, or gag, insert an oral or nasopharyngeal airway.

Abdominal thrust (Heimlich) maneuver administered to unconscious patient.

### BAG AND MASK RESUSCITATION
- Use a resuscitation bag and mask if assisted ventilation is required.
- Apply the mask to the patient's face and create a seal by pressing the thumb of the nondominant hand on the bridge of the nose and the index finger on the chin. Using the rest of the fingers on that hand, pull on the chin and the angle of the mandible to maintain the head in extension. Use the dominant hand to inflate the lungs by squeezing the bag to its full volume.

Resuscitation via bag and mask apparatus.

**FIGURE 25-6.** Endotracheal tube in place. The tube has been inserted using the oral route. The cuff has been inflated to maintain the tube's position and to minimize the risk of aspiration.

Secretions tend to become thicker because the warming and humidifying effect of the upper respiratory tract has been bypassed. The swallowing reflexes, composed of the glottic, pharyngeal, and laryngeal reflexes, are depressed because of prolonged disuse and the mechanical trauma produced by the endotracheal or tracheostomy tube, increasing the risk of aspiration. In addition, ulceration and stricture of the larynx or trachea may develop. Of great concern to the patient is the inability to talk and to communicate needs.

Unintentional or premature removal of the tube is a potentially life-threatening complication of endotracheal intubation. Removal of the tube is a frequent problem in intensive care units and occurs mainly during nursing care or by the patient. It is important that nurses instruct patients and family members about the purpose of the tube and the dangers of removing it. Baseline and ongoing assessment of the patient and of the equipment ensures effective care. Providing comfort measures, including opioid analgesia and sedation, can improve the patient's tolerance of the endotracheal tube.

---

**CHART 25-7**

## Care of the Patient With an Endotracheal Tube

**IMMEDIATELY AFTER INTUBATION**
1. Check symmetry of chest expansion.
   a. Auscultate breath sounds of anterior and lateral chest bilaterally.
   b. Obtain order for chest x-ray to verify proper tube placement.
   c. Check cuff pressure every 8–12 hours.
   d. Monitor for signs and symptoms of aspiration.
2. Ensure high humidity; a visible mist should appear in the T-piece or ventilator tubing.
3. Administer oxygen concentration as prescribed by physician.
4. Secure the tube to the patient's face with tape, and mark the proximal end for position maintenance.
   a. Cut proximal end of tube if it is longer than 7.5 cm (3 inches) to prevent kinking.
   b. Insert an oral airway or mouth device to prevent the patient from biting and obstructing the tube.
5. Use sterile suction technique and airway care to prevent iatrogenic contamination and infection.
6. Continue to reposition patient every 2 hours and as needed to prevent atelectasis and to optimize lung expansion.
7. Provide oral hygiene and suction the oropharynx whenever necessary.

**EXTUBATION (REMOVAL OF ENDOTRACHEAL TUBE)**
1. Explain procedure.
2. Have self-inflating bag and mask ready in case ventilatory assistance is required immediately after extubation.
3. Suction the tracheobronchial tree and oropharynx, remove tape, and then deflate the cuff.
4. Give 100% oxygen for a few breaths, then insert a new, sterile suction catheter inside tube.
5. Have the patient inhale. At peak inspiration remove the tube, suctioning the airway through the tube as it is pulled out.

*Note:* In some hospitals this procedure can be performed by respiratory therapists; in others, by nurses. Check hospital policy.

**CARE OF PATIENT FOLLOWING EXTUBATION**
1. Give heated humidity and oxygen by face mask and maintain the patient in a sitting or high Fowler's position.
2. Monitor respiratory rate and quality of chest excursions. Note stridor, color change, and change in mental alertness or behavior.
3. Monitor the patient's oxygen level using a pulse oximeter.
4. Keep NPO or give only ice chips for next few hours.
5. Provide mouth care.
6. Teach patient how to perform coughing and deep-breathing exercises.

> **NURSING ALERT**
>
> Inadvertent removal of an endotracheal tube can cause laryngeal swelling, hypoxemia, bradycardia, hypotension, and even death. Measures must be taken to prevent premature or inadvertent removal.

To prevent tube removal by the patient, the nurse can use the following strategies: explain to the patient and family the purpose of the tube, distract the patient through one-to-one interaction with the nurse and family or with television, and maintain comfort measures. As a last resort, soft wrist restraints may be used. Discretion and caution must always be used before applying any restraint. If the patient cannot move the arms and hands to the endotracheal tube, restraints are not needed. If the patient is alert, oriented, able to follow directions, and cooperative to the point that it is highly unlikely that he or she will remove the endotracheal tube, restraints are not needed. However, if the nurse determines there is a risk that the patient may try to remove the tube, soft wrist restraints are appropriate with a physician's order (check agency policy). Close monitoring of the patient is essential to ensure safety and prevent harm.

## Tracheostomy

A **tracheotomy** is a surgical procedure in which an opening is made into the trachea. The indwelling tube inserted into the trachea is called a **tracheostomy tube**. A tracheostomy may be either temporary or permanent (Fig. 25-7).

A tracheostomy is used to bypass an upper airway obstruction, to allow removal of tracheobronchial secretions, to permit the long-term use of mechanical ventilation, to prevent aspiration of oral or gastric secretions in the unconscious or paralyzed patient (by closing off the trachea from the esophagus), and to replace an endotracheal tube. There are many disease processes and emergency conditions that make a tracheostomy necessary.

### Procedure

The surgical procedure is usually performed in the operating room or in an intensive care unit, where the patient's ventilation can be well controlled and optimal aseptic technique can be maintained. A surgical opening is made between the second and third tracheal rings. After the trachea is exposed, a cuffed tracheostomy tube of an appropriate size is inserted. The cuff is an inflatable attachment to the tracheostomy tube that is designed to occlude the space between the tracheal walls and the tube, to permit effective mechanical ventilation and to minimize the risk of aspiration. See Figure 25-7 for types of tracheostomy tubes.

The tracheostomy tube is held in place by tapes fastened around the patient's neck. Usually a square of sterile gauze is placed between the tube and the skin to absorb drainage and reduce the risk for infection.

### Complications

Complications may occur early or late in the course of tracheostomy tube management. They may even occur years after the tube has been removed. Early complications include bleeding, pneumothorax, air embolism, aspiration, subcutaneous or mediastinal emphysema, recurrent laryngeal nerve damage, and posterior tracheal wall penetration. Long-term complications include airway obstruction from accumulation of secretions or protrusion of the cuff over the opening of the tube, infection, rupture of the innominate artery, dysphagia, tracheoesophageal fistula, tracheal dilation, and tracheal ischemia and necrosis. Tracheal

A

B

**FIGURE 25-7.** Tracheostomy tubes. (**A**) Fenestrated tube, which allows patient to talk. (**B**) Double-cuffed tube. Inflating the two cuffs alternately can help prevent tracheal damage. Courtesy of Smiths Medical, Keene, NH.

stenosis may develop after the tube is removed. Chart 25-8 outlines measures nurses can take to prevent complications.

## Nursing Management

The patient requires continuous monitoring and assessment. The newly made opening must be kept patent by proper suctioning of secretions. After the vital signs are stable, the patient is placed in a semi-Fowler's position to facilitate ventilation, promote drainage, minimize edema, and prevent strain on the suture lines. Analgesia and sedative agents must be administered with caution because of the risk of suppressing the cough reflex.

Major objectives of nursing care are to alleviate the patient's apprehension and to provide an effective means of communication. The nurse keeps paper and pencil or a Magic Slate and the call light within the patient's reach at all times to ensure a means of communication. The care of the patient with a tracheostomy tube is summarized in Chart 25-9.

### Suctioning the Tracheal Tube (Tracheostomy or Endotracheal Tube)

When a tracheostomy or endotracheal tube is in place, it is usually necessary to suction the patient's secretions because of the decreased effectiveness of the cough mechanism. Tracheal suctioning is performed when adventitious breath sounds are detected or whenever secretions are obviously present. Unnecessary suctioning can initiate bronchospasm and cause mechanical trauma to the tracheal mucosa.

All equipment that comes into direct contact with the patient's lower airway must be sterile to prevent overwhelming pulmonary and systemic infections. The procedure for suctioning a tracheostomy is presented in Chart 25-10. In mechanically ventilated patients, an in-line suction catheter may be used to allow rapid suction when needed and to minimize cross-contamination by airborne pathogens. An in-line suction device allows the patient to be suctioned without being disconnected from the ventilator circuit.

### Managing the Cuff

As a general rule, the cuff on an endotracheal or tracheostomy tube should be inflated. The pressure within the cuff should be the lowest possible pressure that allows delivery of adequate tidal volumes and prevents pulmonary aspiration. Usually the pressure is maintained at less than 25 mm Hg to prevent injury and at more than 15 mm Hg to prevent aspiration. Cuff pressure must be monitored at least every 8 hours by attaching a handheld pressure gauge to the pilot balloon of the tube or by using the minimal leak volume or minimal occlusion volume technique. With long-term intubation, higher pressures may be needed to maintain an adequate seal.

### Promoting Home and Community-Based Care

#### TEACHING PATIENTS SELF-CARE
If the patient is at home with a tracheostomy, the nurse instructs the patient and family about daily care, including techniques to prevent infection, as well as measures to take in an emergency. The nurse provides the patient and family with a list of community contacts for education and support needs.

#### CONTINUING CARE
A referral for home care is indicated for ongoing assessment of the patient and of the ability of the patient and family to provide appropriate and safe care. The home care nurse assesses the patient's and family's ability to cope with the physical changes and psychological issues associated with having a tracheostomy. The nurse also identifies resources and makes referrals for appropriate services to assist the patient and family to manage the tracheostomy at home.

# Mechanical Ventilation

**Mechanical ventilation** may be required for a variety of reasons: to control the patient's respirations during surgery or during treatment of severe head injury, to oxygenate the blood when the patient's ventilatory efforts are inadequate, and to rest the respiratory muscles, among others. Many patients placed on a ventilator can breathe spontaneously, but the effort needed to do so may be exhausting.

A mechanical ventilator is a positive or negative pressure breathing device that can maintain ventilation and oxygen delivery for a prolonged period. Caring for a patient on mechanical ventilation has become an integral part of nursing care in critical care or general medical-surgical units, extended care facilities, and the home. Nurses, physicians, and respiratory therapists must understand each patient's specific pulmonary needs and work together to set realistic goals. Positive patient outcomes depend on an understanding of the principles of mechanical ventilation and the patient's care needs as well as open communication among members of the health care team about the goals of therapy, weaning plans, and the patient's tolerance of changes in ventilator settings.

---

### CHART 25-8

### Preventing Complications Associated With Endotracheal and Tracheostomy Tubes

- Administer adequate warmed humidity.
- Maintain cuff pressure at appropriate level.
- Suction as needed per assessment findings.
- Maintain skin integrity. Change tape and dressing as needed or per protocol.
- Auscultate lung sounds.
- Monitor for signs and symptoms of infection, including temperature and white blood cell count.
- Administer prescribed oxygen and monitor oxygen saturation.
- Monitor for cyanosis.
- Maintain adequate hydration of the patient.
- Use sterile technique when suctioning and performing tracheostomy care.

| CHART 25-9 | Guidelines for Care of the Patient With a Tracheostomy Tube |

| ACTIONS | RATIONALE |
|---|---|
| 1. Gather the needed equipment, including sterile gloves, hydrogen peroxide, normal saline solution or sterile water, cotton-tipped applicators, dressing and twill tape (and the type of tube prescribed, if the tube is to be changed). | Everything needed to care for a tracheostomy should be readily on hand for the most effective care. |
| A cuffed tube (air injected into cuff) is required during mechanical ventilation. A low-pressure cuff is most commonly used. | A cuffed tube prevents air from leaking during positive-pressure ventilation and also prevents tracheal aspiration of gastric contents. An adequate seal is indicated by the disappearance of any air leakage from the mouth or tracheostomy or by the disappearance of the harsh, gurgling sound of air coming from the throat. |
| Patients requiring long-term use of a tracheostomy tube and who can breathe spontaneously commonly use an uncuffed, metal tube. | Low-pressure cuffs exert minimal pressure on the tracheal mucosa and thus reduce the danger of tracheal ulceration and stricture. |
| 2. Provide patient and family instruction on the key points for tracheostomy care, beginning with how to inspect the tracheostomy dressing for moisture or drainage. | The tracheostomy dressing is changed as needed to keep the skin clean and dry. To prevent potential breakdown, moist or soiled dressings should not remain on the skin. |
| 3. Perform hand hygiene. | Hand hygiene reduces bacteria on hands. |
| 4. Explain procedure to patient and family as appropriate. | A patient with a tracheostomy is apprehensive and requires ongoing assurance and support. |
| 5. Put on clean gloves; remove and discard the soiled dressing in a biohazard container. | Observing body substance isolation reduces cross-contamination from soiled dressings. |
| 6. Prepare sterile supplies, including hydrogen peroxide, normal saline solution or sterile water, cotton-tipped applicators, dressing, and tape. | Having necessary supplies and equipment readily available allows the procedure to be completed efficiently. |
| 7. Put on sterile gloves. (Some physicians approve clean technique for long-term tracheostomy patients in the home.) | Sterile equipment minimizes transmission of surface flora to the sterile respiratory tract. Clean technique may be used in the home because of decreased exposure to potential pathogens. |
| 8. Cleanse the wound and the plate of the tracheostomy tube with sterile cotton-tipped applicators moistened with hydrogen peroxide. Rinse with sterile saline solution. | Hydrogen peroxide is effective in loosening crusted secretions. Rinsing prevents skin residue. |
| 9. Soak inner cannula in peroxide or sterile saline, per manufacturer's instructions; rinse with saline solution; and inspect to be sure all dried secretions have been removed. Dry and reinsert inner cannula or replace with a new disposable inner cannula. | Soaking loosens and removes secretions from the inner lumen of the tracheostomy tube. Retained secretions could harbor bacteria, leading to infection. Some plastic tracheostomy tubes may be damaged by using peroxide. |
| 10. Place clean twill tape in position to secure the tracheostomy tube by inserting one end of the tape through the side opening of the outer cannula. Take the tape around the back of the patient's neck and thread it through the opposite opening of the outer cannula. Bring both ends around so that they meet on one side of the neck. Tighten the tape until only two fingers can be comfortably inserted under it. Secure with a knot. For a new tracheostomy, two people should assist with tape changes. Remove soiled twill tape after the new tape is in place. | This taping technique provides a double thickness of tape around the neck, which is needed because the tracheostomy tube can be dislodged by movement or by a forceful cough if left unsecured. A dislodged tracheostomy tube is difficult to reinsert, and respiratory distress may occur. Dislodgement of a new tracheostomy is a medical emergency. |

### CHART 25-9  Guidelines for Care of the Patient With a Tracheostomy Tube, continued

| ACTIONS | RATIONALE |
|---|---|
| 11. Remove old tapes and discard in a biohazard container after the new tape is in place. | Tapes with old secretions may harbor bacteria. |
| 12. Although some long-term tracheostomies with healed stomas may not require a dressing, other tracheostomies do. In such cases, use a sterile tracheostomy dressing, fitting it securely under the twill tapes and flange of tracheostomy tube so that the incision is covered, as shown below. | Healed tracheostomies with minimal secretions do not need a dressing. Dressings that will shred are not used around a tracheostomy because of the risk that pieces of material, lint, or thread may get into the tube, and eventually into the trachea, causing obstruction or abscess formation. Special dressings that do not have a tendency to shred are used. |

(A) The cuff of the tracheostomy tube fits smoothly and snugly in the trachea in a way that promotes circulation but seals off the escape of secretions and air surrounding the tube. (B) For a dressing change, a 4 × 4-inch gauze pad may be folded (cutting would promote shredding, placing the patient at risk for aspiration) around the tracheostomy tube and (C) stabilized by slipping the neck tape ties through the neck plate slots of the tracheostomy tube. The ties may be fastened to the side of the neck to eliminate the discomfort of lying on the knot.

### CHART 25-10  Performing Tracheal Suction

**EQUIPMENT**
- Suction catheters
- Gloves (sterile and nonsterile), gown, mask, and goggles
- Goggles for eye protection
- Basin for sterile normal saline solution for irrigation
- Manual resuscitation bag with supplemental oxygen
- Suction source

**PROCEDURE**
1. Explain the procedure to the patient before beginning and offer reassurance during suctioning; the patient may be apprehensive about choking and about an inability to communicate.
2. Begin by performing hand hygiene. Put on nonsterile gloves, goggles, gown, and mask.
3. Turn on suction source (pressure should not exceed 120 mm Hg).
4. Open suction catheter kit.
5. Fill basin with sterile normal saline solution.
6. Ventilate the patient with manual resuscitation bag and high-flow oxygen.
7. Put sterile glove on dominant hand.
8. Pick up suction catheter in sterile gloved hand and connect to suction.
9. Hyperoxygenate the patient's lungs for several deep breaths. Instill normal saline solution into airway only if there are thick, tenacious secretions.
10. Insert suction catheter at least as far as the end of the tube without applying suction, just far enough to stimulate the cough reflex.
11. Apply suction while withdrawing and gently rotating the catheter 360° (no longer than 10 to 15 seconds, because hypoxia and dysrhythmias may develop, leading to cardiac arrest).
12. Reoxygenate and inflate the patient's lungs for several breaths.
13. Repeat previous three steps until the airway is clear.
14. Rinse catheter by suctioning a few milliliters of sterile saline solution from the basin between suction attempts.
15. Suction oropharyngeal cavity after completing tracheal suctioning.
16. Rinse suction tubing.
17. Discard catheter, gloves, and basin appropriately.

## Indications

If a patient has a continuous decrease in oxygenation ($PaO_2$), an increase in arterial carbon dioxide levels ($PaCO_2$), and a persistent acidosis (decreased pH), mechanical ventilation may be necessary. Conditions such as thoracic or abdominal surgery, drug overdose, neuromuscular disorders, inhalation injury, COPD, multiple trauma, shock, multisystem failure, and coma all may lead to respiratory failure and the need for mechanical ventilation. The criteria for mechanical ventilation (Chart 25-11) guide the decision to place a patient on a ventilator. A patient with apnea that is not readily reversible also is a candidate for mechanical ventilation.

## Classification of Ventilators

Mechanical ventilators are classified according to the method by which they support ventilation. The two general categories are negative-pressure and positive-pressure ventilators. The most common category in use today is the positive-pressure ventilator.

### Negative-Pressure Ventilators

Negative-pressure ventilators exert a negative pressure on the external chest. Decreasing the intrathoracic pressure during inspiration allows air to flow into the lung, filling its volume. Physiologically, this type of assisted ventilation is similar to spontaneous ventilation. It is used mainly in chronic respiratory failure associated with neuromuscular conditions, such as poliomyelitis, muscular dystrophy, amyotrophic lateral sclerosis, and myasthenia gravis. It is inappropriate for the patient whose condition is unstable or complex or who requires frequent ventilatory changes. Negative-pressure ventilators are simple to use and do not require intubation of the airway; consequently, they are especially adaptable for home use.

There are several types of negative-pressure ventilators: iron lung, body wrap, and chest cuirass.

**IRON LUNG (DRINKER RESPIRATOR TANK).** The iron lung is a negative-pressure chamber used for ventilation. It was used extensively during polio epidemics in the past and currently is used by a few polio survivors and patients with other neuromuscular disorders (eg, amyotrophic lateral sclerosis, muscular dystrophy).

**BODY WRAP (PNEUMO-WRAP) AND CHEST CUIRASS (TORTOISE SHELL).** Both of these portable devices require a rigid cage or shell to create a negative-pressure chamber around the thorax and abdomen. Because of problems with proper fit and system leaks, these types of ventilators are used only with carefully selected patients.

### Positive-Pressure Ventilators

Positive-pressure ventilators inflate the lungs by exerting positive pressure on the airway, similar to a bellows mechanism, forcing the alveoli to expand during inspiration. Expiration occurs passively. Endotracheal intubation or tracheostomy is necessary in most cases. These ventilators are widely used in the hospital setting and are increasingly used in the home for patients with primary lung disease. There are three types of positive-pressure ventilators, which are classified by the method of ending the inspiratory phase of respiration: pressure-cycled, time-cycled, and volume-cycled. Another type of positive-pressure ventilator used for selected patients is noninvasive positive-pressure ventilation (NIPPV), which does not require intubation.

#### PRESSURE-CYCLED VENTILATORS

When the pressure-cycled ventilator cycles on, it delivers a flow of air (inspiration) until it reaches a preset pressure, and then cycles off, and expiration occurs passively. Its major limitation is that the volume of air or oxygen can vary as the patient's airway resistance or compliance changes. As a result, the tidal volume delivered may be inconsistent, possibly compromising ventilation. Consequently, in adults, pressure-cycled ventilators are intended only for short-term use. The most common type is the IPPB machine (see earlier discussion).

#### TIME-CYCLED VENTILATORS

Time-cycled ventilators terminate or control inspiration after a preset time. The volume of air the patient receives is regulated by the length of inspiration and the flow rate of the air. Most ventilators have a rate control that determines the respiratory rate, but pure time-cycling is rarely used for adults. These ventilators are used in newborns and infants.

#### VOLUME-CYCLED VENTILATORS

Volume-cycled ventilators are by far the most commonly used positive-pressure ventilators today (Fig. 25-8). With this type of ventilator, the volume of air to be delivered with each inspiration is preset. Once this preset volume is delivered to the patient, the ventilator cycles off and exhalation occurs passively. From breath to breath, the volume of air delivered by the ventilator is relatively constant, ensuring consistent, adequate breaths despite varying airway pressures.

#### NONINVASIVE POSITIVE-PRESSURE VENTILATION

Positive-pressure ventilation can be given via face masks that cover the nose and mouth, nasal masks, or other oral or nasal devices such as the nasal pillow (a small nasal cannula that seals around the nares to maintain the prescribed pressure). NIPPV eliminates the need for endotracheal intubation or tracheostomy and decreases the risk for nosocomial infections such as pneumonia. The most comfortable mode for the patient is pressure-controlled ventilation with pressure support. This eases the work of breathing and enhances gas exchange. The ventilator can be set with a minimum backup rate for patients with periods of apnea.

Patients are considered candidates for noninvasive ventilation if they have acute or chronic respiratory failure, acute pulmonary edema, COPD, chronic heart failure, or a sleep-related breathing disorder. The device also may be used at home to improve tissue oxygenation and to rest the respiratory muscles while the patient sleeps at night. NIPPV is contraindicated for those who have experienced respiratory ar-

---

**CHART 25-11**

### Indications for Mechanical Ventilation

$PaO_2 < 50$ mm Hg with $FiO_2 > 0.60$
$PaO_2 > 50$ mm Hg with pH $< 7.25$
Vital capacity < 2 times tidal volume
Negative inspiratory force < 25 cm $H_2O$
Respiratory rate > 35/min

**FIGURE 25-8.** Positive-pressure ventilators. (**A**) The AVEA can be used to both ventilate and monitor neonatal, pediatric, and adult patients. It can also deliver noninvasive ventilation with Heliox to adult and pediatric patients. Courtesy of VIASYS Healthcare, Inc., Yorba Linda, CA. (**B**) The Puritan-Bennett 840 Ventilator System has volume, pressure, and mixed modes designed for adult, pediatric, and infant ventilation. Courtesy of Tyco Healthcare/Nelicor Puritan Bennett, Pleasanton, CA.

rest, serious dysrhythmias, cognitive impairment, or head or facial trauma. Noninvasive ventilation may also be used for obstructive sleep apnea, for patients at the end of life, and for those who do not want endotracheal intubation but may need short- or long-term ventilatory support.

Continuous positive airway pressure (CPAP) provides positive pressure to the airways throughout the respiratory cycle. Although it can be used as an adjunct to mechanical ventilation with a cuffed endotracheal tube or tracheostomy tube to open the alveoli, it is also used with a leakproof mask to keep alveoli open, thereby preventing respiratory failure. CPAP is the most effective treatment for obstructive sleep apnea, because the positive pressure acts as a splint, keeping the upper airway and trachea open during sleep. To use CPAP, the patient must be breathing independently.

Bilevel positive airway pressure (bi-PAP) ventilation offers independent control of inspiratory and expiratory pressures while providing pressure support ventilation. It delivers two levels of positive airway pressure provided via a nasal or oral mask, nasal pillow, or mouthpiece with a tight seal and a portable ventilator. Each inspiration can be initiated either by the patient or by the machine if it is programmed with a backup rate. The backup rate ensures that the patient will receive a set number of breaths per minute. Bi-PAP is most often used for patients who require ventilatory assistance at night, such as those with severe COPD or sleep apnea. Tolerance is variable; bi-PAP usually is most successful with highly motivated patients.

## Ventilator Modes

Ventilator mode refers to how breaths are delivered to the patient. The most commonly used modes are assist–control, intermittent mandatory ventilation, synchronized intermittent mandatory ventilation, pressure support ventilation, and airway pressure release ventilation (Fig. 25-9).

**Assist–control ventilation** provides full ventilatory support by delivering a preset tidal volume and respiratory rate. If the patient initiates a breath between the machine's breaths, the ventilator delivers at the preset volume (assisted breath). The cycle does not adapt to the patient's spontaneous efforts; every breath is the preset volume.

**Intermittent mandatory ventilation (IMV)** provides a combination of mechanically assisted breaths and spontaneous breaths. Therefore, the patient can increase the respi-

**FIGURE 25-9.** Modes of mechanical ventilation with airflow waveforms.

ratory rate, but each spontaneous breath is limited to the tidal volume the patient generates. Mechanical breaths are delivered at preset intervals and a preselected tidal volume, regardless of the patient's efforts. IMV allows patients to use their own muscles of ventilation to help prevent muscle atrophy. It lowers mean airway pressure, which can assist in preventing barotrauma. However, bucking the ventilator may be increased.

**Synchronized intermittent mandatory ventilation (SIMV)** also delivers a preset tidal volume and number of breaths per minute. Between ventilator-delivered breaths, the patient can breathe spontaneously with no assistance from the ventilator on those extra breaths. As the patient's ability to breathe spontaneously increases, the preset number of ventilator breaths is decreased and the patient does more of the work of breathing. IMV and SIMV can be used to provide full or partial ventilatory support. Nursing interventions for patients receiving IMV or SIMV include monitoring progress by recording respiratory rate, minute volume, spontaneous and machine-generated tidal volume, $FiO_2$, and arterial blood gas levels.

**Pressure support ventilation (PSV)** assists SIMV by applying a pressure plateau to the airway throughout the patient-triggered inspiration to decrease resistance within the tracheal tube and ventilator tubing. Pressure support is reduced gradually as the patient's strength increases. An SIMV backup rate may be added for extra support. The nurse must closely observe the patient's respiratory rate and tidal volumes on initiation of PSV. It may be necessary to adjust the pressure support to avoid tachypnea or large tidal volumes.

**Airway pressure release ventilation (APRV)** produces tidal ventilation by release of airway pressure from an elevated baseline airway pressure to simulate expiration. APRV is a time-triggered, pressure-limited, time-cycled mode of mechanical ventilation that allows unrestricted, spontaneous breathing throughout the ventilatory cycle. It also allows alveolar gas to be expelled through the lungs' natural recoil. Although further research is needed on the effectiveness of this mode of mechanical ventilation, it has been suggested that it has the important advantages of causing less ventilator-induced lung injury and fewer adverse effects on cardiocirculatory function and being associated with lower need for sedation and neuromuscular blockade (Frawley & Habashi, 2001).

A relatively new mode of support, **proportional assist ventilation (PAV)**, provides partial ventilatory support in which the ventilator generates pressure in proportion to the patient's inspiratory efforts. With every breath, the ventilator synchronizes with the patient's ventilatory efforts. The more inspiratory pressure the patient generates, the more pressure the ventilator generates, amplifying the patient's inspiratory effort without any specific preselected target pressure or volume. It generally adds "additional muscle" to the patient's effort; the depth and frequency of breaths are controlled by the patient (Ambrosino & Rossi, 2002).

New modes of mechanical ventilation that incorporate computerized control of ventilation are being developed. In some of these modes, the ventilator constantly monitors many variables and adjusts gas delivery during individual breaths; these within-breath adjustment systems include automatic tube compensation, volume-assured pressure support, and proportional support ventilation. In other modes, the ventilator evaluates gas delivery during one breath and uses that information to adjust the next breath; these between-breath adjustment systems can be made to ensure a preset tidal volume by adjusting pressure, up to a preset maximum, and include pressure volume support, pressure-regulated volume control, and adaptive support ventilation.

## Adjusting the Ventilator

The ventilator is adjusted so that the patient is comfortable and breathes "in sync" with the machine. Minimal alteration of the normal cardiovascular and pulmonary dynamics is desired. Modes of mechanical ventilation are described in Figure 25-9. If the volume ventilator is adjusted appropriately, the patient's arterial blood gas values will be satisfactory and there will be little or no cardiovascular compromise. Chart 25-12 discusses how to achieve adequate mechanical ventilation for each patient.

## Assessing the Equipment

The ventilator needs to be assessed to make sure that it is functioning properly and that the settings are appropriate.

---

**CHART 25-12**

### Initial Ventilator Settings

The following guide is an example of the steps involved in operating a mechanical ventilator. The nurse, in collaboration with the respiratory therapist, always reviews the manufacturer's instructions, which vary according to the equipment, before beginning mechanical ventilation.

1. Set the machine to deliver the tidal volume required (10 to 15 mL/kg).
2. Adjust the machine to deliver the lowest concentration of oxygen to maintain normal $PaO_2$ (80 to 100 mm Hg). This setting may be high initially but will gradually be reduced based on arterial blood gas results.
3. Record peak inspiratory pressure.
4. Set mode (assist–control or synchronized intermittent mandatory ventilation) and rate according to physician order. (See the glossary for definitions of modes of mechanical ventilation.) Set PEEP and pressure support if ordered.
5. Adjust sensitivity so that the patient can trigger the ventilator with a minimal effort (usually 2 mm Hg negative inspiratory force).
6. Record minute volume and obtain ABGs to measure carbon dioxide partial pressure ($PaCO_2$), pH, and $PaO_2$ after 20 minutes of continuous mechanical ventilation.
7. Adjust setting ($FiO_2$ and rate) according to results of arterial blood gas analysis to provide normal values or those set by the physician.
8. If the patient suddenly becomes confused or agitated or begins bucking the ventilator for some unexplained reason, assess for hypoxia and manually ventilate on 100% oxygen with a resuscitation bag.

Even though the nurse may not be primarily responsible for adjusting the settings on the ventilator or measuring ventilator parameters (these are usually responsibilities of the respiratory therapist), the nurse is responsible for the patient and therefore needs to evaluate how the ventilator affects the patient's overall status.

When monitoring the ventilator, the nurse notes the following:

- Type of ventilator (eg, volume-cycled, pressure-cycled, negative-pressure)
- Controlling mode (eg, **controlled ventilation**, assist–control ventilation, synchronized intermittent mandatory ventilation)
- Tidal volume and rate settings (tidal volume is usually set at 6 to 12 mL/kg [ideal body weight]; rate is usually set at 12 to 16 breaths/min)
- $FiO_2$ setting
- Inspiratory pressure reached and pressure limit (normal is 15 to 20 cm $H_2O$; this increases if there is increased airway resistance or decreased compliance)
- Sensitivity (a 2-cm $H_2O$ inspiratory force should trigger the ventilator)
- Inspiratory-to-expiratory ratio (usually 1:3 [1 second of inspiration to 3 seconds of expiration] or 1:2)
- Minute volume (tidal volume × respiratory rate, usually 6 to 8 L/min)
- Sigh settings (usually set at 1.5 times the tidal volume and ranging from 1 to 3 per hour), if applicable
- Water in the tubing, disconnection or kinking of the tubing
- Humidification (humidifier filled with water) and temperature
- Alarms (turned on and functioning properly)
- PEEP and/or pressure support level, if applicable (PEEP is usually set at 5 to 15 cm $H_2O$)

**NURSING ALERT**

**If the ventilator system malfunctions and the problem cannot be identified and corrected immediately, the nurse must ventilate the patient with a manual resuscitation bag until the problem is resolved.**

## Problems With Mechanical Ventilation

Because of the seriousness of the patient's condition and the highly complex and technical nature of mechanical ventilation, a number of problems or complications can occur. Such situations fall into two categories: ventilator problems and patient problems (Table 25-2). In either case,

### TABLE 25-2 Troubleshooting Problems with Mechanical Ventilation

| Problem | Cause | Solution |
|---|---|---|
| **Ventilator Problems** | | |
| Increase in peak airway pressure | Coughing or plugged airway tube | Suction airway for secretions, empty condensation fluid from circuit. |
| | Patient "bucking" ventilator | Adjust sensitivity. |
| | Decreasing lung compliance | Manually ventilate patient. |
| | | Assess for hypoxia or bronchospasm. |
| | | Check arterial blood gas values. |
| | | Sedate only if necessary. |
| | Tubing kinked | Check tubing; reposition patient; insert oral airway if necessary. |
| | Pneumothorax | Manually ventilate patient; notify physician. |
| | Atelectasis or bronchospasm | Clear secretions. |
| Decrease in pressure or loss of volume | Increase in compliance | None |
| | Leak in ventilator or tubing; cuff on tube/humidifier not tight | Check entire ventilator circuit for patency. Correct leak. |
| **Patient Problems** | | |
| Cardiovascular compromise | Decrease in venous return due to application of positive pressure to lungs | Assess for adequate volume status by measuring heart rate, blood pressure, central venous pressure, pulmonary capillary wedge pressure, and urine output. Notify physician if values are abnormal. |
| Barotrauma/pneumothorax | Application of positive pressure to lungs; high mean airway pressures lead to alveolar rupture | Notify physician. Prepare patient for chest tube insertion. Avoid high pressure settings for patients with COPD, ARDS, or history of pneumothorax. |
| Pulmonary infection | Bypass of normal defense mechanisms; frequent breaks in ventilator circuit; decreased mobility; impaired cough reflex | Use meticulous aseptic technique. Provide frequent mouth care. Optimize nutritional status. |

the patient must be supported while the problem is identified and corrected.

### Bucking the Ventilator

The patient is "in sync" with the ventilator when thoracic expansion coincides with the inspiratory phase of the machine and exhalation occurs passively. The patient is said to fight or buck the ventilator when he or she is out of phase with the machine. This is manifested when the patient attempts to breathe out during the ventilator's mechanical inspiratory phase or when there is jerky and increased abdominal muscle effort. The following factors contribute to this problem: anxiety, hypoxia, increased secretions, hypercapnia, inadequate minute volume, and pulmonary edema. These problems must be corrected before resorting to the use of paralyzing agents to reduce bucking; otherwise, the underlying problem is simply masked and the patient's condition will continue to deteriorate.

Muscle relaxants, tranquilizers, analgesic agents, and paralyzing agents are sometimes administered to patients receiving mechanical ventilation. Their purpose is ultimately to increase the patient–machine synchrony by decreasing the patient's anxiety, hyperventilation, or excessive muscle activity. The selection and dose of the appropriate medication are determined carefully and are based on the patient's requirements and the cause of his or her restlessness. Paralyzing agents are always used as a last resort, and always in conjunction with a sedative medication and often an analgesic medication.

## Nursing Management

### Promoting Home and Community-Based Care

Increasingly, patients are being cared for in extended care facilities or at home while receiving mechanical ventilation, with a tracheostomy tube, or receiving oxygen therapy.

## NURSING RESEARCH PROFILE

### Oral Care in the Prevention of Ventilator-Associated Pneumonia

Grap, M. J., Munro, C. L., Elswick, R. K., et al. (2004). Duration of action of a single, early oral application of chlorhexidine on oral microbial flora in mechanically ventilated patients: A pilot study. *Heart & Lung, 33*(2), 83–91.

#### Purpose
Although good oral care has been shown to reduce the incidence of ventilator-associated pneumonia (VAP), oral care is not a high-priority intervention for patients who are intubated on an emergent basis. Therefore, they remain at high risk of VAP. This study was conducted to examine the effect of a single application of chlorhexidine gluconate (CHG) by spray or swab and oral care on subsequent oral microbial flora and on the occurrence of VAP in intubated patients.

#### Design
Thirty-four intubated adults receiving mechanical ventilation were randomly assigned to one of three groups. Adults in two groups received 2 mL of CHG by either oral spray or swab shortly after intubation, and adults in the third group received routine oral care. CHG is a broad-spectrum antibacterial agent used in healthy populations as a daily oral rinse to control plaque and to prevent and treat gingivitis. Oral cultures for specific respiratory pathogens were obtained at baseline, 12 hours, and every 24 hours up to and including 72 hours after intubation. The presence of VAP was assessed using the Clinical Pulmonary Infection Score (CPIS), which is based on six clinical and laboratory variables. Possible scores range from 0 to 12, with a score of 6 or greater considered indicative of pneumonia.

#### Findings
As predicted, there were fewer positive oral cultures and decreased growth of oral respiratory bacteria from baseline to 48 hours (duration of intubation required for a definition of VAP) in the group that received CHG. In contrast, the usual oral care group experienced an increase in positive culture results. Although complete data were available on only 12 patients at 48 hours because of extubation or patient death, important trends were detected. In the two groups treated with CHG, the mean CPIS increased only slightly, from 5.17 to 5.57, whereas the mean CPIS in the usual care group increased from 4.7 to 6.6, a level indicating pneumonia.

#### Nursing Implications
Although statistically significant differences in oral bacterial culture results were not detected, trends in the data suggest that swabbing or spraying the mouth with CHG shortly after intubation may decrease bacterial colonization of the mouth and the risk of VAP. The results of this study suggest the need for early oral care after intubation; however, the study needs to be repeated in a larger group to determine whether oral CHG (or other antibacterial intervention) significantly affects the incidence of VAP.

Patients receiving home ventilator care usually have a chronic neuromuscular condition or COPD. Providing the opportunity for ventilator-dependent patients to return home to live with their families in familiar surroundings can be a positive experience. The ultimate goal of home ventilator therapy is to enhance the patient's quality of life, not simply to support or prolong life.

### TEACHING PATIENTS SELF-CARE

Caring for the patient with mechanical ventilator support at home can be accomplished successfully, but the family must be emotionally, educationally, and physically able to assume the role of primary caregiver. A home care team consisting of the nurse, physician, respiratory therapist, social service or home care agency, and equipment supplier is needed. The home is evaluated to determine whether the electrical equipment needed can be operated safely. A summary of the basic assessment criteria needed for successful home care is presented in Chart 25-13.

Once the decision to initiate mechanical ventilation at home is made, the nurse prepares the patient and family for home care. The nurse teaches the patient and family about the ventilator, suctioning, tracheostomy care, signs of pulmonary infection, cuff inflation and deflation, and assessment of vital signs. Teaching begins in the hospital and continues at home. Nursing responsibilities include evaluating the patient's and family's understanding of the information presented.

The nurse teaches the family cardiopulmonary resuscitation, including mouth-to-tracheostomy tube (instead of mouth-to-mouth) breathing. The nurse also explains how to handle a power failure, which usually involves converting the ventilator from an electrical power source to a battery power source. Conversion is automatic in most types of home ventilators and lasts approximately 1 hour. The nurse instructs the family on the use of a manual self-inflation bag should it be necessary. Some of the patient's and family's responsibilities are listed in Chart 25-14.

### CONTINUING CARE

A home care nurse monitors and evaluates how well the patient and family are adapting to providing care in the home. The nurse assesses the adequacy of the patient's ventilation and oxygenation as well as airway patency. The nurse addresses any unique adaptation problems the patient may have and listens to the patient's and family's anxieties and frustrations, offering support and encouragement where possible. The home care nurse helps identify and contact community resources that may assist in home management of the patient with mechanical ventilation.

The technical aspects of the ventilator are managed by vendor follow-up. A respiratory therapist usually is assigned to the patient and makes frequent home visits to evaluate the patient and perform a maintenance check of the ventilator.

Transportation services are identified in case the patient requires transportation in an emergency. These arrangements must be made before an emergency arises.

---

### CHART 25-13

### Assessment

### Criteria for Successful Home Ventilator Care

The decision to proceed with home ventilation therapy is usually based on the following parameters.

**PATIENT CRITERIA**
- The patient has a chronic underlying pulmonary or neuromuscular disorder.
- The patient's clinical pulmonary status is stable.
- The patient is willing to go home on mechanical ventilation.

**HOME CRITERIA**
- The home environment is conducive to care of the patient.
- The electrical facilities are adequate to operate all equipment safely.
- The home environment is controlled, without drafts in cold weather and with proper ventilation in warm weather.
- Space is available for cleaning and storing ventilator equipment.

**FAMILY CRITERIA**
- Family members are competent, dependable, and willing to spend the time required for proper training with available professional support.
- Family members understand the diagnosis and prognosis.
- Family has sufficient financial and supportive resources.

---

## Nursing Process

### The Patient Receiving Mechanical Ventilation

### Assessment

The nurse plays a vital role in assessing the patient's status and the functioning of the ventilator.

In assessing the patient, the nurse evaluates the patient's physiologic status and how he or she is coping with mechanical ventilation. Physical assessment includes systematic assessment of all body systems, with an in-depth focus on the respiratory system. Respiratory assessment includes vital signs, respiratory rate and pattern, breath sounds, evalua-

### CHART 25-14

## HOME CARE CHECKLIST • Ventilator Care

| At the completion of the home care instruction, the patient or caregiver will be able to: | Patient | Caregiver |
|---|---|---|
| • State proper care of patient on ventilator | | |
|    • Observe physical signs such as color, secretions, breathing pattern, and state of consciousness. | | ✔ |
|    • Perform physical care such as suctioning, postural drainage, and ambulation. | | ✔ |
|    • Observe the tidal volume and pressure manometer regularly. Intervene when they are abnormal (ie, suction if airway pressure increases). | | ✔ |
|    • Provide a communication method for the patient (eg, pad and pencil, electric larynx, talking tracheostomy, sign language). | | ✔ |
|    • Monitor vital signs as directed. | | ✔ |
|    • Use a predetermined signal to indicate when feeling short of breath or in distress. | ✔ | |
| • Care for and maintain equipment properly | | |
|    • Check the ventilator settings twice each day and whenever the patient is removed from the ventilator. | | ✔ |
|    • Adjust the volume and pressure alarms if needed. | | ✔ |
|    • Fill humidifier as needed and check its level three times a day. | | ✔ |
|    • Empty water in tubing as needed. | ✔ | ✔ |
|    • Use a clean humidifier when circuitry is changed. | | ✔ |
|    • Keep exterior of ventilator clean and free of any objects. | | ✔ |
|    • Change external circuitry once a week or more often as indicated. | | ✔ |
|    • Report malfunction or strange noises immediately | ✔ | ✔ |

tion of spontaneous ventilatory effort, and potential evidence of hypoxia (eg, skin color). Increased adventitious breath sounds may indicate a need for suctioning. The nurse also evaluates the settings and functioning of the mechanical ventilator, as described previously.

Assessment also addresses the patient's neurologic status and effectiveness of coping with the need for assisted ventilation and the changes that accompany it. The nurse assesses the patient's comfort level and ability to communicate as well. Because weaning from mechanical ventilation requires adequate nutrition, it is important to assess the patient's gastrointestinal system and nutritional status.

## Diagnosis

### Nursing Diagnoses

Based on the assessment data, the patient's major nursing diagnoses may include:

- Impaired gas exchange related to underlying illness, ventilator setting adjustment during stabilization, or weaning.
- Ineffective airway clearance related to increased mucus production associated with presence of the tube in trachea or continuous positive-pressure mechanical ventilation
- Risk for trauma and infection related to endotracheal intubation or tracheostomy
- Impaired physical mobility related to ventilator dependency
- Impaired verbal communication related to endotracheal tube and attachment to ventilator
- Defensive coping and powerlessness related to ventilator dependency

### Collaborative Problems/ Potential Complications

Based on the assessment data, potential complications may include the following:

- Alterations in cardiac function
- Barotrauma (trauma to the alveoli) and pneumothorax
- Pulmonary infection
- Sepsis

### Planning and Goals

The major goals for the patient may include achievement of optimal gas exchange, maintenance of a patent airway, absence of trauma or infection, attainment of optimal mobility, adjustment to nonverbal methods of communication, acquisition of successful coping measures, and absence of complications.

## Nursing Interventions

Nursing care of the mechanically ventilated patient requires expert technical and interpersonal skills. Nursing interventions are similar regardless of the setting; however, the frequency of interventions and the stability of the patient vary from setting to setting. Nursing interventions for the mechanically ventilated patient are not uniquely different from those for patients with other pulmonary disorders, but astute nursing assessment and a therapeutic nurse–patient relationship are critical. The specific interventions used by the nurse are determined by the underlying disease process and the patient's response.

Two general nursing interventions that are important in the care of the mechanically ventilated patient are pulmonary auscultation and interpretation of arterial blood gas measurements. The nurse is often the first to note changes in physical assessment findings or significant trends in blood gases that signal the development of a serious problem (eg, pneumothorax, tube displacement, pulmonary embolus).

### Enhancing Gas Exchange

The purpose of mechanical ventilation is to optimize gas exchange by maintaining alveolar ventilation and oxygen delivery. The alteration in gas exchange may be caused by the underlying illness or by mechanical factors related to adjustment of the machine to the patient. The health care team, including nurse, physician, and respiratory therapist, continually assesses the patient for adequate gas exchange, signs and symptoms of hypoxia, and response to treatment. Therefore, the nursing diagnosis of impaired gas exchange is, by its complex nature, multidisciplinary and collaborative. The team members must share goals and information freely. All other goals directly or indirectly relate to this primary goal.

Nursing interventions to promote optimal gas exchange include judicious administration of analgesic agents to relieve pain without suppressing the respiratory drive and frequent repositioning to diminish the pulmonary effects of immobility. The nurse also monitors for adequate fluid balance by assessing for the presence of peripheral edema, calculating daily intake and output, and monitoring daily weights. The nurse administers medications prescribed to control the primary disease and monitors for their side effects.

### Promoting Effective Airway Clearance

Continuous positive-pressure ventilation increases the production of secretions regardless of the patient's underlying condition. The nurse assesses for the presence of secretions by lung auscultation at least every 2 to 4 hours. Measures to clear the airway of secretions include suctioning, CPT, frequent position changes, and increased mobility as soon as possible. Frequency of suctioning should be determined by patient assessment. If excessive secretions are identified by inspection or auscultation techniques, suctioning should be performed. Sputum is not produced continuously or every 1 to 2 hours but as a response to a pathologic condition. Therefore, there is no rationale for routine suctioning of all patients every 1 to 2 hours. Although suctioning is used to aid in the clearance of secretions, it can damage the airway mucosa and impair cilia action.

The sigh mechanism on the ventilator may be adjusted to deliver at least 1 to 3 sighs per hour at 1.5 times the tidal volume if the patient is receiving assist–control ventilation. Periodic sighs prevent atelectasis and the further retention of secretions. Because of the risk for hyperventilation and trauma to pulmonary tissue from excess ventilator pressure (barotrauma, pneumothorax), the sigh feature is not used frequently. If the SIMV mode is being used, the mandatory ventilations act as sighs because they are of greater volume than the patient's spontaneous breaths.

Humidification of the airway via the ventilator is maintained to help liquefy secretions so that they are more easily removed. Bronchodilators are administered to dilate the bronchioles and are classified as adrenergic or anticholinergic. Adrenergic bronchodilators are mostly inhaled and work by stimulating the beta-receptor sites, mimicking the effects of epinephrine in the body. The desired effect is smooth muscle relaxation, which dilates the constricted bronchial tubes. Medications include albuterol (Proventil, Ventolin), isoetharine (Bronkosol), isoproterenol (Isuprel), metaproterenol (Alupent, Metaprel), pirbuterol acetate (Maxair), salmeterol (Serevent), and terbutaline (Brethine, Brethaire, Bricanyl). Tachycardia, heart palpitations, and tremors have been reported with use of these medications. Anticholinergic bronchodilators such as ipratropium (Atrovent), tiotropium (Spiriva), and ipratropium with albuterol (Combivent) produce airway relaxation by blocking cholinergic-induced bronchoconstriction. Patients receiving bronchodilator therapy of either type should be monitored for adverse effects, including dizziness, nausea, decreased oxygen saturation, hypokalemia, increased heart rate, and urine retention. Mucolytic agents such as acetylcysteine (Mucomyst) are administered to liquefy secretions so that they are more easily mobilized. Nursing management of patients receiving mucolytic therapy includes assessment for an adequate cough reflex, sputum characteristics, and (in patients not receiving mechanical ventilation) improvement in incentive spirometry. Side effects include nausea, vomiting, bronchospasm, stomatitis (oral ulcers), urticaria, and rhinorrhea (runny nose).

### Preventing Trauma and Infection

Maintaining the endotracheal or tracheostomy tube is an essential part of airway management. The nurse positions the ventilator tubing so that there is minimal pulling or distortion of the tube in the trachea, reducing the risk of trauma to the trachea. Cuff pressure is monitored every 6 to 8 hours to maintain the pressure at less than 25 mm Hg (optimal cuff pressure is 15 to 20 mm Hg). The nurse assesses for the presence of a cuff leak at the same time.

Patients with endotracheal intubation or a tracheostomy tube do not have the normal defenses of the upper airway. In addition, these patients frequently have multiple additional body system disturbances that lead to immunocompromise. Tracheostomy care is performed at least every 8 hours, and more frequently if needed, because of the increased risk for infection. The ventilator circuit tubing and in-line suction tubing are replaced periodically, according to infection control guidelines, to decrease the risk for infection.

The nurse administers oral hygiene frequently, because the oral cavity is a primary source of contamination of the lungs in the intubated and compromised patient. The presence of a nasogastric tube in the intubated patient can increase the risk for aspiration, leading to nosocomial pneumonia. The nurse positions the patient with the head elevated above the stomach as much as possible. Although antiulcer medications such as cimetidine (Tagamet) or ranitidine (Zantac) are sometimes administered, an oral antiulcer medication such as sucralfate (Carafate) is preferable because it maintains normal gastric pH, decreasing the incidence of aspiration pneumonia.

### Promoting Optimal Level of Mobility

Being connected to a ventilator limits the patient's mobility. The nurse helps the patient whose condition has become stable to get out of bed and move to a chair as soon as possible. Mobility and muscle activity are beneficial because they stimulate respirations and improve morale. If the patient is unable to get out of bed, the nurse encourages performance of active range-of-motion exercises every 6 to 8 hours. If the patient cannot perform these exercises, the nurse performs passive range-of-motion exercises every 8 hours to prevent contractures and venous stasis.

### Promoting Optimal Communication

It is important to develop alternative methods of communication for the patient who is receiving mechanical ventilation. The nurse assesses the patient's communication abilities to evaluate for limitations. Questions to consider when assessing the ventilator-dependent patient's ability to communicate include the following:

- Is the patient conscious and able to communicate? Can the patient nod or shake his or her head?
- Is the patient's mouth unobstructed by the tube so that words can be mouthed?
- Is the patient's dominant hand strong and available for writing? For example, if the patient is right-handed, the intravenous (IV) line should be placed in the left arm if possible so that the right hand is free.
- Is the patient a candidate for a Passy-Muir valve, which permits talking?

Once the patient's limitations are known, the nurse offers several appropriate communication approaches: lip reading (use single key words), pad and pencil or Magic Slate, communication board, gesturing, sign language, or electric larynx. Use of a "talking" or fenestrated tracheostomy tube may be suggested to the physician; this allows the patient to talk while on the ventilator. The nurse makes sure that the patient's eyeglasses, hearing aid, sign interpreter, and language translator are available if needed to enhance the patient's ability to communicate.

The patient must be assisted to find the most suitable communication method. Some methods may be frustrating to the patient, family, and nurse; these need to be identified and minimized. A speech therapist can assist in determining the most appropriate method.

### Promoting Coping Ability

Dependence on a ventilator is frightening to both the patient and the family and disrupts even the most stable families. Encouraging the family to verbalize their feelings about the ventilator, the patient's condition, and the environment in general is beneficial. Explaining procedures every time they are performed helps reduce anxiety and familiarizes the patient with ventilator procedures. To restore a sense of control, the nurse encourages the patient to participate in decisions about care, schedules, and treatment when possible. The patient may become withdrawn or depressed while receiving mechanical ventilation, especially if its use is prolonged. To promote effective coping, the nurse informs the patient about progress when appropriate. It is important to provide diversions such as watching television, playing music, or taking a walk (if appropriate and possible). Stress reduction techniques (eg, a back rub, relaxation measures) help relieve tension and help the patient deal with anxieties and fears about both the condition and the dependence on the ventilator.

### Monitoring and Managing Potential Complications

#### ALTERATIONS IN CARDIAC FUNCTION

Alterations in cardiac output may occur as a result of positive-pressure ventilation. The positive intrathoracic pressure during inspiration compresses the heart and great vessels, thereby reducing venous return and cardiac output. This is usually corrected during exhalation when the positive pressure is off. The patient may have decreased cardiac output and resultant decreased tissue perfusion and oxygenation.

To evaluate cardiac function, the nurse first observes for signs and symptoms of hypoxia (restlessness, apprehension, confusion, tachycardia, tachypnea, labored breathing, pallor progressing to cyanosis, diaphoresis, transient hypertension, and decreased urine output). If a pulmonary artery catheter is in place, cardiac output, cardiac index, and other hemodynamic values can be used to assess the patient's status.

### BAROTRAUMA AND PNEUMOTHORAX

Excessive positive pressure can cause barotrauma, which results in a spontaneous **pneumothorax**. This may quickly develop into a tension pneumothorax, further compromising venous return, cardiac output, and blood pressure. The nurse considers any sudden changes in oxygen saturation or the onset of respiratory distress to be a life-threatening emergency requiring immediate action.

### PULMONARY INFECTION

The patient is at high risk for infection, as described earlier. The nurse reports fever or a change in the color or odor of sputum to the physician for follow-up.

## Evaluation

### Expected Patient Outcomes

Expected patient outcomes may include the following:

1. Exhibits adequate gas exchange, as evidenced by normal breath sounds, acceptable arterial blood gas levels, and vital signs
2. Demonstrates adequate ventilation with minimal mucus accumulation
3. Is free of injury or infection, as evidenced by normal temperature, white blood cell count, and clear sputum
4. Is mobile within limits of ability
    a. Gets out of bed to chair, bears weight, or ambulates as soon as possible
    b. Performs range-of-motion exercises every 6 to 8 hours
5. Communicates effectively through written messages, gestures, or other communication strategies
6. Copes effectively
    a. Verbalizes fears and concerns about condition and equipment
    b. Participates in decision making when possible
    c. Uses stress reduction techniques when necessary
7. Absence of complications
    a. Absence of cardiac compromise, as evidenced by stable vital signs and adequate urine output
    b. Absence of pneumothorax, as evidenced by bilateral chest excursion, normal chest x-ray, and adequate oxygenation
    c. Absence of pulmonary infection, as evidenced by normal temperature, clear pulmonary secretions, and negative sputum cultures

## Weaning the Patient From the Ventilator

**Respiratory weaning**, the process of withdrawing the patient from dependence on the ventilator, takes place in three stages: the patient is gradually removed from the ventilator, then from the tube, and finally from oxygen. Weaning from mechanical ventilation is performed at the earliest possible time consistent with patient safety. The decision must be made from a physiologic rather than a mechanical viewpoint. A thorough understanding of the patient's clinical status is required in making this decision. Weaning is started when the patient is recovering from the acute stage of medical and surgical problems and when the cause of respiratory failure is sufficiently reversed.

Successful weaning involves collaboration among the physician, respiratory therapist, and nurse. Each health care provider must understand the scope and function of other team members in relation to patient weaning to conserve the patient's strength, use resources efficiently, and maximize successful outcomes.

### Criteria for Weaning

Careful assessment is required to determine whether the patient is ready to be removed from mechanical ventilation. If the patient is stable and showing signs of improvement or reversal of the disease or condition that caused the need for mechanical ventilation, weaning indices should be assessed. These indices include the following:

- Vital capacity—the amount of air expired after maximum inspiration. It is used to assess the patient's ability to take deep breaths and should be 10 to 15 mL/kg to meet the criteria for weaning.
- Maximum inspiratory pressure—used to assess the patient's respiratory muscle strength. It is also known as negative inspiratory pressure and should be at least −20 cm $H_2O$.
- Tidal volume—the volume of air that is inhaled or exhaled from the lungs during an effortless breath. It should be more than 3.5 mL/kg for weaning (Kacmarek et al., 2005).
- Minute ventilation—equal to the respiratory rate multiplied by tidal volume. Normal is about 6 L/min.
- Rapid/shallow breathing index—calculated by dividing the respiratory rate by the tidal volume. It is used to as-

sess the breathing pattern, and patients with indices lower than 105 breaths/min/L are more likely to be successful at weaning.

Other measurements used to assess readiness for weaning include a $PaO_2$ of greater than 60 mm Hg with an $FiO_2$ of less than 50% (Kacmarek et al., 2005). Stable vital signs and arterial blood gases are also important predictors of successful weaning. Once readiness has been determined, the nurse records baseline measurements of weaning indices to monitor progress.

## Patient Preparation

To maximize the chances of success of weaning, the nurse must consider the patient as a whole, taking into account factors that impair the delivery of oxygen and elimination of carbon dioxide as well as those that increase oxygen demand (eg, sepsis, seizures, thyroid imbalances) or decrease the patient's overall strength (eg, inadequate nutrition, neuromuscular disease). Adequate psychological preparation is necessary before and during the weaning process. Patients need to know what is expected of them during the procedure. They are often frightened by having to breathe on their own again and need reassurance that they are improving and are well enough to handle spontaneous breathing. The nurse explains what will happen during weaning and what role the patient will play in the procedure. The nurse emphasizes that someone will be with or near the patient at all times and answers any questions simply and concisely. Proper preparation of the patient can shorten the time required for successful weaning.

## Methods of Weaning

Successful weaning depends on the combination of adequate patient preparation, available equipment, and an interdisciplinary approach to solving patient problems (Chart 25-15). All usual modes of ventilation can be used for weaning.

When assist–control ventilation is used, the control rate is decreased, so that the patient strengthens the respiratory muscles by triggering progressively more breaths. The nurse assesses the patient for the following signs of distress: rapid/shallow breathing, use of accessory muscles, reduced level of consciousness, increase in carbon dioxide levels, decrease in oxygen saturation, and tachycardia.

SIMV is indicated if the patient satisfies all the criteria for weaning but cannot sustain adequate spontaneous ventilation for long periods. As the patient's respiratory muscles become stronger, the rate is decreased until the patient is breathing spontaneously.

The PAV mode of partial ventilatory support allows the ventilator to generate pressure in proportion to the patient's efforts. With every breath, the ventilator synchronizes with the patient's ventilatory efforts. Nursing assessment includes careful monitoring of the patient's respiratory rate, arterial blood gases, tidal volume, minute ventilation, and breathing pattern.

CPAP allows the patient to breathe spontaneously while applying positive pressure throughout the respiratory cycle to keep the alveoli open and promote oxygenation. Providing CPAP during spontaneous breathing also offers the advantage of an alarm system and may reduce patient anxiety if the patient has been taught that the machine is keeping track of breathing. It also maintains lung volumes and improves the patient's oxygenation status. CPAP is often used in conjunction with PSV. Nurses should carefully assess for tachypnea, tachycardia, reduced tidal volumes, decreasing oxygen saturations, and increasing carbon dioxide levels.

When the patient can breathe spontaneously, weaning trials using a T-piece or tracheostomy mask (see Fig. 25-2) are normally conducted with the patient disconnected from the ventilator, receiving humidified oxygen only, and performing all work of breathing. Because patients do not have to overcome the resistance of the ventilator, they may find this mode more comfortable, or they may become anxious as they breathe with no support from the ventilator. During T-piece trials, the nurse monitors the patient closely and provides encouragement. This method of weaning is usually used when the patient is awake and alert, is breathing without difficulty, has good gag and cough reflexes, and is hemodynamically stable. During the weaning process, the patient is maintained on the same or a higher oxygen concentration than when receiving mechanical ventilation. While the patient is using the T-piece, he or she is observed for signs and symptoms of hypoxia, increasing respiratory muscle fatigue, or systemic fatigue. These include restlessness, increased respiratory rate (greater than 35 breaths/min), use of accessory muscles, tachycardia with premature ventricular contractions, and paradoxical chest movement (asynchronous breathing, chest contraction during inspiration and expansion during expiration). Fatigue or exhaustion is initially manifested by an increased respiratory rate associated with a gradual reduction in tidal volume; later there is a slowing of the respiratory rate.

If the patient appears to be tolerating the T-piece trial, a second set of arterial blood gas measurements is drawn 20 minutes after the patient has been on spontaneous ventilation at a constant $FiO_2$ pressure support ventilation. (Alveolar–arterial equilibration takes 15 to 20 minutes to occur.)

Signs of exhaustion and hypoxia correlated with deterioration in the blood gas measurements indicate the need for ventilatory support. The patient is placed back on the ventilator each time signs of fatigue or deterioration develop.

If clinically stable, the patient usually can be extubated within 2 or 3 hours after weaning and allowed spontaneous ventilation by means of a mask with humidified oxygen. Patients who have had prolonged ventilatory assistance usually require more gradual weaning; it may take days or even weeks. They are weaned primarily during the day and placed back on the ventilator at night to rest.

Because patients respond in different manners to the various weaning methods, there is no definitive way to assess

## CHART 25-15  Guidelines for Care of the Patient Being Weaned From Mechanical Ventilation

### ACTIONS

1. Assess patient for weaning criteria: Vital capacity—10 to 15 mL/kg
   Maximum inspiratory pressure (MIP) at least −20 cm $H_2O$
   Tidal volume—7 to 9 mL/kg
   Minute ventilation—6 L/min
   Rapid/shallow breathing index—below 100 breaths/minute/L
   $PaO_2$ greater than 60 mm Hg with $FiO_2$ less than 40%
2. Monitor activity level, assess dietary intake, and monitor results of laboratory tests of nutritional status.
3. Assess the patient's and family's understanding of the weaning process and address any concerns about the process. Explain that the patient may feel short of breath initially and provide encouragement as needed. Reassure the patient that he or she will be attended closely and that if the weaning attempt is not successful, it can be tried again later.
4. Implement the weaning method prescribed: A/C, IMV, SIMV, PSV, PAV, CPAP, or T-piece.
5. Monitor vital signs, pulse oximetry, ECG, and respiratory pattern constantly for the first 20 to 30 minutes and every 5 minutes after that until weaning is complete.
6. Maintain a patent airway; monitor arterial blood gas levels and pulmonary function tests. Suction the airway as needed.
7. In collaboration with the physician, terminate the weaning process if adverse reactions occur. These include a heart rate increase of 20 beats/min, systolic blood pressure increase of 20 mm Hg, a decrease in oxygen saturation to less than 90%, respiratory rate less than 8 or greater than 20 breaths/minute, ventricular dysrhythmias, fatigue, panic, cyanosis, erratic or labored breathing, paradoxical chest movement.
8. If the weaning process continues, measure tidal volume and minute ventilation every 20 to 30 minutes; compare with the patient's desired values, which have been determined in collaboration with the physician.
9. Assess for psychological dependence if the physiologic parameters indicate weaning is feasible and the patient still resists.

### RATIONALE

1. Careful assessment of multiple weaning indices helps to determine readiness for weaning. When the criteria have been met, the patient's likelihood of successful weaning increases.

2. Reestablishing independent spontaneous ventilation can be physically exhausting. It is crucial that the patient have enough energy reserves to succeed. Providing periods of rest and recommended nutritional intake can increase the likelihood of successful weaning.
3. The weaning process can be psychologically tiring; emotional support can help promote a sense of security. Explaining that weaning will be attempted again later helps reduce the sense of failure if the first attempts are unsuccessful.

4. The prescribed weaning method should reflect the patient's individualized criteria for weaning and weaning history. By having different methods to choose from, the physician can select the one that best fits the patient.
5. Monitoring the patient closely provides ongoing indications of success or failure.

6. These values can be compared to baseline measurements to evaluate weaning. Suctioning helps to reduce the risk of aspiration and maintain the airway.
7. These signs and symptoms indicate an unstable patient at risk for hypoxia and ventricular dysrhythmias. Continuing the weaning process can lead to cardiopulmonary arrest.

8. These values help to determine if weaning is successful and should be continued.

9. Psychological dependence is a common problem after mechanical ventilation. Possible causes include fear of dying and depression from chronic illness. It is important to address this issue before the next weaning attempt.

which method is best. Regardless of the weaning method being used, ongoing assessment of respiratory status is essential to monitor patient progress.

Successful weaning from the ventilator is supplemented by intensive pulmonary care. The following methods are used:

- Oxygen therapy
- Arterial blood gas evaluation
- Pulse oximetry
- Bronchodilator therapy
- CPT
- Adequate nutrition, hydration, and humidification
- Incentive spirometry

These patients still have borderline pulmonary function and need vigorous supportive therapy before their respiratory status returns to a level that supports activities of daily living.

### Weaning From the Tube

Weaning from the tube is considered when the patient can breathe spontaneously, maintain an adequate airway by effectively coughing up secretions, swallow, and move the jaw. If frequent suctioning is needed to clear secretions, tube weaning may be unsuccessful. Secretion clearance and aspiration risks are assessed to determine whether active pharyngeal and laryngeal reflexes are intact.

Once the patient can clear secretions adequately, a trial period of mouth breathing or nose breathing is conducted. This can be accomplished by several methods. The first method requires changing to a smaller size tube to increase the resistance to airflow or plugging the tracheostomy tube (deflating the cuff first). The smaller tube is sometimes replaced by a cuffless tracheostomy tube, which allows the tube to be plugged at lengthening intervals to monitor patient progress. A second method involves changing to a fenestrated tube (a tube with an opening or window in its bend). This permits air to flow around and through the tube to the upper airway and enables talking. A third method involves switching to a smaller tracheostomy button (stoma button). A tracheostomy button is a plastic tube approximately 1 inch long that helps keep the windpipe open after the larger tracheostomy tube has been removed. Finally, when the patient demonstrates the ability to maintain a patent airway, the tube can be removed. An occlusive dressing is placed over the stoma, which heals in several days to weeks.

### Weaning From Oxygen

The patient who has been successfully weaned from the ventilator, cuff, and tube and has adequate respiratory function is then weaned from oxygen. The $FiO_2$ is gradually reduced until the $PaO_2$ is in the range of 70 to 100 mm Hg while the patient is breathing room air. If the $PaO_2$ is less than 70 mm Hg on room air, supplemental oxygen is recommended. To be eligible for financial reimbursement from the Centers for Medicare and Medicaid Services for in-home oxygen, the patient must have a $PaO_2$ of less than 55 mm Hg while awake and at rest.

### Nutrition

Success in weaning the long-term ventilator-dependent patient requires early and aggressive but judicious nutritional support. The respiratory muscles (diaphragm and especially intercostals) become weak or atrophied after just a few days of mechanical ventilation and may be catabolized for energy, especially if nutrition is inadequate. Because the metabolism of fat produces less carbon dioxide than the metabolism of carbohydrate, a high-fat diet may assist patients with respiratory failure, both during mechanical ventilation and while being weaned (Baudouin & Evans, 2003). The evidence on the value of a limited carbohydrate intake versus a carbohydrate-enriched diet is contradictory (Goris, Vermeeren, Wouters, et al., 2003). A high-fat diet may provide as much as 50% of the total daily kilocalories. Adequate protein intake is important in increasing respiratory muscle strength. Protein intake should be approximately 25% of total daily kilocalories, or 1.2 to 1.5 g/kg/day. Care must be taken not to overfeed the patient, because excessive intake can increase the demand for oxygen and the production of carbon dioxide. Daily nutrition should be closely monitored.

Soon after the patient is admitted, a consultation with a dietitian or nutrition support team should be arranged to plan the best form of nutritional replacement. Adequate nutrition may decrease the duration of mechanical ventilation and prevent other complications, especially sepsis. Sepsis can occur if bacteria enter the bloodstream and release toxins that, in turn, cause vasodilation and hypotension, fever, tachycardia, increased respiratory rate, and coma. Aggressive treatment of sepsis is essential to reverse this threat to survival and to promote weaning from the ventilator when the patient's condition improves. Optimal nutritional intake is an essential part of the treatment of sepsis.

# The Patient Undergoing Thoracic Surgery

Assessment and management are particularly important for the patient undergoing thoracic surgery. Frequently, patients undergoing such surgery also have obstructive pulmonary disease with compromised breathing. Preoperative preparation and careful postoperative management are crucial for successful patient outcomes, because these patients may have a narrow range between their physical tolerance for certain activities and their limitations, which, if exceeded, can lead to distress. Various types of thoracic surgical procedures are performed to relieve disease conditions such as lung abscesses, lung cancer, cysts, benign tumors, and emphysema (Chart 25-16). An exploratory **thoracotomy** (creation of a surgical opening into the thoracic cavity) may be performed to diagnose lung or chest disease. A biopsy may be performed in this procedure with a small amount of lung tissue removed for analysis; the chest incision is then closed.

The objectives of preoperative care for the patient undergoing thoracic surgery are to ascertain the patient's

## CHART 25-16 Thoracic Surgeries and Procedures

### PNEUMONECTOMY
The removal of an entire lung (pneumonectomy) is performed chiefly for cancer when the lesion cannot be removed by a less extensive procedure. It also may be performed for lung abscesses, bronchiectasis, or extensive unilateral tuberculosis. The removal of the right lung is more dangerous than the removal of the left, because the right lung has a larger vascular bed and its removal imposes a greater physiologic burden.

A posterolateral or anterolateral thoracotomy incision is made, sometimes with resection of a rib. The pulmonary artery and the pulmonary veins are ligated and severed. The main bronchus is divided and the lung removed. The bronchial stump is stapled, and usually no drains are used because the accumulation of fluid in the empty hemithorax prevents mediastinal shift.

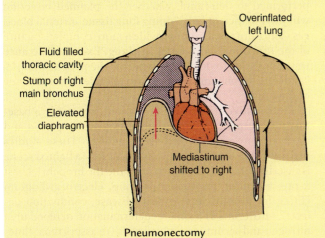

Pneumonectomy

### LOBECTOMY
When the pathology is limited to one area of a lung, a lobectomy (removal of a lobe of a lung) is performed. Lobectomy, which is more common than pneumonectomy, may be carried out for bronchogenic carcinoma, giant emphysematous blebs or bullae, benign tumors, metastatic malignant tumors, bronchiectasis, and fungus infections.

The surgeon makes a thoracotomy incision: its exact location depends on the lobe to be resected. When the pleural space is entered, the involved lung collapses and the lobar vessels and the bronchus are ligated and divided. After the lobe is removed, the remaining lobes of the lung are reexpanded. Usually, two chest catheters are inserted for drainage. The upper tube is for air removal; the lower one is for fluid drainage. Sometimes, only one catheter is needed. The chest tube is connected to a chest drainage apparatus for several days.

Lobectomy

### SEGMENTECTOMY (SEGMENTAL RESECTION)
Some lesions are located in only one segment of the lung. Bronchopulmonary segments are subdivisions of the lung that function as individual units. They are held together by delicate connective tissue. Disease processes may be limited to a single segment. Care is used to preserve as much healthy and functional lung tissue as possible, especially in patients who already have limited cardiopulmonary reserve. Single segments can be removed from any lobe; the right middle lobe, which has only two small segments, invariably is removed entirely. On the left side, corresponding to a middle lobe, is a "lingular" segment of the upper lobe. This can be removed as a single segment or by lingulectomy. This segment frequently is involved in bronchiectasis.

### WEDGE RESECTION
A wedge resection of a small, well-circumscribed lesion may be performed without regard for the location of the intersegmental planes. The pleural cavity usually is drained because of the possibility of an air or blood leak. This procedure is performed for diagnostic lung biopsy and for the excision of small peripheral nodules.

### BRONCHOPLASTIC OR SLEEVE RESECTION
Bronchoplastic resection is a procedure in which only one lobar bronchus, together with a part of the right or left bronchus, is excised. The distal bronchus is reanastomosed to the proximal bronchus or trachea.

### LUNG VOLUME REDUCTION
Lung volume reduction is a surgical procedure involving the removal of 20% to 30% of a patient's lung through a midsternal incision or video thoracoscopy. The diseased lung tissue is identified on a lung perfusion scan. This surgery leads to significant improvements in dyspnea, exercise capacity, quality of life, and survival of a subgroup of people with end-stage emphysema (Naunheim, 2004).

*continued >*

## CHART 25-16 Thoracic Surgeries and Procedures, continued

**VIDEO THORACOSCOPY**
A video thoracoscopy is an endoscopic procedure that allows the surgeon to look into the thorax without making a large incision. The procedure is performed to obtain specimens of tissue for biopsy, to treat recurrent spontaneous pneumothorax, and to diagnose either pleural effusions or pleural masses.

Thoracoscopy has also been found to be an effective diagnostic and therapeutic alternative for the treatment of mediastinal disorders (Cirino, Campos, Jatene, et al., 2000). Some advantages of video thoracoscopy are rapid diagnosis and treatment of some conditions, a decrease in postoperative complications, and a shortened hospital stay (see Chapter 21).

---

functional reserve, to determine whether the patient is likely to survive and recover from the surgery and to ensure that the patient is in optimal condition for surgery.

## Preoperative Management

### Assessment and Diagnostic Findings

The nurse performs chest auscultation to assess breath sounds in all regions of the lungs (see Chapter 21). It is important to note whether breath sounds are normal, indicating a free flow of air in and out of the lungs. (In the patient with emphysema, the breath sounds may be markedly decreased or even absent on auscultation.) The nurse notes crackles and wheezes and assesses for hyperresonance and decreased diaphragmatic motion. Unilateral diminished breath sounds and rhonchi can be the result of occlusion of the bronchi by mucus plugs. The nurse assesses for retained secretions during auscultation by asking the patient to cough. It is important to note any signs of rhonchi or wheezing. The patient history and assessment should include the following questions:

- What signs and symptoms (cough, sputum expectorated [amount and color], hemoptysis, chest pain, dyspnea) are present?
- If there is a smoking history, how long has the patient smoked? Does the patient smoke currently? How many packs a day?
- What is the patient's cardiopulmonary tolerance while resting, eating, bathing, and walking?
- What is the patient's breathing pattern? How much exertion is required to produce dyspnea?
- Does the patient need to sleep in an upright position or with more than two pillows?
- What is the patient's general physiologic status (eg, general appearance, mental alertness, behavior, nutritional status)?
- What other medical conditions exist (eg, allergies, cardiac disorders, diabetes)?

A number of tests are performed to determine the patient's preoperative status and to assess the patient's physical assets and limitations. Many patients are seen by their surgeons in the office, and many tests and examinations are performed on an outpatient basis. The decision to perform any pulmonary resection is based on the patient's cardiovascular status and pulmonary reserve. Pulmonary function studies (especially lung volume and vital capacity) are performed to determine whether the planned resection will leave sufficient functioning lung tissue. Arterial blood gas values are assessed to provide a more complete picture of the functional capacity of the lung. Exercise tolerance tests are useful to determine whether the patient who is a candidate for pneumonectomy can tolerate removal of one of the lungs.

Preoperative studies are performed to provide a baseline for comparison during the postoperative period and to detect any unsuspected abnormalities. These studies may include a bronchoscopic examination (a lighted scope is inserted into the airways to examine the bronchi), chest x-ray, magnetic resonance imaging, electrocardiogram (ECG; for arteriosclerotic heart disease, conduction defects), nutritional assessment, determination of blood urea nitrogen and serum creatinine levels (to assess renal function), determination of glucose tolerance or blood glucose level (to check for diabetes), assessment of serum electrolytes and protein levels, blood volume determinations, and complete blood cell count.

### Preoperative Nursing Management

**IMPROVING AIRWAY CLEARANCE**
The underlying lung condition often is associated with increased respiratory secretions. Before surgery, the airway is cleared of secretions to reduce the possibility of postoperative atelectasis or infection. Risk factors for postoperative atelectasis and pneumonia are listed in Chart 25-17. Strategies to reduce the risk for atelectasis and infection include humidification, postural drainage, and chest percussion after bronchodilators are administered, if prescribed. The nurse estimates the volume of sputum if the patient expectorates large amounts of secretions. Such measurements are carried out to determine whether and when the amount decreases. Antibiotics are

## CHART 25-17  Risk Factors for Surgery-Related Atelectasis and Pneumonia

**PREOPERATIVE RISK FACTORS**
- Increased age
- Obesity
- Poor nutritional status
- Smoking history
- Abnormal pulmonary function tests
- Preexisting lung disease
- Emergency surgery
- History of aspiration
- Comorbid states
- Preexisting disability

**INTRAOPERATIVE RISK FACTORS**
- Thoracic incision
- Prolonged anesthesia

**POSTOPERATIVE RISK FACTORS**
- Immobilization
- Supine position
- Decreased level of consciousness
- Inadequate pain management
- Prolonged intubation/mechanical ventilation
- Presence of nasogastric tube
- Inadequate preoperative education

---

administered as prescribed for infection, which may be causing the excessive secretions.

### TEACHING THE PATIENT

Increasingly, patients are admitted on the day of surgery, which does not provide much time for the acute care nurse to talk with the patient. Nurses in all settings must take an active role in educating the patient and relieving anxiety. The nurse informs the patient what to expect, from administration of anesthesia to thoracotomy and the likely use of chest tubes and a drainage system in the postoperative period. The patient is also informed about the usual postoperative administration of oxygen to facilitate breathing and the possible use of a ventilator. It is essential to explain the importance of frequent turning to promote drainage of lung secretions. Instruction in the use of incentive spirometry begins before surgery to familiarize the patient with its correct use. The nurse teaches diaphragmatic and pursed-lip breathing, and the patient should begin practicing these techniques (see Charts 25-3 and 25-4).

Because a coughing schedule is necessary in the postoperative period to promote the clearance or removal of secretions, the nurse instructs the patient in the technique of coughing and warns the patient that the coughing routine may be uncomfortable. The nurse teaches the patient to splint the incision with the hands, a pillow, or a folded towel (see Chart 25-5).

Another technique, "huffing," may be helpful for the patient with diminished expiratory flow rates or for the patient who refuses to cough because of severe pain. Huffing is the expulsion of air through an open glottis. This type of forced expiration technique (FET) stimulates pulmonary expansion and assists in alveolar inflation. The nurse instructs the patient as follows:

- Take a deep diaphragmatic breath and exhale forcefully against your hand in a quick, distinct pant, or huff.
- Practice doing small huffs and progress to one strong huff during exhalation.

Patients should be informed preoperatively that blood and other fluids may be administered, oxygen will be administered, and vital signs will be checked often for several hours after surgery. If a chest tube is needed, the patient should be informed that it will drain the fluid and air that normally accumulate after chest surgery. The patient and family are informed that the patient may be admitted to the intensive care unit for 1 to 2 days after surgery, that the patient may experience pain at the incision site, and that medication is available to relieve pain and discomfort.

### RELIEVING ANXIETY

The nurse listens to the patient to evaluate his or her feelings about the illness and proposed treatment. The nurse also determines the patient's motivation to return to normal or baseline function. The patient may reveal significant concerns: fear of hemorrhage because of bloody sputum, fear of discomfort from a chronic cough and chest pain, fear of ventilator dependence, or fear of death because of dyspnea and the underlying disease (eg, tumor).

The nurse helps the patient to overcome these fears and to cope with the stress of surgery by correcting any misconceptions, supporting the patient's decision to undergo surgery, reassuring the patient that the incision will "hold," and dealing honestly with questions about pain and discomfort and their treatment. The management and control of pain begin before surgery, when the nurse informs the patient that many postoperative problems can be overcome by following certain routines related to deep breathing, coughing, turning, and moving. If patient-controlled analgesia (PCA) or epidural analgesia is to be used after surgery, the nurse instructs the patient in its use.

## Postoperative Management

After surgery, the vital signs are checked frequently. Oxygen is administered by a mechanical ventilator, nasal cannula, or mask for as long as necessary. A reduction in lung capacity requires a period of physiologic adjustment, and fluids may be given at a low hourly rate to prevent fluid overload and pulmonary edema. After the patient is conscious and the vital signs have stabilized, the head of the bed may be elevated 30 to 45 degrees. Careful positioning of the patient is important. After pneumonectomy, a patient is usually turned every hour from the back to the operative side and should not be completely turned to the unoperated side. This allows the fluid left in the space to consolidate and prevents the remaining lung and the heart from shifting (mediastinal shift) toward the operative side. The patient with a lobectomy may be turned to either side, and a patient with a segmental resection usually is not turned onto the operative side unless the surgeon prescribes this position.

Medication for pain is needed for several days after surgery. Because coughing can be painful, the patient should be taught to splint the chest. Exercises are resumed early in the postoperative period to facilitate lung ventilation. The nurse assesses for signs of complications, including cyanosis, dyspnea, and acute chest pain. These may indicate atelectasis and should be reported immediately. Increased temperature or white blood cell count may indicate an infection, and pallor and increased pulse may indicate internal hemorrhage. Dressings are assessed for fresh bleeding.

## Mechanical Ventilation

Depending on the nature of the surgery, the patient's underlying condition, the intraoperative course, and the depth of anesthesia, the patient may require mechanical ventilation after surgery. The physician is responsible for determining the ventilator settings and modes, as well as determining the overall method and pace of weaning. However, the physician, nurse, and respiratory therapist work together closely to assess the patient's tolerance and weaning progress. Early extubation from mechanical ventilation can also lead to earlier removal of arterial lines.

## Chest Drainage

A crucial intervention for improving gas exchange and breathing in the postoperative period is the proper management of chest drainage and the **chest drainage system**. After thoracic surgery, chest tubes and a closed drainage system are used to re-expand the involved lung and to remove excess air, fluid, and blood. Chest drainage systems also are used in treatment of spontaneous pneumothorax and trauma resulting in pneumothorax. Table 25-3 describes and compares the main features of these systems. Management of chest drainage systems is explained in Chart 25-18. Prevention of cardiopulmonary complications after thoracic surgery is discussed in Chart 25-19.

The normal breathing mechanism operates on the principle of negative pressure; that is, the pressure in the chest

### TABLE 25-3  Comparison of Chest Drainage Systems*

| Types of Chest Drainage Systems | Description | Comments |
|---|---|---|
| **Traditional Water Seal** | | |
| Also referred to as wet suction | Has three chambers: a collection chamber, water seal chamber (middle chamber), and wet suction control chamber | Requires that sterile fluid be instilled into water seal and suction chambers<br>Has positive- and negative-pressure release valves<br>Intermittent bubbling indicates that the system is functioning properly<br>Additional suction can be added by connecting system to a suction source |
| **Dry Suction Water Seal** | | |
| Also referred to as dry suction | Has three chambers: a collection chamber, water seal chamber (middle chamber), and wet suction control chamber | Requires that sterile fluid be instilled in water seal chamber at 2-cm level<br>No need to fill suction chamber with fluid<br>Suction pressure is set with a regulator<br>Has positive- and negative-pressure release valves<br>Has an indicator to signify that the suction pressure is adequate<br>Quieter than traditional water seal systems |
| **Dry Suction** | | |
| Also referred to as one-way valve system | Has a one-way mechanical value that allows air to leave the chest and prevents air from moving back into the chest | No need to fill suction chamber with fluid; thus, can be set up quickly in an emergency<br>Works even if knocked over, making it ideal for patients who are ambulatory |

*If no fluid drainage is expected, a drainage collection device may not be needed.

## CHART 25-18 Guidelines for Managing Chest Drainage Systems

| ACTIONS | RATIONALE |
|---|---|
| 1. If using a chest drainage system with a water seal, fill the water seal chamber with sterile water to the level specified by the manufacturer. | Water seal drainage allows air and fluid to escape into a drainage chamber. The water acts as a seal and keeps the air from being drawn back into the pleural space. The water level regulator dial setting determines the degree of suction applied. |
| 2. When using suction in chest drainage systems with a water seal, fill the suction control chamber with sterile water to the 20-cm level or as prescribed. In systems without a water seal, set the regulator dial at the appropriate suction level. | |
| 3. Attach the drainage catheter exiting the thoracic cavity to the tubing coming from the collection chamber. Tape securely with adhesive tape. | In chest drainage units, the system is closed. The only connection is the one to the patient's catheter. |
| 4. If suction is used, connect the suction control chamber tubing to the suction unit. If using a wet suction system, turn on the suction unit and increase pressure until slow but steady bubbling appears in the suction control chamber. If using a chest drainage system with a dry suction control chamber, turn the regulator dial to 20 cm H$_2$O. | With a wet suction system, the degree of suction is determined by the amount of water in the suction control chamber and is not dependent on the rate of bubbling or the pressure gauge setting on the suction unit. With a dry suction control chamber, the regulator dial replaces the water. |

Example of a disposable chest drainage system.

| | |
|---|---|
| 5. Mark the drainage from the collection chamber with tape on the outside of the drainage unit. Mark hourly/daily increments (date and time) at the drainage level. | This marking shows the amount of fluid loss and how fast fluid is collecting in the drainage chamber. It serves as a basis for determining the need for blood replacement, if the fluid is blood. Visibly bloody drainage will appear in the chamber in the immediate postoperative period but should gradually becomes serous. If the patient is bleeding as heavily as 100 mL every 15 minutes, check the drainage every few minutes. A reoperation or autotransfusion may be needed. The transfusion of blood collected in the drainage chamber must be reinfused within 4 to 6 hours. Usually, however, drainage decreases progressively in the first 24 hours. |

*continued >*

## CHART 25-18 Guidelines for Managing Chest Drainage Systems, continued

| ACTIONS | RATIONALE |
|---|---|
| 6. Ensure that the drainage tubing does not kink, loop, or interfere with the patient's movements. | Kinking, looping, or pressure on the drainage tubing can produce back-pressure, which may force fluid back into the pleural space or impede its drainage. |
| 7. Encourage the patient to assume a comfortable position with good body alignment. With the lateral position, make sure that the patient's body does not compress the tubing. The patient should be turned and repositioned every 1.5 to 2 hours. Provide adequate analgesia. | Frequent position changes promote drainage, and good body alignment helps prevent postural deformities and contractures. Proper positioning also helps breathing and promotes better air exchange. Analgesics may be needed to promote comfort. |
| 8. Assist the patient with range-of-motion exercises for the affected arm and shoulder several times daily. Provide adequate analgesia. | Exercise helps to prevent ankylosis of the shoulder and to reduce postoperative pain and discomfort. Analgesics may be needed to relieve pain. |
| 9. Gently "milk" the tubing in the direction of the drainage chamber as needed. | "Milking" prevents the tubing from becoming obstructed by clots and fibrin. Constant attention to maintaining the patency of the tube facilitates prompt expansion of the lung and minimizes complications. |
| 10. Make sure there is fluctuation ("tidaling") of the fluid level in the water seal chamber (in wet systems), or check the air leak indicator for leaks (in dry systems with a one-way valve). *Note:* Fluid fluctuations in the water seal chamber or air leak indicator area will stop when:<br>a. The lung has reexpanded<br>b. The tubing is obstructed by blood clots, fibrin, or kinks<br>c. A loop of tubing hangs below the rest of the tubing<br>d. Suction motor or wall suction is not working properly | Fluctuation of the water level in the water seal shows effective connection between the pleural cavity and the drainage chamber and indicates that the drainage system remains patent. Fluctuation is also a gauge of intrapleural pressure in systems with a water seal (wet and dry, but not with the one-way valve).<br>An air leak indicator shows changes in intrathoracic pressure in dry systems with a one-way valve. Bubbles will appear if a leak is present. The air leak indicator takes the place of fluid fluctuations in the water seal chamber. |
| 11. With a dry system, assess for the presence of the indicator (bellows or float device) when setting the regulator dial to the desired level of suction. | The indicator shows that the vacuum is adequate to maintain the desired level of suction. |
| 12. Observe for air leaks in the drainage system; they are indicated by constant bubbling in the water seal chamber, or by the air leak indicator in dry systems with a one-way valve. Also assess the chest tube system for correctable external leaks. Notify the physician immediately of excessive bubbling in the water seal chamber not due to external leaks. | Leaking and trapping of air in the pleural space can result in tension pneumothorax. |
| 13. When turning down the dry suction, depress the manual high-negativity vent, and assess for a rise in the water level of the water seal chamber. | A rise in the water level of the water seal chamber indicates high negative pressure in the system that could lead to increased intrathoracic pressure. |
| 14. Observe and immediately report rapid and shallow breathing, cyanosis, pressure in the chest, subcutaneous emphysema, symptoms of hemorrhage, or significant changes in vital signs. | Many clinical conditions can cause these signs and symptoms, including tension pneumothorax, mediastinal shift, hemorrhage, severe incisional pain, pulmonary embolus, and cardiac tamponade. Surgical intervention may be necessary. |
| 15. Encourage the patient to breathe deeply and cough at frequent intervals. Provide adequate analgesia. If needed, request an order for patient-controlled analgesia. Also teach the patient how to perform incentive spirometry. | Deep breathing and coughing help to raise the intrapleural pressure, which promotes drainage of accumulated fluid in the pleural space. Deep breathing and coughing also promote removal of secretions from the tracheobronchial tree, which in turn promotes lung expansion and prevents atelectasis (alveolar collapse). |

## CHART 25-18 Guidelines for Managing Chest Drainage Systems, continued

| ACTIONS | RATIONALE |
|---|---|
| 16. If the patient is lying on a stretcher and must be transported to another area, place the drainage system below the chest level. If the tubing disconnects, cut off the contaminated tips of the chest tube and tubing, insert a sterile connector in the cut ends, and reattach to the drainage system. Do *not* clamp the chest tube during transport. | The drainage apparatus must be kept at a level lower than the patient's chest to prevent fluid from flowing backward into the pleural space. Clamping can result in a tension pneumothorax. |
| 17. When assisting in the chest tube's removal, instruct the patient to perform a gentle Valsalva maneuver or to breathe quietly. The chest tube is then clamped and quickly removed. Simultaneously, a small bandage is applied and made airtight with petrolatum gauze covered by a 4 × 4-inch gauze pad and thoroughly covered and sealed with nonporous tape. | The chest tube is removed as directed when the lung is reexpanded (usually 24 hours to several days), depending on the cause of the pneumothorax. During tube removal, the chief priorities are preventing air from entering the pleural cavity as the tube is withdrawn and preventing infection. |

## CHART 25-19

### Preventing Postoperative Cardiopulmonary Complications After Thoracic Surgery

**PATIENT MANAGEMENT**

- Auscultate lung sounds and assess for rate, rhythm, and depth.
- Monitor oxygenation with pulse oximetry.
- Monitor electrocardiogram for rate and rhythm changes.
- Assess capillary refill, skin color, and status of the surgical dressing.
- Encourage and assist the patient to turn, cough, and take deep breaths.

**CHEST DRAINAGE MANAGEMENT**

- Verify that all connection tubes are patent and connected securely.
- Assess that the water seal is intact when using a wet suction system and assess the regulator dial in dry suction systems.
- Monitor characteristics of drainage including color, amount, and consistency. Assess for significant increases or decreases in drainage output.
- Note fluctuations in the water seal chamber for wet suction systems and the air leak indicator for dry suction systems.
- Keep system below the patient's chest level.
- Assess suction control chamber for bubbling in wet suction systems.
- Keep suction at prescribed level.
- Maintain appropriate fluid in water seal for wet suction systems.
- Keep air vent open when suction is off.

cavity normally is lower than the pressure of the atmosphere, causing air to move into the lungs during inspiration. Whenever the chest is opened, there is a loss of negative pressure, which can result in collapse of the lung. The collection of air, fluid, or other substances in the chest can compromise cardiopulmonary function and can also cause the lung to collapse. Pathologic substances that collect in the pleural space include fibrin or clotted blood, liquids (serous fluids, blood, pus, chyle), and gases (air from the lung, tracheobronchial tree, or esophagus).

Chest tubes may be inserted to drain fluid or air from any of the three compartments of the thorax (the right and left pleural spaces and the mediastinum). The pleural space, located between the visceral and parietal pleura, normally contains 20 mL or less of fluid, which helps lubricate the visceral and parietal pleura. Surgical incision of the chest wall almost always causes some degree of pneumothorax (air accumulating in the pleural space) or hemo-thorax (buildup of serous fluid or blood in the pleural space). Air and fluid collect in the pleural space, restricting lung expansion and reducing gas exchange. Placement of a chest tube in the pleural space restores the negative intrathoracic pressure needed for lung re-expansion after surgery or trauma.

The mediastinal space is an extrapleural space that lies between the right and left thoracic cavities and contains the large blood vessels, heart, mainstem bronchus, and thymus gland. If fluid accumulates here, the heart can become compressed and stop beating, causing death. Mediastinal chest tubes can be inserted either anteriorly or posteriorly to the heart to drain blood after surgery.

There are two types of chest tubes: small-bore and large-bore catheters. Small-bore catheters (7F to 12F) have a one-way valve apparatus to prevent air from moving back into the patient. They can be inserted through a small skin incision. Large-bore catheters, which range in size up to 40F, are usually connected to a chest drainage system to collect any pleural fluid and monitor for air leaks. After the chest tube is positioned, it is sutured to the skin and connected to a drainage apparatus (Fig. 25-10) to remove the residual air and fluid from the pleural or mediastinal space. This results in the re-expansion of remaining lung tissue.

### CHEST DRAINAGE SYSTEMS

Chest drainage systems have a suction source, a collection chamber for pleural drainage, and a mechanism to prevent air from reentering the chest with inhalation. Various types of chest drainage systems are available for use in removal of air and fluid from the pleural space and re-expansion of the lungs. Chest drainage systems come with either wet (water seal) or dry suction control. In wet suction systems, the amount of suction is determined by the amount of water instilled in the suction chamber. The amount of bubbling in the suction chamber indicates how strong the suction is. Wet systems use

**FIGURE 25-10.** Chest drainage systems. (**A**) The Atrium Ocean is an example of a water seal chest drain system composed of a drainage chamber and water seal chamber. The suction control is determined by the height of the water column in that chamber (usually 20 cm). *A*, suction control chamber; *B*, water seal chamber; *C*, air leak zone; *D*, collection chamber. (**B**) The Atrium Oasis is an example of a dry suction water seal system that uses a mechanical regulator for vacuum control, a water seal chamber, and a drainage chamber. *A*, dry suction regulator; *B*, water seal chamber; *C*, air leak monitor; *D*, collection chamber; *E*, suction monitor bellows. Art redrawn with permission from Atrium Medical Corporation, Hudson, NH. Reprinted from Morton P. G., Fontaine, D. K., Hudak, C. M., et al. (2005). *Critical care nursing: A holistic approach* (8th ed.). Philadelphia: Lippincott Williams & Wilkins.

a water seal to prevent air from moving back into the chest on inspiration. Dry systems use a one-way valve and may have a suction control dial in place of the water. Both systems can operate by gravity drainage, without a suction source.

**Water Seal Systems.** The traditional water seal system (or wet suction) for chest drainage has three chambers: a collection chamber, a water seal chamber, and a wet suction control chamber. The collection chamber acts as a reservoir for fluid draining from the chest tube. It is graduated to permit easy measurement of drainage. Suction may be added to create negative pressure and promote drainage of fluid and removal of air. The suction control chamber regulates the amount of negative pressure applied to the chest. The amount of suction is determined by the water level. It is usually set at 20-cm $H_2O$; adding more fluid results in more suction. After the suction is turned on, bubbling appears in the suction chamber. A positive-pressure valve is located at the top of the suction chamber that automatically opens with increases in positive pressure within the system. Air is automatically released through a positive-pressure relief valve if the suction tubing is inadvertently clamped or kinked.

The water seal chamber has a one-way valve or water seal that prevents air from moving back into the chest when the patient inhales. There is an increase in the water level with inspiration and a return to the baseline level during exhalation; this is referred to as tidaling. Intermittent bubbling in the water seal chamber is normal, but continuous bubbling can indicate an air leak. Bubbling and tidaling do not occur when the tube is placed in the mediastinal space; however, fluid may pulsate with the patient's heartbeat. If the chest tube is connected to gravity drainage only, suction is not used. The pressure is equal to the water seal only. Two-chamber chest drainage systems (water seal chamber and collection chamber) are available for use with patients who need only gravity drainage.

The water level in the water seal chamber reflects the negative pressure present in the intrathoracic cavity. A rise in the water level indicates negative pressure in the pleural or mediastinal space. Excessive negative pressure can cause trauma to tissue. Most chest drainage systems have an automatic means to prevent excessive negative pressure. By pressing and holding a manual high-negativity vent (usually located on the top of the chest drainage system) until the water level in the water seal chamber returns to the 2-cm mark, excessive negative pressure is avoided, preventing damage to tissue.

> **NURSING ALERT**
>
> When the wall vacuum is turned off, the drainage system must be open to the atmosphere so that intrapleural air can escape from the system. This can be done by detaching the tubing from the suction port to provide a vent.

> **NURSING ALERT**
>
> If the chest tube and drainage system become disconnected, air can enter the pleural space, producing a pneumothorax. To prevent pneumothorax if the chest tube is inadvertently disconnected from the drainage system, a temporary water seal can be established by immersing the chest tube's open end in a bottle of sterile water.

**Dry Suction Water Seal Systems.** Dry suction water seal systems, also referred to as dry suction, have a collection chamber for drainage, a water seal chamber, and a dry suction control chamber. The water seal chamber is filled with water to the 2-cm level. Bubbling in this area can indicate an air leak. The dry suction control chamber contains a regulator dial that conveniently regulates vacuum to the chest drain. Water is not needed for suction in these systems. Without the bubbling in the suction chamber, the machine is quieter. However, if the container is knocked over, the water seal may be lost.

Once the tube is connected to the suction source, the regulator dial allows the desired level of suction to be dialed in; the suction is increased until an indicator appears. The indicator has the same function as the bubbling in the traditional water seal system; that is, it indicates that the vacuum is adequate to maintain the desired level of suction. Some drainage systems use a bellows (a chamber that can be expanded or contracted) or an orange-colored float device as an indicator of when the suction control regulator is set.

When the water in the water seal rises above the 2-cm level, intrathoracic pressure increases. Dry suction water seal systems have a manual high-negativity vent located on top of the drain. The manual high-negativity vent is pressed until the indicator appears (either a float device or bellows) and the water level in the water seal returns to the desired level, indicating that the intrathoracic pressure is decreased.

> **NURSING ALERT**
>
> The manual vent should not be used to lower the water level in the water seal when the patient is on gravity drainage (no suction) because intrathoracic pressure is equal to the pressure in the water seal.

**Dry Suction Systems with a One-Way Valve.** A third type of chest drainage system is dry suction with a one-way mechanical valve. This system has a collection chamber, a one-way mechanical valve, and a dry suction control chamber. The valve permits air and fluid to leave the chest but prevents their movement back into the pleural space. This model lacks a water seal chamber and therefore can be set up quickly in emergency situations, and the dry control drain still works even if it is knocked over. This makes the dry suction systems useful for the patient who is ambulating or being transported. However, without the water seal chamber, there is no way to tell by inspection whether the pressure in the chest has changed, even though an air leak indicator is present so that the system can be checked. If an air leak is suspected, 30 mL of water is injected into the air leak indicator or the container is tipped so that fluid enters the air leak detection chamber. Bubbles will appear if a leak is present.

If the chest tube has been inserted to re-expand a lung after pneumothorax, or if very little fluid drainage is expected, a one-way valve (Heimlich valve) may be connected to the chest tube. This valve may be attached to a collection bag (Fig. 25-11) or covered with a sterile dressing if no drainage is expected.

## Nursing Process

## The Patient Undergoing Thoracic Surgery

### Postoperative Assessment

The nurse monitors the heart rate and rhythm by auscultation and ECG, because episodes of major dysrhythmias are common after thoracic and cardiac surgery. In the immediate postoperative period, an arterial line may be maintained to allow frequent monitoring of arterial blood gases, serum electrolytes, hemoglobin and hematocrit values, and arterial pressure. Central venous pressure may be monitored to detect early signs of fluid volume disturbances; however, central venous pressure monitoring devices are being used less than in the past. Early extubation from mechanical ventilation can also lead to earlier removal of arterial lines. Another important component of postoperative assessment is to note the results of the preoperative evaluation of the patient's lung reserve by pulmonary function testing. A preoperative $FEV_1$ (the volume of air that the patient can forcibly exhale in 1 second) of more than 2 L or more than 70% of predicted value indicates a good lung reserve. Patients who have a postoperative $FEV_1$ of less than 40% of predicted value have decreased tidal volume, which places them at risk for respiratory failure, other morbidity, and death.

### Diagnosis

#### Nursing Diagnoses

Based on the assessment data, the patient's major postoperative nursing diagnoses may include:

- Impaired gas exchange related to lung impairment and surgery
- Ineffective airway clearance related to lung impairment, anesthesia, and pain
- Acute pain related to incision, drainage tubes, and the surgical procedure
- Impaired physical mobility of the upper extremities related to thoracic surgery
- Risk for imbalanced fluid volume related to the surgical procedure
- Imbalanced nutrition, less than body requirements related to dyspnea and anorexia
- Deficient knowledge about self-care procedures at home

#### Collaborative Problems/ Potential Complications

Based on assessment data, potential complications may include the following:

- Respiratory distress
- Dysrhythmias
- Atelectasis, pneumothorax, and bronchopleural fistula
- Blood loss and hemorrhage
- Pulmonary edema

### Planning and Goals

The major goals for the patient may include improvement of gas exchange and breathing, improvement

**FIGURE 25-11.** One-way (Heimlich) valve, a disposable, single-use chest drainage system with 30 mL collection volume. Used when minimal volume of chest drainage is expected.

of airway clearance, relief of pain and discomfort, increased arm and shoulder mobility, maintenance of adequate fluid volume and nutritional status, understanding of self-care procedures, and absence of complications.

## Nursing Interventions

### Improving Gas Exchange and Breathing

Gas exchange is determined by evaluating oxygenation and ventilation. In the immediate postoperative period, this is achieved by measuring vital signs (blood pressure, pulse, and respirations) at least every 15 minutes for the first 1 to 2 hours, then less frequently as the patient's condition stabilizes.

Pulse oximetry is used for continuous monitoring of the adequacy of oxygenation. It is important to draw blood for arterial blood gas measurements early in the postoperative period, to establish a baseline to assess the adequacy of oxygenation and ventilation and the possible retention of carbon dioxide. The frequency with which postoperative arterial blood gases are measured depends on whether the patient is mechanically ventilated and whether he or she exhibits signs of respiratory distress; these measurements can help determine appropriate therapy. It also is common practice for patients to have an arterial line in place to obtain blood for blood gas measurements and to monitor blood pressure closely. Hemodynamic monitoring may be used to assess hemodynamic stability.

Breathing techniques, such as diaphragmatic and pursed-lip breathing, that were taught before surgery should be performed by the patient every 2 hours to expand the alveoli and prevent atelectasis. Another technique to improve ventilation is sustained maximal inspiration therapy or incentive spirometry. This technique promotes lung inflation, improves the cough mechanism, and allows early assessment of acute pulmonary changes. (See Charts 25-3 and 25-4 for more information.)

Positioning also improves breathing. If the patient is oriented and blood pressure is stabilized, the head of the bed is elevated 30 to 40 degrees during the immediate postoperative period. This facilitates ventilation, promotes chest drainage from the lower chest tube, and helps residual air to rise in the upper portion of the pleural space, where it can be removed through the upper chest tube.

The nurse consults with the surgeon about patient positioning. There is controversy regarding the best side-lying position. In general, the patient should be positioned from back to side frequently and moved from a flat to a semiupright position as soon as tolerated. Most commonly, the patient is instructed to lie on the operative side. However, the patient with unilateral lung pathology may not be able to turn well onto that side because of pain. In addition, positioning the patient with the "good lung" (the nonoperated lung) down allows a better match of ventilation and perfusion and therefore may actually improve oxygenation. The patient's position is changed from flat to semiupright as soon as possible, because remaining in one position tends to promote the retention of secretions in the dependent portion of the lungs, and the upright position increases diaphragmatic excursion, enhancing lung expansion. After a pneumonectomy, the operated side should be dependent so that fluid in the pleural space remains below the level of the bronchial stump and the other lung can fully expand.

The procedure for turning the patient is as follows:

- Instruct the patient to bend the knees and use the feet to push.
- Have the patient shift hips and shoulders to the opposite side of the bed while pushing with the feet.
- Bring the patient's arm over the chest, pointing it in the direction toward which the patient is being turned. Have the patient grasp the side rail with the hand.
- Turn the patient in log-roll fashion to prevent twisting at the waist and pain from possible pulling on the incision.

### Improving Airway Clearance

Retained secretions are a threat to the patient after thoracotomy surgery. Trauma to the tracheobronchial tree during surgery, diminished lung ventilation, and diminished cough reflex all result in the accumulation of excessive secretions. If the secretions are retained, airway obstruction occurs. This, in turn, causes the air in the alveoli distal to the obstruction to become absorbed and the affected portion of the lung to collapse. Atelectasis, pneumonia, and respiratory failure may result.

Several techniques are used to maintain a patent airway. First, secretions are suctioned from the tracheobronchial tree before the endotracheal tube is discontinued. Secretions continue to be removed by suctioning until the patient can cough up secretions effectively. Nasotracheal suctioning may be needed to stimulate a deep cough and aspirate secretions that the patient cannot clear by coughing. However, it should be used only after other methods to raise secretions have been unsuccessful (Chart 25-20).

Coughing technique is another measure used to maintain a patent airway. The patient is encouraged to cough effectively; ineffective coughing results in exhaustion and retention of secretions (see Chart 25-5). To be effective, the cough must be low-pitched, deep, and controlled. Because it is difficult to cough in a supine position, the patient is helped to a sitting position on the edge of the bed, with the feet resting

### CHART 25-20

## Performing Nasotracheal Suction

**STERILE TECHNIQUE TO BE USED**

1. Explain procedure to the patient.
2. Medicate patient for pain if necessary.
3. Place the patient in a sitting or semi-Fowler's position. Make sure the patient's head is not flexed forward. Remove excess pillows if necessary.
4. Oxygenate the patient several minutes before initiating the suctioning procedure. Have oxygen source ready nearby during procedure.
5. Put on sterile gloves.
6. Lubricate catheter with water-soluble gel.
7. Gently pass catheter through the patient's nose to the pharynx. If it is difficult to pass the catheter, and repeated suctioning is expected, a soft rubber nasal trumpet may be placed nasopharyngeally to provide easier catheter passage. Check the position of the tip of the catheter by asking the patient to open the mouth and inspecting it; the tip of the catheter should be in the lower pharynx.
8. Instruct the patient to take a deep breath or stick out the tongue. This action opens the epiglottis and promotes downward movement of the catheter.
9. Advance the catheter into the trachea only during inspiration. Listen for cough or for passage of air through the catheter.
10. Attach the catheter to suction apparatus. Apply intermittent suction while slowly withdrawing the catheter. Do not let suction exceed 120 mm Hg.
11. Do not suction for longer than 10 to 15 seconds, as dysrhythmias, bradycardia, or cardiac arrest may occur in patients with borderline oxygenation.
12. If additional suctioning is needed, withdraw the catheter to the back of the pharynx. Reassure patient and oxygenate for several minutes before resuming suctioning.

on a chair. The patient should cough at least every hour during the first 24 hours and when necessary thereafter. If audible crackles are present, it may be necessary to use chest percussion with the cough routine until the lungs are clear. Aerosol therapy is helpful in humidifying and mobilizing secretions so that they can easily be cleared with coughing. To minimize incisional pain during coughing, the nurse supports the incision or encourages the patient to do so (Fig. 25-12).

After helping the patient to cough, the nurse listens to both lungs, anteriorly and posteriorly, to determine whether there are any changes in breath sounds. Diminished breath sounds may indicate collapsed or hypoventilated alveoli.

CPT is the final technique for maintaining a patent airway. If a patient is identified as being at high risk for postoperative pulmonary complications, then CPT is started immediately (perhaps even before surgery). The techniques of postural drainage, vibration, and percussion help loosen and mobilize the secretions so that they can be coughed up or suctioned.

### Relieving Pain and Discomfort

Pain after a thoracotomy may be severe, depending on the type of incision and the patient's reaction to and ability to cope with pain. Deep inspiration is very painful after thoracotomy. Pain can lead to postoperative complications if it reduces the patient's ability to breathe deeply and cough and if it further limits chest excursions so that ventilation becomes ineffective.

Immediately after the surgical procedure and before the incision is closed, the surgeon may perform a nerve block with a long-acting local anesthetic such as bupivacaine (Marcaine, Sensorcaine). Bupivacaine is titrated to relieve postoperative pain while allowing the patient to cooperate in deep breathing, coughing, and mobilization. However, it is important to avoid depressing the respiratory system with excessive analgesia: the patient should not be so sedated as to be unable to cough. There is controversy about the effectiveness of injections of local anesthetic for pain relief after thoracotomy. Research has shown that local injections of bupivacaine combined with PCA with IV morphine are as effective in relieving pain as epidural analgesia (Concha, Dagnino, Cariaga, et al., 2004).

Lidocaine and prilocaine are local anesthetic agents used to treat pain at the site of the chest tube insertion. These medications are administered as topical transdermal analgesics that penetrate the skin. Lidocaine and prilocaine have also been found to be effective when used together. EMLA cream, which is a mixture of the two medications, has been found to be effective in treating pain from chest tube removal, and one study showed it to be more effective than IV morphine (Valenzuela & Rosen, 1999). However, many physicians prefer not to use analgesia when removing chest tubes because the pain, although severe, is of short duration (usually less than a few minutes) and the analgesia might interfere with respiratory effort.

PCA is often used postoperatively because of the need to maximize patient comfort without depressing the respiratory drive. Opioid analgesic agents such as morphine are commonly used. PCA, administered through an IV pump or an epidural catheter, allows the patient to control the frequency and total dosage. Preset limits on the pump avoid overdosage. With proper instruction, PCA is well

A  The nurse's hands should support the chest incision anteriorly and posteriorly. The patient is instructed to take several deep breaths, inhale, and then cough forcibly.

B  With one hand, the nurse exerts downward pressure on the shoulder of the affected side while firmly supporting the area beneath the wound with the other hand. The patient is instructed to take several deep breaths, inhale, and then cough forcibly.

C  The nurse can wrap a towel or sheet around the patient's chest and hold the ends together, pulling slightly as the patient coughs, and releasing during deep breaths.

**FIGURE 25-12.** Techniques for supporting incision while a patient recovering from thoracic surgery coughs.

D  The patient can be taught to hold a pillow firmly against the incision while coughing. This can be done while lying down or sitting in an upright position.

tolerated and allows earlier mobilization and cooperation with the treatment regimen. (See Chapter 13 for a more extensive discussion of PCA and pain management.)

> **NURSING ALERT**
>
> It is important not to confuse the restlessness of hypoxia with the restlessness caused by pain. Dyspnea, restlessness, increasing respiratory rate, increasing blood pressure, and tachycardia are warning signs of impending respiratory insufficiency. Pulse oximetry is used to monitor oxygenation and to differentiate causes of restlessness.

### Promoting Mobility and Shoulder Exercises

Because large shoulder girdle muscles are transected during a thoracotomy, the arm and shoulder must be mobilized by full range of motion of the shoulder. As soon as physiologically possible, usually within 8 to 12 hours, the patient is helped to get out of bed. Although this may be painful initially, the earlier the patient moves, the sooner the pain will subside. In addition to getting out of bed, the patient begins arm and shoulder exercises to restore movement and prevent painful stiffening of the affected arm and shoulder (Chart 25-21).

### Maintaining Fluid Volume and Nutrition

#### INTRAVENOUS THERAPY
During the surgical procedure or immediately after, the patient may receive a transfusion of blood products, followed by a continuous IV infusion. Because a reduction in lung capacity often occurs after thoracic surgery, a period of physiologic adjustment is needed. Fluids should be administered at a low hourly rate and titrated (as prescribed) to prevent overloading the vascular system and precipitating pulmonary edema. The nurse performs careful respiratory and cardiovascular assessments, as well as intake and output, vital signs, and assessment of jugular vein distention. The nurse also monitors the infusion site for signs of infiltration, including swelling, tenderness, and redness.

#### NUTRITION
It is not unusual for patients undergoing thoracotomy to have poor nutritional status before surgery because of dyspnea, sputum production, and poor appetite. Therefore, it is especially important that adequate nutrition be provided. A liquid diet is provided as soon as bowel sounds return, and the patient is progressed to a full diet as soon as possible. Small, frequent meals are better tolerated and are crucial to the recovery and maintenance of lung function.

### Monitoring and Managing Potential Complications

Complications after thoracic surgery are always a possibility and must be identified and managed early.

## NURSING RESEARCH PROFILE

### Pain Control Strategies for Chest Tube Removal

Puntillo, K. & Ley, S. J. (2004). Appropriately timed analgesics control pain due to chest tube removal. *American Journal of Critical Care, 13*(4), 292–301.

#### Purpose
Patients report moderate to severe pain and distress associated with chest tube removal. This study was conducted to test four approaches to managing pain in postoperative patients who had chest tubes removed. It examined the effects of two analgesic agents (morphine versus ketorolac, a nonsteroidal noninflammatory agent) and two educational approaches (information about the procedure versus the same information about the procedure *plus* information about sensations that could be expected with removal of chest tubes).

#### Design
This double-blind, quasi-experimental study included a sample of 74 patients who had undergone cardiac surgery about 1 day previously. Patients who gave informed consent for the study were randomly assigned to one of four pain relief strategies: (1) intravenous (IV) morphine and procedural information; (2) IV ketorolac and procedural information; (3) IV morphine and procedural plus sensory information; and (4) IV ketorolac and procedural plus sensory information. Patients were instructed on the use of rating scales to assess pain intensity and pain distress. Morphine or ketorolac was administered before removal of the tube at a time that corresponded with the peak effect of each medication (60 minutes before removal for ketorolac, 20 minutes for morphine). To blind the patient and data collector to the analgesic agent used, an injection of normal saline was administered to all patients in addition to the assigned analgesic agent; thus, all patients received injections at both 60 and 20 minutes before removal of the chest tube. Procedural information and sensory information were provided using prepared scripts. Pain intensity and pain distress were measured before administration of the assigned analgesic, immediately after the chest tube was removed, and again 20 minutes later. Level of sedation was also measured before and 20 minutes after chest tube removal. Differences in effectiveness of pain relief strategies and level of sedation were analyzed over time.

#### Findings
Patients reported mild levels of pain and distress during chest tube removal. Sedation levels as assessed by nurses and patients' pain intensity and pain distress scores were not significantly different across the four groups. Patients remained alert, regardless of which analgesic agent was received.

#### Nursing Implications
Many clinicians elect not to medicate patients before removal of chest tubes because the severe pain associated with removal is of short duration and because of the risk of prolonged sedation associated with analgesic agents. The findings of this study indicate that timing the administration of analgesics so that their effect peaks at the time of chest tube removal reduces pain associated with the procedure and does not increase sedation. These findings suggest that nurses should time administration of analgesics so that their effects are beneficial to patients. Furthermore, they suggest that several safe and effective interventions are available to reduce pain and distress associated with chest tube removal.

---

In addition, the nurse monitors the patient at regular intervals for signs of respiratory distress or developing respiratory failure, dysrhythmias, bronchopleural fistula, hemorrhage and shock, atelectasis, and pulmonary infection.

Respiratory distress is treated by identifying and eliminating its cause while providing supplemental oxygen. If the patient progresses to respiratory failure, intubation and mechanical ventilation are necessary.

Dysrhythmias are often related to the effects of hypoxia or the surgical procedure. They are treated with antiarrhythmic medication and supportive therapy (see Chapter 27). Pulmonary infections or effusion, often preceded by atelectasis, may occur a few days into the postoperative course.

Pneumothorax may occur after thoracic surgery if there is an air leak from the surgical site to the pleural cavity or from the pleural cavity to the environment. Failure of the chest drainage system prevents return of negative pressure in the pleural cavity and results in pneumothorax. In the postoperative patient, pneumothorax is often accompanied by hemothorax. The nurse maintains the chest drainage system and monitors the patient for signs and symptoms of pneumothorax: increasing shortness of breath, tachycardia, increased respiratory rate, and increasing respiratory distress.

Bronchopleural fistula is a serious but rare complication that prevents the return of negative intrathoracic pressure and lung re-expansion. Depending on its severity, it is treated with closed chest drainage, me-

## CHART 25-21

### Patient Education

**Performing Arm and Shoulder Exercises**
Arm and shoulder exercises are performed after thoracic surgery to restore movement, prevent painful stiffening of the shoulder, and improve muscle power.

(A) Hold hand of the affected side with the other hand, palms facing in. Raise the arms forward, upward, and then overhead, while taking a deep breath. Exhale while lowering the arms. Repeat five times. (B) Raise arm sideward, upward, and downward in a waving motion. (C) Place arm at side. Raise arm sideward, upward, and over the head. Repeat five times. These exercises can also be performed while lying in bed. (D) Extend the arm up and back, out to the side and back, down at the side and back. (E) Place hands in small of back. Push elbows as far back as possible. (F) Sit erect in an armchair; place the hands on the arms of the chair directly opposite the sides of the body. Press down on hands, consciously pulling the abdomen in and stretching up from the waist. Inhale while raising the body until the elbows are extended completely. Hold this position a moment, and begin exhaling while lowering the body slowly to the original position.

---

chanical ventilation, and possibly talc pleurodesis (described in Chapter 23).

Hemorrhage and shock are managed by treating the underlying cause, whether by reoperation or by administration of blood products or fluids. Pulmonary edema from overinfusion of IV fluids is a significant danger. Early symptoms are dyspnea, crackles, bubbling sounds in the chest, tachycardia, and pink, frothy sputum. This constitutes an emergency and must be reported and treated immediately.

### Promoting Home and Community-Based Care

**TEACHING PATIENTS SELF-CARE**
The nurse instructs the patient and family about postoperative care that will be continued at home. The nurse explains signs and symptoms that should be reported to the physician. These include the following:

- Change in respiratory status: increasing shortness of breath, fever, increased restlessness or other changes in mental or cognitive status, increased respiratory rate, change in respiratory pattern, change in amount or color of sputum
- Bleeding or other drainage from the surgical incision or chest tube exit sites
- Increased chest pain

In addition, respiratory care and other treatment modalities (oxygen, incentive spirometry, CPT, and oral, inhaled, or IV medications) may be continued at home. Therefore, the nurse needs to instruct the patient and family in their correct and safe use.

The nurse emphasizes the importance of progressively increased activity. The nurse instructs the patient to ambulate within limits and explains that return of strength is likely to be very gradual. Another important aspect of patient teaching addresses shoulder exercises. The patient is instructed to do these exercises five times daily. Additional patient teaching is described in Chart 25-22.

**CONTINUING CARE**

Depending on the patient's physical status and the availability of family assistance, a home care referral may be indicated. The home care nurse assesses the patient's recovery from surgery, with special attention to respiratory status, the surgical incision, chest drainage, pain control, ambulation, and nutritional status. The patient's use of respiratory modalities is assessed to ensure that they are being used correctly and safely. In addition, the nurse assesses the patient's adherence to the postoperative treatment plan and identifies acute or late postoperative complications.

The recovery process may take longer than the patient had expected, and providing support to the patient is an important task for the home care nurse. Because of shorter hospital stays, keeping follow-up appointments with the physician is essential. The nurse teaches the patient about the importance of keeping follow-up appointments and completing laboratory tests as prescribed to assist the physician in evaluating recovery. The home care nurse provides continuous encouragement and education to the patient and family during the process. As recovery progresses, the nurse also reminds the patient and family about the importance of participating in health promotion activities and recommended health screening.

## Evaluation

### Expected Patient Outcomes

Expected patient outcomes may include the following:

1. Demonstrates improved gas exchange, as evidenced by improved arterial blood gas measurements.
2. Shows improved airway clearance, as evidenced by deep, controlled coughing and clear breath sounds and decreased or absent adventitious sounds
3. Has decreased pain and discomfort, as evidenced by decreasing use of analgesic medications and increasing activity level
4. Shows improved mobility of shoulder and arm, as evidenced by demonstration of arm and shoulder exercises.
5. Maintains adequate fluid intake and maintains nutrition for healing, as evidenced by adequate urinary output and stable weight.
6. Exhibits less anxiety, as evidenced by use of appropriate coping skills
7. Understands required care, as evidenced by verbalization or demonstration of appropriate use of technology and adherence to therapeutic program
8. Is free of complications, as evidenced by normal vital signs and temperature, improved arterial blood gas measurements, clear lung sounds, and adequate respiratory function

For a detailed plan of nursing care for the patient who has had a thoracotomy, see Chart 25-23.

*(text continues on page 775)*

---

**CHART 25-22**

### HOME CARE CHECKLIST • The Patient With a Thoracotomy

| At the completion of the home care instruction, the patient or caregiver will be able to: | Patient | Caregiver |
|---|:---:|:---:|
| • Use local heat and oral analgesia to relieve intercostal pain. | ✔ | ✔ |
| • Alternate walking and other activities with frequent rest periods, expecting weakness and fatigue for the first 3 weeks. | ✔ | ✔ |
| • Perform breathing exercises several times daily for the first few weeks at home. | ✔ | |
| • Avoid lifting more than 20 pounds until complete healing has taken place; the chest muscles and incision may be weaker than normal for 3 to 6 months after surgery. | ✔ | |
| • Walk at a moderate pace, gradually and persistently extending walking time and distance. | ✔ | |
| • Immediately stop any activity that causes undue fatigue, increased shortness of breath, or chest pain. | ✔ | |
| • Avoid bronchial irritants (smoke, fumes, air pollution, aerosol sprays). | ✔ | ✔ |
| • Avoid others with known colds or lung infections. | ✔ | ✔ |
| • Obtain an annual influenza vaccine and discuss vaccination against pneumonia with the physician. | ✔ | |
| • Report for follow-up care by the surgeon or clinic as necessary. | ✔ | ✔ |
| • Stop smoking, if applicable, and avoid exposure to secondhand smoke. | ✔ | ✔ |

CHART 25-23

## Plan of Nursing Care: Care of the Patient After Thoracotomy

**Nursing Diagnosis:** Impaired gas exchange related to lung impairment and surgery
**Goal:** Improvement of gas exchange and breathing

| NURSING INTERVENTIONS | RATIONALE | EXPECTED OUTCOMES |
|---|---|---|
| 1. Monitor pulmonary status as directed and as needed:<br>  a. Auscultate breath sounds.<br>  b. Check rate, depth, and pattern of respirations.<br>  c. Assess blood gases for signs of hypoxemia or $CO_2$ retention.<br>  d. Evaluate patient's color for cyanosis. | 1. Changes in pulmonary status indicate improvement or onset of complications. | • Lungs are clear on auscultation<br>• Respiratory rate is within acceptable range with no episodes of dyspnea<br>• Vital signs are stable<br>• Dysrhythmias are not present or are under control<br>• Demonstrates deep, controlled, effective breathing to allow maximal lung expansion<br>• Uses incentive spirometer every 2 hours while awake<br>• Demonstrates deep, effective coughing technique<br>• Lungs are expanded to capacity (evidenced by chest x-ray) |
| 2. Monitor and record blood pressure, apical pulse, and temperature every 2–4 hours, central venous pressure (if indicated) every 2 hours. | 2. Aid in evaluating effect of surgery on cardiac status. | |
| 3. Monitor continuous electrocardiogram for pattern and dysrhythmias. | 3. Dysrhythmias (especially atrial fibrillation and atrial flutter) are more frequently seen after thoracic surgery. A patient with total pneumonectomy is especially prone to cardiac irregularity. | |
| 4. Elevate head of bed 30–40 degrees when patient is oriented and hemodynamic status is stable. | 4. Maximum lung excursion is achieved when patient is as close to upright as possible. | |
| 5. Encourage deep-breathing exercises (see section on Breathing Retraining) and effective use of incentive spirometer (sustained maximal inspiration). | 5. Helps to achieve maximal lung inflation and to open closed airways. | |
| 6. Encourage and promote an effective cough routine to be performed every 1–2 hours during first 24 hours. | 6. Coughing is necessary to remove retained secretions. | |
| 7. Assess and monitor the chest drainage system:*<br>  a. Assess for leaks and patency as needed.<br>  b. Monitor amount and character of drainage and document every 2 hours. Notify physician if drainage is 150 mL/h or greater.<br>  c. See Chart 25-18 for summary of nurse's role in management of chest drainage systems. | 7. System is used to eliminate any residual air or fluid after thoracotomy. | |

*A patient with a pneumonectomy usually does not have water seal chest drainage because it is desirable that the pleural space fill with an effusion, which eventually obliterates this space. Some surgeons do use a modified water seal system.

*continued >*

**CHART 25-23**

## Plan of Nursing Care — Care of the Patient After Thoracotomy (Continued)

**Nursing Diagnosis:** Ineffective airway clearance related to lung impairment, anesthesia, and pain
**Goal:** Improvement of airway clearance and achievement of a patent airway

| NURSING INTERVENTIONS | RATIONALE | EXPECTED OUTCOMES |
|---|---|---|
| 1. Maintain an open airway. | 1. Provides for adequate ventilation and gas exchange | • Airway is patent<br>• Coughs effectively<br>• Splints incision while coughing<br>• Sputum is clear or colorless<br>• Lungs are clear on auscultation |
| 2. Perform endotracheal suctioning until patient can raise secretions effectively. | 2. Endotracheal secretions are present in excessive amounts in post-thoracotomy patients due to trauma to the tracheobronchial tree during surgery, diminished lung ventilation, and cough reflex. | |
| 3. Assess and medicate for pain. Encourage deep-breathing and coughing exercises. Help splint incision during coughing. | 3. Helps to achieve maximal lung inflation and to open closed airways. Coughing is painful; incision needs to be supported. | |
| 4. Monitor amount, viscosity, color, and odor of sputum. Notify physician if sputum is excessive or contains bright-red blood. | 4. Changes in sputum suggest presence of infection or change in pulmonary status. Colorless sputum is not unusual; opacification or coloring of sputum may indicate dehydration or infection. | |
| 5. Administer humidification and mini-nebulizer therapy as prescribed. | 5. Secretions must be moistened and thinned if they are to be raised from the chest with the least amount of effort. | |
| 6. Perform postural drainage, percussion, and vibration as prescribed. Do not percuss or vibrate directly over operative site. | 6. Chest physiotherapy uses gravity to help remove secretions from the lung. | |
| 7. Auscultate both sides of chest to determine changes in breath sounds. | 7. Indications for tracheal suctioning are determined by chest auscultation. | |

**Nursing Diagnosis:** Acute pain related to incision, drainage tubes, and the surgical procedure
**Goal:** Relief of pain and discomfort

| NURSING INTERVENTIONS | RATIONALE | EXPECTED OUTCOMES |
|---|---|---|
| 1. Evaluate location, character, quality, and severity of pain. Administer analgesic medication as prescribed and as needed. Observe for respiratory effect of opioid. Is patient too somnolent to cough? Are respirations depressed? | 1. Pain limits chest excursions and thereby decreases ventilation. | • Asks for pain medication, but verbalizes that he or she expects some discomfort while deep breathing and coughing<br>• Verbalizes that he or she is comfortable and not in acute distress<br>• No signs of incisional infection evident |

## CHART 25-23

### Plan of Nursing Care: Care of the Patient After Thoracotomy (Continued)

| NURSING INTERVENTIONS | RATIONALE | EXPECTED OUTCOMES |
|---|---|---|
| 2. Maintain care postoperatively in positioning the patient:<br>　a. Place patient in semi-Fowler's position.<br>　b. Patients with limited respiratory reserve may not be able to turn on unoperated side.<br>　c. Assist or turn patient every 2 hours. | 2. The patient who is comfortable and free of pain will be less likely to splint the chest while breathing. A semi-Fowler's position permits residual air in the pleural space to rise to upper portion of pleural space and be removed via the upper chest catheter. | |
| 3. Assess incision area every 8 hours for redness, heat, induration, swelling, separation, and drainage. | 3. These signs indicate possible infection. | |
| 4. Request order for patient-controlled analgesia pump if appropriate for patient. | 4. Allowing patient control over frequency and dose improves comfort and compliance with treatment regimen. | |

**Nursing Diagnosis:** Anxiety related to outcomes of surgery, pain, technology
**Goal:** Reduction of anxiety to a manageable level

| NURSING INTERVENTIONS | RATIONALE | EXPECTED OUTCOMES |
|---|---|---|
| 1. Explain all procedures in understandable language. | 1. Explaining what can be expected in understandable terms decreases anxiety and increases cooperation. | • States that anxiety is at a manageable level<br>• Participates with health care team in treatment regimen<br>• Uses appropriate coping skills (verbalization, pain relief strategies, use of support systems such as family, clergy)<br>• Demonstrates basic understanding of technology used in care |
| 2. Assess for pain and medicate, especially before potentially painful procedures. | 2. Premedication before painful procedures or activities improves comfort and minimizes undue anxiety. | |
| 3. Silence all *unnecessary* alarms on technology (monitors, ventilators). | 3. *Unnecessary* alarms increase the risk of sensory overload and may increase anxiety. *Essential* alarms must be turned on at all times. | |
| 4. Encourage and support patient while increasing activity level. | 4. Positive reinforcement improves patient motivation and independence. | |
| 5. Mobilize resources (family, clergy, social worker) to help patient cope with outcomes of surgery (diagnosis, change in functional abilities). | 5. A multidisciplinary approach promotes the patient's strengths and coping mechanisms. | |

*continued >*

**CHART 25-23**

## Plan of Nursing Care — Care of the Patient After Thoracotomy (Continued)

**Nursing Diagnosis:** Impaired physical mobility of the upper extremities related to thoracic surgery
**Goal:** Increased mobility of the affected shoulder and arm

| NURSING INTERVENTIONS | RATIONALE | EXPECTED OUTCOMES |
| --- | --- | --- |
| 1. Assist patient with normal range of motion and function of shoulder and trunk:<br>　a. Teach breathing exercises to mobilize thorax.<br>　b. Encourage skeletal exercises to promote abduction and mobilization of shoulder (see Chart 25-21).<br>　c. Assist out of bed to chair as soon as pulmonary and circulatory systems are stable (usually by evening of surgery).<br>2. Encourage progressive activities according to level of fatigue. | 1. Necessary to regain normal mobility of arm and shoulder and to speed recovery and minimize discomfort<br><br>2. Increases patient's use of affected shoulder and arm | • Demonstrates arm and shoulder exercises and verbalizes intent to perform them on discharge<br>• Regains previous range of motion in shoulder and arm |

**Nursing Diagnosis:** Risk for imbalanced fluid volume related to the surgical procedure
**Goal:** Maintenance of adequate fluid volume

| NURSING INTERVENTIONS | RATIONALE | EXPECTED OUTCOMES |
| --- | --- | --- |
| 1. Monitor and record hourly intake and output. Urine output should be at least 30 mL/h after surgery.<br>2. Administer blood component therapy and parenteral fluids and/or diuretics as prescribed to restore and maintain fluid volume. | 1. Fluid management may be altered before, during, and after surgery, and patient's response to and need for fluid management must be assessed.<br>2. Pulmonary edema due to transfusion or fluid overload is an ever-present threat; after pneumonectomy, the pulmonary vascular system has been greatly reduced. | • Patient is adequately hydrated, as evidenced by:<br>　• Urine output greater than 30 mL/h<br>　• Vital signs stable, heart rate, and central venous pressure approaching normal<br>　• No excessive peripheral edema |

**Nursing Diagnosis:** Deficient knowledge of home care procedures
**Goal:** Increased ability to carry out care procedures at home

| NURSING INTERVENTIONS | RATIONALE | EXPECTED OUTCOMES |
| --- | --- | --- |
| 1. Encourage patient to practice arm and shoulder exercises five times daily at home.<br>2. Instruct patient to practice assuming a functionally erect position in front of a full-length mirror. | 1. Exercise accelerates recovery of muscle function and reduces long-term pain and discomfort.<br>2. Practice will help restore normal posture. | • Demonstrates arm and shoulder exercises<br>• Verbalizes need to try to assume an erect posture |

## CHART 25-23

### Plan of Nursing Care: Care of the Patient After Thoracotomy (Continued)

| NURSING INTERVENTIONS | RATIONALE | EXPECTED OUTCOMES |
|---|---|---|
| 3. Instruct patient in following aspects of home care:<br>a. Relieve intercostal pain by local heat or oral analgesia.<br>b. Alternate activities with frequent rest periods.<br>c. Practice breathing exercises at home.<br>d. Avoid heavy lifting until complete healing has occurred.<br>e. Avoid undue fatigue, increased shortness of breath, or chest pain.<br>f. Avoid bronchial irritants.<br>g. Prevent colds or lung infection.<br>h. Get annual influenza vaccine.<br>i. Keep follow-up appointment with physician.<br>j. Stop smoking. | 3. Knowing what to expect facilitates recovery.<br>a. Some soreness may persist for several weeks.<br>b. Weakness and fatigue are common for the first 3 weeks or longer.<br>c. Effective breathing is necessary to prevent splinting of affected side, which may lead to atelectasis.<br>d. Chest muscles and incision may be weaker than normal for 3–6 months.<br>e. Undue stress may prolong the healing process.<br>f. The lung is more susceptible to irritants.<br>g. The lung is more susceptible to infection during the recovery phase.<br>h. Vaccination helps prevent flu.<br>i. This allows timely follow-up assessment.<br>j. Smoking will slow healing process by decreasing oxygen delivery to tissues and make lung susceptible to infection and other complications. | • Verbalizes the importance of relieving discomfort, alternating walking and rest, performing breathing exercises, avoiding heavy lifting, avoiding undue fatigue, avoiding bronchial irritants, preventing colds or lung infections, getting influenza vaccine, keeping follow-up visits, and stopping smoking |

## Critical Thinking Exercises

1. The morning after a man has undergone thoracic surgery, he gets out of bed unassisted and disconnects the chest tube from the drainage system. What immediate complications are of greatest concern, and what actions should the nurse take to prevent these complications? What nursing assessments and nursing interventions are needed to (1) prevent recurrence of this situation and (2) identify and treat other complications?

2. **ebp** A patient with long-standing pulmonary disease is instructed to perform postural drainage three times a day. What is the evidence base for use of postural drainage? What is the strength of that evidence, and what criteria did you use to assess the strength of that evidence? What patient teaching is important for the patient and family member if the patient is to continue postural drainage at home?

3. Oxygen therapy is required for the following patients: a 44-year-old patient who has undergone a right lower lobe lobectomy and requires short-term oxygen therapy; a 68-year-old patient with advanced COPD who has been admitted to the hospital repeatedly in the past 2 years; and a 78-year-old patient with dyspnea secondary to advanced lung cancer. Compare and contrast the similarities and differences in the oxygen therapy necessary for each patient, and discuss teaching and safety precautions indicated for each patient and his or her family. Describe the patient teaching that will be required if each of these patients is discharged from the hospital with a prescription for oxygen therapy.

**4** [ebp] A woman is scheduled to have a tracheostomy performed in the operating room to allow her to continue to receive mechanical ventilation to treat temporary paralysis of her respiratory muscles secondary to a neuromuscular disorder. For the past week, she has been intubated with an endotracheal tube and has been receiving mechanical ventilation. What preprocedure preparation and teaching and what safety precautions are warranted for this patient? Develop an evidence-based protocol for addressing her needs related to tracheostomy care and positive-pressure mechanical ventilation.

**5** Your patient has just returned from the operating room after thoracic surgery. She has an endotracheal tube, two chest tubes, two IV lines, a cardiac monitor, and an indwelling urinary catheter in place. What are your immediate priorities for assessment for this patient? What observations need to be reported to the surgeon immediately? What other nursing interventions are warranted immediately? In 8 hours? At 24 hours and 48 hours postoperatively?

## REFERENCES AND SELECTED READINGS

### BOOKS

Doenges, M. E., Moorhouse, M. F. & Murr, A. C. (2004). *Nurse's pocket guide: Diagnoses, interventions, and rationales* (9th ed.). Philadelphia: F. A. Davis.

Ebersole, P., Hess, P. & Luggen, A. S. (2003). *Toward healthy aging: Human needs and nursing response* (6th ed.). St. Louis: C. V. Mosby.

Grodner, M., Long, S. & Deyoung, S. (2003). *Foundations and clinical application of nutrition: A nursing approach* (3rd ed.). St. Louis: C. V. Mosby.

Hess, D. R. & Kacmarek, R. M. (2002). *Essentials of mechanical ventilation* (2nd ed.): New York: McGraw-Hill Medical.

Kacmarek, R. M., Dimas, S. & Mack, C. W. (2005). *The essentials of respiratory care* (4th ed.). St. Louis: Elsevier Mosby.

Kee, J. L. & Hayes, E. R. (2002). *Pharmacology: A nursing process approach* (4th ed.). Philadelphia: W. B. Saunders.

MacIntyre, N. R., Mishoe, S. C., Galvin, W. F., et al. (2001). *Respiratory care: Principles and practice* (1st ed.). Philadelphia: W. B. Saunders.

Morton, P. G., Fontaine, D. K., Hudak, C. M., et al. (2005). *Critical care nursing: A holistic approach* (8th ed.). Philadelphia: Lippincott Williams & Wilkins.

NHS Quality Improvement Scotland (2003). *Caring for the patient with a tracheostomy: Best practice statement.* Edinburgh: Nursing & Midwifery Practice Development Unit.

Sole, M. L., Klein, D. & Moseley, M. (2004). *Introduction to critical care nursing* (4th ed.). Philadelphia: W. B. Saunders.

Wilkins, R. L., Stoller, J. K. & Scanlon, C. l. (2003). *Egan's fundamentals of respiratory care* (8th ed.). St. Louis: Mosby.

### JOURNALS

*Asterisks indicate nursing research articles.

Allibone, L. (2003). Nursing management of chest drains. *Nursing Standard, 17*(22), 45–54.

Ambrosino, N. & Rossi, A. (2002). Proportional assist ventilation (PAV): A significant advance or a futile struggle between logic and practice. *Thorax, 57*(3), 272–276.

Andrs, K. (2004). Chest drainage to go. *Nursing, 34*(5), 54–55.

Baudouin, S. V. & Evans, T. W. (2003). Nutritional support in critical care. *Clinics in Chest Medicine 24*(3), 633–644.

Benditt, J. O. (2004). Surgical therapies for chronic obstructive pulmonary disease. *Respiratory Care, 49*(1), 53–61.

Bennett, M. & Heard, R. (2004). Hyperbaric oxygen therapy for multiple sclerosis. *Cochrane Database of Systematic Reviews,* CD003057.

Bennett, M. H., Trytko, B. & Jonker, B. (2004). Hyperbaric oxygen therapy for the adjunctive treatment of traumatic brain injury. *Cochrane Database of Systematic Reviews,* CD004609.

Bliss, P. L., McCoy, R. W. & Adams, A. B. (2004). Characteristics of demand oxygen delivery systems: Maximum output and setting recommendations. *Respiratory Care, 49*(2), 160–165.

Bond, P., Grant, F., Coltart, L., et al. (2003). Best practice in the care of patients with a tracheostomy. *Nursing Times, 99*(30), 24–25.

Broussard, C. L. (2003). Hyperbaric oxygenation and wound healing. *Journal of WOCN, 30*(4), 210–216.

Burns, S. M. (2004). The science of weaning: When and how? *Critical Care Nursing Clinics of North America, 16*(3), 379–386.

Cirino, L. M., Campos, L., Jatene, F., et al. (2000). Diagnosis and treatment of mediastinal tumors by thoracoscopy. *Chest, 117*(6), 1787–1792.

Concha, M., Dagnino, J., Cariaga, M., et al. (2004). Analgesia after thoracotomy: Epidural fentanyl/bupivacaine compared with intercostal nerve block plus intravenous morphine. *Journal of Cardiothoracic and Vascular Anesthesia, 18*(3), 322–326.

Dekleva, M., Neskovic, A., Vlahovic, A., et al. (2004). Adjunctive effect of hyperbaric oxygen treatment after thrombolysis on left ventricular function in patients with acute myocardial infarction. *American Heart Journal, 148*(4), E14.

Doherty, D. E. & Briggs, D. D., Jr. (2004). Long-term nonpharmacologic management of patients with chronic obstructive pulmonary disease. *Clinical Cornerstone, 6*(Suppl. 2), S29–S34.

Frawley, P. M. & Habashi, N. M. (2001). Airway pressure release ventilation: Theory and practice. *AACN Clinical Issues, 12*(2), 234–246.

Fuhrman, C., Chouaid, C., Herigault, R., et al. (2004). Comparison of four demand oxygen delivery systems at rest and during exercise for chronic obstructive pulmonary disease. *Respiratory Medicine, 98*(10), 938–944.

*Gelsthorpe, T., & Crocker, C. (2004). A study exploring factors which influence the decision to commence nurse-led weaning. *Nursing in Critical Care, 9*(5), 213–221.

*Goris, A. H., Vermeeren, M. A., Wouters, E. F., et al. (2003). Energy balance in depleted ambulatory patients with chronic obstructive pulmonary disease: The effect of physical activity and oral nutritional supplementation. *British Journal of Nutrition, 89*(5), 725–729.

*Grap, M. J., Munro, C. L., Elswick, R. K., et al. (2004). Duration of action of a single, early oral application of chlorhexidine on oral microbial flora in mechanically ventilated patients: A pilot study. *Heart & Lung, 33*(2), 83–91.

Habashi, N. M. (2005). Other approaches to open-lung ventilation: Airway pressure release ventilation. *Critical Care Medicine, 33*(3 Suppl.), S228–S240.

Harper, A. & Croft-Baker, J. (2004). Carbon monoxide poisoning: Undetected by both patients and their doctors. *Age and Ageing, 33*(2), 105–109.

Hess, D. R. (2005). Facilitating speech in the patient with a tracheostomy. *Respiratory Care, 50*(4), 519–525.

Higgins, D. (2005a). Oxygen therapy. *Nursing Times, 101*(4), 30–31.

Higgins, D. (2005b). Tracheal suction. *Nursing Times, 101*(8), 36–37.

Langenhof, S. & Fichter, J. (2005). Comparison of two demand oxygen delivery devices for administration of oxygen in COPD. *Chest, 128*(4), 2082–2087.

Lindgren, V. A. & Ames, N. J. (2005). Caring for patients on mechanical ventilation. *American Journal of Nursing, 105*(5), 50–60.

*Lorente, L., Lecuona, M., Galvan, R., et al. (2004). Periodically changing ventilator circuits is not necessary to prevent ventilator-associated pneumonia when a heat and moisture exchanger is used. *Infection Control and Hospital Epidemiology, 25*(12), 1077–1082.

*Lorente, L., Lecuona, M., Martin, M. M., et al. (2005). Ventilator-associated pneumonia using a closed versus an open tracheal suction system. *Critical Care Medicine, 33*(1), 115–119.

MacIntyre, N. R. (2004). Evidence-based ventilator weaning and discontinuation. *Respiratory Care, 49*(7), 830–836.

Mathews, P. J., Roark-Sample, B., Schmidt, J., et al. (2004). The latest in respiratory care. *Nursing Management, 20*(Suppl.), 22–24.

McDonagh, M., Helfand, M., Carson, S., et al. (2004). Hyperbaric oxygen therapy for traumatic brain injury: A systematic review of the evidence. *Archives of Physical Medicine and Rehabilitation, 85*(7), 1198–1204.

Moon, R. E. (2002). Mini-forum on multiple sclerosis (MS) and hyperbaric oxygen therapy. *Undersea and Hyperbaric Medicine, 29*(4), 235–236.

Naunheim, K. S. (2004). Update on lung volume reduction. *Journal of Surgical Research, 117*(1), 134–143.

Oermann, C., Sockrider, M. M. D., Giles, D. M. K., et al. (2001). Comparison of high-frequency chest wall oscillation and oscillating positive expiratory pressure in the home management of cystic fibrosis: A pilot study. *Pediatric Pulmonology, 32*(5), 372–377.

Pawson, S. R., & DePriest, J. L. (2004). Are blood gases necessary in mechanically ventilated patients who have successfully completed a spontaneous breathing trial? *Respiratory Care, 49*(11), 1316–1319.

*Puntillo, K., & Ley, S. J. (2004). Appropriately timed analgesics control pain due to chest tube removal. *American Journal of Critical Care, 13*(4), 292–303.

*Robinson, T. (2005). Living with severe hypoxic COPD: The patients' experience. *Nursing Times, 101*(7), 38–42.

Roeckl-Wiedmann, I., Bennett, M. & Kranke, P. (2005). Systematic review of hyperbaric oxygen in the management of chronic wounds. *British Journal of Surgery, 92*(1), 24–32.

Roman, M. (2005). Tracheostomy tubes. *MedSurg Nursing, 14*(2), 143–145.

*Salam, A., Smina, M., Gada, P., et al. (2003). The effect of arterial blood gas values on extubation decisions. *Respiratory Care, 48*(11), 1033–1037.

Schweickert, W. D., Gelbach, B. K., Pohlman, A. S., et al. (2004). Daily interruption of sedative infusions and complications of critical illness in mechanically ventilated patients. *Critical Care Medicine, 32*(6), 1272–1276.

Sharifi, M., Fares, W., Abdel-Karim, I., et al. (2004). Usefulness of hyperbaric oxygen therapy to inhibit restenosis after percutaneous coronary intervention for acute myocardial infarction or unstable angina pectoris. *American Journal of Cardiology, 93*(12), 1533–1535.

Smith, B. (2005). The nursing of a patient following lung volume reduction surgery. *Nursing Times, 101*(6), 61–63.

Spritzer, C. J. (2003). Unraveling the mysteries of mechanical ventilation: A helpful step-by-step guide. *Journal of Emergency Nursing, 29*(1), 29–36.

St. John, R. E. & Malen, J. F. (2004). Contemporary issues in adult tracheostomy management. *Critical Care Nursing Clinics of North America, 16*(3), 413–430.

Stoller, J. K. (2000). Oxygen and air travel. *Respiratory Care, 45*(2), 214–221.

Torres, L. Y. & Sirbegovic, D. J. (2004). Early intervention with a tracheostomy and ventilator speaking valve: Physiological benefits begin in the ICU. *AACN News, 21*(6), 10–13.

Valenzuela, R. & Rosen, D. (1999). Topical lidocaine-prilocaine cream (EMLA) for thoracostomy tube removal. *Anesthesia and Analgesia, 88*(1), 1107–1108.

## RESOURCES

American Association for Respiratory Care, 11030 Ables Lane, Dallas, TX 75229; 972-243-2272; http://www.aarc.org. Accessed April 20, 2006.

American Lung Association, 1740 Broadway, New York, NY 10019; 212-315-8700, 800-LUNG-USA; http://www.lungusa.org. Accessed April 20, 2006.

American Thoracic Society, 1740 Broadway, New York, NY 10019; 212-315-8700; http://www.thoracic.org. Accessed April 20, 2006.

National Heart, Lung and Blood Institute, National Institutes of Health, 9000 Rockville Pike, Bldg 31, Rm 5A52, Bethesda, MD 20892; 301-496-5166 or 301-496-4236; http://www.nhlbi.nih.gov. Accessed April 20, 2006.

# UNIT 6

# Cardiovascular, Circulatory, and Hematologic Function

## Case Study
### Applying Concepts from NANDA, NIC, and NOC

**A Patient Who Has Intermittent Claudication and Ulceration**

**Mr. Black,** age 73 years, has a history of peripheral arterial occlusive disease (2 years), hypertension, hypercholesterolemia, type 2 diabetes, and smoking. He eats low-fat foods and cut back on smoking to half a pack a day. His home-monitored blood glucose levels range from 180 to 215 mg/dL. Because he has severe calf pain after walking, he now walks only two blocks a day: one block from home and one block back. He now receives medical treatment for a nonhealing ulcer on the plantar aspect of his left foot.

 Turn to Appendix C to see a concept map that illustrates the relationships that exist between the nursing diagnoses, interventions, and outcomes for the patient's clinical problems.

## Nursing Classifications and Languages

| NANDA<br>Nursing Diagnoses | NIC<br>Nursing Interventions | NOC<br>Nursing Outcomes<br>Return to functional baseline status, stabilization of, or improvement in: |
|---|---|---|
| **Ineffective Peripheral Tissue Perfusion**—Decrease in oxygen resulting in the failure to nourish tissues at the capillary level | **Circulatory Care: Arterial Insufficiency**—Promotion of arterial circulation<br><br>**Circulatory Precautions**—Protection of localized area with limited perfusion | **Circulation Status**—Unobstructed, unidirectional blood flow at an appropriate pressure through large vessels of the systemic and pulmonary circuits<br><br>**Peripheral Tissue Perfusion**—Adequacy of blood flow through the small vessels of the extremities to maintain tissue function |
| **Chronic Pain**—Unpleasant sensory and emotional experience arising from actual or potential tissue damage or described in terms of such damage; sudden or slow onset of any intensity from mild to severe, constant or recurring without an anticipated or predictable end and a duration of greater than 6 months | **Pain Management**—Alleviation of pain or reduction in pain to a level of comfort that is acceptable to the patient | **Symptom Control**—Personal actions to minimize perceived adverse changes in physical and emotional functioning<br><br>**Comfort Level**—Extent of positive perception of physical and psychological ease |
| **Activity Intolerance**—Insufficient physiological or psychological energy to endure or complete required or desired daily activities | **Exercise Therapy: Ambulation**—Promotion and assistance with walking to maintain or restore autonomic and voluntary body functions during treatment and recovery from illness or injury | **Activity Tolerance**—Physiologic response to energy-consuming movements with daily activities |

NANDA International (2005). *Nursing diagnoses: Definitions & classification 2005–2006*. Philadelphia: North American Nursing Diagnosis Association.
Dochterman, J. M., & Bulechek, G. M. (2004). *Nursing Interventions Classification (NIC)* (4th ed.). St. Louis: Mosby.
Iowa Outcomes Project, 2004. In S. Moorhead, M. Johnson, & M. Maas, eds. (2004). *Nursing outcomes classification (NOC)* (3rd ed.). St. Louis: Mosby.
Dochterman, J. M., & Jones, D. A. (2003). *Unifying nursing languages: The harmonization of NANDA, NIC, and NOC*. Washington, D.C.: American Nurses Association.

"Point, click, learn! Visit thePoint for additional resources."

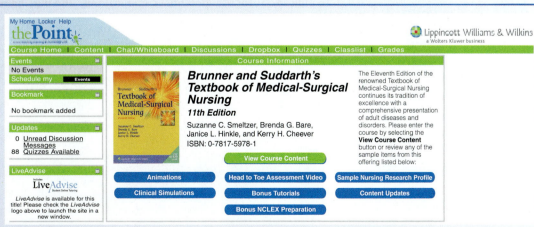

# CHAPTER 26

# Assessment of Cardiovascular Function

## Learning Objectives

*On completion of this chapter, the learner will be able to:*

1. Explain cardiac physiology in relation to cardiac anatomy and the conduction system of the heart.
2. Incorporate assessment of functional health patterns and cardiac risk factors into the health history and physical assessment of the patient with cardiovascular disease.
3. Discuss the clinical indications, patient preparation, and other related nursing implications for common tests and procedures used to assess cardiovascular function and diagnose cardiovascular diseases.
4. Compare the various methods of hemodynamic monitoring (eg, central venous pressure, pulmonary artery pressure, and arterial pressure monitoring) with regard to indications for use, potential complications, and nursing responsibilities.

More than 71 million Americans have one or more types of cardiovascular disease (CVD), including hypertension, coronary artery disease (CAD), heart failure (HF), stroke, and congenital cardiovascular defects (American Heart Association [AHA], 2006). Because of the prevalence of CVD, nurses practicing in any setting across the continuum of care, whether in the home, office, hospital, nursing home, or rehabilitation facility, must be capable of assessing the cardiovascular system. Key components of assessment include a health history, physical examination, and monitoring of a variety of laboratory and diagnostic test results. An accurate and timely assessment of cardiovascular function provides the data necessary to identify nursing diagnoses, formulate an individualized plan of care, evaluate the response of the patient to the care provided, and revise the plan as needed. An understanding of the structure and function of the heart in health and in disease is essential to develop cardiovascular assessment skills.

# Anatomic and Physiologic Overview

The heart is a hollow, muscular organ located in the center of the thorax, where it occupies the space between the lungs (mediastinum) and rests on the diaphragm. It weighs approximately 300 g (10.6 oz); heart weight and size are influenced by age, gender, body weight, extent of physical exercise and conditioning, and heart disease. The heart pumps blood to the tissues, supplying them with oxygen and other nutrients.

The pumping action of the heart is accomplished by the rhythmic contraction and relaxation of its muscular wall. During **systole** (contraction of the muscle), the chambers of the heart become smaller as the blood is ejected. During **diastole** (relaxation of the muscle), the heart chambers fill with blood in preparation for subsequent ejection. A normal

## Glossary

**afterload:** the amount of resistance to ejection of blood from the ventricle

**apical impulse** (also called point of maximum impulse [PMI]): impulse normally palpated at the fifth intercostal space, left midclavicular line; caused by contraction of the left ventricle

**baroreceptors:** nerve fibers located in the aortic arch and carotid arteries that are responsible for reflex control of the blood pressure

**cardiac catheterization:** an invasive procedure used to measure cardiac chamber pressures and assess patency of the coronary arteries

**cardiac conduction system:** specialized heart cells strategically located throughout the heart that are responsible for methodically generating and coordinating the transmission of electrical impulses to the myocardial cells

**cardiac output:** amount of blood pumped by each ventricle in liters per minute; normal cardiac output is 5 L per minute in the resting adult heart

**cardiac stress test:** a test used to evaluate the functioning of the heart during a period of increased oxygen demand

**contractility:** ability of the cardiac muscle to shorten in response to an electrical impulse

**depolarization:** electrical activation of a cell caused by the influx of sodium into the cell while potassium exits the cell

**diastole:** period of ventricular relaxation resulting in ventricular filling

**ejection fraction:** percentage of the end-diastolic blood volume ejected from the ventricle with each heartbeat

**hemodynamic monitoring:** use of monitoring devices to measure cardiovascular function

**hypertension:** blood pressure greater than 140/90 mm Hg

**hypotension:** a decrease in blood pressure to less than 100/60 mm Hg

**international normalized ratio (INR):** a standard method for reporting prothrombin levels, eliminating the variation in test results from laboratory to laboratory

**murmurs:** sounds created by abnormal, turbulent flow of blood in the heart

**myocardial ischemia:** condition in which heart muscle cells receive less oxygen than needed

**myocardium:** muscle layer of the heart responsible for the pumping action of the heart

**normal heart sounds:** sounds produced when the valves close; normal heart sounds are S1 (atrioventricular valves) and S2 (semilunar valves)

**postural (orthostatic) hypotension:** a significant drop in blood pressure (usually 10 mm Hg systolic or more) after an upright posture is assumed

**preload:** degree of stretch of the cardiac muscle fibers at the end of diastole

**pulmonary vascular resistance:** resistance to right ventricle ejection of blood

**radioisotopes:** unstable atoms that emit small amounts of energy in the form of gamma rays; used in cardiac nuclear medicine studies

**repolarization:** return of the cell to resting state, caused by reentry of potassium into the cell while sodium exits the cell

**sinoatrial (SA) node:** primary pacemaker of the heart, located in the right atrium

**stroke volume:** amount of blood ejected from the ventricle per heartbeat; normal stroke volume is 70 mL in the resting heart

**systemic vascular resistance:** resistance to left ventricle ejection

**systole:** period of ventricular contraction resulting in ejection of blood from the ventricles into the pulmonary artery and aorta

**telemetry:** the process of continuous electrocardiographic monitoring by the transmission of radiowaves from a battery-operated transmitter worn by the patient

**venodilating agent:** medication causing dilation of veins resting adult heart beats approximately 60 to 80 times per minute. Each ventricle ejects approximately 70 mL of blood per beat and has an output of approximately 5 L per minute.

## Anatomy of the Heart

The heart is composed of three layers (Fig. 26-1). The inner layer, or endocardium, consists of endothelial tissue and lines the inside of the heart and valves. The middle layer, or **myocardium,** is made up of muscle fibers and is responsible for the pumping action. The exterior layer of the heart is called the epicardium.

The heart is encased in a thin, fibrous sac called the pericardium, which is composed of two layers. Adhering to the epicardium is the visceral pericardium. Enveloping the visceral pericardium is the parietal pericardium, a tough fibrous tissue that attaches to the great vessels, diaphragm, sternum, and vertebral column and supports the heart in the mediastinum. The space between these two layers (pericardial space) is filled with about 30 mL of fluid, which lubricates the surface of the heart and reduces friction during systole.

## Heart Chambers

The four chambers of the heart constitute the right- and left-sided pumping systems. The right side of the heart, made up of the right atrium and right ventricle, distributes venous blood (deoxygenated blood) to the lungs via the pulmonary artery (pulmonary circulation) for oxygenation. The right atrium receives blood returning from the superior vena cava (head, neck, and upper extremities), inferior vena cava (trunk and lower extremities), and coronary sinus (coronary circulation). The left side of the heart, composed of the left atrium and left ventricle, distributes oxygenated blood to the remainder of the body via the aorta (systemic circulation). The left atrium receives oxygenated blood from the pulmonary circulation via the pulmonary veins. The relationships of the four heart chambers are shown in Figure 26-1.

The varying thicknesses of the atrial and ventricular walls relate to the workload required by each chamber. The atria are thin-walled because blood returning to these chambers generates low pressures. In contrast, the ventricular walls are thicker because they generate greater pressures during systole. The right ventricle contracts against low pulmonary

**FIGURE 26-1.** Structure of the heart. Arrows show course of blood flow through the heart chambers.

vascular pressure and has thinner walls than the left ventricle. The left ventricle, with walls two-and-a-half times more muscular than those of the right ventricle, contracts against high systemic pressure.

Because the heart lies in a rotated position within the chest cavity, the right ventricle lies anteriorly (just beneath the sternum) and the left ventricle is situated posteriorly. The left ventricle is responsible for the apical beat or the point of maximum impulse (PMI), which is normally palpable in the left midclavicular line of the chest wall at the fifth intercostal space.

## Heart Valves

The four valves in the heart permit blood to flow in only one direction. The valves, which are composed of thin leaflets of fibrous tissue, open and close in response to the movement of blood and pressure changes within the chambers. There are two types of valves: atrioventricular and semilunar.

### ATRIOVENTRICULAR VALVES

The valves that separate the atria from the ventricles are termed atrioventricular valves. The tricuspid valve, so named because it is composed of three cusps or leaflets, separates the right atrium from the right ventricle. The mitral or bicuspid (two cusps) valve lies between the left atrium and the left ventricle (see Fig. 26-1).

Normally, when the ventricles contract, ventricular pressure increases, closing the atrioventricular valve leaflets. Two additional structures, the papillary muscles and the chordae tendineae, maintain valve closure. The papillary muscles, located on the sides of the ventricular walls, are connected to the valve leaflets by thin fibrous bands called chordae tendineae. During systole, contraction of the papillary muscles causes the chordae tendineae to become taut, keeping the valve leaflets approximated and closed.

### SEMILUNAR VALVES

The two semilunar valves are composed of three half-moon–like leaflets. The valve between the right ventricle and the pulmonary artery is called the pulmonic valve. The valve between the left ventricle and the aorta is called the aortic valve.

## Coronary Arteries

**CONCEPTS** in action **ANIMATION**

The left and right coronary arteries and their branches supply arterial blood to the heart. These arteries originate from the aorta just above the aortic valve leaflets. The heart has large metabolic requirements, extracting approximately 70% to 80% of the oxygen delivered (other organs extract, on average, 25%). Unlike other arteries, the coronary arteries are perfused during diastole. An increase in heart rate shortens diastole and can decrease myocardial perfusion. Patients, particularly those with CAD, can develop **myocardial ischemia** (inadequate oxygen supply) when the heart rate accelerates.

The left coronary artery has three branches. The artery from the point of origin to the first major branch is called the left main coronary artery. Two branches arise off the left main coronary artery: the left anterior descending artery, which courses down the anterior wall of the heart, and the circumflex artery, which circles around to the lateral left wall of the heart.

The right side of the heart is supplied by the right coronary artery, which progresses around to the bottom or inferior wall of the heart. The posterior wall of the heart receives its blood supply by an additional branch from the right coronary artery called the posterior descending artery.

Superficial to the coronary arteries are the coronary veins. Venous blood from these veins returns to the heart primarily through the coronary sinus, which is located posteriorly in the right atrium.

## Cardiac Muscle

The myocardium is the middle, muscular layer of the atrial and ventricular walls. It is composed of specialized cells called myocytes, which form an interconnected network of muscle fibers. These fibers encircle the heart in a figure-of-eight pattern, forming a spiral from the base of the heart to the apex. During contraction, this muscular configuration facilitates a twisting and compressive movement of the heart that begins in the atria and moves to the ventricles. The sequential and rhythmic pattern of contraction, followed by relaxation of the muscle fibers, maximizes the volume of blood ejected with each contraction. This cyclical pattern of myocardial contraction is controlled by the conduction system.

# Physiology of the Heart

## Cardiac Electrophysiology

The **cardiac conduction system** generates and transmits electrical impulses that stimulate contraction of the myocardium. Under normal circumstances, the conduction system first stimulates contraction of the atria and then the ventricles. The synchronization of the atrial and ventricular events allows the ventricles to fill completely before ventricular ejection, thereby maximizing cardiac output. Three physiologic characteristics of two specialized electrical cells, the **nodal cells** and the **Purkinje cells**, provide this synchronization:

*Automaticity*: ability to initiate an electrical impulse
*Excitability*: ability to respond to an electrical impulse
*Conductivity*: ability to transmit an electrical impulse from one cell to another

Both the **sinoatrial (SA) node** and the **atrioventricular (AV) node** are composed of nodal cells. The SA node, the primary pacemaker of the heart, is located at the junction of the superior vena cava and the right atrium (Fig. 26-2). The SA node in a normal resting adult heart has an inherent firing rate of 60 to 100 impulses per minute, but the rate can change in response to the metabolic demands of the body.

The electrical impulses initiated by the SA node are conducted along the myocardial cells of the atria via specialized tracts called internodal pathways. The impulses cause electrical stimulation and subsequent contraction of the atria. The impulses are then conducted to the AV node, which is located in the right atrial wall near the tricuspid valve (see Fig. 26-2). The AV node coordinates the incoming electrical

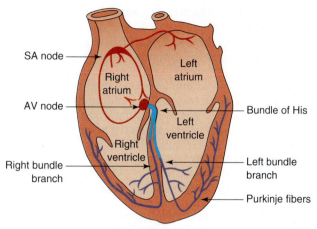

**FIGURE 26-2.** Cardiac conduction system. AV, atrioventricular; SA, sinoatrial.

impulses from the atria and after a slight delay (allowing the atria time to contract and complete ventricular filling) relays the impulse to the ventricles.

Initially, the impulse is conducted through a bundle of specialized conducting tissue, referred to as the bundle of His, which then divides into the right bundle branch (conducting impulses to the right ventricle) and the left bundle branch (conducting impulses to the left ventricle). To transmit impulses to the left ventricle, the largest chamber of the heart, the left bundle branch divides into the left anterior and left posterior bundle branches. Impulses travel through the bundle branches to reach the terminal point in the conduction system, called the Purkinje fibers. These fibers are composed of Purkinje cells, specialized to rapidly conduct the impulses through the thick walls of the ventricles. This is the point at which the myocardial cells are stimulated, causing ventricular contraction.

The heart rate is determined by the myocardial cells with the fastest inherent firing rate. Under normal circumstances, the SA node has the highest inherent rate (60 to 100 impulses per minute), the AV node has the second-highest inherent rate (40 to 60 impulses per minute), and the ventricular pacemaker sites have the lowest inherent rate (30 to 40 impulses per minute). If the SA node malfunctions, the AV node generally takes over the pacemaker function of the heart at its inherently lower rate. Should both the SA and the AV nodes fail in their pacemaker function, a pacemaker site in the ventricle will fire at its inherent bradycardic rate of 30 to 40 impulses per minute.

### CARDIAC ACTION POTENTIAL

The nodal and Purkinje cells (electrical cells) generate and transmit impulses across the heart, stimulating the cardiac myocytes (working cells) to contract. Stimulation of the cardiac working cells occurs due to the exchange of electrically charged particles, called ions, across channels located in the cell membrane. The channels regulate the movement and speed of specific ions, namely sodium, potassium, and calcium, as they enter and exit the cell. Sodium rapidly enters into the cell through sodium fast channels, in contrast to calcium, which enters the cell through calcium slow channels. In the resting or polarized state, sodium is the primary extracellular ion, whereas potassium is the primary intracellular ion. This difference in ion concentration means that the inside of the cell has a negative charge compared to the positive charge on the outside. This relationship changes during cellular stimulation, when sodium or calcium crosses the cell membrane into the cell and potassium ions exit into the extracellular space. This exchange of ions creates a positively charged intracellular space and a negatively charged extracellular space that characterizes the period known as **depolarization**. Once depolarization is complete, the exchange of ions reverts back to its resting state; this period is known as **repolarization**. The repeated cycle of depolarization and repolarization is called the cardiac action potential.

As shown in Figure 26-3, the cardiac action potential has five phases:

- Phase 0: Cellular depolarization is initiated as positive ions influx into the cell. During this phase, the working cells (atrial and ventricular myocytes) rapidly depolarize as sodium moves into the cells through sodium fast channels. The myocytes have a fast response action potential. In contrast, the cells of the SA and AV node depolarize when calcium enters these cells through calcium slow channels. These cells have a slow response action potential.
- Phase 1: Early cellular repolarization begins during this phase as potassium exits the intracellular space.
- Phase 2: This phase is called the plateau phase because the rate of repolarization slows. Calcium ions enter the intracellular space.
- Phase 3: This phase marks the completion of repolarization and return of the cell to its resting state.
- Phase 4: This phase is considered the resting phase before the next depolarization.

Knowledge of the differences between fast- and slow-response action potentials enhances the nurse's understanding of the indications for and actions of antiarrhythmic medications. For example, class I antiarrhythmic medications such as lidocaine (Xylocaine), quinidine (Quinalan), and propafenone (Rythmol) are administered to suppress dysrhythmia formation. These medications act by blocking the influx of sodium into the cells that have a fast-response

**FIGURE 26-3.** Cardiac action potential of a fast-response Purkinje fiber. The arrows indicate the approximate time and direction of movement of each ion influencing membrane potential. $Ca^{++}$ movement out of the cell is not well defined but is thought to occur during phase 4.

action potential. This action prevents rapid depolarization or phase 0, thereby preventing the dysrhythmia. Class II agents or beta-blockers (eg, metoprolol [Lopressor], sotalol [Betapace]) decrease automaticity and help slow tachycardias. Class III agents such as amiodarone (Cordarone) prolong repolarization and are useful in suppressing atrial or ventricular dysrhythmias. Class IV agents or calcium channel blockers (eg, verapamil [Calan], diltiazem [Cardizem]) are used to treat tachycardias. These medications block the influx of calcium in phase 0 of the SA and AV nodes that have a slow-response action potential. This action slows AV node conduction of impulses into the ventricle, resulting in a slower ventricular rate of depolarization and subsequent contraction.

### REFRACTORY PERIODS

Under normal circumstances, the myocardial cell must complete repolarization before it can enter a new phase of depolarization. During this phase, called the refractory period, the cells are incapable of being stimulated. There are two phases of the refractory period of the action potential, commonly referred to as the effective (or absolute) refractory period and the relative refractory period. During the effective refractory period, the cell is completely unresponsive to any electrical stimulus; it is incapable of initiating an early depolarization. The effective refractory period corresponds with the time in phase 0 to the middle of phase 3 of the action potential. The relative refractory period corresponds with the short time at the end of phase 3. During the relative refractory period, if an electrical stimulus is stronger than normal, the cell may depolarize prematurely. Early depolarizations of the atrium or ventricle cause premature contractions, placing the patient at risk for dysrhythmias. Premature ventricular contractions in certain situations, such as the setting of myocardial ischemia, are worrisome because these early ventricular depolarizations can trigger life-threatening dysrhythmias, including ventricular tachycardia or ventricular fibrillation. These dysrhythmias and others are discussed in detail in Chapter 27.

Several circumstances make the heart more susceptible to early depolarization during the relative refractory period, thus increasing the risk for serious dysrhythmias. These conditions include electrolyte disturbances (hypokalemia, hypomagnesemia), hypoxemia, acidosis, hypercarbia, hypothermia, an increase in catecholamines, myocardial injury (eg, acute myocardial infarction [MI]), and chamber enlargement (eg, HF, hypertension, ventricular aneurysm).

## Cardiac Hemodynamics

An important determinant of blood flow in the cardiovascular system is the principle that fluid flows from a region of higher pressure to one of lower pressure. The pressures responsible for blood flow in the normal circulation are generated during systole and diastole. Figure 26-4 depicts the pressure differences in the great vessels and in the four chambers of the heart during systole and diastole.

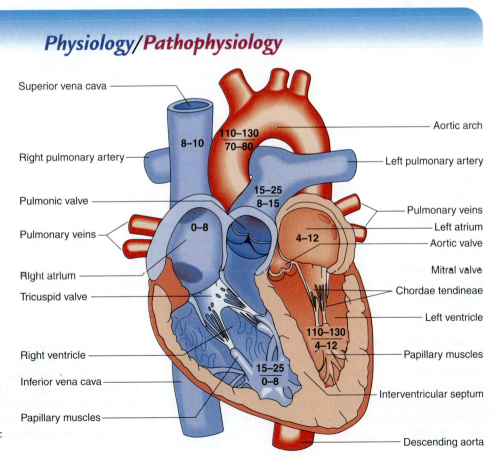

**FIGURE 26-4.** Great vessel and chamber pressures. Pressures are identified in mm Hg as mean pressure or systolic over diastolic pressure.

## CARDIAC CYCLE
**CONCEPTS in action ANIMATION**

Beginning with systole, the pressure inside the ventricles rapidly increases, forcing the atrioventricular valves to close. As a result, blood ceases to flow from the atria into the ventricles, and regurgitation (backflow) of blood into the atria is prevented. The rapid increase of pressure inside the right and left ventricles forces the pulmonic and aortic valves to open, and blood is ejected into the pulmonary artery and aorta, respectively. The exit of blood is at first rapid; then, as the pressure in each ventricle and its corresponding artery equalizes, the flow of blood gradually decreases. At the end of systole, pressure within the right and left ventricles rapidly decreases. This decreases pulmonary artery and aortic pressure, causing closure of the semilunar valves. These events mark the onset of diastole.

During diastole, when the ventricles are relaxed and the atrioventricular valves are open, blood returning from the veins flows into the atria and then into the ventricles. Toward the end of this diastolic period, the atrial muscles contract in response to an electrical impulse initiated by the SA node (atrial systole). The resultant contraction increases the pressure inside the atria, ejecting blood into the ventricles. Atrial systole augments ventricular blood volume by 15% to 25% and is sometimes referred to as the "atrial kick." At this point, ventricular systole begins in response to propagation of the electrical impulse that began in the SA node some milliseconds previously.

**Chamber Pressures.** In the right side of the heart, the pressure generated during ventricular systole (15 to 25 mm Hg) exceeds the pulmonary artery diastolic pressure (8 to 15 mm Hg), and blood is ejected into the pulmonary circulation. During diastole, venous blood flows into the atrium because pressure in the superior and inferior vena cava (8 to 10 mm Hg) is higher than that in the atrium. Blood flows through the open tricuspid valve and into the right ventricle until the two right chamber pressures equalize (0 to 8 mm Hg).

In the left side of the heart, similar events occur, although higher pressures are generated. As pressure mounts in the left ventricle during systole (110 to 130 mm Hg), resting aortic pressure (80 mm Hg) is exceeded and blood is ejected into the aorta. During left ventricular ejection, the resultant aortic pressure (110 to 130 mm Hg) forces blood through the arteries. Forward blood flow into the aorta ceases as the ventricle relaxes and pressure decreases. During diastole, oxygenated blood returning from the pulmonary circulation via the four pulmonary veins flows into the atrium, where pressure remains low. Blood readily flows into the left ventricle because ventricular pressure is also low. At the end of diastole, pressures in the atrium and ventricle equilibrate (4 to 12 mm Hg). Figure 26-4 depicts the systolic and diastolic pressures in the four chambers of the heart.

**Pressure Measurement.** Chamber pressures are measured with the use of special monitoring catheters and equipment. This technique is called hemodynamic monitoring. Nurses caring for critically ill patients must have a sophisticated working knowledge of normal chamber pressures and the hemodynamic changes that occur during serious illnesses. The data obtained from hemodynamic monitoring assist with the diagnosis and management of pathophysiologic conditions affecting critically ill patients. Methods of hemodynamic monitoring are covered in more detail at the end of this chapter.

## Cardiac Output

**Cardiac output** refers to the amount of blood pumped by each ventricle during a given period. The cardiac output in a resting adult is about 5 liters per minute but varies greatly depending on the metabolic needs of the body. Cardiac output is computed by multiplying the stroke volume by the heart rate. **Stroke volume** is the amount of blood ejected per heartbeat. The average resting stroke volume is about 70 mL, and the heart rate is 60 to 80 beats per minute (bpm). Cardiac output can be affected by changes in either stroke volume or heart rate.

### CONTROL OF HEART RATE
Cardiac output must be responsive to changes in the metabolic demands of the tissues. For example, during exercise the total cardiac output may increase fourfold, to 20 liters per minute. This increase is normally accomplished by approximate doubling of both the heart rate and the stroke volume. Changes in heart rate are accomplished by reflex controls mediated by the autonomic nervous system, including its sympathetic and parasympathetic divisions. The parasympathetic impulses, which travel to the heart through the vagus nerve, can slow the cardiac rate, whereas sympathetic impulses increase it. These effects on heart rate result from action on the SA node, to either decrease or increase its inherent rate. The balance between these two reflex control systems normally determines the heart rate. The heart rate is stimulated also by an increased level of circulating catecholamines (secreted by the adrenal gland) and by excess thyroid hormone, which produces a catecholamine-like effect.

In addition, the heart rate is affected by central nervous system and baroreceptor activity. **Baroreceptors** are specialized nerve cells located in the aortic arch and in both right and left internal carotid arteries (at the point of bifurcation from the common carotid arteries). The baroreceptors are sensitive to changes in blood pressure (BP). During elevations in BP (**hypertension**), these cells increase their rate of discharge, transmitting impulses to the medulla. This initiates parasympathetic activity and inhibits sympathetic response, lowering the heart rate and the BP. The opposite is true during **hypotension** (low BP). Hypotension results in less baroreceptor stimulation, which prompts a decrease in parasympathetic inhibitory activity in the SA node, allowing for enhanced sympathetic activity. The resultant vasoconstriction and increased heart rate elevate the BP.

### CONTROL OF STROKE VOLUME
Stroke volume is primarily determined by three factors: preload, afterload, and contractility.

**Preload** refers to the degree of stretch of the cardiac muscle fibers at the end of diastole. The end of diastole is the period when filling volume in the ventricles is the highest and the degree of stretch on the muscle fibers is the greatest. The volume of blood within the ventricle at the end of diastole determines preload, which directly affects stroke volume. As the volume of blood returning to the heart increases, muscle fiber stretch also increases (increased preload), resulting in stronger contraction and a greater stroke volume. This relationship, called the Frank-Starling (or Starling) law of the heart, is maintained until the physiologic limit of the muscle is reached.

The Frank-Starling law is based on the fact that, within limits, the greater the initial length or stretch of the cardiac muscle cells (sarcomeres), the greater the degree of shortening that occurs. This result is caused by increased interaction between the thick and thin filaments within the cardiac muscle cells. Preload is decreased by a reduction in the volume of blood returning to the ventricles. Diuresis, **venodilating agents** (eg, nitrates), and low fluid volume or excessive fluid loss reduce preload. Preload is increased by increasing the return of circulating blood volume to the ventricles. Controlling the loss of blood or body fluids and replacing fluids (ie, blood transfusions and intravenous [IV] fluid administration) are examples of ways to increase preload.

**Afterload,** the amount of resistance to ejection of blood from the ventricle, is the second determinant of stroke volume. The resistance of the systemic BP to left ventricular ejection is called **systemic vascular resistance.** The resistance of the pulmonary BP to right ventricular ejection is called **pulmonary vascular resistance.** There is an inverse relationship between afterload and stroke volume. For example, afterload is increased by arterial vasoconstriction, which leads to decreased stroke volume. The opposite is true with arterial vasodilation: afterload is reduced because there is less resistance to ejection, and stroke volume increases.

**Contractility** refers to the force generated by the contracting myocardium under any given condition. Contractility is enhanced by circulating catecholamines, sympathetic neuronal activity, and certain medications (eg, digoxin [Lanoxin], IV dopamine [Intropin], or dobutamine [Dobutrex]). Increased contractility results in increased stroke volume. Contractility is depressed by hypoxemia, acidosis, and certain medications (eg, beta-adrenergic blocking agents such as atenolol [Tenormin]).

The heart can achieve a greatly increased stroke volume (eg, during exercise) if preload is increased (through increased venous return), if contractility is increased (through sympathetic nervous system discharge), and if afterload is decreased (through peripheral vasodilation with decreased aortic pressure).

The percentage of the end-diastolic volume that is ejected with each stroke is called the **ejection fraction.** With each stroke, about 42% (right ventricle) to 50% (left ventricle) or more of the end-diastolic volume is ejected by the normal heart. The ejection fraction can be used as an index of myocardial contractility: the ejection fraction decreases if contractility is depressed.

### Gerontologic Considerations

Changes in cardiac structure and function are clearly observable in the aging heart. To understand the changes specifically related to aging, it is helpful to distinguish the normal aging process from changes related to CVD. The anatomic and functional changes in the aging heart are summarized in Table 26-1.

The normal aging heart can maintain an adequate cardiac output under ordinary circumstances but may have a limited ability to respond to situations that cause physical or emotional stress. In an elderly person who is less active, the left ventricle may become smaller (atrophy) as a consequence of physical deconditioning. Aging also results in decreased elasticity and widening of the aorta, thickening and rigidity of the cardiac valves, and increased connective tissue in the SA and AV nodes and bundle branches.

These changes lead to decreased myocardial contractility, increased left ventricular ejection time (prolonged systole), and delayed conduction. Therefore, stressful physical and emotional conditions, especially those that occur suddenly, may have adverse effects on the aged person. The heart cannot respond to such conditions with an adequate rate increase and needs more time to return to a normal resting rate after even a minimal increase in heart rate. In some patients, the added stress may precipitate HF.

## Gender Differences in Cardiac Structure and Function

Structural differences between the hearts of men and women have significant implications. Compared with a man's heart, a woman's heart tends to be smaller. It weighs less and has smaller coronary arteries. Because the coronary arteries of a woman are smaller, they occlude from atherosclerosis more easily, making procedures such as cardiac catheterization and angioplasty technically more difficult, with a higher incidence of postprocedural complications. In addition, the resting rate, stroke volume, and ejection fraction of a woman's heart are higher than those of a man's heart, and the conduction time of an electrical impulse coursing from the SA node through the AV node to the Purkinje fibers is briefer.

For many years, it was believed that the female hormone estrogen had cardioprotective effects. Hormone therapy was routinely prescribed for postmenopausal women in the belief that this pharmacologic therapy would deter the onset and progression of coronary atherosclerosis. This belief was supported by anecdotal evidence that the onset of heart disease in women tends to occur later than in men, at a time when most women had experienced menopause and were largely bereft of estrogen. However, data from the Women's Health Initiative refuted this belief (see Chapter 28 for additional information) (Mosca, Appel, Benjamin, et al., 2004).

## Assessment

The frequency and extent of the nursing assessment of cardiovascular function are based on several factors, including the severity of the patient's symptoms, the presence of risk factors, the practice setting, and the purpose

### TABLE 26-1  Age-Related Changes of the Cardiac System

| Cardiovascular System | Structural Changes | Functional Changes | History and Physical Findings |
|---|---|---|---|
| Atria | ↑ Size of left atrium<br>Thickening of the endocardium | ↑ Atrial irritability | Irregular heart rhythm from atrial dysrhythmias |
| Left ventricle | Endocardial fibrosis<br>Myocardial thickening (hypertrophy)<br>Infiltration of fat into myocardium | Left ventricle stiff and less compliant<br>Progressive decline in cardiac output<br>↑ Risk for ventricular dysrhythmias<br>Prolonged systole | Fatigue<br>↓ Exercise tolerance<br>Signs and symptoms of HF or ventricular dysrhythmias<br>Point of maximal impulse palpated lateral to the midclavicular line<br>↓ Intensity $S_1$, $S_2$; split $S_2$<br>$S_4$ may be present |
| Valves | Thickening and rigidity of AV valves<br>Calcification of aortic valve | Abnormal blood flow across valves during cardiac cycle | Murmurs may be present<br>Thrill may be palpated if significant murmur is present |
| Conduction system | Connective tissue collects in SA node, AV node, and bundle branches<br>↓ Number SA node cells<br>↓ Number AV, bundle of His, right and left bundle branch cells | Slower SA node rate of impulse discharge<br>Slowed conduction across AV node and ventricular conduction system | Bradycardia<br>Heart block<br>ECG changes consistent with slowed conduction (↑ PR interval, widened QRS complex) |
| Sympathetic nervous system | ↓ Response to beta-adrenergic stimulation | ↓ Adaptive response to exercise: contractility and heart rate slower to respond to exercise demands<br>Heart rate takes more time to return to baseline | Fatigue<br>Diminished exercise tolerance<br>↓ Ability to respond to stress |
| Aorta and arteries | Stiffening of vasculature<br>↓ Elasticity and widening of aorta<br>Elongation of aorta, displacing the brachiocephalic artery upward | Left ventricular hypertrophy | Progressive increase in systolic BP; slight ↑ in diastolic BP<br>Widening pulse pressure<br>Pulsation visible above right clavicle |
| Baroreceptor response | ↓ Sensitivity of baroreceptors in the carotid artery and aorta to transient episodes of hypertension and hypotension | Baroreceptors unable to regulate heart rate and vascular tone, causing slow response to postural changes in body position | Postural blood pressure changes and reports feeling dizzy, fainting when moving from lying to sitting or standing position |

AV, atrioventricular; BP, blood pressure; ECG, electrocardiographic; HF, heart failure; SA, sinoatrial.

of the assessment. An acutely ill patient with CVD who is admitted to the emergency department or coronary intensive care unit requires a very different assessment than a person who is being examined for a chronic stable condition. Although the key components of the cardiovascular assessment remain the same (health history, physical examination, and monitoring of laboratory and diagnostic test results), the assessment priorities vary according to the needs of the patient. For example, an emergency department nurse caring for a patient who is admitted with symptoms associated with acute coronary syndrome (ACS) performs a rapid and focused assessment because treatment of ACS is time-dependent. The nurse obtains the patient's history of current illness, including the signs and symptoms that prompted the patient to come to the emergency department, cardiac risk factors, and current medications. The physical assessment is ongoing and concentrates on evaluating the patient for ACS complications, such as dysrhythmias and HF, and determining the effectiveness of medical treatment.

## Health History and Clinical Manifestations

The health history allows the nurse to obtain important information about the health status of the patient. In addition, it gives the patient the opportunity to share his or her impressions of relevant symptoms, current state of illness, and experiences associated with managing his or her health (see "Health Perception and Management" later in this chapter). Nurses, physicians, and other health care professionals often obtain health histories from the same patient for similar reasons. It is important for the nurse to be aware of the information obtained by other members of the health care team. This knowledge allows the nurse to validate the findings of others, such as a history of allergies or use of current medications, leaving more time to explore other important topics. Health histories taken by members of each discipline should complement one another and not be repetitive or burdensome to the patient. For example, a patient who is asked about his or her allergies or medications multiple times during the same hospitalization may believe that the nurses and other health care professionals do not communicate with each other.

It is the nurse's responsibility to ensure that the information obtained from the health history accurately reflects the patient's current health. Questions are formulated based on the setting. For example, in the emergency department, the goal of the triage nurse is to assess the patient's major complaint accurately and then rapidly decide what level of care the patient requires. Once the patient's condition stabilizes, a more extensive history can be obtained. In nonemergency situations and with stable patients, it is possible and advisable to obtain a complete health history during the initial contact.

During a health history, the primary source of information is the patient. If the patient does not speak English, a reliable professional interpreter who is cognizant of the importance of confidentiality should be used. It is often helpful to have spouses or partners available during the health history interview. For patients who cannot communicate, the family or the prior medical record are important sources of information. The source of information obtained during the health history is documented in the patient's medical record.

Initially, demographic information regarding age, gender, and ethnic origin is obtained. The family history and the physical examination include assessment for genetic abnormalities associated with cardiovascular disorders. Height and current weight are measured. (If there has been a recent weight loss or gain, the patient is asked about his or her usual weight.) During the interview, the nurse must be sensitive to the cultural background and religious practices of the patient. Having a heightened awareness of cultural diversity prevents barriers to communication that can result

## GENETICS IN NURSING PRACTICE

### Cardiovascular Disorders

Several cardiovascular disorders are associated with genetic abnormalities. Some examples are:
- Familial hypercholesterolemia
- Hypertrophic cardiomyopathy
- Long QT syndrome
- Hereditary hemochromatosis
- Elevated homocysteine levels

### NURSING ASSESSMENTS
#### Family History Assessment
- Assess all patients with cardiovascular symptoms for coronary artery disease (CAD), regardless of age (early-onset CAD occurs).
- Assess family history of sudden death in persons who may or may not have been diagnosed with coronary disease (especially of early onset).
- Ask about sudden death in a previously asymptomatic child, adolescent, or adult.
- Ask about other family members with biochemical or neuromuscular conditions (eg, hemochromatosis or muscular dystrophy).
- Assess whether DNA mutation or other genetic testing has been performed on an affected family member.

#### Patient Assessment
- Assess for signs and symptoms of hyperlipidemias (xanthomas, corneal arcus, abdominal pain of unexplained origin).
- Assess for muscular weakness.

### MANAGEMENT ISSUES SPECIFIC TO GENETICS
- If indicated, refer for further genetic counseling and evaluation so that the family can discuss inheritance, risk to other family members, availability of genetic testing, and gene-based interventions.
- Offer appropriate genetics information and resources (eg, Genetic Alliance website, American Heart Association, Muscular Dystrophy Association).
- Provide support to families newly diagnosed with genetics-related cardiovascular disease.

### GENETICS RESOURCES
Genetic Alliance—a directory of support groups for patients and families with genetic conditions, http://www.geneticalliance.org

Gene Clinics—a listing of common genetic disorders with up-to-date clinical summaries, genetic counseling, and testing information, http://www.geneclinics.org

National Organization of Rare Disorders—a directory of support groups and information for patients and families with rare genetic disorders, http://www.rarediseases.org

OMIM: Online Mendelian Inheritance in Man—a complete listing of inherited genetic conditions, http://www.ncbi.nlm.nih.gov/omim/stats/html

when the interview is based on the nurse's personal frame of reference. For example, patients whose cultural or ethnic norms vary from those of the nurse may differ in their description of symptoms such as pain. In addition, they may engage in nontraditional health practices before seeking formal health care.

The information derived from the history assists in identifying pertinent issues related to the patient's condition and educational and self-care needs. Once these issues are clearly defined and possibly verified through the physical assessment, a plan of care is developed and implemented. During subsequent contacts or visits with the patient, a more focused health history is performed to:

- Determine whether the patient is progressing toward the established goals
- Reevaluate the existing plan of care and revise it as needed
- Evaluate the patient's health status so current issues can be resolved and new issues identified

## Clinical Manifestations

The signs and symptoms experienced by people with CVD are related to dysrhythmias and conduction problems (see Chapter 27); CAD (see Chapter 28); structural, infectious, and inflammatory disorders of the heart (see Chapter 29); and complications of CVD such as HF and cardiogenic shock (see Chapter 30). These disorders have many signs and symptoms in common; therefore, the nurse must be skillful at recognizing these signs and symptoms so that patients are given appropriate and often life-saving care.

CAD, which may be characterized by a history of angina pectoris, MI, or both, is the most prevalent of all forms of CVD and deserves further discussion before common clinical manifestations of CVD are reviewed. More than 13 million Americans have CAD; it is responsible for more than 54% of all CVD-related deaths (AHA, 2006). ACS, a serious manifestation of CAD, develops when an atheromatous plaque in a diseased coronary artery ruptures and forms an obstructive thrombus. The spectrum of diagnoses associated with ACS include unstable angina, non-ST-elevation myocardial infarction (NSTEMI), and ST-elevation myocardial infarction (STEMI) (see Chapter 28). Approximately 50% of people with ACS experience similar symptoms that include chest pain or discomfort associated with myocardial ischemia; therefore, the specific diagnosis cannot be made based on presenting signs and symptoms alone. Further testing with a 12-lead electrocardiogram (ECG) and serum laboratory analysis of cardiac biomarkers is necessary to determine whether the patient has NSTEMI, STEMI, or unstable angina (see Chapter 28).

The following are the most common signs and symptoms of CVD, with related medical diagnoses in parentheses:

- Chest pain or discomfort (angina pectoris, ACS, dysrhythmias, valvular heart disease)
- Shortness of breath or dyspnea (ACS, cardiogenic shock, HF, valvular heart disease)
- Peripheral edema and weight gain (HF)
- Palpitations (tachycardia from a variety of causes, including ACS, caffeine or other stimulants, electrolyte imbalances, stress, valvular heart disease, ventricular aneurysms)
- Fatigue (early warning symptom of ACS, HF, valvular heart disease)
- Dizziness, syncope, or changes in level of consciousness (cardiogenic shock, cerebrovascular disorders, dysrhythmias, hypotension, postural hypotension, vasovagal episode)

Not all chest symptoms, including chest pain or discomfort, reflect myocardial ischemia. When a patient experiences chest pain, the nurse asks questions that aid in differentiating cardiac-related chest symptoms from other sources. Table 26-2 summarizes the characteristics and patterns of the more common cardiac and noncardiac causes of chest symptoms. During the assessment the patient is asked to describe the character or quality of the pain or discomfort and its location. The nurse needs to determine whether there is radiation to or discomfort in other areas and must assess for key signs and symptoms such as diaphoresis or nausea. It is important to identify the events that precipitate symptom onset, the duration of the symptom, and measures that aggravate or relieve the symptom. Chart 26-1 provides examples of questions used to assess common cardiac signs and symptoms. Some of the patient's responses may require clarification and follow-up.

Nurses and other health care professionals must take a patient's complaint of chest pain or discomfort seriously until the cause is determined. The following points should be remembered when assessing patients who may have cardiac symptoms:

- All patients reporting chest symptoms, particularly those at risk for CAD or who have a history of CAD, should be evaluated initially for ACS.
- The location of chest symptoms is not well correlated with the cause of the pain. For example, substernal chest pain can result from a number of causes (see Table 26-2).
- The severity or duration of chest pain or discomfort does not predict the seriousness of its cause. For example, a patient experiencing esophageal spasm may rate chest pain as a "10/10" (eg, the worst pain the patient has ever felt), whereas a patient experiencing an acute MI may report only mild to moderate chest pressure.
- Elderly people and patients with diabetes may not experience chest pain as a typical symptom associated with angina and ACS because of neuropathies. Atypical symptoms, such as fatigue or shortness of breath, are predominant symptoms in these patients.
- Women with ACS are more likely than men to present with atypical symptoms, including shoulder or upper back pain, shortness of breath, or extreme fatigue (Ryan, DeVon, & Zerwic, 2005).
- More than one clinical cardiac condition may occur simultaneously. During an acute MI, patients may report chest pain from myocardial ischemia, shortness of breath from HF, and palpitations from dysrhythmias. Both HF and dysrhythmias are complications of acute MI.

## TABLE 26-2   Assessing Chest Pain

| Location | Character | Duration | Precipitating Events and Aggravating Factors | Alleviating Factors |
|---|---|---|---|---|
| **Angina pectoris—acute coronary syndrome** (unstable angina, myocardial infarction [MI]) *Usual distribution of pain with myocardial ischemia. Less common sites of pain with myocardial ischemia: Jaw, Right side, Epigastrium, Back* | Angina: Uncomfortable pressure, squeezing, or fullness in substernum. Can radiate across chest or to the medial aspect of one or both arms and hands, or to the jaw, shoulders, back, or epigastrium. Radiation to arms and hands is described as numbness, tingling, or aching. | Angina: 5–15 min | Angina: Physical exertion, emotional upset, eating large meal, or exposure to extremes in temperature | Angina: Rest, nitroglycerin, oxygen |
| | MI: Similar symptom presentation as in angina pectoris. Often associated with shortness of breath, diaphoresis, palpitations, fatigue, and nausea or vomiting. | MI: >15 min | MI: Emotional upset or unusual physical exertion occurring within 24 hours of symptom onset. Can occur at rest or while asleep. | MI: Morphine sulfate, reperfusion of coronary artery with thrombolysis or percutaneous coronary intervention |
| **Pericarditis** | Sharp, severe substernal or epigastric pain. Can radiate to neck, arms, and back. Other associated symptoms are fever, malaise, dyspnea, cough, nausea, dizziness, and palpitations. | Intermittent | Sudden onset. Pain increases with inspiration, swallowing, coughing, and rotation of trunk. | Sitting upright, analgesia, anti-inflammatory medications |
| **Pulmonary disorders** (pneumonia, pulmonary embolism) | Sharp, severe substernal or epigastric pain arising from inferior portion of pleura. Patient may be able to localize the pain. | 30+ min | Follows an infectious or noninfectious process (acute MI, cardiac surgery, cancer, immune disorders, uremia). Pleuritic pain increases with inspiration, coughing, movement and supine positioning. Occurs in conjunction with community-acquired or nosocomial lung infections (pneumonia) or deep vein thrombosis (pulmonary embolism). | Treatment of underlying cause |

*continued >*

## TABLE 26-2  Assessing Chest Pain (Continued)

| Location | Character | Duration | Precipitating Events and Aggravating Factors | Alleviating Factors |
|---|---|---|---|---|
| **Esophageal disorders** (hiatal hernia, reflux esophagitis or spasm) | Substernal pain described as sharp, burning, or heavy; often mimics angina; can radiate to neck, arm, or shoulders. | 5–60 min | Recumbency, cold liquids, exercise. | Food, antacid. Nitroglycerin relieves spasm. |
| **Anxiety and panic disorders** | Pain described as stabbing to dull ache. Associated with diaphoresis, palpitations, shortness of breath, tingling of hands or mouth, feeling of unreality, or fear of losing control. | Peaks in 10 min | No associated trigger (unexpected) or situation where symptoms are associated with anticipating or experiencing a specific trigger. | Removal of stimulus, relaxation, medications to treat anxiety or antidepressant medication |
| **Musculoskeletal disorders** (costochondritis) | Sharp or stabbing pain localized in anterior chest. Most often unilateral. Can radiate across chest to epigastrium or back. Patient able to localize pain. | Hours to days | Most often follows respiratory tract infection with significant coughing, vigorous exercise, or post trauma. Some cases are idiopathic. Exacerbated by deep inspiration, coughing, sneezing, and movement of upper torso or arms. | Rest, ice, or heat; analgesic or anti-inflammatory medications |

## Health Perception and Management

In an effort to determine how the patient perceives his or her current health status, the nurse might ask some of the following questions:

- What type of health concerns do you have? Are you able to identify any family history or behaviors (risk factors) that put you at risk for this health problem?
- What are your risk factors for heart disease? What do you do to stay healthy and take care of your heart?
- How is your health? Have you noticed any changes from last year? From 5 years ago?
- Do you have a cardiologist or primary health care provider? How often do you go for checkups?
- Do you use tobacco or consume alcohol?
- What prescription and over-the-counter medications are you taking? Do you take vitamins or herbal supplements?

Some patients may not be aware of their own medical diagnosis. For example, patients may not realize that their heart attack was caused by CAD. Patients who do not understand

## CHART 26-1

### Assessing for Cardiac Signs and Symptoms

| SYMPTOMS | ASSESSMENT QUESTIONS | ASSESSING PATIENT'S CAPACITY FOR SELF-MANAGEMENT |
|---|---|---|
| Chest pain, chest discomfort, angina pain | • Where is your pain? (ask patient to point to location on chest)<br>• What does the pain feel like? (pressure, heaviness, burning)<br>• How severe is it on a scale of 0 to 10?<br>• What causes the pain? (exertion, stress)<br>• Does anything relieve it? (rest, nitroglycerin)<br>• Does it spread to your arms, neck, jaw, shoulders, or back?<br>• How long does the pain last?<br>• Do you have any additional symptoms? (shortness of breath, palpitations, dizziness, sweating) | *Symptom Recognition*<br>• If you have angina, what does it usually feel like?<br>• If you have angina, how do your angina symptoms differ from the discomfort caused by your other medical conditions? (indigestion, GI disorders)<br>• How do you think you would tell the difference between the symptoms of angina and a heart attack?<br>• What were you doing when the pain started?<br>*Symptom Management*<br>• What did you do when the pain started?<br>• How long did you wait before seeking medical attention (calling the doctor, coming to the emergency department, or calling the ambulance)?<br>*Use of Nitroglycerin*<br>• Do you have a prescription for nitroglycerin (NTG) tablets or spray?<br>• At the time of your chest pain, did you use your NTG?<br>• How many tablets or sprays did you use and how frequently?<br>• If you have NTG and did not take it with this angina episode, why do you think you did not take it?<br>• When did you first open your NTG container? Where is it stored? |
| Shortness of breath, edema, weight gain | • When did you first notice feeling short of breath?<br>• What makes you short of breath? Does anything make your breathing better or worse?<br>• What activities are you no longer able to do because you are short of breath?<br>• Do you ever wake up at night feeling short of breath?<br>• Do you have a cough? If yes, what do you cough up?<br>• What is your normal weight?<br>• Have you had a recent weight gain?<br>• Do you get up at night to urinate? Have you noticed an increase or decrease in the amount you usually urinate? | • Has anyone ever told you that you have heart failure? What does this mean to you?<br>• Do you ever forget to take your diuretic medication (water pill) or other heart medicines or decide not to take them? If so, why do you think this happens?<br>• What do you typically eat or drink? Who does the food shopping and meal preparation?<br>• Are you on a sodium- or fluid-restricted diet? Have you been able to follow your special diet?<br>• Do you have a scale to weigh yourself? How often do you weigh yourself?<br>• What are important signs or symptoms to report to your doctor? |

*continued >*

### CHART 26-1

## Assessing for Cardiac Signs and Symptoms, continued

| SYMPTOMS | ASSESSMENT QUESTIONS | ASSESSING PATIENT'S CAPACITY FOR SELF-MANAGEMENT |
|---|---|---|
| | • Have you noticed any weight gain or swelling in your feet, ankles, legs, or abdomen? (sacrum if bedridden) Do your shoes feel tight or clothes feel tight around your waist?<br>• On how many pillows do you sleep, and has this changed recently?<br>• Do you sleep in your bed, or do you breathe easier sleeping in a chair? | |
| Palpitations | • Do you ever feel your heart racing, skipping beats, or pounding? | • What did you do when your symptoms first occurred? |
| | • Do you ever feel lightheaded or dizzy?<br>• Are there any other symptoms that occur at the same time?<br>• How much caffeine do you consume?<br>• Do you use tobacco? (cigarettes, cigars, chew)<br>• Do you use any other stimulants, recreational drugs?<br>• Do you use any nutritional supplements or herbs?<br>• Have there been any changes in the amount of stress you experience? | • Is your primary health care provider aware of these symptoms?<br>• Are you taking medication for this condition, and have you been taking it as directed? |
| Fatigue | • How would you describe your usual activity level?<br>• What is your current activity level?<br>• What were you able to do 1 month and 6 months ago?<br>• What activities can you no longer do because of fatigue?<br>• Do you feel rested when you wake up in the morning?<br>• Can you rest during the day?<br>• How often do you awaken at night, and for what reason? | • Have you spoken with your primary health care provider about decreases in your activity level?<br>• Has anyone ever taught you energy conservation techniques? If so, are you able to use them? |
| Dizziness, syncope (loss of consciousness) | • Do you ever feel dizzy or lightheaded?<br>• Do you ever pass out or have fainting spells?<br>• Does this happen when you move from a lying to a sitting or standing position?<br>• Do you strain while having a bowel movement or when urinating?<br>• Have you been urinating more than usual?<br>• Have you decreased the amount of fluids you normally drink?<br>• Do you have headaches? | • Have you ever been told you have high or low blood pressure? Has it been checked recently?<br>• Are you taking any medications that can lower your blood pressure?<br>• Before standing from a lying position, do you sit for a few minutes? Does that relieve the dizziness?<br>• What are you using to prevent constipation? |

that their behaviors or diagnoses pose a threat to their health may be less motivated to make lifestyle changes or to manage their illness effectively. On the other hand, patients who perceive that their modifiable risk factors for heart disease affect their health and believe that they have the power to modify or change them may be more likely to change these behaviors (Chart 26-2).

The patient's ability to recognize cardiac symptoms and to know what to do when they occur is essential for effective self-care management. All too often, a patient's new symptoms or symptoms of progressing cardiac dysfunction go unrecognized. This results in prolonged delays in seeking life-saving treatment. Major barriers to seeking prompt medical care include lack of knowledge about the symp-

## NURSING RESEARCH PROFILE

### Women and Symptoms of Myocardial Infarction

McSweeney, J. C., Cody, M., O'Sullivan, P., et al. (2003). Women's early warning symptoms of acute myocardial infarction. *Circulation, 108*, 2619–2623.

#### Purpose
Chest pain is referred to as the typical acute symptom of coronary heart disease (CHD), and symptoms other than chest pain are referred to as atypical. However, this determination was based on the results of studies on middle-aged, white men. This study was conducted to determine how women present with acute symptoms of CHD, with a focus on early warning or prodromal symptoms of acute myocardial infarction (MI). The researchers sought to determine the most frequent prodromal symptoms of acute MI among women, how prodromal and acute symptoms relate to comorbidities and risk factors for CHD among women, and whether prodromal symptoms are predictive of acute MI symptomatology among women.

#### Design
Women who were discharged from the hospital after experiencing an acute MI were recruited from five sites in Arkansas, North Carolina, and Ohio. To be eligible for inclusion in the study, participants had to be cognitively intact, speak English, and have telephone access. Once consent was obtained from each participant, nurse research assistants conducted a 60-minute telephone interview using the McSweeney Acute and Prodromal Myocardial Infarction Symptom Survey (MAPMISS). The MAPMISS was developed by the researchers to survey 33 prodromal and 37 acute symptoms of CHD. Prodromal symptoms were defined as symptoms that are intermittent; new or changed in intensity or frequency; or disappear or return to previous levels after the acute MI. Acute symptoms were defined as those that begin at the time of acute MI and resolve after treatment.

Of the 515 women who completed the survey, 93% were white, 6% were black, and 2% were Native American. The mean age was 66.4 ($\pm$ 12) years. A small percentage (13%) of the women had attended school through eighth grade or less, and about 33% had some college education. More than 44% of the subjects reported a yearly income of $20,000 or less.

#### Findings
Women had an average of 5.71 ($\pm$ 4.36) prodromal and 7.3 ($\pm$ 4.8) acute symptoms. Most women (95%) experienced prodromal symptoms such as unusual fatigue (71%), sleep disturbances (48%), and shortness of breath (42%), and they reported the first two symptoms as being severe. These symptoms occurred daily or less frequently at least 1 month before the acute MI. Acute symptoms most frequently reported were shortness of breath (58%), weakness (55%), and fatigue (43%), whereas only 30% described chest discomfort. Prodromal and acute symptom scores were found to be significantly associated with most cardiac risk factors. The prodromal scores were an important predictor of acute symptom scores, more so than cardiac risk factors such as diabetes, hypertension, and hyperlipidemia.

#### Nursing Implications
Although the results of this study are limited by the sample demographics, they provide important contributions to the knowledge of early symptoms of acute MI among women. Symptoms described by women in this study were not the typical symptom of chest pain most commonly associated with acute MI among men. It is important for nurses to be aware of the spectrum of symptoms that can be experienced by women for 1 month or longer before acute MI. A thorough health history should include questions about prodromal symptoms. Women with suspected CHD should be asked about the recent onset of new or changing symptoms, especially fatigue, sleep disturbances, or shortness of breath. Women with these symptoms benefit from further cardiac diagnostic testing. Education targeted at women concerning the symptoms of an acute MI should include information about prodromal symptoms as well as the importance of reporting these symptoms to a health care provider.

---

toms of heart disease, attributing symptoms to a benign source, denying symptom significance, and feeling embarrassed about having symptoms (Zerwic & Ryan, 2004).

An additional issue to consider is the patient's medication history, dosages, and schedules. Is the patient independent in taking medications? Are the medications taken as prescribed? Does the patient understand why the medication regimen is important? Are doses ever forgotten or skipped, or does the patient ever decide to stop taking a medication? An aspirin a day is a common nonprescription medication that improves patient outcomes after an MI. However, if patients are not aware of this benefit, they may be inclined to stop taking aspirin if they think it is a trivial medication. A careful medication history often uncovers common medication errors and causes for nonadherence to the medication regimen.

### Nutrition and Metabolism

Dietary modifications, exercise, weight loss, and careful monitoring are important strategies for managing three major

## CHART 26-2

### Risk Factors for Coronary Artery Disease (CAD)

**Nonmodifiable Risk Factors**

- Family history of CAD
- Increasing age
- Male gender (although postmenopausal women have 2 to 3 times the CAD rates of premenopausal women of the same age)
- Race (higher incidence in African Americans than Caucasians due to greater risk of hypertension)

**Modifiable Risk Factors***

- Hyperlipidemia (LDL < 100 mg/dL and preferably < 70 mg/dL if CAD present; LDL < 160 mg/dL if ≤ 1 risk factor or 130 mg/dL if ≤ 2 risk factors; HDL > 40 mg/dL and triglycerides < 150 mg/dL)
- Hypertension (< 140/90 mm Hg; < 130/80 if diabetes or chronic renal disease present)
- Cigarette smoking, exposure to tobacco smoke (no tobacco use or secondhand exposure)
- Diabetes mellitus (fasting serum glucose < 110 mg/dL and hemoglobin $A_{1c}$ < 7%)
- Obesity (BMI 18.5 to 24.9 $kg/m^2$; waist circumference: male ≤ 40 inches, female ≤ 35 inches)
- Physical inactivity (30 to 60 minutes moderate-intensity aerobic activity on all or most days)

---

*American Heart Association-recommended goals are given in parentheses.

---

cardiovascular risk factors: hyperlipidemia, hypertension, and diabetes mellitus. Diets that are restricted in sodium, fat, cholesterol, and/or calories are commonly prescribed. The nurse obtains the following information:

- The patient's current height and weight (to determine Body Mass Index), waist measurement (assessment for obesity), BP, and any laboratory test results such as blood glucose, glycosylated hemoglobin (diabetes), total blood cholesterol, high-density and low-density lipoprotein levels, and triglyceride levels (hyperlipidemia)
- How often the patient self-monitors BP, blood glucose, and weight as appropriate to the medical diagnoses
- The patient's level of awareness regarding his or her target goals for each of the risk factors, and any problems achieving or maintaining these goals
- What the patient normally eats and drinks in a typical day and any food preferences (including cultural or ethnic preferences)
- Eating habits (canned or commercially prepared foods versus fresh foods, restaurant cooking versus home cooking, assessing for high-sodium foods, dietary intake of fats)
- Who shops for groceries and prepares meals

### Elimination

Typical bowel and bladder habits need to be identified. Nocturia (awakening at night to urinate) is common in patients with HF. Fluid collected in the dependent tissues (extremities) during the day redistributes into the circulatory system once the patient is recumbent at night. The increased circulatory volume is excreted by the kidneys (increased urine production).

When straining during defecation, the patient bears down (the Valsalva maneuver), which momentarily increases pressure on the baroreceptors. This triggers a vagal response, causing the heart rate to slow and resulting in syncope in some patients. Straining during urination can produce the same response.

Because many cardiac medications can cause gastrointestinal side effects or bleeding, the nurse asks about bloating, diarrhea, constipation, stomach upset, heartburn, loss of appetite, nausea, and vomiting. Patients taking platelet-inhibiting medications such as aspirin and clopidogrel (Plavix); platelet aggregation inhibitors such as abciximab (ReoPro), eptifibatide (Integrilin), and tirofiban (Aggrastat); and anticoagulants such as low-molecular-weight heparin (ie, dalteparin [Fragmin], enoxaparin [Lovenox]), heparin, or warfarin (Coumadin) are screened for bloody urine or stools.

### Activity and Exercise

As the nurse assesses the patient's activity and exercise history, it is important to note that decreases in activity tolerance are typically gradual and may go unnoticed by the patient. Therefore, the nurse needs to determine whether there has been a change in the activity pattern during the past 6 to 12 months. The patient's subjective response to activity is an essential assessment parameter. New symptoms or a change in the usual anginal symptoms during activity is a significant finding. Fatigue, associated with a low left ventricular ejection fraction (less than 40%) and certain medications (eg, beta-adrenergic blocking agents), can result in activity intolerance. Patients with fatigue may benefit from having their medications adjusted and learning energy-conservation techniques.

Additional areas to ask about include possible architectural barriers and challenges in the home, and what the patient does for exercise. If the patient exercises, the nurse asks additional questions: What is the intensity, and how long and how often is exercise performed? Has the patient ever participated in a cardiac rehabilitation program? Functional levels are known to improve for almost all patients who participate in a cardiac rehabilitation program, and participation is highly recommended (Leon, Franklin, Costa, et al., 2005; Smith, Allen, Blair, et al., 2006). Patients with disabilities may require an individually tailored exercise program.

### Sleep and Rest

Clues to worsening cardiac disease, especially HF, can be revealed by sleep-related events. Determining where the patient sleeps or rests is important. Recent changes, such as sleeping upright in a chair instead of in bed, increasing the number of pillows used, awakening short of breath at night (paroxysmal nocturnal dyspnea), or awakening with angina (nocturnal angina), are all indicative of worsening HF.

## Cognition and Perception

Evaluating cognitive ability helps determine whether the patient has the mental capacity to manage safe and effective self-care. Is the patient's short-term memory intact? Is there any history of dementia? Is there evidence of depression or anxiety? Can the patient read? Can the patient read English? What is the patient's reading level? What is the patient's preferred learning style? What information does the patient perceive as important? Providing the patient with written information can be a valuable part of patient education, but only if the patient can read and comprehend the information.

Related assessments include possible hearing or visual impairments. If vision is impaired, patients with HF may not be able to weigh themselves independently or keep records of weight, BP, pulse, or other data requested by the health care team.

## Self-Perception and Self-Concept

Personality factors may be associated with the development of and recovery from CAD. Most commonly cited is "type A behavior," which is characterized by competitive, hard-driving behaviors and a sense of time urgency. Although this behavior is not an independent risk factor for CAD, anger and hostility (personality traits common in people with "type A behavior") do affect the heart. People with these traits react to frustrating situations with an increase in BP, heart rate, and neuroendocrine responses. This physiologic activation, called cardiac reactivity, is thought to trigger acute cardiovascular events (Woods, Froelicher, & Motzer, 2004).

During the health history, the nurse discovers how patients feel about themselves by asking questions such as: How would you describe yourself? Do you find that you are easily angered or hostile? How do you feel right now? What helps you manage these feelings? Assistance from a psychiatric advanced practice nurse, psychologist, psychiatrist, or social worker may be necessary.

## Roles and Relationships

Determining the patient's social support systems is important in today's health care environment. Hospital stays for cardiac disorders have shortened, with many invasive diagnostic cardiac procedures, such as cardiac catheterization and percutaneous coronary intervention (PCI), being performed as outpatient procedures.

To assess support systems, the nurse needs to ask: Who is the primary caregiver? With whom does the patient live? Are there adequate services in place to provide a safe home environment? The nurse also assesses for any significant effects the cardiac illness has had on the patient's role in the family. Are there adequate finances and health insurance? The answers to these questions help the nurse develop a plan to meet the patient's home care needs.

## Sexuality and Reproduction

Although people recovering from cardiac illnesses or procedures are often concerned about sexual activity, they are less likely to ask their nurse or other health care provider for information to help them resume their normal sex life. Reduced frequency of and satisfaction with sexual activity are often caused by fear and lack of correct information. Therefore, the nurse needs to initiate a discussion about sexuality with the patient, as opposed to waiting for the patient to bring the subject up in conversation.

The most commonly cited reasons for changes in sexual activity are fear of another heart attack or sudden death; untoward symptoms such as angina, dyspnea, or palpitations; and problems with impotence or depression. In men, impotence may develop as a side effect of cardiac medications (eg, beta-blockers); some men will stop taking their medication as a result. Other medications may be substituted, so patients should be encouraged to discuss this problem with their health care providers. Often, patients and their partners do not have adequate information about the physical demands related to sexual activity and ways in which these demands can be modified. The physiologic demands are greatest during orgasm, reaching 5 or 6 metabolic equivalents (METs). This level of activity is equivalent to walking 3 to 4 miles per hour on a treadmill. The METs expended before and after orgasm are considerably less, at 3.7 METs (Steinke & Swan, 2004). Sharing this information may make the patient and his or her partner more comfortable about resuming sexual activity.

A reproductive history is necessary for women of childbearing age, particularly those with seriously compromised cardiac function. These women may be advised by their physicians not to become pregnant. The reproductive history includes information about previous pregnancies, plans for future pregnancies, oral contraceptive use (especially in women older than 35 years of age who smoke), menopausal status, and use of hormone therapy.

## Coping and Stress Tolerance

It is important to determine the presence of psychosocial factors that adversely affect cardiac health. Anxiety, depression, and stress are known to influence both the development of and recovery from CAD. High levels of anxiety are associated with an increased incidence of CAD and increased in-hospital complication rates after MI. People with depression have an increased risk of MI- and heart disease–related death compared to people without depression. Although the association between depression and CAD is not completely understood, it is postulated that both biologic factors (eg, platelet abnormalities, inflammatory responses) and lifestyle factors contribute to the development of CAD. People who are depressed may be less motivated to adhere to the recommended lifestyle changes and medical regimens necessary to prevent future cardiac events (Glassman, Shapiro, Ford, et al., 2003).

Stress initiates a variety of physiologic responses, including increases in the circulation of catecholamines and cortisol, and has been strongly linked to cardiovascular events. Therefore, the patient needs to be assessed for the presence of labile emotions, as well as sources of stress. This is achieved by asking questions about recent or ongoing stressors, previous coping styles and effectiveness, and the patient's perception of his or her current mood and coping ability. Consultation with a psychiatric advanced practice nurse, psychologist, psychiatrist, or social worker may be indicated.

## Prevention Strategies

Additional features of the health history include identification of risk factors for heart disease and measures taken by the patient to prevent disease. The nurse's questions need to focus on the patient's health promotion practices. Epidemiologic studies show that certain conditions or behaviors (ie, risk factors) are associated with a greater incidence of coronary artery, peripheral vascular, and cerebrovascular disease (AHA, 2006). Risk factors are classified by the extent to which they can be modified by changing one's lifestyle or modifying personal behaviors (see Chart 26-2).

Once a patient's risk factors are determined, the nurse assesses whether the patient has a plan for making necessary behavioral changes and whether assistance is needed to support these lifestyle changes. For example, tobacco use is one of the most commonly implicated and readily modifiable risk factors for CAD. The first step in treating this health risk is to identify patients who use tobacco products and those who have recently quit. Because 70% of people who smoke visit a health care facility each year, nurses have ample opportunities to assess patients for tobacco use and motivation to quit, and to provide referrals to smoking cessation programs as appropriate. For patients who are obese or who have hyperlipidemia, hypertension, or diabetes, the nurse determines any problems the patient may be having following the prescribed management plan (ie, diet, exercise, and medications). It may be necessary to clarify the patient's responsibilities, assist with finding additional resources, or make alternative plans for risk factor modification.

## Physical Assessment

A physical examination is performed to confirm some of the data obtained in the health history. The nurse observes the patient's general appearance and performs a focused cardiac physical examination that includes evaluation of the following:

- Effectiveness of the heart as a pump
- Filling volumes and pressures
- Cardiac output
- Compensatory mechanisms

Indicators that the heart is not functioning effectively as a pump include reduced pulse pressure, cardiac enlargement, and abnormal heart sounds (eg, murmurs or gallop rhythms).

The amount of blood filling the atria and ventricles and the resulting pressures (called filling volumes and pressures) are estimated by the degree of jugular vein distention and the presence or absence of congestion in the lungs, peripheral edema, and postural changes in BP that occur when the patient sits up or stands.

Cardiac output is reflected by cognition, heart rate, pulse pressure, color and texture of the skin, and urine output. Examples of compensatory mechanisms that help maintain cardiac output are increased filling volumes and elevated heart rate. The findings on the physical examination are correlated with data obtained from diagnostic procedures, such as hemodynamic monitoring (discussed later in this chapter).

The examination, which proceeds logically (eg, from head to toe), can be performed in about 10 minutes with practice and covers the following areas: (1) general appearance, (2) cognition, (3) skin, (4) BP, (5) arterial pulses, (6) jugular venous pulsations and pressures, (7) heart, (8) extremities, (9) lungs, and (10) abdomen.

### General Appearance and Cognition

The nurse observes the patient's level of distress, level of consciousness, and thought processes as an indication of the heart's ability to propel oxygen to the brain (cerebral perfusion). The nurse also observes for evidence of anxiety, along with any effects that emotional factors may have on cardiovascular status. The nurse attempts to put the anxious patient at ease throughout the examination.

### Inspection of the Skin

Examination of the skin begins during the evaluation of the patient's general appearance and continues throughout the assessment. It includes all body surfaces, starting with the head and finishing with the lower extremities. Skin color, temperature, and texture are assessed. The more common findings associated with cardiovascular disease are as follows:

- Pallor—a decrease in the color of the skin—is caused by lack of oxyhemoglobin. It is a result of anemia or decreased arterial perfusion. Pallor is best observed around the fingernails, lips, and oral mucosa. In patients with dark skin, the nurse observes the palms of the hands and soles of the feet.
- Peripheral cyanosis—a bluish tinge, most often of the nails and skin of the nose, lips, earlobes, and extremities—suggests decreased blood flow to a particular area, which allows more time for the hemoglobin molecule to become desaturated. This may occur normally in peripheral vasoconstriction associated with a cold environment, in patients with anxiety, or in disease states such as HF.
- Central cyanosis—a bluish tinge observed in the tongue and buccal mucosa—denotes serious cardiac disorders (pulmonary edema and congenital heart disease) in which venous blood passes through the pulmonary circulation without being oxygenated.
- Xanthelasma—yellowish, slightly raised plaques in the skin—may be observed along the nasal portion of one or both eyelids and may indicate elevated cholesterol levels (hypercholesterolemia).
- Reduced skin turgor occurs with dehydration and aging.
- Temperature and moistness are controlled by the autonomic nervous system. Normally the skin is warm and dry. Under stress, the hands may become cool and moist. In cardiogenic shock, sympathetic nervous system stimulation causes vasoconstriction, and the skin becomes cold and clammy. During an acute MI, diaphoresis is common.
- Ecchymosis (bruise)—a purplish-blue color fading to green, yellow, or brown over time—is associated with blood outside of the blood vessels and is usually caused by trauma. Patients who are receiving anticoagulant therapy should be carefully observed for unexplained ecchymosis. In these patients, excessive bruising indicates prolonged clotting times (prothrombin or partial thromboplastin time) caused by an anticoagulant dosage that is too high.

- Wounds, scars, and tissue surrounding implanted devices should also be examined. Wounds are assessed for adequate healing, and any scars from previous surgeries are noted. The skin surrounding a pacemaker or implantable cardioverter–defibrillator generator is examined for thinning, which could indicate erosion of the device through the skin.

## Blood Pressure

Systemic arterial BP is the pressure exerted on the walls of the arteries during ventricular systole and diastole. It is affected by factors such as cardiac output; distention of the arteries; and the volume, velocity, and viscosity of the blood. Normal adult BP values range from 100/60 to 135/85 mm Hg. The average normal BP usually cited is 120/80 mm Hg. An increase in BP above the upper normal range is called hypertension (see Chapter 32 for additional definitions, measurement, and management), whereas a decrease below the lower range is called hypotension.

### PULSE PRESSURE

The difference between the systolic and the diastolic pressures is called the pulse pressure. It is a reflection of stroke volume, ejection velocity, and systemic vascular resistance. Pulse pressure, which normally is 30 to 40 mm Hg, indicates how well the patient maintains cardiac output. The pulse pressure increases in conditions that elevate the stroke volume (anxiety, exercise, bradycardia), reduce systemic vascular resistance (fever), or reduce distensibility of the arteries (atherosclerosis, aging, hypertension). Decreased pulse pressure reflects reduced stroke volume and ejection velocity (shock, HF, hypovolemia, mitral regurgitation) or obstruction to blood flow during systole (mitral or aortic stenosis). A pulse pressure of less than 30 mm Hg signifies a serious reduction in cardiac output and requires further cardiovascular assessment.

### POSTURAL BLOOD PRESSURE CHANGES

**Postural (orthostatic) hypotension** occurs when the BP decreases significantly after the patient assumes an upright posture. It is usually accompanied by dizziness, lightheadedness, or syncope.

Although there are many causes of postural hypotension, the three most common causes in patients with cardiac problems are a reduced volume of fluid or blood in the circulatory system (intravascular volume depletion, dehydration), inadequate vasoconstrictor mechanisms, and insufficient autonomic effect on vascular constriction. Postural changes in BP and an appropriate history help health care providers differentiate among these causes. The following recommendations are important when assessing postural BP changes:

- The patient should be positioned supine and flat (as symptoms permit) for 10 minutes before taking the initial BP and heart rate measurements.
- Supine measurements should be checked before checking upright measurements.
- The BP cuff should not be removed between position changes, but the nurse should check to see that it is still correctly placed.
- Postural BP changes should be assessed with the patient sitting on the edge of the bed with feet dangling and, if appropriate, with the patient standing at the side of the bed.
- One to three minutes should elapse after each postural change before measuring BP and heart rate.
- If the patient exhibits any signs or symptoms of distress, he or she is returned to a supine position before completing the test.
- Both heart rate and BP are recorded. The patient's position (eg, supine, sitting, standing) and any signs or symptoms that accompany the postural change are also noted.

Normal postural responses that occur when a person stands up or changes from a lying to a sitting position include (1) a heart rate increase of 5 to 20 bpm above the resting rate (to offset reduced stroke volume and maintain cardiac output); (2) an unchanged systolic pressure, or a slight decrease of up to 10 mm Hg; and (3) a slight increase of 5 mm Hg in diastolic pressure.

A decrease in the amount of blood or fluid in the circulatory system should be suspected after diuretic therapy or bleeding, when a postural change results in an increased heart rate and either a decrease in systolic pressure by 15 mm Hg or a decrease in diastolic pressure by 10 mm Hg. Vital signs alone do not differentiate between a decrease in intravascular volume and inadequate constriction of the blood vessels as a cause of postural hypotension. With intravascular volume depletion, the reflexes that maintain cardiac output (increased heart rate and peripheral vasoconstriction) function correctly; the heart rate increases and the peripheral vessels constrict. However, because of lost volume, the BP falls. With inadequate vasoconstrictor mechanisms, the heart rate again responds appropriately, but because of diminished peripheral vasoconstriction the BP drops. The following is an example of a postural BP recording showing either intravascular volume depletion or inadequate vasoconstrictor mechanisms:

Supine: BP 120/70 mm Hg, heart rate 70 bpm
Sitting: BP 100/55 mm Hg, heart rate 90 bpm
Standing: BP 98/52 mm Hg, heart rate 94 bpm

In autonomic insufficiency, the heart rate cannot increase to completely compensate for the gravitational effects of an upright posture. Peripheral vasoconstriction may be absent or diminished. Autonomic insufficiency does not rule out a concurrent decrease in intravascular volume. The following is an example of autonomic insufficiency as demonstrated by postural BP changes:

Supine: BP 150/90 mm Hg, heart rate 60 bpm
Sitting: BP 100/60 mm Hg, heart rate 60 bpm

## Arterial Pulses

Factors to be evaluated in examining the pulse are rate, rhythm, quality, configuration of the pulse wave, and quality of the arterial vessel.

### PULSE RATE

The normal pulse rate varies from a low of 50 bpm in healthy, athletic young adults to rates well in excess of 100 bpm after exercise or during times of excitement. Anxiety frequently raises the pulse rate during the physical examination. If the rate is higher than expected, it is appropriate to reassess it near the end of the physical examination, when the patient may be more relaxed.

### PULSE RHYTHM

The rhythm of the pulse is as important to assess as the rate. Minor variations in regularity of the pulse are normal. The pulse rate may increase during inhalation and slow during exhalation. This phenomenon, called sinus arrhythmia, occurs most commonly in children and young adults.

For the initial cardiac examination, or if the pulse rhythm is irregular, the heart rate should be counted by auscultating the apical pulse for a full minute while simultaneously palpating the radial pulse. Any discrepancy between contractions heard and pulses felt is noted. Disturbances of rhythm (dysrhythmias) often result in a pulse deficit, a difference between the apical rate (the heart rate heard at the apex of the heart) and the peripheral rate. Pulse deficits commonly occur with atrial fibrillation, atrial flutter, premature ventricular contractions, and varying degrees of heart block (see Chapter 27 for a detailed discussion of these dysrhythmias).

Understanding the complexity of dysrhythmias requires a sophisticated knowledge of cardiac electrophysiology, which is obtained through advanced education and training.

### PULSE QUALITY

The quality, or amplitude, of the pulse can be described as absent, diminished, normal, or bounding. It should be assessed bilaterally. Scales can be used to rate the strength of the pulse. The following is an example of a 0-to-4 scale:

- 0: pulse not palpable or absent
- +1: weak, thready pulse; difficult to palpate; obliterated with pressure
- +2: diminished pulse; cannot be obliterated
- +3: easy to palpate, full pulse; cannot be obliterated
- +4: strong, bounding pulse; may be abnormal

The numerical classification is quite subjective; therefore, when documenting the pulse quality, it helps to specify a scale range (eg, "left radial +3/+4").

### PULSE CONFIGURATION

The configuration (contour) of the pulse conveys important information. In patients with stenosis of the aortic valve, the valve opening is narrowed, reducing the amount of blood ejected into the aorta. The pulse pressure is narrow, and the pulse feels feeble. In aortic insufficiency, the aortic valve does not close completely, allowing blood to flow back from the aorta into the left ventricle. The rise of the pulse wave is abrupt and strong, and its fall is precipitous—a "collapsing" or "water hammer" pulse. The true configuration of the pulse is best appreciated by palpating over the carotid artery rather than the distal radial artery, because the dramatic characteristics of the pulse wave may be distorted when the pulse is transmitted to smaller vessels.

### EFFECT OF VESSEL QUALITY ON PULSE

The condition of the vessel wall also influences the pulse and is of concern, especially in older patients. Once rate and rhythm have been determined, the nurse assesses the quality of the vessel by palpating along the radial artery and comparing it with normal vessels. Does the vessel wall feel thickened? Is it tortuous?

To assess peripheral circulation, the nurse locates and evaluates all arterial pulses. Arterial pulses are palpated at points where the arteries are near the skin surface and are easily compressed against bones or firm musculature. Pulses are detected over the temporal, carotid, brachial, radial, femoral, popliteal, dorsalis pedis, and posterior tibial arteries. A reliable assessment of the pulses of the lower extremities depends on accurate identification of the location of the artery and careful palpation of the area. Light palpation is essential; firm finger pressure can easily obliterate the dorsalis pedis and posterior tibial pulses and confuse the examiner. In approximately 10% of patients, the dorsalis pedis pulses are not palpable. In such circumstances, both are usually absent together, and the posterior tibial arteries alone provide adequate blood supply to the feet. Arteries in the extremities are often palpated simultaneously to facilitate comparison of quality.

**NURSING ALERT**

**Do not simultaneously palpate the temporal or carotid arteries bilaterally, because it is possible to decrease the blood flow to the brain.**

## Jugular Venous Pulsations

Right-sided heart function can be estimated by observing the pulsations of the jugular veins of the neck and the central venous pressure (CVP), which reflects right atrial or right ventricular end-diastolic pressure (the pressure immediately preceding the contraction of the right ventricle).

Pulsations of the internal jugular veins are most commonly assessed. If they are difficult to see, pulsations of the external jugular veins may be noted. These veins are more superficial and are visible just above the clavicles, adjacent to the sternocleidomastoid muscles. The external jugular veins are frequently distended while the patient lies supine on the examining table or bed. As the patient's head is elevated, distention of the veins normally disappears. The veins normally are not apparent if the patient's head is elevated more than 30 degrees.

Obvious distention of the veins with the patient's head elevated 45 to 90 degrees indicates an abnormal increase in the volume of the venous system. This occurs with right-sided HF, less commonly with obstruction of blood flow in the superior vena cava, and rarely with acute massive pulmonary embolism.

## Heart Inspection and Palpation

The heart is examined indirectly by inspection, palpation, percussion, and auscultation of the chest wall. A systematic approach is used to examine the chest wall in the following six areas (Fig. 26-5):

1. *Aortic area*—second intercostal space to the right of the sternum. To determine the correct intercostal space, start at the angle of Louis by locating the bony ridge near

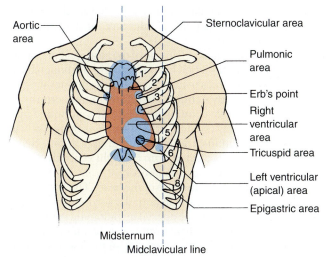

**FIGURE 26-5.** Areas of the precordium to be assessed when evaluating heart function. (Numerals identify ribs of adjacent intercostal spaces.)

**FIGURE 26-6.** Locating (**A**) and palpating (**B**) the apical impulse (also called the point of maximal impulse [PMI]). The apical impulse normally is located at the fifth intercostal space to the left of the sternum at the midclavicular line. The nurse locates the impulse with the palm of the hand and palpates with the fingerpads. © B. Proud in Weber, J. W., & Kelley, J. (2003). *Health assessment in nursing* (2nd ed.). Philadelphia: Lippincott Williams & Wilkins.

the top of the sternum, at the junction of the body and the manubrium. From this angle, locate the second intercostal space by sliding one finger to the left or right of the sternum. Subsequent intercostal spaces are located from this reference point by palpating down the rib cage.
2. *Pulmonic area*—second intercostal space to the left of the sternum
3. *Erb's point*—third intercostal space to the left of the sternum
4. *Right ventricular or tricuspid area*—fourth and fifth intercostal spaces to the left of the sternum
5. *Left ventricular or apical area*—the point of maximal impulse (PMI), the location on the chest where heart contractions can be palpated
6. *Epigastric area*—below the xiphoid process

For most of the examination, the patient lies supine, with the head of the bed slightly elevated. A right-handed examiner stands at the right side of the patient, a left-handed examiner at the left side.

Each area of the precordium is inspected and then palpated. Oblique lighting is used to assist the examiner in identifying subtle pulsation. A normal impulse that is distinct and located over the apex of the heart is called the **apical impulse**, also referred to as the PMI. It may be observed in young people and in older people who are thin. The apical impulse is normally located and auscultated in the left fifth intercostal space at the midclavicular line (Fig. 26-6).

In many cases, the apical impulse is palpable and is normally felt as a light pulsation, 1 to 2 cm in diameter. It is felt at the onset of the first heart sound and lasts for only half of systole (see the next section for a discussion of heart sounds). The nurse uses the palm of the hand to locate the apical impulse initially and the fingerpads to assess its size and quality. A broad and forceful apical impulse is known as a left ventricular heave or lift because it appears to lift the hand from the chest wall during palpation.

An apical impulse below the fifth intercostal space or lateral to the midclavicular line usually denotes left ventricular enlargement from left ventricular failure. Normally, the apical impulse is palpable in only one intercostal space; palpability in two or more adjacent intercostal spaces indicates left ventricular enlargement. If the apical impulse can be palpated in two distinctly separate areas and the pulsation movements are paradoxical (not simultaneous), a ventricular aneurysm may be suspected.

Abnormal, turbulent blood flow within the heart may be palpated with the palm of the hand as a purring sensation. This phenomenon is called a thrill and is associated with a loud murmur. A thrill is always indicative of significant pathology within the heart. Thrills also may be palpated over vessels when blood flow is significantly and substantially obstructed and over the carotid arteries if aortic stenosis is present or if the aortic valve is narrowed.

## Chest Percussion

Normally, only the left border of the heart can be detected by percussion. It extends from the sternum to the midclavicular line in the third to fifth intercostal spaces. The right border lies under the right margin of the sternum and is not detectable. Enlargement of the heart to either the left or right usually can be noted. In people with thick chests, obesity, or emphysema, the heart may lie so deep under the thoracic surface that not even its left border can be noted unless the heart is enlarged. In such cases, unless the nurse detects a displaced apical impulse and suspects cardiac enlargement, percussion is omitted.

## Cardiac Auscultation

All areas identified in Figure 26-5, except the epigastric area, are auscultated. These include the aortic area, the pulmonary area, Erb's point, the tricuspid area, and the apical area. These locations do not correspond to the anatomic locations of the valves within the chest; rather, they reflect the patterns by which heart sounds radiate toward the chest wall. Sound in vessels through which blood is flowing is always reflected downstream. For example, the actions of the mitral valve are usually heard best in the fifth intercostal space at the midclavicular line. This is called the mitral valve area.

### HEART SOUNDS

The **normal heart sounds**, $S_1$ and $S_2$, are produced primarily by the closing of the heart valves. The time between $S_1$ and $S_2$ corresponds to systole (Fig. 26-7). This is normally shorter than the time between $S_2$ and $S_1$ (diastole). As the heart rate increases, diastole shortens.

Normally, the periods of systole and diastole are silent. However, ventricular disease can give rise to transient sounds in systole and diastole that are called gallops, snaps, or clicks. Significant narrowing of the valve orifices at times when they should be open, or residual gapping of valves at times when they should be closed, produces prolonged sounds called **murmurs**.

**$S_1$—First Heart Sound.** Closure of the mitral and tricuspid valves creates the first heart sound ($S_1$), although vibration of the myocardial wall also may contribute to this sound. Although $S_1$ is heard over the entire precordium, it is heard best at the apex of the heart (apical area). Its intensity increases when the valve leaflets are made rigid by calcium in rheumatic heart disease and in any circumstance in which ventricular contraction occurs at a time when the valve is caught wide open (eg, when a premature ventricular contraction interrupts the normal cardiac cycle). $S_1$ varies in intensity from beat to beat when atrial contraction is not synchronous with ventricular contraction because the valve may be fully or partially closed on one beat and open on the next one due to irregular atrial activity. $S_1$ is easily identifiable and serves as the point of reference for the remainder of the cardiac cycle.

**$S_2$—Second Heart Sound.** Closing of the aortic and pulmonic valves produces the second heart sound ($S_2$). Although these two valves close almost simultaneously, the pulmonic valve usually lags slightly behind. Therefore, under certain circumstances, the two components of the second sound may be heard separately (split $S_2$). The splitting is more likely to be accentuated on inspiration and to disappear on exhalation. (More blood is ejected from the right ventricle during inspiration than during exhalation.)

$S_2$ is most audible at the base of the heart. The aortic component of $S_2$ is heard clearly in both the aortic and pulmonic areas and less clearly at the apex. The pulmonic component of $S_2$, if present, may be heard only over the pulmonic area. Therefore, one may hear a "single" $S_2$ in the aortic area and a split $S_2$ in the pulmonic area.

**Gallop Sounds.** If the blood filling the ventricle is impeded during diastole, as occurs in certain disease states, then a temporary vibration may occur in diastole that is similar to, although usually softer than, $S_1$ and $S_2$. The heart sounds then come in triplets and have the acoustic effect of a galloping horse; they are called gallops. This may occur early in diastole, during the rapid-filling phase of the cardiac cycle, or later at the time of atrial contraction.

Gallop sounds are very low-frequency sounds and may be heard only with the bell of the stethoscope placed very lightly against the chest. They are heard best at the apex, although occasionally, when emanating from the right ventricle, they may be heard to the left of the sternum.

A gallop sound that occurs during rapid ventricular filling is called a third heart sound ($S_3$); it may represent a normal finding in children and young adults (Fig. 26-8A). Such a

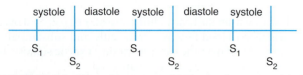

**FIGURE 26-7.** Normal heart sounds. The first heart sound ($S_1$) is produced by the closing of the mitral and tricuspid valves and is best heard at the apex of the heart (left ventricular or apical area). The second heart sound ($S_2$) is produced by the closing of the aortic and pulmonic valves and is loudest at the base of the heart. The time between $S_1$ and $S_2$ corresponds to systole. The time between $S_2$ and $S_1$ is diastole.

**FIGURE 26-8.** Gallops. **(A)** An $S_3$ gallop is heard immediately following the $S_2$ and occurs when the blood filling the ventricle is impeded during diastole, resulting in temporary vibrations. The heart sounds come in triplets and resemble the sound of a galloping horse. Myocardial disease and heart failure are associated with this sound. **(B)** An $S_4$ gallop is heard immediately preceding the $S_1$. The $S_4$ sound occurs during atrial contraction and is often heard when the ventricle is enlarged or hypertrophied. Associated conditions include coronary artery disease, hypertension, and aortic stenosis.

sound is heard in patients who have myocardial disease or in those who have HF and whose ventricles fail to eject all of their blood during systole. An $S_3$ gallop is heard best with the patient lying on the left side.

A gallop sound that occurs during atrial contraction is called a fourth heart sound ($S_4$) (see Fig. 26-8B). An $S_4$ is often heard when the ventricle is enlarged or hypertrophied and therefore resistant to filling. Such a circumstance may be associated with CAD, hypertension, or stenosis of the aortic valve. On rare occasions, all four heart sounds are heard within a single period of cardiac contraction, ejection, refilling, and resting, referred to as a cardiac cycle, giving rise to what is called a quadruple rhythm.

**Snaps and Clicks.** Stenosis of the mitral valve resulting from rheumatic heart disease gives rise to an unusual high-pitched sound very early in diastole that is best heard along the left sternal border. The sound is caused by high pressure in the left atrium with abrupt displacement of a rigid mitral valve. The sound is called an opening snap. It occurs too long after $S_2$ to be mistaken for a split $S_2$ and too early in diastole to be mistaken for a gallop. It almost always is associated with the murmur of mitral stenosis and is specific to this disorder.

In a similar manner, stenosis of the aortic valve gives rise to a short, high-pitched sound immediately after $S_1$ that is called an ejection click. This is caused by very high pressure within the ventricle, displacing a rigid and calcified aortic valve.

**Murmurs.** Murmurs are created by turbulent flow of blood. The causes of the turbulence may be a critically narrowed valve, a malfunctioning valve that allows regurgitant blood flow, a congenital defect of the ventricular wall, a defect between the aorta and the pulmonary artery, or an increased flow of blood through a normal structure (eg, with fever, pregnancy, hyperthyroidism). Murmurs are characterized and consequently described by several characteristics, including their timing in the cardiac cycle, location on the chest wall, intensity, pitch, quality, and pattern of radiation (Chart 26-3).

**Friction Rub.** In pericarditis, a harsh, grating sound that can be heard in both systole and diastole is called a friction rub. It is caused by abrasion of the pericardial surfaces during the cardiac cycle. Because a friction rub may be confused with a murmur, care should be taken to identify the sound and to distinguish it from murmurs that may be heard in both systole and diastole. A pericardial friction rub can be heard best using the diaphragm of the stethoscope, with the patient sitting up and leaning forward.

### AUSCULTATION PROCEDURE

During auscultation, the patient remains supine and the examining room is as quiet as possible. A stethoscope with a diaphragm and a bell is necessary for accurate auscultation of the heart.

Using the diaphragm of the stethoscope, the examiner starts at the apical area and progresses upward along the left sternal border to the pulmonic and aortic areas. Alternatively, the examiner may begin the examination at the aortic and pulmonic areas and progress downward to the apex of the heart. Initially, $S_1$ is identified and evaluated with respect to its intensity and splitting. Next, $S_2$ is identified, and its intensity and any splitting are noted. After

---

**CHART 26-3**

## Characteristics of Heart Murmurs

Heart murmurs are described in terms of location, timing, intensity, pitch, quality, and radiation. These characteristics provide data about the location and nature of the cardiac abnormality.

### Location
The location of the murmur (where it is detected on the chest wall) is crucial. Depending on the type of valvular disorder, a murmur can be heard only at the apex or more widely over the chest wall, or along the left sternal border between the third and fourth interspaces.

### Timing
Timing of the murmur in the cardiac cycle is vital. The examiner first determines whether the murmur is occurring in systole or in diastole. Then, does it begin simultaneously with a heart sound, or is there some delay between the sound and the beginning of the murmur? Does the murmur continue to (or through) the second heart sound, or is there a delay between the end of the murmur and the second heart sound? Are diastolic murmurs (between the second and first heart sounds) continuous, or do they subside in mid- or late diastole?

### Intensity
The intensity of murmurs is conventionally graded from I through VI. Sometimes, grade I murmurs are difficult to hear. However, a grade II cardiac murmur can be easily perceived by the experienced examiner. Murmurs of grades IV or louder are usually associated with thrills that may be palpated on the surface of the chest wall. A grade VI murmur can be heard with the stethoscope off the chest. A murmur may vary in intensity from its beginning to its conclusion. This is very characteristic of certain valvular disorders.

### Pitch
The next important characteristic of a murmur is its pitch, which may be low, often heard only with the bell of the stethoscope placed lightly on the chest wall, or a very high-pitched murmur, heard best with the stethoscope's diaphragm. Other murmurs contain the full spectrum of sound frequency.

### Quality
In addition to the intensity and pitch, noting the character of the sound is vital. A murmur may be described as rumbling, blowing, whistling, harsh, or musical.

### Radiation
The last feature of concern is radiation of the murmur. A murmur can radiate into the axilla, the carotid arteries in the neck, the left shoulder, or the back.

concentrating on $S_1$ and $S_2$, the examiner listens for extra sounds in systole and then in diastole.

Sometimes it helps to ask the following questions: Do I hear snapping or clicking sounds? Do I hear any high-pitched blowing sounds? Is this sound in systole, or diastole, or both? The examiner again proceeds to move the stethoscope to all of the designated areas of the precordium, listening carefully for these sounds. Finally, the patient is turned on the left side and the stethoscope is placed on the apical area, where an $S_3$, an $S_4$, and a mitral murmur are more readily detected.

Once an abnormality is heard, the entire chest surface is reexamined to determine the exact location of the sound and its radiation. The patient may be concerned about the prolonged examination and must be supported and reassured. The auscultatory findings, particularly murmurs, are documented by identifying the following characteristics:

- Location on chest wall
- Timing of sound as either during systole or during diastole; described as early, middle, or late (if heard throughout systole, the sound is often referred to as pansystolic or holosystolic)
- Intensity of the sound (I, very faint; II, quiet; III, moderately loud; IV, loud; V, very loud; or VI, heard with stethoscope removed from the chest)
- Pitch, described as high, medium, or low
- Quality of the sound, commonly described as blowing, harsh, or musical
- Location of radiation of the sound away from where it is heard the loudest

### INTERPRETATION OF CARDIAC SOUNDS

Interpreting cardiac sounds requires detailed knowledge of cardiac physiology and the pathophysiology of cardiac diseases. When nurses evaluate cardiac sounds, they may be expected to perform at different levels. The first level involves simply recognizing that what one is hearing is not normal—such as a third heart sound, a murmur in systole or diastole, a pericardial friction rub over the midsternum, or a second heart sound that is widely split. These findings are reported to the physician and acted on accordingly. This level of function is useful in screening. It is the kind of activity involved in performing physical examinations in schools on normal children or in performing routine physical examinations or screening examinations.

The second level involves recognizing patterns. The nurse correctly observes the findings and recognizes the diagnostic significance of common heart sounds. Highly skilled nurses can differentiate among dysrhythmias and respond accordingly. They can determine the significance of the appearance and disappearance of gallops during the treatment of patients who have had MIs or who have HF. This is the role of coronary care and cardiovascular advanced practice nurses as they work collaboratively with other health care professionals.

## Inspection of the Extremities

The hands, arms, legs, and feet are observed for skin and vascular changes. The most noteworthy changes include the following:

- Decreased capillary refill time indicates a slower peripheral flow rate from sluggish reperfusion and is often observed in patients with hypotension or HF. Capillary refill time provides the basis for estimating the rate of peripheral blood flow. To test capillary refill, the nurse briefly compresses the nailbed so that it blanches, and then releases the pressure. Normally, reperfusion occurs within 3 seconds, as evidenced by the return of color.
- Vascular changes from decreased arterial circulation include a decrease in quality or loss of pulse, discomfort or pain, paresthesia, numbness, decrease in temperature, pallor, and loss of movement. During the first few hours after invasive cardiac procedures (eg, cardiac catheterization), affected extremities should be assessed frequently for vascular changes.
- Hematoma, or a localized collection of clotted blood in the tissue, may be observed in patients who have undergone invasive cardiac procedures such as cardiac catheterization, PCI, or cardiac electrophysiology testing. Major blood vessels of the arms and legs are used for catheter insertion. During these procedures, systemic anticoagulation with heparin is necessary, and minor or small hematomas may occur at the catheter puncture site. However, large hematomas are a serious complication that can compromise circulating blood volume and cardiac output, requiring blood transfusions. Patients who have undergone these procedures must have their puncture sites frequently observed until hemostasis is adequately achieved.
- Peripheral edema is fluid accumulation in dependent areas of the body (feet and legs, sacrum in the bedridden patient). Pitting edema (a depression over an area of pressure) is assessed by pressing firmly for 5 seconds with the thumb over the dorsum of each foot, behind each medial malleolus, and over the shins. It is graded as absent or as present on a scale from slight (1+ = 0 to 2 mm) to very marked (4+ = more than 8 mm). Peripheral edema is observed in patients with HF and in those with peripheral vascular diseases such as deep vein thrombosis or chronic venous insufficiency.
- Clubbing of the fingers and toes implies chronic hemoglobin desaturation, as in congenital heart disease.
- Lower extremity ulcers are observed in patients with arterial or venous insufficiency (see Chapter 31 for a complete description of these conditions).

## Other Systems

### LUNGS

The details of respiratory assessment are described in Chapter 21. Findings frequently exhibited by patients with cardiac disorders include the following:

*Tachypnea:* Rapid, shallow breathing may be noted in patients who have HF, pain, or anxiety.
*Cheyne-Stokes respirations:* Patients with severe left ventricular failure may exhibit Cheyne-Stokes breathing, a pattern of rapid respirations alternating with apnea. It is important to note the duration of the apnea.
*Hemoptysis:* Pink, frothy sputum is indicative of acute pulmonary edema.
*Cough:* A dry, hacking cough from irritation of small airways is common in patients with pulmonary congestion from HF.

*Crackles:* HF or atelectasis associated with bed rest, splinting from ischemic pain, or the effects of analgesics, sedatives, or anesthetic agents often results in the development of crackles. Typically, crackles are first noted at the bases (because of gravity's effect on fluid accumulation and decreased ventilation of basilar tissue), but they may progress to all portions of the lung fields.

*Wheezes:* Compression of the small airways by interstitial pulmonary edema may cause wheezing. Beta-adrenergic blocking agents (beta-blockers), such as propranolol (Inderal), may cause airway narrowing, especially in patients with underlying pulmonary disease.

**ABDOMEN**

For the patient with a cardiovascular disorder, two components of the abdominal examination are relevant:

*Hepatojugular reflux:* Liver engorgement occurs because of decreased venous return secondary to right ventricular failure. The liver is enlarged, firm, nontender, and smooth. The hepatojugular reflux may be demonstrated by pressing firmly over the right upper quadrant of the abdomen for 30 to 60 seconds and noting an increase of 1 cm or more in jugular venous pressure. This increase indicates an inability of the right side of the heart to accommodate increased volume.

*Bladder distention:* Urine output is an important indicator of cardiac function. Reduced urine output may indicate inadequate renal perfusion or a less serious problem such as one caused by urinary retention. When the urine output is decreased, the patient must be assessed for a distended bladder or difficulty voiding. The bladder may be assessed with an ultrasound scanner or the suprapubic area palpated for an oval mass and percussed for dullness, indicative of a full bladder.

### Gerontologic Considerations

When performing a cardiovascular examination on an elderly patient, the nurse may note such differences as more readily palpable peripheral pulses because of decreased elasticity of the arteries and a loss of adjacent connective tissue. Palpation of the precordium in the elderly is affected by the changes in the shape of the chest. For example, a cardiac impulse may not be palpable in patients with chronic obstructive pulmonary disease, because these patients usually have an increased anterior–posterior chest diameter. Kyphoscoliosis, a spinal deformity that occurs frequently in elderly patients, may dislocate the cardiac apex downward so that palpation of the apical impulse is obscured.

Systolic BP increases with age, but diastolic BP usually plateaus after 50 years. Isolated systolic hypertension occurs most commonly among the elderly and is associated with significant cardiovascular morbidity and mortality. Orthostatic hypotension may reflect decreased sensitivity of postural reflexes, which must be considered when medication therapy is prescribed.

An $S_4$ is heard in about 90% of elderly patients and is thought to be due to decreased compliance of the left ventricle. The $S_2$ is usually split. At least 60% of elderly patients have murmurs, the most common being a soft systolic ejection murmur resulting from sclerotic changes of the aortic leaflets (see Table 26-1).

## Diagnostic Evaluation

Diagnostic tests and procedures are used to confirm the data obtained by the history and physical assessment. Some tests are easy to interpret, but others must be interpreted by expert clinicians. All tests should be explained to the patient. Some necessitate special preparation before they are performed and special monitoring by the nurse after the procedure.

### Laboratory Tests

Laboratory tests may be performed for the following reasons:

- To assist in identifying the cause of cardiac-related signs and symptoms
- To identify abnormalities in the blood that affect the prognosis of a patient with CVD
- To assess the degree of inflammation
- To screen for risk factors associated with CAD
- To determine baseline values before initiating therapeutic interventions
- To ensure that therapeutic levels of medications (eg, antiarrhythmic agents and warfarin) are maintained
- To assess the effects of medications (eg, the effects of diuretics on serum potassium levels)
- To screen generally for abnormalities

Because different laboratories use different equipment and different methods of measurements, normal test values may vary depending on the laboratory and the health care institution.

### Cardiac Biomarker Analysis

Plasma analysis of key cardiac isoenzymes and other biomarkers is part of a diagnostic profile for acute MI that also includes the health history, symptoms, and ECG. Enzymes are released from injured cells when the cell membranes rupture. Most enzymes are nonspecific in relation to the particular organ that has been damaged. However, certain isoenzymes come only from myocardial cells and are released when those cells are damaged by sustained hypoxia or trauma that results in infarction. The isoenzymes leak into the interstitial spaces of the myocardium and are carried into the general circulation by the lymphatic system and the coronary circulation, resulting in elevated serum enzyme concentrations.

Because different enzymes move into the blood at varying periods after MI, enzyme levels should be tested in relation to the time of onset of chest discomfort or other symptoms. Creatine kinase (CK) and its isoenzyme CK-MB are the most specific enzymes analyzed in acute MI, and they are the first enzyme levels to increase. Lactic dehydrogenase and its isoenzymes may also be analyzed but only in select patients who have delayed seeking medical attention, because the blood levels of these substances peak in 2 to 3 days, much later than CK levels.

Other important cardiac biomarkers that are assessed include the myoglobin and troponin T or I. Myoglobin, an early marker of MI, is a heme protein with a small molecular weight. This allows it to be rapidly released from damaged myocardial tissue and accounts for its early increase, within 1 to 3 hours after the onset of an acute MI. Myoglobin peaks in 4 to 12 hours and returns to normal in 24 hours. Myoglobin is not used alone to diagnose MI, because elevations can also occur in patients with renal or musculoskeletal disease. However, negative results are helpful in ruling out an early diagnosis of MI.

Troponin T and I are laboratory tests that have several advantages over traditional enzyme studies such as CK-MB. Troponin T and I are proteins found only in cardiac muscle. After myocardial injury, elevated serum troponin T and I concentrations can be detected within 3 to 4 hours; they peak in 4 to 24 hours and remain elevated for 1 to 3 weeks. These early and prolonged elevations make very early diagnosis of MI possible or allow for late diagnosis if the patient has delayed seeking treatment (see Table 28-3 in Chapter 28 for the time course of cardiac biomarkers).

## Blood Chemistry, Hematology, and Coagulation Studies

Table 26-3 provides information about some common serum laboratory tests and the implications for patients with CVD. Lipid measurements are discussed below.

### LIPID PROFILE
Cholesterol, triglycerides, and lipoproteins are measured to evaluate a person's risk of developing atherosclerotic disease, especially if there is a family history of premature heart disease, or to diagnose a specific lipoprotein abnormality. Cholesterol and triglycerides are transported in the blood by combining with protein molecules to form lipoproteins. The lipoproteins are referred to as low-density lipoproteins (LDL) and high-density lipoproteins (HDL). The risk of CAD increases as the ratio of LDL to HDL or the ratio of total cholesterol (LDL + HDL) to HDL increases. Although cholesterol levels remain relatively constant over 24 hours, the blood specimen for the lipid profile should be obtained after a 12-hour fast.

### CHOLESTEROL LEVELS
Cholesterol (normal level is less than 200 mg/dL) is a lipid required for hormone synthesis and cell membrane formation. It is found in large quantities in brain and nerve tissue. Two major sources of cholesterol are diet (animal products) and the liver, where cholesterol is synthesized. Elevated cholesterol levels are known to increase the risk of CAD. Factors that contribute to variations in cholesterol levels include age, gender, diet, exercise patterns, genetics, menopause, tobacco use, and stress levels.

LDLs (normal level is less than 160 mg/dL) are the primary transporters of cholesterol and triglycerides into the cell. One harmful effect of LDL is the deposition of these substances in the walls of arterial vessels. Elevated LDL levels are associated with a greater incidence of CAD. In people with known CAD or diabetes, the primary goal for lipid management is reduction of LDL levels to less than 70 mg/dL.

HDLs (normal range in men is 35 to 70 mg/dL; in women, 35 to 85 mg/dL) have a protective action. They transport cholesterol away from the tissue and cells of the arterial wall to the liver for excretion. Therefore, there is an inverse relationship between HDL levels and risk of CAD. Factors that lower HDL levels include smoking, diabetes, obesity, and physical inactivity. In patients with CAD, a secondary goal of lipid management is the increase of HDL levels to more than 40 mg/dL.

### TRIGLYCERIDES
Triglycerides (normal range is 100 to 200 mg/dL), composed of free fatty acids and glycerol, are stored in the adipose tissue and are a source of energy. Triglyceride levels increase after meals and are affected by stress. Diabetes, alcohol use, and obesity can elevate triglyceride levels. These levels have a direct correlation with LDL and an inverse one with HDL.

## Brain (B-Type) Natriuretic Peptide

Brain (B-type) natriuretic peptide (BNP) is a neurohormone that helps regulate BP and fluid volume. It is primarily secreted from the ventricles in response to increased preload with resulting elevated ventricular pressure. The level of BNP in the blood increases as the ventricular walls expand from increased pressure, making it an excellent diagnostic, monitoring, and prognostic tool in the setting of HF. Because this serum laboratory test can be quickly obtained, BNP levels are useful for prompt diagnosis of HF in settings such as the emergency department. A BNP level of 51.2 pg/mL or greater is correlated with mild HF, and levels greater than 1000 pg/mL are associated with severe HF (Gordon & Rempher, 2003).

## C-Reactive Protein

High-sensitivity assay for C-reactive protein (hs-CRP) is a venous blood test that measures levels of CRP, a protein produced by the liver in response to systemic inflammation. Inflammation is thought to play a role in the development and progression of atherosclerosis. Therefore, hs-CRP is used as an adjunct to other tests to predict CVD risk. People with high levels of hs-CRP (3.0 mg/dL) are at greatest risk for CVD compared to people with moderate (1.0 to 3.0 mg/dL) or low (less than 1.0 mg/dL) levels of hs-CRP. In addition, an elevated hs-CRP places patients with ACS at high risk for recurrent cardiac events, including unstable angina and acute MI, higher mortality, and increased risk of restenosis of coronary arteries after PCI (Koenig, 2005).

## Homocysteine

Determining the homocysteine level enhances the clinician's ability to assess the patient's risk for CVD. An elevated blood level of homocysteine, an amino acid, is thought to indicate a high risk for CAD, stroke, and peripheral vascular disease, although it is not an independent predictor of CAD (AHA, 2005). Homocysteine is linked to the development of atherosclerosis, the underlying disorder in CAD, stroke, and peripheral vascular disease, because it can damage the endothelial lining of arteries and promote thrombus formation. Genetic factors and a diet low in folic acid, vitamin $B_6$, and vitamin $B_{12}$ are associated with elevated homocysteine levels. A 12-hour fast is necessary before drawing a blood sample for an accurate serum measurement. Test results are interpreted as normal (5 to 15 µmol/L), mod-

| TABLE 26-3 | Common Serum Laboratory Tests and Implications for Patients with Cardiovascular Disease (CVD) |
|---|---|
| **Laboratory Test** | **Implications** |
| **Blood Chemistries** | |
| Sodium (Na$^+$) | Low or high serum sodium levels do not directly affect cardiac function.<br>*Hyponatremia:* Decreased sodium levels indicate fluid excess and can be caused by heart failure or administration of thiazide diuretics.<br>*Hypernatremia:* Increased sodium levels indicate fluid deficits and can result from decreased water intake or loss of water through excessive sweating or diarrhea. |
| Potassium (K$^+$) | Potassium has a major role in cardiac electrophysiologic function.<br>*Hypokalemia:* Decreased potassium levels due to administration of potassium-excreting diuretics can cause many forms of dysrhythmias, including life-threatening ventricular tachycardia or ventricular fibrillation, and predispose patients taking digitalis preparations to digitalis toxicity.<br>*Hyperkalemia:* Increased potassium levels can result from an increased intake of potassium (eg, foods high in potassium or potassium supplements), decreased renal excretion of potassium, use of potassium-sparing diuretics (eg, spironolactone), or use of angiotensin-converting enzyme inhibitors (ACE inhibitors) that inhibit aldosterone function. Serious consequences of hyperkalemia include heart block, asystole, and life-threatening ventricular dysrhythmias. |
| Calcium (Ca$^{++}$) | Calcium is necessary for blood coagulability, neuromuscular activity, and automaticity of the nodal cells (sinus and atrioventricular nodes).<br>*Hypocalcemia:* Decreased calcium levels slow nodal function and impair myocardial contractility. The latter effect increases the risk for heart failure.<br>*Hypercalcemia:* Increased calcium levels can occur with the administration of thiazide diuretics because these medications reduce renal excretion of calcium. Hypercalcemia potentiates digitalis toxicity, causes increased myocardial contactility, and increases the risk for varying degrees of heart block and sudden death from ventricular fibrillation. |
| Magnesium (Mg$^{++}$) | Magnesium is necessary for the absorption of calcium, maintenance of potassium stores, and metabolism of adenosine triphosphate. It plays a major role in protein and carbohydrate synthesis and muscular contraction.<br>*Hypomagnesemia:* Decreased magnesium levels are due to enhanced renal excretion of magnesium from the use of diuretic or digitalis therapy. Low magnesium levels predispose patients to atrial or ventricular tachycardias.<br>*Hypermagnesemia:* Increased magnesium levels are commonly caused by the use of cathartics or antacids containing magnesium. Increased magnesium levels depress contractility and excitability of the myocardium, causing heart block and, if severe, asystole. |
| Blood urea nitrogen (BUN) | BUN and creatinine are end products of protein metabolism excreted by the kidneys. |
| Creatinine | Elevated BUN reflects reduced renal perfusion from decreased cardiac output or intravascular fluid volume deficit as a result of diuretic therapy or dehydration.<br>Both laboratory values are used to assess renal function, although creatinine is a more sensitive measure. Renal impairment is detected by an increase in both BUN and creatinine. A normal creatinine level and an elevated BUN detect an intravascular fluid volume deficit. |
| Glucose | Glucose levels are elevated in stressful situations, when mobilization of endogenous epinephrine results in conversion of liver glycogen to glucose. Serum glucose levels are drawn in a fasting state. |
| Glycosylated hemoglobin (hemoglobin A$_{1c}$) | Glycosylated hemoglobin (hemoglobin A$_{1C}$) is monitored in people with diabetes. It reflects the blood glucose levels over 2 to 3 months. The glycemic goal is to maintain the hemoglobin A$_{1C}$ below 7% (normal range 4%–6%), reflecting consistent near-normal blood glucose levels. |
| **Coagulation Studies** | Injury to a vessel wall or tissue initiates the formation of a thrombus. This injury activates the coagulation cascade, the complex interactions among phospholipids, calcium, and clotting factors that convert prothrombin to thrombin. The coagulation cascade has two pathways, the intrinsic and extrinsic pathways. Coagulation studies are routinely performed before invasive procedures, such as cardiac catheterization, electrophysiology testing, and coronary or cardiac surgery. |

*continued >*

| TABLE 26-3 | Common Serum Laboratory Tests and Implications for Patients with Cardiovascular Disease (CVD) (Continued) |
|---|---|
| **Laboratory Test** | **Implications** |
| Partial thromboplastin time (PTT) Activated partial thromboplastin time (aPTT) | PTT or aPTT measures the activity of the intrinsic pathway and is used to assess the effects of unfractionated heparin. A therapeutic range is 1.5 to 2.5 times baseline values. Adjustment of heparin dose is required for aPTT < 50 seconds (↑ dose) or >100 seconds (↓ dose). |
| Prothrombin time (PT) | PT measures the extrinsic pathway activity and is used to monitor the level of anticoagulation with warfarin (Coumadin). |
| International Normalized Ratio (INR) | The INR, reported with the PT, provides a standard method for reporting PT levels and eliminates the variation of PT results from different laboratories. The INR, rather than the PT alone, is used to monitor the effectiveness of warfarin. The therapeutic range for INR is 2.0–3.5, although specific ranges vary based on diagnosis. |
| **Hematologic Studies** | |
| Complete blood count (CBC) | The CBC identifies the total number of white and red blood cells and platelets, and measures hemoglobin and hematocrit. The CBC is carefully monitored in patients with cardiovascular disease. |
| White blood cell (WBC) count | WBC counts are monitored in immunocompromised patients, including patients with heart transplants or in situations where there is concern for infection (eg, after invasive procedures or surgery). |
| Hemoglobin and hematocrit | The hematocrit represents the percentage of red blood cells found in 100 mL of whole blood. The red blood cells contain hemoglobin, which transports oxygen to the cells. Low hemoglobin and hematocrit levels have serious consequences for patients with cardiovascular disease, such as more frequent angina episodes or acute myocardial infarction. |
| Platelets | Platelets are the first line of protection against bleeding. Once activated by blood vessel wall injury or rupture of atherosclerotic plaque, platelets undergo chemical changes that form a thrombus. Several medications inhibit platelet function, including aspirin, clopidogrel (Plavix), and IV GP IIb/IIIa inhibitors (abciximab [ReoPro], eptifibatide [Integrilin], and tirofiban [Aggrastat]). When these medications are administered, it is essential to monitor for thrombocytopenia (low platelet counts). |

erate (16 to 30 μmol/L), intermediate (31 to 100 μmol/L), and severe (more than 100 μmol/L).

## Chest X-Ray and Fluoroscopy

A chest x-ray is obtained to determine the size, contour, and position of the heart. It reveals cardiac and pericardial calcifications and demonstrates physiologic alterations in the pulmonary circulation. Although it does not help diagnose acute MI, it can help diagnose some complications (eg, HF). Correct placement of cardiac catheters, such as pacemakers and pulmonary artery catheters, is also confirmed by chest x-ray.

Fluoroscopy allows visualization of the heart on an x-ray screen. It shows cardiac and vascular pulsations and unusual cardiac contours. Fluoroscopy is useful for positioning IV pacing electrodes and for guiding catheter insertion during cardiac catheterization.

## Electrocardiography

The ECG is a diagnostic tool used in assessing the cardiovascular system. It is a graphic recording of the electrical activity of the heart. The ECG is obtained by placing disposable electrodes in standard positions on the skin of the chest wall and extremities. The heart's electrical impulses are recorded on special graph paper, with 12, 15, or 18 leads, showing the activity from those different reference points.

The standard 12-lead ECG is used to diagnose dysrhythmias, conduction abnormalities, enlarged heart chambers, and myocardial ischemia or infarction and to monitor high or low calcium and potassium levels and the effects of some medications. A 15-lead ECG adds 3 additional chest leads across the right precordium and is used for early diagnosis of right ventricular and posterior left ventricular infarction. The 18-lead ECG adds 3 posterior leads to the 15-lead ECG and is useful for early detection of myocardial ischemia and injury. To enhance interpretation of the ECG, the patient's age, gender, BP, height, weight, symptoms, and medications (especially digitalis and antiarrhythmic agents) are noted on the ECG requisition. The details of electrocardiography are presented in Chapter 27.

### Continuous Electrocardiographic Monitoring

Continuous ECG monitoring to detect abnormalities in heart rate and rhythm is standard for patients who are at high risk for dysrhythmias. In addition, it is often possible to monitor the ST segment of the ECG to identify changes indicative of myocardial ischemia or infarction (see Chapter 28). Two continuous ECG monitoring techniques are hardwire monitoring, found in emergency departments, critical care units, and progressive care units (sometimes called specialty step-down units), and telemetry, found in general nursing care units. Patients monitored continuously need to be informed of the purpose of the monitoring and cautioned that it does not detect symptoms such as dyspnea or chest pain. Therefore, patients need to be advised to report symptoms to the nurse whenever they occur.

## HARDWIRE CARDIAC MONITORING

The patient's ECG can be continuously observed for dysrhythmias and conduction disorders on an oscilloscope at the bedside or at a central monitoring station by a hardwire monitoring system. This system is composed of three to five electrodes positioned on the patient's chest, a lead cable, and a bedside monitor. Hardwire monitoring systems vary in sophistication but in general can do the following:

- Monitor more than one lead simultaneously
- Monitor ST segments (ST-segment depression is a marker of myocardial ischemia; ST-segment elevation provides evidence of an evolving MI)
- Provide graded visual and audible alarms (based on priority, asystole would be highest)
- Computerize rhythm monitoring (dysrhythmias are interpreted and stored in memory)
- Print a rhythm strip
- Record a 12-lead ECG

Two leads commonly used for continuous monitoring are leads II and V1 or a modification of V1 (MCL1) (Fig. 26-9). Lead II provides the best visualization of atrial depolarization (represented by the P wave). Leads V1 and MCL1 best record ventricular depolarization and are most helpful when monitoring for ventricular dysrhythmias (eg, premature ventricular contractions or ventricular tachycardia).

## TELEMETRY

In addition to hardwire monitoring systems, the ECG can be continuously observed by **telemetry**, the transmission of radiowaves from a battery-operated transmitter worn by the patient to a central bank of monitors. Although telemetry systems have the same capabilities as hardwire systems, they are wireless, allowing the patient to ambulate while being monitored. To ensure good conduction and a clear picture of the patient's rhythm on the monitor, it is important to adhere to the following guidelines for electrode placement:

- Clean the skin surface with soap and water and dry well (or as recommended by the manufacturer) before applying the electrodes. If the patient has much hair where the electrodes need to be placed, shave or clip the hair.
- Apply a small amount of benzoin to the skin if the patient is diaphoretic (sweaty) and the electrodes do not adhere well.
- Change the electrodes every 24 to 48 hours and examine the skin for irritation. Apply the electrodes to different locations each time they are changed.
- If the patient is sensitive to the electrodes, use hypoallergenic electrodes.

## SIGNAL-AVERAGED ELECTROCARDIOGRAM

For some patients who are considered to be at high risk for sudden cardiac death, a signal-averaged ECG is performed. This high-resolution ECG assists in identifying the risk for life-threatening dysrhythmias and helps determine the need for invasive diagnostic procedures. Signal averaging works by averaging about 150 to 300 QRS waveforms (QRS waveforms represent depolarization of the ventricle). The resulting averaged QRS complex is analyzed for certain characteristics that are likely to lead to lethal ventricular dysrhythmias. The recording is performed at the bedside and requires about 15 minutes.

## CONTINUOUS AMBULATORY MONITORING

In ambulatory ECG monitoring, which may occur in the hospital but is more commonly used for outpatients, one lead of the patient's ECG is monitored by a Holter monitor. This monitor is a small tape recorder that continuously (for 10 to 24 hours) documents the heart's electrical activity on a magnetic tape. The tape recorder weighs approximately 2 pounds and can be carried over the shoulder or worn around the waist day and night to detect dysrhythmias or evidence of myocardial ischemia during activities of daily living. The patient keeps a diary of activity, noting the time of any symptoms, experiences, or performance of unusual activities. The tape recording is then examined with a special scanner,

**FIGURE 26-9.** Two leads (views of the heart) commonly used for continuous monitoring. To monitor lead II, the negative electrode is placed on the right upper chest; the positive electrode is placed on the left lower chest. To monitor MCL₁, the negative electrode is placed on the left upper chest; the positive electrode is placed in the V1 position. If three electrodes are used, the third electrode, which is the ground electrode, can be placed anywhere on the chest.

LEAD II           MCl₁

analyzed, and interpreted. Evidence obtained in this way helps the physician diagnose dysrhythmias and myocardial ischemia and evaluate therapy, such as antiarrhythmic and antianginal medications or pacemaker function.

### TRANSTELEPHONIC MONITORING

Another method of evaluating the ECG of a patient at home is by transtelephonic monitoring. The patient attaches a specific lead system for transmitting the signals and places a telephone mouthpiece over the transmitter box, and the ECG is recorded and evaluated at another location. This method is often used for diagnosing dysrhythmias and in follow-up evaluation of permanent cardiac pacemakers.

### WIRELESS MOBILE CARDIAC MONITORING SYSTEMS

This emerging technology allows health care professionals to monitor and transmit the ECG of patients outside of the hospital or office setting continuously. The wireless method has a number of advantages compared to Holter and transtelephonic monitoring. It is lightweight, can monitor the patient 24 hours a day 7 days a week, and does not require patients to transmit their ECG by telephone. Patients wear a small sensing device that transmits each heartbeat to a small monitor. When a dysrhythmia is detected, the system automatically transmits the patient's ECG to a monitoring center through either the patient's telephone line when at home or through wireless communications systems when outside of the home. This system enhances detection and early treatment of dysrhythmias that might otherwise be diagnosed only after the patient develops serious symptoms (Frantz, 2003; Tachakra, Wang, Istepanian, et al., 2003).

## Cardiac Stress Testing

Normally, the coronary arteries dilate to four times their usual diameter in response to increased metabolic demands for oxygen and nutrients. However, coronary arteries affected by atherosclerosis dilate much less, compromising blood flow to the myocardium and causing ischemia. Therefore, abnormalities in cardiovascular function are more likely to be detected during times of increased demand, or "stress." The **cardiac stress test** procedures—the exercise stress test, the pharmacologic stress test, and more recently the mental or emotional stress test—are noninvasive ways to evaluate the response of the cardiovascular system to stress. The stress test helps determine the following: (1) presence of CAD, (2) cause of chest pain, (3) functional capacity of the heart after an MI or heart surgery, (4) effectiveness of antianginal or antiarrhythmic medications, (5) dysrhythmias that occur during physical exercise, and (6) specific goals for a physical fitness program. Contraindications to stress testing include severe aortic stenosis, acute myocarditis or pericarditis, severe hypertension, suspected left main CAD, HF, and unstable angina. Because complications associated with stress testing can be life-threatening (MI, cardiac arrest, HF, and severe dysrhythmias), testing facilities must have staff and equipment ready to provide treatment, including advanced cardiac life support.

Mental stress testing uses a mental arithmetic test or simulated public speech to determine whether an ischemic myocardial response occurs, similar to the response evoked by a conventional treadmill exercise test. Although its use for diagnostic purposes in patients with CAD is currently investigational, preliminary results indicate that the ischemic and hemodynamic measures obtained from mental stress testing may be useful in assessing the prognosis of patients with CHD who have had a positive exercise test (Kim, Bartholomew, Mastin, et al., 2003).

Stress testing is often combined with echocardiography or radionuclide imaging (discussed later). These techniques are performed during the resting state and immediately after stress.

### Exercise Stress Testing

In an exercise stress test, the patient walks on a treadmill (most common) or pedals a stationary bicycle or arm crank. Exercise intensity progresses according to established protocols. The Bruce protocol, for example, is a common treadmill protocol in which the speed and grade of the treadmill are increased every 3 minutes. The goal of the test is to increase the heart rate to the "target heart rate." This is 80% to 90% of the maximum predicted heart rate and is based on the patient's age and gender. During the test, the following are monitored: two or more ECG leads for heart rate, rhythm, and ischemic changes; BP; skin temperature; physical appearance; perceived exertion; and symptoms, including chest pain, dyspnea, dizziness, leg cramping, and fatigue. The test is terminated when the target heart rate is achieved or when the patient experiences chest pain, extreme fatigue, a decrease in BP or pulse rate, serious dysrhythmias or ST-segment changes on the ECG, or other complications. When significant ECG abnormalities occur during the stress test (ST-segment depressions or elevations), the test result is reported as positive and further diagnostic testing such as coronary angiography is required.

### NURSING INTERVENTIONS

In preparation for the exercise stress test, the patient is instructed to fast for 4 hours before the test and to avoid stimulants such as tobacco and caffeine. Medications may be taken with sips of water. The physician may instruct the patient not to take certain cardiac medications, such as beta-adrenergic blocking agents, before the test. Clothes and sneakers or rubber-soled shoes suitable for exercising are to be worn. Women are advised to wear a bra that provides adequate support. The nurse describes the equipment used and the sensations and experiences that the patient may have during the test. The nurse explains the monitoring equipment used, the need to have an IV line placed, and the symptoms to report. The type of exercise is reviewed, and the patient is asked to put forth his or her best exercise effort. If the test is to be performed with echocardiography or radionuclide imaging, this information is reviewed as well. After the test, the patient is monitored for 10 to 15 minutes. Once stable, the patient may resume his or her usual activities.

### Pharmacologic Stress Testing

Patients who are physically disabled or deconditioned will not be able to achieve their target heart rate by exercising on a treadmill or bicycle. Two vasodilating agents, dipyridamole (Persantine) and adenosine (Adenocard), administered IV, are used to mimic the effects of exercise by maximally dilating the coronary arteries. The effects of dipyridamole last about 15 to 30 minutes. The side effects are related to its vasodilating action and include chest discomfort, dizziness, headache, flushing, and nausea. Adenosine has similar side effects, although patients report these symptoms as more severe. Adenosine has an extremely short half-life (less than 10 seconds), so any severe effects rapidly subside. Dipyridamole and adenosine are the agents of choice used in conjunction with radionuclide imaging techniques. Theophylline and other xanthines, such as caffeine, block the effects of dipyridamole and adenosine and must be avoided before either of these pharmacologic stress tests.

Dobutamine (Dobutrex) is another medication that may be used if the patient cannot exercise. Dobutamine, a synthetic sympathomimetic, increases heart rate, myocardial contractility, and BP, thereby increasing the metabolic demands of the heart. It is the agent of choice when echocardiography is used because of its effects on altering myocardial wall motion (due to enhanced contractility). Dobutamine is also used for patients who have bronchospasm or pulmonary disease and cannot tolerate having doses of theophylline withheld.

**NURSING INTERVENTIONS**
In preparation for the pharmacologic stress test, the patient is instructed not to eat or drink anything for at least 4 hours before the test. This includes chocolate, caffeine, caffeine-free coffee, tea, carbonated beverages, or medications that contain caffeine (eg, Anacin, Darvon). If caffeine is ingested before a dipyridamole or adenosine stress test, the test will have to be rescheduled. Patients taking aminophylline or theophylline are instructed to stop taking these medications for 24 to 48 hours before the test (if tolerated). Oral doses of dipyridamole are withheld as well. The patient is informed about the transient sensations that may occur during infusion of the vasodilating agent, such as flushing or nausea, which will disappear quickly. The patient is instructed to report any other symptoms occurring during the test to the cardiologist or nurse. An explanation of echocardiography or radionuclide imaging is also provided as necessary. The stress test may take about 1 hour, or up to 3 hours if imaging is performed.

# Echocardiography

## Traditional Echocardiography

Echocardiography is a noninvasive ultrasound test that is used to examine the size, shape, and motion of cardiac structures. It is particularly useful for diagnosing pericardial effusions, determining chamber size and the etiology of heart murmurs, evaluating the function of prosthetic heart valves, and evaluating ventricular wall motion. It involves transmission of high-frequency sound waves into the heart through the chest wall and recording of the return signals. The ultrasound is generated by a hand-held transducer applied to the front of the chest. The transducer picks up the echoes, converts them to electrical impulses, and transmits them to the echocardiography machine for display on an oscilloscope and recording on a videotape. An ECG is recorded simultaneously to assist with interpreting the echocardiogram.

M-mode (motion), the unidimensional mode that was first introduced, provides information about the cardiac structures and their motion. Two-dimensional or cross-sectional echocardiography, an enhancement of the technique, creates a sophisticated, spatially correct image of the heart. Other techniques, such as Doppler and color flow imaging echocardiography, show the direction and velocity of the blood flow through the heart.

Echocardiography may be performed with an exercise or pharmacologic stress test; resting and stress images are obtained. Myocardial ischemia from decreased perfusion during stress causes abnormalities in ventricular wall motion and is easily detected by echocardiography. A stress test using echocardiography is considered positive if abnormalities in ventricular wall motion are detected during stress but not during rest. These findings are highly suggestive of CAD and require further evaluation, such as a cardiac catheterization.

**NURSING INTERVENTIONS**
Before echocardiography, the nurse informs the patient about the test, explaining that it is painless. Echocardiographic monitoring is performed while a transducer that emits the sound waves is moved on the surface of the chest wall. Gel applied to the skin helps transmit the sound waves. Periodically, the patient will have to turn onto the left side or hold a breath. The test takes about 30 to 45 minutes. If the patient is to undergo an exercise or pharmacologic stress test with echocardiography, information on stress testing is also reviewed with the patient.

## Transesophageal Echocardiography (TEE)

A significant limitation of traditional echocardiography has been the poor quality of the images produced. Ultrasound loses its clarity as it passes through tissue, lung, and bone. Another echocardiographic technique involves threading a small transducer through the mouth and into the esophagus. This technique, called transesophageal echocardiography (TEE), provides clearer images because ultrasound waves are passing through less tissue. Pharmacologic stress testing using dobutamine and TEE can also be performed. The high-quality imaging obtained during TEE makes this technique an important first-line diagnostic tool for evaluating patients with many types of CVD, including those with HF, valvular heart disease, and intracardiac thrombi. It is frequently used during cardiac surgery to continuously monitor the response of the heart to the surgical procedure (eg, valve replacement or coronary artery bypass). Complications are uncommon during TEE, but if they do occur they are serious. These complications are caused by sedation and impaired swallowing resulting from the topical anesthesia (respiratory depression and aspiration) and by insertion and manipulation of the transducer into the esophagus and stomach (vasovagal response or esophageal perforation). The patient must be assessed before TEE for a history of dysphagia or radiation therapy to the chest, which increases the risk of complications.

**NURSING INTERVENTIONS**
The following protocol is usually implemented to prepare for a TEE study:

- The patient must fast for 6 hours before the study.
- An IV line is started for administering a sedative and any pharmacologic stress testing medications.

- The patient is maintained on moderate sedation, defined as a state of depressed consciousness during which time the patient responds appropriately to commands and can maintain a patent airway (see Chapter 19).
- The patient's throat is anesthetized before the probe is inserted. The patient is then asked to swallow the probe until it is correctly positioned in the esophagus.
- BP, ECG, respiration, and oxygen saturation ($SpO_2$) are monitored throughout the study.
- During recovery from moderate sedation, frequent assessments of the parameters previously identified are made as well as the patient's level of consciousness. The patient must continue to fast until fully alert and the effects of the topical anesthetic are reversed, usually 2 hours after the procedure. The patient may have a sore throat for the next 24 hours. If the procedure is performed in an outpatient setting, someone must be available to transport the patient home from the test site.

## Radionuclide Imaging

Radionuclide imaging studies involve the use of radioisotopes to evaluate coronary artery perfusion noninvasively, to detect myocardial ischemia and infarction, and to assess left ventricular function. **Radioisotopes** are atoms in an unstable form. Thallium 201 ($Tl^{201}$) and technetium 99m ($Tc^{99m}$) are two radioisotopes used in cardiac nuclear medicine studies. As they decay, they give off small amounts of energy in the form of gamma rays. When they are injected into the bloodstream, the energy emitted can be detected by a gamma scintillation camera positioned over the body. Planar imaging, used with thallium, provides a one-dimensional view of the heart from three locations. Single photon emission computed tomography (SPECT) provides three-dimensional images. With SPECT, the patient is positioned supine with arms raised above the head, while the camera moves around the patient's chest in a 180- to 360-degree arc to identify the areas of decreased myocardial perfusion more precisely.

### Myocardial Perfusion Imaging

The radioisotope $Tl^{201}$ is used to assess myocardial perfusion. It resembles potassium and readily crosses into the cells of healthy myocardium. It is taken up more slowly and in smaller amounts by myocardial cells that are ischemic from decreased blood flow. However, thallium does not cross into the necrotic tissue that results from an MI.

Often, thallium is used with stress testing to assess changes in myocardial perfusion immediately after exercise (or after injection of one of the pharmacologic agents used in stress testing) and at rest. One or two minutes before the end of the stress test, a dose of $Tl^{201}$ is injected into the IV line, allowing the radioisotope to be distributed into the myocardium. Images are taken immediately. Areas that do not show thallium uptake indicate areas of either MI or stress-induced myocardial ischemia. Resting images, taken 3 hours later, help differentiate infarction from ischemia. Infarcted tissue cannot take up thallium regardless of when the scan is taken; the defect remains the same size during exercise or rest. This is called a fixed defect, indicating that there is no perfusion in that area of the myocardium. Ischemic myocardium, on the other hand, recovers in a few hours. If perfusion is restored, thallium crosses into the myocardial cells, and the area of defect on the resting images is either smaller or completely reversed. These reversible defects constitute positive stress test findings. Usually, cardiac catheterization is recommended after a positive test result to determine whether PCI or coronary artery bypass graft surgery is needed.

Another radioisotope used for cardiac imaging is $Tc^{99m}$. Technetium can be combined with various chemical compounds, giving it an affinity for different types of cells. For example, $Tc^{99m}$ sestamibi (Cardiolite) is distributed to myocardial cells in proportion to its perfusion, making this an excellent tracer for assessing perfusion to the myocardium. The procedure for cardiac imaging using $Tc^{99m}$ sestamibi with stress testing is similar to the one using thallium, with two differences. Patients receiving $Tc^{99m}$ sestamibi can have their resting images recorded before or after the exercise images. Timing of the images is not important because the half-life of $Tc^{99m}$ is short, and $Tc^{99m}$ needs to be injected before each scan. Also, SPECT imaging with $Tc^{99m}$ sestamibi provides high-quality images.

#### NURSING INTERVENTIONS

The patient undergoing nuclear imaging techniques with stress testing should be prepared for the type of stressor to be used (exercise or drug) and the type of imaging technique (planar or SPECT). The patient may be concerned about receiving a radioactive substance and needs to be reassured that these tracers are safe—the radiation exposure is similar to that of other diagnostic x-ray studies. No postprocedure radiation precautions are necessary.

When providing teaching for a patient undergoing SPECT, the nurse instructs the patient that the arms will need to be positioned over the head for about 20 to 30 minutes. If the patient is physically unable to do this, thallium with planar imaging can be used.

### Test of Ventricular Function and Wall Motion

Equilibrium radionuclide angiocardiography (ERNA), also known as multiple-gated acquisition (MUGA) scanning, is a common noninvasive technique that uses a conventional scintillation camera interfaced with a computer to record images of the heart during several hundred heartbeats. The computer processes the data and allows for sequential viewing of the functioning heart. The sequential images are analyzed to evaluate left ventricular function, wall motion, and ejection fraction. MUGA scanning can also be used to assess the differences in left ventricular function during rest and exercise.

The patient is reassured that there is no known radiation danger and is instructed to remain motionless during the scan.

### Computed Tomography

Computed tomography (CT), also called computerized axial tomographic (CAT) scanning or electron-beam computed tomography (EBCT), uses x-rays to provide cross-sectional images of the chest, including the heart and great vessels. These techniques are used to evaluate cardiac masses and diseases of the aorta and pericardium.

EBCT, also known as the ultrafast CT, is an especially fast x-ray scanning technique that results in much faster image acquisition with a higher degree of resolution than traditional x-ray or CT scanning provides. It is used to evaluate bypass graft patency, congenital heart lesions, left and right ventricular muscle mass, chamber volumes, cardiac output, and ejection fraction. For people without previous MI, PCI, or coronary artery bypass surgery, the EBCT is used to determine the amount of calcium deposits in the coronary arteries and underlying atherosclerosis. From this scan, a calcium score is derived that predicts the incidence of cardiac events, such as MI or the need for a revascularization procedure within the next 1 to 2 years.

The EBCT is not widely used, but it does show great promise in the early detection of CAD that is not yet clinically significant and that would not be identified by traditional testing methods such as the exercise stress test.

**NURSING INTERVENTIONS**

Patient preparation for these tests is the primary role of the nurse. The nurse explains to the patient that he or she will be positioned on a table during the scan while the scanner rotates around him or her. The procedure is noninvasive and painless. However, to obtain adequate images, the patient must lie perfectly still during the scanning process. An IV access line is necessary if contrast enhancement is to be used.

## Positron Emission Tomography

Positron emission tomography (PET) is a noninvasive scanning method that has been used primarily to study neurologic dysfunction. More recently, and with increasing frequency, PET has been used to diagnose cardiac dysfunction. PET provides more specific information about myocardial perfusion and viability than does TEE or thallium scanning. For cardiac patients, including those without symptoms, PET helps in planning treatment (eg, coronary artery bypass surgery, PCIs). PET also helps evaluate the patency of native and previously grafted vessels and the collateral circulation.

During a PET scan, radioisotopes are administered by injection; one compound is used to determine blood flow in the myocardium, and another shows the metabolic function. The PET camera provides detailed three-dimensional images of the distributed compounds. The viability of the myocardium is determined by comparing the extent of glucose metabolism in the myocardium to the degree of blood flow. For example, ischemic but viable tissue would show decreased blood flow and elevated metabolism. For a patient with this finding, revascularization through surgery or angioplasty would probably be indicated to improve heart function. Restrictions of food intake before the test vary among institutions, but because PET evaluates glucose metabolism, the patient's blood glucose level should be in the normal range before testing. Although PET equipment is costly, it is increasingly available.

**NURSING INTERVENTIONS**

Nurses involved in PET and other scanning procedures may instruct the patient to refrain from using tobacco and ingesting caffeine for 4 hours before the procedure. They should also reassure the patient that radiation exposure is at safe and acceptable levels, similar to those of other diagnostic x-ray studies.

## Magnetic Resonance Imaging

Magnetic resonance imaging (MRI) is a noninvasive, painless technique that is used to examine both the physiologic and anatomic properties of the heart. MRI uses a powerful magnetic field and computer-generated pictures to image the heart and great vessels. It is valuable in diagnosing diseases of the aorta, heart muscle, and pericardium, as well as congenital heart lesions. The application of this technique to the evaluation of coronary artery anatomy, cardiac blood flow, and myocardial viability in conjunction with pharmacologic stress testing is being investigated.

**NURSING INTERVENTIONS**

Because of the strong magnetic field used during MRI, diagnostic centers where these procedures are performed carefully screen patients for contraindications. Standardized questionnaires are commonly used to determine whether the patient has a pacemaker, metal plates, prosthetic joints, or other metallic implants that can become dislodged if exposed to MRI. The patient is instructed to remove any jewelry, watches, or other metal items. Transdermal patches that contain a heat-conducting aluminized layer (eg, NicoDerm, Androderm, Transderm Nitro, Transderm Scop, Catapres-TTS) must be removed before MRI to prevent burning of the skin. During an MRI, the patient is positioned supine on a table that is placed into an enclosed imager or tube containing the magnetic field. People who are claustrophobic may need to receive a mild sedative before undergoing an MRI. As the MRI is performed, there is an intermittent clanking or thumping sound from the magnetic coils that can be annoying to the patient, so patients may be offered headsets to listen to music. The scanner is equipped with a microphone so that the patient can communicate with the staff. The patient is instructed to remain motionless during the scan.

## Cardiac Catheterization

**Cardiac catheterization** is an invasive diagnostic procedure in which radiopaque arterial and venous catheters are introduced into selected blood vessels of the right and left sides of the heart. Catheter advancement is guided by fluoroscopy. Most commonly, the catheters are inserted percutaneously through the blood vessels, or via a cutdown procedure if the patient has poor vascular access. Pressures and oxygen saturation levels in the four heart chambers are measured.

Cardiac catheterization is most frequently used to diagnose CAD, assess coronary artery patency, and determine the extent of atherosclerosis based on the percentage of coronary artery obstruction. These results determine whether revascularization procedures, including PCI or coronary artery bypass surgery, may be of benefit to the patient (see Chapter 28). Cardiac catheterization is also used to diagnose pulmonary arterial hypertension or to treat stenotic heart valves via percutaneous balloon valvuloplasty.

During cardiac catheterization, the patient has an IV line in place for the administration of sedatives, fluids, heparin, and other medications. Noninvasive hemodynamic monitoring that includes BP and multiple ECG tracings is necessary to continuously observe for dysrhythmias or hemodynamic instability. The myocardium can become ischemic and trigger dysrhythmias as catheters are positioned in the coronary arteries or during injection of contrast agents. Resuscitation equipment must be readily available during the procedure. Staff must be prepared to provide advanced cardiac life support measures as necessary.

Radiopaque contrast agents are used to visualize the coronary arteries. Some contrast agents contain iodine, and the patient is assessed before the procedure for previous reactions to contrast agents or allergies to iodine-containing substances (eg, seafood). If the patient has a suspected or known allergy to the substance, antihistamines or methylprednisolone (Solu-Medrol) may be administered before the procedure. In addition, the following blood tests are performed to identify abnormalities that may complicate recovery: blood urea nitrogen (BUN) and creatinine levels, **International Normalized Ratio (INR)** or prothrombin time (PT), activated thromboplastin time (aPTT), hematocrit and hemoglobin values, platelet count, and electrolyte levels.

Patients who have comorbid conditions—including diabetes, renal insufficiency, HF, preexisting renal failure, nephrotic syndrome, hypotension, or dehydration—who undergo cardiac catheterization are at risk for contrast-induced acute renal failure. Preventive strategies under investigation for these patients may include preprocedure administration of IV fluids and the antioxidant acetylcysteine (Mucomyst) (Ferrone, 2004).

Diagnostic cardiac catheterizations are commonly performed on an outpatient basis and require 2 to 6 hours of bed rest after the procedure before the patient ambulates. Variations in time to ambulation are related to the size of the catheter used during the procedure, the site of catheter insertion (femoral or radial artery), the anticoagulation status of the patient, and other patient variables (eg, advanced age, obesity, bleeding disorder). The use of smaller (4 or 6 French) catheters, which are associated with shorter recovery times, is common in diagnostic cardiac catheterizations. Several options to achieve arterial hemostasis after catheter removal, including manual pressure, mechanical compression devices such as the FemoStop (placed over puncture site for 30 minutes), and percutaneously deployed devices, are used. The latter devices are positioned at the femoral arterial puncture site after completion of the procedure. They deploy a saline-soaked gelatin sponge (Quick-Seal), collagen (VasoSeal), sutures (Perclose, Techstar), or a combination of both collagen and sutures (Angio-Seal). Other newer products that expedite arterial hemostasis include external patches (Syvek Patch, Clo-Sur PAD). These products are placed over the puncture site as the catheter is removed and manual pressure is applied for 4 to 10 minutes. Once hemostasis is achieved, the patch is covered with a dressing that remains in place for 24 hours (Hirsch, Reddy, Capasso, et al., 2003).

Major benefits of the vascular closure devices include reliable, immediate hemostasis and a shorter time on bed rest without a significant increase in bleeding or other complications (Hoffer & Block, 2003). A number of factors determine which closure devices are used, such as the physician's preference, the patient's condition, cost, and institutional availability of these devices.

Patients hospitalized for angina or acute MI who require cardiac catheterization usually return to their hospital rooms for recovery. In some cardiac catheterization laboratories, an angioplasty (discussed in Chapter 28) may be performed immediately during the catheterization if indicated.

## Angiography

Cardiac catheterization is usually performed with angiography, a technique in which a contrast agent is injected into the vascular system to outline the heart and blood vessels. When a specific heart chamber or blood vessel is singled out for study, the procedure is known as selective angiography. Angiography makes use of cineangiograms, a series of rapidly changing films on an intensified fluoroscopic screen that record the passage of the contrast agent through the vascular site or sites. The recorded information allows for comparison of data over time.

### Common Sites

Common sites for selective angiography are the aorta, the coronary arteries, and the right and left sides of the heart.

#### AORTOGRAPHY

An aortogram is a form of angiography that outlines the lumen of the aorta and the major arteries arising from it. In thoracic aortography, a contrast agent is used to study the aortic arch and its major branches. The catheter may be introduced into the aorta using the translumbar or retrograde brachial or femoral artery approach.

#### CORONARY ARTERIOGRAPHY

In coronary arteriography, the catheter is introduced into the right or left brachial or femoral artery, then passed into the ascending aorta and manipulated into the right and left coronary arteries. Coronary arteriography is used to evaluate the degree of atherosclerosis and to determine treatment. It is also used to study suspected congenital anomalies of the coronary arteries.

#### RIGHT HEART CATHETERIZATION

Right heart catheterization usually precedes left heart catheterization. It involves the passage of a catheter from an antecubital or femoral vein into the right atrium, right ventricle, pulmonary artery, and pulmonary arterioles. Pressures and oxygen saturation levels from each of these areas are obtained and recorded.

Although right heart catheterization is considered relatively safe, potential complications include cardiac dysrhythmias, venous spasm, infection of the insertion site, cardiac perforation, and, rarely, cardiac arrest.

#### LEFT HEART CATHETERIZATION

Left heart catheterization is performed to evaluate the patency of the coronary arteries and the function of the left ventricle and the mitral and aortic valves. Potential complications include dysrhythmias, MI, perforation of the heart or great vessels, and systemic embolization. Left heart catheterization is performed by retrograde catheterization of the left ventricle. In this approach, the physician usually inserts the catheter into the right brachial artery or a femoral artery and advances it into the aorta and left ventricle.

After the procedure, the catheter is carefully withdrawn and arterial hemostasis is achieved using manual pressure or other techniques previously described. If the physician performed an arterial or venous cutdown, the site is sutured and a sterile dressing is applied.

## Nursing Interventions

Nursing responsibilities before cardiac catheterization include the following:

- The patient is instructed to fast, usually for 8 to 12 hours, before the procedure. If catheterization is to be performed as an outpatient procedure, a friend, family member, or other responsible person must transport the patient home.
- The patient is informed of the expected duration of the procedure and advised that it will involve lying on a hard table for less than 2 hours.
- The patient is reassured that mild sedatives or moderate sedation will be given IV.
- The patient is informed about certain sensations that will be experienced during the catheterization. Knowing what to expect can help the patient cope with the experience. The nurse explains that an occasional pounding sensation (palpitation) may be felt in the chest because of extrasystoles that almost always occur, particularly when the catheter tip touches the myocardium. The patient may be asked to cough and to breathe deeply, especially after the injection of contrast agent. Coughing may help disrupt a dysrhythmia and clear the contrast agent from the arteries. Breathing deeply and holding the breath help lower the diaphragm for better visualization of heart structures. The injection of a contrast agent into either side of the heart may produce a flushed feeling throughout the body and a sensation similar to the need to void, which subsides in 1 minute or less.
- The patient is encouraged to express fears and anxieties. The nurse provides teaching and reassurance to reduce apprehension.

Nursing responsibilities after cardiac catheterization may include the following:

- The catheter access site is observed for bleeding or hematoma formation. Peripheral pulses in the affected extremity (dorsalis pedis and posterior tibial pulses in the lower extremity, radial pulse in the upper extremity) are assessed every 15 minutes for 1 hour, and then every 1 to 2 hours until the pulses are stable.
- Temperature and color of the affected extremity are evaluated, as well as any patient complaints of pain, numbness, or tingling sensations, to detect arterial insufficiency. Any changes are reported promptly.
- Dysrhythmias are carefully assessed by observing the cardiac monitor or by assessing the apical and peripheral pulses for changes in rate and rhythm. A vasovagal reaction, consisting of bradycardia, hypotension, and nausea, can be precipitated by a distended bladder or by discomfort during removal of the arterial catheter, especially if a femoral site has been used. Prompt intervention is critical; this includes raising the feet and legs above the head, administering IV fluids, and administering IV atropine.
- Bed rest must be maintained for 2 to 6 hours after the procedure. If manual or mechanical pressure is used without vascular closure devices, the patient must remain on bed rest for up to 6 hours with the affected leg straight and the head elevated to 30 degrees. For comfort, the patient may be turned from side to side with the affected extremity straight. If the cardiologist used deployed closure devices or patches, the nurse checks local nursing care standards and anticipates that the patient will have fewer activity restrictions, such as elevation of the head of the bed, and that the patient will be allowed to ambulate in 2 hours or less. Analgesic medication is administered as prescribed for discomfort.
- The patient is instructed to report chest pain and bleeding or sudden discomfort from the catheter insertion sites immediately.
- The patient is monitored for contrast agent–induced renal failure that may be suspected if there is an increase in the BUN and creatinine levels. An accurate record of intake and output must be maintained, and both oral and IV fluids are encouraged to increase urinary output and flush the agent from the urinary tract.
- Safety is ensured by instructing the patient to ask for help when getting out of bed the first time after the procedure, because orthostatic hypotension may occur and the patient may feel dizzy and lightheaded.

For patients being discharged from the hospital on the same day as the procedure, additional instructions are provided (Chart 26-4).

### CHART 26-4

### Patient Education

### Self-Management After Cardiac Catheterization

After discharge from the hospital for cardiac catheterization, guidelines for self-care include the following:

- For the next 24 hours, do not bend at the waist (to lift anything), strain, or lift heavy objects.
- Avoid tub baths, but shower as desired.
- Talk with your physician about when you may return to work, drive, or resume strenuous activities.
- Call your physician if any of the following occur: bleeding, swelling, new bruising or pain from your procedure puncture site, temperature of 101.5°F (38.6°C) or more.
- If test results show that you have coronary artery disease, talk with your physician about options for treatment, including cardiac rehabilitation programs in your community.
- Talk with your physician and nurse about lifestyle changes to reduce your risk for further or future heart problems, such as quitting smoking, lowering your cholesterol level, initiating dietary changes, beginning an exercise program, or losing weight.

## Electrophysiologic Testing

The electrophysiology study (EPS) is an invasive procedure that plays a major role in the diagnosis and management of serious dysrhythmias. EPS is indicated for patients with syncope, palpitations, or both, and for survivors of cardiac arrest from ventricular fibrillation (sudden cardiac death). EPS is used to:

- Distinguish atrial from ventricular tachycardias when the determination cannot be made from the 12-lead ECG
- Evaluate how readily a life-threatening dysrhythmia (eg, ventricular tachycardia, ventricular fibrillation) can be induced
- Evaluate AV node function
- Evaluate the effectiveness of antiarrhythmic medications in suppressing the dysrhythmia
- Determine the need for other therapeutic interventions, such as a pacemaker, implantable cardioverter–defibrillator, or radiofrequency ablation (discussed in Chapter 27)

The initial study can take up to 4 hours. The patient receives moderate sedation. Catheters with recording and electrical stimulating (pacing) capabilities are inserted into the heart through the femoral and right subclavian veins to record electrical activity in the right and left atrium, bundle of His, and right ventricle. Fluoroscopy guides the positioning of these catheters. Baseline intracardiac recordings are obtained; programmed electrical stimulations of the atrium or ventricle are then administered in an attempt to induce the patient's dysrhythmia. If the dysrhythmia is induced, various antiarrhythmic medications are administered IV. The study is repeated after each medication to evaluate which medication or combination of medications is most effective in controlling the dysrhythmia.

After the study, the patient receives an equivalent oral antiarrhythmic agent; subsequent studies may be necessary to evaluate the effectiveness of that medication. Results of the study may indicate the need for other therapeutic interventions, such as a pacemaker or implantable cardioverter–defibrillator.

During EPS, lethal dysrhythmias may be induced; therefore, the procedure must be performed in a controlled environment with resuscitation equipment (eg, defibrillator) readily available. Possible complications include bleeding and hematoma from the catheter insertion sites, pneumothorax (air in the pleural cavity that may collapse portions of the lung), deep vein thrombosis, stroke, and sudden death.

### Nursing Interventions

Patients receive nothing to eat or drink for 8 hours before the procedure. Antiarrhythmic medications are withheld for at least 24 hours before the initial study, and the patient's cardiac rate and rhythm are carefully monitored for dysrhythmias. Other medications may be taken with sips of water.

Thorough preparation before EPS helps minimize patient anxiety. The nurse ensures that the patient understands the reason for the study and is aware of the common sensations and experiences expected during and after the study. Often the EPS laboratory has relaxation strategies available for patients, such as headsets with music. Also, the patient needs to be aware that the nurses in the EPS laboratory will be monitoring carefully for signs of discomfort and will offer IV medications to reduce discomfort or anxiety. The patient is reminded to request these medications if necessary. Postprocedure interventions include careful monitoring for complications. The nurse takes vital signs, reviews tracings of continuous ECG monitoring, assesses the apical pulse, auscultates for pericardial friction rub (which indicates bleeding into the pericardial sac), and inspects the catheter insertion sites for bleeding or hematoma formation.

In addition, the nurse assists the patient to maintain bed rest with the affected extremity kept straight and the head of the bed elevated to 30 degrees for 4 to 6 hours. The frequency of assessments and the duration of bed rest may vary based on institutional policy and physician preference.

## Hemodynamic Monitoring

Critically ill patients require continuous assessment of their cardiovascular system to diagnose and manage their complex medical conditions. This is most commonly achieved by the use of direct pressure monitoring systems, often referred to as **hemodynamic monitoring**. CVP, pulmonary artery pressure, and intra-arterial BP monitoring are common forms of hemodynamic monitoring. Patients requiring hemodynamic monitoring are typically cared for in critical care units. Some progressive care units also admit stable patients with CVP or intra-arterial BP monitoring. Noninvasive hemodynamic monitoring is used in some facilities.

To perform invasive hemodynamic monitoring, specialized equipment is necessary, such as the following:

- A CVP, pulmonary artery, or arterial catheter, which is introduced into the appropriate blood vessel or heart chamber
- A flush system composed of IV solution (which may include heparin), tubing, stopcocks, and a flush device, which provides for continuous and manual flushing of the system
- A pressure bag placed around the flush solution that is maintained at 300 mm Hg of pressure; the pressurized flush system delivers 3 to 5 mL of solution per hour through the catheter to prevent clotting and backflow of blood into the pressure monitoring system
- A transducer to convert the pressure coming from the artery or heart chamber into an electrical signal
- An amplifier or monitor, which increases the size of the electrical signal for display on an oscilloscope

Only nurses who have demonstrated knowledge and skill in the use of hemodynamic monitoring should manage patients who require this highly sophisticated type of monitoring. To ensure accuracy of the measurements, an evidence-based approach is necessary. The most important nursing responsibilities when caring for a patient who is undergoing hemodynamic monitoring are the following:

- The nurse makes sure that the system is set up and maintained properly. For example, the connecting tubing used for the monitoring system, called pressure tubing, is specifically manufactured for this purpose. The pressure tubing typically used for adults has a large diameter (7 French) and is no more than 3 to 4 feet long. The pressure monitoring system must be kept patent and free of air bubbles.

- Before the pressure monitoring system is used, the nurse checks to make sure that the stopcock of the transducer is positioned at the level of the right atrium; this is referred to as the phlebostatic level. Figure 26-10 shows how to locate this landmark. The nurse uses a marker to identify this level on the chest wall, which provides a stable reference point for subsequent pressure readings.
- To ensure that the pressure system is properly functioning at atmospheric pressure, the nurse establishes the zero reference point. This process is accomplished by placing the stopcock of the transducer at the phlebostatic level, opening the transducer to air, and activating the zero function key on the bedside monitor. Measurements of CVP, BP, and pulmonary artery pressures can be made with the head of the patient's bed elevated up to 60 degrees, but the system must be repositioned to the phlebostatic level to ensure an accurate reading.

## Central Venous Pressure Monitoring

The CVP, the pressure in the vena cava or right atrium, is used to assess right ventricular function and venous blood return to the right side of the heart. The CVP can be continuously measured by connecting either a catheter positioned in the vena cava or the proximal port of a pulmonary artery catheter to a pressure monitoring system. The pulmonary artery catheter, described in greater detail later, is used for monitoring critically ill patients. Patients in general medical-surgical units who require CVP monitoring may have a single-lumen or multilumen catheter placed into the superior vena cava. Intermittent measurement of the CVP can then be obtained with the use of a water manometer.

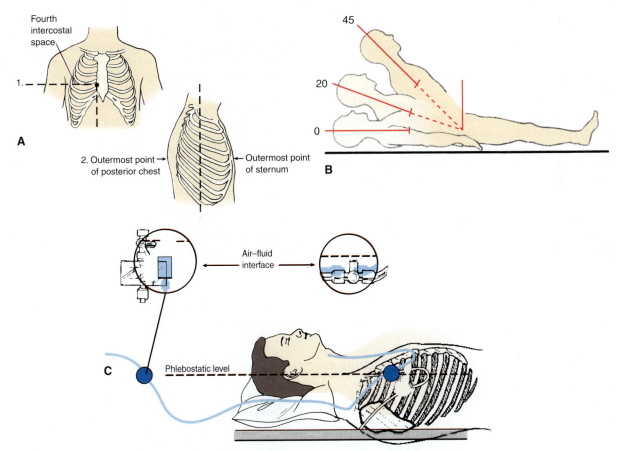

**FIGURE 26-10.** The phlebostatic axis and the phlebostatic level. (**A**) The phlebostatic axis is the crossing of two reference lines: (1) a line from the fourth intercostal space at the point where it joins the sternum, drawn out to the side of the body beneath the axilla; and (2) a line midway between the anterior and posterior surfaces of the chest. (**B**) The phlebostatic level is a horizontal line through the phlebostatic axis. The air–fluid interface of the stopcock of the transducer, or the zero mark on the manometer, must be level with this axis for accurate measurements. When moving from the flat to erect positions, the patient moves the chest and therefore the reference level; the phlebostatic level stays horizontal through the same reference point. (**C**) Two methods for referencing the pressure system to the phlebostatic axis. The system can be referenced by placing the air–fluid interface of either the in-line stopcock or the stopcock on top of the transducer at the phlebostatic level.

Because the pressures in the right atrium and right ventricle are equal at the end of diastole (0 to 8 mm Hg), the CVP is also an indirect method of determining right ventricular filling pressure (preload). This makes the CVP a useful hemodynamic parameter to observe when managing an unstable patient's fluid volume status. CVP monitoring is most valuable when pressures are monitored over time and are correlated with the patient's clinical status. An increasing pressure may be caused by hypervolemia or by a condition such as HF that results in a decrease in myocardial contractility. Pulmonary artery monitoring is preferred for the patient with HF. Decreased CVP indicates reduced right ventricular preload, most often caused by hypovolemia. This diagnosis can be substantiated when a rapid IV infusion causes the CVP to increase. (CVP monitoring is not clinically useful in a patient with HF in whom left ventricular failure precedes right ventricular failure, because in these patients an elevated CVP is a very late sign of HF.)

Before insertion of a CVP catheter, the site is prepared by shaving excessive hair, if necessary, and by cleansing with an antiseptic solution. A local anesthetic is used. The physician threads a single-lumen or multilumen catheter through the external jugular, antecubital, or femoral vein into the vena cava just above or within the right atrium.

### Nursing Interventions

Once the CVP catheter is inserted, it is secured and a dry, sterile dressing is applied. Catheter placement is confirmed by a chest x-ray, and the site is inspected daily for signs of infection. The dressing and pressure monitoring system are changed according to hospital policy. In general, the dressing is kept dry and air occlusive. Dressing changes are performed using sterile technique. CVP catheters can be used for infusing IV fluids, administering IV medications, and drawing blood specimens in addition to monitoring pressure.

To measure the CVP, the transducer must be placed at a standard reference point, called the phlebostatic axis (see Fig. 26-10). When the phlebostatic axis is used, then the CVP can be measured correctly with the patient supine at any backrest position up to 45 degrees. The range for a normal CVP is 0 to 8 mm Hg. The most common complications of CVP monitoring are infection, pneumothorax, and air embolism.

## Pulmonary Artery Pressure Monitoring

Pulmonary artery pressure monitoring is an important tool used in critical care for assessing left ventricular function (cardiac output), diagnosing the etiology of shock, and evaluating the patient's response to medical interventions (eg, fluid administration, vasoactive medications). Pulmonary artery pressure monitoring involves the use of a pulmonary artery catheter and pressure monitoring system. The pressure monitoring system acts as a fluid-filled conduit for detecting pressure changes within the chambers of the heart and the pulmonary arteries.

Pulmonary catheters are available in a variety of models. The type of catheter is selected based on its capabilities, which include cardiac pacing, oximetry, or cardiac output measurement (continuous or intermittent) or a combination of capabilities. Pulmonary artery catheters are balloon-tipped, flow-directed catheters that have distal and proximal lumens (Fig. 26-11). The distal lumen has a port that opens into the pulmonary artery. Once connected by its hub to the pressure monitoring system, it is used to measure continuous pulmonary artery pressures. The proximal lumen has a port that opens into the right atrium. It is used to administer IV medications and fluids or to monitor right atrial pressures (eg, CVP). Each catheter has a balloon inflation hub and valve. A syringe is connected to the hub, which is used to inflate or deflate the balloon with air (1.5-mL capacity). The valve opens and closes the balloon inflation lumen.

A pulmonary artery catheter with specialized capabilities has additional components. For example, the thermodilution

**FIGURE 26-11.** The pulmonary artery monitoring catheter used for obtaining pressure measurements and cardiac output. (**A**) The pressure monitoring system is connected to the distal lumen hub. (**B**) IV solutions are infused through the proximal infusion and injectate lumen hubs. (**C**) An air-filled syringe connected to the balloon inflation valve is used for balloon inflation during catheter insertion and pulmonary artery wedge pressure measurements. (**D**) To obtain cardiac output, the thermistor connector is inserted into the cardiac output component of the bedside cardiac monitor and 5 to 10 mL of normal saline is injected in 4 seconds into the proximal injectate port. (**E**) The thermistor located near the balloon is used to calculate the cardiac output. (Courtesy of Baxter Healthcare Corporation, Edwards Critical Care Division, Santa Ana, CA; used in Woods, S. L., Froelicher, E. S., & Motzer, S. A. [2004]. *Cardiac nursing* [5th ed.]. Philadelphia: Lippincott Williams & Wilkins.)

catheter has three additional features that enable it to measure cardiac output: a thermistor connector attached to the cardiac output computer of the bedside monitor, a proximal injectate port used for injecting fluids when obtaining the cardiac output, and a thermistor (positioned near the distal port) (see Fig. 26-11).

The pulmonary artery catheter, covered with a sterile sleeve, is inserted into a large vein (subclavian, jugular, or femoral) through a sheath. The sheath is equipped with a side port for infusing IV fluids and medications. The catheter is then passed into the vena cava and right atrium. In the right atrium, the balloon tip is inflated, and the catheter is carried rapidly by the flow of blood through the tricuspid valve into the right ventricle, through the pulmonic valve, and into a branch of the pulmonary artery. When the catheter reaches the pulmonary artery, the balloon is deflated and the catheter is secured with sutures (Fig. 26-12). Fluoroscopy may be used during insertion to visualize the progression of the catheter through the heart chambers to the pulmonary artery. This procedure can be performed in the operating room or cardiac catheterization laboratory or at the bedside in the critical care unit. During insertion of the pulmonary artery catheter, the bedside monitor is observed for waveform and ECG changes as the catheter progresses

**FIGURE 26-12.** Pulmonary artery (PA) catheter and pressure monitoring systems. (**A**) Bedside cardiac monitoring. (**B**) Right atria (RA) or central venous pressure monitoring system connected to proximal infusion lumen hub. (**C**) PA monitoring system connected to distal infusion lumen hub. Each system is attached to pressurized IV fluid, a transducer with stopcock and flush device, and pressure tubing. A cable attaches each transducer to the bedside monitor. (**D**) Magnified view of distal end of PA catheter with cross-section of catheter lumen.

through the right-sided heart chambers and into the pulmonary artery.

After the catheter is correctly positioned, the following pressures can be measured: right atrial, pulmonary artery systolic, pulmonary artery diastolic, mean pulmonary artery, and pulmonary artery wedge. Systemic vascular resistance and pulmonary vascular resistance are examples of additional measures that can be calculated.

Normal pulmonary artery pressure is 25/9 mm Hg, with a mean pressure of 15 mm Hg (see Fig. 26-4 for normal ranges). When the balloon tip is inflated, the catheter floats into the pulmonary artery until it becomes wedged. This is an occlusive maneuver that impedes blood flow through that segment of the pulmonary artery. A pressure measurement, called pulmonary artery wedge pressure, is taken within seconds after wedging of the pulmonary artery catheter; then the balloon is immediately deflated and blood flow is restored. The nurse who obtains the wedge reading ensures that the catheter has returned to its normal position in the pulmonary artery by evaluating the pulmonary artery pressure waveform. The pulmonary artery diastolic reading and the pulmonary artery wedge pressure reflect the pressure in the left ventricle at end-diastole. These measures are particularly important to monitor in critically ill patients because they are used to evaluate left ventricular filling pressures (preload). At end-diastole, when the mitral valve is open, the wedge pressure is the same as the pressure in the left atrium and the left ventricle unless the patient has mitral valve disease or pulmonary hypertension. Pulmonary artery wedge pressure is a mean pressure and is normally 4.5 to 13 mm Hg. Critically ill patients usually require higher left ventricular filling pressures to optimize cardiac output. These patients may need to have their wedge pressure maintained as high as 18 mm Hg.

### Nursing Interventions

Catheter site care is essentially the same as for a CVP catheter. As in measuring CVP, the transducer must be positioned at the phlebostatic axis to ensure accurate readings (see Fig. 26-10). Complications of pulmonary artery pressure monitoring include infection, pulmonary artery rupture, pulmonary thromboembolism, pulmonary infarction, catheter kinking, dysrhythmias, and air embolism.

## Intra-arterial Blood Pressure Monitoring

Intra-arterial BP monitoring is used to obtain direct and continuous BP measurements in critically ill patients who have severe hypertension or hypotension (Fig. 26-13). Arterial catheters are also useful when arterial blood gas measurements and blood samples need to be obtained frequently.

Once an arterial site is selected (radial, brachial, femoral, or dorsalis pedis), collateral circulation to the area must be confirmed before the catheter is inserted. This is a safety precaution to prevent compromised arterial perfusion to the area distal to the arterial catheter insertion site. If no collateral circulation existed and the cannulated artery became occluded, ischemia and infarction of the area distal to that artery could occur. Collateral circulation to the hand can be checked by the Allen test to evaluate the radial and ulnar arteries or by an ultrasonic Doppler test for any of the arteries. To perform the

**FIGURE 26-13.** Example of an arterial pressure monitoring system. The arterial catheter is inserted into the radial artery. A three-way stopcock is used for drawing arterial blood samples.

Allen test, the nurse compresses the radial and ulnar arteries simultaneously and asks the patient to make a fist, causing the hand to blanch. After the patient opens the fist, the nurse releases the pressure on the ulnar artery while maintaining pressure on the radial artery. The patient's hand will turn pink if the ulnar artery is patent.

### Nursing Interventions

Site preparation and care are the same as for CVP catheters. The catheter flush solution is the same as for pulmonary artery catheters. A transducer is attached, and pressures are measured in mm Hg. The nurse monitors the patient for complications, which include local obstruction with distal ischemia, external hemorrhage, massive ecchymosis, dissection, air embolism, blood loss, pain, arteriospasm, and infection.

## Critical Thinking Exercises

**1** *ebp* You are caring for a patient who has had an MI. He has stated that he knows he should quit smoking. As you plan for his hospital discharge, you consider the smoking cessation resources that can be made available to him. What is the evidence base regarding smoking cessation strategies in discharge planning? Discuss the strength of the evidence and the effectiveness of smoking cessation strategies and techniques.

**2** The president of a community organization you belong to has asked for your help in organizing a health fair for its members. You are informed that the fair will focus on cardiovascular health. It will take place on a Saturday morning and approximately 200 people will attend. What cardiac risk factors will you screen for? Where will you obtain educational materials needed for distribution at the health fair? What supplies and equipment will you need? How many volunteers will you need to run the health fair? What advice will you give to people who are found to be at risk for heart disease?

**3** To reduce the morbidity and mortality associated with acute MI, patients who experience symptoms of ACS must receive life-saving care as quickly as possible. Chest pain is a common symptom of ACS, but what are some of the other associated symptoms? If chest pain is the primary symptom, what key questions should you ask patients to help determine if the chest pain is cardiac in origin? What physical assessment parameters and tests are needed to reach a rapid and accurate diagnosis? During a home visit, if you suspect that your patient has ACS, what should you do?

## REFERENCES AND SELECTED READINGS

### BOOKS

American Heart Association. (2006). *Heart disease and stroke statistics—2006 update.* Accessed May 31, 2006. http://www.americanheart.org.

Bickley, L. S., & Szilagyi, P. G. (2005). *Bates' guide to physical examination* (9th ed.). Philadelphia: Lippincott Williams & Wilkins.

Chernecky, C. C., & Berger, B. J. (2004). *Laboratory tests and diagnostic procedures* (4th ed.). Philadelphia: W. B. Saunders.

Darovic, G. O. (2004). *Handbook of hemodynamic monitoring* (2nd ed.). Philadelphia: W. B. Saunders.

Kern, M. J. (2004). *The interventional cardiac catheterization handbook* (2nd ed.). St. Louis: C. V. Mosby.

Topol, E. J., Califf, R. M., Isner, J., et al. (2002). *The textbook of cardiovascular medicine* (2nd ed.). Philadelphia: Lippincott Williams & Wilkins.

Weber, J., & Kelley, J. (2003). *Health assessment in nursing* (2nd ed.). Philadelphia: Lippincott Williams & Wilkins.

Woods, S. L., Froelicher, E. S., Motzer, S. A., et al. (2004). *Cardiac nursing* (5th ed.). Philadelphia: Lippincott Williams & Wilkins.

### JOURNALS

*Asterisks indicate nursing research articles.

Anderson, J. E., Jorenby, D. E., Scott, W. J., et al. (2002). Treating tobacco use and dependence: An evidence-based clinical practice guideline for tobacco cessation. *Chest, 121*(3), 932–941.

Drew, B. J., Califf, R. M., Funk, M., et al. (2005). AHA scientific statement: Practice standards for electrocardiographic monitoring in hospital settings: An American Heart Association Scientific Statement from the Councils on Cardiovascular Nursing, Clinical Cardiology, and Cardiovascular Disease in the Young: Endorsed by the International Society of Computerized Electrocardiology and the American Association of Critical-Care Nurses. *Journal of Cardiovascular Nursing, 20*(2), 76–106.

Ferrone, M. (2004). Pharmacotherapeutic options to prevent radiocontrast-induced acute renal failure. *Formulary, 39*(11), 163–185.

Frantz, A. K. (2003). Current issues related to home monitoring. *AACN Clinical Issues, 14*(2), 232–239.

*Funk, M., Chrostowski, V. M., Richards, S., et al. (2005). Feasibility of using ambulatory electrocardiographic monitors following discharge after cardiac surgery. *Home Healthcare Nurse, 23*(7), 441–451.

Glassman, A., Shapiro, P. A., Ford, D. E., et al. (2003). Cardiovascular health and depression. *Journal of Psychiatric Practice, 9*(4), 409–421.

Gordon, C., & Rempher, K. J. (2003). Brain (B-type) natriuretic peptide. Implications for heart failure management. *AACN Clinical Issues, 14*(4), 532–542.

Grundy, S., Howard, B., Smith, S., et al. (2002). Prevention Conference VI: Diabetes and cardiovascular disease executive summary: Conference proceeding for healthcare professionals from a special writing group of the American Heart Association. *Circulation, 105*(18), 2231–2239.

Hirsch, J. A., Reddy, S. A., Capasso, W. E., et al. (2003). Non-invasive hemostatic closure devices: "Patches and pads." *Techniques in Vascular & Interventional Radiology, 6*(2), 92–95.

Hoffer, E. K., & Block, R. D. (2003). Percutaneous arterial closure devices. *Journal of Vascular Interventional Radiology, 14*(7), 865–885.

*Kim, C. K., Bartholomew, B. A., Mastin, S. M., et al. (2003). Detection and reproducibility of mental stress–induced myocardial ischemia with Tc-99m sestamibi SPECT in normal and coronary artery disease populations. *Journal of Nuclear Cardiology, 10*(1), 56–62.

Koenig, W. (2005). Predicting risk and treatment benefit in atherosclerosis: The role of C-reactive protein. *International Journal of Cardiology, 98*(2), 199–206.

Leon, A. S., Franklin, B. A., Costa, F., et al. (2005). Cardiac rehabilitation and secondary prevention of coronary heart disease: An American Heart Association scientific statement from the Council on Clinical Cardiology (Subcommittee on Exercise, Cardiac Rehabilitation, and Prevention) and the Council on Nutrition, Physical Activity, and Metabolism (Subcommittee on Physical Activity), in collaboration with the American Association of Cardiovascular and Pulmonary Rehabilitation. *Circulation, 111*(3), 369–376.

*McSweeney, J. C., Cody, M., O'Sullivan, P., et al. (2003). Women's early warning symptoms of acute myocardial infarction. *Circulation, 108*(21), 2619–2623.

Mosca, L., Appel, L. J., Benjamin, E. J., et al. (2004). Evidence-based guidelines for cardiovascular disease prevention in women. *Journal of the American College of Cardiology, 43*(5), 900–921.

Pearson, T. A., Blair, S. W., Daniel, S. R., et al. (2002). AHA guidelines for primary prevention of cardiovascular disease and stroke: 2002 update. Consensus panel guide to comprehensive risk reduction for adult patients without coronary or other atherosclerotic vascular diseases. *Circulation, 106*(3), 388–391.

Ryan, C. J., DeVon, H. A., & Zerwic, J. J. (2005). Typical and atypical symptoms: Diagnosing acute coronary syndromes accurately. *American Journal of Nursing, 105*(2), 34–36.

Smith, S. C., Allen, G., Blair, S. N., et al. (2006). AHA/ACC guidelines for secondary prevention for patients with coronary and other atherosclerotic vascular disease. *Journal of the American College of Cardiology, 47*(10), 2130–2139.

*Steinke, E. E., & Swan, J. H. (2004). Effectiveness of a videotape for sexual counseling after myocardial infarction. *Research in Nursing & Health, 27*(4), 69–80.

Tachakra, S., Wang, X. H., Istepanian, R. S., et al. (2003). Mobile e-health: The unwired evolution of telemedicine. *Telemedicine Journal & E-Health, 9*(3), 247–257.

Zerwic, J. J., & Ryan, C. J. (2004). Delays in seeking MI treatment. *American Journal of Nursing, 104*(1), 81–83.

### RESOURCES

American Heart Association, 7272 Greenville Avenue, Dallas, TX 75231; 1-800-242-8721; http://www.americanheart.org. Accessed May 30, 2006.

New York Cardiac Center, 467 Sylvan Avenue, Englewood Cliffs, NJ 07632, 201-569-8180; http://nycardiaccenter.org. Accessed May 30, 2006.

Nurse-Beat: Cardiac Nursing Electronic Journal; http://www.nurse-beat.com. Accessed May 30, 2006.

# CHAPTER 27

# Management of Patients With Dysrhythmias and Conduction Problems

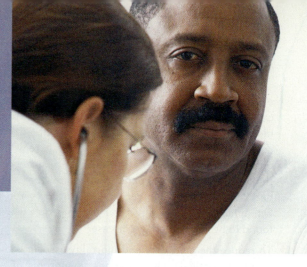

## Learning Objectives

*On completion of this chapter, the learner will be able to:*

1. Correlate the components of the normal electrocardiogram (ECG) with physiologic events of the heart.
2. Define the ECG as a waveform that represents the cardiac electrical event in relation to the lead depicted (placement of electrodes).
3. Analyze elements of an ECG rhythm strip: ventricular and atrial rate, ventricular and atrial rhythm, QRS complex and shape, QRS duration, P wave and shape, PR interval, and P:QRS ratio.
4. Identify the ECG criteria, causes, and management of several dysrhythmias, including conduction disturbances.
5. Use the nursing process as a framework for care of patients with dysrhythmias.
6. Compare the different types of pacemakers, their uses, possible complications, and nursing implications.
7. Use the nursing process as a framework for care of patients with implantable cardiac devices.
8. Describe the key points of using a defibrillator.
9. Describe the purpose of an implantable cardioverter defibrillator, the types available, and the nursing implications.
10. Describe invasive methods to diagnose and treat recurrent dysrhythmias and discuss the nursing implications.

Without a regular rate and rhythm, the heart may not perform efficiently as a pump to circulate oxygenated blood and other life-sustaining nutrients to all of the body's tissues and organs (including the heart itself). With an irregular or erratic rhythm, the heart is considered to be dysrhythmic (sometimes called arrhythmic). This has the potential to be a dangerous condition.

# Dysrhythmias

**Dysrhythmias** are disorders of the formation or conduction (or both) of the electrical impulse within the heart. These disorders can cause disturbances of the heart rate, the heart rhythm, or both. Dysrhythmias may initially be evidenced by the hemodynamic effect they cause (eg, a change in conduction may change the pumping action of the heart and cause decreased blood pressure). Dysrhythmias are diagnosed by analyzing the electrocardiographic (ECG) waveform. They are named according to the site of origin of the impulse and the mechanism of formation or conduction involved (Chart 27-1). For example, an impulse that originates in the sinoatrial (SA) node and that has a slow rate is called sinus bradycardia.

### CHART 27-1

## Identifying Dysrhythmias

**Sites of Origin**
- Sinus (SA) node
- Atria
- Atrioventricular (AV) node or junction
- Ventricles

**Mechanisms of Formation or Conduction**
- Normal (idio) rhythm
- Bradycardia
- Tachycardia
- Dysrhythmia
- Flutter
- Fibrillation
- Premature complexes
- Conduction Blocks

## Glossary

**ablation:** purposeful destruction of heart muscle cells, usually in an attempt to control a dysrhythmia

**antiarrhythmic:** a medication that suppresses or prevents a dysrhythmia

**automaticity:** ability of the cardiac cells to initiate an electrical impulse

**cardioversion:** electrical current administered in synchrony with the patient's own QRS complex to stop a dysrhythmia

**chronotropy:** rate of impulse formation

**conduction:** transmission of electrical impulses from one cell to another

**defibrillation:** electrical current administered to stop a dysrhythmia, not synchronized with the patient's QRS complex

**depolarization:** process by which cardiac muscle cells change from a more negatively charged to a more positively charged intracellular state

**dromotropy:** conduction velocity

**dysrhythmia (also referred to as arrhythmia):** disorder of the formation or conduction (or both) of the electrical impulse within the heart, altering the heart rate, heart rhythm, or both and potentially causing altered blood flow

**implantable cardioverter defibrillator (ICD):** a device implanted into the chest to treat dysrhythmias

**inhibited:** in reference to pacemakers, term used to describe the pacemaker withholding an impulse (not firing)

**inotropy:** force of myocardial contraction

**P wave:** the part of an electrocardiogram (ECG) that reflects conduction of an electrical impulse through the atrium; atrial depolarization

**paroxysmal:** a dysrhythmia that has a sudden onset and/or termination and is usually of short duration

**PP interval:** the duration between the beginning of one P wave and the beginning of the next P wave; used to calculate atrial rate and rhythm

**PR interval:** the part of an ECG that reflects conduction of an electrical impulse from the sinoatrial (SA) node through the atrioventricular (AV) node

**proarrhythmic:** an agent (eg, a medication) that causes or exacerbates a dysrhythmia

**QRS complex:** the part of an ECG that reflects conduction of an electrical impulse through the ventricles; ventricular depolarization

**QT interval:** the part of an ECG that reflects the time from ventricular depolarization through repolarization

**repolarization:** process by which cardiac muscle cells return to a more negatively charged intracellular condition, their resting state

**sinus rhythm:** electrical activity of the heart initiated by the sinoatrial (SA) node

**ST segment:** the part of an ECG that reflects the end of the QRS complex to the beginning of the T wave

**supraventricular tachycardia (SVT):** a rhythm that originates in the conduction system above the ventricles

**TP interval:** the part of an ECG that reflects the time between the end of the T wave and the beginning of the next P wave; used to identify the isoelectric line

**T wave:** the part of an ECG that reflects repolarization of the ventricles

**triggered:** in reference to pacemakers, term used to describe the release of an impulse in response to some stimulus

**U wave:** the part of an ECG that may reflect Purkinje fiber repolarization; usually it is not seen unless a patient's serum potassium level is low

**ventricular tachycardia (VT):** a rhythm that originates in the ventricles

## Normal Electrical Conduction

The electrical impulse that stimulates and paces the cardiac muscle normally originates in the sinus (SA) node, an area located near the superior vena cava in the right atrium. Usually, the electrical impulse occurs at a rate of 60 to 100 times a minute in the adult. The electrical impulse quickly travels from the sinus node through the atria to the atrioventricular (AV) node (Fig. 27-1). The electrical stimulation of the muscle cells of the atria causes them to contract. The structure of the AV node slows the electrical impulse, which allows time for the atria to contract and fill the ventricles with blood. This part of atrial contraction is frequently referred to as the "atrial kick" and accounts for nearly one third of the volume ejected during ventricular contraction. The electrical impulse then travels very quickly through the bundle of His to the right and left bundle branches and the Purkinje fibers, located in the ventricular muscle. The electrical stimulation of the muscle cells of the ventricles in turn causes the mechanical contraction of the ventricles (systole). The cells repolarize and the ventricles then relax (diastole). The electrical impulse causes the mechanical contraction of the heart muscle that follows.

The electrical stimulation is called **depolarization**, and the mechanical contraction is called systole. Electrical relaxation is called **repolarization**, and mechanical relaxation is called

**FIGURE 27-1.** Relationship of electrocardiogram (ECG) complex, lead system, and electrical impulse. The heart conducts electrical activity, which the ECG measures and shows. The configurations of electrical activity displayed on the ECG vary depending on the lead (or view) of the ECG and on the rhythm of the heart. Therefore, the configuration of a normal rhythm tracing from lead I will differ from the configuration of a normal rhythm tracing from lead II, lead II will differ from lead III, and so on. The same is true for abnormal rhythms and cardiac disorders. To make an accurate assessment of the heart's electrical activity or to identify where, when, and what abnormalities occur, the ECG needs to be evaluated from every lead, not just from lead II. Here the different areas of electrical activity are identified by color. RA, right arm; LA, left arm; SA, sinoatrial; AV, atrioventricular; LL, left arm.

diastole. The process from sinus node electrical impulse generation through ventricular repolarization completes the electromechanical circuit, and the cycle begins again. See Chapter 26 for a more complete explanation of cardiac function.

### Influences on Heart Rate and Contractility

The heart rate is influenced by the autonomic nervous system, which consists of sympathetic and parasympathetic fibers. Sympathetic nerve fibers (also referred to as adrenergic fibers) are attached to the heart and arteries as well as several other areas in the body. Stimulation of the sympathetic system increases heart rate (positive **chronotropy**), conduction through the AV node (positive **dromotropy**), and the force of myocardial contraction (positive **inotropy**). Sympathetic stimulation also constricts peripheral blood vessels, therefore increasing blood pressure. Parasympathetic nerve fibers are also attached to the heart and arteries. Parasympathetic stimulation reduces the heart rate (negative chronotropy), AV conduction (negative dromotropy), and the force of atrial myocardial contraction. The decreased sympathetic stimulation results in dilation of arteries, thereby lowering blood pressure.

Manipulation of the autonomic nervous system may increase or decrease the incidence of dysrhythmias. Increased sympathetic stimulation (eg, caused by exercise, anxiety, fever, or administration of catecholamines, such as dopamine [Intropin], aminophylline, or dobutamine [Dobutrex]) may increase the incidence of dysrhythmias. Decreased sympathetic stimulation (eg, with rest, anxiety-reduction methods such as therapeutic communication or meditation, or administration of beta-adrenergic blocking agents) may decrease the incidence of dysrhythmias.

## The Electrocardiogram

The electrical impulse that travels through the heart can be viewed by means of electrocardiography, the end product of which is an electrocardiogram (ECG). Each phase of the cardiac cycle is reflected by specific waveforms on the screen of a cardiac monitor or on a strip of ECG graph paper.

An ECG is obtained by slightly abrading the skin with a clean dry gauze pad and placing electrodes on the body at specific areas. Electrodes come in various shapes and sizes, but all have two components: (1) an adhesive substance that attaches to the skin to secure the electrode in place and (2) a substance that reduces the skin's electrical impedance and promotes detection of the electrical current.

The number and placement of the electrodes depend on the type of ECG needed. Most continuous monitors use two to five electrodes, usually placed on the limbs and the chest. These electrodes create an imaginary line, called a lead, that serves as a reference point from which the electrical activity is viewed. A lead is like an eye of a camera: it has a narrow peripheral field of vision, looking only at the electrical activity directly in front of it. Therefore, the ECG waveforms that appear on the paper or cardiac monitor represent the electrical current in relation to the lead (see Fig. 27-1). A change in the waveform can be caused by a change in the electrical current (where it originates or how it is conducted) or by a change in the lead.

### Obtaining an Electrocardiogram

Electrodes are attached to cable wires, which are connected to one of the following:

- An ECG machine placed at the patient's side for an immediate recording (standard 12-lead ECG)
- A cardiac monitor at the patient's bedside for continuous reading; this kind of monitoring, usually called hardwire monitoring, is associated with intensive care units
- A small box that the patient carries and that continuously transmits the ECG information by radiowaves to a central monitor located elsewhere (called telemetry)
- A small, lightweight tape recorder–like machine (called a Holter monitor) that the patient wears and that continuously records the ECG on a tape, which is later viewed and analyzed with a scanner

The placement of electrodes for continuous monitoring, telemetry, or Holter monitoring varies with the type of technology that is appropriate and available, the purpose of monitoring, and the standards of the institution. For a standard 12-lead ECG, 10 electrodes (6 on the chest and 4 on the limbs) are placed on the body (Fig. 27-2). To prevent interference from the electrical activity of skeletal muscle, the limb electrodes are usually placed on areas that are not bony and that do not have significant movement. These limb electrodes provide the first six leads: leads I, II, III, aVR, aVL, and aVF. The six chest electrodes are attached to the chest at very specific areas. The chest electrodes provide the V or precordial leads, $V_1$ through $V_6$. To locate the fourth intercostal space and the placement of $V_1$, the sternal angle and then the sternal notch, which is about 1 or 2 inches below the sternal angle, are located. When the fingers are moved to the patient's immediate right, the second rib can be palpated. The second intercostal space is the indentation felt just below the second rib.

Locating the specific intercostal space is critical for correct chest electrode placement. Errors in diagnosis can occur if electrodes are incorrectly placed. Sometimes, when the patient is in the hospital and needs to be monitored closely for ECG changes, the chest electrodes are left in place to ensure the same placement for follow-up ECGs.

A standard 12-lead ECG reflects the electrical activity primarily in the left ventricle. Placement of additional electrodes for other leads may be needed to obtain more complete information. For example, in patients with suspected right-sided heart damage, right-sided precordial leads are required to evaluate the right ventricle (see Fig. 27-2).

### Interpreting the Electrocardiogram

The ECG waveform represents the function of the heart's conduction system, which normally initiates and conducts the electrical activity, in relation to the lead. When analyzed accurately, the ECG offers important information about the electrical activity of the heart. ECG waveforms are printed on graph paper that is divided by light and dark vertical and horizontal lines at standard intervals (Fig. 27-3). Time and rate are measured on the horizontal axis of the graph, and amplitude or voltage is measured on the vertical axis. When an ECG waveform moves toward the top of the paper, it is called a positive deflection. When it moves toward the bottom of the paper, it is called a negative deflection. When

**FIGURE 27-2.** ECG electrode placement. The standard left precordial leads are V₁—4th intercostal space, right sternal border; V₂—4th intercostal space, left sternal border; V₃—diagonally between V₂ and V₄; V₄—5th intercostal space, left midclavicular line; V₅—same level as V₄, anterior axillary line; V₆ (not illustrated)—same level as V₄ and V₅, midaxillary line. The right precordial leads, placed across the right side of the chest, are the mirror opposite of the left leads. RA, right arm; LA, left arm; RL, right leg; LL, left leg. Adapted from Molle, E. A., Kronenberger, J., West-Stack, C., & Durham, L. S. (2005). *Lippincott Williams & Wilkins's pocket guide to medical assisting* (2nd ed.). Philadelphia: Lippincott Williams & Wilkins.

reviewing an ECG, each waveform should be examined and compared with the others.

## WAVES, COMPLEXES, AND INTERVALS

The ECG is composed of waveforms (including the P wave, the QRS complex, the T wave, and possibly a U wave) and of segments or intervals (including the PR interval, the ST segment, and the QT interval) (see Fig. 27-3).

The **P wave** represents the electrical impulse starting in the sinus node and spreading through the atria. Therefore, the P wave represents atrial depolarization. It is normally 2.5 mm or less in height and 0.11 seconds or less in duration.

The **QRS complex** represents ventricular depolarization. Not all QRS complexes have all three waveforms. The Q wave is the first negative deflection after the P wave. The Q wave is normally less than 0.04 seconds in duration and less than 25% of the R-wave amplitude. The R wave is the first positive deflection after the P wave, and the S wave is the first negative deflection after the R wave. When a wave is less than 5 mm in height, small letters (q, r, s) are used; when a wave is taller than 5 mm, capital letters (Q, R, S) are used. The QRS complex is normally less than 0.12 seconds in duration.

The **T wave** represents ventricular repolarization (when the cells regain a negative charge; also called the resting state). It follows the QRS complex and is usually the same direction as the QRS complex. Atrial repolarization also occurs but is not visible on the ECG because it occurs at the same time as the QRS.

The **U wave** is thought to represent repolarization of the Purkinje fibers, but it sometimes is seen in patients with hypokalemia (low potassium levels), hypertension, or heart disease. If present, the U wave follows the T wave and is usually smaller than the P wave. If tall, it may be mistaken for an extra P wave.

The **PR interval** is measured from the beginning of the P wave to the beginning of the QRS complex and represents the time needed for sinus node stimulation, atrial depolarization, and conduction through the AV node before ventricular depolarization. In adults, the PR interval normally ranges from 0.12 to 0.20 seconds in duration.

The **ST segment**, which represents early ventricular repolarization, lasts from the end of the QRS complex to the beginning of the T wave. The beginning of the ST segment is usually identified by a change in the thickness or angle of the terminal portion of the QRS complex. The end of the ST segment may be more difficult to identify because it merges into the T wave. The ST segment is normally isoelectric (see discussion of TP interval). It is analyzed to identify whether it is above or below the isoelectric line, which may be, among other signs and symptoms, a sign of cardiac ischemia (see Chapter 28).

The **QT interval**, which represents the total time for ventricular depolarization and repolarization, is measured from the beginning of the QRS complex to the end of the T wave. The QT interval varies with heart rate, gender, and age, and the measured interval needs to be corrected for these variables through specific calculations. Several ECG interpretation books contain charts of these calculations. The QT interval is usually 0.32 to 0.40 seconds in duration if the heart rate is 65 to 95 beats per minute. If the QT interval becomes prolonged, the patient may be at risk for a lethal ventricular dysrhythmia called torsades de pointes.

The **TP interval** is measured from the end of the T wave to the beginning of the next P wave, an isoelectric period (see Fig. 27-3). When no electrical activity is detected, the line on the graph remains flat; this is called the isoelectric line. The ST segment is compared with the TP interval to detect changes from the line on the graph during the isoelectric period.

**FIGURE 27-3.** ECG graph and commonly measured components. Each small box represents 0.04 seconds on the horizontal axis and 1 mm or 0.1 millivolt on the vertical axis. The PR interval is measured from the beginning of the P wave to the beginning of the QRS complex; the QRS complex is measured from the beginning of the Q wave to the end of the S wave; the QT interval is measured from the beginning of the Q wave to the end of the T wave; and the TP interval is measured from the end of the T wave to the beginning of the next P wave.

The **PP interval** is measured from the beginning of one P wave to the beginning of the next. The PP interval is used to determine atrial rhythm and atrial rate. The RR interval is measured from one QRS complex to the next QRS complex. The RR interval is used to determine ventricular rate and rhythm (Fig. 27-4).

### DETERMINING VENTRICULAR HEART RATE FROM THE ELECTROCARDIOGRAM

Heart rate can be obtained from the ECG strip by several methods. A 1-minute strip contains 300 large boxes and 1500 small boxes. Therefore, an easy and accurate method of determining heart rate with a regular rhythm is to count the number of small boxes within an RR interval and divide 1500 by that number. If, for example, there are 10 small boxes between two R waves, the heart rate is 1500/10, or 150; if there are 25 small boxes, the heart rate is 1500/25, or 60 (see Fig. 27-4A).

An alternative but less accurate method for estimating heart rate, which is usually used when the rhythm is irregular, is to count the number of RR intervals in 6 seconds and multiply that number by 10. The top of the ECG paper

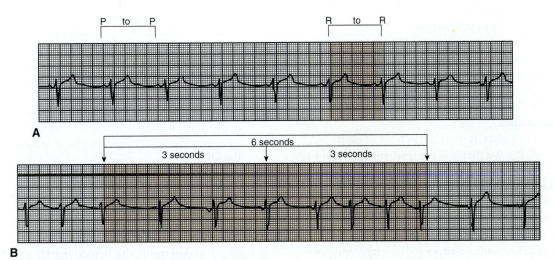

**FIGURE 27-4.** (**A**) Ventricular and atrial heart rate determination with a regular rhythm: 1500 divided by the number of small boxes between two P waves (atrial rate) or between two R waves (ventricular rate). In this example, there are 25 small boxes between both the R waves and the P waves, so the heart rate is 60 beats/minute. (**B**) Heart rate determination if the rhythm is irregular. There are approximately seven RR intervals in 6 seconds, so there are about 70 RR intervals in 60 seconds (7 × 10 = 70). The ventricular heart rate is 70 beats/minute.

is usually marked at 3-second intervals, which is 15 large boxes horizontally (see Fig. 27-4B). The RR intervals are counted, rather than QRS complexes, because a computed heart rate based on the latter might be inaccurately high.

The same methods may be used for determining atrial rate, using the PP interval instead of the RR interval.

### DETERMINING HEART RHYTHM FROM THE ELECTROCARDIOGRAM

The rhythm is often identified at the same time the rate is determined. The RR interval is used to determine ventricular rhythm and the PP interval to determine atrial rhythm. If the intervals are the same or less than 0.8 sec. difference throughout the strip, the rhythm is called regular. If the intervals are different, the rhythm is called irregular.

## Analyzing the Electrocardiogram Rhythm Strip

The ECG must be analyzed in a systematic manner to determine the patient's cardiac rhythm and to detect dysrhythmias and conduction disorders, as well as evidence of myocardial ischemia, injury, and infarction. Chart 27-2 is an example of a method that can be used to analyze the patient's rhythm.

Once the rhythm has been analyzed, the findings are compared with and matched to the ECG criteria for dysrhythmias to determine a diagnosis. It is important for the nurse to assess the patient to determine the physiologic effect of the dysrhythmia and to identify possible causes. Treatment of a dysrhythmia is based on clinical evaluation of the patient with identification of the dysrhythmia's etiology and effect, not on its presence alone.

### *Normal Sinus Rhythm*

Normal **sinus rhythm** occurs when the electrical impulse starts at a regular rate and rhythm in the sinus node and travels through the normal conduction pathway. Normal sinus rhythm has the following characteristics (Fig. 27-5):

*Ventricular and atrial rate:* 60 to 100 in the adult
*Ventricular and atrial rhythm:* Regular
*QRS shape and duration:* Usually normal, but may be regularly abnormal
*P wave:* Normal and consistent shape; always in front of the QRS
*PR interval:* Consistent interval between 0.12 and 0.20 seconds
*P:QRS ratio:* 1:1

### *Types of Dysrhythmias*

Dysrhythmias include sinus, atrial, junctional, and ventricular dysrhythmias and their various subcategories.

#### SINUS NODE DYSRHYTHMIAS

**Sinus Bradycardia.** Sinus bradycardia occurs when the sinus node creates an impulse at a slower-than-normal rate. Causes include lower metabolic needs (eg, sleep, athletic training, hypothyroidism), vagal stimulation (eg, from vomiting, suctioning, severe pain, extreme emotions), medications (eg, calcium channel blockers, amiodarone, beta-blockers), increased intracranial pressure (ICP), and myocardial infarction (MI), especially of the inferior wall. Other possible contributing factors in clinically significant bradycardia include what are referred to as the H's and the T's: hypovolemia, hypoxia, hydrogen ion (acidosis), hypo- or hyperkalemia, hypoglycemia, and hypothermia; toxins, tamponade (cardiac), tension pneumothorax, thrombosis (coronary or pulmonary), and trauma (hypovolemia, increased ICP) (American Heart Association [AHA], 2005). Sinus bradycardia has the following characteristics (Fig. 27-6):

*Ventricular and atrial rate:* Less than 60 in the adult
*Ventricular and atrial rhythm:* Regular
*QRS shape and duration:* Usually normal, but may be regularly abnormal
*P wave:* Normal and consistent shape; always in front of the QRS
*PR interval:* Consistent interval between 0.12 and 0.20 seconds
*P:QRS ratio:* 1:1

All characteristics of sinus bradycardia are the same as those of normal sinus rhythm, except for the rate. The patient is assessed to determine the hemodynamic effect and the possible cause of the dysrhythmia. If the decrease in heart rate results from stimulation of the vagus nerve, such as with bearing down during defecation or vomiting, attempts are made to prevent further vagal stimulation. If the bradycardia is from a medication such as a beta-blocker, the medication may be withheld. If the slow heart rate causes significant

---

### CHART 27-2

#### Interpreting Dysrhythmias: Systematic Analysis of the Electrocardiogram

When examining an ECG rhythm strip to learn more about a patient's dysrhythmia, the nurse conducts the following assessment:
1. Determine the ventricular rate.
2. Determine the ventricular rhythm.
3. Determine QRS duration.
4. Determine whether the QRS duration is consistent throughout the strip. If not, identify other duration.
5. Identify QRS shape; if not consistent, then identify other shapes.
6. Identify P waves; is there a P in front of every QRS?
7. Identify P-wave shape; identify whether it is consistent or not.
8. Determine the atrial rate.
9. Determine the atrial rhythm.
10. Determine each PR interval.
11. Determine if the PR intervals are consistent, irregular but with a pattern to the irregularity, or just irregular.
12. Determine how many P waves for each QRS (P:QRS ratio).

In many cases, the nurse may use a checklist and document the findings next to the appropriate ECG criterion.

**FIGURE 27-5.** Normal sinus rhythm in lead II.

**FIGURE 27-6.** Sinus bradycardia in lead II.

hemodynamic changes, resulting in shortness of breath, acute alteration of mental status, angina, hypotension, ST-segment changes, or premature ventricular complexes, treatment is directed toward increasing the heart rate.

Atropine, 0.5 mg given rapidly as an intravenous (IV) bolus every 3 to 5 minutes to a maximum total dose of 3 mg, is the medication of choice in treating symptomatic sinus bradycardia. It blocks vagal stimulation, thus allowing a normal rate to occur. Rarely, catecholamines and emergency transcutaneous pacing also are implemented.

**Sinus Tachycardia.** Sinus tachycardia occurs when the sinus node creates an impulse at a faster-than-normal rate. Causes may include the following:

- Physiologic or psychological stress (eg, acute blood loss, anemia, shock, hypervolemia, hypovolemia, heart failure, pain, hypermetabolic states, fever, exercise, anxiety)
- Medications that stimulate the sympathetic response (eg, catecholamines, aminophylline, atropine), stimulants (eg, caffeine, alcohol, nicotine), and illicit drugs (eg, amphetamines, cocaine, Ecstasy)
- Enhanced automaticity of the SA node and/or excessive sympathetic tone with reduced parasympathetic tone, a condition called inappropriate sinus tachycardia (Blomström-Lundqvist, Scheinman, Aliot, et al., 2003)
- Autonomic dysfunction, which results in a type of sinus tachycardia called postural orthostatic tachycardia syndrome (POTS). Patients with POTS have tachycardia without hypotension within 5 to 10 minutes of standing or with head-upright tilt testing.

Sinus tachycardia has the following characteristics (Fig. 27-7):

*Ventricular and atrial rate:* Greater than 100 in the adult, but usually less than 120
*Ventricular and atrial rhythm:* Regular
*QRS shape and duration:* Usually normal, but may be regularly abnormal

**FIGURE 27-7.** Sinus tachycardia in lead II.

*P wave:* Normal and consistent shape; always in front of the QRS, but may be buried in the preceding T wave
*PR interval:* Consistent interval between 0.12 and 0.20 seconds
*P:QRS ratio:* 1:1

All aspects of sinus tachycardia are the same as those of normal sinus rhythm, except for the rate. Sinus tachycardia does not start or end suddenly (nonparoxysmal). As the heart rate increases, the diastolic filling time decreases, possibly resulting in reduced cardiac output and subsequent symptoms of syncope and low blood pressure. If the rapid rate persists and the heart cannot compensate for the decreased ventricular filling, the patient may develop acute pulmonary edema.

Treatment of sinus tachycardia is usually determined by the severity of symptoms and directed at identifying and abolishing its cause. Beta-blockers and calcium channel blockers (Table 27-1), although rarely used, may be administered to

### TABLE 27-1  Summary of Antiarrhythmic Medications*

| Class | Action | Drugs: Generic (Trade) Names | Side Effects | Nursing Interventions |
|---|---|---|---|---|
| IA | Moderate depression of depolarization; prolongs repolarization | quinidine (Quinaglute, Quinidex, Cardioquin) | Decreased cardiac contractility Prolonged QRS, QT Proarrhythmic | Observe for HF Monitor BP with IV administration |
|  | Treats and prevents atrial and ventricular dysrhythmias | procainamide (Pronestyl) disopyramide (Norpace) | Hypotension with IV administration Lupus-like syndrome with Pronestyl Anticholinergic effects: dry mouth, decreased urine output | Monitor QRS duration for increase >50% from baseline Monitor for prolonged QT Monitor N-acetyl procainamide (NAPA) laboratory values during procainamide therapy |
| IB | Minimal depression of depolarization; shortened repolarization Treats ventricular dysrhythmias | lidocaine (Xylocaine) mexiletine (Mexitil) tocainide (Tonocard) | CNS changes (eg, confusion, lethargy) | Discuss with physician decreasing the dose in elderly patients and patients with cardiac/liver dysfunction |
| IC | Marked depression of depolarization; little effect on repolarization Treats atrial and ventricular dysrhythmias | flecainide (Tambocor) propafenone (Rythmol) | Proarrhythmic HF Bradycardia AV blocks | Discuss patient's left ventricular function with physician |
| II | Decreases automaticity and conduction Treats atrial and ventricular dysrhythmias | atenolol (Tenormin) bisoprolol/HCTZ (Ziac, Zebeta) esmolol (Brevibloc) labetalol (Trandate) metoprolol (Lopressor, Toprol) propranolol (Inderal, Innopran) sotalol (Betapace; Sorine; also has class III actions) | Bradycardia, AV block Decreased contractility Bronchospasm Hypotension with IV administration Masks hypoglycemia and thyrotoxicosis CNS disturbances | Monitor heart rate, PR interval, signs and symptoms of HF Monitor blood glucose level in patients with type 2 diabetes mellitus |
| III | Prolongs repolarization Treats and prevents ventricular and atrial dysrhythmias, especially in patients with ventricular dysfunction | amiodarone (Cordarone, Pacerone) dofetilide (Tikosyn) ibutilide (Corvert) | Pulmonary toxicity (amiodarone) Corneal microdeposits (amiodarone) Photosensitivity (amiodarone) Hypotension with IV administration Polymorphic ventricular dysrhythmias Nausea and vomiting See beta-blockers (sotalol) | Make sure patient is sent for baseline pulmonary function tests (amiodarone) Closely monitor patient |
| IV | Blocks calcium channel Treats atrial dysrhythmias | verapamil (Calan, Isoptin) diltiazem (Cardizem, Dilacor, Tiazac, Diltia, Cartia) bepridil (Vascor) | Bradycardia, AV blocks Hypotension with IV administration HF, peripheral edema | Monitor heart rate, PR interval Monitor blood pressure closely with IV administration Monitor for signs and symptoms of HF |

*Based on Vaughn-Williams classification.
AV, atrioventricular; BP, blood pressure; CNS, central nervous system; HF, heart failure; IV, intravenous.

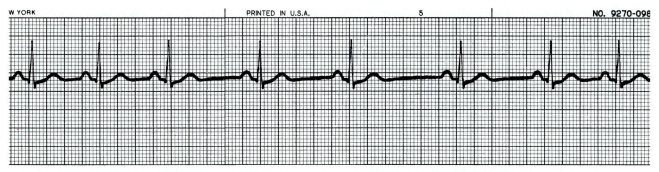

**FIGURE 27-8.** Sinus arrhythmia in lead II. Note irregular RR and PP intervals.

reduce the heart rate quickly. Catheter ablation (discussed later in this chapter) of the SA node may be used in cases of persistent inappropriate sinus tachycardia unresponsive to other treatments. Treatment for POTS may include increased fluid and sodium intake and use of compression stockings to prevent pooling of blood in the lower extremities.

**Sinus Arrhythmia.** Sinus arrhythmia occurs when the sinus node creates an impulse at an irregular rhythm; the rate usually increases with inspiration and decreases with expiration. Nonrespiratory causes include heart disease and valvular disease, but these are rare. Sinus arrhythmia has the following characteristics (Fig. 27-8):

*Ventricular and atrial rate:* 60 to 100 in the adult
*Ventricular and atrial rhythm:* Irregular
*QRS shape and duration:* Usually normal, but may be regularly abnormal
*P wave:* Normal and consistent shape; always in front of the QRS
*PR interval:* Consistent interval between 0.12 and 0.20 seconds
*P:QRS ratio:* 1:1

Sinus arrhythmia does not cause any significant hemodynamic effect and usually is not treated.

## ATRIAL DYSRHYTHMIAS

**Premature Atrial Complex.** A premature atrial complex (PAC) is a single ECG complex that occurs when an electrical impulse starts in the atrium before the next normal impulse of the sinus node. The PAC may be caused by caffeine, alcohol, nicotine, stretched atrial myocardium (eg, as in hypervolemia), anxiety, hypokalemia (low potassium level), hypermetabolic states (eg, with pregnancy), or atrial ischemia, injury, or infarction. PACs are often seen with sinus tachycardia. PACs have the following characteristics (Fig. 27-9):

*Ventricular and atrial rate:* Depends on the underlying rhythm (eg, sinus tachycardia)
*Ventricular and atrial rhythm:* Irregular due to early P waves, creating a PP interval that is shorter than the others. This is sometimes followed by a longer-than-normal PP interval, but one that is less than twice the normal PP interval. This type of interval is called a noncompensatory pause.
*QRS shape and duration:* The QRS that follows the early P wave is usually normal, but it may be abnormal (aberrantly conducted PAC). It may even be absent (blocked PAC).
*P wave:* An early and different P wave may be seen or may be hidden in the T wave; other P waves in the strip are consistent.
*PR interval:* The early P wave has a shorter-than-normal PR interval, but still between 0.12 and 0.20 seconds.
*P:QRS ratio:* usually 1:1

PACs are common in normal hearts. The patient may say, "My heart skipped a beat." A pulse deficit (a difference between the apical and radial pulse rate) may exist.

**FIGURE 27-9.** Premature atrial complexes (PACs) in lead II. Note that the pause following the PAC is longer than the normal PP interval but shorter than twice the normal PP interval.

If PACs are infrequent, no treatment is necessary. If they are frequent (more than six per minute), this may herald a worsening disease state or the onset of more serious dysrhythmias, such as atrial fibrillation. Treatment is directed toward the cause.

**Atrial Flutter.** Atrial flutter occurs in the atrium and creates impulses at a regular atrial rate between 250 and 400 times per minute. Because the atrial rate is faster than the AV node can conduct, not all atrial impulses are conducted into the ventricle, causing a therapeutic block at the AV node. This is an important feature of this dysrhythmia. If all atrial impulses were conducted to the ventricle, the ventricular rate would also be 250 to 400, which would result in ventricular fibrillation, a life-threatening dysrhythmia. Causes are similar to those of atrial fibrillation. Atrial flutter has the following characteristics (Fig. 27-10):

*Ventricular and atrial rate:* Atrial rate ranges between 250 and 400; ventricular rate usually ranges between 75 and 150.
*Ventricular and atrial rhythm:* The atrial rhythm is regular; the ventricular rhythm is usually regular but may be irregular because of a change in the AV conduction.
*QRS shape and duration:* Usually normal, but may be abnormal or may be absent
*P wave:* Saw-toothed shape; these waves are referred to as F waves
*PR interval:* Multiple F waves may make it difficult to determine the PR interval.
*P:QRS ratio:* 2:1, 3:1, or 4:1

Atrial flutter can cause serious signs and symptoms, such as chest pain, shortness of breath, and low blood pressure. If the patient is unstable, electrical cardioversion (discussed later) is usually indicated. In addition, rapid atrial pacing, also called overdrive atrial pacing, in which the atrium is paced at a faster rate than that in atrial flutter, may be considered as an alternative to cardioversion, especially in patients who have undergone cardiac surgery. If the patient is stable, the QRS is narrow, and the RR interval is regular, 6 mg adenosine (Adenocard, Adenoscan) may be rapidly administered IV, followed by a 20-mL saline flush and elevation of the arm to promote rapid circulation of the medication. If the rhythm does not convert to sinus rhythm within 1 to 2 minutes, a 12-mg bolus may be administered and repeated, if needed, within 1 to 2 minutes. If the adenosine fails to convert the rhythm or if the RR interval is irregular, then magnesium, diltiazem (Cardizem), or beta-blockers may be administered IV to slow the ventricular rate. These medications can slow conduction through the AV node. Amiodarone (Cardarone, Pacerone), propafenone (Rhythmol), flecainide (Tambocor), digoxin, clonidine (Catapres), or magnesium may be administered to patients with an acute onset of atrial flutter (see Table 27-1) (AHA, 2005).

If medication therapy is unsuccessful, electrical cardioversion is often successful. If the dysrhythmia has lasted for longer than 48 hours and a transesophageal echocardiogram has not confirmed the absence of atrial clots, then adequate anticoagulation may be indicated before cardioversion (electrical or chemical or ablation). Once conversion has occurred, flecainide, propafenone, amiodarone, or a beta-blocker may be given to prevent a recurrence (see Table 27-1) (AHA, 2005).

**Atrial Fibrillation.** Atrial fibrillation causes a rapid, disorganized, and uncoordinated twitching of atrial musculature. It has been linked to stroke, heart failure, dementia, and premature death and is considered a growing health problem in developed countries (Stewart, 2004). Atrial fibrillation may be transient, starting and stopping suddenly and occurring for a very short time (**paroxysmal**), or it may be persistent, requiring treatment to terminate the rhythm or to control the ventricular rate. Atrial fibrillation is usually associated with advanced age, valvular heart disease, coronary artery disease, hypertension, heart failure, diabetes, hyperthyroidism, pulmonary disease, acute moderate to heavy ingestion of alcohol ("holiday heart" syndrome), or the aftermath of open heart surgery (Stewart, 2004). Atrial fibrillation occurs in 11% to 64% of patients after coronary artery bypass, valvular replacements, and heart transplantation, and it increases the length and cost of the hospital stay and increases the risk for stroke (Kern, 2004). Its onset can also occur after hospital discharge without producing symptoms (Funk, Richards, Desjardins, et al., 2003). Sometimes atrial fibrillation occurs in people without any underlying pathophysiology (termed lone atrial fibrillation).

Atrial fibrillation has the following characteristics (Fig. 27-11):

*Ventricular and atrial rate:* Atrial rate is 300 to 600; ventricular rate is usually 120 to 200 in untreated atrial fibrillation.
*Ventricular and atrial rhythm:* Highly irregular
*QRS shape and duration:* Usually normal, but may be abnormal

**FIGURE 27-10.** Atrial flutter in lead II.

**FIGURE 27-11.** Atrial fibrillation in lead II.

*P wave:* No discernible P waves; irregular undulating waves are seen and are referred to as fibrillatory or f waves
*PR interval:* Cannot be measured
*P:QRS ratio:* Many:1

A rapid ventricular response reduces the time for ventricular filling, resulting in a smaller stroke volume. Because atrial fibrillation causes the atria and ventricles to contract at different times, the atrial kick (the last part of diastole and ventricular filling, which accounts for 25% to 30% of the cardiac output) is also lost. This leads to symptoms of irregular palpitations, fatigue, and malaise. There is usually a pulse deficit, a numeric difference between apical and radial pulse rates. The shorter time in diastole reduces the time available for coronary artery perfusion, thereby increasing the risk for myocardial ischemia. The erratic atrial contraction promotes the formation of a thrombus within the atria, increasing the risk for an embolic event. There is a two- to five-fold increase in the risk of stroke (brain attack).

Treatment of atrial fibrillation depends on its cause and duration and the patient's symptoms, age, and comorbidities. In many patients, atrial fibrillation converts to sinus rhythm within 24 hours and without treatment. Electrical cardioversion is indicated for atrial fibrillation that is hemodynamically unstable. Because of the high risk for embolization of atrial thrombi, cardioversion of atrial fibrillation that has lasted longer than 48 hours should be avoided unless the patient has received anticoagulants.

For atrial fibrillation of acute onset (usually defined as that with an onset within 48 hours), IV adenosine (Adenocard, Adenoscan) has been used to achieve cardioversion to sinus rhythm as well as to assist in the diagnosis. Other medications that may be administered to achieve cardioversion to sinus rhythm include amiodarone (Cardarone), flecainide (Tambocor), ibutilide (Corvert), digoxin, propafenone (Rythmol), clonidine (Catapres), or magnesium (AHA, 2005).

If the QRS is wide and the ventricular rhythm is irregular, atrial fibrillation with an accessory pathway should be suspected. An accessory pathway is congenital tissue between the atrial and ventricular myocardium. Electrical impulses conducted over these pathways bypass the slower-conducting AV node, causing early or pre-excited ventricular depolarization. Medications that block AV conduction (eg, adenosine [Adenocard], digoxin, diltiazem [Cardizem], and verapamil [Calan]) should be avoided.

If prevention of recurrence and maintenance of sinus rhythm are warranted to maintain quality of life, disopyramide, flecainide, propafenone, sotalol, or amiodarone may be prescribed (Kellen, 2004). Angiotensin-converting enzyme (ACE) inhibitors and angiotensin receptor blockers, which block the renin–angiotensin system, have also been found to be effective in preventing the recurrence of atrial fibrillation after cardioversion (Madrid, Bueno, Rebollo, et al., 2002; Ueng, Tsai, Yu, et al., 2003). Calcium channel blockers (diltiazem [Cardizem, Dilacor, Tiazac] and verapamil [Calan, Isoptin, Verelan]) and beta-blockers (see Table 27-1) are used to control the ventricular rate in atrial fibrillation (Kellen, 2004). However, verapamil should not be given to patients with impaired ventricular function. Digoxin may be used as a second-line agent to control the ventricular rate, especially in patients with poor cardiac function (ejection fraction less than 40%) (Snow, Weiss, LeFevre, et al., 2003).

Although control of the rhythm has been the initial treatment of choice, a recent study found that controlling the heart rate (resting heart rate less than 80) is equal to controlling the rhythm in terms of mortality (AFFIRM Investigators, 2002). The study also showed a trend toward increased hospitalization in the rhythm-control group compared to the rate-control group, but this difference was not significant. In a follow-up to the AFFIRM study, beta-blockers were found to be the most effective treatment in promoting adequate rate control (Olshansky, Rosenfeld, Warner, et al., 2004).

Warfarin is indicated if the patient with atrial fibrillation is at high risk for stroke (ie, older than 75 years of age or has hypertension, diabetes, heart failure, or history of stroke). If immediate anticoagulation is necessary, the patient may be placed on heparin until the warfarin level is therapeutic. Aspirin may be substituted for warfarin in patients with contraindications to warfarin and those who are at a lower risk for stroke (without the above stroke risk factors and younger than 75 years of age). Pacemaker implantation or surgery is sometimes indicated for patients who are unresponsive to medications. Several approaches are effective in preventing the occurrence of postoperative atrial fibrillation, including preoperative administration of a beta-blocker, immediate postoperative administration of IV amiodarone, and prophylactic atrial pacing (Kern, 2004).

## JUNCTIONAL DYSRHYTHMIAS

**Premature Junctional Complex.** A premature junctional complex is an impulse that starts in the AV nodal area before the next normal sinus impulse reaches the AV node. Premature junctional complexes are less common than PACs.

**FIGURE 27-12.** Junctional rhythm in lead II; note short PR intervals.

Causes of premature junctional complex include digitalis toxicity, heart failure, and coronary artery disease. The ECG criteria for premature junctional complex are the same as for PACs, except for the P wave and the PR interval. The P wave may be absent, may follow the QRS, or may occur before the QRS but with a PR interval of less than 0.12 seconds. Premature junctional complexes rarely produce significant symptoms. Treatment for frequent premature junctional complexes is the same as for frequent PACs.

**Junctional Rhythm.** Junctional or idionodal rhythm occurs when the AV node, instead of the sinus node, becomes the pacemaker of the heart. When the sinus node slows (eg, from increased vagal tone) or when the impulse cannot be conducted through the AV node (eg, because of complete heart block), the AV node automatically discharges an impulse. Junctional rhythm not caused by complete heart block has the following characteristics (Fig. 27-12):

*Ventricular and atrial rate:* Ventricular rate 40 to 60; atrial rate also 40 to 60 if P waves are discernible
*Ventricular and atrial rhythm:* Regular
*QRS shape and duration:* Usually normal, but may be abnormal
*P wave:* May be absent, after the QRS complex, or before the QRS; may be inverted, especially in lead II
*PR interval:* If the P wave is in front of the QRS, the PR interval is less than 0.12 seconds.
*P:QRS ratio:* 1:1 or 0:1

Junctional rhythm may produce signs and symptoms of reduced cardiac output. If this occurs, the treatment is the same as for sinus bradycardia. Emergency pacing may be needed.

**Nonparoxysmal Junctional Tachycardia.** Junctional tachycardia is caused by enhanced automaticity in the junctional area, resulting in a rhythm similar to junctional rhythm, except at a rate of 70 to 120. Although this rhythm generally does not have any detrimental hemodynamic effect, it may indicate a serious underlying condition, such as digitalis toxicity, myocardial ischemia, hypokalemia, or chronic obstructive pulmonary disease. Because junctional tachycardia is caused by increased automaticity, cardioversion is not an effective treatment; in fact, it causes an increase in the ventricular rate (AHA, 2005).

**Atrioventricular Nodal Reentry Tachycardia.** Atrioventricular nodal reentry tachycardia (AVNRT) occurs when an impulse is conducted to an area in the AV node that causes the impulse to be rerouted back into the same area over and over again at a very fast rate. Each time the impulse is conducted through this area, it is also conducted down into the ventricles, causing a fast ventricular rate. AVNRT that has an abrupt onset and an abrupt cessation with a QRS of normal duration has been termed paroxysmal atrial tachycardia (PAT). AVNRT also occurs when the duration of the QRS complex is 0.12 seconds or greater and a block in the bundle branch is known to be present. Factors associated with the development of AVNRT include caffeine, nicotine, hypoxemia, and stress. Underlying pathologies include coronary artery disease and cardiomyopathy; however, it occurs more often in females and not in association with underlying structural heart disease (Blomström-Lundqvist et al., 2003). AVNRT has the following characteristics (Fig. 27-13):

*Ventricular and atrial rate:* Atrial rate usually 150 to 250; ventricular rate usually 75 to 250

**FIGURE 27-13.** AV nodal reentry tachycardia in lead II.

*Ventricular and atrial rhythm:* Regular; sudden onset and termination of the tachycardia
*QRS shape and duration:* Usually normal, but may be abnormal
*P wave:* Usually very difficult to discern
*PR interval:* If the P wave is in front of the QRS, the PR interval is less than 0.12 seconds
*P:QRS ratio:* 1:1, 2:1

The clinical symptoms vary with the rate and duration of the tachycardia and the patient's underlying condition. The tachycardia usually is of short duration, resulting only in palpitations. A fast rate may also reduce cardiac output, resulting in significant signs and symptoms such as restlessness, chest pain, shortness of breath, pallor, hypotension, and loss of consciousness.

Treatment is aimed at breaking the reentry of the impulse. Vagal maneuvers, such as carotid sinus massage (Fig. 27-14), gag reflex, breath holding, and immersing the face in ice water, increase parasympathetic stimulation, causing slower conduction through the AV node and blocking the reentry of the rerouted impulse. Some patients have learned to use some of these methods to terminate the episode on their own. Because of the risk of a cerebral embolic event, carotid sinus massage is contraindicated in patients with carotid bruits. If the vagal maneuvers are ineffective, the patient may then receive a bolus of adenosine to correct the rhythm or diltiazem or a beta-blocker to control the rate. If the patient is unstable or does not respond to the medications, cardioversion is the treatment of choice. The unstable patient may be given adenosine while preparations for cardioversion are being made. For recurrent sustained AVNRT, the patient may be treated with verapamil, diltiazem, amiodarone, a beta-blocker, or digitalis to prevent a recurrence. Catheter ablation may be used to eliminate the area that permits the rerouting of the impulse that causes the tachycardia. If the rhythm is infrequent and there is no underlying cardiac structural disorder, the patient may be instructed to take a single oral dose of flecainide or a combination of diltiazem and propranolol during an episode of tachycardia.

If P waves cannot be identified, the rhythm may be called **supraventricular tachycardia (SVT)**, or paroxysmal supraventricular tachycardia (PSVT) if it had an abrupt onset, until the underlying rhythm and resulting diagnosis is determined. SVT and PSVT indicate only that the rhythm is not **ventricular tachycardia (VT)**. SVT could be atrial fibrillation, atrial flutter, or AVNRT, among others. Vagal maneuvers and adenosine are used to convert the rhythm or at least slow conduction in the AV node to allow visualization of the P waves. If the ECG does not assist in the differentiation of the dysrhythmia, invasive electrophysiology testing may be necessary to make the diagnosis.

### VENTRICULAR DYSRHYTHMIAS

**Premature Ventricular Complex.** A premature ventricular complex (PVC) is an impulse that starts in a ventricle and is conducted through the ventricles before the next normal sinus impulse. PVCs can occur in healthy people, especially with intake of caffeine, nicotine, or alcohol. They are also caused by cardiac ischemia or infarction, increased workload on the heart (eg, exercise, fever, hypervolemia, heart failure, tachycardia), digitalis toxicity, hypoxia, acidosis, or electrolyte imbalances, especially hypokalemia.

In the absence of disease, PVCs usually are not serious. In the patient with an acute MI, PVCs may indicate the need for more aggressive therapy. In the past, PVCs were considered to be indicative of an increased risk for ensuing VT. However, PVCs that (1) are more frequent than six per minute, (2) are multifocal or polymorphic (having different shapes and rhythms), (3) occur two in a row (pair), and (4) occur on the T wave (the vulnerable period of ventricular depolarization) have not been found to be precursors of VT in patients without structural heart disease (Cardiac Arrhythmia Suppression Trial Investigators, 1989). These PVCs are no longer considered as warning or complex PVCs.

In a rhythm called bigeminy, every other complex is a PVC. In trigeminy, every third complex is a PVC, and in quadrigeminy, every fourth complex is a PVC. PVCs have the following characteristics (Fig. 27-15):

*Ventricular and atrial rate:* Depends on the underlying rhythm (eg, sinus rhythm)
*Ventricular and atrial rhythm:* Irregular due to early QRS, creating one RR interval that is shorter than the others. PP interval may be regular, indicating that the PVC did not depolarize the sinus node.
*QRS shape and duration:* Duration is 0.12 seconds or longer; shape is bizarre and abnormal
*P wave:* Visibility of P wave depends on the timing of the PVC; may be absent (hidden in the QRS or T wave) or in front of the QRS. If the P wave follows the QRS, the shape of the P wave may be different.
*PR interval:* If the P wave is in front of the QRS, the PR interval is less than 0.12 seconds.
*P:QRS ratio:* 0:1; 1:1

The patient may feel nothing or may say that the heart "skipped a beat." The effect of a PVC depends on its timing in the cardiac cycle and how much blood was in the ventricles when they contracted. Initial treatment is aimed at correcting the cause. Long-term pharmacotherapy for only PVCs is not indicated.

**Ventricular Tachycardia.** VT is defined as three or more PVCs in a row, occurring at a rate exceeding 100 beats per minute. The causes are similar to those of PVC. VT is usually associated with coronary artery disease and may precede ventricular fibrillation. VT is an emergency because

**FIGURE 27-14.** Carotid sinus massage.

**FIGURE 27-15.** Multifocal premature ventricular complexes (PVCs) in quadrigeminy in lead V$_1$. Note regular PP interval (P wave within PVC).

the patient is usually (although not always) unresponsive and pulseless. VT has the following characteristics (Fig. 27-16):

*Ventricular and atrial rate:* Ventricular rate is 100 to 200 beats per minute; atrial rate depends on the underlying rhythm (eg, sinus rhythm)
*Ventricular and atrial rhythm:* Usually regular; atrial rhythm may also be regular
*QRS shape and duration:* Duration is 0.12 seconds or more; bizarre, abnormal shape
*P wave:* Very difficult to detect, so atrial rate and rhythm may be indeterminable
*PR interval:* Very irregular, if P waves are seen
*P:QRS ratio:* Difficult to determine, but if P waves are apparent, there are usually more QRS complexes than P waves

The patient's tolerance or lack of tolerance for this rapid rhythm depends on the ventricular rate and underlying disease. Several factors determine the initial treatment, including the following: identifying the rhythm as monomorphic (having a consistent QRS shape and rate) or polymorphic (having varying QRS shapes and rhythms); determining the existence of a prolonged QT interval before the initiation of VT; and ascertaining the patient's heart function (normal or decreased). If the patient is stable, continuing the assessment, especially obtaining a 12-lead ECG, may be the only action necessary. Amiodarone administered IV is the antidysrhythmic medication of choice for a stable patient with VT. Other medications that may be used are procainamide (Pronestyl) and sotalol (Betapace). Although lidocaine (Xylocaine) has been the medication most commonly used for immediate, short-term therapy, it has no proven short- or long-term efficacy in cardiac arrest (AHA, 2005). Cardioversion is the treatment of choice for mono-

phasic VT in a symptomatic patient. Atrial fibrillation should be suspected as the cause of a VT with an irregular rhythm, and it should be treated appropriately. Torsades de pointes is a polymorphic VT preceded by a prolonged QT interval. Because this rhythm is likely to cause the patient to deteriorate and become pulseless, immediate treatment is required: correction of any electrolyte imbalance, administration of isoproterenol (Isuprel) IV, or initiation of ventricular pacing. Magnesium has frequently been used to treat torsades, but its use has not been proven effective (AHA, 2005). Any type of VT in a patient who is unconscious and without a pulse is treated in the same manner as ventricular fibrillation: immediate **defibrillation** is the action of choice.

**Ventricular Fibrillation.** Ventricular fibrillation is a rapid, disorganized ventricular rhythm that causes ineffective quivering of the ventricles. No atrial activity is seen on the ECG. Causes of ventricular fibrillation are the same as for VT; it may also result from untreated or unsuccessfully treated VT. Other causes include electrical shock and Brugada syndrome, in which the patient (frequently of Asian descent) has a structurally normal heart, few or no risk factors for coronary artery disease, and a family history of sudden cardiac death. Ventricular fibrillation has the following characteristics (Fig. 27-17):

*Ventricular rate:* Greater than 300 per minute
*Ventricular rhythm:* Extremely irregular, without a specific pattern
*QRS shape and duration:* Irregular, undulating waves without recognizable QRS complexes

This dysrhythmia is always characterized by the absence of an audible heartbeat, a palpable pulse, and respirations. Because there is no coordinated cardiac activity, cardiac arrest and death are imminent if ventricular fibrillation is not

**FIGURE 27-16.** Ventricular tachycardia in lead V$_1$.

**FIGURE 27-17.** Ventricular fibrillation in lead II.

corrected. Treatment of choice is immediate bystander cardiopulmonary resuscitation (CPR), defibrillation as soon as possible, and activation of emergency services. If the arrest was not witnessed or there was more than a 4-minute delay in emergency services response, five cycles of CPR may be given prior to defibrillation (AHA, 2005). After the initial defibrillation, five cycles of CPR alternating with a rhythm check and defibrillation are the treatments used to convert ventricular fibrillation to an electrical rhythm that produces a pulse. Vasoactive medications (epinephrine, vasopressin, or both) should be administered as soon as possible after the second rhythm check (immediately before or after the second defibrillation). Antidysrhythmic medications (amiodarone, lidocaine, or possibly magnesium) should be administered as soon as possible after the third rhythm check (immediately before or after the third defibrillation). However, once the patient is intubated, CPR should be given continuously, not in cycles, and the rhythm check and medication administration occur every 2 minutes. In addition, underlying and contributing factors are identified and eliminated throughout the event (AHA, 2005).

Inducing hypothermia after a cardiac arrest from ventricular fibrillation was found to be beneficial to neurological outcomes in a select subset of patients. Therefore, current AHA guidelines now recommend inducing mild hypothermia for 12–24 hours in unconscious adults who experience cardiac arrest due to ventricular fibrillation. Hypothermia is defined as a core body temperature of 32°C–34°C (89.6°F–93.2°F). Further studies are needed to determine if hypothermia may be beneficial to other subsets of patients, as well as if the use of other methods of cooling may make this type of therapy more widely beneficial (American Heart Association, 2005).

A nurse caring for a patient with hypothermia (passive or induced) needs to monitor for its complications: pneumonia, sepsis, hyperglycemia, dysrhythmias, and coagulopathy, especially if the temperature drops below the intended goal.

**Idioventricular Rhythm.** Idioventricular rhythm, also called ventricular escape rhythm, occurs when the impulse starts in the conduction system below the AV node. When the sinus node fails to create an impulse (eg, from increased vagal tone) or when the impulse is created but cannot be conducted through the AV node (eg, due to complete AV block), the Purkinje fibers automatically discharge an impulse. When idioventricular rhythm is not caused by AV block, it has the following characteristics (Fig. 27-18):

*Ventricular rate:* 20 and 40; if the rate exceeds 40, the rhythm is known as accelerated idioventricular rhythm (AIVR)
*Ventricular rhythm:* Regular
*QRS shape and duration:* Bizarre, abnormal shape; duration is 0.12 seconds or more

Idioventricular rhythm commonly causes the patient to lose consciousness and experience other signs and symptoms of reduced cardiac output. In such cases, the treatment is the same as for asystole and pulseless electrical activity (PEA) if the patient is in cardiac arrest or for bradycardia if the patient is not in cardiac arrest. Interventions include identifying the underlying cause, administering IV atropine and vasopressor medications, and initiating emergency transcutaneous pacing. In some cases, idioventricular rhythm may cause no symptoms of reduced cardiac output. However, bed rest is prescribed so as not to increase the cardiac workload.

**Ventricular Asystole.** Commonly called flatline, ventricular asystole (Fig. 27-19) is characterized by absent QRS complexes confirmed in two different leads, although P waves may be apparent for a short duration. There is no heartbeat,

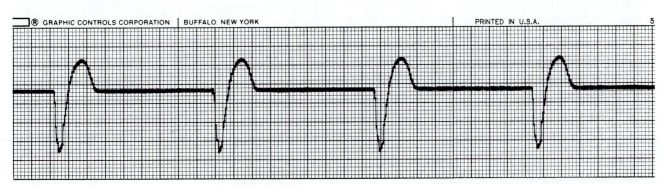

**FIGURE 27-18.** Idioventricular rhythm in lead V₁.

**FIGURE 27-19.** Asystole. Always check two different leads to confirm rhythm.

no palpable pulse, and no respiration. Without immediate treatment, ventricular asystole is fatal. Ventricular asystole is treated the same as PEA, focusing on high-quality CPR with minimal interruptions and identifying underlying and contributing factors. The guidelines for advanced cardiac life support (AHA, 2005) state that the key to successful treatment is rapid assessment to identify a possible cause, which may be hypoxia, acidosis, severe electrolyte imbalance, drug overdose, hypovolemia, cardiac tamponade, tension pneumothorax, coronary or pulmonary thrombosis, trauma, or hypothermia. After the initiation of CPR, intubation and establishment of IV access are the next recommended actions, with no or minimal interruptions in chest compressions. After 2 minutes or five cycles of CPR, a bolus of IV epinephrine is administered and repeated at 3- to 5-minute intervals. One dose of vasopressin may be administered for the first or second dose of epinephrine. A 1-mg bolus of IV atropine may also be administered as soon as possible after the rhythm check (AHA, 2005). Because of the poor prognosis associated with asystole, if the patient does not respond to these actions and others aimed at correcting underlying causes, resuscitation efforts are usually ended ("the code is called") unless special circumstances (eg, hypothermia, transportation to a hospital is required) exist.

## CONDUCTION ABNORMALITIES

When assessing the rhythm strip, the underlying rhythm is first identified (eg, sinus rhythm, sinus arrhythmia). Then the PR interval is assessed for the possibility of an AV block. AV blocks occur when the conduction of the impulse through the AV nodal area is decreased or stopped. These blocks can be caused by medications (eg, digitalis, calcium channel blockers, beta-blockers), myocardial ischemia and infarction, valvular disorders, or myocarditis. If the AV block is caused by increased vagal tone (eg, suctioning, pressure above the eyes or on large vessels, anal stimulation), it is commonly accompanied by sinus bradycardia.

The clinical signs and symptoms of a heart block vary with the resulting ventricular rate and the severity of any underlying disease processes. Whereas first-degree AV block rarely causes any hemodynamic effect, the other blocks may result in decreased heart rate, causing a decrease in perfusion to vital organs, such as the brain, heart, kidneys, lungs, and skin. A patient with third-degree AV block caused by digitalis toxicity may be stable; another patient with the same rhythm caused by acute MI may be unstable. Health care providers must always keep in mind the need to treat the patient, not the rhythm. The treatment is based on the hemodynamic effect of the rhythm.

**First-Degree Atrioventricular Block.** First-degree AV block occurs when all the atrial impulses are conducted through the AV node into the ventricles at a rate slower than normal. This conduction disorder has the following characteristics (Fig. 27-20):

*Ventricular and atrial rate:* Depends on the underlying rhythm
*Ventricular and atrial rhythm:* Depends on the underlying rhythm
*QRS shape and duration:* Usually normal, but may be abnormal
*P wave:* In front of the QRS complex; shows sinus rhythm, regular shape

**FIGURE 27-20.** Sinus rhythm with first-degree AV block in lead II. Note that PR is constant but greater than 0.20 seconds.

**FIGURE 27-21.** Sinus rhythm with second-degree AV block, type I in lead II. Note progressively longer PR durations until there is a nonconducted P wave, indicated by the asterisk.

*PR interval:* Greater than 0.20 seconds; PR interval measurement is constant
*P:QRS ratio:* 1:1

**Second-Degree Atrioventricular Block, Type I.** Second-degree AV block, type I, occurs when there is a repeating pattern in which all but one of a series of atrial impulses are conducted through the AV node into the ventricles (eg, every four of five atrial impulses are conducted). Each atrial impulse takes a longer time for conduction than the one before, until one impulse is fully blocked. Because the AV node is not depolarized by the blocked atrial impulse, the AV node has time to fully repolarize, so that the next atrial impulse can be conducted within the shortest amount of time. Second-degree AV block, type I, has the following characteristics (Fig. 27-21):

*Ventricular and atrial rate:* Depends on the underlying rhythm
*Ventricular and atrial rhythm:* The PP interval is regular if the patient has an underlying normal sinus rhythm; the RR interval characteristically reflects a pattern of change. Starting from the RR that is the longest, the RR interval gradually shortens until there is another long RR interval.
*QRS shape and duration:* Usually normal but may be abnormal
*P wave:* In front of the QRS complex; shape depends on underlying rhythm
*PR interval:* PR interval becomes longer with each succeeding ECG complex until there is a P wave not followed by a QRS. The changes in the PR interval are repeated between each "dropped" QRS, creating a pattern in the irregular PR interval measurements.
*P:QRS ratio:* 3:2, 4:3, 5:4, and so forth

**Second-Degree Atrioventricular Block, Type II.** Second-degree AV block, type II, occurs when only some of the atrial impulses are conducted through the AV node into the ventricles. Second-degree AV block, type II, has the following characteristics (Fig. 27-22):

*Ventricular and atrial rate:* Depends on the underlying rhythm

**FIGURE 27-22.** Sinus rhythm with second-degree AV block, type II in lead $V_1$; note constant PR interval and presence of more P waves than QRS complexes.

*Ventricular and atrial rhythm:* The PP interval is regular if the patient has an underlying normal sinus rhythm. The RR interval is usually regular but may be irregular, depending on the P:QRS ratio.

*QRS shape and duration:* Usually abnormal but may be normal

*P wave:* In front of the QRS complex; shape depends on underlying rhythm

*PR interval:* PR interval is constant for those P waves just before QRS complexes.

*P:QRS ratio:* 2:1, 3:1, 4:1, 5:1, and so forth

**Third-Degree Atrioventricular Block.** Third-degree AV block occurs when no atrial impulse is conducted through the AV node into the ventricles. In third-degree AV block, two impulses stimulate the heart: one stimulates the ventricles (eg, junctional or ventricular escape rhythm), represented by the QRS complex, and one stimulates the atria (eg, sinus rhythm, atrial fibrillation), represented by the P wave. P waves may be seen, but the atrial electrical activity is not conducted down into the ventricles to cause the QRS complex, the ventricular electrical activity. This is called AV dissociation. Complete block (third-degree AV block) has the following characteristics (Fig. 27-23):

*Ventricular and atrial rate:* Depends on the escape and underlying atrial rhythm

*Ventricular and atrial rhythm:* The PP interval is regular and the RR interval is regular, but the PP interval is not equal to the RR interval.

*QRS shape and duration:* Depends on the escape rhythm; in junctional escape, QRS shape and duration are usually normal, and in ventricular escape, QRS shape and duration are usually abnormal

*P wave:* Depends on underlying rhythm

*PR interval:* Very irregular

*P:QRS ratio:* More P waves than QRS complexes

Based on the cause of the AV block and the stability of the patient, treatment is directed toward increasing the heart rate to maintain a normal cardiac output. If the patient is stable and has no symptoms, no treatment is indicated other than decreasing or eliminating the cause (eg, withholding the medication or treatment). If the patient is short of breath or has chest pain, lightheadedness, or low blood pressure, an IV bolus of atropine is the initial treatment of choice. If the patient does not respond to atropine or has had an acute MI, transcutaneous pacing may be started. If the patient has no pulse, treatment is the same as for ventricular asystole. A permanent pacemaker may be necessary if the block persists.

## Nursing Process

### The Patient With a Dysrhythmia

### Assessment

Major areas of assessment include possible causes of the dysrhythmia, contributing factors, and the dysrhythmia's effect on the heart's ability to pump an adequate blood volume. When cardiac output is reduced, the amount of oxygen reaching the tissues and vital organs is diminished. This diminished oxygenation produces the signs and symptoms associated with dysrhythmias. If these signs and symptoms are severe or if they occur frequently, the patient may experience significant distress and disruption of daily life.

A health history is obtained to identify any previous occurrences of decreased cardiac output, such as syncope (fainting), lightheadedness, dizziness, fatigue, chest discomfort, and palpitations. Coexisting conditions that could be a possible cause of the dysrhythmia (eg, heart disease, chronic obstructive pulmonary disease) may also be identified. All medications, prescribed and over-the-counter (including herbs and nutritional supplements), as well as the route of administration, are reviewed. Some medications (eg, digoxin) can cause dysrhythmias. Laboratory results are reviewed to assess levels of medications as well as factors that could contribute to the dysrhythmia (eg, anemia). A thorough psychosocial assessment is performed to identify the possible effects of the dysrhythmia, the patient's perception of the dysrhythmia, and whether anxiety is a significant contributing factor.

The nurse conducts a physical assessment to confirm the data obtained from the history and to observe for signs of diminished cardiac output during the dysrhythmic event, especially changes in level of consciousness. The nurse assesses the patient's skin,

**FIGURE 27-23.** Sinus rhythm with third-degree AV block and idioventricular rhythm in lead V$_1$; note irregular PR intervals.

which may be pale and cool. Signs of fluid retention, such as neck vein distention and crackles and wheezes auscultated in the lungs, may be detected. The rate and rhythm of apical and peripheral pulses are also assessed, and any pulse deficit is noted. The nurse auscultates for extra heart sounds (especially $S_3$ and $S_4$) and for heart murmurs, measures blood pressure, and determines pulse pressures. A declining pulse pressure indicates reduced cardiac output. Just one assessment may not disclose significant changes in cardiac output; therefore, the nurse compares multiple assessment findings over time, especially those that occur with and without the dysrhythmia.

## Diagnosis

### Nursing Diagnoses

Based on assessment data, major nursing diagnoses of the patient may include:

- Decreased cardiac output
- Anxiety related to fear of the unknown
- Deficient knowledge about the dysrhythmia and its treatment

### Collaborative Problems/ Potential Complications

Based on the assessment data, potential complications that may develop include the following:

- Cardiac arrest (see Chapter 30)
- Heart failure (see Chapter 30)
- Thromboembolic event, especially with atrial fibrillation (see Chapter 30)

## Planning and Goals

The major goals for the patient may include eliminating or decreasing the occurrence of the dysrhythmia (by decreasing contributory factors) to maintain cardiac output, minimizing anxiety, and acquiring knowledge about the dysrhythmia and its treatment.

## Nursing Interventions

### Monitoring and Managing the Dysrhythmia

The nurse regularly evaluates the patient's blood pressure, pulse rate and rhythm, rate and depth of respirations, and breath sounds to determine the dysrhythmia's hemodynamic effect. The nurse also asks the patient about episodes of lightheadedness, dizziness, or fainting as part of the ongoing assessment. If a patient with a dysrhythmia is hospitalized, the nurse may obtain a 12-lead ECG, continuously monitor the patient, and analyze rhythm strips to track the dysrhythmia.

Control of the occurrence or the effect of the dysrhythmia, or both, is often achieved by the use of **antiarrhythmic** medications. The nurse assesses and observes for the beneficial and adverse effects of each medication. The nurse also manages medication administration carefully so that a constant serum blood level of the medication is maintained. The nurse may also administer a 6-minute walk test, which is used to identify the patient's ventricular rate in response to exercise. The patient is asked to walk for 6 minutes, covering as much distance as possible. The nurse monitors the patient for symptoms. At the end, the nurse records the distance covered and the pre- and postexercise heart rate as well as the patient's response (Kellen, 2004).

In addition to medication, the nurse assesses for factors that contribute to the dysrhythmia (eg, caffeine, stress, nonadherence to the medication regimen) and assists the patient in developing a plan to make lifestyle changes that eliminate or reduce these factors.

### Minimizing Anxiety

When the patient experiences episodes of dysrhythmia, the nurse maintains a calm and reassuring attitude. This assists in reducing anxiety (reducing the sympathetic response) and fosters a trusting relationship with the patient. Successes are emphasized with the patient to promote a sense of self-management of the dysrhythmia. For example, if a patient is experiencing episodes of dysrhythmia and a medication is administered that begins to reduce the incidence of the dysrhythmia, the nurse communicates that information to the patient. In addition, the nurse can help the patient develop a system to identify possible causative, influencing, and alleviating factors (eg, keeping a diary). The nursing goal is to maximize the patient's control and to make the episode less threatening.

### Promoting Home and Community-Based Care

#### TEACHING PATIENTS SELF-CARE

When teaching patients about dysrhythmias, the nurse presents the information in terms that are understandable and in a manner that is not frightening or threatening. The nurse explains the importance of maintaining therapeutic serum levels of antiarrhythmic medications so that the patient understands why medications should be taken regularly each day. In addition, the relationship between a dysrhythmia and cardiac output is explained so that the patient understands the rationale for the medical regimen. If the patient has a potentially lethal dysrhythmia, it is also important to establish with the patient and family a plan of action to take in case of an emergency. The patient and family should also be taught about potential effects of the dysrhythmia and their signs and symptoms. For example, the patient with chronic atrial fibrillation should be taught about the possibility of an embolic event. This information allows the patient and family to feel more in control and better prepared for possible events.

#### CONTINUING CARE

A referral for home care usually is not necessary for the patient with a dysrhythmia unless the patient is hemodynamically unstable and has significant symptoms of decreased cardiac output. Home care is also warranted if the patient has significant comorbidities, socioeconomic issues, or limited self-management skills that could increase the risk for nonadherence to the therapeutic regimen.

### Evaluation

#### Expected Patient Outcomes

Expected patient outcomes may include:

1. Maintains cardiac output
   a. Demonstrates heart rate, blood pressure, respiratory rate, and level of consciousness within normal ranges
   b. Demonstrates no or decreased episodes of dysrhythmia
2. Experiences reduced anxiety
   a. Expresses a positive attitude about living with the dysrhythmia
   b. Expresses confidence in ability to take appropriate actions in an emergency
3. Expresses understanding of the dysrhythmia and its treatment
   a. Explains the dysrhythmia and its effects
   b. Describes the medication regimen and its rationale
   c. Explains the need to maintain a therapeutic serum level of the medication
   d. Describes a plan to eliminate or limit factors that contribute to the dysrhythmia
   e. States actions to take in the event of an emergency

## Adjunctive Modalities and Management

Dysrhythmia treatments depend on whether the disorder is acute or chronic as well as on the cause of the dysrhythmia and its actual or potential hemodynamic effects.

Acute dysrhythmias may be treated with medications or with external electrical therapy (emergency defibrillation, cardioversion, or pacing). Many antiarrhythmic medications are used to treat atrial and ventricular tachydysrhythmias (see Table 27-1). The choice of medication depends on the specific dysrhythmia and its duration, the presence of heart failure and other diseases, and the patient's response to previous treatment. The nurse is responsible for monitoring and documenting the patient's responses to the medication and for ensuring that the patient has the knowledge and ability to manage the medication regimen.

If medications alone are ineffective in eliminating or decreasing the dysrhythmia, certain adjunctive mechanical therapies are available. The most common are elective cardioversion and defibrillation for acute tachydysrhythmia, and implantable devices (pacemakers for bradycardias and internal cardiodefibrillators for chronic tachydysrhythmias). Surgical treatments, although less common, are also available. The nurse is responsible for assessing the patient's understanding of and response to mechanical therapy, as well as the patient's self-management abilities. The nurse explains that the purpose of the device is to help the patient lead an active and productive life as his or her overall health allows.

### Cardioversion and Defibrillation

Cardioversion and defibrillation are used to treat tachydysrhythmias by delivering an electrical current that depolarizes a critical mass of myocardial cells. When the cells repolarize, the sinus node is usually able to recapture its role as the heart's pacemaker. One major difference between cardioversion and defibrillation is the timing of the delivery of electrical current. In cardioversion, the delivery of the electrical current is synchronized with the patient's electrical events; in defibrillation, the delivery of the current is immediate and unsynchronized.

The electrical current may be delivered externally through the skin with the use of paddles or with conductor pads. Both paddles may be placed on the front of the chest (Fig. 27-24) (standard paddle placement), or one paddle may be placed on the front of the chest and the other connected to an adapter with a long handle and placed under the patient's back (anteroposterior placement) (Fig. 27-25).

**When using paddles, the appropriate conductant is applied between the paddles and the patient's skin. Any other type of conductant, such as ultrasound gel, should not be substituted.**

Instead of paddles, defibrillator multifunction conductor pads may be used (Fig. 27-26). The pads, which contain a conductive medium, are placed in the same position as the paddles. They are connected to the defibrillator and allow for hands-off defibrillation. This method reduces the risk of touching the patient during the procedure and increases electrical safety. Automatic external defibrillators (AEDs), which are now found in public areas such as airports and grocery stores, use this type of delivery for the electrical current.

**FIGURE 27-24.** Standard paddle placement for defibrillation.

**FIGURE 27-25.** Anteroposterior paddle placement for defibrillation.

Whether using pads or paddles, the nurse must observe two safety measures. First, good contact must be maintained between the pads or paddles and the patient's skin (with a conductive medium in between them) to prevent electrical current from leaking into the air (arcing) when the defibrillator is discharged. Second, no one is to be in contact with the patient or with anything that is touching the patient when the defibrillator is discharged, to minimize the chance that electrical current will be conducted to anyone other than the patient.

When assisting with external defibrillation or cardioversion, the nurse should remember these key points:

- Use multifunction conductor pads or paddles with a conducting medium between the paddles and the skin (the conducting medium is available as a sheet, gel, or paste). Do not use gels or pastes with poor electrical conductivity (eg, ultrasound gel) (AHA, 2005).
- Place paddles or pads so that they do not touch the patient's clothing or bed linen and are not near medication patches or direct oxygen flow.
- If cardioverting, ensure that the monitor leads are attached to the patient and that the defibrillator is in the synchronized mode ("in sync"). If defibrillating, ensure that the defibrillator is *not* in the synchronized mode (most machines default to the "not-sync" mode).
- If using paddles, exert 20 to 25 pounds of pressure to ensure good skin contact.
- If using a manual discharge device, do not charge the device until ready to shock; then keep thumbs and fingers off the discharge buttons until paddles or pads are on the chest and ready to deliver the electrical charge.
- Before pressing the discharge button, call "Clear!" three times: As "Clear" is called the first time, ensure that you are not touching the patient, bed, or equipment; as "Clear" is called the second time, ensure that no one is touching the bed, the patient, or equipment, including the endotracheal tube or adjuncts; and as "Clear" is called the third time, perform a final visual check to ensure that you and everyone else are clear of the patient and anything touching the patient.
- Record the delivered energy.
- After the defibrillation, immediately resume CPR, starting with chest compressions.
- After five cycles (about 2 minutes) of CPR, check the cardiac rhythm and deliver another shock if indicated. Administer a vasoactive or antidysrhythmic medication as soon as possible after the rhythm check.
- After the event is complete, inspect the skin under the pads or paddles for burns; if any are detected, consult with the physician or a wound care nurse about treatment.

## Electrical Cardioversion

Electrical **cardioversion** involves the delivery of a "timed" electrical current to terminate a tachydysrhythmia. In cardioversion, the defibrillator is set to synchronize with the ECG on a cardiac monitor so that the electrical impulse discharges during ventricular depolarization (QRS complex). The synchronization prevents the discharge from occurring during the vulnerable period of repolarization (T wave), which could result in VT or ventricular fibrillation. The ECG monitor connected to the external defibrillator usually displays a mark or line that indicates sensing of a QRS complex. Sometimes the lead and the electrodes must be changed for the monitor to recognize the patient's QRS complex. When the synchronizer is on, no electrical current is delivered if the defibrillator does not discern a QRS complex. Because there may be a short delay until recognition of the

**FIGURE 27-26.** Multifunction pads for defibrillation.

QRS, the discharge buttons of an external defibrillator must be held down until the shock has been delivered.

If the cardioversion is elective and the dysrhythmia has lasted longer than 48 hours, anticoagulation for a few weeks before cardioversion may be indicated. Digoxin is usually withheld for 48 hours before cardioversion to ensure the resumption of sinus rhythm with normal conduction. The patient is instructed not to eat or drink for at least 4 hours before the procedure. Gel-covered paddles or conductor pads are positioned front and back (anteroposteriorly) for cardioversion. Before cardioversion, the patient receives IV moderate sedation as well as an analgesic medication or anesthesia. Respiration is then supported with supplemental oxygen delivered by a bag-mask-valve device with suction equipment readily available. Although patients rarely require intubation, equipment is nearby if it is needed. The amount of voltage used varies from 50 to 360 joules, depending on the defibrillator's technology and the type of dysrhythmia. If ventricular fibrillation occurs after cardioversion, the defibrillator is used to defibrillate the patient (sync mode is *not* used).

Indications of a successful response are conversion to sinus rhythm, adequate peripheral pulses, and adequate blood pressure. Because of the sedation, airway patency must be maintained and the patient's state of consciousness assessed. Vital signs and oxygen saturation are monitored and recorded until the patient is stable and recovered from sedation and analgesic medications or anesthesia. ECG monitoring is required during and after cardioversion.

## Defibrillation

Defibrillation is used in emergency situations as the treatment of choice for ventricular fibrillation and pulseless VT, the most common cause of abrupt loss of cardiac function and sudden cardiac death. Defibrillation is not used on patients who are conscious or have a pulse. The sooner defibrillation is used, the better the survival rate: if it is used within 1 minute of the onset of VT or fibrillation, the survival rate is 90%; if it is delayed for 12 minutes, the survival rate is only 2% to 5%. A recent study demonstrated that early defibrillation performed by laypeople in a community setting can increase the survival rate (Hallstrom, Ornato, Weisfeldt, et al., 2004). If immediate CPR is provided and defibrillation is performed within 5 minutes, many adults in ventricular fibrillation may survive with intact neurologic function (AHA, 2005).

Defibrillation depolarizes a critical mass of myocardial cells all at once; when they repolarize, the sinus node usually recaptures its role as the pacemaker. The electrical voltage required to defibrillate the heart is usually greater than that required for cardioversion and may cause more myocardial damage. Defibrillators are classified as monophasic or biphasic. Monophasic defibrillators deliver current in only one direction and require increased energy loads. Newer biphasic defibrillators deliver the electrical charge to the positive paddle, which then reverses back to the originating paddle. This system allows for lower, possibly nonprogressive energy levels (eg, 150 joules with each defibrillation) with potentially less myocardial damage. Studies are being conducted to determine whether these defibrillators significantly improve outcomes (Adgey, Spence, & Walsh, 2005).

If defibrillation was unsuccessful, CPR is immediately initiated and other advanced life support treatments are begun.

Epinephrine or vasopressin is administered after defibrillation to make it easier to convert the dysrhythmia to a normal rhythm with the next defibrillation. These medications may also increase cerebral and coronary artery blood flow. Antiarrhythmic medications such as amiodarone (Cordarone, Pacerone), lidocaine (Xylocaine), or magnesium are administered if ventricular dysrhythmia persists (see Table 27-1). This treatment with continuous CPR, medication administration, and defibrillation continues until a stable rhythm resumes or until it is determined that the patient cannot be revived.

## Pacemaker Therapy

A pacemaker is an electronic device that provides electrical stimuli to the heart muscle. Pacemakers are usually used when a patient has a slower-than-normal impulse formation or a symptomatic AV or ventricular conduction disturbance. They may also be used to control some tachydysrhythmias that do not respond to medication. Biventricular (both ventricles) pacing may be used to treat advanced heart failure that does not respond to medication. Pacemaker technology also may be used in an implantable cardioverter defibrillator (eg, in patients with coronary artery disease and a reduced ejection fraction). (See Chapter 30 for further discussion of heart failure.)

Pacemakers can be permanent or temporary. Temporary pacemakers are used to support patients until they improve or receive a permanent pacemaker (eg, after acute MI or during open heart surgery).

### Pacemaker Design and Types

Pacemakers consist of two components: an electronic pulse generator and pacemaker electrodes, which are located on leads or wires. The generator contains the circuitry and batteries that determine the rate (measured in beats per minute) and the strength or output (measured in milliamperes [mA]) of the electrical stimulus delivered to the heart. The generator also can detect the heart's electrical activity to cause an appropriate response; this component of pacing is called sensitivity and is measured in millivolts (mV). Leads can be threaded through a major vein into the right ventricle (endocardial leads), or they can be lightly sutured onto the outside of the heart and brought through the chest wall during open heart surgery (epicardial wires). The epicardial wires are always temporary and are removed by a gentle tug a few days after surgery. The endocardial leads may be temporarily placed with catheters through a vein (usually the femoral, subclavian, or internal jugular vein [transvenous wires]), usually guided by fluoroscopy. The leads may also be part of a specialized pulmonary artery catheter (see Chapter 30). However, obtaining a pulmonary artery wedge pressure may cause the leads to move out of pacing position. The endocardial and epicardial wires are connected to a temporary generator, which is about the size of a small paperback book. The energy source for a temporary generator is a common household battery. This type of pacemaker therapy necessitates short-term hospitalization of the patient.

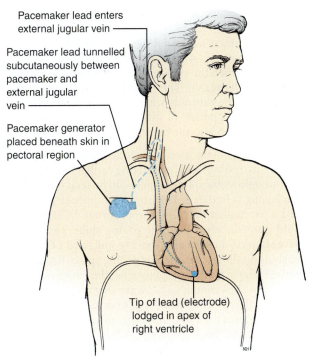

**FIGURE 27-27.** Implanted transvenous pacing lead (with electrode) and pacemaker generator.

Monitoring for pacemaker malfunctioning and battery failure is a nursing responsibility.

The endocardial leads also may be placed permanently, usually through the external jugular vein, and connected to a permanent generator. The generator, which often weighs less than 1 oz, is usually implanted in a subcutaneous pocket created in the pectoral region or below the clavicle (Fig. 27-27). Sometimes an abdominal site is selected. This procedure usually takes about 1 hour, and it is performed in a cardiac catheterization laboratory using a local anesthetic. Permanent pacemaker generators are insulated to protect against body moisture and warmth. While several different energy sources for permanent generators have been used and others have been investigated, lithium cell units are most often used today, and they last approximately 10 years. Some batteries are rechargeable. If the battery is not rechargeable and failure is impending, the leads are disconnected, the old generator is removed, and the new generator is reconnected to the existing leads and reimplanted in the already existing subcutaneous pocket. Battery replacement also is usually performed using a local anesthetic. Hospitalization is necessary for implantation or battery replacement; the patient usually can be discharged the next day.

If a patient suddenly develops a bradycardia, is symptomatic but has a pulse, and is unresponsive to atropine, emergency pacing may be started with transcutaneous pacing, which most defibrillators are now equipped to perform. Automatic external defibrillators (AEDs) are not able to do transcutaneous pacing. Large pacing ECG electrodes (sometimes the same conductive pads used for cardioversion and defibrillation) are placed on the patient's chest and back. The electrodes are connected to the defibrillator, which is the temporary pacemaker generator (Fig. 27-28). Because the impulse must travel through the patient's skin and tissue before reaching the heart, transcutaneous pacing can cause significant discomfort and is intended to be used only in emergencies. This type of pacing necessitates hospitalization. If the patient is alert, sedation and analgesia may be administered. Transcutaneous pacing is not indicated for pulseless bradycardia.

### Pacemaker Generator Functions

Because of the sophistication and wide use of pacemakers, a universal code has been adopted to provide a means of safe communication about their function. The coding is referred to as the NASPE-BPEG code because it is sanctioned by the North American Society of Pacing and Electrophysiology (now called the Heart Rhythm Society) and the British Pacing and Electrophysiology Group. The complete code consists of five letters and was revised in 2002 (Bernstein et al., 2002):

- The first letter of the code identifies the chamber or chambers being paced (ie, the chamber containing a pacing

**FIGURE 27-28.** Transcutaneous pacemaker with electrode pads connected to the anterior and posterior chest walls.

electrode). The letter characters for this code are A (atrium), V (ventricle), or D (dual, meaning both A and V).
- The second letter identifies the chamber or chambers being sensed by the pacemaker generator. Information from the electrode within the chamber is sent to the generator for interpretation and action by the generator. The letter characters are A (atrium), V (ventricle), D (dual), and O (indicating that the sensing function is turned off).
- The third letter of the code describes the type of response that will be made by the pacemaker to what is sensed. The letter characters used to describe this response are I (**inhibited**), T (**triggered**), D (dual, inhibited and triggered), and O (none). Inhibited response means that the response of the pacemaker is controlled by the activity of the patient's heart; that is, when the patient's heart beats the pacemaker will not function, but when the heart does not beat, the pacemaker will function. In contrast, triggered response means that the pacemaker will respond (pace the heart) when it senses intrinsic heart activity.
- The fourth and fifth letters are used only with permanent pacemakers. The fourth letter of the code is related to a permanent generator's ability to vary the heart rate. The possible letters are O, indicating no rate responsiveness, or R, indicating that the generator has rate modulation (ie, the pacemaker has the ability to automatically adjust the pacing rate from moment to moment based on parameters such as physical activity, acid–base changes, temperature, rate and depth of respirations, or oxygen saturation). A pacemaker with rate-responsive ability is capable of improving cardiac output during times of increased cardiac demand, such as exercise. Research has shown that this mode of pacing reduces the incidence of recurrent atrial fibrillation (Glotzer, Hellkamp, Zimmerman, et al., 2003).
- The fifth letter of the code indicates that the permanent generator has multisite pacing capability. The letters are A (atrium), V (ventricle), D (dual), and O (none).

Commonly, only the first three letters are used for a pacing code. An example of a NASPE-BPEG code is DVI:

**D:** Both the atrium and the ventricle have a pacing electrode in place.

**V:** The pacemaker is sensing the activity of the ventricle only.

**I:** The pacemaker's stimulating effect is inhibited by ventricular activity—in other words, it does not create an impulse when the pacemaker senses that the patient's ventricle is active. The pacemaker paces the atrium and then the ventricle when no ventricular activity is sensed for a period of time (the time is individually programmed into the pacemaker for each patient).

The type of generator and its selected settings depend on the patient's dysrhythmia, underlying cardiac function, and age. A straight vertical line usually can be seen on the ECG when pacing is initiated. The line that represents pacing is called a pacemaker spike. The appropriate ECG complex should immediately follow the pacing spike; therefore, a P wave should follow an atrial pacing spike and a QRS complex should follow a ventricular pacing spike. Because the impulse starts in a different place than the patient's normal rhythm, the QRS complex or P wave that responds to pacing looks different from the patient's normal ECG complex. *Capture* is a term used to denote that the appropriate complex followed the pacing spike.

Pacemakers are generally set to sense and respond to intrinsic activity, which is called on-demand pacing (Fig. 27-29). If the pacemaker is set to pace but not to sense, it is called a fixed or asynchronous pacemaker (Fig. 27-30); this is written in pacing code as AOO or VOO. The pacemaker paces at a constant rate, independent of the patient's intrinsic rhythm. Because AOO pacing stimulates only the atrium, it may be used in a patient who has undergone open heart surgery and develops sinus bradycardia. AOO pacing ensures synchrony between atrial stimulation and ventricular stimulation (and therefore contraction), as long as the patient has no conduction disturbances in the AV node. VOO is rare because of the risk that the pacemaker may deliver an impulse during the vulnerable repolarization phase, leading to VT.

VVI (V, paces the ventricle; V, senses ventricular activity; I, paces only if the ventricles do not depolarize) pacing causes loss of AV synchrony and atrial kick, which may cause a decrease in cardiac output and an increase in atrial

**FIGURE 27-29.** Pacing with appropriate sensing (on-demand pacing) in lead $V_1$. Arrows denote pacing spike. Asterisk (*) denotes intrinsic (patient's own) beats, therefore no pacing. F denotes a fusion beat, which is a combination of an intrinsic beat and a paced beat occurring at the same time.

**FIGURE 27-30.** Fixed pacing or total loss of sensing pacing in lead V$_1$; arrows denote pacing spikes.

distention and venous congestion. This can lead to pacemaker syndrome, causing symptoms such as chest discomfort, shortness of breath, fatigue, activity intolerance, and postural hypotension. In addition, atrial pacing and dual chamber pacing have been found to reduce the incidence of atrial fibrillation; however, this reduction has not yet been proven to decrease the incidence of stroke, heart failure, or mortality (Troyman, Kim, & Pinski, 2004).

Synchronized biventricular pacing, also called cardiac resynchronized therapy (CRT), has recently been found to modify the intraventricular, interventricular, and atrial-ventricular conduction defects identified with symptomatic moderate to severe (New York Heart Association Functional Class III and IV) left ventricular dysfunction and heart failure. The generator for biventricular pacing has three leads: one for the right atrium; one for the right ventricle, as with most standard pacemaker generators; and one for the left ventricle, usually placed in the left lateral wall. Recent studies have shown that this therapy improves cardiac function, resulting in decreased heart failure symptoms and an improved quality of life (Trupp, 2004). Biventricular pacing may be used with an implantable cardioverter defibrillator.

### Complications of Pacemaker Use

Complications associated with pacemakers relate to their presence within the body and improper functioning. The following complications may arise from a pacemaker:

- Local infection at the entry site of the leads for temporary pacing, or at the subcutaneous site for permanent generator placement
- Bleeding and hematoma at the lead entry sites for temporary pacing, or at the subcutaneous site for permanent generator placement
- Hemothorax from puncture of the subclavian vein or internal mammary artery
- Ventricular ectopy and tachycardia from irritation of the ventricular wall by the endocardial electrode
- Movement or dislocation of the lead placed transvenously (perforation of the myocardium)
- Phrenic nerve, diaphragmatic (hiccuping may be a sign), or skeletal muscle stimulation if the lead is dislocated or if the delivered energy (mA) is set high
- Rarely, cardiac tamponade from bleeding following removal of epicardial wires used for temporary pacing

In the initial hours after a temporary or permanent pacemaker is inserted, the most common complication is dislodgment of the pacing electrode. Minimizing patient activity can help prevent this complication. If a temporary electrode is in place, the extremity through which the catheter has been advanced is immobilized. With a permanent pacemaker, the patient is instructed initially to restrict activity on the side of the implantation.

The ECG is monitored very carefully to detect pacemaker malfunction. Improper pacemaker function, which can arise from failure in one or more components of the pacing system, is outlined in Table 27-2. The following data should be noted on the patient's record:

- Model of pacemaker
- Type of generator
- Date and time of insertion
- Location of pulse generator
- Stimulation threshold
- Pacer settings (eg, rate, energy output [mA], sensitivity [mV], and duration of interval between atrial and ventricular impulses [AV delay])

This information is important for identifying normal pacemaker function and diagnosing pacemaker malfunction.

A patient experiencing pacemaker malfunction may develop bradycardia as well as signs and symptoms of decreased cardiac output. The degree to which these symptoms become apparent depends on the severity of the malfunction, the patient's level of dependency on the pacemaker, and the patient's underlying condition. Pacemaker malfunction is diagnosed by analyzing the ECG. Manipulating the electrodes, changing the generator's settings, or replacing the pacemaker generator or leads (or both) may be necessary.

Inhibition of permanent pacemakers or reversion to asynchronous fixed rate pacing can occur with exposure to strong electromagnetic fields (electromagnetic interference [EMI]). The incidence of EMI is highest in dual-chambered pacemakers because of their programmed higher sensitivity to electrical stimuli (Yeo & Berg, 2004). However, recent pacemaker technology allows patients to safely use most household electronic appliances and devices (eg, microwave ovens, electric tools). Gas-powered engines should be turned off

### TABLE 27-2  Assessing Pacemaker Malfunction

| Problem | Possible Cause | Intervention |
|---|---|---|
| Loss of capture—complex does *not* follow pacing spike | Inadequate stimulus<br>Catheter malposition<br>Battery depletion<br>Electronic insulation break | Check security of all connections; increase milliamperage.<br>Reposition extremity; turn patient to left side.<br>Change battery.<br>Change generator. |
| Undersensing—pacing spike occurs at preset interval despite patient's intrinsic rhythm | Sensitivity too high<br>Electrical interference (eg, by a magnet)<br>Faulty generator | Decrease sensitivity.<br>Eliminate interference.<br>Replace generator. |
| Oversensing—loss of pacing artifact; pacing does *not* occur at preset interval despite lack of intrinsic rhythm | Sensitivity too low<br>Electrical interference<br>Battery depletion | Increase sensitivity.<br>Eliminate interference.<br>Change battery. |
| Loss of pacing—total absence of pacing spikes | Battery depletion<br>Loose or disconnected wires<br>Perforation | Change battery.<br>Check security of all connections.<br>Obtain 12-lead ECG and portable chest x-ray.<br>Assess for murmur. Contact physician. |
| Change in pacing QRS shape | Septal perforation | Obtain 12-lead ECG and portable chest x-ray.<br>Assess for murmur. Contact physician. |
| Rhythmic diaphragmatic or chest wall twitching or hiccuping | Output too high<br>Myocardial wall perforation | Decrease milliamperage.<br>Turn pacer off. Contact physician at once. Monitor closely for decreased cardiac output. |

before working on them. Objects that contain magnets (eg, the earpiece of a phone; large stereo speakers; magnet therapy products such as mattresses, jewelry, and wraps) should not be near the generator for longer than a few seconds. Patients are advised to keep digital cellular phones at least 6 to 12 inches away from (or on the side opposite of) the pacemaker generator and not to carry them in a shirt pocket. Large electromagnetic fields, such as those produced by magnetic resonance imaging, radio and TV transmitter towers and lines, transmission power lines (these are different from the distribution lines that bring electricity into a home), and electrical substations may cause EMI (electromagnetic interference). Patients should be cautioned to avoid such situations or to simply move farther away from the area if they experience dizziness or a feeling of rapid or irregular heartbeats (palpitations). Welding and the use of a chain saw should be avoided. If such tools are used, precautionary steps such as limiting the welding current to a 60- to 130-ampere range or using electric rather than gasoline-powered chain saws are advised.

In addition, the metal of the pacemaker generator may trigger store and library anti-theft devices as well as airport and building security alarms; however, these alarm systems generally do not interfere with the pacemaker function. Patients should walk through them quickly and avoid standing in or near these devices. The handheld screening devices used in airports may interfere with the pacemaker. Patients should be advised to ask security personnel to perform a hand search instead of using the handheld screening device. Patients also should be instructed to wear or carry medical identification to alert personnel to the presence of the pacemaker.

### Pacemaker Surveillance

Pacemaker clinics have been established to monitor patients and to test pulse generators for impending pacemaker battery failure. A computerized device is held over the generator to "interrogate" it with painless radio signals; it detects the generator's settings, battery status, pacing threshold, sensing function, lead integrity, and other stored information. Several factors, such as lead fracture, muscle inhibition, and insulation disruption, also may be assessed depending on the type of pacemaker and the equipment available. If indicated, the pacemaker is turned off for a few seconds, using a magnet or a programmer, while the ECG is recorded to assess the patient's underlying cardiac rhythm. Transtelephonic transmission of the generator's information is another follow-up method. Special equipment is used to transmit information about the patient's pacemaker over the telephone to a receiving system at a pacemaker clinic. The information is converted into tones; equipment at the clinic converts these tones to an electronic signal and records them on an ECG strip. The pacemaker rate and other data concerning pacemaker function are obtained and evaluated by a cardiologist. This simplifies the diagnosis of a failing generator, reassures the patient, and improves management when the patient is physically remote from pacemaker testing facilities. The frequency of the pacemaker checks varies with the patient's age and underlying condition, the degree of pacemaker dependency, the age and type of the device, and the results from previous pacemaker checks.

## Implantable Cardioverter Defibrillator

The **implantable cardioverter defibrillator (ICD)** is a device that detects and terminates life-threatening episodes of tachycardia or fibrillation, especially those that are ventricular in origin. Patients at high risk of VT or ventricular fibrillation are those who have survived sudden cardiac death syndrome, usually caused by ventricular fibrillation, or have experienced symptomatic VT (syncope secondary to VT). Other people at risk of sudden cardiac death include those with dilated cardiomyopathy, hypertrophic cardiomyopathy, arrhythmogenic right ventricular dysfunction, and prolonged QT syndrome. In addition, patients with moderate to severe left ventricular dysfunction, with or without nonsustained VT, are at high risk for cardiac arrest; therefore, prophylactic implantation may be indicated (Bardy, Lee, Mark, et al., 2005; Moss, Zareba, Hall, et al., 2002). ICDs may also be implanted in patients with symptomatic, recurrent, medication-refractory atrial fibrillation.

An ICD consists of a generator and at least one lead that can sense intrinsic electrical activity and deliver an electrical impulse. The device is usually implanted much like a pacemaker (Fig. 27-31). ICDs are designed to respond to two criteria: a rate that exceeds a predetermined level, and a change in the isoelectric line segments. When a dysrhythmia occurs, rate sensors require a set duration of time to sense the dysrhythmia. Then the device automatically charges and delivers the programmed charge through the lead to the heart. However, in an ICD that has the capability of providing atrial therapies, the device may be programmed to be activated by the patient, giving the patient time to activate the charge at a time and place of his or her choosing. Battery life is about 5 years but varies depending on use of the ICD. ICD surveillance is similar to that of the pacemaker; however, it includes information about the number and frequency of shocks that have been delivered.

Antiarrhythmic medication usually is administered with this technology to minimize the occurrence of the tachydysrhythmia and to reduce the frequency of ICD discharge.

The first defibrillator, which was implanted in 1980 at Johns Hopkins University, simply defibrillated the heart; it was called the automatic internal cardiodefibrillator (AICD). Today, several types of devices are available and may be programmed for multiple treatments (Fuster, Ryden, Asinger, et al., 2001). ICD, the generic name, is now used as the abbreviation for these various devices. Each device offers a different delivery sequence, but all are capable of delivering high-energy (high-intensity) defibrillation to treat a tachycardia (atrial or ventricular). The device may deliver up to six shocks if necessary.

Some ICDs can respond with antitachycardia pacing, in which the device delivers electrical impulses at a fast rate in an attempt to disrupt the tachycardia, by low-energy (low-intensity) cardioversion, by defibrillation, or all three (Fuster, Alexander, & O'Rourke, 2004). Antitachycardia pacing is used to terminate tachycardias caused by a conduction disturbance called reentry, which is repetitive restimulation of the heart by the same impulse. An impulse or a series of impulses is delivered to the heart by the pacemaker at a fast rate to collide with and stop the heart's reentry conduction impulses, and therefore to stop the tachycardia. Some ICDs also have pacemaker capability if the patient develops bradycardia, which sometimes occurs after treatment of the tachycardia. Usually the mode is VVI (V, paces the ventricle; V, senses ventricular activity; I, paces only if the ventricles do not depolarize). Some ICDs also deliver low-energy cardioversion, and some also treat atrial fibrillation (Daoud, Timmermans, Fellows, et al., 2000; Fuster et al., 2004).

Which device is used and how it is programmed depend on the patient's dysrhythmia. As with pacemakers, there is a NASPE-BPEG code for communicating the functions of the ICDs (Berstein, Daubert, Fletcher, et al., 2002). The first letter represents the chamber or chambers shocked (O = none, A = atrium, V = ventricle, D = both atrium and ventricle). The second letter represents the chamber that can be antitachycardia paced (O, A, V, D, meaning the same as the first letter). The third letter indicates the method used by the generator to detect a tachycardia (E = electrogram, H = hemodynamics). The last letter represents the chambers that have antibradycardia pacing (O, A, V, D, meaning the same as the first and second letters of the ICD code).

Complications are similar to those associated with pacemaker insertion. The primary complication associated with the ICD is surgery-related infection. There are a few complications associated with the technical aspects of the equipment, such as premature battery depletion and dislodged or fractured leads.

**FIGURE 27-31.** The implantable cardioverter defibrillator (ICD) consists of a generator and a sensing/pacing/defibrillating electrode.

## Nursing Process

### The Patient with an Implantable Cardiac Device

#### Assessment

After a permanent electronic device (pacemaker or ICD) is inserted, the patient's heart rate and rhythm are monitored by ECG. The device's settings are noted and compared with the ECG recordings to assess the device's function. For example, pacemaker malfunction is detected by examining the pacemaker spike and its relationship to the surrounding ECG complexes (Fig. 27-32). In addition, cardiac output and hemodynamic stability are assessed to identify the patient's response to pacing and the adequacy of pacing. The appearance or increasing frequency of dysrhythmia is observed and reported to the physician. If the patient has an ICD implanted and develops VT or ventricular fibrillation, the ECG should be recorded to note the time between the onset of the dysrhythmia and the onset of the device's shock or antitachycardia pacing.

The incision site where the generator was implanted is observed for bleeding, hematoma formation, or infection, which may be evidenced by swelling, unusual tenderness, drainage, and increased heat. The patient may complain of continuous throbbing or pain. These symptoms are reported to the physician.

The patient should be assessed for anxiety, depression, or anger, which may be symptoms of ineffective coping with the implantation. In addition, the level of knowledge and learning needs of the patient and family and the history of adherence to the therapeutic regimen should be identified. It is especially important to include the family when providing education and support.

#### Diagnosis

##### Nursing Diagnoses

Based on assessment data, the patient's major nursing diagnoses may include the following:

- Risk for infection related to lead or generator insertion
- Risk for ineffective coping
- Deficient knowledge regarding self-care program

##### Collaborative Problems/ Potential Complications

Based on the assessment findings, potential complications that may develop include decreased cardiac output related to device malfunction.

#### Planning and Goals

The major goals for the patient may include absence of infection, adherence to a self-care program, effective coping, and maintenance of device function.

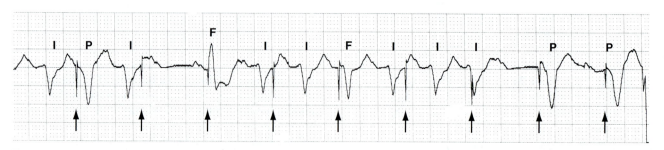

**FIGURE 27-32.** (A) Ventricular pacing with intermittent loss of capture (a pacing spike not followed by a QRS complex). (B) Ventricular pacing with loss of sensing (a pacing spike occurring at an inappropriate time). ↑ = pacing spike; * = loss of capture; P = pacemaker-induced QRS complex; I = patient's intrinsic QRS complex; F = fusion (a QRS complex formed by a merging of the patient's intrinsic QRS complex and the pacemaker-induced QRS complex). Both in lead $V_1$.

## Nursing Interventions

Nursing interventions for the patient with an implantable cardiac device are provided throughout the preoperative, perioperative, and postoperative phases. In addition to providing the patient and family with explanations regarding implantation of the device in the preoperative phase, the nurse may need to manage acute episodes of life-threatening dysrhythmias. In the perioperative and postoperative phases, the nurse carefully observes the patient's responses to the device and provides the patient and family with further teaching as needed (Chart 27-3). The nurse also assists the patient and family in addressing concerns and in making decisions about self-care and lifestyle changes necessitated by the dysrhythmia and resulting device implantation (Dougherty, Pyper, & Benoliel, 2004; Dougherty, Pyper, & Fransz, 2004).

### Preventing Infection

The nurse changes the dressing as needed and inspects the insertion site for redness, swelling, soreness, or any unusual drainage. An increase in the patient's temperature should be reported to the physician. Changes in wound appearance are also reported to the physician.

### Promoting Effective Coping

The patient treated with an electronic device experiences not only lifestyle and physical changes but also emotional changes. At different times during the healing process, the patient may feel angry, depressed, fearful, anxious, or a combination of these emotions. Although each patient uses individual coping strategies (eg, humor, prayer, communication with a significant other) to manage emotional distress, some strategies may work better than others. Signs that may indicate ineffective coping include social isolation, increased or prolonged irritability or depression, and difficulty in relationships.

To promote effective coping strategies, the nurse must recognize the patient's as well as the family's emotional state and assist them to explore their feelings. Because of the unpredictable and painful ICD discharge, patients with ICDs are most vulnerable to feelings of helplessness, leading to depression (Edelman, Lemon, & Kidman, 2003). The nurse may help the patient identify perceived changes (eg, loss of ability to participate in contact sports), the emotional response to the change (eg, anger), and how the patient responds to that emotion (eg, quickly becomes angry when talking with spouse). The nurse reassures the patient that the responses are normal and then helps the patient identify realistic goals (eg, develop interest in another activity) and develop a plan to attain these goals. The patient and family should be encouraged to talk about their experiences and emotions with each other and the health care team. The nurse may refer the patient and family to a hospital, community, or online support group. The nurse may also teach the patient easy-to-use stress reduction techniques (eg, deep-breathing exercises) to facilitate coping. Instructing the patient about the ICD may help the patient to cope with changes that occur as a result of device implantation (Chart 27-4).

### Promoting Home and Community-Based Care

#### TEACHING PATIENTS SELF-CARE

After device insertion, the patient's hospital stay may be 1 day or less, and follow-up in an outpatient clinic or office is common. The patient's anxiety and feelings of vulnerability may interfere with the ability to learn information provided. The nurse needs to include caregivers in the teaching and provide printed materials for use by the patient and caregiver. The nurse establishes priorities for learning with the patient and caregiver. Teaching may include the importance of periodic device monitoring, promoting safety, avoiding infection, and avoiding EMI (see Chart 27-3). In addition, the educational plan should include information about activities that are safe and those that may be dangerous. The nurse discusses with the patient and family what they are to do when a shock is delivered. They may wish to learn CPR.

## Evaluation

### Expected Patient Outcomes

Expected patient outcomes may include:

1. Remains free of infection
    a. Has normal temperature
    b. Has white blood cell count within normal range (5000 to 10,000/mm$^3$)
    c. Exhibits no redness or swelling of pacemaker insertion site
2. Adheres to a self-care program
    a. Responds appropriately when queried about the signs and symptoms of infection
    b. Identifies when to seek medical attention (as demonstrated in responses to signs and symptoms)
    c. Adheres to monitoring schedule
    d. Describes appropriate methods to avoid EMI
    e. Identifies activities that are safe and those to avoid
    f. For those with an ICD, describes how they will manage an ICD shock event
3. Maintains device function (see Chart 27-3)
    a. Measures and records pulse rate at regular intervals
    b. For those with pacemakers, experiences no abrupt changes in pulse rate or rhythm
4. Demonstrates and/or describes an effective coping strategy

## Electrophysiologic Studies

An electrophysiology (EP) study is an invasive procedure used to evaluate and treat various dysrhythmias that have caused cardiac arrest or significant symptoms. It also is indicated for patients with symptoms that suggest a dysrhythmia

## CHART 27-3

# HOME CARE CHECKLIST • The Patient With an ICD Implantable Cardioverter Defibrillator

| At the completion of home care instructions, the patient and significant other will be able to: | Patient | Caregiver |
|---|---|---|
| **Avoid infection at the ICD insertion site.** | | |
| • Observe incision site daily for redness, swelling, and heat. | ✔ | ✔ |
| • Take temperature; report any increase. | ✔ | ✔ |
| • Avoid tight restrictive clothing that may cause friction over the insertion site. | ✔ | ✔ |
| **Adhere to activity restrictions.** | | |
| • Restrict movement of arm until incision heals if the ICD was implanted in pectoral region. | ✔ | |
| • Avoid heavy lifting. | ✔ | |
| • Discuss safety of activities (eg, driving) with physician. | ✔ | ✔ |
| • Avoid contact sports. | ✔ | |
| **Electromagnetic interference: Understand the importance of the following:** | | |
| • Avoid large magnetic fields such as those created by magnetic resonance imaging, large motors, arc welding, electrical substations, and so forth. Magnetic fields may deactivate the ICD, negating any effect on a dysrhythmia. | ✔ | |
| • At security gates at airports, government buildings, or other secured areas, show identification card and request a hand (not handheld device) search. | ✔ | |
| • Some electrical and small motor devices, as well as products that contain magnets (eg, cellular phones), may interfere with the functioning of the ICD if placed very close to the ICD. Avoid leaning directly over devices, or ensure contact is of brief duration; place cellular phone on opposite side of ICD. | ✔ | |
| • Household appliances (eg, microwave ovens) should not cause any concern. | ✔ | ✔ |
| **Promote safety.** | | |
| • Describe what to do if symptoms occur and notify physician if any discharges seem unusual. | ✔ | ✔ |
| • Maintain a log that records discharges. Record events that precipitate the sensation of shock. This provides important data for the physician to use in readjusting the medical regimen. | ✔ | ✔ |
| • Encourage family members to attend a CPR class. | | ✔ |
| • Call 911 for emergency assistance if feeling of dizziness occurs. | ✔ | ✔ |
| • Wear medical identification (eg, Medic-Alert) that includes physician information. | ✔ | |
| • Avoid frightening family or friends with unexpected shocks, which will not harm them. Inform family and friends that in the event they are in contact with the patient when a shock is delivered, they may also feel the shock. It is especially important to warn sexual partners that this may occur. | ✔ | ✔ |
| **Follow-up care** | | |
| • Discuss psychological responses to the ICD implantation, such as changes in self-image, depression due to loss of mobility secondary to driving restrictions, fear of shocks, increased anxiety, concerns that sexual activity may trigger the ICD, and changes in partner relationship. | ✔ | ✔ |
| • Adhere to appointments that are scheduled to test electronic performance of ICD. Remember to take log of ICD discharges to review with physician. | ✔ | ✔ |
| • Attend an ICD support group within the area. | ✔ | |

that has gone undetected and undiagnosed by other methods. An EP study is used to do the following:

- Identify the impulse formation and propagation through the cardiac electrical conduction system
- Assess the function or dysfunction of the SA and AV nodal areas
- Identify the location (called mapping) and mechanism of dysrhythmogenic foci
- Assess the effectiveness of antiarrhythmic medications and devices for the patient with a dysrhythmia
- Treat certain dysrhythmias through the destruction of the causative cells (**ablation**)

An EP procedure is a type of cardiac catheterization that is performed in a specially equipped cardiac catheterization laboratory by an electrophysiologist, who is a cardiologist with specialized training, assisted by other EP laboratory personnel. The patient is conscious but lightly sedated. Usually a catheter with multiple electrodes is inserted through a small incision in the femoral vein, threaded through the inferior vena cava, and advanced into the heart; however, a catheter may also be inserted into the femoral artery, depending on the type of study and the information needed. The electrodes are positioned within the heart at specific locations—for instance, in the right atrium near the sinus node, in the coronary sinus, near the tricuspid valve, and at the apex of

### CHART 27-4

## HOME CARE CHECKLIST • The Patient With an Implantable Cardiac Device

| At the completion of home care instructions, the patient and significant other will be able to: | Patient | Caregiver |
|---|---|---|
| **Monitor pacemaker function.** | | |
| • Describe the importance of reporting to physician or pacemaker clinic periodically as prescribed, so that the pacemaker's rate and function can be monitored. This is especially important during the first month after implantation. | ✔ | |
| • Adhere to monitoring schedule as instructed after implantation. | ✔ | |
| • Check pulse daily. Report *immediately* any sudden slowing or increasing of the pulse rate. This may indicate pacemaker malfunction. | ✔ | ✔ |
| • Resume more frequent monitoring when battery depletion is anticipated. (The time for reimplantation depends on the type of battery in use.) | ✔ | |
| **Promote safety and avoid infection.** | | |
| • Wear loose-fitting clothing around the area of the pacemaker. | ✔ | |
| • State the reason for the slight bulge over the pacemaker implant. | ✔ | ✔ |
| • Notify physician if the pacemaker area becomes red or painful. | ✔ | ✔ |
| • Avoid trauma to the area of the pacemaker generator. | ✔ | |
| • Study the manufacturer's instructions and become familiar with the pacemaker. | ✔ | ✔ |
| • Recognize that physical activity does not usually have to be curtailed, with the exception of contact sports. | ✔ | |
| • Carry medical identification indicating physician's name, type and model number of pacemaker, manufacturer's name, pacemaker rate, and hospital where pacemaker was inserted. | ✔ | |
| **Electromagnetic interference: Understand the importance of the following:** | | |
| • Avoid large magnetic fields such as those surrounding magnetic resonance imaging, large motors, arc welding, electrical substations. Magnetic fields can deactivate the pacemaker. | ✔ | |
| • Some electrical and small motor devices, as well as products that contain magnets (eg, cellular phones), may interfere with pacemaker function if placed very close to the generator. Avoid leaning directly over devices, or ensure that contact is brief; place cellular phone on opposite side of generator and do not carry in a shirt pocket. | ✔ | ✔ |
| • Household items, such as microwave ovens, should not cause any concern. | ✔ | ✔ |
| • When going through security gates (eg, at airports, government buildings) show identification card and request hand (not handheld device) search. | ✔ | ✔ |
| • Hospitalization may be necessary periodically to change battery or replace pacemaker unit. | ✔ | ✔ |

the right ventricle. The number and placement of electrodes depend on the type of study being conducted. These electrodes allow the electrical signal to be recorded from within the heart (intracardiogram).

The electrodes also allow the clinician to introduce a pacing stimulus to the intracardiac area at a precisely timed interval and rate, thereby stimulating the area (programmed stimulation). An area of the heart may be paced at a rate much faster than the normal rate of **automaticity**, the rate at which impulses are spontaneously formed (eg, in the sinus node). This allows the pacemaker to become an artificial focus of automaticity and to assume control (overdrive suppression). Then the pacemaker is stopped suddenly, and the time it takes for the sinus node to resume control is assessed. A prolonged time indicates dysfunction of the sinus node.

One of the main purposes of programmed stimulation is to assess the ability of the area surrounding the electrode to cause a reentry dysrhythmia. One or a series of premature impulses is delivered to an area in an attempt to cause the tachydysrhythmia. Because the precise location of the suspected area and the specific timing of the pacing needed are unknown, the electrophysiologist uses several different techniques to cause the dysrhythmia during the study. If the dysrhythmia can be reproduced by programmed stimulation, it is called inducible. Once a dysrhythmia is induced, a treatment plan is determined and implemented. If, on the follow-up EP study, the tachydysrhythmia cannot be induced, then the treatment is determined to be effective. Different medications may be administered and combined with electrical devices (pacemaker, ICD) to determine the most effective treatment to suppress the dysrhythmia.

Patient care, patient teaching, and associated complications of an EP study are the same as those associated with cardiac catheterization (see Chapter 26). The study is usually about 2 hours in length; however, if the electrophysiologist conducts not only a diagnostic procedure but also treatment, the study can take up to 6 hours. During the procedure, patients benefit from a calm, reassuring approach.

Patients who are to undergo an EP study may be anxious about the procedure and its outcome. A detailed discussion involving the patient, the family, and the electrophysiologist usually occurs to ensure that the patient can give informed consent and to reduce the patient's anxiety about the procedure. Before the procedure, the patient should receive instructions about the procedure and its usual duration, the environment where the procedure is performed, and what to expect. Although an EP study is not painful, it does cause discomfort and can be tiring. It may also cause feelings that were experienced when the dysrhythmia occurred in the past. In addition, patients are taught what will be expected of them (eg, lying very still during the procedure, reporting symptoms or concerns).

The patient should also know that the dysrhythmia may occur during the procedure. It often stops on its own; if it does not, treatment is given to restore the patient's normal rhythm. The dysrhythmia may have to be terminated using cardioversion or defibrillation, but this is performed under more controlled circumstances than if performed in an emergency.

Postprocedural care is similar to that for cardiac catheterization, including restriction of activity to promote hemostasis at the insertion site. To identify any complications and to ensure healing, the patient's vital signs and the appearance of the insertion site are assessed frequently. Because an artery is not always used, there is a lower incidence of vascular complications than with other catheterization procedures. Cardiac arrest may occur, but the incidence is low (less than 1%) (Fuster et al., 2004).

## Cardiac Conduction Surgery

Atrial tachycardias and ventricular tachycardias that do not respond to medications and are not suitable for antitachycardia pacing may be treated by methods that include a maze procedure and ablation. Hospitalization is required for both procedures.

### Maze Procedure

The maze procedure is an open heart surgical procedure for refractory atrial fibrillation. Small transmural incisions are made throughout the atria. The resulting formation of scar tissue prevents reentry conduction of the electrical impulse. Although the procedure has been found to be about 95% effective, it usually requires significant time and cardiopulmonary bypass (Gaynor, Diodato, Prasad, et al., 2004). In addition, some patients need a permanent pacemaker after the surgery. Use of catheter ablation to perform the maze procedure using minimally invasive surgery is being studied. This less invasive procedure does not require cardiopulmonary bypass and is performed with catheters inserted through small sternal keyhole-type incisions.

### Catheter Ablation Therapy

Catheter ablation destroys specific cells that are the cause or central conduction route of a tachydysrhythmia. It is performed with or after an EP study. Usual indications for ablation are AVNRT, a recurrent atrial dysrhythmia (especially atrial fibrillation), or VT unresponsive to previous therapy (or for which the therapy produced significant side effects).

Ablation is also indicated to eliminate accessory AV pathways or bypass tracts that exist in the hearts of patients with preexcitation syndromes such as Wolff-Parkinson-White (WPW) syndrome. During normal embryonic development, all connections between the atrium and ventricles disappear, except for that between the AV node and the bundle of His. In some people, embryonic connections of normal heart muscle between the atrium and ventricles remain, providing an accessory pathway or a tract through which the electrical impulse can bypass the AV node. These pathways can be located in several different areas. If the patient develops atrial fibrillation, the impulse may be conducted into the ventricle at a rate of 300 times per minute or more, which can lead to ventricular fibrillation and sudden cardiac death. Preexcitation syndromes are identified by specific ECG findings. For example, in WPW syndrome there is a shortened PR interval, slurring (called a delta wave) of the initial QRS deflection, and prolonged QRS duration (Fig. 27-33).

Ablation is most often accomplished by using radiofrequency, which involves placing a special catheter at or near the origin of the dysrhythmia. High-frequency, low-energy sound waves are passed through the catheter, causing thermal injury and cellular changes that result in localized de-

**FIGURE 27-33.** Wolff-Parkinson-White syndrome. (**A**) Sinus rhythm. Note the short PR interval, slurred initial upstroke of the QRS complex (delta wave, at the arrow), and prolonged QRS duration, upper lead II, lower lead $V_1$. (**B**) Rhythm strip of same patient following ablation, upper lead $V_1$, lower lead II. ECG strips courtesy of Linda Ardini and Catherine Berkmeyer, Inova Fairfax Hospital, Falls Church, VA.

struction and scarring. The tissue damage is more specific to the dysrhythmic tissue, with less trauma to the surrounding cardiac tissue than occurs with cryoablation or electrical ablation.

During the ablation procedure, defibrillation pads, an automatic blood pressure cuff, and a pulse oximeter are used, and an indwelling urinary catheter is inserted. The patient is usually given moderate sedation. An EP study is performed and attempts to induce the dysrhythmia are made. The ablation catheter is placed at the origin of the dysrhythmia, and the ablation procedure is performed. Multiple ablations may be necessary. Successful ablation is achieved when the dysrhythmia can no longer be induced. The patient is monitored for another 30 to 60 minutes and then retested to ensure that the dysrhythmia will not recur.

Postprocedural care on a step-down unit is similar to that for an EP study, except that the patient is monitored more closely, depending on the time needed for recovery from sedation.

## Critical Thinking Exercises

**1** [ebp] You are caring for a 79-year-old woman who had coronary artery bypass surgery 3 days ago. Her recovery had been uneventful until today, when her heart rate increased and the heart rhythm became irregular. Your analysis of the ECG strip indicates that she has developed sinus tachycardia with frequent PACs. What are some of the possible causes of this dysrhythmia? Identify some of the key factors that would need to be included in your assessment to assist in identification of the cause of the dysrhythmia. What nursing interventions are needed? What is the evidence base that supports these nursing interventions? Discuss the strength of the evidence and the criteria used to evaluate the strength of the evidence.

**2** You are caring for a 40-year-old man who recently had an AV sequential pacemaker inserted, with the rate set at 72 beats per minute. When taking his pulse, you note that his heart rate is 66 beats per minute. Describe the possible causes of this difference in heart rates and the nursing actions that are needed.

**3** [ebp] The wife of this same patient tells you that her husband has informed her that now that he has a pacemaker, they must get rid of their microwave oven. What would you say to the wife? How would you discuss this with the patient? What other education would you provide to this patient and his wife about safety in relation to the pacemaker? What is the evidence base that supports this education? Discuss the strength of the evidence and the criteria used to evaluate the strength of the evidence.

**4** You are caring for a 65-year-old man with heart failure, chronic renal insufficiency, and chronic obstructive pulmonary disease. He has an ICD that was implanted 5 years ago. He was admitted 2 weeks ago for progressive dyspnea, peripheral edema, and intermittent delirium. He requests that only comfort measures now be given; he and his family have asked for withdrawal of the ICD support. Is this ethically permissible? How would you respond? What discussion should occur, and with whom?

## REFERENCES AND SELECTED READINGS

### BOOKS

Chulay, M., & Burns, S. (2005). *AACN essentials of critical care nursing.* New York: McGraw-Hill.

Conover, M. B. (2003). *Understanding electrocardiography.* St. Louis: Mosby.

Fuster, V., Alexander R. W., & O'Rourke, R. A. (Eds.). (2004). *Hurst's the heart* (11th ed.). New York: McGraw-Hill.

Kinney, M., Brooks-Brunn, J. A., Molter, N., et al. (Eds.). (1998). *AACN clinical reference for critical care nursing* (4th ed.). St. Louis: Mosby.

*Management of new onset atrial fibrillation.* Evidence Report/Technology Assessment: Number 12. AHRQ Publication No. 01-E026. (2001). Rockville, MD: Agency for Healthcare Research and Quality.

Marriott, H. J., & Conover, M. B. (1998). *Advanced concepts in arrhythmias.* St. Louis: Mosby.

McEvoy, G. K. (Ed.). (2005). *AHFS drug information.* Bethesda, MD: American Society of Health System Pharmacists.

McNamara, R. L., Bass, E. B., Miller, M. R., et al. (2001). *Management of new onset atrial fibrillation.* Evidence Report/Technology Assessment No. 12 (prepared by the Johns Hopkins University Evidence-Based Practice Center in Baltimore, MD, under Contract No. 290-97-0006). AHRQ Publication Number 01-E026. Rockville, MD: Agency for Healthcare Research and Quality.

Zipes, D. P., Libby, P., Bonow, R. O., et al. (Eds.). (2005). *Braunwald's heart disease: A textbook of cardiovascular medicine* (7th ed.) Philadelphia: W. B. Saunders.

### JOURNALS

*Asterisks indicate nursing research articles.

Adgey, A. A., Spence, M. S., & Walsh, S. J. (2005). Theory and practice of defibrillation: Defibrillation for ventricular fibrillation. *Heart,* 9(1), 118–125.

American Heart Association (2005). 2005 American Heart Association guidelines for cardiopulmonary resuscitation and emergency cardiovascular care. *Circulation,* 112(24 Supplement), 1–211.

Atrial Fibrillation Follow-up Investigation of Rhythm Management (AFFIRM) Investigators. (2002). A comparison of rate control and rhythm control in patients with atrial fibrillation. *New England Journal of Medicine,* 347(23), 1825–1833.

Bardy, G. H., Lee, K. L., Mark, D. B., et al. (2005). Amiodarone or an implantable cardioverter-defibrillator for congestive heart failure. *New England Journal of Medicine,* 352(3), 225–237.

Bernstein, A. D., Daubert, J-C., Fletcher, R. D., et al. (2002) The Revised NASPE/BPEG Generic Code for antibradycardia, adaptive-rate, and multisite pacing. *Journal of Pacing and Clinical Electrophysiology,* 25(2), 260–264.

Blomström-Lundqvist, C., Scheinman, M. M, Aliot, E. M., et al. (2003). ACC/AHA/ESC guidelines for the management of patients with supraventricular arrhythmias: A report of the American College of Cardiology/American Heart Association Task Force on Practice Guidelines and the European Society of Cardiology Committee for Practice Guidelines. (Writing Committee to Develop Guidelines for the Management of Patients with Supraventricular Arrhythmias. American College of Cardiology Web Site: Available at: http://www.acc.org/clinical/guidelines/arrhythmias/sva_index.pdf. Accessed June 2, 2006).

Cardiac Arrhythmia Suppression Trial Investigators. (1989). The Cardiac Arrhythmia Suppression Trial. *New England Journal of Medicine,* 321(25), 1754–1756.

Daoud, E. G., Timmermans, C., Fellows, C., et al. (2000). Initial clinical experience with ambulatory use of an implantable atrial defibrillator for conversion of atrial fibrillation. Metrix Investigators. *Circulation,* 102(12), 1407–1413.

*Dougherty, C. M., Pyper, G. P., & Benoliel, J. Q. (2004). Domains of concern of intimate partners of sudden cardiac arrest survivors after ICD implantation. *Journal of Cardiovascular Nursing,* 19(1), 21–31.

Dougherty, C. M., Pyper, G. P., & Frasz, H. A. (2004). Description of a nursing intervention program after an implantable cardioverter defibrillator. *Heart & Lung,* 33(3), 183–190.

Drew, B. J., & Krucoff, M. W. (1999). Multilead ST-segment monitoring in patients with acute coronary syndromes: A consensus statement for healthcare professionals. *American Journal of Critical Care,* 8(6), 372–386.

Edelman, S., Lemon, J., & Kidman, A. (2003). Psychological therapies for recipients of implantable cardioverter defibrillators. *Heart & Lung,* 32(4), 234–240.

Fenton, J. M. (2001). The clinician's approach to evaluating patients with dysrhythmias. *AACN Clinical Issues: Advanced Practice Acute Critical Care,* 12(1), 72–86.

*Funk, M., Richards, S. B., Desjardins J., et al. (2003). Incidence, timing, symptoms, and risk factors for atrial fibrillation after cardiac surgery. *American Journal of Critical Care,* 12(5), 424–435.

Fuster, V., Rydén, A., Asinger, R. W., et al (2001). ACC/AHA/ESC Guidelines for the management of patients with atrial fibrillation. *Journal of American College of Cardiology,* 38, 2118–2150.

Gaynor, S. L., Diodato, M. D., Prasad, S. M., et al. (2004). A prospective, single-center clinical trial of a modified Cox maze procedure with bipolar radiofrequency ablation. *Journal of Thoracic & Cardiovascular Surgery,* 128(4), 535–542.

Glotzer, T. V., Hellkamp, A. S., Zimmerman, J., et al. (2003). Atrial high rate episodes detected by pacemaker diagnostics predict death and stroke: Report of the Atrial Diagnostics Ancillary Study of the Mode Selection Trial (MOST). *Circulation,* 107(12), 1614–1619.

Gregoratos, G., Abrams, J., Epstein, A. E., et al. (2002). ACC/AHA/NASPE 2002 guideline update for implantation of cardiac pacemakers and antiarrhythmia devices: A report of the American College of Cardiology/American Heart Association Task Force on Practice Guidelines (ACC/AHA/NASPE). Committee to Pacemaker Implantation. *Circulation,* 106(16), 2145–2161.

Hallstrom, A. P., Ornato, J. P., Weisfeldt, M., et al. Public Access Defibrillation Trial Investigators (2004). Public-access defibrillation and survival after out-of-hospital cardiac arrest. *New England Journal of Medicine,* 351(7), 637–646.

Hirsh, J., Fuster, V., Ansell, J., et al. (2003). American Heart Association/American College of Cardiology Foundation guide to warfarin therapy. *Circulation,* 107(12), 1692–1711.

Kellen, J. C. (2004). Implications for nursing care of patients with atrial fibrillation. *Journal of Cardiovascular Nursing,* 19(2), 128–137.

Kellen, J. C., Ettinger, A., Todd, L., et al. (1996). The Cardiac Arrhythmia Suppression Trial: Implications for nursing practice. *American Journal of Critical Care,* 5(1), 19–25.

Kern, L. (2004). Postoperative atrial fibrillation: New directions in prevention and treatment. *Journal of Cardiovascular Nursing,* 19(2), 103–115.

Knight, B. P., Gersh, B. J., Carlson, M. D., et al. for the AHA Writing Group. (2005). Role of permanent pacing to prevent atrial fibrillation. *Circulation,* 111(2), 240–243.

Madrid, A. H., Bueno, M. G., Rebollo, J. M. G, et al. (2002). Use of irbesartan to maintain sinus rhythm in patients with long-lasting persistent atrial fibrillation: A prospective and randomized study. *Circulation, 106,* 331–336.

Moss, A. J., Zareba, W., Hall, J., et al. for the Multicenter Automatic Defibrillator Implantation Trial II Investigators (2002). Prophylactic implantation of a defibrillator in patients with myocardial infarction and reduced ejection fraction. *New England Journal of Medicine, 346*(8), 877–883.

Obias-Manno, D., & Wijetunga, M. (2004). Risk stratification and primary prevention of sudden cardiac death: Sudden death prevention. *AACN Clinical Issues, 15*(3), 404–418.

Ocampo, C. M. (2000). Living with an implantable cardioverter defibrillator: Impact on the patient, family and society. *Nursing Clinics of North America, 35*(4), 1019–1030.

Olshansky, B., Rosenfeld, L. E., Warner, A. L., et al. (2004). The Atrial Fibrillation Follow-up Investigation of RhMthm management (AFFIRM) study: Approaches to control rate in atrial fibrillation. *Journal of American College of Cardiology, 43*(7), 1201–1208.

Shaffer, R. S. (2002). ICD therapy: The patient's perspective. *American Journal of Nursing, 102*(2), 46–49.

Snow, V., Weiss, K. B., LeFevre, M., et al. AAFP Panel on Atrial Fibrillation. ACP Panel on Atrial Fibrillation. (2003). Management of newly detected atrial fibrillation: A clinical practice guideline from the American Academy of Family Physicians and the American College of Physicians. *Annals of Internal Medicine. 139*(12), 1009–1017.

Stevenson, W. G., Chaitman, B. R., Ellenbogen, K. A., et al. for the Subcommittee on Electrocardiography and Arrhythmias of the American Heart Association Council on Clinical Cardiology, in collaboration with the Heart Rhythm Society. (2004). Clinical assessment and management of patients with implanted cardioverter-defibrillators presenting to nonelectrophysiologists. *Circulation, 110*(25), 3866–3869.

Stewart, S. (2004). Epidemiology and economic impact of atrial fibrillation. *Journal of Cardiovascular Nursing, 19*(2), 94–102.

Thomas, S. A., Friedmann, E., & Kelley, F. J. (2001). Living with an implantable cardioverter-defibrillator: A review of the current literature related to psychosocial factors. *AACN Clinical Issues: Advanced Practice Acute Critical Care, 12*(1), 156–163.

Troyman, R. G., Kim, M. H., & Pinski, S. L. (2004) Cardiac pacing: The state of the art. *Lancet, 364*(9446), 1701–1719.

Trupp, R. J. (2004). Cardiac resynchronization therapy: Optimizing the device, optimizing the patient. *Journal of Cardiovascular Nursing, 19*(4), 223–233.

Ueng, K. C., Tsai, T. P., Yu, W. C., et al. (2003). Use of enalapril to facilitate sinus rhythm maintenance after external cardioversion of long-standing persistent atrial fibrillation. Results of a prospective and controlled study. *European Heart, 24*(23), 2090–2098.

Yeo, T. P., & Berg, N. C. (2004). Counseling patients with implanted cardiac devices. *Nurse Practitioner, 29*(12), 58–65.

## RESOURCES

American Association of Critical Care Nurses, 101 Columbia, Aliso Viejo, CA 92656-4109; 800-899-2226; http://www.aacn.org. Accessed June 2, 2006.

American College of Cardiology, 911 Old Georgetown Road, Bethesda, MD 20814; 800-253-4636; http://www.acc.org. Accessed June 2, 2006.

American Heart Association, National Center, 7272 Greenville Ave., Dallas, TX 75231; 1-800-242-8721; http://www.americanheart.org. Accessed June 2, 2006.

Heart Rhythm Society, 1400 K Street, N.W., Suite 500, Washington D.C. 20005; 202-464-3400; http://www.hrsonline.org. Accessed June 2, 2006.

National Heart, Lung, Blood Institute, Health Information Center, National Institutes of Health, PO Box 30105, Bethesda, MD 20824; 301-592-8573; http://www.nhlbi.nih.gov. Accessed June 2, 2006.

National Institute on Aging, Building 31, Room 5C27, 31 Center Drive, MSC 2292, Bethesda, MD 20892; 301-496-1752; http://www.nia.nih.gov. Accessed June 2, 2006.

# CHAPTER 28

# Management of Patients With Coronary Vascular Disorders

## Learning Objectives

*On completion of this chapter, the learner will be able to:*

1. Describe the pathophysiology, clinical manifestations, and treatment of coronary atherosclerosis.
2. Describe the pathophysiology, clinical manifestations, and treatment of angina pectoris.
3. Use the nursing process as a framework for care of patients with angina pectoris.
4. Describe the pathophysiology, clinical manifestations, and treatment of myocardial infarction.
5. Use the nursing process as a framework for care of a patient with acute coronary syndrome.
6. Describe percutaneous coronary interventional and coronary artery revascularization procedures.
7. Describe the nursing care of a patient who has had a percutaneous coronary interventional procedure for treatment of coronary artery disease.
8. Describe the nursing care of a patient who has undergone cardiac surgery.

Cardiovascular disease is the leading cause of death in the United States for men and women of all racial and ethnic groups (American Heart Association [AHA], 2004). Research related to the identification and treatment of cardiovascular disease now includes all segments of the population affected by cardiac conditions, including women, children, and people of diverse racial and ethnic backgrounds.

# Coronary Artery Disease

Coronary artery disease (CAD) is the most prevalent type of cardiovascular disease in adults. For this reason, it is important for nurses to become familiar with various manifestations of coronary artery conditions and methods for assessing, preventing, and treating these disorders medically and surgically.

## Coronary Atherosclerosis

The most common cause of cardiovascular disease in the United States is **atherosclerosis**, an abnormal accumulation of lipid, or fatty, substances and fibrous tissue in the lining of arterial blood vessel walls. These substances create blockages and narrow the coronary vessels in a way that reduces blood flow to the myocardium. It is now known that atherosclerosis involves a repetitious inflammatory response to injury to the artery wall and subsequent alteration in the structural and biochemical properties of the arterial walls. New information that relates to the development of atherosclerosis has increased understanding of treatment and prevention of this progressive and potentially life-threatening process.

## Pathophysiology

Atherosclerosis is thought to begin as fatty streaks of lipids that are deposited in the intima of the arterial wall. These lesions commonly begin early in life, perhaps even in childhood. Not all fatty streaks later develop into more advanced lesions. Genetics and environmental factors are involved in the progression of these lesions. The continued development of atherosclerosis involves an inflammatory response, which begins with injury to the vascular endothelium. The injury may be initiated by smoking, hypertension, and other factors. The presence of inflammation has multiple effects on the arterial wall, including the attraction of inflammatory cells (including macrophages) (Moustapha & Anderson, 2003). The macrophages infiltrate the injured vascular endothelium and ingest lipids, which turns them into what are called foam cells. Activated macrophages also

## Glossary

**acute coronary syndrome (ACS):** signs and symptoms that indicate unstable angina or acute myocardial infarction

**angina pectoris:** chest pain brought about by myocardial ischemia

**angiotensin-converting enzyme (ACE) inhibitors:** medications that inhibit the angiotensin-converting enzyme

**atherosclerosis:** abnormal accumulation of lipid deposits and fibrous tissue within arterial walls and lumen

**atheroma:** fibrous cap composed of smooth muscle cells that forms over lipid deposits within arterial vessels and that protrudes into the lumen of the vessel, narrowing the lumen and obstructing blood flow; also called plaque

**contractility:** ability of the cardiac muscle to shorten in response to an electrical impulse

**coronary artery bypass graft (CABG):** a surgical procedure in which a blood vessel from another part of the body is grafted onto the occluded coronary artery below the occlusion in such a way that blood flow bypasses the blockage

**creatine kinase (CK):** an enzyme found in human tissues; one of the three types of CK is specific to heart muscle and may be used as an indicator of heart muscle injury

**high-density lipoprotein (HDL):** a protein-bound lipid that transports cholesterol to the liver for excretion in the bile; composed of a higher proportion of protein to lipid than low-density lipoprotein; exerts a beneficial effect on the arterial wall

**ischemia:** insufficient tissue oxygenation

**low-density lipoprotein (LDL):** a protein-bound lipid that transports cholesterol to tissues in the body; composed of a lower proportion of protein to lipid than high-density lipoprotein; exerts a harmful effect on the arterial wall

**metabolic syndrome:** a cluster of metabolic abnormalities including insulin resistance, obesity, dyslipidemia, and hypertension that increase the risk of cardiovascular disease

**myocardial infarction (MI):** death of heart tissue caused by lack of oxygenated blood flow; if acute, abbreviated as AMI

**percutaneous coronary intervention (PCI):** an invasive procedure in which a catheter is placed in a coronary artery, and one of several methods is employed to remove or reduce a blockage within the artery

**percutaneous transluminal coronary angioplasty (PTCA):** a type of percutaneous coronary intervention in which a balloon is inflated within a coronary artery to break an atheroma and open the vessel lumen, improving coronary artery blood flow

**primary prevention:** interventions taken to prevent the development of coronary artery disease

**secondary prevention:** interventions taken to prevent the advancement of existing coronary artery disease

**stent:** a woven mesh that provides structural support to a coronary vessel, preventing its closure

**sudden cardiac death:** immediate cessation of effective heart activity

**thrombolytic:** an agent or process that breaks down blood clots

**troponin:** myocardial protein; measurement is used to assess heart muscle injury release biochemical substances that can further damage the endothelium, attracting platelets and initiating clotting.

Smooth muscle cells within the vessel wall subsequently proliferate and form a fibrous cap over a core filled with lipid and inflammatory infiltrate. These deposits, called **atheromas** or plaques, protrude into the lumen of the vessel, narrowing it and obstructing blood flow (Fig. 28-1). Plaque may be stable or unstable, depending on the degree of inflammation and consequent thickness of the fibrous cap. If the fibrous cap of the plaque is thick and the lipid pool remains relatively stable, it can resist the stress from blood flow and vessel movement. If the cap is thin and inflammation is ongoing, the lipid core may grow, causing it to rupture and hemorrhage into the plaque. A ruptured plaque is a focus for thrombus formation. The thrombus may then obstruct blood flow, leading to sudden cardiac death or an acute **myocardial infarction (MI)**, which is the death of a portion of the heart muscle.

The anatomic structure of the coronary arteries makes them particularly susceptible to the mechanisms of atherosclerosis. As Figure 28-2 shows, the three major coronary arteries have multiple branches. Atherosclerotic lesions most often form where the vessels branch, suggesting a hemodynamic component that favors their formation (Porth, 2005). Although heart disease is most often caused by atherosclerosis of the coronary arteries, other phenomena may also decrease blood flow to the heart. Examples include vasospasm (sudden constriction or narrowing) of a coronary artery, myocardial trauma from internal or external forces, structural disease, congenital anomalies, decreased oxygen supply (eg, from acute blood loss, anemia, or low blood pressure), and increased oxygen demand (eg, from rapid heart rate, thyrotoxicosis, or use of cocaine).

## Clinical Manifestations

Coronary atherosclerosis produces symptoms and complications according to the location and degree of narrowing of the arterial lumen, thrombus formation, and obstruction of blood flow to the myocardium. This impediment to blood flow is usually progressive, causing an inadequate blood supply that deprives the cardiac muscle cells of oxygen needed for their survival. The condition is known as **ischemia**. **Angina pectoris** refers to chest pain that is brought about by myocardial ischemia. Angina pectoris usually is caused by significant coronary atherosclerosis. If the decrease in blood supply is great enough, of long enough duration, or both, irreversible damage and death of myocardial cells, or MI, may result. Over time, irreversibly damaged myocardium undergoes degeneration and is replaced by scar tissue, causing various degrees of myocardial dysfunction. Significant myocardial damage may result in persistently low cardiac output, and the heart cannot support the body's needs for blood, which is called heart failure. A decrease in blood supply from CAD may even cause the heart to abruptly stop beating (**sudden cardiac death**).

The most common manifestation of myocardial ischemia is acute onset of chest pain. However, the classic epidemiologic study of the people in Framingham, Massachusetts, showed that nearly 15% of men and women who had MIs were totally asymptomatic (Kannel, 1986). Patients with myocardial ischemia may present to an emergency department or clinic with a variety of symptoms other than chest pain. Patients who are older or have a history of diabetes or heart failure may report symptoms such as shortness of breath. Many women have been found to have atypical symptoms, including dyspnea, nausea, and weakness (DeVon & Zerwic, 2003). Prodromal symptoms may occur (ie, angina a few hours to days before the acute episode), or a major cardiac event may be the first indication of coronary atherosclerosis.

**FIGURE 28-1.** Atherosclerosis begins as monocytes and lipids enter the intima of an injured vessel (**A, B**). Smooth muscle cells proliferate within the vessel wall (**C**) contributing to the development of fatty accumulations and atheroma (**D**). As the plaque enlarges, the vessel narrows and blood flow decreases (**E**). The plaque may rupture and a thrombus might form, obstructing blood flow.

## Risk Factors

Epidemiologic studies point to several factors that increase the probability that heart disease will develop in a person.

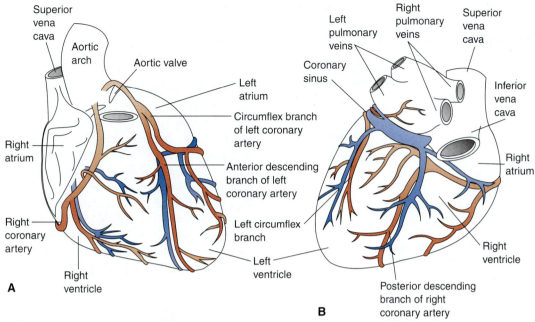

**FIGURE 28-2.** The coronary arteries supply the heart muscle with oxygenated blood, adjusting the flow according to metabolic needs. (**A**) Anterior view, and (**B**) posterior view of heart.

Major risk factors include elevated blood lipid levels, smoking, hypertension, diabetes mellitus, obesity, family history of premature cardiovascular disease (first-degree relative with cardiovascular disease at 55 years of age or younger for men and at 65 years of age or younger for women), and age (more than 45 years for men; more than 55 years for women). Some people do not have classic risk factors. The Third Report of the Expert Panel on Detection, Evaluation, and Treatment of High Blood Cholesterol in Adults (ATP III; Expert Panel, 2001) lists the clinical guidelines for cholesterol testing and management. ATP III guidelines address **primary prevention** (preventing the occurrence of CAD) and **secondary prevention** (preventing the progression of CAD). Elevated **low-density lipoprotein (LDL)** cholesterol, also known as the "bad cholesterol," is the primary target of cholesterol-lowering therapy. Those at highest risk for having a cardiac event within 10 years are those with existing CAD or those with diabetes, peripheral arterial disease, abdominal aortic aneurysm, or carotid artery disease. The latter diseases are called CAD risk equivalents, because patients with these diseases have the same risk for a cardiac event as patients with CAD (Chart 28-1). The possibility of having a cardiac event within 10 years is also determined by factors such as age, systolic blood pressure, smoking history, level of total cholesterol, level of LDL, and level of **high-density lipoprotein (HDL)**, also known as the "good cholesterol."

In addition, a cluster of metabolic abnormalities known as **metabolic syndrome** has emerged as a major risk factor for cardiovascular disease (Haffner & Taegtmeyer, 2003; Wilson & Grundy, 2003). A diagnosis of this syndrome includes three of the following conditions:

- Insulin resistance (fasting glucose more than 100 mg/dL or abnormal glucose tolerance test)
- Abdominal obesity (waist circumference more than 35 inches in women, more than 40 inches in men)
- Dyslipidemia (triglycerides more than 150 mg/dL, HDL less than 50 mg/dL in women, less than 40 mg/dL in men)
- Hypertension
- Proinflammatory state (high levels of C-reactive protein)
- Prothrombotic state (high fibrinogen)

Many people with type 2 diabetes mellitus fit this clinical picture. It is theorized that in obese patients, excessive adipose tissue may secrete mediators that lead to metabolic changes (Reilly & Rader, 2003). Immune mechanisms are activated and contribute to atherogenic changes in the cardiovascular system (Fig. 28-3).

Measurement of lipoprotein(a) [Lp(a)] and homocysteine (an amino acid associated with cardiac disease)

---

### CHART 28-1

### Coronary Artery Disease Risk Equivalents

Individuals at highest risk for a cardiac event within 10 years are those with existing coronary artery disease (CAD) and those with any of the following diseases, which are called CAD risk equivalents:

- Diabetes
- Peripheral arterial disease
- Abdominal aortic aneurysm
- Carotid artery disease

From Expert Panel on Detection, Evaluation, and Treatment of High Blood Cholesterol in Adults. (2001). Executive summary of the third report of the National Cholesterol Education Program (NCEP) Expert Panel on Detection, Evaluation, and Treatment of High Blood Cholesterol in Adults (Adult Treatment Panel III). *Journal of the American Medical Association, 285*(19), 2486–2497.

**FIGURE 28-3.** Pathophysiology of cardiovascular disease in metabolic syndrome. Both central adiposity and the immune system play a role in the development of metabolic syndrome. Adipokines (such as leptin) and cytokines (such as tumor necrosis factor) are thought to contribute to the development of metabolic abnormalities. The eventual effect of these processes is the promotion of atherosclerosis. Adapted from Reilly, M. P., & Rader, D. J. (2003). The metabolic syndrome: More than the sum of its parts? *Circulation, 108*(13), 1546–1551.

---

**CHART 28-2**

### Risk Factors for Coronary Artery Disease

A modifiable risk factor is one over which a person may exercise control, such as by changing a lifestyle or personal habit or by using medication. A nonmodifiable risk factor is a circumstance over which a person has no control, such as age or heredity. A risk factor may operate independently or in tandem with other risk factors. The more risk factors a person has, the greater the likelihood of coronary artery disease. Those at risk are advised to seek regular medical examinations and to engage in "heart-healthy" behavior (a deliberate effort to reduce the number and extent of risks).

**Nonmodifiable Risk Factors**

Family history of coronary heart disease
Increasing age
Gender (men develop CAD at an earlier age than women)
Race (higher incidence of heart disease in African Americans than in Caucasians)

**Modifiable Risk Factors**

Hyperlipidemia
Cigarette smoking, tobacco use
Hypertension
Diabetes mellitus
Lack of estrogen in women
Obesity
Physical inactivity

---

may also be appropriate in some people (Pearson, Mensah, & Alexander, 2003).

## Prevention

Four modifiable risk factors—cholesterol abnormalities, tobacco use, hypertension, and diabetes mellitus—have been cited as major risk factors for CAD and its complications. As a result, they receive much attention in health promotion programs (Chart 28-2).

### Controlling Cholesterol Abnormalities

The association of a high blood cholesterol level with heart disease is well established. The metabolism of fats is an important contributor to the development of heart disease. Fats, which are insoluble in water, are encased in water-soluble lipoproteins that allow them to be transported within the circulatory system. The various lipoproteins are categorized by their protein content, which is measured in density. The density increases when more protein is present. Four elements of fat metabolism—total cholesterol, LDL, HDL, and triglycerides—affect the development of heart disease. Cholesterol is processed by the gastrointestinal tract into lipoprotein globules called chylomicrons. These are reprocessed by the liver as lipoproteins (Fig. 28-4). This is a physiologic process necessary for the formation of lipoprotein-based cell membranes and other important metabolic processes. When an excess of LDL is produced, LDL particles adhere to vulnerable points in the arterial endothelium. Here macrophages ingest them, leading to the formation of foam cells and the beginning of plaque formation.

All adults 20 years of age or older should have a fasting lipid profile (total cholesterol, LDL, HDL, and triglyceride) performed at least once every 5 years and more often if the profile is abnormal. Patients who have had an acute event (eg, MI), a **percutaneous coronary intervention (PCI)**, or a **coronary artery bypass graft (CABG)** require assessment of the LDL cholesterol level within a few months of the event or procedure, because LDL levels may be low immediately after the acute event or procedure. Subsequently, lipids should be monitored every 6 weeks until the desired level is achieved and then every 4 to 6 months (ATP III, 2001).

LDL exerts a harmful effect on the coronary vasculature because the small LDL particles can be easily transported into the vessel lining. In contrast, HDL promotes the use of total cholesterol by transporting LDL to the liver, where it is biodegraded and then excreted. The goal is to have low LDL values and high HDL values. The desired level of LDL depends on the patient:

- Less than 160 mg/dL for patients with one or no risk factors

**FIGURE 28-4.** Lipoproteins and the development of atherosclerosis. As dietary cholesterol and saturated fat are processed by the gastrointestinal tract, chylomicrons enter the blood. They are broken down into chylomicron remnants in the capillaries. The liver processes them into lipoproteins. When these are released into the circulation, excess low-density lipoproteins (LDLs) adhere to receptors on the intimal wall. Macrophages also ingest LDLs and transport them into the vessel wall, beginning the process of plaque formation (Porth, 2005). HDLs, high-density lipoproteins; VLDL, very low density lipoprotein.

- Less than 130 mg/dL for patients with two or more risk factors
- Less than 100 mg/dL for patients with CAD or at high risk for CAD. Less than 70 mg/dL is desirable for patients at very high risk for an acute coronary event (Grundy, Cleeman, Merz, et al., 2004).

Serum cholesterol and LDL levels can often be controlled by diet and physical activity. Depending on the patient's LDL level and risk of CAD, medication may also be prescribed.

The level of HDL should exceed 40 mg/dL and should ideally be more than 60 mg/dL. A high HDL level is a strong negative risk factor for heart disease (ie, it protects against disease).

Triglyceride is another fatty substance, made up of fatty acids, that is transported through the blood by a lipoprotein. Although an elevated triglyceride level (more than 200 mg/dL) may be genetic in origin, it also can be caused by obesity, physical inactivity, excessive alcohol intake, high-carbohydrate diets, diabetes mellitus, kidney disease, and certain medications, such as oral contraceptives, corticosteroids, and beta-adrenergic blockers when given in higher doses. Management of an elevated triglyceride level focuses on weight reduction and increased physical activity. Medications such as nicotinic acid and fibric acids (eg, fenofibrate [Tricor], clofibrate [Atromid-S]) may also be prescribed, especially if the triglyceride level is greater than 500 mg/dL (ATP III, 2001).

### DIETARY MEASURES

Table 28-1 provides recommendations of the Therapeutic Lifestyle Changes (TLC) diet (ATP III, 2001). These general recommendations may need to be adjusted for the individual patient who has other nutritional needs, such as the patient who is pregnant or has diabetes. To assist in following the appropriate TLC diet, the patient should be referred to a registered dietitian. Other TLC recommendations include weight loss, cessation of tobacco use, and increased physical activity.

| TABLE 28-1 | Nutrient Content of the Therapeutic Lifestyle Changes (TLC) Diet |
|---|---|
| **Nutrient** | **Recommended Intake** |
| Total calories* | Balance intake and expenditure to maintain desirable weight |
| Total fat | 25%–35% of total calories |
|   Saturated fat† | <7% of total calories |
|   Polyunsaturated fat | Up to 10% of total calories |
|   Monounsaturated fat | Up to 20% of total calories |
| Carbohydrate‡ | 50%–60% of total calories |
| Fiber | 20–30 g/day |
| Protein | Approximately 15% of total calories |
| Cholesterol | <200 mg/day |

*Daily energy expenditure should include at least moderate physical activity (contributing approximately 200 kcal per day).

†Trans-fatty acids are formed from the processing (manufacturing, hydrogenation) of vegetable oils into a more solid form. The effects of trans-fatty acids are similar to saturated fats (ie, raising low-density lipoprotein and lowering high-density lipoprotein). Intake of trans-fatty acids should be minimized.

‡Carbohydrates should be derived predominately from foods rich in complex carbohydrates, including grains, especially whole grains, fruits, and vegetables.

From Expert Panel on Detection, Evaluation, and Treatment of High Blood Cholesterol in Adults. (2001). Executive summary of the third report of the National Cholesterol Education Program (NCEP) Expert Panel on Detection, Evaluation, and Treatment of High Blood Cholesterol in Adults (Adult Treatment Panel III). *Journal of the American Medical Association, 285*(19), 2486–2497.

Soluble dietary fiber may also help reduce cholesterol levels. Soluble fibers, which are found in fresh fruit, cereal grains, vegetables, and legumes, enhance the excretion of metabolized cholesterol. The ability of fiber to reduce serum cholesterol continues to be investigated. Intake of at least 20 to 30 grams of fiber each day is recommended (ATP III, 2001).

Many resources are available to assist people to control their cholesterol levels. The National Heart, Lung, and Blood Institute (NHLBI) and its National Cholesterol Education Program (NCEP), the AHA, and the American Diabetes Association, as well as CAD support groups and reliable Internet sources, are a few examples of the available resources. Cookbooks and recipes that include the nutritional contents of foods can be included as resources for patients. Dietary control has been made easier because food manufacturers are required to provide comprehensive nutritional data on product labels. The label information of interest to a person attempting to eat a heart-healthy diet is as follows:

- Serving size, expressed in household measures
- Amount of total fat per serving
- Amount of saturated fat and trans fat per serving
- Amount of cholesterol per serving
- Amount of fiber per serving

Patients who adopt strict vegetarian dietary guidelines, such as those recommended by the Ornish Heart Disease Reversing Program, have significant reduction in blood lipids, blood glucose, body mass index, and blood pressure (Aldana, Whitmer, Greenlaw, et al., 2003). However, a program this intensive is not acceptable to all people who should modify risk factors. The effects of low-carbohydrate diets on blood lipid levels are under study.

## PHYSICAL ACTIVITY

Regular, moderate physical activity increases HDL levels and reduces triglyceride levels. The goal for the average person is a total of 30 minutes of moderate exercise (such as brisk walking) on most days (Mosca, 2004). The nurse helps the patient set realistic goals for physical activity. For example, the inactive patient can start with activity that lasts 3 minutes, such as parking farther from a building to increase daily walking time. For sustained activity, patients should begin with a 5-minute warm-up period to stretch and prepare the body for exercise. They should end the exercise with a 5-minute cool-down period in which they gradually reduce the intensity of the activity to prevent a sudden decrease in cardiac output. Patients should be instructed to engage in an activity or variety of activities that interest them, to maintain motivation. They should also be taught to exercise to an intensity that does not preclude their ability to talk; if they cannot have a conversation while exercising, they should slow down or switch to a less intensive activity. When the weather is hot and humid, the patient should exercise during the early morning, or indoors, and wear loose-fitting clothing. When the weather is cold, the patient should layer clothing and wear a hat. The nurse can also suggest walking in large stores or shopping malls in bad weather. The patient should stop any activity if chest pain, unusual shortness of breath, dizziness, lightheadedness, or nausea occurs.

## MEDICATIONS

Medications are used in some instances to control cholesterol levels (Table 28-2). If diet alone cannot normalize serum cholesterol levels, medications can have a synergistic effect with the prescribed diet. Lipid-lowering medications can reduce CAD mortality in patients with elevated lipid levels and in at-risk patients with normal lipid levels. The lipid-lowering agents affect the different lipid components and are usually grouped into four types:

- 3-Hydroxy-3-methylglutaryl coenzyme A (HMG-CoA) reductase inhibitors or statins (eg, atorvastatin [Lipitor], simvastatin [Zocor]; see Table 28-2) block cholesterol synthesis, lower LDL and triglyceride levels, and increase HDL levels. These medications are frequently the initial medication therapy for significantly elevated cholesterol and LDL levels. Because of their effect on the liver, results of hepatic function tests are monitored.
- Nicotinic acids (niacin [Niacor, Niaspan]; see Table 28-2) decrease lipoprotein synthesis, lower LDL and triglyceride levels, and increase HDL levels. The dose of niacin needs to be titrated weekly to achieve therapeutic dosage. Niacin may be used for minimally elevated cholesterol and LDL levels or as an adjunct to a statin when the lipid goal has not been achieved and triglycerides are elevated. Side effects include gastrointestinal upset, gout, and flushing. Because of the effect of niacin on the liver, hepatic function is monitored.

### TABLE 28-2  Medications Affecting Lipoprotein Metabolism

| Medication and Daily Dosage | Lipid/Lipoprotein Effects | Side Effects | Contraindications |
|---|---|---|---|
| **HMG-CoA Reductase Inhibitors (statins)** | | | |
| Lovastatin (Mevacor)<br>Prevastatin (Pravachol)<br>Simvastatin (Zocor)<br>Fluvastatin (Lescol)<br>Atorvastatin calcium (Lipitor)<br>Rosuvastatin (Crestor) | LDL ↓ 18–55%<br>HDL ↑ 5–15%<br>TG ↓ 7–30% | Myopathy, increased liver enzyme levels | Absolute: active or chronic liver disease<br>Relative: concomitant use of certain drugs* |
| **Nicotinic Acid** | | | |
| Niacin (Niacor, Niaspan)<br>Immediate-release nicotinic acid<br>Extended-release nicotinic acid<br>Sustained-release nicotinic acid | LDL ↓ 5–25%<br>HDL ↑ 15–35%<br>TG ↓ 20–50% | Flushing, hyperglycemia, hyperuricemia (or gout), upper gastrointestinal distress, hepatotoxicity | Absolute: chronic liver disease, severe gout<br>Relative: diabetes, hyperuricemia, peptic ulcer disease |
| **Fibric Acids** | | | |
| Fenofibrate (Tricor)<br>Clofibrate (Atromid-S) | LDL ↓ 5–20% (may be increased in patients with high TG)<br>HDL ↑ 10–20%<br>TG ↓ 20–50% | Dyspepsia, gallstones, myopathy, unexplained non-CHD deaths | Absolute: severe renal disease, severe hepatic disease |
| **Bile Acid Sequestrants** | | | |
| Cholestyramine (LoCholest, Questran, Prevalite)<br>Colesevelam (Welchol)<br>Colestipol HCl (Colestid) | LDL ↓ 15–30%<br>HDL ↑ 3–5%<br>TG no change or increase | Gastrointestinal distress, constipation, decreased absorption of other drugs | Absolute: dysbetalipoproteinemia, TG >400 mg/dL<br>Relative: TG >200 mg/dL |

HMG-CoA, 3-hydroxy-3-methylglutaryl coenzyme A; LDL, low-density lipoprotein; HDL, high-density lipoprotein; TG, triglycerides; ↓ decrease, ↑ increase; CHD, coronary heart disease

*Cyclosporine (Neoral, Sandimmune, SangCya); macrolide antibiotics (azithromycin [Zithromax], clarithromycin [Biaxin]; dirithromycin [Dynabac]; erythromycin [Aknemycin, E-mycin, Ery-Tab]; various antifungal agents and cytochrome P-450 inhibitors; fibrates; and niacin should be used with appropriate caution).

From Expert Panel on Detection, Evaluation, and Treatment of High Blood Cholesterol in Adults. (2001). Executive summary of the third report of the National Cholesterol Education Program (NCEP) Expert Panel on Detection, Evaluation, and Treatment of High Blood Cholesterol in Adults (Adult Treatment Panel III). *Journal of the American Medical Association, 285*(19), 2486–2497.

- Fibric acid or fibrates (eg, clofibrate [Atromid-S], fenofibrate [Tricor]; see Table 28-2) decrease the synthesis of cholesterol, reduce triglyceride levels, and increase HDL levels. They have the potential to increase LDLs and may be used in patients with triglyceride levels above 400 mg/dL. Because of the risk of myopathy and acute renal failure, fibrates should be used with caution in patients who are also taking a statin.
- Bile acid sequestrants or resins (eg, cholestyramine [LoCholest, Questran, Prevalite]; see Table 28-2) bind cholesterol in the intestine, increase its breakdown, and lower LDL levels with minimal effect on HDLs and no effect (or minimal increase) on triglyceride levels. These medications are more often used as adjunct therapy when statins alone have not been effective in controlling lipid levels and triglyceride levels are less than 200 mg/dL. Significant side effects, such as gastric distention and constipation, can occur with use of these medications.

Medication therapy is reserved for at-risk patients and is not regarded as a substitute for dietary modification. All of these medications have been shown to reduce major coronary events (ATP III, 2001).

Patients with elevated cholesterol levels should be monitored for adherence to the therapeutic plan, the effect of cholesterol-lowering medications, and the development of side effects. Lipid levels are obtained and adjustments made to the diet and medication every 6 weeks until the lipid goal or maximum dose is achieved and then every 6 months thereafter.

## Promoting Cessation of Tobacco Use

Cigarette smoking contributes to the development and severity of CAD in the following three ways:

- First, the inhalation of smoke increases the blood carbon monoxide level, and hemoglobin, the oxygen-carrying component of blood, combines more readily with carbon monoxide than with oxygen. A decreased amount of available oxygen may decrease the heart's ability to pump.
- Second, the nicotinic acid in tobacco triggers the release of catecholamines, which raise the heart rate and blood pressure. Nicotinic acid can also cause the coronary arteries to constrict. Smokers have a tenfold increase in risk for sudden cardiac death. The increase in catecholamines may be a factor in sudden cardiac death.
- Third, use of tobacco causes a detrimental vascular response and increases platelet adhesion, leading to a higher probability of thrombus formation.

A person with increased risk for heart disease is encouraged to stop tobacco use through any means possible: educational programs, counseling, consistent motivation and reinforcement messages, support groups, and medications. Some people have found complementary therapies (eg, acupuncture, guided imagery, hypnosis) to be helpful. People who stop smoking reduce their risk of heart disease by 30% to 50% within the first year, and the risk continues to decline as long as they refrain from smoking.

Exposure to other smokers' smoke (passive or secondhand smoke) is believed to cause heart disease in nonsmokers. Oral contraceptive use by women who smoke is inadvisable because these medications significantly increase the risk for CAD and sudden cardiac death.

Use of medications such as the nicotine patch (Nicotrol, NicoDerm CQ, Habitrol) or the antidepressant bupropion (Zyban) may assist with stopping use of tobacco. Products containing nicotine have some of the same effects as smoking: catecholamine release (increasing heart rate and blood pressure) and increased platelet adhesion. These medications should be used for a short time and at the lowest effective doses.

## Managing Hypertension

Hypertension is defined as blood pressure measurements that repeatedly exceed 140/90 mm Hg. The risk of cardiovascular disease increases as blood pressure increases, and people with a blood pressure greater than 120/80 mm Hg are considered prehypertensive and at risk (Chobanian, Bakris, Cushman, et al., 2003). Long-standing elevated blood pressure may result in increased stiffness of the vessel walls, leading to vessel injury and a resulting inflammatory response within the intima. Inflammatory mediators then lead to the release of growth-promoting factors that cause vessel hypertrophy and hyperresponsiveness. These changes result in acceleration and aggravation of atherosclerosis. Hypertension also increases the work of the left ventricle, which must pump harder to eject blood into the arteries. Over time, the increased workload causes the heart to enlarge and thicken (ie, hypertrophy) and may eventually lead to cardiac failure.

Early detection of high blood pressure and adherence to a therapeutic regimen can prevent the serious consequences associated with untreated elevated blood pressure. Hypertension is discussed in detail in Chapter 32.

## Controlling Diabetes Mellitus

The relationship between diabetes mellitus and heart disease has been confirmed. For 65% to 75% of patients with diabetes, cardiovascular disease is identified as the cause of death (Zipes, Libby, Bonow, et al., 2005). Hyperglycemia fosters dyslipidemia, increased platelet aggregation, and altered red blood cell function, which can lead to thrombus formation. It has been suggested that these metabolic alterations impair endothelial cell–dependent vasodilation and smooth muscle function. Treatment with insulin (eg, Humalog, Humulin, Novolin) and metformin (Glucophage) has shown improvement in endothelial function and improved endothelial-dependent dilation (Gaenzer, Neumayr, Marschang, et al., 2002). Diabetes is considered equivalent to existing CAD as a risk factor for a cardiac event within 10 years (ATP III, 2001). Diabetes is discussed in detail in Chapter 41.

## Gender

Because heart disease had been considered to primarily affect Caucasian men, the disease has not been as readily recognized and treated in women. However, in the United States, it is reported that more than 500,000 women die of cardiovascular disease each year, a number that exceeds that for men and is higher than the next seven causes of death combined (AHA, 2004). For women, cardiovascular events occur an average of 10 years later in life than in men, but overall, women tend to have a higher incidence of complications from cardiovascular disease and a higher mortality. African-American women have a mortality rate nearly twice that of Caucasian women (AHA, 2004). Women tend not to recognize the symptoms as early as men and to wait longer to report their symptoms and seek medical assistance (Nabel & Selker, 2004). In the past, women were less likely than men to be referred for coronary artery diagnostic procedures, to receive medical therapy (eg, **thrombolytic** therapy to break down the blood clots that cause acute MI, or nitroglycerin), and to be treated with invasive interventions (eg, angioplasty) (Sheifer, Escarce, & Schulman, 2000). With better education of health care professionals and the general public, gender differences now have less influence on diagnosis and treatment. A recent analysis of procedures used for acute MI found that women were as likely as men to undergo cardiac catheterization and PCIs but were less likely to undergo coronary bypass surgery (Bertoni, Bonds, Lovato, et al., 2004).

In women younger than 55 years of age, the incidence of CAD is significantly lower than in men. However, in women older than 55 years of age, the incidence of CAD is approximately equal to that in men. The age difference between women and men newly diagnosed with CAD was traditionally thought to be related to estrogen. It is now recognized that menopause is a milestone in the aging process during which risk factors tend to accumulate. Cardiovascular disease may be well developed by the time of menopause, despite the supposed protective effects of estrogen (Mosca, 2004). Although hormone therapy (HT)—formerly referred to as hormone replacement therapy (HRT)—for menopausal women was once promoted as preventive therapy for CAD, research studies do not support HT as an effective means of prevention. HT decreases menopausal symptoms and the risk for osteoporosis-related bone fractures, but HT also has been associated with an increased incidence of CAD, breast cancer, deep vein thrombosis, stroke, and pulmonary embolism. The Women's Health Initiative demonstrated that long-term HT use may have more risks than benefits, and that HT should not be initiated or continued for primary prevention of CAD. The U.S. Preventive Services Task Force (2003) concurred with these recommendations.

## Behavior Patterns

Many clinicians believe that stress and certain behaviors contribute to the pathogenesis of CAD and cardiac events. Psychological and epidemiologic studies have identified behaviors that characterize people who are prone to heart disease: excessive competitiveness, a sense of time urgency or impatience, aggressiveness, and hostility. A person with these behaviors is classified as having a type A personality.

The type A personality may not be as significant as was once thought; evidence of its precise role remains inconclusive. Current predictors of coronary events focus on physiologic factors (Moustapha & Anderson, 2003). However, it has long been recognized that emotional stress can lead to a release of catecholamines and subsequent coronary ischemia. Thus, people with type A traits are advised to alter behaviors and responses to triggering events and to reduce other risk factors. Nurses can assist by teaching cognitive restructuring and relaxation techniques. Because depression is associated with negative outcomes, patients should also be assessed for depression and appropriately treated.

## *Angina Pectoris*

Angina pectoris is a clinical syndrome usually characterized by episodes or paroxysms of pain or pressure in the anterior chest. The cause is insufficient coronary blood flow, resulting in a decreased oxygen supply when there is increased myocardial demand for oxygen in response to physical exertion or emotional stress. In other words, the need for oxygen exceeds the supply. The severity of angina is based on the precipitating activity and its effect on activities of daily living.

## Pathophysiology

Angina is usually caused by atherosclerotic disease. Almost invariably, angina is associated with a significant obstruction of a major coronary artery. Normally, the myocardium extracts a large amount of oxygen from the coronary circulation to meet its continuous demands. When there is an increase in demand, flow through the coronary arteries needs to be increased. When there is blockage in a coronary artery, flow cannot be increased, and ischemia results. The types of angina are listed in Chart 28-3. Several factors are associated with typical anginal pain:

- Physical exertion, which can precipitate an attack by increasing myocardial oxygen demand

### CHART 28-3

### Types of Angina

- **Stable angina:** predictable and consistent pain that occurs on exertion and is relieved by rest
- **Unstable angina** (also called preinfarction angina or crescendo angina): symptoms occur more frequently and last longer than stable angina. The threshold for pain is lower, and pain may occur at rest.
- **Intractable or refractory angina:** severe incapacitating chest pain
- **Variant angina** (also called Prinzmetal's angina): pain at rest with reversible ST-segment elevation; thought to be caused by coronary artery vasospasm
- **Silent ischemia:** objective evidence of ischemia (such as ECG changes with a stress test), but patient reports no symptoms

- Exposure to cold, which can cause vasoconstriction and elevated blood pressure, with increased oxygen demand
- Eating a heavy meal, which increases the blood flow to the mesenteric area for digestion, thereby reducing the blood supply available to the heart muscle. In a severely compromised heart, shunting of blood for digestion can be sufficient to induce anginal pain.
- Stress or any emotion-provoking situation, causing the release of catecholamines, which increases blood pressure, heart rate, and myocardial workload

Atypical angina is not associated with these listed factors. It may occur at rest.

## Clinical Manifestations

Ischemia of the heart muscle may produce pain or other symptoms, varying in severity from mild indigestion to a choking or heavy sensation in the upper chest that ranges from discomfort to agonizing pain accompanied by severe apprehension and a feeling of impending death. The pain is often felt deep in the chest behind the sternum (retrosternal area). Typically, the pain or discomfort is poorly localized and may radiate to the neck, jaw, shoulders, and inner aspects of the upper arms, usually the left arm. The patient often feels tightness or a heavy, choking, or strangling sensation that has a viselike, insistent quality. The patient with diabetes mellitus may not have severe pain with angina because diabetic neuropathy can blunt nociceptors' transmission, dulling the perception of pain. A woman may have different symptoms than a man, because coronary disease in women tends to be more diffuse and affects long segments of the artery rather than discrete segments.

A feeling of weakness or numbness in the arms, wrists, and hands, as well as shortness of breath, pallor, diaphoresis, dizziness or lightheadedness, and nausea and vomiting, may accompany the pain. Anxiety may occur with angina. An important characteristic of angina is that it subsides with

## NURSING RESEARCH PROFILE

### Recognizing the Symptoms of Unstable Angina

DeVon, H. A., & Zerwic, J. J. (2003). The symptoms of unstable angina—do women and men differ? *Nursing Research, 52*(2), 108–118.

**Purpose**
Previous research has identified differences in the epidemiology, presentation, and outcomes of women and men with coronary artery disease. The purpose of this study was to determine whether there are gender differences in the symptoms of unstable angina, and if so, whether these differences remain after controlling for age, diabetes, anxiety, depression, and functional status.

**Design**
A convenience sample of 50 women and 50 men hospitalized with unstable angina was recruited from two medical centers. A quantitative, nonexperimental design was used. Subjects were interviewed in their hospital rooms. Three instruments (the Unstable Angina Symptoms Questionnaire [UASQ], the Canadian Cardiovascular Society [CCS] classification of angina, and the Hospital Anxiety and Depression Scale [HADS]) were used to assess anginal symptoms, anxiety, and depression.

**Findings**
The most frequently reported symptoms for both genders were chest pain and shortness of breath. More women than men experienced shortness of breath (74% versus 60%), weakness (74% versus 48%), difficulty breathing (66% versus 38%), nausea (42% versus 22%), and loss of appetite (40% versus 10%). Women also experienced more back pain, stabbing pain, and depression. The researchers concluded that during episodes of unstable angina, women have similar symptoms to those of men, but a higher proportion of women also have symptoms considered to be less typical, including upper back pain, stabbing pain, and knife-like pain.

**Nursing Implications**
The results of this study are consistent with previous studies that focused on gender differences in symptoms of acute myocardial infarction. Nurses should be aware that women with unstable angina frequently present with typical symptoms but may also present with a number of less typical symptoms. Patient assessment should include a careful history to elicit these symptoms. In addition, women should be educated about both typical and atypical symptoms of acute coronary events.

---

rest or nitroglycerin. In many patients, anginal symptoms follow a stable, predictable pattern.

Unstable angina is characterized by attacks that increase in frequency and severity and are not relieved by rest and nitroglycerin. Patients with unstable angina require medical intervention.

### Gerontologic Considerations

The elderly person with angina may not exhibit the typical pain profile because of the diminished responses of neurotransmitters that occur with aging. Often, the presenting symptom in the elderly is dyspnea. If pain occurs, it is atypical pain that radiates to both arms rather than just the left arm. Sometimes, there are no symptoms ("silent" CAD), making recognition and diagnosis a clinical challenge. Elderly patients should be encouraged to recognize their chest pain–like symptom (eg, weakness) as an indication that they should rest or take prescribed medications. Pharmacologic stress testing may be used to diagnose CAD in elderly patients because other conditions (eg, peripheral vascular disease, arthritis, degenerative disk disease, physical disability, foot problems) may limit the patient's ability to exercise (Chart 28-4).

## Assessment and Diagnostic Findings

The diagnosis of angina begins with the patient's history related to the clinical manifestations of ischemia. A 12-lead electrocardiogram (ECG) and blood laboratory values help in making the diagnosis. The patient may undergo an exercise or pharmacologic stress test in which the heart is monitored by ECG, echocardiogram, or both. The patient may also be referred for a nuclear scan or invasive procedure (eg, cardiac catheterization, coronary artery angiography).

Because CAD is believed to result from inflammation of the arterial endothelium, C-reactive protein (CRP), a marker for inflammation of vascular endothelium, may be measured. High blood levels of CRP have been associated with increased coronary artery calcification and risk of an acute cardiovascular event (eg, MI) in seemingly healthy people (Ridker, Rifai, Rose, et al., 2002). There is interest in using CRP levels as an additional risk factor for cardiovascular disease in clinical evaluation and research, but the predictive value of CRP levels has not yet been fully established (Pearson et al., 2003).

## Medical Management

The objectives of the medical management of angina are to decrease the oxygen demand of the myocardium and to increase the oxygen supply. Medically, these objectives are met through pharmacologic therapy and control of risk factors. Alternatively, reperfusion procedures may be used to restore the blood supply to the myocardium. These include PCI procedures (eg, **percutaneous transluminal coronary angioplasty [PTCA]**, intracoronary stents, and atherectomy) and CABG.

## CHART 28-4 Ethics and Related Issues

### Should Aggressive Treatment be Recommended for the Elderly With Acute Coronary Syndrome (ACS)?

**SITUATION**

Many patients who present with acute coronary events are elderly. They often have chronic conditions such as diabetes or arthritis. Elderly patients have traditionally been managed conservatively with medications, but currently interventions such as cardiac catheterization may be recommended. These patients look to their family members for help with treatment decisions.

**DILEMMA**

An 80-year-old woman is hospitalized with unstable angina. The cardiologist discusses the situation with her two adult sons. He recommends cardiac catheterization with possible PTCA and stent placement. The patient is oriented but lethargic. She defers to her sons regarding treatment decisions. One son worries that she will be subjected to an invasive procedure that is potentially high risk, painful, expensive, and possibly futile. The second son feels that if there is hope of success, she should have the procedure.

**DISCUSSION**

Research on the risks and benefits of treatment for ACS now includes the elderly as a subgroup. One study reports that the elderly may benefit as much, if not more, than younger patients from coronary reperfusion procedures in terms of reduction of death or myocardial infarction (Bach, Cannon, Weintraub, et al., 2004)

1. What arguments would you offer that support or discourage aggressive treatment for ACS in the elderly?
2. What assistance can you offer to enhance the patient and family's autonomy regarding decision making as well as their sense of justice regarding the allocation of resources?

## Pharmacologic Therapy

### NITROGLYCERIN

Nitrates remain the mainstay for treatment of angina pectoris. A vasoactive agent, nitroglycerin (Nitrostat, Nitrol, Nitro-Bid) is administered to reduce myocardial oxygen consumption, which decreases ischemia and relieves pain. Nitroglycerin dilates primarily the veins and, in higher doses, also the arteries. Dilation of the veins causes venous pooling of blood throughout the body. As a result, less blood returns to the heart, and filling pressure (preload) is reduced. If the patient is hypovolemic (does not have adequate circulating blood volume), the decrease in filling pressure can cause a significant decrease in cardiac output and blood pressure.

Nitrates in higher doses also relax the systemic arteriolar bed, lowering blood pressure and decreasing afterload. These effects decrease myocardial oxygen requirements and increase oxygen supply, bringing about a more favorable balance between supply and demand.

Nitroglycerin may be given by several routes: sublingual tablet or spray, oral capsule, topical agent, and intravenous (IV) administration. Sublingual nitroglycerin is generally placed under the tongue or in the cheek (buccal pouch) and alleviates the pain of ischemia within 3 minutes. Chart 28-5 provides more information on self-administration of sublingual nitroglycerin. Oral preparations and topical patches are used to provide sustained effects. The patches are often applied in the morning and removed at bedtime. This regimen allows for a nitrate-free period to prevent the development of tolerance.

A continuous or intermittent IV infusion of nitroglycerin may be administered to the hospitalized patient with recurring signs and symptoms of ischemia or after a revascularization procedure. The amount of nitroglycerin administered is based on the patient's symptoms while avoiding side effects such as hypotension. It usually is not administered if the systolic blood pressure is 90 mm Hg or less. Generally, after the patient is symptom-free, the nitroglycerin may be switched to a topical preparation within 24 hours.

### BETA-ADRENERGIC BLOCKING AGENTS

Beta-blockers such as metoprolol (Lopressor, Toprol) and atenolol (Tenormin) reduce myocardial oxygen consumption by blocking beta-adrenergic sympathetic stimulation to the heart. The result is a reduction in heart rate, slowed conduction of impulses through the conduction system, decreased blood pressure, and reduced myocardial **contractility** (force of contraction) to balance the myocardial oxygen needs (demands) and the amount of oxygen available (supply). This helps control chest pain and delays the onset of ischemia during work or exercise. Beta-blockers reduce the incidence of recurrent angina, infarction, and cardiac mortality. The dose can be titrated to achieve a resting heart rate of 50 to 60 beats per minute.

Cardiac side effects and possible contraindications include hypotension, bradycardia, advanced atrioventricular block, and decompensated heart failure. If a beta-blocker is given IV for an acute cardiac event, the ECG, blood pressure, and heart rate are monitored closely after the medication has been administered. Because some beta-blockers also affect the beta-adrenergic receptors in the bronchioles, causing bronchoconstriction, they are contraindicated in patients with significant pulmonary obstructive diseases, such as asthma. Other side effects include depression, fatigue, decreased libido, and masking of symptoms of hypoglycemia. Patients taking beta-blockers are cautioned not to stop taking them abruptly, because angina may worsen and MI may develop. Beta-blocker therapy should be decreased gradually over several days before being discontinued. Patients with

### CHART 28-5  PHARMACOLOGY · Self-Administration of Nitroglycerin

Most patients with angina pectoris must self-administer nitroglycerin on an as-needed basis. A key nursing role in such cases is educating patients about the medication and how to take it. Sublingual nitroglycerin comes in tablet and spray forms.

- Instruct the patient to make sure the mouth is moist, the tongue is still, and saliva is not swallowed until the nitroglycerin tablet dissolves. If the pain is severe, the patient can crush the tablet between the teeth to hasten sublingual absorption.
- Advise the patient to carry the medication at all times as a precaution. However, because nitroglycerin is very unstable, it should be carried securely in its original container (eg, capped dark glass bottle); tablets should never be removed and stored in metal or plastic pillboxes.
- Explain that nitroglycerin is volatile and is inactivated by heat, moisture, air, light, and time. Instruct the patient to renew the nitroglycerin supply every 6 months.
- Inform the patient that the medication should be taken in anticipation of any activity that may produce pain. Because nitroglycerin increases tolerance for exercise and stress when taken prophylactically (ie, before angina-producing activity, such as exercise, stair-climbing, or sexual intercourse), it is best taken before pain develops.
- Recommend that the patient note how long it takes for the nitroglycerin to relieve the discomfort. Advise the patient that if pain persists after taking three sublingual tablets at 5-minute intervals, emergency medical services should be called.
- Discuss possible side effects of nitroglycerin, including flushing, throbbing headache, hypotension, and tachycardia.
- Advise the patient to sit down for a few minutes when taking nitroglycerin to avoid hypotension and syncope.

---

diabetes who take beta-blockers are instructed to monitor their blood glucose levels often and to observe for signs and symptoms of hypoglycemia.

### CALCIUM CHANNEL BLOCKING AGENTS

Calcium channel blockers (calcium ion antagonists) have a variety of effects. These agents decrease sinoatrial node automaticity and atrioventricular node conduction, resulting in a slower heart rate and a decrease in the strength of the heart muscle contraction (negative inotropic effect). These effects decrease the workload of the heart. Calcium channel blockers also relax the blood vessels, causing a decrease in blood pressure and an increase in coronary artery perfusion. Calcium channel blockers increase myocardial oxygen supply by dilating the smooth muscle wall of the coronary arterioles; they decrease myocardial oxygen demand by reducing systemic arterial pressure and the workload of the left ventricle.

The calcium channel blockers most commonly used are amlodipine (Norvasc) and diltiazem (Cardizem, Tiazac). They may be used by patients who cannot take beta-blockers, who develop significant side effects from beta-blockers or nitrates, or who still have pain despite beta-blocker and nitroglycerin therapy. Calcium channel blockers are also used to prevent and treat vasospasm, which commonly occurs after an invasive interventional procedure.

First-generation calcium channel blockers such as nifedipine should be avoided or used with great caution in people with heart failure, because they decrease myocardial contractility. Amlodipine and felodipine (Plendil) are the calcium channel blockers of choice for patients with heart failure. Hypotension may occur after the IV administration of any of the calcium channel blockers. Other side effects may include atrioventricular block, bradycardia, constipation, and gastric distress.

### ANTIPLATELET AND ANTICOAGULANT MEDICATIONS

Antiplatelet medications are administered to prevent platelet aggregation and subsequent thrombosis, which impedes blood flow.

**Aspirin.** Aspirin prevents platelet activation and reduces the incidence of MI and death in patients with CAD. A 160- to 325-mg dose of aspirin should be given to the patient with angina as soon as the diagnosis is made (eg, in the emergency department or physician's office) and then continued with 81 to 325 mg daily. Although aspirin may be one of the most important medications in the treatment of CAD, it may be overlooked because of its low cost and common use. Patients should be advised to continue aspirin even if they concurrently take nonsteroidal anti-inflammatory drugs (NSAIDs) or other analgesics. Because aspirin may cause gastrointestinal upset and bleeding, the use of $H_2$-blockers (eg, famotidine [Pepcid], ranitidine [Zantac]) or proton pump inhibitors (eg, omeprazole [Prilosec]) should be considered to allow continued aspirin therapy.

**Clopidogrel and Ticlopidine.** Clopidogrel (Plavix) or ticlopidine (Ticlid) is given to patients who are allergic to aspirin or given in addition to aspirin in patients at high risk for MI. Unlike aspirin, these medications take a few days to achieve their antiplatelet effect. They also cause gastrointestinal upset.

**Heparin.** IV unfractionated heparin prevents the formation of new blood clots. Treating patients with unstable angina with heparin reduces the occurrence of MI. If the patient's signs and symptoms indicate a significant risk for a cardiac event, the patient is hospitalized and may be given an IV bolus of heparin and started on a continuous infusion. The amount of heparin administered is based on the results of the activated partial thromboplastin time (aPTT). Heparin therapy is usually considered therapeutic when the aPTT is 2 to 2.5 times the normal aPTT value.

A subcutaneous injection of low-molecular-weight heparin (LMWH; enoxaparin [Lovenox] or dalteparin [Fragmin]) may be used instead of IV unfractionated heparin to treat patients with unstable angina or non–ST-segment elevation MIs (Antman, Anbe, Armstrong, et al., 2004). LMWH provides effective and stable anticoagulation, potentially reducing the risk of rebound ischemic events, and it eliminates the need to monitor aPTT results. LMWH may be beneficial before and during PCIs and for ST-segment elevation MIs.

Because unfractionated heparin and LMWH increase the risk of bleeding, the patient is monitored for signs and symptoms of external and internal bleeding, such as low blood pressure, increased heart rate, and decreased serum hemoglobin and hematocrit. The patient receiving heparin is placed on bleeding precautions, which include:

- Applying pressure to the site of any needle puncture for a longer time than usual
- Avoiding intramuscular (IM) injections
- Avoiding tissue injury and bruising from trauma or use of constrictive devices (eg, continuous use of an automatic blood pressure cuff)

A decrease in platelet count or evidence of thrombosis may indicate heparin-induced thrombocytopenia (HIT), an antibody-mediated reaction to heparin that may result in thrombosis (Cleveland, 2003). Patients who have received heparin within the past 3 months and those who have been receiving unfractionated heparin for 5 to 15 days are at high risk for HIT.

**Glycoprotein IIb/IIIa Agents.** IV administration of glycoprotein *(GP) IIb/IIIa agents* (abciximab [ReoPro], tirofiban [Aggrastat], eptifibatide [Integrilin]) is indicated for hospitalized patients with unstable angina and as adjunct therapy for PCI. These agents prevent platelet aggregation by blocking the GPIIb/IIIa receptors on the platelets, preventing adhesion of fibrinogen and other factors that crosslink platelets to each other and thereby allow platelets to form a thrombus (clot). As with heparin, bleeding is the major side effect, and bleeding precautions should be initiated.

### OXYGEN ADMINISTRATION

Oxygen therapy is usually initiated at the onset of chest pain in an attempt to increase the amount of oxygen delivered to the myocardium and to decrease pain. The therapeutic effectiveness of oxygen is determined by observing the rate and rhythm of respirations. Blood oxygen saturation is monitored by pulse oximetry; the normal oxygen saturation ($SpO_2$) level is greater than 93%.

## The Patient With Angina Pectoris

### Assessment

The nurse gathers information about the patient's symptoms and activities, especially those that precede and precipitate attacks of angina pectoris. Appropriate questions are listed in Chart 28-6, using a PQRST format. Other helpful questions may be asked: How long

### CHART 28-6

### Assessing for Symptoms Associated With Angina

| ACRONYM | FACTORS ABOUT PAIN THAT NEED TO BE ASSESSED | ASSESSMENT QUESTIONS |
|---|---|---|
| P | Position/Location | "Where is the pain? Can you point to it?" |
|   | Provocation | "What were you doing when the pain began?" |
| Q | Quality | "How would you describe the pain?" |
|   |         | "Is it like the pain you had before?" |
|   | Quantity | "Has the pain been constant?" |
| R | Radiation | "Can you feel the pain anywhere else?" |
|   | Relief | "Did anything make the pain better?" |
| S | Severity | "How would you rate the pain on a 0–10 scale with 0 being no pain and 10 being the most amount of pain?" (or use visual analog scale or adjective rating scale) |
|   | Symptoms | "Did you notice any other symptoms with the pain?" |
| T | Timing | "How long ago did the pain start?" |

Jarvis, C. (2004) *Physical examination and health assessment* (4th ed.) St. Louis: Saunders.

does the angina usually last? Does nitroglycerin relieve the angina? If so, how many tablets or sprays are needed to achieve relief? How long does it takes for relief to occur?

The answers to these questions form a basis for designing an effective program of treatment and prevention. In addition to assessing angina pectoris or its equivalent, the nurse also assesses the patient's risk factors for CAD, the patient's response to angina, the patient's and family's understanding of the diagnosis, and adherence to the current treatment plan.

## Diagnosis

### Nursing Diagnoses

Based on the assessment data, major nursing diagnoses may include:

- Ineffective cardiac tissue perfusion secondary to CAD, as evidenced by chest pain or equivalent symptoms
- Death anxiety
- Deficient knowledge about the underlying disease and methods for avoiding complications
- Noncompliance, ineffective management of therapeutic regimen related to failure to accept necessary lifestyle changes

### Collaborative Problems/ Potential Complications

Potential complications that may develop include the following, which are discussed in the chapters indicated:

- Acute pulmonary edema (see Chapter 30)
- Heart failure (see Chapter 30)
- Cardiogenic shock (see Chapter 30)
- Dysrhythmias and cardiac arrest (see Chapters 27 and 30)
- MI (described later in this chapter)

## Planning and Goals

Major patient goals include immediate and appropriate treatment when angina occurs, prevention of angina, reduction of anxiety, awareness of the disease process and understanding of the prescribed care, adherence to the self-care program, and absence of complications.

## Nursing Interventions

### Treating Angina

If the patient reports pain (or the person's equivalent to pain), the nurse takes immediate action. When a patient experiences angina, the nurse directs the patient to stop all activities and sit or rest in bed in a semi-Fowler's position to reduce the oxygen requirements of the ischemic myocardium. The nurse assesses the patient's angina, asking questions to determine whether the angina is the same as the patient typically experiences. A change may indicate a worsening of the disease or a different cause. The nurse then continues to assess the patient, measuring vital signs and observing for signs of respiratory distress. If the patient is in the hospital, a 12-lead ECG is usually obtained and scrutinized for ST-segment and T-wave changes. If the patient has been placed on cardiac monitoring with continuous ST-segment monitoring, the ST segment is assessed for changes.

Nitroglycerin is administered sublingually, and the patient's response is assessed (relief of chest pain and effect on blood pressure and heart rate). If the chest pain is unchanged or is lessened but still present, nitroglycerin administration is repeated up to three doses. Each time blood pressure, heart rate, and the ST segment (if the patient is on a monitor with ST-segment monitoring capability) are assessed. The nurse administers oxygen therapy if the patient's respiratory rate is increased or if the oxygen saturation level is decreased. Oxygen is usually administered at 2 L/min by nasal cannula, even without evidence of respiratory distress, although there is no documentation of its effect on outcome. If the pain is significant and continues after these interventions, the patient is further evaluated for acute MI and may be transferred to a higher-acuity nursing unit.

### Reducing Anxiety

Patients with angina often fear loss of their roles within society and the family. They may also fear that the pain may lead to an MI or death. Exploring the implications that the diagnosis has for the patient and providing information about the illness, its treatment, and methods of preventing its progression are important nursing interventions. Various stress reduction methods should be explored with the patient. For example, music therapy, in which patients listen to selected music through headphones, has been shown to reduce anxiety in patients who are in a coronary care unit and may serve as an adjunct to therapeutic communication (Evans, 2002). Addressing the spiritual needs of the patient and family may also assist in allaying anxieties and fears.

### Preventing Pain

The nurse reviews the assessment findings, identifies the level of activity that causes the patient's pain, and plans the patient's activities accordingly. If the patient has pain frequently or with minimal activity, the nurse alternates the patient's activities with rest periods. Balancing activity and rest is an important aspect of the educational plan for the patient and family.

### Promoting Home and Community-Based Care

#### TEACHING PATIENTS SELF-CARE
Learning about the modifiable risk factors that contribute to the development of CAD and resulting

angina is essential. Exploring what the patient and family see as their priorities in managing the disease and developing a plan based on those priorities can assist with patient adherence to the therapeutic regimen. It is important to explore with the patient methods to avoid, modify, or adapt the triggers for anginal pain. The teaching program for the patient with angina is designed so that the patient and family understand the illness, identify the symptoms of myocardial ischemia, state the actions to take when symptoms develop, and discuss methods to prevent chest pain and the advancement of CAD. The goals of the educational program are to reduce the frequency and severity of anginal attacks, to delay the progress of the underlying disease if possible, and to prevent complications. The factors outlined in Chart 28-7 are important in educating the patient with angina pectoris.

The self-care program is prepared in collaboration with the patient and family or friends. Activities should be planned to minimize the occurrence of angina episodes. The patient needs to understand that any pain unrelieved within 15 minutes by the usual methods, including nitroglycerin (see Chart 28-5), should be treated at the closest emergency center; the patient should call 911 for assistance.

### CONTINUING CARE

Arrangements are made for a home care nurse when appropriate. The home care nurse assists the patient with scheduling and keeping follow-up appointments. The patient may need reminders about follow-up monitoring, including periodic blood laboratory testing and ECGs. In addition, the home care nurse may monitor the patient's adherence to dietary restrictions and to prescribed antianginal medications, including nitroglycerin. If the patient has severe anginal symptoms, the nurse may assess the home environment and recommend modifications that diminish the occurrence of anginal episodes. For instance, if a patient cannot climb stairs without experiencing ischemia, the home care nurse may help the patient plan daily activities that minimize stair climbing. Some patients may benefit from moving the bedroom to a lower level in the home.

## Evaluation

### Expected Patient Outcomes

Expected patient outcomes may include:

1. Reports that pain is relieved promptly
   a. Recognizes symptoms
   b. Takes immediate action
   c. Seeks medical assistance if pain persists or changes in quality
2. Reports decreased anxiety
   a. Expresses acceptance of diagnosis
   b. Expresses control over choices within medical regimen
   c. Does not exhibit signs and symptoms that indicate a high level of anxiety

---

### CHART 28-7

### HOME CARE CHECKLIST • Managing Angina Pectoris

| At the completion of home care instructions, the patient and significant other will be able to: | Patient | Caregiver |
|---|---|---|
| • Reduce the probability of an episode of anginal pain by balancing rest with activity: | | |
| – Participate in a regular daily program of activities that do not produce chest discomfort, shortness of breath, or undue fatigue. | ✔ | |
| – Avoid exercises requiring sudden bursts of activity; avoid isometric exercise. | ✔ | |
| – State that temperature extremes (particularly cold) may induce anginal pain; therefore, avoid exercise in temperature extremes. | ✔ | |
| – Alternate activity with periods of rest. | ✔ | |
| – Use appropriate resources for support during emotionally stressful times (eg, counselor, nurse, clergy, physician). | ✔ | ✔ |
| • Avoid using medications or any over-the-counter substances (eg, diet pills, nasal decongestants) that can increase the heart rate and blood pressure without first discussing with a health care provider. | ✔ | ✔ |
| • Stop smoking and other use of tobacco, and avoid second-hand smoke (because smoking increases the heart rate, blood pressure, and blood carbon monoxide levels). | ✔ | ✔ |
| • Eat a diet low in saturated fat, high in fiber, and if indicated, lower in calories. | ✔ | ✔ |
| • Achieve and maintain normal blood pressure. | ✔ | |
| • Achieve and maintain normal blood glucose levels. | ✔ | |
| • Take medications, especially aspirin and beta-blockers, as prescribed. | ✔ | |
| • Carry nitroglycerin at all times; state when and how to use it; identify its side effects. | ✔ | ✔ |

3. Understands ways to avoid complications and is free of complications
   a. Describes the process of angina
   b. Explains reasons for measures to prevent complications
   c. Exhibits normal ECG and cardiac biomarkers
   d. Experiences no signs and symptoms of acute MI
4. Adheres to self-care program
   a. Takes medications as prescribed
   b. Keeps health care appointments
   c. Implements plan to reduce risk factors

# Myocardial Infarction (MI)

## Pathophysiology

In an MI, an area of the myocardium is permanently destroyed. MI is usually caused by reduced blood flow in a coronary artery due to rupture of an atherosclerotic plaque and subsequent occlusion of the artery by a thrombus. In unstable angina, the plaque ruptures but the artery is not completely occluded. Because unstable angina and acute MI are considered to be the same process but different points along a continuum, the term **acute coronary syndrome** (ACS) may be used in lieu of these diagnoses. Other causes of MI include vasospasm (sudden constriction or narrowing) of a coronary artery, decreased oxygen supply (eg, from acute blood loss, anemia, or low blood pressure), and increased demand for oxygen (eg, from a rapid heart rate, thyrotoxicosis, or ingestion of cocaine). In each case, a profound imbalance exists between myocardial oxygen supply and demand.

Coronary occlusion, heart attack, and MI are terms used synonymously, but the preferred term is MI. The area of infarction develops over minutes to hours. As the cells are deprived of oxygen, ischemia develops, cellular injury occurs, and the lack of oxygen results in infarction, or the death of cells. The expression "time is muscle" reflects the urgency of appropriate treatment to improve patient outcomes. Each year in the United States, nearly 900,000 people have acute MIs; one fourth of these people die of MI (AHA, 2004). Half of those who die never reach a hospital.

Various descriptions are used to further identify an MI: the type of MI (ST-segment elevation, non–ST-segment elevation), the location of the injury to the ventricular wall (anterior, inferior, posterior, or lateral wall), and the point in time within the process of infarction (acute, evolving, or old).

The ECG usually identifies the type and location, and other ECG indicators such as a Q wave and patient history identify the timing. Regardless of the location of the infarction of cardiac muscle, the goal of medical therapy is to prevent or minimize myocardial tissue death and to prevent complications. The pathophysiology of heart disease and the risk factors involved were discussed earlier in this chapter.

## Clinical Manifestations

Chest pain that occurs suddenly and continues despite rest and medication is the presenting symptom in most patients with an MI (Chart 28-8). Some of these patients have prodromal symptoms or a previous diagnosis of CAD, but about half report no previous symptoms (AHA, 2004). Patients may

---

### CHART 28-8

### Assessing for Acute Myocardial Infarction (MI) or Acute Coronary Syndrome (ACS)

Be on the alert for the following signs and symptoms:

**Cardiovascular**
- Chest pain or discomfort, palpitations. Heart sounds may include $S_3$, $S_4$, and new onset of a murmur.
- Increased jugular venous distention may be seen if the MI has caused heart failure.
- Blood pressure may be elevated because of sympathetic stimulation or decreased because of decreased contractility, impending cardiogenic shock, or medications.
- Pulse deficit may indicate atrial fibrillation.
- In addition to ST-segment and T-wave changes, ECG may show tachycardia, bradycardia, or dysrhythmias.

**Respiratory**
Shortness of breath, dyspnea, tachypnea, and crackles if MI has caused pulmonary congestion. Pulmonary edema may be present.

**Gastrointestinal**
Nausea and vomiting.

**Genitourinary**
Decreased urinary output may indicate cardiogenic shock.

**Skin**
Cool, clammy, diaphoretic, and pale appearance due to sympathetic stimulation may indicate cardiogenic shock.

**Neurologic**
Anxiety, restlessness, and light-headedness may indicate increased sympathetic stimulation or a decrease in contractility and cerebral oxygenation. The same symptoms may also herald cardiogenic shock.

**Psychological**
Fear with feeling of impending doom, or patient may deny that anything is wrong.

---

present with a combination of symptoms, including chest pain, shortness of breath, indigestion, nausea, and anxiety. They may have cool, pale, and moist skin. Their heart rate and respiratory rate may be faster than normal. These signs and symptoms, which are caused by stimulation of the sympathetic nervous system, may be present for only a short time or may persist. In many cases, the signs and symptoms of MI cannot be distinguished from those of unstable angina.

## Assessment and Diagnostic Findings

The diagnosis of MI is generally based on the presenting symptoms, the ECG, and laboratory test results (eg, serial cardiac biomarker values). The prognosis depends on the severity of coronary artery obstruction and the extent of myocardial damage. Physical examination is always conducted, but the examination alone does not confirm the diagnosis.

## Patient History

The patient history has two parts: the description of the presenting symptom (eg, pain) and the history of previous illnesses and family history of heart disease. Previous history should also include information about the patient's risk factors for heart disease.

## Electrocardiogram

The ECG provides information that assists in diagnosing acute MI. It should be obtained within 10 minutes from the time a patient reports pain or arrives in the emergency department. By monitoring serial ECG changes over time, the location, evolution, and resolution of an MI can be identified and monitored.

The ECG changes that occur with an MI are seen in the leads that view the involved surface of the heart. The classic ECG changes are T-wave inversion, ST-segment elevation, and development of an abnormal Q wave (Fig. 28-5). Because infarction evolves over time, the ECG also changes over time. The first ECG signs of an acute MI occur as a result of myocardial ischemia and injury. Myocardial injury causes the T wave to become enlarged and symmetric. As the area of injury becomes ischemic, myocardial repolarization is altered and delayed, causing the T wave to invert. The ischemic region may remain depolarized while adjacent areas of the myocardium return to the resting state. Myocardial injury also causes ST-segment changes. The injured myocardial cells depolarize normally but repolarize more rapidly than normal cells, causing the ST segment to rise at least 1 mm above the isoelectric line (area between the T wave and the next P wave is used as the reference for the isoelectric line) when measured 0.06 to 0.08 seconds after the end of the QRS, a point called the J point (Fig. 28-6). This elevation in the ST segment in two contiguous leads is a key diagnostic indicator for MI.

The appearance of abnormal Q waves is another indication of MI. Q waves develop within 1 to 3 days because there is no depolarization current conducted from necrotic tissue. The lead system then views the flow of current from other parts of the heart. An abnormal Q wave is 0.04 seconds or longer, 25% of the R-wave depth (provided the R wave exceeds a depth of 5 mm), or did not exist before the event. An acute MI may also cause a significant decrease in the height of the R wave. During an acute MI, injury and ischemic changes are usually present. An abnormal Q wave may be present without ST-segment and T-wave changes, which indicates an old, not acute, MI. For some patients, there are no persistent ECG changes, and the MI is diagnosed by blood levels of cardiac biomarkers.

Using the above information, patients are diagnosed with one of the following forms of ACS:

- Unstable angina: The patient has clinical manifestations of coronary ischemia, but ECG or cardiac biomarkers show no evidence of acute MI.
- ST-segment elevation MI: The patient has ECG evidence of acute MI with characteristic changes in two contiguous leads on a 12-lead ECG. In this type of MI, there is significant damage to the myocardium.
- Non–ST-segment elevation MI: The patient has elevated cardiac biomarkers but no definite ECG evidence of acute MI.

During recovery from an MI, the ST segment often is the first ECG indicator to return to normal (1 to 6 weeks). The T wave becomes large and symmetric for 24 hours, and it then inverts within 1 to 3 days for 1 to 2 weeks. Q-wave alterations are usually permanent. An old ST-segment elevation MI is usually indicated by an abnormal Q wave or decreased height of the R wave without ST-segment and T-wave changes.

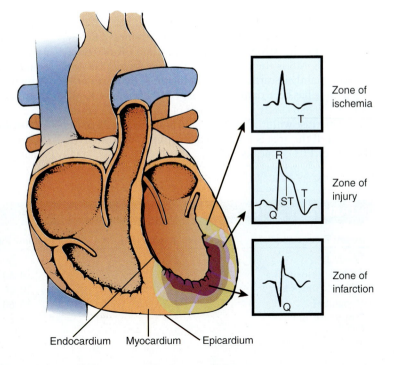

**FIGURE 28-5.** Effects of ischemia, injury, and infarction on an ECG recording. Ischemia causes inversion of the T wave because of altered repolarization. Cardiac muscle injury causes elevation of the ST segment and tall, symmetrical T waves. Later, Q waves develop because of the absence of depolarization current from the necrotic tissue and opposing currents from other parts of the heart.

**FIGURE 28-6.** Using the ECG to diagnose acute myocardial infarction (MI). (ST-segment elevation is measured 0.06 to 0.08 seconds after the J point. An elevation of more than 1 mm in contiguous leads is indicative of acute MI.)

### Echocardiogram

The echocardiogram is used to evaluate ventricular function. It may be used to assist in diagnosing an MI, especially when the ECG is nondiagnostic. The echocardiogram can detect hypokinetic and akinetic wall motion and can determine the ejection fraction (see Chapter 26).

### Laboratory Tests

Laboratory tests called cardiac biomarkers are used to diagnose an MI. Newer laboratory tests with faster results, resulting in earlier diagnosis, include myoglobin and troponin analysis. These tests are based on the release of cellular contents into the circulation when myocardial cells die. Table 28-3 shows the time courses of cardiac biomarkers.

#### CREATINE KINASE AND ITS ISOENZYMES

There are three **creatine kinase** (CK) isoenzymes: CK-MM (skeletal muscle), CK-MB (heart muscle), and CK-BB (brain tissue). CK-MB is the cardiac-specific isoenzyme; CK-MB is found mainly in cardiac cells and therefore increases only when there has been damage to these cells. Elevated CK-MB assessed by mass assay is an indicator of acute MI; its level begins to increase within a few hours and peaks within 24 hours of an MI. If the area is reperfused (eg, due to thrombolytic therapy or PCI), it peaks earlier.

#### MYOGLOBIN

Myoglobin is a heme protein that helps transport oxygen. Like CK-MB enzyme, myoglobin is found in cardiac and skeletal muscle. The myoglobin level starts to increase within 1 to 3 hours and peaks within 12 hours after the onset of symptoms. An increase in myoglobin is not very specific in indicating an acute cardiac event; however, negative results are an excellent parameter for ruling out an acute MI.

#### TROPONIN

**Troponin**, a protein found in the myocardium, regulates the myocardial contractile process. There are three isomers of troponin: C, I, and T. Troponins I and T are specific for cardiac muscle, and these tests are currently recognized as reliable and critical markers of myocardial injury. An increase in the level of troponin in the serum can be detected within a few hours during acute MI. It remains elevated for a long period, often as long as 3 weeks, and it therefore can be used to detect recent myocardial damage.

## Medical Management

The goal of medical management is to minimize myocardial damage, preserve myocardial function, and prevent complications. These goals are facilitated by the use of guidelines developed by the American College of Cardiology and American Heart Association (Chart 28-9). These goals may be achieved by reperfusing the area with the emergency use of thrombolytic medications or by PCI. Minimizing myocardial damage is also accomplished by reducing myocardial oxygen demand and increasing oxygen supply with medications, oxygen administration, and bed rest. The resolution of pain and ECG changes indicate that demand and supply are in equilibrium; they may also indicate reperfusion. Visualization of blood flow through an open vessel in the catheterization laboratory is evidence of reperfusion.

### Pharmacologic Therapy

The patient with suspected MI is given aspirin, nitroglycerin, morphine, a beta-blocker, and other medications as indicated while the diagnosis is being confirmed. Patients should receive a beta-blocker initially, throughout the hospitalization, and after hospital discharge. Long-term therapy with beta-blockers can decrease the incidence of future cardiac events.

#### THROMBOLYTICS

Thrombolytics are usually administered IV, although some may also be given directly into the coronary artery in the

| TABLE 28-3 | Biomarkers of Acute Myocardial Infarction | | | |
|---|---|---|---|---|
| Serum Test | Earliest Increase (hr) | Test Running Time (min) | Peak (hr) | Return to Normal |
| Total CK | 3–6 | 30–60 | 24–36 | 3 days |
| CK-MB: isoenzyme | 4–8 | 30–60 | 12–24 | 3–4 days |
| mass assay | 2–3 | 30–60 | 10–18 | 3–4 days |
| Myoglobin | 1–3 | 30–60 | 4–12 | 12 hr |
| Troponin T or I | 3–4 | 30–60 | 4–24 | 1–3 wk |

> **CHART 28-9**
>
> ### Medical Treatment Guidelines for Acute Myocardial Infarction
>
> Use rapid transit to the hospital.
> Obtain 12-lead ECG to be read within 10 minutes.
> Obtain laboratory blood specimens of cardiac biomarkers, including troponin.
> Obtain other diagnostics to clarify the diagnosis.
>
> Begin routine medical interventions:
> - Supplemental oxygen
> - Nitroglycerin
> - Morphine
> - Aspirin 162–325 mg
> - Beta-blocker
> - Angiotensin-converting enzyme inhibitor within 24 hours
>
> Evaluate for indications for reperfusion therapy:
> - Percutaneous coronary intervention
> - Thrombolytic therapy
>
> Continue therapy as indicated:
> - Intravenous heparin or low-molecular-weight heparin
> - Clopidogrel (Plavix) or ticlopidine (Ticlid)
> - Glycoprotein IIb/IIIa inhibitor
> - Bed rest for a minimum of 12 to 24 hours
>
> Antman, E. M. et al. (2004). ACC/AHA Guidelines for the management of patients with ST-elevation myocardial infarction. *Circulation, 110*(5), 1–49.

their ability to administer these medications within 30 minutes from the time the patient arrives in the emergency department. This is called *door-to-needle time*. The thrombolytic agents used most often are alteplase (t-PA, Activase) and reteplase (r-PA, TNKase).

Alteplase is a tissue plasminogen activator (t-PA) that activates the plasminogen present on the blood clot. An IV bolus dose is given and followed by an infusion. Aspirin and unfractionated heparin or LMWH may be used with t-PA to prevent another clot from forming at the same lesion site.

Reteplase, a newer recombinant thrombolytic, is very similar to alteplase and has similar effects. It is administered in two bolus doses, followed with a heparin infusion.

### ANALGESICS

The analgesic of choice for acute MI is morphine sulfate administered in IV boluses to reduce pain and anxiety. It reduces preload and afterload, which decreases the workload of the heart. Morphine also relaxes bronchioles to enhance oxygenation. The cardiovascular response to morphine is monitored carefully, particularly the blood pressure, which can decrease, and the respiratory rate, which can be depressed. Because morphine decreases the sensation of pain, ST-segment monitoring may be a better indicator of subsequent ischemia than assessment of pain.

### ANGIOTENSIN-CONVERTING ENZYME INHIBITORS

**Angiotensin-converting enzyme (ACE) inhibitors** prevent the conversion of angiotensin I to angiotensin II. In the absence of angiotensin II, the blood pressure decreases and the kidneys excrete sodium and fluid (diuresis), decreasing the oxygen demand of the heart. Use of ACE inhibitors in patients after MI decreases mortality rates and prevents remodeling of myocardial cells that is associated with the onset of heart failure. It is important to ensure that the patient is not hypotensive, hyponatremic, hypovolemic, or hyperkalemic before administering ACE inhibitors. Blood pressure, urine output, and serum sodium, potassium, and creatinine levels need to be monitored closely.

## Emergent Percutaneous Coronary Intervention

The patient in whom an acute MI is suspected may be referred for an immediate PCI. PCI may be used to open the occluded coronary artery in an acute MI and promote reperfusion to the area that has been deprived of oxygen. Superior outcomes have been reported with use of PCI compared to thrombolytics (Antman, Anbe, Armstrong, et al., 2004). Early PCI has been shown to be effective in patients of all ages, including those older than 75 years (Bach, Cannon, Weintraub, et al., 2004). PCI treats the underlying atherosclerotic lesion. Because the duration of oxygen deprivation is directly related to the number of cells that die, the time from the patient's arrival in the emergency department to the time PCI is performed should be less than 60 minutes (time is muscle). This is frequently referred to as *door-to-balloon time*. A cardiac catheterization laboratory and staff must be available if an emergent PCI is to be performed within this short time.

## Cardiac Rehabilitation

After the MI patient is free of symptoms, an active rehabilitation program is initiated. Cardiac rehabilitation is a program

cardiac catheterization laboratory (Chart 28-10). The purpose of thrombolytics is to dissolve and lyse the thrombus in a coronary artery (thrombolysis), allowing blood to flow through the coronary artery again (reperfusion), minimizing the size of the infarction, and preserving ventricular function. Even though thrombolytics may dissolve the thrombus, they do not affect the underlying atherosclerotic lesion. The patient may be referred for a cardiac catheterization and other invasive interventions.

Thrombolytics dissolve all clots, not just the one in the coronary artery. Thus they should not be used if the patient has formed a protective clot elsewhere, such as after major surgery or hemorrhagic stroke. Because thrombolytics reduce the patient's ability to form a clot, the patient is at risk for bleeding. Thrombolytics should not be used if the patient is bleeding or has a bleeding disorder. All patients who receive thrombolytic therapy are placed on bleeding precautions to minimize the risk for bleeding. This means minimizing the number of punctures for inserting IV lines, avoiding IM injections, preventing tissue trauma, and applying pressure for longer than usual after any puncture.

To be effective, thrombolytics must be administered as early as possible after the onset of symptoms that indicate an acute MI, generally within 3 to 6 hours. They are given to patients with ECG evidence of acute MI. Hospitals monitor

### CHART 28-10

#  PHARMACOLOGY · Administration of Thrombolytic Therapy

**Indications**
- Chest pain for longer than 20 minutes, unrelieved by nitroglycerin
- ST-segment elevation in at least two leads that face the same area of the heart
- Less than 6 hours from onset of pain

**Absolute Contraindications**
- Active bleeding
- Known bleeding disorder
- History of hemorrhagic stroke
- History of intracranial vessel malformation
- Recent major surgery or trauma
- Uncontrolled hypertension
- Pregnancy

**Nursing Considerations**
- Minimize the number of times the patient's skin is punctured.
- Avoid intramuscular injections.
- Draw blood for laboratory tests when starting the IV line.
- Start IV lines before thrombolytic therapy; designate one line to use for blood draws.
- Avoid continual use of noninvasive blood pressure cuff.
- Monitor for acute dysrhythmias and hypotension.
- Monitor for reperfusion: resolution of angina or acute ST-segment changes.
- Check for signs and symptoms of bleeding: decrease in hematocrit and hemoglobin values, decrease in blood pressure, increase in heart rate, oozing or bulging at invasive procedure sites, back pain, muscle weakness, changes in level of consciousness, complaints of headache
- Treat major bleeding by discontinuing thrombolytic therapy and any anticoagulants; apply direct pressure and notify the physician immediately.
- Treat minor bleeding by applying direct pressure if accessible and appropriate; continue to monitor.

---

that targets risk reduction by means of education, individual and group support, and physical activity. Most insurance programs, including Medicare, cover the cost of cardiac rehabilitation, although only 8% to 39% of patients who are candidates for cardiac rehabilitation services participate in these programs (Williams, Fleg, Ades, et al., 2002).

The goals of rehabilitation for the patient who has had an MI are to extend life and improve the quality of life. The immediate objectives are to limit the effects and progression of atherosclerosis, return the patient to work and pre-illness lifestyle, enhance the psychosocial and vocational status of the patient, and prevent another cardiac event. These objectives are accomplished by encouraging physical activity and physical conditioning, educating the patient and family, and providing counseling and behavioral interventions.

Throughout all phases of rehabilitation, the goals of activity and exercise tolerance are achieved through gradual physical conditioning, aimed at improving cardiac efficiency over time. Cardiac efficiency is achieved when work and activities of daily living can be performed at a lower heart rate and lower blood pressure, thereby reducing the heart's oxygen requirements and reducing cardiac workload.

Physical conditioning is achieved gradually over time. It is not unusual for patients to "overdo it" in an attempt to achieve their goals too rapidly. Patients are observed for chest pain, dyspnea, weakness, fatigue, and palpitations and are instructed to stop exercise if any of these develop. In a monitored program, they are also monitored for an increase in heart rate above the target heart rate, an increase in systolic or diastolic blood pressure of more than 20 mm Hg, a decrease in systolic blood pressure, onset or worsening of dysrhythmias, or ST-segment changes on the ECG.

The target heart rate during hospitalization is an increase of less than 10% from the resting heart rate, or 120 beats per minute. Following discharge, the target heart rate is based on the patient's stress test results (usually 60% to 85% of the heart rate at which symptoms occurred), medications, and underlying condition. Oxygen saturation may also be assessed through pulse oximetry to ensure that it remains higher than 93%. If signs or symptoms occur, the patient is instructed to slow down or stop exercising. If the patient is exercising in an unmonitored program, he or she is cautioned to cease activity immediately if signs or symptoms occur and to seek appropriate medical attention.

Patients who are able to walk at 3 to 4 miles per hour can usually resume sexual activities. The nurse recommends that the patient be well rested and in a familiar setting, wait at least 1 hour after eating or drinking alcohol, and use a comfortable position. Sexual dysfunction or cardiac symptoms should be reported to the health care provider.

### Phases of Cardiac Rehabilitation

Cardiac rehabilitation occurs along the continuum of the disease. It is typically categorized in three phases.

Phase I begins with the diagnosis of atherosclerosis, which may occur when the patient is admitted to the hospital for ACS (eg, unstable angina or acute MI). It consists of low-level activities and initial education for the patient and family. Because of today's brief hospital stays, mobilization occurs earlier and patient teaching focuses on the essentials of self-care, rather than instituting behavioral changes for risk reduction. Priorities for in-hospital teaching include the signs and symptoms that indicate the need to call 911 (seek emergency assistance), the medication regimen, rest–activity balance, and follow-up appointments with the physician. The nurse needs to reassure the patient that although CAD is a lifelong disease and must be treated as such, most patients can resume a normal life after an MI. This positive approach while in the hospital helps to motivate and teach the patient to continue the education and lifestyle changes that are usually needed after discharge. The amount of activity recommended at discharge depends on the age of the patient, his or her condition before the cardiac event, the extent of the disease, the course of the hospital stay, and the development of any complications.

Phase II occurs after the patient has been discharged. It usually lasts for 4 to 6 weeks but may last as long as 6 months. This outpatient program consists of supervised, often ECG-monitored, exercise training that is individualized based on the results of an exercise stress test. Support and guidance related to the treatment of the disease and teaching and counseling related to lifestyle modification for risk factor reduction are a part of this phase. Short-term and long-range goals are collaboratively determined based on the patient's needs. At each session, the patient is assessed for the effectiveness of and adherence to the medical plan. To prevent complications and another hospitalization, the cardiac rehabilitation staff alerts the referring physician to any problems.

Outpatient cardiac rehabilitation programs are designed to encourage patients and families to support each other. Many programs offer support sessions for spouses and significant others while the patients exercise. The programs involve group educational sessions for both patients and families that are given by cardiologists, exercise physiologists, dietitians, nurses, and other health care professionals. These sessions may take place outside a traditional classroom setting. For instance, a dietitian may take a group of patients and their families to a grocery store to examine labels and meat selections or to a restaurant to discuss menu offerings for a "heart-healthy" diet.

Phase III focuses on maintaining cardiovascular stability and long-term conditioning. The patient is usually self-directed during this phase and does not require a supervised program, although it may be offered. The goals of each phase build on the accomplishments of the previous phase.

## The Patient With Myocardial Infarction

### Assessment

One of the most important aspects of care of the patient with an MI is the assessment. It establishes the baseline for the patient so that any deviations may be identified, systematically identifies the patient's needs, and helps determine the priority of those needs. Systematic assessment includes a careful history, particularly as it relates to symptoms: chest pain or discomfort, difficulty breathing (dyspnea), palpitations, unusual fatigue, faintness (syncope), or sweating (diaphoresis). Each symptom must be evaluated with regard to time, duration, and the factors that precipitate the symptom and relieve it, and in comparison with previous symptoms. A precise and complete physical assessment is critical to detect complications and any change in patient status. Chart 28-8 identifies important assessments and possible findings.

IV sites are examined frequently. Two IV lines are typically placed for any patient with ACS to ensure that access is available for administering emergency medications. Medications are administered IV to achieve rapid onset and to allow for timely adjustment. After the patient's condition stabilizes, IV lines may be changed to a saline lock to maintain IV access.

### Diagnosis

#### Nursing Diagnoses

Based on the clinical manifestations, history, and diagnostic assessment data, major nursing diagnoses may include:

- Ineffective cardiac tissue perfusion related to reduced coronary blood flow from coronary thrombus and atherosclerotic plaque
- Risk for imbalanced fluid volume
- Risk for ineffective peripheral tissue perfusion related to decreased cardiac output from left ventricular dysfunction
- Death anxiety
- Deficient knowledge about post-MI self-care

#### Collaborative Problems/ Potential Complications

Based on the assessment data, potential complications that may develop include the following:

- Acute pulmonary edema (see Chapter 30)
- Heart failure (see Chapter 30)
- Cardiogenic shock (see Chapter 30)
- Dysrhythmias and cardiac arrest (see Chapters 27 and 30)
- Pericardial effusion and cardiac tamponade (see Chapter 30)

### Planning and Goals

The major goals for the patient include relief of pain or ischemic signs and symptoms (eg, ST-segment changes), prevention of further myocardial damage, absence of respiratory dysfunction, maintenance or attainment of adequate tissue perfusion by decreasing the heart's workload, reduced anxiety, adherence to the self-care program, and absence or early recognition of complications. Care of the patient with an uncomplicated MI is summarized in the Plan of Nursing Care (Chart 28-11).

*(text continues on page 883)*

### CHART 28-11

## Plan of Nursing Care: Care of the Patient With an Uncomplicated Myocardial Infarction

**Nursing Diagnosis:** Ineffective cardiac tissue perfusion related to reduced coronary blood flow.
**Goal:** Relief of chest pain/discomfort

| NURSING INTERVENTIONS | RATIONALE | EXPECTED OUTCOMES |
|---|---|---|
| 1. Initially assess, document, and report to the physician the following: | 1. These data assist in determining the cause and effect of the chest discomfort and provide a baseline with which post-therapy symptoms can be compared. | • Reports beginning relief of chest discomfort and symptoms<br>• Appears comfortable and is free of pain and other signs or symptoms:<br>  Respiratory rate, cardiac rate, and blood pressure return to prediscomfort level<br>  Skin warm and dry |
|   a. The patient's description of chest discomfort, including location, intensity, radiation, duration, and factors that affect it. Other symptoms such as nausea, diaphoresis, or complaints of unusual fatigue. |   a. There are many conditions associated with chest discomfort. There are characteristic clinical findings of ischemic pain and symptoms. | • Adequate cardiac output as evidenced by: stable/improving<br>  ECG<br>  Heart rate and rhythm<br>  Blood pressure<br>  Mentation<br>  Urine output<br>  Serum BUN and creatinine<br>  Skin color, temperature, and moisture |
|   b. The effect of chest discomfort on cardiovascular perfusion—to the heart (eg, change in blood pressure, heart sounds), to the brain (eg, changes in LOC), to the kidneys (eg, decrease in urine output), and to the skin (eg, color, temperature). |   b. MI decreases myocardial contractility and ventricular compliance and may produce dysrhythmias. Cardiac output is reduced, resulting in reduced blood pressure and decreased organ perfusion. The heart rate may increase as a compensatory mechanism to maintain cardiac output. | |
| 2. Obtain a 12-lead ECG recording during the symptomatic event, as prescribed, to determine extension of infarction. | 2. An ECG during symptoms may be useful in the diagnosis of an extension of MI. | |
| 3. Administer oxygen as prescribed. | 3. Oxygen therapy increases the oxygen supply to the myocardium if actual oxygen saturation is less than normal. | |
| 4. Administer medication therapy as prescribed and evaluate the patient's response continuously. | 4. Medication therapy (nitroglycerin, morphine, beta blocker, aspirin) is the first line of defense in preserving myocardial tissue. The side effects of these medications can be hazardous and the patient's status must be assessed. | |
| 5. Ensure physical rest: use of the bedside commode with assistance; backrest elevated to promote comfort; diet as tolerated; arms supported during upper extremity activity; use of stool | 5. Physical rest reduces myocardial oxygen consumption. Fear and anxiety precipitate the stress response; this results in increased levels of endogenous catecholamines, which increase myo- | |

# CHART 28-11

## Plan of Nursing Care: Care of the Patient With an Uncomplicated Myocardial Infarction (Continued)

| NURSING INTERVENTIONS | RATIONALE | EXPECTED OUTCOMES |
|---|---|---|
| softener to prevent straining at stool. Provide a restful environment, and allay fears and anxiety by being supportive, calm, and competent. Individualize visitation, based on patient response. | cardial oxygen consumption. Also, with increased epinephrine, the pain threshold is decreased, and pain increases myocardial oxygen consumption. | |

**Nursing Diagnosis:** Potential impaired gas exchange related to fluid overload
**Goal:** Absence of respiratory difficulties

| NURSING INTERVENTIONS | RATIONALE | EXPECTED OUTCOMES |
|---|---|---|
| 1. Initially, every 4 hours, and with chest discomfort or symptoms, assess, document, and report to the physician abnormal heart sounds (particularly $S_3$ and $S_4$ gallops and the holosystolic murmur of left ventricular papillary muscle dysfunction), abnormal breath sounds (particularly crackles), and patient intolerance to specific activities. | 1. These data are useful in diagnosing left ventricular failure. Diastolic filling sounds ($S_3$ and $S_4$ gallop) result from decreased left ventricular compliance associated with MI. Papillary muscle dysfunction (from infarction of the papillary muscle) can result in mitral regurgitation and a reduction in stroke volume, leading to left ventricular failure. The presence of crackles (usually at the lung bases) may indicate pulmonary congestion from increased left heart pressures. The association of symptoms and activity can be used as a guide for activity prescription and a basis for patient teaching. | • No shortness of breath, dyspnea on exertion, orthopnea, or paroxysmal nocturnal dyspnea<br>• Respiratory rate less than 20 breaths/min with physical activity and 16 breaths/min with rest<br>• Skin color normal<br>• $PaO_2$ and $PaCO_2$ within normal range<br>• Heart rate less than 100 beats/min and greater than 60 beats/min, with blood pressure within patient's normal limits<br>• Chest x-ray normal<br>• Relief of chest discomfort<br>• Appears comfortable:<br>  Appears rested<br>  Respiratory rate, cardiac rate, and blood pressure return to prediscomfort level<br>  Skin warm and dry |
| 2. Teach patient:<br> a. To adhere to the diet prescribed (for example, explain low-sodium, low-calorie diet)<br><br> b. To adhere to activity prescription | 2.<br> a. Low-sodium diet may reduce extracellular volume, thus reducing preload and afterload, and thus myocardial oxygen consumption. In the obese patient, weight reduction may decrease cardiac work and improve tidal volume.<br> b. The activity prescription is determined individually to maintain the heart rate and blood pressure within safe limits. | |

*continued >*

### CHART 28-11

## Plan of Nursing Care
## Care of the Patient With an Uncomplicated Myocardial Infarction (Continued)

**Nursing Diagnosis:** Risk for ineffective peripheral tissue perfusion related to decreased cardiac output
**Goal:** Maintenance/attainment of adequate tissue perfusion

| NURSING INTERVENTIONS | RATIONALE | EXPECTED OUTCOMES |
|---|---|---|
| 1. Initially, every 4 hours, and with chest discomfort, assess, document, and report to the physician the following:<br>  a. Hypotension<br>  b. Tachycardia and other dysrhythmia<br>  c. Activity intolerance<br>  d. Mentation changes (use family input)<br>  e. Reduced urine output (less than 200 mL per 8 hours)<br>  f. Cool, moist, cyanotic extremities | 1. These data are useful in determining a low cardiac output state. An ECG with pain may be useful in the diagnosis of an extension of myocardial ischemia, injury, and infarction, and of variant angina. | • Blood pressure within the patient's normal range<br>• Ideally, normal sinus rhythm without dysrhythmia is maintained, or patient's baseline rhythm is maintained between 60 and 100 beats/min without further dysrhythmia.<br>• No complaints of fatigue with prescribed activity<br>• Remains fully alert and oriented and without cognitive or behavioral change<br>• Appears comfortable<br>• Urine output greater than 30 mL/hr<br>• Extremities warm and dry with normal color |

**Nursing Diagnosis:** Death anxiety
**Goal:** Reduction of anxiety

| NURSING INTERVENTIONS | RATIONALE | EXPECTED OUTCOMES |
|---|---|---|
| 1. Assess, document, and report to the physician the patient's and family's level of anxiety and coping mechanisms.<br><br><br>2. Assess the need for spiritual counseling and refer as appropriate.<br><br>3. Assess the need for social service referral. | 1. These data provide information about the psychological well-being and a baseline so that post-therapy symptoms can be compared. Causes of anxiety are variable and individual, and may include acute illness, hospitalization, pain, disruption of activities of daily living at home and at work, changes in role and self-image due to illness, and financial concerns. Because anxious family members can transmit anxiety to the patient, the nurse must also identify strategies to reduce the family's fear and anxiety.<br>2. If a patient finds support in a religion, spiritual counseling may assist in reducing anxiety and fear.<br>3. Social services can assist with post-hospital care and financial concerns. | • Reports less anxiety<br>• Patient and family discuss their anxieties and fears about death<br>• Patient and family appear less anxious<br>• Appears restful, respiratory rate less than 16/min, heart rate less than 100/min without ectopic beats, blood pressure within patient's normal limits, skin warm and dry<br>• Participates actively in a progressive rehabilitation program<br>• Practices stress reduction techniques |

## CHART 28-11 Plan of Nursing Care: Care of the Patient With an Uncomplicated Myocardial Infarction (Continued)

| NURSING INTERVENTIONS | RATIONALE | EXPECTED OUTCOMES |
|---|---|---|
| 4. Allow patient (and family) to express anxiety and fear:<br>  a. By showing genuine interest and concern<br>  b. By facilitating communication (listening, reflecting, guiding)<br>  c. By answering questions | 4. Unresolved anxiety (the stress response) increases myocardial oxygen consumption. | |
| 5. Use of flexible visiting hours allows the presence of a supportive family to assist in reducing the patient's level of anxiety. | 5. The presence of supportive family members may reduce both patient's and family's anxiety. | |
| 6. Encourage active participation in a cardiac rehabilitation program. | 6. Prescribed cardiac rehabilitation may help reduce anxiety, enhance feelings of well-being, and facilitate compliance with risk factor recommendations. | |
| 7. Teach stress reduction techniques. | 7. Stress reduction may help to reduce myocardial oxygen consumption and may enhance feelings of well-being. | |

**Nursing Diagnosis:** Deficient knowledge about post-MI self-care
**Goal:** Adheres to the home health care program
Chooses lifestyle consistent with heart-healthy recommendations.

(See Chart 28-12, Promoting Health After MI)

## Nursing Interventions

### Relieving Pain and Other Signs and Symptoms of Ischemia

Balancing myocardial oxygen supply with demand (eg, as evidenced by the relief of chest pain) is the top priority in the care of the patient with an acute MI. Although medication therapy is required to accomplish this goal, nursing interventions are also important. Collaboration among the patient, nurse, and physician is critical in assessing the patient's response to therapy and in altering the interventions accordingly.

The recommended treatment for acute MI is reperfusion with thrombolytic therapy or emergent PCI for patients who present to the health care facility immediately and who have no major contraindications. These therapies are important because, in addition to relieving symptoms, they aid in minimizing or avoiding permanent injury to the myocardium. With or without reperfusion, administration of aspirin, an IV beta-blocker, and nitroglycerin is indicated. Use of a GPIIb/IIIa agent or heparin may also be indicated. The nurse administers morphine to relieve pain and anxiety and to promote vasodilation, reducing preload and afterload.

Oxygen should be administered along with medication therapy to assist with relief of symptoms. Administration of oxygen even in low doses raises the circulating level of oxygen to reduce pain associated with low levels of myocardial oxygen. The route of administration, usually by nasal cannula, and the oxygen flow rate are documented. A flow rate of 2 to 4 L/min is usually adequate to maintain oxygen saturation levels of 96% to 100% if no other disease is present.

Vital signs are assessed frequently as long as the patient is experiencing pain and other signs or symptoms of acute ischemia. Physical rest in bed with the backrest elevated or in a cardiac chair helps decrease chest discomfort and dyspnea. Elevation of the head and torso is beneficial for the following reasons:

- Tidal volume improves because of reduced pressure from abdominal contents on the diaphragm and better lung expansion and gas exchange.
- Drainage of the upper lung lobes improves.
- Venous return to the heart (preload) decreases, reducing the work of the heart.

### Improving Respiratory Function

Regular and careful assessment of respiratory function can help the nurse detect early signs of pulmonary complications. Scrupulous attention to fluid volume status prevents overloading the heart and lungs. Encouraging the patient to breathe deeply and change position frequently helps keep fluid from pooling in the bases of the lungs.

### Promoting Adequate Tissue Perfusion

Limiting the patient to bed or chair rest during the initial phase of treatment is particularly helpful in reducing myocardial oxygen consumption. This limitation should remain until the patient is pain-free and hemodynamically stable. Checking skin temperature and peripheral pulses frequently is important to monitor tissue perfusion. Oxygen may be administered.

### Reducing Anxiety

Alleviating anxiety and decreasing fear are important nursing functions that reduce the sympathetic stress response. Decreased sympathetic stimulation decreases the workload of the heart, which may relieve pain and other signs and symptoms of ischemia.

Developing a trusting and caring relationship with the patient is critical in reducing anxiety. Providing information to the patient and family in an honest and supportive manner encourages the patient to be a partner in care and greatly assists in developing a positive relationship. Ensuring a quiet environment, preventing interruptions that disturb sleep, using a caring and appropriate touch, teaching the patient relaxation techniques, using humor and encouraging laughter, and providing the appropriate prayer book and helping the patient pray if consistent with the patient's beliefs are other nursing interventions that can be used to reduce anxiety. Frequent opportunities are provided for the patient to privately share concerns and fears. An atmosphere of acceptance helps the patient know that these concerns and fears are both realistic and normal. Music therapy is an effective method of reducing anxiety and managing stress (Evans, 2002). Pet therapy, in which animals are brought to the patient, appears to provide emotional support and reduce anxiety. Hospitals may have a procedure that has been developed based on research and infection control standards pertaining to the animals and their animal handlers and the patients who are eligible for pet therapy.

### Monitoring and Managing Potential Complications

Complications that can occur after acute MI are caused by the damage that occurs to the myocardium and to the conduction system as a result of the reduced coronary blood flow. Because these complications can be life-threatening, close monitoring for and early identification of their signs and symptoms are critical (see the Plan of Nursing Care in Chart 28-11).

The nurse monitors the patient closely for changes in cardiac rate and rhythm, heart sounds, blood pressure, chest pain, respiratory status, urinary output, skin color and temperature, sensorium, ECG changes, and laboratory values. Any changes in the patient's condition are reported promptly to the physician, and emergency measures are instituted when necessary.

### Promoting Home and Community-Based Care

#### TEACHING PATIENTS SELF-CARE

The most effective way to increase the probability that the patient will implement a self-care regimen after discharge is to identify the priorities as perceived by the patient, provide adequate education about heart-healthy living, and facilitate the patient's involvement in a cardiac rehabilitation program. Working with patients in developing plans to meet their specific needs further enhances the potential for an effective treatment plan (Chart 28-12).

#### CONTINUING CARE

Depending on the patient's condition and the availability of family assistance, a home care referral may be indicated. The home care nurse assists the patient with scheduling and keeping follow-up appointments and with adhering to the prescribed cardiac rehabilitation regimen. The patient may need reminders about follow-up monitoring, including periodic blood laboratory testing and ECGs. In addition, the home care nurse may monitor the patient's adherence to dietary restrictions and to prescribed medications. If the patient is receiving home oxygen, the nurse ensures that the patient is using the oxygen as prescribed and that appropriate home safety measures are maintained. If the patient has evidence of heart failure secondary to the myocardial infarction, appropriate home care guidelines for the patient with heart failure are followed (see Chapter 30, Continuing Care section).

## Evaluation

### Expected Patient Outcomes

Expected patient outcomes may include the following:

1. Relief of angina
2. No signs of respiratory difficulties
3. Adequate tissue perfusion
4. Decreased anxiety
5. Adherence to a self-care program
6. Absence of complications

## CHART 28-12  Health Promotion

### Promoting Health After Myocardial Infarction and Other Acute Coronary Syndromes

To extend and improve the quality of life, a patient who has had an MI must learn to adjust his or her lifestyle to promote heart-healthy living. With this in mind, the nurse and patient develop a program to help the patient achieve desired outcomes.

#### Changing Lifestyle During Convalescence and Healing

Adaptation to an MI is an ongoing process and usually requires some modification of lifestyle. Some specific modifications include:
- Avoiding any activity that produces chest pain, extreme dyspnea, or undue fatigue
- Avoiding extremes of heat and cold and walking against the wind
- Losing weight, if indicated
- Stopping smoking and use of tobacco; avoiding second-hand smoke
- Using personal strengths to support lifestyle changes
- Developing heart-healthy eating patterns and avoiding large meals and hurrying while eating
- Modifying meals to align with the Therapeutic Lifestyle Changes (TLC) or the Dietary Approaches to Stopping Hypertension (DASH) diet
- Adhering to medical regimen, especially in taking medications
- Following recommendations that ensure blood pressure and blood glucose are in control
- Pursuing activities that relieve and reduce stress

#### Adopting an Activity Program

Additionally, the patient needs to undertake an *orderly* program of increasing activity and exercise for long-term rehabilitation as follows:
- Engaging in a regimen of physical conditioning with a gradual increase in activity duration and then a gradual increase in activity intensity
- Walking daily, increasing distance and time as prescribed
- Monitoring pulse rate during physical activity until the maximum level of activity is attained
- Avoiding activities that tense the muscles: isometric exercise, weight-lifting, any activity that requires sudden bursts of energy
- Avoiding physical exercise immediately after a meal
- Alternating activity with rest periods (some fatigue is normal and expected during convalescence)
- Participating in a daily program of exercise that develops into a program of regular exercise for a lifetime

#### Managing Symptoms

The patient must learn to recognize and take appropriate action for possible recurrences of symptoms as follows:
- Call 911 if chest pressure or pain (or anginal equivalent) is not relieved in 15 minutes by nitroglycerin
- Contacting the physician if any of the following occur: shortness of breath, fainting, slow or rapid heartbeat, swelling of feet and ankles

## Invasive Coronary Artery Procedures

### Percutaneous Coronary Interventions (PCIs)

Invasive interventional procedures to treat angina and CAD include PTCA, intracoronary stent implantation, atherectomy, and brachytherapy. All of these procedures are classified as PCIs.

### Percutaneous Transluminal Coronary Angioplasty (PTCA)

In PTCA, an invasive interventional procedure, a balloon-tipped catheter is used to open blocked coronary vessels and resolve ischemia. It is used in patients with angina and as an intervention for acute MI. Catheter-based interventions can also be used to open blocked CABGs. The purpose of PTCA is to improve blood flow within a coronary artery by compressing and "cracking" the atheroma. The procedure is attempted when the cardiologist believes that PTCA can improve blood flow to the myocardium.

PTCA is carried out in the cardiac catheterization laboratory. Hollow catheters called sheaths are inserted, usually in the femoral artery (and sometimes femoral vein), providing a conduit for other catheters. Catheters are then threaded through the femoral artery, up through the aorta, and into the coronary arteries. Angiography is performed using injected radiopaque contrast agents (commonly called dye) to identify the location and extent of the blockage. A balloon-tipped dilation catheter is passed through the sheath and positioned over the lesion. The physician determines the catheter position by examining markers on the balloon that can be seen with fluoroscopy. When the catheter is properly positioned, the balloon is inflated with high pressure for several seconds and then deflated. The pressure compresses and possibly "cracks" the atheroma (Fig. 28-7). The media and adventitia of the coronary artery are also stretched.

Several inflations and several balloon sizes may be required to achieve the goal, usually defined as an improvement in blood flow and a residual stenosis of less than 20%. Other measures of the success of a PTCA are an increase in the artery's lumen, a difference of less than 20 mm Hg in blood pressure from one side of the lesion to the other, and no clinically obvious arterial trauma. Because the blood supply to the coronary artery decreases while the balloon is inflated, the patient may complain of chest pain and the ECG may display significant ST-segment changes. Intracoronary stents are usually positioned in the intima of the vessel to maintain patency after the balloon is withdrawn.

### Coronary Artery Stent

After PTCA, the area that has been treated may close off partially or completely, a process called restenosis. The intima of the coronary artery has been injured and responds by initiating an acute inflammatory process. This process may include release of mediators that lead to vasoconstriction, clotting, and scar tissue formation. A coronary artery stent is placed to overcome these risks. A **stent** is a metal mesh that provides structural support to a vessel at risk of acute closure. The stent is positioned over the angioplasty balloon. When the balloon is inflated, the mesh expands and presses against the vessel wall, holding the artery open. The balloon is withdrawn, but the stent is left permanently in place within the artery (see Fig. 28-7). Eventually, endothelium covers the stent and it is incorporated into the vessel wall. Because of the risk of thrombus formation in the stent, the patient receives antiplatelet medications (eg, clopidogrel [Plavix] and aspirin). These medications are routinely continued for at least 3 to 6 months to decrease the risk of thrombus formation (Schwertz & Vaitkus, 2003).

Some stents are coated with medications, such as sirolimus or paclitaxel, which may minimize the formation of thrombi or scar tissue within the stent. These drug-eluting stents have increased the success of PCI (Schwertz & Vaitkus, 2003).

### Atherectomy

Atherectomy is an invasive interventional procedure that involves the removal of the atheroma, or plaque, from a coronary artery by cutting, shaving, or grinding (Fink, Abraham, Vincent, et al., 2005). It may be used in conjunction with PTCA. Directional coronary atherectomy and transluminal extraction catheter procedures involve the use of a catheter that removes the lesion and its fragments. Another procedure called rotational atherectomy uses a catheter with diamond chips impregnated on the tip (called a bur) that rotates like a dentist's drill at 130,000 to 180,000 rpm, pulverizing the lesion. Usually, several passes of these catheters are needed to achieve satisfactory results. Postprocedural patient care is the same as for a patient after PTCA.

### Brachytherapy

PTCA and stent implantation cause a cellular reaction in the coronary artery that promotes proliferation of the intima of the artery, increasing the possibility of arterial obstruction. Brachytherapy reduces the recurrence of obstruction, preventing vessel restenosis by inhibiting smooth muscle cell proliferation. Brachytherapy (from the Greek word *brachys*, meaning *short*) involves the delivery of gamma or beta radiation by placing a radioisotope close to the lesion. The radioisotope may be delivered by a catheter or implanted with the stent. Long-term studies are needed to determine

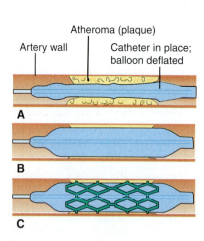

**FIGURE 28-7.** Percutaneous transluminal coronary angioplasty. (**A**) A balloon-tipped catheter is passed into the affected coronary artery and placed across the area of the atheroma (plaque). (**B**) The balloon is then rapidly inflated and deflated with controlled pressure. (**C**) A stent is placed to maintain patency of the artery, and the balloon is removed.

(1) whether the beneficial effects of radiation therapy are sustained and (2) the optimal dose and type of isotope to use for brachytherapy.

## Complications

Complications that can occur during a PCI procedure include dissection, perforation, abrupt closure, or vasospasm of the coronary artery, acute MI, acute dysrhythmias (eg, ventricular tachycardia), and cardiac arrest. These may require emergency surgical treatment. Complications after the procedure may include abrupt closure of the coronary artery and vascular complications, such as bleeding at the insertion site, retroperitoneal bleeding, hematoma, pseudoaneurysm, arteriovenous fistula, or arterial thrombosis and distal embolization, as well as acute renal failure (Table 28-4) (Thompson & King, 2003).

## Postprocedure Care

Patient care is similar to that for a cardiac catheterization (see Chapter 26). Many patients are admitted to the hospital the day of the PCI. Those with no complications go home the next day. When the PCI is performed emergently to relieve ACS, the patient will usually go to a critical care unit and stay in the hospital for a few days. During the PCI, patients receive IV heparin and are monitored closely for signs of bleeding. Patients may also receive a GPIIb/IIIa agent (eg, eptifibatide [Integrilin]) for several hours following the PCI to prevent platelet aggregation and thrombus formation in the coronary artery. Hemostasis is achieved, and femoral sheaths may be removed at the end of the procedure by using a vascular closure device (eg, Angio-Seal, VasoSeal) or a device that sutures the vessels. Hemostasis after sheath removal may also be achieved by direct manual pressure, a mechanical compression device (eg, C-shaped clamp), or a pneumatic compression device (eg, FemoStop).

The patient may return to the nursing unit with the large peripheral vascular access sheaths in place. The sheaths are then removed after blood studies (eg, activated clotting time) indicate that the heparin is no longer active and the clotting time is within an acceptable range. This usually takes a few hours, depending on the amount of heparin given during the procedure. The patient must remain flat in bed and keep the affected leg straight until the sheaths are removed and then for a few hours afterward to maintain hemostasis. Because the immobility and bed rest may cause discomfort, treatment may include analgesics and sedation. Sheath removal and the application of pressure on the vessel insertion site may cause the heart rate to slow and the blood pressure to decrease (vasovagal response). An IV bolus of atropine is usually given to treat this response.

Some patients with unstable lesions and at high risk for abrupt vessel closure are restarted on heparin after sheath removal, or they receive an IV infusion of a GPIIb/IIIa inhibitor. These patients are monitored more closely and may recover more slowly.

After hemostasis is achieved, a pressure dressing is applied to the site. Patients resume self-care and ambulate unassisted

### TABLE 28-4 Complications After Percutaneous Transluminal Coronary Angioplasty (PTCA)

| Complication | Signs and Symptoms | Possible Causes | Nursing Actions |
|---|---|---|---|
| Bleeding or hematoma | Hard lump or bluish tinge at sheath insertion site | Anticoagulant therapy, coughing, vomiting, bending leg or hip, obesity, bladder distention, high blood pressure | Keep the patient on bedrest. Apply manual pressure at site of sheath insertion. Outline extent of hematoma with a marking pen. If bleeding does not stop, notify physician or nurse practitioner. |
| Lost or weakened pulse distal to sheath insertion site | Extremity cool, cyanotic, pale, or painful | Arterial thrombus or embolus | Notify physician or nurse practitioner. Anticipate surgery and anticoagulation or thrombolytic therapy. |
| Pseudoaneurysm and arteriovenous fistula | Pulsatile mass felt or bruit heard near sheath insertion site | Vessel trauma during procedure | Notify physician or nurse practitioner. Anticipate ultrasound-guided compression. Prepare patient for surgery to close fistula. |
| Retroperitoneal bleeding | Back or flank pain, Low blood pressure, Tachycardia, Restlessness and agitation, Decreased hematocrit | Arterial tear causing bleeding into flank area | Notify physician or nurse practitioner immediately. Stop any anticoagulation medication. Anticipate need for intravenous fluids and/or administration of blood. |
| Acute renal failure | Decreased urine output, Elevated BUN, creatinine | Nephrotoxic contrast agent | Monitor urine output. Monitor BUN and creatinine. Provide adequate hydration. Administer renal protective agents (eg acetylcysteine) before and after procedure as prescribed. |

Adapted from Washington Adventist Hospital. Care of the interventional cardiology patient nursing protocol, based on communication from Amy Dukovic, Cardiac Interventional Nurse Practitioner.

within a few hours of the procedure. The duration of immobilization depends on the size of the sheath inserted, the amount of anticoagulant administered, the method of hemostasis, the patient's underlying condition, and the physician's preference. On the day after the procedure, the site is inspected and the dressing replaced with an adhesive bandage. The nurse teaches the patient to monitor the site for bleeding or development of a hard mass indicative of hematoma.

## Surgical Procedures: Coronary Artery Revascularization

Advances in diagnostics, medical management, surgical and anesthesia techniques, as well as the care provided in critical care and surgical units, home care, and rehabilitation programs, have continued to make surgery a viable treatment option for patients with CAD. CAD has been treated by myocardial revascularization since the 1960s, and the most common CABG techniques have been performed for approximately 35 years. CABG is a surgical procedure in which a blood vessel is grafted to the occluded coronary artery so that blood can flow beyond the occlusion; it is also called a bypass graft.

The major indications for CABG are as follows (Eagle & Guyton, 2004; Rihal, Raco, Gersh, et al., 2003):

- Alleviation of angina that cannot be controlled with medication or PCI
- Treatment of left main coronary artery stenosis or multi-vessel CAD
- Prevention and treatment of MI, dysrhythmias, or heart failure
- Treatment for complications from an unsuccessful PCI

The recommendation for CABG is determined by a number of factors, including the number of diseased coronary vessels, the degree of left ventricular dysfunction, the presence of other health problems, the patient's symptoms, and any previous treatment. Studies have shown that CABG may be the preferred treatment for high-risk patients such as those with severe triple-vessel CAD, ventricular dysfunction, and diabetes (Rihal et al., 2003). Studies continue to compare clinical outcomes of CABG and PCI in patients with CAD (Berger, Sketch, & Califf, 2004).

For a patient to be considered for CABG, the coronary arteries to be bypassed must have approximately a 70% occlusion (60% if in the left main coronary artery). If significant blockage is not present, the flow through the artery will compete with the flow through the bypass, and circulation to the ischemic area of myocardium may not be improved. It is also necessary that the artery be patent beyond the area of blockage, or the flow through the bypass will be impeded.

A vessel commonly used for CABG is the greater saphenous vein, followed by the lesser saphenous vein (Fig. 28-8). Cephalic and basilic veins are used also. The vein is removed from the leg (or arm) and grafted to the ascending aorta and to the coronary artery distal to the lesion. The saphenous veins are used in emergency CABG procedures because they can be obtained quickly by one surgeon while

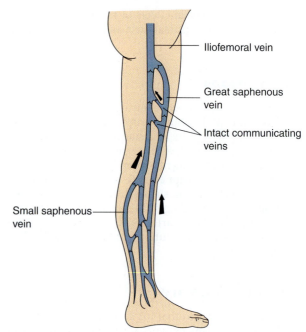

**FIGURE 28-8.** The greater and lesser saphenous veins are commonly used in bypass graft procedures.

another performs the chest surgery. A common adverse effect of vein removal is edema in the extremity from which the vein was taken. The degree of edema varies and usually diminishes over time. Within 5 to 10 years, atherosclerotic changes often develop in saphenous vein grafts.

The right and left internal mammary arteries and occasionally the radial arteries are also used for CABG. Arterial grafts are preferred to venous grafts because they do not develop atherosclerotic changes as quickly and remain patent longer. The surgeon leaves the proximal end of the mammary artery intact and detaches the distal end of the artery from the chest wall. This end of the artery is then grafted to the coronary artery distal to the occlusion. The internal mammary arteries may not be long enough to use for multiple bypasses. Because of this, many CABG procedures are performed with a combination of venous and arterial grafts.

## Traditional Coronary Artery Bypass Graft

The traditional CABG procedure is performed with the patient under general anesthesia. The surgeon makes a median sternotomy incision and connects the patient to the cardiopulmonary bypass (CPB) machine. Next, a blood vessel from another part of the patient's body (eg, saphenous vein, left internal mammary artery) is grafted distal to the coronary artery lesion, bypassing the obstruction (Fig. 28-9). CPB is then discontinued, chest tubes and epicardial pacing wires are placed, and the incision is closed. The patient then is admitted to a critical care unit.

### Cardiopulmonary Bypass

Many cardiac surgical procedures are possible because of CPB (ie, extracorporeal circulation). The procedure me-

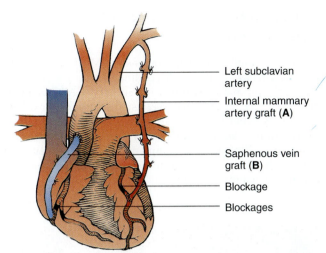

**FIGURE 28-9.** Coronary artery bypass grafts. One or more procedures may be performed using various veins and arteries. (**A**) Left internal mammary artery, used frequently because of its functional longevity. (**B**) Saphenous vein, also used as bypass graft.

chanically circulates and oxygenates blood for the body while bypassing the heart and lungs. CPB maintains perfusion to body organs and tissues and allows the surgeon to complete the anastomoses in a motionless, bloodless surgical field.

CPB is accomplished by placing a cannula in the right atrium, vena cava, or femoral vein to withdraw blood from the body. The cannula is connected to tubing filled with an isotonic crystalloid solution (usually 5% dextrose in lactated Ringer's solution). Venous blood removed from the body by the cannula is filtered, oxygenated, cooled or warmed by the machine, and then returned to the body. The cannula used to return the oxygenated blood is usually inserted in the ascending aorta, or it may be inserted in the femoral artery (Fig. 28-10). The heart is stopped by the injection of cardioplegia solution, which is high in potassium, into the coronary arteries. The patient receives heparin to prevent clotting and thrombus formation in the bypass circuit when blood comes in contact with the foreign surfaces of the tubing. At the end of the procedure when the patient is disconnected from the bypass machine, protamine sulfate is administered to reverse the effects of heparin.

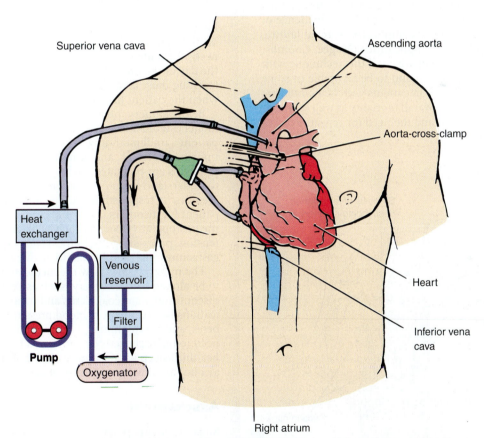

**FIGURE 28-10.** The cardiopulmonary bypass (CPB) system, in which cannulas are placed through the right atrium into the superior and inferior vena cavae to divert blood from the body and into the bypass system. The pump system creates a vacuum, pulling blood into the venous reservoir. The blood is cleared of air bubbles, clots, and particulates by the filter and then is passed through the oxygenator, releasing carbon dioxide and obtaining oxygen. Next, the blood is pulled to the pump and pushed out to the heat exchanger, where its temperature is regulated. The blood is then returned to the body via the ascending aorta.

During the procedure, hypothermia is maintained, usually 28°C to 32°C (82.4°F to 89.6°F). The blood is cooled during CPB and returned to the body. The cooled blood slows the body's basal metabolic rate, thereby decreasing the demand for oxygen. Cooled blood usually has a higher viscosity, but the crystalloid solution used to prime the bypass tubing dilutes the blood. When the surgical procedure is completed, the blood is rewarmed as it passes through the CPB circuit. Urine output, arterial blood gases, electrolytes, and coagulation studies are monitored to assess the patient's status during CPB.

## Alternative Coronary Artery Bypass Graft Techniques

A number of alternative CABG techniques have been developed that may have fewer complications for some groups of patients. Off-pump CABG (OPCAB) surgery has been used successfully in many patients since the 1990s. OPCAB involves a standard median sternotomy incision, but the surgery is performed without CPB. A beta-adrenergic blocker may be used to slow the heart rate. The surgeon also uses a myocardial stabilization device to hold the site still for the anastomosis of the bypass graft into the coronary artery while the heart continues to beat (Fig. 28-11). The potential benefits of OPCAB include a decrease in the incidence of stroke and other neurologic complications, renal failure, and other postoperative complications (Magee, Coombs, Peterson, et al., 2003). Comparison of this technique with traditional CABG has been found to be favorable in some patient groups, particularly in patients with hemodynamic instability, with regard to overall mortality as well as the incidence of stroke and MI and the need for repeat revascularization (Rose, 2003).

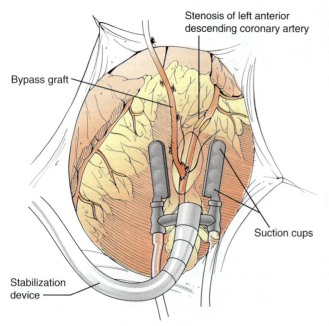

**FIGURE 28-11.** Stabilizer device for off-pump coronary artery bypass surgery.

## Complications of Coronary Artery Bypass Graft

CABG may result in complications such as MI, dysrhythmias, and hemorrhage (Table 28-5). Although most patients improve symptomatically following surgery, CABG is not a cure for CAD, and angina, exercise intolerance, or other symptoms experienced before CABG may recur. Medications required before surgery may need to be continued. Lifestyle modifications recommended before surgery remain important to treat the underlying CAD and for the continued viability of the newly implanted grafts.

### ◀◀▶▶ Nursing Process

## The Preoperative Cardiac Surgery Patient

Cardiac surgery patients have many of the same needs and require the same perioperative care as other surgical patients (see Chapters 18 through 20). These patients and their families are experiencing a major life crisis. The association of the heart with life and death intensifies their emotional and psychological needs. Patients frequently are admitted to the hospital the day of the procedure. Therefore, preoperative teaching must take place at an earlier time, usually when the patient has preadmission testing.

Before surgery, physical and psychological assessments establish baselines for future reference. The patient's understanding of the surgical procedure, informed consent, and adherence to treatment protocols are evaluated. Helping the patient to cope, to understand the procedure, and to maintain dignity are nursing responsibilities. The nurse assesses the patient for disorders that could complicate or affect the postoperative course, such as diabetes, hypertension, preexisting disabilities, and respiratory, gastrointestinal, and hematologic diseases.

The nurse clarifies how the medication regimen is to be altered before surgery, such as decreasing or discontinuing anticoagulants and maintaining medications for treatment of blood pressure, angina, diabetes, and dysrhythmias. The nurse also clarifies the need to maintain activity patterns, a healthy diet, healthful sleep habits, and cessation of smoking and alcohol to minimize the risks of surgery.

### Assessment

Most of the preoperative evaluation is completed before the patient enters the hospital. Many surgeons' offices or hospitals mail an information packet to the patient's home.

A history and physical examination are performed by nursing and medical personnel. A chest x-ray, ECG, laboratory tests, blood typing and cross-matching, and

*(text continues on page 894)*

## TABLE 28-5 Potential Complications of Cardiac Surgery

| Complication | Description | Assessment and Management |
|---|---|---|
| **Cardiac Complications** (The patient may require interventions for more than one complication at a time. Collaboration among nurses, physicians, pharmacists, respiratory therapists, and dietitians is necessary to achieve the desired patient outcomes.) | | |
| **Decreased Cardiac Output** | | |
| Hypovolemia (most common cause of decreased cardiac output after cardiac surgery) | • Net loss of blood and intravascular volume<br>• Surgical hypothermia (As the reduced body temperature rises after surgery, blood vessels dilate, and more volume is needed to fill the vessels.)<br>• Intravenous fluid loss to the interstitial spaces because surgery and anesthesia make capillary beds more permeable<br>• Increased heart rate, arterial hypotension, low pulmonary artery wedge pressure (PAWP), and low central venous pressures (CVP) often are seen | • Fluid replacement may be prescribed. Replacement fluids include: colloid (albumin, hetastarch), packed red blood cells, or crystalloid solution (normal saline, lactated Ringer's solution). |
| Persistent bleeding | • Cardiopulmonary bypass may cause platelet dysfunction, and hypothermia alters clotting mechanisms<br>• Surgical trauma causing tissues and blood vessels to ooze bloody drainage<br>• Intraoperative anticoagulant (heparin) therapy<br>• Postoperative coagulopathy may also result from liver dysfunction and depletion of clotting components | • Accurate measurement of wound bleeding and chest tube blood is essential. Bloody drainage should not exceed 200 mL/h for the first 4 to 6 hours. Drainage should decrease and stop within a few days, while progressing from sanguineous to serosanguineous and serous drainage.<br>• Protamine sulfate may be administered to neutralize unfractionated heparin; vitamin K and blood products may be used to treat hematologic deficiencies.<br>• If bleeding persists, the patient may return to the operating room. |
| Cardiac tamponade | • Fluid and clots accumulate in the pericardial sac, which compresses the heart, preventing blood from filling the ventricles.<br>• Signs and symptoms include arterial hypotension, tachycardia, muffled heart sounds, decreasing urine output, and ↑ CVP. Additional signs and symptoms: arterial pressure waveform demonstrating a pulsus paradoxus (decrease of more than 10 mm Hg during inspiration) and decreased chest tube drainage (suggesting that the drainage is trapped or clotted in the mediastinum). | • The chest drainage system is checked to eliminate possible kinks or obstructions in the tubing.<br>• Drainage system patency may be reestablished by milking the tubing (taking care not to strip the tubing, creating negative pressure within the chest, which may harm the surgical repair or trigger a dysrhythmia).<br>• Chest x-ray may show a widening mediastinum.<br>• Emergency medical management is required; may include pericardiocentesis or return to surgery. |
| Fluid overload | • High PAWP, CVP, and pulmonary artery diastolic pressures as well as crackles indicate fluid overload. | • Diuretics are prescribed and the rate of IV fluid administration is reduced.<br>• Alternative treatments include continuous renal replacement therapy and dialysis. |
| Hypothermia | • Low body temperature leads to vasoconstriction, shivering, and arterial hypertension. | • Patient is rewarmed gradually after surgery, decreasing vasoconstriction |
| Hypertension | • Results from postoperative vasoconstriction. It may stretch suture lines and cause postoperative bleeding. The condition may be transient. | • Vasodilators (nitroglycerin [Tridil], nitroprusside [Nipride, Nitropress]) may be used to treat hypertension. Administer cautiously to avoid hypotension. |

*continued >*

### TABLE 28-5 Potential Complications of Cardiac Surgery (Continued)

| Complication | Description | Assessment and Management |
|---|---|---|
| Tachydysrhythmias | • Increased heart rate is common with perioperative volume changes. Uncontrolled atrial fibrillation commonly occurs during the first few days postoperatively. | • If a tachydysrhythmia is the primary problem, the heart rhythm is assessed and medications (eg, adenosine [Adenocard, Adenoscan], amiodarone [Cordarone], digoxin [Lanoxin], diltiazem [Cardizem], esmolol [Brevibloc], lidocaine [Xylocaine], procainamide [Pronestyl]), may be prescribed. Patients may be prescribed antiarrhythmics before CABG to minimize the risk of postoperative tachydysrhythmias.<br>• Carotid massage may be performed by a physician to assist with diagnosing or treating the dysrhythmia.<br>• Cardioversion and defibrillation are alternatives for symptomatic tachydysrhythmias.<br>• For patients who cannot attain normal sinus rhythm, an alternate goal may be to establish a stable rhythm that produces a sufficient cardiac output. |
| Bradycardias | • Decreased heart rate | • Many postoperative patients will have temporary pacer wires that can be attached to a pulse generator (pacemaker) to stimulate the heart to beat faster. Less commonly, atropine, epinephrine, or isoproterenol may be used to increase heart rate. |
| Cardiac failure | • Myocardial contractility may be decreased perioperatively. | • The nurse observes for and reports falling mean arterial pressure; rising PAWP, pulmonary artery diastolic pressure, and CVP; increasing tachycardia; restlessness and agitation; peripheral cyanosis; venous distention; labored respirations; and edema.<br>• Medical management includes diuretics, digoxin, and IV inotropic agents. |
| Myocardial infarction (may occur intraoperatively or postoperatively) | • Portion of the cardiac muscle dies; therefore, contractility decreases. Impaired ventricular wall motion further decreases cardiac output. Symptoms may be masked by the postoperative surgical discomfort or the anesthesia–analgesia regimen. | • Careful assessment to determine the type of pain the patient is experiencing; MI suspected if the mean blood pressure is low with normal preload.<br>• Serial ECGs and cardiac biomarkers assist in making the diagnosis (alterations may be due to the surgical intervention). Analgesics are prescribed in small amounts while the patient's blood pressure and respiratory rate are monitored (because vasodilation secondary to analgesics or decreasing pain may occur and compound the hypotension).<br>• Activity progression depends on the patient's activity tolerance. |

| TABLE 28-5 | Potential Complications of Cardiac Surgery (Continued) | |
|---|---|---|
| Complication | Description | Assessment and Management |
| **Pulmonary Complications** | | |
| Impaired gas exchange | • During and after anesthesia, patients require mechanical assistance to breathe.<br>• Potential for postoperative atelectasis.<br>• Anesthetic agents stimulate production of mucus and chest incision pain may decrease the effectiveness of ventilation. | • Pulmonary complications are often detected during assessment of breath sounds, oxygen saturation levels, arterial blood gases, and when monitoring peak pressure and exhaled tidal volumes on the ventilator.<br>• Extended periods of mechanical ventilation may be required while complications are treated. |
| **Fluid Volume Complications** | | |
| Hemorrhage | • Untoward and excessive bleeding may be life-threatening. | • Serial hemoglobin, hematocrit, and coagulation studies are performed to guide therapy.<br>• Administration of fluids, colloids, and blood products: packed red blood cells, fresh frozen plasma, platelet concentrate.<br>• Administration of aprotinin (Trasylol) perioperatively to reduce blood transfusion needs.<br>• Administration of desmopressin acetate (DDAVP) to enhance platelet function. |
| **Neurologic Complications** | | |
| Neurologic changes; stroke | • Inability to follow simple command within 6 hours of recovery from anesthetic; different capabilities on right or left side of body | • Neurologically, most patients begin to recover from anesthesia in the operating room.<br>• Patients who are elderly or who have renal or hepatic failure may take longer to recover.<br>• Patient should be evaluated for stroke when neurologic changes are evident. |
| **Pain (see Chapter 13)** | | |
| **Renal Failure and Electrolyte Imbalance** | | |
| Renal failure | • Usually acute and resolves within 3 months, but may become chronic and require ongoing dialysis | • May respond to diuretics or may require continuous renal replacement therapy (CRRT) or dialysis |
| Acute tubular necrosis | • Often results from hypoperfusion of the kidneys or from injury to the renal tubules by nephrotoxic medications | • Fluids, electrolytes, and urine output are monitored frequently. |
| Electrolyte imbalance | • Postoperative imbalances in potassium, magnesium, sodium, calcium, and blood glucose are related to surgical losses, metabolic changes, and the administration of medications and IV fluids. | • Monitor electrolytes and basic metabolic studies frequently.<br>• Implement treatment to correct electrolyte imbalance promptly (see Chart 28-13). |

*continued >*

### TABLE 28-5　Potential Complications of Cardiac Surgery (Continued)

| Complication | Description | Assessment and Management |
|---|---|---|
| **Other Complications** | | |
| Hepatic failure | • Most common in patients with cirrhosis, hepatitis, or prolonged right-sided heart failure | • Use of medications metabolized by the liver must be minimized.<br>• Bilirubin, albumin, and amylase levels are monitored, and nutritional support must be provided. |
| Infection | • Surgery and anesthesia alter the patient's immune system. Many invasive devices are used to monitor and support the patient's recovery and may serve as a source of infection. | • The following must be monitored to detect signs of possible infection: body temperature, white blood cell counts and differential counts, incision and puncture sites, cardiac output and systemic vascular resistance, urine (clarity, color, and odor), bilateral breath sounds, sputum (color, odor, amount), as well as nasogastric secretions.<br>• Antibiotic therapy may be expanded or modified as necessary.<br>• Invasive devices must be discontinued as soon as they are no longer required. Institutional protocols for maintaining and replacing invasive lines and devices must be followed to minimize the patient's risk for infection. |

autologous blood donation (patient's own blood) may also be performed. The health assessment focuses on obtaining baseline physiologic, psychological, and social information. The patient's and family's learning needs are identified and addressed as necessary. Of particular importance are the patient's usual functional level, coping mechanisms, and support systems. These are important because the support of the family or significant others affects the patient's postoperative course and rehabilitation. Discharge plans are influenced by the lifestyle demands of the home situation and the physical environment of the home.

### Health History

The preoperative history and health assessment should be thorough and well documented because they provide a basis for postoperative comparison. A systematic assessment of all systems is performed, with emphasis on cardiovascular functioning.

The functional status of the cardiovascular system is determined by reviewing the patient's symptoms, including past and present experiences with chest pain, hypertension, palpitations, cyanosis, breathing difficulty (dyspnea), leg pain that occurs with walking (intermittent claudication), orthopnea, paroxysmal nocturnal dyspnea, and peripheral edema. Because alterations in cardiac output can affect renal, respiratory, gastrointestinal, integumentary, hematologic, and neurologic functioning, a history of these systems is also reviewed. The patient's history of major illnesses, previous surgeries, medication therapies, and use of drugs, alcohol, and tobacco is also obtained.

Particular attention is paid to blood glucose control in patients with diabetes, because there is a higher incidence of postoperative complications when glycemic control is poor (Goldrick, 2003).

### Physical Assessment

A complete physical examination is performed, with special emphasis on the following:

- General appearance and behavior
- Vital signs
- Nutritional and fluid status, weight, and height
- Inspection and palpation of the heart, noting the point of maximal impulse, abnormal pulsations, and thrills
- Auscultation of the heart, noting pulse rate, rhythm, and quality; $S_3$ and $S_4$, snaps, clicks, murmurs, and friction rub
- Jugular venous pressure
- Peripheral pulses
- Peripheral edema

### Psychosocial Assessment

The psychosocial assessment and the assessment of the patient's and family's learning needs are as important as the physical examination. Anticipation of cardiac surgery is a source of great stress to the patient and family. They are anxious and fearful and often have many unanswered questions. Their anxiety usually increases with the patient's admission to the hospital and the immediacy of surgery. An assessment of the level of anxiety is important. If it is low, it may indicate denial. If it is extremely high, it may interfere with the use of effective coping mechanisms and with preoperative teaching. Questions may be asked to obtain the following information:

- Meaning of the surgery to the patient and family
- Coping mechanisms that are being used
- Measures used in the past to deal with stress
- Anticipated changes in lifestyle
- Support systems in effect
- Fears regarding the present and the future
- Knowledge and understanding of the surgical procedure, postoperative course, and long-term rehabilitation

The nurse allows adequate time for the patient and family to express their fears. Those most often expressed are fear of the unknown, fear of pain, fear of body image change, and fear of dying. During the assessment, the nurse determines how much the patient and family know about the impending surgery and the expected postoperative events. They are encouraged to ask questions and to indicate how much information they wish to receive. Some patients prefer not to have detailed information, whereas others want to know as much as possible. Patients are approached as unique individuals with their own specific learning needs, learning styles, and levels of understanding.

Patients requiring emergency heart surgery may have cardiac catheterization and surgery within several hours of admission. The nurse has little opportunity to assess and meet their emotional and learning needs before surgery. As a result, patients require extra help after surgery to adjust to the situation.

## Diagnosis

### Preoperative Nursing Diagnoses

Nursing diagnoses for patients awaiting cardiac surgery vary according to each patient's cardiac disease and symptoms. Preoperative nursing diagnoses may include:

- Fear related to the surgical procedure, its uncertain outcome, and the threat to well-being
- Deficient knowledge regarding the surgical procedure and the postoperative course
- Ineffective cardiac tissue perfusion related to reduced coronary blood flow

### Collaborative Problems/ Potential Complications

The stress of impending cardiac surgery may precipitate complications that require collaborative management with the physician. Based on the assessment data, potential complications that may develop include:

- Angina
- Severe anxiety requiring an anxiolytic (anxiety-reducing) medication
- Cardiac dysrhythmias

## Planning and Goals

The major goals for the patient may include reducing fear, learning about the surgical procedure and postoperative course, and avoiding perioperative complications.

## Nursing Interventions

During the preoperative phase of cardiac surgery, the nurse develops a plan of care that includes emotional support and teaching for the patient and family. Establishing rapport, answering questions, listening to fears and concerns, clarifying misconceptions, and providing information about what to expect are interventions the nurse uses to prepare the patient and family emotionally for the surgery and the postoperative events.

### Reducing Fear

The patient and family are given time and opportunities to express their fears. If there is fear of the unknown, other surgical experiences that the patient has had can be compared with the impending surgery. It is often helpful to describe to the patient the sensations that he or she can expect. If the patient has already had a cardiac catheterization, the similarities and differences between that procedure and the surgery may be compared. The patient is encouraged to talk about any concerns related to previous experiences.

A discussion of the patient's fears about pain is initiated. A comparison is made between the pain experienced with cardiac surgery and other pain experiences. The preoperative sedation, the anesthetic, and the postoperative pain medications are described. The nurse reassures the patient that the fear of pain is normal, that some pain will be experienced, that medication to relieve pain will be provided, and that the patient will be closely observed. The patient is encouraged to take the analgesic medication before the pain becomes severe. Positioning and relaxation often make the pain more tolerable. Patients who have concern about scarring from surgery are encouraged to discuss this concern, and misconceptions are corrected. It may be helpful to indicate that the health care team members will keep the patient informed about the healing process.

The patient and family are encouraged to talk about their fear of the patient dying. They should be reassured that this fear is normal. For those who only hint about this concern despite efforts to encourage them to talk about it, coaching may be helpful (eg, "Are you worrying about not making it through surgery? Most people who have heart surgery at least think about the possibility of dying."). After the fear is expressed, the nurse can help the patient and family explore their feelings.

By alleviating undue anxiety and fear, preparing the patient emotionally for surgery decreases the chance of preoperative problems, promotes smooth anesthesia induction, and enhances the patient's involvement in care and recovery after surgery. Preparing the family for the usual postoperative events helps them to cope, support the patient, and participate in postoperative and rehabilitative care.

### Monitoring and Managing Potential Complications

Angina may occur because of increased stress and anxiety related to the forthcoming surgery. The patient who develops angina usually responds to normal angina therapy, most commonly nitroglycerin. Some patients require oxygen and IV nitroglycerin infusions (see the Angina Pectoris section). Physiologically unstable patients may require management in a critical care unit preoperatively.

For patients with extreme anxiety or fear and for whom emotional support and education are not successful, medication therapy may be helpful. The anxiolytic agents most commonly used before cardiac surgery are lorazepam (Ativan) and diazepam (Valium).

### Promoting Home and Community-Based Care

**TEACHING PATIENTS SELF-CARE**
Patient and family teaching is based on assessed learning needs. Teaching usually includes information about hospitalization, surgery (eg, preoperative and postoperative care, length of surgery, pain and discomfort that can be expected, visiting hours and procedures in the critical care unit), the recovery phase (eg, length of hospitalization, what to expect from home care and rehabilitation, when normal activities such as housework, shopping, and work can be resumed), and ongoing lifestyle habits. Any changes made in medical therapy and preoperative preparations need to be explained and reinforced.

The patient is informed that physical preparation usually involves showering with an antiseptic solution. A sedative may be prescribed the night before and the morning of surgery. Most cardiac surgical teams use prophylactic antibiotic therapy, and this is initiated immediately before surgery.

Teaching the patient and family together may be most effective. Anxiety often increases with the admission process and impending surgery. Teaching the patient and family together capitalizes on their established support relationship.

The patient may be offered a tour of the critical care unit, the postanesthesia care unit (PACU), or both. (In some hospitals, the patient initially goes to the PACU.) The patient recovering from anesthesia may be reassured by having already seen the surroundings and having met someone from the unit. The patient and family are informed about the equipment, tubes, and lines that will be present after surgery and their purposes. They should know to expect monitors, several IV lines, chest tubes, and a urinary catheter. Explaining the purpose and the approximate time that these devices will be in place helps to reassure the patient. Most patients remain intubated and on mechanical ventilation for 2 to 24 hours after surgery. They should be aware that this prevents them from talking, and they should be reassured that the staff will be able to assist them with other means of communication.

The nurse takes care to answer the patient's questions about postoperative care and procedures. Deep breathing and coughing, use of the incentive spirometer, and foot exercises are explained and practiced by the patient before surgery. The family's questions at this time usually focus on the length of the surgery, who will discuss the results of the procedure with them after surgery and when this may occur, where to wait during the surgery, the visiting procedures for the critical care unit, and how they can support the patient before surgery and in the critical care unit.

### Evaluation

#### Expected Patient Outcomes

Expected patient outcomes may include:

1. Demonstrates reduced fear
   a. Identifies fears
   b. Discusses fears with family
   c. Uses past experiences as a focus for comparison
   d. Expresses positive attitude about outcome of surgery
   e. Expresses confidence in measures to be used to relieve pain
2. Learns about the surgical procedure and postoperative course
   a. Identifies the purposes of the preoperative preparation procedure
   b. Tours the critical care unit, if desired
   c. Identifies limitations expected after surgery
   d. Discusses expected immediate postoperative environment (eg, tubes, machines, nursing surveillance)
   e. Demonstrates expected activities after surgery (eg, deep breathing, coughing, early ambulation)
3. Shows no evidence of complications
   a. Reports anginal pain is relieved with medications and rest
   b. Takes medications as prescribed

## Intraoperative Nursing Management

The perioperative nurse performs an assessment and prepares the patient for the operating room and recovery experience. Any changes in the patient's status and the need for changes in therapy are identified. Procedures are explained before they are performed, such as the application of electrodes and use of continuous monitoring, indwelling catheters, and an $SpO_2$ probe. IV lines are inserted to administer fluids, medications, and blood products. The patient receives general anesthesia, is intubated, and is placed on mechanical ventilation. In addition to assisting with the surgical procedures, perioperative nurses are responsible for the comfort and safety of the patient. Some of the areas of intervention include positioning, skin care, wound care, and emotional support of the patient and family.

Before the chest incision is closed, chest tubes are inserted to evacuate air and drainage from the mediastinum and the thorax. Temporary epicardial pacemaker electrodes may be implanted on the surface of the right atrium and the right ventricle. These epicardial electrodes can be connected to an external pacemaker if the patient has persistent bradycardia perioperatively. Possible intraoperative complications include low cardiac output, dysrhythmias, hemorrhage, MI, stroke, embolization, and organ failure from shock, embolus, or adverse drug reactions. Astute intraoperative patient assessment is critical to prevent, detect, and initiate prompt intervention for these complications.

## Nursing Process

### The Postoperative Cardiac Surgery Patient

Initial postoperative care focuses on achieving or maintaining hemodynamic stability and recovery from general anesthesia. Care may be provided in the PACU or intensive care unit. After the patient's cardiac status and respiratory status are stable, the patient is transferred to a surgical progressive care unit with telemetry. Care focuses on the monitoring of cardiopulmonary status, pain management, wound care, progressive activity, and nutrition. Education about medications and risk factor modification is emphasized. Discharge from the hospital may occur 3 to 5 days after CABG in patients without complications. Following recovery from the surgery, patients can expect fewer symptoms from CAD and an improved quality of life. CABG has been shown to increase the lifespan of high-risk patients, including those with left main artery blockages and left ventricular dysfunction with multivessel blockages (Magee et al., 2003).

The immediate postoperative period for the patient who has undergone cardiac surgery presents many challenges to the health care team. All efforts are made to facilitate the transition from the operating room to the critical care unit or PACU with minimal risk. Specific information about the surgical procedure and important factors about postoperative management are communicated by the surgical team and anesthesia personnel to the critical care nurse, who then assumes responsibility for the patient's care. Figure 28-12 presents an overview of the many aspects of postoperative care of the cardiac surgical patient.

### Assessment

When the patient is admitted to the critical care unit or PACU, and hourly for at least every 12 hours thereafter, a complete assessment of all systems is performed to determine the postoperative status of the patient compared with the preoperative baseline and to identify anticipated changes since surgery. The following parameters are assessed:

- *Neurologic status:* level of responsiveness, pupil size and reaction to light, reflexes, facial symmetry, movement of the extremities, and hand grip strength
- *Cardiac status:* heart rate and rhythm, heart sounds, pacemaker status, arterial blood pressure, central venous pressure (CVP), pulmonary artery pressure, pulmonary artery wedge pressure (PAWP), waveforms from the invasive blood pressure lines, cardiac output or index, systemic and pulmonary vascular resistance, pulmonary artery oxygen saturation ($SvO_2$) (see Chapter 26 for a detailed description of hemodynamic monitoring)
- *Respiratory status:* chest movement, breath sounds, ventilator settings (eg, rate, tidal volume, oxygen concentration, mode such as synchronized intermittent mandatory ventilation, positive end-expiratory pressure, pressure support), respiratory rate, peak inspiratory pressure, arterial oxygen saturation ($SaO_2$), percutaneous oxygen saturation ($SpO_2$), end-tidal $CO_2$, pleural chest tube drainage, arterial blood gases
- *Peripheral vascular status:* peripheral pulses; color of skin, nail beds, mucosa, lips, and earlobes; skin temperature; edema; condition of dressings and invasive lines
- *Renal function:* urinary output; urine specific gravity and osmolality may be assessed
- *Fluid and electrolyte status:* intake, output from all drainage tubes, all cardiac output parameters, and indications of electrolyte imbalance
- *Pain:* nature, type, location, and duration (incisional pain must be differentiated from anginal pain); apprehension; response to analgesics

Assessment also includes observing all equipment and tubes to determine whether they are functioning properly: endotracheal tube, ventilator, end-tidal $CO_2$ monitor, $SpO_2$ monitor, pulmonary artery catheter, $SvO_2$ monitor, arterial and IV lines, IV infusion devices and tubing, cardiac monitor, pacemaker, chest tubes, and urinary drainage system.

As the patient regains consciousness and progresses through the postoperative period, the nurse also assesses indicators of psychological and emotional status. The patient may exhibit behavior that reflects denial or depression or may experience postcardiotomy delirium. Characteristic signs of delirium include transient perceptual illusions, visual and auditory hallucinations, disorientation, and paranoid delusions.

It is also necessary to assess the family's needs. The nurse ascertains how family members are coping with the situation; determines their psychological, emotional, and spiritual needs; and finds out whether they are receiving adequate information about the patient's condition.

**FIGURE 28-12.** Postoperative care of the cardiac surgical patient requires the nurse to be proficient in interpreting hemodynamics, correlating physical assessments with laboratory results, sequencing interventions, and evaluating progress toward desired outcomes.

Labels (clockwise from upper left):
- Nasogastric tube to decompress stomach.
- Endotracheal tube for providing ventilatory assistance, suctioning, and use of end-tidal $CO_2$ monitor.
- Swan-Ganz catheter for monitoring central venous pressure, pulmonary artery and pulmonary artery wedge pressures, temperature, $SVO_2$. Can be used for determining cardiac output, for venous and pulmonary artery blood sampling, and for medication administration. Venous lines can be used for fluid administration.
- ECG electrodes for monitoring heart rate and rhythm.
- $SpO_2$ monitor for measuring arterial oxygen saturation.
- Assess peripheral pulses: radial, posterior tibial, dorsalis pedis.
- Neurological assessment:
  - Level of responsiveness
  - Hand grasp
  - Pupils
  - Pain
  - Movement
- Assess skin color and temperature, color of lips, and color and capillary refill of nail beds.
- Epicardial pacing electrodes to temporarily pace the heart.
- Mediastinal and pleural chest tubes attached to suction; drainage and wound healing are monitored.
- Radial arterial line; used for monitoring arterial blood pressure and for blood sampling.
- Indwelling catheter to closed drainage system for accurate measurement of urine output; a temperature probe may be part of the indwelling catheter.

## Assessing for Complications

The patient is continuously assessed for indications of impending complications (see Table 28-5). The nurse and the surgeon function collaboratively to prevent complications, to identify early signs and symptoms of complications, and to institute measures to reverse their progression.

### DECREASED CARDIAC OUTPUT

A decrease in cardiac output is always a threat to the patient who has had cardiac surgery. It can have a variety of causes:

- Preload alterations: too little blood volume returning to the heart as a result of hypovolemia, persistent bleeding, or cardiac tamponade; or too much blood volume returning to the heart from fluid overload
- Afterload alteration: constricted arteries from postoperative hypertension or hypothermic vasoconstriction impede left ventricular emptying, increasing the workload of the heart
- Heart rate alterations: too fast, too slow, or dysrhythmias
- Contractility alterations: cardiac failure, MI, electrolyte imbalances, hypoxia

### FLUID VOLUME AND ELECTROLYTE IMBALANCE

Fluid and electrolyte imbalance may occur after cardiac surgery. Nursing assessment for these complications includes monitoring of intake and output, weight, hemodynamic parameters, hematocrit levels, distention of neck veins, edema, liver size, breath sounds (eg, fine crackles, wheezing), and electrolyte levels. Changes in serum electrolytes are reported promptly so that treatment can be instituted. Especially important are dangerously high or dangerously low levels of potassium, magnesium, sodium, and calcium. Elevated blood glucose levels are common in the postoperative period. Administration of IV insulin may be required in patients both with and without diabetes to achieve the glycemic control necessary for promoting wound healing (Van den Berghe, Wouters, Bouillon, et al., 2003).

### IMPAIRED GAS EXCHANGE

Impaired gas exchange is another possible complication after cardiac surgery. All body tissues require an adequate supply of oxygen for survival. To achieve this after surgery, an endotracheal tube with ventilator assistance may be used for 24 hours or more. The assisted ventilation is continued until the patient's blood gas measurements are acceptable and the patient demonstrates the ability to breathe independently. Patients who are stable after surgery may be extubated as early as 2 to 4 hours after surgery, which reduces their discomfort and anxiety regarding their limited ability to communicate.

The patient is continuously assessed for signs of impaired gas exchange: restlessness, anxiety, cyanosis of mucous membranes and peripheral tissues, tachycardia, and fighting the ventilator. Breath sounds are assessed often to detect fluid in the lungs and monitor lung expansion. Arterial blood gases, $SpO_2$, and end-tidal $CO_2$ are assessed for decreased oxygen and increased carbon dioxide. Following extubation, aggressive pulmonary interventions, such as turning, coughing, and deep breathing, are necessary to prevent atelectasis and pneumonia.

### IMPAIRED CEREBRAL CIRCULATION

Brain function depends on a continuous supply of oxygenated blood. The brain does not have the capacity to store oxygen and must rely on adequate continuous perfusion by the heart. It is important to observe the patient for any symptoms of hypoxia: restlessness, headache, confusion, dyspnea, hypotension, and cyanosis. An assessment of the patient's neurologic status includes level of consciousness, response to verbal commands and painful stimuli, pupil size and reaction to light, facial symmetry, movement of the extremities, hand grip strength, presence of pedal and popliteal pulses, and temperature and color of extremities. Any indication of a change in status is documented, and abnormal findings are reported to the surgeon because they may signal the onset of a complication. Hypoperfusion or microemboli may produce central nervous system injury after cardiac surgery.

## Diagnosis

### Nursing Diagnoses

Based on the assessment data and the type of surgical procedure performed, major nursing diagnoses may include:

- Decreased cardiac output related to blood loss, compromised myocardial function, and dysrhythmias
- Impaired gas exchange related to the trauma of chest surgery
- Risk for imbalanced fluid volume (and electrolyte imbalance) related to alteration in circulating blood volume
- Disturbed sensory perception (visual or auditory) related to excessive environmental stimuli (critical care environment, surgical experience), insufficient sleep, psychological stress, altered sensory integration, and electrolyte imbalances
- Acute pain related to surgical trauma and pleural irritation caused by chest tubes
- Ineffective tissue perfusion (renal, cerebral, cardiopulmonary, gastrointestinal, peripheral) related to decreased cardiac output, hemolysis, vasopressor drug therapy, embolization, underlying atherosclerotic disease, or coagulation problems
- Ineffective thermoregulation related to infection or postpericardiotomy syndrome
- Deficient knowledge about self-care activities

### Collaborative Problems/ Potential Complications

Based on the assessment data, potential complications that may develop include:

- Cardiac complications: heart failure, MI, stunned myocardium, dysrhythmias, tamponade, cardiac arrest
- Pulmonary complications: pulmonary edema, pulmonary emboli, pleural effusions, pneumothorax or hemothorax, respiratory failure, acute respiratory distress syndrome
- Hemorrhage/coagulopathy
- Neurologic complications: embolic or hemorrhagic stroke
- Renal failure
- Electrolyte imbalances
- Hepatic failure
- Infection/sepsis

## Planning and Goals

The major goals for the patient include restoration of cardiac output, adequate gas exchange, maintenance of fluid and electrolyte balance, reduction of symptoms of sensory-perception alterations, relief of pain, maintenance of adequate tissue perfusion, maintenance of normal body temperature, learning self-care activities, and absence of complications.

## Nursing Interventions

### Restoring Cardiac Output

To evaluate the patient's cardiac status, the nurse primarily determines the effectiveness of cardiac output through clinical observations and routine measurements: serial readings of blood pressure, heart rate, CVP, arterial pressure, and pulmonary artery pressures.

Renal function is related to cardiac function, as blood pressure and heart rate drive glomerular filtration; therefore, urinary output is measured and recorded. Urine output of less than 30 mL/hr may indicate a decrease in cardiac output. Urine specific gravity may also be assessed (normal is 1.010 to 1.025), as may urine osmolality. Inadequate fluid volume may be manifested by low urinary output and high specific gravity, whereas overhydration is manifested by high urine output and low specific gravity.

Body tissues depend on adequate cardiac output to provide a continuous supply of oxygenated blood to meet the changing demands of the organs and body systems. Because the buccal mucosa, nail beds, lips, and earlobes are sites with rich capillary beds, they should be observed for cyanosis or duskiness as possible signs of reduced cardiac output. Moist or dry skin may indicate vasodilation or vasoconstriction, respectively. Distention of the neck veins or of the dorsal surface of the hand raised to heart level may signal right-sided heart failure. If cardiac output has decreased, the skin becomes cool, moist, and cyanotic or mottled.

Dysrhythmias may develop when perfusion of the heart is poor. The most common dysrhythmias encountered during the postoperative period are atrial fibrillation, bradycardias, tachycardias, and ectopic beats. Continuous observation of the cardiac monitor for dysrhythmias is essential.

Any indications of decreased cardiac output are reported promptly to the physician. These assessment data and results of diagnostic tests are used by the physician to determine the cause of the problem. After a diagnosis has been made, the physician and the nurse work collaboratively to restore cardiac output and prevent further complications. When indicated, the physician prescribes blood components, fluids, digitalis or other antidysrhythmics, diuretics, vasodilators, or vasopressors. If additional surgery is necessary, the patient and family are prepared for the procedure.

### Promoting Adequate Gas Exchange

To ensure adequate gas exchange, the nurse assesses and maintains the patency of the endotracheal tube. The patient is suctioned when wheezes, coarse crackles, or rhonchi are present. Routinely, 100% oxygen is delivered to the patient from the ventilator or by a manual resuscitation bag (eg, Ambu-Bag) before and after suctioning to minimize the risk of hypoxia that can result from the suctioning procedure. Arterial blood gas determinations are compared with baseline data, and changes are reported to the physician promptly.

Because a patent airway is essential for oxygen and carbon dioxide exchange, the endotracheal tube must be secured to prevent it from slipping into the right mainstem bronchus and occluding the left bronchus. When the patient's condition stabilizes, body position is changed every 1 to 2 hours. Frequent changes of patient position provide for optimal pulmonary ventilation and perfusion by allowing the lungs to expand more fully. The nurse assesses breath sounds to detect crackles, wheezes, and fluid in the lungs.

The patient is usually weaned from the ventilator and extubated within 24 hours of CABG. Physical assessment and arterial blood gas results guide the process. Before being extubated, the patient should have cough and gag reflexes and stable vital signs; be able to lift the head off the bed or give firm hand grasps; have adequate vital capacity, negative inspiratory force, and minute volume appropriate for body size; and have acceptable arterial blood gas levels while breathing warmed humidified oxygen without the assistance of the ventilator.

During this time, the nurse assists with the weaning process and eventually with removal of the endotracheal tube. Deep breathing and coughing are encouraged at least every 1 to 2 hours after extubation to open the alveolar sacs and provide for increased ventilation, and to clear secretions.

### Maintaining Fluid and Electrolyte Balance

To promote fluid and electrolyte balance, the nurse carefully assesses intake and output. Flow sheets are used to determine positive or negative fluid balance. All fluid intake is recorded, including IV, nasogastric tube, and oral fluids. All output is recorded, including urine, nasogastric drainage, and chest drainage.

Hemodynamic parameters (ie, blood pressure, CVP, PAWP) are correlated with intake, output, and weight to determine the adequacy of hydration and cardiac output. Serum electrolytes are monitored, and the patient is observed for signs of potassium, magnesium, sodium, or calcium imbalance.

Any indications of dehydration, fluid overload, or electrolyte imbalance are reported promptly, and the physician and nurse work collaboratively to restore fluid and electrolyte balance. The patient's response is monitored.

### Minimizing Sensory-Perception Imbalance

Some patients exhibit abnormal behaviors that occur with varying intensity and duration. In the early years of cardiac surgery, this phenomenon occurred more frequently than it does today. Advances in surgical techniques and in the delivery of anesthetic agents have significantly decreased the incidence of postoperative delirium. When it occurs today, it is thought to be caused by anxiety, sleep deprivation, increased sensory input, medications, and physiologic problems such as hypoxemia (Marshall & Soucy, 2003). Delirium may appear after a 2- to 5-day stay in an intensive care environment.

Basic comfort measures are used in conjunction with prescribed analgesics and sedatives to promote rest. Because of safety concerns, lines and tubes are discontinued as soon as possible. Patient care is coordinated to provide undisturbed periods of rest. As the patient's condition stabilizes and the patient is disturbed less frequently for monitoring and therapeutic procedures, rest periods can be extended. As much uninterrupted sleep as possible is provided, especially during the patient's normal hours of sleep.

Careful explanations of all procedures and of the need for cooperation help keep the patient oriented throughout the postoperative course. Continuity of care is desirable; a familiar face and a nursing staff with a consistent approach help the patient feel safe. The patient's family should be welcomed at the bedside. A well-designed and individualized plan of nursing care can assist the nursing team in coordinating their efforts for the emotional well-being of the patient.

### Relieving Pain

Deep pain may not be felt in the peri-incisional area but may occur in a broader, more diffuse area. Patients who have had cardiac surgery experience pain caused by the interruption of intercostal nerves along the incision route and irritation of the pleura by the chest catheters. Incisional pain may also be experienced from peripheral vein or artery graft harvest sites.

It is essential to observe and listen to the patient for verbal and nonverbal clues about pain. The nurse accurately records the nature, type, location, and duration of the pain (chest incisional pain must be differentiated from anginal pain). The patient is encouraged to use patient-controlled analgesia (PCA) or accept medication as often as it is prescribed to reduce the amount of pain. The addition of IV and oral NSAIDs (or other adjunctive pain relievers) to opioids has decreased the amount of opioids required for pain relief and increased patient comfort. Patients report the most pain during coughing, turning, and moving (Milgrom, Brooks, Qi, et al., 2004). Physical support of the incision with a folded bath blanket or small pillow during deep breathing and coughing helps to minimize pain. The patient should then be able to participate in respiratory exercises and to increase self-care progressively. Patient comfort improves after removal of the chest tubes.

Pain produces tension, which may stimulate the central nervous system to release catecholamines, resulting in constriction of the arterioles and increased heart rate. This can cause increased afterload and decreased cardiac output. Opioids alleviate pain and induce sleep and feelings of euphoria, which reduces the metabolic rate and oxygen demands. After the administration of opioids, any observations indicating relief of apprehension and pain are documented in the patient's record. The patient is observed for any adverse effects of opioids, which may include respiratory depression, hypotension, ileus, or urinary retention. If serious side effects occur, an opioid antagonist (eg, naloxone [Narcan]) may be used. However, continuous titration of low hourly doses of an opioid via either IV drip or PCA pump, as opposed to periodic IV or IM boluses, until the pain is tolerable decreases the occurrence of adverse effects.

### Maintaining Adequate Tissue Perfusion

Peripheral pulses (eg, pedal, tibial, femoral, radial, brachial) are routinely palpated to assess for arterial obstruction. If a pulse is absent in any extremity, the cause may be prior catheterization of that extremity or chronic peripheral vascular disease. The newly identified absence of any pulse is immediately reported to the physician.

Thromboemboli formation also can result from injury to the intima of the blood vessels, dislodging a clot from a damaged valve, loosening of mural thrombi, or coagulation problems. Air embolism can result from CPB or central venous cannulation. Symptoms of embolization vary according to site. The usual embolic sites are the lungs, coronary arteries, mesentery, spleen, extremities, kidneys, and brain. The patient is observed for onset of the following:

- Chest pain and respiratory distress from pulmonary embolus or MI
- Abdominal or back pain from mesenteric emboli
- Pain, cessation of pulses, blanching, numbness, or coldness in an extremity
- Decreased urine output from renal emboli
- One-sided weakness and pupillary changes, as occur in stroke

All such symptoms are promptly reported to the physician.

After surgery, the following measures are taken to prevent venous stasis, which can cause deep venous thrombosis and subsequent pulmonary embolism:

- Applying elastic compression stockings or elastic bandage wraps and sequential pneumatic compression wraps
- Discouraging crossing of legs
- Avoiding use of the knee gatch on the bed
- Omitting pillows in the popliteal space
- Instituting passive exercises followed by active exercises to promote circulation and prevent venous stasis

Inadequate renal perfusion can occur as a complication of cardiac surgery. One possible cause is low cardiac output. Trauma to blood cells during CPB can cause hemolysis of red blood cells, which then occlude the renal glomeruli. Use of vasopressor agents to increase blood pressure may constrict the renal arterioles and reduce blood flow to the kidneys.

Nursing management includes accurate measurement of urine output. An output of less than 30 mL/hr may indicate hypovolemia or renal insufficiency. Urine specific gravity can be monitored to determine the kidneys' ability to concentrate urine in the renal tubules. Fluids may be prescribed to increase cardiac output and renal blood flow. IV diuretics may be administered to increase urine output. The nurse should be aware of the patient's blood urea nitrogen, serum creatinine, and urine and serum electrolyte levels. Abnormal levels are reported promptly because it may be necessary to adjust fluids and the dose or type of medication administered. If efforts to maintain renal perfusion are ineffective, the patient may require continuous renal replacement therapy or dialysis (see Chapter 44).

## Maintaining Normal Body Temperature

Patients are usually hypothermic when admitted to the critical care unit following the cardiac surgical procedure. The patient must be gradually warmed to a normal temperature. This is accomplished partially by the patient's own basal metabolic processes and often with the assistance of warmed ventilator air, warm air or warm cotton blankets, or heat lamps. While the patient is hypothermic, the clotting process is less efficient, the heart is prone to dysrhythmias, and oxygen does not readily transfer from the hemoglobin to the tissues. Because anesthesia and hypothermia suppress normal basal metabolism, oxygen supply usually meets the cellular demand.

After cardiac surgery, the patient is at risk for developing elevated body temperature caused by infection or postpericardiotomy syndrome. The resultant increase in metabolic rate increases tissue oxygen demands and increases cardiac workload. Measures are taken to prevent this sequence of events or to halt it as soon as it is recognized.

Common sites of infection include the lungs, urinary tract, incisions, and intravascular catheters. Meticulous care is used to prevent contamination at the sites of catheter and tube insertions. Aseptic technique is used when changing dressings and when providing endotracheal tube and catheter care. Clearance of pulmonary secretions is accomplished by frequent repositioning of the patient, suctioning, and chest physical therapy, as well as teaching and encouraging the patient to breathe deeply and cough. Closed systems are used to maintain all IV and arterial lines. All invasive equipment is discontinued as soon as possible after surgery.

Postpericardiotomy syndrome may occur in patients who undergo cardiac surgery (Porth, 2005). The syndrome is characterized by fever, pericardial pain, pleural pain, dyspnea, pericardial effusion, pericardial friction rub, and arthralgia. These signs and symptoms may occur in combination. Leukocytosis occurs, along with elevation of the erythrocyte sedimentation rate. These signs frequently appear after the patient is discharged from the hospital.

It is necessary to differentiate postpericardiotomy syndrome from other postoperative complications (eg, infection, incisional pain, MI, pulmonary embolus, bacterial endocarditis, pneumonia, atelectasis). Treatment depends on the severity of the symptoms. Anti-inflammatory agents often produce a dramatic improvement in symptoms.

## Promoting Home and Community-Based Care

### TEACHING PATIENTS SELF-CARE

Depending on the type of surgery and postoperative progress, the patient may be discharged from the hospital a few days after surgery. Although the patient may be eager to return home, the patient and family usually are apprehensive about this transition. The family members often express the fear that they are not capable of caring for the patient at home. They often are concerned that complications will occur that they are unprepared to handle.

The nurse helps the patient and family set realistic, achievable goals. A teaching plan that meets the patient's individual needs is developed with the patient and family. This is started before admission and reviewed each shift through the hospital stay or with each home care and rehabilitation contact. Specific instructions are provided about incision care; signs and symptoms of infection; diet; activity progression and exercise; deep breathing, incentive spirometry, and smoking cessation; weight and temperature monitoring; the medication regimen; and follow-up visits with home care nurses, the rehabilitation personnel, the surgeon, and the cardiologist or internist.

Some patients have difficulty learning and retaining information after cardiac surgery. Many patients have difficulties in cognitive function after cardiac surgery that do not occur after other types of major surgery. The patient may experience recent memory loss, short attention span, difficulty with simple math, poor handwriting, and visual disturbances. Patients with these difficulties often become frustrated when they try to resume normal activities and learn how to care for themselves at home. The patient and family are reassured that the difficulty is almost always temporary and will subside, usually in 6 to 8 weeks. In the meantime, instructions are given to the patient at a much slower pace than normal, and a family member assumes responsibility for making sure that the prescribed regimen is followed. All information is provided in writing in the patient's primary language; alternate formats (eg, large print, Braille, audiotapes) are used if indicated.

## NURSING RESEARCH PROFILE

### Recovery of Women Following CABG

DiMattio, M. K., & Tulman, L. (2003). A longitudinal study of functional status and correlates following coronary artery bypass graft surgery in women. *Nursing Research, 52*(2), 98–107.

#### Purpose
Only limited information is available to help women gauge their functional status following coronary artery bypass grafts (CABGs). These women tend to be older and more likely to have age-related comorbidities than men. In addition, they have a greater frequency of symptoms related to the surgery and often have less social support than men. The purpose of this study was to describe women's functional recovery during the first 6 weeks at home following CABG procedures.

#### Design
This longitudinal study enrolled 81 participants in five medical centers, where they all had CABGs. Of this number, 61 completed the study. Participants who dropped out were more likely to be older and readmitted to the hospital. Data were collected by an initial face-to-face interview in the hospital followed by phone interviews at 2, 4, and 6 weeks after discharge. A number of scales and subscales were used to rate functional status, including the Inventory of Functional Status in the Elderly, select subscales of the Sickness Impact Profile, and the Energy/Fatigue and Pain Severity subscales of the Medical Outcomes Study Patient Assessment Questionnaire.

#### Findings
Women had significant gains in functional status over the 6 weeks, especially between weeks 2 and 4. They engaged most frequently in personal care and low-level household activity. None of the women recovered completely or regained their baseline functional status within 6 weeks. Although fatigue and pain decreased over time, these symptoms were still experienced at 6 weeks.

#### Nursing Implications
The study gives nurses valuable information to use with discharge planning and follow-up for women after CABGs. Women should not expect to be fully recovered at 6 weeks after discharge.

### CONTINUING CARE

Arrangements are made for a home care nurse when appropriate. Because the hospital stay is relatively short, it is particularly important for the nurse to assess the patient's and family's ability to manage care in the home. Teaching is continued by the home care nurse. Vital signs and incisions are monitored, the patient is assessed for signs and symptoms of complications, and support for the patient and family is provided. Additional interventions may include dressing changes, IV antibiotic administration, diet counseling, and tobacco use cessation strategies. Patients and families need to know that cardiac surgery did not cure the patient's underlying heart disease. Lifestyle changes for risk factor reduction must be made, and medications taken before surgery may still be needed after surgery.

Patient teaching does not end at the time of discharge from home healthcare. The patient is encouraged to contact the surgeon, cardiologist, and nurse if he or she has problems or questions. This provides the patient and family with reassurance that professional support is available. The patient is expected to have at least one follow-up visit with the surgeon.

Many patients and families benefit from supportive programs such as the postcardiac surgery rehabilitation programs offered by many medical centers. These programs provide exercise monitoring; instructions about diet and stress reduction; information about resuming exercise, work, driving, and sexual activity; assistance with tobacco use cessation; and support groups for patients and families. The AHA sponsors the Mended Hearts Club, which provides information as well as an opportunity for families to share experiences.

## Evaluation

### Expected Patient Outcomes

Expected patient outcomes may include:

1. Maintains adequate cardiac output
2. Maintains adequate gas exchange
3. Maintains fluid (and electrolyte) balance
4. Experiences decreased symptoms of sensory-perception disturbances
5. Experiences relief of pain
6. Maintains adequate tissue perfusion
7. Maintains normal body temperature
8. Incisions are well healed
9. Performs self-care activities
10. Engages in follow-up care with health care providers and cardiac rehabilitation services
11. Adheres to recommendations for diet and lifestyle changes to maintain optimal future health
12. Exhibits no complications

A typical plan of postoperative nursing care and more detailed expected outcomes for the cardiac surgery patient are presented in Chart 28-13.

*(text continues on page 912)*

### CHART 28-13

## Plan of Nursing Care — Care of the Patient After Cardiac Surgery

**Nursing Diagnosis:** Decreased cardiac output related to blood loss and compromised myocardial function
**Goal:** Restoration of cardiac output to maintain organ and tissue perfusion

| NURSING INTERVENTIONS | RATIONALE | EXPECTED OUTCOMES |
|---|---|---|
| 1. Monitor cardiovascular status. Serial readings of blood pressures (arterial, pulmonary artery, pulmonary artery wedge pressure [PAWP], central venous pressure [CVP]), cardiac output/index, systemic and pulmonary vascular resistance, and cardiac rhythm and rate are obtained, recorded, and correlated with the patient's condition. | 1. Effectiveness of cardiac output is determined by hemodynamic monitoring. | The following parameters are within the patient's normal ranges: <br> • Arterial pressure <br> • PAWP <br> • Pulmonary artery pressures <br> • CVP <br> • Heart sounds <br> • Pulmonary and systemic vascular resistance <br> • Cardiac output and cardiac index <br> • Peripheral pulses <br> • Cardiac rate and rhythm <br> • Cardiac biomarkers <br> • Urine output <br> • Skin and mucosal color <br> • Skin temperature |
| a. Assess arterial blood pressure every 15 minutes until stable; then arterial or cuff blood pressure every 1–4 hours × 24 hours; then every 8–12 hours until hospital discharge; then every visit. | a. Blood pressure is one of the most important physiologic parameters to follow; vasoconstriction after cardiopulmonary bypass may require treatment with an IV vasodilator. | |
| b. Auscultate for heart sounds and rhythm. | b. Auscultation provides evidence of cardiac tamponade (muffled distant heart sounds), pericarditis (precordial rub), dysrhythmias. | |
| c. Assess peripheral pulses (pedal, tibial, radial). | c. Presence or absence and quality of pulses provide data about cardiac output as well as obstructive lesions. | |
| d. Measure pulmonary artery diastolic (PAD) pressure and PAWP to determine left ventricular end-diastolic volume and to assess cardiac output. | d. Rising pressures may indicate congestive heart failure or pulmonary edema. Low pressures may indicate need for volume replacement. | |
| e. Monitor PAWP, PAD, and CVP to assess blood volume, vascular tone, and pumping effectiveness of the heart. *Trends are more important than isolated readings.* Mechanical ventilation may alter hemodynamics. | e. High PAWP, PAD, or CVP may result from hypervolemia, heart failure, or cardiac tamponade. If blood pressure drop is due to low blood volume, PAWP, PAD, and CVP will show corresponding drop. | |
| f. Monitor ECG pattern for cardiac dysrhythmias (see Chap. 27 for discussion of dysrhythmias). | f. Dysrhythmias may occur with coronary ischemia, hypoxia, alterations in serum potassium, edema, bleeding, acid-base or electrolyte disturbances, digitalis toxicity, cardiac failure. ST-segment | |

## CHART 28-13 Plan of Nursing Care: Care of the Patient After Cardiac Surgery (Continued)

| NURSING INTERVENTIONS | RATIONALE | EXPECTED OUTCOMES |
|---|---|---|
| g. Assess cardiac biomarker results when available.<br>h. Measure urine output every ½ hour to 1 hour at first, then with vital signs.<br>i. Observe buccal mucosa, nailbeds, lips, earlobes, and extremities.<br>j. Assess skin; note temperature and color.<br><br>2. Observe for persistent bleeding: steady, continuous drainage of blood; hypotension; low CVP; tachycardia. Prepare to administer blood products, IV solutions.<br>3. Observe for cardiac tamponade: hypotension; rising PAWP, PAD, CVP, or pulsus paradoxus; muffled heart sounds; weak, thready pulse; jugular vein distention; decreasing urinary output. Check for diminished amount of blood in chest drainage collection system. Prepare for reoperation.<br>4. Observe for cardiac failure: hypotension, rising PAWP, PAD, CVP, tachycardia, restlessness, agitation, cyanosis, venous distention, dyspnea, moist crackles, ascites. Prepare to administer diuretics, digoxin, IV inotropic agents.<br>5. Observe for myocardial infarction: ST-segment elevations, T-wave changes, decreased cardiac output in the presence of normal circulating volume and filling pressures. Monitor serial ECGs and cardiac biomarkers. Differentiate myocardial pain from incisional pain. | changes may indicate myocardial ischemia. Pacemaker capture and antiarrhythmic medications are used to maintain a heart rate and rhythm and to support stable blood pressures.<br>g. Elevations may indicate myocardial infarction.<br>h. Urine output less than 30 mL/h indicates decreased renal perfusion and may reflect decreased cardiac output.<br>i. Duskiness and cyanosis may indicate decreased cardiac output.<br>j. Cool moist skin indicates vasoconstriction and decreased cardiac output.<br><br>2. Bleeding can result from cardiac incisions, tissue fragility, trauma to tissues, clotting defects.<br><br>3. Cardiac tamponade results from bleeding into the pericardial sac or accumulation of fluid in the sac, which compresses the heart and prevents adequate filling of the ventricles. Decrease in chest drainage may indicate that fluid and clots are accumulating in the pericardial sac.<br>4. Cardiac failure results from decreased pumping action of the heart; can cause deficient perfusion to vital organs.<br><br>5. Symptoms may be masked by the patient's level of consciousness and pain medication. | • Less than 200 mL/hr of drainage through chest tubes during first 4 to 6 hours<br>• Vital signs stable<br><br>• CVP and other hemodynamic parameters within normal limits<br>• Urinary output within normal limits<br>• Skin color normal<br>• Respirations unlabored, clear breath sounds<br>• Pain limited to incision<br>• ECG and cardiac biomarkers negative for ischemic changes |

*continued >*

## CHART 28-13

### Plan of Nursing Care — Care of the Patient After Cardiac Surgery (Continued)

**Nursing Diagnosis:** Impaired gas exchange related to trauma of extensive chest surgery
**Goal:** Adequate gas exchange

| NURSING INTERVENTIONS | RATIONALE | EXPECTED OUTCOMES |
|---|---|---|
| 1. Maintain mechanical ventilation until the patient is able to breathe independently. | 1. Ventilatory support may be used to decrease work of the heart, to maintain effective ventilation, and to provide an airway in the event of complications. | • Airway patent<br>• ABGs within normal range<br>• Endotracheal tube correctly placed, as evidenced by x-ray<br>• Breath sounds clear<br>• Ventilator synchronous with respirations<br>• Breath sounds clear after suctioning/coughing<br>• Nailbeds and mucous membranes pink<br>• Mental acuity consistent with amount of sedatives and analgesics received<br>• Oriented to person; able to respond yes and no appropriately<br>• Able to be weaned successfully from ventilator |
| 2. Monitor arterial blood gases, tidal volume, peak inspiratory pressure, and extubation parameters. | 2. ABGs and ventilator parameters indicate effectiveness of ventilator and changes that need to be made to improve gas exchange. | |
| 3. Auscultate chest for breath sounds. | 3. Crackles indicate pulmonary congestion; decreased or absent breath sounds may indicate pneumothorax, hemothorax, dislodgement of tube. | |
| 4. Sedate patient adequately, as prescribed, and monitor respiratory rate and depth if ventilations are not "controlled" by ventilator. | 4. Sedation helps the patient to tolerate the endotracheal tube and to cope with ventilatory sensations; sedatives can depress respiratory rate and depth. | |
| 5. Suction tracheobronchial secretions as needed, using strict aseptic technique. | 5. Retention of secretions leads to hypoxia and possible infection. | |
| 6. Assist in weaning and endotracheal tube removal. | 6. Decreased risk of pulmonary infections and enhanced ability of patient to communicate without an endotracheal tube. | |
| 7. After extubation, promote deep breathing, coughing, and turning. Encourage use of the incentive spirometer and compliance with breathing treatments. Teach incisional splinting with a "cough pillow" to decrease discomfort. | 7. Aids in keeping airway patent, preventing atelectasis, and facilitating lung expansion. | |

**Nursing Diagnosis:** Risk for imbalanced fluid volume and electrolyte imbalance related to alterations in blood volume
**Goal:** Fluid and electrolyte balance

| NURSING INTERVENTIONS | RATIONALE | EXPECTED OUTCOMES |
|---|---|---|
| 1. Maintain fluid and electrolyte balance. | 1. Adequate circulating blood volume is necessary for optimal cellular activity; metabolic acidosis and electrolyte imbalance can occur after surgery. | • Fluid intake and output balanced<br>• Hemodynamic assessment parameters negative for fluid overload or hypovolemia<br>• Normal blood pressure with position changes<br>• Absence of dysrhythmia |

## CHART 28-13

### Plan of Nursing Care — Care of the Patient After Cardiac Surgery (Continued)

| NURSING INTERVENTIONS | RATIONALE | EXPECTED OUTCOMES |
|---|---|---|
| a. Keep intake and output flow sheets; record urine volume every ½ hour to 4 hours while in critical care unit; then every 8 to 12 hours while hospitalized.<br>b. Assess blood pressure, hemodynamic parameters, weight, electrolytes, hematocrit, jugular venous pressure, tissue turgor, breath sounds, urinary output, and nasogastric tube drainage.<br>c. Measure postoperative chest drainage (should not exceed 200 mL/hr for first 4 to 6 hours); cessation of drainage may indicate kinked or blocked chest tube. Ensure patency and integrity of the drainage system. Maintain autotransfusion system if in use.<br>d. Weigh daily. Notify physician if weight gain of 2 lb or more in 24 hours.<br>2. Be alert to changes in serum electrolyte levels.<br><br>   a. Hypokalemia (low potassium) *Effects:* dysrhythmias: PVCs, ventricular tachycardia<br>     Observe for specific ECG changes. Administer IV potassium replacement as prescribed.<br>   b. Hyperkalemia (high potassium) *Effects:* ECG changes, tall peaked T waves, wide QRS, brachycardia<br>     Be prepared to administer diuretic or an ion-exchange resin (sodium polystyrene sulfonate [Kayexalate]); IV sodium bicarbonate, or IV insulin and glucose. | a. Provides a method to determine positive or negative fluid balance and fluid requirements.<br><br>b. Provides information about state of hydration.<br><br><br><br><br><br>c. Excessive blood loss from chest cavity can cause hypovolemia.<br><br><br><br><br><br><br><br>d. Indicator of fluid balance.<br><br>2. A specific concentration of electrolytes is necessary in both extracellular and intracellular body fluids to sustain life.<br>   a. *Causes:* inadequate intake, diuretics, vomiting, excessive nasogastric drainage, stress from surgery<br><br><br><br>   b. *Causes:* increased intake, hemolysis from cardiopulmonary bypass/mechanical assist devices, acidosis, renal insufficiency, tissue necrosis, adrenal cortical insufficiency.<br>     The resin binds potassium and promotes intestinal excretion of it.<br>     IV sodium bicarbonate drives potassium into the cells from extracellular fluid. | • Stable weight<br>• Blood pH 7.35 to 7.45<br>• Serum potassium 3.5 to 5.0 mEq/L (3.5 to 5.0 mmol/L)<br>• Serum magnesium 1.3 to 2.3 mg/dL (0.62 to 0.95 mmol/L)<br>• Serum sodium 135 to 145 mEq/L (135 to 145 mmol/L)<br>• Serum calcium 8.6 to 10.2 mg/dL (2.15 to 2.55 mmol/L)<br>• Serum glucose <110mg/dL |

*continued >*

## CHART 28-13

### Plan of Nursing Care: Care of the Patient After Cardiac Surgery (Continued)

| NURSING INTERVENTIONS | RATIONALE | EXPECTED OUTCOMES |
|---|---|---|
| | Insulin assists the cells with glucose and potassium absorption. | |
| c. Hypomagnesemia (low magnesium) *Effects:* dysrhythmias: PVCs, ventricular tachycardia, paresthesias, carpopedal spasm, muscle cramps, tetany, irritability, tremors, hyperexcitability, hyperreflexia, seizures. Be prepared to treat the cause. Magnesium supplements may be given (oral route preferred, IV administered with caution). | c. *Causes:* decreased intake, impaired absorption, increased excretion normal for 24 hours after major surgery and diuretic therapy. | |
| d. Hyponatremia (low sodium) *Effects:* weakness, fatigue, confusion, seizures, coma Administer sodium or diuretics as prescribed. | d. *Causes:* reduction of total body sodium, or increased water intake causing dilution of sodium | |
| e. Hypocalcemia (low calcium) *Effects:* numbness and tingling; carpal spasm; muscle cramps; tetany, hypotension, dysrhythmias Administer oral or IV replacement therapy as prescribed. | e. *Causes:* alkalosis, multiple blood transfusions of citrated blood products | |
| f. Hypercalcemia (high calcium) *Effects:* dysrhythmias Institute treatment as prescribed. | f. *Causes:* diuretic therapy, prolonged immobility | |
| g. Hyperglycemia (high blood glucose) *Effects:* increased urine output, thirst, metabolic acidosis Administer insulin as prescribed. | g. *Cause:* stress response to surgery | |

**Nursing Diagnosis:** Disturbed sensory perception related to excessive environmental stimulation, sleep deprivation, electrolyte imbalance
**Goal:** Reduction of symptoms of sensory perceptual imbalance; prevention of postcardiotomy delirium

| NURSING INTERVENTIONS | RATIONALE | EXPECTED OUTCOMES |
|---|---|---|
| 1. Use measures to prevent postcardiotomy delirium:<br>a. Explain all procedures and the need for patient cooperation. | 1. Postcardiotomy delirium may result from anxiety, sleep deprivation, increased sensory input, disorientation to night and day. | • Cooperates with procedures<br>• Sleeps for long, uninterrupted intervals<br>• Oriented to person, place, time |

**CHART 28-13**

## Plan of Nursing Care — Care of the Patient After Cardiac Surgery (Continued)

| NURSING INTERVENTIONS | RATIONALE | EXPECTED OUTCOMES |
|---|---|---|
| b. Plan nursing care to provide for periods of uninterrupted sleep with patient's normal day–night pattern.<br>c. Decrease sleep-preventing environmental stimuli as much as possible.<br>d. Promote continuity of care.<br>e. Orient to time and place frequently. Encourage family to visit.<br>f. Assess for medications that may contribute to delirium.<br>g. Teach relaxation techniques and diversions.<br>h. Encourage self-care as much as tolerated to enhance self-control. Assess support systems and coping mechanisms<br>2. Observe for perceptual distortions, hallucinations, disorientation, and paranoid delusions. | Normally, sleep cycles are at least 50 min long. The first cycle may be as long as 90 to 120 min and then shorten during successive cycles. Sleep deprivation results when the sleep cycles are interrupted or inadequate in number. | • Experiences no perceptual distortions, hallucinations, disorientation, delusions |

**Nursing Diagnosis:** Acute pain related to surgical trauma and pleural irritation caused by chest tubes
**Goal:** Relief of pain

| NURSING INTERVENTIONS | RATIONALE | EXPECTED OUTCOMES |
|---|---|---|
| 1. Record nature, type, location, intensity, and duration of pain.<br>2. Assist patient to differentiate between surgical pain and anginal pain.<br>3. Encourage routine pain medication dosing for the first 24 to 72 hours and observe for side effects of lethargy, hypotension, tachycardia, respiratory depression. | 1. Pain and anxiety increase pulse rate, oxygen consumption, and cardiac workload.<br>2. Anginal pain requires immediate assessment and treatment.<br>3. Analgesia promotes rest, decreases oxygen consumption caused by pain, and aids patient in performing deep-breathing and coughing exercises; pain medications is more effective when taken before pain is severe. | • States pain is decreasing in severity<br>• Reports absence of pain<br>• Restlessness decreased<br>• Vital signs stable<br>• Participates in deep-breathing and coughing exercises<br>• Verbalizes fewer complaints of pain each day<br>• Positions self; participates in care activities<br>• Gradually increases activity |

*continued >*

## CHART 28-13 Plan of Nursing Care: Care of the Patient After Cardiac Surgery (Continued)

**Nursing Diagnosis:** Ineffective renal tissue perfusion related to decreased cardiac output, hemolysis, or vasopressor drug therapy
**Goal:** Maintenance of adequate renal perfusion

| NURSING INTERVENTIONS | RATIONALE | EXPECTED OUTCOMES |
| --- | --- | --- |
| 1. Assess renal function: | 1. Renal injury can be caused by deficient perfusion, hemolysis, low cardiac output, and use of vasopressor agents to increase blood pressure. | • Urine output consistent with fluid intake; greater than 30 mL/hr<br>• Urine specific gravity 1.003 to 1.030<br>• BUN, creatinine, electrolytes within normal limits |
|   a. Measure urine output every ½ hour to 4 hours in critical care then every 8–12 hours until hospital discharge. |   a. Less than 30 mL/h indicates decreased renal function. | |
|   b. Measure urine specific gravity. |   b. Indicates kidneys' ability to concentrate urine in renal tubules. | |
|   c. Monitor and report lab results: BUN, serum creatinine, urine and serum electrolytes. |   c. Indicate kidneys' ability to excrete waste products. | |
| 2. Prepare to administer rapid-acting diuretics or inotropic drugs (eg, dobutamine). | 2. Promote renal function and increase cardiac output and renal blood flow. | |
| 3. Prepare patient for dialysis or continuous renal replacement therapy if indicated. | 3. Provides patient with the opportunity to ask questions and prepare for the procedure. | |

**Nursing Diagnosis:** Ineffective thermoregulation related to infection or postpericardiotomy syndrome
**Goal:** Maintenance of normal body temperature

| NURSING INTERVENTIONS | RATIONALE | EXPECTED OUTCOMES |
| --- | --- | --- |
| 1. Assess temperature every hour. | 1. Fever can indicate infectious or inflammatory process. | • Normal body temperature<br>• Incisions are free of infection and are healing<br>• Absence of symptoms of postpericardiotomy syndrome |
| 2. Use aseptic technique when changing dressings, suctioning endotracheal tube; maintain closed systems for all intravenous and arterial lines and for indwelling urinary catheter. | 2. Decreases risk of infection. | |
| 3. Observe for symptoms of postpericardiotomy syndrome: fever, malaise, pericardial effusion, pericardial friction rub, arthralgia. | 3. Occurs in approximately 10% of patients after cardiac surgery. | |
| 4. Obtain cultures and other labwork (CBC, ESR); administer antibiotics as prescribed | 4. Antibiotics treat documented infection. | |

## CHART 28-13 · Plan of Nursing Care: Care of the Patient After Cardiac Surgery (Continued)

| NURSING INTERVENTIONS | RATIONALE | EXPECTED OUTCOMES |
|---|---|---|
| 5. Administer anti-inflammatory agents as directed. | 5. Relieve symptoms of inflammation (eg, warm or flushed sensation, swelling, fullness, stiffness or aching sensation, and fatigue). | |

**Nursing Diagnosis:** Deficient knowledge about self-care activities
**Goal:** Ability to perform self-care activities

| NURSING INTERVENTIONS | RATIONALE | EXPECTED OUTCOMES |
|---|---|---|
| 1. Develop teaching plan for patient and family. Provide specific instructions for the following:<br>• Diet and daily weights<br>• Activity progression<br>• Exercise<br>• Deep breathing, coughing, lung expansion exercises<br>• Temperature monitoring<br>• Medication regimen<br>• Pulse taking<br>• Access to the emergency medical system<br>• Need for MedicAlert identification | 1. Each patient will have unique learning needs. | • Patient and family members explain and comply with therapeutic regimen<br>• Patient and family members identify necessary lifestyle changes<br>• Has copy of discharge instructions (in the patient's primary language and at appropriate reading level; has an alternate format if indicated)<br>• Keeps follow-up appointments |
| 2. Provide verbal and written instructions; provide several teaching sessions for reinforcement and answering questions. | 2. Repetition promotes learning by allowing for clarification of misinformation. After cardiac surgery, patients have short-term memory difficulty; information written in the patient's primary language and appropriate reading level is essential because it can be used as a resource after discharge. | |
| 3. Involve family in teaching sessions. | 3. Family members responsible for home care are usually anxious and require adequate time for learning. | |
| 4. Provide contact information for surgeon and cardiologist and instructions about follow-up visit with surgeon. | 4. Arrangements for contacts with health care personnel help to allay anxieties. | |
| 5. Make appropriate referrals: home care agency, cardiac rehabilitation program, community support groups, Mended Hearts Club. | 5. Learning and lifestyle changes continue after discharge from the hospital. | |

## Critical Thinking Exercises

1. **[ebp]** You are working in a cardiology office and you receive a phone call from a patient who had an MI 2 years ago. She reports that she is experiencing some shortness of breath and mild back pain. What evidence base is there to suggest that symptoms of an MI may be different for women than men? Discuss the strength of this evidence and its significance in determining assessment criteria to be used for women and men. What questions would you ask this patient? What would you instruct her to do? Provide rationale for your instructions.

2. You are taking over the care of a patient who returned from the catheterization laboratory 2 hours ago following a successful PCI. He was reported to be stable on bed rest, with no bleeding from the right femoral site. The patient appears very pale and complains of right flank pain. Identify the key parameters that need to be assessed. Describe the actions you would take and state why.

3. You are caring for a patient who has been hospitalized awaiting CABG surgery. As you deliver his morning medications, he states that he is feeling "pressure" in the lower sternal area, but he thinks it is just "nerves." What questions would you ask and what would you assess? What would your next actions be?

## REFERENCES AND SELECTED READINGS

### BOOKS

American Heart Association (2004). *Heart disease and stroke statistics—2004 update.* Dallas, TX: American Heart Association.
Carpenito, L. J. (2004). *Nursing diagnosis: Application to clinical practice* (10th ed.). Philadelphia: Lippincott Williams & Wilkins.
Cummins, R. O. (Ed.) (2003) *ACLS: Principles and practice.* Dallas, TX: American Heart Association.
Fink, M. P., Abraham, E., Vincent, J. L., et al. (2005). *Textbook of critical care* (5th ed.). Philadelphia: Elsevier.
Morton, P. G., Fontaine, D. K., Hudak, C. M., et al. (2005). *Critical care nursing* (8th ed.). Philadelphia: Lippincott Williams & Wilkins.
Porth, C. M. (2005). *Pathophysiology: Concepts of altered health states* (7th ed.). Philadelphia: Lippincott Williams & Wilkins.
Zipes, D. P., Libby, P., Bonow, R. D., et al. (2005). *Braunwald's heart disease* (10th ed.). Philadelphia: Saunders.

### JOURNALS

*Asterisks indicate nursing research articles.

Aldana, S. G., Whitmer, W. R., Greenlaw, R., et al. (2003). Cardiovascular risk reductions associated with aggressive lifestyle modification and cardiac rehabilitation. *Heart & Lung, 32*(6), 374–382.
American College of Cardiology Foundation and American Heart Association. (2002). ACC/AHA 2002 guideline update for exercise testing: A report of the American College of Cardiology/American Heart Association Task Force on Practice Guidelines (Committee on Exercise Testing). *Circulation, 106*(14), 1883–1892.
Antman, E. M., Anbe, D. T., Armstrong, P. W., et al. (2004). ACC/AHA Guidelines for the management of patients with ST-elevation myocardial infarction—executive summary. *Circulation, 110*(5), 1–49.
Bach, R. G., Cannon, C. P., Weintraub, W. S., et al. (2004). The effect of routine, early invasive management on outcome for elderly patients with non-ST-segment elevation acute coronary syndromes. *Annals of Internal Medicine, 141*(3), 186–195.
Berger, P. B., Sketch, M. H., & Califf, R. M. (2004). Choosing between percutaneous coronary intervention and coronary artery bypass grafting for patients with multivessel disease: What can we learn from the arterial revascularization therapy study (ARTS)? *Circulation, 109*(9), 1079–1081.
Bertoni, A. G., Bonds, D. E., Lovato, J., et al. (2004). Sex disparities in procedure use for acute myocardial infarction in the United States, 1995–2001. *American Heart Journal, 147*(6), 1054–1060.
Braunwald, E., Antman, E. M., Beasley, J. W., et al. (2002). ACC/AHA Guideline update for the management of patients with unstable angina and non-ST-segment elevation myocardial infarction—2002: Summary article. *Circulation, 106*(14), 1893–1900.
Chobanian, A. V., Bakris, G. L., Cushman, W. C., et al. (2003). The Seventh Report of the Joint National Committee on Prevention, Detection, Evaluation, and Treatment of High Blood Pressure: The JNC 7 Report. *Journal of the American Medical Association, 289*(19), 2560–2571.
Cleveland, K. W. (2003). Argatroban: A new treatment option for heparin-induced thrombocytopenia. *Critical Care Nurse, 23*(6), 61–69.
*DeVon, H. A., & Zerwic, J. J. (2003). The symptoms of unstable angina. Do women and men differ? *Nursing Research, 52*(2), 108–118.
*DeVon, H. A., & Zerwic, J. J. (2004) Differences in the symptoms associated with unstable angina and myocardial infarction. *Progress in Cardiovascular Nursing, 19*(1), 6–11.
*DiMattio, M. K., & Tulman, L. (2003). A longitudinal study of functional status and correlates following coronary artery bypass graft surgery in women. *Nursing Research, 52*(2), 98–107.
Eagle, K. A., & Guyton, R. A. (2004). ACC/AHA 2004 guideline update for coronary artery bypass graft surgery: Summary article. A report of the American College of Cardiology/American Heart Association Task Force on Practice Guidelines (Committee to update the 1999 Guidelines for Coronary Artery Bypass Graft Surgery). *Circulation, 110*(14), 1–9.
Evans, D. (2002). The effectiveness of music as an intervention for hospital patients: A systematic review. *Journal of Advanced Nursing, 37*(1), 8–18.
Expert Panel on Detection, Evaluation, and Treatment of High Blood Cholesterol in Adults. (2001). Executive summary of the third report of the National Cholesterol Education Program (NCEP) Expert Panel on Detection, Evaluation, and Treatment of High Blood Cholesterol in Adults (Adult Treatment Panel III). *JAMA, 285*(19), 2486–2497.
Gaenzer, H., Neumayr, G., Marschang, P., et al. (2002). Effects of insulin therapy on endothelium-dependent dilation in type 2 diabetes mellitus. *American Journal of Cardiology, 89*(4), 431–434.
Gibbons, R. J. (2003). ACC/AHA 2002 guideline update for the management of patients with chronic stable angina: A report of the American College of Cardiology/American Heart Association Task Force on Practice Guidelines. *Circulation, 107*(1), 149–158.
Goldrick, B. A. (2003). Surgical-site infections: Obesity, diabetes among risk factors for infections within 30 days of surgery. *American Journal of Nursing, 103*(4), 64AA.
Grundy, S. M., Cleeman, J. I., Merz, N. B., et al. (2004). Implications of recent clinical trials for the national cholesterol education program Adult Treatment Panel III guidelines. *Circulation, 110*(2), 227–239.
Haffner, S., & Taegtmeyer, H. (2003). Epidemic obesity and the metabolic syndrome. *Circulation 108*(13), 1541–1545.
Kannel, W. B. (1986). Silent myocardial ischemia and infarction: Insights from the Framingham Study. *Cardiology Clinics, 4*(4), 583–591.
Magee, M. J., Coombs, L. P., Peterson, E. D., et al. (2003). Patient selection and current practice for off-pump coronary artery bypass surgery. *Circulation, 108*(10, supp), II-9–II-14.
Marshall, M. C., & Soucy, M. D. (2003). Delirium in the intensive care unit. *Critical Care Nursing Quarterly, 26*(3), 172–178.

*Milgrom, L. B., Brooks, J. A., Qi, R., et al. (2004). Pain levels experienced with activities after cardiac surgery. *American Journal of Critical Care, 13*(2), 116–125.

Mosca, L. (2004). Evidence-based guidelines for cardiovascular disease prevention in women. *Circulation, 109*(5), 672–693.

Moustapha, A., & Anderson, V. (2003). Contemporary view of the acute coronary syndromes. *Journal of Invasive Cardiology, 15*(2), 71–79.

Nabel, E. G., & Selker, H. P. (2004). Women's ischemic syndrome evaluation. *Circulation, 109*(6), e50–e52.

Pearson, T., Mensah, G. A., & Alexander, R. W. (2003). Markers of inflammation and cardiovascular disease. A statement for health care professionals from the Centers for Disease Control and Prevention and the American Heart Association. *Circulation, 107*(3), 499–511.

Regar, E., Lemos, P. A., & Saia, F. (2004) Incidence of thrombotic stent occlusion during the first three months after sirolimus-eluting stent implantation in 500 consecutive patients. *American Journal of Cardiology, 93*(10), 1271–1275.

Reilly, M. P., & Rader, D. J. (2003). The metabolic syndrome: More than the sum of its parts? *Circulation, 108*(13), 1546–1551.

Ridker, P. M., Rifai, N., Rose, L., et al. (2002). Comparison of C-reactive protein and low-density lipoprotein cholesterol levels in the prediction of first cardiovascular events. *New England Journal of Medicine, 347*(20), 1557–1565.

Rihal, C. S., Raco, D. L., Gersh, B. J., et al. (2003). Indications for coronary artery bypass surgery and percutaneous coronary intervention in chronic stable angina: Review of the evidence and methodological considerations. *Circulation, 108*(20), 2439–2445.

Rose, E. S. (2003). Off-pump coronary artery bypass surgery. *New England Journal of Medicine, 348*(5), 379–380.

Schwertz, D. W., & Vaitkus, P. (2003). Drug-eluting stents to prevent reblockage of coronary arteries. *Journal of Cardiovascular Nursing, 18*(1), 11–16.

Sheifer, S. E., Escarce, J. J., & Schulman, K. A. (2000). Race and sex differences in the management of coronary artery disease. *American Heart Journal, 139*(5), 848–857.

Thompson, E. J., & King, S. L. (2003). Acetylcysteine and fenoldopam. *Critical Care Nurse, 23*(3), 39–46.

U.S. Preventive Services Task Force. (2003). Postmenopausal hormone replacement therapy for the primary prevention of chronic conditions: Recommendations and rationale. *American Journal of Nursing, 103*(6), 83–91.

Van den Berghe, G., Wouters, P. J., Bouillon, R., et al. (2003). Outcome benefit of intensive insulin therapy in the critically ill: Insulin dose versus glycemic control. *Critical Care Medicine, 31*(2), 359–366.

Williams, M. A., Fleg, J. L., Ades, P. A., & American Heart Association Council on Clinical Cardiology Subcommittee on Exercise, Cardiac Rehabilitation, and Prevention. (2002). Secondary prevention of coronary heart disease in the elderly (with emphasis on patients ≥75 years of age): An American Heart Association scientific statement from the Council on Clinical Cardiology Subcommittee on Exercise, Cardiac Rehabilitation, and Prevention. *Circulation, 105*(14), 1735–1743.

Wilson, P. W., & Grundy, S. M. (2003). The metabolic syndrome: Practical guide to origins and treatment: part I. *Circulation, 108*(12), 1422–1425.

## RESOURCES

American Dietetic Association, 216 W. Jackson Blvd., Chicago, IL 60606; 1-800-366-1644; http://www.eatright.org. Accessed May 30, 2006.

American Heart Association, 7272 Greenville Ave., Dallas, TX 75231; 1-800-AHA-USA1 (1-800-242-8721); http://www.americanheart.org. Accessed May 30, 2006.

Healthy People 2010, Office of Disease Prevention and Health Promotion, U.S. Department of Health and Human Services, 200 Independence Ave., SW, Washington, DC 20201; 1-800-877-696-6775; http://www.health.gov/healthypeople. Accessed May 30, 2006.

Heartmates, P.O. Box 16202, Minneapolis, MN 55416; 952-929-3331; http://www.heartmates.com. Accessed May 30, 2006.

National Heart, Lung, and Blood Institute, National Institutes of Health, Building 31, Room 5A52, Bethesda, MD 20892; 301-592-8593; http://www.nhlbi.nih.gov. Accessed May 30, 2006.

# CHAPTER 29

# Management of Patients With Structural, Infectious, and Inflammatory Cardiac Disorders

## Learning Objectives

*On completion of this chapter, the learner will be able to:*

1. Define valvular disorders of the heart and describe the pathophysiology, clinical manifestations, and management of patients with mitral and aortic disorders.
2. Describe types of cardiac valve repair and replacement procedures used to treat valvular problems and the care needed by patients who undergo these procedures.
3. Describe the pathophysiology, clinical manifestations, and management of patients with cardiomyopathies.
4. Describe the pathophysiology, clinical manifestations, and management of patients with infections of the heart.
5. Describe the rationale for prophylactic antibiotic therapy for patients with mitral valve prolapse, valvular heart disease, rheumatic endocarditis, infective endocarditis, and myocarditis.

Structural disorders of the heart present many challenges for the patient, family, and health care team, as do the conduction and vascular disorders discussed in Chapters 27 and 28. Problems with the heart valves, holes in the intracardiac septum, cardiomyopathies, and infectious diseases of the heart muscle alter cardiac output. Treatments for these disorders may be noninvasive, such as medication therapy and activity and dietary modification. Invasive treatments, such as valve repair or replacement, septal repair, ventricular assist devices, total artificial hearts, cardiac transplantation, and other procedures, may also be used. Nurses play an integral role in the care of patients with structural, infectious, and inflammatory cardiac conditions.

## Valvular Disorders

The valves of the heart control the flow of blood through the heart into the pulmonary artery and aorta by opening and closing in response to the blood pressure changes as the heart contracts and relaxes through the cardiac cycle.

The atrioventricular valves separate the atria from the ventricles and include the **tricuspid valve**, which separates the right atrium from the right ventricle, and the **mitral valve**, which separates the left atrium from the left ventricle. The tricuspid valve has three leaflets; the mitral valve has two. Both valves have chordae tendineae that anchor the valve leaflets to the papillary muscles and ventricular wall.

The semilunar valves are located between the ventricles and their corresponding arteries. The **pulmonic valve** lies between the right ventricle and the pulmonary artery; the **aortic valve** lies between the left ventricle and the aorta. Figure 29-1 shows valves in the closed position.

When any of the heart valves do not close or open properly, blood flow is affected. When valves do not close completely, blood flows backward through the valve in a process called **regurgitation**. When valves do not open completely, a condition called **stenosis**, the flow of blood through the valve is reduced.

Disorders of the mitral valve fall into the following categories: mitral valve **prolapse** (ie, stretching of the valve leaflet into the atrium during systole), mitral regurgitation, and mitral stenosis. Disorders of the aortic valve are categorized as aortic regurgitation and aortic stenosis. These valvular disorders may require surgical repair or replacement of the valve to correct the problem, depending on severity of symptoms (Fig. 29-2). Tricuspid and pulmonic valve disorders also occur, usually with fewer symptoms and complications. Regurgitation and stenosis may occur at the same time in the same or different valves.

### Mitral Valve Prolapse

Mitral valve prolapse, formerly known as mitral prolapse syndrome, is a deformity that usually produces no symptoms. Rarely, it progresses and can result in sudden death. Mitral valve prolapse occurs more frequently in women than in men, and it is now being diagnosed more frequently than it once was, probably because of improved diagnostic methods. The cause of mitral valve prolapse is usually an inherited connective tissue disorder resulting in enlargement of one or

## Glossary

**allograft:** heart valve replacement made from a human heart valve (synonym: homograft)
**annuloplasty:** repair of a cardiac valve's outer ring
**aortic valve:** semilunar valve located between the left ventricle and the aorta
**autograft:** heart valve replacement made from the patient's own heart valve (eg, the pulmonic valve is excised and used as an aortic valve)
**cardiomyopathy:** disease of the heart muscle
**chordoplasty:** repair of the stringy, tendinous fibers that connect the free edges of the atrioventricular valve leaflets to the papillary muscles
**commissurotomy:** splitting or separating fused cardiac valve leaflets
**heterograft:** heart valve replacement made of tissue from an animal heart valve (synonym: xenograft)
**homograft:** heart valve replacement made from a human heart valve (synonym: allograft)
**leaflet repair:** repair of a cardiac valve's movable "flaps" (leaflets)
**mitral valve:** atrioventricular valve located between the left atrium and left ventricle
**orthotopic transplantation:** the recipient's heart is removed, and a donor heart is grafted into the same site; the patient has one heart

**prolapse** (of a valve): stretching of an atrioventricular heart valve leaflet into the atrium during systole
**pulmonic valve:** semilunar valve located between the right ventricle and the pulmonary artery
**regurgitation:** backward flow of blood through a heart valve
**stenosis:** narrowing or obstruction of a cardiac valve's orifice
**total artificial heart:** mechanical device used to aid a failing heart, assisting the right and left ventricles
**tricuspid valve:** atrioventricular valve located between the right atrium and right ventricle
**valve replacement:** insertion of a device at the site of a malfunctioning heart valve to restore blood flow in one direction through the heart
**valvuloplasty:** repair of a stenosed or regurgitant cardiac valve by commissurotomy, annuloplasty, leaflet repair, or chordoplasty (or a combination of procedures)
**ventricular assist device:** mechanical device used to aid a failing right or left ventricle
**xenograft:** heart valve replacement made of tissue from an animal heart valve (synonym: heterograft)

FIGURE 29-1. The valves of the heart (aortic or semilunar, tricuspid, and mitral) in the closed position.

both of the mitral valve leaflets. The annulus often dilates. The chordae tendineae and papillary muscles may elongate.

## Pathophysiology

In mitral valve prolapse, a portion of one or both mitral valve leaflets balloons back into the atrium during systole. Rarely, the ballooning stretches the leaflet to the point that the valve does not remain closed during systole (ie, ventricular contraction). Blood then regurgitates from the left ventricle back into the left atrium. About 15% of patients who develop murmurs eventually experience heart enlargement, atrial fibrillation, pulmonary hypertension, or congestive heart failure (Zipes, Libby, Bonow, et al., 2005).

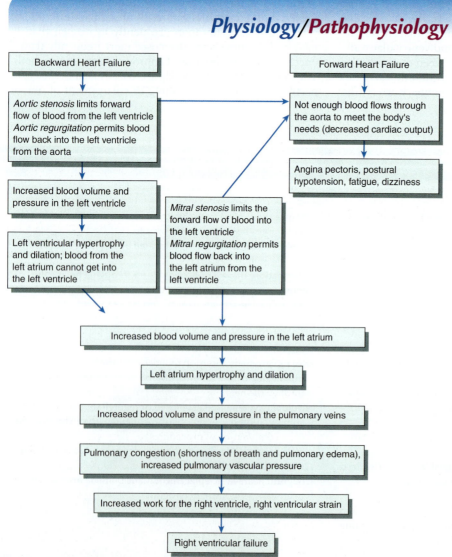

FIGURE 29-2. Pathophysiology: left-sided heart failure as a result of aortic and mitral valvular heart disease and the development of right ventricular failure.

## Clinical Manifestations

Most people who have mitral valve prolapse never have symptoms. A few have symptoms of fatigue, shortness of breath, lightheadedness, dizziness, syncope, palpitations, chest pain, and anxiety (Fuster, Alexander, & O'Rourke, 2004; Woods, Froelicher, Motzer, et al., 2005; Zipes et al., 2005). Fatigue may occur regardless of activity level and amount of rest or sleep. Shortness of breath is not correlated with activity levels or pulmonary function. Atrial or ventricular dysrhythmias may produce the sensation of palpitations, but palpitations have been reported while the heart has been beating normally. Chest pain, which is often localized to the chest, is not correlated with activity and may last for days.

Anxiety may be a response to the symptoms; however, some patients report anxiety as the only symptom. Some clinicians speculate that the symptoms may be explained by dysautonomia (a dysfunction of the autonomic nervous system resulting in increased excretion of catecholamines), although no consensus exists about the cause of the symptoms experienced by some patients.

## Assessment and Diagnostic Findings

Often, the first and only sign of mitral valve prolapse is identified when a physical examination of the heart reveals an extra heart sound, referred to as a mitral click. A systolic click is an early sign that a valve leaflet is ballooning into the left atrium. In addition to the mitral click, a murmur of mitral regurgitation may be heard if progressive valve leaflet stretching and regurgitation have occurred. A few patients experience signs and symptoms of heart failure if mitral regurgitation exists. Doppler echocardiography may be used to diagnose and monitor the progression of mitral valve prolapse.

## Medical Management

Medical management is directed at controlling symptoms. If dysrhythmias are documented and cause symptoms, the patient is advised to eliminate caffeine and alcohol from the diet and to stop smoking, and antidysrhythmic medications may be prescribed.

Chest pain that does not respond to nitrates may respond to calcium channel blockers or beta-blockers. Heart failure is treated the same as it would be for any other case of heart failure (see Chapter 30). In advanced stages of disease, mitral valve repair or replacement may be necessary.

## Nursing Management

The nurse educates the patient about the diagnosis and the possibility that the condition is hereditary. First-degree relatives (eg, parents, siblings) may be advised to have echocardiograms. Because most patients with mitral valve prolapse are asymptomatic, the nurse explains the need to inform the health care provider about any symptoms that may develop. The nurse also instructs the patient about the need for prophylactic antibiotic therapy before undergoing invasive procedures (eg, dental work, genitourinary or gastrointestinal procedures) that may introduce infectious agents systemically. This therapy is prescribed for symptomatic patients and for asymptomatic patients who have both a systolic click and murmur or mitral regurgitation. If the patient is in doubt about risk factors and the need for antibiotics, he or she should consult the physician. Women diagnosed with mitral valve prolapse without mitral regurgitation or other complications may complete pregnancies and have vaginal deliveries.

To minimize symptoms, the nurse teaches the patient to avoid caffeine and alcohol. The nurse encourages the patient to read product labels, particularly on over-the-counter products such as cough medicine, because these products may contain alcohol, caffeine, ephedrine, and epinephrine, which may produce dysrhythmias and other symptoms. Treatment of dysrhythmias, chest pain, heart failure, or other complications of mitral valve prolapse is described in Chapter 30. In addition, the nurse also explores possible diet, activity, sleep, and other lifestyle factors that may correlate with symptoms.

## *Mitral Regurgitation*

Mitral regurgitation involves blood flowing back from the left ventricle into the left atrium during systole. Often, the margins of the mitral valve cannot close during systole. The leaflets cannot close because of the thickening and fibrosis of the leaflets and chordae tendineae, resulting in their contraction. The most common causes of mitral valve regurgitation in developed countries are degenerative changes of the mitral valve and ischemia of the left ventricle (Fuster et al., 2004). The most common causes in developing countries are rheumatic heart disease and its sequelae (Fuster et al., 2004).

Other conditions leading to mitral regurgitation include myxomatous changes, which enlarge and stretch the left atrium and ventricle, causing leaflets and chordae tendineae to stretch or rupture. Infective endocarditis may cause perforation of a leaflet, or the scarring following the infection may cause retraction of the leaflets or chordae tendineae. Collagen-vascular diseases (eg, systemic lupus erythematosus), cardiomyopathy, and ischemic heart disease may also result in changes in the left ventricle, causing the papillary muscles, chordae tendineae, or leaflets to stretch, shorten, or rupture.

## Pathophysiology

Mitral regurgitation may result from problems with one or more of the leaflets, the chordae tendineae, the annulus, or the papillary muscles. As previously stated, a mitral valve leaflet may shorten or tear, and the chordae tendineae may elongate, shorten, or tear. The annulus may be stretched by heart enlargement or deformed by calcification. The papillary muscle may rupture, stretch, or be pulled out of position by changes in the ventricular wall (eg, scar from a myocardial infarction or ventricular dilation). The papillary muscles may be unable to contract because of ischemia. Regardless of the cause, blood regurgitates back into the atrium during systole.

With each beat of the left ventricle, some of the blood is forced back into the left atrium. Because this blood is added to the blood flowing in from the lungs, the left atrium must stretch. It eventually hypertrophies and dilates. The backward flow of blood from the ventricle diminishes the volume of blood flowing into the atrium from the lungs. As a result, the lungs become congested, eventually adding extra strain on the right ventricle. Mitral regurgitation ultimately involves the lungs and the right ventricle.

## Clinical Manifestations

Chronic mitral regurgitation is often asymptomatic, but acute mitral regurgitation (eg, that resulting from a myocardial infarction) usually manifests as severe congestive heart failure. Dyspnea, fatigue, and weakness are the most common symptoms. Palpitations, shortness of breath on exertion, and cough from pulmonary congestion also occur.

## Assessment and Diagnostic Findings

A systolic murmur is heard as a high-pitched, blowing sound at the apex. The pulse may be regular and of good volume, or it may be irregular as a result of extrasystolic beats or atrial fibrillation. Doppler echocardiography is used to diagnose and monitor the progression of mitral regurgitation. Transesophageal echocardiography (TEE) provides the best images of the mitral valve.

## Medical Management

Management of mitral regurgitation is the same as that for congestive heart failure (see Chapter 30). Usually, patients with mitral regurgitation benefit from afterload reduction (arterial dilation) by treatment with angiotensin-converting enzyme (ACE) inhibitors, such as captopril (Capoten), enalapril (Vasotec), lisinopril (Prinivil, Zestril), ramipril (Altace), or hydralazine (Apresoline). Once symptoms of heart failure develop, the patient needs to restrict his or her activity level. Antibiotic prophylaxis therapy is instituted to prevent infectious endocarditis. Surgical intervention consists of mitral valvuloplasty (ie, surgical repair of the heart valve) or valve replacement.

## *Mitral Stenosis*

Mitral stenosis is an obstruction of blood flowing from the left atrium into the left ventricle. It is most often caused by rheumatic endocarditis, which progressively thickens the mitral valve leaflets and chordae tendineae. The leaflets often fuse together. Eventually, the mitral valve orifice narrows and progressively obstructs blood flow into the ventricle.

## Pathophysiology

Normally, the mitral valve opening is as wide as the diameter of three fingers. In cases of marked stenosis, the opening narrows to the width of a pencil. The left atrium has great difficulty moving blood into the ventricle because of the increased resistance of the narrowed orifice. The left atrium dilates (stretches) and hypertrophies (thickens) because of the increased blood volume it holds. Because there is no valve to protect the pulmonary veins from the backward flow of blood from the atrium, the pulmonary circulation becomes congested. As a result, the right ventricle must contract against an abnormally high pulmonary arterial pressure and is subjected to excessive strain. Eventually, the right ventricle fails. The enlarged left atrium may create pressure on the left bronchial tree, resulting in a dry cough or wheezing.

## Clinical Manifestations

The first symptom of mitral stenosis is often breathing difficulty (ie, dyspnea) on exertion as a result of pulmonary venous hypertension. Symptoms usually develop after the valve opening is reduced by one-third to one-half its usual size. Patients are likely to show progressive fatigue as a result of low cardiac output. They may expectorate blood (ie, hemoptysis); cough; wheeze; and experience palpitations, orthopnea, paroxysmal nocturnal dyspnea (PND), and repeated respiratory infections.

## Assessment and Diagnostic Findings

The pulse is weak and often irregular because of atrial fibrillation (caused by the strain on the atrium). A low-pitched, rumbling, diastolic murmur is heard at the apex. As a result of the increased blood volume and pressure, the atrium dilates, hypertrophies, and becomes electrically unstable, and patients experience atrial dysrhythmias. Doppler echocardiography is used to diagnose mitral stenosis. Electrocardiography (ECG) and cardiac catheterization with angiography may be used to help determine the severity of the mitral stenosis.

## Medical Management

Congestive heart failure is treated as described in Chapter 30. Patients with mitral stenosis may benefit from anticoagulants to decrease the risk for developing atrial thrombus and may also require treatment for anemia. Antibiotic prophylaxis is instituted to prevent infectious endocarditits.

Patients with mitral stenosis are advised to avoid strenuous activities and competitive sports, both of which increase the heart rate. Mitral stenosis decreases the amount of blood that can flow from the left atrium to the left ventricle during diastole. When the heart rate increases, diastole is shortened, and thus the amount of time for the forward flow of blood is less. Therefore, as the heart rate increases, cardiac output decreases and pulmonary pressures increase with the backup of blood from the left atrium into the pulmonary veins.

Surgical intervention consists of valvuloplasty, usually a commissurotomy to open or rupture the fused commissures of the mitral valve. Percutaneous transluminal valvuloplasty or mitral valve replacement may be performed.

## *Aortic Regurgitation*

Aortic regurgitation is the flow of blood back into the left ventricle from the aorta during diastole. It may be caused by inflammatory lesions that deform the leaflets of the aortic valve, preventing them from completely closing the aortic valve orifice. This valvular defect also may result from infective or rheumatic endocarditis, congenital abnormalities, diseases such as syphilis, a dissecting aneurysm that causes dilation or tearing of the ascending aorta, blunt chest trauma, or deterioration of an aortic valve replacement. In many cases, the cause is unknown and is classified as idiopathic.

## Pathophysiology

Blood from the aorta returns to the left ventricle during diastole, in addition to the blood normally delivered by the left atrium. The left ventricle dilates in an attempt to accommodate the increased volume of blood. It also hypertrophies in an attempt to increase muscle strength to expel more blood with above-normal force, thus increasing systolic blood pressure. The arteries attempt to compensate for the higher pressures by reflex vasodilation; the peripheral arterioles relax, reducing peripheral resistance and diastolic blood pressure.

## Clinical Manifestations

Aortic insufficiency develops without symptoms in most patients. Some patients are aware of a forceful heartbeat, especially in the head or neck. Marked arterial pulsations that are visible or palpable at the carotid or temporal arteries may be present as a result of the increased force and volume of the blood ejected from the hypertrophied left ventricle. Exertional dyspnea and fatigue follow. Progressive signs and symptoms of left ventricular failure include breathing difficulties (eg, orthopnea, PND).

## Assessment and Diagnostic Findings

A diastolic murmur is heard as a high-pitched, blowing sound at the third or fourth intercostal space at the left sternal border. The pulse pressure (ie, difference between systolic and diastolic pressures) is considerably widened in patients with aortic regurgitation. One characteristic sign of the disease is the water-hammer (Corrigan's) pulse, in which the pulse strikes the palpating finger with a quick, sharp stroke and then suddenly collapses. The diagnosis may be confirmed by Doppler echocardiography (preferably transesophageal), radionuclide imaging, ECG, magnetic resonance imaging (MRI), and cardiac catheterization. Patients with symptoms usually have echocardiograms every 4 to 6 months, and those without symptoms have echocardiograms every 2 to 3 years.

## Medical Management

Before the patient undergoes invasive or dental procedures, antibiotic prophylaxis is needed to prevent endocarditis. The patient is advised to avoid physical exertion, competitive sports, and isometric exercise. Dysrhythmias and heart failure are treated as described in Chapters 27 and 30.

The medications usually prescribed first for patients with symptoms of aortic regurgitation are vasodilators such as calcium channel blockers (eg, nifedipine [Adalat, Procardia]) and ACE inhibitors (eg, captopril [Capoten], enalapril [Vasotec], lisinopril [Prinivil, Zestril], ramipril [Altace]) or hydralazine (Apresoline). The treatment of choice is aortic valvuloplasty or valve replacement, preferably performed before left ventricular failure occurs. Surgery is recommended for any patient with left ventricular hypertrophy, regardless of the presence or absence of symptoms.

## *Aortic Stenosis*

Aortic valve stenosis is narrowing of the orifice between the left ventricle and the aorta. In adults, the stenosis is often a result of degenerative calcifications. Calcifications begin on the flexion lines of the leaflets (cusps) at the base (ring, annulus) of the valve and progressively extend outward over the cusps. The calcification may be caused by inflammatory changes that occur in response to years of normal mechanical stress. Diabetes mellitus, hypercholesterolemia, hypertension, and low levels of high-density lipoprotein cholesterol may be risk factors for degenerative changes of the valve. Congenital leaflet malformations or an abnormal number of leaflets (ie, one or two rather than three) may be involved. Rarely, rheumatic endocarditis may cause adhesions or fusion of the commissures and valve ring, stiffening of the cusps, and calcific nodules on the cusps. However, the cause of cusp calcification may be unknown.

## Pathophysiology

Progressive narrowing of the valve orifice occurs, usually over several years to several decades. The left ventricle overcomes the obstruction to circulation by contracting more slowly but with greater energy than normal, forcibly squeezing the blood through the smaller orifice. The obstruction to left ventricular outflow increases pressure on the left ventricle. The ventricular wall thickens, or hypertrophies. When these compensatory mechanisms of the heart begin to fail, clinical signs and symptoms develop.

## Clinical Manifestations

Many patients with aortic stenosis are asymptomatic. When symptoms develop, patients usually first have exertional dyspnea, caused by increased pulmonary venous pressure due to left ventricular failure. Orthopnea, PND, and pulmonary edema may also occur. Other symptoms are dizziness and syncope because of reduced blood flow to the brain. Angina pectoris is a frequent symptom resulting from the increased oxygen demands of the hypertrophied left ventricle, the decreased time in diastole for myocardial perfusion, and the decreased blood flow into the coronary arteries. Blood pressure may be low but is usually normal. Pulse pressure may be low (30 mm Hg or less) because of diminished blood flow.

## Assessment and Diagnostic Findings

On physical examination, a loud, rough systolic murmur may be heard over the aortic area. The sound to listen for is a systolic crescendo–decrescendo murmur, which may radiate into the carotid arteries and to the apex of the left ventricle. The murmur is low-pitched, rough, rasping, and vibrating. An $S_4$ sound may be heard. If the examiner rests a hand over the base of the heart (second intercostal space next to the sternum and above the suprasternal notch up along the carotid arteries), a vibration may be felt. The vibration is caused by turbulent blood flow across the narrowed valve orifice. By having the patient lean forward during auscultation and palpation, especially during exhalation, it is possible to accentuate the signs of aortic stenosis.

Doppler echocardiography is used to diagnose and monitor the progression of aortic stenosis. Patients with symptoms usually have echocardiograms every 6 to 12 months, and those without symptoms have echocardiograms every 2 to 5 years. Evidence of left ventricular hypertrophy may be seen on a 12-lead ECG and an echocardiogram. After stenosis progresses to the point that surgical intervention is considered, left-sided heart catheterization is necessary to measure the severity of the valvular abnormality and to evaluate the coronary arteries. Pressure tracings are taken from the left ventricle and from the base of the aorta. The systolic pressure in the left ventricle is considerably higher than that in the aorta during systole. Graded exercise studies (stress tests) are not usually prescribed for patients with aortic stenosis because of the high risk of precipitating ventricular tachycardia or fibrillation.

## Medical Management

Antibiotic prophylaxis to prevent endocarditis is essential for anyone with aortic stenosis undergoing invasive procedures. After dysrhythmia or left ventricular failure occurs, medications are prescribed (see Chapters 27 and 30). Definitive treatment for aortic stenosis is surgical replacement of the aortic valve. Patients who are symptomatic and are not surgical candidates may benefit from one- or two-balloon percutaneous valvuloplasty procedures.

## Nursing Management: Valvular Heart Disorders

The nurse teaches the patient with valvular heart disease about the diagnosis, the progressive nature of valvular heart disease, and the treatment plan. The patient is taught to report new symptoms or changes in symptoms to the health care provider. In addition, the nurse emphasizes the need for prophylactic antibiotic therapy before any invasive procedure (eg, dental work, genitourinary or gastrointestinal procedure) that may introduce infectious agents into the bloodstream. The nurse teaches the patient that the infectious agent, usually a bacterium, is able to adhere to the diseased heart valve more readily than to a normal valve. Once attached to the valve, the infectious agent multiplies, resulting in endocarditis and further damage to the valve.

The nurse measures the patient's heart rate, blood pressure, and respiratory rate, compares these results with previous data, and notes any changes. Heart and lung sounds are auscultated and peripheral pulses palpated. The nurse assesses the patient with valvular heart disease for the following conditions:

- Signs and symptoms of heart failure, such as fatigue, dyspnea on exertion, an increase in coughing, hemoptysis, multiple respiratory infections, orthopnea, and PND (see Chapter 30)
- Dysrhythmias, by palpating the patient's pulse for strength and rhythm (ie, regular or irregular) and asking whether the patient has experienced palpitations or felt forceful heartbeats (see Chapter 27)
- Symptoms such as dizziness, syncope, increased weakness, or angina pectoris (see Chapter 28)

The nurse collaborates with the patient to develop a medication schedule and teaches about the name, dosage, actions, adverse effects, and any drug–drug or drug–food interactions of the prescribed medications for heart failure, dysrhythmias, angina pectoris, or other symptoms. Particular precautions are emphasized, such as the risk to patients with aortic stenosis who experience angina pectoris and take nitroglycerin. The venous dilation that results from nitroglycerin decreases blood return to the heart, thus decreasing cardiac output and increasing the risk of syncope and decreased coronary artery blood flow. The nurse teaches the patient about the importance of attempting to relieve the symptoms of angina with rest and relaxation before taking nitroglycerin and to anticipate the potential adverse effects.

In addition, the nurse teaches the patient to weigh himself or herself daily and report gains of 2 pounds in 1 day or 5 pounds in 1 week to the health care provider. The nurse may assist the patient with planning activity and rest periods to achieve an acceptable lifestyle. The patient may need to be advised to rest and sleep sitting in a chair or bed with the head elevated when experiencing symptoms of pulmonary congestion. Care of patients treated with valvuloplasty or surgical valve replacement is described later in this chapter.

# Valve Repair and Replacement Procedures

## Valvuloplasty

The repair, rather than replacement, of a cardiac valve is referred to as **valvuloplasty**. In general, valves that undergo valvuloplasty function longer than prosthetic valve replacements, and patients do not require continuous anticoagulation. The type of valvuloplasty depends on the cause and type of valve dysfunction. Repair may be made to the commissures between the leaflets in a procedure known as **commissurotomy**, to the annulus of the valve by annuloplasty, to the leaflets, or to the chordae by chordoplasty. Transesophageal echocardiography (TEE) is usually performed at the conclusion of a valvuloplasty to evaluate the effectiveness of the procedure.

Most valvuloplasty procedures require general anesthesia and often require cardiopulmonary bypass. However, some procedures can be performed in the cardiac catheterization laboratory and do not always require general anesthesia or cardiopulmonary bypass. Percutaneous partial cardiopulmonary bypass is used in some cardiac catheterization laboratories. Cardiopulmonary bypass is achieved by inserting a large catheter (ie, cannula) into two peripheral blood vessels, usually a femoral vein and an artery. Blood is diverted from the body through the venous catheter to the cardiopulmonary bypass machine (see Chapter 28) and returned to the patient through the arterial catheter.

## Commissurotomy

The most common valvuloplasty procedure is commissurotomy. Each valve has leaflets; the site where the leaflets meet is called the *commissure*. The leaflets may adhere to one another and close the commissure (ie, stenosis). Less commonly, the leaflets fuse in such a way that in addition to stenosis, the leaflets are also prevented from closing completely, resulting in a backward flow of blood (ie, regurgitation). A commissurotomy is the procedure performed to separate the fused leaflets.

### Closed Commissurotomy

Closed commissurotomies do not require cardiopulmonary bypass. The valve is not directly visualized. The most common commissurotomy procedure is percutaneous balloon valvuloplasty. Some closed commissurotomies are performed using a surgical technique.

#### BALLOON VALVULOPLASTY

Balloon valvuloplasty (Fig. 29-3) is beneficial for mitral valve stenosis in younger patients, for aortic valve stenosis in elderly patients, and for patients with complex medical conditions that place them at high risk for the complications of more extensive surgical procedures. Most commonly used for mitral and aortic valve stenosis, balloon valvuloplasty also has been used for tricuspid and pulmonic valve stenosis. The procedure is contraindicated for patients with left atrial or ventricular thrombus, severe aortic root dilation, significant mitral valve regurgitation, thoracolumbar scoliosis, rotation of the great vessels, and other cardiac conditions that require open heart surgery.

Balloon valvuloplasty is performed in the cardiac catheterization laboratory. The patient may receive light or moderate sedation or just a local anesthetic. Mitral balloon valvuloplasty involves advancing one or two catheters into the right atrium, through the atrial septum into the left atrium, across the mitral valve into the left ventricle, and out into the aorta. A guide wire is placed through each catheter, and the original catheter is removed. A large balloon catheter is then placed over the guide wire and positioned with the balloon across the mitral valve. The balloon is then inflated with a dilute angiographic solution. When two balloons are used, they are inflated simultaneously. The advantage of two balloons is that they are each smaller than the one large balloon often used, making smaller atrial septal defects. As the balloons are inflated, they usually do not completely occlude the mitral valve, thereby permitting some forward flow of blood during the inflation period. The balloons are usually inflated for 10 to 30 seconds. Multiple inflations are usually required to achieve the desired results.

All patients have some degree of mitral regurgitation after the procedure. Other possible complications include bleeding from the catheter insertion sites, emboli resulting in complications such as strokes, and rarely, left-to-right atrial shunts through an atrial septal defect caused by the procedure.

Aortic balloon valvuloplasty is performed most commonly by introducing a catheter through the aorta, across the aortic valve, and into the left ventricle, although it also may be performed by passing the balloon or balloons through the atrial septum. The one-balloon or the two-balloon technique can be used for treating aortic stenosis. Balloons are inflated for 15 to 60 seconds, and inflation is usually repeated multiple times. The aortic valve procedure is not as effective as the mitral valve procedure, and the rate of restenosis is 36% to 80% in the first 12 months after the procedure (Zipes et al., 2005). Possible complications include aortic regurgitation, emboli, ventricular perforation, rupture of the aortic valve annulus, ventricular dysrhythmia, mitral valve damage, and bleeding from the catheter insertion sites.

#### CLOSED SURGICAL VALVULOPLASTY

Closed surgical valvuloplasty has been performed for mitral, aortic, tricuspid, and pulmonary valve stenosis. The procedure is performed in the operating room with the patient under general anesthesia. A midsternal incision is made, a small hole is cut into the heart, and the surgeon's finger or a dilator is used to open the commissure.

### Open Commissurotomy

Open commissurotomies are performed with direct visualization of the valve. The patient is under general anesthesia.

**FIGURE 29-3.** Balloon valvuloplasty: cross-section of heart illustrating the guide wire and dilation catheter placed through an atrial transseptal puncture and across the mitral valve. The guide wire is extended out from the aortic valve into the aorta for catheter support.

**FIGURE 29-4.** Annuloplasty ring insertion. (**A**) Mitral valve regurgitation; leaflets do not close. (**B**) Insertion of an annuloplasty ring. (**C**) Completed valvuloplasty; leaflets close.

A midsternal or left thoracic incision is made. Cardiopulmonary bypass is initiated, and an incision is made into the heart. The valve is exposed, and the surgeon uses a finger, scalpel, balloon, or dilator to open the commissures.

An added advantage of direct visualization of the valve is that thrombus and calcifications may be identified and removed. If the valve has chordae or papillary muscles, they may be inspected and surgically repaired as necessary (chordoplasty is discussed later in this chapter).

## Annuloplasty

**Annuloplasty** is the repair of the valve annulus (ie, junction of the valve leaflets and the muscular heart wall). General anesthesia and cardiopulmonary bypass are required for all annuloplasties. The procedure narrows the diameter of the valve's orifice and is useful for the treatment of valvular regurgitation.

There are two annuloplasty techniques. One technique uses an annuloplasty ring (Fig. 29-4), which may be preshaped (rigid/semirigid) or flexible. The leaflets of the valve are sutured to a ring, creating an annulus of the desired size. When the ring is in place, the tension created by the moving blood and contracting heart is borne by the ring rather than by the valve or a suture line, and progressive regurgitation is prevented by the repair. The second technique involves tacking the valve leaflets to the atrium with sutures or taking tucks to tighten the annulus. Because the valve's leaflets and the suture lines are subjected to the direct forces of the blood and heart muscle movement, the repair may degenerate more quickly than one using the annuloplasty ring technique.

## Leaflet Repair

Damage to cardiac valve leaflets may result from stretching, shortening, or tearing. **Leaflet repair** for elongated, ballooning, or other excess tissue leaflets is removal of the extra tissue. The elongated tissue may be folded over onto itself (ie, tucked) and sutured (ie, leaflet plication). A wedge of tissue may be cut from the middle of the leaflet and the gap sutured closed (ie, leaflet resection) (Fig. 29-5). Short

**FIGURE 29-5.** Valve leaflet resection and repair with a ring annuloplasty. (**A**) Mitral valve regurgitation; the section indicated by dashed lines is excised. (**B**) Approximation of edges and suturing. (**C**) Completed valvuloplasty, leaflet repair, and annuloplasty ring.

leaflets are most often repaired by chordoplasty. After the short chordae are released, the leaflets often unfurl and can resume their normal function (closing the valve during systole). A piece of pericardium may also be sutured to extend the leaflet. A pericardial or synthetic patch may be used to repair holes in the leaflets.

## Chordoplasty

**Chordoplasty** is repair of the chordae tendineae. The mitral valve is involved with chordoplasty (because it has the chordae tendineae), and chordoplasty is seldom required for the tricuspid valve. Regurgitation may be caused by stretched, torn, or shortened chordae tendineae. Stretched chordae tendineae can be shortened, transposed to the other leaflet, or replaced with synthetic chordae. Torn chordae can be reattached to the leaflet and shortened chordae can be elongated. Regurgitation may also be caused by stretched papillary muscles, which can be shortened.

## Valve Replacement

Prosthetic **valve replacement** began in the 1960s. When valvuloplasty or valve repair is not a viable alternative, such as when the annulus or leaflets of the valve are immobilized by calcifications, valve replacement is performed. General anesthesia and cardiopulmonary bypass are used for valve replacements. Most procedures are performed through a median sternotomy (ie, incision through the sternum), although the mitral valve may be approached through a right thoracotomy incision. Mitral, and more rarely aortic, valve replacements may be performed with minimally invasive techniques that do not involve cutting through the length of the sternum. Instead, incisions are made in only the upper or lower half of the sternum or between ribs; these incisions are only 2 to 4 inches long. Some of these minimally invasive procedures are robot-assisted; the surgical instruments are connected to a robot, and the surgeon, watching a video display, uses a joystick to control the robot and surgical instruments. With these procedures, patients have less bleeding, pain, risk for infection, and scarring. Hospital stays average 3 days, and recovery may be as short as 3 weeks (Aazami & Schafers, 2003; Fuster et al., 2004; Mitka, 2003).

After the valve is visualized, the leaflets of the aortic or pulmonic valve are removed, but some or all of the mitral valve structures (leaflets, chordae, and papillary muscles) are left in place to help maintain the shape and function of the left ventricle after mitral valve replacement. Sutures are placed around the annulus and then through the valve prosthesis. The replacement valve is slid down the suture into position and tied into place (Fig. 29-6). The incision is closed, and the surgeon evaluates the function of the heart and the quality of the prosthetic repair. The patient is weaned from cardiopulmonary bypass, the surgical repair is often assessed with color flow Doppler TEE, and surgery is completed.

Before surgery, the heart had gradually adjusted to the pathology, but the surgery abruptly "corrects" the way blood flows through the heart. Complications unique to

**FIGURE 29-6.** Valve replacement. (**A**) The native valve is trimmed, and the prosthetic valve is sutured in place. (**B**) Once all sutures are placed through the ring, the surgeon slides the prosthetic valve down the sutures and into the natural orifice. The sutures are then tied off and trimmed.

valve replacement are related to the sudden changes in intracardiac blood pressures. All prosthetic valve replacements create a degree of stenosis when they are implanted in the heart. Usually, the stenosis is mild and does not affect heart function. If valve replacement was for a stenotic valve, blood flow through the heart is often improved. The signs and symptoms of the backward heart failure resolve in a few hours or days. If valve replacement was for a regurgitant valve, it may take months for the chamber into which blood had been regurgitating to achieve its optimal postoperative function. The signs and symptoms of heart failure resolve gradually as the heart function improves. Patients are at risk for many postoperative complications, such as bleeding, thromboembolism, infection, congestive heart failure, hypertension, dysrhythmias, hemolysis, and mechanical obstruction of the valve.

## Types of Valve Prostheses

Two types of valve prostheses may be used: mechanical and tissue (ie, biologic) valves (Fig. 29-7).

### Mechanical Valves

Mechanical valves are of the ball-and-cage or disk design and are thought to be more durable than tissue prosthetic valves; therefore, they are often used for younger patients. Mechanical valves are used for patients with renal failure, hypercalcemia, endocarditis, or sepsis who require valve replacement. The mechanical valves do not deteriorate or become infected as easily as the tissue valves used for patients with these conditions. Significant complications associated with mechanical valves are thromboemboli requiring long-term use of anticoagulants. Some amount of hemolysis also occurs with mechanical valves; usually it is not clinically significant.

**FIGURE 29-7.** Common mechanical and tissue valve replacements. (**A**) Caged ball valve (Starr-Edwards, mechanical). (**B**) Tilting-disk valve (Medtronic-Hall, mechanical). (**C**) Porcine heterograft valve (Carpenter-Edwards, tissue).

### Tissue (Biologic) Valves

Tissue (ie, biologic) valves are of three types: xenografts, homografts, and autografts. Tissue valves are less likely to generate thromboemboli, and long-term anticoagulation is not required. Tissue valves are not as durable as mechanical valves and require replacement more frequently.

#### XENOGRAFTS

**Xenografts** are tissue valves (eg, bioprostheses, **heterografts**) that are used for all tricuspid valve replacements. They are used for women of childbearing age because the potential complications of long-term anticoagulation associated with menses, placental transfer to a fetus, and delivery of a child do not exist. They also are used for patients older than 70 years of age, patients with a history of peptic ulcer disease, and others who cannot tolerate long-term anticoagulation. Most xenografts are from pigs (porcine), but valves from cows (bovine) may also be used. Viability is 7 to 10 years. Xenografts do not generate thrombi, thereby eliminating the need for long-term anticoagulation.

#### HOMOGRAFTS

**Homografts,** or **allografts** (ie, human valves), are obtained from cadaver tissue donations and are used for aortic and pulmonic valve replacement. The aortic valve and a portion of the aorta or the pulmonic valve and a portion of the pulmonary artery are harvested and stored cryogenically. Homografts are not always available and are very expensive. They last for about 10 to 15 years, somewhat longer than xenografts. They are not thrombogenic and are resistant to subacute bacterial endocarditis.

#### AUTOGRAFTS

**Autografts** (ie, autologous valves) are obtained by excising the patient's own pulmonic valve and a portion of the pulmonary artery for use as the aortic valve. Anticoagulation is unnecessary because the valve is the patient's own tissue and is not thrombogenic. The autograft is an alternative for children (it may grow as the child grows), women of childbearing age, young adults, patients with a history of peptic ulcer disease, and people who cannot tolerate anticoagulation. Aortic valve autografts have remained viable for more than 20 years.

Most aortic valve autograft procedures are double valve-replacement procedures; a homograft also is performed for pulmonic valve replacement. If pulmonary vascular pressures are normal, some surgeons elect not to replace the pulmonic valve. Patients can recover without a valve between the right ventricle and the pulmonary artery.

## Nursing Management: Valvuloplasty and Replacement

Patients who have had percutaneous balloon valvuloplasty procedures may be admitted to a telemetry or intensive care unit. The nurse assesses for signs and symptoms of heart failure and emboli (see Chapter 30), listens for any changes in heart sounds at least every 4 hours, and provides the patient with the same care as for postprocedure cardiac catheterization or percutaneous transluminal coronary angioplasty (PTCA) (see Chapter 28). After undergoing percutaneous balloon valvuloplasty, the patient usually remains in the hospital for 24 to 48 hours.

Patients who have had surgical valvuloplasty or valve replacements are admitted to the intensive care unit. Care focuses on recovery from anesthesia and hemodynamic stability. Vital signs are assessed every 5 to 15 minutes and as needed until the patient recovers from anesthesia or sedation, and then are assessed every 2 to 4 hours and as needed. Intravenous (IV) medications to increase or decrease blood pressure and to treat dysrhythmias or altered heart rates are administered and their effects monitored. The medications are gradually decreased until they are no longer required or the patient can take the needed medication by another route (eg, oral, topical). Patient assessments are conducted every 1 to 4 hours and as needed, with particular attention to neurologic, respiratory, and cardiovascular systems. (See Chapter 28, Chart 28-13, which presents a plan of nursing care for a patient recovering from cardiac surgery.)

After the patient has recovered from anesthesia and sedation, is hemodynamically stable without IV medications, and has stable physical assessment parameters, he or she is usually transferred to a telemetry unit, typically within 24 to 72 hours of surgery. Nursing care continues as for most postoperative patients, including wound care and patient teaching regarding diet, activity, medications, and self-care.

The nurse educates the patient about long-term anticoagulant therapy, explaining the need for frequent follow-up appointments and blood laboratory studies. Patients who take warfarin (Coumadin) usually have individualized target International Normalized Ratios (INRs) between 2 and 3.5. Patients who have been treated with an annuloplasty ring or a tissue valve replacement usually require anticoagulation for only 3 months, unless there are other risk factors such as atrial fibrillation or a history of thromboembolism. Aspirin may be prescribed with warfarin for some patients. The nurse provides teaching about all prescribed medications: the name of the medication, dosage, its actions, prescribed schedule, potential adverse effects, and any drug–drug or drug–food interactions. Patients with a mechanical valve prosthesis (including annuloplasty rings and other prosthetic materials used in valvuloplasty) or a history of rheumatic heart disease require education to prevent infective endocarditis with antibiotic prophylaxis, which is prescribed before all dental and surgical procedures.

The patient is usually discharged from the hospital in 3 to 7 days. Home care and office or clinic nurses reinforce all new information and self-care instructions with patients and families for 4 to 8 weeks after the procedure. Doppler echocardiograms are usually performed 3 to 4 weeks after discharge from the hospital to further evaluate the effects and results of the surgery. The echocardiogram also provides a baseline for future comparison should cardiac symptoms or complications develop. Doppler echocardiograms are usually repeated every 1 to 2 years.

## Septal Repair

The atrial or ventricular septum may have an abnormal opening between the right and left sides of the heart (ie, septal defect). Although most septal defects are congenital and are repaired during infancy or childhood, adults may not have undergone early repair or may develop septal defects as a result of myocardial infarctions or diagnostic and treatment procedures.

Repair of septal defects requires general anesthesia and cardiopulmonary bypass. The heart is opened, and a pericardial or synthetic (usually polyester or Dacron) patch is used to close the opening. Atrial septal defect repairs have low morbidity and mortality rates. When the mitral or tricuspid valve is involved, however, the procedure is more complicated because valve repair or replacement may be required and the heart failure may be more severe. Generally, ventricular septal defect repairs are uncomplicated, but close proximity of the defect to the intraventricular conduction system and the valves may make this repair more complex. (See Chapter 28, Chart 28-13, which presents a plan of nursing care for a patient recovering from cardiac surgery.) Patients should be taught the importance of infective endocarditis antibiotic prophylaxis for 6 months after the repair. If minimal or no hemodynamic abnormality is evident by Doppler echocardiography after 6 months, antibiotic prophylaxis may be discontinued.

## Cardiomyopathy

**Cardiomyopathy** is a heart muscle disease associated with cardiac dysfunction. It is classified according to the structural and functional abnormalities of the heart muscle: dilated cardiomyopathy (DCM), hypertrophic cardiomyopathy (HCM), restrictive or constrictive cardiomyopathy (RCM), arrhythmogenic right ventricular cardiomyopathy (ARVC), and unclassified cardiomyopathy (Richardson, McKenna, Bristow, et al., 1996). The patient may have pathology representing more than one of these classifications, such as a patient with HCM developing dilation and symptoms of DCM. *Ischemic cardiomyopathy* is a term frequently used to describe an enlarged heart caused by coronary artery disease, which is usually accompanied by heart failure (see Chapter 30).

Regardless of type and cause, cardiomyopathy may lead to severe heart failure, lethal dysrhythmias, and death. The mortality rate is highest for African Americans and the elderly.

### Pathophysiology

The pathophysiology of all cardiomyopathies is a series of events that culminate in impaired cardiac output. Decreased stroke volume stimulates the sympathetic nervous system and the renin–angiotensin–aldosterone response, resulting in increased systemic vascular resistance and increased sodium and fluid retention, which places an increased workload on the heart. These alterations can lead to heart failure (see Chapter 30).

### Dilated Cardiomyopathy (DCM)

DCM is the most common form of cardiomyopathy, with an incidence of 5 to 8 cases per 100,000 people per year and increasing. DCM occurs more often in men and African

Americans, who also have higher mortality rates (Zipes et al., 2005). DCM is distinguished by significant dilation of the ventricles without simultaneous hypertrophy (ie, increased muscle wall thickness) and systolic dysfunction (Fig. 29-8). The ventricles have elevated systolic and diastolic volumes but a decreased ejection fraction (EF). DCM was formerly named *congestive cardiomyopathy,* but it may exist without signs and symptoms of congestion.

More than 75 conditions and diseases may cause DCM, including pregnancy, heavy alcohol intake, viral infection (eg, influenza), and Chagas disease. When the causative factor cannot be identified, the diagnosis is *idiopathic DCM.* Idiopathic DCM accounts for approximately 25% of all heart failure cases. Because genetic factors may be involved, echocardiography and ECG should be used to screen all first-degree blood relatives (eg, parents, siblings, children) for DCM (Zipes et al., 2005).

Microscopic examination of the muscle tissue shows diminished contractile elements (actin and myosin filaments) of the muscle fibers and diffuse necrosis of myocardial cells. The result is poor systolic function. The structural changes decrease the amount of blood ejected from the ventricle with systole, increasing the amount of blood remaining in the ventricle after contraction. Less blood is then able to enter the ventricle during diastole, increasing end-diastolic pressure and eventually increasing pulmonary and systemic venous pressures. Altered valve function, usually regurgitation, can result from an enlarged stretched ventricle. Poor blood flow through the ventricle may also cause ventricular or atrial thrombi, which may embolize to other locations in the body. Early diagnosis and treatment can prevent or delay significant symptoms and sudden death from DCM.

### Hypertrophic Cardiomyopathy (HCM)

HCM is a rare autosomal dominant condition, occurring in men, women, and children (often detected after puberty) with an estimated prevalence rate of 0.05% to 0.2% (Berul & Zevitz, 2002). Echocardiograms may be performed every year from 12 to 18 years of age and then every 5 years from 18 to 70 years of age. HCM also may be idiopathic (ie, no known cause).

In HCM, the heart muscle asymmetrically increases in size and mass, especially along the septum (see Fig. 29-8). HCM often affects nonadjacent areas of the ventricle. The increased thickness of the heart muscle reduces the size of the ventricular cavities and causes the ventricles to take a longer time to relax after systole. During the first part of diastole it is more difficult for the ventricles to fill with blood. The atrial contraction at the end of diastole becomes critical for ventricular filling and systolic contraction.

HCM may be nonobstructive or obstructive. If the increased septal size causes misalignment of the papillary muscles of the left ventricle, the septum and mitral valve can obstruct the flow of blood from the left ventricle into the aorta during ventricular contraction. Because of the structural changes, HCM had also been called idiopathic hypertrophic subaortic stenosis (IHSS) and asymmetric septal hypertrophy (ASH). The structural changes that result in the smaller-than-normal ventricular cavity also create a higher-velocity flow of blood out of the left ventricle into the aorta. HCM may cause significant diastolic dysfunction, but systolic function is usually normal or high, resulting in a higher-than-normal ejection fraction. Doppler echocardiography is used to detect the HCM and blood flow alterations (Zipes et al., 2005).

Cardiac muscle cells normally lie parallel to and end-to-end with each other. The hypertrophied cardiac muscle cells are oblique and perpendicular to each other, decreasing the effectiveness of contractions and possibly increasing the risk for dysrhythmias such as ventricular tachycardia and ventricular fibrillation. In HCM the coronary arteriole walls are thickened, which decreases the internal diameter of the arterioles. The narrow arterioles restrict the blood supply to the myocardium, causing numerous small areas of ischemia and necrosis. The necrotic areas of the myocardium ultimately fibrose and scar, further impeding ventricular contraction.

### Restrictive Cardiomyopathy

RCM is characterized by diastolic dysfunction caused by rigid ventricular walls that impair diastolic filling and ventricular stretch (see Fig. 29-8). Systolic function is usually normal. Because RCM is the least common cardiomyopathy, representing approximately 5% of cases of pediatric

**FIGURE 29-8.** Cardiomyopathies that lead to congestive heart failure. From Anatomical Chart Company (2006). *Atlas of pathophysiology* (2nd ed.). Ambler, PA: Lippincott Williams & Wilkins.

cardiomyopathies, its pathogenesis is the least understood (Shaddy, 2004). RCM may be associated with amyloidosis (amyloid, a protein substance, is deposited within cells) and other such infiltrative diseases. However, the cause is unknown (ie, idiopathic) in most cases. Signs and symptoms are similar to constrictive pericarditis: dyspnea, nonproductive cough, and chest pain. Echocardiography is used to differentiate the two conditions. In addition, patients with RCM usually have pulmonary artery systolic (PAS) pressures of at least 50 mm Hg and pulmonary artery wedge pressures (PAWPs) at least 5 mm Hg greater than central venous pressures (CVPs), and computed tomography (CT) or MRI scans usually show normal thickness of the pericardium. Patients with constrictive pericarditis usually have PAS pressures less than 50 mm Hg and PAWP and CVP within 5 mm Hg of each other, and CT or MRI scans show thickening of the pericardium.

### *Arrhythmogenic Right Ventricular Cardiomyopathy*

ARVC occurs when the myocardium of the right ventricle is progressively infiltrated and replaced by fibrous scar and adipose tissue. Initially, only localized areas of the right ventricle are affected, but as the disease progresses, the entire heart is affected. Eventually, the right ventricle dilates and develops poor contractility, right ventricular wall abnormalities, and dysrhythmias. The prevalence of ARVC is unknown because many cases are not recognized. Palpitations or syncope may develop between 15 and 40 years of age. ARVC should be suspected in patients with ventricular tachycardia originating in the right ventricle (ie, a left bundle branch block configuration on ECG) or sudden death, especially among previously symptom-free athletes (McRae, Chung, Asher et al., 2001). ARVC may be genetic (ie, autosomal dominant) (Richardson et al., 1996). First-degree blood relatives (eg, parents, siblings, children) should be screened for the disease with a 12-lead ECG, Holter monitor, and echocardiography.

### *Unclassified Cardiomyopathies*

Unclassified cardiomyopathies are different from or have characteristics of more than one of the previously described types. Examples of unclassified cardiomyopathies include fibroelastosis, noncompacted myocardium, systolic dysfunction with minimal dilation, and mitochondrial involvement (Richardson et al., 1996).

## Clinical Manifestations

Patients with cardiomyopathy may remain stable and without symptoms for many years. As the disease progresses, so do symptoms. Frequently, dilated or restrictive cardiomyopathy is first diagnosed when the patient presents with signs and symptoms of heart failure (eg, dyspnea on exertion, fatigue). Patients with cardiomyopathy may also report PND, cough (especially with exertion), and orthopnea, which may lead to a misdiagnosis of bronchitis or pneumonia. Other symptoms include fluid retention, peripheral edema, and nausea, which is caused by poor perfusion of the gastrointestinal system. The patient also may experience chest pain, palpitations, dizziness, nausea, and syncope with exertion. However, with HCM, cardiac arrest (ie, sudden cardiac death) may be the initial manifestation in young people, including athletes (Maron, McKenna, Danielson, et al., 2003).

## Assessment and Diagnostic Findings

Physical examination in the early stage may reveal tachycardia and extra heart sounds (eg, $S_3$, $S_4$). Patients with DCM may have diastolic murmurs, and patients with DCM and HCM may have systolic murmurs. With disease progression, examination also reveals signs and symptoms of heart failure (eg, crackles on pulmonary auscultation, jugular vein distention, pitting edema of dependent body parts, enlarged liver).

Diagnosis is usually made from findings disclosed by the patient history and by ruling out other causes of heart failure such as myocardial infarction. The echocardiogram is one of the most helpful diagnostic tools because the structure and function of the ventricles can be observed easily. ECG demonstrates dysrhythmias (atrial fibrillation, ventricular dysrhythmias) and changes consistent with left ventricular hypertrophy (left axis deviation, wide QRS, ST changes, inverted T waves). In ARVC, there often is a small deflection, an epsilon wave, at the end of the QRS. The chest x-ray reveals heart enlargement and possibly pulmonary congestion. Cardiac catheterization is sometimes used to rule out coronary artery disease as a causative factor. Endomyocardial biopsy may be performed to analyze myocardial tissue cells.

## Medical Management

Medical management is directed toward determining and managing possible underlying or precipitating causes; correcting the heart failure with medications, a low-sodium diet, and an exercise/rest regimen (see Chapter 30); and controlling dysrhythmias with antiarrhythmic medications and possibly with an implanted electronic device, such as an implantable cardioverter defibrillator (see Chapter 27). Infective endocarditis prophylaxis and systemic anticoagulation to prevent thromboembolic events are usually recommended. If the patient has signs and symptoms of congestion, fluid intake may be limited to 2 liters each day. Patients with HCM should avoid dehydration and may need beta-blockers [atenolol (Tenormin), metoprolol (Lopressor), nadolol (Corgard), propranolol (Inderal)] to maintain cardiac output and minimize the risk of left ventricular outflow tract obstruction during systole. Patients with HCM or RCM may need to limit physical activity to avoid a life-threatening dysrhythmia.

A pacemaker may be implanted to alter the electrical stimulation of the muscle and prevent the forceful hyperdynamic contractions that occur with HCM. Atrial-ventricular and biventricular pacing have been used to decrease symptoms and obstruction of the left ventricular outflow tract. For some patients with DCM and HCM, biventricular pacing increases the ejection fraction and reverses some of the structural changes in the myocardium.

Nonsurgical septal reduction therapy, also called alcohol septal ablation, has been used to treat obstructive HCM. In the cardiac catheterization laboratory, a percutaneous catheter is positioned in one or more of the septal coronary arteries. Once the position is verified, 2 to 5 mL of ethanol (ethyl alcohol) is injected at a rate of about 1 mL/minute to kill the myocardial cells; it is believed that the ethanol causes dehydration of the cardiac cells (Cruickshank, 2004; Maron, 2002). The slow rate of injection minimizes the risk of heart block and premature ventricular contractions (PVCs). The procedure produces a septal myocardial infarction. The resulting scar is thinner than the living myocardium would have been, so the obstruction is decreased. The patient may develop a left anterior hemibranch block or left bundle branch block. If the patient experiences pain, hydrocodone/acetaminophen (Vicodin) is usually administered. Nitrates and morphine are not used, because coronary artery dilation is contraindicated.

## *Surgical Management*

When heart failure progresses and medical treatment is no longer effective, surgical intervention, including heart transplantation, is considered. However, because of the limited number of organ donors, many patients die waiting for transplantation. In some cases, a left ventricular assist device is implanted to support the failing heart until a suitable donor heart becomes available (mechanical assist devices and total artificial hearts are discussed later in this chapter).

### LEFT VENTRICULAR OUTFLOW TRACT SURGERY

When patients with HCM become symptomatic despite medical therapy and a difference in pressure of 50 mm Hg or more exists between the left ventricle and the aorta, surgery is considered. The most common procedure is a myectomy (sometimes referred to as a myotomy-myectomy), in which some of the heart tissue is excised. Septal tissue approximately 1 cm wide and deep is cut from the enlarged septum below the aortic valve. The length of septum removed depends on the degree of obstruction caused by the hypertrophied muscle.

Instead of a septal myectomy, the surgeon may open the left ventricular outflow tract to the aortic valve by mitral valvuloplasty involving the leaflets, chordae, or papillary muscles, or the patient's mitral valve may be replaced with a low-profile disk valve. The space taken up by the mitral valve is substantially reduced by the valvuloplasty or prosthetic valve, allowing blood to move around the enlarged septum to the aortic valve through the area the mitral valve once occupied. The primary complication of all the procedures is dysrhythmias. Additional complications include postoperative surgical complications such as pain, ineffective airway clearance, deep vein thrombosis, risk for infection, and delayed surgical recovery.

### LATISSIMUS DORSI MUSCLE WRAP

DCM may be treated with a latissimus dorsi muscle wrap, also called dynamic cardiomyoplasty (Rigatelli, Barbiero, Cotogni, et al., 2003; Woods et al., 2005; Zipes et al., 2005). The left latissimus dorsi muscle is dissected from the lateral side and back of the chest, leaving the medial end of the muscle and the blood supply intact, and the lateral end of the muscle is pulled through the pleural space into the pericardium. The latissimus dorsi muscle flap is then wrapped around the ventricles and sutured in place. Pacemaker leads are implanted into the muscle flap, and a pacemaker generator is implanted in the chest wall. For at least 2 weeks following surgery, the pacemaker remains turned off to facilitate the development of adhesions between the muscle wrap and the ventricles. Eventually, the pacemaker is turned on and used to stimulate latissimus dorsi muscle contraction. Several weeks of training, or conditioning, are necessary before this skeletal muscle functions effectively. The ultimate goal is for the latissimus dorsi muscle wrap to augment ventricular contraction and increase cardiac output. This skeletal muscle loses its contractility over time, and the patient may be evaluated for heart transplantation.

### HEART TRANSPLANTATION

The first human-to-human heart transplant was performed in 1967. Since then, transplant procedures, equipment, and medications have continued to improve. In 1983, when cyclosporine became available, heart transplantation became a therapeutic option for patients with end-stage heart disease. Cyclosporine (Neoral, Sandimmune, SangCya) is an immunosuppressant that greatly decreases the body's rejection of foreign proteins, such as transplanted organs. Unfortunately, cyclosporine also decreases the body's ability to resist infections, and a satisfactory balance must be achieved between suppressing rejection and avoiding infection.

Cardiomyopathy, ischemic heart disease, valvular disease, rejection of previously transplanted hearts, and congenital heart disease are the most common indications for transplantation (Taylor, Edwards, Mohacsi, et al., 2003; Woods et al., 2005). Typical candidates have severe symptoms uncontrolled by medical therapy, no other surgical options, and a prognosis of less than 12 months to live. A multidisciplinary team screens the candidate before recommending the transplantation procedure. The person's age, pulmonary status, other chronic health conditions, psychosocial status, family support, infections, history of other transplantations, compliance, and current health status are considered.

When a donor heart becomes available, a computer generates a list of potential recipients on the basis of ABO blood group compatibility, the body sizes of the donor and the potential recipient, and the geographic locations of the donor and potential recipient. Distance is a factor, because postoperative function depends on the heart being implanted within 6 hours of harvest from the donor. Some patients are candidates for more than one organ transplant: (eg, heart–lung, heart–pancreas, heart–kidney, heart–liver).

**Orthotopic Transplantation.** Orthotopic transplantation is the most common surgical procedure for cardiac transplantation (Fig. 29-9). The recipient's heart is removed, and the donor heart is implanted at the vena cava and pulmonary veins. Some surgeons prefer to remove the recipient's heart leaving a portion of the recipient's atria (with the vena cava and pulmonary veins) in place. The donor heart, which usually has been preserved in ice, is prepared for implant by cutting away a small section of the atria that corresponds with the sections of the recipient's heart that were left in place. The donor heart is implanted by suturing the donor atria to the residual atrial tissue of the recipient's heart. After the venous or atrial anastomoses are complete, the recipient's pulmonary artery and aorta are sutured to those of the donor heart.

**Postoperative Course.** Patients who have had heart transplants are constantly balancing the risk of rejection with the risk of infection. They must adhere to a complex regimen of diet, medications, activity, follow-up laboratory studies, biopsies of the transplanted heart (to diagnose rejection),

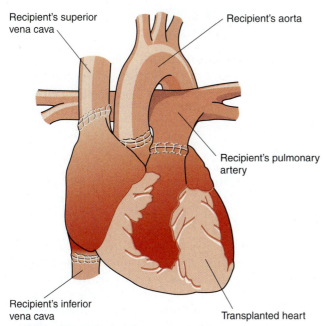

**FIGURE 29-9.** Orthotopic method of heart transplantation.

and clinic visits. Most commonly, patients receive cyclosporine or tacrolimus (Prograf), azathioprine (Imuran) or mycophenolate mofetil (CellCept), and corticosteroids (ie, prednisone) to minimize rejection.

The transplanted heart has no nerve connections to the recipient's body (ie, denervated heart), and the sympathetic and vagus nerves do not affect the transplanted heart. The resting rate of the transplanted heart is approximately 70 to 90 beats per minute, but it increases gradually if catecholamines are in the circulation. Patients must gradually increase and decrease their exercise (ie, extended warm-up and cool-down periods), because 20 to 30 minutes may be required to achieve the desired heart rate. Atropine does not increase the heart rate of transplanted hearts.

In addition to rejection and infection, complications may include accelerated atherosclerosis of the coronary arteries (ie, cardiac allograft vasculopathy or accelerated graft atherosclerosis). Both immunologic and nonimmunologic factors cause arterial injury and inflammation of the coronary arteries, which contribute to the accelerated atherosclerosis along the entire length of the coronary arteries (Deng, 2002; Woods et al., 2005). Hypertension may occur in patients taking cyclosporine or tacrolimus; the cause has not been identified. Osteoporosis frequently occurs as a side effect of the antirejection medications and pretransplantation dietary insufficiency and medications as well as the long-term sedentary lifestyle. Posttransplantation lymphoproliferative disease and cancer of the skin and lips are the most common malignancies after transplantation, possibly caused by immunosuppression. Weight gain; obesity; diabetes; dyslipidemias (eg, hypercholesterolemia); hypotension; renal failure; and central nervous system, respiratory, and gastrointestinal disturbances may be adverse effects of the corticosteroids or other immunosuppressants. Toxicity from immunosuppressant medications may occur. The 1-year survival rate for patients with transplanted hearts is approximately 80% to 90%, and the 5-year survival rate is approximately 60% to 70% (Deng, 2002; Fuster et al., 2004; Zipes, et al., 2005).

Patients respond to the psychosocial stresses imposed by organ transplantation in various ways. They may experience guilt that someone had to die for them to be able to live, have anxiety about the new heart, experience depression or fear about rejection, or have difficulty with family role changes before and after transplantation (Evangelista, Doering, & Dracup et al., 2003; Fuster et al., 2004; Woods et al., 2004).

## MECHANICAL ASSIST DEVICES AND TOTAL ARTIFICIAL HEARTS

The use of cardiopulmonary bypass for cardiovascular surgery and the possibility of performing heart transplantation for end-stage cardiac disease have increased the need for mechanical assist devices. Patients who cannot be weaned from cardiopulmonary bypass and patients in cardiogenic shock may benefit from a period of mechanical heart assistance. The most commonly used device is the intra-aortic balloon pump (see Chapter 30). This pump decreases the work of the heart during contraction but does not perform the actual work of the heart.

**Ventricular Assist Devices.** More complex devices that actually perform some or all of the pumping function for the heart also are being used. These more sophisticated **ventricular assist devices** (VADs) can circulate as much blood per minute as the heart, if not more (Fig. 29-10). Each VAD is used to support one ventricle. Some VADs can be combined with an oxygenator; the combination is called extracorporeal membrane oxygenation (ECMO). The oxygenator–VAD combination is used for the patient whose heart cannot pump adequate blood through the lungs or the body.

There are two basic types of VADs: pneumatic and electric or electromagnetic. Pneumatic VADs are external or implanted pulsatile devices with a flexible reservoir housed in a rigid exterior. The reservoir usually fills with blood drained from the patient's atrium or ventricle. The device then forces pressurized air into the rigid housing, compressing the reservoir and returning the blood to the patient's circulation, usually into the aorta. Electric or electromagnetic VADs are similar to the pneumatic VADs, but instead of using pressurized air to return the blood to the patient's circulation, one or more flat metal plates are pushed against the reservoir.

**Total Artificial Hearts.** **Total artificial hearts** are designed to replace both ventricles. Some require the removal of the patient's heart to implant the total artificial heart, and others do not. All of these devices are experimental. Although there has been some short-term success, the long-term results have been disappointing. Researchers hope to develop a device that can be permanently implanted and that will eliminate the need for donated human heart transplantation for end-stage cardiac disease (Fuster et al., 2004; Kherani & Oz, 2004; Zipes et al., 2005).

Most VADs and total artificial hearts are temporary treatments while the patient's own heart recovers or until a donor heart becomes available for transplantation (ie, "bridge to transplant"). Some devices are being investigated for permanent use. Complications of VADs and total artificial hearts include bleeding disorders, hemorrhage, thrombus, emboli, hemolysis, infection, renal failure, right-sided heart failure, multisystem failure, and mechanical failure (Zipes et al., 2005). Nursing care for these patients focuses on assessing for and minimizing these complications and providing emotional support and education about the mechanical assist device and about the underlying cardiac disease.

## NURSING RESEARCH PROFILE

### Perspectives of Women After Heart Transplantation

Evangelista, L. S., Doering, L., & Dracup, K. (2003). Meaning and life purpose: The perspectives of post-transplant women. *Heart & Lung, 32*(4), 250–257.

#### Purpose
Studies have shown that psychological distress is experienced following heart transplant surgery. However, few studies have explored how heart transplant recipients have perceived their transplant experiences and how their lives have been affected by the transplant. The majority of studies that have been conducted have been limited to male subjects. The purpose of this descriptive, exploratory study was to examine women's perceptions and psychosocial responses to the experiences of end-stage heart failure and heart transplant surgery.

#### Design
Participants were women who had had a heart transplant. Thirty-three participants, who had a mean age of 62.3 years and who were a mean of 4.6 years since heart transplant, were recruited from an outpatient posttransplant clinic to complete two standardized questionnaires (Life Attitudes Profile; Multiple Affect Adjective Checklist) and participate in a semistructured interview with a researcher. The data collection took place in the participants' homes. The Life Attitudes Profile was used to measure the participants' perceptions of their life's meaning, goals, anxiety, fulfillment, and satisfaction with life. The Multiple Affect Adjective Checklist was used to measure participants' mood states of anxiety, depression, and hostility. During the interviews the participants were asked to describe their perceptions about their illness and health condition and how their lives had been affected by their health experiences, including their heart transplant surgery. Analysis of the data included correlations between life's meaning, life purpose, and psychological mood states. Content analysis was used to identify common themes that emerged in the interviews.

#### Findings
The study participants had an average meaning score of 30.64 (range, 10–43) and an average life purpose score of 40.12 (range, 17–63)—the higher the scores, the higher or better are the perceptions of meaning and life purpose. The participants reported that they experienced high levels of psychological distress, including anxiety, depression, and hostility, both before and after the transplant surgery. They reported experiencing pretransplant fears about dying while asleep, the shortage of donated organs, and not having enough strength to manage their conditions, and they reported experiencing posttransplant fears about physiologic rejection of the new heart and about the continuing possibility of dying. These data validated the results of previous studies.

The participants reported that they had experienced feelings of lack of control over their health and lives, and this lack of control caused some participants to become depressed or angry. The women's perceptions of lack of control were important findings among heart transplant patients. The majority of the women had positive attitudes about their transplant surgery.

#### Nursing Implications
Nurses need to provide psychological support and counseling to women before and after heart transplant surgery. The counseling should address individual concerns, promote positive meaning in life, and encourage optimistic behaviors. Discussions about life's meaning and purpose may decrease a woman's psychological distress. Women need to be assisted to identify their fears and develop strategies to retain a sense of control.

## Nursing Process

### The Patient with Cardiomyopathy

#### Assessment

Nursing assessment for the patient with cardiomyopathy begins with a detailed history of the presenting signs and symptoms. The nurse identifies possible etiologic factors, such as heavy alcohol intake, recent illness or pregnancy, or history of the disease in immediate family members. If the patient reports chest pain, a thorough review of the pain, including its precipitating factors, is warranted. The review of systems includes the presence of orthopnea, PND, and syncope or dyspnea with exertion. The number of pillows needed to sleep, usual weight, any weight change, and limitations on activities of daily living are assessed. The New York Heart Association Classification for heart failure is determined. The patient's usual diet is evaluated to determine whether alterations are needed to reduce sodium intake.

Because of the chronicity of cardiomyopathy, the nurse conducts a careful psychosocial history, exploring the impact of the disease on the patient's role within the family and community. Identification of per-

**FIGURE 29-10.** Left ventricular assist device.

ceived stressors helps the patient and the health care team to implement activities to relieve anxiety related to changes in health status. Very early on, the patient's support systems are identified, and members become involved in the patient's care and therapeutic regimen. The assessment addresses the effect the diagnosis has had on the patient and members of his or her support system and the patient's emotional status. Depression is not uncommon in a patient with cardiomyopathy who has developed heart failure.

The physical assessment focuses on signs and symptoms of heart failure. The baseline assessment includes such key components as:

- Vital signs
- Calculation of pulse pressure and identification of pulsus paradoxus
- Current weight and any weight gain or loss
- Detection by palpation of the point of maximal impulse, often shifted to the left
- Cardiac auscultation for a systolic murmur and $S_3$ and $S_4$ heart sounds
- Pulmonary auscultation for crackles
- Measurement of jugular vein distention
- Assessment of edema and its severity

## Diagnosis

### Nursing Diagnoses

Based on the assessment data, major nursing diagnoses may include:

- Decreased cardiac output related to structural disorders caused by cardiomyopathy or to dysrhythmia from the disease process and medical treatments
- Ineffective cardiopulmonary, cerebral, peripheral, and renal tissue perfusion related to decreased peripheral blood flow (resulting from decreased cardiac output)
- Impaired gas exchange related to pulmonary congestion caused by myocardial failure (resulting from decreased cardiac output)
- Activity intolerance related to decreased cardiac output or excessive fluid volume, or both
- Anxiety related to the change in health status and in role functioning
- Powerlessness related to disease process
- Noncompliance with medication and diet therapies

### Collaborative Problems/ Potential Complications

Based on the assessment data, potential complications include:

- Congestive heart failure
- Ventricular dysrhythmias
- Atrial dysrhythmias
- Cardiac conduction defects
- Pulmonary or cerebral embolism
- Valvular dysfunction

These complications are discussed earlier in this chapter and in Chapters 27 and 30.

## Planning and Goals

The major goals for patients include improvement or maintenance of cardiac output, increased activity tolerance, reduction of anxiety, adherence to the self-care program, increased sense of power with decision making, and absence of complications.

## Nursing Interventions

### Improving Cardiac Output

During a symptomatic episode, rest is indicated. Many patients with DCM find that sitting up with their legs down is more comfortable than lying down in a bed. This position is helpful in pooling venous blood in the periphery and reducing preload. Assessing the patient's oxygen saturation at rest and during activity may assist with determining a need for supplemental oxygen. Oxygen is usually administered through a nasal cannula when indicated.

Ensuring that medications are taken as prescribed is important to preserving adequate cardiac output. The nurse may assist the patient with planning a schedule for taking medications and identifying methods to remember to follow it, such as associating the time to take a medication with an activity (eg, eating a meal, brushing teeth). It is important to ensure that patients with DCM avoid verapamil (Calan, Isoptin), patients with HCM avoid diuretics, and patients with RCM avoid nifedipine (Adalat, Procardia) to maintain contractility. In patients with HCM, the inotropic action of digoxin may create or worsen left ventricular outflow track obstruction. Patients with RCM have increased sensitivity to digoxin, and the nurse must anticipate that low doses will be prescribed and assess for digoxin toxicity.

It is also important to ensure that the patient receives or chooses food selections that are appropriate for a low-sodium diet. One way to monitor a patient's response to treatment is to determine the patient's weight every day and identify any significant change. Another indication of the effect of treatment involves assessment of shortness of breath after activity and comparison to before treatment. Patients with low cardiac output may need assistance keeping warm and frequently changing position to stimulate circulation and reduce the possibility of skin breakdown. Patients with HCM must be taught to avoid dehydration. One guideline for patients to use for self-assessment is to anticipate the urge to void at least every 4 hours while awake; if the urge to void is not present or the urine is a deep yellow color, more fluid intake is necessary.

### Increasing Activity Tolerance

The nurse plans the patient's activities so that they occur in cycles, alternating rest with activity periods. This benefits the patient's physiologic status, and it helps teach the patient about the need for planned cycles of rest and activity. For example, after taking a bath or shower, the patient should plan to sit and read a newspaper or engage in other relaxing activities. Suggesting that the patient sit while chopping vegetables, drying his or her hair, or shaving helps the patient identify methods to balance rest with activity. The nurse also makes sure that the patient recognizes the symptoms indicating the need for rest and actions to take when the symptoms occur. Patients with HCM or RCM must avoid strenuous activity, isometric exercises, and competitive sports.

### Reducing Anxiety

Spiritual, psychological, and emotional support may be indicated for patients, families, and significant others. Interventions are directed toward eradicating or alleviating perceived stressors. Patients receive appropriate information about cardiomyopathy and self-management activities. It is important to provide an atmosphere in which patients feel free to verbalize concerns and receive assurance that their concerns are legitimate. If the patient is awaiting transplantation or facing death, it is necessary to allow time to discuss these issues. Providing the patient with realistic hope helps reduce anxiety while he or she awaits a donor heart. The nurse helps the patient, family, and significant others with anticipatory grieving.

### Decreasing the Sense of Powerlessness

Patients must recognize that they go through a grieving process when given a diagnosis of cardiomyopathy. The patient is assisted in identifying the things in life that he or she has lost (eg, foods that the patient enjoyed eating but are high in sodium, the ability to engage in an active lifestyle, the ability to play sports, the ability to lift grandchildren). The patient also is assisted in identifying his or her emotional responses to the loss (eg, anger, depression). The nurse then assists the patient in identifying the amount of control that the patient has over his or her life, such as making food choices, managing medications, and working with health care providers to achieve the best possible outcomes. The use of tools that track behaviors with the resulting symptoms may be helpful. For example, a diary in which the patient records his or her food selections and weight may help the patient understand the relationship between sodium intake and weight gain. Some patients can manage a self-titrating diuretic regimen in which they adjust the dose of diuretic to their symptoms.

### Promoting Home and Community-Based Care

#### TEACHING PATIENTS SELF-CARE

A key part of the plan of nursing care involves teaching patients about the medication regimen, symptom monitoring, and symptom management. The nurse plays an integral role as the patient learns to balance his or her lifestyle and work while accomplishing therapeutic activities. Helping patients cope with their disease status helps them adjust their lifestyles and implement a self-care program at home. Attainment of a goal, no matter how small, also promotes the patient's sense of well-being.

#### CONTINUING CARE

The nurse reinforces previous teaching and performs ongoing assessment of the patient's symptoms and progress. The nurse also assists the patient and family to adjust to lifestyle changes. It often helps to teach patients to read nutrition labels, to maintain a record of daily weights and symptoms, and to organize daily activities to increase activity tolerance. In addition, the nurse assesses the patient's response to recommendations about diet and fluid intake and to the medication regimen, and stresses the signs and symptoms that should be reported to the physician. Because of the risk of dysrhythmia, it may be necessary to teach the patient's family cardiopulmonary resuscitation. Women are often advised to avoid pregnancy, but each case is assessed individually. The nurse assesses the psychosocial needs of the patient and family on an ongoing basis. There may be concerns and fears about the prognosis, changes in lifestyle, effects of medications, and the possibility of others in the family having the same condition, and these often increase the patient's anxiety and interfere with effective coping strategies. Establishing trust is vital to the nurse's relationship with these chronically ill patients and their families. This is particularly significant when the nurse is involved with a patient and family in discussions about end-of-life decisions. Patients who have significant symptoms of heart failure or other complications of cardiomyopathy may need a home care referral.

## Evaluation

### Expected Patient Outcomes

Expected patient outcomes may include:

1. Maintains or improves cardiac function
    a. Exhibits heart and respiratory rates within normal limits
    b. Reports decreased dyspnea and increased comfort; maintains or improves gas exchange
    c. Reports no weight gain; appropriate weight for height
    d. Maintains or improves peripheral blood flow
2. Maintains or increases activity tolerance
    a. Carries out activities of daily living (eg, brushes teeth, feeds self)
    b. Reports increased tolerance to activity
3. Is less anxious
    a. Discusses prognosis freely
    b. Verbalizes fears and concerns
    c. Participates in support groups if appropriate
4. Decreases sense of powerlessness
    a. Identifies emotional response to diagnosis
    b. Discusses control that he or she has
5. Adheres to self-care program
    a. Takes medications according to prescribed schedule
    b. Modifies diet to accommodate sodium and fluid recommendations
    c. Modifies lifestyle to accommodate recommended activity and rest behaviors
    d. Identifies signs and symptoms to be reported to health care professionals

# Infectious Diseases of the Heart

Any of the heart's three layers may be affected by an infectious process. The diseases are named for the layer of the heart most involved in the infectious process: infective endocarditis (endocardium), myocarditis (myocardium), and pericarditis (pericardium). Rheumatic endocarditis is a unique infective endocarditis syndrome. The diagnosis is made primarily on the basis of the patient's symptoms and echocardiography. The ideal management for all infectious diseases is prevention. IV antibiotics are usually necessary once an infection in the heart has developed.

## Rheumatic Endocarditis

Acute rheumatic fever, which occurs most often in school-age children, may develop after an episode of group A beta-hemolytic streptococcal pharyngitis (Chart 29-1). Patients with rheumatic fever may develop rheumatic heart disease as evidenced by a new heart murmur, cardiomegaly, peri-

---

**CHART 29-1**

### Rheumatic Fever

Rheumatic fever is a preventable disease. Diagnosing and treating streptococcal pharyngitis can prevent rheumatic fever and, therefore, rheumatic heart disease. Signs and symptoms of streptococcal pharyngitis include:

- Fever (38.9° to 40°C [101° to 104°F])
- Chills
- Sore throat (sudden in onset)
- Diffuse redness of throat with exudate on oropharynx (may not appear until after the first day)
- Enlarged and tender lymph nodes
- Abdominal pain (more common in children)
- Acute sinusitis and acute otitis media (may cause or result from streptococcal pharyngitis)

If signs and symptoms of streptococcal pharyngitis are present, a throat culture is necessary to make an accurate diagnosis. All patients with throat cultures positive for streptococcal pharyngitis must adhere to the prescribed antibiotic treatment. Penicillin is the most common antibiotic prescribed. Completing the course of prescribed antibiotics minimizes the risk of developing rheumatic fever (and subsequent rheumatic heart disease).

---

carditis, and heart failure. Prompt treatment of "strep" throat with antibiotics can prevent the development of rheumatic fever. The streptococcus is spread by direct contact with oral or respiratory secretions. Although the bacteria are the causative agents, malnutrition, overcrowding, and lower socioeconomic status may predispose individuals to rheumatic fever (Chin & Worley, 2003). The incidence of rheumatic fever in the United States and other developed countries is believed to have steadily decreased, but the exact incidence is difficult to determine because the infection may go unrecognized, and people may not seek treatment (Zipes et al., 2005). Clinical diagnostic criteria are not standardized, and autopsies are not routinely performed.

## Pathophysiology

Rheumatic endocarditis is not infectious in the sense that tissues are not invaded and directly damaged by the streptococci. Injury is caused by an inflammatory or sensitivity reaction to streptococci. Leukocytes accumulate in the affected tissues and form nodules, which eventually are replaced by scar tissue. The myocardium is involved in the inflammatory process. Rheumatic myocarditis develops, which temporarily weakens the contractile power of the heart. The pericardium is affected, and rheumatic pericarditis occurs during the acute illness. Myocardial and pericardial involvement usually resolves without serious sequelae. However, rheumatic endocarditis results in permanent and often crippling adverse effects.

Rheumatic endocarditis first manifests anatomically as tiny translucent vegetations or growths, which resemble pinhead-sized beads arranged in a row along the free margins of the valve leaflets. These tiny beads look harmless and may disappear without injuring the leaflet. However, more often they have serious effects. They are the starting point of a process that gradually thickens the leaflets, causing them to shorten and thicken, preventing them from closing completely. As a result, blood flows backward through the valve; this is called *valvular regurgitation*. The most common site of valvular regurgitation is the mitral valve. In some patients, the inflamed margins of the valve leaflets become adherent or the chordae tendineae fuse, resulting in valvular stenosis, a narrowed or stenotic valvular orifice. Regurgitation and stenosis may occur in the same valve.

## Clinical Manifestations

The Jones criteria are one set of diagnostic criteria for rheumatic fever. According to these criteria, patients who have had a group A beta-hemolytic streptococcal infection are diagnosed with rheumatic fever if they develop at least two of the following: carditis, polyarthritis, subcutaneous nodules, erythema marginatum, or chorea (Special Writing Group of the Committee on Rheumatic Fever, Endocarditis, and Kawasaki's Disease of the Council on Cardiovascular Disease in the Young of the American Heart Association, 1992). Carditis, the inflammatory process of the disease, affects all three layers of the heart and may also affect bone joints, producing polyarthritis that may last for up to 4 weeks. Round, firm, painless, free-moving, subcutaneous nodules may develop over bony surfaces and tendons. These nodules usually disappear after 1 to 2 weeks. Patients may also develop a macular or papular, nonitchy rash on the trunk and proximal extremities, called erythema marginatum. The rash blanches with pressure, is not indurated, and does not leave a scar. Individual lesions may come and go over a few minutes, moving from place to place on the body. Patients may develop chorea (rapid, purposeless, erratic, jerky, uncoordinated, involuntary movements of the extremities and face) during the acute phase and up to several months afterward. The chorea usually resolves completely within 6 months. Rheumatic heart disease may cause valvular insufficiency, heart failure, and death.

Most patients with rheumatic fever recover within 3 to 4 weeks. However, a few patients become critically ill with intractable heart failure, serious dysrhythmias, and pneumonia. Once the symptoms of rheumatic fever subside, residual effects of rheumatic endocarditis may lead to progressive valvular deformities. The existence and extent of cardiac damage may not be apparent in clinical examinations during the acute phase of the disease. However, eventually the heart murmurs characteristic of valvular regurgitation, stenosis, or both become audible on auscultation. In some patients, thrills are detectable on palpation. Usually, the myocardium can compensate for these valvular defects for a time, and the patient remains in good health. As the valvular pathology progresses, the myocardium is no longer able to compensate (see Fig. 29-2), and the signs and symptoms of heart failure develop (see Chapter 30).

## Assessment and Diagnostic Findings

A sore throat, or a history of one within 5 weeks, is a first symptom of possible rheumatic fever. Other symptoms include those described in Clinical Manifestations as well as fever, headache, weight loss, fatigue, malaise, diaphoresis, and pallor. More rarely, chest pain, abdominal pain, or vomiting may also occur.

Throat cultures are necessary to diagnose the presence of a group A beta-hemolytic streptococcal infection. Results from a rapid antigen detection test for group A beta-hemolytic streptococci may be used until the throat culture results are available. Rapid antigen detection tests have a 95% specificity but only 60% to 90% sensitivity; thus, throat cultures are used in addition to the rapid antigen tests (Chin & Worley, 2003). (See Chapter 22 for additional information.)

During assessment for rheumatic heart disease, the nurse should keep in mind that no diagnostic studies are specific for rheumatic endocarditis and that symptoms may not develop until years after the rheumatic fever. The symptoms depend on which side of the heart is involved. The mitral valve is most often affected, producing symptoms of left-sided heart failure—shortness of breath with crackles and wheezes in the lungs (see Chapter 30 for a discussion of left-sided versus right-sided failure). The severity of the symptoms depends on the size and location of the lesion in the heart. The systemic symptoms are proportional to the virulence of the invading organism. When a new murmur is detected in a patient with a systemic infection, infectious endocarditis should be suspected. Patients are also at risk for sequelae associated with embolic phenomena of the lung, kidney, spleen, heart, brain, or peripheral vessels.

The ECG may show sinus tachycardia, sinus bradycardia, sinus dysrhythmia, first-degree heart block, and atrial fibrillation or atrial flutter. The erythrocyte sedimentation rate (ESR) or serum C-reactive protein level may be elevated.

## Prevention

Rheumatic fever and rheumatic endocarditis may be prevented through early and adequate treatment of oropharyngeal streptococcal infections. A first-line approach in preventing initial attacks of rheumatic fever is recognition of oropharyngeal streptococcal infections, adequate treatment, and control of epidemics in the community. Every nurse should be familiar with the signs and symptoms of streptococcal pharyngitis: high fever (38.9°C to 40°C [101°F to 104°F]), chills, sore throat, redness of the throat with exudate, enlarged lymph nodes, abdominal pain, and acute rhinitis (see Chart 29-1).

## Medical Management

The objectives of medical management for oropharyngeal infections are to identify and eradicate the causative organism and prevent additional complications, such as rheumatic fever and rheumatic endocarditis. Throat cultures are used to identify the causative organism, if any, for the pharyngitis. If group A beta-hemolytic streptococcus is suspected, a one-time intramuscular injection of penicillin or a 10-day course of oral penicillin is prescribed. Erythromycin or cephalosporin may be prescribed for patients who are allergic to penicillin.

Initially, patients diagnosed with rheumatic fever are treated like patients with oropharyngeal group A beta-hemolytic streptococcal infections. After the initial antibiotic treatment, the patient should receive a prophylactic intramuscular dose of penicillin every 3 to 4 weeks to prevent recurrence of rheumatic fever and rheumatic heart disease. Prophylactic antibiotics are prescribed for 5 years (or until age 21, whichever is longer) if the patient did not experience carditis, or for 10 years (or until age 40, whichever is longer) if the patient had carditis or develops valvular heart disease. Oral erythromycin is prescribed for patients who are allergic to penicillin. For other symptoms except chorea, anti-inflammatory medications (eg, salicylates [aspirin], corticosteroids [prednisone]) may be prescribed. Although the chorea usually does not require treatment, patients may be treated with diazepam (Valium) or phenobarbital if the condition is severe. Symptoms of heart failure are treated as described in Chapter 30.

Patients also require prophylactic antibiotics for invasive procedures. Clindamycin (Cleocin), azithromycin (Zithromax), and clarithromycin (Biaxin) are often prescribed because the bacteria may be resistant to the antibiotic used for recurrent rheumatic fever prophylaxis (Chin & Worley, 2003; Dajani, Taubert, Wilson, et al., 1997).

## Nursing Management

A key nursing role in the care of patients with rheumatic fever and rheumatic endocarditis is teaching patients about the disease, its treatment, and the preventive steps needed to minimize recurrence and potential complications. After acute treatment with antibiotics, patients must take prophylactic antibiotics on a regular schedule and before invasive procedures. It is important to have long-term cardiac reevaluations, to maintain hydration, and to report any signs of thromboemboli or heart failure to health care providers.

Patients who have rheumatic endocarditis and whose valvular dysfunction is mild may require no further treatment. Nevertheless, the danger exists for recurrent attacks of acute rheumatic fever, bacterial endocarditis, embolism from vegetations or mural thrombi in the heart, and eventual cardiac failure. The nurse monitors the patient for signs and symptoms of valvular disease, heart failure, pulmonary hypertension, thromboemboli, and dysrhythmias.

## Infective Endocarditis

Infective endocarditis is a microbial infection of the endothelial surface of the heart. It usually develops in people with prosthetic heart valves, structural cardiac defects (eg, valve disorders, HCM) (Chart 29-2). It is more common in older people, who are more likely to have degenerative or calcific valve lesions, reduced immunologic response to infection, and the metabolic alterations associated with aging. Staphylococcal endocarditis infections of the valves in the right side of the heart are common among injection drug users (Miro, del Rio, & Mestres, 2003; Zipes et al., 2005). Hospital-acquired infective endocarditis occurs most often in patients with debilitating disease or indwelling catheters and

### CHART 29-2

### Risk Factors for Infective Endocarditis

**High Risk**
- Prosthetic cardiac valves
- History of bacterial endocarditis (even without heart disease)
- Complex cyanotic congenital malformations
- Surgically constructed systemic or pulmonary shunts or conduits
- Aortic valve disease
- Mitral regurgitation
- Combined mitral regurgitation and stenosis
- Patent ductus arteriosus
- Ventricular septal defect
- Coarctation of the aorta

**Moderate Risk**
- Mitral valve prolapse with valvular regurgitation or thickened leaflets
- Hypertrophic cardiomyopathy
- Acquired valvular dysfunction
- Most congenital cardiac malformations (other than those listed above)
- Atrial septal defect (unrepaired or repaired)
- Ventricular septal defect (repaired)
- Patent ductus arteriosus (repaired)
- Parenteral nutrition lines or IV lines into the right atrium
- Nonvalvular cardiac implants
- Degenerative valve disease

in patients who are receiving prolonged IV fluid or antibiotic therapy. Patients taking immunosuppressive medications or corticosteroids are more susceptible to fungal endocarditis.

Invasive procedures, particularly those involving mucosal surfaces, can cause a bacteremia, which rarely lasts for more than 15 minutes. If a patient has any anatomic cardiac defects, however, bacteremia can cause bacterial endocarditis. From 1950 to the mid-1980s, the incidence of infective endocarditis remained steady at about 4.2 cases per 100,000 patients. The incidence then increased, partially attributed to increased IV/injection drug abuse (Zipes et al., 2005).

## Pathophysiology

A deformity or injury of the endocardium leads to accumulation on the endocardium of fibrin and platelets and clot formation. Infectious organisms, usually streptococci, staphylococci, enterococci, or pneumococci, invade the clot and endocardial lesion. Other causative microorganisms include fungi (eg, *Candida*, *Aspergillus*) and Rickettsiae. The infection most frequently results in platelets, fibrin, blood cells, and microorganisms that cluster as vegetations on the endocardium. The vegetations may embolize to other tissues throughout the body. As the clot on the endocardium continues to expand, the infecting organism is covered by the new clot and concealed from the body's normal defenses. The infection may erode through the endocardium into the underlying structures (eg, valve leaflets), causing tears or other deformities of valve leaflets, dehiscence of prosthetic valves, deformity of the chordae tendineae, or mural abscesses.

A diagnosis of *acute* bacterial (infective) endocarditis (ABE) is made when the onset of infection and resulting valvular destruction is rapid, occurring within days to weeks. A diagnosis of *subacute* bacterial (infective) endocarditis (SBE) is made when the onset of infection and resulting valvular destruction takes 2 weeks to months to occur (Zipes et al., 2005).

Usually, the onset of infective endocarditis is insidious. The signs and symptoms develop from the toxic effect of the infection, from destruction of the heart valves, and from embolization of fragments of vegetative growths on the heart. Systemic emboli occur with left-sided heart infective endocarditis; pulmonary emboli occur with right-sided heart infective endocarditis (Crawford & Durack, 2003; Zipes et al., 2005).

## Clinical Manifestations

The primary presenting symptoms of infective endocarditis are fever and a heart murmur. The fever may be intermittent or absent, especially in patients who are receiving antibiotics or corticosteroids, in those who are elderly, or those who have heart failure or renal failure. A heart murmur may be absent initially but develops in almost all patients. Murmurs that worsen over time indicate progressive damage from vegetations or perforation of the valve or the chordae tendineae.

In addition to the fever and heart murmur, clusters of petechiae may be found on the body. Small, painful nodules (Osler nodes) may be present in the pads of fingers or toes. Irregular, red or purple, painless, flat macules (Janeway lesions) may be present on the palms, fingers, hands, soles, and toes. Hemorrhages with pale centers (Roth spots) caused by emboli in the nerve fiber layer of the eye may be observed in the fundi of the eyes. Splinter hemorrhages (ie, reddish-brown lines and streaks) may be seen under the fingernails and toenails, and petechiae may appear in the conjunctiva and mucous membranes. There may be cardiomegaly, heart failure, tachycardia, or splenomegaly.

Central nervous system manifestations of infective endocarditis include headache; temporary or transient cerebral ischemia; and strokes, which may be caused by emboli to the cerebral arteries. Embolization may be a presenting symptom, and it may occur at any time and may involve other organ systems. Embolic phenomena may occur, as discussed in the previous section on rheumatic endocarditis.

## Assessment and Diagnostic Findings

Although the previously described characteristics may indicate infective endocarditis, the signs and symptoms may indicate other diseases as well. Vague complaints of malaise, anorexia, weight loss, cough, and back and joint pain may be mistaken for influenza. A definitive diagnosis is made when a microorganism is found in two separate blood cultures, in a vegetation, or in an abscess. Three sets of blood cultures (with each set including one aerobic and one anaerobic culture) drawn 1 hour apart should be obtained before administration of any antimicrobial agents. Negative blood cultures do not definitely rule out infective endocarditis. Patients may have elevated white blood cell (WBC) counts. In addition, patients may be anemic and have an elevated ESR and a positive rheumatoid factor. Microscopic hematuria may be present on urinalysis.

Doppler echocardiography may assist in the diagnosis by demonstrating a mass on the valve, prosthetic valve, or supporting structures and by identification of vegetations, abscesses, new prosthetic valve dehiscence, or new regurgitation (Moss & Munt, 2003; Zipes et al., 2005). The echocardiogram may reveal the development of heart failure. TEE may provide better data than transthoracic imaging.

## Prevention

Although rare, bacterial endocarditis may be life-threatening. A key strategy is primary prevention in moderate- and high-risk patients (ie, those with rheumatic heart disease, mitral valve prolapse, or prosthetic heart valves). Antibiotic prophylaxis is recommended for moderate- and high-risk patients immediately before and sometimes after the following procedures:

- Dental procedures that induce gingival or mucosal bleeding, including professional cleaning and placement of orthodontic bands (not brackets)
- Tonsillectomy or adenoidectomy
- Surgical procedures that involve intestinal or respiratory mucosa
- Bronchoscopy with a rigid bronchoscope
- Sclerotherapy for esophageal varices
- Esophageal dilation
- Endoscopic retrograde cholangiography with biliary obstruction
- Gallbladder surgery
- Cystoscopy
- Urethral dilation
- Urethral catheterization if urinary tract infection is present
- Urinary tract surgery if urinary tract infection is present
- Prostatic surgery
- Incision and drainage of infected tissue
- Vaginal hysterectomy

The type of antibiotic used for prophylaxis varies with the type of procedure and the degree of risk. Patients are usually instructed to take 2 g of amoxicillin (Amoxil) orally 1 hour before dental, oral, respiratory, or esophageal procedures. If patients are allergic to penicillin, clindamycin (Cleocin), cephalexin (Keflex), cefadroxil (Duricef), azithromycin (Zithromax), or clarithromycin (Biaxin) may be used. Antibiotic recommendations for gastrointestinal or genitourinary procedures are ampicillin and gentamicin (Garamycin) for high-risk patients, and amoxicillin or ampicillin for moderate-risk patients; only patients allergic to ampicillin or amoxicillin should receive vancomycin (Vancocin) as a substitute.

The severity of oral inflammation and infection is a significant factor in the incidence and degree of bacteremia.

Poor dental hygiene can lead to bacteremia, particularly in the setting of a dental procedure. Regular professional oral care combined with personal oral care may reduce the risk of bacteremia. Personal oral care includes using a soft toothbrush and toothpaste to brush the teeth, gums, tongue, and oral mucosa at least twice a day, as well as rinsing the mouth for 30 seconds intermittently between tooth brushing with an antiseptic mouthwash. Patients must be advised to avoid nail biting and to minimize outbreaks of acne and psoriasis. Female patients are advised not to use intrauterine devices (IUDs).

Increased vigilance is also required in patients with IV catheters and during invasive procedures. To minimize the risk of infection, nurses must ensure meticulous hand hygiene, site preparation, and aseptic technique during insertion and maintenance procedures. All catheters, tubes, drains, and other devices are removed as soon as they are no longer needed or no longer function.

## Complications

Even if the patient responds to therapy, endocarditis can be destructive to the heart and other organs. Heart failure and cerebral vascular complications, such as stroke (i.e., cerebrovascular accident or brain attack), may occur before, during, or after therapy. Heart failure, which may result from perforation of a valve leaflet, rupture of chordae, blood flow obstruction due to vegetations, or intracardiac shunts from dehiscence of prosthetic valves, indicates a poor prognosis with medical therapy alone and a higher surgical risk (Zipes et al., 2005). Valvular stenosis or regurgitation, myocardial damage, and mycotic (fungal) aneurysms are potential cardiac complications. First-, second-, and third-degree atrioventricular blocks may occur and are often a sign of a valve ring abscess. Septic or nonseptic emboli, immunologic responses, abscess of the spleen, mycotic aneurysms, cerebritis, and hemodynamic deterioration may cause complications in other organs.

## Medical Management

The causative organism may be identified by serial blood cultures. The objective of treatment is to eradicate the invading organism through adequate doses of an appropriate antimicrobial agent.

### Pharmacologic Therapy

Antibiotic therapy is usually administered parenterally in a continuous IV infusion for 2 to 6 weeks. Parenteral therapy is administered in doses that produce a high serum concentration and for a significant period to ensure eradication of the dormant bacteria within the dense vegetations. This therapy is often delivered in the patient's home and is monitored by a home care nurse. Serum levels of the selected antibiotic are monitored. If the serum does not demonstrate bactericidal activity, increased dosages of the antibiotic are prescribed or a different antibiotic is used. Numerous antimicrobial regimens are in use, but penicillin is usually the medication of choice. Blood cultures are taken periodically to monitor the effect of therapy. In fungal endocarditis, an antifungal agent, such as amphotericin B (Abelcet, Amphocin, Fungizone), is the usual treatment.

The patient's temperature is monitored at regular intervals, because the course of the fever is one indication of the effectiveness of treatment. However, febrile reactions also may occur as a result of medication. After adequate antimicrobial therapy is initiated, the infective organism is usually eliminated. The patient should begin to feel better, regain an appetite, and have less fatigue. During this time, patients require psychosocial support, because although they feel well, they may find themselves confined to the hospital or home with restrictive IV therapy.

### Surgical Management

Surgical interventions include valve débridement or excision, débridement of vegetations, débridement and closure of an abscess, and closure of a fistula. Aortic or mitral valve débridement, excision, or replacement is required in patients who develop congestive heart failure despite adequate medical treatment; those who have more than one serious systemic embolic episode, valve obstruction, a periannular (heart valve) or myocardial abscess, or aortic abscess; and those with uncontrolled infection, persistent or recurrent infection, or fungal endocarditis. Surgical valve replacement greatly improves the prognosis for patients with severe symptoms from damaged heart valves. The aortic valve may be best treated with an autograft, as previously described. Most patients who have prosthetic valve endocarditis (ie, infected valve replacements) require valve replacement.

## Nursing Management

The nurse monitors the patient's temperature. The patient may have a fever for weeks. Heart sounds are assessed. A new or worsening murmur may indicate dehiscence of a prosthetic valve, rupture of an abscess, or injury to valve leaflets or chordae tendineae. The nurse monitors for signs and symptoms of systemic embolization, or, for patients with right-sided heart endocarditis, for signs and symptoms of pulmonary infarction and infiltrates. In addition, the nurse assesses signs and symptoms of organ damage such as stroke (ie, cerebrovascular accident or brain attack), meningitis, heart failure, myocardial infarction, glomerulonephritis, and splenomegaly.

Patient care is directed toward management of infection. The patient is started on antibiotics as soon as blood cultures have been obtained. Long-term IV antimicrobial therapy is often necessary; therefore, many patients have peripherally inserted central catheters or other long-term IV access. All invasive lines and wounds must be assessed daily for redness, tenderness, warmth, swelling, drainage, or other signs of infection. The patient and family are instructed about activity restrictions, medications, and signs and symptoms of infection. The nurse instructs the patient and family about the need for prophylactic antibiotics not only before, but possibly after, dental, respiratory, gastrointestinal, or genitourinary procedures. The home care nurse supervises and monitors IV antibiotic therapy delivered in the home setting and educates the patient and family about prevention and health promotion. The nurse provides the patient and family with emotional support and facilitates coping strategies during the prolonged course of the infection and antibiotic treatment. If the patient has undergone surgical treatment, the nurse provides postoperative care and instructions.

## Myocarditis

Myocarditis, an inflammatory process involving the myocardium, can cause heart dilation, thrombi on the heart wall (mural thrombi), infiltration of circulating blood cells around the coronary vessels and between the muscle fibers, and degeneration of the muscle fibers themselves. Mortality varies with the severity of symptoms. Most patients with mild symptoms recover completely, but some patients develop cardiomyopathy and heart failure.

### Pathophysiology

Myocarditis usually results from viral (coxsackievirus A and B), rickettsial, fungal, parasitic, metazoal, protozoal, or spirochetal infection. It also may occur after acute systemic infections such as rheumatic fever or Chagas disease; in patients receiving immunosuppressive therapy; or in patients with infective endocarditis, Crohn disease, or systemic lupus erythematosus. Myocarditis may result from an immune reaction to pharmacologic agents used in the treatment of other diseases or radiation (especially to the left chest or upper back). It may begin in one small area of the myocardium and then spread throughout the myocardium. The degree of myocardial involvement determines the degree of hemodynamic effect and the resulting signs and symptoms. It is theorized that DCM is a latent manifestation of myocarditis (Calabrese & Thiene, 2003; Zipes et al., 2005).

### Clinical Manifestations

The symptoms of acute myocarditis depend on the type of infection, the degree of myocardial damage, and the capacity of the myocardium to recover. Patients may be asymptomatic, and the infection resolves on its own. However, they may develop mild to moderate symptoms and seek medical attention, often reporting fatigue and dyspnea, palpitations, and occasional discomfort in the chest and upper abdomen. The most common symptoms are flu-like. Patients may also sustain sudden cardiac death or quickly develop severe congestive heart failure.

### Assessment and Diagnostic Findings

Assessment of the patient may reveal no detectable abnormalities; as a result, the entire illness can go undiagnosed. Patients may be tachycardic or may report chest pain (with a subsequent cardiac catheterization demonstrating normal coronary arteries). Endocardial biopsies may be diagnostic for an organism, immune process, or radiation reaction causing the myocarditis. Patients without any abnormal heart structure (at least initially) may suddenly develop dysrhythmias or ST-T wave changes. If the patient has structural heart abnormalities (eg, systolic dysfunction), a clinical assessment may disclose cardiac enlargement, faint heart sounds (especially $S_1$), a gallop rhythm, or a systolic murmur. The WBC count and ESR may be elevated.

### Prevention

Prevention of infectious diseases by means of appropriate immunizations (eg, influenza, hepatitis) and early treatment appears to be important in decreasing the incidence of myocarditis (Zipes et al., 2005).

### Medical Management

Patients are given specific treatment for the underlying cause if it is known (eg, penicillin for hemolytic streptococci) and are placed on bed rest to decrease cardiac workload. Bed rest also helps decrease myocardial damage and the complications of myocarditis. In young patients with myocarditis, activities, especially athletics, should be limited for a 6-month period or at least until heart size and function have returned to normal. Physical activity is increased slowly, and the patient is instructed to report any symptoms that occur with increasing activity, such as a rapidly beating heart. The use of corticosteroids in treating myocarditis remains controversial (Zipes et al., 2005). Nonsteroidal anti-inflammatory drugs (NSAIDs) such as aspirin and ibuprofen should not be used during the acute phase or if heart failure develops, because these medications can cause further myocardial damage. If heart failure or dysrhythmia develops, management is essentially the same as for all causes of heart failure and dysrhythmias (see Chapters 27 and 30), except that beta-blockers are avoided because they decrease the strength of ventricular contraction (have a negative inotropic effect).

### Nursing Management

The nurse assesses for resolution of tachycardia, fever, and any other clinical manifestations. The cardiovascular assessment focuses on signs and symptoms of heart failure and dysrhythmias. Patients with dysrhythmias should have continuous cardiac monitoring with personnel and equipment readily available to treat life-threatening dysrhythmias.

**Patients with myocarditis are sensitive to digitalis. Nurses must closely monitor these patients for digitalis toxicity, which is evidenced by dysrhythmia, anorexia, nausea, vomiting, headache, and malaise.**

Elastic compression stockings and passive and active exercises should be used because embolization from venous thrombosis and mural thrombi can occur, especially in patients on bed rest.

# Pericarditis

Pericarditis refers to an inflammation of the pericardium, the membranous sac enveloping the heart. It may be a primary illness or it may develop during various medical and surgical disorders. For example, pericarditis may occur after pericardectomy (opening of the pericardium) following cardiac surgery. Pericarditis also may occur 10 days to 2 months after acute myocardial infarction (Dressler syndrome). Pericarditis may be subacute, acute, or chronic. It is classified either as adhesive (or constrictive) because the layers of the pericardium become attached to each other and restrict ventricular filling, or by what accumulates in the pericardial sac: serous (serum), purulent (pus), calcific (calcium deposits), fibrinous (clotting proteins), or sanguinous (blood). Pericarditis also may be described as exudative or noneffusive.

## Pathophysiology

Causes underlying or associated with pericarditis are listed in Chart 29-3. Pericarditis may lead to an accumulation of fluid in the pericardial sac (pericardial effusion) and increased pressure on the heart, leading to cardiac tamponade (see Chapter 30). Frequent or prolonged episodes of pericarditis may also lead to thickening and decreased elasticity of the pericardium, or scarring may fuse the visceral and parietal pericardium. These conditions restrict the heart's ability to fill with blood (constrictive pericarditis). The pericardium may become calcified, further restricting ventricular expansion during ventricular filling (diastole). With less filling, the ventricles pump less blood, leading to decreased cardiac output and signs and symptoms of heart failure. Restricted diastolic filling may result in increased systemic venous pressure, causing peripheral edema and hepatic failure.

## Clinical Manifestations

Pericarditis may be asymptomatic. The most characteristic symptom of pericarditis is chest pain, although pain also may be located beneath the clavicle, in the neck, or in the left trapezius (scapula) region. The pain or discomfort usually remains fairly constant, but it may worsen with deep inspiration and when lying down or turning. It may be relieved with a forward-leaning or sitting position. The most characteristic sign of pericarditis is a creaky or scratchy friction rub heard most clearly at the left lower sternal border. Other signs may include a mild fever, increased WBC count, anemia, and an elevated ESR or C-reactive protein level. Patients may have a nonproductive cough. Dyspnea and other signs and symptoms of heart failure may occur as the result of pericardial compression due to constrictive pericarditis or cardiac tamponade.

## Assessment and Diagnostic Findings

The diagnosis is most often made on the basis of the history, signs, and symptoms. An echocardiogram may detect inflammation, pericardial effusion or tamponade, and heart failure. It may help confirm the diagnosis and may be used to guide pericardiocentesis (needle or catheter drainage of the pericardium). TEE may be useful in diagnosis but may underestimate the extent of pericardial effusions. CT may be the best diagnostic tool for determining the size, shape, and location of pericardial effusions and may be used to guide pericardiocentesis. MRI may assist with detection of inflammation and adhesions. Occasionally, a video-assisted pericardioscope-guided biopsy of the pericardium or epicardium is performed to obtain tissue samples for culture and microscopic examination. Because the pericardial sac surrounds the heart, a 12-lead ECG may show concave ST elevations in many, if not all, leads (with no reciprocal changes) and may show depressed PR segments or atrial dysrhythmias.

## Medical Management

The objectives of management of pericarditis are to determine the cause, administer therapy for treatment and symptom relief, and detect signs and symptoms of cardiac tamponade. When cardiac output is impaired, the patient is placed on bed rest until the fever, chest pain, and friction rub have subsided.

Analgesics and NSAIDs such as aspirin or ibuprofen (Motrin) may be prescribed for pain relief during the acute phase. These agents also hasten the reabsorption of fluid in patients with rheumatic pericarditis. Indomethacin (Indocin) is contraindicated, because it may decrease coronary blood flow. Corticosteroids (eg, prednisone) may be prescribed

### CHART 29-3

### Causes of Pericarditis

- Idiopathic or nonspecific causes
- Infection: usually viral (eg, human immunodeficiency virus, coxsackievirus, influenza); rarely bacterial (eg, streptococci, staphylococci, meningococci, gonococci, gram-negative rods); and mycotic (fungal)
- Disorders of connective tissue: systemic lupus erythematosus, rheumatic fever, rheumatoid arthritis, polyarteritis, scleroderma
- Hypersensitivity states: immune reactions, medication reactions, serum sickness
- Disorders of adjacent structures: myocardial infarction, dissecting aneurysm, pleural and pulmonary disease (pneumonia)
- Neoplastic disease: caused by metastasis from lung cancer or breast cancer, leukemia, and primary (mesothelioma) neoplasms
- Radiation therapy of chest and upper torso (peak occurrence 5–9 months after treatment)
- Trauma: chest injury, cardiac surgery, cardiac catheterization, implantation of pacemaker or implantable cardioverter defibrillator (ICD)
- Renal failure and uremia
- Tuberculosis

if the pericarditis is severe or if the patient does not respond to NSAIDs. Colchicine may also be used as alternative therapy.

Pericardiocentesis, a procedure in which some of the pericardial fluid is removed, is rarely necessary. It may be performed to assist in the identification of the cause or relieve symptoms, especially if there are signs and symptoms of heart failure or tamponade. Pericardial fluid is cultured if bacterial, tubercular, or fungal disease is suspected, and a sample is sent for cytology if neoplastic disease is suspected. A pericardial window, a small opening made in the pericardium, may be performed to allow continuous drainage into the chest cavity. Surgical removal of the tough encasing pericardium (pericardiectomy) may be necessary to release both ventricles from the constrictive and restrictive inflammation and scarring.

## Nursing Management

Patients with acute pericarditis require pain management with analgesics, positioning, and psychological support. Patients with chest pain often benefit from education and reassurance that the pain is not a heart attack. To minimize complications, the nurse helps the patient with activity restrictions until the pain and fever subside. As the patient's condition improves, the nurse encourages gradual increases of activity. However, if pain, fever, or friction rub reappear, activity restrictions must be resumed. The nurse educates the patient and family about a healthy lifestyle to enhance the patient's immune system.

Nurses caring for patients with pericarditis must be alert to cardiac tamponade (see Chapter 30). The nurse monitors the patient for heart failure. Patients with hemodynamic instability or pulmonary congestion are treated as they would be if they had heart failure (see Chapter 30).

## Nursing Process

### The Patient With Pericarditis

### Assessment

The primary symptom of the patient with pericarditis is pain, which is assessed by evaluating the patient in various positions. The nurse tries to identify whether the pain is influenced by respiratory movements, while holding an inhaled breath or holding an exhaled breath; by flexion, extension, or rotation of the spine, including the neck; by movements of the shoulders and arms; by coughing; or by swallowing. Recognizing the events that precipitate or intensify pain may help establish a diagnosis and differentiate the pain of pericarditis from the pain of myocardial infarction.

A pericardial friction rub occurs when the pericardial surfaces lose their lubricating fluid because of inflammation. The rub is audible on auscultation and is synchronous with the heartbeat. However, it may be elusive and difficult to detect.

**NURSING ALERT**

A pericardial friction rub is diagnostic of pericarditis. It has a creaky or scratchy sound and is louder at the end of exhalation. Nurses should search diligently for the pericardial friction rub by placing the diaphragm of the stethoscope tightly against the thorax and auscultating the left sternal edge in the fourth intercostal space, the site where the pericardium comes into contact with the left chest wall. The rub may be heard best when a patient is sitting and leaning forward.

If there is difficulty in distinguishing a pericardial friction rub from a pleural friction rub, the patient is asked to hold his or her breath; a pericardial friction rub will continue.

The patient's temperature is monitored frequently. Pericarditis may cause an abrupt onset of fever in a patient who has been afebrile.

### Diagnosis

#### Nursing Diagnosis

Based on the assessment data, the major nursing diagnosis may be:

- Acute pain related to inflammation of the pericardium

#### Collaborative Problems/ Potential Complications

Based on the assessment data, potential complications that may develop include:

- Pericardial effusion
- Cardiac tamponade

### Planning and Goals

The patient's major goals may include relief of pain and absence of complications.

### Nursing Interventions

#### Relieving Pain

Relief of pain is achieved by rest. Because sitting upright and leaning forward is the posture that tends to relieve pain, chair rest may be more comfortable. It is important to instruct the patient to restrict activity until the pain subsides. As the chest pain and friction rub abate, activities of daily living may be resumed gradually. If the patient is taking analgesics, antibiotics, or corticosteroids for the pericarditis, his or her responses are monitored and recorded. Patients taking NSAIDs are assessed for gastrointestinal adverse effects. If chest pain and friction rub recur, bed rest or chair rest is resumed.

## Monitoring and Managing Potential Complications

### PERICARDIAL EFFUSION

Fluid may accumulate between the pericardial linings or in the pericardial sac, a condition called *pericardial effusion* (see Chapter 30). The fluid can constrict the myocardium and impair its ability to pump. Cardiac output declines further with each contraction. Failure to identify and treat this problem can lead to the development of cardiac tamponade and possible sudden death.

### CARDIAC TAMPONADE

The signs and symptoms of cardiac tamponade may begin with the patient reporting shortness of breath, chest tightness, or dizziness. The nurse may observe that the patient is becoming progressively more restless. Assessment of blood pressure may reveal a decrease of 10 mm Hg or more in the systolic blood pressure during inspiration (pulsus paradoxus). Usually, the systolic pressure decreases and the diastolic pressure remains stable; hence, the pulse pressure narrows. The patient may have tachycardia, and the ECG voltage may be decreased or the QRS complexes may alternate in height (electrical alternans). Heart sounds may progress from distant to imperceptible. Neck vein distention and other signs of rising central venous pressure develop. These signs and symptoms occur because as the fluid-filled pericardial sac compresses the myocardium. Blood continues to return to the heart from the periphery but cannot flow into the heart to be pumped back into the circulation.

In such situations, the nurse notifies the physician immediately and prepares to assist with diagnostic echocardiography and pericardiocentesis (see Chapter 30). The nurse stays with the patient and continues to assess and record signs and symptoms while intervening to decrease patient anxiety.

## Evaluation

### Expected Patient Outcomes

Expected patient outcomes may include:

1. Freedom from pain
    a. Performs activities of daily living without pain, fatigue, or shortness of breath
    b. Temperature returns to normal range
    c. Exhibits no pericardial friction rub
2. Absence of complications
    a. Sustains blood pressure in normal range
    b. Has heart sounds that are strong and can be auscultated
    c. Shows absence of neck vein distention

## Critical Thinking Exercises

1. **ebp** A friend tells you she does not like to take drugs and does not plan to adhere to advice from her health care providers to use antibiotics before routine dental checkups. You know your friend has had a mitral valvuloplasty that included use of an annuloplasty ring. How would you respond to your friend? On what evidence do you base your response? What is the strength of that evidence?

2. A 19-year-old man with hypertrophic cardiomyopathy is being discharged from the hospital. He lives alone and states he really needs to get back to the gym to resume his weight training. Based on your knowledge about the developmental tasks of 19-year-olds, what do you anticipate his psychosocial needs would be? His family came to the hospital during the first 2 days of his hospital stay, but they live out of town and have returned home. Should they be included in the plan of care? The cardiologist has requested a consult with transplant services. How will this consult be included in the plan of care?

3. A 68-year-old man with atrial fibrillation, who is recovering from an aortic valve replacement for aortic stenosis and three coronary artery bypass grafts, has been prescribed a beta-blocker, an ACE inhibitor, digoxin, and warfarin. The cardiologist advises the patient to continue to carry nitroglycerin spray for treatment of angina, should it occur. What are this patient's teaching and discharge planning needs? As you care for the patient on the third postoperative day, you assess that the patient has short-term memory deficits. What are your plans to achieve discharge as expected on postoperative day 5 to 7?

4. You are caring for a 34-year-old man with infective endocarditis. He reports difficulty breathing. As you enter the room, you find a very anxious patient sitting upright in bed, breathing very rapidly with audible moist/bubbling respiratory sounds. Perspiration on his face is noticeable. Describe the actions you would take and explain why.

## REFERENCES AND SELECTED READINGS

### BOOKS

American Heart Association. (2004). *Heart and stroke statistical update.* Dallas, TX: American Heart Association.

Beers, M. H., Berkow, R., & Burs, M. (Eds.) (1999). *The Merck manual of diagnosis and therapy* (17th ed.). Whitehouse Station, NJ: Merck & Co.

Bickley, L. S., & Szilagyi, P. G. (2003). *Bates's guide to physical examination and history taking* (8th ed.). Philadelphia: Lippincott Williams & Wilkins.

Fuster, V., Alexander, R. W., & O'Rourke, R. A. (Eds.). (2004). *Hurst's the heart* (11th ed.). New York: McGraw-Hill.

Lynn-McHale Wiegand, D. J., & Carlson, K. K. (2005). *AACN procedure manual for critical care* (5th ed.). Philadelphia: Elsevier.

Morton, P. G., Fontaine, D. K., Hudak, C. M., & Gallo, B. M. (2005). *Critical care nursing: A holistic approach* (8th ed.). Philadelphia: Lippincott Williams & Wilkins.

Schakenbach, L. H. (2001). Care of the patient with a ventricular assist device. In M. Chulay & S. Wingate (Eds.), *Care of the cardiovascular patient series*. Aliso Viejo, CA: American Association of Critical-Care Nurses.

Woods, S. L., Froelicher, E. S. S., Motzer, S. A., et al. (2005). *Cardiac nursing* (5th ed.). Philadelphia: Lippincott Williams & Wilkins.

Zipes, D. P., Libby, P., Bonow, E.T, et al. (Eds.). (2005). *Braunwald's heart disease: A textbook of cardiovascular medicine* (7th ed.). Philadelphia: W. B. Saunders.

## JOURNALS

*Asterisks indicate nursing research articles.

Aazami, M., & Schafers, H. J. (2003). Advances in heart valve surgery. *Journal of Interventional Cardiology, 16*(6), 535–541.

Avery, R. K. (2003). Cardiac allograft vasculopathy. *New England Journal of Medicine, 349*(9), 829–830.

Bahruth, A. J. (2004). What every patient should . . . pretransplantation and posttransplantation. *Critical Care Nursing Quarterly, 27*(1), 31–60.

Baptiste, M. M. (2001). Aortic valve replacement. *RN, 64*(1), 58–64.

Berul, C., & Zevitz, M. E. (2004). Cardiomyopathy, hypertrophic. *eMedicine*. Retrieved from http://www.emedicine.com/PED/topic1102.htm. Accessed June 11, 2006.

Bond, A. E., Nelson, K., Germany, C. L., et al. (2003). The left ventricular assist device. *American Journal of Nursing, 103*(1), 32–40.

Borer, J. S., & Bonow, R. O. (2003). Contemporary approach to aortic and mitral regurgitation. *Circulation, 108*(20), 2432–2438.

Braunwald, E., Seidman, C. E., & Sigwart, U. (2003). Contemporary evaluation and management of hypertrophic cardiomyopathy. *Circulation, 106*(11), 1312–1316.

Calabrese, F., & Thiene, G. (2003). Myocarditis and inflammatory cardiomyopathy: Microbiological and molecular biological aspects. *Cardiovascular Research, 60*(1), 11–25.

Camp, D. (2000). The left ventricular assist device (LVAD). *Critical Care Nursing Clinics of North America, 12*(1), 61–68.

Cheitlin, M. D., Armstrong, W. F., Aurigemma, G. P., et al. (2003). ACC/AHA/ASE 2003 guideline update for the clinical application of echocardiography: Summary article: A report of the American College of Cardiology/American Heart Association Task Force on Practice Guidelines (ACC/AHA/ASE Committee to Update the 1997 Guidelines for the Clinical Application of Echocardiography). *Circulation, 108*(9), 1146–1162.

Chin, T. K., & Worley, C. (2003). Rheumatic fever. *eMedicine*. Retrieved from http://www.emedicine.com/ped/topic2006.htm. Accessed June 11, 2006.

Christensen, D. M. (2000). The ventricular assist device: An overview. *Nursing Clinics of North America, 35*(4), 945–959.

Christensen, T. D., Andersen, N. T., Attermann, J., et al. (2003). Mechanical heart valve patients can manage oral anticoagulant therapy themselves. *European Journal of Cardio-Thoracic Surgery, 23*(3), 292–298.

Cilliers, A. M., Manyemba, J., & Saloojee, H. (2004). Anti-inflammatory treatment for carditis in acute rheumatic fever. *Cochrane Database of Systematic Reviews, 2*.

Crawford, M. H., & Durack, D. T. (2003). Clinical presentation of infective endocarditis. *Cardiology Clinics, 21*(2), 159–166.

Cruickshank, S. (2004). Cardiomyopathy. *Nursing Standard, 18*(23), 46–55.

Dajani, A. S., Taubert, K. A., Wilson, W., et al. (1997). Prevention of bacterial endocarditis. *Circulation, 96*(1), 358–366.

Deng, M. C. (2002). Cardiac transplantation. *Heart, 87*(2), 177–184.

Deng, M. C., Edwards, L. B., Hertz, M. I., et al. (2003). Mechanical circulatory support device database of the International Society for Heart and Lung Transplantation: First annual report, 2003. *Journal of Heart & Lung Transplantation, 22*(6), 653–662.

Dhawan, V. K. (2003). Infective endocarditis. *Topics in Emergency Medicine, 25*(2), 123–133.

Durack, D., Lukes, A. S., & Bright, D. K. (1994). New criteria for diagnosis of infective endocarditis: Utilization of specific echocardiographic findings. *American Journal of Medicine, 96*(3), 200–209.

*Evangelista, L. S., Doering, L., & Dracup, K. (2003). Meaning and life purpose: Perspectives of post-transplant women. *Heart & Lung, 32*(4), 250–257.

Freed, L. A., Levy, D., Levine, R. A., et al. (1999). Prevalence and clinical outcome of mitral-valve prolapse. *New England Journal of Medicine, 34*(1), 1–7.

Freedman, R. (2001). Use of implantable pacemakers and implantable defibrillators in hypertrophic cardiomyopathy. *Current Opinion in Cardiology, 16*(1), 58–65.

Goldsmith, I., Alexander, G. G., & Lip, G. Y. H. (2002). Valvar heart disease and prosthetic heart valves. *British Medical Journal, 325*(7374), 1228–1231.

Granowitz, E. V. (2003). Risk stratification and bedside prognostication in infective endocarditis. *Journal of the American Medical Association, 289*(15), 1991–1993.

Gulbins, H., Kreuzer, E., & Reichart, B. (2003). Homografts: A review. *Expert Review of Cardiovascular Therapy, 1*(4), 533–539.

Haley, J. H., Tajik, A. J., Danielson, G. K., et al. (2004). Transient constrictive pericarditis: Causes and natural history. *Journal of the American College of Cardiology, 43*(2), 271–275.

Hasbun, R., Vikram, H. R., Barakat, L. A., et al. (2003). Complicated left-sided native valve endocarditis in adults: Risk classification for mortality. *Journal of the American Medical Association, 289*(15), 1933–1940.

Kherani, A. R., & Oz, M. C. (2004). Ventricular assistance to bridge to transplantation. *Surgical Clinics of North America, 84*(1), 75–89, viii–ix.

Lewis, P. S., Boyd, C. M., Hubert, N. E., et al. (2001). Ethanol-induced therapeutic myocardial infarction to treat hypertrophic obstructive cardiomyopathy. *Critical Care Nurse, 21*(2), 20–34.

Maron, B., Estes, N. A. M., III, Maron, M., et al. (2003). Primary prevention of sudden death as a novel treatment strategy in hypertrophic cardiomyopathy. *Circulation, 107*(23), 2872–2875.

Maron, B. J. (2002). Hypertrophic cardiomyopathy: A systematic review. *Journal of the American Medical Association, 287*(10), 1308–1320.

Maron, B. J., McKenna, W. J., Danielson, G. K., et al. (2003). American College of Cardiology/European Society of Cardiology clinical expert consensus document on hypertrophic cardiomyopathy: A report of the American College of Cardiology Foundation Task Force on Clinical Expert Consensus Documents and the European Society of Cardiology Committee for Practice Guidelines. *Journal of the American College of Cardiology, 42*(9), 1687–1713.

Mason, J. W. (2003). Myocarditis and dilated cardiomyopathy: An inflammatory link. *Cardiovascular Research, 60*(1), 5–10.

Mason, V. F., & Konicki, A. J. (2003). Left ventricular assist devices as destination therapy. *AACN Clinical Issues, 14*(4), 488–497.

McKenna, W., & Behr, E. (2002). Hypertrophic cardiomyopathy: Management, risk stratification, and prevention of sudden death. *Heart, 87*(2), 169–176.

McRae, A. I., Chung, M. K., & Asher, C. R. (2001). Arrhythmogenic right ventricular cardiomyopathy: A cause of sudden death in young people. *Cleveland Clinic Journal of Medicine, 68*(5), 459–467.

Miro, J. M., del Rio, A., & Mestres, C. A. (2003). Infective endocarditis and cardiac surgery in IV drug abusers and HIV-1 infected patients. *Cardiology Clinics, 21*(2), 167–184.

Mitka, M. (2003). Trials planned for testing nonsurgical approach to replacing heart valves. *Journal of the American Medical Association, 289*(11), 1366–1367.

Moreillon, P., & Que, Y. A. (2004). Infective endocarditis. *Lancet, 363*(9403), 139–149.

Morse, C. J. (2001). Advanced practice nursing in heart transplantation. *Progress in Cardiovascular Nursing, 16*(1), 21–24, 38.

Moss, R., & Munt, B. (2003). Injection drug use and right sided endocarditis. *Heart, 89*(5), 577–581.

Murtagh, B., Frazier, O. H. & Letsou, G. V. (2003). Diagnosis and management of bacterial endocarditis in 2003. *Current Opinions in Cardiology, 18*(2), 106–110.

Nauer, K. A., Schouchoff, B., & Demitras, K. (2000). Minimally invasive aortic valve surgery. *Critical Care in Nursing Quarterly, 23*(1), 66–71.

Neuner, J. M., Hamel, M. B., Phillips, R. S., et al. (2003). Diagnosis and management of adults with pharyngitis. A cost-effectiveness analysis. *Annals of Internal Medicine, 139*(2), 113–122.

Nishimura, R. A., & Holmes, D. R., Jr. (2004). Hypertrophic obstructive cardiomyopathy. *New England Journal of Medicine, 350*(13), 1320–1327.

Olaison, L., & Pettersson, G. (2003). Current best practices and guidelines. Indications for surgical intervention in infective endocarditis. *Cardiology Clinics, 21*(2), 235–251, vii.

Poston, R. S., & Griffith, B. P. (2004). Heart transplantation. *Journal of Intensive Care Medicine, 19*(1), 3–12.

Rahimtoola, S. H. (2003). Choice of prosthetic heart valve for adult patients. *Journal of the American College of Cardiology, 41*(6), 893–904.

Rhodes, L. R. (2004). Cardiac allograft vasculopathy. *Critical Care Nursing Quarterly, 27*(1), 10–16.

Richardson, P., McKenna, W., Bristow, M., et al. (1996). Report of the 1995 World Health Organization/International Society and Federation of Cardiology Task Force on the Definition and Classification of Cardiomyopathies. *Circulation, 93*(5), 841–842.

Rigatelli, G., Rigatelli, G., Barbiero, M., et al. (2003). "Demand" stimulation of latissimus dorsi heart wrap: Experience in humans and comparison with adynamic girdling. *Annals of Thoracic Surgery, 76*(5), 1587–1592.

Rose, E. A., Gelijns, A. S., Moskowitz, A. J., et al. (2001). Long-term use of a left ventricular assist device for end-stage heart failure. *New England Journal of Medicine, 345*(20), 1435–1443.

Rosenhek, R., Binder, T., & Maurer, G. (2002). Intraoperative transesophageal echocardiography in valve replacement surgery. *Echocardiography, 19*(8), 701–707.

Savage, L. (2003). Quality of life among patients with a left ventricular assist device: What is new? *AACN Clinical Issues: Advanced Practice in Acute Critical Care, 14*(1), 64–72.

Schmid, M. W. (2000). Risks and complications of peripherally and centrally inserted IV catheters. *Critical Care Nursing Clinics of North America, 12*(2), 165–174.

Sexton, D. J., & Spelman, D. (2003). Current best practices and guidelines. Assessment and management of complications in infective endocarditis. *Cardiology Clinics, 21*(2), 273–282, vii–viii.

Shaddy, R. E. (2004). Cardiomyopathy, restrictive. *eMedicine*. Retrieved from http://www.emedicine.com/PED/topic2503.htm. Accessed June 11, 2006.

Soler, R., Rodriguez, E., Remuinan, C., et al. (2003). Magnetic resonance imaging of primary cardiomyopathies. *Journal of Computer Assisted Tomography, 27*(5), 724–734.

Special Writing Group of the Committee on Rheumatic Fever, Endocarditis, and Kawasaki's Disease of the Council on Cardiovascular Disease in the Young of the American Heart Association. (1992). Guidelines for the diagnosis of rheumatic fever. Jones Criteria, 1992 update. *Journal of the American Medical Association, 268*(15), 2069–2973.

Starr, A., Fessler, C. L., Grunkemeier, G., et al. (2002). Heart valve replacement surgery: Past, present and future. *Clinical & Experimental Pharmacology & Physiology, 29*(8), 735–738.

Stewart, K. J., Badenhop, D., Brubaker, P. H., et al. (2003). Cardiac rehabilitation following percutaneous revascularization, heart transplant, heart valve surgery, and for chronic heart failure. *Chest, 123*(6), 2104–2111.

Tam, J., Shaikh, N., & Sutherland, E. (2002). Echocardiographic assessment of patients with hypertrophic and restrictive cardiomyopathy: Imaging and echocardiography. *Current Opinion in Cardiology, 17*(5), 470–477.

Taylor, D. O., Edwards, L. B., Mohacsi, P. J., et al. (2003). The registry of the International Society for Heart and Lung Transplantation: Twentieth official adult heart transplant report—2003. *Journal of Heart and Lung Transplantation, 22*(6), 616–624.

Wade, C. R., Reith, K. K., Sikora, J. H., et al. (2004). Postoperative nursing care of the cardiac transplant recipient. *Critical Care Nursing Quarterly, 27*(1), 17–28.

Wiegand, D. L. (2003). Cardiovascular surgery. Advances in cardiac surgery: Valve repair. *Critical Care Nurse, 23*(2), 72–91.

## RESOURCES

American Heart Association, National Center, 7272 Greenville Avenue, Dallas, TX 75231; 1-800-242-8721; http://www.americanheart.org. Accessed June 2, 2006.

Cardiomyopathy Association, 40 Metro Center, Tolpits Lane, Watford, Herts, WD18 9SB, United Kingdom; 44-(0)-1923-249-977; www.cardiomyopathy.org. Accessed June 2, 2006.

Heartmates, Inc., P.O. Box 16202, Minneapolis, MN 55416; 612-558-3331; http://www.heartmates.com. Accessed June 2, 2006.

National Heart, Lung, and Blood Institute, Health Information Center, National Institutes of Health, P.O. Box 30105, Bethesda, MD 20824-0105; 301-592-8573; http://www.nhlbi.nih.gov. Accessed June 2, 2006.

# CHAPTER 30

# Management of Patients With Complications From Heart Disease

## Learning Objectives

*On completion of this chapter, the learner will be able to:*

1. Describe the management of patients with heart failure (HF).
2. Use the nursing process as a framework for care of patients with HF.
3. Develop a teaching plan for patients with HF.
4. Describe the management of patients with pulmonary edema and cardiogenic shock.
5. Describe the management of patients with thromboembolism, pericardial effusion, and sudden cardiac death.

Today, the patient with heart disease can be assisted to live longer and achieve a higher quality of life than even a decade ago. Through advances in diagnostic procedures that allow earlier and more accurate diagnoses, treatment can begin well before significant debilitation occurs. Newer treatments, technologies, and pharmacotherapies are being developed rapidly. However, heart disease remains a chronic condition, and complications may develop. This chapter presents the complications most often resulting from heart diseases and the treatments provided by the health care team for these complications.

## Cardiac Hemodynamics

The basic function of the heart is to pump blood. The heart's ability to pump is measured by **cardiac output (CO)**, the amount of blood pumped per minute. CO is determined by measuring the heart rate (HR) and multiplying it by the **stroke volume (SV)**, the amount of blood pumped out of the ventricle with each contraction. CO usually is calculated using the equation $CO = HR \times SV$.

The HR is primarily controlled by the autonomic nervous system. When SV decreases, the nervous system is stimulated to increase HR and thereby maintain adequate CO. HR is easily measured, but SV is more difficult to measure precisely. SV depends on three factors: preload, afterload, and contractility (Fig. 30-1). Precise measurement of these factors requires hemodynamic monitoring.

**Preload** is the amount of blood presented to the ventricle just before systole. It increases pressure in the ventricle, which stretches the ventricular wall. Like a rubber band, the ventricular muscle fibers need to be stretched (by blood volume) to produce optimal ejection of blood. Too little or too much muscle fiber stretch decreases the volume of blood ejected. The major factor that determines preload is venous return, the volume of blood that enters the ventricle during diastole. Another factor that determines preload is ventricular **compliance**, the elasticity or amount of "give" when blood enters the ventricle. Elasticity is decreased when the muscle thickens, as in hypertrophic cardiomyopathy (see Chapter 29) or when there is increased fibrotic tissue within the ventricle. Fibrotic tissue replaces dead myocardial cells, such as after a myocardial infarction (MI) (see Chapter 28). Fibrotic tissue has little compliance, making the ventricle stiff. Given the same volume of blood, a noncompliant ventricle has a higher intraventricular pressure than a compliant one. Higher pressure increases the workload of the heart and can lead to **heart failure (HF)** if it is sustained.

## Glossary

**afterload:** the amount of resistance to ejection of blood from a ventricle

**anuria:** urine output of less than 50 mL per 24 hours

**ascites:** an accumulation of serous fluid in the peritoneal cavity

**cardiac output (CO):** the amount of blood pumped out of the heart in 1 minute

**cardiac resynchronization therapy (CRT):** a treatment for heart failure in which a device paces both ventricles to synchronize contractions

**compliance:** the elasticity or amount of "give" when blood enters the ventricle

**congestive heart failure (CHF):** a fluid overload condition (congestion) associated with heart failure

**contractility:** the force of ventricular contraction; related to the number and state of myocardial cells

**diastolic heart failure:** the inability of the heart to pump sufficiently because of an alteration in the ability of the heart to fill; current term used to describe a type of heart failure

**dyspnea on exertion (DOE):** shortness of breath that occurs with exertion

**ejection fraction (EF):** percentage of blood volume in the ventricles at the end of diastole that is ejected during systole; a measurement of contractility

**heart failure (HF):** the inability of the heart to pump sufficient blood to meet the needs of the tissues for oxygen and nutrients; signs and symptoms of pulmonary and systemic congestion may or may not be present

**implantable cardioverter defibrillator (ICD):** a device implanted in patients with ventricular dysrhythmias that detects and treats dysrhythmias

**left-sided heart failure (left ventricular failure):** inability of the left ventricle to fill or pump (empty) sufficient blood to meet the needs of the tissues for oxygen and nutrients; traditional term used to describe patient's symptoms of heart failure

**oliguria:** diminished urine output; less than 400 mL per 24 hours

**orthopnea:** shortness of breath when lying flat

**paroxysmal nocturnal dyspnea (PND):** shortness of breath that occurs suddenly during sleep

**pericardiocentesis:** procedure that involves aspiration of fluid from the pericardial sac

**pericardiotomy:** surgically created opening of the pericardium

**preload:** the amount of myocardial stretch just before systole caused by the volume of blood presented to the ventricle

**pulmonary edema:** abnormal accumulation of fluid in the interstitial spaces or in the alveoli of the lungs

**pulseless electrical activity (PEA):** condition in which electrical activity is present but there is not an adequate pulse or blood pressure because of ineffective cardiac contraction or circulating blood volume

**pulsus paradoxus:** systolic blood pressure of more than 10 mm Hg higher during exhalation than during inspiration; difference is normally less than 10 mm Hg

**right-sided heart failure (right ventricular failure):** inability of the right ventricle to fill or pump (empty) sufficient blood to the pulmonary circulation

**stroke volume (SV):** amount of blood pumped out of the ventricle with each contraction

**systolic heart failure:** inability of the heart to pump sufficiently because of an alteration in the ability of the heart to contract; current term used to describe a type of heart failure

**FIGURE 30-1.** The determinants of stroke volume (SV). The SV is determined by the amount of preload presented to the ventricle, the amount of afterload or resistance to ventricular ejection, and the strength of cardiac contractility. The cardiac output is the product of SV and heart rate. Redrawn from Porth, C. M. (2005). *Pathophysiology: Concepts of altered health states* (7th ed.). Philadelphia: Lippincott Williams & Wilkins.

**Afterload** refers to the amount of resistance to the ejection of blood from the ventricle. To eject blood, the ventricle must overcome the resistance caused by tension in the aorta and systemic vessels. Afterload is inversely related to SV, and an increase in afterload causes the ventricle to work harder and may decrease the amount of blood ejected. The major factors that determine afterload are the diameter and distensibility of the great vessels (aorta and pulmonary artery) and the opening and competence of the semilunar valves (pulmonic and aortic valves). When the valves open easily, resistance is lower. If the patient has significant vasoconstriction, hypertension, or a narrowed valvular opening from stenosis, resistance (afterload) increases. When afterload increases, the workload of the heart must increase to overcome the resistance and eject blood.

**Contractility**, the force of contraction, is related to the status of the myocardium. Catecholamines, released by sympathetic stimulation during exercise or from administration of positive inotropic medications, can increase contractility and SV. MI causes necrosis and subsequent fibrosis of some myocardial cells, shifting the workload to the remaining cells. Significant loss of myocardial cells can decrease contractility and cause HF. Afterload can be reduced by medications to match the lower contractility and maintain adequate CO.

## Noninvasive Assessment of Cardiac Hemodynamics

Several noninvasive assessment findings can indicate cardiac hemodynamic status, although the findings do not directly correlate to preload, afterload, or contractility. Right ventricular preload may be estimated by measuring jugular venous distention (JVD). Elevated left ventricular preload may be identified by a positive hepatojugular test. Mean arterial blood pressure is an approximate indicator of left ventricular afterload. Activity tolerance may be used as an indicator of overall cardiac functioning. These assessments are described in more detail later in this chapter.

## Invasive Assessment of Cardiac Hemodynamics

An important tool for evaluating the components of SV in a hemodynamically unstable patient is the pulmonary artery catheter, which is used to obtain the hemodynamic data essential for diagnosis and treatment (see Chapter 26). Measurements of intracardiac pressures, pulmonary artery pressures, and cardiac output are made at intervals. Therapy, especially intravenous (IV) medication, is adjusted based on the assessment and diagnostic findings. The patient with an invasive hemodynamic catheter is usually managed in an intensive care environment because of the need for frequent nursing assessments and interventions.

## Heart Failure

HF is the inability of the heart to pump sufficient blood to meet the needs of the tissues for oxygen and nutrients. In the past, HF was often referred to as **congestive heart failure (CHF)**, because many patients experience pulmonary or peripheral congestion. Currently HF is recognized as a clinical syndrome characterized by signs and symptoms of fluid overload or of inadequate tissue perfusion. Fluid overload and decreased tissue perfusion result when the heart cannot generate a CO sufficient to meet the body's demands. The term HF indicates myocardial disease in which there is a problem with contraction of the heart (systolic dysfunction) or filling of the heart (diastolic dysfunction) that may or may not cause pulmonary or systemic congestion. Some cases of HF are reversible, depending on the cause. Most often, HF is a progressive, life-long diagnosis that is managed with lifestyle changes and medications to prevent acute congestive episodes.

## Chronic Heart Failure

As with coronary artery disease, the incidence of HF increases with age. At least 5 million people in the United States have HF, and 550,000 new cases are diagnosed each year (American Heart Association [AHA], 2004). Although HF can affect people of all ages, the prevalence in people older than 75 years of age is about 10%, and as the U.S. population ages, HF has become an epidemic that challenges the country's health care resources (AHA, 2004). HF is the most common reason for hospitalization of people older than 65 years of age and the second most common reason for visits to a physician's office. The rate of hospital readmission remains staggeringly high. The economic burden caused by HF is estimated to be more than $25 billion in direct and indirect costs and is expected to increase (AHA, 2004).

The increase in the incidence of HF reflects the increased number of elderly people and improvements in treatment of cardiac diseases, resulting in increased survival rates. Many hospitalizations could be prevented by appropriate outpatient care. Prevention and early intervention to arrest the progression of HF are major health initiatives in the United States.

There are two types of HF, which are identified by assessment of left ventricular functioning, usually by echocardiogram. The more common type is an alteration in ventricular contraction called **systolic heart failure**, which is characterized by a weakened heart muscle. The less common alteration is **diastolic heart failure**, which is characterized by a stiff and noncompliant heart muscle, making it difficult for the ventricle to fill. An assessment of the **ejection fraction (EF)** is performed to assist in determining the type of HF. EF, an indication of the volume of blood ejected with each contraction, is calculated by subtracting the amount of blood at the end of systole from the amount at the end of diastole and calculating the percentage of blood that is ejected. A normal EF is 55% to 65% of the ventricular volume; the ventricle does not completely empty between contractions. The EF is normal in diastolic HF but severely reduced in systolic HF.

Although a low EF is a hallmark of HF, the severity of HF is frequently classified according to the patient's symptoms. The New York Heart Association (NYHA) Classification is described in Table 30-1, and the causes are explained in subsequent sections of this chapter. The American College of Cardiology and the American Heart Association (ACC/AHA) have proposed a new HF classification system (Institute for Clinical Systems Improvement [ICSI], 2004). This system (Table 30-2) takes into consideration the natural history and progressive nature of HF. Treatment guidelines have been developed for each stage.

## Pathophysiology

HF results from a variety of cardiovascular conditions, including chronic hypertension, coronary artery disease, and valvular disease. These conditions can result in decreased contraction (systole), decreased filling (diastole), or both. Significant myocardial dysfunction most often occurs before the patient experiences signs and symptoms of HF such as shortness of breath, edema, or fatigue.

As HF develops, the body activates neurohormonal compensatory mechanisms. These mechanisms represent the

| TABLE 30-1 | New York Heart Association (NYHA) Classification of Heart Failure | |
|---|---|---|
| Classification | Symptoms | Prognosis |
| I | Ordinary physical activity does not cause undue fatigue, dyspnea, palpitations, or chest pain<br>No pulmonary congestion or peripheral hypotension<br>Patient is considered asymptomatic<br>Usually no limitations of activities of daily living (ADLs) | Good |
| II | Slight limitation on ADLs<br>Patient reports no symptoms at rest but increased physical activity will cause symptoms<br>Basilar crackles and $S_3$ murmur may be detected | Good |
| III | Marked limitation on ADL<br>Patient feels comfortable at rest but less than ordinary activity will cause symptoms | Fair |
| IV | Symptoms of cardiac insufficiency at rest | Poor |

| TABLE 30-2 | American College of Cardiology and American Heart Association (ACC/AHA) Classification of Heart Failure |
|---|---|
| Classification | Symptoms |
| Stage A | Patients at high risk of developing left ventricular dysfunction |
| Stage B | Patients with left ventricular dysfunction who have not developed symptoms |
| Stage C | Patients with left ventricular dysfunction with current or prior symptoms |
| Stage D | Patients with refractory end-stage heart failure |

body's attempt to cope with the HF and are responsible for the signs and symptoms that eventually develop. Understanding these mechanisms is important because the treatment of HF is aimed at relieving them.

Systolic HF results in decreased blood volume being ejected from the ventricle. The decreased ventricular stretch is sensed by baroreceptors in the aortic and carotid bodies (Piano & Prasun, 2003). The sympathetic nervous system is then stimulated to release epinephrine and norepinephrine (Fig. 30-2). The purpose of this initial response is to increase heart rate and contractility and support the failing myocardium, but the continued response has multiple negative effects. Sympathetic stimulation causes vasoconstriction of the skin, gastrointestinal tract, and kidneys. A decrease in renal perfusion due to low CO and vasoconstriction then causes the release of renin by the kidney. Renin promotes the formation of angiotensin I, a benign, inactive substance. Angiotensin-converting enzyme (ACE) in the lumen of pulmonary blood vessels converts angiotensin I to angiotensin II, a potent vasoconstrictor, which then increases the blood pressure and afterload. Angiotensin II also stimulates the release of aldosterone from the adrenal cortex, resulting in sodium and fluid retention by the renal tubules and stimulating the thirst center. This leads to the fluid volume overload commonly seen in HF. Angiotensin, aldosterone, and other neurohormones (eg, endothelin, prostacyclin) lead to an increase in preload and afterload, which increases stress on the ventricular wall, causing an increase in the workload of the heart. A counterregulatory mechanism is attempted through the release of natriuretic peptides. Atrial natriuretic peptide (ANP) and B-type natriuretic peptide (BNP) are released from the overdistended cardiac chambers. These substances promote vasodilation and diuresis. However, their effect is usually not strong enough to overcome the negative effects of the other mechanisms.

As the heart's workload increases, contractility of the myocardial muscle fibers decreases. Decreased contractility results in an increase in end-diastolic blood volume in the ventricle, stretching the myocardial muscle fibers and increasing the size of the ventricle (ventricular dilation). The increased size of the ventricle further increases the stress on the ventricular wall, adding to the workload of the heart. One way the heart compensates for the increased workload is to increase the thickness of the heart muscle (ventricular hypertrophy). However, hypertrophy results in an abnormal proliferation of myocardial cells, a process known as ventricular remodeling. Under the influence of neurohormones (eg, angiotensin II), large myocardial cells are produced that are dysfunctional and die early, leaving the other normal myocardial cells to struggle to maintain CO (Ammon, 2001). The compensatory mechanisms of HF have been called the "vicious cycle of HF" because the heart does not pump sufficient blood to the body, which causes the body to stimulate the heart to work harder; the heart cannot respond and failure becomes worse.

Diastolic HF develops because of continued increased workload on the heart, which responds by increasing the number and size of myocardial cells (ie, ventricular hypertrophy and altered cellular functioning). These responses cause resistance to ventricular filling, which increases ventricular filling pressures despite a normal or reduced blood volume. Less blood in the ventricles causes decreased CO.

The low CO and high ventricular filling pressures can cause the same neurohormonal responses as described for systolic HF.

## Etiology

Myocardial dysfunction is most often caused by coronary artery disease, cardiomyopathy, hypertension, or valvular disorders. Patients with diabetes mellitus are also at high risk for HF. Atherosclerosis of the coronary arteries is the primary cause of HF, and coronary artery disease is found in more than 60% of the patients with HF (Zipes, Libby, & Bonow, 2005). Ischemia causes myocardial dysfunction because of resulting hypoxia and acidosis from the accumulation of lactic acid. MI causes focal heart muscle necrosis, the death of myocardial cells, and a loss of contractility; the extent of the infarction correlates with the severity of HF. Revascularization of the coronary artery by a percutaneous coronary intervention or by coronary artery bypass surgery may improve myocardial oxygenation and ventricular function.

Cardiomyopathy is a disease of the myocardium. There are three types: dilated, hypertrophic, and restrictive (see Chapter 29). Dilated cardiomyopathy, the most common type of cardiomyopathy, causes diffuse cellular necrosis and fibrosis, leading to decreased contractility (systolic failure). Dilated cardiomyopathy can be idiopathic (unknown cause), or it can result from an inflammatory process, such as myocarditis, or from a cytotoxic agent, such as alcohol or doxorubicin (Adriamycin). Hypertrophic cardiomyopathy and restrictive cardiomyopathy lead to decreased distensibility and ventricular filling (diastolic failure). Usually, HF due to cardiomyopathy becomes chronic and progressive. However, cardiomyopathy and HF may resolve following removal of the causative agent, such as with the cessation of alcohol ingestion.

Systemic or pulmonary hypertension increases afterload (resistance to ejection), which increases the workload of the heart and leads to hypertrophy of myocardial muscle fibers; this can be considered a compensatory mechanism because it increases contractility. However, the hypertrophy may impair the heart's ability to fill properly during diastole, and the hypertrophied ventricle may eventually fail.

Valvular heart disease is also a cause of HF. The valves ensure that blood flows in one direction. With valvular dysfunction, blood has increasing difficulty moving forward, increasing pressure within the heart and increasing cardiac workload, leading to HF. Chapter 29 discusses the effects of valvular heart disease.

Several systemic conditions contribute to the development and severity of HF, including increased metabolic rate (eg, fever, thyrotoxicosis), iron overload (eg, from hemochromatosis), hypoxia, and severe anemia (serum hematocrit less than 25%). All of these conditions require an increase in CO to satisfy the systemic oxygen demand. Hypoxia or anemia also may decrease the supply of oxygen to the myocardium. Cardiac dysrhythmias may cause HF or may be a result of HF; either way, the altered electrical stimulation impairs myocardial contraction and decreases the overall efficiency of myocardial function. Other factors, such as acidosis (respiratory or metabolic), electrolyte abnormalities, and antiarrhythmic medications, can worsen myocardial function.

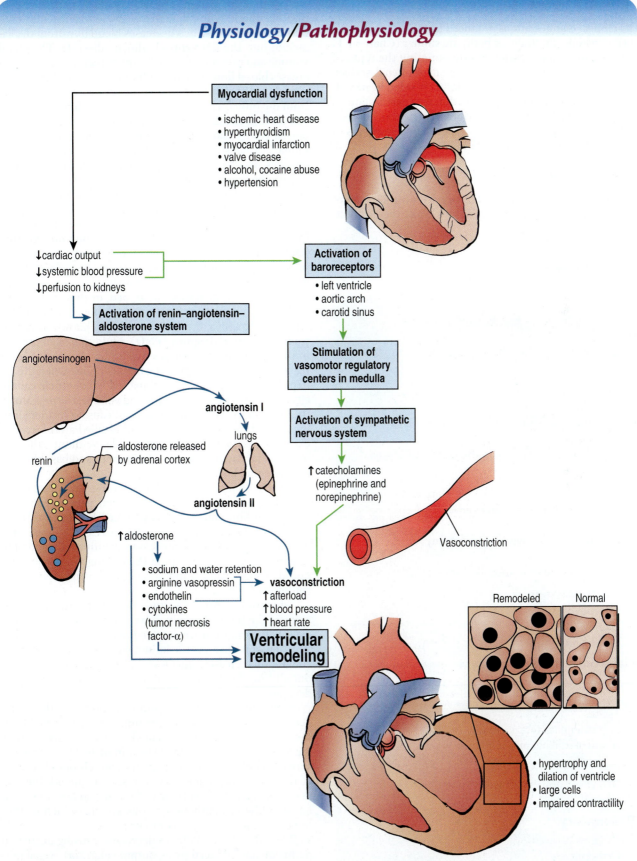

**FIGURE 30-2.** The pathophysiology of heart failure. A decrease in cardiac output activates multiple neurohormonal mechanisms that ultimately result in the signs and symptoms of heart failure.

## Clinical Manifestations

The clinical manifestations produced by the different types of HF (systolic, diastolic, or both) are similar (Chart 30-1) and therefore do not assist in differentiating the types of HF. The signs and symptoms of HF are most often described in terms of the effect on the ventricles. **Left-sided heart failure (left ventricular failure)** causes different manifestations than **right-sided heart failure (right ventricular failure)**. In chronic HF, patients may have signs and symptoms of both left and right ventricular failure.

### Left-Sided Heart Failure

Pulmonary congestion occurs when the left ventricle cannot effectively pump blood out of the ventricle into the aorta and the systemic circulation. The increased left ventricular end-diastolic blood volume increases the left ventricular end-diastolic pressure, which decreases blood flow from the left atrium into the left ventricle during diastole. The blood volume and pressure in the left atrium increases, which decreases blood flow from the pulmonary vessels. Pulmonary venous blood volume and pressure increase, forcing fluid from the pulmonary capillaries into the pulmonary tissues and alveoli, causing pulmonary interstitial edema and impaired gas exchange. The clinical manifestations of pulmonary congestion include dyspnea, cough, pulmonary crackles, and low oxygen saturation levels. An extra heart sound, the $S_3$, or ventricular "gallop," may be detected on auscultation. It is caused by a large volume of fluid entering the ventricle at the beginning of diastole.

Dyspnea, or shortness of breath, may be precipitated by minimal to moderate activity (**dyspnea on exertion [DOE]**); dyspnea also can occur at rest. The patient may report **orthopnea**, difficulty breathing when lying flat. Patients with orthopnea usually prefer not to lie flat. They may need pillows to prop themselves up in bed, or they may sit in a chair and even sleep sitting up. Some patients have sudden attacks of dyspnea at night, a condition known as **paroxysmal nocturnal dyspnea (PND)**. Fluid that accumulated in the dependent extremities during the day begins to be reabsorbed into the circulating blood volume when the patient lies down. Because the impaired left ventricle cannot eject the increased circulating blood volume, the pressure in the pulmonary circulation increases, causing further shifting of fluid into the alveoli. The fluid-filled alveoli cannot exchange oxygen and carbon dioxide. Without sufficient oxygen, the patient experiences dyspnea and has difficulty getting enough sleep.

The cough associated with left ventricular failure is initially dry and nonproductive. Most often, patients complain of a dry hacking cough that may be mislabeled as asthma or chronic obstructive pulmonary disease (COPD). The cough may become moist over time. Large quantities of frothy sputum, which is sometimes pink (blood-tinged), may be produced, usually indicating severe pulmonary congestion (pulmonary edema).

Adventitious breath sounds may be heard in various areas of the lungs. Usually, bibasilar crackles that do not clear with coughing are detected in the early phase of left ventricular failure. As the failure worsens and pulmonary congestion increases, crackles may be auscultated throughout all lung fields. At this point, oxygen saturation may decrease.

In addition to increased pulmonary pressures that cause decreased oxygenation, the amount of blood ejected from the left ventricle decreases. The dominant feature in HF is inadequate tissue perfusion. The diminished CO has widespread manifestations because not enough blood reaches all the tissues and organs (low perfusion) to provide the necessary oxygen. The decrease in SV can also lead to stimulation of the sympathetic nervous system, which further impedes perfusion to many organs.

Blood flow to the kidneys decreases, causing decreased perfusion and reduced urine output (**oliguria**). Renal perfusion pressure falls, which results in the release of renin from the kidney. Release of renin leads to aldosterone secretion and increased intravascular volume. However, when the patient is sleeping, the cardiac workload is decreased,

---

### CHART 30-1 — Assessing for Heart Failure

Be on the alert for the following signs and symptoms:

**General**
- Pale, cyanotic skin (with decreased perfusion to extremities)
- Dependent edema (with increased venous pressure)
- Decreased activity tolerance
- Unexplained confusion or altered mental status

**Cardiovascular**
- Apical impulse, enlarged and left lateral displacement (with cardiac enlargement)
- Third heart sound ($S_3$)
- Murmurs (with valvular dysfunction)
- Tachycardia
- Increased jugular venous distention (JVD)

**Cerebrovascular**
- Lightheadedness
- Dizziness
- Confusion

**Gastrointestinal**
- Nausea and anorexia
- Enlarged liver
- Ascites
- Hepatojugular test, increased (with increased right ventricular filling pressure)

**Renal**
- Decreased urinary frequency during the day
- Nocturia

**Respiratory**
- Dyspnea on exertion
- Orthopnea
- Paroxysmal nocturnal dyspnea
- Bilateral crackles that do not clear with cough
- Cough on exertion or when supine

improving renal perfusion, which may then lead to frequent urination at night (nocturia).

As HF progresses, decreased CO may cause other symptoms. Decreased gastrointestinal perfusion causes altered digestion. Decreased brain perfusion causes dizziness, lightheadedness, confusion, restlessness, and anxiety due to decreased oxygenation and blood flow. As anxiety increases, so does dyspnea, increasing anxiety and creating a vicious cycle. Stimulation of the sympathetic system also causes the peripheral blood vessels to constrict, so the skin appears pale or ashen and feels cool and clammy.

Decreases in ejected ventricular volume cause the sympathetic nervous system to increase the heart rate (tachycardia), often causing the patient to complain of palpitations. The pulses become weak and thready. Without adequate CO, the body cannot respond to increased energy demands, and the patient becomes easily fatigued and has decreased activity tolerance. Fatigue also results from the increased energy expended in breathing and the insomnia that results from respiratory distress, coughing, and nocturia.

### Right-Sided Heart Failure

When the right ventricle fails, congestion in the peripheral tissues and the viscera predominates. This occurs because the right side of the heart cannot eject blood and cannot accommodate all the blood that normally returns to it from the venous circulation. Increased venous pressure leads to JVD and increased hydrostatic pressure throughout the venous system.

The systemic clinical manifestations include edema of the lower extremities (dependent edema), hepatomegaly (enlargement of the liver), **ascites** (accumulation of fluid in the peritoneal cavity), anorexia and nausea, and weakness and weight gain due to retention of fluid.

Edema usually affects the feet and ankles and worsens when the patient stands or dangles the legs. The edema decreases when the patient elevates the legs. The edema can gradually progress up the legs and thighs and eventually into the external genitalia and lower trunk. Edema in the abdomen, as evidenced by increased abdominal girth, may be the only edema present. Sacral edema is not uncommon in patients who are on bed rest, because the sacral area is dependent. Pitting edema, in which indentations in the skin remain after even slight compression with the fingertips (Fig. 30-3), is obvious only after retention of at least 4.5 kg (10 lb) of fluid (4.5 L).

Hepatomegaly and tenderness in the right upper quadrant of the abdomen result from venous engorgement of the liver. The increased pressure may interfere with the liver's ability to function (secondary liver dysfunction). As hepatic dysfunction progresses, increased pressure within the portal vessels may force fluid into the abdominal cavity, a condition known as ascites. Ascites may increase pressure on the stomach and intestines and cause gastrointestinal distress. Hepatomegaly may also increase pressure on the diaphragm, causing respiratory distress.

Anorexia (loss of appetite) and nausea or abdominal pain results from the venous engorgement and venous stasis within the abdominal organs. The weakness that accompanies right-sided HF results from reduced CO, impaired circulation, and inadequate removal of catabolic waste products from the tissues.

**FIGURE 30-3.** Example of pitting edema. (**A**) The nurse applies finger pressure to an area near the ankle. (**B**) When the pressure is released, an indentation remains in the edematous tissue. From Bickley, L. S. & Szilagyi, P. G. (2005). *Bates' guide to physical examination and history taking* (9th ed). Philadelphia: Lippincott Williams & Wilkins.

## Assessment and Diagnostic Findings

HF may go undetected until the patient presents with signs and symptoms of pulmonary and peripheral edema. However, the physical signs that suggest HF may also occur with other diseases, such as renal failure, liver failure, oncologic conditions, and COPD. If further assessment and evaluation are not completed, these patients may be treated for HF inappropriately. Assessment of ventricular function is an essential part of the initial diagnostic workup.

An echocardiogram is usually performed to confirm the diagnosis of HF, help identify the underlying cause, and determine the EF, which helps identify the type and severity of HF. This information may also be obtained noninvasively by radionuclide ventriculography or invasively by ventriculography as part of a cardiac catheterization procedure. A chest x-ray and an electrocardiogram (ECG) are obtained to assist in the diagnosis and to determine the underlying cause of HF. Laboratory studies usually completed in the initial workup include serum electrolytes, blood urea nitrogen (BUN), creatinine, thyroid-stimulating hormone, complete blood cell count, B-type natriuretic peptide (BNP), and routine urinalysis. The BNP level is a key diagnostic indicator of HF. High levels of BNP are a sign of high cardiac filling pressure and can aid in the diagnosis of HF (ICSI, 2004). The results of these laboratory studies assist in determining the underlying cause and can also be used to establish a baseline to assess effects of treatment. Exercise testing or cardiac catheterization may be performed to determine whether coronary artery disease and cardiac ischemia are causing the HF.

In patients with acute MI who are at risk for HF, ventricular function is assessed before discharge from the hospital. Quantifying the degree of left-ventricular dysfunction is important to determine appropriate medical management. Evaluation of ventricular function may also be performed if the initial assessment of HF suggested noncardiac causes but treatment failed to produce a response.

## Medical Management

The overall goals of management of HF are to relieve patient symptoms, to improve functional status and quality of life, and to extend survival. Medical management is based on the type, severity, and cause of HF. Specific objectives of medical management include the following:

- Eliminate or reduce any etiologic contributory factors, especially those that may be reversible (eg, atrial fibrillation, excessive alcohol ingestion)
- Reduce the workload on the heart by reducing afterload and preload
- Optimize all therapeutic regimens
- Prevent exacerbations of HF

Treatment options vary according to the severity of the patient's condition and may include basic lifestyle changes, oral and IV pharmacologic management, supplemental oxygen, implantation of assistive devices, and surgical approaches, including cardiac transplantation.

Managing the patient with HF includes providing general education and counseling to the patient and family. It is important that the patient and family understand the nature of HF and the importance of their participation in the treatment regimen. Lifestyle recommendations include restriction of dietary sodium; avoidance of excessive fluid intake, alcohol, and smoking; weight reduction when indicated; and regular exercise. The patient must know how to recognize signs and symptoms that need to be reported to the health care professional.

### Pharmacologic Therapy

Several medications are routinely prescribed for systolic HF, including ACE inhibitors, beta-blockers, diuretics, and digitalis. Medications for diastolic failure depend on the underlying condition, such as hypertension (see Chapter 32) or valvular dysfunction (see Chapter 29).

#### ANGIOTENSIN-CONVERTING ENZYME INHIBITORS

ACE inhibitors play a pivotal role in the management of HF due to systolic dysfunction. They have been found to relieve the signs and symptoms of HF and significantly decrease mortality and morbidity. ACE inhibitors slow the progression of HF, improve exercise tolerance, and decrease the number of hospitalizations for HF (Moser & Biddle, 2003). Available as oral and IV medications, ACE inhibitors promote vasodilation and diuresis by decreasing afterload and preload. By doing so, they decrease the workload of the heart. Vasodilation reduces resistance to left ventricular ejection of blood, diminishing the heart's workload and improving ventricular emptying. In promoting diuresis, ACE inhibitors decrease the secretion of aldosterone, a hormone that causes the kidneys to retain sodium and water. ACE inhibitors stimulate the kidneys to excrete sodium and fluid (while retaining potassium), thereby reducing left ventricular filling pressure and decreasing pulmonary congestion. ACE inhibitors may be the first medication prescribed for patients in mild failure—patients with fatigue or DOE but without signs of fluid overload and pulmonary congestion.

ACE inhibitors are started at a low dose that is increased every 2 weeks until the optimal dose is achieved and the patient is hemodynamically stable. The final maintenance dose depends on the patient's blood pressure, fluid status, and renal status and on the severity of the HF.

Patients receiving ACE inhibitors are monitored for hypotension, hypovolemia, hyperkalemia, and alterations in renal function, especially if they are also receiving diuretics. When to observe for these effects and for how long depends on the onset, peak, and duration of the medication. Table 30-3 identifies several types of ACE inhibitors and their pharmacokinetics. Hypotension is most likely to develop from ACE inhibitor therapy in patients older than 75 years of age and in those with a systolic blood pressure of 100 mm Hg or less, a serum sodium level of lower than 135 mEq/L, or severe heart failure. Adjusting the dose or type of diuretic in response to the patient's blood pressure and renal function may allow for continued increases in the dosage of ACE inhibitors.

Because ACE inhibitors cause the kidneys to retain potassium, the patient who is also receiving a diuretic may not need to take oral potassium supplements. However, patients receiving potassium-sparing diuretics (which do not cause potassium loss with diuresis) must be carefully monitored for hyperkalemia, an increased level of potassium in the

### TABLE 30-3 Angiotensin-Converting Enzyme (ACE) Inhibitors

| ACE Inhibitor | Pharmacokinetics | | | Nursing Considerations |
|---|---|---|---|---|
| | Onset | Peak (hr) | Duration (hr) | |
| benazepril (Lotensin) | within 1 hr | 2–4 | 24 | Monitor blood pressure, urine output, and electrolyte levels. |
| captopril (Capoten) | 15–60 min | 1–1.5 | 6–12* | |
| enalapril (Vasotec) | 1 hr | 4–6 | 24 | Monitor serum creatinine and urine creatinine clearance. |
| enalaprilat (Vasotec I.V.) | 15 min | 1–4 | 6 | |
| fosinopril (Monopril) | within 1 hr | 2–6 | 24 | Monitor for development of cough that is resistant to cough suppressants. |
| lisinopril (Prinival, Zestril) | 1 hr | 6 | 24 | |
| moexipril (Univasc) | 1 hr | 3–6 | 24 | Teach patient to change positions gradually and to report signs of dizziness or lethargy. |
| quinapril (Accupril) | within 1 hr | 2–4 | up to 24* | |
| ramipril (Altace) | 1–2 hr | 4–6 | 24 | Instruct patient to weigh self daily and to report rapid weight gain and significant feet and hand swelling. |
| trandolapril (Mavik) | within 30 min | 2–4 | > 8 days | |

*Duration of effect is related to the dose.

blood. Before the initiation of the ACE inhibitor, hyperkalemic and hypovolemic states must be corrected. ACE inhibitors may be discontinued if the potassium level remains greater than 5.0 mEq/L or if the serum creatinine is 3.0 mg/dL or more.

Other side effects of ACE inhibitors include a dry, persistent cough that may not respond to cough suppressants. However, the cough could also indicate a worsening of ventricular function and failure. Rarely, the cough indicates angioedema. If angioedema affects the oropharyngeal area and impairs breathing, the ACE inhibitor must be stopped immediately.

If the patient cannot continue taking an ACE inhibitor because of development of cough, an elevated creatinine level, or hyperkalemia, an angiotensin II receptor blocker (ARB) or hydralazine (Apresoline) and isosorbide dinitrate (Dilatrate SR, Isordil, Sorbitrate) are prescribed.

### ANGIOTENSIN II RECEPTOR BLOCKERS

Although the action of ARBs is different than that of ACE inhibitors, ARBs (eg, valsartan [Diovan]) have similar hemodynamic effects: decreased blood pressure, decreased systemic vascular resistance, and improved cardiac output (ICSI, 2004). Whereas ACE inhibitors block the conversion of angiotensin I to angiotensin II, ARBs block the effects of angiotensin II at the angiotensin II receptor. ACE inhibitors and ARBs also have similar side effects: hyperkalemia, hypotension, and renal dysfunction. ARBs are usually prescribed as an alternative to ACE inhibitors, especially when patients cannot tolerate ACE inhibitors because of cough.

### HYDRALAZINE AND ISOSORBIDE DINITRATE

A combination of hydralazine (Apresoline) and isosorbide dinitrate (Dilatrate SR, Isordil, Sorbitrate) may be another alternative for patients who cannot take ACE inhibitors. Nitrates (eg, isosorbide dinitrate) cause venous dilation, which reduces the amount of blood return to the heart and lowers preload. Hydralazine lowers systemic vascular resistance and left ventricular afterload. This combination of medications is usually used when patients cannot tolerate ACE inhibitors.

### BETA-BLOCKERS

Beta-blockers, such as carvedilol (Coreg) and metoprolol (Lopressor, Toprol), have been found to reduce mortality and morbidity in patients with NYHA Class II or III HF by reducing the adverse effects from the constant stimulation of the sympathetic nervous system. Beta-blockers are routinely prescribed in addition to ACE inhibitors, diuretics, and digitalis (ICSI, 2004) and have also been recommended for patients with asymptomatic systolic dysfunction, such as those with a decreased EF, to prevent the onset of symptoms of HF.

Beta-blockers may produce many side effects and may exacerbate symptoms of HF. Side effects are most common in the initial few weeks of treatment. The most frequent side effects are dizziness, hypotension, and bradycardia. Because of these side effects, beta-blockers are started only after the patient is stabilized and euvolemic (eg, state of normal volume). The dose is titrated slowly (every 2 weeks), with close monitoring at each increase. If symptoms of HF increase during the titration phase, treatment options include increasing the dose of the diuretic, reducing the dose of the ACE inhibitor, or decreasing the dose of the beta-blocker.

An important nursing role during titration is educating the patient about the potential worsening of symptoms during the early phase of treatment and stressing that improvement may take several weeks. It is very important for nurses to provide support to patients going through this symptom-provoking phase of treatment. Because beta-blockade can cause bronchiole constriction, a beta-1–selective beta-blocker (ie, one that primarily blocks the beta-adrenergic receptor sites in the heart) such as metoprolol (Lopressor, Toprol) is recommended for patients with well-controlled, mild to moderate asthma. Patients need to be monitored closely for increased asthma symptoms nonetheless, as even cardioselective beta-blockers retain some modest beta-2 effects. Any type of beta-blocker is contraindicated in patients with severe or uncontrolled asthma.

### DIURETICS

Diuretics are prescribed to remove excess extracellular fluid by increasing the rate of urine produced in patients with signs and symptoms of fluid overload. Of the types of diuretics prescribed for patients with edema from HF, three are most common: thiazide, loop, and potassium-sparing diuretics. These medications are classified according to their site of action in the kidney and their effects on renal electrolyte excretion and reabsorption.

Thiazide diuretics, such as metolazone (Zaroxolyn), inhibit sodium and chloride reabsorption mainly in the early distal tubules. They also increase potassium and bicarbonate excretion. Loop diuretics, such as furosemide (Lasix), inhibit sodium and chloride reabsorption mainly in the ascending loop of Henle. Both of these types of diuretics may be used for patients in severe HF who are unresponsive to a single diuretic. Diuretics may be most effective if the patient assumes a supine position for 1 or 2 hours after taking them. These medications may not be necessary if the patient responds to activity recommendations, avoids excessive fluid intake (eg, more than 2 quarts/day), and adheres to a low-sodium diet (eg, less than 2 g/day).

Spironolactone (Aldactone) is a potassium-sparing diuretic that inhibits sodium reabsorption in the late distal tubule and collecting duct. It has been found to be effective in reducing mortality and morbidity in patients with moderate to severe HF when taken along with ACE inhibitors, loop diuretics, and digoxin (ICSI, 2004). Serum creatinine and potassium levels are monitored frequently (eg, within the first week and then every 4 weeks) when this medication is first administered.

Side effects of diuretics include electrolyte imbalances, symptomatic hypotension (especially with overdiuresis), hyperuricemia (causing gout), and ototoxicity. The dose depends on the indications, patient age, clinical signs and symptoms, and renal function. Table 30-4 lists commonly used diuretics and their recommended doses and pharmacokinetic properties. Careful patient monitoring and dose adjustments are necessary to balance the effectiveness of these medications with the side effects (Chart 30-2). Diuretics are administered IV for exacerbations of HF when rapid diuresis is necessary. Diuretics tend to improve the patient's symptoms, provided that renal function is adequate (ICSI, 2004).

### TABLE 30-4  Diuretic Medications Used to Treat Heart Failure

| Diuretic | Usual Adult Dose | Onset (hr) | Peak (hr) | Duration (hr) |
|---|---|---|---|---|
| **Thiazide Diuretics** | | | | |
| bendroflumethiazide (Naturetin) | 2.5–20 mg in single or divided dose, once a day, once every other day, or once a day for 3–5 days per week | 2 | 4 | 12–16 |
| benzthiazide (Exna) | 12.5–200 mg in single or divided dose | 2 | 4–6 | 16–18 |
| chlorothiazide (Diuril) | Oral: 0.25–2 g as single or divided dose; may be given on alternate days | 2 | 4 | 16–18 |
|  | IV: 0.5–1 g in single or divided dose (note: avoid extravasation) | 15 min | 30 min | |
| chlorthalidone (Hygroton) | 12.5–200 mg once a day, once every other day, or once a day for 3 days per week | 2 | 2–6 | 24–72 |
| hydrochlorothiazide (HydroDIURIL, Esidrix, Oretic) | 12.5–200 mg as single or divided dose once a day, once every other day, or once a day for 3–5 days per week | 2 | 4–6 | 12–16 |
| hydroflumethiazide (Diucardin, Saluron) | 25–200 mg as single or divided dose once a day, once every other day, or once a day for 3–5 days per week | 2 | 4 | 12–16 |
| methyclothiazide (Enduron) | 2.5–10 mg once a day | 2 | 6 | 24 |
| metolazone (Zaroxolyn, Mykrox) | Zaroxolyn: 2.5–20 mg once a day; Mykrox: 0.5–1 mg once a day | 1 | 2 | 12–24 |
| polythiazide (Renese) | 1–4 mg once a day, once every other day, or once a day for 3–5 days per week | 2 | 6 | 24–28 |
| quinethazone (Hydromox) | 25–100 mg as single or divided dose; rarely, 200 mg once a day | 2 | 6 | 18–24 |
| trichlormethiazide (Metahydrin, Naqua) | 1–4 mg once or twice a day | 2 | 6 | 24 |
| **Loop Diuretics** | | | | |
| bumetanide (Bumex) | 0.5–2 mg once, twice, or three times a day; may be given on alternate days or once every 3 days | 30–60 min | 1–2 | 4–6 |
|  | 0.5–1 mg over 2 min; repeat every 2–3 h; a continuous infusion may be given at a rate of 1 mg/h | 5–10 min | 15–30 min | ½–1 |
| ethacrynic acid (Edecrin) | 50–400 mg as single or divided dose | <30 min | 2 | 6–8 |
|  | 0.5–1 mg/kg (max 100 mg) over several min; may be repeated within 2–6 h; repeat every hour in emergencies | <5 min | 15–30 min | 2 |
| furosemide (Lasix) | 20–600 mg as single daily dose, divided daily dose, as a dose given every other day or given once a day for 2–4 days per week | <1 | 1–2 | 6–8 |
|  | 20–200 mg (max 6 mg/kg) given at a rate of 4 mg/min; after response obtained, given once or twice a day | <5 min | 30 min | 2 |
| torsemide (Demadex) | 5–200 mg as a daily single dose | <1 | 1–2 | 6–8 |
|  | IV and oral doses are equivalent; give IV over 2 min. | <10 min | <1 | 6–8 |
| **Potassium-Sparing Diuretics** | | | | |
| amiloride (Midamor) | 5–20 mg daily as single dose | 2 | 6–10 | 24 |
| spironolactone (Aldactone) | 25–400 mg as single dose or divided up to 4 doses | 24–48 | 48–72 | 48–72 |
| triamterene (Dyrenium) | 50–300 mg as single dose | 2–4 | 6–8 | 12–16 |

## DIGITALIS

The most commonly prescribed form of digitalis for patients with HF is digoxin (Lanoxin). This medication increases the force of myocardial contraction and slows conduction through the atrioventricular node. It improves contractility, increasing left ventricular output, which also results in enhanced diuresis. The effect of a given dose of digoxin depends on the state of the myocardium, electrolyte and fluid balance, and renal function. Although the use of digitalis does not result in decreased mortality rates among patients with HF, it is effective in decreasing the symptoms of systolic HF and in increasing the patient's ability to perform activities of daily living (Spencer, 2003).

A key concern associated with digitalis therapy is digitalis toxicity. Chart 30-3 summarizes the actions and uses of digoxin along with the nursing surveillance required when it is administered. The patient is observed for indications that digitalis therapy is effective: lessening dyspnea and orthopnea, decrease in pulmonary crackles on auscultation, relief of peripheral edema, weight loss, and increase in activity tolerance. The serum potassium level is measured at

## CHART 30-2

# PHARMACOLOGY · Administering and Monitoring Diuretic Therapy

When nursing care involves diuretic therapy for conditions such as heart failure, the nurse needs to administer the medication and monitor the patient's response carefully, as follows:

- Administer the diuretic at a time conducive to the patient's lifestyle; for example, early in the day to avoid nocturia.
- Give supplementary potassium with thiazide and loop diuretics as prescribed to replace potassium loss.
- Check laboratory results for electrolyte depletion, especially potassium, magnesium, and sodium; and for electrolyte elevation, especially potassium with potassium-sparing agents.
- Monitor daily weights, intake and output to assess response. Monitor serum blood urea nitrogen and creatinine. Notify health care provider if renal impairment is suspected.
- Assess lung sounds, jugular vein distention, daily weight, and peripheral, abdominal, or sacral edema to identify response to therapy.
- Monitor for adverse reactions, such as nausea and gastrointestinal distress, vomiting, diarrhea, weakness, headache, fatigue, anxiety or agitation, and cardiac dysrhythmias.
- Assess for signs of volume depletion, such as postural hypotension, dizziness, and balance problems.
- Monitor for glucose intolerance in patients with and without diabetes mellitus who are receiving thiazide diuretics.
- Monitor for potential ototoxicity in patients, especially those with renal failure, who are receiving a loop diuretic.
- Advise patients to avoid prolonged exposure to the sun because of the risk of photosensitivity.
- Monitor for elevated serum uric acid levels and the development of gout.
- Implement nursing actions to facilitate effect of medication, such as positioning patient supine after dose is taken.

---

intervals because diuresis may cause hypokalemia. The effect of digoxin is enhanced in the presence of hypokalemia, so digoxin toxicity may occur. Serum digoxin levels are obtained if there have been changes in the patient's medications, renal function, or symptoms.

### CALCIUM CHANNEL BLOCKERS

First-generation calcium channel blockers, such as verapamil (Calan, Isoptin), nifedipine (Adalat, Procardia), and diltiazem (Cardizem, Tiazac), are contraindicated in patients with systolic dysfunction, although they may be used in patients with diastolic dysfunction. Amlodipine (Norvasc) and felodipine (Plendil), which are dihydropyridine calcium channel blockers, cause vasodilation, reducing systemic vascular resistance. They may be used to improve symptoms, especially in patients with nonischemic cardiomyopathy.

### INTRAVENOUS INFUSIONS

**Nesiritide.** Nesiritide (Natrecor), a BNP made using recombinant technology, is indicated for patients with acutely decompensated HF. BNPs are produced by the myocardium to mount a compensatory response in the presence of the myocardial demands, including increased ventricular end-diastolic pressure, myocardial wall stress, and increased release of neurohormones (eg, norepinephrine, renin, aldosterone), that occur with HF. Specifically, BNP binds to vascular smooth muscle and endothelial cells, causing dilation of arteries and veins. It also suppresses the neurohormones responsible for fluid retention, thus promoting diuresis. The result is reduced preload and afterload and increased SV (Hachey & Smith, 2003).

Nesiritide causes rapid improvement in the symptoms of HF. It may be used to treat hospitalized patients with acute exacerbations or to prevent exacerbations in outpatients when given as a series of intermittent IV infusions. The most common side effect is dose-related hypotension.

**Milrinone.** Milrinone (Primacor) is a phosphodiesterase inhibitor that delays the release of calcium from intracellular reservoirs and prevents the uptake of extracellular calcium by the cells. This promotes vasodilation, resulting in decreased preload and afterload and reduced cardiac workload. Milrinone is administered IV if the patient has not responded to other therapies. The major side effects are hypotension (usually asymptomatic), gastrointestinal dysfunction, increased ventricular dysrhythmias, and, rarely, decreased platelet counts. Blood pressure is monitored closely.

**Dobutamine.** Dobutamine (Dobutrex) is an IV medication administered to patients with significant left ventricular dysfunction. A catecholamine, dobutamine stimulates the beta-1–adrenergic receptors. Its major action is to increase cardiac contractility. However, at high doses, it also increases the heart rate and the incidence of ectopic beats and tachydysrhythmias. Because it also increases atrioventricular conduction, care must be taken in patients who have underlying atrial fibrillation.

Patients receiving continuous IV infusions of any of these vasoactive medications are routinely monitored continuously via ECG, and their vital signs are assessed frequently.

### MEDICATIONS FOR DIASTOLIC DYSFUNCTION

Patients with predominant diastolic dysfunction may be treated with different pharmacologic agents than indicated for patients with systolic dysfunction. After contributing causes such as hypertension and ischemic heart disease are evaluated and treated, patients may be started on ACE inhibitors and diuretics. Beta-blockers are also used in

## CHART 30-3

#  PHARMACOLOGY · Digoxin Use and Toxicity in Heart Failure

Digoxin, a cardiac glycoside derived from digitalis, is used for patients with systolic HF, atrial fibrillation, and atrial flutter. Digoxin improves cardiac function as follows:
- Increases the force of myocardial contraction
- Slows cardiac conduction through the AV node and therefore slows the ventricular rate in instances of supraventricular dysrhythmias
- Increases cardiac output by enhancing the force of ventricular contraction
- Promotes diuresis by increasing cardiac output.

The therapeutic level is usually 0.5 to 2.0 ng/mL. Blood samples are usually obtained and analyzed to determine digitalis concentration at least 6 to 10 hours after the last dose. Toxicity may occur despite normal serum levels, and recommended dosages vary considerably.

### Preparations

**DIGOXIN**
- Tablets: 0.125, 0.25, 0.5 mg (Lanoxin)
- Capsules: 0.05, 0.1, 0.2 mg (Lanoxicaps)
- Elixir: 0.05 mg/mL (Lanoxin Pediatric elixir)
- Injection: 0.25 mg/mL, 0.1 mg/mL (Lanoxin)

### Digoxin Toxicity

A serious complication of digoxin therapy is toxicity. Diagnosis of digoxin toxicity is based on the patient's clinical symptoms, which include the following:
- Anorexia, nausea, vomiting, fatigue, depression, and malaise (early effects of digitalis toxicity)
- Changes in heart rate or rhythm; onset of irregular rhythm.
- ECG changes indicating SA or AV block; new onset of irregular rhythm indicating ventricular dysrhythmias; and atrial tachycardia with block, junctional tachycardia, and ventricular tachycardia

### Reversal of Toxicity

Digoxin toxicity is treated by holding the medication while monitoring the patient's symptoms and serum digoxin level. If the toxicity is severe, digoxin immune FAB (Digibind) may be prescribed. Digibind binds with digoxin and makes it unavailable for use. The Digibind dosage is based on the digoxin level and the patient's weight. Serum digoxin values are not accurate for several days after administration of Digibind because they do not differentiate between bound and unbound digoxin. Because Digibind quickly decreases the amount of available digoxin, an increase in ventricular rate due to atrial fibrillation and worsening of symptoms of HF may ensue shortly after its administration.

### Nursing Considerations and Actions

1. Assess the patient's clinical response to digoxin therapy by evaluating relief of symptoms such as dyspnea, orthopnea, crackles, hepatomegaly, and peripheral edema.
2. Monitor the patient for factors that increase the risk of toxicity:
   - Decreased potassium level (hypokalemia), which may be caused by diuretics. Hypokalemia increases the action of digoxin and predisposes patients to digoxin toxicity and dysrhythmias.
   - Use of medications that enhance the effects of digoxin, including oral antibiotics and cardiac drugs that slow AV conduction and can further decrease heart rate
   - Impaired renal function, particularly in patients age 65 and older. Because digoxin is eliminated by the kidneys, renal function (serum creatinine) is monitored and doses of digoxin are adjusted accordingly.
3. Before administering digoxin, it is standard nursing practice to assess apical heart rate. When the patient's rhythm is atrial fibrillation and the heart rate is less than 60, or the rhythm becomes regular, the nurse may withhold the medication and notify the physician, because these signs indicate the development of AV conduction block. Although withholding digoxin is a common practice, the medication does not need to be withheld for a heart rate of less than 60 if the patient is in sinus rhythm because digoxin does not affect sinoatrial node automaticity. Measuring the PR interval for a patient with cardiac monitoring is more important than the apical pulse in determining whether digoxin should be held.
4. Monitor for gastrointestinal side effects: anorexia, nausea, vomiting, abdominal pain and distention.
5. Monitor for neurologic side effects: headache, malaise, nightmares, forgetfulness, social withdrawal, depression, agitation, confusion, paranoia, hallucinations, decreased visual acuity, yellow or green halo around objects (especially lights), or "snowy" vision.

---

these patients if they have concomitant atrial fibrillation (ICSI, 2004).

**OTHER MEDICATIONS**

Anticoagulants may be prescribed, especially if the patient has a history of an embolic event or atrial fibrillation or a mural thrombus is present. Other medications, such as antianginal medications, may be administered to treat the underlying cause of HF. Nonsteroidal anti-inflammatory drugs (NSAIDs) such as ibuprofen (Advil, Motrin) should be avoided, because they increase systemic vascular resistance and decrease renal perfusion, especially in the elderly. For similar reasons, use of decongestants should be avoided.

## Nutritional Therapy

A low-sodium (2 to 3 g/day) diet and avoidance of excessive amounts of fluid are usually recommended. Dietary restriction of sodium reduces fluid retention and the symptoms of peripheral and pulmonary congestion. The purpose of sodium restriction is to decrease the amount of circulating blood volume, which would decrease the need for the heart to pump that volume. A balance needs to be achieved between the ability of the patient to comply with the diet and the recommended dietary restriction. Any change in diet needs to be made with consideration of good nutrition as well as the patient's likes, dislikes, and cultural food patterns. Patient compliance is important because dietary indiscretions may result in severe exacerbations of HF requiring hospitalization. However, behavioral changes in this area are difficult for many patients (Sneed & Paul, 2003).

**NURSING ALERT**

The sources of sodium should be specified in describing the regimen, rather than simply saying "low-salt" or "salt-free," and the quantity should be indicated in milligrams. Salt is not 100% sodium; there are 393 mg of sodium in 1 g (1000 mg) of salt.

## Additional Therapy

### SUPPLEMENTAL OXYGEN

Oxygen therapy may become necessary as heart failure progresses. The need is based on the degree of pulmonary congestion and resulting hypoxia. Some patients require supplemental oxygen only during activity.

### OTHER INTERVENTIONS

A number of procedures and surgical approaches may benefit patients with HF. If the patient has underlying coronary artery disease, coronary artery revascularization with percutaneous coronary intervention or coronary artery bypass surgery (see Chapter 28) may be considered. Ventricular function may improve in some patients when coronary flow is increased (Albert, 2003b).

Patients with HF are at high risk for dysrhythmias. Sudden cardiac death accounts for half of all deaths from heart failure (Young, Abraham, & Smith, 2003). In patients with life-threatening dysrhythmias, placement of an **implantable cardioverter defibrillator (ICD)** can prevent sudden cardiac death and extend survival.

In the patient with HF who does not improve with standard therapy, **cardiac resynchronization therapy (CRT)** is another treatment that may be beneficial. CRT involves the use of a biventricular pacemaker to treat electrical conduction defects. Left bundle branch block is a feature of delayed conduction that is frequently seen in patients with HF that results in dyssynchronous conduction and contraction of the right and left ventricles, which can further decrease EF (Albert, 2003a). Use of a pacing device with leads placed in the right atrium, right ventricle, and left ventricular cardiac vein can synchronize the contractions of the right and left ventricles. This intervention has been shown to improve cardiac output, optimize myocardial energy consumption, reduce mitral regurgitation, and slow the ventricular remodeling process. For selected patients, this results in fewer symptoms and increased functional status (Bradley, Bradley, & Baughman, 2003). For patients who require CRT and an ICD, combination devices are available.

For some patients with end-stage HF, cardiac transplantation is the only option for long-term survival (Tokarczyk, 2003). Some of these patients require mechanical circulatory assistance with an implanted ventricular assist device as a bridge therapy to cardiac transplantation (see Chapter 29). Research continues toward perfection of a totally implantable artificial heart that may be used as an alternative to transplantation.

## Nursing Management

Despite advances in medical and surgical approaches to HF, mortality remains high. Nurses can make a major difference in promoting positive outcomes. In both inpatient and outpatient settings, nursing interventions for the patient with HF include the following:

- Administering medications and assessing the patient's response to the pharmacologic regimen
- Assessing fluid balance, including intake and output, with a goal of optimizing volume status
- Weighing the patient daily at the same time and on the same scale, usually in the morning after urination; monitoring for a 2- to 3-lb gain in a day or 5-lb gain in a week
- Auscultating lung sounds to detect an increase or decrease in pulmonary crackles
- Determining the degree of jugular venous distention (JVD)
- Identifying and evaluating the severity of dependent edema
- Monitoring pulse rate and blood pressure; checking for postural hypotension due to dehydration
- Examining skin turgor and mucous membranes for signs of dehydration
- Assessing for symptoms of fluid overload (eg, orthopnea, PND, DOE)

### Monitoring and Managing Potential Complications

Many potential problems associated with HF therapy relate to the use of diuretics:

- Profuse and repeated diuresis can lead to hypokalemia (ie, potassium depletion). Signs include ventricular dysrhythmias, hypotension, muscle weakness, diminished deep tendon reflexes, and generalized weakness. Hypokalemia poses problems for the patient with HF because it markedly weakens cardiac contractions. In patients receiving digoxin, hypokalemia can lead to digitalis toxicity. Digitalis toxicity and hypokalemia increase the likelihood of dangerous dysrhythmias (see Chart 30-3). Patients with HF may also develop low levels of magnesium, which can add to the risk of dysrhythmias.

- Hyperkalemia may occur, especially with the use of ACE inhibitors, ARBs, or spironolactone.
- Prolonged diuretic therapy may produce hyponatremia (deficiency of sodium in the blood), which results in disorientation, apprehension, weakness, fatigue, malaise, and muscle cramps.
- Other problems associated with diuretic administration are hyperuricemia (excessive uric acid in the blood) and gout, plus volume depletion from excessive fluid loss.

> **NURSING ALERT**
>
> Grapefruit (fresh and juice) is a good dietary source of potassium but has serious drug–food interactions. Patients are advised to consult their physician or pharmacist before including grapefruit in their diet.

## Gerontologic Considerations

Several normal changes that occur with aging increase the frequency of HF: increased systolic blood pressure, increased ventricular wall thickness, increased atrial size, and increased myocardial fibrosis. Elderly people may present with atypical signs and symptoms: fatigue, weakness, and somnolence. Decreased renal function makes the elderly patient resistant to diuretics and more sensitive to changes in volume, especially with diastolic dysfunction. The administration of diuretics to elderly men requires nursing surveillance for bladder distention caused by urethral obstruction from an enlarged prostate gland. The bladder may be assessed with an ultrasound scanner, or the suprapubic area palpated for an oval mass and percussed for dullness, indicative of bladder fullness. Frequency and urgency from diuretics may be particularly stressful to the elderly patient.

# Nursing Process

## The Patient With Heart Failure

### Assessment

The nursing assessment for the patient with HF focuses on observing for effectiveness of therapy and for the patient's ability to understand and implement self-management strategies. Signs and symptoms of pulmonary and systemic fluid overload are recorded and reported immediately so that adjustments can be made in therapy. The nurse also explores the patient's emotional response to the diagnosis of HF, a chronic and often progressive condition.

### Health History

The health history focuses on the signs and symptoms of HF, such as dyspnea, shortness of breath, and cough. Sleep disturbances, particularly sleep suddenly interrupted by shortness of breath, may be reported. The nurse also asks about the number of pillows needed for sleep (an indication of orthopnea), edema, abdominal symptoms, altered mental status, activities of daily living, and the activities that cause fatigue. The nurse explores the patient's understanding of HF, self-management strategies, and the desire to adhere to those strategies. The nurse helps patients identify the impact the illness has had on their quality of life and successful coping skills that they have used. Family and significant others are often included in these discussions.

### Physical Examination

The lungs are auscultated to detect crackles and wheezes. Crackles, which are produced by the sudden opening of edematous small airways and alveoli that have adhered together by exudate, may be heard at the end of inspiration and are not cleared with coughing. Wheezing may also be heard in some patients. The rate and depth of respirations are also documented.

The heart is auscultated for an $S_3$ heart sound, a sign that the heart is beginning to fail and that increased blood volume fills the ventricle with each beat. HR and rhythm are also documented. When the heart rate is rapid, the SV decreases because the ventricle has less time to fill. This in turn produces increased pressure in the atria and eventually in the pulmonary vascular bed.

JVD is also assessed; distention greater than 3 cm above the sternal angle is considered abnormal. This is an estimate, not a precise measurement, of central venous pressure.

Sensorium and level of consciousness must be evaluated. As the volume of blood ejected by the heart decreases, so does the amount of oxygen transported to the brain.

The nurse assesses dependent parts of the patient's body for perfusion and edema. With significant decreases in SV, there is a decrease in perfusion to the periphery, causing the skin to feel cool and appear pale or cyanotic. If the patient is sitting upright, the feet and lower legs are examined for edema; if the patient is supine in bed, the sacrum and back are also assessed for edema. Fingers and hands may also become edematous.

The liver is assessed for hepatojugular reflux. The patient is asked to breathe normally while manual pressure is applied over the right upper quadrant of the abdomen for 30 to 60 seconds. If neck vein distention increases more than 1 cm, the finding is positive for increased venous pressure.

If the patient is hospitalized, the nurse measures output carefully to establish a baseline against which to assess the effectiveness of diuretic therapy. Intake and output records are rigorously maintained. It is important to know whether the patient has ingested more fluid than he or she has excreted (positive fluid balance), which is then correlated with a gain in weight. The patient must be monitored for oliguria (diminished urine output, less than 400 mL/24 hours) or **anuria** (urine output less than 50 mL/24 hours).

The patient is weighed daily in the hospital or at home, at the same time of day, with the same type of clothing, and on the same scale. If there is a significant change in weight (ie, 2- to 3-lb increase in a day or 5-lb increase in a week), the patient is instructed to notify the physician or to adjust the medications (eg, increase the diuretic dose).

## Diagnosis

### Nursing Diagnoses

Based on the assessment data, major nursing diagnoses for the patient with HF may include the following:

- Activity intolerance and fatigue related to imbalance between oxygen supply and demand because of decreased CO
- Excess fluid volume related to excess fluid or sodium intake, and retention of fluid related to the HF syndrome
- Anxiety related to breathlessness and restlessness from inadequate oxygenation
- Powerlessness related to inability to perform role responsibilities because of chronic illness and hospitalizations
- Noncompliance related to lack of knowledge

### Collaborative Problems/ Potential Complications

Based on the assessment data, potential complications that may develop include the following:

- Cardiogenic shock (see also Chapter 15)
- Dysrhythmias (see Chapter 27)
- Thromboembolism (see Chapter 31)
- Pericardial effusion and cardiac tamponade (see Chapter 29)

## Planning and Goals

Major goals for the patient may include promoting activity and reducing fatigue, relieving fluid overload symptoms, decreasing the incidence of anxiety or increasing the patient's ability to manage anxiety, encouraging the patient to verbalize his or her ability to make decisions and influence outcomes, and teaching the patient about the self-care program.

## Nursing Interventions

### Promoting Activity Tolerance

Although prolonged bed rest and even short periods of recumbency promote diuresis by improving renal perfusion, they also decrease activity tolerance. Prolonged bed rest, which may be self-imposed, should be avoided because of its deconditioning effects and risks such as pressure ulcers (especially in edematous patients), venous thrombosis, and pulmonary embolism. An acute illness that exacerbates HF symptoms or that requires hospitalization may be an indication for temporary bed rest. Otherwise, a total of 30 to 45 minutes of physical activity every day should be encouraged (Pina, Apstein, Balady, et al., 2003). Exercise training has many favorable effects for HF, including increasing functional capacity and decreasing dyspnea. The exercise regimen should include 10 to 15 minutes of warm-up activities, followed by about 30 minutes of exercise at the prescribed intensity level. A typical program for a patient with HF might include a daily walking regimen, with duration increased over a 6-week period. The physician, nurse, and patient collaborate to develop a schedule that promotes pacing and prioritization of activities. The schedule should alternate activities with periods of rest and avoid having two significant energy-consuming activities occur on the same day or in immediate succession.

Before undertaking physical activity, the patient should be given the following safety guidelines:

- Begin with a few minutes of warm-up activities.
- Avoid performing physical activities outside in extreme hot, cold, or humid weather.
- Ensure that you are able to talk during the physical activity; if you cannot do so, decrease the intensity of activity.
- Wait 2 hours after eating a meal before performing the physical activity.
- Stop the activity if severe shortness of breath, pain, or dizziness develops.
- End with cool-down activities and a cool-down period.

Because some patients may be severely debilitated, they may need to limit physical activities to only 3 to 5 minutes at a time, one to four times per day. The patient should increase the duration of the activity, then the frequency, before increasing the intensity of the activity.

Barriers to performing other activities are identified, and methods of adjusting an activity are discussed. For example, vegetables can be chopped or peeled while sitting at the kitchen table rather than standing at the kitchen counter. Small, frequent meals decrease the amount of energy needed for digestion while providing adequate nutrition. The nurse helps the patient identify peak and low periods of energy, planning energy-consuming activities for peak periods. For example, the patient may prepare the meals for the entire day in the morning. Pacing and prioritizing activities help maintain the patient's energy to allow participation in regular physical activity.

The patient's response to activities needs to be monitored. If the patient is hospitalized, vital signs and oxygen saturation level are monitored before, during, and immediately after an activity to identify whether they are within the desired range. HR should return to baseline within 3 minutes following the activity. If the patient is at home, the degree of fatigue felt after the activity can be used to assess the response. If the patient tolerates the activity, short-term and long-term

## NURSING RESEARCH PROFILE

### Readiness for Behavioral Changes in Patients with Heart Failure

Sneed, N. V., & Paul., S. C. (2003). Readiness for behavioral changes in patients with heart failure. *American Journal of Critical Care, 12*(5), 444–453.

#### Purpose
Patient education for patients with heart failure (HF) focuses on the lifestyle changes that are necessary to control signs and symptoms. Important changes include avoiding sodium, alcohol, and tobacco; regular exercise; and weight loss. However, education does not guarantee changes in behavior. The purpose of this study was to identify stages of readiness for change pertaining to six important behaviors and to determine self-reported differences in patients who made the changes and in those who did not.

#### Design
A total of 178 patients with HF completed a survey rating their readiness for change. The survey questions were based on the five stages of change described by the Transtheoretical Model for Change (ie, whether patients planned to make a change, had already made the change). The survey also assessed patients' knowledge of the signs and symptoms of HF, as well as their adherence to recommendations for sodium restriction, fluid restriction, exercise, and (if applicable) weight loss, smoking cessation, and alcohol cessation. Participants were also asked to report their signs and symptoms of HF, such as shortness of breath and fatigue.

#### Findings
Participants generally reported adherence to the major lifestyle recommendations. However, only 38% reported engaging in a regular exercise program, and 92% had eaten foods high in sodium within the preceding 24 hours. Knowledge about HF was low and did not differ by the stage of change. The findings did not support the hypothesis that patients who had made the recommended lifestyle changes would report fewer signs and symptoms of HF.

#### Nursing Implications
Actual patient behaviors did not demonstrate that patients adhered to the recommended lifestyle changes, even when patients thought they were following them. The authors suggest that the scale for rating readiness for change may not work well in patients with HF. The lack of knowledge identified by patients may be related to the number of changes these patients are asked to make. Nurses continue to be challenged to find effective ways to educate patients with HF.

---

goals can be developed to gradually increase the intensity, duration, and frequency of activity.

Adherence to exercise training is essential if the patient is to benefit from it, but it may be difficult for patients with multiple other conditions (eg, arthritis) and longer duration of heart failure (Corvera-Tindel, Doering, Gomez, et al., 2004). Referral to a cardiac rehabilitation program may be needed, especially for HF patients with recent myocardial infarction, recent open heart surgery, or increased anxiety. A supervised program may also benefit those who need a structured environment, significant educational support, regular encouragement, and interpersonal contact.

### Managing Fluid Volume

Patients with severe HF may receive IV diuretic therapy, but patients with less severe symptoms may receive oral diuretic medication (see Table 30-4 for a summary of common diuretics). Oral diuretics should be administered early in the morning so that diuresis does not interfere with the patient's nighttime rest. Discussing the timing of medication administration is especially important for elderly patients who may have urinary urgency or incontinence. A single dose of a diuretic may cause the patient to excrete a large volume of fluid shortly after its administration.

The nurse monitors the patient's fluid status closely, auscultating the lungs, monitoring daily body weights, and assisting the patient to adhere to a low-sodium diet by reading food labels and avoiding high-sodium foods such as canned, processed, and convenience foods (Chart 30-4). If the diet includes fluid restriction, the nurse can assist the patient to plan fluid intake throughout the day while respecting the patient's dietary preferences. If the patient is receiving IV fluids, the amount of fluid needs to be monitored closely, and the physician or pharmacist can be consulted about the possibility of maximizing the amount of medication in the same amount of IV fluid (eg, double-concentrating to decrease the fluid volume administered).

 **NURSING ALERT**

Periodic assessment of the patient's electrolyte levels alerts health team members to hypokalemia, hypomagnesemia, and hyponatremia. Serum levels are assessed frequently when the patient starts diuretic therapy and then usually every 3 to 12 months. It is important to remember that serum potassium levels do not always indicate the total amount of potassium within the body.

## CHART 30-4

### Facts About Dietary Sodium

Although the major source of sodium in the average American diet is salt, many types of natural foods contain varying amounts of sodium. Even if no salt is added in cooking and if salty foods are avoided, the daily diet will still contain about 2000 mg of sodium.

#### Additives in Food

In general, food prepared at home is lower in sodium than restaurant or processed foods. Added food substances (additives), such as sodium alginate, which improves food texture; sodium benzoate, which acts as a preservative; and disodium phosphate, which improves cooking quality in certain foods, increase the sodium intake when included in the daily diet. Therefore, patients on low-sodium diets should be advised to check labels carefully for such words as "salt" or "sodium," especially on canned foods. For example, without looking at the sodium content per serving found on the nutrition labels, when given a choice between a serving of potato chips and a cup of canned cream of mushroom soup, most would think that soup is lower in sodium. However, when the labels are examined, the lower sodium choice is found to be the chips. Although potato chips are *not* recommended in a low sodium diet, this example illustrates that it is important to read food labels to determine both sodium content and serving size.

#### Nonfood Sodium Sources

Sodium is also contained in municipal water. Patients on sodium-restricted diets should be cautioned against using nonprescription medications such as antacids, cough syrups, and laxatives. Salt substitutes may be allowed, but it is recognized that they are high in potassium. Over-the-counter medications should not be used without first consulting the physician.

#### Promoting Dietary Adherence

If patients find food unpalatable because of the dietary sodium restrictions and/or the taste disturbances caused by the medications, they may refuse to eat or to comply with the dietary regimen. For this reason, severe sodium restrictions should be avoided and the amount of medication should be balanced with the patient's ability to restrict dietary sodium. A variety of flavorings, such as lemon juice, vinegar, and herbs, may be used to improve the taste of the food and increase acceptance of the diet. The patient's food preferences should be taken into account—diet counseling and educational handouts can be geared to individual and ethnic preferences. It is very important to involve the family in the dietary teaching.

---

The nurse positions the patient or teaches the patient how to assume a position that facilitates breathing. The number of pillows may be increased, the head of the bed may be elevated, or the patient may sit in a comfortable armchair. In this position, the venous return to the heart (preload) is reduced, pulmonary congestion is alleviated, and pressure on the diaphragm is minimized. The lower arms are supported with pillows to eliminate the fatigue caused by the constant pull of their weight on the shoulder muscles.

Because decreased circulation in edematous areas increases the risk of skin injury, the nurse assesses for skin breakdown and institutes preventive measures. Frequent changes of position, positioning to avoid pressure, the use of elastic compression stockings, and leg exercises may help prevent skin injury.

### Controlling Anxiety

Because patients with HF have difficulty maintaining adequate oxygenation, they are likely to be restless and anxious and feel overwhelmed by breathlessness. These symptoms tend to intensify at night. Emotional stress stimulates the sympathetic nervous system, which causes vasoconstriction, elevated arterial pressure, and increased heart rate. This sympathetic response increases the cardiac workload. By decreasing anxiety, the patient's cardiac workload also is decreased. Oxygen may be administered during an acute event to diminish the work of breathing and to increase the patient's comfort.

When the patient exhibits anxiety, the nurse takes steps to promote physical comfort and psychological support. In many cases, a family member's presence provides reassurance. To help decrease the patient's anxiety, the nurse should speak in a slow, calm, and confident manner and maintain eye contact.

Once the patient is comfortable, the nurse can begin teaching ways to control anxiety and to avoid anxiety-provoking situations. The nurse explains how to use relaxation techniques and helps the patient identify factors that contribute to anxiety. Lack of sleep may increase anxiety, which may prevent adequate rest. Other contributing factors may include misinformation, lack of information, or poor nutritional status. Promoting physical comfort, providing accurate information, and teaching the patient to perform relaxation techniques and to avoid anxiety-triggering situations may relax the patient.

In cases of confusion and anxiety reactions that affect the patient's safety, the use of restraints should be avoided. Restraints are likely to be resisted, and resistance inevitably increases the cardiac workload. The patient who insists on getting out of bed at night can be seated comfortably in an armchair. As cerebral and systemic circulation improves, the degree of anxiety decreases and the quality of sleep improves.

**NURSING ALERT**

Cerebral hypoxia with superimposed carbon dioxide retention may be a problem in HF, causing the patient to react to sedative–hypnotic medications with confusion and increased anxiety. Hepatic congestion may slow the liver's metabolism of medication, leading to toxicity. Sedative–hypnotic medications must be administered with caution.

In addition to anxiety, patients with HF have a high incidence of depression and should be screened for this condition (Artinian, 2003).

### Minimizing Powerlessness

Patients need to recognize that they are not helpless and that they can influence the direction of their lives and the outcomes of treatment. The nurse assesses for factors that contribute to a sense of powerlessness and intervenes accordingly. Contributing factors may include lack of knowledge and lack of opportunities to make decisions, particularly if health care providers and family members behave in maternalistic or paternalistic ways. If the patient is hospitalized, hospital policies may promote standardization and limit the patient's ability to make decisions (eg, what time to have meals or to take medications).

Taking time to listen actively to patients often encourages them to express their concerns and ask questions. Other strategies include providing the patient with decision-making opportunities, such as when activities are to occur or where objects are to be placed, and increasing the frequency and significance of those opportunities over time; providing encouragement while identifying the patient's progress; and assisting the patient to differentiate between factors that can be controlled and those that cannot. In some cases, the nurse may want to review hospital policies and standards that tend to promote powerlessness and advocate for their elimination or change (eg, limited visiting hours, prohibition of food from home).

### Promoting Home and Community-Based Care

#### TEACHING PATIENTS SELF-CARE

The nurse provides patient education and involves the patient in the therapeutic regimen to promote understanding and adherence to the plan. When the patient recognizes that the diagnosis of HF can be successfully managed with lifestyle changes and medications, recurrences of acute HF lessen, unnecessary hospitalizations decrease, and life expectancy increases. Patients and their families are taught to follow the medication regimen as prescribed, maintain a low-sodium diet, perform and record daily weights, engage in routine physical activity, and recognize and report symptoms that indicate worsening HF. Although noncompliance is not well understood, interventions that may promote adherence include teaching to ensure accurate understanding. A summary of teaching points for the patient with HF is presented in Chart 30-5.

The patient and family members are supported and encouraged to ask questions so that information can be clarified and understanding enhanced. The nurse should be aware of cultural factors and adapt the teaching plan accordingly. Patients and their families need to be informed that the progression of the disease is influenced in part by choices made about health care and the decisions about following the treatment plan. They also need to be informed that health care providers are there to assist them in reaching their health care goals. Patients and family members need to make the decisions about the treatment plan and need to understand the possible outcomes of those decisions. The treatment plan then will be based on the patient's goals rather than on what health care providers think is needed. The nurse conveys that monitoring symptoms and daily weights, restricting sodium intake, avoiding excess fluids, preventing infection through influenza and pneumococcal immunizations, avoiding noxious agents (eg, alcohol, tobacco), and participating in regular exercise all aid in preventing exacerbations of HF.

#### CONTINUING CARE

Success in management of HF requires a complex medical regimen and multiple lifestyle changes that the patient may find difficult. Assistance may be provided through home health care, a heart failure clinic, or telehealth management.

Depending on the patient's physical status and the availability of family assistance, a home care referral may be indicated for a patient who has been hospitalized. Elderly patients and those who have long-standing heart disease with compromised physical stamina often require assistance with the transition to home after hospitalization for an acute episode of HF. It is important for the home care nurse to assess the physical environment of the home. Suggestions for adapting the home environment to meet the patient's activity limitations are important. If stairs are a concern, the patient can plan the day's activities so that stair climbing is minimized; for some patients, a temporary bedroom may be set up on the main level of the home. The home care nurse works with the patient and family to maximize the benefits of these changes.

The home care nurse also reinforces and clarifies information about dietary changes and fluid restrictions, the need to monitor symptoms and daily body weights, and the importance of obtaining follow-up health care. Assistance may be given in scheduling and keeping appointments as well. The patient is encouraged to gradually increase his or her self-care and responsibility for accomplishing the therapeutic regimen.

Heart failure clinics offer disease management strategies for patients with HF. Referral to a heart failure

## CHART 30-5

### HOME CARE CHECKLIST • The Patient With Heart Failure

| At the completion of the home care instruction, the patient or caregiver will be able to: | Patient | Caregiver |
|---|---|---|
| • Identify heart failure as a chronic disease that can be managed with medications and specific self-management behaviors. | ✔ | ✔ |
| • Take or administer medications daily, exactly as prescribed. | ✔ | ✔ |
| • Monitor effects of medication. | ✔ | ✔ |
| • Know signs and symptoms of orthostatic hypotension and how to prevent it. | ✔ | ✔ |
| • Weigh self daily.<br>– Obtain weight at the same time each day (eg, every morning after urination). | ✔ | |
| • Restrict sodium intake to 2–3 g daily: adapt diet by examining nutrition labels to check sodium content per serving; avoid canned or processed foods; eat fresh or frozen foods; consult the written diet plan and the list of permitted and restricted foods; avoid salt use; and avoid excesses in eating and drinking. | ✔ | ✔ |
| • Review activity program.<br>– Participate in a daily exercise program.<br>– Increase walking and other activities gradually, provided they do not cause unusual fatigue or dyspnea.<br>– Conserve energies by balancing activity with rest periods.<br>– Avoid activity in extremes of heat and cold, which increase the work of the heart.<br>– Recognize that air conditioning may be essential in a hot, humid environment. | ✔ | |
| • Develop methods to manage and prevent stress.<br>– Avoid tobacco.<br>– Avoid alcohol.<br>– Engage in meditation, guided imagery, or music therapy. | ✔ | |
| • Keep regular appointments with physician or clinic. | ✔ | ✔ |
| • Be alert for symptoms that may indicate recurring heart failure.<br>– Know how to reach healthcare provider. | ✔ | ✔ |
| • Report immediately to the physician or clinic any of the following:<br>– Gain in weight of ≥ 2–3 lb (0.9–1.4 kg) in 1 day, or 5 lb (2.3 kg) in 1 week<br>– Loss of appetite<br>– Unusual shortness of breath with activity<br>– Swelling of ankles, feet, or abdomen<br>– Persistent cough<br>– Development of restless sleep; increase in number of pillows needed to sleep | ✔ | ✔ |

clinic gives the patient access to education, professional staff, and individualized treatment regimens. Research has shown that patients managed through HF clinics have fewer exacerbations of HF, fewer hospitalizations, decreased costs of medical care, and increased quality of life (Silver, Pisano, & Cianci, 2004).

Telehealth management can provide the frequent contact necessary to manage HF without requiring frequent visits to health care providers. A variety of techniques ranging from simple telephone monitoring to sophisticated computer and video connections that monitor daily weight, vital signs, and symptoms may be used. Studies have shown that telehealth management decreases costs and hospitalizations for exacerbations of HF (Gramsky, Josephson, Langford, et al., 2003).

## Evaluation

### Expected Patient Outcomes

Expected patient outcomes may include the following:

1. Demonstrates tolerance for increased activity
    a. Describes adaptive methods for usual activities
    b. Stops any activity that causes symptoms of intolerance
    c. Maintains vital signs (pulse, blood pressure, respiratory rate, and pulse oximetry) within the targeted range
    d. Identifies factors that contribute to activity intolerance and takes actions to avoid them
    e. Establishes priorities for activities
    f. Schedules activities to conserve energy and to reduce fatigue and dyspnea

2. Maintains fluid balance
    a. Exhibits decreased peripheral and sacral edema
    b. Demonstrates methods for preventing edema
3. Is less anxious
    a. Avoids situations that produce stress
    b. Sleeps comfortably at night
    c. Reports decreased stress and anxiety
4. Makes decisions regarding care and treatment
    a. States ability to influence outcomes
5. Adheres to self-care regimen
    a. Performs and records daily weights
    b. Ensures dietary intake includes no more than 2 to 3 g of sodium per day
    c. Takes medications as prescribed
    d. Reports any unusual symptoms or side effects

## Acute Heart Failure (Pulmonary Edema)

**Pulmonary edema** is the abnormal accumulation of fluid in the lungs. The fluid may accumulate in the interstitial spaces and in the alveoli.

## Pathophysiology

Pulmonary edema is an acute event that results from HF. It can occur acutely, such as with MI, or it can occur as an exacerbation of chronic HF. Myocardial scarring as a result of ischemia can limit the distensibility of the ventricle and render it vulnerable to a sudden increase in workload. With increased resistance to left ventricular filling, blood backs up into the pulmonary circulation. The patient quickly develops pulmonary edema, sometimes called flash pulmonary edema, from the blood volume overload in the lungs. Pulmonary edema can also be caused by noncardiac disorders, such as renal failure, liver failure, and oncologic conditions that cause the body to retain fluid. The pathophysiology is similar to that seen in HF, in that the left ventricle cannot handle the volume overload and blood volume and pressure build up in the left atrium. The rapid increase in atrial pressure results in an acute increase in pulmonary venous pressure, which produces an increase in hydrostatic pressure that forces fluid out of the pulmonary capillaries into the interstitial spaces and alveoli.

Impaired lymphatic drainage also contributes to the accumulation of fluid in the lung tissues. The fluid within the alveoli mixes with air, creating "bubbles" that are expelled from the mouth and nose, producing the classic symptom of pulmonary edema: frothy pink (blood-tinged) sputum. Because of the fluid within the alveoli, air cannot enter, and gas exchange is impaired. The result is hypoxemia, which is often severe. The onset may be preceded by premonitory symptoms of pulmonary congestion, but it also may develop quickly in the patient with a ventricle that has little reserve to meet increased oxygen needs.

## Clinical Manifestations

As a result of decreased cerebral oxygenation, the patient becomes increasingly restless and anxious. Along with a sudden onset of breathlessness and a sense of suffocation, the patient's hands become cold and moist, the nail beds become cyanotic (bluish), and the skin turns ashen (gray). The pulse is weak and rapid, and the neck veins are distended. Incessant coughing may occur, producing increasing quantities of mucoid sputum. As pulmonary edema progresses, the patient's anxiety and restlessness increase; the patient becomes confused, then stuporous. Breathing is rapid, noisy, and moist-sounding. The patient's oxygen saturation is significantly decreased. The patient, nearly suffocated by the blood-tinged, frothy fluid filling the alveoli, is literally drowning in secretions. The situation demands immediate action.

## Assessment and Diagnostic Findings

The diagnosis is made by evaluating the clinical manifestations resulting from pulmonary congestion. A chest x-ray may be obtained to confirm that the pulmonary veins are engorged. Abrupt onset of signs of left-sided HF (eg, crackles on auscultation of the lungs, flash pulmonary edema) may occur without evidence of right-sided HF (eg, no JVD, no dependent edema).

## Prevention

Like most complications, pulmonary edema is easier to prevent than to treat. To recognize it in its early stages, the nurse auscultates the lung fields and heart sounds, measures JVD, and assesses the degree of peripheral edema and the severity of breathlessness. A dry, hacking cough; fatigue; weight gain; development or worsening of edema; and decreased activity tolerance may be early indicators of developing pulmonary edema.

In an early stage, the condition may be alleviated by placing the patient in an upright position with the feet and legs dependent, eliminating overexertion, and minimizing emotional stress to reduce the left ventricular load. The treatment regimen and the patient's understanding of and adherence to it are re-examined. The long-range approach to preventing pulmonary edema must be directed at identifying its precipitating factors.

## Medical Management

Clinical management of a patient with acute pulmonary edema due to left ventricular failure is directed toward reducing volume overload, improving ventricular function, and increasing respiratory exchange. These goals are accomplished through a combination of oxygen and ventilatory support, IV medications, and nursing interventions.

### Oxygen Therapy

Oxygen is administered in concentrations adequate to relieve hypoxemia and dyspnea. Usually, a face mask or nonrebreathing mask is initially used. If respiratory failure is severe or persists, continuous positive airway pressure may be delivered by a face mask with a tight seal. For some patients, endotracheal intubation and mechanical ventilation are required. The ventilator can provide positive end-expiratory pressure, which is effective in reducing venous return, decreasing fluid movement from the pulmonary capillaries to the alveoli, and improving oxygenation. Oxygenation is monitored by pulse oximetry and by measurement of arterial blood gases.

### Morphine

Morphine is titrated IV in small doses (2 to 5 mg) to reduce peripheral resistance and venous return so that blood can be redistributed from the pulmonary circulation to other parts of the body. This decreases pressure in the pulmonary capillaries and seepage of fluid into the lung tissue. The effect of morphine in decreasing anxiety is also beneficial.

### Diuretics

Diuretics promote the excretion of sodium and water by the kidneys. Furosemide (Lasix), for example, is administered IV to produce a rapid diuretic effect. Furosemide also causes vasodilation and pooling of blood in peripheral blood vessels, which reduces the amount of blood returned to the heart. Some physicians prescribe bumetanide (Bumex) and metolazone (Zaroxolyn) in place of furosemide.

### Intravenous Infusions

As described earlier in this chapter, continuous IV infusions of nesiritide, dobutamine, and milrinone may be indicated for the patient with acutely decompensated heart function.

## Nursing Management

### Positioning the Patient to Promote Circulation

Proper positioning can help reduce venous return to the heart. The patient is positioned upright, preferably with the legs dangling over the side of the bed. This has the immediate effect of decreasing venous return, lowering the output of the right ventricle, and decreasing lung congestion. Patients who cannot sit with the lower extremities dependent may be placed in an upright position in bed.

### Providing Psychological Support

As the ability to breathe decreases, the patient's fear and anxiety rise proportionately, making the condition more severe. Reassuring the patient and providing skillful anticipatory nursing care are integral parts of the therapy. Because the patient feels a sense of impending doom and has an unstable condition, the nurse must remain with the patient. The nurse gives the patient simple, concise information in a reassuring voice about what is being done to treat the condition and the expected results. The nurse also identifies any anxiety-inducing factors (eg, a pet left alone at home, presence of an unwelcome family member at the bedside, unpaid household bills) and initiates strategies to eliminate the concern or reduce its effect.

### Monitoring Medications

The patient receiving morphine is observed for respiratory depression, hypotension, and vomiting; a morphine antagonist, such as naloxone hydrochloride (Narcan), is kept available and given to the patient who exhibits any serious side effects.

The patient receiving diuretic therapy may excrete a large volume of urine within minutes after a potent diuretic is administered. A bedside commode may be used to decrease the energy required by the patient and to reduce the resultant increase in cardiac workload induced by getting on and off a bedpan. If necessary, an indwelling urinary catheter may be inserted.

The patient receiving continuous IV infusions of vasoactive drugs requires ECG monitoring and frequent measurement of vital signs.

## Other Complications

### Cardiogenic Shock

Cardiogenic shock occurs when decreased CO leads to inadequate tissue perfusion and initiation of the shock syndrome. Cardiogenic shock may occur following MI when a large area of myocardium becomes ischemic, necrotic, and hypokinetic. It also can occur as a result of end-stage HF, cardiac tamponade, pulmonary embolism, cardiomyopathy, and dysrhythmias. Cardiogenic shock is a life-threatening condition with a high mortality rate (for further information see Chapter 15).

### Pathophysiology

The signs and symptoms of cardiogenic shock reflect the circular nature of the pathophysiology of HF. The degree of shock is proportional to the extent of left ventricular dysfunction. The heart muscle loses its contractile power, resulting in a marked reduction in SV and CO. The decreased CO in turn reduces arterial blood pressure and tissue perfusion in the vital organs (heart, brain, lung, kidneys). Flow to the coronary arteries is reduced, resulting in decreased oxygen supply to the myocardium, which increases ischemia and further reduces the heart's ability to pump. Inadequate emptying of the ventricle also leads to increased pulmonary pressures, pulmonary congestion, and pulmonary edema, exacerbating the hypoxia, causing ischemia of vital organs, and setting a vicious cycle in motion (Fig. 30-4).

### Clinical Manifestations

The classic signs of cardiogenic shock are those of tissue hypoperfusion and result from HF and the overall shock state. They include cerebral hypoxia (restlessness, confusion, agitation), low blood pressure, rapid and weak pulse, cold and clammy skin, tachypnea with respiratory crackles, and decreased urinary output. Initially, arterial blood gas analysis may show respiratory alkalosis. Dysrhythmias are common and result from myocardial ischemia.

### Assessment and Diagnostic Findings

The patient with cardiogenic shock is managed in an intensive care unit. A pulmonary artery catheter may be inserted

**FIGURE 30-4.** Pathophysiology of cardiogenic shock.

to measure CO and other hemodynamic parameters that are used to assess the severity of the problem and to guide patient management. The pulmonary artery wedge pressure is elevated and the CO is decreased as the left ventricle loses its ability to pump. The systemic vascular resistance is elevated because of the sympathetic nervous system stimulation that occurs as a compensatory response to the decrease in blood pressure. The decreased blood flow to the kidneys causes a hormonal response (ie, activation of the renin–angiotensin–aldosterone system) that causes fluid retention and further vasoconstriction. Increases in HR, circulating volume, and vasoconstriction occur to maintain circulation to the brain, heart, kidneys, and lungs, but at a cost: an increase in the workload of the heart.

The reduction in blood volume delivered to the tissues results in an increase in the amount of oxygen extracted from the blood that is delivered to the tissues (to try to meet the cellular demand for oxygen). The increased systemic oxygen extraction results in decreased venous (mixed and central) oxygen saturation. When the cellular oxygen needs cannot be met, anaerobic metabolism and buildup of lactic acid occur. Continuous central venous oximetry and measurement of blood lactic acid levels may help assess the severity of the shock as well as the effectiveness of treatment.

Continued cellular hypoperfusion eventually results in organ failure. The patient becomes unresponsive, severe hypotension ensues, and the patient develops shallow respirations and cold, cyanotic, or mottled skin. Arterial blood gas analysis shows metabolic acidosis, and all laboratory test results indicate organ dysfunction. Chapter 15 presents more detail about the pathophysiology and management of cardiogenic shock.

## Medical Management

The most important approach to treating cardiogenic shock is to correct the underlying problem, reduce any further demand on the heart, improve oxygenation, and restore tissue perfusion. For example, if the ventricular failure is the result of an acute MI, emergency percutaneous coronary intervention may be indicated. Major dysrhythmias are corrected because they may have caused or contributed to the shock. If the patient has hypervolemia, diuresis is indicated. Diuretics, vasodilators, and mechanical therapies, such as continuous renal replacement therapy, have been used to reduce the circulating blood volume. If hypovolemia (low intravascular volume) is suspected or detected through hemodynamic pressure readings, the patient is given IV volume expanders (eg, normal saline solution, lactated Ringer's solution, albumin) to increase the amount of circulating fluid. The patient is placed on strict bed rest to conserve energy. If the patient has hypoxemia, as detected by pulse oximetry or arterial blood gas analysis, oxygen administration is increased, often under positive pressure when regular flow is insufficient to meet tissue demands. Intubation and sedation may be necessary to maintain oxygenation. The settings for mechanical ventilation are adjusted according to the patient's oxygenation status and the need for conserving energy.

### Pharmacologic Therapy

Medication therapy is selected and guided according to CO, other cardiac parameters, and mean arterial blood pressure. Because of the decreased perfusion to the gastrointestinal system and the need to adjust the dosage quickly, most medications are administered IV.

Diuretics may be administered to decrease preload and afterload, reducing the workload of the heart. They are administered carefully to avoid worsening tissue hypoperfusion. Vasodilators such as milrinone (Primacor), sodium nitroprusside (Nipride), and nitroglycerin (Tridil) reduce the volume returning to the heart, decrease blood pressure, and decrease cardiac workload. They cause the arteries and veins to dilate, thereby shunting much of the intravascular volume to the periphery and causing a reduction in preload and afterload.

Positive inotropic medications are administered to increase myocardial contractility. Dobutamine (Dobutrex), dopamine (Intropin), and epinephrine (Adrenalin) can each cause tachydysrhythmias because they increase automaticity with increasing dosage. Therefore, monitoring baseline HR is important. As the baseline HR increases, so does the risk of developing tachydysrhythmias.

Vasopressors, or pressor agents, are used to increase blood pressure and increase CO. Many pressor medications are catecholamines, such as norepinephrine (Levophed) and high-dose dopamine (Intropin). Their purpose is to promote perfusion to the heart and brain, but they compromise circulation to other organs (eg, kidney). They also tend to increase the workload of the heart by increasing oxygen demand; thus, they are not administered early in cardiogenic shock.

### Other Treatments

Other therapeutic modalities for cardiogenic shock include use of circulatory assist devices. The most frequently used mechanical support device is the intra-aortic balloon pump (IABP). The IABP is a catheter with an inflatable balloon at the end. The catheter is usually inserted through the femoral artery, and the balloon is positioned in the descending thoracic aorta (Fig. 30-5). The IABP uses internal counterpulsation through the regular inflation and deflation of the balloon to augment the pumping action of the heart. It inflates during diastole, increasing the pressure in the aorta during diastole and therefore increasing blood flow through the coronary and peripheral arteries. It deflates just before systole, lessening the pressure within the aorta before left ventricular contraction, decreasing the amount of resistance the heart has to overcome to eject blood and therefore decreasing the amount of work the heart must put forth to eject blood. The device is connected to a console that synchronizes the inflation and deflation of the balloon with the ECG or the arterial pressure (as indicators for systole and diastole). Hemodynamic monitoring is essential to determine the patient's response to the IABP.

Other ventricular assist devices for long-term support of the failing heart are described in Chapter 29.

## Nursing Management

The patient in cardiogenic shock requires constant monitoring. Because of the frequency of nursing interventions and the technology required for effective patient management, the patient is treated in an intensive care unit. The critical care nurse must carefully assess the patient, observe the cardiac rhythm, monitor hemodynamic parameters, monitor fluid status, and adjust medications and therapies based on the assessment data. The patient is continuously evaluated for responses to the medical interventions and for the development of complications, so that problems can be addressed immediately.

## Thromboembolism

The decreased mobility of the patient with cardiac disease and the impaired circulation that accompany these disorders contribute to the development of intracardiac and intravascular thrombosis. Intracardiac thrombus is especially common in patients with atrial fibrillation, because the atria do not contract forcefully and blood flows slowly and turbulently, increasing the likelihood of thrombus formation. Intracardiac thrombus is detected by an echocardiogram and treated with anticoagulants, such as heparin and warfarin (Coumadin). Adverse effects of thromboemboli are discussed in detail in Chapter 31.

### Pulmonary Embolism

Pulmonary embolism is the most common thromboembolic problem among patients with HF. It poses a particular threat to people with cardiovascular disease (Koschel, 2004). Blood clots may form in the deep veins of the legs and embolize to the pulmonary vasculature, causing a life-threatening embolic event. Emboli mechanically obstruct the pulmonary vessels, cutting off the blood supply to sections of the lung (Fig. 30-6).

Clinical indicators of pulmonary embolism can vary but typically include dyspnea, chest pain, hemoptysis, tachycardia, and symptoms of deep venous thrombosis. Diagnostic tests often include a chest x-ray, ventilation–perfusion lung scan, or high-resolution helical computed tomography. A blood D-dimer assay is helpful to determine whether fibrinolysis of clots is taking place somewhere in the body.

Patient management begins with cardiopulmonary assessment and intervention. Emboli can cause hypoxic vasoconstriction and the release of inflammatory mediators in the pulmonary vessels, which can ultimately lead to right heart failure and respiratory failure (Goldhaber & Elliott, 2003). Anticoagulant therapy with unfractionated IV heparin or low-molecular-weight heparin is started when pulmonary embolism is suspected. Thrombolytic therapy may be used in patients with massive pulmonary emboli accompanied by hypotension and shock. Following initial therapy, patients are placed on warfarin (Coumadin) for at least 6 months. Prevention of deep vein thrombosis and pulmonary emboli is an important aspect of patient management. Both pharmacologic and mechanical means (eg, pneumatic compression devices) have proven effective in at-risk patients. Care for patients with pulmonary embolism is further discussed in Chapter 23.

**FIGURE 30-5.** The intra-aortic balloon pump inflates at the beginning of diastole, which results in increased perfusion of the coronary and peripheral arteries. It deflates just before systole, which results in a decrease in afterload (resistance to ejection) and in the left ventricular workload.

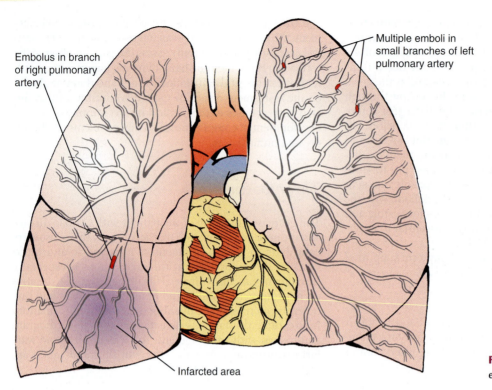

**FIGURE 30-6.** Pulmonary emboli may be single or multiple.

## Pericardial Effusion and Cardiac Tamponade

### Pathophysiology

Pericardial effusion (accumulation of fluid in the pericardial sac) may accompany pericarditis (see Chapter 29), advanced HF, metastatic carcinoma, cardiac surgery, or trauma.

> **NURSING ALERT**
>
> Cardiac tamponade is a life-threatening situation, demanding immediate intervention.

Normally, the pericardial sac contains less than 50 mL of fluid, which is needed to decrease friction for the beating heart. An increase in pericardial fluid raises the pressure within the pericardial sac and compresses the heart. This has the following effects:

- Increased right and left ventricular end-diastolic pressures
- Decreased venous return
- Inability of the ventricles to distend and fill adequately

Pericardial fluid may accumulate slowly without causing noticeable symptoms until a large amount accumulates. However, a rapidly developing effusion can stretch the pericardium to its maximum size and, because of increased pericardial pressure, reduce venous return to the heart and decrease CO. The result is cardiac tamponade (eg, compression of the heart).

### Clinical Manifestations

The patient may report a feeling of fullness within the chest or may have substantial or ill-defined pain. The feeling of pressure in the chest may result from stretching of the pericardial sac. Because of increased pressure within the pericardium, venous pressure tends to increase, as evidenced by engorged neck veins. Other signs include shortness of breath and labile or low blood pressure. Systolic blood pressure that is markedly lower during inhalation is called **pulsus paradoxus.** The difference in systolic pressure between the point that is heard during exhalation and the point that it is heard during inhalation is measured. Pulsus paradoxus exceeding 10 mm Hg is abnormal. The cardinal signs of cardiac tamponade are falling systolic blood pressure, narrowing pulse pressure, rising venous pressure (increased JVD), and distant (muffled) heart sounds (Chart 30-6).

### Assessment and Diagnostic Findings

A chest x-ray shows a large pericardial effusion. An echocardiogram is performed to confirm the diagnosis.

### Medical Management

#### Pericardiocentesis

If cardiac function becomes seriously impaired, **pericardiocentesis** (puncture of the pericardial sac to aspirate pericardial fluid) is performed to remove fluid from the peri-

## CHART 30-6

### Assessing for Cardiac Tamponade

Assessment findings in cardiac tamponade resulting from pericardial effusion include feelings of faintness, shortness of breath, anxiety, and pain from decreased cardiac output, cough from pressure created in the trachea from swelling of the pericardial sac, distended neck veins from rising venous pressure, paradoxical pulse, and muffled or distant heart sounds.

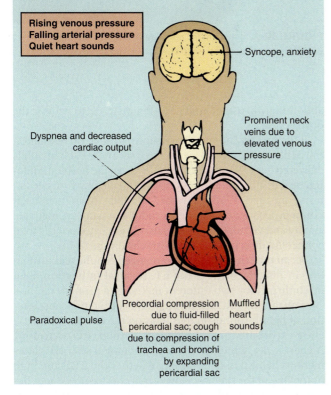

cardial sac. The major goal is to prevent cardiac tamponade, which restricts normal heart filling and contraction.

During the procedure, the patient is monitored by ECG and hemodynamic pressure measurements. Emergency resuscitation equipment should be readily available. The head of the bed is elevated to 45 to 60 degrees, placing the heart in proximity to the chest wall so that the needle can be inserted into the pericardial sac more easily. If a peripheral IV line is not already in place, one is inserted, and a slow IV infusion is started in case it becomes necessary to administer emergency medications or blood products.

The pericardial aspiration needle is attached to a 50-mL syringe by a three-way stopcock. Several possible sites are used for pericardial aspiration. Typically, ultrasound imaging is used to guide placement of the needle into the pericardial space. The needle is advanced slowly until it has entered the pericardium and fluid is obtained.

A resulting decrease in central venous pressure and an associated increase in blood pressure after withdrawal of pericardial fluid indicate that the cardiac tamponade has been relieved. The patient almost always feels immediate relief. If there is a substantial amount of pericardial fluid, a small catheter may be left in place to drain recurrent accumulation of blood or fluid. Pericardial fluid is sent to the laboratory for examination for tumor cells, bacterial culture, chemical and serologic analysis, and differential blood cell count.

Complications of pericardiocentesis include ventricular or coronary artery puncture, dysrhythmias, pleural laceration, gastric puncture, and myocardial trauma. After pericardiocentesis, the patient's heart rhythm, blood pressure, venous pressure, and heart sounds are monitored to detect possible recurrence of cardiac tamponade. If it recurs, repeated aspiration is necessary. Cardiac tamponade may require treatment by open pericardial drainage (pericardiotomy) (see Chapter 23).

### Pericardiotomy

Recurrent pericardial effusions, usually associated with neoplastic disease, may be treated by a **pericardiotomy** (pericardial window). Under general anesthesia, a portion of the pericardium is excised to permit the pericardial fluid to drain into the lymphatic system. The nursing care is the same as that for other cardiac surgery (see Chapter 28).

## Cardiac Arrest

Cardiac arrest occurs when the heart ceases to produce an effective pulse and circulate blood. It may be caused by a cardiac electrical event such as ventricular fibrillation, progressive profound bradycardia, or when there is no heart rhythm at all (asystole). Cardiac arrest may follow respiratory arrest; it may also occur when electrical activity is present but there is ineffective cardiac contraction or circulating volume, which is called **pulseless electrical activity (PEA)**. Formerly called electrical-mechanical dissociation (EMD), PEA can be caused by hypovolemia (eg, with excessive bleeding), hypoxia, hypothermia, hyperkalemia, massive pulmonary embolism, myocardial infarction, and medication overdose (eg, beta-blockers, calcium channel blockers).

### Clinical Manifestations

In cardiac arrest, consciousness, pulse, and blood pressure are lost immediately. Ineffective respiratory gasping may occur. The pupils of the eyes begin dilating within 45 seconds. Seizures may or may not occur.

> **NURSING ALERT**
>
> The most reliable sign of cardiac arrest is the absence of a pulse. In the adult and the child, the carotid pulse is assessed. In an infant, the brachial pulse is assessed. Valuable time should not be wasted taking the blood pressure, listening for the heartbeat, or checking proper contact of electrodes.

The risk of irreversible brain damage and death increases with every minute from the time that circulation ceases. The interval varies with the age and underlying condition of the patient. During this period, the diagnosis of cardiac arrest must be made and measures must be taken immediately to restore circulation.

## Emergency Management: Cardiopulmonary Resuscitation

Cardiopulmonary resuscitation (CPR) provides blood flow to vital organs until effective circulation can be re-established. The ABCDs of basic CPR are *a*irway, *b*reathing, *c*irculation, and *d*efibrillation (AHA, 2005). Once loss of consciousness has been established, the resuscitation priority for the adult in most cases is placing a phone call to activate the code team or the emergency medical system (EMS). Exceptions to this include near drowning, drug or medication overdose, and respiratory arrest situations, for which 2 minutes of CPR should be performed before activating the EMS. Because the underlying cause of arrest in an infant or child is usually respiratory, the priority is to begin CPR and then activate the EMS after 2 minutes of CPR. Because the care of the pediatric patient is individualized, the following discussion on the care of a cardiac arrest patient applies mainly to adults.

Resuscitation consists of the following steps:

1. Airway: maintaining an open airway
2. Breathing: providing artificial ventilation by rescue breathing
3. Circulation: promoting artificial circulation by external cardiac compression; administer medication therapy (eg, epinephrine for asystole)
4. Defibrillation with standard defibrillator or automatic external defibrillator (AED) for ventricular tachycardia and ventricular fibrillation

If the patient is already being monitored or is immediately placed on the monitor using the multifunction pads or the quick-look paddles (found on most defibrillators) and the ECG shows ventricular tachycardia or ventricular fibrillation, immediate defibrillation rather than CPR is the treatment of choice. In this scenario, CPR is performed initially only if the defibrillator is not immediately available. The survival rate decreases for every minute that defibrillation is delayed (AHA, 2005). If the patient has not been defibrillated within 10 minutes, the chance of survival is close to zero. More information on defibrillation can be found in Chapter 27.

### Maintaining Airway and Breathing

The first step in CPR is to establish an open airway. Any obvious material in the mouth or throat should be removed. The airway should be opened using a head-tilt chin-lift maneuver. The rescuer "looks, listens, and feels" for air movement. An oropharyngeal airway is inserted if available. Two rescue ventilations are provided using a bag-mask or mouth-mask device (Fig. 30-7). An obstructed airway should be suspected when the rescuer cannot give the initial ventilations, and the Heimlich maneuver or abdominal thrusts should be administered to relieve the obstruction.

**FIGURE 30-7.** The chin lift and bag-and-mask technique for ventilating patients who need cardiopulmonary resuscitation.

If the first rescue ventilations meet little or no resistance, the patient is ventilated every 5 to 6 seconds. Each breath is delivered over 1 second. If the patient is in the hospital, endotracheal intubation is frequently performed by a physician, nurse anesthetist, or respiratory therapist during a resuscitation procedure (also called a code) to ensure an adequate airway and ventilation. The resuscitation bag device is then connected directly to the endotracheal tube (ET).

Because of the risk of unrecognized esophageal intubation or dislodgement of the ET, tracheal intubation must be confirmed by two different methods: a primary method (visualization of the ET through the vocal cords, auscultation of breath sounds in five areas on the chest, or bilateral chest expansion) and a secondary method ($CO_2$ detector). A chest x-ray, which is frequently obtained after ET placement, is helpful in determining whether the ET is too high or too low in the trachea. However, a chest x-ray cannot definitively confirm placement of an ET: an ET in the esophagus or the trachea produces the same appearance on the x-ray. Arterial blood gas levels are measured to guide oxygen therapy.

### Restoring Circulation

After performing ventilation, the carotid pulse is assessed, and external cardiac compressions are provided if no pulse is detected. If a defibrillator is not yet available but a process has been put into place to obtain one, chest compressions are initiated. Compressions are performed with the patient on a firm surface, such as the floor, a cardiac board, or a meal tray. The rescuer (facing the patient's side) places the heel of one hand on the lower half of the sternum, two fingerwidths (3.8 cm [1.5 inches]) from the tip of the xiphoid, and positions the other hand on top of the first hand (Fig. 30-8). The fingers should not touch the chest wall (AHA, 2003).

Using the force of body weight while keeping the elbows straight, the rescuer presses quickly downward from the shoulder area to deliver a forceful compression to the victim's lower sternum about 3.8 to 5 cm (1.5 to 2 inches) toward the

**FIGURE 30-8.** Chest compressions in cardiopulmonary resuscitation (CPR) are performed by placing the heel of one hand on the lower half of the sternum and the other hand on top of the first hand. Elbows are kept straight and body weight is used to apply quick, forceful compressions to the lower sternum. For the most effective hand placement and outcome, the patient's chest should be bare.

spine. The chest compression rate is approximately 100 times per minute. A compression to ventilation ratio of 30 to 2 is recommended without pause for ventilations.

When the code team or emergency medical personnel arrive, the patient is quickly assessed to determine cardiac rhythm and respiratory status, as well as possible causes of the arrest. The specific subsequent advanced life support interventions depend on the assessment results. For example, after the patient is placed on a cardiac monitor and ventricular fibrillation is detected, the patient is defibrillated up to three times, and then CPR is resumed. However, if asystole is detected on the monitor, CPR is resumed immediately while trying to identify the underlying cause, such as hypovolemia, hypothermia, or hypoxia. CPR may be stopped when the patient responds and begins to breathe, rescuers are too exhausted or at risk (eg, a building is at risk of collapsing) to continue CPR, or signs of death are obvious. If the patient does not respond to therapies given during the arrest, the resuscitation effort may be stopped or "called" by the physician. The decision to terminate resuscitation is based on medical considerations and takes into account the underlying condition of the patient and the chances for survival.

### Follow-Up Monitoring and Care

Once resuscitated, the patient is transferred to an intensive care unit for close monitoring. Continuous ECG monitoring and frequent blood pressure assessments are essential until hemodynamic stability is re-established. Etiologic factors that precipitated the arrest, such as metabolic or rhythm abnormalities, must be identified and treated. Possible contributing factors, such as electrolyte or acid–base imbalances, need to be identified and corrected. Selected medications (Table 30-5) may be used during and after resuscitation.

## NURSING RESEARCH PROFILE

### Family Presence During Cardiopulmonary Resuscitation

MacLean, S. L., Guzzetta, C. E., White, C., et al. (2003). Family presence during cardiopulmonary resuscitation and invasive procedures: Practices of critical care and emergency nurses. *Journal of Emergency Nursing, 29*(3), 208–221.

#### Purpose
In hospitals and urgent care facilities, there is a growing trend to allow families to be present during CPR and invasive procedures. Among nurses there is variable support and controversy regarding this change in practice. The purpose of this study was to identify facility policies and nurse preferences and practices related to allowing family members to be present at the bedside during CPR and invasive procedures.

#### Design
A 30-item survey was randomly mailed to critical care and emergency department nurses who belong to various national specialty organizations. The survey included questions about written policies and the nurses' preferences as to whether there should be written policies. Nurses were also asked about their personal experiences with family presence. A total of 984 surveys were returned, for a response rate of 32.8%.

#### Findings
Only 5% of the nurses worked on units with written policies allowing family presence during CPR and invasive procedures. About 50% worked on units that permitted the presence of family members during these events but did not have written policies. Many nurses reported that they had taken family members to the bedside for CPR and other procedures (36% and 44%, respectively) or would do so in the future. They also reported that family members had requested to be present for CPR and invasive procedures (31% and 61%, respectively).

#### Nursing Implications
Most critical care and emergency department nurses support the option of family presence, provided that staff members are available to guide, educate, and support families. This reflects the trend toward family-centered care and the desire to meet the holistic needs of patients and family members. Written policies or guidelines are recommended.

## TABLE 30-5 Medications Used in Cardiopulmonary Resuscitation

| Agent and Action | Indications | Nursing Considerations |
|---|---|---|
| Oxygen—improves tissue oxygenation and corrects hypoxemia | Administered to all patients with acute cardiac ischemia or suspected hypoxemia, including those with COPD | • Use 100% $FiO_2$ during resuscitation.<br>• Recognize that no lung damage occurs when used for less than 24 hours.<br>• Monitor dose by pulse oximeter. |
| Epinephrine (Adrenalin)—increases systemic vascular resistance and blood pressure; improves coronary and cerebral perfusion and myocardial contractility | Given to patients in cardiac arrest, especially caused by asystole or pulseless electrical activity; may be given if caused by ventricular tachycardia or ventricular fibrillation | • Administer 1 mg every 3–5 minutes by IV push or through the endotracheal (ET) tube.<br>• Avoid adding to IV lines that contain alkaline solution (eg, bicarbonate). |
| Vasopressin (Pitressin)—increases systemic vascular resistance and blood pressure | An alternative to epinephrine | • Give 40 U IV one time only. |
| Atropine—blocks parasympathetic action; increases SA node automaticity and AV conduction | Given to patients with symptomatic bradycardia (hemodynamically unstable, frequent premature ventricular contractions and symptoms of ischemia) | • Give rapidly as 2.0 to 2.5 mg IV push or through the ET tube.<br>• Be aware that less than 0.5 mg in the adult can cause the heart rate to decrease to a worse bradycardia.<br>• Monitor patient for reflexive tachycardia. |
| Sodium bicarbonate ($NaHCO_3$)—corrects metabolic acidosis | Given to correct metabolic acidosis that is refractory to standard advanced cardiac life support interventions (cardiopulmonary resuscitation, intubation, and respiratory management) | • Administer initial dose of 1 mEq/kg IV; then administer the dose based on the base deficit calculated from arterial blood gas values.<br>• Recognize that to prevent development of rebound metabolic alkalosis, complete correction of acidosis is not indicated |
| Magnesium—promotes adequate functioning of the cellular sodium–potassium pump | Given to patients with torsades de pointes | • May give diluted over 1–2 min or intravenous push.<br>• Monitor for hypotension, asystole, bradycardia, respiratory paralysis. |

COPD, chronic obstructive pulmonary disease

## Critical Thinking Exercises

**1** You are assessing a 72-year-old woman with a 3-year history of HF. Her medications include carvedilol, valsartan, furosemide, and potassium. She reports two episodes of severe dizziness. What are possible causes of dizziness in this patient? What questions would you include in your assessment? What medical and nursing interventions would be appropriate for each possible cause?

**2** [ebp] On an inpatient progressive care unit, you are assigned to care for a 60-year-old man who has been readmitted for the third time with severe HF and widespread edema. According to the patient's chart, he has a history of noncompliance with diet and medications. What are your immediate priorities and short-term goals for this patient? What medical interventions are indicated? Develop an evidence-based plan of care for this patient in the future. Describe your planned interaction with the patient (ie, communication technique, behaviors) that would encourage the patient to participate in the plan.

**3** [ebp] On an inpatient progressive care unit, you receive a 55-year-old man who just been transferred from the cardiac intensive care unit. You realize that he is at risk of complications after a large anterior wall MI, which was treated with emergent cardiac catheterization and percutaneous coronary intervention. His medications include aspirin, clopidogrel, metoprolol, and lisinopril. During your initial assessment, you notice that the patient appears weak and pale. You have trouble hearing his blood pressure, but think you hear a systolic pressure of about 80 mm Hg. List the possible complications this patient may be experiencing. What assessment parameters would you check next? Discuss the strength of the evidence that supports priority nursing interventions and expected outcomes. Describe your communication with the patient during the interventions.

# REFERENCES AND SELECTED READINGS

## BOOKS

American Heart Association. (2004). *2004 Heart and stroke statistics.* Dallas, TX: Author.

Carpenito, L. J. (2004). *Nursing diagnosis: Application to clinical practice* (10th ed.). Philadelphia: Lippincott Williams & Wilkins.

Fink, M. P., Abraham, E., Vincent, J. L., et al. (Eds.). (2005). *Textbook of critical care* (5th ed.). Philadelphia: Elsevier.

Morton, P. G., Fontaine, D. K., Hudak, C. M., et al. (Eds.). (2005). *Critical care nursing* (8th ed.). Philadelphia: Lippincott Williams & Wilkins.

Porth, C. M. (2005). *Pathophysiology: Concepts of altered health states* (7th ed.). Philadelphia: Lippincott Williams & Wilkins.

Silver, M. A., Pisano, C., & Cianci, P. (2004). *Outpatient management of heart failure.* Littleton, CO: Postgraduate Institute for Medicine.

Zipes, D. P., Libby, P., & Bonow, R. D. (Eds.). (2005). *Braunwald's heart disease* (7th ed.). Philadelphia: Saunders.

## JOURNALS

*Asterisks indicate nursing research articles.

Albert, N. M. (2003a). Cardiac resynchronization therapy through biventricular pacing in patients with heart failure and ventricular dyssynchrony. *Critical Care Nurse, 23*(Supp), 2–13.

Albert, N. M. (2003b). Surgical management of heart failure. *Critical Care Nursing Clinics of North America, 15*(4), 477–487.

American Heart Association. (2005). Guidelines for cardiopulmonary resuscitation and emergency cardiovascular care. *Circulation, 112*(24), 1–203.

Ammon, S. (2001). Managing patients with heart failure. *American Journal of Nursing, 101*(12), 34–40.

Artinian, N. T. (2003). The psychosocial aspects of heart failure. *American Journal of Nursing, 103*(12), 32–43.

Bradley, D. J., Bradley, E. A., & Baughman, K. L. (2003). Cardiac resynchronization and death from progressive heart failure: A meta-analysis of randomized controlled trials. *Journal of the American Medical Association, 289*(6), 730–740.

*Corvera-Tindel, T., Doering, L. V., Gomez, T., et al. (2004). Predictors of noncompliance to exercise training in heart failure. *Journal of Cardiovascular Nursing, 19*(4), 269–277.

Goldhaber, S. Z., & Elliott, C. G. (2003). Acute pulmonary embolism. Part I: Epidemiology, pathophysiology, and diagnosis. *Circulation, 108*(22), 2726–2729.

Gramsky, C., Josephson, S., Langford, M., et al. (2003). Outpatient management of heart failure. *Critical Care Nursing Clinics of North America, 15*(4), 501–509.

Hachey, D. M., & Smith, T. (2003). Use of neseritide to treat acute decompensated heart failure. *Critical Care Nurse, 23*(1), 53–55.

Hunt, S. A., Baker, D. W., Chin, M. H., et al., American College of Cardiology/American Heart Association Task Force on Practice Guidelines (Committee to Revise the 1995 Guidelines for the Evaluation and Management of Heart Failure), International Society for Heart and Lung Transplantation, & Heart Failure Society of America. (2001). ACC/AHA guidelines for the evaluation and management of chronic heart failure in the adult: A report of the American College of Cardiology/American Heart Association Task Force on Practice Guidelines (Committee to Revise the 1995 Guidelines for the Evaluation and Management of Heart Failure). *Journal of the American College of Cardiology, 38*(7), 2101–2113.

Institute for Clinical Systems Improvement (ICSI) (2004). *Heart failure in adults.* Bloomington, MN: ICSI. Available at http://www.AHRQ.gov/summary/summary.aspx?doc_id=7657+ss=1. Accessed May 31, 2006.

Koschel, M. J. (2004). Pulmonary embolism. *American Journal of Nursing, 104*(6), 46–50.

*MacLean, S. L., Guzzetta, C. E., White, C., et al. (2003). Family presence during cardiopulmonary resuscitation and invasive procedures: Practices of critical care and emergency nurses. *Journal of Emergency Nursing, 29*(3), 208–221.

Moser, D. K., & Biddle, M. J. (2003). Angiotensin-converting enzyme inhibitors and angiotensin II receptor blockers. *Critical Care Nursing Clinics of North America, 15*(4), 423–437.

Piano, M. R., & Prasun, M. (2003). Neurohormone activation. *Critical Care Nursing Clinics of North America, 15*(4), 413–421.

Pina, I. L., Apstein, C. S., Balady, G. J., et al. (2003). Exercise and heart failure. *Circulation, 107*(8), 1210.

Smith, A. L., & Brown, C. S. (2003). New advances and novel treatments in heart failure. *Critical Care Nurse, 23*(Supp), 11–18.

*Sneed, N. V., & Paul, S. C. (2003). Readiness for behavioral changes in patients with heart failure. *American Journal of Critical Care, 12*(5), 444–453.

Spencer, A. P. (2003). Digoxin in heart failure. *Critical Care Nursing Clinics of North America, 15*(4), 447–452.

Tokarczyk, T. R. (2003). Cardiac transplantation as a treatment option for the heart failure patient. *Critical Care Nursing Quarterly, 26*(1), 61–68.

Trypp, R. J., Abraham, W. T., & Lamba, S. (2003). Future therapies for heart failure. *Critical Care Nursing Clinics of North America, 15*(4), 525–530.

Young, J. B., Abraham, W. T., & Smith, A. L. (2003). Combined cardiac resynchronization and implantable cardioversion defibrillation in advanced chronic heart failure. *Journal of the American Medical Association, 289*(20), 2685–2694.

## RESOURCES

American Heart Association, 7320 Greenville Ave., Dallas, TX 75231; 1-800-242-8721; http://www.americanheart.org. Accessed May 31, 2006.

Heart Failure Society of America, Court International, Suite 238-N, 2550 University Avenue West, Saint Paul, MN 55144; 651-642-1633; http://www.abouthf.org. Accessed May 31, 2006.

Heartmates, Inc., P.O. Box 16202, Minneapolis, MN 55416; 952-929-3331; http://www.heartmates.com. Accessed May 31, 2006.

National Heart, Lung, and Blood Institute, National Institutes of Health, Building 31, Room 5A52, Bethesda, MD 20892; 301-592-8573; http://www.nhlbi.nih.gov. Accessed May 31, 2006.

# CHAPTER 31

# Assessment and Management of Patients With Vascular Disorders and Problems of Peripheral Circulation

## Learning Objectives

*On completion of this chapter, the learner will be able to:*

1. Identify anatomic and physiologic factors that affect peripheral blood flow and tissue oxygenation.
2. Use appropriate parameters for assessment of peripheral circulation.
3. Use the nursing process as a framework of care for patients with vascular insufficiency of the extremities.
4. Compare the various diseases of the arteries and their causes, pathologic and physiologic changes, clinical manifestations, management, and prevention.
5. Describe the prevention and management of venous thrombosis.
6. Compare strategies to prevent venous insufficiency, leg ulcers, and varicose veins.
7. Use the nursing process as a framework of care for patients with leg ulcers.
8. Describe nursing and medical management of cellulitis.
9. Describe the relationship between lymphangitis and lymphedema.

Adequate perfusion ensures oxygenation and nourishment of body tissues, and it depends in part on a properly functioning cardiovascular system. Adequate blood flow depends on the efficiency of the heart as a pump, the patency and responsiveness of the blood vessels, and the adequacy of circulating blood volume. Nervous system activity, blood viscosity, and the metabolic needs of tissues influence the rate and adequacy of blood flow.

# Anatomic and Physiologic Overview

The vascular system consists of two interdependent systems. The right side of the heart pumps blood through the lungs to the pulmonary circulation, and the left side of the heart pumps blood to all other body tissues through the systemic circulation. The blood vessels in both systems channel the blood from the heart to the tissues and back to the heart (Fig. 31-1). Contraction of the ventricles is the driving force that moves blood through the vascular system.

Arteries distribute oxygenated blood from the left side of the heart to the tissues, whereas the veins carry deoxygenated blood from the tissues to the right side of the heart. Capillary vessels located within the tissues connect the arterial and venous systems. These vessels permit the exchange of nutrients and metabolic wastes between the circulatory system and the tissues. Arterioles and venules immediately adjacent to the capillaries, together with the capillaries, make up the microcirculation.

The lymphatic system complements the function of the circulatory system. Lymphatic vessels transport lymph (a fluid similar to plasma) and tissue fluids (containing proteins, cells, and cellular debris) from the interstitial space to systemic veins.

## Anatomy of the Vascular System

### Arteries and Arterioles

Arteries are thick-walled structures that carry blood from the heart to the tissues. The aorta, which has a diameter of approximately 25 mm (1 inch) in the average-sized adult, gives rise to numerous branches, which continue to divide into progressively smaller arteries that are 4 mm (0.16 inch) in diameter. The vessels divide further, diminishing in size to approximately 30 μm in diameter. These smallest arteries, called the arterioles, are generally embedded within the tissues.

The walls of the arteries and arterioles are composed of three layers: the intima, an inner endothelial cell layer; the media, a middle layer of smooth muscle and elastic tissue; and the adventitia, an outer layer of connective tissue. The intima, a very thin layer, provides a smooth surface for contact with the flowing blood. The media makes up most of the vessel wall in the aorta and other large arteries of the body. This layer is composed chiefly of elastic and connective tissue fibers that give the vessels considerable strength and allow them to constrict and dilate to accommodate the blood ejected from the heart during each cardiac cycle (stroke volume) and maintain an even, steady flow of blood. The adventitia is a layer of connective tissue that anchors the vessel to its surroundings. There is much less elastic tissue in the smaller arteries and arterioles, and the media in these vessels is composed primarily of smooth muscle (Porth, 2005).

Smooth muscle controls the diameter of the vessels by contracting and relaxing. Chemical, hormonal, and neuronal factors influence the activity of smooth muscle. Because arterioles offer resistance to blood flow by altering their diameter, they are often referred to as *resistance vessels*. Arterioles regulate the volume and pressure in the arterial system and the rate of blood flow to the capillaries. Because

# Glossary

**anastomosis:** junction of two vessels
**aneurysm:** a localized sac or dilation of an artery formed at a weak point in the vessel wall
**ankle-brachial index (ABI) or ankle-arm index (AAI):** ratio of the ankle systolic pressure to the arm systolic pressure; an objective measurement of arterial disease that provides quantification of the degree of stenosis
**angioplasty:** an invasive procedure that uses a balloon-tipped catheter to dilate a stenotic area of a blood vessel
**arteriosclerosis:** diffuse process whereby the muscle fibers and the endothelial lining of the walls of small arteries and arterioles thicken
**atherosclerosis:** disease process involving the accumulation of lipids, calcium, blood components, carbohydrates, and fibrous tissue on the intimal layer of a large or medium-sized artery
**bruit:** sound produced by turbulent blood flow through an irregular, tortuous, stenotic, or dilated vessel
**dissection:** separation of the weakened elastic and fibromuscular elements in the medial layer of an artery
**duplex ultrasonography:** combines B-mode gray-scale imaging of tissue, organs, and blood vessels with capabilities of estimating velocity changes by use of a pulsed Doppler
**intermittent claudication:** a muscular, cramp-like pain in the extremities consistently reproduced with the same degree of exercise or activity and relieved by rest
**international normalized ratio (INR):** method of measuring anticoagulation levels, such as warfarin (Coumadin); devised to bring a universal standard to monitoring of anticoagulation achieved by oral medications
**ischemia:** deficient blood supply
**rest pain:** persistent pain in the foot or digits when the patient is resting, indicating a severe degree of arterial insufficiency
**rubor:** reddish blue discoloration of the extremities; indicative of severe peripheral arterial damage in vessels that remain dilated and unable to constrict
**stenosis:** narrowing or constriction of a vessel

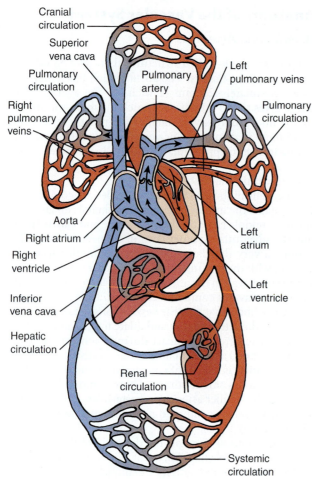

**FIGURE 31-1.** Systemic and pulmonary circulation. Oxygen-rich blood from the pulmonary circulation is pumped from the left heart into the aorta and the systemic arteries to the capillaries, where the exchange of nutrients and waste products takes place. The deoxygenated blood returns to the right heart by way of the systemic veins and is pumped into the pulmonary circulation. From *Stedman's Medical Dictionary* (28th ed.). (2006). Philadelphia: Lippincott Williams & Wilkins.

of the large amount of smooth muscle in the media, the walls of the arteries are relatively thick, accounting for approximately 25% of the total diameter of the artery.

The intima and the inner third of the smooth muscle layer of the media are in such close contact with the blood that the blood vessel receives its nourishment by direct diffusion. The adventitia and the outer media layers have a limited vascular system for nourishment and require their own blood supply to meet metabolic needs.

## Capillaries

The walls of the capillaries, which lack smooth muscle and adventitia, are composed of a single layer of endothelial cells. This thin-walled structure permits rapid and efficient transport of nutrients to the cells and removal of metabolic wastes. The diameter of capillaries ranges from 5 to 10 μm; this means that red blood cells must alter their shape to pass through these vessels. Changes in a capillary's diameter are passive and are influenced by contractile changes in the blood vessels that carry blood to and from a capillary. The capillary's diameter also changes in response to chemical stimuli. In some tissues, a cuff of smooth muscle, called the precapillary sphincter, is located at the arteriolar end of the capillary and is responsible, along with the arteriole, for controlling capillary blood flow (Porth, 2005).

Some capillary beds, such as those in the fingertips, contain arteriovenous anastomoses, through which blood passes directly from the arterial to the venous system. These vessels are believed to regulate heat exchange between the body and the external environment.

The distribution of capillaries varies with the type of tissue. For example, skeletal tissue, which has high metabolic requirements, has a denser capillary network than cartilage, which has low metabolic needs.

## Veins and Venules

Capillaries join to form larger vessels called venules, which join to form veins. The venous system is therefore structurally analogous to the arterial system; venules correspond to arterioles, veins to arteries, and the vena cava to the aorta. Analogous types of vessels in the arterial and venous systems have approximately the same diameters (see Fig. 31-1).

The walls of the veins, in contrast to those of the arteries, are thinner and considerably less muscular. In most veins, the wall makes up only 10% of the diameter, in contrast to 25% in most arteries. In veins, the walls are composed of three layers, like those of arteries, although in veins, these layers are not as well defined.

The thin, less muscular structure of the vein wall allows these vessels to distend more than arteries. Greater distensibility and compliance permit large volumes of blood to remain in the veins under low pressure. For this reason, veins are referred to as *capacitance vessels*. Approximately 75% of total blood volume is contained in the veins. The sympathetic nervous system, which innervates the vein musculature, can stimulate the veins to constrict (venoconstriction), thereby reducing venous volume and increasing the volume of blood in the general circulation. Contraction of skeletal muscles in the extremities creates the primary pumping action to facilitate venous blood flow back to the heart (Porth, 2005).

Some veins, unlike arteries, are equipped with valves. In general, veins that transport blood against the force of gravity, as in the lower extremities, have one-way bicuspid valves that prevent blood from seeping backward as it is propelled toward the heart. Valves are composed of endothelial leaflets, the competency of which depends on the integrity of the vein wall.

## Lymphatic Vessels

The lymphatic vessels are a complex network of thin-walled vessels similar to the blood capillaries. This network collects lymphatic fluid from tissues and organs and transports the fluid to the venous circulation. The lymphatic vessels converge into two main structures: the thoracic duct and the right lymphatic duct. These ducts empty into the junction of the subclavian and the internal jugular veins. The right lymphatic duct conveys lymph primarily from the right side of the head, neck, thorax, and upper arms. The thoracic duct conveys lymph from the remainder of the body.

Peripheral lymphatic vessels join larger lymph vessels and pass through regional lymph nodes before entering the venous circulation. The lymph nodes play an important role in filtering foreign particles.

The lymphatic vessels are permeable to large molecules and provide the only means by which interstitial proteins can return to the venous system. With muscular contraction, lymph vessels become distorted to create spaces between the endothelial cells, allowing protein and particles to enter. Muscular contraction of the lymphatic walls and surrounding tissues aids in propelling the lymph toward the venous drainage points (Porth, 2005).

## Function of the Vascular System

### Circulatory Needs of Tissues

The amount of blood flow needed by body tissues constantly changes. The percentage of blood flow received by individual organs or tissues is determined by the rate of tissue metabolism, the availability of oxygen, and the function of the tissues. When metabolic requirements increase, blood vessels dilate to increase the flow of oxygen and nutrients to the tissues. When metabolic needs decrease, vessels constrict and blood flow to the tissues decreases. Metabolic demands of tissues increase with physical activity or exercise, local heat application, fever, and infection. Reduced metabolic requirements of tissues accompany rest or decreased physical activity, local cold application, and cooling of the body. If the blood vessels fail to dilate in response to the need for increased blood flow, tissue **ischemia** (deficient blood supply to a body part) results. The mechanism by which blood vessels dilate and constrict to adjust for metabolic changes ensures that normal arterial pressure is maintained (Porth, 2005).

As blood passes through tissue capillaries, oxygen is removed and carbon dioxide is added. The amount of oxygen extracted by each tissue differs. For example, the myocardium tends to extract about 50% of the oxygen from arterial blood in one pass through its capillary bed, whereas the kidneys extract only about 7% of the oxygen from the blood that passes through them. The average amount of oxygen removed collectively by all of the body tissues is about 25%. This means that the blood in the vena cava contains about 25% less oxygen than aortic blood. This is known as the *systemic arteriovenous oxygen difference* (Porth, 2005). This difference becomes greater when less oxygen is delivered to the tissues than they need.

### Blood Flow

Blood flow through the cardiovascular system always proceeds in the same direction: left side of the heart to the aorta, arteries, arterioles, capillaries, venules, veins, vena cava, and right side of the heart. This unidirectional flow is caused by a pressure difference that exists between the arterial and venous systems. Because arterial pressure (approximately 100 mm Hg) is greater than venous pressure (approximately 40 mm Hg) and fluid always flows from an area of higher pressure to an area of lower pressure, blood flows from the arterial to the venous system.

The pressure difference ($\Delta P$) between the two ends of the vessel propels the blood. Impediments to blood flow offer the opposing force, which is known as resistance (R). The rate of blood flow is determined by dividing the pressure difference by the resistance:

$$\text{Flow rate} = \Delta P/R$$

This equation clearly shows that when resistance increases, a greater driving pressure is required to maintain the same degree of flow (Porth, 2005). In the body, an increase in driving pressure is accomplished by an increase in the force of contraction of the heart. If arterial resistance is chronically elevated, the myocardium hypertrophies (enlarges) to sustain the greater contractile force.

In most long smooth blood vessels, flow is laminar or streamlined, with blood in the center of the vessel moving slightly faster than the blood near the vessel walls. Laminar flow becomes turbulent when the blood flow rate increases, when blood viscosity increases, when the diameter of the vessel becomes greater than normal, or when segments of the vessel are narrowed or constricted (Porth, 2005). Turbulent blood flow creates a sound, called a **bruit**, that can be heard with a stethoscope.

### Blood Pressure

Chapters 26 and 32 provide more information on the physiology and measurement of blood pressure.

### Capillary Filtration and Reabsorption

Fluid exchange across the capillary wall is continuous. This fluid, which has the same composition as plasma without the proteins, forms the interstitial fluid. The equilibrium between hydrostatic and osmotic forces of the blood and interstitium, as well as capillary permeability, determines the amount and direction of fluid movement across the capillary. Hydrostatic force is a driving pressure that is generated by the blood pressure. Osmotic pressure is the pulling force created by plasma proteins. Normally, the hydrostatic pressure at the arterial end of the capillary is relatively high compared with that at the venous end. This high pressure at the arterial end of the capillaries tends to drive fluid out of the capillary and into the tissue space. Osmotic pressure tends to pull fluid back into the capillary from the tissue space, but this osmotic force cannot overcome the high hydrostatic pressure at the arterial end of the capillary. However, at the venous end of the capillary, the osmotic force predominates over the low hydrostatic pressure, and there is a net reabsorption of fluid from the tissue space back into the capillary (Porth, 2005).

Except for a very small amount, fluid that is filtered out at the arterial end of the capillary bed is reabsorbed at the venous end. The excess filtered fluid enters the lymphatic circulation. These processes of filtration, reabsorption, and lymph formation aid in maintaining tissue fluid volume and removing tissue waste and debris. Under normal conditions, capillary permeability remains constant.

Under certain abnormal conditions, the fluid filtered out of the capillaries may greatly exceed the amounts reabsorbed and carried away by the lymphatic vessels. This imbalance can result from damage to capillary walls and subsequent increased permeability, obstruction of lymphatic drainage, elevation of venous pressure, or decrease in plasma protein osmotic force. Accumulation of excess interstitial fluid that results from these processes is known as *edema*.

## Hemodynamic Resistance

The most important factor that determines resistance in the vascular system is the vessel radius. Small changes in vessel radius lead to large changes in resistance. The predominant sites of change in the caliber or width of blood vessels, and therefore in resistance, are the arterioles and the precapillary sphincter. Peripheral vascular resistance is the opposition to blood flow provided by the blood vessels. This resistance is proportional to the viscosity or thickness of the blood and the length of the vessel and is influenced by the diameter of the vessels. Under normal conditions, blood viscosity and vessel length do not change significantly, and these factors do not usually play an important role in blood flow. However, a large increase in hematocrit may increase blood viscosity and reduce capillary blood flow.

## Peripheral Vascular Regulating Mechanisms

Even at rest, the metabolic needs of body tissues are continuously changing. Therefore, an integrated and coordinated regulatory system is necessary so that blood flow to individual tissues is maintained in proportion to the needs of those tissues. This regulatory mechanism is complex and consists of central nervous system influences, circulating hormones and chemicals, and independent activity of the arterial wall itself.

Sympathetic (adrenergic) nervous system activity, mediated by the hypothalamus, is the most important factor in regulating the caliber and therefore the blood flow of peripheral blood vessels. All vessels are innervated by the sympathetic nervous system except the capillary and precapillary sphincters. Stimulation of the sympathetic nervous system causes vasoconstriction. The neurotransmitter responsible for sympathetic vasoconstriction is norepinephrine (Porth, 2005). Sympathetic activation occurs in response to physiologic and psychological stressors. Diminution of sympathetic activity by medications or sympathectomy results in vasodilation.

Other hormonal substances affect peripheral vascular resistance. Epinephrine, released from the adrenal medulla, acts like norepinephrine in constricting peripheral blood vessels in most tissue beds. However, in low concentrations, epinephrine causes vasodilation in skeletal muscles, the heart, and the brain. Angiotensin I, which is formed from the interaction of renin (synthesized by the kidney) and angiotensinogen, a circulating serum protein, is then converted to angiotensin II by an enzyme secreted by the pulmonary vasculature, called angiotensin-converting enzyme (ACE). Angiotensin II is a potent vasoconstrictor, particularly of the arterioles. Although the amount of angiotensin II concentrated in the blood is usually small, its profound vasoconstrictive effects are important in certain abnormal states, such as heart failure and hypovolemia (Porth, 2005).

Alterations in local blood flow are influenced by various circulating substances that have vasoactive properties. Potent vasodilators include nitric oxide, prostacyclin, histamine, bradykinin, prostaglandin, and certain muscle metabolites. A reduction in available oxygen and nutrients and changes in local pH also affect local blood flow. Thromboxane $A_2$ and serotonin are substances liberated from platelets that aggregate at the site of damaged vessels, causing arteriolar vasoconstriction and continued platelet aggregation at the site of injury (Porth, 2005). The application of heat to parts of the body surface causes local vasodilation, whereas the application of cold causes vasoconstriction.

## Pathophysiology of the Vascular System

Reduced blood flow through peripheral blood vessels characterizes all peripheral vascular diseases. The physiologic effects of altered blood flow depend on the extent to which tissue demands exceed the supply of oxygen and nutrients available. If tissue needs are high, even modestly reduced blood flow may be inadequate to maintain tissue integrity. Tissues then fall prey to ischemia, become malnourished, and ultimately die unless adequate blood flow is restored.

### Pump Failure

Inadequate peripheral blood flow occurs when the heart's pumping action becomes inefficient. Left-sided heart failure (left ventricular failure) causes an accumulation of blood in the lungs and a reduction in forward flow or cardiac output, which results in inadequate arterial blood flow to the tissues. Right-sided heart failure (right ventricular failure) causes systemic venous congestion and a reduction in forward flow (see Chapter 30).

### Alterations in Blood and Lymphatic Vessels

Intact, patent, and responsive blood vessels are necessary to deliver adequate amounts of oxygen to tissues and to remove metabolic wastes. Arteries can become damaged or obstructed as a result of atherosclerotic plaque, thromboemboli, chemical or mechanical trauma, infections or inflammatory processes, vasospastic disorders, and congenital malformations. A sudden arterial occlusion causes profound and often irreversible tissue ischemia and tissue death. When arterial occlusions develop gradually, there is less risk of sudden tissue death because collateral circulation may develop, giving that tissue the opportunity to adapt to gradually decreased blood flow.

Venous blood flow can be reduced by a thromboembolus obstructing the vein, by incompetent venous valves, or by a reduction in the effectiveness of the pumping action of surrounding muscles. Decreased venous blood flow results in increased venous pressure, a subsequent increase in capillary hydrostatic pressure, net filtration of fluid out of the capillaries into the interstitial space, and subsequent edema. Edematous tissues cannot receive adequate nutrition from the blood and consequently are more susceptible to breakdown, injury, and infection. Obstruction of lymphatic vessels also results in edema. Lymphatic vessels can become obstructed by a tumor or by damage from mechanical trauma or inflammatory processes.

### Circulatory Insufficiency of the Extremities

Although many types of peripheral vascular diseases exist, most result in ischemia and produce some of the same symptoms: pain, skin changes, diminished pulse, and possible edema. The type and severity of symptoms depend in part on the type, stage, and extent of the disease process and on the speed with which the disorder develops. Table 31-1 highlights the distinguishing features of arterial and venous insufficiency. In this chapter, peripheral vascular disease is categorized as arterial, venous, or lymphatic.

### Gerontologic Considerations

Aging produces changes in the walls of the blood vessels that affect the transport of oxygen and nutrients to the tissues. The intima thickens as a result of cellular proliferation and fibrosis. Elastin fibers of the media become calcified, thin, and fragmented, and collagen accumulates in the intima and the media. These changes cause the vessels to stiffen, which results in increased peripheral resistance, impaired blood flow, and increased left ventricular workload.

## Assessment and Diagnostic Evaluation

### Health History and Clinical Manifestations

An in-depth description from the patient of any pain and its precipitating factors, a thorough assessment of the patient's skin color and temperature, and the character of the peripheral pulses are all important in the diagnosis of arterial disorders.

#### Intermittent Claudication

A muscular, cramp-type pain in the extremities consistently reproduced with the same degree of exercise or activity and relieved by rest is experienced by patients with peripheral arterial insufficiency. Referred to as **intermittent claudication**, this pain is caused by the inability of the arterial system to provide adequate blood flow to the tissues in the face of increased demands for nutrients and oxygen during exercise. As the tissues are forced to complete the energy cycle without adequate nutrients and oxygen, muscle metabolites and lactic acid are produced. Pain is experienced as the metabolites aggravate the nerve endings of the surrounding tissue. Typically, about 50% of the arterial lumen or 75% of the cross-sectional area must be obstructed before intermittent claudication is experienced. When the patient rests and thereby decreases the metabolic needs of the muscles, the pain subsides. The progression of the arterial disease can be monitored by documenting the amount of exercise or the distance the patient can walk before pain is produced. Persistent pain in the forefoot (ie, the anterior portion of the foot) when the patient is resting indicates a severe degree of arterial insufficiency and a critical state of ischemia. Known as **rest pain**, this discomfort is often worse at night and may interfere with sleep. This pain frequently requires that the extremity be lowered to a dependent position to improve perfusion to the distal tissues.

The site of arterial disease can be deduced from the location of claudication, because pain occurs in muscle groups distal to the diseased vessel. Calf pain may accompany reduced blood flow through the superficial femoral or popliteal artery, whereas pain in the hip or buttock may result from reduced blood flow in the abdominal aorta or the common iliac or hypogastric arteries.

#### Changes in Skin Appearance and Temperature

Adequate blood flow warms the extremities and gives them a rosy coloring. Inadequate blood flow results in cool and pale extremities. Further reduction of blood flow to these tissues, which occurs when the extremity is elevated, for example, results in an even whiter or more blanched appearance

| TABLE 31-1 | Characteristics of Arterial and Venous Insufficiency | |
|---|---|---|
| **Characteristic** | **Arterial** | **Venous** |
| **Pain** | Intermittent claudication to sharp, unrelenting, constant | Aching, cramping |
| **Pulses** | Diminished or absent | Present, but may be difficult to palpate through edema |
| **Skin characteristics** | Dependent rubor—elevation pallor of foot, dry, shiny skin, cool-to-cold temperature, loss of hair over toes and dorsum of foot, nails thickened and ridged | Pigmentation in gaitor area (area of medial and lateral malleolus), skin thickened and tough, may be reddish blue, frequently with associated dermatitis |
| **Ulcer characteristics** | | |
|   Location | Tip of toes, toe webs, heel or other pressure areas if confined to bed | Medial malleolus; infrequently lateral malleolus or anterior tibial area |
|   Pain | Very painful | Minimal pain if superficial or may be very painful |
|   Depth of ulcer | Deep, often involving joint space | Superficial |
|   Shape | Circular | Irregular border |
|   Ulcer base | Pale to black and dry gangrene | Granulation tissue—beefy red to yellow fibrinous in chronic long-term ulcer |
| **Leg edema** | Minimal unless extremity kept in dependent position constantly to relieve pain | Moderate to severe |

(eg, pallor). **Rubor**, a reddish-blue discoloration of the extremities, may be observed within 20 seconds to 2 minutes after the extremity is placed in the dependent position. Rubor suggests severe peripheral arterial damage in which vessels that cannot constrict remain dilated. Even with rubor, the extremity begins to turn pale with elevation. Cyanosis, a bluish tint of the skin, is manifested when the amount of oxygenated hemoglobin contained in the blood is reduced.

Additional changes resulting from a chronically reduced nutrient supply include loss of hair, brittle nails, dry or scaling skin, atrophy, and ulcerations. Edema may be apparent bilaterally or unilaterally and is related to the affected extremity's chronically dependent position because of severe rest pain. Gangrenous changes appear after prolonged, severe ischemia and represent tissue necrosis. In elderly patients who are inactive, gangrene may be the first sign of disease. These patients may have adjusted their lifestyle to accommodate the limitations imposed by the disease and may not walk far enough to develop symptoms of claudication. Circulation is decreased, but this is not apparent to the patient until trauma occurs. At this point, gangrene develops when minimal arterial flow is impaired further by edema formation resulting from the traumatic event.

### Pulses

Determining the presence or absence, as well as the quality, of peripheral pulses is important in assessing the status of peripheral arterial circulation (Fig. 31-2). Absence of a pulse may indicate that the site of **stenosis** (narrowing or constriction) is proximal to that location. Occlusive arterial disease impairs blood flow and can reduce or obliterate palpable pulsations in the extremities. Pulses should be palpated bilaterally and simultaneously, comparing both sides for symmetry in rate, rhythm, and quality.

### *Gerontologic Considerations*

In elderly people, symptoms of peripheral arterial disease may be more pronounced than in younger people. Intermittent claudication may occur after walking only a few blocks or after walking up a slight incline. Any prolonged pressure on the foot can cause pressure areas that become ulcerated, infected, and gangrenous. The outcomes of arterial insufficiency can include reduced mobility and activity as well as a loss of independence.

## Diagnostic Evaluation

Various tests may be performed to identify and diagnose abnormalities that can affect the vascular structures (arteries, veins, and lymphatics).

### Doppler Ultrasound Flow Studies

Palpation of pulses is subjective, and the examiner may mistake his or her own pulse for that of the patient. To prevent

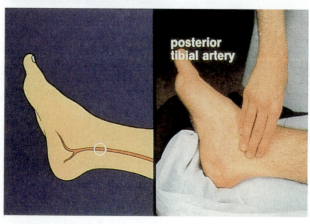

**FIGURE 31-2.** Assessing peripheral pulses. (*Left*) Popliteal pulse. (*Right*) Dorsalis pedis pulse. (*Bottom*) Posterior tibial pulse.

this, the examiner should use light touch and avoid using only the index finger for palpation because this finger has the strongest arterial pulsation of all the fingers. The thumb should not be used for the same reason. When pulses cannot be reliably palpated, a hand-held continuous wave (CW) Doppler ultrasound device may be used to hear (insonate) the blood flow in vessels. This hand-held device emits a continuous signal through the patient's tissues. The signals are reflected by ("echo off") the moving blood cells and are received by the device. The filtered-output Doppler signal is then transmitted to a loudspeaker or headphones, where it can be heard for interpretation. Because CW Doppler emits a continuous signal, all vascular structures in the path of the sound beam are insonated, and differentiating arterial from venous flow and detecting the site of a stenosis may be difficult. The depth at which blood flow can be detected by Doppler is determined by the frequency (in megahertz [MHz]) it generates. The lower the frequency, the deeper the tissue penetration; a 5- to 10-MHz probe may be used to evaluate the peripheral arteries.

To evaluate the lower extremities, the patient is placed in the supine position with the head of the bed elevated 20 to 30 degrees; the legs are externally rotated, if possible, to permit adequate access to the medial malleolus. Acoustic gel is applied to the patient's skin to permit uniform transmission of the ultrasound wave (electrocardiogram gel is not used because it contains sodium, which may dissolve the epoxy that covers the transducer's tip). The tip of the Doppler transducer is positioned at a 45- to 60-degree angle over the expected location of the artery and angled slowly to identify arterial blood flow. Excessive pressure is avoided because severely diseased arteries can collapse with even minimal pressure.

Because the transducer can detect blood flow in advanced arterial disease states, especially if collateral circulation has developed, identifying a signal documents only the presence of blood flow. The patient's primary care provider must be notified of the absence of a signal if one had been detected previously.

CW Doppler is more useful as a clinical tool when combined with ankle blood pressures, which are used to determine the **ankle-brachial index (ABI)**, also called the **ankle-arm index (AAI)** (Fig. 31-3). The ABI is the ratio of the systolic blood pressure in the ankle to the systolic blood pressure in the arm. It is an objective indicator of arterial disease that allows the examiner to quantify the degree of stenosis. With increasing degrees of arterial narrowing, there is a progressive decrease in systolic pressure distal to the involved sites.

The first step in determining the ABI is to have the patient rest in a supine position (not seated) for at least 5 minutes. An appropriate-sized blood pressure cuff (typically, a 10-cm cuff) is applied to the patient's ankle above the malleolus. After identifying an arterial signal at the posterior tibial and dorsalis pedis arteries, the systolic pressures are obtained in both ankles. Diastolic pressures in the ankles cannot be measured with a Doppler. If pressure in these arteries cannot be measured, pressure can be measured in the peroneal artery, which can also be assessed at the ankle (Fig. 31-4).

Doppler ultrasonography is used to measure brachial pressures in both arms. Both arms are evaluated because the patient may have an asymptomatic stenosis in the sub-

**FIGURE 31-3.** Continuous-wave (CW) Doppler ultrasound detects blood flow in peripheral vessels. Combined with computation of ankle or arm pressures, this diagnostic technique helps health care providers characterize the nature of peripheral vascular disease. Photograph reprinted with permission from Cantwell-Gab, K. (1996). Identifying chronic PAD. *American Journal of Nursing, 96*(7), 40–46.

clavian artery, causing brachial pressure on the affected side to be 20 mm Hg or more lower than systemic pressure. The abnormally low pressure should not be used for assessment.

To calculate ABI, the ankle systolic pressure for each foot is divided by the higher of the two brachial systolic pressures (Chart 31-1). The ABI can be computed for a patient with the following systolic pressures:

*Right brachial:* 160 mm Hg
*Left brachial:* 120 mm Hg
*Right posterior tibial:* 80 mm Hg
*Right dorsalis pedis:* 60 mm Hg
*Left posterior tibial:* 100 mm Hg
*Left dorsalis pedis:* 120 mm Hg

**FIGURE 31-4.** Location of peroneal artery; lateral malleolus. Photograph reprinted with permission from Cantwell-Gab, K. (1996). Identifying chronic PAD. *American Journal of Nursing, 96*(7), 40–46.

### CHART 31-1

### Avoiding Common Errors in Calculating Ankle-Brachial Index (ABI)

Take the following precautions to ensure an accurate ABI calculation:

- *Use the correctly sized blood pressure (BP) cuffs.* To obtain accurate BP measurements, use a cuff with a bladder width at least 40% and length at least 80% of the limb circumference.
- *On the nursing plan of care, document the BP cuff sizes used* (for example, "12-cm BP cuff used for brachial pressures; 10-cm BP cuff used for ankle pressures"). This minimizes the risk of shift-to-shift discrepancies in ABIs.
- *Use sufficient BP cuff inflation.* To ensure complete closure of the artery and the most accurate measurements, inflate cuffs 20 to 30 mm Hg beyond the point at which the last arterial signal is detected.
- *Do not deflate BP cuffs too rapidly.* Try to maintain a deflation rate of 2 to 4 mm Hg/second for patients without dysrhythmias and 2 mm Hg/second or slower for patients with dysrhythmias. Deflating the cuff more rapidly may miss the patient's highest pressure and result in recording an erroneous (low) BP measurement.
- *Be suspicious of arterial pressures recorded at less than 40 mm Hg.* This may mean the venous signal has been mistaken for the arterial signal. If the arterial pressure, which is normally 120 mm Hg, is measured at less than 40 mm Hg, ask a colleague to double-check the findings before recording this as an arterial pressure.
- *Suspect medial calcific sclerosis anytime an ABI is 1.3 or greater or ankle pressure is more than 300 mm Hg.* Medial calcific sclerosis is associated with diabetes mellitus, chronic renal failure, and hyperparathyroidism. It produces falsely elevated ankle pressures by hardening the media of the arteries, making the vessels noncompressible.

(From Cantwell-Gab, K. [1996]. Identifying chronic PAD. *American Journal of Nursing*, 96[1] 40–46, with permission.)

The highest systolic pressure for each ankle (80 mm Hg for the right, 120 mm Hg for the left) would be divided by the highest brachial pressure (160 mm Hg).

Right: 80/160 mm Hg = 0.50 ABI
Left: 120/160 mm Hg = 0.75 ABI

In general, systolic pressure in the ankle of a healthy person is the same or slightly higher than the brachial systolic pressure, resulting in an ABI of about 1.0 (no arterial insufficiency). Patients with claudication usually have an ABI of 0.95 to 0.50 (mild to moderate insufficiency); patients with ischemic rest pain have an ABI of less than 0.50; patients with severe ischemia or tissue loss have an ABI of 0.25 or less.

### Exercise Testing

Exercise testing is used to determine how long a patient can walk and to measure the ankle systolic blood pressure in response to walking. The patient walks on a treadmill at 1.5 mph with a 10% incline for a maximum of 5 minutes. Most patients can complete the test unless they have severe cardiac, pulmonary, or orthopedic problems or a physical disability. A normal response to the test is little or no drop in ankle systolic pressure after exercise. However, in a patient with true claudication, ankle pressure drops. Combining this hemodynamic information with the walking time helps the physician determine whether intervention is necessary.

### Duplex Ultrasonography

**Duplex ultrasonography** involves B-mode gray-scale imaging of the tissue, organs, and blood vessels (arterial and venous) and permits estimation of velocity changes by use of a pulsed Doppler (Fig. 31-5). Color flow techniques, which can identify vessels, may be used to shorten the examination time. The procedure primarily helps determine the level and extent of venous disease. The technique makes it possible to image and assess blood flow, evaluate flow of the distal vessels, locate the disease (stenosis versus occlusion), and determine anatomic morphology and the hemodynamic significance of plaque causing stenosis. Duplex ultrasound findings help in planning therapy and monitoring its outcomes. The test is noninvasive and usually requires no patient preparation. The equipment is portable, making it useful anywhere for initial diagnosis, screening, or follow-up evaluations.

### Computed Tomography

Computed tomography (CT) provides cross-sectional images of soft tissue and visualizes the area of volume changes to an extremity and the compartment where changes take place. CT of a lymphedematous arm or leg, for example,

**FIGURE 31-5.** Color flow duplex image of popliteal artery with normal triphasic Doppler flow.

demonstrates a characteristic honeycomb pattern in the subcutaneous tissue.

In spiral (also called helical) CT, the scan head moves circumferentially around the patient as the patient passes through the scanner, creating a series of overlapping images that are connected to one another in a continuous spiral. In 1998, multidetector CT (MDCT) scanners capable of providing four "slices" or visual pictures per x-ray tube rotation became available. Currently, 9- and 16-slice scanners are available in some imaging centers and hospitals; these provide improved volume coverage speed and/or longitudinal spatial resolution, resulting in improved images (Fishman & Jeffrey, 2004). Scan times are short; however, the patient is exposed to x-rays, and a contrast agent usually must be injected to adequately visualize the blood vessels. Using computer software, the slice-like images are reconstructed into three-dimensional images that can be rotated and viewed from multiple angles.

### Computed Tomography Angiography

In computed tomography angiography (CTA), a spiral CT scanner and rapid intravenous (IV) infusion of contrast agent are used to image very thin (between 1.0 and 1.25 mm) sections of the target area, and the results are configured in three dimensions so that the image closely resembles a regular angiogram. CTA shows the aorta and main arteries better than it shows smaller vessels. Scan times are usually between 20 and 30 seconds. The high volume of contrast agent injected into a peripheral vein limits the usefulness of this study in children and in patients with significantly impaired renal function (Fishman & Jeffrey, 2004).

### Magnetic Resonance Angiography

Magnetic resonance angiography is performed with a standard magnetic resonance imaging (MRI) scanner, but with image-processing software specifically programmed to isolate the blood vessels. The images are reconstructed to resemble a standard angiogram, but because the images are reassembled in three dimensions, they can be rotated and viewed from multiple angles. Because a contrast agent may not be necessary, this study is useful in patients with poor renal function or allergy to contrast agent. The scan time can be long, and motion artifacts are common, requiring postprocessing methods and display techniques not available at every facility (Haaga, Lanziere, & Gilkeson, 2003).

### Angiography

An arteriogram produced by angiography may be used to confirm the diagnosis of occlusive arterial disease when considering surgery or other interventions. It involves injecting a radiopaque contrast agent directly into the vascular system to visualize the vessels. The location of a vascular obstruction or an **aneurysm** (abnormal dilation of a blood vessel) and the collateral circulation can be demonstrated. Typically, the patient experiences a temporary sensation of warmth as the contrast agent is injected, and local irritation may occur at the injection site. Infrequently, a patient may have an immediate or delayed allergic reaction to the iodine contained in the contrast agent. Manifestations include dyspnea, nausea and vomiting, sweating, tachycardia, and numbness of the extremities. Any such reaction must be reported to the physician at once; treatment may include the administration of epinephrine, antihistamines, or corticosteroids. Additional risks include vessel injury, bleeding, and cerebrovascular accident (CVA, brain attack, stroke).

### Air Plethysmography

Air plethysmography is used to quantify venous reflux and calf muscle pump ejection. Changes in leg volumes are measured with the patient's legs elevated, with the patient supine and standing, and after the patient performs toe-ups (the patient extends the ankle while standing; stands on his or her toes) by an air-filled device wrapped around the feet and legs. Air plethysmography provides information about venous filling time, functional venous volume, ejected volume, and residual volume. It is useful in evaluating patients with suspected valvular incompetence or chronic venous insufficiency.

### Contrast Phlebography

Also known as venography, contrast phlebography involves injecting a radiopaque contrast agent into the venous system. If a thrombus exists, the x-ray image reveals an unfilled segment of vein in an otherwise completely filled vein. Injection of the contrast agent may cause brief but painful inflammation of the vein. The test is generally performed if the patient is to undergo thrombolytic therapy, but duplex ultrasonography is now accepted as the standard for diagnosing venous thrombosis.

### Lymphangiography

Lymphangiography provides a way of detecting lymph node involvement resulting from metastatic carcinoma, lymphoma, or infection in sites that are otherwise inaccessible to the examiner except by surgery. In this test, a lymphatic vessel in each foot (or hand) is injected with contrast agent. A series of x-rays are taken at the conclusion of the injection, 24 hours later, and periodically thereafter, as indicated. The failure to identify subcutaneous lymphatic collection of contrast agent and the persistence of contrast agent in the tissue for days afterward help confirm a diagnosis of lymphedema.

### Lymphoscintigraphy

Lymphoscintigraphy is a reliable alternative to lymphangiography. A radioactively labeled colloid is injected subcutaneously in the second interdigital space. The extremity is then exercised to facilitate the uptake of the colloid by the lymphatic system, and serial images are obtained at preset intervals.

## Arterial Disorders

## Arteriosclerosis and Atherosclerosis

**Arteriosclerosis** is the most common disease of the arteries; the term means "hardening of the arteries." It is a diffuse process whereby the muscle fibers and the endothelial lining of the walls of small arteries and arterioles become thickened. **Atherosclerosis** involves a different process, affecting the intima of the large and medium-sized arteries. These changes consist of the accumulation of lipids, calcium, blood components, carbohydrates, and fibrous tissue on the intimal layer of the artery. These accumulations are referred to as atheromas or plaques.

Although the pathologic processes of arteriosclerosis and atherosclerosis differ, rarely does one occur without the other, and the terms are often used interchangeably. Atherosclerosis is a generalized disease of the arteries, and when it is present in the extremities, it is usually present elsewhere in the body.

## Pathophysiology

The most common direct results of atherosclerosis in arteries include narrowing (stenosis) of the lumen, obstruction by thrombosis, aneurysm, ulceration, and rupture. Its indirect results are malnutrition and the subsequent fibrosis of the organs that the sclerotic arteries supply with blood. All actively functioning tissue cells require an abundant supply of nutrients and oxygen and are sensitive to any reduction in the supply of these nutrients. If such reductions are severe and permanent, the cells undergo ischemic necrosis (death of cells due to deficient blood flow) and are replaced by fibrous tissue, which requires much less blood flow.

Atherosclerosis can develop at any point in the body, but certain sites are more vulnerable, such as regions where arteries bifurcate or branch areas. In the proximal lower extremity, these include the distal abdominal aorta, the common iliac arteries, the orifice of the superficial femoral and profunda femoris arteries, and the superficial femoral artery in the adductor canal, which is particularly narrow. Distal to the knee, atherosclerosis can occur anywhere along the artery.

Although many theories exist about the development of atherosclerosis, no single theory explains the pathogenesis completely; however, tenets of several theories are incorporated into the reaction-to-injury theory. According to this theory, vascular endothelial cell injury results from prolonged hemodynamic forces, such as shearing stresses and turbulent flow, irradiation, chemical exposure, or chronic hyperlipidemia. Injury to the endothelium increases the aggregation of platelets and monocytes at the site of the injury. Smooth muscle cells migrate and proliferate, allowing a matrix of collagen and elastic fibers to form. Multiple processes may be involved (Moore, 2002).

Atherosclerotic lesions are of two types: fatty streaks and fibrous plaque:

- Fatty streaks are yellow and smooth, protrude slightly into the lumen of the artery, and are composed of lipids and elongated smooth muscle cells. These lesions have been found in the arteries of people of all age groups, including infants. It is not clear whether fatty streaks predispose a person to the formation of fibrous plaques or whether they are reversible. They do not usually cause clinical symptoms.
- Fibrous plaques are composed of smooth muscle cells, collagen fibers, plasma components, and lipids. They are white to white-yellow and protrude in various degrees into the arterial lumen, sometimes completely obstructing it. These plaques are found predominantly in the abdominal aorta and the coronary, popliteal, and internal carotid arteries, and they are believed to be progressive, irreversible lesions (Fig. 31-6).

Gradual narrowing of the arterial lumen stimulates the development of collateral circulation (Fig. 31-7). Collateral circulation arises from preexisting vessels that enlarge to reroute blood flow around a hemodynamically significant stenosis or occlusion. Collateral flow allows continued per-

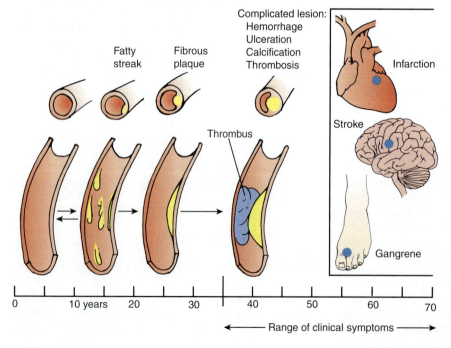

**FIGURE 31-6.** Schematic concept of the progression of atherosclerosis. Fatty streaks constitute one of the earliest lesions of atherosclerosis. Many fatty streaks regress, whereas others progress to fibrous plaques and eventually to atheroma, which may be complicated by hemorrhage, ulceration, calcification, or thrombosis and may produce myocardial infarction, stroke, or gangrene.

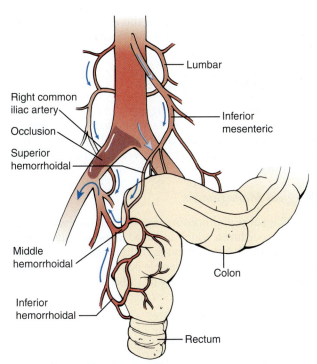

**FIGURE 31-7.** Development of channels for collateral blood flow in response to occlusion of the right common iliac artery and the terminal aortic bifurcation.

fusion to the tissues, but it is often inadequate to meet increased metabolic demand, and ischemia results.

## Risk Factors

Many risk factors are associated with atherosclerosis (Chart 31-2). Although it is not entirely clear whether modification of these risk factors prevents the development of cardiovascular disease, evidence indicates that it may slow the disease process. Some risk factors, such as age, gender, and genetics, cannot be modified (Moore, 2002).

The use of tobacco products may be one of the most important risk factors in the development of atherosclerotic lesions. Nicotine in tobacco decreases blood flow to the extremities and increases heart rate and blood pressure by stimulating the sympathetic nervous system, causing vasoconstriction. It also increases the risk for clot formation by increasing the aggregation of platelets. Carbon monoxide, a toxin produced by burning tobacco, combines more readily with hemoglobin than oxygen does, depriving the tissues of oxygen. The amount of tobacco used is directly related to the extent of the disease, and cessation of tobacco use reduces the risks. Many other factors, such as obesity, stress, and lack of exercise, have been identified as contributing to the disease process.

C-reactive protein (CRP) is a sensitive marker of cardiovascular inflammation, both systemically and locally. Slight increases in serum CRP levels are associated with an increased risk of damage in the vasculature, especially if these increases are accompanied by other risk factors, including increasing age, female gender, hypertension, hypercholesterolemia, obesity, elevated blood glucose levels, smoking, or a positive family history of cardiovascular disease (Stuveling, Hillege, Bakker, et al., 2004).

Hyperhomocysteinemia has been demonstrated in patients with peripheral, cerebrovascular, and coronary artery disease and is now considered an independent risk factor for atherosclerosis. Homocysteine is a protein that promotes coagulation by increasing factor V and factor XI activity while depressing protein C activation and increasing the binding of lipoprotein (a) in fibrin. These processes increase thrombin formation and increase the propensity for thrombosis (Kohlman-Trigoboff, 2003). Some patients may benefit from the combined supplementation of vitamins $B_6$ and $B_{12}$ as well as folate, which may lower homocysteine levels (Fletcher & Fairfield, 2005). However, it is not yet known whether this therapy changes the risk for atherosclerosis associated with hyperhomocysteinemia.

## Prevention

Intermittent claudication is a symptom of generalized atherosclerosis and may be a marker of occult coronary artery disease. Because it is suspected that a high-fat diet contributes to atherosclerosis, it is reasonable to measure serum cholesterol and to begin disease prevention efforts that include diet modification. The American Heart Association recommends reducing the amount of fat ingested in a healthy diet, substituting unsaturated fats for saturated fats, and decreasing cholesterol intake to reduce the risk of cardiovascular disease.

Certain medications that supplement dietary modification and exercise are used to reduce blood lipid levels. The National Cholesterol Education Program (NCEP) has established guidelines for treating hyperlipidemia, with the primary goal of low-density lipoprotein (LDL) levels of less than 100 mg/dL. LDL levels of less than 70 mg/dL are recommended for patients with a history of diabetes, cigarette smoking, atherosclerosis, or hypertension (Grundy, Cleeman, Berz, et al., 2004). Secondary goals include

---

### CHART 31-2

**Risk Factors for Atherosclerosis and Peripheral Arterial Disease**

**Modifiable Risk Factors**
- Nicotine use (ie, tobacco smoking or chewing)
- Diet (contributing to hyperlipidemia)
- Hypertension
- Diabetes mellitus (speeds the atherosclerotic process by thickening the basement membranes of both large and small vessels)
- Obesity
- Stress
- Sedentary lifestyle
- Elevated C-reactive protein
- Hyperhomocysteinemia

**Nonmodifiable Risk Factors**
- Age
- Gender
- Familial predisposition/genetics

achieving total cholesterol levels of less than 200 mg/dL and triglyceride levels less than 150 mg/dL. Medications classified as HMG-CoA reductase inhibitors or "statins," including atorvastatin (Lipitor), lovastatin (Mevacor), pravastatin (Pravachol), and simvastatin (Zocor), are currently first-line treatment and reduce the incidence of major cardiovascular events (Cote, Ligeti, Cutler, et al., 2003). Several other classes of medications used to reduce lipid levels include bile acid sequestrants (cholestyramine [Questran, Prevalite], colesevelam [Welchol], colestipol [Colestid]), nicotinic acid (niacin [Niacor, Niaspan]), fibric acid inhibitors (gemfibrozil [Lopid]), and cholesterol absorption inhibitors (ezetimibe [Zetia]). Patients receiving long-term therapy with these medications require close medical supervision.

Hypertension, which may accelerate the rate at which atherosclerotic lesions form in high-pressure vessels, can lead to CVA (brain attack, stroke), ischemic renal disease, severe peripheral arterial disease, or coronary artery disease. Hypertension is a major risk factor for the development of peripheral arterial disease (PAD), resulting in a twofold risk of development of claudication. All patients with PAD should achieve blood pressure control consistent with the Seventh Report of the Joint National Committee on Prevention, Detection, Evaluation and Treatment of High Blood Pressure (JNC 7) guidelines (systolic blood pressure less than 130 mm Hg; diastolic blood pressure less than 90 mm Hg) (Chobanian, Bakris, Black, et al., 2003).

Although no single risk factor has been identified as the primary contributor to the development of atherosclerotic cardiovascular disease, it is clear that the greater the number of risk factors, the greater the risk of atherosclerosis. Elimination of all controllable risk factors, particularly the use of tobacco products, is strongly recommended.

## Clinical Manifestations

The clinical signs and symptoms resulting from atherosclerosis depend on the organ or tissue affected. Coronary atherosclerosis (heart disease), angina, and acute myocardial infarction are discussed in Chapter 28. Cerebrovascular diseases, including transient cerebral ischemic attacks and stroke, are discussed in Chapter 62. Atherosclerosis of the aorta, including aneurysm, and atherosclerotic lesions of the extremities are discussed later in this chapter. Renovascular disease (renal artery stenosis and end-stage renal disease) is discussed in Chapter 45.

## Medical Management

The traditional medical management of atherosclerosis involves modification of risk factors, a controlled exercise program to improve circulation and its functioning capacity, medication therapy, and interventional or surgical graft procedures.

### Surgical Management

Vascular surgical procedures are divided into two groups: inflow procedures, which improve blood supply from the aorta into the femoral artery, and outflow procedures, which provide blood supply to vessels below the femoral artery. Inflow surgical procedures are described with diseases of the aorta and outflow procedures with peripheral arterial occlusive disease.

### Radiologic Interventions

Several interventional radiologic techniques are important adjunctive therapies to surgical procedures. If an isolated lesion or lesions are identified during the arteriogram, **angioplasty**, also called percutaneous transluminal angioplasty (PTA), may be performed. After the patient receives a local anesthetic, a balloon-tipped catheter is maneuvered across the area of stenosis. Although some clinicians theorize that PTA improves blood flow by overstretching (and thereby dilating) the elastic fibers of the nondiseased arterial segment, most believe that the procedure widens the arterial lumen by "cracking" and flattening the plaque against the vessel wall (see Chapter 28). Complications from PTA include hematoma formation, embolus, **dissection** (separation of the intima) of the vessel, and bleeding. To decrease the risk of reocclusion, stents (small, mesh tubes made of nitinol, titanium, or stainless steel) may be inserted to support the walls of blood vessels and prevent collapse immediately after balloon inflation (Fig. 31-8). A variety of stents and stent-grafts may be used for short-segment stenoses. Complications associated with stent or stent-graft use include

**FIGURE 31-8.** (A) Flexible stent. Courtesy of Medtronics, Peripheral Division, Santa Rosa, California. (B) Representation of a common iliac artery with a Wallstent (Boston Scientific).

distal embolization, intimal damage (dissection), and dislodgment. The advantage of angioplasty, stents, and stent-grafts is the decreased length of hospital stay required for the treatment; many of the procedures are performed on an outpatient basis.

# Nursing Process

## The Patient With Peripheral Arterial Insufficiency of the Extremities

### Assessment

The nursing assessment includes a complete health and medication history and identification of risk factors for PAD. Signs and symptoms detected during the nursing assessment may include claudication pain; rest pain in the forefoot; pallor, rubor, or cyanosis; weak or absent peripheral pulses; and skin breakdown or ulcerations.

### Nursing Diagnosis

Based on assessment data, major nursing diagnoses for the patient may include the following:

- Altered peripheral tissue perfusion related to compromised circulation
- Chronic pain related to impaired ability of peripheral vessels to supply tissues with oxygen
- Risk for impaired skin integrity related to compromised circulation
- Deficient knowledge regarding self-care activities

### Planning and Goals

The major goals for the patient may include increased arterial blood supply to the extremities, promotion of vasodilation, prevention of vascular compression, relief of pain, attainment or maintenance of tissue integrity, and adherence to the self-care program. An overview of the care of a patient with peripheral arterial problems is provided in the Plan of Nursing Care: The Patient With Peripheral Vascular Problems (Chart 31-3).

### Nursing Interventions

#### Improving Peripheral Arterial Circulation

Arterial blood supply to a body part can be enhanced by positioning the part below the level of the heart. For the lower extremities, this is accomplished by elevating the head of the patient's bed on 15-cm (6-inch) blocks or by having the patient use a reclining chair or sit with the feet resting on the floor.

The nurse can assist the patient with walking or other moderate or graded isometric exercises that may be prescribed to promote blood flow and encourage the development of collateral circulation. The nurse instructs the patient to walk to the point of pain, rest until the pain subsides, and then resume walking so that endurance can be increased as collateral circulation develops. Pain can serve as a guide in determining the amount of exercise appropriate for a person. The onset of pain indicates that the tissues are not receiving adequate oxygen, signaling the patient to rest before continuing activity. However, a regular exercise program can result in increased walking distance before the onset of claudication. The amount of exercise a patient can tolerate before the onset of pain is determined to provide a baseline for evaluation.

Not all patients with peripheral vascular disease should exercise. Before recommending any exercise program, the primary health care provider should be consulted. Conditions that worsen with exercise include leg ulcers, cellulitis, gangrene, or acute thrombotic occlusions.

#### Promoting Vasodilation and Preventing Vascular Compression

Arterial dilation promotes increased blood flow to the extremities and is therefore a goal for patients with PAD. However, if the arteries are severely sclerosed, inelastic, or damaged, dilation is not possible. For this reason, measures to promote vasodilation, such as medications or surgery, may be only minimally effective.

Nursing interventions may involve applications of warmth to promote arterial flow and instructions to the patient to avoid exposure to cold temperatures, which causes vasoconstriction. Adequate clothing and warm temperatures protect the patient from chilling. If chilling occurs, a warm bath or drink is helpful. A hot water bottle or heating pad may be applied to the patient's abdomen, causing vasodilation throughout the lower extremities.

In patients with vasospastic disorders (eg, Raynaud's disease), heat may be applied directly to ischemic extremities using a warmed or electric blanket; however, the temperature of the heat source must not exceed body temperature. Even at low temperatures, trauma to the tissues can occur in ischemic extremities. Excess heat may increase the metabolic rate of the extremities and increase the need for oxygen beyond that provided by the reduced arterial flow through the diseased artery.

> **NURSING ALERT**
>
> **Patients are instructed to test the temperature of bath water and to avoid using hot water bottles and heating pads on the extremities. Applying a hot water bottle or a heating pad to the abdomen can cause reflex vasodilation in the extremities and is safer than direct application of heat to affected extremities.**

*(text continues on page 990)*

### CHART 31-3
## Plan of Nursing Care: The Patient With Peripheral Vascular Problems

**Nursing Diagnosis:** Ineffective peripheral tissue perfusion related to compromised circulation
**Goal:** Increased arterial blood supply to extremities

| NURSING INTERVENTIONS | RATIONALE | EXPECTED OUTCOMES |
|---|---|---|
| 1. Lower the extremities below the level of the heart (if condition is arterial in nature). | 1. Dependency of lower extremities enhances arterial blood supply. | • Extremities warm to touch<br>• Color of extremities improved<br>• Experiences decreased muscle pain with exercise |
| 2. Encourage moderate amount of walking or graded extremity exercises if no contraindications exist | 2. Muscular exercise promotes blood flow and the development of collateral circulation. | |

**Goal:** Decrease in venous congestion

| NURSING INTERVENTIONS | RATIONALE | EXPECTED OUTCOMES |
|---|---|---|
| 1. Elevate extremities above heart level (if condition is venous in nature). | 1. Elevation of extremities counteracts gravity, promotes venous return, and prevents venous stasis. | • Elevates lower extremities as prescribed<br>• Decreased edema of extremities<br>• Avoids prolonged standing still or sitting<br>• Gradually increases walking time daily |
| 2. Discourage standing still or sitting for prolonged periods. | 2. Prolonged standing still or sitting promotes venous stasis. | |
| 3. Encourage walking. | 3. Walking promotes venous return by activating the "muscle pump." | |

**Goal:** Promotion of vasodilation and prevention of vascular compression

| NURSING INTERVENTIONS | RATIONALE | EXPECTED OUTCOMES |
|---|---|---|
| 1. Maintain warm temperature and avoid chilling. | 1. Warmth promotes arterial flow by preventing the vasoconstriction effects of chilling. | • Protects extremities from exposure to cold<br>• Avoids all tobacco products<br>• Uses stress-management program to minimize emotional upset<br>• Avoids constricting clothing and accessories<br>• Avoids leg crossing<br>• Takes medication as prescribed |
| 2. Discourage use of tobacco products. | 2. Nicotine in all tobacco products causes vasospasm, which impedes peripheral circulation. | |
| 3. Counsel in ways to avoid emotional upsets; stress management. | 3. Emotional stress causes peripheral vasoconstriction by stimulating the sympathetic nervous system. | |
| 4. Encourage avoidance of constrictive clothing and accessories. | 4. Constrictive clothing and accessories impede circulation and promote venous stasis. | |
| 5. Encourage avoidance of leg crossing. | 5. Leg crossing causes compression of vessels with subsequent impediment of circulation, resulting in venous stasis. | |
| 6. Administer vasodilator medications and adrenergic blocking agents as prescribed, with appropriate nursing considerations. | 6. Vasodilators relax smooth muscle; adrenergic blocking agents block the response to sympathetic nerve impulses or circulating catecholamines. | |

## CHART 31-3

## Plan of Nursing Care: The Patient With Peripheral Vascular Problems (Continued)

**Nursing Diagnosis:** Chronic pain related to impaired ability of peripheral vessels to supply tissues with oxygen
**Goal:** Relief of pain

| NURSING INTERVENTIONS | RATIONALE | EXPECTED OUTCOMES |
|---|---|---|
| 1. Promote increased circulation. | 1. Enhancement of peripheral circulation increases the oxygen supplied to the muscle and decreases the accumulation of metabolites that cause muscle spasms. | • Uses measures to increase arterial blood supply to extremities<br>• Uses analgesics as prescribed |
| 2. Administer analgesics as prescribed, with appropriate nursing considerations. | 2. Analgesics help to reduce pain and allow the patient to participate in activities and exercises that promote circulation. | |

**Nursing Diagnosis:** Risk for impaired skin integrity related to compromised circulation
**Goal:** Attainment/maintenance of tissue integrity

| NURSING INTERVENTIONS | RATIONALE | EXPECTED OUTCOMES |
|---|---|---|
| 1. Instruct in ways to avoid trauma to extremities. | 1. Poorly nourished tissues are susceptible to trauma and bacterial invasion; healing of wounds is delayed or inhibited due to poor tissue perfusion. | • Inspects skin daily for evidence of injury or ulceration<br>• Avoids trauma and irritation to skin<br>• Wears protective shoes<br>• Adheres to meticulous hygiene regimen<br>• Eats a healthy diet that contains adequate protein and vitamins A and C |
| 2. Encourage wearing protective shoes and padding for pressure areas. | 2. Protective shoes and padding prevent foot injuries and blisters. | |
| 3. Encourage meticulous hygiene; bathing with neutral soaps, applying lotions, carefully trimming nails. | 3. Neutral soaps and lotions prevent drying and cracking of skin. | |
| 4. Caution to avoid scratching or vigorous rubbing. | 4. Scratching and rubbing can cause skin abrasions and bacterial invasion. | |
| 5. Promote good nutrition; adequate intake of vitamins A and C, protein, and zinc; control of obesity. | 5. Good nutrition promotes healing and prevents tissue breakdown. | |

**Nursing Diagnosis:** Deficient knowledge regarding self-care activities
**Goal:** Adherence to the self-care program

| NURSING INTERVENTIONS | RATIONALE | EXPECTED OUTCOMES |
|---|---|---|
| 1. Include family/significant others in teaching program. | 1. Adherence to the self-care program is enhanced when the patient receives support from family and from appropriate self-help groups and agencies. | • Practices frequent position changes as prescribed<br>• Practices postural exercises as prescribed<br>• Takes medications as prescribed |

continued >

### CHART 31-3

## Plan of Nursing Care: The Patient With Peripheral Vascular Problems (Continued)

| NURSING INTERVENTIONS | RATIONALE | EXPECTED OUTCOMES |
|---|---|---|
| 2. Provide written instructions about foot care, leg care, and exercise program. | 2. Written instructions serve as reminder and reinforcement of information. | • Avoids vasoconstrictors<br>• Uses measures to prevent trauma<br>• Uses stress management program<br>• Accepts condition as chronic but amenable to therapies that will decrease symptoms |
| 3. Assist to obtain properly fitting clothing, shoes, stockings. | 3. Constrictive clothing and accessories impede circulation and promote venous stasis. | |
| 4. Refer to self-help groups as indicated, such as smoking cessation clinics, stress management, weight management, and exercise program. | 4. Reducing risk factors may reduce symptoms or slow disease progression. | |

Nicotine from tobacco products causes vasospasm and can thereby dramatically reduce circulation to the extremities. Tobacco smoke also impairs transport and cellular use of oxygen and increases blood viscosity. Patients with arterial insufficiency who use tobacco (ie, smoke, chew) must be fully informed of the effects of nicotine on circulation and encouraged to stop using tobacco.

Emotional upsets stimulate the sympathetic nervous system, resulting in peripheral vasoconstriction. Emotional stress can be minimized to some degree by avoiding stressful situations when possible or by consistently following a stress-management program. Counseling services or relaxation training may be indicated for people who cannot cope effectively with situational stressors.

Constrictive clothing and accessories such as tight socks, panty girdles, and shoelaces impede circulation to the extremities and promote venous stasis and therefore should be avoided. Crossing the legs should be discouraged because it compresses vessels in the legs.

### Relieving Pain

Frequently, the pain associated with peripheral arterial insufficiency is chronic, continuous, and disabling. It limits activities, affects work and responsibilities, disturbs sleep, and alters the patient's sense of well-being. Patients are often depressed, irritable, and unable to exert the energy necessary to execute prescribed therapies, making pain relief even more difficult. Analgesics such as oxycodone plus acetylsalicylic acid (Percodan) or oxycodone plus acetaminophen (Percocet) may be helpful in reducing pain so that the patient can participate in therapies that can increase circulation and ultimately relieve pain more effectively.

### Maintaining Tissue Integrity

Poorly perfused tissues are susceptible to damage and infection. When lesions develop, healing may be delayed or inhibited because of the poor blood supply to the area. Infected, nonhealing ulcerations of the extremities can be debilitating and may require prolonged and often expensive treatments. Amputation of an ischemic limb may eventually be necessary. Measures to prevent these complications must be a high priority and vigorously implemented.

Trauma to the extremities must be avoided. Advising the patient to wear sturdy, well-fitting shoes or slippers to prevent foot injury and blisters may be helpful, and recommending neutral soaps and body lotions may prevent drying and cracking of skin. Scratching and vigorous rubbing can abrade skin and create sites for bacterial invasion; therefore, feet should be patted dry. Stockings should be clean and dry. Fingernails and toenails should be carefully trimmed straight across and sharp corners filed to follow the contour of the nail. If nails are thick and brittle and cannot be trimmed safely, a podiatrist must be consulted. Corns and calluses need to be removed by a health care professional. Special shoe inserts may be needed to prevent calluses from recurring. All signs of blisters, ingrown toenails, infection, or other problems should be reported to health care professionals for treatment and follow-up. Patients with diminished vision and those with disorders that limit mobility of the arms or legs may require assistance in periodically examining the lower extremities for trauma or evidence of inflammation or infection.

Good nutrition promotes healing and prevents tissue breakdown and is therefore included in the overall therapeutic program for patients with peripheral vascular disease. Eating a well-balanced diet that contains adequate protein and vitamins is necessary for patients with arterial insufficiency. Key nutrients play specific roles in wound healing. Vitamin C is essential for collagen synthesis and capillary development. Vitamin A enhances epithelialization. Zinc is necessary for cell mitosis and cell proliferation. Obesity strains the heart, increases venous congestion, and reduces circulation;

# CHAPTER 31 • Assessment and Management of Patients With Vascular Disorders and Problems of Peripheral Circulation

therefore, a weight-reduction plan may be necessary for some patients. A diet low in lipids may be indicated for patients with atherosclerosis.

## Promoting Home and Community-Based Care

The self-care program is planned with the patient so that activities that promote arterial and venous circulation, relieve pain, and promote tissue integrity are acceptable. The patient and family are helped to understand the reasons for each aspect of the program, the possible consequences of nonadherence, and the importance of keeping follow-up appointments. Long-term care of the feet and legs is of prime importance in the prevention of trauma, ulceration, and gangrene. Chart 31-3 describes nursing care for patients with peripheral vascular disease. Chart 31-4 provides detailed patient instructions for foot and leg care.

## Evaluation

### Expected Patient Outcomes

Expected patient outcomes may include:

1. Demonstrates an increase in arterial blood supply to extremities
   a. Exhibits extremities warm to touch
   b. Has improved color of extremities (ie, free of rubor or cyanosis)

---

### CHART 31-4

### HOME CARE CHECKLIST • Foot and Leg Care in Peripheral Vascular Disease

| At the completion of the home care instruction, the patient or caregiver will be able to: | Patient | Caregiver |
|---|:---:|:---:|
| • Demonstrate daily foot bathing: Wash between toes with mild soap and lukewarm water, then rinse thoroughly and pat rather than rub dry. | ✓ | ✓ |
| • Recognize the dangers of thermal injury:<br>– Wear clean, loose, soft cotton socks (they are comfortable, allow air to circulate, and absorb moisture)<br>– In cold weather, wear extra socks in extra-large shoes.<br>– Avoid heating pads, whirlpools, and hot tubs.<br>– Avoid sunburn. | ✓ | |
| • Identify safety concerns:<br>– Inspect feet daily with a mirror for redness, dryness, cuts, blisters, etc.<br>– Always wear soft shoes or slippers when out of bed.<br>– Trim nails straight across after showering.<br>– Consult podiatrist to trim nails if vision is decreased; also for care of corns, blisters, ingrown nails.<br>– Clear pathways in house to prevent injury.<br>– Avoid wearing thong sandals.<br>– Use lamb's wool between toes if they overlap or rub each other. | ✓ | ✓ |
| • Demonstrate use of comfort measures:<br>– Wear leather shoes with an extra-depth toebox. Synthetic shoes do not allow air to circulate.<br>– If feet become dry and scaly, use cream with lanolin. Never put cream between toes.<br>– If feet perspire, especially between toes, use powder daily and/or lamb's wool between toes to promote drying. | ✓ | |
| • Demonstrate strategies to decrease risk of constricting blood vessels:<br>– Avoid circular compression around feet or knees—for example, by applying knee-high stockings or tight socks.<br>– Do not cross legs at knees.<br>– Stop using all tobacco products (ie, smoking or chewing) because nicotine causes vasoconstriction and vasospasm.<br>– Avoid applying tight, constricting bandages.<br>– Participate in a regular walking exercise program to stimulate circulation. | ✓ | |
| • Recognize when to seek medical attention:<br>– Contact health care provider at the onset of skin breakdown such as abrasions, blisters, fungus infection (athlete's foot), or pain.<br>– Do not use any medication on feet or legs unless prescribed.<br>– Avoid using iodine, alcohol, corn/wart-removing compound, or adhesive products before checking with health care provider. | ✓ | ✓ |

c. Experiences decreased muscle pain with exercise
   d. Demonstrates an increase in walking distance or duration
2. Promotes vasodilation; prevents vascular compression
   a. Protects extremities from exposure to cold
   b. Avoids use of tobacco
   c. Uses stress-management strategies to minimize emotional upset
   d. Wears nonconstricting clothing
   e. Avoids leg crossing
   f. Takes medications as prescribed
3. Has decrease in severity and duration of pain
4. Attains or maintains tissue integrity
   a. Avoids trauma and irritation to skin
   b. Wears protective shoes
   c. Adheres to meticulous hygiene regimen
   d. Eats a healthy diet that contains adequate protein, vitamins A and C, and zinc
   e. Performs self-care activities

## Peripheral Arterial Occlusive Disease

Arterial insufficiency of the extremities occurs most often in men and is a common cause of disability. The legs are most frequently affected; however, the upper extremities may be involved. The age of onset and the severity are influenced by the type and number of atherosclerotic risk factors (see Chart 31-2). In PAD, obstructive lesions are predominantly confined to segments of the arterial system extending from the aorta below the renal arteries to the popliteal artery (Fig. 31-9). Distal occlusive disease is frequently seen in patients with diabetes mellitus and in elderly patients.

## Clinical Manifestations

The hallmark symptom is intermittent claudication. This pain may be described as aching, cramping, or inducing fatigue or weakness that occurs with the same degree of exercise or activity and is relieved with rest. The pain commonly occurs in muscle groups distal to the area of stenosis or occlusion. As the disease progresses, the patient may have a decreased ability to walk the same distance as previously or may notice increased pain with ambulation. When the arterial insufficiency becomes severe, the patient has rest pain. This pain is associated with critical ischemia of the distal extremity and is persistent, aching, or boring; it may be so excruciating that it is unrelieved by opioids and is disabling. Ischemic rest pain is usually worse at night and often wakes the patient. Elevating the extremity or placing it in a horizontal position increases the pain, whereas placing the extremity in a dependent position reduces the pain. Some patients sleep with the affected leg hanging over the side of the bed. Some patients sleep in a reclining chair in an attempt to prevent or relieve the pain.

## Assessment and Diagnostic Findings

A sensation of coldness or numbness in the extremities may accompany intermittent claudication and is a result of reduced arterial flow. The extremity is cool and pale when elevated or ruddy and cyanotic when placed in a dependent position. Skin and nail changes, ulcerations, gangrene, and muscle atrophy may be evident. Bruits may be auscultated with a stethoscope. Peripheral pulses may be diminished or absent.

Examination of the peripheral pulses is an important part of assessing arterial occlusive disease. Unequal pulses between extremities or the absence of a normally palpable pulse is a sign of PAD.

The presence, location, and extent of arterial occlusive disease are determined by a careful history of the symptoms and by physical examination. The color and temperature of the extremity are noted and the pulses palpated. The nails may be thickened and opaque, and the skin may be shiny, atrophic, and dry, with sparse hair growth. The assessment includes comparison of the right and left extremities.

The diagnosis of peripheral arterial occlusive disease may be made using CW Doppler and ABIs, treadmill testing for claudication, duplex ultrasonography, or other imaging studies previously described.

## Medical Management

Generally, patients feel better with some type of exercise program. If this program is combined with weight reduction and cessation of tobacco use, patients often can improve their activity tolerance. Patients should not be promised that their symptoms will be relieved if they stop tobacco use, because claudication may persist, and they may lose their motivation to stop using tobacco.

### Pharmacologic Therapy

Pentoxifylline (Trental) and cilostazol (Pletal) are the only medications specifically indicated for the treatment of claudication. Pentoxifylline increases erythrocyte flexibility, lowers blood fibrinogen concentrations, and has antiplatelet effects. However, recent meta-analyses have questioned the overall efficacy of this medication (Treat-Jacobson & Walsh, 2003). Cilostazol is a phosphodiesterase III inhibitor that is a vasodilator and that thwarts platelet aggregation.

Antiplatelet agents such as aspirin or clopidogrel (Plavix) help prevent the formation of thromboemboli, which can lead to myocardial infarction and stroke. Aspirin has been shown to reduce the risk of myocardial infarction, stroke, and death in patients with vascular disease; however, adverse events associated with aspirin use include gastrointestinal upset or bleeding. Clopidogrel is indicated for the prevention of cardiovascular ischemic events in patients with PAD but not for the treatment of claudication symptoms.

### Surgical Management

In most patients, when intermittent claudication becomes severe and disabling or when the limb is at risk for amputation because of tissue necrosis, vascular grafting or endarterectomy is the treatment of choice. The choice of the surgical procedure depends on the degree and location of the stenosis or occlusion. Other important considerations are the overall health of the patient and the length of the procedure that can be tolerated. It is sometimes necessary

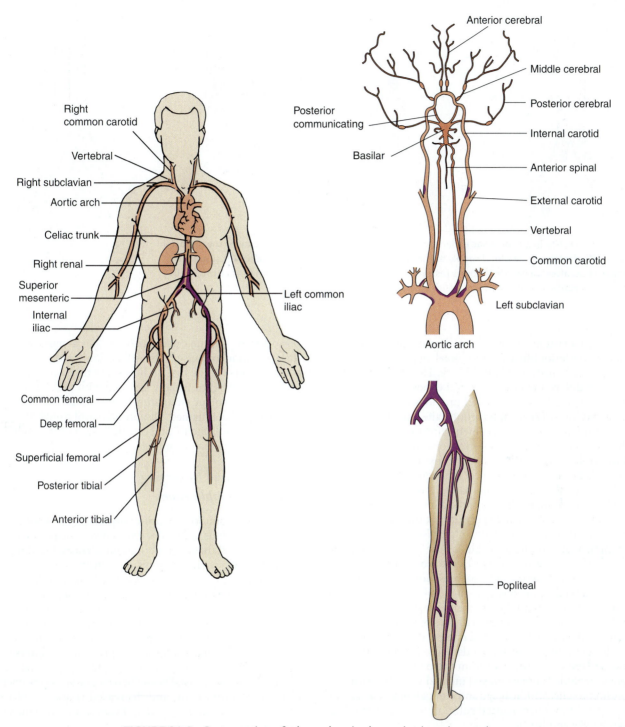

**FIGURE 31-9.** Common sites of atherosclerotic obstruction in major arteries.

to provide the palliative therapy of primary amputation rather than an arterial bypass. If endarterectomy is performed, an incision is made into the artery and the atheromatous obstruction is removed (Fig. 31-10).

Bypass grafts are performed to reroute the blood flow around the stenosis or occlusion. Before bypass grafting, the surgeon determines where the distal **anastomosis** (site where the vessels are surgically joined) will be placed. The distal outflow vessel must be at least 50% patent for the graft to remain patent. A higher bypass graft patency rate is associated with keeping the length of the bypass as short as possible (Rutherford, 2005).

If the atherosclerotic occlusion is below the inguinal ligament in the superficial femoral artery, the surgical procedure of choice is the femoral-to-popliteal graft. This procedure is further classified as above-knee and below-knee grafts, referring to the location of the distal anastomosis.

Lower leg or ankle vessels with occlusions may also require grafts. Occasionally, the popliteal artery is completely occluded and only collateral vessels maintain perfusion.

**FIGURE 31-10.** In an aortoiliac endarterectomy, the vascular surgeon (**A**) identifies the diseased area, (**B**) clamps off the blood supply to the vessel, (**C**) removes the plaque, and (**D**) sutures the vessel shut, after which blood flow is restored. Adapted with permission from Rutherford, R. B. (2005). *Vascular surgery: Vol. 1 and 2* (6th ed.). Philadelphia: Elsevier.

The distal anastomosis may be made onto any of the tibial arteries (posterior tibial, anterior tibial, or peroneal arteries) or the dorsalis pedis or plantar artery. The distal anastomosis site is determined by the ease of exposure of the vessel in surgery and by which vessel provides the best flow to the distal limb. These grafts require the use of native vein (ie, autologous; the patient's own vein) to ensure patency. The greater or lesser saphenous vein or a combination of one of the saphenous veins and an upper extremity vein such as the cephalic vein is used to meet the required length.

How long the graft remains patent is determined by several factors, including the size of the graft, graft location, and development of intimal hyperplasia at anastomosis sites. Bypass grafts may be synthetic or autologous vein. Several synthetic materials are available for use as a peripheral bypass graft: woven or knitted Dacron or expanded polytetrafluoroethylene (ePTFE, such as Gore-Tex or Impra). Cryopreserved saphenous veins and umbilical veins are also available. Infection can be a problem that threatens survival of the graft and almost always requires removal of the graft.

If a vein graft is the surgical choice, care must be taken in the operating room not to damage the vein after harvesting (removing the vein from the patient's body). The vein is occluded at one end and inflated with a heparinized solution to check for leakage and competency. The graft is then placed in a heparinized solution to keep it from becoming dry and brittle.

## Nursing Management

### Maintaining Circulation

The primary objective in the postoperative period is to maintain adequate circulation through the arterial repair. Pulses, Doppler assessment, color and temperature, capillary refill, and sensory and motor function of the affected extremity are checked and compared with those of the other extremity; these values are recorded every hour for the first 8 hours and then every 2 hours for 24 hours. Doppler evaluation of the vessels distal to the bypass graft should be performed for all postoperative vascular patients because it is more sensitive than palpation for pulses. The ABI is monitored at least once every 8 hours for the first 24 hours and then once each day until discharge (not usually assessed with pedal artery bypasses). An adequate circulating blood volume should be established and maintained. Disappearance of a pulse that was present may indicate thrombotic occlusion of the graft; the surgeon is immediately notified.

### Monitoring and Managing Potential Complications

Continuous monitoring of urine output, central venous pressure, mental status, and pulse rate and volume permits early recognition and treatment of fluid imbalances. Bleeding can result from the heparin administered during surgery or from an anastomotic leak. A hematoma may form as well.

Leg crossing and prolonged extremity dependency are avoided to prevent thrombosis. Edema is a normal postoperative finding; however, elevating the extremities and encouraging the patient to exercise the extremities while in bed reduces edema. Elastic compression stockings may be prescribed for some patients, but care must be taken to avoid compressing distal vessel bypass grafts. Severe edema of the extremity, pain, and decreased sensation of toes or fingers can be an indication of compartment syndrome (see Chapter 69).

### Promoting Home and Community-Based Care

Discharge planning includes assessing the patient's ability to manage activities of daily living (ADLs) independently. The nurse determines whether the patient has a network of family and friends to assist with ADLs. The patient is encouraged to make the lifestyle changes necessitated by the onset of a chronic disease, including pain management and modifications in diet, activity, and hygiene (skin care). The nurse ensures that the patient has the knowledge and ability to assess for any postoperative complications such as infection, occlusion of the artery or graft, and decreased blood flow.

The nurse assists the patient in developing and implementing a plan to stop using tobacco. Nursing care for patients with peripheral vascular disease is described in Chart 31-3.

## Upper Extremity Arterial Occlusive Disease

Arterial occlusions occur less frequently in the upper extremities (arms) than in the legs and cause less severe symptoms because the collateral circulation is significantly better in the arms. The arms also have less muscle mass and are not subjected to the workload of the legs.

### Clinical Manifestations

Stenosis and occlusions in the upper extremity result from atherosclerosis or trauma. The stenosis usually occurs at the origin of the vessel proximal to the vertebral artery, setting up the vertebral artery as the major contributor of flow. The patient typically complains of arm fatigue and pain with exercise (forearm claudication) and inability to hold or grasp objects (eg, painting, combing hair, placing objects on shelves above the head) and occasionally difficulty driving.

The patient may develop a "subclavian steal" syndrome characterized by reverse flow in the vertebral and basilar artery to provide blood flow to the arm. This syndrome may cause vertebrobasilar (cerebral) symptoms, including vertigo, ataxia, syncope, or bilateral visual changes.

### Assessment and Diagnostic Findings

Assessment findings include coolness and pallor of the affected extremity, decreased capillary refill, and a difference in arm blood pressures of more than 20 mm Hg. Noninvasive studies performed to evaluate for upper extremity arterial occlusions include upper and forearm blood pressure determinations and duplex ultrasonography to identify the anatomic location of the lesion and to evaluate the hemodynamics of the blood flow. Transcranial Doppler evaluation is performed to evaluate the intracranial circulation and to detect any siphoning of blood flow from the posterior circulation to provide blood flow to the affected arm. If a surgical or interventional procedure is planned, an arteriogram may be necessary.

### Medical Management

If a short, focal lesion is identified in an upper extremity artery, a PTA may be performed. If the lesion involves the subclavian artery with documented siphoning of blood flow from the intracranial circulation, several surgical procedures are available: carotid–to–subclavian artery bypass, axillary–to–axillary artery bypass, and autogenous reimplantation of the subclavian to the carotid artery.

### Nursing Management

Nursing assessment involves bilateral comparison of upper arm blood pressures (obtained by stethoscope and Doppler); radial, ulnar, and brachial pulses; motor and sensory function; temperature; color changes; and capillary refill every 2 hours. Disappearance of a pulse or Doppler flow that had been present may indicate an acute occlusion of the vessel, and the physician is notified immediately.

After surgery, the arm is kept at heart level or elevated, with the fingers at the highest level. Pulses are monitored with Doppler assessment of the arterial flow every hour for 8 hours and then every 2 hours for 24 hours. Blood pressure (obtained by stethoscope and Doppler) is also assessed every hour for 8 hours and then every 2 hours for 24 hours. Motor and sensory function, warmth, color, and capillary refill are monitored with each arterial flow (pulse) assessment.

> **NURSING ALERT**
>
> Before and for 24 hours after surgery, the patient's arm is kept at heart level and protected from cold, venipunctures or arterial sticks, tape, and constrictive dressings.

Discharge planning includes assessing the patient's ability to manage ADLs independently. The nurse determines whether the patient has a network of family and friends to assist with ADLs. The patient may need to make the lifestyle changes necessary to accommodate a chronic disease, including pain management and modifications in diet, activity, and hygiene (skin care). The nurse ensures that the patient has the knowledge and ability to assess for any postoperative complications such as infection, reocclusion of the artery or occlusion of the graft, and decreased blood flow. The patient is assisted in developing and implementing a plan to stop using tobacco. Chart 31-3 describes nursing care for patients with peripheral vascular disease.

## Thromboangiitis Obliterans (Buerger's Disease)

Buerger's disease is characterized by recurring inflammation of the intermediate and small arteries and veins of the lower and (in rare cases) upper extremities. It results in thrombus formation and occlusion of the vessels. It is differentiated from other vessel diseases by its microscopic appearance. In contrast to atherosclerosis, Buerger's disease is believed to be an autoimmune disease that results in occlusion of distal vessels.

The cause of Buerger's disease is unknown, but it is believed to be an autoimmune vasculitis. It occurs most often in men between 20 and 35 years of age, and it has been reported in all races and in many areas of the world. There is considerable evidence that heavy smoking or chewing of tobacco is a causative or an aggravating factor (Mills, 2003). Generally, the lower extremities are affected, but arteries in the upper extremities or viscera can also be involved. Buerger's disease is generally bilateral and symmetric with focal lesions. Superficial thrombophlebitis may be present.

## Clinical Manifestations

Pain is the outstanding symptom of Buerger's disease. The patient complains of foot cramps, especially of the arch (instep claudication), after exercise. The pain is relieved by rest; often, a burning pain is aggravated by emotional disturbances, nicotine, or chilling. Cold sensitivity of the Raynaud type is found in half the patients and is frequently confined to the hands. Digital rest pain is constant, and the characteristics of the pain do not change between activity and rest.

Physical signs include intense rubor (reddish-blue discoloration) of the foot and absence of the pedal pulse, but with normal femoral and popliteal pulses. Radial and ulnar artery pulses are absent or diminished. Various types of paresthesias may develop.

As the disease progresses, definite redness or cyanosis of the part appears when the extremity is in a dependent position. Involvement is generally bilateral, but color changes may affect only one extremity or only certain digits. Color changes may progress to ulceration, and ulceration with gangrene eventually occurs.

## Assessment and Diagnostic Findings

Segmental limb blood pressures are taken to demonstrate the distal location of the lesions or occlusions. Duplex ultrasonography is used to document patency of the proximal vessels and to visualize the extent of distal disease. Contrast angiography is used to identify the diseased portion of the anatomy.

### Gerontologic Considerations

Although Buerger's disease is different from atherosclerosis, it may be accompanied by atherosclerosis of the larger vessels. The patient's ability to walk may be severely limited. Patients are at higher risk for nonhealing wounds because of impaired circulation.

## Medical Management

The treatment of Buerger's disease is essentially the same as that for atherosclerotic peripheral arterial disease. The main objectives are to improve circulation to the extremities, prevent the progression of the disease, and protect the extremities from trauma and infection. Treatment of ulceration and gangrene is directed toward minimizing infection and conservative débridement of necrotic tissue. Tobacco use is highly detrimental, and patients are strongly advised to completely stop using tobacco. Symptoms are often relieved by cessation of tobacco use.

Vasodilators are rarely prescribed because these medications cause dilation of only healthy vessels; vasodilators may divert blood away from the partially occluded vessels, thus exacerbating the manifestations of the disease. A regional sympathetic block or ganglionectomy may be useful in some instances to produce vasodilation and increase blood flow.

If gangrene of a toe develops as a result of arterial occlusive disease in the leg, it is unlikely that toe amputation or even transmetatarsal amputation will be sufficient; often, a below-knee amputation or occasionally an above-knee amputation is necessary. The indications for amputation include gangrene, especially if the infected area is moist; severe rest pain; or fulminating sepsis.

## Nursing Management

The patient is assisted in developing and implementing a plan to stop using tobacco and to manage pain. The patient may need to be encouraged to make the lifestyle changes necessary to adequately manage a chronic disease, including modifications in diet, activity, and hygiene (skin care). The nurse determines whether the patient has a network of family and friends to assist with ADLs. The nurse ensures that the patient has the knowledge and ability to assess for any postoperative complications such as infection and decreased blood flow. Chart 31-3 describes nursing care for patients with peripheral vascular disease. Nursing management during the immediate postoperative phase after amputation and through the rehabilitation phase is described in Chapter 69.

## *Aortitis*

The aorta, which is the main trunk of the arterial system, is divided into the ascending aorta (contained in the pericardium), the aortic arch (extending upward, backward, and downward), and the descending aorta. The thoracic aorta is located above the diaphragm; the abdominal aorta is located below the diaphragm. The abdominal aorta is further designated as suprarenal (above renal artery level), perirenal level (at renal artery level), and infrarenal (below renal artery level).

Aortitis is inflammation of the aorta, particularly of the aortic arch. Two types are known to occur: Takayasu's disease (occlusive thromboaortopathy) and syphilitic aortitis. Both are rare.

Takayasu's disease, a chronic inflammatory disease of the aortic arch and its branches, primarily affects young or middle-aged women and is more common in those of Asian descent. It is nonatherosclerotic; the exact pathologic mechanism is unknown but is thought to be immune complex mediated. It progresses from a systemic inflammatory response with localized arteritis to end-organ ischemia because of large vessel stenosis or obstruction. Magnetic resonance angiography (MRA), CT, duplex ultrasonography, or arteriography is used to diagnose and evaluate the lesions, which are typically long, smooth areas of narrowing with or without aneurysms. The primary goal of treatment is to suppress the vascular inflammatory response. This may be achieved by administering a corticosteroid such as prednisone (Deltasone), 45 to 60 mg orally daily. Selective PTA and surgical revascularization may be performed after suppression of the systemic vascular inflammation.

## *Aortoiliac Disease*

If collateral circulation has developed, patients with a stenosis or occlusion of the aortoiliac segment may be asymptomatic, or they may complain of buttock or low back discomfort associated with walking. Men may experience impotence. These patients may have decreased or absent femoral pulses.

## Medical Management

The treatment of aortoiliac disease is essentially the same as that for atherosclerotic peripheral arterial occlusive disease. The surgical procedure of choice is the aortoiliac graft. If possible, the distal graft is anastomosed to the iliac artery, and the entire surgical procedure is performed within the abdomen. If the iliac vessels are diseased, the distal anastomosis is made to the femoral arteries (aortobifemoral graft). Bifurcated woven or knitted Dacron grafts are preferred for this surgical procedure.

## Nursing Management

Preoperative assessment, in addition to the standard parameters (see Chapter 18), includes evaluating the brachial, radial, ulnar, femoral, posterior tibial, and dorsalis pedis pulses to establish a baseline for follow-up after arterial lines are placed and postoperatively. Patient teaching includes an overview of the procedure to be performed, the preparation for surgery, and the anticipated postoperative plan of care. Sights, sounds, and sensations that the patient may experience are discussed.

Postoperative care includes monitoring for signs of thrombosis in arteries distal to the surgical site. The nurse assesses color and temperature of the extremity, capillary refill time, sensory and motor function, and pulses by palpation and Doppler every hour for the first 8 hours and then every 2 hours for the first 24 hours. Any dusky or bluish discoloration, coolness, capillary refill time greater than 2 seconds, decrease in sensory or motor function, or decrease in pulse quality is reported immediately to the physician.

Postoperative care also includes monitoring urine output and ensuring that output is at least 30 mL/hour. Renal function may be impaired as a result of hypoperfusion from hypotension, ischemia to the renal arteries during the surgical procedure, hypovolemia, or embolization of the renal artery or renal parenchyma. Vital signs, pain, and intake and output are monitored with the pulse and extremity assessments. Results of laboratory tests are monitored and reported to the physician. Abdominal assessment for bowel sounds and paralytic ileus is performed at least every 8 hours. Bowel sounds may not return before the third postoperative day. The absence of bowel sounds, absence of flatus, and abdominal distention are indications of paralytic ileus. Manual manipulation of the bowel during surgery may have caused bruising, resulting in decreased peristalsis. Nasogastric suction may be necessary to decompress the bowel until peristalsis returns. A liquid bowel movement before the third postoperative day may indicate bowel ischemia, which may occur when the mesenteric blood supply (celiac, superior mesenteric, or inferior mesenteric arteries) is occluded. Ischemic bowel usually causes increased pain and a markedly elevated white blood cell count (20,000 to 30,000 cells/mm$^3$).

## Aneurysm

An aneurysm is a localized sac or dilation formed at a weak point in the wall of the artery (Fig. 31-11). It may be classified by its shape or form. The most common forms of aneurysms are saccular and fusiform. A saccular aneurysm projects from one side of the vessel only. If an entire arterial segment becomes dilated, a fusiform aneurysm develops. Very small aneurysms due to localized infection are called mycotic aneurysms.

Historically, the cause of abdominal aortic aneurysm, the most common type of degenerative aneurysm, has been attributed to atherosclerotic changes in the aorta. Other causes of aneurysm formation are listed in Chart 31-5. Aneurysms are serious because they can rupture, leading to hemorrhage and death.

## Thoracic Aortic Aneurysm

Approximately 85% of all cases of thoracic aortic aneurysm are caused by atherosclerosis. They occur most frequently in men between the ages of 40 and 70 years. The thoracic area is the most common site for a dissecting aneurysm. About one third of patients with thoracic aneurysms die of rupture of the aneurysm (Rutherford, 2005).

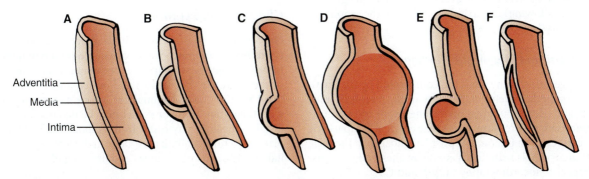

**FIGURE 31-11.** Characteristics of arterial aneurysm. (**A**) Normal artery. (**B**) False aneurysm—actually a pulsating hematoma. The clot and connective tissue are outside the arterial wall. (**C**) True aneurysm. One, two, or all three layers of the artery may be involved. (**D**) Fusiform aneurysm—symmetric, spindle-shaped expansion of entire circumference of involved vessel. (**E**) Saccular aneurysm—a bulbous protrusion of one side of the arterial wall. (**F**) Dissecting aneurysm—this usually is a hematoma that splits the layers of the arterial wall.

> **CHART 31-5**
>
> ### Etiologic Classification of Arterial Aneurysms
>
> **Congenital:** Primary connective tissue disorders (Marfan's syndrome, Ehlers-Danlos syndrome) and other diseases (focal medial agenesis, tuberous sclerosis, Turner's syndrome, Menkes' syndrome)
>
> **Mechanical (hemodynamic):** Poststenotic and arteriovenous fistula and amputation-related
>
> **Traumatic (pseudoaneurysms):** Penetrating arterial injuries, blunt arterial injuries, pseudoaneurysms
>
> **Inflammatory (noninfectious):** Associated with arteritis (Takayasu's disease, giant cell arteritis, systemic lupus erythematosus, Behçet's syndrome, Kawasaki's disease) and periarterial inflammation (ie, pancreatitis)
>
> **Infectious (mycotic):** Bacterial, fungal, spirochetal infections
>
> **Pregnancy-related degenerative:** Nonspecific, inflammatory variant
>
> **Anastomotic (postarteriotomy) and graft aneurysms:** Infection, arterial wall failure, suture failure, graft failure
>
> Adapted with permission from Rutherford, R. B. (2005). *Vascular surgery* (Vols. 1 and 2, 6th ed.). Philadelphia: W. B. Saunders.

## Clinical Manifestations

Symptoms are variable and depend on how rapidly the aneurysm dilates and how the pulsating mass affects surrounding intrathoracic structures. Some patients are asymptomatic. In most cases, pain is the most prominent symptom. The pain is usually constant and boring but may occur only when the person is supine. Other conspicuous symptoms are dyspnea, the result of pressure of the aneurysm sac against the trachea, a main bronchus, or the lung itself; cough, frequently paroxysmal and with a brassy quality; hoarseness, stridor, or weakness or complete loss of the voice (aphonia), resulting from pressure against the laryngeal nerve; and dysphagia (difficulty in swallowing) due to impingement on the esophagus by the aneurysm.

## Assessment and Diagnostic Findings

When large veins in the chest are compressed by the aneurysm, the superficial veins of the chest, neck, or arms become dilated, and edematous areas on the chest wall and cyanosis are often evident. Pressure against the cervical sympathetic chain can result in unequal pupils. Diagnosis of a thoracic aortic aneurysm is principally made by chest x-ray, transesophageal echocardiography (TEE), and CT.

## Medical Management

In most cases, an aneurysm is treated by surgical repair. General measures such as controlling blood pressure and correcting risk factors may be helpful. It is important to control blood pressure in patients with dissecting aneurysms. Systolic pressure is maintained at about 100 to 120 mm Hg with antihypertensive medications (eg, hydralazine [Apresoline], or a beta-blocker such as esmolol [Brevibloc] or metoprolol [Lopressor]). Sodium nitroprusside (Nipride) may be used by continuous IV drip to emergently lower the blood pressure. The goal of surgery is to repair the aneurysm and restore vascular continuity with a vascular graft (Fig. 31-12). Intensive monitoring is usually required after this type of surgery, and the patient is cared for in the critical care unit. Repair of thoracic aneurysms using endovascular grafts implanted (deployed) percutaneously in an interventional suite (eg, interventional radiology, cardiac catheterization laboratory) or an operating room may decrease postoperative recovery time and decrease complications compared with traditional surgical techniques. Thoracic endografts are made of similar materials as in aortic endografts, such as Gore-Tex or PTFE material reinforced with stents (nitinol, titanium). These endovascular grafts are inserted into the thoracic aorta via various vascular access routes, including the femoral or iliac artery. Because a large operative incision is not necessary to gain vascular access, the overall patient recovery time tends to be shorter than if the patient had open surgical repair.

# Abdominal Aortic Aneurysm

The most common cause of abdominal aortic aneurysm is atherosclerosis. The condition, which is more common among Caucasians, affects men four times more often than women and is most prevalent in elderly patients (Rutherford, 2005). Most of these aneurysms occur below the renal arteries (infrarenal aneurysms). Untreated, the eventual outcome may be rupture and death.

## Pathophysiology

All aneurysms involve a damaged media layer of the vessel. This may be caused by congenital weakness, trauma, or disease. After an aneurysm develops, it tends to enlarge. Risk factors include genetic predisposition, tobacco use, and hypertension; more than half of patients with aneurysms have hypertension.

## Clinical Manifestations

Only about 40% of patients with abdominal aortic aneurysms have symptoms. Some patients complain that they can feel their heart beating in their abdomen when lying down, or they may say they feel an abdominal mass or abdominal throbbing. If the abdominal aortic aneurysm is associated with thrombus, a major vessel may be occluded or smaller distal occlusions may result from emboli. Small cholesterol, platelet, or fibrin emboli may lodge in the interosseous or digital arteries, causing cyanosis and mottling of the toes.

## Assessment and Diagnostic Findings

The most important diagnostic indication of an abdominal aortic aneurysm is a pulsatile mass in the middle and upper abdomen. About 80% of these aneurysms can be palpated. A systolic bruit may be heard over the mass. Duplex ultra-

**FIGURE 31-12.** Repair of an ascending aortic aneurysm and aortic valve replacement. (**A**) Incision into aortic aneurysm. (**B**) Aortic valve replacement with aortic graft implant to repair ascending aortic aneurysm. (**C**) Aortic aneurysm trimmed and closed over graft.

sonography or CT is used to determine the size, length, and location of the aneurysm (Fig. 31-13). When the aneurysm is small, ultrasonography is conducted at 6-month intervals until the aneurysm reaches a size so that surgery to prevent rupture is of more benefit than the possible complications of a surgical procedure. Some aneurysms remain stable over many years of observation.

### GERONTOLOGIC CONSIDERATIONS

Most abdominal aortic aneurysms occur in patients between 60 and 90 years of age. Rupture is likely with co-existing hypertension and with aneurysms more than 6 cm wide. In most cases at this point, the chances of rupture are greater than the chance of death during surgical repair. If the elderly patient is considered at moderate risk of complications related to surgery or anesthesia, the aneurysm is not repaired until it is at least 5.5 cm (2 inches) wide.

## Medical Management

### PHARMACOLOGIC THERAPY

If the aneurysm is stable in size based on serial duplex ultrasound scans, the blood pressure is closely monitored over time, because there is an association between increased diastolic blood pressure (above 100 mm Hg) and aneurysm rupture (Rutherford, 2005). Antihypertensive agents, including diuretics, beta-blockers, ACE inhibitors, angiotensin II receptor antagonists, and calcium channel blockers, are frequently prescribed to maintain the patient's blood pressure within acceptable limits (see Chapter 32).

### SURGICAL MANAGEMENT

An expanding or enlarging abdominal aortic aneurysm is likely to rupture. Surgery is the treatment of choice for abdominal aortic aneurysms more than 5.5 cm (2 inches) wide or those that are enlarging; the standard treatment has been open surgical repair of the aneurysm by resecting the vessel and sewing a bypass graft in place. The mortality rate associated with elective aneurysm repair, a major surgical procedure, is reported to be 1% to 4%. The prognosis for a patient with a ruptured aneurysm is poor, and surgery is performed immediately (Rutherford, 2005).

An alternative for treating an infrarenal abdominal aortic aneurysm is endovascular grafting, which involves the transluminal placement and attachment of a sutureless aortic graft prosthesis across an aneurysm (Fig. 31-14).

**FIGURE 31-13.** Duplex ultrasonic image of abdominal aortic aneurysm at the perirenal level. Cross-sectional image documents the location of right and left renal arteries.

**FIGURE 31-14.** AneuRx Endograft repair of an abdominal aortic aneurysm (Medtronic).

This procedure can be performed under local or regional anesthesia. Endovascular grafting of abdominal aortic aneurysms may be performed if the patient's abdominal aorta and iliac arteries are not extremely tortuous and if the aneurysm does not begin at the level of the renal arteries. Clinical trials are being conducted to evaluate endograft treatment of abdominal aortic aneurysms at or above the level of the renal arteries and the thoracic aorta. Potential complications include bleeding, hematoma, or wound infection at the femoral insertion site; distal ischemia or embolization; dissection or perforation of the aorta; graft thrombosis or infection; break of the attachment system; graft migration; proximal or distal graft leaks; delayed rupture; and bowel ischemia.

### Nursing Management

Before surgery, nursing assessment is guided by anticipating a rupture and by recognizing that the patient may have cardiovascular, cerebral, pulmonary, and renal impairment from atherosclerosis. The functional capacity of all organ systems should be assessed. Medical therapies designed to stabilize physiologic function should be promptly implemented.

Signs of impending rupture include severe back or abdominal pain, which may be persistent or intermittent. Abdominal pain is often localized in the middle or lower abdomen to the left of the midline. Low back pain may be present because of pressure of the aneurysm on the lumbar nerves. This is a significant symptom, usually indicating that the aneurysm is expanding rapidly and is about to rupture. Indications of a rupturing abdominal aortic aneurysm include constant, intense back pain; falling blood pressure; and decreasing hematocrit. Rupture into the peritoneal cavity is rapidly fatal. A retroperitoneal rupture of an aneurysm may result in hematomas in the scrotum, perineum, flank, or penis. Signs of heart failure or a loud bruit may suggest a rupture into the vena cava. If the aneurysm adheres to the adjacent vena cava, the vena cava may become damaged when rupture or leak of the aneurysm occurs. Rupture into the vena cava results in higher-pressure arterial blood entering the lower-pressure venous system and causing turbulence, which is heard as a bruit. The high blood pressure and increased blood volume returning to the right side of the heart from the vena cava may cause right-sided heart failure. The overall surgical mortality rate associated with a ruptured aneurysm is 50% to 75%.

Postoperative care requires intense monitoring of pulmonary, cardiovascular, renal, and neurologic status. Possible complications of surgery include arterial occlusion, hemorrhage, infection, ischemic bowel, renal failure, and impotence.

## Other Aneurysms

Aneurysms may also arise in the peripheral vessels, most often as a result of atherosclerosis. These may involve such vessels as the subclavian artery, renal artery, femoral artery, or (most frequently) popliteal artery. Between 50% and 60% of popliteal aneurysms are bilateral and may be associated with abdominal aortic aneurysms.

The aneurysm produces a pulsating mass and disturbs peripheral circulation distal to it. Pain and swelling develop because of pressure on adjacent nerves and veins. Diagnosis is made by duplex ultrasonography and CT to determine the size, length, and extent of the aneurysm. Arteriography may be performed to evaluate the level of proximal and distal involvement.

### Medical Management

Surgical repair is performed with replacement grafts or endovascular repair using a stent-graft or wall graft, which is a Dacron or PTFE graft with external structures made from a variety of materials (nitinol, titanium, stainless steel) for additional support.

### Nursing Management

The patient who has had an endovascular repair must lie supine for 6 hours; the head of the bed may be elevated up to 45 degrees after 2 hours. The patient needs to use a bedpan or urinal while on bed rest, or an indwelling urinary catheter may be used. Vital signs and Doppler assessment of peripheral pulses are performed every 15 minutes for four times, then every 30 minutes for four times, then every hour for four times, and then as directed by the physician or agency policy. The access site (usually the femoral or iliac artery) is assessed when vital signs and pulses are monitored. The nurse assesses for bleeding, pulsation, swelling, pain, and hematoma formation. Skin changes of the lower extremity, lumbar area, or buttocks that might indicate signs of embolization, such as extremely tender, irregularly shaped, cyanotic areas, as well as any changes in vital signs, pulse quality, bleeding, swelling, pain, or hematoma, are immediately reported to the physician.

The patient's temperature should be monitored every 4 hours, and any signs of postimplantation syndrome should be reported. Postimplantation syndrome typically begins within 24 hours of stent-graft placement and consists of a spontaneously occurring fever, leukocytosis, and, occasionally, transient thrombocytopenia. The exact etiology is unknown, but the symptoms are thought to be related to the activation of cytokines, which results from thrombosis in the repaired aneurysm that occurs because of the release of coagulation proteins and platelets (Latessa, 2002). These symptoms can be managed with mild analgesics or anti-inflammatory agents, such as acetaminophen or ibuprofen, and usually subside within a week.

Because of the increased risk for hemorrhage, the physician is also notified of persistent coughing, sneezing, vomiting, or systolic blood pressure greater than 180 mm Hg. Most patients can resume their preprocedure diet and are encouraged to drink fluids. An IV infusion may be continued until the patient can drink normally. Fluids are important to maintain blood flow through the arterial repair site and to assist the kidneys with excreting IV contrast agent and other medications used during the procedure. Six hours after the procedure, the patient may be able to roll from side to side and may be able to ambulate with assistance to the bathroom. After the patient can take adequate fluids orally, the IV infusion may be discontinued and the IV access converted to a saline lock.

## *Dissecting Aorta*

Occasionally, in an aorta diseased by arteriosclerosis, a tear develops in the intima or the media degenerates, resulting in a dissection (see Fig. 31-11). Arterial dissections are three times more common in men than in women and occur most commonly in the 50- to 70-year-old age group (Rutherford, 2005).

## Pathophysiology

Arterial dissections (separations) are commonly associated with poorly controlled hypertension, blunt chest trauma, and cocaine use. The profound increase in sympathetic response caused by cocaine use creates an increase in the force of left ventricular contraction that causes heightened shear forces upon the aortic wall (Rutherford, 2005). Dissection is caused by rupture in the intimal layer. A rupture may occur through adventitia or into the lumen through the intima, allowing blood to re-enter the main channel and resulting in chronic dissection (eg, pseudoaneurysm) or occlusion of branches of the aorta.

As the separation progresses, the arteries branching from the involved area of the aorta shear and occlude. The tear occurs most commonly in the region of the aortic arch, with the highest mortality rate associated with ascending aortic dissection. The dissection of the aorta may progress backward in the direction of the heart, obstructing the openings to the coronary arteries or producing hemopericardium (effusion of blood into the pericardial sac) or aortic insufficiency, or it may extend in the opposite direction, causing occlusion of the arteries supplying the gastrointestinal tract, kidneys, spinal cord, and legs.

## Clinical Manifestations

Onset of symptoms is usually sudden. Severe and persistent pain, described as tearing or ripping, may be reported. The pain is in the anterior chest or back and extends to the shoulders, epigastric area, or abdomen. Aortic dissection may be mistaken for an acute myocardial infarction, which could confuse the clinical picture and initial treatment. Cardiovascular, neurologic, and gastrointestinal symptoms are responsible for other clinical manifestations, depending on the location and extent of the dissection. The patient may appear pale. Sweating and tachycardia may be detected. Blood pressure may be elevated or markedly different from one arm to the other if dissection involves the orifice of the subclavian artery on one side. Because of the variable clinical picture associated with this condition, early diagnosis is usually difficult.

## Assessment and Diagnostic Findings

Arteriography, CT, transesophageal echocardiography, duplex ultrasonography, and MRI aid in the diagnosis.

## Medical Management

The medical or surgical treatment of a dissecting aorta depends on the type of dissection present and follows the general principles outlined for the treatment of thoracic aortic aneurysms.

## Nursing Management

A patient with a dissecting aorta requires the same nursing care as a patient with an aortic aneurysm requiring surgical intervention, as described earlier in this chapter. Interventions described in Chart 31-3 are also appropriate.

## *Arterial Embolism and Arterial Thrombosis*

Acute vascular occlusion may be caused by an embolus or acute thrombosis. Acute arterial occlusions may result from iatrogenic injury, which can occur during insertion of invasive catheters such as those used for arteriography, PTA or stent placement, or an intra-aortic balloon pump. Other causes include trauma from a fracture, crush injury, and penetrating wounds that disrupt the arterial intima. The accurate diagnosis of an arterial occlusion as embolic or thrombotic in origin is necessary to initiate appropriate treatment.

## Pathophysiology

Arterial emboli arise most commonly from thrombi that develop in the chambers of the heart as a result of atrial fibrillation, myocardial infarction, infective endocarditis, or chronic heart failure. These thrombi become detached and are carried from the left side of the heart into the arterial system, where they lodge in and obstruct an artery that is smaller than the embolus. Emboli may also develop in advanced aortic atherosclerosis because the atheromatous plaques ulcerate or become rough. Acute thrombosis frequently occurs in patients with preexisting ischemic symptoms.

## Clinical Manifestations

The symptoms of arterial emboli depend primarily on the size of the embolus, the organ involved, and the state of the collateral vessels. The immediate effect is cessation of distal blood flow. The blockage can progress distal and proximal to the site of the obstruction. Secondary vasospasm can contribute to the ischemia. The embolus can fragment or break apart, resulting in occlusion of distal vessels. Emboli tend to lodge at arterial bifurcations and areas narrowed by atherosclerosis. Cerebral, mesenteric, renal, and coronary arteries are often involved in addition to the large arteries of the extremities.

The symptoms of acute arterial embolism in extremities with poor collateral flow are acute, severe pain and a gradual loss of sensory and motor function. The six *P*s associated with acute arterial embolism are *p*ain, *p*allor, *p*ulselessness, *p*aresthesia, *p*oikilothermia (coldness), and *p*aralysis. Eventually, superficial veins may collapse because of decreased blood flow to the extremity. Because of ischemia, the part of the extremity distal to the occlusion is markedly colder and paler than the part proximal to the occlusion.

Arterial thrombosis can also acutely occlude an artery. A thrombosis is a slowly developing clot that usually occurs where the arterial wall has become damaged, generally as a result of atherosclerosis. Thrombi may also develop in an arterial aneurysm. The manifestations of an acute thrombotic arterial occlusion are similar to those described for embolic occlusion. However, treatment is more difficult with a thrombus because the arterial occlusion has occurred in a degenerated vessel and requires more extensive reconstructive surgery to restore flow than is required with an embolic event.

## Assessment and Diagnostic Findings

An arterial embolus is usually diagnosed on the basis of the sudden nature of the onset of symptoms and an apparent source for the embolus. Two-dimensional transthoracic echocardiography or transesophageal echocardiography (TEE), chest x-ray, and electrocardiography may reveal underlying cardiac disease. Noninvasive duplex and Doppler ultrasonography can determine the presence and extent of underlying atherosclerosis, and arteriography may be performed.

## Medical Management

Management of arterial thrombosis depends on its cause. Management of acute embolic occlusion usually requires surgery because time is of the essence. Because the onset of the event is acute, collateral circulation has not developed, and the patient quickly moves through the list of six *P*s to paralysis, the most advanced stage. Heparin therapy is initiated immediately to prevent further development of emboli and to hamper the extension of existing thrombi. Typically, an initial IV bolus of 5000 to 10,000 units is administered, followed by a continuous infusion of 1000 units per hour until the patient undergoes surgery.

### Surgical Management

Emergency embolectomy is the procedure of choice if the involved extremity is viable (Fig. 31-15). Arterial emboli are usually treated by insertion of an embolectomy catheter. The catheter is passed through a groin incision into the affected artery and advanced past the occlusion. The catheter balloon is inflated with sterile saline solution, and the thrombus is extracted as the catheter is withdrawn. This procedure involves incising the vessel and removing the clot.

### Endovascular Management

Percutaneous thrombectomy devices may also be used for the treatment of an acute thrombosis. All endovascular devices necessitate obtaining access to the patient's arterial system and inserting a catheter into the patient's artery to obtain access to the thrombus. The approach is similar to that used for angiograms in that it is made through the groin to the femoral artery. Some devices require that a small incision be made into the patient's artery. Available endovascular devices include:

- The AngioJet, which uses a backward-pointing jet of fluid flow to disrupt the thrombus. It then aspirates the particles into the device's catheter and deposits them in a collection device. Use of this device typically results in

**FIGURE 31-15.** Extraction of an embolus by balloon-tipped embolectomy catheter. The deflated balloon-tipped catheter is advanced past the embolus, inflated, and then gently withdrawn, carrying the embolic material with it. Adapted with permission from Rutherford, R. B. (2005). *Vascular surgery: Vol. 1 and 2* (6th ed.). Philadelphia: Elsevier.

only 50% to 70% patency of the vessel, so many patients require additional thrombolytic therapy for dissolving the residual thrombus.
- The Bacchus Trellis device, which uses pharmacologic thrombolysis to produce clot dissolution. This device is placed into the patient's artery, with the tip at the location where the thrombus has occurred. A rotating, sinusoidal-shaped wire mixes the thrombolytic agent and simultaneously dissolves the clot, and the resultant particles are aspirated through the catheter into a collection device to prevent distal embolization.
- Therapeutic ultrasonic devices, which are inserted into the patient's artery through a catheter (eg, OmniSonics, Ekos catheter), use high-frequency, low-energy ultrasound to dissolve an occlusive thrombus. The thrombus is dissolved into particles small enough to traverse the distal capillary bed without causing further obstructive embolization. Clinical trials are underway to determine the long-term efficacy of these devices (Ouriel, 2003).

Complications arising from the use of any of the endovascular devices may include arterial dissection or distal artery embolization.

### Pharmacologic Therapy

When the patient has collateral circulation, treatment may include IV anticoagulation with heparin, which can prevent the thrombus from spreading and reduce muscle necrosis. Intra-arterial thrombolytic medications are used to dissolve the embolus. Fibrin-specific thrombolytic medications (eg, tissue plasminogen activator [t-PA, Alteplase, Activase] and single-chain urokinase-type plasminogen activator [scu-PA, prourokinase]) do not deplete circulating fibrinogen and plasminogen, which prevents the development of systemic fibrinolysis. Other thrombolytic medications are reteplase (r-PA, Retavase), tenecteplase (TNKase), and staphylokinase (Moore, 2002). Although these agents differ in their pharmacokinetics, they are administered in a similar manner: a catheter is advanced under x-ray visualization to the clot, and the thrombolytic agent is infused.

Thrombolytic therapy should not be used when there are known contraindications to therapy or when the extremity cannot tolerate the several additional hours of ischemia that it takes for the agent to lyse (disintegrate) the clot. Contraindications to thrombolytic therapy include active internal bleeding, CVA (brain attack, stroke), recent major surgery, uncontrolled hypertension, and pregnancy.

### Nursing Management

Before surgery, the patient remains on bed rest with the affected extremity level or slightly dependent (15 degrees). The affected part is kept at room temperature and protected from trauma. Heating and cooling pads are contraindicated because ischemic extremities are easily traumatized by alterations in temperature. If possible, tape and electrocardiogram electrodes should not be used on the extremity; sheepskin and foot cradles are used to protect an affected leg from mechanical trauma.

If the patient is treated with thrombolytic therapy, the dose of thrombolytic therapy is based on the patient's weight. The patient is admitted to a critical care unit for continuous monitoring. Vital signs are taken every 15 minutes for 2 hours, then every 30 minutes for the next 6 hours, and then every hour for 16 hours. Bleeding is the most common side effect of thrombolytic therapy, and the patient is closely monitored for any signs of bleeding. The nurse minimizes the number of punctures for inserting IV lines and obtaining blood samples, avoids intramuscular injections, prevents any possible tissue trauma, and applies pressure at least twice as long as usual after any puncture that is performed. If t-PA is used for the treatment, heparin is usually administered to prevent another thrombus from forming at the site of the lesion. The t-PA activates plasminogen on the thrombus more than circulating plasminogen, but it does not decrease the clotting factors as much as other thrombolytic therapies, so patients receiving t-PA can make new thrombi more readily than with some of the other thrombolytics.

During the postoperative period, the nurse collaborates with the surgeon about the patient's appropriate activity level based on the patient's condition. Generally, every effort is made to encourage the patient to move the extremity to stimulate circulation and prevent stasis. Anticoagulant therapy may be continued after surgery to prevent thrombosis of the affected artery and to diminish the development of subsequent thrombi at the initiating site. The nurse assesses for evidence of local and systemic hemorrhage, including mental status changes, which can occur when anticoagulants are administered. Pulses, Doppler signals, ABI, and motor and sensory function are assessed every hour for the first 24 hours, because significant changes may indicate reocclusion. Metabolic abnormalities, renal failure, and compartment syndrome may be complications after an acute arterial occlusion.

## Raynaud's Disease

Raynaud's disease is a form of intermittent arteriolar vasoconstriction that results in coldness, pain, and pallor of the fingertips or toes. The cause is unknown, although many patients with the disease have immunologic disorders. Symptoms may result from a defect in basal heat production that eventually decreases the ability of cutaneous vessels to dilate. Episodes may be triggered by emotional factors or by unusual sensitivity to cold. The disease is most common in women between the ages of 16 and 40 years, and it occurs more frequently in cold climates and during the winter.

The term *Raynaud's phenomenon* is used to refer to localized, intermittent episodes of vasoconstriction of small arteries of the feet and hands that cause color and temperature changes. Generally unilateral and affecting only one or two digits, the phenomenon is always associated with underlying systemic disease. It may occur with scleroderma, systemic lupus erythematosus, rheumatoid arthritis, obstructive arterial disease, or trauma.

The prognosis for patients with Raynaud's disease varies; some slowly improve, some become progressively worse, and others show no change. Ulceration and gangrene are rare; however, chronic disease may cause atrophy of the skin and muscles. With appropriate patient teaching and lifestyle modifications, the disorder is generally benign and self-limiting.

## Clinical Manifestations

The classic clinical picture reveals pallor brought on by sudden vasoconstriction. The skin then becomes bluish (cyanotic) due to pooling of deoxygenated blood during vasospasm. As a result of exaggerated reflow (hyperemia) due to vasodilation, a red color (rubor) is produced when oxygenated blood returns to the digits after the vasospasm stops. The characteristic sequence of color change of Raynaud's phenomenon is described as white, blue, and red. Numbness, tingling, and burning pain occur as the color changes. The involvement tends to be bilateral and symmetric.

## Medical Management

Avoiding the particular stimuli (eg, cold, tobacco) that provoke vasoconstriction is a primary factor in controlling Raynaud's disease. Calcium channel blockers (nifedipine [Procardia, Adalat]) may be effective in relieving symptoms. Sympathectomy (interrupting the sympathetic nerves by removing the sympathetic ganglia or dividing their branches) may help some patients.

## Nursing Management

The nurse teaches the patient to avoid situations that may be stressful or unsafe. Stress-management classes may be helpful. Exposure to cold must be minimized, and in areas where the fall and winter months are cold, the patient should remain indoors as much as possible and wear layers of clothing when outdoors. Hats and mittens or gloves should be worn at all times when outside. Fabrics specially designed for cold climates (eg, Thinsulate) are recommended. Patients should warm up their vehicles before getting in so that they can avoid touching a cold steering wheel or door handle, which could elicit an attack. During summer, a sweater should be available when entering air-conditioned rooms.

Patients are often concerned about serious complications, such as gangrene and amputation, but these complications are uncommon. Patients should avoid all forms of nicotine; the nicotine gum or patches used to help people quit smoking may induce attacks.

Patients should be cautioned to handle sharp objects carefully to avoid injuring the fingers. Patients should be informed about the postural hypotension that may result from medications, such as calcium channel blockers, used to treat Raynaud's disease. The nurse also discusses safety precautions related to alcohol, exercise, and hot weather.

# Venous Disorders

## Venous Thrombosis, Deep Vein Thrombosis, Thrombophlebitis, and Phlebothrombosis

Although the terms *venous thrombosis*, *deep vein thrombosis* (DVT), *thrombophlebitis*, and *phlebothrombosis* do not necessarily reflect identical disease processes, for clinical purposes they are often used interchangeably.

## Pathophysiology

Superficial veins, such as the greater saphenous, lesser saphenous, cephalic, basilic, and external jugular veins, are thick-walled muscular structures that lie just under the skin. Deep veins are thin-walled and have less muscle in the media. They run parallel to arteries and bear the same names as the arteries. Deep and superficial veins have valves that permit unidirectional flow back to the heart. The valves lie at the base of a segment of the vein that is expanded into a sinus. This arrangement permits the valves to open without coming into contact with the wall of the vein, permitting rapid closure when the blood starts to flow backward. Other kinds of veins are known as perforating veins. These vessels have valves that allow one-way blood flow from the superficial system to the deep system.

Although the exact cause of venous thrombosis remains unclear, three factors, known as Virchow's triad, are believed to play a significant role in its development: stasis of blood (venous stasis), vessel wall injury, and altered blood coagulation (Chart 31-6). Venous stasis occurs when blood

---

**CHART 31-6**

### Risk Factors for Deep Vein Thrombosis (DVT) and Pulmonary Embolism

**Endothelial Damage**
- Trauma
- Surgery
- Pacing wires
- Central venous catheters
- Dialysis access catheters
- Local vein damage
- Repetitive motion injury

**Venous Stasis**
- Bed rest or immobilization
- Obesity
- History of varicosities
- Spinal cord injury
- Age (greater than 65 years)

**Altered Coagulation**
- Cancer
- Pregnancy
- Oral contraceptive use
- Proteins C deficiency
- Protein S deficiency
- Antiphospholipid antibody syndrome
- Factor V Leiden defect
- Prothrombin 20210A defect
- Hyperhomocysteinemia
- Elevated factors II, VIII, IX, XI
- Antithrombin III deficiency
- Polycythemia
- Septicemia

flow is reduced, as in heart failure or shock; when veins are dilated, as with some medication therapies; and when skeletal muscle contraction is reduced, as in immobility, paralysis of the extremities, or anesthesia. Moreover, bed rest reduces blood flow in the legs by at least 50% (Porth, 2005). Damage to the intimal lining of blood vessels creates a site for clot formation. Direct trauma to the vessels, as with fractures or dislocation, diseases of the veins, and chemical irritation of the vein from IV medications or solutions, can damage veins. Increased blood coagulability occurs most commonly in patients for whom anticoagulant medications have been abruptly withdrawn. Oral contraceptive use and several blood dyscrasias (abnormalities) also can lead to hypercoagulability.

Formation of a thrombus frequently accompanies thrombophlebitis, which is an inflammation of the vein walls. When a thrombus develops initially in the veins as a result of stasis or hypercoagulability but without inflammation, the process is referred to as phlebothrombosis. Venous thrombosis can occur in any vein, but it occurs more in the veins of the lower extremities. The superficial and deep veins of the extremities may be affected.

Upper extremity venous thrombosis is not as common as lower extremity thrombosis. Upper extremity venous thrombosis is more common in patients with IV catheters or in patients with an underlying disease that causes hypercoagulability. Internal trauma to the vessels may result from pacemaker leads, chemotherapy ports, dialysis catheters, or parenteral nutrition lines. The lumen of the vein may be decreased as a result of the catheter or from external compression, such as by neoplasms or an extra cervical rib. Effort thrombosis of the upper extremity is caused by repetitive motion (as in competitive swimmers, tennis players, and construction workers) that irritates the vessel wall, causing inflammation and subsequent thrombosis.

Venous thrombi are aggregates of platelets attached to the vein wall that have a tail-like appendage containing fibrin, white blood cells, and many red blood cells. The "tail" can grow or can propagate in the direction of blood flow as successive layers of the thrombus form. A propagating venous thrombosis is dangerous because parts of the thrombus can break off and produce an embolic occlusion of the pulmonary blood vessels. Fragmentation of the thrombus can occur spontaneously as it dissolves naturally, or it can occur in association with an elevation in venous pressure, as occurs when a person stands suddenly or engages in muscular activity after prolonged inactivity. After an episode of acute DVT, recanalization (ie, reestablishment of the lumen of the vessel) typically occurs. The time required for complete recanalization is an important determinant of venous valvular incompetence, which is one complication of venous thrombosis (Tran & Meissner, 2002). Other complications of venous thrombosis are listed in Chart 31-7.

## Clinical Manifestations

A major problem associated with recognizing DVT is that the signs and symptoms are nonspecific. The exception is phlegmasia cerulea dolens (massive iliofemoral venous thrombosis), in which the entire extremity becomes massively swollen, tense, painful, and cool to the touch. Despite this variability, clinical signs should always be investigated.

---

**CHART 31-7**

### Complications of Venous Thrombosis

**Chronic venous occlusion**
**Pulmonary emboli from dislodged thrombi**
**Valvular destruction**
- Chronic venous insufficiency
- Increased venous pressure
- Varicosities
- Venous ulcers

**Venous obstruction**
- Increased distal pressure
- Fluid stasis
- Edema
- Venous gangrene

---

### Deep Veins

With obstruction of the deep veins comes edema and swelling of the extremity because the outflow of venous blood is inhibited. The amount of swelling can be determined by measuring the circumference of the affected extremity at various levels with a tape measure and comparing one extremity with the other at the same level to determine size differences. If both extremities are swollen, a size difference may be difficult to detect. The affected extremity may feel warmer than the unaffected extremity, and the superficial veins may appear more prominent.

Tenderness, which usually occurs later, is produced by inflammation of the vein wall and can be detected by gently palpating the affected extremity. Homans' sign (pain in the calf after the foot is sharply dorsiflexed) is not specific for DVT because it can be elicited in any painful condition of the calf. In some cases, signs and symptoms of a pulmonary embolus are the first indication of DVT.

### Superficial Veins

Thrombosis of superficial veins produces pain or tenderness, redness, and warmth in the involved area. The risk of the superficial venous thrombi becoming dislodged or fragmenting into emboli is very low because most of them dissolve spontaneously. This condition can be treated at home with bed rest, elevation of the leg, analgesics, and possibly anti-inflammatory medication.

### Assessment and Diagnostic Findings

Careful assessment is invaluable in detecting early signs of venous disorders of the lower extremities. Patients with a history of varicose veins, hypercoagulation, neoplastic disease, cardiovascular disease, or recent major surgery or injury are at high risk. Other patients at high risk include those who are obese or elderly and women taking oral contraceptives.

When performing the nursing assessment, key concerns include limb pain, a feeling of heaviness, functional impairment, ankle engorgement, and edema; differences in leg circumference bilaterally from thigh to ankle; increase in the surface temperature of the leg, particularly the calf or ankle; and areas of tenderness or superficial thrombosis (ie, cord-like venous segment). Although Homans' sign has been used historically to assess for DVT, it is not a reliable or valid sign and has no clinical value in assessment for DVT (Gupta & Stouffer, 2001).

## Prevention

Venous thrombosis, thrombophlebitis, and DVT can be prevented, especially if patients who are considered at high risk are identified and preventive measures are instituted without delay. Preventive measures include the application of elastic compression stockings, the use of intermittent pneumatic compression devices, and special body positioning and exercise (discussed later in the section on nursing management). An additional method to prevent venous thrombosis in surgical patients is administration of subcutaneous unfractionated or low-molecular-weight heparin (LMWH).

## Medical Management

The objectives of treatment for DVT are to prevent the thrombus from growing and fragmenting (risking pulmonary embolism) and to prevent recurrent thromboemboli. Anticoagulant therapy (administration of a medication to delay the clotting time of blood, prevent the formation of a thrombus in postoperative patients, and forestall the extension of a thrombus after it has formed) can meet these objectives, although anticoagulants cannot dissolve a thrombus that has already formed.

### Pharmacologic Therapy

Measures for preventing or reducing blood clotting within the vascular system are indicated in patients with thrombophlebitis, recurrent embolus formation, and persistent leg edema from heart failure. They are also indicated in elderly patients with a hip fracture that may result in lengthy immobilization. Contraindications for anticoagulant therapy are noted in Chart 31-8.

#### UNFRACTIONATED HEPARIN

Unfractionated heparin is administered subcutaneously to prevent development of DVT, or by intermittent or continuous IV infusion for 5 to 7 days to prevent the extension of a thrombus and the development of new thrombi. Oral anticoagulants, such as warfarin (Coumadin), are administered with heparin therapy. Medication dosage is regulated by monitoring the activated partial thromboplastin time (aPTT), the **international normalized ratio** (INR), and the platelet count.

#### LOW-MOLECULAR-WEIGHT HEPARIN

Subcutaneous LMWHs that may include medications such as dalteparin (Fragmin) and enoxaparin (Lovenox) are effective treatments for some cases of DVT. These agents have longer half-lives than unfractionated heparin, so doses can be given in one or two subcutaneous injections each day. Doses are adjusted according to weight. LMWHs prevent the extension of a thrombus and development of new thrombi, and they are associated with fewer bleeding complications and lower risks of heparin-induced thrombocytopenia (HIT) than unfractionated heparin. Because there are several preparations, the dosing schedule must be based on the product used and the protocol at each institution. The cost of LMWH is higher than that of unfractionated heparin; however, LMWH may be used safely in pregnant women, and patients who take it may be more mobile and have an improved quality of life.

#### THROMBOLYTIC THERAPY

Unlike the heparins, thrombolytic (fibrinolytic) therapy lyses and dissolves thrombi in 50% of patients. Thrombolytic therapy (eg, t-PA [Alteplase, Activase], reteplase [r-PA, Retavase], tenecteplase [TNKase], staphylokinase, urokinase, streptokinase) is given within the first 3 days after acute thrombosis. Therapy initiated beyond 5 days after the onset of symptoms is significantly less effective (Moore, 2002). The advantages of thrombolytic therapy include less long-term damage to the venous valves and a reduced incidence of postthrombotic syndrome and chronic venous insufficiency. However, thrombolytic therapy results in a threefold greater incidence of bleeding than heparin. If bleeding occurs and cannot be stopped, the thrombolytic agent is discontinued.

---

CHART 31-8

# PHARMACOLOGY · Contraindications to Anticoagulant Therapy

- Lack of patient cooperation
- Bleeding from the following systems:
    Gastrointestinal
    Genitourinary
    Respiratory
    Reproductive
- Hemorrhagic blood dyscrasias
- Aneurysms
- Severe trauma
- Alcoholism

- Recent or impending surgery of:
    Eye
    Spinal cord
    Brain
- Severe hepatic or renal disease
- Recent cerebrovascular hemorrhage
- Infections
- Open ulcerative wounds
- Occupations that involve a significant hazard for injury
- Recent delivery of a baby

## FACTOR XA INHIBITOR

Fondaparinux (Arixtra) selectively inhibits factor Xa. This agent is given daily subcutaneously at a fixed dose, has a half-life of 17 hours, and is excreted unchanged via the kidneys (and therefore must be used with caution in patients with renal insufficiency). Fondaparinux has no effect on routine tests of coagulation, such as the aPTT or activated clotting time (ACT), so routine coagulation monitoring is unnecessary (Weitz, 2004). Fondaparinux is approved for prophylaxis during major orthopedic surgery, such as hip or knee arthroplasties.

## ORAL ANTICOAGULANTS

Warfarin (Coumadin) is a vitamin K antagonist that is frequently used for extended therapy. Routine coagulation monitoring is essential to ensure that a therapeutic response is obtained and maintained over time. Interactions with a range of other medications can reduce or enhance the anticoagulant effects of warfarin, as can variable intake of foods containing vitamin K (see Chapter 33, Chart 33-15, for a review of agents that interact with warfarin). Warfarin has a narrow therapeutic window, and there is a slow onset of action. Treatment is initially supported with concomitant parenteral anticoagulation with heparin until the warfarin demonstrates anticoagulant effectiveness.

## Surgical Management

Surgery is necessary for DVT when anticoagulant or thrombolytic therapy is contraindicated (see Chart 31-8), the danger of pulmonary embolism is extreme, or the venous drainage is so severely compromised that permanent damage to the extremity is likely. A thrombectomy (removal of the thrombosis) is the procedure of choice. A vena cava filter may be placed at the time of the thrombectomy; this filter traps large emboli and prevents pulmonary emboli (see Chapter 23). Balloon angioplasty and stent placement are being used in the iliac veins of patients with acute and chronic venous disease.

## Nursing Management

If the patient is receiving anticoagulant therapy, the nurse must frequently monitor the aPTT, prothrombin time (PT), INR, ACT, hemoglobin and hematocrit values, platelet count, and fibrinogen level, depending on which medication is being given. Close observation is also required to detect bleeding; if bleeding occurs, it must be reported immediately and anticoagulant therapy discontinued.

## Assessing and Monitoring Anticoagulant Therapy

To prevent inadvertent infusion of large volumes of unfractionated heparin, which could cause hemorrhage, continuous IV infusion by an electronic infusion device is the preferred method of administering unfractionated heparin. Dosage calculations are based on the patient's weight, and any possible bleeding tendencies are detected by a pretreatment clotting profile. If renal insufficiency exists, lower doses of heparin are required. Periodic coagulation tests and hematocrit levels are obtained. Heparin is in the effective, or therapeutic, range when the aPTT is 1.5 times the control.

Oral anticoagulants, such as warfarin (Coumadin), are monitored by the PT or the INR. Because the full anticoagulant effect of warfarin is delayed for 3 to 5 days, it is usually administered concurrently with heparin until desired anticoagulation has been achieved (ie, when the PT is 1.5 to 2 times normal or the INR is 2.0 to 3.0).

## Monitoring and Managing Potential Complications

### BLEEDING

The principal complication of anticoagulant therapy is spontaneous bleeding anywhere in the body. Bleeding from the kidneys is detected by microscopic examination of the urine and is often the first sign of excessive dosage. Bruises, nosebleeds, and bleeding gums are also early signs. To promptly reverse the effects of heparin, IV injections of protamine sulfate may be administered. Risks of protamine administration include bradycardia and hypotension, which can be minimized by slow administration. Protamine sulfate can be used in patients receiving LMWH, but it is less effective with LMWH than with unfractionated heparin. Reversing the anticoagulation effects of warfarin is more difficult, but effective measures that may be prescribed include administration of vitamin K and/or infusion of fresh-frozen plasma or prothrombin concentrate. Oral vitamin K significantly reduces the INR within 24 hours. Low-dose IV vitamin K is also effective.

### THROMBOCYTOPENIA

Another complication of therapy may be HIT, which is defined as a sudden decrease in the platelet count by at least 30% of baseline levels in patients receiving heparin. Patients at greatest risk are those who receive unfractionated heparin for a long period of time (ie, several days or weeks). Therefore, it is preferable not to anticoagulate patients with unfractionated heparin over the long term. Beginning warfarin concomitantly with heparin can provide a stable INR or PT by day 5 of heparin treatment, at which time the heparin may be discontinued.

The administration of LMWH is less frequently associated with HIT. The thrombocytopenia is thought to result from an autoimmune mechanism that causes destruction of platelets. If the process is not arrested, platelets may aggregate, initiating inappropriate clotting, and thrombosis may occur. This serious complication results in thromboembolic manifestations known as HIT with thrombosis, and the prognosis is extremely guarded.

Prevention of thrombocytopenia depends on regular monitoring of platelet counts. Early signs include a decreasing platelet count, the need for increasing doses of heparin to maintain the therapeutic level, and thromboembolic or hemorrhagic complications (appearance of skin necrosis, either at the site of injection or at distal sites where thromboses occur; skin discoloration consisting of large hemorrhagic areas; hematomas; purpura; and blistering) (Miller, 2003). If thrombocytopenia does occur, platelet aggregation studies are conducted, the heparin is discontinued, and alternate anticoagulant therapy is rapidly initiated because the continued prothrombotic state poses an ongoing threat of continuous clot development.

Lepirudin (Refludan) and argatroban are direct thrombin inhibitors approved for treatment of HIT. Lepirudin has a half-life of 1.3 hours, is excreted by the kidneys, and can be monitored using the aPTT. An initial IV bolus infusion followed by a continuous infusion with subsequent adjustments to maintain the aPTT between 1.5 and 2.5 times baseline has been recommended. Strict dosage adjustment in renal failure is required, because the clearance of lepirudin is proportional to the patient's creatinine clearance. Argatroban has a half-life of 30 to 45 minutes, is metabolized by the liver, and is unaffected by renal function. The anticoagulant effect of argatroban is predictable, with low variability between patients, but it is dose-dependent and requires monitoring with either the aPTT or ACT.

There is no safe, rapidly acting antidote if the patient develops bleeding complications from direct thrombin inhibitors. Recombinant factor VIIa may reverse the anticoagulant effects, but it may not be available in all hospitals, and it is very expensive. The safety profile of the direct thrombin inhibitors is not known in patients with cancer or in women who are pregnant (Weitz, 2004).

### DRUG INTERACTIONS

Because oral anticoagulants interact with many other medications and herbal and nutritional supplements, close monitoring of the patient's medication schedule is necessary. Many medications and supplements potentiate or inhibit oral anticoagulants; it is always wise to check to see if any medications or supplements are contraindicated with warfarin (see Chapter 33, Chart 33-15). Contraindications to anticoagulant therapy are summarized in Chart 31-8.

## Providing Comfort

Bed rest, elevation of the affected extremity, elastic compression stockings, and analgesics for pain relief are adjuncts to therapy. They help improve circulation and increase comfort. Depending on the extent and location of a venous thrombosis, bed rest may be required for 5 to 7 days after diagnosis. This is approximately the time necessary for the thrombus to adhere to the vein wall, preventing embolization.

Warm, moist packs applied to the affected extremity reduce the discomfort associated with DVT, as do mild analgesics prescribed for pain control. When the patient begins to ambulate, elastic compression stockings are used. Walking is better than standing or sitting for long periods. Bed exercises, such as repetitive dorsiflexion of the foot, are also recommended.

## Compression Therapy

### STOCKINGS

Elastic compression stockings usually are prescribed for patients with venous insufficiency. These stockings exert a sustained, evenly distributed pressure over the entire surface of the calves, reducing the caliber of the superficial veins in the legs and resulting in increased flow in the deeper veins. The stockings may be knee-high, thigh-high, or panty hose. Thigh-high stockings are difficult for the patient to wear because they tend to roll down. The roll of the stocking further restricts blood flow rather than providing evenly distributed pressure over the thigh.

> **NURSING ALERT**
>
> Any type of stocking, including the elastic type, can inadvertently become a tourniquet if applied incorrectly (ie, rolled tightly at the top). In such instances, the stockings produce stasis rather than prevent it. For ambulatory patients, elastic compression stockings are removed at night and reapplied before the legs are lowered from the bed to the floor in the morning.

When the stockings are off, the skin is inspected for signs of irritation, and the calves are examined for tenderness. Any skin changes or signs of tenderness are reported. Stockings are contraindicated in patients with severe pitting edema because they can produce severe pitting at the knee.

 **Gerontologic Considerations.** Because of decreased strength and manual dexterity, elderly patients may be unable to apply elastic compression stockings properly. If this is the case, a family member or friend should be taught to assist the patient to apply the stockings so that they do not cause undue pressure on any part of the feet or legs.

### WRAPS

Short stretch elastic wraps may be applied from the toes to the knee in a 50% spiral overlap. These wraps are available in a two-layer system, which includes an inner layer of soft padding. These wraps are rectangular and become squares on stretching, indicating the appropriate degree of stretch and reducing the possibility of wrapping a leg too loosely or too tightly. Three- and four-layer systems are also available (Profore, Dynacare), but these may be used only once compared to the two-wrap system, which can be used multiple times.

Other types of compression are available. The Unna boot, which consists of a paste bandage impregnated with zinc oxide, glycerin, gelatin, and sometimes calamine, is applied without tension in a circular fashion from the base of the toes to the tibial tuberosity with a 50% spiral overlap. It is important to keep the foot dorsiflexed at a 90-degree angle to the leg, thus avoiding excess pressure or trauma to the anterior ankle area. This type of compression may remain in place for as long as 1 week. The CirCaid, a nonelastic leg wrap with a series of overlapping, interlocking Velcro straps, augments the effect of the muscle pump while the patient is walking. The CirCaid is usually worn during the day. Patients may find the CirCaid easier to apply and wear than the Unna boot.

### INTERMITTENT PNEUMATIC COMPRESSION DEVICES

These devices can be used with elastic compression stockings to prevent DVT. They consist of an electric controller that is attached by air hoses to plastic knee-high or thigh-high sleeves. The leg sleeves are divided into compartments,

## NURSING RESEARCH PROFILE

### What is the Evidence for Choosing Either Below-Knee or Thigh-Length Graduated Compression Stockings to Prevent DVT?

Byrne, B. (2002). Deep vein thrombosis prophylaxis: The effectiveness and implications of using below-knee or thigh-length graduated compression stockings. *Journal of Vascular Nursing, 20*(2), 53–59.

#### Purpose
Patients with DVTs have an increased incidence of recurrent DVTs as well as chronic limb ischemia, venous insufficiency, and ulceration. Ambulation is well known as an effective way to prevent DVT, but for those who cannot walk, graduated compression stockings reduce the incidence of DVT. Thigh-length and below-knee graduated compression stockings are the lengths most commonly used in clinical practice. Thigh-length graduated compression stockings tend to be associated with less patient comfort and compliance, cost more, and are more difficult to apply. This review examined published research-based evidence for choosing one length of graduated compression stocking over the other in terms of DVT prophylaxis. In addition, it examined nursing implications of stocking length.

#### Design
A literature review was conducted using Medline, Cumulative Index to Nursing and Allied Health Literature (CINAHL), School of Health and Related Research, and the Cochrane Library databases with English and human subject restrictions. Thirty-two of 428 research articles were identified that studied graduated compression stockings in the prevention of DVT. Of these articles, only 10 specifically studied the benefits of the lengths of the stockings in DVT prophylaxis.

In addition to these methods, telephone interviews of nurse managers, clinical nurse teachers, or charge nurses employed in the intensive care units of 10 tertiary care hospitals in Victoria, Australia, were conducted to determine whether graduated compression stockings were routinely used in these units, and if so, to identify the preferred length of stockings used in these units and the rationale for the length chosen. Furthermore, two companies that produce graduated compression stockings in Australia were contacted and asked to provide the literature-based evidence that they used when making purchase recommendations.

#### Findings
Nine out of the 10 selected research articles reported that there was no difference in overall efficacy between below-knee and thigh-length stockings in preventing DVTs. These research studies used small samples that represented groups with specific diagnoses. Thus, findings from these studies were limited in terms of their generalizability.

Findings yielded from interviewing the nurses revealed that 5 of the 10 hospitals routinely used graduated compression stockings. When these facilities used the stockings (routinely or otherwise), 4 used thigh-length, 5 used below-knee, and 1 never used them. None of the nurses interviewed was able to refer to evidence on which their units' practices were based.

The two companies that manufactured graduated compression stockings provided either outdated references (eg, 25 years old) to support the use of their products or references already identified via the literature search independently conducted by this study's author.

#### Nursing Implications
Nursing care of patients determined to be "at risk" for DVT should include prevention, which includes wearing graduated compression stockings. The evidence in the literature to date suggests that below-knee stockings and thigh-length stockings are equally effective in DVT prophylaxis. Although more studies are needed to draw generalizable conclusions, it seems prudent to recommend that below-knee graduated compression stockings should be included in nursing DVT prophylaxis manuals as the standard of care, because they are easier to apply, more tolerable, and less costly than thigh-length graduated compression stockings.

---

which sequentially fill to apply pressure to the ankle, calf, and thigh at 35 to 55 mm Hg of pressure. These devices can increase blood velocity beyond that produced by the stockings. Nursing measures include ensuring that prescribed pressures are not exceeded and assessing for patient comfort.

### Positioning the Body and Encouraging Exercise

When the patient is on bed rest, the feet and lower legs should be elevated periodically above the level of the heart. This position allows the superficial and tibial veins to empty rapidly and to remain collapsed. Active and passive leg exercises, particularly those involving calf muscles, should be performed to increase venous flow. Early ambulation is most effective in preventing venous stasis. Deep-breathing exercises are beneficial because they produce increased negative pressure in the thorax, which assists in emptying the large veins. Once ambulatory, the patient is instructed to avoid sitting for more than 2 hours at a time. The goal is to walk at least 10 minutes every 1 to 2 hours. The patient is also instructed to perform active and passive leg exercises as frequently as necessary when he or she cannot ambulate, such as during long car, train, and plane trips.

### Promoting Home and Community-Based Care

In addition to teaching the patient how to apply elastic compression stockings and explaining the importance of elevating the legs and exercising adequately, the nurse teaches about the medication, its purpose, and the need to take the correct amount at the specific times prescribed (Chart 31-9). The patient should also be aware that periodic blood tests are necessary to determine if a change in medication or dosage is required. If the patient fails to adhere to the therapeutic regimen, continuation of the medication therapy should be questioned. A person who refuses to discontinue the use of alcohol should not receive anticoagulants because chronic alcohol use decreases their effectiveness. In patients with liver disease, the potential for bleeding may be exacerbated by anticoagulant therapy.

## Chronic Venous Insufficiency

Venous insufficiency results from obstruction of the venous valves in the legs or a reflux of blood through the valves. Superficial and deep leg veins can be involved. Resultant venous hypertension can occur whenever there has been a prolonged increase in venous pressure, such as occurs with DVT. Because the walls of veins are thinner and more elastic than the walls of arteries, they distend readily when venous pressure is consistently elevated. In this state, leaflets of the venous valves are stretched and prevented from closing completely, allowing a backflow or reflux of blood in the veins. Duplex ultrasonography confirms the obstruction and identifies the level of valvular incompetence.

### Clinical Manifestations

When the valves in the deep veins become incompetent after a thrombus has formed, postthrombotic syndrome may develop (Fig. 31-16). This disorder is characterized by chronic venous stasis, resulting in edema, altered pigmentation, pain, and stasis dermatitis. The patient may notice the symptoms less in the morning and more in the evening. Obstruction or poor calf muscle pumping in addition to valvular reflux must be present for the development of severe postthrombotic syndrome and stasis ulcers. Superficial veins may be dilated. The disorder is longstanding, difficult to treat, and often disabling.

Stasis ulcers develop as a result of the rupture of small skin veins and subsequent ulcerations. When these vessels rupture, red blood cells escape into surrounding tissues and then degenerate, leaving a brownish discoloration of the tissues. The pigmentation and ulcerations usually occur in the lower part of the extremity, in the area of the medial malleolus of the ankle. The skin becomes dry, cracks, and itches; subcutaneous tissues fibrose and atrophy. The risk for injury and infection of the extremities is increased.

---

**CHART 31-9**

### Patient Education

#### Taking Anticoagulant Medications

- Take the anticoagulant at the same time each day, usually between 8:00 and 9:00 am.
- Wear or carry identification indicating the anticoagulant being taken.
- Keep all appointments for blood tests.
- Because other medications affect the action of the anticoagulant, do not take any of the following medications or supplements without consulting with the primary health care provider: vitamins, cold medicines, antibiotics, aspirin, mineral oil, and anti-inflammatory agents, such as ibuprofen (Motrin) and similar medications or herbal or nutritional supplements. The primary health care provider should be contacted before taking any over-the-counter drugs.
- Avoid alcohol, because it may change the body's response to an anticoagulant.
- Avoid food fads, crash diets, or marked changes in eating habits.
- Do not take warfarin (Coumadin) unless directed.
- Do not stop taking Coumadin (when prescribed) unless directed.
- When seeking treatment from physician, a dentist, a podiatrist, or another health care provider, be sure to inform the caregiver that you are taking an anticoagulant.
- Contact your primary health care provider before having dental work or elective surgery.
- If any of the following signs appear, report them immediately to the primary health care provider:
    Faintness, dizziness, or increased weakness
    Severe headaches or abdominal pain
    Reddish or brownish urine
    Any bleeding—for example, cuts that do not stop bleeding
    Bruises that enlarge, nosebleeds, or unusual bleeding from any part of the body
    Red or black bowel movements
    Rash
- Avoid injury that can cause bleeding.
- For women: Notify the primary health care provider if you suspect pregnancy.

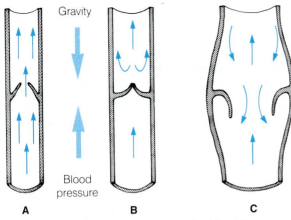

**FIGURE 31-16.** Competent valves showing blood flow patterns when the valve is open (**A**) and closed (**B**), allowing blood to flow against gravity. (**C**) With faulty or incompetent valves, the blood cannot move toward the heart.

## Complications

Venous ulceration is the most serious complication of chronic venous insufficiency and can be associated with other conditions affecting the circulation of the lower extremities. Cellulitis or dermatitis may complicate the care of chronic venous insufficiency and venous ulcerations.

## Management

Management of the patient with venous insufficiency is directed at reducing venous stasis and preventing ulcerations. Measures that increase venous blood flow are antigravity activities, such as elevating the leg, and compression of superficial veins with elastic compression stockings.

Elevating the legs decreases edema, promotes venous return, and provides symptomatic relief. The legs should be elevated frequently throughout the day (at least 15 to 30 minutes every 2 hours). At night, the patient should sleep with the foot of the bed elevated about 15 cm (6 inches). Prolonged sitting or standing in one position is detrimental; walking should be encouraged. When sitting, the patient should avoid placing pressure on the popliteal spaces, as occurs when crossing the legs or sitting with the legs dangling over the side of the bed. Constricting garments such as panty girdles or socks that are too tight at the top or that leave marks on the skin should be avoided.

Compression of the legs with elastic compression stockings reduces the pooling of venous blood and enhances venous return to the heart. Elastic compression stockings are recommended for people with venous insufficiency. The stocking should fit so that pressure is greater at the foot and ankle and then gradually declines to a lesser pressure at the knee or groin. If the top of the stocking is too tight or becomes twisted, a tourniquet effect is created, which worsens venous pooling. Stockings should be applied after the legs have been elevated for a period, when the amount of blood in the leg veins is at its lowest.

Extremities with venous insufficiency must be carefully protected from trauma; the skin is kept clean, dry, and soft. Signs of ulceration are immediately reported to the health care provider for treatment and follow-up.

## Leg Ulcers

A leg ulcer is an excavation of the skin surface that occurs when inflamed necrotic tissue sloughs off. About 75% of all leg ulcers result from chronic venous insufficiency. Lesions due to arterial insufficiency account for approximately 20%; the remaining 5% are caused by burns, sickle cell anemia, and other factors (Gloviczki & Yao, 2001).

## Pathophysiology

Inadequate exchange of oxygen and other nutrients in the tissue is the metabolic abnormality that underlies the development of leg ulcers. When cellular metabolism cannot maintain energy balance, cell death (necrosis) results. Alterations in blood vessels at the arterial, capillary, and venous levels may affect cellular processes and lead to the formation of ulcers.

## Clinical Manifestations

The characteristics of leg ulcers are determined by the cause of the ulcer. Most ulcers, especially in elderly patients, have more than one cause. The symptoms depend on whether the problem is arterial or venous in origin (see Table 31-1). The severity of the symptoms depends on the extent and duration of the vascular insufficiency. The ulcer itself appears as an open, inflamed sore. The area may be draining or covered by eschar (dark, hard crust).

### Arterial Ulcers

Chronic arterial disease is characterized by intermittent claudication, which is pain caused by activity and relieved after a few minutes of rest. The patient may also complain of digital or forefoot pain at rest. If the onset of arterial occlusion is acute, ischemic pain is unrelenting and rarely relieved even with opioid analgesics. Typically, arterial ulcers are small, circular, deep ulcerations on the tips of toes or in the web spaces between the toes. Ulcers often occur on the medial side of the hallux or lateral fifth toe and may be caused by a combination of ischemia and pressure (Fig. 31-17).

Arterial insufficiency may result in gangrene of the toe (digital gangrene), which usually is caused by trauma. The toe is stubbed and then turns black (see Fig. 31-17). Usually, patients with this problem are elderly people without adequate circulation to provide revascularization. Débridement is contraindicated in these instances. Although the toe is gangrenous, it is dry. Managing dry gangrene is preferable to débriding the toe and causing an open wound that will not heal because of insufficient circulation. If the toe were to be amputated, the lack of adequate circulation would prevent healing and might make further amputation necessary—a below-knee or an above-knee amputation. A higher-level amputation in an elderly person could result in a loss of independence and possibly the need for institutional care. Dry gangrene of the toe in an elderly person with poor cir-

**FIGURE 31-17.** (A) Ulcers resulting from arterial emboli. (B) Gangrene of the toes resulting from severe arterial ischemia. (C) Ulcer from venous stasis.

culation is usually left undisturbed. The nurse keeps the toe clean and dry until it separates (without creating an open wound).

### Venous Ulcers

Chronic venous insufficiency is characterized by pain described as aching or heaviness. The foot and ankle may be edematous. Ulcerations are in the area of the medial or lateral malleolus (gaiter area) and are typically large, superficial, and highly exudative. Venous hypertension causes extravasation of blood, which discolors the area (see Fig. 31-17). Patients with neuropathy frequently have ulcerations on the side of the foot over the metatarsal heads. These ulcers are painless and are described in further detail in Chapter 41.

## Assessment and Diagnostic Findings

Because ulcers have many causes, the cause of each ulcer needs to be identified so appropriate therapy can be prescribed. The history of the condition is important in determining venous or arterial insufficiency. The pulses of the lower extremities (femoral, popliteal, posterior tibial, and dorsalis pedis) are carefully examined. More conclusive diagnostic aids are Doppler and duplex ultrasound studies, arteriography, and venography. Cultures of the ulcer bed may be necessary to determine whether an infecting agent is the primary cause of the ulcer.

## Medical Management

Patients with ulcers can be effectively managed by advanced practice nurses or wound-ostomy-continence nurses in collaboration with physicians. All ulcers have the potential to become infected.

### Pharmacologic Therapy

Antibiotic therapy is prescribed when the ulcer is infected; the specific antibiotic agent is based on culture and sensitivity test results. Oral antibiotics usually are prescribed because topical antibiotics have not proven to be effective for leg ulcers.

### Compression Therapy

Adequate compression therapy involves the application of external or counter pressure to the lower extremity to facilitate venous return to the heart. The pressure should be applied in a gradient or graduated fashion with the pressure being somewhat higher at the ankle. One form is the compression stocking; some of these are custom-made to the patient's anatomic specifications. The patient should be instructed to wear the stockings at all times except at night and to reapply the stockings in the morning before getting out of bed. Short stretch elastic wraps, Unna boots, and CirCaids may be other effective options. (See previous section on Compression Therapy.)

### Débridement

To promote healing, the wound is kept clean of drainage and necrotic tissue. The usual method is to flush the area with normal saline solution or clean it with a noncytotoxic wound-cleansing agent (Saf-Clens, Biolex, Restore). If this is unsuccessful, débridement may be necessary. Débridement is the removal of nonviable tissue from wounds. Removing the dead tissue is important, particularly in instances of infection. Débridement can be accomplished by several different methods:

- Surgical débridement is the fastest method and can be performed by a physician, skilled advanced practice nurse, or wound-ostomy-continence nurse in collaboration with the physician.
- Nonselective débridement can be accomplished by applying isotonic saline dressings of fine-mesh gauze to the ulcer. When the dressing dries, it is removed (dry), along with the debris adhering to the gauze. Pain management is usually necessary.
- Enzymatic débridement with the application of enzyme ointments may be prescribed to treat the ulcer. The ointment is applied to the lesion but not to normal surrounding skin. Most enzymatic ointments are covered with saline-soaked gauze that has been thoroughly wrung out. A dry gauze dressing and a loose bandage are then applied. The enzymatic ointment is discontinued when the necrotic tissue has been débrided, and an appropriate wound dressing is applied.

- Calcium alginate dressings (Kaltostat, Sorbsan, Aquacel Hydrofiber) may be used for débridement when absorption of exudate is needed. These dressings are changed when the exudate seeps through the cover dressing or at least every 7 days. The dressing can also be used on areas that are bleeding, because the material helps stop the bleeding. As the dry fibers absorb exudate, they become a gel that is painlessly removed from the ulcer bed. Calcium alginate dressings should not be used on dry or nonexudative wounds.

### Topical Therapy

A variety of topical agents can be used in conjunction with cleansing and débridement therapies to promote healing of leg ulcers. The goals of treatment are to remove devitalized tissue and to keep the ulcer clean and moist while healing takes place. The treatment should not destroy developing tissue. For topical treatments to be successful, adequate nutritional therapy must be maintained.

### Wound Dressing

After the circulatory status has been assessed and determined to be adequate for healing (ABI of more than 0.5), surgical dressings can be used to promote a moist environment. The simplest method is to use a wound contact material next to the wound bed and cover it with gauze. Other available options that promote the growth of granulation tissue and re-epithelialization include the hydrocolloids (eg, Comfeel, DuoDerm CGF, Restore, Tegasorb). These materials also provide a barrier for protection because they adhere to the wound bed and surrounding tissue. However, these dressings may not be effective treatment for deep wounds and infected wounds.

Knowledge deficit, frustration, fear, and depression can result in the patient's and family's decreased compliance with the prescribed therapy; therefore, patient and family education is necessary before beginning and throughout the wound care program.

### Stimulated Healing

Tissue-engineered human skin equivalent (Apligraf [Graftskin]) is a skin product cultured from human dermal fibroblasts and keratinocytes used in combination with therapeutic compression. When applied, it seems to react to factors in the wound and may interact with the patient's cells to stimulate the production of growth factors. Application is not difficult, no suturing is involved, and the procedure is painless.

### Hyperbaric Oxygenation

Hyperbaric oxygenation (HBO) may be beneficial as an adjunct treatment in patients with diabetes who evidence no signs of wound healing after 30 days of standard wound treatment. HBO is accomplished by placing the patient into a chamber that increases barometric pressure while the patient is breathing 100% oxygen. The process by which HBO is thought to work involves several factors. The edema in the wound area is decreased because high oxygen tension facilitates vasoconstriction and enhances the ability of leukocytes to phagocytize and kill bacteria. In addition, HBO is thought to increase diffusion of oxygen to the hypoxic wound, thereby enhancing epithelial migration and improving collagen production. The two most common adverse effects of HBO are middle ear barotrauma and confinement anxiety (Broussard, 2004).

## ◀◀▼▶▶ Nursing Process

## The Patient With Leg Ulcers

### Assessment

A careful nursing history and assessment of symptoms are important. The extent and type of pain are carefully assessed, as are the appearance and temperature of the skin of both legs. The quality of all peripheral pulses is assessed, and the pulses in both legs are compared. The legs are checked for edema. If the extremity is edematous, the degree of edema is determined. Any limitation of mobility and activity that results from vascular insufficiency is identified. The patient's nutritional status is assessed, and a history of diabetes, collagen disease, or varicose veins is obtained.

### Diagnosis

#### Nursing Diagnoses

Based on the assessment data, major nursing diagnoses for the patient may include:

- Impaired skin integrity related to vascular insufficiency
- Impaired physical mobility related to activity restrictions of the therapeutic regimen and pain
- Imbalanced nutrition: less than body requirements, related to increased need for nutrients that promote wound healing

#### Collaborative Problems/ Potential Complications

Based on the assessment data, potential complications that may develop include:

- Infection
- Gangrene

### Planning and Goals

The major goals for the patient may include restoration of skin integrity, improved physical mobility, adequate nutrition, and absence of complications.

### Nursing Interventions

The nursing challenge in caring for these patients is great, whether the patient is in the hospital, in a long-term care facility, or at home. The physical problem is often a long-term and disabling one that causes a substantial drain on the patient's physical, emotional, and economic resources.

### Restoring Skin Integrity

To promote wound healing, measures are used to keep the area clean. Cleansing requires very gentle handling, a mild soap, and lukewarm water. Positioning of the legs depends on whether the ulcer is of arterial or venous origin. If there is arterial insufficiency, the patient should be referred to be evaluated for vascular reconstruction. If there is venous insufficiency, dependent edema can be avoided by elevating the lower extremities. A decrease in edema promotes the exchange of cellular nutrients and waste products in the area of the ulcer, promoting healing.

Avoiding trauma to the lower extremities is imperative in promoting skin integrity. Protective boots may be used (eg, Rooke Vascular boot); they are soft and provide warmth and protection from injury and displace tissue pressure to prevent ulcer formation. If the patient is on bed rest, it is important to relieve pressure on the heels to prevent pressure ulcerations. When the patient is in bed, a bed cradle can be used to relieve pressure from bed linens and to prevent anything from touching the legs. When the patient is ambulatory, all obstacles are moved from the patient's path so that the patient's legs will not be bumped. Heating pads, hot water bottles, or hot baths are avoided, because they increase the oxygen demands and thus the blood flow demands of the already compromised tissue. The patient with diabetes mellitus suffers from neuropathy with decreased sensation, and heating pads may produce injury before the patient is aware of being burned.

### Improving Physical Mobility

Generally, physical activity is initially restricted to promote healing. When infection resolves and healing begins, ambulation should resume gradually and progressively. Activity promotes arterial flow and venous return and is encouraged after the acute phase of the ulcer process. Until full activity is resumed, the patient is encouraged to move about when in bed, to turn from side to side frequently, and to exercise the upper extremities to maintain muscle tone and strength. Meanwhile, diversional activities are encouraged. Consultation with an occupational therapist may be helpful if prolonged immobility and inactivity are anticipated.

If pain limits the patient's activity, analgesics may be prescribed by the physician. The pain of peripheral vascular disease is typically chronic and often disabling. Analgesics may be taken before scheduled activities to help the patient participate more comfortably.

### Promoting Adequate Nutrition

Nutritional deficiencies are common, requiring dietary alterations to remedy deficiencies. A diet that is high in protein, vitamins C and A, iron, and zinc is encouraged to promote healing. Many patients with peripheral vascular disease are elderly. Particular consideration should be given to their iron intake, because many elderly people are anemic. After a dietary plan has been developed that meets the patient's nutritional needs and promotes healing, diet instruction is provided to the patient and family.

### Promoting Home and Community-Based Care

The self-care program is planned with the patient so that activities that promote arterial and venous circulation, relieve pain, and promote tissue integrity are encouraged. Reasons for each aspect of the program are explained to the patient and family. Leg ulcers are often chronic and difficult to heal; they frequently recur, even when the patient rigorously follows the plan of care. Long-term care of the feet and legs to promote healing of wounds and prevent recurrence of ulcerations is the primary goal. Leg ulcers increase the patient's risk of infection, may be painful, and may limit mobility, necessitating lifestyle changes. Participation of family members and home health care providers may be necessary for treatments such as dressing changes, reassessments, reinforcement of instruction, and evaluation of the effectiveness of the plan of care. Regular follow-up with a primary health care provider is necessary.

## Evaluation

### Expected Patient Outcomes

Expected patient outcomes may include:

1. Demonstrates restored skin integrity
    a. Exhibits absence of inflammation
    b. Exhibits absence of drainage; negative wound culture
    c. Avoids trauma to the legs
2. Increases physical mobility
    a. Progresses gradually to optimal level of activity
    b. Reports that pain does not impede activity
3. Attains adequate nutrition
    a. Selects foods high in protein, vitamins, iron, and zinc
    b. Discusses with family members dietary modifications that need to be made at home
    c. Plans, with the family, a diet that is nutritionally sound

## Varicose Veins

Varicose veins (varicosities) are abnormally dilated, tortuous, superficial veins caused by incompetent venous valves (see Fig. 31-16). Most commonly, this condition occurs in the lower extremities, the saphenous veins, or the lower trunk, but it can occur elsewhere in the body, such as the esophagus (eg, esophageal varices; see Chapter 39).

It is estimated that varicose veins occur in up to 60% of the adult population in the United States, with an increased incidence correlated with increased age (Johnson, 1997). The condition is most common in women and in people whose occupations require prolonged standing, such as salespeople, hair stylists, teachers, nurses and ancillary medical personnel, and construction workers. A hereditary weakness of the vein wall may contribute to the development of varicosities, and it commonly occurs in several members of the same family. Varicose veins are rare before puberty. Pregnancy may cause varicosities because of hormonal effects related to distensibility, increased pressure by the gravid uterus, and increased blood volume (Johnson, 1997).

## Pathophysiology

Varicose veins may be primary (without involvement of deep veins) or secondary (resulting from obstruction of deep veins). A reflux of venous blood in the veins results in venous stasis. If only the superficial veins are affected, the person may have no symptoms but may be troubled by their appearance.

## Clinical Manifestations

Symptoms, if present, may include dull aches, muscle cramps, increased muscle fatigue in the lower legs, ankle edema, and a feeling of heaviness of the legs. Nocturnal cramps are common. When deep venous obstruction results in varicose veins, the patient may develop the signs and symptoms of chronic venous insufficiency: edema, pain, pigmentation, and ulcerations. Susceptibility to injury and infection is increased.

## Assessment and Diagnostic Findings

Diagnostic tests for varicose veins include the duplex scan, which documents the anatomic site of reflux and provides a quantitative measure of the severity of valvular reflux. Air plethysmography measures the changes in venous blood volume. Venography is not routinely performed to evaluate for valvular reflux. However, when it is used, it involves injecting a radiopaque contrast agent into the leg veins so that the vein anatomy can be visualized by x-ray studies during various leg movements.

## Prevention

The patient should avoid activities that cause venous stasis, such as wearing a constricting panty girdle or socks that are too tight at the top or that leave marks on the skin; crossing the legs at the thighs; and sitting or standing for long periods. Changing position frequently, elevating the legs when they are tired, and getting up to walk for several minutes of every hour promote circulation. The patient is encouraged to walk 1 or 2 miles each day if there are no contraindications. Walking up the stairs rather than using the elevator or escalator is helpful, and swimming is good exercise.

Elastic compression stockings, especially knee-high stockings, are useful. The overweight patient should be encouraged to begin a weight-reduction plan.

## Medical Management

### Ligation and Stripping

Surgery for varicose veins requires that the deep veins be patent and functional. The saphenous vein is ligated and divided. The vein is ligated high in the groin, where the saphenous vein meets the femoral vein. Also, the vein may be removed (stripped). After the vein is ligated, an incision is made 2 to 3 cm below the knee, and a metal or plastic wire is passed the full length of the vein to the point of ligation. The wire is then withdrawn, pulling (removing, stripping) the vein as it is removed. Pressure and elevation minimize bleeding during surgery.

### Thermal Ablation

Thermal ablation is a nonsurgical approach using thermal energy. Radiofrequency ablation uses an electrical contact inside the vein. As the device is withdrawn, the vein is sealed. Laser ablation uses a laser fiber tip that seals the vein (decompressed). Topical gel may be used first to numb the skin along the course of the saphenous vein. To protect the surrounding tissue, a series of small punctures are made along the vein, and 100 to 200 mL of dilute lidocaine is delivered to the perivenous space using ultrasound guidance. The goal of this tumescent anesthesia (ie, anesthesia that causes localized swelling) is to provide analgesia, thermal protection (the cuff of fluid surrounds the veins and accompanying nerves), and extrinsic compression of the vein. The saphenous vein is entered percutaneously near the knee using ultrasound guidance. A catheter is introduced into the saphenous vein and advanced to the saphenofemoral junction. The device is then activated and withdrawn, sealing the vein. Small bandages and compression stockings are applied after the procedure. The patient is asked not to remove the stockings for at least 48 hours and then to rewrap the legs and wear the compression stockings while ambulatory for at least 3 weeks. Patients are ambulatory prior to being discharged from the outpatient facility and have no activity restrictions, except that swimming is discouraged for 3 weeks. Nonsteroidal anti-inflammatory drugs such as acetaminophen (Tylenol) or ibuprofen (Motrin) are used as needed for pain. The patient is informed that he or she may bruise along the course of the saphenous vein, may experience leg cramps for a few days, and may find it difficult to straighten the knees for up to 1.5 weeks.

### Sclerotherapy

Sclerotherapy involves injection of an irritating chemical into a vein to produce localized phlebitis and fibrosis, thereby obliterating the lumen of the vein. This treatment may be performed alone for small varicosities or may follow vein ablation, ligation, or stripping. Sclerosing is palliative rather than curative. Sclerotherapy is typically performed in an examination or procedure room and does not require any sedation. After the sclerosing agent is injected, elastic compression bandages are applied to the leg and are worn for approximately 5 days after the procedure. Elastic compression stockings are then worn for an additional 5 weeks. After sclerotherapy, walking activities are encouraged as prescribed to maintain blood flow in the leg and to dilute the sclerosing agent.

## Nursing Management

Ligation and stripping can be performed in an outpatient setting, or the patient can be admitted to the hospital on the day of surgery and discharged the next day if a bilateral procedure is to be performed and the patient is at high risk for postoperative complications. If the procedure is performed in an outpatient setting, nursing measures are the same as if the patient were hospitalized. Bed rest is discouraged and the patient is encouraged to become ambulatory as soon as sedation has worn off. The patient is instructed to walk every hour for 5 to 10 minutes while awake for the first 24 hours if he or she can tolerate the discomfort, and then to increase walking and activity as tolerated. Elastic compression stockings are worn continuously for about 1 week after vein stripping. The nurse assists the patient to perform exercises and move the legs. The foot of the bed should be elevated. Standing and sitting are discouraged.

### Promoting Comfort and Understanding

Analgesics are prescribed to help the patient move the affected extremities more comfortably. Dressings are inspected for bleeding, particularly at the groin, where the risk of bleeding is greatest. The nurse is alert for reported sensations of "pins and needles." Hypersensitivity to touch in the involved extremity may indicate a temporary or permanent nerve injury resulting from surgery, because the saphenous vein and nerve are close to each other in the leg.

Usually, the patient may shower after the first 24 hours. The patient is instructed to dry the incisions well with a clean towel using a patting technique, rather than rubbing. Alternatively, the patient may be instructed to dry the area using a blow-dryer. Application of skin lotion is avoided until the incisions are completely healed to avoid infection. The patient is instructed to apply sunscreen or zinc oxide to the incisional area prior to sun exposure; otherwise, hyperpigmentation of the incision, scarring, or both may occur.

If the patient underwent sclerotherapy, a burning sensation in the injected leg may be experienced for 1 or 2 days. The nurse may encourage the use of a mild analgesic as prescribed and walking to provide relief.

### Promoting Home and Community-Based Care

Long-term leg elastic support is essential after discharge, and the patient needs to obtain adequate supplies of elastic compression stockings or bandages. Exercise of the legs is necessary; the development of an individualized plan requires consultation with the patient and the health care team.

# Lymphatic Disorders

The lymphatic system consists of a set of vessels that spread throughout most of the body. These vessels start as lymph capillaries that drain unabsorbed plasma from the interstitial spaces (spaces between the cells). The lymphatic capillaries unite to form the lymph vessels, which pass through the lymph nodes and then empty into the large thoracic duct that joins the jugular vein on the left side of the neck.

The fluid drained from the interstitial space by the lymphatic system is called lymph. The flow of lymph depends on the intrinsic contractions of the lymph vessels, the contraction of muscles, respiratory movements, and gravity. The lymphatic system of the abdominal cavity maintains a steady flow of digested fatty food (chyle) from the intestinal mucosa to the thoracic duct. In other parts of the body, the lymphatic system's function is regional; the lymphatic vessels of the head, for example, empty into clusters of lymph nodes located in the neck, and those of the extremities empty into nodes of the axillae and the groin.

## Lymphangitis and Lymphadenitis

Lymphangitis is an acute inflammation of the lymphatic channels. It arises most commonly from a focus of infection in an extremity. Usually, the infectious organism is a hemolytic streptococcus. The characteristic red streaks that extend up the arm or the leg from an infected wound outline the course of the lymphatic vessels as they drain.

The lymph nodes located along the course of the lymphatic channels also become enlarged, red, and tender (acute lymphadenitis). They can also become necrotic and form an abscess (suppurative lymphadenitis). The nodes involved most often are those in the groin, axilla, or cervical region.

Because these infections are nearly always caused by organisms that are sensitive to antibiotics, it is unusual to see abscess formation. Recurrent episodes of lymphangitis are often associated with progressive lymphedema. After acute attacks, an elastic compression stocking or sleeve should be worn on the affected extremity for several months to prevent long-term edema.

## Lymphedema and Elephantiasis

Lymphedemas are classified as primary (congenital malformations) or secondary (acquired obstructions). Tissue swelling occurs in the extremities because of an increased quantity of lymph that results from obstruction of lymphatic vessels. It is especially marked when the extremity is in a dependent position. Initially, the edema is soft and pitting. As the condition progresses, the edema becomes firm, nonpitting, and unresponsive to treatment. The most common type is congenital lymphedema (lymphedema praecox), which is caused by hypoplasia of the lymphatic system of the lower extremity. This disorder is usually seen in women and first appears between 15 and 25 years of age.

The obstruction may be in the lymph nodes and the lymphatic vessels. Sometimes, it is seen in the arm after an axillary node dissection (eg, for breast cancer) and in the leg in association with varicose veins or chronic thrombophlebitis. In the latter case, the lymphatic obstruction usually is caused by chronic lymphangitis. Lymphatic obstruction caused by a parasite (filaria) is seen frequently in the tropics. When chronic swelling is present, there may be frequent bouts of acute infection characterized by high fever and chills and increased residual edema after the inflammation has resolved. These lead to chronic fibrosis, thickening of the subcutaneous tissues, and hypertrophy of the skin. This condition, in which chronic swelling of the extremity recedes only slightly with elevation, is referred to as elephantiasis.

## Medical Management

The goal of therapy is to reduce and control the edema and prevent infection. Active and passive exercises assist in moving lymphatic fluid into the bloodstream. External compression devices milk the fluid proximally from the foot to the hip or from the hand to the axilla. When the patient is ambulatory, custom-fitted elastic compression stockings or sleeves are worn; those with the highest compression strength (exceeding 40 mm Hg) are required. When the leg is affected, continuous bed rest with the leg elevated may aid in mobilizing the fluids. Manual lymphatic drainage is a highly specialized massage technique designed to direct or shift the congested lymph through functioning lymphatics that have preserved drainage. Manual lymphatic drainage is incorporated in a sequential treatment approach used in combination with compression bandages, exercises, skin care, pressure gradient sleeves, and pneumatic pumps, depending on the severity and stage of the lymphedema (Cheville, McGarvery, Petrek, et al., 2003).

### Pharmacologic Therapy

As initial therapy, the diuretic furosemide (Lasix) may be prescribed to prevent fluid overload due to mobilization of extracellular fluid. Diuretics have also been used along with elevation of the leg and the use of elastic compression stockings or sleeves. However, the use of diuretics alone has little benefit, because their main action is to limit capillary filtration by decreasing the circulating blood volume. If lymphangitis or cellulitis is present, antibiotic therapy is initiated. The patient is taught to inspect the skin for evidence of infection.

### Surgical Management

Surgery is performed if the edema is severe and uncontrolled by medical therapy, if mobility is severely compromised, or if infection persists. One surgical approach involves the excision of the affected subcutaneous tissue and fascia, with skin grafting to cover the defect. Another procedure involves the surgical relocation of superficial lymphatic vessels into the deep lymphatic system by means of a buried dermal flap to provide a conduit for lymphatic drainage.

## Nursing Management

After surgery, the management of skin grafts and flaps is the same as when these therapies are used for other conditions. Antibiotics may be prescribed for 5 to 7 days. Constant elevation of the affected extremity and observation for complications are essential. Complications may include flap necrosis, hematoma or abscess under the flap, and cellulitis. The nurse instructs the patient or caregiver to inspect the dressing daily. Unusual drainage or any inflammation around the wound margin suggests infection and should be reported to the physician. The patient is informed that there may be a loss of sensation in the skin graft area. The patient is also instructed to avoid the application of heating pads or exposure to sun to prevent burns or trauma to the area.

# Cellulitis

Cellulitis is the most common infectious cause of limb swelling. Cellulitis can occur as a single isolated event or a series of recurrent events. It is often misdiagnosed, usually as recurrent thrombophlebitis or chronic venous insufficiency.

## Pathophysiology

Cellulitis occurs when an entry point through normal skin barriers allows bacteria to enter and release their toxins in the subcutaneous tissues.

## Clinical Manifestations

The acute onset of swelling, localized redness, and pain is frequently associated with systemic signs of fever, chills, and sweating. The redness may not be uniform and often skips areas. Regional lymph nodes may also be tender and enlarged.

## Medical Management

Mild cases of cellulitis can be treated on an outpatient basis with oral antibiotic therapy. If the cellulitis is severe, the patient is treated with IV antibiotics for at least 7 to 14 days. The key to preventing recurrent episodes of cellulitis lies in adequate antibiotic therapy for the initial event and in identifying the site of bacterial entry. The most commonly overlooked areas are the cracks and fissures that occur in the skin between the toes. Other possible locations are drug use injection sites, contusions, abrasions, ulcerations, ingrown toenails, and hangnails.

## Nursing Management

The patient is instructed to elevate the affected area above heart level and apply warm, moist packs to the site every 2 to 4 hours. Patients with sensory and circulatory deficits, such as those caused by diabetes and paralysis, should use caution when applying warm packs because burns may occur; it is advisable to use a thermometer or have a caregiver ensure that the temperature is not more than lukewarm. Education should focus on preventing a recurrent episode. The patient with peripheral vascular disease or diabetes mellitus should receive education or reinforcement about skin and foot care.

---

### Critical Thinking Exercises

**1** Your 75-year-old patient has been diagnosed with a stenosis of his external iliac artery and is scheduled for an angiogram with a possible balloon angioplasty and stent placement. What factors would you consider when planning his postprocedure care, continuing care, and home care? If the patient is taking warfarin (Coumadin) for atrial fibrillation and has renal insufficiency (creatinine of 1.8 mg/dL) as a complication of diabetes, how would you address these factors in the plan of care?

**2** Your 96-year-old patient presents with a 2-year history of chronic stasis ulceration of the left lower extremity requiring weekly placement of an Unna boot. The patient lives alone, six blocks from any mass transit or shopping area, and no longer drives a vehicle. The patient wants to continue living at his current location. What options and plan of care would you discuss with the patient?

**3** **ebp** Your patient has been diagnosed with a recurrent DVT of the femoral vein. The patient has been treated previously with unfractionated heparin and developed HIT. What is the strength of the evidence that promotes the efficacy of alternative anticoagulants (eg, pharmacologic agents other than unfractionated heparin) in treating his DVT? Discuss strategies for DVT prophylaxis that you will include in your teaching plan with this patient. What is the strength of the evidence for each of these preventive strategies?

## REFERENCES AND SELECTED READINGS

## BOOKS

Ascher, E., & Haimovici, H. (2004). *Haimovici's vascular surgery* (5th ed). Malden, MA: Blackwell Publishers.
Bickley, L. S., & Szilagyi, P. G. (2003). *Bates' guide to physical examination and history taking* (8th ed.). Philadelphia: Lippincott Williams & Wilkins.
Coleman, R. W., Hirsch, J., Marder, V. J., et al. (2001). *Hemostasis and thrombosis: Basic principles and clinical practice* (4th ed.). Philadelphia: Lippincott Williams & Wilkins.
Fahey, V. (1999). *Vascular nursing* (3rd ed.). Philadelphia: W. B. Saunders.
Fishman, E. K., & Jeffrey, R. B. (2004). *Multidetector CT—Principles, techniques, and clinical applications*. Philadelphia: Lippincott Williams & Wilkins.
Gloviczki, P., & Yao, J. T. (2001). *Handbook of venous disorders—Guidelines of the American Venous Forum* (2nd ed.). New York: Oxford University Press.
Guyton, A., & Hall, J. (2005). *Textbook of medical physiology* (11th ed.). Philadelphia: Elsevier.
Haaga, J. R., Lanziere, C. F., & Gilkeson, R. C. (2003). *CT and MR imaging of the whole body* (Vol. 1, 4th ed.). St. Louis: Mosby.
Jarvis, C. (2004). *Physical examination and health assessment* (4th ed.). St. Louis: W. B. Saunders.
Lynn-McHale Wiegand, D. J. & Carlson, K. K. (2005). *AACN procedure manual for critical care nurses* (5th ed.). St. Louis: Mosby.
Moore, W. S. (2002). *Vascular surgery: A comprehensive review* (6th ed.). Philadelphia: W. B. Saunders.
Parodi, J. C., Veith, F. J., & Marin, M. (1999). *Endovascular grafting techniques*. Baltimore: Williams & Wilkins.
Porth, C. M. (2005). *Pathophysiology: Concepts of altered health states* (7th ed.). Philadelphia: Lippincott Williams & Wilkins.
Rutherford, R. B. (2005). *Vascular surgery* (6th ed., Vols. I and II). Philadelphia: Elsevier.
Strandness, D. E. (2002). *Duplex scanning in vascular disorders* (3rd ed.). Philadelphia: Lippincott Williams & Wilkins.
White, R. A., & Fogarty, T. J. (1999). *Peripheral endovascular interventions* (2nd ed.). New York: Springer-Verlag.
Yao, J. T., & Pearce, W. H. (1999). *Practical vascular surgery*. Stamford, CT: Appleton & Lange.

## JOURNALS

*Asterisk indicates nursing research article.

Bonham, P. A. (2003). Assessment and management of patients with venous, arterial and diabetic/neurotrophic lower extremity wounds. *AACN Clinical Issues, 14*(4), 442–456.
Brady, A. R., Thompson, S. G., Fowkes, G. R., et al. (2004). Abdominal aortic aneurysm: Expansion risk factors and time intervals for surveillance. *Circulation, 110*(1), 16–21.
Brem, H., Kirsner, R. S., & Falanga, V. (2004). Protocol for the successful treatment of venous ulcers. *American Journal of Surgery, 188*(1), 1–8.
Broussard, C. L. (2004). Hyperbaric oxygenation and wound healing. *Journal of Vascular Nursing, 22*(2), 42–48.
*Byrne, B. (2002). Deep vein thrombosis prophylaxis: The effectiveness and implications of using below-knee or thigh-high graduated compression stockings. *Journal of Vascular Nursing, 20*(2), 53–59.
Caprini, J. A., Glase C. J., Anderson, C. B., et al. (2004). Laboratory markers in the diagnosis of venous thromboembolism. *Circulation, 109*(12) [suppl I]:I-4–I-8.
Cheanvechai, V., Harthum, N. L., Graham, L. M., et al. (2004). Incidence of peripheral vascular disease in women: Is it different from that in men? *Journal of Thoracic and Cardiovascular Surgery, 127*(2), 314–317.
Cheville, A. L., McGarvery, C. L., Petrek, J. A., et al. (2003). Lymphedema management. *Seminars in Radiation Oncology, 13*(3), 290–301.
Chobanian, A. V., Bakris, G. L., Black, H. R., et al. (2003). The seventh report of the Joint National Committee on Prevention, Detection, Evaluation, and Treatment of High Blood Pressure: The JNC 7 report. *Journal of the American Medical Association, 289*(19), 2560–2572.
Cote, M. C., Ligeti, R., Cutler, B. S., et al. (2003). Management of hyperlipidemia in patients with vascular disease. *Journal of Vascular Nursing, 21*(2), 63–67.
Fletcher, R. H., & Fairfield, K. M. (2005). Vitamin supplementation in disease prevention. Available at http://www.UpToDate.com. Accessed January 30, 2006.
Grundy, S. M., Cleeman, C. N., Berz, B., et al. (2004). National Cholesterol Education Program (NCEP) Report: Implications of recent clinical trials for National Cholesterol Education Program Adult Treatment Panel III Guidelines. *Circulation, 110*(2), 227–239.
Gupta, R., & Stouffer, G. A. (2001). Deep venous thrombosis: A review of the pathophysiology, clinical features, and diagnostic modalities. *American Journal of the Medical Sciences, 322*(6), 358–364.
Johnson, M. T. (1997). Treatment and prevention of varicose veins. *Journal of Vascular Nursing, 15*(3), 97–103.
Kohlman-Trigoboff, D. (2003). Hyperhomcysteinemia and vascular disease. *Journal of Vascular Nursing, 21*(1), 30–31.
Kohlman-Trigoboff, D. (2004). Hypertension management in patients with vascular disease. *Journal of Vascular Nursing, 22*(2), 53–56.
Latessa, V. (2002). Endovascular stent-graft repair of descending thoracic aortic aneurysms: The nursing implications of care. *Journal of Vascular Nursing, 20*(2), 86–93.
Markel, A., Meissner, M., Manzo, R. A., et al. (2003). Deep venous thrombosis: Rate of spontaneous lysis and thrombus extension. *International Angiology, 22*(4), 376–382.
Miller, P. L. (2003). Heparin-induced thrombocytopenia—Recognition and treatment. *AORN Journal, 78*(1), 79–89.
Mills, J. L. (2003). Buerger's disease in the 21st century: Diagnosis, clinical features and therapy. *Seminars in Vascular Surgery, 16*(3), 179–189.

Ouriel, K. (2003). Endovascular techniques in the treatment of acute limb ischemia: Thrombolytic agents, trials, and percutaneous mechanical thrombectomy techniques. *Seminars in Vascular Surgery, 16*(4), 270–279.

Rutherford, R. B., & Krupski, W. C. (2004). Current status of open versus endovascular stent-graft repair of abdominal aortic aneurysm. *Journal of Vascular Surgery, 39*(5), 1129–1139.

Selvin, E., & Erlinger, T. P. (2004). Prevalence of and risk factors for peripheral arterial disease in the United States: Results from the National Health and Nutrition Examination Survey, 1999–2000. *Circulation, 110*(6), 738–743.

Stuveling, E. M., Hillege, H. L., Bakker, S. L., et al. (2004). C-reactive protein and microalbuminuria differ in their associations with various domains of vascular disease. *Atherosclerosis, 172*(1), 107–114.

Tran, N. T., & Meissner, M. H. (2002). Epidemiology, pathophysiology and natural history of chronic venous disease. *Seminars in Vascular Surgery, 15*(1), 5–12.

Treat-Jacobson, D., & Walsh, M. E. (2003). Treating patients with peripheral arterial disease and claudication. *Journal of Vascular Nursing, 21*(1), 5–14.

Weitz, J. I. (2004). New anticoagulants for treatment of venous thromboembolism. *Circulation, 110*(9 suppl I), I-19–I-26.

## RESOURCES

Agency for Healthcare Research and Quality, 540 Gaither Road, Rockville, MD 20850; 301-427-1364; http://www.ahrq.gov. Accessed May 31, 2006.

American Venous Forum, 900 Cummings Center, #221-U, Beverly, MA 01915; 978-927-8330; http://www.venous-info.com. Accessed May 31, 2006.

National Heart, Lung, and Blood Institute, Health Information Center, P.O. Box 30105, Bethesda, MD 20824-0105; 301-592-8573; http://www.nhlbi.nih.gov. Accessed May 31, 2006.

Society for Vascular Surgery, 633 N. St. Clair, 24th Floor, Chicago, IL 60611; 1-800-258-7188; http://www.vascularweb.org. Accessed May 31, 2006.

Society of Vascular Nursing, 7794 Grow Drive, Pensacola, FL 32514; 888-536-4786; http://www.svnnet.org. Accessed May 31, 2006.

Society of Vascular Ultrasound, 4601 Presidents Drive, Suite 260, Lanham, MD 20706-4831; 1-800-788-8346; http://www.svunet.org. Accessed May 31, 2006.

Vascular Disease Foundation, 3333 S. Wadsworth Boulevard, #B104-37, Lakewood, CO 80227; 1-866-723-4636; http://www.vdf.org. Accessed May 31, 2006.

# CHAPTER 32

# Assessment and Management of Patients With Hypertension

## Learning Objectives

*On completion of this chapter, the learner will be able to:*

1. Define normal blood pressure and categories of abnormal pressures.
2. Identify risk factors for hypertension.
3. Explain the differences between normal blood pressure and hypertension and discuss the significance of hypertension.
4. Describe treatment approaches for hypertension, including lifestyle changes and medication therapy.
5. Use the nursing process as a framework for care of the patient with hypertension.
6. Describe hypertensive crises and their treatment.

Blood pressure is the product of cardiac output multiplied by peripheral resistance. *Cardiac output* is the product of the heart rate multiplied by the stroke volume. In normal circulation, pressure is exerted by the flow of blood through the heart and blood vessels. High blood pressure, known as *hypertension*, can result from a change in cardiac output, a change in peripheral resistance, or both. The medications used for treating hypertension decrease peripheral resistance, blood volume, or the strength and rate of myocardial contraction.

Hypertension is defined by the Seventh Report of the Joint National Committee on Prevention, Detection, Evaluation, and Treatment of High Blood Pressure (**JNC 7**) as a systolic blood pressure greater than 140 mm Hg and a diastolic pressure greater than 90 mm Hg based on the average of two or more accurate blood pressure measurements taken during two or more contacts with a health care provider (Chobanian, Bakris, Black, et al., 2003). Table 32-1 shows the classification of blood pressure established by JNC 7 in 2003. The categories of blood pressure, from normal to stage 2 hypertension, emphasize the direct relationship between the risk of morbidity and mortality from increasing levels of blood pressure and the specific levels of both the systolic and diastolic blood pressures. The higher either the systolic or diastolic pressure, the greater the health risk (Lewington, Clark, Qizilbash, et al., 2002).

JNC 7 defines a blood pressure of less than 120/80 mm Hg diastolic as normal, 120 to 129/80 to 89 mm Hg as prehypertension, and 140/90 mm Hg or higher as hypertension (see Table 32-1) (Chobanian et al., 2003). The term *stage* is used to define two levels of hypertension so that it is similar to the terms used to describe cancer progression; thus, the public and health care professionals will understand that consistently higher elevations in blood pressure from stage 1 to stage 2 are associated with greater health risks. JNC 7 introduced a new category, *prehypertension*, into the categorization of blood pressure levels to emphasize that people whose blood pressure begins to rise above 120/80 mm Hg are more likely to become hypertensive. To prevent or delay progression to hypertension, JNC 7 urged health care providers to encourage people with blood pressures in the prehypertension category to begin lifestyle modifications such as nutritional changes and exercise. JNC 7 recommended that people with stage 1 hypertension be treated with drugs and be seen by their health care provider about every month until their blood pressure goal is reached and subsequently about every 3 to 6 months. People with stage 2 hypertension or with other complicating conditions need to be seen more frequently.

**TABLE 32-1 Classification of Blood Pressure for Adults Age 18 and Older***

| BP Classification* | Systolic BP (mm Hg) | | Diastolic BP (mm Hg) |
|---|---|---|---|
| Normal | <120 | and | <80 |
| Prehypertension | 120–139 | or | or 80–89 |
| Stage 1 hypertension | 140–159 | or | 90–99 |
| Stage 2 hypertension | ≥160 | or | ≥100 |

* Based on the average of two or more properly measured, seated readings taken on each of two or more office visits.

From the Seventh Report of the Joint National Committee on Prevention, Detection, Evaluation, and Treatment of High Blood Pressure. (2003). *Hypertension, 42*(6), 1206–1252.

## Hypertension

Between 28% and 31% of the adults in the United States have hypertension (Fields, Burt, Cutler, et al., 2004). Of this population, 90% to 95% have **primary hypertension**, high blood pressure from an unidentified cause (Oparil, Zaman, & Calhoun, 2003). The remaining 5% to 10% of this group have **secondary hypertension**, high blood pressure related to identified causes. These causes include narrowing of the renal arteries, renal parenchymal disease, hyperaldosteronism (mineralocorticoid hypertension), certain medications, pregnancy, and coarctation of the aorta (Kaplan, Lieberman, & Neal, 2002).

## Glossary

**BMI:** body mass index, which is calculated by dividing body weight (in kilograms) by height (in meters) squared; a body mass index of greater than 30 is considered to indicate obesity

**dyslipidemia:** abnormal blood lipid levels, including high total, LDL, and triglyceride levels as well as low HDL levels

**GFR:** glomerular filtration rate, an indicator of renal function

**HDL:** high-density lipoprotein

**hypertensive emergency:** a situation in which blood pressure is severely elevated and there is evidence of actual or probable target organ damage

**hypertensive urgency:** a situation in which blood pressure is severely elevated but there is no evidence of target organ damage

**JNC 7:** Seventh Joint National Committee on the Prevention, Detection, Evaluation and Treatment of High Blood Pressure; committee established to study and make recommendations about hypertension in the United States; findings and recommendations of JNC 7 are contained in an extensive report published in 2003

**LDL:** low-density lipoprotein

**monotherapy:** medication therapy with a single medication

**primary hypertension:** also called essential hypertension; denotes high blood pressure from an unidentified cause

**rebound hypertension:** pressure that is controlled with therapy and that becomes uncontrolled (abnormally high) with the discontinuation of therapy

**secondary hypertension:** high blood pressure from an identified cause, such as renal disease

Hypertension is sometimes called "the silent killer" because people who have it are often symptom-free. In a national survey conducted from 1999 to 2000, 31% of people who had pressures exceeding 140/90 mm Hg were unaware of their elevated blood pressure (Hajjar & Kotchen, 2003). Once identified, elevated blood pressure should be monitored at regular intervals, because hypertension is a lifelong condition.

Hypertension often accompanies other risk factors for atherosclerotic heart disease, such as **dyslipidemia** (abnormal blood fat levels), obesity, diabetes mellitus, metabolic syndrome, and a sedentary lifestyle. The incidence of hypertension is higher in the southeastern United States, particularly among African Americans (Casper, Barnett, Williams, et al., 2003). Cigarette smoking does not cause high blood pressure; however, if a person with hypertension smokes, his or her risk of dying from heart disease or related disorders increases significantly.

High blood pressure can be viewed in three ways: as a sign, a risk factor for atherosclerotic cardiovascular disease, or a disease. As a sign, nurses and other health care professionals use blood pressure to monitor a patient's clinical status. Elevated pressure may indicate an excessive dose of vasoconstrictive medication or other problems. As a risk factor, hypertension contributes to the rate at which atherosclerotic plaque accumulates within arterial walls. As a disease, hypertension is a major contributor to death from cardiac, renal, and peripheral vascular disease.

Prolonged blood pressure elevation eventually damages blood vessels throughout the body, particularly in target organs such as the heart, kidneys, brain, and eyes. The usual consequences of prolonged, uncontrolled hypertension are myocardial infarction, heart failure, renal failure, strokes, and impaired vision. Hypertrophy (enlargement) of the left ventricle of the heart may occur as it works to pump blood against the elevated pressure. An echocardiogram is the recommended method of determining whether hypertrophy has occurred.

## Pathophysiology

CONCEPTS in action ANIMATION

Although no precise cause can be identified for most cases of hypertension, it is understood that hypertension is a multifactorial condition. Because hypertension is a sign, it is most likely to have many causes, just as fever has many causes. For hypertension to occur, there must be a change in one or more factors affecting peripheral resistance or cardiac output (Fig. 32-1). In addition, there must also be a problem with the body's control systems that monitor or regulate pressure. Single gene mutations have been identified for a few rare types of hypertension, but most

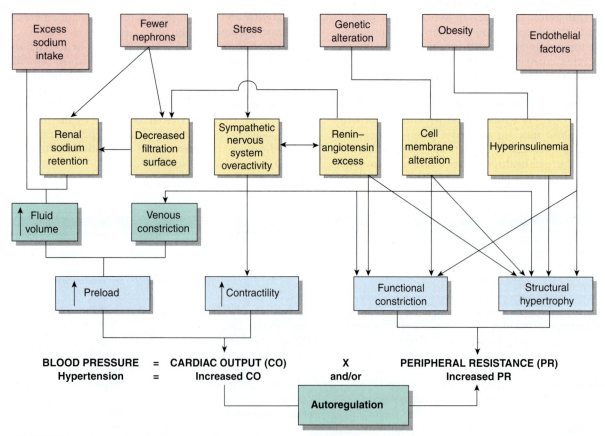

**FIGURE 32-1.** Factors involved in control of blood pressure. Adapted from Kaplan, N. M., Lieberman, E., & Neal, W. (2002). *Kaplan's clinical hypertension* (8th ed.). Philadelphia: Lippincott Williams & Wilkins.

types of high blood pressure are thought to be polygenic (mutations in more than one gene) (Dominiczak, Negrin, Clark, et al., 2000).

Many factors have been implicated as causes of hypertension:

- Increased sympathetic nervous system activity related to dysfunction of the autonomic nervous system
- Increased renal reabsorption of sodium, chloride, and water related to a genetic variation in the pathways by which the kidneys handle sodium
- Increased activity of the renin-angiotensin-aldosterone system, resulting in expansion of extracellular fluid volume and increased systemic vascular resistance
- Decreased vasodilation of the arterioles related to dysfunction of the vascular endothelium
- Resistance to insulin action, which may be a common factor linking hypertension, type 2 diabetes mellitus, hypertriglyceridemia, obesity, and glucose intolerance

### Gerontologic Considerations

Structural and functional changes in the heart and blood vessels contribute to increases in blood pressure that occur with age. These changes include accumulation of atherosclerotic plaque, fragmentation of arterial elastins, increased collagen deposits, and impaired vasodilation. The result of these changes is a decrease in the elasticity of the major blood vessels. Consequently, the aorta and large arteries are less able to accommodate the volume of blood pumped out by the heart (stroke volume), and the energy that would have stretched the vessels instead elevates the systolic blood pressure. Isolated systolic hypertension is more common in older adults and is associated with significant cardiovascular and cerebrovascular morbidity and mortality.

## Clinical Manifestations

Physical examination may reveal no abnormalities other than high blood pressure. Occasionally, retinal changes such as hemorrhages, exudates (fluid accumulation), arteriolar narrowing, and cotton-wool spots (small infarctions) occur. In severe hypertension, papilledema (swelling of the optic disc) may be seen. People with hypertension may be asymptomatic and remain so for many years. However, when specific signs and symptoms appear, they usually indicate vascular damage, with specific manifestations related to the organs served by the involved vessels. Coronary artery disease with angina or myocardial infarction is a common consequence of hypertension. Left ventricular hypertrophy occurs in response to the increased workload placed on the ventricle as it contracts against higher systemic pressure. When heart damage is extensive, heart failure follows. Pathologic changes in the kidneys (indicated by increased blood urea nitrogen [BUN] and serum creatinine levels) may manifest as nocturia. Cerebrovascular involvement may lead to a stroke or transient ischemic attack (TIA), manifested by alterations in vision or speech, dizziness, weakness, a sudden fall, or temporary paralysis on one side (hemiplegia). Cerebral infarctions account for most of the strokes and TIAs in patients with hypertension.

## Assessment and Diagnostic Evaluation

A thorough health history and physical examination are necessary. The retinas are examined and laboratory studies are performed to assess possible target organ damage. Routine laboratory tests include urinalysis, blood chemistry (ie, analysis of sodium, potassium, creatinine, fasting glucose, and total and high density lipoprotein [HDL] cholesterol levels), and a 12-lead electrocardiogram (ECG). Left ventricular hypertrophy can be assessed by echocardiography. Renal damage may be suggested by elevations in BUN and creatinine levels or by microalbuminuria or macroalbuminuria. Additional studies, such as creatinine clearance, renin level, urine tests, and 24-hour urine protein, may be performed.

A risk factor assessment, as advocated by JNC 7, is needed to classify and guide the treatment of hypertensive people at risk for cardiovascular damage. Risk factors and cardiovascular problems related to hypertension are presented in Chart 32-1.

### CHART 32-1

### Risk Factors for Cardiovascular Problems in Hypertensive Patients

**Major Risk Factors (in Addition to Hypertension)**

- Smoking
- Dyslipidemia (elevated **LDL** [or total] cholesterol and/or low HDL cholesterol)*
- Diabetes mellitus*
- Impaired renal function (GFR < 60 mL/min and/or microalbuminuria)
- Obesity (body mass index [**BMI**] ≥ 30 kg/m$^2$)*
- Physical inactivity
- Age (older than 55 years for men, 65 years for women)
- Family history of cardiovascular disease (in female relative younger than 65 years or male relative younger than 55 years)

**Target Organ Damage or Clinical Cardiovascular Disease**

- Heart disease (left ventricular hypertrophy, angina or previous myocardial infarction, previous coronary revascularization, heart failure)
- Stroke (cerebrovascular accident, brain attack) or TIA
- Chronic kidney disease
- Peripheral arterial disease
- Retinopathy

---

* These risk factors plus hypertension, elevated triglyceride levels, and abdominal obesity are components of the metabolic syndrome.

Adapted from Table 6 of the Seventh Report of the Joint National Committee on Prevention, Detection, Evaluation, and Treatment of High Blood Pressure. (2003). *Hypertension, 42*(6), 1206–1252.

## Medical Management

The goal of hypertension treatment is to prevent complications and death by achieving and maintaining the arterial blood pressure at 140/90 mm Hg or lower. JNC 7 specifies a lower goal pressure of 130/80 mm Hg for people with diabetes mellitus or chronic kidney disease, which is defined as either a reduced glomerular filtration rate (**GFR**) resulting in a serum creatinine of greater than 1.3 mg per dL in women or greater than 1.5 mg per dL in men, or albuminuria of greater than 300 mg per day (Chobanian et al., 2003). The optimal management plan would be one that is inexpensive and simple and causes the least possible disruption in the patient's life.

The management options for hypertension are summarized in the treatment algorithm issued by JNC 7 (Fig. 32-2). Table 32-2 summarizes recommended lifestyle modifications. The clinician uses the algorithm with the risk factor assessment data and the patient's blood pressure category to choose the initial and subsequent treatment plans for the

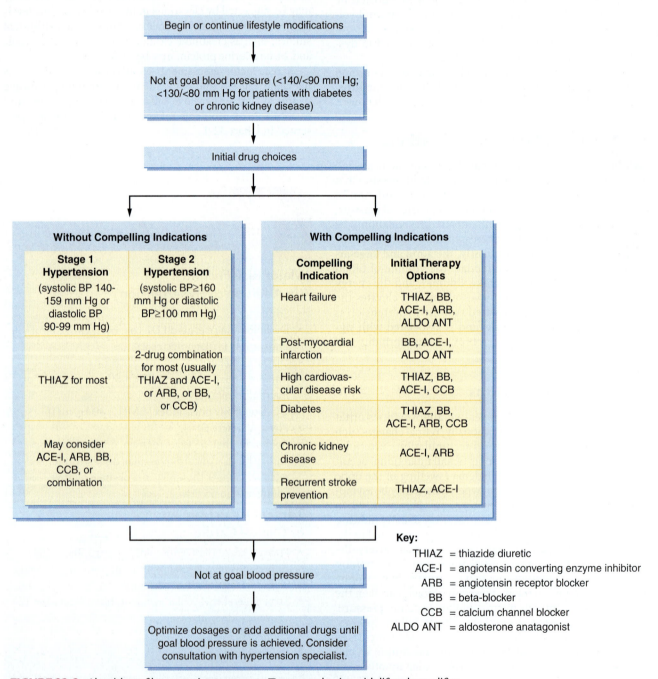

**FIGURE 32-2.** Algorithm of hypertension treatment. Treatment begins with lifestyle modifications and continues with various medication regimens. From the Seventh Report of the Joint National Committee on Prevention, Detection, Evaluation, and Treatment of High Blood Pressure (JNC 7). Reference card available from the National, Heart, Lung, and Blood Institute (NHLBI), available at http://www.nhlbi.nih.gov.

### TABLE 32-2  Lifestyle Modifications To Prevent and Manage Hypertension*

| Modification | Recommendation | Goal of SBP† Reduction (Range)‡ |
|---|---|---|
| Weight reduction | Maintain normal body weight (body mass index 18.5–24.9 kg/m$^2$). | 5–20 mm Hg/10 kg |
| Adopt DASH (Dietary Approaches to Stop Hypertension) eating plan | Consume a diet rich in fruits, vegetables, and low-fat dairy products with a reduced content of saturated and total fat. | 8–14 mm Hg |
| Dietary sodium reduction | Reduce dietary sodium intake to no more than 100 mmol per day (2.4 g sodium or 6 g sodium chloride). | 2–8 mm Hg |
| Physical activity | Engage in regular aerobic physical activity such as brisk walking (at least 30 minutes per day, most days of the week). | 4–9 mm Hg |
| Moderation of alcohol consumption | Limit consumption to no more than 2 drinks (eg, 24 oz beer, 10 oz wine, or 3 oz 80-proof whiskey) per day in most men and to no more than 1 drink per day in women and lighter-weight people. | 2–4 mm Hg |

\* For overall cardiovascular risk reduction, stop smoking.
† SBP = Systolic blood pressure.
‡ The effects of implementing these modifications are dose- and time-dependent and could be greater for some individuals.
From the Seventh Report of the Joint National Committee on Prevention, Detection, Evaluation, and Treatment of High Blood Pressure. (2003). *Hypertension, 42*(6), 1206–1252.

patient. Research findings demonstrate that weight loss, reduced alcohol and sodium intake, and regular physical activity are effective lifestyle adaptations to reduce blood pressure (Appel, Champagne, Harsha, et al., 2003; Appel, Espeland, Easter, et al., 2001; Cushman, Cutler, Hanna, et al., 1998; Hagberg, Park, & Brown, 2000; Sacks, Svetkey, & Vollmer, 2001; Stranges, Wu, Dorn, et al., 2004). Studies also show that diets high in fruits, vegetables, and low-fat dairy products can prevent the development of hypertension and can lower elevated blood pressure (Sacks et al., 2001). Table 32-3 shows the Dietary Approaches to Stop Hypertension (DASH) diet, which has been shown to lower blood pressure in people who follow it (Appel et al., 2003).

## Pharmacologic Therapy

For patients with uncomplicated hypertension and no specific indications for another medication, the recommended initial medications include diuretics, beta-blockers, or both. Patients are first given low doses of medication. If blood pressure does not fall to less than 140/90 mm Hg, the dose is increased gradually, and additional medications are included as necessary to achieve control. Table 32-4 describes the various pharmacologic agents that are recommended for the treatment of hypertension. When the blood pressure is less than 140/90 mm Hg for at least 1 year, gradual reduction of the types and doses of medication is indicated. To promote compliance, clinicians try to prescribe the simplest treatment schedule possible, ideally one pill once each day.

### Gerontologic Considerations

Hypertension, particularly elevated systolic blood pressure, increases the risk of death and complications in people older than 50 years (Chobanian et al., 2003). Treatment reduces this risk. Like younger patients, older patients should begin treatment with lifestyle modifications. If medications are needed to achieve the blood pressure goal of less than 140/90 mm Hg, the starting dose should be half that used in younger patients.

### TABLE 32-3  The DASH (Dietary Approaches to Stop Hypertension) Diet

| Food Group | Number of Servings Per Day |
|---|---|
| Grains and grain products | 7 or 8 |
| Vegetables | 4 or 5 |
| Fruits | 4 or 5 |
| Low-fat or fat-free dairy foods | 2 or 3 |
| Meat, fish, and poultry | 2 or fewer |
| Nuts, seeds, and dry beans | 4 or 5 weekly |

The diet is based on 2,000 calories per day.
Source: www.nhlbi.nih.gov/health/public/heart/hbp/dash/index.htm

## Nursing Process

### The Patient With Hypertension

#### Assessment

When hypertension is initially detected, nursing assessment involves carefully monitoring the blood pressure at frequent intervals and then,

*(text continues on page 1030)*

## TABLE 32-4 Medication Therapy for Hypertension

| Medications | Major Action | Advantages and Contraindications | Effects and Nursing Considerations |
|---|---|---|---|
| **Diuretics and Related Drugs** | | | |
| *Thiazide Diuretics* | | | |
| chlorthalidone (Hygroton) chlorothiazide (Diuril) hydrochlorothiazide (Esidrix; HydroDIURIL) indapamide (Lozol) methyclothiazide (Enduron) metolazone (Mylerox, Zaroxolyn) | Decrease of blood volume, renal blood flow, and cardiac output Depletion of extracellular fluid Negative sodium balance (from natriuresis), mild hypokalemia Directly affect vascular smooth muscle | Relatively Inexpensive Effective orally Effective during long-term administration Mild side effects Enhance other antihypertensive medications Counter sodium retention effects of other antihypertensive medications *Contraindications:* Gout, known sensitivity to sulfonamide-derived medications, severely impaired kidney function, and history of hyponatremia | Side effects include dry mouth, thirst, weakness, drowsiness, lethargy, muscle aches, muscular fatigue, tachycardia, GI disturbance. Postural hypotension may be potentiated by alcohol, barbiturates, opioids, or hot weather. Because thiazides cause loss of sodium, potassium, and magnesium, monitor for signs of electrolyte imbalance. Encourage intake of potassium-rich foods (eg, fruits). *Gerontologic Considerations:* Risk of postural hypotension is significant because of volume depletion; measure blood pressure in three positions; caution patient to rise slowly. |
| *Loop Diuretics* | | | |
| furosemide (Lasix) bumetanide (Bumex) forsemide (Demadex) | Volume depletion Blocks reabsorption of sodium, chloride, and water in kidney | Action rapid Potent Used when thiazides fail or patient needs rapid diuresis *Contraindications:* Same as for thiazides | Risk of volume and electrolyte depletion from the profound diuresis that can occur Fluid and electrolyte replacement may be required *Gerontologic Considerations:* Same as for thiazides. |
| *Potassium-Sparing Diuretics* | | | |
| amiloride (Midamor) triamterene (Dyrenium) | Blocks sodium reabsorption Acts on distal tubule independently of aldosterone | Causes potassium retention *Contraindications:* Renal disease, azotemia, severe hepatic disease, hyperkalemia | Drowsiness, lethargy, headache Monitor for hyperkalemia if given with ACE inhibitor or angiotensin receptor blocker. Diarrhea and other GI symptoms—administer medication after meals. |
| **Aldosterone Receptor Blockers** | | | |
| eplerenone (Inspra) spironolactone (Aldactone) | Competitive inhibitors of aldosterone binding | Indicated for patients with a history of myocardial infarction or symptomatic ventricular dysfunction *Contraindications:* Hyperkalemia and impaired renal function Epleronone is contraindicated in diabetes mellitus with micro-albuminuria | Drowsiness, lethargy, headache Monitor for hyperkalemia if given with ACE inhibitor or angiotensin receptor blocker (ARB) Diarrhea and other GI symptoms—administer medication after meals. Avoid use of potassium supplements or salt substitutes. Teach patients, families, and caregivers signs and symptoms of hyperkalemia. Spironolactone may cause gynecomastia. |

## TABLE 32-4  Medication Therapy for Hypertension (Continued)

| Medications | Major Action | Advantages and Contraindications | Effects and Nursing Considerations |
|---|---|---|---|
| **Central Alpha₂-Agonists and Other Centrally Acting Drugs** | | | |
| reserpine (Serpasil) | Impairs synthesis and re-uptake of norepinephrine | Slows pulse, which counteracts tachycardia of hydralazine<br>*Contraindications:* History of depression, psychosis, obesity, chronic sinusitis, peptic ulcer | May cause severe depression; report manifestations, as this may require that drug be omitted.<br>Nasal congestion.<br>Use with caution if history of gallbladder, renal, or cardiac disease, or seizure disorder.<br>*Gerontologic Considerations:* Depression and postural hypotension common in elderly |
| methyldopa (Aldomet) | Dopa-decarboxylase inhibitor; displaces norepinephrine from storage sites | Drug of choice for pregnant women with hypertension<br>Useful in patients with renal failure or prostate disease<br>Does not decrease cardiac output or renal blood flow<br>Does not induce oliguria<br>*Contraindications:* Liver disease | Drowsiness, dizziness<br>Dry mouth; nasal congestion (troublesome at first but then tends to disappear)<br>Use with caution with renal disease.<br>*Gerontologic Considerations:* May produce mental and behavioral changes in the elderly. |
| clonidine (Catapres)<br>clonidine patch (Catapres-TTs) | Exact mode of action not understood, but acts through the central nervous system, apparently through centrally mediated alpha-adrenergic stimulation in the brain, producing blood pressure reduction | Little or no orthostatic effect. Moderately potent, and sometimes is effective when other medications fail to lower blood pressure.<br>*Contraindications:* Severe coronary artery disease, pregnancy; contraindicated in children | Dry mouth, drowsiness, sedation, and occasional headaches and fatigue. Anorexia, malaise, and vomiting with mild disturbance of liver function have been reported.<br>Rebound or withdrawal hypertension is relatively common; monitor blood pressure when stopping medication. |
| guanfacine (Tenex) | Stimulates central alpha-2 adrenergic receptors | Reduces heart rate and causes vasodilation. Serious adverse reactions are uncommon. Use with caution in persons with diminished liver function, recent myocardial infarction, or known cardiovascular disease. | Common side effects include dry mouth, dizziness, sleepiness, fatigue, headache, constipation, and impotence. |
| **Beta Blockers** | | | |
| atenolol (Tenormin)<br>betaxolol (Kerlone)<br>bisoprolol (Zebeta)<br>propranolol (Inderal)<br>propranolol long-acting (Inderal LA)<br>metoprolol (Lopressor)<br>metoprolol extended-release (Toprol XL)<br>nadolol (Corgard)<br>timolol (Blocadren) | Block the sympathetic nervous system (beta-adrenergic receptors), especially the sympathetics to the heart, producing a slower heart rate and lowered blood pressure | Reduce pulse rate in patients with tachycardia and blood pressure elevation<br>Indicated for patients who also have stable angina pectoris and silent ischemia<br>*Contraindications:* Bronchial asthma, allergic rhinitis, right ventricular failure from pulmonary hypertension, heart failure, depression, diabetes mellitus, dyslipidemia, heart block, peripheral vascular disease, heart rate less than 60 bpm | Mental depression manifested by insomnia, lassitude, weakness, and fatigue<br>Avoid sudden discontinuation.<br>Lightheadedness and occasional nausea, vomiting, and epigastric distress<br>Check heart rate before giving.<br>*Gerontologic Considerations:* Risk of toxicity is increased for elderly patients with decreased renal and liver function. Take blood pressure in three positions and observe for hypotension. |

*continued >*

## TABLE 32-4 Medication Therapy for Hypertension (Continued)

| Medications | Major Action | Advantages and Contraindications | Effects and Nursing Considerations |
|---|---|---|---|
| **Beta-Blockers with Intrinsic Sympathomimetic Activity** | | | |
| acebutolol (Sectral)<br>penbutolol (Levatrol)<br>pindolol (Visken) | Block both cardiac beta$_1$ and beta$_2$ receptors<br>Also have antiarrhythmic activity by slowing atrioventricular conduction | *Advantages:* Similar to beta-blockers<br>*Contraindications:* Similar to beta-blockers | Avoid sudden discontinuation.<br>Withhold if bradycardia or heart block is present.<br>Use with caution with COPD, diabetes mellitus.<br>Similar to beta-blockers. |
| **Alpha$_1$-Blockers** | | | |
| doxazosin (Cardura)<br>prazosin hydrochloride (Minipress)<br>terazosin (Hytrin) | Peripheral vasodilator acting directly on the blood vessel; similar to hydralazine | Act directly on the blood vessels and are effective agents in patients with adverse reactions to hydralazine<br>*Contraindications:* Angina pectoris and coronary artery disease. Induces tachycardia if not preceded by administration of propranolol and a diuretic. | Occasional vomiting and diarrhea, urinary frequency, and cardiovascular collapse, especially if given in addition to hydralazine without lowering the dose of the latter. Patients occasionally experience drowsiness, lack of energy, and weakness. |
| **Combined Alpha and Beta Blockers** | | | |
| carvedilol (Coreg)<br>labetalol hydrochloride (Normodyne, Trandate) | Block alpha- and beta-adrenergic receptors; cause peripheral dilation and decrease peripheral vascular resistance | Fast-acting<br>No decrease in renal blood flow<br>*Contraindications:* Asthma, cardiogenic shock, severe tachycardia, heart block | Orthostatic hypotension, tachycardia |
| **Vasodilators** | | | |
| fenoldopam mesylate (Corlopam) | Stimulates dopamine and alpha$_2$-adrenergic receptors | Given intravenously for hypertensive emergencies. Use with caution in patients with glaucoma, recent stroke (brain attack), asthma, hypokalemia, or diminished liver function. | Headache, flushing, hypotension, sweating, tachycardia caused by vasodilation<br>Observe for local reactions at the injection site. |
| hydralazine (Apresoline) | Decreases peripheral resistance but concurrently elevates cardiac output<br>Acts directly on smooth muscle of blood vessels | Not used as initial therapy; used in combination with other medications.<br>Used also in pregnancy-induced hypertension<br>*Contraindications:* Angina or coronary disease, heart failure, hypersensitivity | Headache, tachycardia, flushing, and dyspnea may occur—can be prevented by pretreating with reserpine<br>Peripheral edema may require diuretics.<br>May produce lupus erythematosus–like syndrome |
| minoxidil (Loniten) | Direct vasodilating action on arteriolar vessels, causing decreased peripheral vascular resistance; reduces systolic and diastolic pressures | Hypotensive effect more pronounced than with hydralazine<br>No effect on vasomotor reflexes so does not cause postural hypotension<br>*Contraindications:* Pheochromocytoma | Tachycardia, angina pectoris, ECG changes, edema<br>Take blood pressure and apical pulse before administration.<br>Monitor intake and output and daily weights.<br>Causes hirsutism |
| sodium nitroprusside (Nipride, Nitropress)<br>nitroglycerin (NitroBid IV, Tridil) | Peripheral vasodilation by relaxation of smooth muscle | Fast-acting<br>Used only in hypertensive emergencies<br>*Contraindications:* Sepsis, azotemia, high intracranial pressure | Dizziness, headache, nausea, edema, tachycardia, palpitations<br>Can cause thiocyanate and cyanide intoxication. |

### TABLE 32-4  Medication Therapy for Hypertension (Continued)

| Medications | Major Action | Advantages and Contraindications | Effects and Nursing Considerations |
|---|---|---|---|
| **Angiotensin-Converting Enzyme (ACE) Inhibitors** | | | |
| benazepril (Lotensin)<br>captopril (Capoten)<br>enalaprilat (Vasotec IV)<br>enalapril (Vasotec)<br>fosinopril (Monopril)<br>lisinopril (Prinivil, Zestril)<br>moexipril (Univasc)<br>perindopril (Accon)<br>quinapril (Accupril)<br>ramipril (Altace)<br>trandolapril (Mavik) | Inhibit conversion of angiotensin I to angiotensin II<br>Lower total peripheral resistance | Fewer cardiovascular side effects<br>Can be used with thiazide diuretic and digitalis<br>Hypotension can be reversed by fluid replacement.<br>Angioedema is a rare but potentially life-threatening complication.<br>*Contraindications:* Renal impairment, pregnancy | *Gerontologic Considerations:*<br>Require reduced dosages and the addition of loop diuretics when there is renal dysfunction |
| **Angiotensin II Receptor Blockers (ARBs)** | | | |
| candesartan (Atacand)<br>eprosartan (Teveten)<br>irbesartan (Avapro)<br>losartan (Cozaar)<br>olmesartan (Benicar)<br>telmisartan (Micardis)<br>valsartan (Diovan) | Block the effects of angiotensin II at the receptor<br>Reduce peripheral resistance | Minimal side effects<br>*Contraindications:* Pregnancy, renovascular disease | Monitor for hyperkalemia. |
| **Calcium Channel Blockers** | | | |
| *Nondihydropyridines* | | | |
| diltiazem extended release (Cardizem CV, Dilacor XT, Tiazac)<br>diltiazem long-acting (Cardizem LA) | Inhibit calcium ion influx<br>Reduce cardiac afterload | Inhibit coronary artery spasm not controlled by beta-blockers or nitrates<br>*Contraindications:* Sick sinus syndrome; AV block; hypotension; heart failure | Do not discontinue suddenly.<br>Observe for hypotension.<br>Report irregular heartbeat, dizziness, edema.<br>Instruct on regular dental care because of potential gingivitis. |
| verapamil immediate release (Calan, Isoptin)<br>verapamil long-acting (Calan SR, Isoptin SR)<br>verapamil (Covera HS, Verelan PM) | Inhibits calcium ion influx<br>Slows velocity of conduction of cardiac impulse | Effective antiarrhythmic<br>Rapid IV onset<br>Blocks SA and AV node channels<br>*Contraindications:* Sinus or AV node disease; severe heart failure; severe hypotension | Administer on empty stomach or before meal.<br>Do not discontinue suddenly. Depression may subside when medication is discontinued.<br>To relieve headaches, reduce noise, monitor electrolytes.<br>Decrease dose for patients with liver or renal failure. |
| *Dihydropyridines* | | | |
| amlodipine (Norvasc)<br>felodipine (Plendil)<br>isradipine (Dynacirc CR)<br>nicardipine (Cardene)<br>nifedipine long-acting (Procardia XL, Adalat CC)<br>nisoldipine (Sular) | Inhibit calcium ion influx across membranes<br>Vasodilating effects on coronary and peripheral arteriole<br>Decrease cardiac work and energy consumption, increase delivery of oxygen to myocardium | Rapid action<br>Effective by oral or sublingual route<br>No tendency to slow SA nodal activity or prolong AV node conduction<br>Isolated systolic hypertension<br>*Contraindications:* None (except heart failure for nifedipine) | Administer on empty stomach.<br>Use with caution in diabetic patients with diabetes.<br>Small frequent meals if nausea<br>Muscle cramps, joint stiffness, sexual difficulties may disappear when dose decreased.<br>Report irregular heartbeat, constipation, shortness of breath, edema.<br>May cause dizziness |

after diagnosis, at routinely scheduled intervals. The American Heart Association has defined the standards for blood pressure measurement, including conditions required before measurements are made, equipment specifications, and techniques for measuring blood pressure to obtain accurate and reliable readings (Chart 32-2) (Pickering, Hall, Appel, et al., 2005). When the patient begins an antihypertensive treatment regimen, blood pressure assessments are needed to determine the effectiveness of medication therapy and to detect any changes in blood pressure that indicate the need for a change in the treatment plan.

A complete history is obtained to assess for signs and symptoms that indicate target organ damage (ie, whether specific tissues are damaged by the elevated blood pressure). Such manifestations may include anginal pain; shortness of breath; alterations in speech, vision, or balance; nosebleeds; headaches; dizziness; or nocturia.

During the physical examination, the nurse must also pay specific attention to the rate, rhythm, and character of the apical and peripheral pulses to detect effects of hypertension on the heart and blood vessels. A thorough assessment can yield valuable information about the extent to which the hypertension has affected the body and about any other personal, social, or financial factors related to the condition. For example, some patients' ability to adhere to an antihypertensive medication regimen may be thwarted if they lack the financial resources to buy the medication.

## Diagnosis

### Nursing Diagnoses

Based on the assessment data, nursing diagnoses for the patient may include the following:

- Deficient knowledge regarding the relation between the treatment regimen and control of the disease process
- Noncompliance with therapeutic regimen related to side effects of prescribed therapy

### Collaborative Problems/ Potential Complications

Based on the assessment data, potential complications that may develop include the following:

- Left ventricular hypertrophy
- Myocardial infarction

---

### CHART 32-2

### Measuring Blood Pressure (BP)

**EQUIPMENT**

*For the Patient at Home*
- Automatic or semiautomatic device with digital display of readings

*For the Practitioner*
- Mercury sphygmomanometer, recently calibrated aneroid manometer, or validated electronic device
- Cuff

**INSTRUCTIONS FOR THE PATIENT**
- Avoid smoking cigarettes or drinking caffeine for 30 minutes before BP is measured.
- Sit quietly for 5 minutes before the measurement.
- Sit comfortably with the forearm supported at heart level on a firm surface, with both feet on the ground; avoid talking while the measurement is being taken.

**INSTRUCTIONS FOR THE PRACTITIONER**
- Select the size of the cuff based upon the size of the patient. (The cuff size should have a bladder width of at least 40% of limb circumference and length at least 80% of limb circumference.) The average adult cuff is 12 to 14 cm wide and 30 cm long. Using a cuff that is too small will give a higher BP measurement, and using a cuff that is too large results in a lower BP measurement compared to one taken with a properly sized cuff.
- Routinely calibrate the sphygmomanometer.
- Wrap the cuff firmly around the arm. Center the cuff bladder directly over the brachial artery.
- Position the patient's arm at the level of the heart.
- Palpate the systolic pressure before auscultating. This technique helps to detect the presence of an auscultatory gap more readily.
- Ask the patient to sit quietly while the BP is measured because the BP can increase when the patient is engaged in conversation.
- Initially, record BP results of both arms and take subsequent measurements from the arm with the higher BP. Normally, the BP should vary by no more than 5 mm Hg between arms.
- Record the site where the BP was measured and the position of the patient (eg, right arm).
- Inform the patient of his or her BP value and what it means. Emphasize the need for periodic reassessment, and encourage patients who measure BP at home to keep a written record of readings.

**INTERPRETATION**

Assessment is based on the average of at least two readings. (If two readings differ by more than 5 mm Hg, additional readings are taken and an average reading is calculated from the results.)

- Heart failure
- TIAs
- Cerebrovascular accident (stroke or brain attack)
- Renal insufficiency and failure
- Retinal hemorrhage

## Planning and Goals

The major goals for the patient include understanding of the disease process and its treatment, participation in a self-care program, and absence of complications.

## Nursing Interventions

The objective of nursing care for hypertensive patients focuses on lowering and controlling the blood pressure without adverse effects and without undue cost. To achieve these goals, the nurse must support and teach the patient to adhere to the treatment regimen by implementing necessary lifestyle changes, taking medications as prescribed, and scheduling regular follow-up appointments with the health care provider to monitor progress or identify and treat any complications of disease or therapy.

### Increasing Knowledge

The patient needs to understand the disease process and how lifestyle changes and medications can control hypertension. The nurse needs to emphasize the concept of controlling hypertension rather than curing it. The nurse can encourage the patient to consult a dietitian to help develop a plan for weight loss. The program usually consists of restricting sodium and fat intake, increasing intake of fruits and vegetables, and implementing regular physical activity. Explaining that it takes 2 to 3 months for the taste buds to adapt to changes in salt intake may help the patient adjust to reduced salt intake. The patient should be advised to limit alcohol intake (see Table 32-2 for specific recommendations) and tobacco should be avoided—not because smoking is related to hypertension, but because anyone with high blood pressure is already at increased risk for heart disease, and smoking amplifies this risk. Support groups for weight control, smoking cessation, and stress reduction may be beneficial for some patients; others can benefit from the support of family and friends. The nurse assists the patient to develop and adhere to an appropriate exercise regimen, because regular activity is a significant factor in weight reduction and a blood pressure–reducing intervention in the absence of any loss in weight (Chobanian et al., 2003).

### Promoting Home and Community-Based Care

Blood pressure screenings with the sole purpose of case finding are not recommended by the National High Blood Pressure Education Program because approximately 70% of people with hypertension are already aware of their blood pressure levels (Chobanian et al., 2003). If asked to participate in a blood pressure screening, the nurse should be sure that proper blood pressure measurement technique is being used (see Chart 32-2), that the manometers used are calibrated (Pickering et al., 2005), and that provision has been made to provide follow-up for any person identified as having an elevated blood pressure level. Adequate time should also be allowed to teach people what the blood pressure numbers mean. Each person should be given a written record of his or her blood pressure at the screening.

#### TEACHING PATIENTS SELF-CARE

The therapeutic regimen is the responsibility of the patient in collaboration with the health care provider. The nurse can help the patient achieve blood pressure control through education about high blood pressure and how to manage it through medication, lifestyle changes of diet, weight control, and exercise (see Table 32-2), setting goal blood pressures, and providing assistance with social support. Involving family members in education programs enables them to support the patient's efforts to control hypertension. The American Heart Association and the National Heart, Lung, and Blood Institute provide printed and electronic patient education materials.

Providing written information about the expected effects and side effects of medications is important. When side effects occur, patients need to understand the importance of reporting them and to whom they should be reported. Patients need to be informed that **rebound hypertension** can occur if antihypertensive medications are suddenly stopped. Both female and male patients should be informed that some medications, such as beta-blockers, may cause sexual dysfunction and that other medications are available if a problem with sexual function or satisfaction occurs. The nurse can encourage and teach patients to measure their blood pressure at home. This practice involves patients in their own care and emphasizes that failing to take medications may result in an identifiable rise in blood pressure. Patients need to know that blood pressure varies continuously and that the range within which their pressure varies should be monitored.

#### GERONTOLOGIC CONSIDERATIONS

Compliance with the therapeutic program may be more difficult for elderly people. The medication regimen can be difficult to remember, and the expense can be a problem. **Monotherapy** (treatment with a single agent), if appropriate, may simplify the medication regimen and make it less expensive. Special care must be taken to ensure that the elderly patient understands the regimen and can see and read instructions, open the medication container, and get the prescription refilled. The elderly person's family or caregivers should be included in the teaching program so that they understand the patient's needs, encourage adherence to the treatment plan, and know when and whom to call if problems arise or information is needed.

## CONTINUING CARE

Regular follow-up care is imperative so that the disease process can be assessed and treated, depending on whether control or progression is found, as shown in Table 32-5. A history and physical examination should be completed at each clinic visit. The history should include all data pertaining to any potential problem, specifically medication-related problems such as postural (orthostatic) hypotension (experienced as dizziness or lightheadedness).

Deviation from the therapeutic program is a significant problem for people with hypertension and other chronic conditions requiring lifetime management. An estimated 50% of patients discontinue their medications within 1 year of beginning to take them. Blood pressure control is achieved by only 34% (Chobanian et al., 2003). Compliance increases, however, when patients actively participate in self-care, including self-monitoring of blood pressure and diet—possibly because patients receive immediate feedback and have a greater sense of control.

Patients with hypertension must make considerable effort to adhere to recommended lifestyle modifications and to take regularly prescribed medications. The effort needed to follow the therapeutic plan may seem unreasonable to some, particularly when they have no symptoms without medications but do have side effects with medications. The recommended lifestyle changes are listed in Table 32-2. Continued education and encouragement are usually needed to enable patients to formulate an acceptable plan that helps them live with their hypertension and adhere to the treatment plan. Compromises may have to be made about some aspects of therapy to achieve higher-priority goals.

The nurse can assist with behavior change by supporting patients in making small changes with each visit that move them toward their goals. Another important factor is following up at each visit to see how the patient has progressed with the plans made at the prior visit. If the patient has had difficulty with a particular aspect of the plan, the patient and nurse can work together to develop an alternative or modification to the plan that the patient believes will be more successful.

### Monitoring and Managing Potential Complications

Symptoms suggesting that hypertension is progressing to the extent that target organ damage is occurring must be detected early so that appropriate treatment can be initiated. When the patient returns for follow-up care, all body systems must be assessed to detect any evidence of vascular damage. An eye examination with an ophthalmoscope is particularly important because retinal blood vessel damage indicates similar damage elsewhere in the vascular system. The patient is questioned about blurred vision, spots in front of the eyes, and diminished visual acuity. The heart, nervous system, and kidneys are also carefully assessed. Any significant findings are promptly reported to determine whether additional diagnostic studies are required. Based on the findings, medications may be changed to improve blood pressure control.

> **NURSING ALERT**
>
> The patient and caregivers should be cautioned that antihypertensive medications can cause hypotension. Low blood pressure or postural hypotension should be reported immediately. Elderly people have impaired cardiovascular reflexes and thus are more sensitive to the extracellular volume depletion caused by diuretics and to the sympathetic inhibition caused by adrenergic antagonists. The nurse teaches patients to change positions slowly when moving from a lying or sitting position to a standing position. The nurse also counsels elderly patients to use supportive devices such as hand rails and walkers as necessary to prevent falls that could result from dizziness.

**TABLE 32-5 Recommendations for Follow-Up Based on Initial Blood Pressure Measurements for Adults Without Acute End Organ Damage**

| Initial BP (mm Hg)* | Follow-Up Recommended† |
|---|---|
| Normal | Recheck in 2 years |
| Prehypertension | Recheck in 1 year‡ |
| Stage 1 hypertension | Confirm within 2 months‡ |
| Stage 2 hypertension | Evaluate or refer to source of care within 1 month |
| | For those with higher pressures (eg, >180/100 mm Hg), evaluate and treat immediately or within 1 week, depending on clinical situation and complications. |

* If systolic and diastolic values fall into different categories, follow recommendations for shorter follow-up (eg, 160/86 mm Hg should be evaluated or referred to source of care within 1 month).
† Modify the scheduling of follow-up according to reliable information about past blood pressure measurements, other cardiovascular risk factors, or target organ disease.
‡ Provide advice about lifestyle modifications.

From the Seventh Report of the Joint National Committee on Prevention, Detection, Evaluation, and Treatment of High Blood Pressure. (2003). Hypertension, 42(6), 1206–1252.

## Evaluation

### EXPECTED PATIENT OUTCOMES

Expected patient outcomes may include the following:

1. Maintains adequate tissue perfusion:
   a. Maintains blood pressure at less than 140/90 mm Hg (or less than 130/80 mm Hg for people with diabetes mellitus or chronic kidney disease) with lifestyle modifications, medications, or both
   b. Demonstrates no symptoms of angina, palpitations, or vision changes
   c. Has stable BUN and serum creatinine levels
   d. Has palpable peripheral pulses
2. Complies with the self-care program:
   a. Adheres to the dietary regimen as prescribed: reduces calorie, sodium, and fat intake; increases fruit and vegetable intake
   b. Exercises regularly
   c. Takes medications as prescribed and reports any side effects
   d. Measures blood pressure routinely
   e. Abstains from tobacco and excessive alcohol intake
   f. Keeps follow-up appointments
3. Has no complications:
   a. Reports no changes in vision
   b. Exhibits no retinal damage on vision testing
   c. Maintains pulse rate and rhythm and respiratory rate within normal ranges
   d. Reports no dyspnea or edema
   e. Maintains urine output consistent with intake
   f. Has renal function test results within normal range
   g. Demonstrates no motor, speech, or sensory deficits
   h. Reports no headaches, dizziness, weakness, changes in gait, or falls

# Hypertensive Crises

JNC 7 describes two classes of hypertensive crisis that require immediate intervention: hypertensive emergency and hypertensive urgency (Chobanian et al., 2003). Hypertensive emergencies and urgencies may occur in patients whose hypertension has been poorly controlled or in those who have abruptly discontinued their medications. Once the hypertensive crisis has been managed, a complete evaluation is performed to review the patient's ongoing treatment plan and strategies to minimize the occurrence of subsequent hypertensive crises. The current recommendations for management of both hypertensive emergencies and urgencies are based on expert opinions because there are not clinical trial data comparing treatment options or identifying the impact of treatment on morbidity and mortality (Cherney & Straus, 2002).

**Hypertensive emergency** is a situation in which blood pressure is extremely elevated (more than 180/120 mm Hg) and must be lowered immediately (not necessarily to less than 140/90 mm Hg) to halt or prevent damage to the target organs (Chobanian et al., 2003). Assessment will reveal actual or developing clinical dysfunction of the target organ. Conditions associated with hypertensive emergency include hypertension of pregnancy, acute myocardial infarction, dissecting aortic aneurysm, and intracranial hemorrhage. Hypertensive emergencies are acute, life-threatening blood pressure elevations that require prompt treatment in an intensive care setting because of the serious target organ damage that may occur. The therapeutic goals are reduction of the mean blood pressure by up to 25% within the first hour of treatment, a further reduction to a goal pressure of about 160/100 mm Hg over a period of up to 6 hours, and then a more gradual reduction in pressure over a period of days. The exceptions to these goals are the treatment of ischemic stroke (in which there is no evidence of benefit from immediate pressure reduction) and treatment of aortic dissection (in which the goal is to lower systolic pressure to less than 100 mm Hg if the patient can tolerate the reduction) (Chobanian et al., 2003).

The medications of choice in hypertensive emergencies are those that have an immediate effect. Intravenous vasodilators, including sodium nitroprusside (Nipride, Nitropress), nicardipine hydrochloride (Cardene), fenoldopam mesylate (Corlopam), enalaprilat (Vasotec), and nitroglycerin (Nitro-Bid, Tridil) have immediate actions that are short-lived (minutes to 4 hours), and they are therefore used for initial treatment. For more information about these medications, see Table 32-4.

**Hypertensive urgency** describes a situation in which blood pressure is very elevated but there is no evidence of impending or progressive target organ damage (Chobanian et al., 2003). Elevated blood pressures associated with severe headaches, nosebleeds, or anxiety are classified as urgencies. Oral doses of fast-acting agents such as beta-adrenergic blocking agents (eg, labetalol [Normodyne, Trandate]), angiotensin-converting enzyme inhibitors (eg, captopril [Capoten]), or alpha$_2$-agonists (eg, clonidine [Catapres]) are recommended for the treatment of hypertensive urgencies (see Table 32-4).

Extremely close hemodynamic monitoring of the patient's blood pressure and cardiovascular status is required during treatment of hypertensive emergencies and urgencies (see Chapter 26). The exact frequency of monitoring is a matter of clinical judgment and varies with the patient's condition. Taking vital signs every 5 minutes is appropriate if the blood pressure is changing rapidly; taking vital signs at 15- or 30-minute intervals in a more stable situation may be sufficient. A precipitous drop in blood pressure can occur that would require immediate action to restore blood pressure to an acceptable level.

## Critical Thinking Exercises

**1** You are a charge nurse in an emergency department. A 72-year-old man arrives one evening with a laceration of his right forearm from a minor gardening injury. The laceration will require suturing. When you take the patient's blood pressure on his left arm, you note that it is 164/78. You tell the patient his blood pressure and express concern that his systolic blood pressure is high. He shrugs and tells you, "The top number is always elevated, but it's nothing to worry about." What is the evidence base that indicates that untreated isolated systolic hypertension can cause disability and death? What other information do you plan to gather from this patient? What plan of action might you initiate?

**2** **ebp** You are volunteering at a church-sponsored blood pressure screening clinic that is being offered after Sunday services, in tandem with a fund-raising buffet breakfast. The pastor approaches you and notes that the breakfast buffet serves a variety of egg dishes, hash browns, sausage patties, bacon, and pastries. He asks you what effects, if any, this food may have on his parishioners' blood pressures. What effect might this type of diet have on the parishioners' blood pressures today? Discuss the strength of the evidence that supports specific dietary strategies aimed at preventing and treating hypertension.

## REFERENCES AND SELECTED READINGS

### BOOKS

Kaplan, N., Lieberman, E., & Neal, W. (2002). *Kaplan's clinical hypertension* (8th ed.). Philadelphia: Lippincott Williams & Wilkins.

Zipes, D. P., Libby, P., Bonow, R. O., et al. (Eds.) (2005). *Heart disease: A textbook of cardiovascular medicine* (7th ed.). Philadelphia: W. B. Saunders.

### JOURNALS

Appel, L. J., Champagne, C. M., Harsha, D. W., et al. (2003). Effects of comprehensive lifestyle modification on blood pressure control: Main results of the premier clinical trial. *Journal of the American Medical Association, 289*(16), 2083–2093.

Appel, L. J., Espeland, M. A., Easter, L., et al. (2001). Effects of reduced sodium intake on hypertension control in older individuals: Results from the trial of nonpharmacologic interventions in the elderly (TONE). *Archives of Internal Medicine, 161*(5), 685–693.

Casper, M. L., Barnett, E., Williams, G. I., et al. Atlas of stroke mortality: Racial, ethnic, and geographic disparities in the United States. www.cdc.gov/cvh/maps/strokeatlas/index.htm. Accessed March 24, 2005.

Cherney, D., & Straus, S. (2002). Management of patients with hypertensive urgencies and emergencies: A systematic review of the literature. *Journal of General Internal Medicine, 17*(12), 937–945.

Chobanian, A. V., Bakris, G. L., Black, H. R., et al. (2003). The Seventh Report of the Joint National Committee on Prevention, Detection, Evaluation, and Treatment of High Blood Pressure: The JNC 7 Report (erratum in: *Journal of the American Medical Association,* 2003; 290(2):197). *Journal of the American Medical Association, 289*(19), 2560–2572.

Cushman, W. C., Cutler, J. A., Hanna, E., et al. (1998). Prevention and treatment of hypertension study (PATHS): Effects of an alcohol treatment program on blood pressure. *Archives of Internal Medicine, 158*(11), 1197–1207.

Dominiczak, A. F., Negrin, D. C., Clark, J. S., et al. (2000). Genes and hypertension: From gene mapping in experimental models to vascular gene transfer strategies. *Hypertension, 35*(1 Pt 2), 164–172.

Fields, L. E., Burt, V. L., Cutler, J. A., et al. (2004). The burden of adult hypertension in the United States 1999 to 2000: A rising tide. *Hypertension, 44*(4), 398–404.

Hagberg, J. M., Park, J. J., & Brown, M. D. (2000). The role of exercise training in the treatment of hypertension: An update. *Sports Medicine, 30*(3), 193–206.

Hajjar, I., & Kotchen, T. A. (2003). Trends in prevalence, awareness, treatment, and control of hypertension in the United States, 1988–2000. *JAMA, 290*(2), 199–206.

Lewington, S., Clarke, R., Qizilbash, N., et al. (2002). Age-specific relevance of usual blood pressure to vascular mortality: A meta-analysis of individual data for one million adults in 61 prospective studies. *Lancet, 360*(9349), 1903–1913.

Oparil, S., Zaman, M. A., & Calhoun, D. A. (2003). Pathogenesis of hypertension. *Annals of Internal Medicine, 139*(9), 761–776.

Pickering, T. G., Hall, J. E., Appel, L. J., et al. (2005). Recommendations for blood pressure measurement in humans and experimental animals: Part 1: Blood pressure measurement in humans: A statement for professionals from the Subcommittee of Professional and Public Education of the American Heart Association Council on High Blood Pressure Research. *Hypertension, 45*(1), 142–161.

Sacks, F. M., Svetkey, L. P., Vollmer, W. M., et al. (2001). Effects on blood pressure of reduced dietary sodium and the Dietary Approaches to Stop Hypertension (DASH) diet. DASH-Sodium Collaborative Research Group. *New England Journal of Medicine, 344*(1), 3–10.

Stranges, S., Wu, T., Dorn, J. M., et al. (2004). Relationship of alcohol drinking pattern to risk of hypertension: A population-based study. *Hypertension, 44*(6), 813–819.

### RESOURCES

American Heart Association National Center, 7272 Greenville Ave., Dallas, TX 75231-4596; 1-214-373-6300; fax, 1-214-706-1191; http://www.americanheart.org/. Accessed April 1, 2006.

Centers for Disease Control and Prevention (CDC), 600 Clifton Rd., Atlanta, GA 30333; Cardiovascular Health Program: 1-404-639-3534 or 1-800-311-3435; http://www.cdc.gov/cvh. Accessed April 1, 2006.

Heart and Stroke Foundation of Canada, 222 Queen St., Suite 1402, Ottawa, Ontario K1P5V9, 1-613-569-4361; fax 1-613-569-3278; http://www.heartandstroke.ca/. Accessed April 1, 2006.

National Heart, Lung, and Blood Institute, NHLBI Information Center, P.O. Box 30105, Bethesda, MD 20824-0105; http://www.nhlbi.nih.gov. Accessed April 1, 2006.

World Health Association (WHO), Avenue Appia 20, 1211 Geneva, 27 Switzerland; Cardiovascular Disease Information: http://www.who.int/entity/cardiovascular_diseases/en. Accessed April 1, 2006.

# CHAPTER 33

# Assessment and Management of Patients With Hematologic Disorders

## Learning Objectives

*On completion of this chapter, the learner will be able to:*

1. Describe the process of hematopoiesis.
2. Describe the processes involved in maintaining hemostasis.
3. Differentiate between the hypoproliferative and the hemolytic anemias and compare and contrast the physiologic mechanisms, clinical manifestations, medical management, and nursing interventions for each.
4. Use the nursing process as a framework for care of patients with anemia.
5. Compare the leukemias in terms of their incidence, physiologic alterations, clinical manifestations, management, and prognosis.
6. Use the nursing process as a framework for care of patients with acute leukemia.
7. Use the nursing process as a framework for care of patients with lymphoma or multiple myeloma.
8. Use the nursing process as a framework for care of patients with bleeding or thrombotic disorders.
9. Identify therapies for blood disorders, including the nursing implications for the administration of blood components.

# Glossary

**absolute neutrophil count (ANC):** a mathematical calculation of the actual number of neutrophils in the circulation, derived from the total WBCs and the percentage of neutrophils counted in a microscope's visual field; provides a rough indication of infection risk

**anemia:** decreased RBC count

**anergy:** diminished reactivity to antigens (transient or complete)

**angiogenesis:** formation of new blood vessels, such as in a healing wound or in a malignant tumor

**angular cheilosis:** cracking sore at corner of mouth

**aplasia:** lack of cellular development (eg, of cells within the bone marrow)

**apoptosis:** complex process of programmed cell death

**band cell:** slightly immature neutrophil

**blast cell:** primitive WBC

**cytokines:** hormones produced by leukocytes that are vital to regulation of hematopoiesis, apoptosis, and immune responses

**D-dimer:** test that measures fibrin breakdown; considered to be more specific than fibrin degradation products in the diagnosis of disseminated intravascular coagulation (DIC)

**differentiation:** development of functions and characteristics that are different from those of the parent stem cell

**dysplasia:** abnormal development (eg, of blood cells); size, shape and appearance of cells are altered

**ecchymosis:** bruise

**erythrocyte:** see RBC

**erythrocyte sedimentation rate (ESR):** laboratory test that measures the rate of settling of RBCs; elevation is indicative of inflammation; also called the "sed rate"

**erythroid cells:** broad term used in reference to any cell that is or will become a mature RBC

**erythropoiesis:** process of formation of RBCs

**erythropoietin:** hormone produced primarily by the kidney; necessary for erythropoiesis

**fibrin:** filamentous protein; basis of thrombus and blood clot

**fibrinogen:** protein converted into fibrin to form thrombus and clot

**fibrinolysis:** process of breakdown of fibrin clot

**granulocyte:** granulated WBC (neutrophil, eosinophil, basophil); sometimes used synonymously with neutrophil

**granulocytopenia:** fewer than normal granulocytes

**hematocrit:** percentage of total blood volume consisting of RBCs

**hematopoiesis:** complex process of the formation and maturation of blood cells

**hemoglobin:** iron-containing protein of RBCs; delivers oxygen to tissues

**hemolysis:** destruction of RBCs; can occur within or outside of the vasculature

**hemosiderin:** iron-containing pigment derived from breakdown of hemoglobin

**hemostasis:** intricate balance between clot formation and clot dissolution

**histiocytes:** cells present in all loose connective tissue, capable of phagocytosis; part of the RES

**hyperplasia:** abnormally increased proliferation of normal cells

**hypochromia:** pallor within the RBC caused by decreased hemoglobin content

**left shift,** or **shift to the left:** increased release of immature forms of WBCs from the bone marrow in response to need

**leukocyte:** see WBC

**leukemia:** uncontrolled proliferation of WBCs, often immature

**leukopenia:** less than normal amount of WBCs in circulation

**lymphoid:** pertaining to lymphocytes

**lymphocyte:** form of WBC involved in immune functions

**lysis:** destruction of cells

**macrocytosis:** larger than normal RBCs

**macrophage:** cells of the RES that are capable of phagocytosis

**mast cell:** cells found in connective tissue involved in defense of the body and coagulation

**microcytosis:** smaller than normal RBCs

**monocyte:** large WBC that becomes a macrophage when it leaves the circulation and moves into body tissues

**myeloid:** pertaining to nonlymphoid blood cells that differentiate into RBCs, platelets, monocytes and macrophages, neutrophils, eosinophils, basophils, and mast cells

**myelopoiesis:** formation and maturation of cells derived from myeloid stem cell

**neutropenia:** lower than normal number of neutrophils

**neutrophil:** fully mature WBC capable of phagocytosis; primary defense against bacterial infection

**normochromic:** normal RBC color, indicating normal amount of hemoglobin

**normocytic:** normal size of RBC

**nucleated RBC:** immature form of RBC; portion of nucleus remains within the red cell; not normally seen in circulating blood

**oxyhemoglobin:** combined form of oxygen and hemoglobin; found in arterial blood

**pancytopenia:** abnormal decrease in WBCs, RBCs, and platelets

**petechiae:** tiny capillary hemorrhages

**phagocytosis:** process of ingestion and digestion of bacteria by cells

**plasma:** liquid portion of blood

**plasminogen:** protein that is converted to plasmin to dissolve thrombi and clots

**platelet:** thrombocyte; a cellular component of blood involved in blood coagulation

**poikilocytosis:** variation in shape of RBCs

**polycythemia:** excess RBCs

**RBC:** red blood cell, erythrocyte; a cellular component of blood involved in the transport of oxygen and carbon dioxide

**red blood cell:** see RBC

**reticulocytes:** slightly immature RBCs, usually only 1% of total circulating RBCs

**reticuloendothelial system (RES):** complex system of cells throughout body capable of phagocytosis

**serum:** portion of blood remaining after coagulation occurs

**stem cell:** primitive cell, capable of self-replication and differentiation into myeloid or lymphoid stem cell

**thrombin:** enzyme necessary to convert fibrinogen into fibrin clot

**thrombocyte:** see platelet

**thrombocytopenia:** lower than normal platelet count

**thrombocytosis:** higher than normal platelet count

**WBC:** white blood cells, leukocytes; cellular components of blood involved in defense of the body; subtypes include neutrophils, eosinophils, monocytes, and lymphocytes

**white blood cell:** see WBC

Unlike many other body systems, the hematologic system truly encompasses the entire human body. Patients with hematologic disorders often have significant abnormalities in blood tests but few or no symptoms. Therefore, the nurse must have a good understanding of the pathophysiology of the patient's condition and the ability to make a thorough assessment that relies heavily on the interpretation of laboratory tests. It is equally important for the nurse to anticipate potential patient needs and to target nursing interventions accordingly. Because it is so important to the understanding of most hematologic diseases, a basic appreciation of blood cells and bone marrow function is necessary.

# Anatomic and Physiologic Overview

The hematologic system consists of the blood and the sites where blood is produced, including the bone marrow and the **reticuloendothelial system** (RES). Blood is a specialized organ that differs from other organs in that it exists in a fluid state. Blood is composed of plasma and various types of cells. **Plasma** is the fluid portion of blood; it contains various proteins, such as albumin, globulin, **fibrinogen**, and other factors necessary for clotting, as well as electrolytes, waste products, and nutrients. About 55% of blood volume is plasma.

## Blood

The cellular component of blood consists of three primary cell types (Table 33-1): **erythrocytes (red blood cells [RBCs], red cells), leukocytes (white blood cells [WBCs]),** and **thrombocytes (platelets).** These cellular components of blood normally make up 40% to 45% of the blood volume. Because most blood cells have a short life span, the need for the body to replenish its supply of cells is continuous; this process is termed **hematopoiesis.** The primary site for hematopoiesis is the bone marrow. During embryonic development and in other conditions, the liver and spleen may also be involved.

Under normal conditions, the adult bone marrow produces about 175 billion erythrocytes, 70 billion **neutrophils** (a mature type of WBC), and 175 billion platelets each day. When the body needs more blood cells, as in infection (when neutrophils are needed to fight the invading pathogen) or in bleeding (when more RBCs are required), the marrow increases its production of the cells required. Thus, under normal conditions, the marrow responds to increased demand and releases adequate numbers of cells into the circulation.

Blood makes up approximately 7% to 10% of the normal body weight and amounts to 5 to 6 L of volume. Circulating through the vascular system and serving as a link between body organs, blood carries oxygen absorbed from the lungs and nutrients absorbed from the gastrointestinal (GI) tract to the body cells for cellular metabolism. Blood also carries hormones, antibodies, and other substances to their sites of action or use. In addition, blood carries waste products produced by cellular metabolism to the lungs, skin, liver, and kidneys, where they are transformed and eliminated from the body.

Blood is fluid; therefore, the danger always exists that trauma can lead to loss of blood from the vascular system. To prevent this, an intricate clotting mechanism is activated when necessary to seal any leak in the blood vessels. Excessive clotting is equally dangerous, because it can obstruct blood flow to vital tissues. To prevent this, the body has a fibrinolytic mechanism that eventually dissolves clots (thrombi) formed within blood vessels. The balance between these two systems, clot (thrombus) formation and clot (thrombus) dissolution or **fibrinolysis,** is called **hemostasis.**

## Bone Marrow

The bone marrow is the site of hematopoiesis, or blood cell formation (Fig. 33-1). All skeletal bones are involved in children, but as children age, marrow activity decreases. Marrow activity is usually limited to the pelvis, ribs, vertebrae, and sternum in adults.

Marrow is one of the largest organs of the body, making up 4% to 5% of total body weight. It consists of islands of cellular components (red marrow) separated by fat (yellow marrow). As the adult ages, the proportion of active marrow

| TABLE 33-1 | Blood Cells |
|---|---|
| Cell Type | Major Function |
| **WBC (Leukocyte)** | Fights infection |
| Neutrophil | Essential in preventing or limiting bacterial infection via phagocytosis |
| Monocyte | Enters tissue as macrophage; highly phagocytic, especially against fungus; immune surveillance |
| Eosinophil | Involved in allergic reactions (neutralizes histamine); digests foreign proteins |
| Basophil | Contains histamine; integral part of hypersensitivity reactions |
| Lymphocyte | Integral component of immune system |
|   T lymphocyte | Responsible for cell-mediated immunity; recognizes material as "foreign" (surveillance system) |
|   B lymphocyte | Responsible for humoral immunity; many mature into plasma cells to form antibodies |
| Plasma cell | Secretes immunoglobulin (Ig, antibody); most mature form of B lymphocyte |
| **RBC (Erythrocyte)** | Carries hemoglobin to provide oxygen to tissues; average life span is 120 days |
| **Platelet (Thrombocyte)** | Fragment of megakaryocyte; provides basis for coagulation to occur; maintains hemostasis; average life span is 10 days |

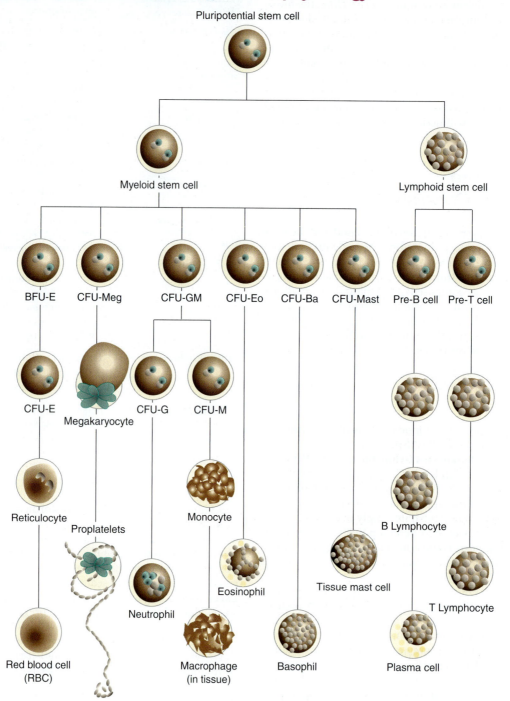

**FIGURE 33-1.** Hematopoiesis. Uncommitted (pluripotent) stem cells can differentiate into myeloid or lymphoid stem cells. These stem cells then undergo a complex process of differentiation and maturation into normal cells that are released into the circulation. The myeloid stem cell is responsible not only for all nonlymphoid white blood cells (WBCs) but also for the production of red blood cells (RBCs) and platelets. Each step of the differentiation process depends in part on the presence of specific growth factors for each cell type. When the stem cells are dysfunctional, they may respond inadequately to the need for more cells, or they may respond excessively, sometimes uncontrollably, as in leukemia. Adapted from Amgen, Inc., 1995, Thousand Oaks, CA.

is gradually replaced by fat; however, in the healthy person, the fat can again be replaced by active marrow when more blood cell production is required. In adults with disease that causes marrow destruction, fibrosis, or scarring, the liver and spleen can also resume production of blood cells by a process known as extramedullary hematopoiesis.

The marrow is highly vascular. Within it are primitive cells called **stem cells.** The stem cells have the ability to self-replicate, thereby ensuring a continuous supply of stem cells throughout the life cycle. When stimulated to do so, stem cells can begin a process of **differentiation** into either **myeloid** or **lymphoid** stem cells. These stem cells are committed to produce specific types of blood cells. Lymphoid stem cells produce either T or B **lymphocytes.** Myeloid stem cells differentiate into three broad cell types: erythrocytes, leukocytes, and platelets. Thus, with the exception of lymphocytes, all blood cells are derived from myeloid stem cells. A defect in a myeloid stem cell can cause problems with erythrocyte, leukocyte, and platelet production. Many complex mechanisms are involved in hematopoiesis, often at the molecular level. A thorough description of these processes is beyond the scope of this textbook; however, some mechanisms against which a specific treatment is targeted are briefly described in the relevant disease-specific sections of this chapter.

## Blood Cells

### Erythrocytes (Red Blood Cells)

The normal erythrocyte is a biconcave disk that resembles a soft ball compressed between two fingers (Fig. 33-2). It has a diameter of about 8 μm and is so flexible that it can pass easily through capillaries that may be as small as 2.8 μm in diameter. The membrane of the red cell is very thin so that gases, such as oxygen and carbon dioxide, can easily diffuse across it; the disk shape provides a large surface area that facilitates the absorption and release of oxygen molecules.

Mature erythrocytes consist primarily of **hemoglobin,** which contains iron and makes up 95% of the cell mass. Mature erythrocytes have no nuclei, and they have many fewer metabolic enzymes than do most other cells. The presence of a large amount of hemoglobin enables the red cell to perform its principal function, the transport of oxygen between the lungs and tissues. Occasionally the marrow releases slightly immature forms of erythrocytes, called **reticulocytes,** into the circulation. This occurs as a normal response to an increased demand for erythrocytes (as in bleeding) or in some disease states.

The oxygen-carrying hemoglobin molecule is made up of four subunits, each containing a heme portion attached to a globin chain. Iron is present in the heme component of the molecule. An important property of heme is its ability to bind to oxygen loosely and reversibly. Oxygen readily binds to hemoglobin in the lungs and is carried as **oxyhemoglobin** in arterial blood. Oxyhemoglobin is a brighter red than hemoglobin that does not contain oxygen (reduced hemoglobin), which is why arterial blood is a brighter red than venous blood. The oxygen readily dissociates (detaches) from hemoglobin in the tissues, where the oxygen is needed for cellular metabolism. In venous blood, hemoglobin combines with hydrogen ions produced by cellular metabolism and thus buffers excessive acid. Whole blood normally contains about 15 g of hemoglobin per 100 mL of blood.

### ERYTHROPOIESIS

Erythroblasts arise from the primitive myeloid stem cells in bone marrow. The erythroblast is an immature nucleated cell that accumulates hemoglobin and then gradually loses its nucleus. At this stage, the cell is known as a reticulocyte. Further maturation into an erythrocyte entails the loss of the dark-staining material within the cell and slight shrinkage. The mature erythrocyte is then released into the circulation. Under conditions of rapid **erythropoiesis** (erythrocyte production), reticulocytes and other immature cells (eg, **nucleated RBCs**) may be released prematurely into the circulation. This is often seen when the liver or spleen takes over as the site of erythropoiesis and more nucleated red cells are seen within the circulation.

Differentiation of the primitive myeloid stem cell of the marrow into an erythroblast is stimulated by **erythropoietin,** a hormone produced primarily by the kidney. If the kidney detects low levels of oxygen (as would occur in **anemia,** in which fewer red cells are available to bind oxygen, or in people living at high altitudes), the release of erythropoietin is increased. The increased erythropoietin then stimulates the marrow to increase production of erythrocytes. The entire process typically takes 5 days.

For normal erythrocyte production, the bone marrow also requires iron, vitamin $B_{12}$, folic acid, pyridoxine (vitamin $B_6$), protein, and other factors. A deficiency of these factors during erythropoiesis can result in decreased red cell production and anemia.

**Iron Stores and Metabolism.** The average daily diet in the United States contains 10 to 15 mg of elemental iron, but only 0.5 to 1 mg of ingested iron is normally absorbed from the small intestine. The rate of iron absorption is regulated by the amount of iron already stored in the body and by the rate of erythrocyte production. Additional amounts of iron, up to 2 mg daily, must be absorbed by women of childbearing age to replace that lost during menstruation. Total body iron content in the average adult is approximately 3 g, most of which is present in hemoglobin or in one of its breakdown products. Iron is stored in the small intestine as ferritin and in reticuloendothelial cells. When required, the iron is released into the plasma, binds to transferrin, and is transported into the membranes of the normoblasts (erythrocyte precursor cells) within the marrow, where it is incorporated into hemoglobin. Iron is lost in the feces, either in bile, blood, or mucosal cells from the intestine.

The concentration of iron in blood is normally about 75 to 175 μg/dL (13 to 31 μmol/L) for men and 65 to 165 μg/dL (11 to 29 μmol/L) for women. With iron deficiency, bone marrow iron stores are rapidly depleted; hemoglobin synthesis is depressed, and the erythrocytes produced by the marrow are small and low in hemoglobin. Iron deficiency in the adult generally indicates that blood has been lost from the body (eg, from bleeding in the GI tract or heavy menstrual flow). In the adult, lack of dietary iron is rarely the sole cause of iron deficiency anemia. The source of iron deficiency should be investigated promptly, because iron deficiency in an adult may be a sign of bleeding in the GI tract or colon cancer.

**FIGURE 33-2.** Normal types of blood cells. From Cohen, B. J. (2005). *Memmler's the human body in health and disease* (10th ed.). Philadelphia: Lippincott Williams & Wilkins.

**Vitamin $B_{12}$ and Folic Acid Metabolism.** Vitamin $B_{12}$ and folic acid are required for the synthesis of DNA in many tissues, but deficiencies of either of these vitamins have the greatest effect on erythropoiesis. Both vitamin $B_{12}$ and folic acid are derived from the diet. Folic acid is absorbed in the proximal small intestine, but only small amounts are stored within the body. If the diet is deficient in folic acid, stores within the body quickly become depleted. Because vitamin $B_{12}$ is found only in foods of animal origin, strict vegetarians may ingest little vitamin $B_{12}$. Vitamin $B_{12}$ combines with intrinsic factor produced in the stomach. The vitamin $B_{12}$–intrinsic factor complex is absorbed in the distal ileum. People who have had a partial or total gastrectomy may have limited amounts of intrinsic factor, and therefore the absorption of vitamin $B_{12}$ may be diminished. The effects of either decreased absorption or decreased intake of vitamin $B_{12}$ are not apparent for 2 to 4 years.

Vitamin $B_{12}$ and folic acid deficiencies are characterized by the production of abnormally large erythrocytes called megaloblasts. Because these cells are abnormal, many are sequestered (trapped) while still in the bone marrow, and their rate of release is decreased. Some of these cells actually die in the marrow before they can be released into the circulation. This results in megaloblastic anemia.

## RED BLOOD CELL DESTRUCTION

The average life span of a normal circulating erythrocyte is 120 days. Aged erythrocytes lose their elasticity and become trapped in small blood vessels and the spleen. They are removed from the blood by the reticuloendothelial cells, particularly in the liver and the spleen. As the erythrocytes are destroyed, most of their hemoglobin is recycled. Some hemoglobin also breaks down to form bilirubin and is secreted in the bile. Most of the iron is recycled to form new hemoglobin molecules within the bone marrow; small amounts are lost daily in the feces and urine and monthly in menstrual flow.

## Leukocytes (White Blood Cells)

Leukocytes are divided into two general categories: granulocytes and lymphocytes. In normal blood, the total leukocyte count is 5,000 to 10,000 cells per cubic millimeter. Of these, approximately 60% to 70% are granulocytes and 30% to 40% are lymphocytes. Both of these types of leukocytes primarily protect the body against infection and tissue injury.

### GRANULOCYTES

**Granulocytes** are defined by the presence of granules in the cytoplasm of the cell. Granulocytes are divided into three main subgroups, which are characterized by the staining properties of these granules (see Fig. 33-2). Eosinophils have bright-red granules in their cytoplasm, whereas the granules in basophils stain deep blue. The third and by far the most numerous cell in this class is the neutrophil, with granules that stain a pink to violet hue. Neutrophils are also called polymorphonuclear neutrophils (PMNs, or polys) or segmented neutrophils (segs).

The nucleus of the mature neutrophil has multiple lobes (usually two to five) that are connected by thin filaments of nuclear material, or a "segmented" nucleus; it is usually twice the size of an erythrocyte. The somewhat less mature granulocyte has a single-lobed, elongated nucleus and is called a **band cell**. Ordinarily, band cells account for only a small percentage of circulating granulocytes, although their percentage can increase greatly under conditions in which neutrophil production increases, such as infection. An increased number of band cells is sometimes called a **left shift** or **shift to the left**. (Traditionally, the diagram of neutrophil maturation showed the myeloid stem cell on the left with progressive maturation stages toward the right, ending with a fully mature neutrophil on the far right side. A shift to the left indicates that more immature cells are present in the blood than normal.)

Fully mature neutrophils result from the gradual differentiation of myeloid stem cells, specifically myeloid **blast cells**. The process, called **myelopoiesis**, is highly complex and depends on many factors. These factors, including specific **cytokines** such as growth factors, are normally present within the marrow itself. As the blast cell matures, the cytoplasm of the cell changes in color (from blue to violet) and granules begin to form with the cytoplasm. The shape of the nucleus also changes. The entire process of maturation and differentiation takes about 10 days (see Fig. 33-1). Once the neutrophil is released into the circulation from the marrow, it stays there for only about 6 hours before it migrates into the body tissues to perform its function of **phagocytosis** (ingestion and digestion of bacteria and particles) (Fig. 33-3). Here, neutrophils last no more than 1 to 2 days before they die. The number of circulating granulocytes found in the healthy person is relatively constant, but in infection large numbers of these cells are rapidly released into the circulation.

### AGRANULOCYTES

**Monocytes.** Monocytes (also called mononuclear leukocytes) are leukocytes with a single-lobed nucleus and a granule-free cytoplasm—hence the term *agranulocyte* (see Fig. 33-2). In normal adult blood, monocytes account for

## Physiology/Pathophysiology

**FIGURE 33-3.** Phagocytosis. When foreign matter (eg, bacteria or dead tissue) comes in contact with the cell membrane of the neutrophil, the membrane surrounds and pinches off the area, leaving the membrane intact. Thus, the engulfed material is left in a vacuole within the neutrophil, where enzymes within the cell destroy the foreign material.

approximately 5% of the total leukocytes. Monocytes are the largest of the leukocytes. Produced by the bone marrow, they remain in the circulation for a short time before entering the tissues and transforming into **macrophages**. Macrophages are particularly active in the spleen, liver, peritoneum, and the alveoli; they remove debris from these areas and phagocytize bacteria within the tissues.

**Lymphocytes.** Mature lymphocytes are small cells with scanty cytoplasm (see Fig. 33-2). Immature lymphocytes are produced in the marrow from the lymphoid stem cells. A second major source of production is the cortex of the thymus. Cells derived from the thymus are known as T lymphocytes (or T cells); those derived from the marrow can also be T cells but are more commonly B lymphocytes (or B cells). Lymphocytes complete their differentiation and maturation primarily in the lymph nodes and in the lymphoid tissue of the intestine and spleen after exposure to a specific antigen. Mature lymphocytes are the principal cells of the immune system, producing antibodies and identifying other cells and organisms as "foreign."

### FUNCTION OF LEUKOCYTES

Leukocytes protect the body from invasion by bacteria and other foreign entities. The major function of neutrophils is phagocytosis (see Fig. 33-3). Neutrophils arrive at a given site within 1 hour after the onset of an inflammatory reaction and initiate phagocytosis, but they are short-lived. An influx of monocytes follows; these cells continue their phagocytic activities for long periods as macrophages. This process constitutes a second line of defense for the body against inflammation and infection. Although neutrophils can often work adequately against bacteria without the help of macrophages, macrophages are particularly effective against fungi and viruses. Macrophages also digest senescent (aging or aged) blood cells, such as erythrocytes, primarily within the spleen.

The primary function of lymphocytes is to produce substances that aid in attacking foreign material. One group of lymphocytes (T lymphocytes) kills foreign cells directly or releases a variety of lymphokines, substances that enhance the activity of phagocytic cells. T lymphocytes are responsible for delayed allergic reactions, rejection of foreign tissue (eg, transplanted organs), and destruction of tumor cells. This process is known as *cellular immunity*. The other group of lymphocytes (B lymphocytes) is capable of differentiating into plasma cells. Plasma cells, in turn, produce antibodies called immunoglobulin (Ig), which are protein molecules that destroy foreign material by several mechanisms. This process is known as *humoral immunity*.

Eosinophils and basophils function in hypersensitivity reactions. Eosinophils are important in the phagocytosis of parasites. The increase in eosinophil levels in allergic states indicates that these cells are involved in the hypersensitivity reaction; they neutralize histamine. Basophils produce and store histamine as well as other substances involved in hypersensitivity reactions. The release of these substances provokes allergic reactions.

## Platelets (Thrombocytes)

Platelets, or thrombocytes, are not technically cells; rather, they are granular fragments of giant cells in the bone marrow called megakaryocytes. Platelet production in the marrow is regulated in part by the hormone thrombopoietin, which stimulates the production and differentiation of megakaryocytes from the myeloid stem cell.

Platelets play an essential role in the control of bleeding. They circulate freely in the blood in an inactive state, where they nurture the endothelium of the blood vessels, maintaining the integrity of the vessel. When vascular injury occurs, platelets collect at the site and are activated. They adhere to the site of injury and to each other, forming a platelet plug that temporarily stops bleeding. Substances released from platelet granules activate coagulation factors in the blood plasma and initiate the formation of a stable clot composed of **fibrin**, a filamentous protein. Platelets have a normal life span of 7 to 10 days.

## Plasma and Plasma Proteins

After cellular elements are removed from blood, the remaining liquid portion is called plasma. More than 90% of plasma is water. The remainder consists primarily of plasma proteins, clotting factors (particularly fibrinogen), and small amounts of other substances such as nutrients, enzymes, waste products, and gases. If plasma is allowed to clot, the remaining fluid is called **serum**. Serum has essentially the same composition as plasma, except that fibrinogen and several clotting factors have been removed in the clotting process.

Plasma proteins consist primarily of albumin and the globulins. The globulins can be separated into three main fractions (alpha, beta, and gamma), each of which consists of distinct proteins that have different functions. Important proteins in the alpha and beta fractions are the transport globulins and the clotting factors that are made in the liver. The transport globulins carry various substances in bound form in the circulation. For example, thyroid-binding globulin carries thyroxin, and transferrin carries iron. The clotting factors, including fibrinogen, remain in an inactive form in the blood plasma until activated by the clotting cascade. The gamma globulin fraction refers to the immunoglobulins, or antibodies. These proteins are produced by the well-differentiated lymphocytes and plasma cells. The actual fractionation of the globulins can be seen on a specific laboratory test (serum protein electrophoresis).

Albumin is particularly important for the maintenance of fluid balance within the vascular system. Capillary walls are impermeable to albumin, so its presence in the plasma creates an osmotic force that keeps fluid within the vascular space. Albumin, which is produced by the liver, has the capacity to bind to several substances that are transported in plasma (eg, certain medications, bilirubin, some hormones). People with poor hepatic function may have low concentrations of albumin, with a resultant decrease in osmotic pressure and the development of edema.

## Reticuloendothelial System

The reticuloendothelial system (RES) is composed of special tissue macrophages, which are derived from monocytes. When released from the marrow, monocytes spend a short time in the circulation (about 24 hours) and then enter the body tissues. Within the tissues, the monocytes continue to differentiate into macrophages, which can survive for months. Macrophages have a variety of important functions. They defend the body against foreign invaders (ie, bacteria and other pathogens) via phagocytosis. They remove old or damaged cells from the circulation. They stimulate the inflammatory process and present antigens to the immune system (see Chapter 50). Macrophages give rise to tissue **histiocytes,** including Kupffer cells of the liver, peritoneal macrophages, alveolar macrophages, and other components of the RES. Thus, the RES is a component of many other organs within the body, particularly the spleen, lymph nodes, lungs, and liver.

The spleen is the site of activity for most macrophages. Most of the spleen (75%) is made of red pulp; here the blood enters the venous sinuses through capillaries that are surrounded by macrophages. Within the red pulp are tiny aggregates of white pulp, consisting of B and T lymphocytes. The spleen sequesters newly released reticulocytes from the marrow, removing nuclear fragments and other materials (eg, denatured hemoglobin, iron) before the now fully mature erythrocyte returns to the circulation. Although a minority of erythrocytes (less than 5%) is pooled in the spleen, a significant proportion of platelets (20% to 40%) is pooled here. If the spleen is enlarged, a greater proportion of red cells and platelets can be sequestered. The spleen is a major source of hematopoiesis in fetal life. It can resume hematopoiesis later in adulthood if necessary, particularly when marrow function is compromised (eg, in bone marrow fibrosis). The spleen has important immunologic functions as well. It forms substances called opsonins that promote the phagocytosis of neutrophils; it also forms the antibody IgM after exposure to an antigen.

## Hemostasis

Hemostasis is the process of preventing blood loss from intact vessels and of stopping bleeding from a severed vessel. The prevention of blood loss from intact vessels requires adequate numbers of functional platelets. Platelets nurture the endothelium and thereby maintain the structural integrity of the vessel wall. Two processes are involved in arresting bleeding: primary and secondary hemostasis (Fig. 33-4).

In primary hemostasis, the severed blood vessel constricts. Circulating platelets aggregate at the site and adhere to the vessel and to one another. An unstable hemostatic plug is formed. For the coagulation process to be correctly activated, circulating inactive coagulation factors must be converted to active forms. This process occurs on the surface of the aggregated platelets at the site of vessel injury. The end result is the formation of fibrin, which reinforces the platelet plug and anchors it to the injury site. This process is termed secondary hemostasis. The process of blood coagulation is highly complex. It can be activated by the intrinsic or the extrinsic pathway. Both pathways are needed for maintenance of normal hemostasis.

Many factors are involved in the reaction cascade that forms fibrin. When tissue is injured, the extrinsic pathway is activated by the release of thromboplastin from the tissue. As the result of a series of reactions, prothrombin is converted to **thrombin,** which in turn catalyzes the conversion of fibrinogen to fibrin. Clotting by the intrinsic pathway is activated when the collagen that lines blood vessels is exposed. Clotting factors are activated sequentially until, as with the extrinsic pathway, fibrin is ultimately formed. Although the intrinsic pathway is slower, this sequence is probably most often responsible for clotting in vivo.

As the injured vessel is repaired and again covered with endothelial cells, the fibrin clot is no longer needed. The fibrin is digested via two systems: the plasma fibrinolytic system and the cellular fibrinolytic system. The substance **plasminogen** is required to lyse (break down) the fibrin. Plasminogen, which is present in all body fluids, circulates with fibrinogen and is therefore incorporated into the fibrin clot as it forms. When the clot is no longer needed (eg, after an injured blood vessel has healed), the plasminogen is activated to form plasmin. Plasmin digests the fibrinogen and fibrin. The breakdown particles of the clot, called fibrin degradation products, are released into the circulation. Through this system, clots are dissolved as tissue is repaired, and the vascular system returns to its normal baseline state.

### Gerontologic Considerations

In elderly patients, the bone marrow's ability to respond to the body's need for blood cells (erythrocytes, leukocytes, and platelets) may be decreased. This decreased ability is a result of many factors, including diminished production of the growth factors necessary for hematopoiesis by stromal cells within the marrow or a diminished response to the growth factors (in the case of erythropoietin). In addition, in elderly patients, the bone marrow may be more susceptible to the myelosuppressive effects of medications. As a result of these factors, when an elderly person needs more blood cells (eg, leukocytes in infection, erythrocytes in anemia), the bone marrow may not be able to increase production of these cells adequately. **Leukopenia** (a decreased number of circulating leukocytes) or anemia can result.

Anemia is the most common hematologic condition affecting elderly patients; with each successive decade of life, the incidence of anemia increases. Anemia frequently results from iron deficiency (in the case of blood loss) or from a nutritional deficiency, particularly folate or vitamin $B_{12}$ deficiency or protein-calorie malnutrition; it may also result from inflammation or chronic disease. Management of the disorder varies depending on the etiology. Therefore, it is important to identify the cause of the anemia rather than to consider it an inevitable consequence of aging. Elderly people with concurrent cardiac or pulmonary problems may not tolerate anemia very well, and a prompt, thorough evaluation is warranted.

## Assessment of Hematologic Disorders

Most hematologic diseases reflect a defect in the hematopoietic, hemostatic, or reticuloendothelial system. The defect can be quantitative (eg, increased or decreased production of cells), qualitative (eg, the cells that are produced are defective in their normal functional capacity), or both.

Initially, many hematologic conditions cause few symptoms. Therefore, extensive laboratory tests are often required to diagnose a hematologic disorder. For most hematologic

## Physiology/Pathophysiology

**FIGURE 33-4.** Hemostasis. When the endothelial surface of a blood vessel is injured, several processes occur. In primary hemostasis, platelets within the circulation are attracted to the exposed layer of collagen at the site of injury. They adhere to the site of injury, releasing factors that stimulate other platelets to aggregate at the site, forming an unstable platelet plug. In secondary hemostasis, based on the type of stimulus, one of two clotting pathways is initiated—the intrinsic or extrinsic pathway—and the clotting factors within that pathway are activated. The end result from either pathway is the conversion of prothrombin to thrombin. Thrombin is necessary for fibrinogen to be converted into fibrin, the stabilizing protein that anchors the fragile platelet plug to the site of injury to prevent further bleeding and permit the injuring vessel or site to heal. Modified from www.irvingcrowley.com/cls/clotting.gif.

conditions, continued monitoring via specific blood tests is required because it is very important to assess for changes in test results over time. In general, it is important to assess trends in blood counts because these trends help the clinician decide whether the patient is responding appropriately to interventions.

## Hematologic Studies

The most common tests used are the complete blood count (CBC) and the peripheral blood smear (see Appendix A). The CBC identifies the total number of blood cells (leukocytes, erythrocytes, and platelets) as well as the hemoglobin, **hematocrit** (percentage of blood volume consisting of erythrocytes), and RBC indices. Because cellular morphology (shape and appearance of the cells) is particularly important in most hematologic disorders, the blood cells involved must be examined. This process is referred to as the manual examination of the peripheral smear, which may be part of the CBC. In this test, a drop of blood is spread on a glass slide, stained, and examined under a microscope. The shape and size of the erythrocytes and platelets, as well as the actual appearance of the leukocytes, provide useful information in identifying hematologic conditions. Blood for the CBC is typically obtained by venipuncture.

## Bone Marrow Aspiration and Biopsy

The bone marrow aspiration and biopsy are crucial when additional information is needed to assess how a person's blood cells are being formed and to assess the quantity and quality of each type of cell produced within the marrow. These tests are also used to document infection or tumor within the marrow.

Normal bone marrow is in a semifluid state and can be aspirated through a special large needle. In adults, bone marrow is usually aspirated from the iliac crest and occasionally from the sternum. The aspirate provides only a sample of cells. Aspirate alone may be adequate for evaluating certain conditions, such as anemia. However, when more information is required, a biopsy is also performed. Biopsy samples are taken from the posterior iliac crest; occasionally, an anterior approach is required. A marrow biopsy shows the architecture of the bone marrow as well as its degree of cellularity.

Most patients need no more preparation than a careful explanation of the procedure, but for some very anxious patients, an antianxiety agent may be useful. It is always important for the physician or nurse to describe and explain to the patient the procedure and the sensations that will be experienced. The risks, benefits, and alternatives are also discussed. A signed informed consent is needed before the procedure is performed.

Before aspiration, the skin is cleansed as for any minor surgery, using aseptic technique. Then a small area is anesthetized with a local anesthetic through the skin and subcutaneous tissue to the periosteum of the bone. It is not possible to anesthetize the bone itself. The bone marrow needle is introduced with a stylet in place. When the needle is felt to go through the outer cortex of bone and enter the marrow cavity, the stylet is removed, a syringe is attached, and a small volume (0.5 mL) of blood and marrow is aspirated. Patients typically feel a pressure sensation as the needle is advanced into position. The actual aspiration always causes sharp but brief pain, resulting from the suction exerted as the marrow is aspirated into the syringe; the patient should be warned about this. Taking deep breaths or using relaxation techniques often helps ease the discomfort.

If a bone marrow biopsy is necessary, it is best performed after the aspiration and in a slightly different location, because the marrow structure may be altered after aspiration. A special biopsy needle is used. Because these needles are large, the skin is punctured first with a surgical blade to make a 3- or 4-mm incision. The biopsy needle is advanced well into the marrow cavity. When the needle is properly positioned, a portion of marrow is cored out, using a twisting or gentle rocking motion to free the sample and permit its removal within the biopsy needle. The patient feels a pressure sensation but should not feel actual pain. The nurse should instruct the patient to inform the physician if pain occurs so that an additional anesthetic can be administered.

Hazards of either bone marrow aspiration or biopsy include bleeding and infection. The risk for bleeding is somewhat increased if the patient's platelet count is low or if the patient has been taking a medication (eg, aspirin) that alters platelet function. After the marrow sample is obtained, pressure is applied to the site for several minutes. The site is then covered with a sterile dressing. Most patients have no discomfort after a bone marrow aspiration, but the site of a biopsy may ache for 1 or 2 days. Warm tub baths and a mild analgesic (eg, acetaminophen) may be useful. Aspirin-containing analgesics should be avoided because they can aggravate or potentiate bleeding.

# Anemia

## Overview

Anemia, a condition in which the hemoglobin concentration is lower than normal, reflects the presence of fewer than normal erythrocytes within the circulation. As a result, the amount of oxygen delivered to body tissues is also diminished. Anemia is not a specific disease state per se but a sign of an underlying disorder. It is by far the most common hematologic condition (Table 33-2). A common

### TABLE 33-2 Classification of Anemias

| Type of Anemia | Laboratory Findings |
|---|---|
| **Hypoproliferative (Resulting From Defective RBC Production)** | |
| Iron deficiency | Decreased reticulocytes, iron, ferritin, iron saturation, MCV; increased TIBC |
| Vitamin $B_{12}$ deficiency (megaloblastic) | Decreased vitamin $B_{12}$ level; increased MCV |
| Folate deficiency (megaloblastic) | Decreased folate level; increased MCV |
| Decreased erythropoietin production (eg, from renal dysfunction) | Decreased erythropoietin level; normal MCV and MCH; increased creatinine level |
| Cancer/inflammation | Normal MCV, MCH, normal or decreased erythropoietin level; increased % of iron saturation, ferritin level; decreased iron, TIBC |
| **Bleeding (Resulting From RBC Loss)** | |
| Bleeding from gastrointestinal tract, menorrhagia (excessive menstrual flow), epistaxis (nosebleed), trauma | Increased reticulocyte level; normal Hgb and Hct if measured soon after bleeding starts, but levels decrease thereafter; normal MCV initially but later decreases; decreased ferritin and iron levels (later) |
| **Hemolytic (Resulting From RBC Destruction)** | |
| Altered erythropoiesis (sickle cell anemia, thalassemia, other hemoglobinopathies) | Decreased MCV; fragmented RBCs; increased reticulocyte level |
| Hypersplenism (hemolysis) | Increased MCV |
| Drug-induced anemia | Increased spherocyte level |
| Autoimmune anemia | Increased spherocyte level |
| Mechanical heart valve–related anemia | Fragmented red cells |

Hct, hematocrit; Hgb, hemoglobin concentration; MCH, mean corpuscular hemoglobin; MCV, mean corpuscular volume; RBCs, red blood cells; TIBC, total iron-binding capacity.

occurrence among all age groups, it is particularly prevalent among the elderly. A recent study documented the prevalence of anemia in elderly residents of skilled nursing facilities to be 48% (Artz et al., 2004).

## Classification of Anemias

Anemia may be classified in several ways. A physiologic approach classifies anemia according to whether the deficiency in erythrocytes is caused by a defect in their production (hypoproliferative anemia), by their destruction (hemolytic anemia), or by their loss (bleeding).

In hypoproliferative anemias, the marrow cannot produce adequate numbers of erythrocytes. Decreased erythrocyte production is reflected by an inappropriately normal or low reticulocyte count. Inadequate production of erythrocytes may result from marrow damage due to medications (eg, chloramphenicol) or chemicals (eg, benzene) or from a lack of factors (eg, iron, vitamin $B_{12}$, folic acid, erythropoietin) necessary for erythrocyte formation.

In hemolytic anemias, premature destruction of erythrocytes results in the liberation of hemoglobin from the erythrocytes into the plasma. The increased erythrocyte destruction leads to tissue hypoxia, which in turn stimulates erythropoietin production. This increased production is reflected in an increased reticulocyte count as the bone marrow responds to the loss of erythrocytes. The released hemoglobin is converted in large part to bilirubin; therefore, the bilirubin concentration rises. **Hemolysis** can result from an abnormality within the erythrocyte itself (eg, sickle cell anemia, glucose-6-phosphate dehydrogenase [G-6-PD] deficiency) or within the plasma (eg, immune hemolytic anemias), or from direct injury to the erythrocyte within the circulation (eg, hemolysis caused by mechanical heart valve). Chart 33-1 identifies the causes of hemolytic anemia.

It is usually possible to determine whether the presence of anemia in a given patient is caused by destruction or by inadequate production of erythrocytes on the basis of the following factors:

- The marrow's ability to respond to decreased erythrocytes (as evidenced by an increased reticulocyte count in the circulating blood)
- The degree to which young erythrocytes proliferate in the bone marrow and the manner in which they mature (as observed on bone marrow biopsy)
- The presence or absence of end products of erythrocyte destruction within the circulation (eg, increased bilirubin level, decreased haptoglobin level)

## Clinical Manifestations

Aside from the severity of the anemia itself, several factors influence the development of anemia-associated symptoms:

- The rapidity with which the anemia has developed
- The duration of the anemia (ie, its chronicity)
- The metabolic requirements of the patient
- Other concurrent disorders or disabilities (eg, cardiopulmonary disease)
- Special complications or concomitant features of the condition that produced the anemia

---

**CHART 33-1**

### Causes of Hemolytic Anemias

**Inherited Hemolytic Anemia**

Abnormal hemoglobin
   Sickle cell anemia*
   Thalassemia*
Red blood cell membrane abnormality
   Hereditary spherocytosis*
   Hereditary elliptocytosis
   Acanthocytosis
   Stomatocytosis
Enzyme deficiencies
   Glucose-6-phosphate dehydrogenase (G-6-PD) deficiency*

**Acquired Hemolytic Anemia**

Antibody-related
   Iso-antibody/transfusion reaction*
   Autoimmune hemolytic anemia (AIHA)*
   Cold agglutinin disease*
Not antibody-related
   Red blood cell membrane defects
   Paroxysmal nocturnal hemoglobinuria (PNH)
   Liver disease
   Uremia
   Trauma
   Mechanical heart valve
   Microangiopathic hemolytic anemia
   Infection
      Bacterial
      Parasitic
   Disseminated intravascular coagulation (DIC)*
   Toxins
   Hypersplenism*

*Discussed in text.

---

In general, the more rapidly an anemia develops, the more severe its symptoms. An otherwise healthy person can often tolerate as much as a 50% gradual reduction in hemoglobin without pronounced symptoms or significant incapacity, whereas the rapid loss of as little as 30% may precipitate profound vascular collapse in the same person. A person who has become gradually anemic, with hemoglobin levels between 9 and 11 g/dL, usually has few or no symptoms other than slight tachycardia on exertion and fatigue.

People who customarily are very active or who have significant demands on their lives (eg, a single, working mother of small children) are more likely to have symptoms, and those symptoms are more likely to be pronounced than in more sedentary people. Patients with hypothyroidism with decreased oxygen needs may be completely asymptomatic, without tachycardia or increased cardiac output, at a hemoglobin level of 10 g/dL. Similarly, patients with coexistent cardiac, vascular, or pulmonary disease may develop more pronounced symptoms of anemia (eg, dyspnea, chest pain, muscle pain or cramping) at a higher hemoglobin level than those without these concurrent health problems.

Finally, some anemic disorders are complicated by various other abnormalities that do not result from the anemia but are inherently associated with these particular diseases. These abnormalities may give rise to symptoms that completely overshadow those of the anemia, as in the painful crises of sickle cell anemia.

## Assessment and Diagnostic Findings

A variety of hematologic studies are performed to determine the type and cause of the anemia. In an initial evaluation, the hemoglobin, hematocrit, reticulocyte count, and RBC indices, particularly the mean corpuscular volume (MCV) and red cell distribution width (RDW), are particularly useful. Iron studies (serum iron level, total iron-binding capacity [TIBC], percent saturation, and ferritin), as well as serum vitamin $B_{12}$ and folate levels, are also frequently obtained. Other tests include haptoglobin and erythropoietin levels. The remaining CBC values are useful in determining whether the anemia is an isolated problem or part of another hematologic condition, such as **leukemia** or myelodysplastic syndrome (MDS). Bone marrow aspiration may be performed. In addition, other diagnostic studies may be performed to determine the presence of underlying chronic illness, such as malignancy, or the source of any blood loss, such as polyps or ulcers within the GI tract.

## Complications

General complications of severe anemia include heart failure, paresthesias, and confusion. At any given level of anemia, patients with underlying heart disease are far more likely to have angina or symptoms of heart failure than those without heart disease. Complications associated with specific types of anemia are included in the description of each type.

## Medical Management

Management of anemia is directed toward correcting or controlling the cause of the anemia; if the anemia is severe, the erythrocytes that are lost or destroyed may be replaced with a transfusion of packed red blood cells (PRBCs). The management of the various types of anemia is covered in the discussions that follow.

# Nursing Process

## The Patient With Anemia

### Assessment

The health history and physical examination provide important data about the type of anemia involved, the extent and type of symptoms it produces, and the impact of those symptoms on the patient's life. Weakness, fatigue, and general malaise are common, as are pallor of the skin and mucous membranes (conjunctivae, oral mucosa).

Jaundice may be present in patients with megaloblastic anemia or hemolytic anemia. The tongue may be smooth and red (in iron deficiency anemia) or beefy red and sore (in megaloblastic anemia); the corners of the mouth may be ulcerated (**angular cheilosis**) in both types of anemia. People with iron deficiency anemia may crave ice, starch, or dirt; this craving is known as pica. The nails may be brittle, ridged, and concave.

The health history should include a medication history, because some medications can depress bone marrow activity, induce hemolysis, or interfere with folate metabolism. An accurate history of alcohol intake, including the amount and duration, should be obtained. Family history is important, because certain anemias are inherited. Athletic endeavors should be assessed, because extreme exercise can decrease erythropoiesis and erythrocyte survival.

A nutritional assessment is important, because it may indicate deficiencies in essential nutrients such as iron, vitamin $B_{12}$, and folic acid. Children of indigent families may be at higher risk for anemia because of nutritional deficiencies. Strict vegetarians are also at risk for megaloblastic types of anemia if they do not supplement their diet with vitamin $B_{12}$.

Cardiac status should be carefully assessed. When the hemoglobin level is low, the heart attempts to compensate by pumping faster and harder in an effort to deliver more blood to hypoxic tissue. This increased cardiac workload can result in such symptoms as tachycardia, palpitations, dyspnea, dizziness, orthopnea, and exertional dyspnea. Heart failure may eventually develop, as evidenced by an enlarged heart (cardiomegaly) and liver (hepatomegaly) and by peripheral edema.

Assessment of the GI system may disclose complaints of nausea, vomiting (with specific questions about the appearance of any emesis [eg, looks like "coffee grounds"]), melena or dark stools, diarrhea, anorexia, and glossitis (inflammation of the tongue). Stools should be tested for occult blood. Women should be questioned about their menstrual periods (eg, excessive menstrual flow, other vaginal bleeding) and the use of iron supplements during pregnancy.

The neurologic examination is also important because of the effect of pernicious anemia on the central and peripheral nervous systems. Assessment should include the presence and extent of peripheral numbness and paresthesias, ataxia, poor coordination, and confusion. Finally, it is important to monitor relevant laboratory test results and to note any changes over time.

### Diagnosis

#### Nursing Diagnoses

Based on the assessment data, major nursing diagnoses for the patient with anemia may include:

- Fatigue related to decreased hemoglobin and diminished oxygen-carrying capacity of the blood

- Altered nutrition, less than body requirements, related to inadequate intake of essential nutrients
- Altered tissue perfusion related to inadequate blood volume or hematocrit
- Noncompliance with prescribed therapy

## Collaborative Problems/ Potential Complications

Based on the assessment data, potential complications that may develop include:

- Heart failure
- Angina
- Paresthesias
- Confusion

## Planning and Goals

The major goals for the patient may include decreased fatigue, attainment or maintenance of adequate nutrition, maintenance of adequate tissue perfusion, compliance with prescribed therapy, and absence of complications.

## Nursing Interventions

### Managing Fatigue

The most common symptom and complication of anemia is fatigue. This distressing symptom is too often minimized by health care providers. Fatigue is often the symptom that has the greatest negative impact on a patient's level of functioning and consequent quality of life. Patients often describe the fatigue from anemia as oppressive. Fatigue can be significant, yet the anemia may not be severe enough to warrant transfusion. Fatigue can interfere with a person's ability to work, both inside and outside the home. It can harm relationships with family and friends. Patients often lose interest in hobbies and activities, including sexual activity. The distress from fatigue is often related to a person's responsibilities and life demands as well as the amount of assistance and support received from others.

Nursing interventions can focus on assisting the patient to prioritize activities and to establish a balance between activity and rest that is realistic and feasible from the patient's perspective. Patients with chronic anemia need to maintain some physical activity and exercise to prevent the deconditioning that results from inactivity.

### Maintaining Adequate Nutrition

Inadequate intake of essential nutrients, such as iron, vitamin $B_{12}$, folic acid, and protein, can cause some anemias. The symptoms associated with anemia (eg, fatigue, anorexia) can in turn interfere with maintaining adequate nutrition. A healthy diet should be encouraged. The nurse should inform the patient that alcohol interferes with the utilization of essential nutrients and should advise the patient to avoid alcoholic beverages or to limit their intake. Dietary teaching sessions should be individualized and include cultural aspects related to food preferences and food preparation. The involvement of family members enhances compliance with dietary recommendations. Dietary supplements (eg, vitamins, iron, folate, protein) may be prescribed as well.

Equally important, the patient and family must understand the role of nutritional supplements in the proper context, because many forms of anemia are not the result of a nutritional deficiency. In such cases, even an excessive intake of nutritional supplements will not improve the anemia. A potential problem in patients with chronic transfusion requirements occurs with the indiscriminate use of iron supplements. Unless an aggressive program of chelation therapy is implemented, these people are at risk for iron overload from their transfusions. The addition of an iron supplement only exacerbates the situation.

### Maintaining Adequate Perfusion

Patients with acute blood loss or severe hemolysis may have decreased tissue perfusion from decreased blood volume or reduced circulating erythrocytes (decreased hematocrit). Lost volume is replaced with transfusions or intravenous (IV) fluids, based on the symptoms and the laboratory test results. Supplemental oxygen may be necessary, but it is rarely needed on a long-term basis unless there is underlying severe cardiac or pulmonary disease. The nurse monitors the patient's vital signs and pulse oximeter readings closely; other medications, such as antihypertensive agents, may need to be adjusted or withheld.

### Promoting Compliance With Prescribed Therapy

For patients with anemia, medications or nutritional supplements are often prescribed to alleviate or correct the condition. These patients need to understand the purpose of the medication, how to take the medication and over what time period, and how to manage any side effects of therapy. To enhance compliance, the nurse assists the patient to develop ways to incorporate the therapeutic plan into everyday activities, rather than merely giving the patient a list of instructions. For example, many patients have difficulty taking iron supplements because of related GI effects. Rather than seeking assistance from a health care provider in managing the problem, some patients simply stop taking the iron.

Abruptly stopping some medications can have serious consequences, as in the case of high-dose corticosteroids to manage hemolytic anemias. Some medications, such as growth factors, are extremely expensive. Patients receiving these medications may need assistance to obtain needed insurance coverage or to explore alternative ways to obtain these medications.

## Monitoring and Managing Potential Complications

A significant complication of anemia is heart failure from chronic diminished blood volume and the heart's compensatory effort to increase cardiac output. Patients with anemia should be assessed for signs and symptoms of heart failure. A daily record of body weight can be more useful and accurate than a record of intake and output. Diuretics may be required if fluid retention results from heart failure.

In megaloblastic forms of anemia, the significant potential complications are neurologic. A neurologic assessment should be performed for patients with known or suspected megaloblastic anemia. Patients may initially complain of paresthesias in their lower extremities. These paresthesias are usually manifested as numbness and tingling on the bottom of the foot, and they gradually progress. As the anemia progresses, other signs become apparent. Position and vibration sense may be diminished; difficulty maintaining balance is not uncommon, and some patients have gait disturbances as well. Initially mild confusion may develop; it may become severe.

## Evaluation

### Expected Patient Outcomes

Expected patient outcomes may include:

1. Reports less fatigue
    a. Follows a progressive plan of rest, activity, and exercise
    b. Prioritizes activities
    c. Paces activities according to energy level
2. Attains and maintains adequate nutrition
    a. Eats a healthy diet
    b. Develops a meal plan that promotes optimal nutrition
    c. Maintains adequate amounts of iron, vitamins, and protein from diet or supplements
    d. Adheres to nutritional supplement therapy when prescribed
    e. Verbalizes understanding of rationale for using recommended nutritional supplements
    f. Verbalizes understanding of rationale for avoiding nonrecommended nutritional supplements
3. Maintains adequate perfusion
    a. Has vital signs within baseline for patient
    b. Has pulse oximetry (arterial oxygenation) value within normal limits
4. Absence of complications
    a. Avoids or limits activities that cause dyspnea, palpitations, dizziness, or tachycardia
    b. Uses rest and comfort measures to alleviate dyspnea
    c. Has vital signs within baseline for patient
    d. Has no signs of increasing fluid retention (eg, peripheral edema, decreased urine output, neck vein distention)
    e. Remains oriented to time, place, and situation
    f. Ambulates safely, using assistive devices as necessary
    g. Remains free of injury
    h. Verbalizes understanding of importance of serial CBC measurements
    i. Maintains safe home environment; obtains assistance as necessary

# Hypoproliferative Anemias

## Iron Deficiency Anemia

Iron deficiency anemia typically results when the intake of dietary iron is inadequate for hemoglobin synthesis. The body can store about one fourth to one third of its iron, and it is not until those stores are depleted that iron deficiency anemia actually begins to develop. Iron deficiency anemia is the most common type of anemia in all age groups, and it is the most common anemia in the world. It is particularly prevalent in developing countries, where inadequate iron stores can result from inadequate intake of iron (seen with vegetarian diets) or from blood loss (eg, from intestinal hookworm). Iron deficiency is also common in the United States. In children, adolescents, and pregnant women, the cause is typically inadequate iron in the diet to keep up with increased growth. However, for most adults with iron deficiency anemia, the cause is blood loss. In fact, in adults, the cause of iron deficiency anemia should be considered to be bleeding until proven otherwise.

The most common cause of iron deficiency anemia in men and postmenopausal women is bleeding (from ulcers, gastritis, inflammatory bowel disease, or GI tumors). The most common cause of iron deficiency anemia in premenopausal women is menorrhagia (excessive menstrual bleeding) and pregnancy with inadequate iron supplementation. Patients with chronic alcoholism often have chronic blood loss from the GI tract, which causes iron loss and eventual anemia. Other causes include iron malabsorption, as is seen after gastrectomy or with celiac disease.

### Clinical Manifestations

Patients with iron deficiency primarily have the symptoms of anemia. If the deficiency is severe or prolonged, they may also have a smooth, sore tongue; brittle and ridged nails; and angular cheilosis (an ulceration of the corner of the mouth). These signs subside after iron replacement therapy. The health history may be significant for multiple pregnancies, gastrointestinal bleeding, and pica (a craving for unusual substances).

### Assessment and Diagnostic Findings

The definitive method of establishing the diagnosis of iron deficiency anemia is bone marrow aspiration. The aspirate is stained to detect iron, which is at a low level or even absent. However, few patients with suspected iron deficiency anemia undergo bone marrow aspiration. In many patients, the diagnosis can be established with other tests, particularly in patients with a history of conditions that predispose them to this type of anemia.

There is a strong correlation between laboratory values that measure iron stores and hemoglobin levels. After iron stores are depleted (as reflected by low serum ferritin levels), the hemoglobin level falls. The diminished iron stores cause small erythrocytes to be produced by the marrow. Therefore, as the anemia progresses, the MCV, which measures the size of the erythrocytes, also decreases. Hematocrit and RBC levels are also low in relation to the hemoglobin level. Other laboratory tests that measure iron stores are useful but are not as consistent indicators as a low ferritin level, which reflects low iron stores. Typically, patients with iron deficiency anemia have a low serum iron level and an elevated TIBC, which measures the transport protein supplying the marrow with iron as needed (also referred to as transferrin). However, other disease states, such as infection and inflammatory conditions, can also cause a low serum iron level and TIBC, as well as an elevated ferritin level. Currently, the most reliable and clinically useful laboratory findings in evaluating iron deficiency anemia are the ferritin and hemoglobin values.

## Medical Management

Except in the case of pregnancy, the cause of iron deficiency should be investigated. Anemia may be a sign of a curable GI cancer or of uterine fibroid tumors. Stool specimens should be tested for occult blood. People 50 years of age or older should have periodic colonoscopy, endoscopy, or x-ray examination of the GI tract to detect ulcerations, gastritis, polyps, or cancer. Several oral iron preparations—ferrous sulfate, ferrous gluconate, and ferrous fumarate—are available for treating iron deficiency anemia. The hemoglobin level may increase in only a few weeks, and the anemia can be corrected in a few months. Iron store replenishment takes much longer, so it is important that the patient continue taking the iron for as long as 6 to 12 months. Vitamin C facilitates the absorption of iron.

In some cases, oral iron is poorly absorbed or poorly tolerated, or iron supplementation is needed in large amounts. In these situations, IV or intramuscular (IM) administration of iron dextran may be needed. Before parenteral administration of a full dose, a small test dose should be administered parenterally to avoid the risk of anaphylaxis with either IV or IM injections. Emergency medications (eg, epinephrine) should be close at hand. If no signs of allergic reaction have occurred after 30 minutes, the remaining dose of iron may be administered. Several doses are required to replenish the patient's iron stores.

## Nursing Management

Preventive education is important, because iron deficiency anemia is common in menstruating and pregnant women. Food sources high in iron include organ meats (beef or calf's liver, chicken liver), other meats, beans (black, pinto, and garbanzo), leafy green vegetables, raisins, and molasses. Taking iron-rich foods with a source of vitamin C (eg, orange juice) enhances the absorption of iron.

The nurse helps the patient select a healthy diet. Nutritional counseling can be provided for those whose usual diet is inadequate. Patients with a history of eating fad diets or strict vegetarian diets are counseled that such diets often contain inadequate amounts of absorbable iron. The nurse encourages the patient to continue iron therapy as long as it is prescribed, although the patient may no longer feel fatigued.

Because iron is best absorbed on an empty stomach, the patient is instructed to take the supplement an hour before meals. Iron supplements are usually given in the oral form, typically as ferrous sulfate. Most patients can use the less expensive, more standard forms of ferrous sulfate. Tablets with enteric coating may be poorly absorbed and should be avoided. Many patients have difficulty tolerating iron supplements because of GI side effects (primarily constipation, but also cramping, nausea, and vomiting). Some iron formulations are designed to limit GI side effects by the addition of a stool softener or use of sustained-release formulations to limit nausea or gastritis. Specific patient teaching aids (Chart 33-2) can assist patients with the use of iron supplements.

If taking iron on an empty stomach causes gastric distress, the patient may need to take it with meals. However, doing so diminishes iron absorption by as much as 50%, thus prolonging the time required to replenish iron stores. Antacids or dairy products should not be taken with iron, because they greatly diminish its absorption. Polysaccharide iron complex forms that have less GI toxicity are also available, but they are more expensive.

Liquid forms of iron that cause less GI distress are available. However, they can stain the teeth; the patient should be instructed to take this medication through a straw, to rinse the mouth with water, and to practice good oral hygiene

---

**CHART 33-2**

### Patient Education

### Taking Oral Iron Supplements

- Take iron on an empty stomach (1 hour before or 2 hours after a meal). Iron absorption is reduced with food, especially dairy products.
- To prevent gastrointestinal distress, the following schedule may work better if more than one tablet a day is prescribed: Start with only one tablet per day for a few days, then increase to two tablets per day, then three tablets per day. This method permits the body to adjust gradually to the iron.
- Increase the intake of vitamin C (citrus fruits and juices, strawberries, tomatoes, broccoli), to enhance iron absorption.
- Eat foods high in fiber to minimize problems with constipation.
- Remember that stools will become dark in color.
- To prevent staining the teeth with a liquid preparation, use a straw or place a spoon at the back of the mouth to take the supplement. Rinse the mouth thoroughly afterward.

after taking this medication. Finally, the patient should be informed that iron salts may color the stool dark green or black. However, iron replacement therapy does not cause a false-positive result on stool analyses for occult blood.

IV supplementation may be used when the patient's iron stores are completely depleted, the patient cannot tolerate oral forms of iron supplementation (see Medical Management), or both. IM supplementation is used infrequently. The volume of iron required when administered IM may be excessive. The IM injection causes some local pain and can stain the skin. These side effects are minimized by using the Z-track technique for administering iron dextran deep into the gluteus maximus muscle (buttock). The nurse avoids vigorously rubbing the injection site after the injection. Because of the problems with IM administration, the IV route is preferred for administration of iron dextran.

## Anemias in Renal Disease

The degree of anemia in patients with end-stage renal disease varies greatly, but in general patients do not become significantly anemic until the serum creatinine level exceeds 3 mg/100 mL. The symptoms of anemia are often the most disturbing of the patient's symptoms. If untreated, the hematocrit usually falls to between 20% and 30%, although in rare cases it may fall to less than 15%. The erythrocytes appear normal on the peripheral smear.

This anemia is caused by both a mild shortening of erythrocyte life span and a deficiency of erythropoietin (necessary for erythropoiesis). As renal function decreases, erythropoietin, which is produced by the kidney, also decreases. Because erythropoietin is also produced outside the kidney, some erythropoiesis continues, even in patients whose kidneys have been removed. However, the number of red blood cells produced is small and the degree of erythropoiesis is inadequate.

Patients undergoing long-term hemodialysis lose blood into the dialyzer and therefore may become iron deficient. Folic acid deficiency develops because this vitamin passes into the dialysate. Therefore, patients who receive hemodialysis and who have anemia should be evaluated for iron and folate deficiency and treated appropriately.

The availability of recombinant erythropoietin (epoetin alfa [Epogen, Procrit]; darbepoetin alfa [Aranesp]) has dramatically altered the management of anemia in end-stage renal disease by decreasing the need for RBC transfusion, with its associated risks. Erythropoietin, in combination with oral iron supplements, can raise and maintain hematocrit levels to between 33% and 38%. This treatment has been successful with dialysis patients. Hypertension is the most serious side effect in this patient population when the hematocrit rapidly increases to a high level. Therefore, the hematocrit should be checked frequently when a patient with renal disease begins erythropoietin therapy. The dose of erythropoietin should be titrated to the hematocrit. In some patients, the elevated hematocrit and associated hypertension may necessitate antihypertensive therapy.

## Anemia of Chronic Disease

The term "anemia of chronic disease" is a misnomer in that only the chronic diseases of inflammation, infection, and malignancy cause this type of anemia. Many chronic inflammatory diseases are associated with a **normochromic, normocytic** anemia (ie, the erythrocytes are normal in color and size). These disorders include rheumatoid arthritis; severe, chronic infections; and many cancers. It is therefore imperative that the "chronic disease" be diagnosed when this form of anemia is identified so that it can be appropriately managed.

The anemia is usually mild to moderate and nonprogressive. It develops gradually over 6 to 8 weeks and then stabilizes at a hematocrit seldom less than 25%. The hemoglobin level rarely falls below 9 g/dL, and the bone marrow has normal cellularity with increased stores of iron as the iron is diverted from the serum. Erythropoietin levels are low, perhaps because of decreased production, and iron use is blocked by **erythroid cells** (cells that are or will become mature erythrocytes). A moderate shortening of erythrocyte survival also occurs.

Most of these patients have few symptoms and do not require treatment for the anemia. With successful treatment of the underlying disorder, the bone marrow iron is used to make erythrocytes and the hemoglobin level rises.

## Aplastic Anemia

Aplastic anemia is a rare disease caused by a decrease in or damage to marrow stem cells, damage to the microenvironment within the marrow, and replacement of the marrow with fat. The precise etiology is unknown, but it is hypothesized that the body's T cells mediate an inappropriate attack against the bone marrow (Bevans & Shalabi, 2004), resulting in bone marrow **aplasia** (markedly reduced hematopoiesis). Therefore, in addition to severe anemia, significant **neutropenia** and thrombocytopenia (a deficiency of platelets) are also seen.

### Pathophysiology

Aplastic anemia can be congenital or acquired, but most cases are idiopathic (ie, without apparent cause). Infections and pregnancy can trigger it, or it may be caused by certain medications, chemicals, or radiation damage. Agents that regularly produce marrow aplasia include benzene and benzene derivatives (eg, airplane glue). Certain toxic materials, such as inorganic arsenic and several pesticides (including dichlorodiphenyltrichloroethane [DDT], which is no longer used or available in the United States), have also been implicated as potential causes.

### Clinical Manifestations

The manifestations of aplastic anemia are often insidious. Complications resulting from bone marrow failure may occur before the diagnosis is established. Typical complications are infection and symptoms of anemia (eg, fatigue, pallor, dyspnea). Purpura (bruising) may develop later and should trigger a CBC and hematologic evaluation if these were not performed initially. If the patient has had repeated throat infections, cervical lymphadenopathy may be seen. Other lymphadenopathies and splenomegaly sometimes occur. Retinal hemorrhages are common.

## Assessment and Diagnostic Findings

In many situations, aplastic anemia occurs when a medication or chemical is ingested in toxic amounts. However, in a few people, it develops after a medication has been taken at the recommended dosage. This may be considered an idiosyncratic reaction in those who are highly susceptible, possibly caused by a genetic defect in the medication biotransformation or elimination process. A bone marrow aspirate shows an extremely hypoplastic or even aplastic (very few to no cells) marrow replaced with fat.

## Medical Management

It is presumed that the lymphocytes of patients with aplastic anemia destroy the stem cells and consequently impair the production of erythrocytes, leukocytes, and platelets. Despite its severity, aplastic anemia can be treated in most people. Those who are younger than 60 years, who are otherwise healthy, and who have a compatible donor can be cured of the disease by a bone marrow transplant (BMT) or peripheral blood stem cell transplant (PBSCT). In others, the disease can be managed with immunosuppressive therapy, commonly using a combination of antithymocyte globulin (ATG) and cyclosporine. ATG, a purified gamma globulin solution, is obtained from horses or rabbits immunized with human T lymphocytes (Bevans & Shalabi, 2004). Side effects during the infusion are common and may include fever and chills. The sudden onset of a rash or bronchospasm may herald anaphylaxis and requires prompt management (see Chapters 53 and 71). Serum sickness, as evidenced by fever, rash, arthralgias, and pruritus, may develop in some patients; it may take weeks to resolve. A recent study showed that 122 patients receiving this immunosuppressive treatment had a 55% 7-year survival rate (Rosenfeld et al., 2003).

Immunosuppressants prevent the patient's lymphocytes from destroying the stem cells. If relapse occurs (ie, the patient becomes pancytopenic again), reinstitution of the same immunologic agents may induce another remission. Corticosteroids are not very useful as immunosuppressive agents, because patients with aplastic anemia are particularly susceptible to the development of bone complications from corticosteroids (ie, aseptic necrosis of the head of the femur).

Supportive therapy plays a major role in the management of aplastic anemia. Any offending agent is discontinued. The patient is supported with transfusions of PRBCs and platelets as necessary. Death usually is caused by hemorrhage or infection.

## Nursing Management

Patients with aplastic anemia are vulnerable to problems related to erythrocyte, leukocyte, and platelet deficiencies. They should be assessed carefully for signs of infection and bleeding. Specific interventions are delineated in the sections on neutropenia and thrombocytopenia.

## Megaloblastic Anemias

In the anemias caused by deficiencies of vitamin $B_{12}$ or folic acid, identical bone marrow and peripheral blood changes occur because both vitamins are essential for normal DNA synthesis. In either anemia, the erythrocytes that are produced are abnormally large and are called megaloblastic red cells. Other cells derived from the myeloid stem cell (nonlymphoid leukocytes, platelets) are also abnormal. A bone marrow analysis reveals **hyperplasia** (abnormal increase in the number of cells), and the precursor erythroid and myeloid cells are large and bizarre in appearance. However, many of these abnormal erythroid and myeloid cells are destroyed within the marrow, so the mature cells that do leave the marrow are actually fewer in number. Thus, **pancytopenia** (a decrease in all myeloid-derived cells) can develop. In advanced stages of disease, the hemoglobin value may be as low as 4 to 5 g/dL, the leukocyte count 2,000 to 3,000/mm$^3$, and the platelet count less than 50,000/mm$^3$. Those cells that are released into the circulation are often abnormally shaped. The neutrophils are hypersegmented. The platelets may be abnormally large. The erythrocytes are abnormally shaped, and the shapes may vary widely (**poikilocytosis**). Because the erythrocytes are very large, the MCV is very high, usually exceeding 110 µm$^3$.

### Pathophysiology

#### FOLIC ACID DEFICIENCY

Folic acid is stored as compounds referred to as folates. The folate stores in the body are much smaller than those of vitamin $B_{12}$, and they are quickly depleted when the dietary intake of folate is deficient (within 4 months). Folate is found in green vegetables and liver. Folate deficiency occurs in people who rarely eat uncooked vegetables. Alcohol increases folic acid requirements, and at the same time patients with alcoholism usually have a diet that is deficient in the vitamin. Folic acid requirements are also increased in patients with chronic hemolytic anemias and in women who are pregnant, because the need for erythrocyte production is increased in these conditions. Some patients with malabsorptive diseases of the small bowel, such as sprue, may not absorb folic acid normally.

#### VITAMIN $B_{12}$ DEFICIENCY

A deficiency of vitamin $B_{12}$ can occur in several ways. Inadequate dietary intake is rare but can develop in strict vegetarians who consume no meat or dairy products. Faulty absorption from the GI tract is more common. This occurs in conditions such as Crohn's disease, or after ileal resection or gastrectomy. Another cause is the absence of intrinsic factor, as in pernicious anemia. Intrinsic factor is normally secreted by cells within the gastric mucosa; normally it binds with the dietary vitamin $B_{12}$ and travels with it to the ileum, where the vitamin is absorbed. Without intrinsic factor, orally consumed vitamin $B_{12}$ cannot be absorbed, and erythrocyte production is eventually diminished. Even if adequate vitamin $B_{12}$ and intrinsic factor are present, a deficiency may occur if disease involving the ileum or pancreas impairs absorption. Pernicious anemia, which tends to run in families, is primarily a disorder of adults, particularly the elderly. The abnormality is in the gastric mucosa: the stomach wall atrophies and fails to secrete intrinsic factor. Therefore, the absorption of vitamin $B_{12}$ is significantly impaired.

The body normally has large stores of vitamin $B_{12}$, so years may pass before the deficiency results in anemia. Because the body compensates so well, the anemia can be severe before the patient becomes symptomatic. For unknown reasons, patients with pernicious anemia have a higher incidence of gastric cancer than the general population; these patients should have endoscopies at regular intervals (every 1 to 2 years) to screen for early gastric cancer.

## Clinical Manifestations

Symptoms of folic acid and vitamin $B_{12}$ deficiencies are similar, and the two anemias may coexist. However, the neurologic manifestations of vitamin $B_{12}$ deficiency do not occur with folic acid deficiency, and they persist if vitamin $B_{12}$ is not replaced. Therefore, careful distinction between the two anemias must be made. Serum levels of both vitamins can be measured. In the case of folic acid deficiency, even small amounts of folate increase the serum folate level, sometimes to normal. Measuring the amount of folate within the red cell itself (red cell folate) is therefore a more sensitive test in determining true folate deficiency.

After the body stores of vitamin $B_{12}$ are depleted, the patient may begin to show signs and symptoms of the anemia. However, because the onset and progression of the anemia are so gradual, the body can compensate very well until the anemia is severe, so that the typical manifestations of anemia (weakness, listlessness, fatigue) may not be apparent initially. The hematologic effects of deficiency are accompanied by effects on other organ systems, particularly the GI tract and nervous system. Patients with pernicious anemia develop a smooth, sore, red tongue and mild diarrhea. They are extremely pale, particularly in the mucous membranes. They may become confused; more often they have paresthesias in the extremities (particularly numbness and tingling in the feet and lower legs). They may have difficulty maintaining their balance because of damage to the spinal cord, and they also lose position sense (proprioception). These symptoms are progressive, although the course of illness may be marked by spontaneous partial remissions and exacerbations. Without treatment, patients can die after several years, usually from heart failure secondary to anemia.

## Assessment and Diagnostic Findings

The classic method of determining the cause of vitamin $B_{12}$ deficiency is the Schilling test, in which the patient receives a small oral dose of radioactive vitamin $B_{12}$, followed in a few hours by a large, nonradioactive parenteral dose of vitamin $B_{12}$ (this aids in renal excretion of the radioactive dose). If the oral vitamin is absorbed, more than 8% will be excreted in the urine within 24 hours; therefore, if no radioactivity is present in the urine (ie, the radioactive vitamin $B_{12}$ stays within the GI tract), the cause is GI malabsorption of the vitamin $B_{12}$. Conversely, if radioactivity is detected in the urine, the cause of the deficiency is not ileal disease or pernicious anemia. Later, the same procedure is repeated, but this time intrinsic factor is added to the oral radioactive vitamin $B_{12}$. If radioactivity is now detected in the urine (ie, the vitamin $B_{12}$ was absorbed from the GI tract in the presence of intrinsic factor), the diagnosis of pernicious anemia can be made. The Schilling test is useful only if the urine collections are complete; therefore, the nurse must promote the patient's understanding and compliance with this collection.

Other methods of establishing the diagnosis are more frequently used. Although it is possible to measure methylmalonic acid levels in vitamin $B_{12}$ deficiency, these levels also increase in the setting of renal insufficiency. Furthermore, it is expensive to measure these levels, which also limits the utility of the test. A more useful, easier test is the intrinsic factor antibody test. A positive test indicates the presence of antibodies that bind the vitamin $B_{12}$–intrinsic factor complex and prevent it from binding to receptors in the ileum, thus preventing its absorption. Unfortunately, this test is not specific for pernicious anemia alone, but it can aid in the diagnosis.

## Medical Management

Folate deficiency is treated by increasing the amount of folic acid in the diet and administering 1 mg of folic acid daily. Folic acid is administered IM only to people with malabsorption problems. With the exception of the vitamins administered during pregnancy, most proprietary vitamin preparations do not contain folic acid, so it must be administered as a separate tablet. After the hemoglobin level returns to normal, the folic acid replacement can be stopped. However, patients with alcoholism should continue receiving folic acid as long as they continue to consume alcohol.

Vitamin $B_{12}$ deficiency is treated by vitamin $B_{12}$ replacement. Vegetarians can prevent or treat deficiency with oral supplements with vitamins or fortified soy milk. When the deficiency is due to the more common defect in absorption or the absence of intrinsic factor, replacement is by monthly IM injections of vitamin $B_{12}$. Even in the absence of intrinsic factor, a small amount of an oral dose of vitamin $B_{12}$ can be absorbed by passive diffusion, but large doses (2 mg/day) are required if vitamin $B_{12}$ is to be replaced orally.

As vitamin $B_{12}$ is replaced, the reticulocyte count rises within 1 week, and in several weeks the blood counts are all normal. The tongue feels better and appears less red in several days. However, the neurologic manifestations require more time for recovery; if there is severe neuropathy, the patient may never recover fully. To prevent recurrence of pernicious anemia, vitamin $B_{12}$ therapy must be continued for life.

### NURSING ALERT

**Even when the megaloblastic anemia is severe, RBC transfusions may not be used because the patient's body has compensated over time by expanding the total blood volume. Administration of blood transfusions to such patients, particularly those who are elderly or who have cardiac dysfunction, can precipitate pulmonary edema. If transfusions are required, the RBCs should be transfused slowly, with careful attention to signs and symptoms of fluid overload.**

## Nursing Management

Assessment of patients who have or are at risk of megaloblastic anemia includes inspection of the skin and mucous membranes. Mild jaundice may be apparent and is best seen in the sclera without using fluorescent lights. Vitiligo (patchy loss of skin pigmentation) and premature graying of the hair are often seen in patients with pernicious anemia. The tongue is smooth, red, and sore. Because of the neurologic complications associated with these anemias, a careful neurologic assessment is important, including tests of position and vibration sense.

The nurse needs to pay particular attention to ambulation and should assess the patient's gait and stability as well as the need for assistive devices (eg, canes, walkers) and for assistance in managing daily activities. Of particular concern is ensuring safety when position sense, coordination, and gait are affected. Physical and occupational therapy referrals may be needed. If sensation is altered, the patient needs to be instructed to avoid excessive heat and cold.

Because mouth and tongue soreness may restrict nutritional intake, the nurse advises the patient to eat small amounts of bland, soft foods frequently. The nurse also may explain that other nutritional deficiencies, such as alcohol-induced anemia, can induce neurologic problems.

**PROMOTING HOME AND COMMUNITY-BASED CARE**

The patient must be taught about the chronicity of the disorder and the need for monthly vitamin $B_{12}$ injections or daily oral vitamin $B_{12}$ even in the absence of symptoms. If parenteral replacement is used, many patients can be taught to self-administer their injections. The gastric atrophy associated with pernicious anemia increases the risk for gastric carcinoma, so the patient needs to understand that ongoing medical follow-up and screening are important.

## Myelodysplastic Syndrome (MDS)

Myelodysplastic syndrome (MDS) is a group of disorders of the myeloid stem cell that causes **dysplasia** (abnormal development) in one or more types of cell lines. The most common feature of MDS—dysplasia of the erythrocytes—is manifested as a macrocytic anemia; however, the leukocytes (myeloid cells, particularly neutrophils) and platelets can also be affected. Although the bone marrow is actually hypercellular, many of the cells within it die before being released into the circulation. Therefore, the actual number of cells in the circulation is typically lower than normal. In addition to the quantitative defect (ie, fewer cells than normal), there is also a qualitative defect: the cells are not as functional as normal. The neutrophils have diminished ability to destroy bacteria by phagocytosis; platelets are less able to aggregate and are less adhesive than usual. The result of these qualitative defects is an increased risk of infection and bleeding, even when the actual number of circulating cells may not be excessively low. A significant proportion of MDS cases evolve into acute myeloid leukemia (AML); this type of leukemia tends to be nonresponsive to standard therapy.

Primary MDS tends to be a disease of the elderly: more than 80% of patients with MDS are older than 60 years. Secondary MDS may occur at any age and results from prior toxic exposure to chemicals, including chemotherapeutic medications (particularly alkylating agents). Secondary MDS tends to have a poorer prognosis than does primary MDS.

### Clinical Manifestations

The manifestations of MDS can vary widely. Many patients are asymptomatic, with the illness being discovered incidentally when a CBC is performed for other purposes. Other patients have profound symptoms and complications from the illness. Fatigue is often present, at varying levels. Neutrophil dysfunction puts the person at risk for infection; recurrent pneumonias are common. Because platelet function can also be altered, bleeding can occur. These problems may persist in a fairly steady state for months, even years. They may also progress over time; as the dysplasia evolves into a leukemic state, the complications increase in severity.

### Assessment and Diagnostic Findings

The CBC typically reveals a macrocytic anemia; leukocyte and platelet counts may be diminished as well. Serum erythropoietin levels may be inappropriately low, as is the reticulocyte count. As the disease evolves into AML, more immature blast cells are noted on the CBC.

### Medical Management

With the exception of allogeneic bone marrow transplant (BMT), there is no known cure for MDS. Chemotherapy has been used, particularly in patients with more aggressive forms of the illness, but typically with disappointing results (Giralt, 2004). Recently, new agents, 5-azacytadine, lenolidomide, and decifibine, were approved by the U.S. Food and Drug Administration (FDA) for use in patients with MDS. Research studies indicated that patients who responded to these agents had decreased transfusion requirements, decreased evolution toward AML, and improved quality of life (Estey, 2004; Foss, 2004; List, Kurtin, Roe, et al., 2005; Silverman, 2004).

However, patients with mild cytopenias (low blood counts) often require no therapy. For most patients with MDS, transfusions of red cells may be required to control the anemia and its symptoms. These patients can develop significant problems with iron overload from the repeated transfusions; this problem can be diminished with prompt initiation of chelation therapy to remove the excess iron (see Nursing Management). In some patients, the use of erythropoietin can be successful in reducing the need for transfusions and their attendant complications. Some patients may require ongoing platelet transfusions to prevent significant bleeding. Over time, these patients often develop iso-sensitization to donor platelets, resulting in suboptimal increases in the platelet count after platelets are transfused. Infections need to be managed aggressively and promptly. Administration of growth factors, particularly granulocyte colony-stimulating factor (G-CSF), erythropoietin, or both, has been successful in increasing neutrophils and diminishing anemia in certain patients; however, these agents are expensive and the effect is lost if the medications are stopped.

Because MDS tends to occur in elderly people, other chronic conditions may limit treatment options. Secondary MDS and MDS that evolves into AML tend to be much more refractory to conventional therapy for leukemia.

## Nursing Management

Caring for patients with MDS can be challenging because the illness is unpredictable. As with other hematologic conditions, some patients (especially those with no symptoms) have difficulty perceiving that they have a serious illness that can place them at risk of life-threatening complications. At the other extreme, many patients have tremendous difficulty coping with the uncertain trajectory of the illness and fear that the illness will evolve into AML at a time when they are feeling very well physically.

Patients with MDS need extensive instruction about infection risk, measures to avoid it, signs and symptoms of developing infection, and appropriate actions to take should such symptoms occur. Instruction should also be given regarding the risk of bleeding. Patients with MDS who are hospitalized may require neutropenic precautions.

Laboratory values need to be monitored closely to anticipate the need for transfusion and to determine response to treatment with growth factors. Patients with chronic transfusion requirements usually benefit from the insertion of a vascular access device for this purpose. Patients receiving growth factors or chelation therapy need instruction about these medications, their side effects, and administration techniques.

Chelation therapy is a process that is used to remove excess iron acquired from chronic transfusions. Iron is bound to a substance, the chelating agent, and then excreted in the urine. Oral forms of chelating agents have not previously been successful (due to either diminished efficacy or excessive toxicity), but new formulations are now available (Vanorden & Hagemann, 2006). Chelation therapy is most effective as a subcutaneous infusion administered over 8 to 12 hours; most patients prefer to do this at night. Because chelation therapy removes only a small amount of iron with each treatment, patients with chronic transfusion requirements (and iron overload) need to continue chelation therapy as long as the iron overload exists, potentially for the rest of their lives. Patients who are embarking on chelation therapy must be highly motivated and need instruction in the subcutaneous infusion technique, infusion pump maintenance, and side effect management. Local erythema at the injection site is the most common reaction and typically requires no intervention. Patients should have baseline and annual auditory and eye examinations, because hearing loss and visual changes can occur with chelation treatment.

## Hemolytic Anemias

In hemolytic anemias, the erythrocytes have a shortened life span; thus, their number in the circulation is reduced. Fewer erythrocytes result in decreased available oxygen, causing hypoxia, which in turn stimulates an increase in erythropoietin release from the kidney. The erythropoietin stimulates the bone marrow to compensate by producing new erythrocytes and releasing some of them into the circulation somewhat prematurely as reticulocytes. If the red cell destruction persists, the hemoglobin is broken down excessively; about 80% of the heme is converted to bilirubin, conjugated in the liver, and excreted in the bile.

The mechanism of erythrocyte destruction varies, but all types of hemolytic anemia share certain laboratory features: the reticulocyte count is elevated, the fraction of indirect (unconjugated) bilirubin is increased, and the supply of haptoglobin (a binding protein for free hemoglobin) is depleted as more hemoglobin is released. As a result, the plasma haptoglobin level is low. If the marrow cannot compensate to replace the erythrocytes (indicated by a decreased reticulocyte count), the anemia will progress.

Hemolytic anemia has various forms. Among the inherited forms are sickle cell anemia, thalassemia and thalassemia major, G-6-PD deficiency, and hereditary spherocytosis. Acquired forms include autoimmune hemolytic anemia, non-immune-mediated paroxysmal nocturnal hemoglobinuria, microangiopathic hemolytic anemia, and heart valve hemolysis, as well as anemias associated with hypersplenism.

### Sickle Cell Anemia

Sickle cell anemia is a severe hemolytic anemia that results from inheritance of the sickle hemoglobin gene. This gene causes the hemoglobin molecule to be defective. The sickle hemoglobin (HbS) acquires a crystal-like formation when exposed to low oxygen tension. The oxygen level in venous blood can be low enough to cause this change; consequently, the erythrocyte containing HbS loses its round, pliable, biconcave disk shape and becomes deformed, rigid, and sickle-shaped (Fig. 33-5). These long, rigid erythrocytes can adhere to the endothelium of small vessels; when they adhere to each other, blood flow to a region or an organ may be reduced. If ischemia or infarction results, the patient may have pain, swelling, and fever. The sickling process takes time; if the erythrocyte is again exposed to adequate amounts of oxygen (eg, when it travels through the pulmonary circulation) before the membrane becomes too rigid, it can revert to a normal shape. For this reason, the "sickling crises" are intermittent. Cold can aggravate the sickling process, because vasoconstriction slows the blood flow. Oxygen delivery can also be impaired by an increased

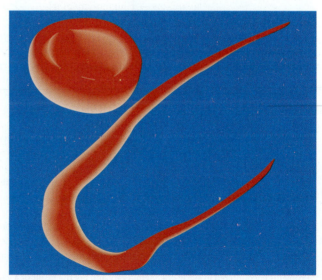

**FIGURE 33-5.** A normal red blood cell (*upper left*) and a sickled red blood cell.

blood viscosity, with or without occlusion due to adhesion of sickled cells; in this situation, the effects are seen in larger vessels, such as arterioles.

The *HbS* gene is inherited in people of African descent and to a lesser extent in people from the Middle East, the Mediterranean area, and aboriginal tribes in India. Sickle cell anemia is the most severe form of sickle cell disease. Less severe forms include sickle cell hemoglobin C (SC) disease, sickle cell hemoglobin D (SD) disease, and sickle cell beta-thalassemia. The clinical manifestations and management are the same as for sickle cell anemia. The term "sickle cell trait" refers to the carrier state for SC diseases; it is the most benign type of SC disease, in that less than 50% of the hemoglobin within an erythrocyte is HbS. However, in terms of genetic counseling, it is still an important condition. If two people with sickle cell trait have children, the children may inherit two abnormal genes. These children will produce only HbS and therefore will have sickle cell anemia. (Refer to Chapter 9 for additional discussion of genetic diseases.)

## Clinical Manifestations

Symptoms of sickle cell anemia vary and are only somewhat based on the amount of HbS. Symptoms and complications result from chronic hemolysis or thrombosis. The sickled erythrocytes have a shortened life span. Anemia is always present; usually hemoglobin values are 7 to 10 g/dL. Jaundice is characteristic and is usually obvious in the sclerae. The bone marrow expands in childhood in a compensatory effort to offset the anemia, sometimes leading to enlargement of the bones of the face and skull. The chronic anemia is associated with tachycardia, cardiac murmurs, and often an enlarged heart (cardiomegaly). Dysrhythmias and heart failure may occur in adults.

Virtually any organ may be affected by thrombosis, but the primary sites involve those areas with normally slower circulation, such as the spleen, lungs, and central nervous system. All the tissues and organs are constantly vulnerable to microcirculatory interruptions by the sickling process and therefore are susceptible to hypoxic damage or true ischemic necrosis. Patients with sickle cell anemia are unusually susceptible to infection, particularly pneumonia and osteomyelitis. Complications of sickle cell anemia include infection, stroke, renal failure, impotence, heart failure, and pulmonary hypertension (Table 33-3).

### SICKLE CELL CRISIS

There are three types of sickle cell crisis in the adult population. The most common is the very painful *sickle crisis*, which results from tissue hypoxia and necrosis due to inadequate blood flow to a specific region of tissue or organ. *Aplastic crisis* results from infection with the human parvovirus. The hemoglobin level falls rapidly and the marrow cannot compensate, as evidenced by an absence of reticulocytes. *Sequestration crisis* results when other organs pool the sickled cells. Although the spleen is the most common organ responsible for sequestration in children, most children with sickle cell anemia have had a splenic infarction by 10 years of age, and the spleen is then no longer functional (autosplenectomy). In adults, the common organs involved in sequestration are the liver and, more seriously, the lungs.

### TABLE 33-3  Complications in Sickle Cell Anemia*

| Organ Involved | Mechanisms* | Diagnostic Findings | Signs and Symptoms |
|---|---|---|---|
| Spleen | Primary site of sickling → infarctions → ↓ phagocytic function of macrophages | Autosplenectomy; ↑ infection (esp. pneumonia, osteomyelitis) | Abdominal pain; fever, signs of infection |
| Lungs | Infection<br>Infarction → ↑ pulmonary pressure → pulmonary hypertension | Pulmonary infiltrate<br>↑ sPLA$_2$† | Chest pain; dyspnea |
| Central Nervous System | Infarction | Cerebral vascular accident (stroke, brain attack) | Weakness (if severe); learning difficulties (if mild) |
| Kidney | Sickling → damage to renal medulla | Hematuria; inability to concentrate urine; renal failure | Dehydration |
| Heart | Anemia | Tachycardia; cardiomegaly → heart failure | Weakness, fatigue, dyspnea |
| Bone | ↑ Erythroid production | Widening of medullary spaces and cortical thinning | Ache, arthralgias |
|  | Infarction of bone | Osteosclerosis → avascular necrosis | Bone pain, especially hips |
| Liver | Hemolysis | Jaundice and gallstone formation; hepatomegaly | Abdominal pain |
| Skin and peripheral vasculature | ↑ Viscosity/stasis → infarction → skin ulcers | Skin ulcers; ↓ wound healing | Pain |
| Eye | Infarction | Scarring, hemorrhage, retinal detachment | ↓ Vision; blindness |
| Penis | Sickling → vascular thrombosis | Priapism → impotence | Pain, impotence |

*Problems encountered in sickle cell anemia vary and are the result of a variety of mechanisms, as depicted in this table. Common physical findings and symptoms are also variable.
†sPLA$_2$: Secretory phospholipase A$_2$, a laboratory test that can predict impending acute chest syndrome (see text).

## ACUTE CHEST SYNDROME

Acute chest syndrome is manifested by a rapidly decreasing hemoglobin level, tachycardia, fever, and bilateral infiltrates seen on the chest x-ray. These signs often mimic infection, but in fact the most common cause appears to be infarction within the pulmonary vasculature (Hammerman & Faber, 2004). Another common cause is pulmonary fat embolism. Increased secretory phospholipase $A_2$ concentration has been identified as a predictor of impending acute chest syndrome; the increased amounts of free fatty acids can cause increased permeability of the pulmonary endothelium and leakage of the pulmonary capillaries (Hammerman & Faber, 2004). Although this syndrome is potentially lethal, prompt intervention can result in a favorable outcome.

## PULMONARY HYPERTENSION

Pulmonary hypertension is a common sequela of sickle cell disease. Patients with sickle cell anemia are most likely to die of either pulmonary hypertension or chronic lung disease (Vichinsky, 2004). Unfortunately, diagnosing pulmonary hypertension is difficult because clinical symptoms rarely occur until damage is irreversible. Although changes are not evident on chest x-ray, high-resolution computed tomography (CT) of the chest often demonstrates microvascular occlusion and diminished perfusion of the lung. Pulse oximetry measurements are typically normal, and breath sounds are clear to auscultation until the disease has progressed to later stages (Vichinsky, 2004). A recent study demonstrated an improvement in diagnosis of pulmonary hypertension by screening patients with sickle cell disease with Doppler echocardiography (Gladwin, Sachdev, & Jison, 2004).

## *Assessment and Diagnostic Findings*

The patient with sickle cell trait usually has a normal hemoglobin level, a normal hematocrit, and a normal blood smear. In contrast, the patient with sickle cell anemia has a low hematocrit and sickled cells on the smear. The diagnosis is confirmed by hemoglobin electrophoresis.

## *Prognosis*

Patients with sickle cell anemia are usually diagnosed in childhood, because they become anemic in infancy and begin to have sickle cell crises at 1 or 2 years of age. Some children die in the first years of life, typically of infection, but antibiotic use and parent teaching strategies have greatly improved the outcomes for these children. However, with current management strategies, the average life expectancy is still suboptimal, at 42 to 48 years. Young adults are often forced to live with multiple, often severe, complications from their disease. In some patients, the symptoms and complications diminish by 30 years of age; these patients live into the sixth decade or longer. Currently, there is no way to predict which patients will fall into this subgroup.

## *Medical Management*

Treatment for sickle cell anemia is the focus of continued research (Cao, 2004; Stuart & Nagel, 2004). Many trials of medications that have antisickling properties are being conducted, as is research using antiadhesion treatment for vasoocclusive crises. However, aside from the equally important aggressive management of symptoms and complications, currently there are only four primary treatment modalities for sickle cell diseases: bone marrow transplant (BMT), hydroxyurea, arginine, and long-term RBC transfusion.

BMT offers the potential for cure for this disease. However, this treatment modality is available to only a small subset of affected patients, because of either the lack of a compatible donor or the severe organ damage (eg, renal, liver, lung) already present in the patient.

### PHARMACOLOGIC THERAPY

Hydroxyurea (Hydrea), a chemotherapy agent, has been shown to be effective in increasing hemoglobin F levels in patients with sickle cell anemia, thereby decreasing the permanent formation of sickled cells. Patients who receive hydroxyurea appear to have fewer painful episodes of sickle cell crisis, a lower incidence of acute chest syndrome, and less need for transfusions. However, whether hydroxyurea can prevent or reverse actual organ damage remains unknown. Side effects of hydroxyurea include chronic suppression of leukocyte formation, teratogenesis, and potential for later development of a malignancy. Patient response to this agent varies significantly. The incidence and severity of side effects are also highly variable within a dose range. Some patients have toxicity with a very small dose (5 mg/kg per day), whereas others have little toxicity with a much higher dose (35 mg/kg per day). More research is needed to identify specific patient subgroups that are more likely to respond to this medication.

Arginine has antisickling properties and can enhance the availability of nitric oxide, a potent vasodilator, resulting in decreased pulmonary artery pressure. Arginine is synergistic with hydroxyurea and can be useful as combination therapy for managing pulmonary hypertension (Vichinsky, 2004).

### TRANSFUSION THERAPY

Chronic RBC transfusions have been shown to be highly effective in several situations: in an acute exacerbation of anemia (eg, aplastic crisis), in the prevention of severe complications from anesthesia and surgery, and in improving the response to infection (when it results in exacerbated anemia). Chronic transfusions have also been shown to be effective in diminishing episodes of sickle cell crisis in pregnant women, but these transfusions have not been shown to improve fetal survival. Transfusion therapy may be effective in preventing complications from sickle cell disease. Although controversial, some data support the use of chronic transfusions in patients with cerebral ischemic injury (as seen on magnetic resonance imaging [MRI] or Doppler studies) to prevent more severe injury (eg, cerebrovascular accident [CVA, brain attack, or stroke]) (Adams et al., 2004). More than 50% of asymptomatic patients have some cerebral ischemia documented by MRI. In a pivotal study, chronic transfusion with packed red blood cells (PRBCs) resulted in a 90% reduction of stroke in children at risk of this complication, defined by elevated blood viscosity on transcranial Doppler ultrasonography (Gebreyohanns & Adams, 2004). Transfusions may also be useful in the management of severe cases of acute chest syndrome (Liem et al., 2004).

The risk of complications from transfusion is important to consider. These risks include iron overload, which necessitates chronic chelation therapy (see Myelodysplastic Syndrome, Nursing Management); poor venous access, which necessitates a vascular access device (and its attendant risk of infection or thrombosis); infections (hepatitis, human immunodeficiency virus [HIV]); and alloimmunization (an immune response to antigens from donor cells) from repeated transfusions. Another complication from transfusion is increased blood viscosity without reduction in the concentration of hemoglobin S. Exchange transfusion (in which the patient's own blood is removed and replaced via transfusion) may be performed to diminish the risk of increasing the viscosity excessively; the objective is to reduce the hematocrit to less than 30%, with transfusions supplying more than 80% of the patient's blood volume. Finally, it is important to consider the significant financial cost of an aggressive transfusion and chelation program.

Patients with sickle cell anemia require daily folic acid replacements to maintain the supply required for increased erythropoiesis from hemolysis. Infections must be treated promptly with appropriate antibiotics; infection, particularly pneumococcal infection, remains a major cause of death. These patients should receive pneumococcal vaccines (Davies et al., 2004).

Acute chest syndrome is managed by prompt initiation of antibiotic therapy. Incentive spirometry has been shown to decrease the incidence of pulmonary complications significantly. In severe cases, bronchoscopy may be required to identify the source of pulmonary disease. Fluid restriction may be more beneficial than aggressive hydration. Corticosteroids may also be useful. Transfusions reverse the hypoxia and decrease the level of secretory phospholipase $A_2$. Pulmonary function should be monitored regularly to detect pulmonary hypertension early, when therapy (hydroxyurea, arginine, transfusions, or BMT) may have a positive impact.

Because repeated blood transfusions are necessary, patients may develop multiple autoantibodies, making cross-matching difficult. In this patient population, a hemolytic transfusion reaction (see later discussion) may mimic the signs and symptoms of a sickle cell crisis. The classic distinguishing factor is that with a hemolytic transfusion reaction, the patient becomes *more* anemic after being transfused. These patients need very close observation. Further transfusion is avoided if possible until the hemolytic process abates. If possible, the patient is supported with corticosteroids (prednisone), IV immunoglobulin (IVIG; Gammagard, Sandoglobulin, Venoglobulin), and erythropoietin (Epogen, Procrit).

### SUPPORTIVE THERAPY

Supportive care is equally important. Pain management is a significant issue. The incidence of painful sickle cell crises is highly variable; many patients have pain on a daily basis. The severity of the pain may not be enough to cause the patient to seek assistance from health care providers but severe enough to interfere with the ability to work and function within the family unit. Acute pain episodes tend to be self-limited, lasting hours to days. If the patient cannot manage the pain at home, intervention is frequently sought in the acute care setting, usually at an urgent care facility or emergency department. Adequate hydration is important during a painful sickling episode. Oral hydration is acceptable if the patient can maintain adequate amounts of fluids; IV hydration with dextrose 5% in water ($D_5W$) or dextrose 5% in 0.25 normal saline solution (3 L/m²/24 hours) is usually required for sickle crisis. Supplemental oxygen may also be needed.

The use of medication to relieve pain is important (see Chapter 13 for a discussion of pain management). Aspirin is very useful in diminishing mild to moderate pain; it also diminishes inflammation and potential thrombosis (due to its ability to diminish platelet adhesion). Nonsteroidal anti-inflammatory drugs (NSAIDs) are useful for moderate pain or in combination with opioid analgesics. Although no tolerance develops with NSAIDs, a "ceiling effect" does develop whereby an increase in dosage does not increase analgesia. NSAID use must be carefully monitored, because these medications can precipitate renal dysfunction. When opioid analgesics are used, morphine is the medication of choice for acute pain. Patient-controlled analgesia (PCA) is frequently used. A recent study of 40 adults with sickle cell disease found that PCA was beneficial in managing pain due to sickling crises because it restored the patient's control over analgesia during hospitalization, provided quicker pain relief, and provided increased independence from health care providers (Johnson, 2003).

Chronic pain increases in incidence as the patient ages. Here, the pain is caused by complications (eg, avascular necrosis of the hip) from the sickling. With chronic pain management, the principal goal is to maximize functioning; pain may not be completely eliminated without sacrificing function. This concept may be difficult for patients to accept; they may need repeated explanations and support from nonjudgmental health care providers. Nonpharmacologic approaches to pain management are crucial in this setting. Examples include physical and occupational therapy, physiotherapy (including the use of heat, massage, and exercise), cognitive and behavioral intervention (including distraction, relaxation, and motivational therapy), and support groups.

Working with patients who have multiple episodes of severe pain can be challenging. It is important for health care providers to realize that patients with sickle cell disease must face a lifelong experience with severe and unpredictable pain. Such pain is disruptive to the person's level of functioning, including social functioning, and may result in a feeling of helplessness. Patients with inadequate social support systems may have more difficulty coping with chronic pain.

## Nursing Process

### The Patient With Sickle Cell Crisis

A patient in sickle cell crisis should be assessed for factors that could have precipitated the crisis, such as symptoms of infection or dehydration, or situations that promote fatigue or emotional stress.

## Assessment

The patient is asked to recall factors that precipitated previous crises and measures he or she uses to prevent and manage crises. Pain levels should always be monitored using a pain intensity scale, such as a 0-to-10 scale. The quality of the pain (eg, sharp, dull, burning), the frequency of the pain (constant versus intermittent), and factors that aggravate or alleviate the pain are included in this assessment. If a sickle cell crisis is suspected, the nurse needs to determine whether the pain currently experienced is the same as or different from the pain typically encountered in crisis.

Because the sickling process can interrupt circulation in any tissue or organ, with resultant hypoxia and ischemia, a careful assessment of all body systems is necessary. Particular emphasis is placed on pain, swelling, and fever. All joint areas are carefully examined for pain and swelling. The abdomen is assessed for pain and tenderness because of the possibility of splenic infarction.

The respiratory system must be assessed carefully, including auscultation of breath sounds, measurement of oxygen saturation levels, and signs of cardiac failure, such as the presence and extent of dependent edema, an increased point of maximal impulse (PMI), and cardiomegaly (as seen on a chest x-ray). The patient is assessed for signs of dehydration by a history of fluid intake and careful examination of mucous membranes, skin turgor, urine output, and serum creatinine and blood urea nitrogen values.

A careful neurologic examination is important to elicit symptoms of cerebral hypoxia. However, ischemic findings on MRI or Doppler studies may significantly precede the findings on the physical examination. MRI and Doppler studies are used for early diagnosis and may result in improved patient outcome because therapy can be initiated more promptly.

Because patients with sickle cell anemia are so susceptible to infections, they are assessed for the presence of any infectious process. Particular attention is given to examination of the chest, long bones, and femoral head, because pneumonia and osteomyelitis are especially common. Leg ulcers, which may be infected and are slow to heal, are common.

The extent of anemia (as measured by the hemoglobin level and the hematocrit) and the ability of the marrow to replenish erythrocytes (as measured by the reticulocyte count) are monitored and compared with the patient's baseline values. The patient's current and past history of medical management is also obtained, particularly chronic transfusion therapy, hydroxyurea use, and prior treatment for infection.

## Diagnosis

### Nursing Diagnoses

Based on the assessment data, major nursing diagnoses for the patient with sickle cell crisis may include:

- Acute pain related to tissue hypoxia due to agglutination of sickled cells within blood vessels
- Risk for infection
- Risk for powerlessness related to illness-induced helplessness
- Deficient knowledge regarding sickle crisis prevention

### Collaborative Problems/ Potential Complications

Based on the assessment data, potential complications may include:

- Hypoxia, ischemia, infection, and poor wound healing leading to skin breakdown and ulcers
- Dehydration
- Cerebrovascular accident (CVA, brain attack, stroke)
- Anemia
- Renal dysfunction
- Heart failure, pulmonary hypertension, and acute chest syndrome
- Impotence
- Poor compliance
- Substance abuse related to poorly managed chronic pain

## Planning and Goals

The major goals for the patient are relief of pain, decreased incidence of crisis, enhanced sense of self-esteem and power, and absence of complications.

## Nursing Interventions

### Managing Pain

Acute pain during a sickle cell crisis can be severe and unpredictable. The patient's subjective description and rating of pain on a pain scale must guide the use of analgesics, which are valuable in controlling the acute pain of a sickle crisis. Any joint that is acutely swollen should be supported and elevated until the swelling diminishes. Relaxation techniques, breathing exercises, and distraction are helpful for some patients. After the acute painful episode has diminished, aggressive measures should be implemented to preserve function. Physical therapy, whirlpool baths, and transcutaneous nerve stimulation (TENS) are examples of such modalities.

### Preventing and Managing Infection

Nursing care focuses on monitoring the patient for signs and symptoms of infection. Prescribed antibiotics should be initiated promptly, and the patient should be assessed for signs of dehydration. If the patient is to take prescribed oral antibiotics at home, he or she must understand the need to complete the entire course of antibiotic therapy and must be able to identify a feasible administration schedule.

### Promoting Coping Skills

This illness frequently leaves the patient feeling powerless and with decreased self-esteem because its acute exacerbations often result in chronic health problems. These feelings can be exacerbated by inadequate pain management, and enhancing pain management can be extremely useful in establishing a therapeutic relationship based on mutual trust. Nursing care that focuses on the patient's strengths rather than deficits can enhance effective coping skills. Providing the patient with opportunities to make decisions about daily care may increase the patient's feelings of control.

### Minimizing Deficient Knowledge

Patients with sickle cell anemia benefit from understanding what situations can precipitate a sickle cell crisis and the steps they can take to prevent or diminish such crises. Keeping warm and maintaining adequate hydration can be very effective in diminishing the occurrence and severity of attacks. Avoiding stressful situations is more challenging. Group education may be more effective if it is carried out by members of the community who are from the same ethnic group as those with the disease.

### Monitoring and Managing Potential Complications

Management measures for many of the potential complications were delineated in previous sections. Other measures follow.

#### LEG ULCERS

Leg ulcers require careful management and protection from trauma and contamination. Referral to a wound-ostomy-continence nurse may facilitate healing and assist with prevention. If leg ulcers fail to heal, skin grafting may be necessary. Scrupulous aseptic technique is warranted to prevent nosocomial infections.

#### PRIAPISM LEADING TO IMPOTENCE

Male patients may develop sudden, painful episodes of priapism (persistent penile erection). The patient is taught to empty his bladder at the onset of the attack, exercise, and take a warm bath. If an episode persists longer than 3 hours, medical attention, which consists of IV hydration, administration of analgesics, and possible penile intracavernosal aspiration, is recommended. Repeated episodes may lead to extensive vascular thrombosis, resulting in impotence.

#### CHRONIC PAIN AND SUBSTANCE ABUSE

Many patients have considerable difficulty coping with chronic pain and repeated episodes of sickle cell crisis. Those who feel they have little control over their health and the physical complications that result from this illness may find it difficult to adhere to a prescribed treatment plan. Being nonjudgmental and actively seeking involvement from the patient in establishing a treatment plan are useful strategies.

Some patients with sickle cell anemia develop problems with substance abuse. For many, this abuse results from inadequate management of acute pain during episodes of crisis. Some clinicians suggest that abuse may result from prescribing insufficient amounts of opioid analgesics. The patient's pain may never be adequately relieved, promoting mistrust of the health care system and (from the patient's perspective) the need to seek care from a variety of sources when the pain is not severe. This cycle is best managed by prevention. Receiving care from a single provider over time is much more beneficial than receiving care from rotating physicians and staff in an emergency department. When crises occur, the staff in the emergency department should be in contact with the patient's primary health care provider so that optimal management can be achieved. Once a pattern of substance abuse is established, it is very difficult to manage, but continuity of care and establishing written contracts with the patient can be useful management strategies.

### Promoting Home and Community-Based Care

#### TEACHING PATIENTS SELF-CARE

Because patients with sickle cell anemia are typically diagnosed as children, parents participate in the initial education. Based on the parents' knowledge, socioeconomic level, and interest, teaching focuses on the disease process (including some pathophysiology), treatment, and the assessment and monitoring skills needed to identify potential complications. As the child ages, educational interventions prepare the child to assume more responsibility for self-care.

Vascular access device management and chelation therapy can be taught to most families. Follow-up care for patients with vascular access devices may also need to be provided by nurses in an outpatient facility or by a home care nurse.

#### CONTINUING CARE

The illness trajectory of sickle cell anemia is highly varied, with unpredictable episodes of complications and crises. Care is often provided on an emergency basis, especially for some patients with pain management problems (see previous section). All health care providers who provide services to patients with sickle cell disease and their families need to communicate regularly with each other. Patients need to learn which parameters are important for them to monitor and how to monitor them. Guidelines should also be given regarding when it is appropriate to seek urgent care.

## Evaluation

### Expected Patient Outcomes

Expected patient outcomes may include:
1. Control of pain
    a. Acute pain is controlled with analgesics
    b. Uses relaxation techniques, breathing exercises, distraction to help relieve pain

2. Is free of infection
   a. Has normal temperature
   b. Leukocyte count within normal range (5000 to 10,000/mm³)
   c. Identifies importance of continuing antibiotics at home (if applicable)
3. Expresses improved sense of control
   a. Participates in goal setting and in planning and implementing daily activities
   b. Participates in decisions about care
4. Increases knowledge about disease process
   a. Identifies situations and factors that can precipitate sickle cell crisis
   b. Describes lifestyle changes needed to prevent crisis
   c. Describes the importance of warmth, adequate hydration, and prevention of infection in preventing crisis
5. Absence of complications

## Thalassemia

The thalassemias are a group of hereditary anemias characterized by **hypochromia** (an abnormal decrease in the hemoglobin content of erythrocytes), extreme **microcytosis** (smaller-than-normal erythrocytes), destruction of blood elements (hemolysis), and variable degrees of anemia. The thalassemias occur worldwide, but the highest prevalence is found in people of Mediterranean, African, and Southeast Asian ancestry.

Thalassemias are associated with defective synthesis of the hemoglobin chain; the production of one or more globulin chains within the hemoglobin molecule is reduced. When this occurs, the imbalance in the configuration of the hemoglobin causes it to precipitate in the erythroid precursors or the erythrocytes themselves. This increases the rigidity of the erythrocytes and thus the premature destruction of these cells.

Thalassemias are classified into two major groups according to which hemoglobin chain is diminished: alpha or beta. The alpha-thalassemias occur mainly in people from Asia and the Middle East, and the beta-thalassemias are most prevalent in people from Mediterranean regions but also occur in those from the Middle East or Asia. The alpha-thalassemias are milder than the beta forms and often occur without symptoms; the erythrocytes are extremely microcytic, but the anemia, if present, is mild.

The severity of beta-thalassemia varies depending on the extent to which the hemoglobin chains are affected. Patients with mild forms have a microcytosis and mild anemia. If left untreated, severe beta-thalassemia (thalassemia major, or Cooley's anemia) can be fatal within the first few years of life. Bone marrow transplant (BMT) offers a chance of cure, but when this is not possible, the disease is usually treated with transfusion of PRBCs. Patients may survive into their 20s and 30s. Patient teaching during the reproductive years should include preconception counseling about the risk of thalassemia major.

### Thalassemia Major

Thalassemia major (Cooley's anemia) is characterized by severe anemia, marked hemolysis, and ineffective erythropoiesis (production of erythrocytes). With early regular transfusion therapy, growth and development through childhood are facilitated. Organ dysfunction due to iron overload results from the excessive amounts of iron in multiple PRBC transfusions. Regular chelation therapy (eg, subcutaneous deferoxamine) has reduced the complications of iron overload and prolonged the life of these patients. This disease is potentially curable by BMT if the procedure can be performed before liver damage occurs (ie, during childhood).

## Glucose-6-Phosphate Dehydrogenase Deficiency

The G-6-PD gene is the source of the abnormality in this disorder; this gene produces an enzyme within the erythrocyte that is essential for membrane stability. A few patients have inherited an enzyme so defective that they have a chronic hemolytic anemia; however, the most common type of defect results in hemolysis only when the erythrocytes are stressed by certain situations, such as fever or the use of certain medications. The disorder came to the attention of researchers during World War II, when some soldiers developed hemolysis while taking primaquine, an antimalarial agent. African Americans and people of Greek or Italian origin are those primarily affected by this disorder. The type of deficiency found in the Mediterranean population is more severe than that in the African Caribbean population, resulting in greater hemolysis and sometimes in life-threatening anemia. All types of G-6-PD deficiency are inherited as X-linked defects; therefore, many more men are at risk than women. In the United States, about 12% of African American males are affected. The deficiency is also common in those of Asian ancestry and in certain Jewish populations.

Oxidant drugs have hemolytic effects for people with G-6-PD deficiency. These medications include antimalarial agents (eg, chloroquine [Aralen]), sulfonamides (eg, trimethoprim/sulfamethoxazole [Bactrim, Septra]), nitrofurantoin (eg, Macrodantin), common coal tar analgesics (including aspirin in high doses), thiazide diuretics (eg, hydrochlorothiazide [HydroDIURIL], chlorothiazide [Diuril]), oral hypoglycemic agents (eg, glyburide [Micronase], metformin [Glucophage]), chloramphenicol (Chloromycetin), and vitamin K (phytonadione [AquaMEPHYTON]). In affected people, a severe hemolytic episode can also result from ingestion of fava beans.

### Clinical Manifestations

Patients are asymptomatic and have normal hemoglobin levels and reticulocyte counts most of the time. However, several days after exposure to an offending medication, they may develop pallor, jaundice, and hemoglobinuria (hemoglobin in the urine). The reticulocyte count increases, and symptoms of hemolysis develop. Special stains of the peripheral blood may then disclose Heinz bodies (degraded hemoglobin) within the erythrocytes. Hemolysis is often mild and self-limited. However, in the more severe Mediterranean type of G-6-PD deficiency, spontaneous recovery may not occur, and transfusions may be necessary.

### Assessment and Diagnostic Findings

The diagnosis is made by a screening test or by a quantitative assay of G-6-PD.

### Medical Management

The treatment is to stop the offending medication. Transfusion is necessary only in the severe hemolytic state, which is more commonly seen in the Mediterranean variety of G-6-PD deficiency.

### Nursing Management

The patient is educated about the disease and given a list of medications to avoid. If hemolysis does develop, nursing interventions are the same as for hemolysis from other causes. Patients should be instructed to wear MedicAlert bracelets that identify that they have G-6-PD deficiency.

## Hereditary Spherocytosis

Hereditary spherocytosis is a relatively common (1 in 5000 people) hemolytic anemia characterized by an abnormal permeability of the erythrocyte membrane; this causes the cells to change into a spherical shape. These erythrocytes are destroyed prematurely in the spleen. The severity of this hemolytic anemia varies; jaundice can be intermittent, and splenomegaly (enlarged spleen) also can occur. Surgical removal of the spleen is the principal treatment for this disorder.

## Immune Hemolytic Anemia

Hemolytic anemias can result from exposure of the erythrocyte to antibodies. Alloantibodies (ie, antibodies against the host, or "self") result from the immunization of a person with foreign antigens (eg, the immunization of an Rh-negative person with Rh-positive blood). Alloantibodies tend to be large (IgM type) and cause immediate destruction of the sensitized erythrocytes, either within the blood vessel (intravascular hemolysis) or within the liver. The most common type of alloimmune hemolytic anemia in adults results from a hemolytic transfusion reaction.

Autoantibodies may develop for many reasons. In many instances, the person's immune system is dysfunctional, so that it falsely recognizes its own erythrocytes as foreign and produces antibodies against them. This mechanism is seen in people with chronic lymphocytic leukemia (CLL). Another mechanism is a deficiency in suppressor lymphocytes, which normally prevent antibody formation against a person's own antigens. Autoantibodies tend to be of the IgG type. The erythrocytes are sequestered in the spleen and destroyed by the macrophages outside the blood vessel (extravascular hemolysis).

Autoimmune hemolytic anemias can be classified based on the body temperature involved when the antibodies react with the red blood cell antigen. Warm-body antibodies bind to erythrocytes most actively in warm conditions (37°C); cold-body antibodies react in cold conditions (0°C). Most autoimmune hemolytic anemias are the warm-body type. Autoimmune hemolytic anemia is associated with other disorders in most cases (eg, medication exposure, lymphoma, CLL, other malignancy, collagen vascular disease, autoimmune disease, infection). In idiopathic autoimmune hemolytic states, the reason why the immune system produces the antibodies is not known. All ages and both genders are equally vulnerable to this form, whereas the incidence of secondary forms is greater in people older than 45 years of age and in females.

### Clinical Manifestations

Clinical manifestations can vary, and they usually reflect the degree of anemia. The hemolysis may be very mild, so that the patient's marrow compensates adequately and the patient is asymptomatic. At the other extreme, the hemolysis can be so severe that the resultant anemia is life-threatening. Most patients complain of fatigue and dizziness. Splenomegaly is the most common physical finding, occurring in more than 80% of patients; hepatomegaly, lymphadenopathy, and jaundice are also common.

### Assessment and Diagnostic Findings

Laboratory tests show a low hemoglobin level and hematocrit, most often with an accompanying increase in the reticulocyte count. Erythrocytes appear abnormal; spherocytes are common. The serum bilirubin level is elevated, and if the hemolysis is severe, the haptoglobin level is low or absent. The Coombs test (also referred to as the direct antiglobulin test [DAT]), which detects antibodies on the surface of erythrocytes, shows a positive result.

### Medical Management

Any possible offending medication should be immediately discontinued. The treatment consists of high doses of corticosteroids until hemolysis decreases. Corticosteroids decrease the macrophage's ability to clear the antibody-coated erythrocytes. If the hemoglobin level returns toward normal, usually after several weeks, the corticosteroid dose can be lowered or, in some cases, tapered and discontinued. However, corticosteroids rarely produce a lasting remission. In severe cases, blood transfusions may be required. Because the antibody may react with all possible donor cells, careful blood typing is necessary, and the transfusion should be administered slowly and cautiously.

Splenectomy (removal of the spleen) removes the major site of erythrocyte destruction; therefore, splenectomy may be performed if corticosteroids do not produce a remission. If neither corticosteroid therapy nor splenectomy is successful, immunosuppressive agents may be administered. The two immunosuppressive agents most frequently used are cyclophosphamide (Cytoxan), which has a more rapid effect but more toxicity, and azathioprine (Imuran), which has a less rapid effect but less toxicity. The synthetic androgen danazol can be useful in some patients, particularly in combination with corticosteroids. The mechanism for this success is unclear. If corticosteroids or immunosuppressive agents are used, the taper must be very gradual to prevent a rebound "hyperimmune" response and exacerbation of the hemolysis. Immunoglobulin administration is effective in about one third of patients, but the effect is transient and the medication is expensive. Transfusions may be necessary if the anemia is severe; it may be extremely difficult to cross-match samples of available units of PRBCs with that of the patient.

For patients with cold-antibody hemolytic anemia, no treatment may be required other than to advise the patient to keep warm; relocation to a warm climate may be necessary.

## Nursing Management

Patients may have great difficulty understanding the pathologic mechanisms underlying the disease and may need repeated explanations in terms they can understand. Patients who have had a splenectomy should be vaccinated against pneumococcal infections (eg, Pneumovax) and informed that they are permanently at greater risk for infection. Patients receiving long-term corticosteroid therapy, particularly those with concurrent diabetes or hypertension, need careful monitoring. They must understand the need for the medication and the importance of never abruptly discontinuing it. A written explanation and a tapering schedule should be provided, and adjustments based on hemoglobin levels should be emphasized. Similar teaching should be provided when immunosuppressive agents are used. Corticosteroid therapy is not without significant risk, and patients need to be monitored closely for complications. The short- and long-term complications of corticosteroid therapy are presented in Chart 33-3 and in Chapter 42.

**NURSING ALERT**

It can be difficult to cross-match blood when antibodies are present. If imperfectly cross-matched RBCs must be transfused, the nurse should begin the infusion very slowly (10 to 15 mL over 20 to 30 minutes) and monitor the patient very closely for signs and symptoms of a hemolytic transfusion reaction.

## Hereditary Hemochromatosis

Hemochromatosis is a genetic condition in which iron is abnormally (excessively) absorbed from the GI tract. Normally the GI tract absorbs 1 to 2 mg of iron/day, but in those with hereditary hemochromatosis, this rate increases to 8 to 10 mg/day (Pietrangelo, 2004). The excessive iron is deposited in various organs, particularly the liver, myocardium, testes, thyroid, and pancreas. Eventually, the affected organs become dysfunctional. Although hereditary hemochromatosis is diagnosed in 0.5% of the population in the United States (ie, 1 million people), the actual prevalence is unknown because it is not always diagnosed. However, the genetic defect associated with hemochromatosis is most commonly seen as a specific mutation (C282Y homozygosity) of the *HFE* gene, with a prevalence of 5:1000 people of northern European descent (Pietrangelo, 2004). Women are less affected than men because of the natural loss of iron through menses.

Often there is no evidence of tissue damage until middle age, because the accumulation of iron in body organs occurs gradually. Symptoms of weakness, lethargy, arthralgia, weight loss, and loss of libido are common and occur earlier in the illness trajectory. The skin may be hyperpigmented with melanin deposits (occasionally **hemosiderin**, an iron-containing pigment) and appears bronze in color. Cardiac dysrhythmias and cardiomyopathy can occur, with resulting dyspnea and edema. Endocrine dysfunction is manifested as hypothyroidism, diabetes mellitus, and hypogonadism (testicular atrophy, diminished libido, and impotence). Cirrhosis is very common; thus, hemochromatosis should be considered in patients with cirrhosis who also have diabetes (Beutler et al., 2003). Development of hepatocellular carcinoma in one third of patients is a significant effect of the hemochromatosis.

The most useful laboratory findings are an elevated serum iron level and high transferrin saturation (more than 60% in men, more than 50% in women). CBC values are typically normal. The definitive diagnostic test for hemochromatosis has been liver biopsy, but testing for the *HFE* gene mutation is now more commonly used. Patients who are homozygous for the gene are at high risk for the disorder (Pietrangelo, 2004).

## Medical Management

Therapy involves the removal of excess iron via therapeutic phlebotomy (removal of whole blood from a vein). Each unit of blood removed results in a decrease of 200 to 250 mg of iron. The objective is to reduce the serum ferritin to less than 50 µg/L and the transferrin saturation to 30% or less. To achieve this, frequent phlebotomy is required (1 to 2 units weekly), with a gradual reduction in frequency of phlebotomies over a 1- to 3-year period. After 1 to 3 years, the frequency of phlebotomy can be reduced to 1 unit of blood every several months to prevent reaccumulation of iron deposits. The goal is to maintain an iron saturation of less than 50% and a serum ferritin of less than 100 µg/L. Aggressive removal of excess iron can prevent end-organ dysfunction. However, if end-organ damage has already occurred (ie, destructive arthritis, cirrhosis, hypogonadism, type 1 diabetes mellitus), phlebotomy slows rather than reverses organ dysfunction (Pietrangelo, 2004).

## Nursing Management

Patients with hemochromatosis often limit their dietary intake of iron, although this is not effective and is not encouraged. However, it is important for these patients to avoid any additional insults to the liver, such as alcohol abuse. Serial screening tests for hepatoma (ie, alpha-fetoprotein) are important. Other body systems should be monitored for signs of organ dysfunction, particularly the endocrine and cardiac systems, so that appropriate management can be implemented quickly. Because patients with hemochromatosis require frequent phlebotomies,

## CHART 33-3

# PHARMACOLOGY · Complications Associated with Corticosteroid Therapy

Whenever a patient begins a course of corticosteroid therapy, the potential for complications is great. Dosing regimens vary widely, depending on the underlying hematologic condition and the patient's response to the medication. For example, several chemotherapy protocols include high doses of corticosteroids for a period of several days. After that time, the medication is stopped abruptly without tapering the dosage. In other conditions, such as idiopathic thrombocytopenic purpura or hemolytic anemias, the corticosteroids are very carefully tapered to prevent a flare up of the underlying disease. With the exception of patients with preexisting conditions such as diabetes, hypertension, and osteoporosis, it is difficult to predict which complications will occur in a given patient. Patients who receive high doses of corticosteroids for longer than a few weeks should be screened for symptoms related to the potential complications listed here. If at all possible, patients who require long-term corticosteroid use should be switched to an alternate-day dosing schedule; this method may diminish the severity of complications that arise.

### Short-Term Complications

*Fluid and Electrolyte Complications*
Fluid retention
Sodium retention
Potassium loss
Hypokalemic alkalosis
Hypertension

*Endocrine Complications*
Decreased carbohydrate tolerance
Diabetes mellitus
Persistent hyperglycemia in diabetes mellitus

*Neurologic Complications*
Headache

*Musculoskeletal Complications*
Muscle weakness

*Psychological Complications*
Depression
Euphoria
Mood swings
Insomnia
Psychosis

### Long-Term Complications

*Endocrine Complications*
Decreased adrenocortical activity
Decreased ability to respond to stress
Decreased carbohydrate tolerance
Decreased growth rate (children)
Cushingoid state
Menstrual irregularities
Increased sweating

*Metabolic Complications*
Protein catabolism causing negative nitrogen balance

*Gastrointestinal Complications*
Gastritis
Ulcerative esophagitis
Peptic ulcer
Pancreatitis

*Musculoskeletal Complications*
Decreased muscle mass
Osteoporosis
Vertebral compression fracture
Pathologic fracture
Aseptic necrosis of femoral and humeral heads

*Neurologic Complications*
Vertigo
Increased intracranial pressure
Seizures

*Ophthalmic Complications*
Cataract formation
Glaucoma
Exophthalmos

*Dermatologic Complications*
Impaired wound healing
Ecchymoses
Increased skin fragility
Decreased skin thickness
Petechiae

*Immunologic Complications*
Decreased response to infection
Masked signs of early stages of infection
Suppressed reaction to skin tests
Increased risk for opportunistic infection (eg, *Pneumocystis*, herpes zoster)

---

problems with venous access are common. All children of patients who are homozygous for the *HFE* gene mutation should be screened for the mutation as well. Patients who are heterozygous for the *HFE* do not develop the disease but need to be counseled that they can transmit the gene to their children.

## Polycythemia

**Polycythemia**, literally meaning "too many cells in the blood," refers to an increased volume of erythrocytes. It is a term used when the hematocrit is elevated (to more than 55% in males, more than 50% in females). Dehydration (decreased volume of plasma) can cause an elevated hematocrit, but not typically to the level to be considered polycythemia. Polycythemia is classified as either primary or secondary (Prchal, 2003).

## Polycythemia Vera

Polycythemia vera, or primary polycythemia, is a proliferative disorder in which the myeloid stem cells seem to have escaped normal control mechanisms. The bone marrow is hypercellular, and the erythrocyte, leukocyte, and platelet counts in the peripheral blood are elevated. However, the erythrocyte elevation is predominant; the hematocrit can exceed 60%. This phase can last for an extended period (10 years or longer). Over time, the spleen resumes its embryonic function of hematopoiesis and enlarges. Eventually, the bone marrow may become fibrotic, with a resultant inability to produce as many cells ("burnt out" or spent phase). The disease evolves into myeloid metaplasia with myelofibrosis, MDS, or AML in a significant proportion of patients; this form of AML is usually refractory to standard treatments (Chomienne et al., 2004). The incidence of polycythemia has been estimated at 2.3 per 100,000 people. The median age at onset is 60 years (Prchal, 2003). Median survival exceeds 10 years with treatment but is only 6 to 18 months without treatment (Terreri, 2004).

### Clinical Manifestations

Patients typically have a ruddy complexion and splenomegaly (enlarged spleen). Symptoms result from increased blood volume (headache, dizziness, tinnitus, fatigue, paresthesias, and blurred vision) or from increased blood viscosity (angina, claudication, dyspnea, and thrombophlebitis), particularly if the patient has atherosclerotic blood vessels. For this reason, blood pressure is often elevated. Uric acid may be elevated, resulting in gout and renal stone formation. Another common and bothersome problem is generalized pruritus, which may be caused by histamine release due to the increased number of basophils. Erythromelalgia, a burning sensation in the fingers and toes, may be reported and is only partially relieved by cooling.

### Assessment and Diagnostic Findings

Diagnosis is based on an elevated erythrocyte mass (a nuclear medicine procedure), a normal oxygen saturation level, and often an enlarged spleen. Other factors useful in establishing the diagnosis include elevated leukocyte and platelet counts. The erythropoietin level is not as low as would be expected with an elevated hematocrit; it is normal or only slightly low. Causes of secondary erythrocytosis should not be present (see later discussion).

### Complications

Patients with polycythemia vera are at increased risk for thromboses resulting in a CVA (brain attack, stroke) or myocardial infarction (MI); thrombotic complications are the most common cause of death. Bleeding is also a complication, possibly because the platelets (often very large) are somewhat dysfunctional. The bleeding can be significant and can occur in the form of nosebleeds, ulcers, frank GI bleeding, hematuria, and intracranial hemorrhage.

### Medical Management

The objective of management is to reduce the high blood cell mass. Phlebotomy is an important part of therapy. It involves removing enough blood (initially 500 mL once or twice weekly) to diminish the blood viscosity and to deplete the patient's iron stores, thereby rendering the patient iron deficient and consequently unable to continue to manufacture erythrocytes excessively. Many patients are managed by routine phlebotomy on an intermittent basis. Radioactive phosphorus ($^{32}$P) or chemotherapeutic agents (eg, hydroxyurea [Hydrea]) can be used to suppress marrow function, but this may increase the risk for leukemia. Patients receiving hydroxyurea appear to have a lower incidence of thrombotic complications than those treated by phlebotomy alone; this may result from a more controlled platelet count. Anagrelide (Agrylin), which inhibits platelet aggregation, can also be useful in controlling the thrombocytosis associated with polycythemia vera. However, many patients have difficulty tolerating the medication; it can cause significant side effects, including headache, fluid retention, cardiac dysrhythmias, and heart failure. Furthermore, anagrelide is now considered leukemogenic (ie, may cause leukemia) (Berlin, 2003). Interferon alfa-2b (Intron-A) is the most effective treatment for managing the pruritus associated with polycythemia vera (Berlin, 2003) but may be difficult for patients to tolerate because of its frequent side effects (eg, flu-like syndrome, depression). Antihistamines, including histamine-2 blockers, are not particularly effective in controlling itching. Allopurinol (Zyloprim) is used to prevent gouty attacks in patients with elevated uric acid concentrations.

The use of aspirin to prevent thrombotic complications is controversial. A recent study comparing low-dose aspirin (100 mg) to placebo in 518 patients with polycythemia vera found that aspirin decreased the risk for significant thrombotic complications (deep vein thrombosis [DVT], pulmonary embolism, MI, stroke) (Landolfi et al., 2004). Low-dose aspirin is frequently used in patients with cardiovascular disease, but even this dose may be avoided in patients with prior bleeding, especially bleeding from the GI tract. Aspirin is also useful in reducing the pain associated with erythromelalgia.

### Nursing Management

The nurse's role is primarily that of educator. Risk factors for thrombotic complications, particularly smoking, obesity, and poorly controlled hypertension, should be assessed, and the patient should be instructed about the signs and symptoms of thrombosis. To reduce the likelihood of DVT, avoidance of tight or restrictive clothing (particularly stockings), crossing the legs, and sedentary behavior should be encouraged. Patients with a history of bleeding are usually advised to avoid aspirin and aspirin-containing medications, because these medications alter platelet function. Minimizing alcohol intake should also be emphasized to further diminish the risk of bleeding. The patient needs to be instructed to avoid iron supplements, including those within multivitamin supplements, because the iron can further stimulate RBC production. For pruritus, the nurse may recommend bathing in tepid or cool water and avoiding vigorous toweling-off after bathing. Sodium bicarbonate dissolved in bath water may also be effective (Golden, 2003), along with applications of cocoa butter– or oatmeal-based lotions and bath products.

## Secondary Polycythemia

Secondary polycythemia is caused by excessive production of erythropoietin. This may occur in response to a reduced amount of oxygen, which acts as a hypoxic stimulus, as in cigarette smoking, chronic obstructive pulmonary disease, or cyanotic heart disease, or in nonpathologic conditions such as living at a high altitude. It can also result from certain hemoglobinopathies (eg, hemoglobin Chesapeake), in which the hemoglobin has an abnormally high affinity for oxygen. Secondary polycythemia can also occur from neoplasms (eg, renal cell carcinoma) that stimulate erythropoietin production.

### Medical Management

Management of secondary polycythemia may not be necessary; when it is, it involves treating the primary conditions. If the cause cannot be corrected (eg, by treating the renal cell carcinoma or improving pulmonary function), therapeutic phlebotomy may be necessary in symptomatic patients to reduce blood viscosity and volume.

## Leukopenia

Leukopenia, a condition in which there are fewer leukocytes than normal, results from neutropenia (diminished neutrophils) or lymphopenia (diminished lymphocytes). Even if other types of leukocytes (eg, monocytes, basophils) are diminished, their numbers are too few to reduce the total leukocyte count significantly.

## Neutropenia

**Neutropenia** (a neutrophil count of less than 2,000/mm$^3$) results from decreased production of neutrophils or increased destruction of these cells (Chart 33-4). Neutrophils are essential in preventing and limiting bacterial infection. A patient with neutropenia is at increased risk for infection from both exogenous and endogenous sources. (The GI tract and skin are common endogenous sources.) The risk of infection is based not only on the severity of the neutropenia (low neutrophil count) but also on the duration of the neutropenia. The actual number of neutrophils, known as the **absolute neutrophil count** (ANC), is determined by a simple mathematical calculation using data obtained from the CBC and differential (Chart 33-5). The risk for infection increases proportionally with the decrease in neutrophil count. The risk is significant when the ANC is less than 1000/mm$^3$, is high when it is less than 500/mm$^3$, and is almost certain when it is less than 100/mm$^3$. The risk of developing infection also increases with the length of time during which neutropenia persists, even if it is fairly mild. Conversely, even a severe neutropenia may not result in infection if the duration of the neutropenia is brief, as is often seen after chemotherapy (Chart 33-6).

> **CHART 33-4**
>
> ### Causes of Neutropenia
>
> **Decreased Production of Neutrophils**
> - Aplastic anemia, due to medications or toxins
> - Metastatic cancer, lymphoma, leukemia
> - Myelodysplastic syndromes
> - Chemotherapy
> - Radiation therapy
>
> **Ineffective Granulocytopoiesis**
> - Megaloblastic anemia
>
> **Increased Destruction of Neutrophils**
> - Hypersplenism
> - Medication-induced*
> - Immunologic disease (eg, systemic lupus erythematosus)
> - Viral disease (eg, infectious hepatitis, mononucleosis)
> - Bacterial infections
>
> *Formation of antibody to medication, leading to a rapid decrease in neutrophils.

### Clinical Manifestations

There are no definite symptoms of neutropenia until the patient becomes infected. A routine CBC with differential, as obtained after chemotherapy treatment, can reveal neutropenia before the onset of infection.

### Medical Management

Treatment of the neutropenia varies depending on its cause. If the neutropenia is medication-induced, the offending agent is stopped immediately, if possible. Treatment of an underlying neoplasm can temporarily make the neutropenia worse, but with bone marrow recovery, treatment may actually improve it. Corticosteroids may be used if the cause is an immunologic disorder. The use of growth factors such as G-CSF or granulocyte-macrophage colony-stimulating factor (GM-CSF) can be effective in increasing neutrophil production when the cause of the neutropenia is decreased production. Withholding or reducing the dose of chemotherapy or radiation therapy may be required when the neutropenia is caused by these treatments; however, in the case of potentially curative therapy, administration of growth

## CHART 33-5

### Calculating the Absolute Neutrophil Count (ANC)

$$ANC = \frac{\text{Total WBC count} \times (\%\text{ neutrophils} + \%\text{ bands})}{100}$$

Normally, the neutrophil count is greater than 2000/mm$^3$. The actual (or absolute) neutrophil count (ANC) is calculated using the above formula.

For example, if the total white blood cell (WBC) count is 3000/mm$^3$ with 72% neutrophils and 3% bands, the ANC would be calculated as follows:

$$ANC = \frac{3000(72 + 3)}{100} = 2250$$

This result is not indicative of neutropenia, because the ANC is greater than 2000 despite the low total WBC count (3000/mm$^3$).

Conversely, in the following example, neutropenia is evident despite a normal WBC count (5500/mm$^3$) with 8% neutrophils and 0% bands:

$$ANC = \frac{5500(8 + 0)}{100} = 440$$

Here, the ANC is severely low (440) despite the normal total WBC count (5500/mm$^3$).

When evaluating neutropenia, it is important to calculate the ANC and not to rely solely on the total WBCs and percentage of neutrophils alone.

---

factor is considered to be preferable, so that the maximum antitumor effect can be achieved by maintaining the chemotherapy regimen as originally planned.

If the neutropenia is accompanied by fever, the patient is considered to have an infection and usually is admitted to the hospital. Cultures of blood, urine, and sputum and a chest x-ray are obtained. To ensure adequate therapy against the infectious organisms, broad-spectrum antibiotics are initiated as soon as the cultures are obtained, although the antibiotics may be changed after culture and sensitivity results are available.

### Nursing Management

Nurses in all settings have a crucial role in assessing the severity of neutropenia and in preventing and managing complications, which most often include infections. Patient teaching is equally important, particularly in the outpatient setting, so that the patient can implement appropriate self-care measures and know when and how to seek medical care (Chart 33-7). Patients at risk of neutropenia should have blood drawn for a CBC with differential; the frequency is based on the suspected severity and duration of the neutropenia. Nurses need to be able to calculate the ANC (see Chart 33-5) and to assess the severity of neutropenia and the risk of infection. Chart 33-8 identifies nursing interventions related to neutropenia.

## Lymphopenia

Lymphopenia (a lymphocyte count less than 1500/mm$^3$) can result from ionizing radiation, long-term use of corticosteroids, uremia, some neoplasms (eg, breast and lung cancers, advanced Hodgkin's disease), and some protein-losing enteropathies (in which the lymphocytes within the intestines are lost).

## Leukemia

The term *leukocytosis* refers to an increased level of leukocytes in the circulation. Typically, only one specific cell type is increased. Usually, because the proportions of several types of leukocytes (eg, eosinophils, basophils, monocytes) are small, only an increase in neutrophils or lymphocytes can be great enough to elevate the total leukocyte count. Although leukocytosis can be a normal response to increased need (eg, in acute infection), the elevation in leukocytes should decrease as the physiologic need decreases. A prolonged or progressively increasing elevation in leukocytes is abnormal and should be evaluated. A significant cause for persistent leukocytosis is malignancy.

Hematopoiesis is characterized by a rapid, continuous turnover of cells. Normally, production of specific blood cells from their stem cell precursors is carefully regulated according to the body's needs. If the mechanisms that control the production of these cells are disrupted, the cells can proliferate excessively. Hematopoietic malignancies are often classified by the cells involved. **Leukemia**, literally "white blood," is a neoplastic proliferation of one particular cell type (granulocytes, monocytes, lymphocytes, or infrequently erythrocytes or megakaryocytes). The defect originates in the hematopoietic stem cell, the myeloid, or the lymphoid stem cell. The lymphomas are neoplasms of lymphoid tissue, usually derived from B lymphocytes. Multiple myeloma is a malignancy of the most mature form of B lymphocyte, the plasma cell.

The common feature of the leukemias is an unregulated proliferation of leukocytes in the bone marrow. In acute forms (or late stages of chronic forms), the proliferation of leukemic cells leaves little room for normal cell production. There can also be a proliferation of cells in the liver and spleen (extramedullary hematopoiesis). With acute forms, there can be infiltration of other organs, such as the meninges, lymph nodes, gums, and skin. The cause of leukemia is not fully known, but there is some evidence that genetic influences and viral pathogenesis may be involved. Bone marrow damage from radiation exposure or from chemicals such as benzene and alkylating agents (eg, melphalan [Alkeran]) can cause leukemia.

*(text continues on page 1071)*

### CHART 33-6

## Risk Factors for Development of Infection and Bleeding in Patients with Hematologic Disorders

### Risk for Infection

- *Severity of neutropenia:* Risk of infection is proportional to duration and severity of neutropenia
- *Duration of neutropenia:* Increased duration leads to increased risk of infection
- *Nutritional status:* Decreased protein stores lead to decreased immune response and anergy
- *Deconditioning:* Decreased mobility leads to decreased respiratory effort, leading to increased pooling of secretions
- *Lymphocytopenia; disorders of lymphoid system (chronic lymphocytic leukemia [CLL], lymphoma, myeloma):* Decreased cell-mediated and humoral immunity
- *Invasive procedures:* Break in skin integrity leads to increased opportunity for organisms to enter blood system
- *Hypogammaglobulinemia:* Decreased antibody formation
- *Poor hygiene:* Increased organisms on skin and mucous membranes
- *Poor dentition; mucositis:* Decreased endothelial integrity leads to increased opportunity for organisms to enter blood system
- *Antibiotic therapy:* Increased risk for superinfection, often fungal
- *Certain medications:* See text

### Risk for Bleeding

- *Severity of thrombocytopenia:* Risk increases when platelet count decreases; usually not a significant risk until platelet count is lower than 20,000/mm$^3$ or lower than 50,000/mm$^3$ when invasive procedure performed
- *Duration of thrombocytopenia:* Risk increases when duration increases (eg, risk is less when duration is transient after chemotherapy than when duration is permanent with poor marrow production)
- *Sepsis:* Mechanism unknown; appears to cause increased platelet consumption
- *Increased intracranial pressure:* Increased blood pressure leads to rupture of blood vessels
- *Liver dysfunction:* Decreased synthesis of clotting factors
- *Renal dysfunction:* Decreased platelet function
- *Dysproteinemia:* Protein coats surface of platelet, leading to decreased platelet function; protein causes increased viscosity, which leads to increased stretching of capillaries and thus increased bleeding
- *Alcohol abuse:* Suppressive effect on marrow leads to decreased platelet production and decreased ability to function; decreased liver function results in decreased production of clotting factors
- *Splenomegaly:* Increased platelet destruction; spleen traps circulating platelets
- *Concurrent medications:* See text

### CHART 33-7

## HOME CARE CHECKLIST • The Patient at Risk for Infection

| At the completion of the home care instruction, the patient or caregiver will be able to: | Patient | Caregiver |
|---|---|---|
| • Describe consequences of alterations in neutrophils, lymphocytes, immunoglobulins, or their sources. | ✓ | ✓ |
| • Verbalize the reason for being at risk for infection. | ✓ | ✓ |
| • Identify signs and symptoms of infection. | ✓ | ✓ |
| • Demonstrate how to monitor for signs of infection. | ✓ | ✓ |
| • Describe to whom, how, and when to report signs of infection. | ✓ | ✓ |
| • Identify appropriate behaviors to take to prevent infection:<br>–Maintain good hand hygiene technique, total body hygiene, and skin integrity.<br>–Avoid fresh flowers, plants, garden work (soil), bird cages, and litter boxes.<br>–Avoid fresh salads and unpeeled fruits or vegetables.<br>–Maintain a high-calorie, high-protein diet, with fluid intake of 3,000 mL daily (unless fluids are restricted).<br>–Avoid people with infections, crowds.<br>–Perform deep breathing, use incentive spirometer every 4 hr while awake.<br>–Provide adequate lubrication with gentle vaginal manipulation during sexual intercourse; avoid anal intercourse. | ✓ | ✓ |
| • Describe appropriate actions to take should infection occur. | ✓ | ✓ |

## CHART 33-8 Neutropenia Precautions

### Nursing Diagnosis
Risk for infection secondary to impaired immunocompetence due to:
- Diminished neutrophil count (see below) secondary to bone marrow invasion or hypocellularity secondary to treatment
- Dysfunctional neutrophils (eg, secondary to myelodysplastic syndrome [MDS])
- Dysfunctional or diminished lymphocytes
- Hypogammaglobulinemia
- Diminished immune response or anergy
- Malnutrition
- Surgery or invasive procedures
- Antibiotic therapy (increased risk for superimposed infection)
  - Neutropenic, infected patients often do *not* exhibit the classic signs of inflammation/infection (ie, redness, cloudiness of any drainage); the only initial sign may be fever (and it often occurs later in the infectious process with neutropenia).
  - Skin and mucous membranes are the body's first line of defense against infection; loss of endothelial cell integrity allows organisms to enter the blood and lymph systems.

### Assessment
#### PATIENT
Assess the following areas thoroughly every shift or visit (with spot checks throughout shift if the patient is hospitalized) and notify physician of any signs of infection or worsening of status:
- *Skin:* Check for tenderness, edema, breaks in skin integrity, moisture, drainage, lesions (especially under breasts, axillae, groin, skin folds, bony prominences, perineum); check all puncture sites (eg, intravenous sites) for signs and symptoms of inflammation/infection.
- *Oral mucosa:* Check for moisture, lesions, color (check palate, tongue, buccal mucosa, gums, lips, oropharynx).
- *Respiratory:* Check for presence of cough, sore throat; auscultate breath sounds.
- *Gastrointestinal:* Check for abdominal discomfort/distention, nausea, change in bowel pattern; auscultate bowel sounds.
- *Genitourinary:* Check for dysuria, urgency, frequency; check urine for color, clarity, odor.
- *Neurologic:* Check for complaints of headache, neck stiffness, visual disturbances; assess level of consciousness, orientation, behavior.
- *Temperature:* Check every 4 hr or every visit; call primary health care provider if temperature is >38°C (>101°F), fever is unresponsive to acetaminophen, or patient shows a decline in hemodynamic status.

### DIAGNOSTIC STUDIES
- Monitor complete blood count (CBC) and differential daily (especially absolute neutrophil count [ANC], lymphocyte count).
- Call physician if ANC is <1,000, significantly different from previous count, or whenever patient becomes symptomatic (eg, febrile).
- Monitor globulin, albumin, total protein levels.
- Monitor all culture and sensitivity reports.
- Monitor x-ray reports.

### Nursing Interventions
#### ENVIRONMENT AND STAFF
- **Thorough hand hygiene must be performed by everyone before entering patient's room each and every time**.
- Allow no one with a cold or sore throat to care for the patient or to enter room, or come in contact with patient at home.
- Care for neutropenic patients before caring for other patients (as much as possible).
- Use private room for patient if ANC is <1,000.
- Allow no fresh flowers (stagnant water).
- Change water in containers every shift (include $O_2$ humidification systems every 24 hr).
- Ensure room is cleaned daily.

#### DIETARY
- Provide low microbial diet.
- Eliminate fresh salads and unpeeled fresh fruits or vegetables.

#### PATIENT
- Avoid suppositories, enemas, rectal temperatures.
- Practice deep breathing (with incentive spirometer) every 4 hr while awake.
- Ambulate; wear high-efficiency particulate air (HEPA) filter mask if neutropenia is severe.
- Prevent skin dryness with water-soluble lubricants, especially in high-risk areas (eg, lips, corners of mouth, elbows, feet, bony prominences).

#### HYGIENE
- Provide meticulous total body hygiene daily (preferably with antimicrobial solution), including perineal care after every bowel movement.

*continued >*

## CHART 33-8 Neutropenia Precautions, continued

- Provide thorough oral hygiene after meals and every 4 hr while awake; warm saline, or salt and soda solution, is effective; avoid use of lemon-glycerine swabs, commercial mouthwashes, and hydrogen peroxide.

### INTRAVENOUS (IV) THERAPY
- Do not use plastic cannulas for peripheral IVs when ANC is <500; a central vascular access device is preferred for long-term or intensive IV therapy.
- Inspect IV sites every shift; monitor closely for any discomfort; erythema may not be present.
- Maintain meticulous IV site care.
- Cleanse skin with antimicrobial solution before venipuncture (unless patient is allergic).
- Moisture-vapor–permeable dressings are permissible with strict adherence to institutional protocol.
- Change IV tubing per institution policy, using aseptic technique.
- Administer antimicrobial agents on time.

### Expected Patient Outcomes
- Patient demonstrates an absence of infection as evidenced by an absence of fever, chills, inflammation, drainage, cough, dyspnea, sore throat, dysuria, or urinary frequency.
- Patient demonstrates an absence of infection as evidenced by the presence of vital signs within normal limits, including intact neurologic status and intact skin.

### Duration of Evaluation
Until patient is no longer neutropenic and any infection is resolved.

---

## NURSING RESEARCH PROFILE

### Timeliness of Antimicrobial Administration in Emergency Departments for Patients With Cancer and Febrile Neutropenia

Niremberg, A., Mulhearn, L., Lin, S., et al. (2004). Emergency department waiting times for patients with cancer and febrile neutropenia: A pilot study. Oncology Nursing Forum, 31(4), 711–715.

#### Purpose
Fever and neutropenia are potentially serious complications of chemotherapy treatment for cancer. Prompt initiation of antimicrobial therapy may diminish the risk of developing a serious outcome (eg, sepsis or septic shock). Because most patients require prompt treatment when clinics are closed, they typically use the emergency department (ED) for evaluation of these complications and initiation of antimicrobial therapy. The purpose of this study was to determine the length of time involved in the evaluation and treatment of febrile neutropenia among cancer patients in the ED.

#### Design
This prospective, descriptive study had a convenience sample of 19 adults with cancer and febrile neutropenia who sought ED treatment. Patients who presented to the ED during the night, weekends, or holidays (eg, times when the ambulatory unit was closed) were eligible to participate. There were 10 male (53%) and 9 female (47%) participants, who were mostly middle-aged (mean age 56 years), had family support for assistance (74%), had mostly private insurance coverage (79%), and most often received chemotherapy for multiple myeloma or lymphoma (53%). Participants were interviewed and their medical records examined to determine the time lapsed between initiation of the fever to arrival at the ED; the time of triage, or initial patient assessment; the time that laboratory results were completed; the time to initiation of antimicrobial therapy; and the time of admission to the hospital.

#### Findings
Thirty-three episodes of febrile neutropenia in the 19 study participants were evaluated. On average, participants had a fever for 21 hours (range, 1 to 72 hours) prior to entering the ED. Forty-eight percent had an indwelling vascular access device, and 17% had other indwelling devices (eg, stent). Thirty percent had oral mucositis. Both invasive devices and oral mucositis are risk factors for bacterial infection in patients with neutropenia.

The median waiting time in the ED was 75 minutes for evaluation and 210 minutes for administration of antimicrobial agents. The average time spent in the ED until hospital admission was 5.5 hours (range, 2 to 11.6 hours).

#### Nursing Implications
Patients receiving chemotherapy, particularly for hematologic malignancies, are typically taught about infection and the importance of seeking prompt medical care if they become febrile. Nurses are responsible for providing this education. Results of this study suggest that current educational interventions may be inadequate.

Nurses in the ED are responsible for the initial triage of patients and need to facilitate a thorough and expedient workup of patients with cancer and febrile neutropenia who have received chemotherapy. Nurses must serve as advocates for these patients so that antimicrobial therapy is initiated promptly.

The leukemias are commonly classified according to the stem cell line involved, either lymphoid or myeloid. They are also classified as either acute or chronic, based on the time it takes for symptoms to evolve and the phase of cell development that is halted (ie, with few leukocytes differentiating beyond that phase).

In acute leukemia, the onset of symptoms is abrupt, often occurring within a few weeks. Leukocyte development is halted at the blast phase, so that most leukocytes are undifferentiated cells or are blasts. Acute leukemia progresses very rapidly; death occurs within weeks to months without aggressive treatment.

In chronic leukemia, symptoms evolve over a period of months to years, and the majority of leukocytes produced are mature. Chronic leukemia progresses more slowly; the disease trajectory can extend for years.

## Acute Myeloid Leukemia

Acute myeloid leukemia (AML) results from a defect in the hematopoietic stem cell that differentiates into all myeloid cells: monocytes, granulocytes (neutrophils, basophils, eosinophils), erythrocytes, and platelets. All age groups are affected; the incidence rises with age, with a peak incidence at age 60 years. AML is the most common nonlymphocytic leukemia.

The prognosis is highly variable. Patient age may be a factor; patients who are younger may survive for 5 years or more after diagnosis of AML. However, patients who are older or have a more undifferentiated form of AML tend to have a worse prognosis. Those who have leukemia stemming from preexisting MDS or who previously received alkylating agents for cancer (secondary AML) have a much worse prognosis; the leukemia tends to be more resistant to treatment, resulting in a much shorter duration of remission. With treatment, patients with secondary AML survive an average of less than 1 year, with death usually a result of infection or hemorrhage. Patients receiving supportive care also usually survive less than 1 year, dying of infection or bleeding. The 5-year survival rate for patients with AML who are 65 years or younger is 33%; it drops to 4% for those older than 65 years (American Cancer Society, 2006).

### Clinical Manifestations

Most signs and symptoms of AML result from insufficient production of normal blood cells. Fever and infection result from neutropenia, weakness and fatigue from anemia, and bleeding tendencies from thrombocytopenia. The proliferation of leukemic cells within organs leads to a variety of additional symptoms: pain from an enlarged liver or spleen, hyperplasia of the gums, and bone pain from expansion of marrow.

### Assessment and Diagnostic Findings

AML develops without warning, with symptoms occurring over a period of weeks to months. The CBC shows a decrease in both erythrocytes and platelets. Although the total leukocyte count can be low, normal, or high, the percentage of normal cells is usually vastly decreased. A bone marrow analysis shows an excess of immature blast cells (more than 30%). AML can be further classified into seven different subgroups, based on cytogenetics, histology, and morphology (appearance) of the blasts. The actual prognosis varies somewhat between subgroups, but the clinical course and treatment differ substantially. Patients with acute promyelocytic leukemia (APL, or AML-M3) often have significantly more problems with bleeding, in that they have underlying coagulopathy and a higher incidence of disseminated intravascular coagulation (DIC).

### Complications

Complications of AML include bleeding and infection, the major causes of death. The risk of bleeding correlates with the level of platelet deficiency (thrombocytopenia). The low platelet count can result in **ecchymoses** (bruises) and **petechiae** (pinpoint red or purple hemorrhagic spots on the skin). Major hemorrhages also may develop when the platelet count drops to less than 10,000/mm$^3$. The most common sites of bleeding are GI, pulmonary, and intracranial. For undetermined reasons, fever and infection also increase the likelihood of bleeding.

Because of the lack of mature and normal granulocytes, patients with leukemia are always threatened by infection. The likelihood of infection increases with the degree and duration of neutropenia; neutrophil counts that persist at less than 100/mm$^3$ make the chances of systemic infection extremely high. As the duration of severe neutropenia increases, the patient's risk of developing fungal infection also increases.

### Medical Management

The overall objective of treatment is to achieve complete remission, in which there is no evidence of residual leukemia in the bone marrow. Attempts are made to achieve remission by the aggressive administration of chemotherapy, called induction therapy, which usually requires hospitalization for several weeks. Induction therapy typically involves high doses of cytarabine (Cytosar, Ara-C) and daunorubicin (Cerubidine) or mitoxantrone (Novantrone) or idarubicin (Idamycin); sometimes etoposide (VP-16, VePesid) is added to the regimen. The choice of agents is based on the patient's physical status and history of prior antineoplastic treatment.

The aim of induction therapy is to eradicate the leukemic cells, but this is often accompanied by the eradication of normal types of myeloid cells. Thus, the patient becomes severely neutropenic (an ANC of 0 is not uncommon), anemic, and thrombocytopenic (a platelet count of less than 10,000/mm$^3$ is common). During this time, the patient is typically very ill, with bacterial, fungal, and occasionally viral infections, bleeding, and severe mucositis, which causes diarrhea and a marked decline in the ability to maintain adequate nutrition. Supportive care consists of administering blood products (PRBCs and platelets) and promptly treating infections. The use of granulocytic growth factors, either G-CSF (filgrastim [Neupogen]) or GM-CSF (sargramostim [Leukine]), can shorten the period of significant neutropenia by stimulating the bone marrow to produce leukocytes more quickly; these agents do not appear to increase the risk of producing more leukemic cells.

When the patient has recovered from the induction therapy (ie, the neutrophil and platelet counts have returned to normal and any infection has resolved), he or she typically receives consolidation therapy (postremission therapy) to eliminate any residual leukemia cells that are not clinically detectable and to reduce the chance for recurrence. Multiple treatment cycles of various agents are used, usually containing some form of cytarabine (eg, Cytosar, Ara-C). Frequently, the patient receives one cycle of treatment that is almost the same, if not identical, to the induction treatment but at lower dosages, therefore resulting in less toxicity.

Another aggressive treatment option is BMT or PBSCT. When a suitable tissue match can be obtained, the patient embarks on an even more aggressive regimen of chemotherapy (sometimes in combination with radiation therapy), with the treatment goal of destroying the hematopoietic function of the patient's bone marrow. The patient is then "rescued" with the infusion of the donor stem cells to reinitiate blood cell production. Patients who undergo PBSCT have a significant risk for infection, graft-versus-host disease (GVHD, in which the donor's lymphocytes [graft] recognize the patient's body as "foreign" and set up reactions to attack the "foreign" host), and other complications. The most appropriate use and timing of PBSCT remain unclear. Patients with a poorer prognosis may benefit from early PBSCT; those with a good prognosis may not need transplant at all. (See Chapter 16 for a discussion of nursing management in bone marrow transplantation.)

Another important option for the patient to consider is supportive care alone. In fact, supportive care may be the only option if the patient has significant comorbidity, such as extremely poor cardiac, pulmonary, renal, or hepatic function. In such cases, aggressive antileukemia therapy is not used; occasionally, hydroxyurea (Hydrea) may be used briefly to control the increase of blast cells. Patients are more commonly supported with antimicrobial therapy and transfusions as needed. This treatment approach provides the patient with some additional time at home; however, death frequently occurs within months, typically from infection or bleeding. (Refer to Chapter 17 for a discussion of end-of-life care.)

### Complications of Treatment

Massive leukemic cell destruction from chemotherapy results in the release of intracellular electrolytes and fluids into the systemic circulation. Increases in uric acid levels, potassium, and phosphate are seen; this process is referred to as tumor **lysis** syndrome (see Chapter 16). The increased uric acid and phosphorus levels make the patient vulnerable to renal stone formation and renal colic, which can progress to acute renal failure. Hyperkalemia and hypocalcemia can lead to cardiac dysrhythmias; hypotension; neuromuscular effects such as muscle cramps, weakness, and spasm/tetany; confusion; and seizures. Patients require a high fluid intake, alkalization of the urine, and prophylaxis with allopurinol to prevent crystallization of uric acid and subsequent stone formation. GI problems may result from the infiltration of abnormal leukocytes into the abdominal organs and from the toxicity of the chemotherapeutic agents.

Anorexia, nausea, vomiting, diarrhea, and severe mucositis are common. Because of the profound myelosuppressive effects of chemotherapy, significant neutropenia and thrombocytopenia typically result in serious infection and increased risk of bleeding.

### Nursing Management

Nursing management of the patient with acute leukemia is presented at the end of the leukemia section in this chapter.

## Chronic Myeloid Leukemia

Chronic myeloid leukemia (CML) arises from a mutation in the myeloid stem cell. Normal myeloid cells continue to be produced, but there is a pathologic increase in the production of forms of blast cells. Therefore, a wide spectrum of cell types exists within the blood, from blast forms through mature neutrophils. Because there is an uncontrolled proliferation of cells, the marrow expands into the cavities of long bones (eg, the femur), and cells are also formed in the liver and spleen (extramedullary hematopoiesis), resulting in enlargement of these organs that is sometimes painful. In 90% to 95% of patients with CML, a section of DNA is missing from chromosome 22 (the Philadelphia chromosome [Ph1]); it is translocated onto chromosome 9. The specific location of these changes is on the *BCR* gene of chromosome 22 and the *ABL* gene on chromosome 9. When these two genes fuse (*BCR-ABL* gene), they produce an abnormal protein (a tyrosine kinase protein) that causes leukocytes to divide rapidly. This *BCR-ABL* gene is present in virtually all patients with this disease.

CML is uncommon in people younger than 20 years; the incidence increases with age (median age, 55 to 60 years) (Cortes, 2004). Patients diagnosed with CML in the chronic phase have an overall median life expectancy of 3 to 5 years. During that time, they have few symptoms and complications from the disease itself. Problems with infections and bleeding are rare. However, once the disease transforms to the acute phase (blast crisis), the overall survival rarely exceeds several months.

### Clinical Manifestations

The clinical picture of CML varies. Many patients are asymptomatic, and leukocytosis is detected by a CBC performed for some other reason. The leukocyte count commonly exceeds 100,000/mm$^3$. Patients with extremely high leukocyte counts may be somewhat short of breath or slightly confused due to decreased capillary perfusion to the lungs and brain from leukostasis (the excessive volume of leukocytes inhibits blood flow through the capillaries). The patient may have an enlarged, tender spleen. The liver may also be enlarged. Some patients have insidious symptoms, such as malaise, anorexia, and weight loss. Lymphadenopathy is rare. There are three stages in CML: chronic, transformation, and accelerated or blast crisis. Patients develop more symptoms and complications as the disease progresses.

## Medical Management

Advances in understanding of the pathology of CML at a molecular level have led to dramatic changes in its treatment. An oral formulation of a tyrosine kinase inhibitor, imatinib mesylate (Gleevec), works by blocking signals within the leukemia cells that express the *BCR-ABL* protein, thus preventing a series of chemical reactions that cause the cell to grow and divide. Imatinib appears to be more useful in the chronic phase of the illness; clinical trials are in process to determine combination strategies with imatinib and other agents to improve response rates in the accelerated phase and blast crisis (Giles et al., 2004). Antacids and grapefruit juice may limit drug absorption, and large doses of acetaminophen can cause hepatotoxicity. The long-term effects of imatinib, its impact on survival, and the optimal length of treatment are being studied.

Other therapy depends on the stage of disease. In the chronic phase, the expected outcome is correction of the chromosomal abnormality (ie, conversion of the malignant stem cell population back to normal). Agents that have been used successfully for this purpose are interferon-alfa (Roferon-A) and cytosine, often in combination. These agents are administered daily as subcutaneous injections. This therapy is not benign; many patients cannot tolerate the profound fatigue, depression, anorexia, mucositis, and inability to concentrate. A less aggressive therapeutic approach focuses on reducing the leukocyte count to a more normal level but does not alter cytogenetic changes. This goal can be achieved by using oral chemotherapeutic agents, typically hydroxyurea (Hydrea) or busulfan (Myleran). In the case of an extreme leukocytosis at diagnosis (eg, leukocyte count greater than 300,000/mm$^3$), a more emergent treatment may be required. In this instance, leukapheresis (in which the patient's blood is removed and separated, with the leukocytes withdrawn, and the remaining blood returned to the patient) can temporarily reduce the number of leukocytes. An anthracycline chemotherapeutic agent (eg, daunomycin) may also be used to bring the leukocyte count down quickly to a safer level, where more conservative therapy can be instituted.

The transformation phase can be insidious or rapid; it marks the process of evolution (or transformation) to the acute form of leukemia (blast crisis). In the transformation phase, the patient may complain of bone pain and may report fevers (without any obvious sign of infection) and weight loss. Even with chemotherapy, the spleen may continue to enlarge. The patient may become more anemic and thrombocytopenic; an increased basophil level is detected by the CBC.

In the acute form of CML (blast crisis), treatment may resemble induction therapy for acute leukemia, using the same medications as for AML or ALL. Patients whose disease evolves into a "lymphoid" blast crisis are more likely to be able to reenter a chronic phase after induction therapy. For those whose disease evolves into AML, therapy is largely ineffective in achieving a second chronic phase. Life-threatening infections and bleeding occur frequently in this phase.

CML is a disease that can potentially be cured with BMT or PBSCT. Patients who receive such transplants while still in the chronic phase of the illness tend to have a greater chance for cure than those who receive them in the acute phase. The transplantation procedure may be considered for otherwise healthy patients who are younger than 65 years. More recently, research has shown that nonmyeloablative types of transplantation are effective and have diminished morbidity (Qazilbash et al., 2004). The use of imatinib therapy may decrease the need for transplantation in CML; however, the long-term efficacy of imatinib as well as its effects on transplant morbidity, mortality, and risk of relapse remain unknown (Radich et al., 2004).

## *Acute Lymphocytic Leukemia*

Acute lymphocytic leukemia (ALL) results from an uncontrolled proliferation of immature cells (lymphoblasts) derived from the lymphoid stem cell. The cell of origin is the precursor to the B lymphocyte in approximately 75% of ALL cases; T-lymphocyte ALL occurs in approximately 25% of ALL cases. The *BCR-ABL* translocation (see earlier discussion) is found in 20% of ALL blast cells. ALL is most common in young children, with boys affected more often than girls; the peak incidence is 4 years of age. After 15 years of age, ALL is relatively uncommon. Increasing age appears to be associated with diminished survival; the 5-year event-free survival rate is almost 80% for children with ALL but drops to 40% for adults (Larson, 2004; Pui et al., 2004). Yet even if relapse occurs, resumption of induction therapy can often achieve a second complete remission. Moreover, BMT may be successful even after a second relapse, particularly in certain subsets of patients (eg, those with Philadelphia chromosome–positive ALL [Ph+ ALL]) (Larson, 2004).

## Clinical Manifestations

Immature lymphocytes proliferate in the marrow and impede the development of normal myeloid cells. As a result, normal hematopoiesis is inhibited, resulting in reduced numbers of leukocytes, erythrocytes, and platelets. Leukocyte counts may be either low or high, but there is always a high proportion of immature cells. Manifestations of leukemic cell infiltration into other organs are more common with ALL than with other forms of leukemia and include pain from an enlarged liver or spleen and bone pain. The central nervous system is frequently a site for leukemic cells; thus, patients may exhibit headache and vomiting because of meningeal involvement.

## Medical Management

The expected outcome of treatment is complete remission. Lymphoid blast cells are typically very sensitive to corticosteroids and to vinca alkaloids; therefore, these medications are an integral part of the initial induction therapy. Because ALL frequently invades the central nervous system, prophylaxis with cranial irradiation or intrathecal chemotherapy (eg, methotrexate) or both is also a key part of the treatment plan.

Treatment protocols for ALL tend to be complex, using a wide variety of chemotherapeutic agents. They often include a maintenance phase, when lower doses of medications are given for up to 3 years. Despite the complexity, treatment can be provided in the outpatient setting in some circumstances until severe complications develop. Imatinib appears effective in those with Philadelphia chromosome–positive ALL. Monoclonal antibodies, in which the antibody specific for the antigen expressed on the ALL blast cell is selected, are also being studied (Larson, 2004). For example, the CD52 antigen is expressed on approximately 70% of ALL cells; thus, alemtuzumab (Campath), a monoclonal antibody with specific affinity for the CD52 antigen, may be effective therapy for this subset of patients.

Infections, especially viral infections, are common. The use of corticosteroids to treat ALL increases the patient's susceptibility to infection. Patients with ALL tend to have a better response to treatment than do patients with AML. BMT or PBSCT offers a chance for prolonged remission, or even cure, if the illness recurs after therapy.

## Nursing Management

Nursing management of the patient with acute leukemia is presented at the end of the leukemia section in this chapter.

## Chronic Lymphocytic Leukemia

Chronic lymphocytic leukemia (CLL) is a common malignancy of older adults; two thirds of all patients with CLL are older than 60 years at diagnosis. It is the most common form of leukemia in the United States and Europe, affecting more than 120,000 people, but it is rarely seen in Asia. The average survival for patients with CLL ranges from 14 years (early stage) to 2 years (late stage) (Rai et al., 2004). CLL occurs more often in males (1.5:1 male–female ratio), and survival tends to be shorter in males (Rai et al., 2004).

## Pathophysiology

CLL is typically derived from a malignant clone of B lymphocytes (T-lymphocyte CLL is rare). In contrast to the acute forms of leukemia, most of the leukemia cells in CLL are fully mature. It appears that these cells can escape **apoptosis** (programmed cell death), resulting in an excessive accumulation of the cells in the marrow and circulation. The antigen CD52 is prevalent on the surface of many of these leukemic B cells. The disease is classified into three or four stages (two classification systems are in use). In the early stage, an elevated lymphocyte count is seen; it can exceed 100,000/mm$^3$. Because the lymphocytes are small, they can easily travel through the small capillaries within the circulation, and the pulmonary and cerebral complications of leukocytosis (as seen with myeloid leukemias) typically are not found in CLL.

Lymphadenopathy occurs as the lymphocytes are trapped within the lymph nodes. The nodes can become very large and are sometimes painful. Hepatomegaly and splenomegaly then develop.

In later stages, anemia and thrombocytopenia may develop. Treatment is typically initiated in the later stages; earlier treatment does not appear to increase survival (Zent & Kay, 2004). Autoimmune complications can also occur at any stage, as either autoimmune hemolytic anemia or idiopathic thrombocytopenic purpura (ITP). In the autoimmune process, the reticuloendothelial system (RES) destroys the body's own erythrocytes or platelets.

## Clinical Manifestations

Many patients are asymptomatic and are diagnosed incidentally during routine physical examinations or during treatment for another disease. An increased lymphocyte count (lymphocytosis) is always present. The erythrocyte and platelet counts may be normal or, in later stages of the illness, decreased. Enlargement of lymph nodes (lymphadenopathy) is common; this can be severe and sometimes painful. The spleen can also be enlarged (splenomegaly).

Patients with CLL can develop "B symptoms," a constellation of symptoms including fevers, drenching sweats (especially at night), and unintentional weight loss. Patients with CLL have defects in their humoral and cell-mediated immune systems; therefore, infections are common. The defect in cellular immunity is evidenced by an absent or decreased reaction to skin sensitivity tests (eg, *Candida*, mumps), which is known as **anergy**. Life-threatening infections are common. Viral infections, such as herpes zoster, can become widely disseminated.

## Medical Management

In early stages, CLL may require no treatment. When symptoms are severe (drenching night sweats, painful lymphadenopathy) or when the disease progresses to later stages (with resultant anemia and thrombocytopenia), chemotherapy with fludarabine (Fludara) or corticosteroids and chlorambucil (Leukeran) is often used. The major side effect of fludarabine is prolonged bone marrow suppression, manifested by prolonged periods of neutropenia, lymphopenia, and thrombocytopenia. Patients are then at risk of such infections as *Pneumocystis jiroveci*, *Listeria*, mycobacteria, herpes viruses, and cytomegalovirus (CMV). Other useful agents include cyclophosphamide (Cytoxan), vincristine (Oncovin), and doxorubicin (Adriamycin).

The use of monoclonal antibodies is gaining popularity; these are effective and less toxic agents (Zent & Kay, 2004). The monoclonal antibody rituximab (Rituxan) has efficacy in CLL therapy and is often used in combination with other chemotherapeutic medications. The monoclonal antibody alemtuzumab (Campath) targets the CD52 antigen commonly found on CLL cells and is effective in clearing the marrow and circulation of these cells without affecting the stem cells. Because CD52 is present on both B and T lymphocytes, patients receiving alemtuzumab are at significant risk for infection; prophylactic use of antiviral agents and antibiotics (eg, trimethoprim/sulfamethoxazole [Bactrim, Septra]) is important and needs to continue for at least 2 months after treatment ends. Bacterial infections are common in patients with CLL, and IV treatment with immunoglobulin may be given to selected patients.

The disease trajectory of CLL is variable; thus, it is difficult to determine the best time to initiate treatment. Patients with early-stage disease are often monitored without treatment. In contrast, patients with signs of more aggressive disease or those who have developed an associated autoimmune disorder (autoimmune hemolytic anemia or ITP) are treated promptly (Ferrajoli & Keating, 2004).

# Nursing Process

## The Patient With Acute Leukemia

### Assessment

Although the clinical picture varies with the type of leukemia as well as the treatment implemented, the health history may reveal a range of subtle symptoms reported by the patient before the problem is detectable on physical examination. Weakness and fatigue are common manifestations, not only of the leukemia, but also of the resulting complications of anemia and infection. If the patient is hospitalized, the assessments should be performed daily, or more frequently as warranted. Because the physical findings may be subtle initially, a thorough, systematic assessment incorporating all body systems is essential. For example, a dry cough, mild dyspnea, and diminished breath sounds may indicate a pulmonary infection. However, the infection may not be seen initially on the chest x-ray; the absence of neutrophils delays the inflammatory response against the pulmonary infection, and it is the inflammatory response that produces the x-ray changes. The platelet count can become dangerously low, leaving the patient at risk for significant bleeding. The specific body system assessments are delineated in the neutropenic precautions and bleeding precautions found in Charts 33-8 and 33-9, respectively. When serial assessments are performed, current findings are compared with previous findings to evaluate improvement or worsening.

The nurse also must closely monitor the results of laboratory studies. Flow sheets and spreadsheets are particularly useful in tracking the leukocyte count, ANC, hematocrit, platelet, creatinine and electrolyte levels, and hepatic function tests. Culture results need to be reported immediately so that appropriate antimicrobial therapy can begin or be modified.

### Diagnosis

#### Nursing Diagnoses

Based on the assessment data, major nursing diagnoses for the patient with acute leukemia may include:

- Risk for infection and bleeding
- Risk for impaired skin integrity related to toxic effects of chemotherapy, alteration in nutrition, and impaired mobility
- Impaired gas exchange
- Impaired mucous membranes due to changes in epithelial lining of the GI tract from chemotherapy or prolonged use of antimicrobial medications
- Imbalanced nutrition, less than body requirements, related to hypermetabolic state, anorexia, mucositis, pain, and nausea
- Acute pain and discomfort related to mucositis, leukocyte infiltration of systemic tissues, fever, and infection
- Hyperthermia related to tumor lysis or infection
- Fatigue and activity intolerance related to anemia or infection
- Impaired physical mobility due to anemia and protective isolation
- Risk for excess fluid volume related to renal dysfunction, hypoproteinemia, need for multiple IV medications and blood products
- Diarrhea due to altered GI flora, mucosal denudation
- Risk for deficient fluid volume related to potential for diarrhea, bleeding, infection, and increased metabolic rate
- Self-care deficit due to fatigue, malaise, and protective isolation
- Anxiety due to knowledge deficit and uncertainty about future
- Disturbed body image related to change in appearance, function, and roles
- Grieving related to anticipatory loss and altered role functioning
- Potential for spiritual distress
- Deficient knowledge about disease process, treatment, complication management, and self-care measures

#### Collaborative Problems/ Potential Complications

Based on the assessment data, potential complications that may develop include:

- Infection
- Bleeding
- Renal dysfunction
- Tumor lysis syndrome
- Nutritional depletion
- Mucositis
- Depression

### Planning and Goals

The major goals for the patient may include absence of complications and pain, attainment and maintenance of adequate nutrition, activity tolerance, ability to provide self-care and to cope with the diagnosis and prognosis, positive body image, and an understanding of the disease process and its treatment.

### Nursing Interventions

#### Preventing or Managing Infection and Bleeding

The nursing interventions related to diminishing the risk of infection and for bleeding are delineated in Charts 33-8 and 33-9.

## CHART 33-9

# Bleeding Precautions

**Nursing Diagnosis**

Risk for injury/bleeding secondary to thrombocytopenia/altered coagulation due to:
- Malignant invasion in bone marrow
- Bone marrow suppression resulting from chemotherapy (particularly alkylators, antitumor antibiotics, antimetabolites) and radiation therapy
- Hypersplenism
- Disseminated intravascular coagulation (DIC)
- Altered coagulation

**Assessment**

PATIENT

Assess the following areas thoroughly every shift (with spot checks throughout the shift if patient is hospitalized), and notify physician if there is new onset of the following and/or worsening of status:
- *Integument:* Petechiae (usually located on trunk, legs), ecchymoses or hematomas, conjunctival hemorrhages, bleeding gums, bleeding at puncture sites (venipuncture, lumbar puncture, bone marrow)
- *Cardiovascular:* Hypotension, tachycardia, dizziness, epistaxis
- *Pulmonary:* Respiratory distress, tachypnea
- *Gastrointestinal:* Hemoptysis, abdominal distention, rectal bleeding
- *Genitourinary:* Vaginal or urethral bleeding
- *Neurologic:* Headache, blurred vision, mental status changes

**Laboratory Tests**
- Monitor complete blood count (CBC), platelets daily (at least); coagulation panel.
- Notify physician if platelet count is <10,000/mm$^3$ or if count has changed significantly from previous count (including coagulation), or whenever patient becomes symptomatic.
- Ensure patient's blood was human leukocyte antigen (HLA) typed before transfusions or chemotherapy begins if admitted for induction therapy (eg, for acute leukemia).
- Obtain 1-hour posttransfusion platelet count if prescribed.
- Test all urine, emesis, stools for occult blood.

**Nursing Interventions**

PREVENT COMPLICATIONS
- Avoid aspirin and aspirin-containing medications or other medications known to inhibit platelet function, if possible.
- Do not give intramuscular injections.
- Do not insert indwelling catheters.
- Take no rectal temperatures; do not give suppositories, enemas.
- Use stool softeners, oral laxatives to prevent constipation.
- Use smallest possible needles when performing venipuncture.
- Apply pressure to venipuncture sites for 5 min or until bleeding has stopped.
- Permit no flossing of teeth and no commercial mouthwashes.
- Use only soft-bristled toothbrush for mouth care.
- Use only toothettes for mouth care if platelet count is <10,000/mm$^3$, or if gums bleed.
- Lubricate lips with water-soluble lubricant every 2 hr while awake.
- Avoid suctioning if at all possible; if unavoidable, use only gentle suctioning.
- Discourage vigorous coughing or blowing of the nose.
- Use only electric razor for shaving.
- Pad side rails as needed.
- Prevent falls by ambulating with patient as necessary.

CONTROL BLEEDING
- Apply direct pressure.
- For epistaxis, position patient in high Fowler's position; apply ice pack to back of neck and direct pressure to nose.
- Notify physician for prolonged bleeding (eg, unable to stop within 10 min).
- Administer platelets, fresh frozen plasma, packed red blood cells, as prescribed.

**Evaluation and Expected Patient Outcomes**
- Patient demonstrates an absence of bleeding as evidenced by absence of spontaneous petechiae, ecchymoses, epistaxis, hemoptysis, bleeding gums, conjunctival hemorrhage, vaginal bleeding, hematuria, guaiac positive stool, blurred vision, orthostatic hypotension, and prolonged bleeding from puncture sites.
- Patient demonstrates an absence of bleeding as evidenced by the presence of vital signs within normal limits and intact neurologic status.

*Serious hemorrhage is unusual in mildly thrombocytopenic patients in absence of local lesions (peptic ulcer, bleeding from hemorrhoids, cystitis).

### Managing Mucositis

Although emphasis is placed on the oral mucosa, the entire GI mucosa can be altered, not only by the effects of chemotherapy but also from prolonged administration of antibiotics. Assessment of the oral mucosa must be thorough; therefore, dentures must be removed. Areas to assess include the palate, buccal mucosa, tongue, gums, lips, oropharynx, and the area under the tongue. In addition to identifying and describing lesions, the color and moisture of the mucosa should be noted.

Oral hygiene is very important to diminish the bacteria within the mouth, maintain moisture, and provide comfort. Soft-bristled toothbrushes should be used until the neutrophil and platelet counts become very low; at that time, sponge-tipped applicators may be substituted if necessary. Lemon-glycerin swabs and commercial mouthwashes should never be used because the glycerin and alcohol in them are extremely drying to the tissues. Simple rinses with saline (or saline and baking soda) solutions are inexpensive but effective in cleaning and moistening the oral mucosa. Because the risk for yeast or fungal infection in the mouth is great, other medications are often prescribed, such as chlorhexidine rinses (Peridex), clotrimazole troches (Mycelex), or fluconazole (Diflucan). The nurse reminds the patient about the importance of these medications to enhance adherence to the therapeutic regimen. Rinsing with chlorhexidine may discolor the teeth, and its efficacy is unclear.

To diminish perineal–rectal complications, it is important to cleanse this area thoroughly after each bowel movement. Women are instructed to cleanse the perineum from front to back. Sitz baths are a comfortable method of cleansing; the perineal–anal region and buttocks must be carefully dried afterward to minimize the chance of excoriation. Stool softeners should be used to increase the moisture of bowel movements; however, the stool texture must be monitored so that the softeners can be decreased or stopped if the stool becomes too loose.

### Improving Nutritional Intake

The disease process can increase the patient's metabolic rate and nutritional requirements. (Sepsis further increases them.) Nutritional intake is often reduced because of pain and discomfort associated with stomatitis. Mouth care before and after meals and the administration of analgesics before eating can help increase intake. If oral anesthetics are used, the patient must be warned to chew with extreme care to avoid inadvertently biting the tongue or buccal mucosa.

Nausea should not be a major contributing factor, because recent advances in antiemetic therapy are highly effective. However, nausea can result from antimicrobial therapy, so some antiemetic therapy may still be required after the chemotherapy has been completed.

Small, frequent feedings of foods that are soft in texture and moderate in temperature may be better tolerated. Low-microbial diets are typically prescribed (avoiding uncooked fruits or vegetables and those without a peelable skin). Nutritional supplements are frequently used. Daily body weights (as well as intake and output measurements) are useful in monitoring fluid status. Both calorie counts and more formal nutritional assessments are useful. Parenteral nutrition is often required to maintain adequate nutrition.

### Easing Pain and Discomfort

Recurrent fevers are common in acute leukemia; at times, they are accompanied by shaking chills (rigors), which can be severe. Myalgias and arthralgias can result. Acetaminophen is typically given to decrease fever, but it does so by increasing diaphoresis. Sponging with cool water may be useful, but cold water or ice packs should be avoided because the heat cannot dissipate from constricted blood vessels. Bedclothes need frequent changing as well. Gentle back and shoulder massage may provide comfort.

Stomatitis can also cause significant discomfort. In addition to oral hygiene practices, PCA can be effective in controlling the pain (see Chapter 13). With the exception of severe mucositis, less pain is associated with acute leukemia than with many other forms of cancer. However, the amount of psychological suffering that the patient must endure can be immense. Patients greatly benefit from active listening.

Because patients with acute leukemia require hospitalization for extensive nursing care (either during induction or consolidation therapy or during resultant complications), sleep deprivation frequently results. Nurses need to implement creative strategies that permit uninterrupted sleep for at least a few hours while still administering necessary medications on time.

### Decreasing Fatigue and Deconditioning

Fatigue is a common and oppressive problem. Nursing interventions should focus on assisting the patient to establish a balance between activity and rest. Patients with acute leukemia need to maintain some physical activity and exercise to prevent the deconditioning that results from inactivity. Use of a high-efficiency particulate air (HEPA) filter mask can permit the patient to ambulate outside the room despite severe neutropenia. Although many patients lack the motivation or energy to use them, stationary bicycles within the room can also be used. At a minimum, patients should be encouraged to sit up in a chair while awake rather than staying in bed; even this simple activity can improve the patient's tidal volume and enhance circulation. Physical therapy can also be beneficial.

### Maintaining Fluid and Electrolyte Balance

Febrile episodes, bleeding, and inadequate or overly aggressive fluid replacement can alter the patient's fluid status. Similarly, persistent diarrhea, vomiting, and long-term use of certain antimicrobial agents can cause significant deficits in electrolytes. Intake and output need to be measured accurately, and daily weights should also be monitored. The patient should be assessed for signs of dehydration as well as fluid overload, with particular attention to pulmonary status and the development of dependent edema. Laboratory test results, particularly electrolytes, blood urea nitrogen, creatinine, and hematocrit, should be monitored and compared with previous results. Replacement of electrolytes, particularly potassium and magnesium, is commonly required. Patients receiving amphotericin or certain antibiotics are at increased risk for electrolyte depletion.

### Improving Self-Care

Because hygiene measures are so important in this patient population, they must be performed by the nurse when the patient cannot do so. However, the patient should be encouraged to do as much as possible to preserve mobility and function as well as self-esteem. Patients may have negative feelings, even disgust, because they can no longer care for themselves. Empathetic listening is helpful, as is realistic reassurance that these deficits are temporary. As the patient recovers, it is important to assist him or her to resume more self-care. Patients are usually discharged from the hospital with a central vascular access device (eg, Hickman catheter, peripherally inserted central catheter [PICC]), and most patients can care for the catheter with adequate instruction and practice under observation.

### Managing Anxiety and Grief

Being diagnosed with acute leukemia can be extremely frightening. In many instances, the need to begin treatment is emergent, and the patient has little time to process the fact that he or she has the illness before making decisions about therapy. Providing emotional support and discussing the uncertain future are crucial. The nurse also needs to assess how much information the patient wants to have regarding the illness, its treatment, and potential complications. This desire should be reassessed at intervals, because needs and interest in information change throughout the course of the disease and treatment. Priorities must be identified so that procedures, assessments, and self-care expectations are adequately explained even to those who do not wish extensive information.

Many patients become depressed and begin to grieve for the losses they feel, such as normal family functioning, professional roles and responsibilities, and social roles, as well as physical functioning. The nurse can assist the patient to identify the source of the grief and encourage him or her to allow time to adjust to the major life changes produced by the illness. Role restructuring, in both family and professional life, may be required. Again, when possible, encouraging the patient to identify options and to take time making significant decisions regarding such restructuring is helpful.

Discharge from the hospital can also provoke anxiety. Although most patients are extremely eager to go home, they may lack confidence in their ability to manage potential complications and to resume their normal activity. Close communication between nurses across care settings can reassure patients that they will not be abandoned.

### Encouraging Spiritual Well-Being

Because acute leukemia is a serious, potentially life-threatening illness, the nurse may offer support to enhance the patient's spiritual well-being. The patient's spiritual and religious practices should be assessed and pastoral services offered. Throughout the patient's illness, it is important that the nurse assist the patient to maintain hope. However, that hope should be realistic and will certainly change over the course of the illness. For example, the patient may initially hope to be cured, but with repeated relapses and a change to hospice or palliative care the same patient may hope for a quiet, dignified death. (Refer to Chapter 17 for a discussion of end-of-life care.)

### Monitoring and Managing Potential Complications

Nursing interventions for potential complications were described previously.

### Promoting Home and Community-Based Care

#### TEACHING PATIENTS SELF-CARE

Most patients cope better when they have an understanding of what is happening to them. Based on their education, literacy level, and interest, teaching of patient and family should focus on the disease (including some pathophysiology), its treatment, and certainly the significant risk for infection and bleeding (see Charts 33-8 and 33-9) that results.

Management of a vascular access device can be taught to most patients or family members. Follow-up and care for the devices may also need to be provided by nurses in an outpatient facility or by a home care agency.

#### CONTINUING CARE

Shortened hospital stays and outpatient care have significantly altered care for patients with acute leukemia. In many instances, when the patient is clinically stable but still requires parenteral antibiotics or blood products, these procedures can be performed in an outpatient setting. Nurses in these various settings must communicate regularly. The patient needs to learn which parameters are important to monitor and how to monitor them. Specific instructions need to be given about when the patient should seek care from the physician or other health care provider.

The patient and family need to have a clear understanding of the disease and the prognosis. The nurse acts as an advocate to ensure that this information is provided. When the patient no longer responds to therapy, it is important to respect the patient's choices about treatment, including measures to prolong life and other end-of-life measures. Advance directives, including living wills, provide patients with some measure of control during terminal illness.

Many patients in this stage still choose to be cared for at home, and families often need support when considering this option. Coordination of home care services and instruction can help alleviate anxiety about managing the patient's care in the home. As the patient becomes weaker, the caregivers must assume more of the patient's care. In addition, caregivers often need to be encouraged to take care of themselves, allowing time for rest and accepting emotional support. Hospice staff can assist in providing respite for family members as well as care for the patient. Patients and families also need assistance to cope with changes in their roles and responsibilities. Anticipatory grieving is an essential task during this time (see Chapter 17).

In patients with acute leukemia, death typically occurs from infection or bleeding. Family members need to have information about these complications and the measures to take should either occur. Many family members cannot cope with the care required when a patient begins to bleed actively. It is important to delineate alternatives to keeping the patient at home, such as inpatient hospice units. Should another option be sought, family members who may feel guilty that they could not keep the patient at home will require support from the nurse.

## Evaluation

### Expected Patient Outcomes

Expected patient outcomes may include:

1. Shows no evidence of infection
2. Experiences no bleeding
3. Has intact oral mucous membranes
   a. Participates in oral hygiene regimen
   b. Reports no discomfort in mouth
4. Attains optimal level of nutrition
   a. Maintains weight with increased food and fluid intake
   b. Maintains adequate protein stores (albumin)
5. Reports satisfaction with pain and comfort levels
6. Has less fatigue and increased activity
7. Maintains fluid and electrolyte balance
8. Participates in self-care
9. Copes with anxiety and grief
   a. Discusses concerns and fears
   b. Uses stress management strategies appropriately
   c. Participates in decisions regarding end-of-life care
   d. Discusses hope for peaceful death
10. Absence of complications

# Agnogenic Myeloid Metaplasia

Agnogenic myeloid metaplasia (AMM), also known as myelofibrosis, is a chronic myeloproliferative disorder that arises from neoplastic transformation of an early hematopoietic stem cell. The disease is characterized by marrow fibrosis or scarring, splenomegaly, extramedullary hematopoiesis (typically spleen, liver, or both), leukocytosis and thrombocytosis, and anemia. Some patients have suppressed leukocyte and platelet counts as well as anemia (pancytopenia). Patients with AMM have increased **angiogenesis** (formation of new blood vessels) within the marrow. Early forms of blood cells (including nucleated RBCs and megakaryocyte fragments) are frequently found in the circulation.

AMM is a disease of the elderly, with a median age at diagnosis of 60 to 65 years. Survival varies from as little as 1 year to more than 30 years; the average is 3.5 to 5.5 years (Barosi, 2003). Heart failure, complications of marrow failure, and transformation to AML are the common causes of death.

## Medical Management

For those unable to undergo stem cell transplant, medical management is directed toward palliation, reducing symptoms related to cytopenias, splenomegaly, and hypermetabolic state. Although one third of anemic patients respond to the combination of an androgen plus a corticosteroid, the primary treatment remains PRBC transfusion. Because of the prolonged requirement for these transfusions, iron overload is a common problem. Iron chelation therapy should be initiated in patients in whom survival is expected to exceed a few years. Hydroxyurea is often used to control high leukocyte and platelet counts and to reduce the size of the spleen. Splenic irradiation or splenectomy may also be used to control the significant splenomegaly that can develop. However, both modalities render the patient at significant risk of development of infection. Alpha-interferon has been useful in controlling the disease, particularly in younger patients. Thalidomide (Thalomid) has been tried in an attempt to diminish the angiogenesis within the marrow; unfortunately, most patients cannot tolerate the drug for more than several months (Barosi, 2003). BMT or PBSCT may be a useful treatment modality in younger, otherwise healthy people.

## Nursing Management

Splenomegaly can be profound in patients with AMM, with enlargement of the spleen that extends to the pelvic rim. This condition is extremely uncomfortable and can severely limit nutritional intake. Analgesics are often ineffective. Methods to reduce the size of the spleen are usually more effective in controlling pain. Splenomegaly, coupled with a hypermetabolic state, results in weight loss (often severe) and muscle wasting. Patients benefit from very small, frequent meals of foods that are high in calories and protein. Weakness, fatigue, and altered body image are other significant problems. Energy conservation methods and active listening are important nursing interventions. The patient needs to be educated about signs and symptoms of infection as well as appropriate interventions when an infection is suspected.

# Lymphoma

The lymphomas are neoplasms of cells of lymphoid origin. These tumors usually start in lymph nodes but can involve lymphoid tissue in the spleen, the GI tract (eg, the wall of the stomach), the liver, or the bone marrow. They are often classified according to the degree of cell differentiation and the origin of the predominant malignant cell. Lymphomas can be broadly classified into two categories: Hodgkin's disease and non-Hodgkin's lymphoma (NHL).

## Hodgkin's Disease

Hodgkin's disease is a relatively rare malignancy that has an impressive cure rate. It is somewhat more common in men than women and has two peaks of incidence: one in the early 20s and the other after 50 years of age. Disease occurrence has a familial pattern: first-degree relatives have a higher-than-normal frequency of disease, but the actual incidence of this pattern is low. No increased incidence for non-blood relatives (eg, spouses) has been documented. Hodgkin's disease is seen more commonly in patients receiving chronic immunosuppressive therapy (eg, for renal transplant) and in woodworkers. It is also seen in veterans of the military who were exposed to the herbicide Agent Orange.

### Pathophysiology

Unlike other lymphomas, Hodgkin's disease is unicentric in origin in that it initiates in a single node. The disease spreads by contiguous extension along the lymphatic system. The malignant cell of Hodgkin's disease is the Reed-Sternberg cell, a gigantic tumor cell that is morphologically unique and is thought to be of immature lymphoid origin. It is the pathologic hallmark and essential diagnostic criterion for Hodgkin's disease. However, the tumor is very heterogeneous and may actually contain few Reed-Sternberg cells. Repeated biopsies may be required to establish the diagnosis.

The cause of Hodgkin's disease is unknown but a viral etiology is suspected. In fact, fragments of the Epstein-Barr virus have been found in some Reed-Sternberg cells.

Hodgkin's disease is customarily classified into five subgroups based on pathologic analyses that reflect the natural history of the malignancy and suggest the prognosis. For example, when lymphocytes predominate, with few Reed-Sternberg cells and minimal involvement of the lymph nodes, the prognosis is much more favorable than when the lymphocyte count is low and the lymph nodes are virtually replaced by tumor cells of the most primitive type. Most patients with Hodgkin's disease have the types currently designated "nodular sclerosis" or "mixed cellularity." The nodular sclerosis type tends to occur more often in young women, at an earlier stage but with a worse prognosis than the mixed cellularity subgroup, which occurs more commonly in men and causes more constitutional symptoms but has a better prognosis.

### Clinical Manifestations

Hodgkin's disease usually begins as a painless enlargement of one or more lymph nodes on one side of the neck. The individual nodes are painless and firm but not hard. The most common sites for lymphadenopathy are the cervical, supraclavicular, and mediastinal nodes; involvement of the iliac or inguinal nodes or spleen is much less common. A mediastinal mass may be seen on chest x-ray; occasionally, the mass is large enough to compress the trachea and cause dyspnea. Pruritus is common; it can be extremely distressing, and the cause is unknown. Some patients experience brief but severe pain after drinking alcohol, usually at the site of the tumor. Again, the cause of this is unknown.

All organs are vulnerable to invasion by Hodgkin's disease. The symptoms result from compression of organs by the tumor, such as cough and pulmonary effusion (from pulmonary infiltrates), jaundice (from hepatic involvement or bile duct obstruction), abdominal pain (from splenomegaly or retroperitoneal adenopathy), or bone pain (from skeletal involvement). Herpes zoster infections are common. A cluster of constitutional symptoms has important prognostic implications. Referred to as "B symptoms," they include fever (without chills), drenching sweats (particularly at night), and unintentional weight loss of more than 10%. "B symptoms" are found in 40% of patients and are more common in advanced disease.

A mild anemia is the most common hematologic finding. The leukocyte count may be elevated or decreased. The platelet count is typically normal, unless the tumor has invaded the bone marrow, suppressing hematopoiesis. The **erythrocyte sedimentation rate** (ESR) and the serum copper level are used by some clinicians to assess disease activity. Patients with Hodgkin's disease have impaired cellular immunity, as evidenced by an absent or decreased reaction to skin sensitivity tests (eg, *Candida,* mumps).

### Assessment and Diagnostic Findings

Because many manifestations are similar to those occurring with infection, diagnostic studies are performed to rule out an infectious origin for the disease. The diagnosis is made by means of an excisional lymph node biopsy and the finding of the Reed-Sternberg cell. Once the diagnosis is confirmed and the histologic type is established, it is necessary to assess the extent of the disease, a process referred to as staging.

During the health history, the patient is assessed for any "B symptoms." Physical examination requires a careful, systematic evaluation of the lymph node chains, as well as the size of the spleen and liver. A chest x-ray and a CT scan of the chest, abdomen, and pelvis are crucial to identify the extent of lymphadenopathy within these regions. A positron emission tomography (PET) scan may be the most sensitive imaging test in identifying residual disease. Laboratory tests include CBC, platelet count, ESR, and liver and renal function studies. A bone marrow biopsy is performed if there are signs of marrow involvement, and some physicians routinely perform bilateral biopsies. Bone scans may be performed to identify any involvement in these areas. A staging laparotomy and lymphangiography are no longer considered mandatory, primarily because of the accuracy of CT and PET.

## Medical Management

The general goal in treatment of Hodgkin's disease, regardless of stage, is cure. Treatment is determined primarily by the stage of the disease, not the histologic type; however, extensive research is ongoing to target treatment regimens to histologic subtypes or prognostic features. Traditionally, early Hodgkin's disease was treated by a staging laparotomy followed by radiation therapy. This treatment method has commonly been replaced by a short course (2 to 4 months) of chemotherapy followed by radiation therapy in certain subsets of early-stage disease (IA and IIA) (Bonadonna et al., 2004; Diehl et al., 2004). Some patients with early-stage disease and good prognostic features may receive radiation therapy alone. Combination chemotherapy, for example with doxorubicin (Adriamycin), bleomycin (Blenoxane), vinblastine (Velban), and dacarbazine (DTIC), referred to as ABVD, is now the standard treatment for more advanced disease (stages III and IV and all B stages).

Radiation therapy is still very useful for patients with extensive adenopathy (often termed bulky disease). In this group, residual disease often persists after the chemotherapy treatment is finished; radiation therapy to the areas of remaining adenopathy has been shown to improve survival.

Even when Hodgkin's disease does recur, the use of high doses of chemotherapeutic agents, followed by autologous BMT or stem cell transplantation, can be very effective in controlling the disease and extending survival time.

### Long-Term Complications of Therapy

Much is now known about the long-term effects of chemotherapy and radiation therapy, primarily from the large numbers of people who were cured of Hodgkin's disease by these treatments. The various complications of treatment are listed in Chart 33-10. Risk factors for other cancers should be assessed, and long-term surveillance is crucial. Lung cancer is the most common type of second malignancy in patients with Hodgkin's disease, particularly following combination chemotherapy and radiation (Mauch, Aleman, Carde, et al., 2003). Breast cancer appears to be more common in women, particularly in those who were treated before age 30 years, and in those who received radiation therapy alone (Mauch et al., 2003). The potential development of a second malignancy is obviously of concern to the patient, and this potential should be addressed with the patient when treatment decisions are made. However, it is important to consider that Hodgkin's disease is curable. Patients should be encouraged to reduce other factors that increase the risk of developing second cancers, such as use of tobacco and alcohol and exposure to environmental carcinogens. Revised treatment approaches are aimed at diminishing the risk for complications without sacrificing the potential for cure.

## Non-Hodgkin's Lymphomas (NHLs)

The NHLs are a heterogeneous group of cancers that originate from the neoplastic growth of lymphoid tissue. As in CLL, the neoplastic cells are thought to arise from a single clone of lymphocytes; however, in NHL, the cells may vary morphologically. Most NHLs involve malignant B lymphocytes; only 5% involve T lymphocytes. In contrast to Hodgkin's disease, the lymphoid tissues involved are largely infiltrated with malignant cells. The spread of these malignant lymphoid cells occurs unpredictably, and true localized disease is uncommon. Lymph nodes from multiple sites may be infiltrated, as may sites outside the lymphoid system (extranodal tissue).

There has been a threefold increase in incidence of NHL in recent years (Lister, 2004). It is now the sixth most common type of cancer diagnosed in the United States and the sixth most common cause of cancer death (Jemal, Siegal, Ward, et al., 2006). The incidence increases with each decade of life; the average age at diagnosis is 50 to 60 years. Although no common etiologic factor has been identified, the incidence of NHL has increased in people with immunodeficiencies or autoimmune disorders; prior treatment for cancer; prior organ transplant; viral infections (including Epstein-Barr virus and HIV); and exposure to pesticides, solvents, dyes, or defoliating agents, including Agent Orange. Prognosis varies greatly among the various types of NHL. Long-term survival (more than 10 years) is commonly achieved in low-grade, localized lymphomas. Even with aggressive disease forms, cure is possible in at least one third of patients who receive aggressive treatment.

### Clinical Manifestations

Symptoms are highly variable, reflecting the diverse nature of the NHLs. Lymphadenopathy is most common (66%); however, in more indolent (less aggressive) types of lymphomas, the lymphadenopathy can wax and wane (Freedman, 2004).

---

**CHART 33-10**

### Potential Long-Term Complications of Therapy for Hodgkin's Disease

- Immune dysfunction
- Herpes infections (zoster and varicella)
- Pneumococcal sepsis
- Acute myeloid leukemia (AML)
- Myelodysplastic syndromes (MDS)
- Non-Hodgkin's lymphoma
- Solid tumors
- Thyroid cancer
- Thymic hyperplasia
- Hypothyroidism
- Pericarditis (acute or chronic)
- Cardiomyopathy
- Pneumonitis (acute or chronic)
- Avascular necrosis
- Growth retardation
- Infertility
- Decreased libido
- Dental caries

With early-stage disease, or with the types that are considered more indolent, symptoms may be virtually absent or very minor, and the illness typically is not diagnosed until it progresses to a later stage, when the patient is symptomatic. At these stages (III or IV), lymphadenopathy is distinctly noticeable. One third of patients with NHLs have "B symptoms" (recurrent fever, drenching night sweats, and unintentional weight loss of 10% or more). Lymphomatous masses can compromise organ function. For example, a mass in the mediastinum can cause respiratory distress; abdominal masses can compromise the ureters, leading to renal dysfunction; and splenomegaly can cause abdominal discomfort, nausea, early satiety, anorexia, and weight loss. Involvement of the central nervous system with lymphoma is increasing in frequency (Freedman, 2004).

## Assessment and Diagnostic Findings

The actual diagnosis of NHL is categorized into a highly complex classification system based on histopathology, immunophenotyping, and cytogenetic analyses of the malignant cells. The specific histopathologic type of the disease has important prognostic implications. Treatment also varies and is based on these features. Indolent types tend to have small cells that are distributed in a follicular pattern. Aggressive types tend to have large or immature cells distributed through the nodes in a diffuse pattern. Staging, also an important factor, is typically based on data obtained from CT and PET scans, bone marrow biopsies, and occasionally cerebrospinal fluid analysis. The stage is based on the site of disease and its spread to other sites. For example, in stage I disease, only one area of involvement is detected; thus, stage I disease is highly localized and may respond well to localized therapy (eg, radiation therapy). In contrast, in stage IV disease at least one extranodal site is detected.

Low-grade lymphomas may not require treatment until the disease progresses to a later stage, but historically they have also been relatively unresponsive to treatment, and in most cases, use of therapeutic modalities did not improve overall survival. More aggressive types of NHL (eg, lymphoblastic lymphoma, Burkitt's lymphoma) require prompt initiation of chemotherapy; however, these types tend to be more responsive to treatment.

## Medical Management

Treatment is based on the actual classification of disease, the stage of disease, prior treatment (if any), and the patient's ability to tolerate therapy. If the disease is not an aggressive form and is truly localized, radiation alone may be the treatment of choice. With aggressive types of NHL, aggressive combinations of chemotherapeutic agents are given even in early stages. More intermediate forms are commonly treated with combination chemotherapy and radiation therapy for stage I and II disease. The biologic agent interferon has been approved for the treatment of follicular low-grade lymphomas, and an antibody to CD20, rituximab (Rituxan), has been effective in achieving partial responses in patients with recurrent low-grade lymphoma. In fact, the combination of rituximab with conventional chemotherapy (Cytoxan, doxorubicin, vincristine, and prednisone [CHOP]) is now considered standard treatment for common, aggressive lymphomas (Lister, 2004). Unfortunately, in most situations, relapse is commonly seen in patients with low-grade lymphomas. A recent study documented the effectiveness of maintenance therapy with rituximab in reducing progression of disease (Hochster et al., 2004). Central nervous system involvement is common with some aggressive forms of NHL; in this situation, cranial radiation or intrathecal chemotherapy is used in addition to systemic chemotherapy.

Treatment after relapse is controversial. BMT or PBSCT may be considered for patients younger than 60 years (see Chapter 16). Other treatment options include yttrium 90 ibritumomab tiuxetan (Zevalin) (Riley & Byar, 2004) or proteasome inhibitors (eg, bortezomib [Velcade]) (Goy et al., 2004).

## Nursing Management

Lymphoma is a highly complex constellation of diseases. When caring for patients with lymphoma, it is extremely important to know the specific disease type, stage of disease, treatment history, and current treatment plan. Most of the care for patients with Hodgkin's disease or NHL takes place in the outpatient setting, unless complications occur (eg, infection, respiratory compromise due to mediastinal mass). The most commonly used treatment methods are chemotherapy and radiation therapy. Chemotherapy causes systemic side effects (eg, myelosuppression, nausea, hair loss, risk of infection), whereas radiation therapy causes specific effects that are limited to the area being irradiated. For example, patients receiving abdominal radiation therapy may experience nausea and diarrhea but not hair loss. Regardless of the type of treatment, all patients may experience fatigue.

The risk for infection is significant for these patients, not only from treatment-related myelosuppression but also from the defective immune response that results from the disease itself. Patients need to be taught to minimize the risks of infection, to recognize signs of possible infection, and to contact the health care professional should such signs develop (see Chart 33-7).

Additional complications depend on the location of the lymphoma. Therefore, it is important for the nurse to know the tumor location so that assessments can be targeted appropriately. For example, patients with lymphomatous masses in the upper chest should be assessed for superior vena cava obstruction or airway obstruction, if the mass is near the bronchus or trachea.

Many lymphomas can be cured with current treatments. However, as survival rates increase, the incidence of second malignancies, particularly AML or MDS, also increases. Therefore, survivors should be screened regularly for the development of second malignancies.

## Multiple Myeloma

Multiple myeloma is a malignant disease of the most mature form of B lymphocyte, the plasma cell. It is not classified as a lymphoma. Plasma cells secrete immunoglobulins, proteins necessary for antibody production to fight infection.

Median survival time for patients with multiple myeloma is 3 to 5 years. Death usually results from infection.

## Pathophysiology

In multiple myeloma, the malignant plasma cells produce an increased amount of a specific immunoglobulin that is nonfunctional. Functional types of immunoglobulin are still produced by nonmalignant plasma cells, but in lower-than-normal quantity. The specific immunoglobulin secreted by the myeloma cells is detectable in the blood or urine and is referred to as the monoclonal protein, or M protein. This protein serves as a useful marker to monitor the extent of disease and the patient's response to therapy. It is commonly measured by serum or urine protein electrophoresis. Moreover, the patient's total protein level is typically elevated, again due to the production of M protein. Malignant plasma cells also secrete certain substances to stimulate the creation of new blood vessels to enhance the growth of these clusters of plasma cells; this process is referred to as angiogenesis. Occasionally the plasma cells infiltrate other tissue, in which case they are referred to as plasmacytomas. Plasmacytomas can occur in the sinuses, spinal cord, and soft tissues.

## Clinical Manifestations

The classic presenting symptom of multiple myeloma is bone pain, usually in the back or ribs. Bone pain is reported by two thirds of all patients at diagnosis. Unlike arthritic pain, the bone pain associated with myeloma increases with movement and decreases with rest; patients may report that they have less pain on awakening but the pain intensity increases during the day. In myeloma, a substance secreted by the plasma cells, osteoclast activating factor, and other substances (eg, interleukin-6 [IL-6]) are involved in stimulating osteoclasts. Both mechanisms appear to be involved in the process of bone breakdown. Thus, lytic lesions as well as osteoporosis may be seen on bone x-rays. (They are not well visualized on bone scans.) The bone destruction can be severe enough to cause vertebral collapse and fractures, including spinal fractures, which can impinge on the spinal cord and result in spinal cord compression. It is this bone destruction that causes significant pain.

If the bone destruction is fairly extensive, excessive ionized calcium is lost from the bone and enters the serum; hypercalcemia may therefore develop (frequently manifested by excessive thirst, dehydration, constipation, altered mental status, confusion, and perhaps coma). Renal failure may also occur; the configuration of the circulating immunoglobulin molecule (particularly the shape of lambda light chains) can damage the renal tubules.

> **! NURSING ALERT**
>
> Any elderly patient whose chief complaint is back pain and who has an elevated total protein level should be evaluated for possible myeloma.

As more and more malignant plasma cells are produced, the marrow has less space for erythrocyte production, and anemia may develop. This anemia is also caused to a great extent by a diminished production of erythropoietin (a glycoprotein necessary for erythrocyte production) by the kidney. The patient may complain of fatigue and weakness due to the anemia. In the late stage of the disease, a reduced number of leukocytes and platelets may also be seen because the bone marrow is infiltrated by malignant plasma cells.

When plasma cells secrete excessive amounts of immunoglobulin, the serum viscosity can increase. Hyperviscosity may be manifested by bleeding from the nose or mouth, headache, blurred vision, paresthesias, or heart failure.

## Assessment and Diagnostic Findings

Finding an elevated monoclonal protein spike in the serum (via serum protein electrophoresis) or urine (via urine protein electrophoresis) or light chain in the urine (sometimes referred to as Bence Jones protein) is considered to be a major criterion in the diagnosis of multiple myeloma. The presence of lytic bone lesions on x-ray studies aids in the diagnosis, as does the presence of anemia or hypercalcemia. The diagnosis of myeloma can be confirmed by bone marrow biopsy; the presence of sheets of plasma cells is the hallmark diagnostic criterion. Because the infiltration of the marrow by these malignant plasma cells is not uniform, the plasma cells may not be increased in a given sample (a false-negative result).

## Medical Management

There is no cure for multiple myeloma. Even BMT or PBSCT is considered to extend remission rather than provide a cure. However, for many patients, it is possible to control the illness and maintain their level of functioning quite well for several years or longer. Chemotherapy is the primary treatment; corticosteroids, particularly dexamethasone (Decadron), are especially effective and are often combined with other agents (eg, melphalan [Alkeran], cyclophosphamide [Cytoxan], doxorubicin [Adriamycin], vincristine [Oncovin], and carmustine [BCNU]).

Radiation therapy is very useful in strengthening the bone at a specific lesion, particularly one at risk for bone fracture or spinal cord compression. It is also useful in relieving bone pain and reducing the size of plasma cell tumors that occur outside the skeletal system. However, because it is a nonsystemic form of treatment, it does not diminish the source of the bone conditions (ie, the production of malignant plasma cells). Therefore, radiation therapy is typically used in combination with systemic treatment such as chemotherapy.

When lytic lesions result in vertebral compression fractures, vertebroplasty is often performed. This procedure is performed under fluoroscopy. A hollow needle is positioned within the fractured vertebra, and when the precise location is confirmed, an orthopedic cement is infiltrated into the vertebra to stabilize the fracture and strengthen the vertebra. For most patients, relief from pain is almost immediate. This procedure has been enhanced by concomitant kyphoplasty, the use of a special inflatable balloon inserted into the vertebra to increase the height of the vertebra prior to injecting the cement.

Newer forms of bisphosphonates, such as pamidronate (Aredia) and zoledronic acid (Zometa), have been shown to strengthen bone in multiple myeloma by diminishing the secretion of osteoclast activating factor, thus controlling bone pain and potentially preventing bone fracture. These agents are also effective in managing and preventing hypercalcemia. Some evidence suggests that bisphosphonates may actually have activity against the myeloma cells themselves by inhibiting a growth factor necessary for myeloma cell survival (Lipton, 2004; Terpos & Rahemtulla, 2004). Recently, an increased incidence of osteonecrosis of the jaw has been found in people with and without multiple myeloma receiving long-term bisphosphonate therapy (Lugassy et al., 2004; Ruggiero et al., 2004). This association between bisphosphonates and osteonecrosis has not yet been proved, and the incidence of osteonecrosis appears to be very low. Nonetheless, careful assessment for this complication should be performed, and it may be prudent to warn patients to have any necessary invasive dental procedure performed prior to initiating bisphosphonate therapy.

When patients have signs and symptoms of hyperviscosity, plasmapheresis may be used to lower the immunoglobulin level. Symptoms may be more useful than serum viscosity levels in determining the need for this intervention.

Recent advances in the understanding of the process of angiogenesis have resulted in new therapeutic options. The sedative thalidomide (Thalomid), initially used as an antiemetic, has significant antimyeloma effects. It inhibits cytokines necessary for new vascular generation, such as vascular endothelial growth factor, and for myeloma cell growth and survival, such as IL-6 and tumor necrosis factor, by boosting the body's immune response against the tumor and by creating favorable conditions for apoptosis (programmed cell death) of the myeloma cells. Thalidomide is effective in refractory myeloma and in "smoldering" disease states and may prevent progression to a more active state. Thalidomide is not a typical chemotherapeutic agent and has a unique side effect profile. Fatigue, dizziness, constipation, rash, and peripheral neuropathy are commonly encountered; myelosuppression is not. There is also an increased incidence of DVT; prophylactic anticoagulation may be prescribed to prevent this complication (Kyle & Rajkumar, 2004). Thalidomide is contraindicated in pregnancy because of associated severe birth defects. Thus, the patient must be counseled and agree to use approved methods of birth control prior to taking this drug.

More recently, the use of a proteasome inhibiting agent, bortezomib (Velcade), has been approved by the FDA for use in refractory disease (Devenney, 2004). Side effects include transient thrombocytopenia, orthostatic hypotension, nausea and vomiting, skin rash, and neuropathy.

Further research has documented the efficacy of a thalidomide analogue, known as CC-5013, or Revlimid (lenalidomide). This agent inhibits angiogenesis and promotes apoptosis and cytotoxicity (Kyle & Rajkuman, 2004). The side effect profile is quite different from thalidomide: myelosuppression is common, whereas sedation, neuropathy, and constipation are not.

## Nursing Management

Pain management is very important in patients with multiple myeloma. NSAIDs can be very useful for mild pain or can be administered in combination with opioid analgesics. Because NSAIDs can cause gastritis and renal dysfunction, renal function must be carefully monitored. The patient needs to be educated about activity restrictions (eg, lifting no more than 10 pounds, use of proper body mechanics). Braces are occasionally needed to support the spinal column.

The patient also needs to be instructed about the signs and symptoms of hypercalcemia. Maintaining mobility and hydration is important to diminish exacerbations of this complication; however, the primary cause is the disease itself. Renal function should also be monitored closely. Renal failure can become severe, and dialysis may be needed. Maintaining high urine output (3 L/day) can be very useful in preventing or limiting this complication.

Because antibody production is impaired, infections, particularly bacterial infections, are common and can be life-threatening. The patient needs to be instructed in appropriate infection prevention measures (see Chart 33-7) and should be advised to contact the health care provider immediately if he or she has a fever or other signs and symptoms of infection. The patient should receive pneumonia (Pneumovax) and influenza vaccines. Prophylactic antibiotics are sometimes used. IV immune globulin (IVIG) can be useful for patients with recurrent infections.

### Gerontologic Considerations

The incidence of multiple myeloma increases with age; the disease rarely occurs in patients younger than 40 years of age. Because of the increasing older population, more patients are seeking treatment for this disease. Back pain, which is often a presenting symptom in this disease, should be closely investigated in older patients. BMT or PBSCT is an option that can prolong remission and potentially cure some patients, but it is unavailable to most older people because of age limitations.

## Bleeding Disorders

### Overview

Normal hemostatic mechanisms can control bleeding from vessels and prevent spontaneous bleeding. The bleeding vessel constricts and platelets aggregate at the site, forming an unstable hemostatic plug. Circulating coagulation factors are activated on the surface of these aggregated platelets, forming fibrin, which anchors the platelet plug to the site of injury.

The failure of normal hemostatic mechanisms can result in bleeding, which is severe at times. This bleeding is commonly provoked by trauma, but in certain circumstances it can occur spontaneously. When the source is platelet or coagulation factor abnormalities, the site of bleeding can be anywhere in the body. When the source is vascular abnormalities, the site of bleeding may be more localized. Some patients have defects in more than one hemostatic mechanism simultaneously.

In a variety of situations, the bone marrow may be stimulated to increase platelet production (thrombopoiesis). The increased production may be a reactive response, as in a compensatory response to significant bleeding, or a more general response to increased hematopoiesis, as in iron deficiency anemia. Sometimes, the increase in platelets does not result from increased production but from a loss in platelet pooling within the spleen. The spleen typically holds about one third of the circulating platelets at any time. If the spleen is absent (eg, splenectomy), the platelet reservoir is also lost, and an abnormally high number of platelets enters the circulation. In time, the rate of thrombopoiesis slows to reestablish a more normal platelet level.

## Clinical Manifestations

Signs and symptoms of bleeding disorders vary depending on the type of defect. A careful history and physical examination can be very useful in determining the source of the hemostatic defect. Abnormalities of the vascular system give rise to local bleeding, usually into the skin. Because platelets are primarily responsible for stopping bleeding from small vessels, patients with platelet defects develop petechiae, often in clusters; these are seen on the skin and mucous membranes but also occur throughout the body. Bleeding from platelet disorders can be severe. Unless the platelet disorder is severe, bleeding can often be stopped promptly when local pressure is applied; it does not typically recur when the pressure is released.

In contrast, coagulation factor defects do not tend to cause superficial bleeding, because the primary hemostatic mechanisms are still intact. Instead, bleeding occurs deeper within the body (eg, subcutaneous or IM hematomas, hemorrhage into joint spaces). External bleeding diminishes very slowly when local pressure is applied; it often recurs several hours after pressure is removed. For example, severe bleeding may start several hours after a tooth extraction. Risk factors for bleeding are listed in Chart 33-6.

## Medical Management

Management varies based on the underlying cause of the bleeding disorder. If bleeding is significant, transfusions of blood products are indicated. The specific blood product used is determined by the underlying defect. If fibrinolysis is excessive, hemostatic agents such as aminocaproic acid (Amicar) can be used to inhibit this process. This agent must be used with caution, because excessive inhibition of fibrinolysis can result in thrombosis.

## Nursing Management

Patients who have bleeding disorders or who have the potential for development of such disorders as a result of disease or therapeutic agents must be taught to observe themselves carefully and frequently for bleeding (Chart 33-11). They need to understand the importance of avoiding activities that increase the risk of bleeding, such as contact sports. The skin is observed for petechiae and ecchymoses (bruises) and the nose and gums for bleeding. Hospitalized patients may be monitored for bleeding by testing all drainage and excreta (feces, urine, emesis, and gastric drainage) for occult as well as obvious blood. Outpatients are often given fecal occult blood screening cards to detect occult blood in stools.

## *Primary Thrombocythemia*

Primary thrombocythemia (also called essential thrombocythemia) is a stem cell disorder within the bone marrow. A marked increase in platelet production occurs, with the platelet count consistently greater than 600,000/mm$^3$. Platelet size may be abnormal, but platelet survival is typically normal. Occasionally, the platelet increase is accompanied by an increase in erythrocytes, leukocytes, or both; however, these cells are not increased to the extent that they are in polycythemia vera, CML, or myelofibrosis. Although

---

**CHART 33-11**

### HOME CARE CHECKLIST • The Patient at Risk for Bleeding

| At the completion of the home care instruction, the patient or caregiver will be able to: | Patient | Caregiver |
|---|---|---|
| • Describe the source and function of platelets and clotting factors. | ✔ | ✔ |
| • Verbalize the rationale for being at risk for bleeding. | ✔ | ✔ |
| • Identify medications and other substances to avoid (eg, aspirin-containing medications, alcohol). | ✔ | ✔ |
| • Demonstrate how to monitor for signs of bleeding. | ✔ | ✔ |
| • Describe to whom, how, and when to report signs of bleeding. | ✔ | ✔ |
| • Notify health care professional before having dental work. | ✔ | ✔ |
| • Describe appropriate ways to prevent bleeding (avoid use of suppositories, enemas, tampons; avoid constipation, vigorous sexual intercourse, anal sex; use only electric razor for shaving and a soft-bristled toothbrush for teeth). | ✔ | ✔ |
| • Demonstrate appropriate actions to take should bleeding occur. | ✔ | ✔ |

the exact cause is unknown, primary thrombocythemia is similar to other myeloproliferative disorders, particularly polycythemia vera. However, unlike the other myeloproliferative disorders, it rarely evolves into acute leukemia.

Primary thrombocythemia, which affects men and women equally, tends to occur in late middle age. The median survival exceeds 10 years.

## Clinical Manifestations

Many patients with primary thrombocythemia are asymptomatic; the illness is diagnosed as the result of finding an elevated platelet count on a CBC. Symptoms, when they do occur, result primarily from hemorrhage or vasoocclusion in the microvasculature. Symptoms occur most often when the platelet count exceeds 1 million/mm$^3$. However, symptoms do not always correlate with the extent to which the platelet count is elevated. Thrombosis is common and can be either arterial or venous; arterial thrombosis is more common (Harrison & Green, 2003). Because these platelets can be dysfunctional, minor or major hemorrhage can also occur. Bleeding from the mucous membranes of the nose and mouth is common, and significant GI bleeding is also possible. Bleeding typically does not occur unless the platelet count exceeds 1.5 million/mm$^3$.

Vasoocclusive manifestations are most frequently seen in the form of erythromelalgia. The toxic effects of platelet substances include painful burning, warmth, and redness in a localized distal area of the extremities. Neurologic manifestations occur in 25% of patients (Schafer, 2004). Numbness, tingling, chronic headache, and visual disturbance may be seen; these occlusive manifestations can progress to stroke and seizure and, less commonly, to MI. More common forms of venous thrombosis include DVT and pulmonary embolism. The spleen may be enlarged but usually not to a significant extent.

## Assessment and Diagnostic Findings

The diagnosis of primary thrombocythemia is made by ruling out other potential disorders—either other myeloproliferative disorders or underlying illnesses that cause a reactive or secondary thrombocytosis (see below). Iron deficiency should be excluded, because a reactive increase in the platelet count often accompanies this deficiency. Occult malignancy should be excluded. The CBC shows markedly large and abnormal platelets. Analysis of the bone marrow (by aspiration and biopsy) may not be particularly useful.

No data reliably predict the development of complications. Risk factors for the development of thrombotic complications are age older than 60 years, prior thrombotic or bleeding events, and preexisting cardiovascular risk factors (Schafer, 2004). Major bleeding tends to occur when the platelet count is very high.

## Medical Management

The management of primary thrombocythemia is highly controversial. The risk for significant thrombotic or hemorrhagic complications may not be increased until the platelet count exceeds 1.5 million/mm$^3$ (Schafer, 2004). A careful assessment of other risk factors, such as history of peripheral vascular disease, history of tobacco use, atherosclerosis, and prior thrombotic events, should be used in making the decision as to when to initiate therapy.

In younger patients with no risk factors, low-dose aspirin therapy may be sufficient to prevent thrombotic complications. However, the use of aspirin can increase the risk of hemorrhagic complications and is typically a contraindication in patients with a history of GI bleeding. Aspirin can relieve the neurologic symptoms (eg, headache), erythromelalgia, and visual symptoms of primary thrombocythemia.

In older patients and in those with concurrent risk factors, more aggressive measures may be necessary. Hydroxyurea (Hydrea), a chemotherapeutic medication, is effective in lowering the platelet count. This agent is taken orally and causes minimal side effects other than dose-related leukopenia. (However, its potential for leukogenesis diminishes its efficacy in younger patients with risk factors.) The medication anagrelide (Agrylin) is more specific in lowering the platelet count than hydroxyurea but has more side effects. Severe headaches cause many patients to stop taking the medication. Tachycardia and chest pain may also occur, and anagrelide is contraindicated in patients with concurrent cardiac problems. Interferon-alfa-2b (Intron-A) has been shown to lower platelet counts by an unknown mechanism. The medication is administered subcutaneously at varying frequency, commonly three times per week. Significant side effects, such as fatigue, weakness, memory deficits, dizziness, anemia, and liver dysfunction, limit its usefulness.

Rarely, the occlusive symptoms are so great that the platelet count must be reduced immediately. When necessary, platelet pheresis (see later discussion) can reduce the amount of circulating platelets, but only transiently. The extent to which symptoms and complications (eg, thromboses) are reduced by pheresis remains unclear.

## Nursing Management

Patients with primary thrombocythemia need to be instructed about the accompanying risks of hemorrhage and thrombosis. The patient is informed about signs and symptoms of thrombosis, particularly the neurologic manifestations, such as visual changes, numbness, tingling, and weakness. Risk factors for thrombosis are assessed, and measures to diminish risk factors (particularly cessation of tobacco use) are encouraged. Patients receiving aspirin therapy should be informed about the increased risk of bleeding. Patients who are at risk for bleeding should be instructed about medications (eg, aspirin, NSAIDs) and other substances (eg, alcohol) that can alter platelet function. Patients receiving interferon therapy are taught to self-administer the medication and manage side effects.

## *Secondary Thrombocytosis*

Increased platelet production is the primary mechanism of secondary, or reactive, **thrombocytosis**. The platelet count is above normal, but, in contrast to primary thrombocythemia, an increase to more than 1 million/mm$^3$ is rare. Platelet function is normal; the platelet survival time is normal or decreased. Consequently, symptoms associated with hemorrhage or thrombosis are rare. Many disorders or conditions can cause a reactive increase in platelets, including infection, chronic inflammatory disorders, iron deficiency, malignant disease, acute hemorrhage, and splenectomy (see previous discussion of primary thrombocythemia). Treatment is aimed at the underlying disorder. With successful management, the platelet count usually returns to normal.

# Thrombocytopenia

**Thrombocytopenia** (low platelet level) can result from various factors: decreased production of platelets within the bone marrow, increased destruction of platelets, or increased consumption of platelets. Causes and treatments are summarized in Table 33-4.

### TABLE 33-4  Causes and Management of Thrombocytopenia

| Cause | Management |
|---|---|
| **Decreased Platelet Production** | |
| Hematologic malignancy, especially acute leukemias | Treat leukemia; platelet transfusion |
| Myelodysplastic syndromes (MDS) | Treat MDS; platelet transfusion |
| Metastatic involvement of bone marrow from solid tumors | Treat solid tumor |
| Aplastic anemia | Treat underlying condition |
| Megaloblastic anemia | Treat underlying anemia |
| Toxins | Remove toxin |
| Medications | Stop medication |
| Infection (esp. septicemia, viral infection, tuberculosis) | Treat infection |
| Alcohol | Refrain from alcohol consumption |
| Chemotherapy | Delay or decrease dose; growth factor; platelet transfusion |
| **Increased Platelet Destruction** | |
| Due to antibodies: | Treat condition |
|   Idiopathic thrombocytopenic purpura (ITP) | |
|   Lupus erythematosus | |
|   Malignant lymphoma | |
|   Chronic lymphocytic leukemia (CLL) | Treat CLL and/or treat as ITP |
|   Medications | Stop medication |
| Due to infection: | Treat infection |
|   Bacteremia | |
|   Postviral infection | |
| Sequestration of platelets in an enlarged spleen | If thrombocytopenia is severe, splenectomy may be needed |
| **Increased Platelet Consumption** | |
| Disseminated intravascular coagulation (DIC) | Treat underlying condition triggering DIC; administer heparin, EACA, blood products |

## Clinical Manifestations

Bleeding and petechiae usually do not occur with platelet counts greater than 50,000/mm$^3$, although excessive bleeding can follow surgery or other trauma. When the platelet count drops to less than 20,000/mm$^3$, petechiae can appear, along with nasal and gingival bleeding, excessive menstrual bleeding, and excessive bleeding after surgery or dental extractions. When the platelet count is less than 5000/mm$^3$, spontaneous, potentially fatal central nervous system or GI hemorrhage can occur. If the platelets are dysfunctional due to disease (eg, MDS) or medications (eg, aspirin), the risk for bleeding may be much greater even when the actual platelet count is not significantly reduced.

## Assessment and Diagnostic Findings

A platelet deficiency that results from decreased production (eg, leukemia, MDS) can usually be diagnosed by examining the bone marrow via aspiration and biopsy. Infections, either viral or bacterial, as well as alcoholism can also suppress platelet production. When platelet destruction is the cause of thrombocytopenia, the marrow shows increased megakaryocytes (the cells from which the platelets originate) and normal or even increased platelet production as the body attempts to compensate for the decreased platelets in circulation. Another cause of thrombocytopenia is sequestration. Approximately one third of the circulating platelets are within the spleen, and a greatly enlarged spleen results in increased sequestration of platelets. Many medications (eg, sulfa drugs, methotrexate) can either decrease platelet production or shorten their life span. Numerous genetic causes of thrombocytopenia have been discovered, including autosomal dominant, autosomal recessive, and X-linked mutations (Drachman, 2004).

An important cause to exclude is "pseudothrombocytopenia." Here, platelets aggregate and clump in the presence of ethylenediamine tetra-acetic acid (EDTA), the anticoagulant present in the tube used for CBC collection. This clumping accounts for up to 20% of instances of isolated thrombocytopenia (Drachman, 2004). A manual examination of the peripheral smear can easily determine platelet clumping as the cause of thrombocytopenia; newer cell counter machines can also detect this.

## Medical Management

The management of secondary thrombocytopenia is usually treatment of the underlying disease. If platelet production is impaired, platelet transfusions may increase the platelet count and stop bleeding or prevent spontaneous hemorrhage. If excessive platelet destruction occurs, transfused platelets are also destroyed, and the platelet count does not increase. The most common cause of excessive platelet destruction is ITP (see the following discussion). In some instances splenectomy can be a useful therapeutic intervention, but often it is not an option; for example, in patients in whom the enlarged spleen is due to portal hypertension related to cirrhosis, splenectomy may cause more bleeding disorders.

## Nursing Management

The interventions for a patient with thrombocytopenia are listed in Chart 33-9.

## Idiopathic Thrombocytopenic Purpura

ITP is a disease that affects people of all ages, but it is more common among children and young women. There are two forms of ITP: acute and chronic. Acute ITP, which occurs predominantly in children, often appears 1 to 6 weeks after a viral illness. This form is self-limited; remission often occurs spontaneously within 6 months. Chronic ITP is often diagnosed by exclusion of other causes of thrombocytopenia.

### Pathophysiology

Although the precise cause of ITP remains unknown, viral infections sometimes precede the disease in children. Occasionally medications such as sulfa drugs can induce ITP. Other conditions, such as systemic lupus erythematosus or pregnancy, can also induce ITP. Antiplatelet autoantibodies that bind to the patient's platelets are found in the blood of patients with ITP. When the platelets are bound by the antibodies, the RES or tissue macrophage system ingests the platelets, destroying them. The body attempts to compensate for this destruction by increasing platelet production within the marrow.

### Clinical Manifestations

Many patients have no symptoms, and the low platelet count (often less than 20,000/mm$^3$; less than 5000/mm$^3$ is not uncommon) is an incidental finding. Common physical manifestations are easy bruising, heavy menses, and petechiae on the extremities or trunk. Patients with simple bruising or petechiae ("dry purpura") tend to have fewer complications from bleeding than those with bleeding from mucosal surfaces, such as the GI tract (including the mouth) and pulmonary system (eg, hemoptysis), which is termed "wet purpura." Patients with wet purpura have a greater risk of intracranial bleeding than do those with dry purpura. Despite low platelet counts, the platelets are young and very functional. They adhere to endothelial surfaces and to one another, so spontaneous bleeding does not always occur. Thus, treatment may not be initiated unless bleeding becomes severe or life-threatening, or the platelet count is extremely low (less than 10,000/mm$^3$) (Stasi & Provan, 2004).

### Assessment and Diagnostic Findings

Patients may have an isolated decrease in platelets (less than 20,000/mm$^3$ is common), but they may also have an increase in megakaryocytes (platelet precursors) within the marrow, as detected on bone marrow aspirate. Although many patients are found to be infected with *Helicobacter pylori*, it is currently unknown whether treatment of this infection will improve platelet counts (Franchini & Veneri, 2004). It is unclear why *H. pylori* and ITP are correlated. It is thought that *H. pylori* may cause an autoimmune reaction or that it binds von Willebrand factor (vWF), both of which may result in accelerated platelet demise.

### Medical Management

The primary goal of treatment is a "safe" platelet count. Because the risk for bleeding typically does not increase until the platelet count is less than 10,000/mm$^3$, a patient whose count exceeds 30,000/mm$^3$ to 50,000/mm$^3$ may be carefully observed without additional intervention. However, if the count is less than 20,000/mm$^3$ or if bleeding occurs, the goal is to improve the patient's platelet count rather than to cure the disease. The decision to treat should not be made merely on the basis of the patient's platelet count, but also on his or her lifestyle and activity level. A person with a sedentary lifestyle can tolerate a low platelet count more safely than one with a more active lifestyle.

Treatment for ITP usually involves several approaches. If the patient is taking a medication known to cause ITP (eg, quinine, sulfa-containing medications), that medication must be stopped immediately. The mainstay of short-term therapy is the use of immunosuppressive agents. These agents block the binding receptors on macrophages so that the platelets are not destroyed. Prednisone is the agent typically used, and it is effective in about 80% of patients (Zimmer et al., 2004). Cyclophosphamide (Cytoxan) and azathioprine (Imuran) can also be used, and dexamethasone (Decadron) may be effective. Platelet counts typically begin to rise within a few days after institution of corticosteroid therapy; this effect takes longer with azathioprine. Because of the associated side effects, patients cannot take high doses of corticosteroids indefinitely. It is not unusual for the platelet count to drop once the corticosteroid dose is tapered. Some patients can be successfully maintained on low doses of prednisone.

IV immune globulin (IVIG) is also commonly used to treat ITP. It is effective in binding the receptors on the macrophages; however, high doses are required, the drug is very expensive, and the effect is transient. Splenectomy is an alternative treatment but results in a sustained normal platelet count only 50% of the time; however, many patients can maintain a "safe" platelet count of more than 30,000/mm$^3$ after removal of the spleen. Even those who do respond to splenectomy may have recurrences of severe thrombocytopenia months or years later. Patients who have undergone splenectomy are permanently at risk for sepsis; these patients should receive pneumonia (Pneumovax), *Haemophilus influenzae* B, and meningococcal vaccines, preferably 2 to 3 weeks before the splenectomy is performed. The Pneumovax vaccine should be repeated at 5- to 10-year intervals.

Other management options include the chemotherapy agent vincristine (Oncovin). Vincristine appears to work by blocking the receptors on the macrophages and therefore inhibiting platelet destruction; it may also stimulate thrombopoiesis. Some data support the efficacy of certain monoclonal antibodies (eg, rituximab) in increasing platelet counts, but more research on their effects is needed (Robak, 2004).

Another approach to the management of chronic ITP involves the use of anti-D (WinRho) in patients who are Rh(D)-positive. The actual mechanism of action is unknown. One theory is that the anti-D binds to the patient's erythrocytes, which are in turn destroyed by the body's macrophages. The receptors in the RES may become saturated with the sensitized erythrocytes, diminishing removal of antibody-coated platelets. Anti-D produces a transient decreased hematocrit and increased platelet count in many, but not all, patients with ITP. Anti-D appears to be most effective in children with ITP and least effective in patients who have undergone splenectomy.

Despite the extremely low platelet count, platelet transfusions are usually avoided. Transfusions tend to be ineffective because the patient's antiplatelet antibodies bind with the transfused platelets, causing them to be destroyed. Platelet counts can actually drop after platelet transfusion. Occasionally, transfusion of platelets may protect against catastrophic bleeding in patients with severe wet purpura. Aminocaproic acid (EACA, Amicar), a fibrinolytic enzyme inhibitor that slows the dissolution of clots, may be useful for patients with significant mucosal bleeding refractory to other treatments.

## Nursing Management

Nursing care includes an assessment of the patient's lifestyle to determine the risk of bleeding from activity. A careful medication history is also obtained, including use of over-the-counter medications, herbs, and nutritional supplements. The nurse must be alert for sulfa-containing medications and others that alter platelet function (eg, aspirin-based or other NSAIDs). The nurse assesses for any history of recent viral illness and reports of headache or visual disturbances, which could be initial symptoms of intracranial bleeding. Patients who are admitted to the hospital with wet purpura and low platelet counts should have a neurologic assessment incorporated into their routine vital sign measurements. All injections or rectal medications should be avoided, and rectal temperature measurements should not be performed, because they can stimulate bleeding.

Patient teaching addresses signs of exacerbation of disease (petechiae, ecchymoses); how to contact appropriate health care personnel; the name and type of medication inducing ITP (if appropriate); current medical treatment (medications, tapering schedule if relevant, side effects); and the frequency of monitoring the platelet count. The patient is instructed to avoid all agents that interfere with platelet function. The patient should avoid constipation, the Valsalva maneuver (eg, straining at stool), and flossing of the teeth. Electric razors should be used for shaving, and soft-bristled toothbrushes should replace stiff-bristled ones. The patient is also counseled to refrain from vigorous sexual intercourse when the platelet count is less than 10,000/mm$^3$. Patients who are receiving corticosteroids long term are at risk for complications including osteoporosis, proximal muscle wasting, cataract formation, and dental caries (see Chart 33-3). Bone mineral density should be monitored, and these patients may benefit from calcium and vitamin D supplementation and bisphosphonate therapy to prevent significant bone disease.

# Platelet Defects

Quantitative platelet defects are relatively common (thrombocytopenia), but qualitative defects can also occur. With qualitative defects, the number of platelets may be normal, but the platelets do not function normally. In the past, platelet function was most commonly evaluated by the bleeding time; however, this test was a crude measurement. Now other tests using a platelet function analyzer exist; this method is particularly valuable for rapid and simple screening (Harrison & Green, 2003).

An important functional platelet disorder is that induced by aspirin. Even small amounts of aspirin reduce normal platelet aggregation, and the prolonged bleeding time lasts for several days after aspirin ingestion. Although this does not cause bleeding in most people, patients with a coagulation disorder (eg, hemophilia) or thrombocytopenia can have significant bleeding after taking aspirin, particularly if invasive procedures or trauma has occurred.

NSAIDs can also inhibit platelet function, but the effect is not as prolonged as with aspirin (about 5 days versus 7 to 10 days). Other causes of platelet dysfunction include end-stage renal disease, possibly from metabolic products affecting platelet function; MDS; multiple myeloma (due to abnormal protein interfering with platelet function); cardiopulmonary bypass; and other medications (Chart 33-12).

## Clinical Manifestations

Bleeding may be mild or severe. Its extent is not necessarily correlated with the platelet count or with tests that measure coagulation (prothrombin time [PT], partial thromboplastin time [PTT]). Ecchymoses are common, particularly on the extremities. Patients with platelet dysfunction may be at risk for significant bleeding after trauma or invasive procedures (eg, biopsy, dental extraction).

## Medical Management

If the platelet dysfunction is caused by medication, use of the offending medication should be stopped, if possible, particularly when bleeding occurs. If platelet dysfunction is marked, bleeding can often be prevented by transfusion of normal platelets before invasive procedures. Aminocaproic acid (EACA, Amicar) may be required to prevent significant bleeding after such procedures.

## Nursing Management

Patients with significant platelet dysfunction need to be instructed to avoid substances that can diminish platelet function, such as certain over-the-counter medications, herbs, nutritional supplements, and alcohol. They also need to serve as their own advocates and to inform their health care providers (including dentists) of the underlying condition before any invasive procedure is performed, so that appropriate steps can be initiated to diminish the risk of bleeding. Bleeding precautions should be initiated as appropriate (see Chart 33-9).

### CHART 33-12  PHARMACOLOGY · Medications and Substances That Impair Platelet Function

**Anesthetic Agents**
Local anesthetics
Halothane

**Antibiotics**
Beta-lactam antibiotics
  Penicillins
  Cephalosporins
Nitrofurantoin
Sulfonamides

**Anticoagulation Agents**
Heparin
Fibrinolytic agents

**Anti-inflammatory Agents (Nonsteroidal)**
Aspirin
Ibuprofen
Naproxen

**Antineoplastic Agents**
Carmustine
Daunorubicin
Mithramycin

**Cardiovascular Drugs**
Beta-blockers
Calcium channel blockers
Isosorbide
Nitroglycerine
Nitroprusside
Quinidine

**Medications That Increase Platelet cAMP**
Dipyridamole
Prostacycline
Theophylline

**Food and Food Additives**
Caffeine
Chinese black tree fungus
Clove
Cumin
Ethanol
Fish oils
Garlic
Onion extract
Turmeric

**Plasma Expanders**
Dextrans
Hydroxyethyl starch

**Psychotropic Agents**
Tricyclic antidepressants
Phenothiazines

**Miscellaneous**
Antihistamines
Clofibrate
Furosemide
Heroin
Contrast agents
Ticlopidine
Vitamin E

**Herbal Supplements**
Feverfew
Ginger
Gingko
Ginseng
Kava kava

## Hemophilia

Two inherited bleeding disorders—hemophilia A and hemophilia B—are clinically indistinguishable, although they can be distinguished by laboratory tests. Hemophilia A is caused by a genetic defect that results in deficient or defective factor VIII. Hemophilia B (also called Christmas disease) stems from a genetic defect that causes deficient or defective factor IX. Hemophilia is a relatively rare disease; hemophilia A, which occurs in 1 of every 10,000 births, is three times more common than hemophilia B. Both types of hemophilia are inherited as X-linked traits, so almost all affected people are males; females can be carriers but are almost always asymptomatic. The disease is recognized in early childhood, usually in the toddler age group. However, patients with mild hemophilia may not be diagnosed until they experience severe trauma (eg, a high-school football injury) or surgery. Hemophilia occurs in all ethnic groups.

### Clinical Manifestations

Hemophilia, which can be severe, is manifested by hemorrhages into various parts of the body. Hemorrhage can occur even after minimal trauma. The frequency and severity of the bleeding depend on the degree of factor deficiency as well as the intensity of the precipitating trauma. For example, patients with a mild factor VIII deficiency (ie, 6% to 50% of normal levels) rarely develop hemorrhage spontaneously; hemorrhage tends to occur secondary to trauma. In contrast, spontaneous hemorrhages, particularly hemarthroses and hematomas, can frequently occur in patients with severe factor VIII deficiency (ie, less than 1% of normal levels). These patients require frequent factor VIII replacement therapy.

About 75% of all bleeding in patients with hemophilia occurs into joints. The most commonly affected joints are the knees, elbows, ankles, shoulders, wrists, and hips. Patients often note pain in a joint before they are aware of swelling and limitation of motion. Recurrent joint hemorrhages can result in damage so severe that chronic pain or ankylosis (fixation) of the joint occurs. Many patients with severe factor deficiency are crippled by the joint damage before they become adults. Hematomas can be superficial or deep hemorrhages into muscle or subcutaneous tissue. With severe factor VIII deficiency, hematomas can occur without known trauma and progressively extend in all directions. When the hematomas occur within muscle, particularly in the extremities, peripheral nerves can be compressed. Over time, this compression results in decreased sensation, weakness, and atrophy of the area involved.

Bleeding is not limited to the joint areas. Spontaneous hematuria and GI bleeding can occur. Bleeding is also common in other mucous membranes, such as the nasal passages. The most dangerous site of hemorrhage is in the head (intracranial or extracranial). Any head trauma requires prompt evaluation and treatment. Surgical procedures typically result in excessive bleeding at the surgical site. Because clot formation is poor, wound healing is also poor. Such bleeding is most commonly associated with dental extraction.

## Medical Management

In the past, the only treatment for hemophilia was infusion of fresh frozen plasma, which had to be administered in such large quantities that patients experienced fluid volume overload. Now factor VIII and factor IX concentrates are available to all blood banks. Recombinant forms of these factors have been made available and may diminish the use of factor concentrates. Patients are given concentrates when they are actively bleeding or as a preventive measure before traumatic procedures (eg, lumbar puncture, dental extraction, surgery). The patient and family are taught how to administer the concentrate by IV at home at the first sign of bleeding. It is crucial to initiate treatment as soon as possible so that bleeding complications can be avoided. A few patients eventually develop antibodies to the concentrates, so their factor levels cannot be increased. Recombinant factor VIIa is approved by the FDA for patients with acquired antibodies to factors VIII and IX (Carr & Martin, 2004), but treatment is often unsuccessful.

Aminocaproic acid (EACA, Amicar) is very effective as an adjunctive measure after oral surgery. It is also useful in treating mucosal bleeding. Another agent, desmopressin (DDAVP), induces a transient rise in factor VIII levels; the mechanism for this response is unknown. In patients with mild forms of hemophilia A, desmopressin is extremely useful, significantly reducing the amount of blood products required. However, desmopressin is not effective in patients with severe factor VIII deficiency.

## Nursing Management

Most patients with hemophilia are diagnosed as children. They often require assistance in coping with the condition because it is chronic, places restrictions on their lives, and is an inherited disorder that can be passed to future generations. From childhood, patients are helped to cope with the disease and to identify the positive aspects of their lives. They are encouraged to be self-sufficient and to maintain independence by preventing unnecessary trauma that can cause acute bleeding episodes and temporarily interfere with normal activities. As they work through their feelings about the condition and progress to accepting it, they can assume more and more responsibility for maintaining optimal health.

Patients with mild factor deficiency may not be diagnosed until adulthood if they do not experience significant trauma or surgery as children. These patients need extensive teaching about activity restrictions and self-care measures to diminish the chance of hemorrhage and complications of bleeding. The nurse should emphasize safety at home and in the workplace.

Patients with hemophilia are instructed to avoid any agents that interfere with platelet aggregation, such as aspirin, NSAIDs, herbs, nutritional supplements, and alcohol. This restriction applies to over-the-counter medications such as cold remedies. Dental hygiene is very important as a preventive measure because dental extractions are so hazardous. Applying pressure may be sufficient to control bleeding resulting from minor trauma if the factor deficiency is not severe. Nasal packing should be avoided, because bleeding frequently resumes when the packing is removed. Splints and other orthopedic devices may be useful in patients with joint or muscle hemorrhages. All injections should be avoided; invasive procedures (eg, endoscopy, lumbar puncture) should be minimized or performed after administration of appropriate factor replacement. Patients with hemophilia should be encouraged to carry or wear medical identification.

During hemorrhagic episodes, the extent of bleeding must be assessed carefully. Patients who are at risk for significant compromise (eg, bleeding into the respiratory tract or brain) warrant close observation and systematic assessment for emergent complications (eg, respiratory distress, altered level of consciousness). If the patient has had recent surgery, the nurse frequently and carefully assesses the surgical site for bleeding. Frequent vital sign monitoring is needed until the nurse is certain that there is no excessive postoperative bleeding.

Analgesics are commonly required to alleviate the pain associated with hematomas and hemorrhage into joints. Many patients report that warm baths promote relaxation, improve mobility, and lessen pain. However, during bleeding episodes, heat, which can accentuate bleeding, is avoided; applications of cold are used instead.

Although recent technology (ie, the formulation of heat-solvent or detergent-treated factor concentrates) has rendered factor VIII and IX preparations free of viruses such as HIV and hepatitis, many patients have already been exposed to these infections through previous transfusions. These patients and their families may need assistance in coping with the diagnosis and the consequences of these infections.

Between 20% and 30% of patients with hemophilia A and between 1% and 3% of patients with hemophilia B develop antibodies (inhibitors) to factor concentrates (Chehab, 2002). Although one third of such inhibitors are transient, their effects can be significant and induce partial or complete refractoriness to factor replacement and result in increased risk of bleeding. Patients may require plasmapheresis or concurrent immunosuppressive therapy, particularly in the setting of significant bleeding. Factor VIIa can be administered, although it is very expensive and requires frequent administration because of its short half-life. Occasionally, tolerance to the antibody can be induced by repeated daily exposure to factor VIII. Patients receiving daily administration of factor VIII can take months or longer for tolerance to develop; however, it can be successful 60% to 80% of the time (Key, 2004). Patients with severe factor deficiency should be screened for antibodies, particularly before major surgery.

## Von Willebrand's Disease

Von Willebrand's disease, a common bleeding disorder affecting males and females equally, is usually inherited as a dominant trait. The prevalence of this disease is estimated to be 1%; thus, it is 50 times more prevalent than hemophilia (Tarantino & Aledort, 2004). The disease is caused by a deficiency of vWF, which is necessary for factor VIII activity. vWF is also necessary for platelet adhesion at the site of vascular injury. Although synthesis of factor VIII is normal, its half-life is shortened; therefore, factor VIII levels commonly are mildly low (15% to 50% of normal).

There are three types of von Willebrand's disease (Mannucci, 2004). Type 1, the most common, is characterized by decreases in structurally normal vWF. Type 2 shows variable qualitative defects based on the specific vWF subtype involved. Type 3 is very rare and is characterized by a severe vWF deficiency as well as significant deficiency of factor VIII.

### Clinical Manifestations

Patients commonly have nosebleeds, heavy menses, prolonged bleeding from cuts, and postoperative bleeding, although they do not have massive soft tissue or joint hemorrhages. As the laboratory values fluctuate (see Assessment and Diagnostic Findings), so does the bleeding. For example, a careful history of prior bleeding may show little problem with postoperative bleeding on one occasion but significant bleeding from a dental extraction at another time.

### Assessment and Diagnostic Findings

Laboratory test results show a normal platelet count but a prolonged bleeding time and a slightly prolonged PTT. These defects are not static, and laboratory test results can vary widely within the same patient over time. More important tests include the ristocetin cofactor, or vWF collagen binding assay, which measures vWF activity. Other tests include vWF antigen, factor VIII, and, for patients with suspected type 2 defects, vWF multimers (Paper, 2003).

### Medical Management

The goal of treatment is to replace the deficient protein (eg, vWF or factor VIII) at the time of spontaneous bleeding or prior to an invasive procedure. Replacement products include Humate-P, a commercial concentrate of vWF and factor VIII, and Alphanate, which contains similar amounts of these factors (Mannucci, 2004). Replacement continues for several days to ensure correction of the factor VIII deficiency. Up to 7 to 10 days of treatment may be necessary after major surgery, and the dosage and frequency of administration depend on factor VIII levels. Antibody (inhibitor) formation is usually seen only in patients with type 3 von Willebrand's disease, when large amounts of replacement products have been administered. Desmopressin (DDAVP), a synthetic vasopressin analogue, can be used to prevent bleeding associated with dental or surgical procedures or to manage mild bleeding after surgery. Desmopressin provides a transient increase in factor VIII coagulant activity and may also correct the bleeding time. It can be administered as an IV infusion or intranasally. With major surgery or invasive procedures, IV administration is preferable. DDAVP is contraindicated in patients with unstable coronary artery disease, because it can induce platelet aggregation and cause MI. Side effects include headache, facial flushing, tachycardia, hyponatremia, and rarely seizures.

Other agents may be effective in reducing the bleeding. Aminocaproic acid (EACA, Amicar) is useful in managing mild forms of mucosal bleeding. Estrogen-progesterone compounds may diminish the extent of menses. Platelet transfusions are useful when there is significant bleeding.

## Acquired Coagulation Disorders

### Liver Disease

With the exception of factor VIII, most blood coagulation factors are synthesized in the liver. Therefore, hepatic dysfunction (due to cirrhosis, tumor, or hepatitis; see Chapter 39) can result in diminished amounts of the factors needed to maintain coagulation and hemostasis. Prolongation of the PT, unless it is caused by vitamin K deficiency, may indicate severe hepatic dysfunction. Although minor bleeding is common (eg, ecchymoses), these patients are also at risk for significant bleeding, related especially to trauma or surgery. Transfusion of fresh frozen plasma may be required to replace clotting factors and to prevent or stop bleeding. Patients may also have life-threatening hemorrhage from peptic ulcers or esophageal varices. In these cases, replacement with fresh frozen plasma, PRBCs, and platelets is usually required.

### Vitamin K Deficiency

The synthesis of many coagulation factors depends on vitamin K. Vitamin K deficiency is common in malnourished patients, and some antibiotics decrease the intestinal flora that produce vitamin K, depleting vitamin K stores. Administration of vitamin K (phytonadione [Mephyton], either orally or as a subcutaneous injection) can correct the deficiency quickly; adequate synthesis of coagulation factors is reflected by normalization of the PT.

# Complications of Anticoagulant Therapy

Anticoagulants are used in the treatment or prevention of thrombosis. These agents, particularly warfarin or heparin, can cause bleeding. If the PT or PTT is longer than desired and bleeding has not occurred, the medication can be stopped or the dose decreased. Vitamin K is administered as an antidote for warfarin toxicity. Protamine sulfate is rarely needed for heparin toxicity, because the half-life of heparin is very short. With significant bleeding, fresh frozen plasma is needed to replace the vitamin K–dependent coagulation factors. Other complications of anticoagulant therapy are discussed in Chapter 31.

# Disseminated Intravascular Coagulation (DIC)

Disseminated intravascular coagulation (DIC), formerly termed disseminated intravascular coagulopathy, is not a disease but a sign of an underlying condition. DIC may be triggered by sepsis, trauma, cancer, shock, abruptio placentae, toxins, or allergic reactions. The severity of DIC is variable, but it is potentially life-threatening.

## Pathophysiology

Normal hemostatic mechanisms are altered in DIC so that a massive amount of tiny clots forms in the microcirculation. Initially, the coagulation time is normal. However, as the platelets and clotting factors are consumed to form the microthrombi, coagulation fails. Thus, the paradoxical result of excessive clotting is bleeding. The clinical manifestations of DIC are reflected in the organs, which are affected either by excessive clot formation (with resultant ischemia to all or part of the organ) or by bleeding. The excessive clotting triggers the fibrinolytic system to release fibrin degradation products, which are potent anticoagulants, furthering the bleeding. The bleeding is characterized by low platelet and fibrinogen levels; prolonged PT, PTT, and thrombin time; and elevated fibrin degradation products (**D-dimers**) (Table 33-5).

The mortality rate can exceed 80% of patients who develop severe DIC with ischemic thrombosis and frank hemorrhage. Identification of patients who are at risk for DIC and recognition of the early clinical manifestations of this syndrome can result in earlier medical intervention, which may improve the prognosis. However, the primary prognostic factor is the ability to treat the underlying condition that precipitated DIC.

## Clinical Manifestations

Patients with frank DIC may bleed from mucous membranes, venipuncture sites, and the GI and urinary tracts. The bleeding can range from minimal occult internal bleeding to profuse hemorrhage from all orifices. The patient may also develop organ dysfunction, such as renal failure and pulmonary and multifocal central nervous system infarctions, as a result of microthromboses, macrothromboses, or hemorrhages.

During the initial process of DIC, the patient may have no new symptoms, the only manifestation being a progressive decrease in the platelet count. As the thrombosis becomes more extensive, the patient exhibits signs and symptoms of thrombosis in the organs involved. Then, as the clotting factors and platelets are consumed to form these thrombi, bleeding occurs. Initially the bleeding is subtle, but it can develop into frank hemorrhage. Signs and symptoms, which depend on the organs involved, are listed in Chart 33-13.

## Medical Management

The most important management factor in DIC is treating the underlying cause; until the cause is controlled, the DIC will persist. Correcting the secondary effects of tissue ischemia by improving oxygenation, replacing fluids, correcting electrolyte imbalances, and administering vasopressor medications is also important. If serious hemorrhage occurs, the depleted coagulation factors and platelets may be replaced to reestablish the potential for normal hemostasis and thereby diminish bleeding. Cryoprecipitate is given to replace fibrinogen and factors V and VII; fresh frozen plasma is administered to replace other coagulation factors.

A controversial treatment strategy is to interrupt the thrombosis process through the use of heparin infusion. Heparin may inhibit the formation of microthrombi and thus permit perfusion of the organs (skin, kidneys, or brain) to resume. Heparin use was traditionally reserved for patients in whom thrombotic manifestations predom-

## TABLE 33-5 Laboratory Values Commonly Found in Disseminated Intravascular Coagulation (DIC)*

| Test | Function Evaluated | Normal Range | Changes in DIC |
|---|---|---|---|
| Platelet count | Platelet number | 150,000–450,000/mm$_3$ | ↓ |
| Prothrombin time (PT) | Extrinsic pathway | 11–12.5 sec | ↑ |
| Partial thromboplastin time (PTT) | Intrinsic pathway | 23–35 sec | ↑ |
| Thrombin time (TT) | Clot formation | 8–11 sec | ↑ |
| Fibrinogen | Amount available for coagulation | 170–340 mg/dL | ↓ |
| D-dimer | Local fibrinolysis | 0–250 ng/mL | ↑ |
| Fibrin degradation products (FDPs) | Fibrinolysis | 0–5 μg/mL | ↑ |
| Euglobulin clot lysis | Fibrinolytic activity | ≥2 hours | ≤1 hour |

*Because DIC is a dynamic condition, the laboratory values measured will change over time. Therefore, a progressive increase or decrease in a given laboratory value is likely to be more important than the actual value of a test at a single point in time.

### CHART 33-13

## Assessing for Recognizing Thrombosis and Bleeding in Disseminated Intravascular Coagulation (DIC)*

| SYSTEM | SIGNS AND SYMPTOMS OF MICROVASCULAR THROMBOSIS | SIGNS AND SYMPTOMS OF MICROVASCULAR AND FRANK BLEEDING |
|---|---|---|
| Integumentary system (skin) | ↓ Temperature, sensation; ↑ pain; cyanosis in extremities, nose, earlobes; focal ischemia, superficial gangrene | Petechiae, including periorbital and oral mucosa; bleeding: gums, oozing from wounds, previous injection sites, around catheters (IVs, tracheostomies); epistaxis; diffuse ecchymoses; subcutaneous hemorrhage; joint pain |
| Circulatory system | ↓ Pulses; capillary filling time > 3 sec | Tachycardia |
| Respiratory system | Hypoxia (secondary to clot in lung); dyspnea; chest pain with deep inspiration; ↓ breath sounds over areas of large embolism | High-pitched bronchial breath sounds; tachypnea; ↑ consolidation; signs and symptoms of acute respiratory distress syndrome |
| Gastrointestinal system | Gastric pain; "heartburn" | Hematemesis (heme⊕† NG output) melena (heme⊕ stools → tarry stools → bright-red blood from rectum) retroperitoneal bleeding (abdomen firm and tender to palpation; distended; ↑ abdominal girth) |
| Renal system | ↓ Urine output; ↑ creatinine, ↑ blood urea nitrogen | Hematuria |
| Neurologic system | ↓ Alertness and orientation; ↓ pupillary reaction; ↓ response to commands; ↓ strength and movement ability | Anxiety; restlessness; ↓ mentation, altered level of consciousness; headache; visual disturbances; conjunctival hemorrhage |

*Note: Signs of microvascular thrombosis are the result of an inappropriate activation of the coagulation system, causing thrombotic occlusion of small vessels within all body organs. As the clotting factors and platelets are consumed, signs of microvascular bleeding appear. This bleeding can quickly extend into frank hemorrhage. Treatment must be aimed at the disorder underlying the DIC; otherwise, the stimulus for the syndrome will persist.

†heme⊕, positive for hemoglobin

---

inated or in whom extensive blood component replacement failed to halt the hemorrhage or increased fibrinogen and other clotting levels. Heparin is now considered also applicable for use in less acute forms of DIC (Leung, 2004). The effectiveness of heparin can best be determined by observing for normalization of the plasma fibrinogen concentration and diminishing signs of bleeding. Fibrinolytic inhibitors, such as aminocaproic acid (EACA, Amicar), may be used with heparin.

Other therapies include recombinant activated protein C (APC; drotrecogin alfa [Xigris]), which is effective in diminishing inflammatory responses on the surface of the vessels as well as having anticoagulant properties (Aird, 2004). Bleeding is common, can occur at any site, and can be significant. Antithrombin (AT) infusions can also be used for their anticoagulant and anti-inflammatory properties. Bleeding can be significant, particularly when administered in association with heparin.

## ◀▶ Nursing Process

### The Patient With Disseminated Intravascular Coagulation

#### Assessment

Nurses need to be aware of which patients are at risk of DIC. Sepsis and acute promyelocytic leukemia are the most common causes of DIC. Patients need to be assessed thoroughly and frequently for signs and symptoms of thrombi and bleeding and monitored for any progression of these signs (see Chart 33-13).

## Diagnosis

### Nursing Diagnoses

Based on the assessment data, major nursing diagnoses for the patient with DIC may include the following:

- Risk for deficient fluid volume related to bleeding
- Risk for impaired skin integrity related to ischemia or bleeding
- Risk for imbalanced fluid volume related to excessive blood/factor component replacement
- Ineffective tissue perfusion related to microthrombi
- Death anxiety

### Collaborative Problems/Potential Complications

Collaborative problems include the clinical conditions that precipitated the DIC. Based on the assessment data, potential complications may include:

- Renal failure
- Gangrene
- Pulmonary embolism or hemorrhage
- Altered level of consciousness
- Acute respiratory distress syndrome
- Stroke

## Planning and Goals

Major patient goals include maintenance of hemodynamic status, maintenance of intact skin and oral mucosa, maintenance of fluid balance, maintenance of tissue perfusion, enhanced coping, and absence of complications, as described in the Plan of Nursing Care for the Patient with DIC (Chart 33-14).

## Nursing Interventions

See Chart 33-14.

### Monitoring and Managing Potential Complications

Assessment and interventions should target potential sites of end-organ damage. As organs are inadequately perfused from the microthrombi, organ function diminishes; the kidneys, lungs, brain, and skin are particularly vulnerable, and renal dysfunction is common. Lack of renal perfusion may result in acute tubular necrosis and renal failure, sometimes requiring dialysis. Placement of a large-bore dialysis catheter is extremely hazardous for this patient population and should be accompanied by adequate platelet and plasma transfusions. Hepatic dysfunction is also relatively common, reflected in altered liver function tests, depleted albumin stores, and diminished synthesis of clotting factors. Respiratory function warrants careful monitoring and aggressive measures to diminish alveolar compromise, such as incentive spirometry. Suctioning should be performed as gently as possible to diminish the risk for additional bleeding. Central nervous system involvement can be manifested as headache, visual changes, and alteration in level of consciousness.

## Evaluation

See Chart 33-14 for evaluation and expected outcomes for the patient with DIC.

# Thrombotic Disorders

As in many bleeding disorders, several conditions can alter the balance within the normal hemostasis process and cause excessive thrombosis. Abnormalities that predispose a person to thrombotic events include decreased clotting inhibitors within the circulation (which enhances coagulation), altered hepatic function (which may decrease production of clotting factors or clearance of activated coagulation factors), lack of fibrinolytic enzymes, and tortuous vessels (which promote platelet aggregation). Thrombosis can be caused by more than one predisposing factor. Several conditions can result from thrombosis, such as MI (see Chapter 28), CVA (brain attack or stroke; see Chapter 62), and peripheral arterial occlusion (see Chapter 31). Several inherited or acquired deficiency conditions, including hyperhomocysteinemia, AT III deficiency, protein C deficiency, APC resistance, factor V Leiden, and protein S deficiency can predispose a patient to repeated episodes of thrombosis; they are referred to as hypercoagulable states or thrombophilia. Table 33-6 lists these disorders, their abnormal laboratory values, and the need for family testing.

Thrombosis requires anticoagulation therapy. The duration of therapy varies with the location and extent of the thrombosis, precipitating events (eg, trauma, immobilization), and concurrent risk factors (eg, use of oral contraceptives, tortuous blood vessels, history of thrombotic events). With some conditions, lifelong anticoagulant therapy is necessary.

## Hyperhomocysteinemia

Increased plasma levels of homocysteine are a significant risk factor not only for venous thrombosis (eg, DVT, pulmonary embolism) but also for arterial thrombosis (eg, stroke, MI). Hyperhomocysteinemia can be hereditary, or it can result from a nutritional deficiency of folic acid and, to a lesser extent, of vitamins $B_{12}$ and $B_6$, because these vitamins are cofactors in homocysteine metabolism. For unknown reasons, people who are elderly, those with renal failure, and smokers may also have elevated levels of homocysteine in the absence of nutritional deficiencies of these vitamins. Although a simple fasting measurement of plasma homocysteine can serve as a useful screening test, people with genetically inherited hyperhomocysteinemia and those who are vitamin $B_6$ deficient may have normal or minimally elevated levels. A much more sensitive method involves obtaining a second measurement 4 hours after the patient consumes methionine; the hyperhomocysteinemia is found twice as often when this method is used. In hyperhomocys-

*(text continues on page 1098)*

CHART 33-14

# Plan of Nursing Care: The Patient With Disseminated Intravascular Coagulation (DIC)

**Nursing Diagnosis:** Risk for deficient fluid volume related to bleeding
**Goals:** Hemodynamic status maintained; urine output ≥30 mL/hr

| NURSING INTERVENTIONS | RATIONALE | EXPECTED OUTCOMES |
|---|---|---|
| 1. Avoid procedures/activities that can increase intracranial pressure (eg, coughing, straining to have a bowel movement). | 1. Prevents intracranial bleeding. | • Level of consciousness (LOC) stable<br>• CVP 5–12 cm H$_2$O, systolic BP ≥70 mm Hg<br>• Urine output ≥30 mL/hour<br>• Decreased bleeding<br>• Decreased oozing<br>• Decreased ecchymoses<br>• Amenorrhea<br>• Absence of oral and bronchial bleeding<br>• Oral mucosa clean, moist, intact |
| 2. Monitor vital signs closely, including neurologic checks:<br>  a. Monitor hemodynamics<br>  b. Monitor abdominal girth<br>  c. Monitor urine output | 2. Identifies signs of hemorrhage/shock quickly. | |
| 3. Avoid medications that interfere with platelet function if possible (eg, ASA, NSAIDs, beta-lactam antibiotics). | 3. Decreases problems with platelet aggregation and adhesion. | |
| 4. Avoid rectal probes, rectal medications. | 4. Decreases chance for rectal bleeding. | |
| 5. Avoid IM injections. | 5. Decreases chance for intramuscular bleeding. | |
| 6. Monitor amount of external bleeding carefully<br>  a. Monitor number of dressings, % of dressing saturated; time to saturate a dressing is more objective than "dressing saturated a moderate amount."<br>  b. Assess suction output, all excreta for frank or occult blood.<br>  c. Monitor pad counts in women with vaginal bleeding.<br>  d. Females may receive progesterone to prevent menses. | 6.<br>  a. Provides accurate, objective assessment of extent of bleeding.<br><br><br><br>  b. Identifies presence of or quantifies extent of bleeding.<br>  c. Quantifies extent of bleeding.<br>  d. Decreases chance for gynecologic source of hemorrhage. | |
| 7. Use low pressure with any suctioning needed. | 7. Prevents excessive trauma that could cause bleeding. | |
| 8. Administer oral hygiene carefully.<br>  a. Avoid lemon-glycerine swabs, hydrogen peroxide, commercial mouthwashes.<br>  b. Use sponge-tipped swabs, salt/baking soda (bicarbonate of soda) mouth rinses. | 8. Prevents excessive trauma that could cause bleeding. Glycerin and alcohol (in commercial mouthwashes) will dry mucosa, increasing risk for bleeding. | |
| 9. Avoid dislodging any clots, including those around IV sites and injection sites. | 9. Prevents excessive bleeding at sites. | |

## CHART 33-14

### Plan of Nursing Care: The Patient With Disseminated Intravascular Coagulation (DIC) (Continued)

**Nursing Diagnosis:** Risk for impaired skin integrity related to ischemia or bleeding
**Goals:** Skin integrity remains intact; oral mucosa remains intact

| NURSING INTERVENTIONS | RATIONALE | EXPECTED OUTCOMES |
|---|---|---|
| 1. Assess skin, with particular attention to bony prominences, skin folds. | 1. Prompt identification of any area at risk for skin breakdown or showing early signs of breakdown can facilitate prompt intervention and thus prevent complications. | • Skin integrity remains intact; skin is warm, and of normal color<br>• Oral mucosa is intact, pink, moist, without bleeding |
| 2. Reposition carefully; use pressure-reducing mattress.<br>3. Perform careful skin care every 2 hr, emphasizing dependent areas, all bony prominences, perineum.<br>4. Use lamb's wool between digits, around ears, as needed. | 2–4. Meticulous skin care and use of measures to prevent pressure on bony prominences decrease the risk of skin trauma. | |
| 5. Use prolonged pressure after injection or procedure when such measures must be performed (at least 5 min) | 5. Initial platelet plug is very unstable and easily dislodged, which can lead to increased bleeding. | |
| 6. Perform oral hygiene carefully (see above). | 6. Meticulous care is needed to decrease trauma, bleeding, and risk of infection. | |

**Nursing Diagnosis:** Risk for imbalanced fluid volume related to excessive blood and/or factor component replacement
**Goals:** Absence of edema; absence of rales; intake not greater than output

| NURSING INTERVENTIONS | RATIONALE | EXPECTED OUTCOMES |
|---|---|---|
| 1. Auscultate breath sounds every 2–4 hr. | 1. Crackles can develop quickly. | • Breath sounds clear<br>• Absence of edema<br>• Intake does not exceed output<br>• Weight stable |
| 2. Monitor extent of edema | 2. Fluid may extend beyond intravascular system. | |
| 3. Monitor volume of IVs, blood products; decrease volume of IV medications if indicated. | 3. Helps prevent fluid overload. | |
| 4. Administer diuretics as prescribed | 4. Decreases fluid volume. | |

**Nursing Diagnosis:** Ineffective tissue perfusion related to microthrombi
**Goals:** Neurologic status remains intact; absence of hypoxemia; peripheral pulses remain intact; skin integrity remains intact; urine output remains ≥30 mL/hr

*continued >*

| CHART 33-14 Plan of Nursing Care | The Patient With Disseminated Intravascular Coagulation (DIC) (Continued) | |
|---|---|---|
| **NURSING INTERVENTIONS** | **RATIONALE** | **EXPECTED OUTCOMES** |
| 1. Assess neurologic, pulmonary, integumentary systems.<br>2. Monitor response to heparin therapy.<br>3. Assess extent of bleeding.<br><br>4. Monitor fibrinogen levels.<br><br>5. Stop aminocaproic acid (EACA) if symptoms of thrombosis occur (see Table 33-7). | 1. Initial signs of thrombosis can be subtle.<br>2. Response to heparin is most accurately reflected in fibrinogen level.<br>3. Objective measurements of all sites of bleeding are crucial to accurately assess extent of blood loss.<br>4. Response to heparin is most accurately reflected in fibrinogen level.<br>5. EACA should be used only in setting of extensive hemorrhage not responding to replacement therapy. | • Arterial blood gases, $O_2$ saturation, pulse oximetry, LOC within normal limits.<br>• Breath sounds clear<br>• Absence of edema<br>• Intake does not exceed output<br>• Weight stable |

**Nursing Diagnosis:** Death anxiety
**Goals:** Fears verbalized/identified; realistic hope maintained

| **NURSING INTERVENTIONS** | **RATIONALE** | **EXPECTED OUTCOMES** |
|---|---|---|
| 1. Identify previous coping mechanisms, if possible; encourage patient to use them as appropriate.<br>2. Explain all procedures and rationale for these in terms patient and family can understand.<br>3. Assist family in supporting patient.<br>4. Use services from behavioral medicine, chaplain as needed. | 1. Identifying previous stressful situations can aid in recall of successful coping mechanisms.<br>2. Decreased knowledge and uncertainty can increase anxiety.<br><br>3. Family can be useful in assisting patient to use coping strategies and to maintain hope.<br>4. Additional professional intervention may be necessary, particularly if previous coping mechanisms are maladaptive or ineffective. Spiritual dimension should be supported. | • Previously used coping strategies identified and tried, to extent patient is able to do so<br>• Patient indicates understanding of procedures and situation as condition permits |

teinemia, the endothelial lining of the vessel walls is denuded; this can precipitate thrombus formation. Patients who are found to have hyperhomocysteinemia should receive folic acid, vitamin $B_6$, and/or vitamin $B_{12}$ supplements and should understand the rationale for their use.

## Antithrombin (AT) Deficiency

AT is a protein that inhibits thrombin and certain coagulation factors, and AT deficiency is a hereditary condition that can cause venous thrombosis, particularly when the AT level is less than 60% of normal. Patients with AT deficiency can develop venous thrombosis as young adults; by 50 years of age, two thirds of patients with AT deficiency have venous thrombosis. The most common sites for thrombosis are the deep veins of the leg and the mesentery. Recurrent thrombosis often occurs. There is an increased resistance to heparin anticoagulation, which means that these patients may require greater amounts of heparin to achieve adequate anticoagulation. Patients with AT deficiency should be encouraged to have their family members tested for the deficiency.

AT deficiency can also be acquired by four mechanisms: accelerated consumption of AT (as in DIC), re-

| TABLE 33-6 | Hypercoagulable States |
|---|---|
| **Disorder** | **Abnormal Laboratory Value*** |
| **Inherited Disorders (Family Testing Necessary)** | |
| Hyperhomocysteinemia | Homocysteine ↑ after methionine load |
| Antithrombin III (AT III) deficiency | AT III ↓ |
| Protein C deficiency | Protein C activity ↓ (must be measured off warfarin [Coumadin]) |
| Activated protein C (APC) resistance | Must be measured off anticoagulant; <2× prolongation of PTT when APC added. Patients with APC resistance have a smaller increase in clotting time than normal (ie, the prolongation of clotting time is less than normal). |
| Factor V Leiden | Positive |
| Protein S deficiency | Protein S activity ↓; must be measured off warfarin (Coumadin) |
| Dysfibrinogenemia | ↑ thrombin time; ↑ reptilase time; ↓ functional fibrinogen; often requires special fibrinogen assays |
| **Acquired Disorders (Family Testing Unnecessary)** | |
| Anticardiolipin antibody | Positive |
| Cancer | Varied, depending on disorder |
| Lupus anticoagulant | Positive |
| Hyperhomocysteinemia | Homocystine ↑ after methionine load |
| AT III deficiency | AT III ↓ |
| Paroxysmal nocturnal hemoglobinuria | + Hamm's test; acid hemolysis |
| Myeloproliferative disorders | Varied, depending on disorder |
| Nephrotic syndrome | Varied, depending on disorder |
| Cancer chemotherapy | Varied, depending on disorder |

*Protein C and protein S are vitamin K–dependent proteins. Warfarin (Coumadin) interferes with the hepatic synthesis of vitamin K–dependent factors, which may decrease levels of protein C or protein S; therefore, protein C and protein S should be measured while the patient is off warfarin.

duced synthesis of AT (as in hepatic dysfunction), increased excretion of AT (as in nephrotic syndrome), and medication-inducted (eg, estrogens, L-asparaginase) (Bauer, 2004).

## Protein C Deficiency

Protein C is an enzyme that, when activated, inhibits coagulation. When levels of protein C are deficient, the risk for thrombosis increases, and thrombosis can often occur spontaneously. Protein C deficiency is at least as prevalent as AT deficiency, and people who are deficient in protein C can develop thrombosis early in life, as early as 15 years of age. A rare but significant complication of anticoagulation management in patients with protein C deficiency is warfarin-induced skin necrosis. This complication appears to result from progressive thrombosis in the capillaries within the skin; the extent of the necrosis can be extreme.

## Activated Protein C (APC) Resistance and Factor V Leiden Mutation

APC resistance is a common condition that can occur with other hypercoagulable states. APC is an anticoagulant, and resistance to APC increases the risk for venous thrombosis. A molecular defect in the factor V gene has been identified in most (90%) of those with APC resistance; this defect is called factor V Leiden mutation. It has been identified as the most common cause of inherited hypercoagulability in Caucasians, but its incidence appears to be much lower in other ethnic groups. Factor V Leiden mutation synergistically increases the risk of thrombosis in patients with other risk factors (eg, use of oral contraceptives, hyperhomocysteinemia, increased age). It does not appear that the use of postmenopausal hormone therapy in women increases the risk of thrombotic events as does the use of oral contraceptives; the dose of estrogen in the former situation is much lower than in the latter. People who are homozygous for the factor V Leiden mutation are at extremely high risk of thrombosis and need life-long anticoagulation.

## Protein S Deficiency

Protein S is another natural anticoagulant normally produced in the liver. APC requires protein S to inactivate certain clotting factors. When the level of protein S is deficient, this inactivation process is diminished, and the risk of thrombosis can be increased. Like patients with protein C deficiency, those with protein S deficiency have a greater risk of recurrent venous thrombosis at a young age, as young as 15 years.

## Acquired Thrombophilia

Antibodies to phospholipids are common acquired causes for thrombophilia (hypercoagulable states). The most common antibodies present against phospholipids are either lupus or anticardiolipin antibodies. Both of these antibodies can be transient, resulting from infection or certain medications. Most thrombotic events are venous, but arterial thrombosis can occur in up to one third of the cases. Patients who persistently test positive for either antibody and who have had a thrombotic event are at significant risk of recurrent thrombosis (greater than 50%). Recurrent thromboses tend to be of the same type—that is, venous thrombosis after an initial venous thrombosis, arterial thrombosis after an initial arterial thrombosis. Thrombi typically occur in larger vessels.

Another common acquired cause of thrombophilia is cancer. Specific types of stomach, pancreatic, lung, and ovarian cancers are most commonly associated with thrombophilia. The type of thrombosis that results is unusual. Rather than DVT or pulmonary embolism, the thrombosis occurs in unusual sites, such as the portal, hepatic, or renal vein or the inferior vena cava. Migratory superficial thrombophlebitis or nonbacterial thrombotic endocarditis can also occur. In these patients, anticoagulation can be difficult to manage and the thrombosis can progress despite standard doses of anticoagulants.

## Medical Management

The primary method of treating thrombotic disorders is anticoagulation. However, in thrombophilic conditions, when to treat (prophylaxis or not) and how long to treat (lifelong or not) can be controversial. Anticoagulation therapy is not without risks; the most significant risk is bleeding. Risks of anticoagulation therapy are identified in Chapter 31. The most common anticoagulant medications are identified in the following section.

### Pharmacologic Therapy

Along with administering anticoagulant therapy, concerns include minimizing any risk factors that predispose a patient to thrombosis. When risk factors (eg, immobility after surgery, pregnancy) cannot be avoided, prophylactic anticoagulation may be necessary.

#### UNFRACTIONATED HEPARIN THERAPY

Heparin is a naturally occurring anticoagulant that enhances AT III and inhibits platelet function. To prevent thrombosis, heparin is typically given as a subcutaneous injection, two or three times daily. To treat thrombosis, heparin is usually administered IV. The therapeutic effect of heparin is monitored by serial measurements of the activated PTT; the dose is adjusted to maintain the range at 1.5 to 2.5 times the laboratory control. Oral forms are being evaluated in clinical trials (Nutescu et al., 2004).

**Heparin-induced Thrombocytopenia.** Heparin-induced thrombocytopenia (HIT) is a significant complication of heparin-based therapy, and any patient beginning heparin therapy should have the platelet count monitored. In HIT, antibodies are formed against the heparin complex. The actual incidence of HIT is unknown, but it has been shown to occur in as many as 5% of orthopedic patients receiving heparin (Warkentin, 2003). The type of heparin used and the duration of therapy appear to be risk factors for developing HIT: bovine preparations are more likely to lead to HIT than porcine preparations, and low-molecular-weight heparin (LMWH) formulations carry a lower risk. Prolonged use of heparin (beyond 4 days) and immobility are also risk factors (Warkentin, 2003). Neither the dose nor the route of administration (IV versus subcutaneous) is a risk (McIntosh, 2004). A decline in platelet count is a hallmark sign which typically occurs after 4 to 14 days of heparin therapy. The platelet count can drop significantly, usually by 50% of baseline. Interestingly, affected patients are at increased risk for thrombosis, either venous or arterial, and the thrombosis can range from DVT, MI, CVA (brain attack, stroke), to ischemic damage to an extremity necessitating amputation. The risk for fatal thrombosis is 4% to 5% (Warkentin, 2003). A mild form of HIT, HIT-1, is actually more common than HIT; HIT-1 results only in a mild decline in platelet count and usually occurs 1 to 4 days after heparin is initiated (Viale & Schwartz, 2004).

Treatment of HIT includes prompt cessation of heparin and initiation of an alternative means of anticoagulation. If the heparin is stopped without providing additional anticoagulation, the patient is at increased risk for developing new thrombi (McIntosh, 2004). Two inhibitors of thrombin, lepirudin (Refludan) and argatroban, are FDA-approved anticoagulants for the treatment of HIT.

#### LOW-MOLECULAR-WEIGHT HEPARIN THERAPY

LMWHs (eg, Dalteparin [Fragmin], Enoxaparin [Lovenox]) are special forms of heparin that have more selective effects on coagulation. Based on their biochemical properties, LMWHs have a longer half-life and a less variable anticoagulant response than standard heparin. These differences permit LMWHs to be safely administered only once or twice daily, without the need for laboratory monitoring for dose adjustments. The incidence of HIT is much lower when a LMWH is used; however, LMWH is 100% cross-reactive with HIT antibodies and therefore contraindicated in HIT (McIntosh, 2004). In certain conditions, the use of a LMWH has allowed anticoagulation therapy to be moved entirely to the outpatient setting. Many cases of uncomplicated DVT are being managed outside the hospital. LMWHs are also being increasingly used as "bridge therapy" when patients receiving anticoagulation therapy (warfarin) require an invasive procedure (eg, biopsy, surgery) (Spyropoulos et al., 2004). In this situation, warfarin is stopped and an LMWH is used in its place until the procedure is completed. After the procedure, warfarin therapy is resumed. The LMWH is discontinued after a therapeutic level of warfarin is achieved.

#### WARFARIN (COUMADIN) THERAPY

Coumarin anticoagulants (warfarin [Coumadin]) are antagonists of vitamin K and therefore interfere with the synthesis of vitamin K–dependent clotting factors. Coumarin anticoagulants bind to albumin, are metabolized in the liver, and have an extremely long half-life. Typically, a patient with a venous thromboembolus is initially treated with both heparin (either the unfractionated form or LMWH) and warfarin. When the international normalized ratio (INR), which is a standard method of reporting prothrombin time (PT), reaches the desired therapeutic range, the heparin is stopped. The dosage required to maintain the therapeutic range (typically an INR of 2.0 to 3.0) varies widely among patients and even within the same patient, depending on the diagnosis and the rationale for anticoagulation. Frequent monitoring of the INR is extremely important so that the dosage of warfarin can be adjusted as needed. Warfarin is affected by many medications; consultation with a pharmacist is important to assess the extent to which concurrently administered medications, herbs, and nutritional supplements may interact with warfarin. It is also affected by many foods, so patients need dietary instruction and may benefit from consultation with a dietitian. In particular, foods with high vitamin K content antagonize the effects of warfarin. Some of these foods include spinach, asparagus, and yogurt. Chart 33-15 lists agents that interact with warfarin.

## Nursing Management

Patients with thrombotic disorders should avoid activities that promote circulatory stasis (eg, immobility, crossing the legs). Exercise, especially ambulation, should be per-

## CHART 33-15

# PHARMACOLOGY · Agents That Interact with Warfarin (Coumadin)

Although warfarin (Coumadin), an anticoagulant medication, is commonly used to treat and prevent thrombosis, many drug–drug and drug–food interactions are associated with its use. A careful medication history (including over-the-counter medications, herbs, and other substances, such as vitamins and minerals) is important when oral anticoagulation therapy is prescribed. Consultation with a pharmacist is recommended to assess the extent to which concurrent medications may affect the anticoagulant and for appropriate dosage adjustments. The following list contains a few examples of agents that interact with warfarin.

### Agents That Inhibit Warfarin Function

- Barbiturates
- Carbamazepine
- Cholestyramine
- Corticosteroids
- Digitalis
- Estrogens
- Ethanol
- Glutethimide
- Griseofulvin
- Haloperidol
- Oral contraceptives
- Phenytoin
- Rifampin
- Spironolactone

### Agents That Potentiate Warfarin Function

- Acetaminophen
- Allopurinol
- Amiodarone
- Anabolic steroids
- Anti-inflammatory agents
- Antimalarial agents
- Aspirin
- Broad-spectrum antibiotics
- Chloral hydrate
- Chloramphenicol
- Cimetidine
- Colchicine
- Clofibrate
- Chlorpromazine
- Danazol
- Disulfiram
- Ethacrynic acid
- Feprazone
- Herbal medicines: feverfew, garlic, gingko, ginseng
- Vitamin C (in very large doses)
- Vitamin E (in very large doses)
- Isoniazid
- Mefenamic acid
- Methotrexate
- Metronidazole
- Oral hypoglycemic agents
- Oxyphenbutazone
- Phenytoin
- Probenecid
- Propylthiouracil
- Quinidine
- Quinine
- Salicylates
- Sulfinpyrazone
- Sulfonamides (long-acting)
- Thyroxine
- Triclofos
- Tricyclic antidepressants

---

formed frequently throughout the day, particularly during long trips by car or plane. Surgery further increases the risk for thrombosis. Medications that alter platelet aggregation, such as low-dose aspirin, may be prescribed. Some patients require life-long therapy with anticoagulants such as warfarin (Coumadin).

In addition, patients with thrombotic disorders, particularly those with thrombophilia, should be assessed for concurrent risk factors for thrombosis and should avoid concomitant risk factors if possible. For example, use of tobacco and nicotine products exacerbates the problem and should be avoided. Just as for other conditions, patients should know the name of their specific condition and understand its significance. In many instances, younger patients with thrombophilia may not require prophylactic anticoagulation; however, with concomitant risk factors (eg, pregnancy), increasing age, or subsequent thrombotic events, prophylactic or long-term anticoagulation therapy may be required. Being able to provide the health care provider with an accurate health history can be extremely useful and can help guide the selection of appropriate therapeutic interventions. Patients with hereditary disorders should encourage their siblings and children to be tested for the disorder.

When a patient with a thrombotic disorder is hospitalized, frequent assessments should be performed for signs and symptoms of beginning thrombus formation, particularly in the legs (DVT) and lungs (pulmonary embolism). Ambulation or range-of-motion exercises as well as the use of elastic compression stockings should be initiated promptly to decrease stasis. Prophylactic anticoagulants are commonly prescribed.

## Therapies for Blood Disorders

### Splenectomy

The surgical removal of the spleen (splenectomy) is sometimes necessary after trauma to the abdomen. Because the spleen is very vascular, severe hemorrhage can result if the spleen is ruptured. Under such circumstances, splenectomy becomes an emergency procedure.

Splenectomy is also a possible treatment for other hematologic disorders. For example, an enlarged spleen may be the site of excessive destruction of blood cells. If the destruction is life-threatening, surgery may be lifesaving. This is the case in autoimmune hemolytic anemia and ITP when these disorders do not respond to more conservative measures, such as corticosteroid therapy. Some patients with grossly enlarged spleens develop severe thrombocytopenia due to the platelets being sequestered in the spleen; splenectomy removes the "trap," and platelet counts may normalize over time.

In general, the mortality rate after splenectomy is low. Laparoscopic splenectomy can be performed in selected patients, with a resultant decrease in postoperative morbidity. Complications that may result from surgery are atelectasis, pneumonia, abdominal distention, and abscess formation. Although young children are at the highest risk after splenectomy, all age groups are vulnerable to overwhelming lethal infections and should receive the pneumonia vaccine (Pneumovax) before undergoing splenectomy, if possible.

The patient is instructed to seek prompt medical attention if even relatively minor symptoms of infection occur. Often, patients with high platelet counts have even higher counts after splenectomy (more than 1 million/mm$^3$), which can predispose them to serious thrombotic or hemorrhagic problems. However, this increase is transient and usually does not warrant additional treatment.

### Therapeutic Apheresis

*Apheresis* is a Greek word meaning separation. In therapeutic apheresis (or pheresis), blood is taken from the patient and passed through a centrifuge, where a specific component is separated from the blood and removed (Table 33-7). The remaining blood is then returned to the patient. The entire system is closed, so the risk of bacterial contamination is extremely low. When platelets or leukocytes are removed, the decrease in these cells within the circulation is temporary. However, the temporary decrease provides a window of time until suppressive medications (eg, chemotherapy) can have therapeutic effects. Sometimes plasma is removed rather than blood cells—typically so that specific, abnormal proteins within the plasma are transiently lowered until a long-term therapy can be initiated.

Apheresis is also used to obtain larger amounts of platelets from a donor than can be provided from a single unit of whole blood. A unit of platelets obtained in this way is equivalent to six to eight units of platelets obtained from six to eight separate donors via standard blood donation methods. Platelet donors can have their platelets apheresed as often as every 14 days. Leukocytes can be obtained similarly, typically after the donor has received growth factors (G-CSF, GM-CSF) to stimulate the formation of additional leukocytes and thereby increase the leukocyte count. The use of these growth factors also stimulates the release of stem cells within the circulation. Apheresis is used to harvest these stem cells (typically over a period of several days) for use in PBSCT.

### Therapeutic Phlebotomy

Therapeutic phlebotomy is the removal of a certain amount of blood under controlled conditions. Patients with elevated hematocrits (eg, those with polycythemia vera) or excessive iron absorption (eg, hemochromatosis) can usually be managed by periodically removing 1 unit (about 500 mL) of

| TABLE 33-7 | Types of Apheresis* | |
|---|---|---|
| **Procedure** | **Purpose** | **Examples of Clinical Use** |
| Platelet pheresis | Remove platelets | Extreme thrombocytosis, essential thrombocythemia (temporary measure); single-donor platelets transfusion |
| Leukapheresis | Remove WBCs (can be specific to neutrophils or lymphocytes) | Extreme leukocytosis (eg, AML, CML) (very temporary measure); harvest WBCs for transfusion |
| Erythrocytapheresis (RBC exchange) | Remove RBCs | RBC dyscrasias (eg, sickle cell disease); RBCs replaced via transfusion |
| Plasmapheresis (plasma exchange) | Remove plasma proteins | Hyperviscosity syndromes; treatment for some renal and neurologic diseases (eg, Goodpasture's syndrome, Guillain-Barré, myasthenia gravis) |
| Stem cell harvest | Remove circulating stem cells | Transplantation (donor harvest or autologous) |

*Therapeutic apheresis can be used to treat a wide variety of conditions. When it is used to treat a disease that causes an increase in a specific cell type with a short life in circulation (ie, WBCs, platelets), the reduction in those cells is temporary. However, this temporary reduction permits a margin of safety while waiting for a longer-lasting treatment modality (eg, chemotherapy) to take effect. Apheresis can also be used to obtain stem cells for transplantation, either from a matched donor (allogenic) or from the patient (autologous).

AML, acute myeloid leukemia; CML, chronic myeloid leukemia; RBC, red blood cell; WBC, white blood cell.

whole blood (Parker et al., 2004). Eventually this process can produce iron deficiency, leaving the patient unable to produce as many erythrocytes. The actual procedure for therapeutic phlebotomy is similar to that for blood donation (see later discussion).

## Blood Component Therapy

A single unit of whole blood contains 450 mL of blood and 50 mL of an anticoagulant. A unit of whole blood can be processed and dispensed for administration. However, it is more appropriate, economical, and practical to separate that unit of whole blood into its primary components: erythrocytes, platelets, and plasma (leukocytes are rarely used; see later discussion). Because the plasma is removed, a unit of PRBCs is very concentrated (hematocrit approximately 70%). Each component must be processed and stored differently to maximize the longevity of the viable cells and factors within it; each individual blood component has a different storage life. PRBCs are stored at 4°C. With special preservatives, they can be stored safely for up to 42 days before they must be discarded. In contrast, platelets must be stored at room temperature because they cannot withstand cold temperatures, and they last for only 5 days before they must be discarded. To prevent clumping, platelets are gently agitated while stored. Plasma is immediately frozen to maintain the activity of the clotting factors within; it lasts for 1 year if it remains frozen. Alternatively, plasma can be further pooled and processed into blood derivatives, such as albumin, immune globulin, factor VIII, and factor IX. Table 33-8 describes each blood component and how it is commonly used.

**TABLE 33-8 Blood and Blood Components Commonly Used in Transfusion Therapy***

| | Composition | Indications and Considerations |
|---|---|---|
| **Whole blood** | Cells and plasma, hematocrit about 40% | Volume replacement and oxygen-carrying capacity; usually used only in significant bleeding (>25% blood volume lost) |
| **Packed red blood cells (PRBCs)** | RBCs with little plasma (hematocrit about 75%); some platelets and WBCs remain | ↑ RBC mass<br>Symptomatic anemia: platelets in the unit are not functional; WBCs in the unit may cause reaction and are not functional |
| **Platelets—random** | Platelets ($5.5 \times 10^{10}$ platelets/unit)<br>Plasma; some RBCs, WBCs | Bleeding due to severe ↓ platelets<br>Prevent bleeding when platelets <5,000–10,000/mm³<br>Survival ↓ in presence of fever, chills, infection<br>Repeated treatment → ↓ survival due to alloimmunization |
| **Platelets—single donor** | Platelets ($3 \times 10^{11}$ platelets/unit)<br>1 unit is equivalent to 6–8 units of random platelets | Used for repeated treatment: ↓ alloimmunization risk by limiting exposure to multiple donors |
| **Plasma** | Plasma; all coagulation factors<br>Complement | Bleeding in patients with coagulation factor deficiencies; plasmapheresis |
| **Granulocytes** | Neutrophils (>$1 \times 10^{10}$/unit); lymphocytes; some RBCs and platelets | Severe neutropenia in selected patients; controversial |
| **Lymphocytes (WBCs)** | Lymphocytes (number varies) | Stimulate graft-versus-disease effect |
| **Cryoprecipitate** | Fibrinogen ≥150 mg/bag, AHF (VIII:C) 80–110 units/bag, von Willebrand factor; fibronectin | von Willebrand's disease<br>Hypofibrinogenemia<br>Hemophilia A |
| **Antihemophilic factor (AHF)** | Factor VIII | Hemophilia A |
| **Factor IX concentrate** | Factor IX | Hemophilia B (Christmas disease) |
| **Factor IX complex** | Factors II, VII, IX, X | Hereditary factor VII, IX, X deficiency; hemophilia A with factor VII inhibitors |
| **Albumin** | Albumin 5%, 25% | Hypoproteinemia; burns; volume expansion by 5% to ↑ blood volume; 25% → ↓ hematocrit |
| **Intravenous gamma globulin** | IgG antibodies | Hypogammaglobulinemia (in CLL, recurrent infections); ITP; primary immunodeficiency states |
| **Antithrombin III concentrate (AT III)** | AT III (trace amounts of other plasma proteins) | AT III deficiency with or at risk for thrombosis |

*The composition of each type of blood component is described as well as the most common indications for using a given blood component. RBCs, platelets, and fresh frozen plasma are the blood products most commonly used. When transfusing these blood products, it is important to realize that the individual product is always "contaminated" with very small amounts of other blood products (eg, WBCs mixed in a unit of platelets). This contamination can cause some difficulties, particularly isosensitization, in certain patients.

AHF, antihemophilic factor; CLL, chronic lymphocytic leukemia; ITP, idiopathic thrombocytopenic purpura.

## Special Preparations

Factor VIII concentrate (antihemophilic factor) is a lyophilized, freeze-dried concentrate of pooled fractionated human plasma. It is used in treating hemophilia A. Factor IX concentrate (prothrombin complex) is similarly prepared and contains factors II, VII, IX, and X. It is used primarily for treatment of factor IX deficiency (hemophilia B). Factor IX concentrate is also useful in treating congenital factor VII and factor X deficiencies. Recombinant forms of factor VIII, such as Humate-P or Alphanate, are also useful. Because they contain vWF, these agents are used in von Willebrand's disease as well as in hemophilia A, particularly when patients develop acquired factor VIII inhibitors (eg, antibodies).

Plasma albumin is a large protein molecule that usually stays within vessels and is a major contributor to plasma oncotic pressure. This protein is used to expand the blood volume of patients in hypovolemic shock and, rarely, to increase the concentration of circulating albumin in patients with hypoalbuminemia.

Immune globulin is a concentrated solution of the antibody IgG; it contains very little IgA or IgM. It is prepared from large pools of plasma. The IV form (IVIG) is used in various clinical situations to replace inadequate amounts of IgG in patients who are at risk for recurrent bacterial infection (eg, those with CLL, those receiving BMT or PBSCT). It is also used in certain autoimmune disorders, such as ITP. IVIG, in contrast to all other fractions of human blood, cells, or plasma, can survive being subjected to heating at 60°C (140°F) for 10 hours to free it of the viral contaminants that may be present (Chart 33-16).

## Procuring Blood and Blood Products

### Blood Donation

To protect both the donor and the recipients, all prospective donors are examined and interviewed before they are allowed to donate their blood. The intent of the interview is to assess the general health status of the donor and to identify risk factors that might harm a recipient of the donor's blood. Donors should be in good health and without any of the following:

- A history of viral hepatitis at any time in the past, or a history of close contact with a patient who had hepatitis or was undergoing dialysis within 6 months
- A history of receiving a blood transfusion or an infusion of any blood derivative (other than serum albumin) within 12 months. (People previously transfused in the United Kingdom, Gibraltar, or Falkland Islands are not allowed to donate blood in the United States because they have an increased likelihood of transmitting Creutzfeldt-Jakob disease.)
- A history of untreated syphilis or malaria, because these diseases can be transmitted by transfusion even years later. A person who has been free of symptoms and off therapy for 3 years after malaria may be a donor.
- A history or evidence of drug abuse in which illicit drugs were self-injected, because many IV/injection drug abusers are carriers of hepatitis and because the risk of HIV is high in this group
- A history of possible exposure to HIV; the population at risk includes people who engage in anal sex, people with multiple sexual partners, IV drug abusers, sexual partners of people at risk of HIV, and people with hemophilia

---

**CHART 33-16**

### Diseases Transmitted by Blood Transfusion

**Hepatitis (Viral Hepatitis B, C)**
- Greater risk from pooled blood products and blood of paid donors than from volunteer donors
- Screening test detects most hepatitis B and C
- Transmittal risk estimated at 1:10,000

**AIDS (HIV and HTLV)**
- Donated blood screened for antibodies to HIV
- Transmittal risk estimated at 1:670,000
- People with high-risk behaviors (multiple sex partners, anal sex, IV/injection drug use) and people with signs and symptoms that suggest AIDS should not donate blood

**Cytomegalovirus (CMV)**
- Transmittal risk greater for premature newborns with CMV antibody-negative mothers and for immunocompromised recipients who are CMV-negative (eg, those with acute leukemia, organ or tissue transplant recipients).
- Blood products rendered "leukocyte-reduced" help reduce transmission of virus.

**Graft-Versus-Host Disease (GVHD)**
- Occurs only in severely immunocompromised recipients (eg, Hodgkin's disease, bone marrow transplantation).
- Transfused lymphocytes engraft in recipient and attack host lymphocytes or body tissues; signs and symptoms are fever, diffuse reddened skin rash, nausea, vomiting, diarrhea.
- Preventive measures include irradiating blood products to inactivate donor lymphocytes (no known radiation risks to transfusion recipient) and processing donor blood with leukocyte reduction filters.

**Creutzfeldt-Jakob Disease (CJD)**
- Rare, fatal disease causing irreversible brain damage
- No evidence of transmittal by transfusion, but hemophiliacs and others are concerned that transmittal is possible
- All blood donors must be screened for positive family history of CJD.
- Potential donors who spent 6 months or more in the United Kingdom (or Europe) from 1980 to 1996 cannot donate blood; blood products from a donor who develops CJD are recalled.

- A skin infection, because of the possibility of contaminating the phlebotomy needle, and subsequently the blood itself
- A recent history of asthma, urticaria, or allergy to medications, because hypersensitivity can be transferred passively to the recipient
- Pregnancy, because of the nutritional demands of pregnancy on the mother
- A history of tooth extraction or oral surgery within 72 hours, because such procedures are frequently associated with transient bacteremia
- A history of untreated exposure to infectious disease within the past 3 weeks, because of the risk of transmission to the recipient
- Recent immunizations, because of the risk of transmitting live organisms (2-week waiting period for live, attenuated organisms; 1 month for rubella, mumps, varicella; 1 year for rabies)
- A history of recent tattoo, because of the risk of bloodborne infections (eg, hepatitis, HIV)
- Cancer, because of the uncertainty about transmission of the disease. People who have a history of a nonhematologic cancer treated with surgery or radiation and who are without evidence of recurrence for at least 5 years are eligible to donate.
- A diagnosis of hemochromatosis (although this exclusion is under debate)
- A history of whole blood donation within the past 56 days

Potential donors should be asked whether they have consumed any aspirin or aspirin-containing medications within the past 3 days. Although aspirin use does not render the donor ineligible, the platelets obtained would be dysfunctional and therefore not useful; aspirin usage within 48 to 72 hours contraindicates platelet donation. Aspirin does not affect the erythrocytes or plasma obtained from the donor.

All donors are expected to meet the following minimal requirements:

- Body weight should exceed 50 kg (110 pounds) for a standard 450-mL donation. Donors weighing less than 50 kg donate proportionately less blood. People younger than 17 years of age are disqualified from donation.
- The oral temperature should not exceed 37.5°C (99.6°F).
- The pulse rate should be regular and between 50 and 100 beats per minute.
- The systolic arterial blood pressure should be 90 to 180 mm Hg, and the diastolic pressure should be 50 to 100 mm Hg.
- The hemoglobin level should be at least 12.5 g/dL for women and 13.5 g/dL for men.

### Directed Donation

At times, friends and family of a patient wish to donate blood for that person. These blood donations are termed directed donations. These donations are not any safer than those provided by random donors, because directed donors may not be as willing to identify themselves as having a history of any of the risk factors that disqualify a person from donating blood.

### Standard Donation

Phlebotomy consists of venipuncture and blood withdrawal. Standard precautions are used. Donors are placed in a semi-recumbent position. The skin over the antecubital fossa is carefully cleansed with an antiseptic preparation, a tourniquet is applied, and venipuncture is performed. Withdrawal of 450 mL of blood usually takes less than 15 minutes. After the needle is removed, donors are asked to hold the involved arm straight up, and firm pressure is applied with sterile gauze for 2 to 3 minutes or until bleeding stops. A firm bandage is then applied. The donor remains recumbent until he or she feels able to sit up, usually within a few minutes. Donors who experience weakness or faintness should rest for a longer period. The donor then receives food and fluids and is asked to remain another 15 minutes.

The donor is instructed to leave the dressing on and to avoid heavy lifting for several hours, to avoid smoking for 1 hour, to avoid drinking alcoholic beverages for 3 hours, to increase fluid intake for 2 days, and to eat healthy meals for 2 weeks. Specimens from this donated blood are tested to detect infections and to identify the specific blood type (see later discussion).

### Autologous Donation

A patient's own blood may be collected for future transfusion; this method is useful for many elective surgeries where the potential need for transfusion is high (eg, orthopedic surgery). Preoperative donations are ideally collected 4 to 6 weeks before surgery. Iron supplements are prescribed during this period to prevent depletion of iron stores. Occasionally, erythropoietin (epoetin-alfa [Epogen, Procrit]) is given to stimulate erythropoiesis so that the donor's hematocrit remains high enough to be eligible for donation. Typically, 1 unit of blood is drawn each week; the number of units obtained varies with the type of surgical procedure to be performed (ie, the amount of blood anticipated to be transfused). Phlebotomies are not performed within 72 hours of surgery. Individual blood components can also be collected.

The primary advantage of autologous transfusions is the prevention of viral infections from another person's blood. Other advantages include safe transfusion for patients with a history of transfusion reactions, prevention of alloimmunization, and avoidance of complications in patients with alloantibodies. It is the policy of the American Red Cross that autologous blood be transfused only to the donor. If the blood is not required, it can be frozen until the donor needs it in the future (for up to 10 years). The blood is never returned to the general donor supply of blood products to be used by another person.

The disadvantage of autologous donation is that it may be performed even when the likelihood that the anticipated procedure will necessitate a transfusion is small. Needless autologous donation is expensive, takes time, and uses resources inappropriately. Moreover, in an emergency situation, the autologous units available may be inadequate, and the patient may still require additional units from the general donor supply. Furthermore, although autologous transfusion can eliminate the risk of viral contamination, the risk for bacterial contamination is the same as that in transfusion from random donors.

Contraindications to donation of blood for autologous transfusion are acute infection, severely debilitating chronic disease, hemoglobin level less than 12.5 g/dL, hematocrit less than 38%, unstable angina, and acute cardiovascular or cerebrovascular disease. A history of poorly controlled epilepsy may be considered a contraindication in some centers. Patients with cancer may donate for themselves.

### Intraoperative Blood Salvage

This transfusion method provides replacement for patients who cannot donate before surgery and for those undergoing vascular, orthopedic, or thoracic surgery. During a surgical procedure, blood lost into a sterile cavity (eg, hip joint) is suctioned into a cell-saver machine. The whole blood or PRBCs are washed, often with saline solution, filtered, and then returned to the patient as an IV infusion. Salvaged blood cannot be stored, because bacteria cannot be completely removed from the blood and it cannot be used when it is contaminated with bacteria (Kirschman, 2004).

### Hemodilution

This transfusion method may be initiated before or after induction of anesthesia. About 1 to 2 units of blood are removed from the patient through a venous or arterial line and simultaneously replaced with a colloid or crystalloid solution. The blood obtained is then reinfused after surgery. The advantage of this method is that the patient loses fewer erythrocytes during surgery, because the added IV solutions dilute the concentration of erythrocytes and lower the hematocrit. However, patients who are at risk of myocardial injury should not be further stressed by hemodilution.

## Complications of Blood Donation

Excessive bleeding at the donor's venipuncture site is sometimes caused by a bleeding disorder in the donor but more often results from a technique error: laceration of the vein, excessive tourniquet pressure, or failure to apply enough pressure after the needle is withdrawn.

Fainting is common after blood donation and may be related to emotional factors, a vasovagal reaction, or prolonged fasting before donation. Because of the loss of blood volume, hypotension and syncope may occur when the donor assumes an erect position. A donor who appears pale or complains of faintness should immediately lie down or sit with the head lowered below the knees. He or she should be observed for another 30 minutes.

Anginal chest pain may be precipitated in patients with unsuspected coronary artery disease. Seizures can occur in donors with epilepsy, although the incidence is very low. Both angina and seizures require further medical evaluation.

Many people have the misconception that donating blood can cause acquired immunodeficiency syndrome (AIDS) and other infections. Potential donors need to be educated that the equipment used in donation is sterile, a closed system, and not reusable; they are at no risk for acquiring infections such as AIDS from donating blood.

## Blood Processing

Samples of the unit of blood are always taken immediately after donation so that the blood can be typed and tested. Each donation is tested for antibodies to HIV 1 and 2, hepatitis B core antibody (anti-HBc), hepatitis C virus (HCV), and human T-cell lymphotropic virus, type I (anti-HTLV-I/II). The blood is also tested for hepatitis B surface antigen (HbsAG) and for syphilis. Negative reactions are required for the blood to be used, and each unit of blood is labeled to certify the results. A new testing method, nucleic acid amplification testing, has increased the ability to detect the presence of HCV, HIV, and West Nile virus infection, because it directly tests for genomic nucleic acids of the viruses rather than for the presence of antibodies to the viruses. This testing significantly shortens the "window" of inability to detect HIV and HCV from a donated unit, further ensuring the safety of the blood; the risk of transmission of HIV or HCV is now estimated at 1 in 2 million blood units (Goodman, 2004). Blood is also screened for CMV; if it tests positive for CMV, it can still be used, except in recipients who are negative for CMV and who are immunocompromised (eg, BMT or PBSCT recipients).

Equally important to viral testing is accurate determination of the blood type. More than 200 antigens have been identified on the surface of RBC membranes. Of these, the most important for safe transfusion are the ABO and Rh systems. The ABO system identifies which sugars are present on the membrane of a person's erythrocytes: A, B, both A and B, or neither A nor B (type O). To prevent a significant reaction, the same type of PRBCs should be transfused. Previously, it was thought that in an emergency situation in which the patient's blood type was not known, type O blood could be safely transfused. This practice is no longer advised by the American Red Cross.

The Rh antigen (also called D) is present on the surface of erythrocytes in 85% of the population (Rh-positive). Those who lack the D antigen are called Rh-negative. PRBCs are routinely tested for the D antigen as well as ABO. Patients should receive PRBCs with a compatible Rh type.

The majority of transfusion reactions (other than those due to procedural error) are due to the presence of donor leukocytes within the blood component unit (PRBCs or platelets); the recipient may form antibodies to the antigens present on these leukocytes. PRBC components typically have 1 to $3 \times 10^9$ leukocytes remaining in each unit. Leukocytes from the blood product are frequently filtered to diminish the likelihood of developing reactions and refractoriness to transfusions, particularly in patients who have chronic transfusion needs. The process of leukocyte filtration renders the blood component "leukocyte-poor" (leukopoor). Filtration can occur at the time the unit is collected from the donor and processed, which achieves better results but is more expensive, or at the time the blood component is transfused by attaching a leukocyte filter to the blood administration tubing. Many centers advocate routinely using leukopoor filtered blood components for people who have or are likely to develop chronic transfusion requirements.

When a patient is extremely immunocompromised, as in the case of bone or stem cell transplant, any donor lymphocytes must be removed from the blood components. In this situation, the blood component is exposed to low amounts of radiation (25 Gy) that kill any lymphocytes within the blood component. Irradiated blood products are highly effective in preventing transfusion-associated GVHD, which is fatal in most cases. Irradiated blood products have a shorter shelf life.

# Transfusion

Administration of blood and blood components requires knowledge of correct administration techniques and possible complications. It is very important to be familiar with the agency's policies and procedures for transfusion therapy. Methods for transfusing blood components are presented in Charts 33-17 and 33-18.

## Setting

Although most blood transfusions are performed in the acute care setting, patients with chronic transfusion requirements often can receive transfusions in other settings. Free-standing infusion centers, ambulatory care clinics, physicians' offices, and even patients' homes may be appropriate settings for transfusion. Typically, patients who need chronic transfusions but are otherwise stable physically are appropriate candidates for outpatient therapy. Verification and administration of the blood product are performed as in a hospital setting. Although most blood products can be transfused in the outpatient setting, the home is typically

---

**CHART 33-17**

### Transfusion of Packed Red Blood Cells (PRBCs)

**Preprocedure**

1. Confirm that the transfusion has been prescribed.
2. Check that patient's blood has been typed and cross-matched.
3. Verify that patient has signed a written consent form per institution or agency policy.
4. Explain the procedure to the patient. Instruct patient in signs and symptoms of transfusion reaction (itching, hives, swelling, shortness of breath, fever, chills).
5. Take patient's temperature, pulse, respiration, and blood pressure to establish a baseline for comparing vital signs during transfusion.
6. Use hand hygiene and wear gloves in accordance with Standard Precautions.
7. Use a 20-gauge or larger needle for insertion in a large vein. Use special tubing that contains a blood filter to screen out fibrin clots and other particulate matter. Do not vent the blood container.

**Procedure**

1. Obtain the PRBCs from the blood bank *after* the intravenous line is started. (Institution policy may limit release to only 1 unit at a time.)
2. Double-check the labels with another nurse or physician to make sure that the ABO group and Rh type agree with the compatibility record. Check to see that the number and type on the donor blood label and on the patient's chart are correct. Check the patient's identification by asking the patient's name and checking the identification wristband.
3. Check the blood for gas bubbles and any unusual color or cloudiness. (Gas bubbles may indicate bacterial growth. Abnormal color or cloudiness may be a sign of hemolysis.)
4. Make sure PRBC transfusion is initiated within 30 min after removal of the PRBCs from the blood bank refrigerator.
5. For first 15 minutes, run the transfusion slowly—no faster than 5 mL/min. Observe the patient carefully for adverse effects. If no adverse effects occur during the first 15 min, increase the flow rate unless the patient is at high risk for circulatory overload.
6. Monitor closely for 15–30 min to detect signs of reaction. Monitor vital signs at regular intervals per institution or agency policy; compare results with baseline measurements. Increase frequency of measurements based on patient's condition. Observe the patient frequently throughout the transfusion for any signs of adverse reaction, including restlessness, hives, nausea, vomiting, torso or back pain, shortness of breath, flushing, hematuria, fever, or chills. Should any adverse reaction occur, stop infusion immediately, notify physician, and follow the agency's transfusion reaction standard.
7. Note that administration time does not exceed 4 hr because of the increased risk for bacterial proliferation.
8. Be alert for signs of adverse reactions: circulatory overload, sepsis, febrile reaction, allergic reaction, and acute hemolytic reaction.
9. Change blood tubing after every 2 units transfused, to decrease chance of bacterial contamination.

**Postprocedure**

1. Obtain vital signs and compare with baseline measurements.
2. Dispose of used materials properly.
3. Document procedure in patient's medical record, including patient assessment findings and tolerance to procedure.
4. Monitor patient for response to and effectiveness of the procedure.

---

*Note:* Never add medications to blood or blood products; if blood is too thick to run freely, normal saline may be added to the unit. If blood must be warmed, use an in-line blood warmer with a monitoring system.

## CHART 33-18

### Transfusion of Platelets or Fresh Frozen Plasma (FFP)

**Preprocedure**
1. Confirm that the transfusion has been prescribed.
2. Verify that patient has signed a written consent form per institution policy.
3. Explain the procedure to the patient. Instruct patient in signs and symptoms of transfusion reaction (itching, hives, swelling, shortness of breath, fever, chills).
4. Take patient's temperature, pulse, respiration, and blood pressure to establish a baseline for comparing vital signs during transfusion.
5. Use hand hygiene and wear gloves in accordance with Standard Precautions.
6. Use a 22-gauge or larger needle for placement in a large vein, if possible. Use appropriate tubing per institution policy (platelets often require different tubing from that used for other blood products).

**Procedure**
1. Obtain the platelets or FFP from the blood bank (only *after* the intravenous line is started.)
2. Double-check the labels with another nurse or physician to make sure that the ABO group matches the compatibility record (not usually necessary for platelets; here only if compatible platelets are ordered). Check to see that the number and type on the donor blood label and on the patient's chart are correct. Check the patient's identification by asking the patient's name and checking the identification wristband.
3. Check the blood product for any unusual color or clumps (excessive redness indicates contamination with larger amounts of red blood cells).
4. Make sure platelets or FFP units are administered immediately after they are obtained.
5. Infuse each unit as fast as patient can tolerate to diminish platelet clumping during administration. Observe the patient carefully for adverse effects, including circulatory overload. Decrease rate of infusion if necessary.
6. Observe the patient closely throughout the transfusion for any signs of adverse reaction, including restlessness, hives, nausea, vomiting, torso or back pain, shortness of breath, flushing, hematuria, fever, or chills. Should any adverse reaction occur, stop infusion immediately, notify physician, and follow the agency's transfusion reaction standard.
7. Monitor vital signs at end of transfusion per institution policy; compare results with baseline measurements.
8. Flush line with saline after transfusion to remove blood component from tubing.

**Postprocedure**
1. Obtain vital signs and compare with baseline measurements.
2. Dispose of used materials properly.
3. Document procedure in patient's medical record, including patient assessment findings and tolerance to procedure.
4. Monitor patient for response to and effectiveness of procedure. A platelet count may be ordered 1 hr after platelet transfusion to facilitate this evaluation.

*Note:* FFP requires ABO but not Rh compatibility. Platelets are not typically cross-matched for ABO compatibility. Never add medications to blood or blood products.

---

limited to transfusions of PRBCs and factor components (eg, factor VIII for patients with hemophilia).

## Pretransfusion Assessment

### Patient History

Patient history is an important component of the pretransfusion assessment to determine the history of previous transfusions as well as previous reactions to transfusion. The history should include the type of reaction, its manifestations, the interventions required, and whether any preventive interventions were used in subsequent transfusions. It is important to assess the number of pregnancies a woman has had, because a high number can increase her risk for reaction due to antibodies developed from exposure to fetal circulation. Other concurrent health problems should be noted, with careful attention to cardiac, pulmonary, and vascular disease.

### Physical Assessment

A systematic physical assessment and measurement of baseline vital signs are important before transfusing any blood product. The respiratory system should be assessed, including careful auscultation of the lungs and the patient's use of accessory muscles. Cardiac system assessment should include careful inspection for any edema as well as other signs of cardiac failure (eg, jugular venous distention). The skin should be observed for rashes, petechiae, and ecchymoses. The sclera should be examined for icterus. In the event of a transfusion reaction, a comparison of findings can help differentiate between types of reactions.

## Patient Teaching

Reviewing the signs and symptoms of a transfusion reaction is crucial for patients who have not received a transfusion before. Even for patients who have received prior transfusions, a brief review of the signs and symptoms of transfusion reactions is advised. Signs and symptoms of a reaction include fever, chills, respiratory distress, low back pain, nausea, pain at the IV site, or anything "unusual." Although a thorough review is very important, it is also important to reassure the patient that the blood is carefully tested against the patient's own blood (cross-matched) to diminish the likelihood of any untoward reaction. Such assurance can be extremely beneficial in allaying anxiety. Similarly, the patient can be reassured about the very low possibility of contracting HIV from the transfusion; this fear persists among many people.

## Complications

Any patient who receives a blood transfusion may develop complications from that transfusion. When explaining the reasons for the transfusion, it is important to include the risks and benefits and what to expect during and after the transfusion. Patients must be informed that the supply of blood is not completely risk-free, although it has been tested carefully. Nursing management is directed toward preventing complications, promptly recognizing complications if they develop, and promptly initiating measures to control complications. The following sections describe the most common or potentially severe transfusion-related complications.

### Febrile Nonhemolytic Reaction

A febrile nonhemolytic reaction is caused by antibodies to donor leukocytes that remain in the unit of blood or blood component; it is the most common type of transfusion reaction, accounting for more than 90% of reactions. It occurs more frequently in patients who have had previous transfusions (exposure to multiple antigens from previous blood products) and in Rh-negative women who have borne Rh-positive children (exposure to an Rh-positive fetus raises antibody levels in the mother). These reactions occur in 1% of PRBC transfusions and 20% of platelet transfusions. More than 10% of patients with chronic transfusion requirements develop this type of reaction.

The diagnosis of a febrile nonhemolytic reaction is made by excluding other potential causes, such as a hemolytic reaction or bacterial contamination of the blood product. The signs and symptoms of a febrile nonhemolytic transfusion reaction are chills (minimal to severe) followed by fever (more than 1°C elevation). The fever typically begins within 2 hours after the transfusion is begun. Although the reaction is not life-threatening, the fever, and particularly the chills and muscle stiffness, can be frightening to the patient.

This reaction can be diminished, even prevented, by further depleting the blood component of donor leukocytes; this is accomplished by a leukocyte reduction filter. Antipyretics can be given to prevent fever, but routine premedication is not advised because it can mask the beginning of a more serious transfusion reaction.

### Acute Hemolytic Reaction

The most dangerous, and potentially life-threatening, type of transfusion reaction occurs when the donor blood is incompatible with that of the recipient. Antibodies already present in the recipient's plasma rapidly combine with antigens on donor erythrocytes, and the erythrocytes are hemolyzed (destroyed) in the circulation (intravascular hemolysis). The most rapid hemolysis occurs in ABO incompatibility. This reaction can occur after transfusion of as little as 10 mL of PRBCs. Rh incompatibility often causes a less severe reaction. The most common causes of acute hemolytic reaction are errors in blood component labeling and patient identification that result in the administration of an ABO-incompatible transfusion.

Symptoms consist of fever, chills, low back pain, nausea, chest tightness, dyspnea, and anxiety. As the erythrocytes are destroyed, the hemoglobin is released from the cells and excreted by the kidneys; therefore, hemoglobin appears in the urine (hemoglobinuria). Hypotension, bronchospasm, and vascular collapse may result. Diminished renal perfusion results in acute renal failure, and DIC may also occur.

The reaction must be recognized promptly and the transfusion discontinued immediately. Blood and urine specimens must be obtained and analyzed for evidence of hemolysis. Treatment goals include maintaining blood volume and renal perfusion and preventing and managing DIC.

Acute hemolytic transfusion reactions are preventable. Meticulous attention to detail in labeling blood samples and blood components and accurately identifying the recipient cannot be overemphasized.

### Allergic Reaction

Some patients develop urticaria (hives) or generalized itching during a transfusion. The cause of these reactions is thought to be a sensitivity reaction to a plasma protein within the blood component being transfused. Symptoms of an allergic reaction are urticaria, itching, and flushing. The reactions are usually mild and respond to antihistamines. If the symptoms resolve after administration of an antihistamine (eg, diphenhydramine [Benadryl]), the transfusion may be resumed. Rarely, the allergic reaction is severe, with bronchospasm, laryngeal edema, and shock. These reactions are managed with epinephrine, corticosteroids, and pressor support, if necessary.

Giving the patient antihistamines before the transfusion may prevent future reactions. For severe reactions, future blood components are washed to remove any remaining plasma proteins. Leukocyte filters are not useful to prevent such reactions, because the offending plasma proteins can pass through the filter.

### Circulatory Overload

If too much blood is infused too quickly, hypervolemia can occur. This condition can be aggravated in patients who already have increased circulatory volume (eg, those with heart failure). PRBCs are safer to use than whole blood. If the administration rate is sufficiently slow, circulatory overload may be prevented. For patients who are at risk of, or already in, circulatory overload, diuretics are administered after the transfusion or between units of PRBCs. Patients receiving fresh frozen plasma or even platelets may also develop circulatory overload. The infusion rate of these blood components must also be titrated to the patient's tolerance.

Signs of circulatory overload include dyspnea, orthopnea, tachycardia, and sudden anxiety. Jugular vein distention, crackles at the base of the lungs, and an increase in blood pressure can also occur. If the transfusion is continued, pulmonary edema can develop, as manifested by severe dyspnea and coughing of pink, frothy sputum.

If fluid overload is mild, the transfusion can often be continued after slowing the rate of infusion and administering diuretics. However, if the overload is severe, the patient is placed in an upright position with the feet in a dependent position, the transfusion is discontinued, and the physician is notified. The IV line is kept patent with a very slow infusion of normal saline solution or a saline or heparin lock device to maintain access to the vein in case IV medications are necessary. Oxygen and morphine may be needed to treat severe dyspnea.

### Bacterial Contamination

The incidence of bacterial contamination of blood components is very low; however, administration of contaminated products puts the patient at great risk. Contamination can occur at any point during procurement or processing but is usually due to organisms on the donor's skin (Goodman, 2004). Many bacteria cannot survive in the cold temperatures used to store PRBCs, but some organisms can survive cold temperatures. Platelets are at greater risk of contamination because they are stored at room temperature. Recently, blood centers have developed rapid methods of culturing the platelet unit (Goodman, 2004), thereby diminishing the risk of using a contaminated platelet unit for transfusion.

Preventive measures include meticulous care in the procurement and processing of blood components. When PRBCs or whole blood is transfused, it should be administered within a 4-hour period, because warm room temperatures promote bacterial growth. A contaminated unit of blood product may appear normal, or it may have an abnormal color.

The signs of bacterial contamination are fever, chills, and hypotension. These signs may not occur until the transfusion is complete, occasionally not until several hours after the transfusion. If the condition is not treated immediately with fluids and broad-spectrum antibiotics, shock can occur. Even with aggressive management, including vasopressor support, the mortality rate is high.

As soon as the reaction is recognized, any remaining transfusion is discontinued, and the IV line is kept open with normal saline solution. The physician and the blood bank are notified, and the blood container is returned to the blood bank for testing and culture. Septicemia is treated with IV fluids and antibiotics; corticosteroids and vasopressors are often also necessary.

### Transfusion-Related Acute Lung Injury

This potentially fatal, idiosyncratic reaction occurs in fewer than 1 in 5000 transfusions. Antibodies (usually in the donor's plasma) that are present in the blood component stimulate the recipient's leukocytes; aggregates of these leukocytes form and occlude the microvasculature within the lungs or damage the endothelium in the lungs (Kopko, 2004). The precise pathologic mechanism is not yet completely understood, but the lung injury is manifested as pulmonary edema that can occur within 4 hours after the transfusion.

Signs and symptoms include fever, chills, acute respiratory distress (in the absence of other signs of left ventricular failure, such as elevated central venous pressure), and bilateral pulmonary infiltrates. Aggressive supportive therapy (oxygen, intubation, diuretics) may prevent death.

### Delayed Hemolytic Reaction

Delayed hemolytic reactions usually occur within 14 days after transfusion, when the level of antibody has been increased to the extent that a reaction can occur. The hemolysis of the erythrocytes is extravascular via the RES and occurs gradually.

Signs and symptoms of a delayed hemolytic reaction are fever, anemia, increased bilirubin level, decreased or absent haptoglobin, and possibly jaundice. Rarely is there hemoglobinuria. Generally, these reactions are not dangerous, but it is useful to recognize them, because subsequent transfusions with blood products containing these antibodies may cause a more severe hemolytic reaction. However, recognition is also difficult, because the patient may not be in a health care setting to be tested for this reaction, and even if the patient is hospitalized, the reaction may be too mild to be recognized clinically. Because the amount of antibody present can be too low to detect, it is difficult to prevent delayed hemolytic reactions. Fortunately, the reaction is usually mild and requires no intervention.

### Disease Acquisition

Despite advances in donor screening and blood testing, certain diseases can still be transmitted by transfusion of blood components (see Chart 33-16).

## Complications of Long-Term Transfusion Therapy

The complications that have been described represent a real risk to any patient any time a blood component is administered. However, patients with long-term transfusion requirements (eg, those with MDS, thalassemia, aplastic anemia, sickle cell anemia) are at greater risk for infection transmission and for becoming more sensitized to donor antigens, simply because they are exposed to more units of blood and, consequently, more donors. A summary of complications associated with long-term transfusion therapy is given in Table 33-9.

Iron overload is a complication unique to people who have had long-term PRBC transfusions. One unit of PRBCs contains 250 mg of iron. Patients with chronic transfusion requirements can quickly acquire more iron than they can use, leading to iron overload. Over time, the excess iron deposits in body tissues and can cause organ damage, particularly in the liver, heart, testes, and pancreas. Promptly initiating a program of iron chelation therapy (eg, with deferoxamine [Desferal]) can prevent end-organ damage from iron toxicity (see Myelodysplastic Syndrome, Nursing Management, and Hereditary Hemochromatosis, Nursing Management). Chelation is a cumbersome process for the patient, necessitating chronic infusions, most often subcutaneously, at least several times per week. An oral formulation of chelating agents is now available.

## Nursing Management for Transfusion Reactions

If a transfusion reaction is suspected, the transfusion must be immediately stopped and the physician notified. A thorough patient assessment is crucial, because many complications have similar signs and symptoms. The following steps are taken to determine the type and severity of the reaction:

- Stop the transfusion. Maintain the IV line with normal saline solution through new IV tubing, administered at a slow rate.
- Assess the patient carefully. Compare the vital signs with baseline. Assess the patient's respiratory status carefully. Note the presence of adventitious breath sounds, use of accessory muscles, extent of dyspnea, and changes in mental status, including anxiety and confusion. Note any chills, diaphoresis, jugular vein distention, and reports of back pain or urticaria.
- Notify the physician of the assessment findings, and implement any treatments prescribed. Continue to monitor the patient's vital signs and respiratory, cardiovascular, and renal status.
- Notify the blood bank that a suspected transfusion reaction has occurred.
- Send the blood container and tubing to the blood bank for repeat typing and culture. The identifying tags and numbers are verified.

If a hemolytic transfusion reaction or bacterial infection is suspected, the nurse does the following:

- Obtain appropriate blood specimens from the patient.
- Collect a urine sample as soon as possible for a hemoglobin determination.
- Document the reaction according to the institution's policy.

## Pharmacologic Alternatives to Blood Transfusions

Pharmacologic agents that stimulate production of one or more types of blood cells by the marrow are commonly used (Chart 33-19).

Researchers continue to seek a blood substitute that is practical and safe (Klein, 2005). Manufacturing artificial blood is problematic, given the myriad functions of blood components. Recent research has focused on the role of blood in oxygen transport or its role as an oxygen carrier and the manufacturing of a suitable RBC substitute. Current artificial RBC products undergoing clinical trials have distinct advantages and disadvantages compared with human RBCs. These products can be rendered essentially

### TABLE 33-9 Common Complications Resulting from Long-Term PRBC Transfusion Therapy*

| | Manifestation | Management |
|---|---|---|
| Infection | Hepatitis (B,C) | May immunize against hepatitis B; give alpha-interferon for hepatitis C; monitor hepatic function |
| | Cytomegalovirus (CMV) | WBC filters to protect against CMV |
| Iron overload | Heart failure | Prevent by chelation therapy |
| | Endocrine failure (diabetes, hypothyroidism, hypoparathyroidism, hypogonadism) | |
| Transfusion reaction | Sensitization | Diminish by RBC phenotyping, using WBC-filtered products |
| | Febrile reactions | Diminish by using WBC-filtered products |

*Patients with long-term transfusion therapy requirements are at risk not only for the transfusion reactions discussed in the text but also for the complications noted above. In many cases, the use of WBC-filtered (eg, leukocyte-poor) blood products is standard for patients who receive long-term PRBC transfusion therapy. An aggressive chelation program initiated early in the course of therapy can prevent problems with iron overload.

PRBC, packed red blood cells; WBC, white blood cell; RBC, red blood cell.

## CHART 33-19

### Pharmacologic Alternatives to Blood Transfusions

#### Growth Factors
Recombinant technology has provided a means to produce hematopoietic growth factors necessary for the production of blood cells within the bone marrow. By increasing the body's production of blood cells, transfusions and complications resulting from diminished blood cells (eg, infection from neutropenia or transfusions) may be avoided. However, the successful use of growth factors requires functional bone marrow.

#### Erythropoietin
Erythropoietin (epoetin alpha [eg, Epogen, Procrit]) is an effective alternative treatment for patients with chronic anemia secondary to diminished levels of erythropoietin, as in chronic renal disease. This medication stimulates erythropoiesis. It also has been used for patients who are anemic from chemotherapy or zidovudine (AZT) therapy and for those who have diseases involving bone marrow suppression, such as myelodysplastic syndrome (MDS). The use of erythropoietin can also enable a patient to donate several units of blood for future use (eg, preoperative autologous donation). The medication can be administered intravenously or subcutaneously, although plasma levels are better sustained with the subcutaneous route. Side effects are rare, but erythropoietin can cause or exacerbate hypertension. If the anemia is corrected too quickly or is overcorrected, the elevated hematocrit can cause headache and, potentially, seizures. These adverse effects are rare except for patients with renal failure. Serial complete blood counts (CBCs) should be performed to evaluate the response to the medication. The dose and frequency of administration are titrated to the hematocrit.

#### Granulocyte-Colony Stimulating Factor (G-CSF)
G-CSF (filgrastim [Neupogen]) is a cytokine that stimulates the proliferation and differentiation of myeloid stem cells; a rapid increase in neutrophils is seen within the circulation. G-CSF is effective in improving transient but severe neutropenia after chemotherapy or in some forms of MDS. It is particularly useful in preventing bacterial infections that would be likely to occur with neutropenia. G-CSF is administered subcutaneously on a daily basis. The primary side effect is bone pain; this probably reflects the increase in hematopoiesis within the marrow. Serial CBCs should be performed to evaluate the response to the medication and to ensure that the rise in white blood cells is not excessive. The effect of G-CSF on myelopoiesis is short; the neutrophil count drops once the medication is stopped.

#### Granulocyte-Macrophage Colony Stimulating Factor (GM-CSF)
GM-CSF (sargramostim [Leukine]) is a cytokine that is naturally produced by a variety of cells, including monocytes and endothelial cells. It works either directly or synergistically with other growth factors to stimulate myelopoiesis. GM-CSF is not as specific to neutrophils as is G-CSF; thus, an increase in erythroid (RBC) and megakaryocytic (platelet) production may also be seen. GM-CSF serves the same purpose as G-CSF. However, it may have a greater effect on macrophage function and therefore may be more useful against fungal infections, whereas G-CSF may be better used to fight bacterial infections. GM-CSF is also administered subcutaneously. Side effects include bone pain, fevers, and myalgias.

#### Thrombopoietin
Thrombopoietin (TPO) is a cytokine that is necessary for the proliferation of megakaryocytes and subsequent platelet formation. Unfortunately, clinical studies have not consistently demonstrated effectiveness of TPO in the setting of chemotherapy-induced thrombocytopenia, but it is effective in facilitating platelet collection via apheresis (Vadhan-Raj, Cohen, & Bueso-Ramos, 2005). Further studies are ongoing to assess the efficacy of TPO in other, more chronic conditions associated with thrombocytopenia (Vadhan-Raj et al., 2005).

---

sterile, resulting in fewer immunity-related transfusion problems. They require no refrigeration, have approximately 12 times the shelf-life of PRBCs, and require no cross-matching. Their most significant disadvantage is their short half-life: approximately 1 day, versus the normal 120-day lifespan of a normal erythrocyte. Therefore, the usefulness of these products would likely be limited to situations where the need is short term (eg, surgery or trauma).

## Peripheral Blood Stem Cell Transplantation and Bone Marrow Transplantation

PBSCT and BMT are therapeutic modalities that offer the possibility of cure for some patients with hematologic disorders such as severe aplastic anemia, some forms of leukemia, and thalassemia. Because most hematologic disease states arise from some form of bone marrow dysfunction, an autologous transplantation (receiving one's own stem cells) is not as common an option as is allogeneic transplantation. A patient receives intensive chemotherapy (sometimes with radiation therapy as well), with the goal being complete ablation of the patient's bone marrow. Stem cells from the donor (ideally, from a matched sibling) or actual marrow from the donor are then infused into the patient using a process similar to a PRBC transfusion. The stem cells travel to the marrow and slowly begin the process of resuming hematopoiesis. The advantage of autologous transplantation is the reduced likelihood of complications and mortality; however, the risk for relapse is also higher.

A relatively new strategy is based on transplantation for adoptive cell therapy using certain immune mechanisms derived from the donor's lymphocytes (Baron & Storb, 2004). In nonmyeloablative stem cell or marrow transplantation, also referred to as a "minitransplant," the conditioning regimen involves much less myelosuppression than in conventional regimens, rendering the patient immunosuppressed but for a shorter period of time. Consequently, the procedure is less toxic to the patient, and there is a significant decrease in morbidity.

After the deconditioning regimen (ie, during the time the patient is immunosuppressed), the allogeneic transplantation is performed, using either marrow or stem cells. The goal is for the donor's lymphocytes to react against any residual malignant cells within the patient and destroy them. This process is typically augmented by infusion of the donor's lymphocytes as well (referred to as donor lymphocyte infusion [DLI]). If relapse occurs, repeated DLI has been effective in reestablishing remission in many patients. This approach has great promise, particularly in the setting of hematologic malignancy, and may increase the utility of transplantation for more patients than is possible with conventional methods.

Recent research has focused on improving methods to utilize stem cells from cord blood as a source for allogeneic transplantation (Chao et al., 2004). These techniques have proved useful in children, but the amount of stem cells obtained from cord blood has been too small for use in adults. Methods to expand the stem cells harvested are being studied. An important advantage to using stem cells from cord blood is that precise tissue matching is not required because the donor's immune system is immature—yet it is that immaturity of immune function (ie, T-cell development) that renders the recipient more prone to infection and other complications.

The success of transplantation depends on tissue compatibility and the patient's tolerance of the immunosuppression that results from the ablative therapy. Patients require intensive nursing care that is directed toward preventing infection and assessing for early signs and symptoms of complications. One common complication involves the activation of donor T lymphocytes; these lymphocytes respond to their new host (ie, the patient) as foreign and mount a reaction against the body. This process (GVHD) can involve the skin, GI tract, and liver and can be life-threatening. Acute GVHD occurs in about 60% of patients receiving a matched related donor transplant; mortality can be as high as 50% (Bolanos-Meade & Vogelsang, 2004). GVHD is a significant complication in nonmyeloablative transplantation therapy as well as in conventional allotransplantation. In hematologic malignancies, some GVHD is actually desirable in that the donor lymphocytes can also mount a reaction against any lingering tumor cells; this process is referred to as graft-versus-disease effect. Late complications (occurring more than 100 days after transplantation) are common; these patients, particularly those who receive an allogeneic transplant, require careful follow-up for years after transplantation. (Refer to Chapter 16 for further discussion.)

## Critical Thinking Exercises

1. You are working in a hematology-oncology clinic. The laboratory reports a critical laboratory result for one of your patients with possible MDS: the leukocyte count is 1200/mm³ with 40% neutrophils. What other laboratory results would be important to review or consider? The patient is also anemic (hemoglobin 8.2 mg/dL) and platelets are 110,000/mm³. What observations will you include in your assessment of this patient? Determine the extent to which this patient is neutropenic. What medical treatments would you anticipate? How would you educate the patient about neutropenia precautions? What information do you need to obtain about the patient's home setting that will assist you in determining the patient's risk of developing an infection at home? How will you modify this education if the patient has mild dementia? Lives alone? Does not understand or speak English well?

2. **ebp** You are caring for a 22-year-old-man who has had repeated hospitalizations for sickle cell crisis. What is the evidence base that indicates which factors should be assessed to determine the patient's educational, coping, and pain management needs? Identify the evidence base that supports concepts that you will incorporate into the patient's discharge plan.

3. You are caring for a man with a chronic transfusion requirement (typically 2 to 3 units of PRBCs each month). He asks you how he should modify his diet so that "I don't need so much blood." How would you respond? What role do iron supplements play in patients with chronic transfusion needs? How would you assess this patient for iron overload?

4. You are caring for a patient who is septic and is now receiving a transfusion of 2 units of PRBCs. The patient's temperature spikes to 101.3°F (38.5°C) after half of the second unit has been transfused. What are the possible causes of the fever? What are the appropriate nursing interventions?

# REFERENCES AND SELECTED READINGS

## BOOKS

Abrams, A. C. (2003). *Clinical drug therapy: Rationales for nursing practice* (7th ed.). Philadelphia: Lippincott Williams & Wilkins.

Anderson, K. C., & Ness, P. M. (2000). *Scientific basis of transfusion medicine: Implications for clinical practice.* Philadelphia: W. B. Saunders.

Berger, A., Portenoy, R., & Weissman, D. (2002). *Principles and practice of palliative care and supportive oncology* (2nd ed.). Philadelphia: Lippincott Williams & Wilkins.

Beutler, E., Lichtman, M. A., Coller, B. S., et al. (2005). *Williams hematology* (7th ed.). New York: McGraw Hill.

Bick, R. (2002). *Disorders of thrombosis and hemostasis: Clinical and laboratory practice* (3rd ed.). Philadelphia: Lippincott Williams & Wilkins.

Blumenthal, M., Goldberg, A., & Brinkman, J. (Eds.). (2000). *Herbal medicine.* Newton, MA: Integrative Medicine Communications.

Coleman, R. W., Hirsh, J., Marder, V. J., et al. (2000). *Hemostasis and thrombosis: Basic principles and clinical practice* (3rd ed.). Baltimore: Lippincott Williams & Wilkins.

Fisch, M. J., & Bruera, E. (2003). *Handbook of advanced cancer care.* New York: Cambridge.

Fischer, D., Knobf, M. T., Durivgage, H. J., et al. (2003). *The cancer chemotherapy handbook* (6th ed.). St. Louis: Mosby.

Greer, J., Foerster J., Lukens, J., et al. (2003). *Wintrobe's clinical hematology* (11th ed.). Philadelphia: Lippincott Williams & Wilkins.

Hoffman, R., Benz, E. J., Shattil, S. J., et al. (Eds.). (2005). *Hematology: Basic principles and practice* (4th ed.). New York: Churchill Livingstone.

McCullough, J. (2005). *Transfusion medicine* (2nd ed.). London, UK: Churchill Livingstone.

Mintz, P. D. (2005). *Transfusion therapy: Clinical principles and practice* (2nd ed.). Bethesda, MD: American Association of Blood Banks Press.

Skeel, R. (2003). *Handbook of cancer chemotherapy* (6th ed.). Philadelphia: Lippincott Williams & Wilkins.

Triulzi, D. J. (2002). *Blood transfusion therapy: A physician's handbook* (7th ed.). Bethesda, MD: American Association of Blood Banks.

Wilkes, G. M., & Barton-Burke, M. (2004). *2005 oncology nursing drug handbook.* Boston: Jones and Bartlett.

Winningham, M. L., & Barton-Burke, M. (2000). *Fatigue in cancer: A multidimensional approach.* Boston: Jones and Bartlett.

## JOURNALS

*Asterisks indicate nursing research articles.

### Anemia

Adams, R. J., Brambilla, D. J., & Granger, S. (2004). Stroke and conversion to high risk in children screened with transcranial Doppler ultrasound during the STOP study. *Blood, 103*(10), 3689–3694.

Artz, A. S., Fergusson, D., Drink, P., et al. (2004). Prevalence of anemia in skilled-nursing home residents. *Archives in Gerontology and Geriatrics, 39*(3), 201–206.

Cao, H. (2004). Pharmacological induction of fetal hemoglobin synthesis using histone deacetylase inhibitors. *Hematology, 9*(3), 223–233.

Davies, E. G., Riddington, C. Lottenberg, R., et al. (2004). Pneumococcal vaccines for sickle cell disease. *Cochrane Database Systematic Review* (1), CD003885.

Gebreyohanns, M., & Adams, R. J. (2004). Sickle cell disease: Primary stroke prevention. *CNS Spectrums, 9*(6), 445–449.

Gladwin, M., Sachdev, V., & Jison, M. (2004). Pulmonary hypertension as a risk factor for death in patients with sickle cell disease. *New England Journal of Medicine, 350*(9), 886–895.

Hammerman, S. I., & Faber, H. W. (2004). Pulmonary complications of sickle cell disease. Available at http://www.UpToDate.com. Accessed June 1, 2006.

*Johnson, L. (2003). Sickle cell disease patients and patient-controlled analgesia. *British Journal of Nursing, 12*(3), 144–153.

Liem, R. I., O'Gorman, M. K., & Brown, D. L. (2004). Effect of red cell exchange transfusion on plasma levels of inflammatory mediators in sickle cell patients with acute chest syndromes. *American Journal of Hematology, 76*(1), 19–25.

Rosenfeld, S., Follmann, D. Nunez, O., et al. (2003). Antithymocyte globulin and cyclosporine for severe aplastic anemia: association between hematologic response and long-term outcome. *Journal of the American Medical Association, 289*(9), 1130–1135.

Stuart, M. J., & Nagel, R. L. (2004). Sickle-cell disease. *Lancet, 364*(9442), 1343–1360.

Vichinsky, E. P. (2004). Pulmonary hypertension in sickle cell disease. *New England Journal of Medicine, 350*(9), 857–859.

### Hemochromatosis

Beutler, E., Hoffbrand, V., & Cook, J. D. (2003). Iron deficiency and overload. *Hematology (American Society of Hematology Educational Program),* 40–61.

Parker, D. M., Deel, P. C., & Arner, S. S. (2004). Iron out the details of therapeutic phlebotomy. *Nursing, 34*(2), 46–47.

Pietrangelo, A. (2004). Hereditary hemochromatosis: A new look at an old disease. *New England Journal of Medicine, 350*(23), 2383–2397.

### Myelodysplastic Syndromes

Bevans, M. F., & Shalabi, R. A. (2004). Management of patients receiving antithymocyte globulin for aplastic anemia and myelodysplastic syndrome. *Clinical Journal of Oncology Nursing, 8*(4), 377–382.

Estey, E. H. (2004). Modulation of angiogenesis in patients with myelodysplastic syndrome. *Best Practice and Research. Clinical Haematology, 17*(4), 623–639.

Foss, F. M. (2004). Nucleoside analogs and antimetabolite therapies for myelodysplastic syndrome. *Best Practice and Research: Clinical Haematology, 17*(4), 573–584.

Giralt, S. A. (2004). Bone marrow transplant in myelodysplastic syndromes: New technologies, same questions. *Current Hematology Reports, 3*(3), 165–172.

Kantarjan, H., Issa, J. P., Rosenfeld, C. S., et al. (2006). Decitibine improves patient outcomes in myelodysplastic syndromes: Results of a phase III randomized study. *Cancer, 106*(8), 1794–1803.

List, A., Kurtin, S., Roe, D., et al. (2005). Efficacy of lenalidomide in myelodysplastic syndromes. *New England Journal of Medicine, 352*(6), 549–557.

Silverman, L. R. (2004). DNA methyltransferase inhibitors in myelodysplastic syndrome. *Best Practice and Research: Clinical Haematology, 17*(4), 585–594.

Vanorden, H. E., & Hagemann, T. M. (2006). Deferasirox—an oral agent for chronic iron overload. *Annals of Pharmacotherapy,* in press.

### Polycythemia Vera

Berlin, N. I. (2003). Polycythemia vera. *Hematology/Oncology Clinics of North America, 17*(5), 1191–1210.

Chomienne, C., Rain, J. D., Briere, J., et al. (2004). Risk of leukemic transformation in PV and ET patients. *Pathologie Biologie, 52*(5), 289–293.

Golden, C. (2003). Polycythemia vera: A review. *Clinical Journal of Oncology Nursing, 7*(5), 553–556.

Landolfi, R., Marchioli, R., Kutti, J., et al. (2004). Efficacy and safety of low-dose aspirin in polycythemia vera. *New England Journal of Medicine, 350*(2), 114–124.

Prchal, J. T. (2003). Classification and molecular biology of polycythemias (erythrocytoses) and thrombocytosis. *Hematology/Oncology Clinics of North America, 17*(5), 1151–1158.

Terreri, A. (2004). Diagnostic approach to the patient with suspected polycythemia vera, Available at http://www.UptoDate.com. Accessed June 1, 2006.

### Leukopenia/Neutropenia

Larson, E., & Nirenberg, A. (2004). Evidence-based nursing practice to prevent infection in hospitalized neutropenic patients with cancer. *Oncology Nursing Forum, 31*(4), 717–723.

*Nirenberg, A., Mulhearn, L., Lin, S., et al. (2004). Emergency department waiting times for patients with cancer with febrile neutropenia: A pilot study. *Oncology Nursing Forum, 31*(4), 711–715.

### Leukemia/Myelofibrosis

American Cancer Society (2006). *What are the key statistics about acute myeloid leukemia?* Available at http://www.cancer.org/docroot/CRI/content/CRI_2_4_1x_What_Are_the_Key_Statistics_About_Acute_Myeloid_Leukemia_AML.asp?sitearea=. Accessed June 1, 2006.

Barosi, G. (2003). Myelofibrosis with myeloid metaplasia. *Hematology/Oncology Clinics of North America, 17*(5), 1211–1226.

Cortes, J. (2004). Natural history and staging of chronic myelogenous leukemia. *Hematology/Oncology Clinics of North America, 18*(3), 569–584.

Ferrajoli, A., & Keating, M. J. (2004). Current guidelines in defining therapeutic strategies. *Hematology/Oncology Clinics of North America, 18*(4), 881–893.

Giles, F. J., Cortes, E., Kantarjian, H. M., et al. (2004). Accelerated and blastic phases of chronic myelogenous leukemia. *Hematology/Oncology Clinics of North America, 18*(3), 753–774.

Iovino, C. S., & Camacho, L. H. (2003). Acute myeloid leukemia: A classification and treatment update. *Clinical Journal of Oncology Nursing, 7*(5), 535–540.

Larson, R. A. (2004). Adult ALL: Where are we and where are we going? *Clinical Advances in Hematology & Oncology, 2*(6), 342–344.

*Molassiotis, A. (2003). Research in brief: Anorexia and weight loss in long-term survivors of haematological malignancies. *Journal of Clinical Nursing, 12*(6), 925–927.

Pui, C. H., Relling, M. V., & Downing, J. R. (2004). Acute lymphoblastic leukemia. *New England Journal of Medicine, 350*(15), 1135–1148.

Qazilbash, M. H., Giralt, S. A., & Champlin, R. E. (2004). Nonmyeloblative stem cell transplantation for chronic myeloid leukemia. *Hematology/Oncology Clinics of North America, 18*(3), 703–713.

Radich, J. P., Olavarria, E., & Apperley, J. F. (2004). Allogeneic hematopoietic stem cell transplantation for chronic myeloid leukemia. *Hematology/Oncology Clinics of North America, 18*(3), 685–702.

Rai, K. R., Wasil, T., Iqbal, U., et al. (2004). Clinical staging and prognostic markers in chronic lymphocytic leukemia. *Hematology/Oncology Clinics of North America, 18*(4), 795–805.

Zent, C. S., & Kay, N. E. (2004). Update on monoclonal antibody therapy in chronic lymphocytic leukemia. *Clinical Advances in Hematology & Oncology, 2*(2), 107–113.

### Lymphoma/Myeloma

Bonadonna, G., Bonfante, V., Viviani, S., et al. (2004). ABVD plus subtotal nodal versus involved-field radiotherapy in early-stage Hodgkin's disease: Long-term results. *Journal of Clinical Oncology, 22*(14), 2835–2841.

Devenney, B. (2004). Multiple myeloma: An overview. *Clinical Journal of Oncology Nursing, 8*(4), 401–405.

Diehl, V., Thomas, R. K., & Re, D. (2004). Part II: Hodgkin's lymphoma—diagnosis and treatment. *Lancet Oncology, 5*(1), 19–26.

Freedman, A. S. (2004). Approach to the diagnosis, staging, and prognosis of non-Hodgkin's lymphoma. Available at http://www.UptoDate.com. Accessed June 1, 2006.

Goy, A., Younces, A., McLaughlin, P., et al. (2004). Update on a phase II study of bortezomib in patients with relapsed or refractory indolent or aggressive non-Hodgkin's lymphomas. *Clinical Advances in Hematology & Oncology, 2*(10), 4–6.

Hochster, H. S., Weller, E., Ryan, T., et al. (2004). Results of E1496: A phase III trial of CVP with or without maintenance rituximab in advanced indolent lymphoma. Paper presented at the 40th ASCO Annual Meeting, New Orleans, American Society of Clinical Oncology.

Jemal, A., Siegal, R., Ward, E., et al. (2006). Cacer statistics. *CA: A Cancer Journal for Clinicians, 56*(2), 106–130.

Kyle, R. A., & Rajkumar, S. V. (2004). Multiple myeloma. *New England Journal of Medicine, 351*(18), 1860–1873.

Lipton, A. (2004). Pathophysiology of bone metastases: How this knowledge may lead to therapeutic intervention. *Journal of Supportive Oncology, 2*(3), 205–213.

Lister, T. A. (2004). Who should receive myeloablative therapy for lymphoma? *New England Journal of Medicine, 350*(13), 1277–1278.

Lugassy, G., Shaham, R., Nemets, A., et al. (2004). Severe osteomyelitis of the jaw in long-term survivors of multiple myeloma: A new clinical entity. *American Journal of Medicine, 117*(6), 440–441.

Mauch, P., Aleman, B., Carde, P., et al. (2003). Report from the Rockefeller Foundation–sponsored international workshop on reducing mortality and improving quality of life in long-term survivors of Hodgkin's disease. *European Journal of Haemotology, 66*(Suppl.), 68–76.

Riley, M. B., & Byar, K. (2004). The rationale for and background of radioimmunotherapy: An emerging therapy for B-cell non-Hodgkin's lymphoma. *Seminars in Oncology Nursing, 20*(suppl 1), 1–8.

Ruggiero, S. L., Mehrotra, B., Rosenberg, T. J., et al. (2004). Osteonecrosis of the jaw associated with the use of bisphosphonates: A review of 63 cases. *Journal of Oral Maxillofacial Surgery, 62*(5), 527–534.

Terpos, E., & Rahemtulla A. (2004). Bisphosphonate treatment for multiple myeloma. *Drugs Today, 40*(1), 29–40.

### Platelet Disorders

Chomienne, C., Rain, J. D., Briere, J., et al. (2004). Risk of leukemic transformation in PV and ET patients. *Pathologie Biologie, 52*(5), 289–293.

Drachman, J. G. (2004). Inherited thrombocytopenia: When a low platelet count does not mean ITP. *Blood, 103*(2), 390–398.

Franchini, M., & Veneri D. (2004). *Helicobacter pylori* infection and immune thrombocytopenic purpura: An update. *Helicobacter, 9*(4), 342–346.

Harrison, C. N., & Green, A. R. (2003). Essential thrombocytopenia. *Hematology/Oncology Clinics of North America, 17*(5), 1175–1190.

Robak, T. (2004). Monoclonal antibodies in the treatment of autoimmune cytopenias. *European Journal of Haemotology, 72*(2), 79–88.

Schafer, A. I. (2004). Thrombocytosis. *New England Journal of Medicine, 350*(12), 1211–1219.

Stasi, R., & Provan D. (2004). Management of immune thrombocytopenic purpura in adults. *Mayo Clinic Proceedings, 79*(4), 504–522.

Vadhan-Raj, S., Cohen, V., & Bueso-Ramos, C. (2005). Thrombotic growth factors and cytokines. *Current Hematology Reports, 4*(2), 137–144.

Zimmer, J., Andres, E., Noel, E., et al. (2004). Current management of adult idiopathic thrombocytopenia purpura in practice: A cohort study of 201 patients from a single center. *Clinical Laboratory, Haematology, 26*(2), 137 142.

### Bleeding Disorders

Aird, W. C. (2004). Natural anticoagulant inhibitors: Activated protein C. *Clinical Haematology, 17*(1), 161–182.

Carr, M. E., & Martin, E. J. (2004). Recombinant factor VIIa: Clinical applications for an intravenous hemostatic agent with broad-spectrum potential. *Expert Review of Cardiovascular Therapy, 2*(5), 661–674.

Chehab, N. (2002). *A review of coagulation products used in the treatment of hemophilia.* The Cleveland Clinic Center for Continuing Education. Available at http://www.clevelandclinicmeded.com. Accessed June 1, 2006.

Harrison, P. (2003). Platelet function testing. Available at http://www.UpToDate.com. Accessed June 1, 2006.

Key, N. S. (2004). Inhibitors in congenital coagulation disorders. *British Journal of Hematology, 127*(4), 379–391.

Leung, L. (2004). Clinical features, diagnosis, and treatment of disseminated intravascular coagulation. Available at http://www.UpToDate.com. Accessed June 1, 2006.

Mannucci, P. M. (2004). Treatment of von Willebrand's disease. *New England Journal of Medicine, 351*(7), 683–694.

Paper, R. (2003). Can you recognize and respond to von Willebrand disease? *Nursing, 33*(7), 54–56.

Tarantino, M. D., & Aledort, L. M. (2004). Advances in clotting factor treatment for congenital hemorrhagic disorders. *Clinical Advances in Hematology & Oncology, 2*(6), 363–368.

### Thrombotic Disorders

Bauer, K. A. (2004). Antithrombin (ATIII) deficiency. Available at http://www.UpToDate.com. Accessed June 1, 2006.

*Christian, J. B., Lapane, K. L., & Toppa, R. S. (2003). Racial disparities in receipt of secondary stroke prevention agents among US nursing home residents. *Stroke, 34*(11), 2693–2697.

Linkins, L. A., & Weitz, J. I. (2005). New anticoagulant therapy. *Annual Review of Medicine, 56*(1), 63–72.

McIntosh, B. A. (2004). Developing an algorithm for treating heparin-induced thrombocytopenia. *Clinical Advances in Hematology & Oncology, 2*(4), 216–222.

Nutescu, E. A., Helgason, C. M., Briller, J., et al. (2004). New blood thinner offers first potential alternative in 50 years: Ximelagatran. *Journal of Cardiovascular Nursing, 19*(6), 374–383.

Spyropoulos, A. C., Jenkins, P., & Bornikova, L. (2004). A disease management protocol for outpatient perioperative bridge therapy with enoxaparin in patients requiring temporary interruption of long-term oral anticoagulation. *Pharmacotherapy, 24*(5), 649–658.

Viale, P., & Schwartz, R. (2004). Venous thromboembolism in patients with cancer part II: Current treatment strategies. *Clinical Journal of Oncology Nursing, 8*(5), 465–469.

Warkentin, T. E. (2003). New approaches to the diagnosis of heparin-induced thrombocytopenia. *Chest, 127*(suppl. 2), 35S–45S.

*Wilson, F. L., Racine, E., Tekieli, V., et al. (2003). Literacy, readability and cultural barriers: Critical factors to consider when educating older African Americans about anticoagulation therapy. *Journal of Clinical Nursing, 12*(2), 275–282.

### Bone Marrow/Stem Cell Transplantation

Baron, F., & Storb S. (2004). Allogeneic hematopoietic cell transplantation as treatment for hematological malignancies: A review. *Springer Seminars in Immunopathology, 26*(1–2), 71–94.

Bolanos-Meade, J., & Vogelsang, G. B. (2004). Acute graft-versus-host disease. *Clinical Advances in Hematology/Oncology, 2*(10), 672–682.

Chao, N. J., Emerson, S. G., & Weinberg, K. I. (2004). Stem cell transplantation (cord blood transplants). *Hematology, 9*(4), 354–371.

*El-Banna, M. N., Berger, A. M., Farr, L., et al. (2004). Fatigue and depression in patients with lymphoma undergoing autologous peripheral blood stem cell transplantation. *Oncology Nursing Forum, 31*(5), 937–944.

*Hacker, E. D. (2003). Quantitative measurement of quality of life in adult patients undergoing bone marrow transplant or peripheral blood stem cell transplant: A decade review. *Oncology Nursing Forum, 30*(4), 613–631.

*Larsen, J., Nordstrom, G., Bjorkstrand, B., et al. (2003). Symptom distress, functional status and health-related quality of life before high-dose chemotherapy with stem-cell transplantation. *European Journal of Cancer Care, 12*(1), 71–80.

### Transfusion

Goodman, J. L. (2004). The safety and availability of blood and tissues: Progress and challenges. *New England Journal of Medicine, 351*(8), 819–822.

Kirschman, R. A. (2004). Finding alternatives to blood transfusion. *Nursing, 34*(6), 58–62.

Klein, H. G. (2005). Blood substitutes: How close to a solution? *Developmental Biology, 120*(1), 45–52.

Kopko, P. M. (2004). Leukocyte antibodies and biologically active mediators in the pathogenesis of transfusion-related acute lung injury. *Current Hematology Reports, 3*(6), 456–461.

Simmons, P. (2003). A primer for nurses who administer blood products. *MedSurg Nursing, 12*(3), 184–190.

### General References

*Bulsara, C., Ward, A., & Joske, D. (2004). Haematological cancer patients: Achieving a sense of empowerment by use of strategies to control illness. *Journal of Clinical Nursing, 13*(2), 251–258.

Hessig, R. E., Arcand, L. L., & Frost, M. H. (2004). The effects of an educational intervention on oncology nurses' attitude, perceived knowledge, and self-reported application of complementary therapies. *Oncology Nursing Forum, 31*(1), 71–78.

## RESOURCES

Alternative Medicine Foundation, Inc., 5411 W. Cedar Lane, Suite 205A, Bethesda, MD 20814; 301-340-1960; http://www.amfoundation.org. Accessed June 1, 2006.

American Association of Blood Banks (AABB), 8101 Glenbrook Road, Bethesda, MD 20814; 301-907-6977; http://www.aabb.org. Accessed June 1, 2006.

American Cancer Society, 1599 Clifton Rd., N.E., Atlanta, GA 30329; 800-227-2345; http://www.cancer.org. Accessed June 1, 2006.

American Hemochromatosis Society, 777 E. Atlantic Ave., PMB Z-363, Delray Beach, FL 33483; 1-888-655-4766; http://www.americanhs.org. Accessed June 1, 2006.

American Pain Society, 4700 W. Lake Ave., Glenview, IL 60025; 1-847-375-4715; http://www.ampainsoc.org. Accessed June 1, 2006.

American Red Cross, 1730 E Street NW, Washington, DC 20006; 1-202-639-3520; http://www.redcross.org. Accessed June 1, 2006.

American Society of Clinical Oncology (ASCO), 1900 Duke Street, Suite 200, Alexandria, VA, 22314; 1-703-299-0150; http://www.asco.org. Accessed June 1, 2006.

Aplastic Anemia and MDS International Foundation, P.O. Box 613, Annapolis, MD 21404; 1-800-747-2820; http://www.aplastic.org. Accessed June 1, 2006.

Blood and Marrow Transplant Newsletter, 1985 Spruce Ave., Highland Park, IL 60036.

International Myeloma Foundation, 12650 Riverside Drive, Suite 206, North Hollywood, CA 91607; 1-800-452-2873; http://www.myeloma.org. Accessed June 1, 2006.

Leukemia and Lymphoma Society, 1311 Mamaroneck Ave. White Plains, NY 10605; 1-800-955-4572; http://www.leukemia-lymphoma.org. Accessed June 1, 2006.

Myelodysplastic Syndromes Foundation, P.O. Box 477, 464 Main St., Crosswicks, NJ 08515; 1-800-637-0839; http://www.mds-foundation.org. Accessed June 1, 2006.

National Association of Vascular Access Networks, 11417 S. 700 East, Suite 205, Draper, UT 84020; 1-888-576-2826; http://www.navannet.org. Accessed June 1, 2006.

National Cancer Institute Cancer Information Service, 31 Center Drive, MSC 2580, Building 31, Room 10A16, Bethesda, MD 20892-2580; 1-800-4-CANCER; http://cis.nci.nih.gov. Accessed June 1, 2006.

National Center for Complementary and Alternative Medicine (NCCAM), National Institute of Health, Bethesda, MD, 20892, 1-888-644-6226; http://www.nccam.nih.gov. Accessed June 1, 2006.

National Hemophilia Foundation, 116 W. 32nd St., 11th Floor, New York, NY 10001; 1-800-424-2634; http://www.hemophilia.org. Accessed June 1, 2006.

National Library of Medicine, Health Information for Consumers, 8600 Rockville Pike, Bethesda, MD, 20894; 1-888-346-3656; http://www.nlm.nih.gov. Accessed June 1, 2006.

National Marrow Donor Program, Suite 500, 3001 Broadway St. N.E., Minneapolis, MN 55413; 1-800-627-7692; http://www.marrow.org. Accessed June 1, 2006.

Office of Dietary Supplements, National Institutes of Health, 6100 Executive Blvd., Rm 3B01, MSC 7517, Bethesda, MD 20892; 301-435-2920; http://ods.od.nih.gov. Accessed June 1, 2006.

Oncology Nursing Society, 501 Holiday Dr., Pittsburgh, PA 15220; http://www.ons.org. Accessed June 1, 2006.

Platelet Disorder Support Association, P.O. Box 61533, Potomac, MD 20859; 1-977-528-3538; http://www.pdsa.org. Accessed June 1, 2006.

Sickle Cell Disease Association of America, Inc., 200 Corporate Pointe, Suite 495, Culver City, CA 90230; http://www.sicklecelldisease.org. Accessed June 1, 2006.

# UNIT 7

# Digestive and Gastrointestinal Function

## Case Study
### Applying Concepts from NANDA, NIC, and NOC

**A Patient With Nausea, Vomiting, and Diarrhea**

**Mr. Doyle** is a 32-year-old man who has had several episodes of bloody diarrhea with severe cramping, nausea, and vomiting after attending a party 12 hours earlier where he drank eggnog and ate foods from a buffet table. Vital signs are: Temp 103°F; HR 108; B/P 118/80; Resp 20. Because Mr. Doyle is a kidney transplant recipient and is on immunosuppressive medications, he is admitted to the hospital; his diagnosis is salmonellosis.

 Turn to Appendix C to see a concept map that illustrates the relationships that exist between the nursing diagnoses, interventions, and outcomes for the patient's clinical problems.

## Nursing Classifications and Languages

| NANDA<br>Nursing Diagnoses | NIC<br>Nursing Interventions | NOC<br>Nursing Outcomes<br>Return to functional baseline status, stabilization of, or improvement in: |
|---|---|---|
| **Nausea**—Unpleasant wavelike sensation in the back of the throat, epigastrium, or abdomen that may lead to the urge or need to vomit | **Nausea Management**—Prevention and alleviation of nausea | **Symptom Severity**—Severity of perceived adverse changes in physical, emotional, and social functioning |
| **Diarrhea**—Passage of loose, unformed stools | **Diarrhea Management**—Prevention and alleviation of diarrhea | **Comfort Level**—Extent of physical and psychological ease |
| **Risk for Deficient Fluid Volume**—At risk for experiencing vascular, cellular, or intracellular dehydration | **Fluid/Electrolyte Management**—Regulation and prevention of complications from altered fluid and/or electrolyte levels | **Hydration**—Adequate water in the intracellular and extracellular compartments of the body |
|  | **Vomiting Management**—Prevention and alleviation of vomiting |  |

NANDA International (2005). *Nursing diagnoses: Definitions & classification 2005–2006*. Philadelphia: North American Nursing Diagnosis Association.
Dochterman, J. M., & Bulechek, G. M. (2004). *Nursing Interventions Classification (NIC)* (4th ed.). St. Louis: Mosby.
Iowa Outcomes Project, 2004. In S. Moorhead, M. Johnson, & M. Maas, M. (2004). *Nursing outcomes classification (NOC)* (3rd ed.). St. Louis: Mosby.
Dochterman, J. M., & Jones, D. A. (2003). *Unifying nursing languages: The harmonization of NANDA, NIC, and NOC.* Washington, D.C.: American Nurses Association.

"Point, click, learn! Visit thePoint for additional resources."

# CHAPTER 34

# Assessment of Digestive and Gastrointestinal Function

## Learning Objectives

*On completion of this chapter, the learner will be able to:*

1. Describe the structure and function of the organs of the gastrointestinal (GI) tract.
2. Describe the mechanical and chemical processes involved in digesting and absorbing foods and eliminating waste products.
3. Use assessment parameters appropriate for determining the status of GI function.
4. Describe the appropriate preparation, teaching, and follow-up care for patients who are undergoing diagnostic testing of the GI tract.

# Anatomic and Physiologic Overview

## Anatomy of the Gastrointestinal Tract

The gastrointestinal (GI) tract is a 23- to 26-foot-long pathway that extends from the **mouth** to the esophagus, stomach, small and large intestines, and rectum, to the terminal structure, the anus (Fig. 34-1). The **esophagus** is located in the mediastinum anterior to the spine and posterior to the trachea and heart. This hollow muscular tube, which is approximately 25 cm in length, passes through the diaphragm at an opening called the diaphragmatic hiatus.

The remaining portion of the GI tract is located within the peritoneal cavity. The **stomach** is situated in the left upper portion of the abdomen under the left lobe of the liver and the diaphragm, overlaying most of the pancreas (see Fig. 34-1). A hollow muscular organ with a capacity of approximately 1500 mL, the stomach stores food during eating, secretes digestive fluids, and propels the partially digested food, or chyme, into the small intestine. The gastroesophageal junction is the inlet to the stomach. The stomach has four anatomic regions: the cardia (entrance), fundus, body, and pylorus (outlet). Circular smooth muscle in the wall of the pylorus forms the pyloric sphincter and controls the opening between the stomach and the small intestine.

The **small intestine** is the longest segment of the GI tract, accounting for about two thirds of the total length. It folds back and forth on itself, providing approximately 7000 cm of surface area for secretion and **absorption**, the process by which nutrients enter the bloodstream through the intestinal walls. It has three sections: the most proximal section is the duodenum, the middle section is the jejunum, and the distal section is the ileum. They terminate at the ileocecal valve. This valve, or sphincter, controls the flow of digested material from the ileum into the cecal portion of the large intestine and prevents reflux of bacteria into the small intestine. Attached to the cecum is the vermiform appendix, an appendage that has little or no physiologic function. Emptying into the duodenum at the ampulla of Vater is the common bile duct, which allows for the passage of both bile and pancreatic secretions.

The **large intestine** consists of an ascending segment on the right side of the abdomen, a transverse segment that extends from right to left in the upper abdomen, and a descending segment on the left side of the abdomen. Completing the terminal portion of the large intestine are the sigmoid colon, the rectum, and the anus. Regulating the anal outlet is a network of striated muscle that forms both the internal and the external anal sphincters.

The GI tract receives blood from arteries that originate along the entire length of the thoracic and abdominal aorta and veins that return blood from the digestive organs and the spleen. This portal venous system is composed of five large veins: the superior mesenteric, inferior mesenteric, gastric, splenic, and cystic veins, which eventually form the vena portae that enters the liver. Once in the liver, the blood is distributed throughout and collected into the hepatic veins that then terminate in the inferior vena cava. Of particular importance are the gastric artery and the superior and inferior mesenteric arteries. Oxygen and nutrients are supplied to the stomach by the gastric artery and to the intestine by the

# Glossary

**absorption:** phase of the digestive process that occurs when small molecules, vitamins, and minerals pass through the walls of the small and large intestine and into the bloodstream

**amylase:** an enzyme that aids in the digestion of starch

**anus:** last section of the GI tract; outlet for waste products from the system

**chyme:** mixture of food with saliva, salivary enzymes, and gastric secretions that is produced as the food passes through the mouth, esophagus, and stomach

**digestion:** phase of the digestive process that occurs when digestive enzymes and secretions mix with ingested food and when proteins, fats, and sugars are broken down into their component smaller molecules

**elimination:** phase of digestive process that occurs after digestion and absorption, when waste products are evacuated from the body

**esophagus:** collapsible tube connecting the mouth to the stomach, through which food passes as it is ingested

**fibroscopy (gastrointestinal):** intubation of a part of the GI system with a flexible, lighted tube to assist in diagnosis and treatment of diseases of that area

**hydrochloric acid:** acid secreted by the glands in the stomach; mixes with chyme to break it down into absorbable molecules and to aid in the destruction of bacteria

**ingestion:** phase of the digestive process that occurs when food is taken into the GI tract via the mouth and esophagus

**intrinsic factor:** a gastric secretion that combines with vitamin $B_{12}$ so that the vitamin can be absorbed

**large intestine:** the portion of the GI tract into which waste material from the small intestine passes as absorption continues and elimination begins; consists of several parts—ascending segment, transverse segment, descending segment, sigmoid colon, and rectum

**lipase:** an enzyme that aids in the digestion of fats

**mouth:** first portion of the GI tract, through which food is ingested

**pepsin:** a gastric enzyme that is important in protein digestion

**small intestine:** longest portion of the GI tract, consisting of three parts—duodenum, jejunum, and ileum—through which food mixed with all secretions and enzymes passes as it continues to be digested and begins to be absorbed into the bloodstream

**stomach:** distensible pouch into which the food bolus passes to be digested by gastric enzymes

**trypsin:** enzyme that aids in the digestion of protein

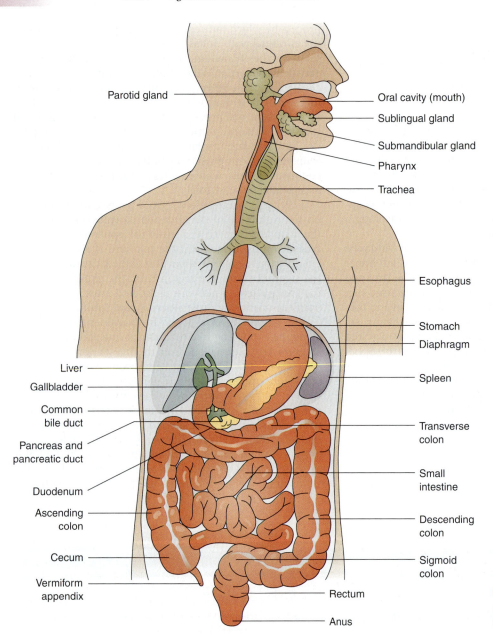

**FIGURE 34-1.** Organs of the digestive system and associated structures.

mesenteric arteries (Fig. 34-2). Venous blood is returned from the small intestine, cecum, and the ascending and transverse portions of the colon by the superior mesenteric vein, which corresponds with the distribution of the branches of the superior mesenteric artery. Blood flow to the GI tract is about 20% of the total cardiac output and increases significantly after eating.

Both the sympathetic and parasympathetic portions of the autonomic nervous system innervate the GI tract. In general, sympathetic nerves exert an inhibitory effect on the GI tract, decreasing gastric secretion and motility and causing the sphincters and blood vessels to constrict. Parasympathetic nerve stimulation causes peristalsis and increases secretory activities. The sphincters relax under the influence of parasympathetic stimulation except for the sphincter of the upper esophagus and the external anal sphincter, which are under voluntary control.

## Functions of the Digestive System

All cells of the body require nutrients. These nutrients are derived from the intake of food that contains proteins, fats, carbohydrates, vitamins, minerals, and cellulose fibers and other vegetable matter, some of which has no nutritional value. Primary functions of the GI tract are the following:

- The breakdown of food particles into the molecular form for **digestion**
- The absorption into the bloodstream of small nutrient molecules produced by digestion
- The **elimination** of undigested unabsorbed foodstuffs and other waste products

After food is ingested, it is propelled through the GI tract, coming into contact with a wide variety of secretions that aid in its digestion, absorption, or elimination from the GI tract.

# CHAPTER 34 • Assessment of Digestive and Gastrointestinal Function

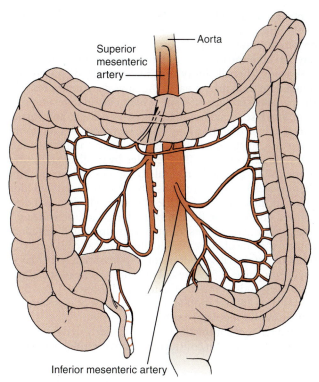

**FIGURE 34-2.** Anatomy and blood supply of the large intestine.

## Chewing and Swallowing

The process of digestion begins with the act of chewing, in which food is broken down into small particles that can be swallowed and mixed with digestive enzymes. Eating—or even the sight, smell, or taste of food—can cause reflex salivation. Approximately 1.5 L of saliva is secreted daily from the parotid, the submaxillary, and the sublingual glands. Ptyalin, or salivary amylase, is an enzyme that begins the digestion of starches. Water and mucus, also contained in saliva, help lubricate the food as it is chewed, thereby facilitating swallowing.

Swallowing begins as a voluntary act that is regulated by the swallowing center in the medulla oblongata of the central nervous system (CNS). As a bolus of food is swallowed, the epiglottis moves to cover the tracheal opening and prevent aspiration of food into the lungs. Swallowing, which propels the bolus of food into the upper esophagus, thus ends as a reflex action. The smooth muscle in the wall of the esophagus contracts in a rhythmic sequence from the upper esophagus toward the stomach to propel the bolus of food along the tract. During this process of esophageal peristalsis, the lower esophageal sphincter relaxes and permits the bolus of food to enter the stomach. Subsequently, the lower esophageal sphincter closes tightly to prevent reflux of stomach contents into the esophagus.

## Gastric Function

The stomach, which stores and mixes food with secretions, secretes a highly acidic fluid in response to the presence or anticipated **ingestion** of food. This fluid, which can total 2.4 L/day, can have a pH as low as 1 and derives its acidity from **hydrochloric acid** (HCl) secreted by the glands of the stomach. The function of this gastric secretion is twofold: to break down food into more absorbable components and to aid in the destruction of most ingested bacteria. **Pepsin,** an important enzyme for protein digestion, is the end product of the conversion of pepsinogen from the chief cells (Table 34-1). **Intrinsic factor,** also secreted by the gastric mucosa, combines with dietary vitamin $B_{12}$ so that the

| TABLE 34-1 | The Major Digestive Enzymes and Secretions | |
|---|---|---|
| **Enzyme/Secretion** | **Enzyme Source** | **Digestive Action** |
| **Action of Enzymes That Digest Carbohydrates** | | |
| Ptyalin (salivary amylase) | Salivary glands | Starch→dextrin, maltose, glucose |
| Amylase | Pancreas and intestinal mucosa | Starch→dextrin, maltose, glucose |
| | | Dextrin→maltose, glucose |
| Maltase | Intestinal mucosa | Maltose→glucose |
| Sucrase | Intestinal mucosa | Sucrose→glucose, fructose |
| Lactase | Intestinal mucosa | Lactose→glucose, galactose |
| **Action of Enzymes/Secretions That Digest Protein** | | |
| Pepsin | Gastric mucosa | Protein→polypeptides |
| Trypsin | Pancreas | Proteins and polypeptides→polypeptides, dipeptides, amino acids |
| Aminopeptidase | Intestinal mucosa | Polypeptides→dipeptides, amino acids |
| Dipeptidase | Intestinal mucosa | Dipeptides→amino acids |
| Hydrochloric acid | Gastric mucosa | Protein→polypeptides, amino acids |
| **Action of Enzymes Secretions That Digest Fat (Triglyceride)** | | |
| Pharyngeal lipase | Pharynx mucosa | Triglycerides→fatty acids, diglycerides, monoglycerides |
| Steapsin | Gastric mucosa | Triglycerides→fatty acids, diglycerides, monoglycerides |
| Pancreatic lipase | Pancreas | Triglycerides→fatty acids, diglycerides, monoglycerides |
| Bile | Liver and gallbladder | Fat emulsification |

vitamin can be absorbed in the ileum. In the absence of intrinsic factor, vitamin $B_{12}$ cannot be absorbed, and pernicious anemia results (see Chapter 33).

Peristaltic contractions in the stomach propel the stomach's contents toward the pylorus. Because large food particles cannot pass through the pyloric sphincter, they are churned back into the body of the stomach. In this way, food in the stomach is agitated mechanically and broken down into smaller particles. Food remains in the stomach for a variable length of time, from 30 minutes to several hours, depending on the volume, osmotic pressure, and chemical composition of the gastric contents. Peristalsis in the stomach and contractions of the pyloric sphincter allow the partially digested food to enter the small intestine at a rate that permits efficient absorption of nutrients. This partially digested food mixed with gastric secretions is called **chyme**. Hormones, neuroregulators, and local regulators found in the gastric secretions control the rate of gastric secretions and influence gastric motility (Table 34-2).

## Small Intestine Function

The digestive process continues in the duodenum. Duodenal secretions come from the accessory digestive organs—the pancreas, liver, and gallbladder—and the glands in the wall of the intestine itself. These secretions contain digestive enzymes: amylase, lipase, and bile. Pancreatic secretions have an alkaline pH due to their high concentration of bicarbonate. This alkalinity neutralizes the acid entering the duodenum from the stomach. Digestive enzymes secreted by the pancreas include **trypsin**, which aids in digesting protein; **amylase**, which aids in digesting starch; and **lipase**, which aids in digesting fats. These secretions drain into the pancreatic duct, which empties into the common bile duct at the ampulla of Vater. Bile, secreted by the liver and stored in the gallbladder, aids in emulsifying ingested fats, making them easier to digest and absorb. The sphincter of Oddi, found at the confluence of the common bile duct and duodenum, controls the flow of bile. Hormones, neuroregulators, and local regulators found in these intestinal secretions control the rate of intestinal secretions and also influence GI motility. Intestinal secretions total approximately 1 L/day of pancreatic juice, 0.5 L/day of bile, and 3 L/day of secretions from the glands of the small intestine. Tables 34-1 and 34-2 give further information about the actions of digestive enzymes and GI regulatory substances.

Two types of contractions occur regularly in the small intestine: segmentation contractions and intestinal peristalsis.

### TABLE 34-2 The Major Gastrointestinal Regulatory Substances

| Substance | Stimulus for Production | Target Tissue | Effect on Secretions | Effect on Motility |
|---|---|---|---|---|
| **Neuroregulators** | | | | |
| Acetylcholine | Sight, smell, chewing food, stomach distention | Gastric glands, other secretory glands, gastric and intestinal muscle | Increased gastric acid | Generally increased; decreased sphincter tone |
| Norepinephrine | Stress, other various stimuli | Secretory glands, gastric and intestinal muscle | Generally inhibitory | Generally decreased; increased sphincter tone |
| **Hormonal Regulators** | | | | |
| Gastrin | Stomach distention with food | Gastric glands | Increased secretion of gastric juice, which is rich in HCl | Increased motility of stomach, decreased time required for gastric emptying Relaxation of ileocecal sphincter Excitation of colon Constriction of gastroesophageal sphincter |
| Cholecystokinin | Fat in duodenum | Gallbladder | Release of bile into duodenum | |
| | | Pancreas | Increased production of enzyme-rich pancreatic secretions | |
| | | Stomach | Inhibits gastric secretion somewhat | |
| Secretin | pH of chyme in duodenum below 4–5 | Stomach | Inhibits gastric secretion somewhat | Inhibits stomach contractions |
| | | Pancreas | Increased production of bicarbonate-rich pancreatic juice | |
| **Local Regulator** | | | | |
| Histamine | Unclear; substances in food | Gastric glands | Increased gastric acid production | |

*Segmentation contractions* produce mixing waves that move the intestinal contents back and forth in a churning motion. *Intestinal peristalsis* propels the contents of the small intestine toward the colon. Both movements are stimulated by the presence of chyme.

Food, initially ingested in the form of fats, proteins, and carbohydrates, is broken down into absorbable particles (constituent nutrients) by the process of digestion. Carbohydrates are broken down into disaccharides (eg, sucrose, maltose, and galactose) and monosaccharides (eg, glucose, fructose). Glucose is the major carbohydrate that tissue cells use as fuel. Proteins are a source of energy after they are broken down into amino acids and peptides. Ingested fats become monoglycerides and fatty acid by the process of emulsification, which makes them smaller and therefore easier to absorb. Chyme stays in the small intestine for 3 to 6 hours, allowing for continued breakdown and absorption of nutrients.

Small, finger-like projections called villi are present throughout the entire intestine and function to produce digestive enzymes as well as to absorb nutrients. Absorption is the primary function of the small intestine. Vitamins and minerals are not digested but rather absorbed essentially unchanged. The process of absorption begins in the jejunum and is accomplished by both active transport and diffusion across the intestinal wall into the circulation. Nutrients are absorbed at specific locations throughout the small intestine and duodenum, whereas fats, proteins, carbohydrates, sodium, and chloride are absorbed in the jejunum. Vitamin $B_{12}$ and bile salts are absorbed in the ileum. Magnesium, phosphate, and potassium are absorbed throughout the small intestine.

## Colonic Function

Within 4 hours after eating, residual waste material passes into the terminal ileum and slowly into the proximal portion of the right colon through the ileocecal valve. With each peristaltic wave of the small intestine, the valve opens briefly and permits some of the contents to pass into the colon.

Bacteria, which make up a major component of the contents of the large intestine, assist in completing the breakdown of waste material, especially of undigested or unabsorbed proteins and bile salts. Two types of colonic secretions are added to the residual material: an electrolyte solution and mucus. The electrolyte solution is chiefly a bicarbonate solution that acts to neutralize the end products formed by the colonic bacterial action, whereas the mucus protects the colonic mucosa from the interluminal contents and provides adherence for the fecal mass.

Slow, weak peristaltic activity moves the colonic contents along the tract. This slow transport allows for efficient reabsorption of water and electrolytes, which is the primary purpose of the colon. Intermittent strong peristaltic waves propel the contents for considerable distances. This generally occurs after another meal is eaten, when intestine-stimulating hormones are released. The waste materials from a meal eventually reach and distend the rectum, usually in about 12 hours. As much as one fourth of the waste materials from a meal may still be in the rectum 3 days after the meal was ingested.

## Waste Products of Digestion

Feces consist of undigested foodstuffs, inorganic materials, water, and bacteria. Fecal matter is about 75% fluid and 25% solid material. The composition is relatively unaffected by alterations in diet because a large portion of the fecal mass is of nondietary origin, derived from the secretions of the GI tract. The brown color of the feces results from the breakdown of bile by the intestinal bacteria. Chemicals formed by intestinal bacteria are responsible in large part for the fecal odor. Gases formed contain methane, hydrogen sulfide, and ammonia, among others. The GI tract normally contains approximately 150 mL of these gases, which are either absorbed into the portal circulation and detoxified by the liver or expelled from the rectum as flatus.

Elimination of stool begins with distention of the rectum, which reflexively initiates contractions of the rectal musculature and relaxes the normally closed internal anal sphincter. The internal sphincter is controlled by the autonomic nervous system; the external sphincter is under the conscious control of the cerebral cortex. During defecation, the external anal sphincter voluntarily relaxes to allow colonic contents to be expelled. Normally, the external anal sphincter is maintained in a state of tonic contraction. Thus, defecation is seen to be a spinal reflex (involving the parasympathetic nerve fibers) that can be inhibited voluntarily by keeping the external anal sphincter closed. Contracting the abdominal muscles (straining) facilitates emptying of the colon. The average frequency of defecation in humans is once daily, but this varies among people.

## Gerontologic Considerations

Although an increased prevalence of several common GI disorders occurs in the elderly population, aging per se appears to have minimal direct effect on most GI functions, in large part because of the functional reserve of the GI tract. Normal physiologic changes of the GI system that occur with aging are identified in Chart 34-1. Careful assessment and monitoring of signs and symptoms related to these changes are imperative.

Age-related changes in the mouth include loss of teeth, diminished number of taste buds, decreased production of saliva, and atrophy of gingival tissue. These changes cause difficulty in chewing and swallowing. Changes in the esophagus include decreased muscle tone and weakness in the lower esophageal sphincter, leading to reflux and heartburn.

Although irritable bowel symptoms decrease with aging, there seems to be an increase in many GI disorders of function and motility. The gastroenterologist frequently encounters elderly patients who have complaints of dysphagia, anorexia, dyspepsia, and disorders of colonic function (Prather, 2002). Decreased gastric motility leads to delayed gastric emptying. Atrophy of the mucosa causes a decrease in HCl production, and this can lead to food intolerances, malabsorption, or decrease in vitamin $B_{12}$ absorption. Changes in the small and large intestine are evidenced largely by decreased motility and decreased transit time, which lead to complaints of indigestion and constipation. Other changes lead to decreased absorption of nutrients (dextrose, fats, calcium, and iron) in the large intestine. Fecal incontinence can result from decrease or loss of sphincter control.

## CHART 34-1

### Gerontologic Considerations

**Age-Related Changes of the Gastrointestinal System**

**Oral Cavity and Pharynx**
- Injury/loss or decay of teeth
- Atrophy of taste buds
- Decreased saliva production
- Reduced ptyalin and amylase in saliva

**Esophagus**
- Decreased motility and emptying
- Weakened gag reflex
- Decreased resting pressure of lower esophageal sphincter

**Stomach**
- Degeneration and atrophy of gastric mucosal surfaces with decreased production of HCl
- Decreased secretion of gastric acids and most digestive enzymes
- Decreased motility and emptying

**Small Intestine**
- Atrophy of muscle and mucosal surfaces
- Thinning of villi and epithelial cells

**Large Intestine**
- Decrease in mucus secretion
- Decrease in elasticity of rectal wall
- Decreased tone of internal anal sphincter
- Slower and duller nerve impulses in rectal area

## Assessment

### Health History and Clinical Manifestations

A focused GI assessment begins with a complete history. Information about abdominal pain, dyspepsia, gas, nausea and vomiting, diarrhea, constipation, fecal incontinence, jaundice, and previous GI disease is investigated. Past and current medication use and any previous diagnostic studies, treatments, or surgery are noted. Current nutritional status is ascertained via history, and serum values (complete metabolic panel including liver function studies, triglyceride, iron studies, and complete blood count [CBC]) are obtained. Questioning about the use of tobacco and alcohol includes details about type, amount, length of use, and the date of discontinuation, if any. The nurse and patient discuss changes in appetite or eating patterns and any unexplained weight gain or loss over the past year. It is also important to include questions about psychosocial, spiritual, or cultural factors that may be affecting the patient.

#### Pain

Pain can be a major symptom of GI disease. The character, duration, pattern, frequency, location, distribution of referred pain (Fig. 34-3), and time of the pain vary greatly depending on the underlying cause. Other factors such as meals, rest, activity, and defecation patterns may directly affect this pain.

#### Dyspepsia

Dyspepsia, upper abdominal discomfort, or distress associated with eating (commonly called *indigestion*) is the most common symptom of patients with GI dysfunction.

**FIGURE 34-3.** Common sites of referred abdominal pain.

Indigestion is an imprecise term that refers to a host of upper abdominal or epigastric symptoms such as pain, discomfort, fullness, bloating, early satiety, belching, heartburn, or regurgitation; it occurs in approximately 25% of the adult population. Typically, fatty foods cause the most discomfort because they remain in the stomach for digestion longer than proteins or carbohydrates. Salads and coarse vegetables as well as highly seasoned foods may also cause considerable GI distress.

### Intestinal Gas

The accumulation of gas in the GI tract may result in belching (expulsion of gas from the stomach through the mouth) or flatulence (expulsion of gas from the rectum). Usually, gases in the small intestine pass into the colon and are released as flatus. Patients often complain of bloating, distention, or feeling "full of gas" with excessive flatulence as a symptom of food intolerance or gallbladder disease.

### Nausea and Vomiting

Nausea is a vague, intensely unsettling sensation of sickness or "queasiness" that may or may not be followed by vomiting. It can be triggered by odors, activity, medications, or food intake. The emesis, or vomitus, may vary in color and content and may contain undigested food particles, blood (hematemesis), or bilious material mixed with gastric juices. The causes of nausea and vomiting are many; they may result from (1) visceral afferent stimulation (ie, dysmotility, peritoneal irritation, infections, hepatobiliary or pancreatic disorders, mechanical obstruction); (2) CNS disorders (ie, vestibular disorders, increased intracranial pressure, infections, psychogenic); and/or (3) irritation of the chemoreceptor trigger zone from radiation therapy, systemic disorders, and antitumor chemotherapy medications.

### Change in Bowel Habits and Stool Characteristics

Changes in bowel habits may signal colonic dysfunction or disease. Diarrhea, an abnormal increase in the frequency and liquidity of the stool or in daily stool weight or volume, commonly occurs when the contents move so rapidly through the intestine and colon that there is inadequate time for the GI secretions and oral contents to be absorbed. This physiologic function is typically associated with abdominal pain or cramping and nausea or vomiting. Constipation, a decrease in the frequency of stool, or stools that are hard, dry, and of smaller volume than normal, may be associated with anal discomfort and rectal bleeding. See Chapter 38 for further discussion of diarrhea and constipation.

The characteristics of the stool can vary greatly. Stool is normally light to dark brown; however, specific disease processes and ingestion of certain foods and medications may change the appearance of stool (Table 34-3). Blood in the stool can present in various ways and must be investigated. If blood is shed in sufficient quantities into the upper GI tract, it produces a tarry-black color (melena), whereas blood entering the lower portion of the GI tract or passing rapidly through it will appear bright or dark red. Lower rectal or anal bleeding is suspected if there is streaking of blood on the surface of the stool or if blood is noted on toilet tissue. Other common abnormalities in stool characteristics described by the patient may include:

- Bulky, greasy, foamy stools that are foul in odor and may or may not float
- Light-gray or clay-colored stool, caused by a decrease or absence of conjugated bilirubin
- Stool with mucus threads or pus that may be visible on gross inspection of the stool
- Small, dry, rock-hard masses occasionally streaked with blood
- Loose, watery stool that may or may not be streaked with blood

### TABLE 34-3 Foods and Medications That Alter Stool Color

| Altering Substance | Color |
|---|---|
| Meat protein | Dark brown |
| Spinach | Green |
| Carrots and beets | Red |
| Cocoa | Dark red or brown |
| Senna | Yellow |
| Bismuth, iron, licorice, and charcoal | Black |
| Barium | Milky white |

## Physical Assessment

The physical examination includes assessment of the mouth, abdomen, and rectum and requires a good source of light, full exposure of the abdomen, warm hands with short fingernails, and a comfortable, relaxed patient with an empty bladder. The mouth, tongue, buccal mucosa, teeth, and gums are inspected, noting any ulcers, nodules, swelling, discoloration, or inflammation. Dentures should be removed to allow good visualization of the entire oral cavity.

The patient lies supine with knees flexed slightly for inspection, auscultation, palpation, and percussion of the abdomen (Fig. 34-4). For the purposes of examination and documentation, the abdomen can be divided into either four quadrants or nine regions (Fig. 34-5). Choosing one of these mapping methods and using it consistently results in a thorough evaluation of the abdomen and appropriate corresponding documentation. The four-quadrant method involves the use of an imaginary line drawn vertically from the sternum to the pubis through the umbilicus and a second line drawn perpendicular to the first horizontally across the abdomen through the umbilicus. Inspection is performed first, noting skin changes, nodules, lesions, scarring, discolorations, inflammation, bruising, or striae. Lesions are of particular importance, because GI diseases often produce skin changes. The contour and symmetry of the abdomen are noted and any localized bulging, distention, or peristaltic waves are identified. Expected contours of the anterior abdominal wall can be described as flat, rounded, or scaphoid.

Inspecting the abdomen

Auscultating the abdomen

Palpating the abdomen

Percussing the abdomen

**FIGURE 34-4.** Examination of the abdomen includes inspection, auscultation, palpation, and percussion.

**A. Four quadrants**

1 - right upper quadrant (RUQ)
2 - right lower quadrant (RLQ)
3 - left upper quadrant (LUQ)
4 - left lower quadrant (LLQ)

**B. Nine regions**

1 - epigastric region
2 - umbilical region
3 - hypogastric or suprapubic region
4 - right hypochondriac region
5 - left hypochondriac region
6 - right lumbar region
7 - left lumbar region
8 - right inguinal region
9 - left inguinal region

**FIGURE 34-5.** Division of the abdomen into (**A**) four quadrants or (**B**) nine regions.

Auscultation, which always precedes percussion and palpitation, is used to determine the character, location, and frequency of bowel sounds and to identify vascular sounds. Bowel sounds are assessed in all four quadrants using the diaphragm of the stethoscope, which affords greatest auscultation of high-pitched and gurgling sounds. The frequency and character of the sounds are usually heard as clicks and gurgles that occur irregularly and range from 5 to 35 per minute. The terms *normal* (sounds heard about every 5 to 20 seconds), *hypoactive* (one or two sounds in 2 minutes), *hyperactive* (5 to 6 sounds heard in less than 30 seconds), or *absent* (no sounds in 3 to 5 minutes) are frequently used in documentation, but these assessments are highly subjective. Using the bell of the stethoscope, any bruits in the aortic, renal, iliac, and femoral arteries are noted. Friction rubs are high-pitched and can be heard over the liver and spleen during respiration. Borborygmi or "stomach growling" is heard as a loud prolonged gurgle.

Percussion is used to assess the size and density of the abdominal organs and to detect the presence of air-filled, fluid-filled, or solid masses. Percussion is used either independently or concurrently with palpation because it can validate palpation findings. Use of light palpation is appropriate for identifying areas of tenderness or muscular resistance, and deep palpation is used to identify masses. All quadrants are percussed for a sense of overall tympani and dullness. Tympani is the predominant sound that results from the presence of air in the stomach and small intestines; dullness is heard over organs and solid masses. Testing for rebound tenderness is not performed by many examiners because it can cause severe pain; light percussion is used instead to produce a mild localized response when peritoneal irritation is present.

The final part of the examination is evaluation of the terminal portions of the GI tract, the rectum, perianal region, and anus. The anal canal is approximately 2.5 to 4 cm in length and opens into the perineum. Concentric rings of muscle, the internal and external sphincters, normally keep the anal canal securely closed. Gloves, water-soluble lubrication, a penlight, and drapes are necessary tools for the evaluation. Although the rectal examination is generally uncomfortable and often embarrassing for the patient, it is a mandatory part of every thorough examination. For women, the rectal examination may be part of the gynecologic examination. Positions for the rectal examination include knee-chest, left lateral with hips and knees flexed, or standing with hips flexed and upper body supported by the examination table. Most patients are comfortable on the right side with knees brought up to the chest. External examination includes inspection for lumps, rashes, inflammation, excoriation, tears, scars, pilonidal dimpling, and tufts of hair at the pilonidal area. The discovery of tenderness, inflammation, or both should alert the examiner to the possibility of a pilonidal cyst, perianal abscess, or anorectal fistula or fissure. The patient's buttocks are carefully spread and visually inspected until the patient has relaxed the external sphincter control. The patient is asked to bear down, thus allowing the ready appearance of fistulas, fissures, rectal prolapse, polyps, and internal hemorrhoids. Internal examination is performed with a lubricated index finger inserted into the anal canal while the patient bears down. The tone of the sphincter is noted, as are any nodules or irregularities of the anal ring. Because this is an uncomfortable part of the examination for most patients, the patient is encouraged to focus on deep breathing and visualization of a pleasant setting during the brief examination.

# Diagnostic Evaluation

Initial diagnostic tests begin with serum laboratory studies, including but not limited to CBC, complete metabolic panel, prothrombin time/partial thromboplastin time, triglycerides, liver function tests, amylase, and lipase, with the possibility of more specific studies such as carcinoembryonic antigen (CEA), cancer antigen (CA) 19-9, and alpha-fetoprotein, indicating sensitivity and specificity for colorectal and hepatocellular carcinomas, respectively. CEA is a protein that is normally not detected in the blood of a healthy person; therefore, when detected it indicates that cancer is present, but not what type of cancer is present. Practitioners can use CEA results to determine the stage and extent of the disease and the prognosis for patients with cancer, especially GI and in particular colorectal cancer (Porth, 2005). CA 19-9 is also a protein that exists on the surface of certain cells and is shed by tumor cells, making it useful as a tumor marker to follow the course of the cancer. CA 19-9 levels are elevated in most patients with advanced pancreatic cancer, but it may also be elevated in other conditions such as colorectal, lung, and gallbladder cancers, gallstones, pancreatitis, cystic fibrosis, and liver disease.

Many other modalities are available for diagnostic assessment of the GI tract. The majority of these tests and procedures are performed on an outpatient basis in special settings designed for this purpose (eg, endoscopy suite or GI laboratory). In the past, patients who required such tests frequently were elderly; however, within the past 5 years, in part due to heightened media exposure and early diagnosis of colorectal cancer, the median age of patients evaluated for colorectal cancer has decreased significantly. Preparation for many of these studies includes clear liquid diets, fasting, ingestion of a liquid bowel preparation, the use of laxatives or enemas, and ingestion or injection of a contrast agent or a radiopaque dye. These measures are poorly tolerated by some patients and are especially problematic in the elderly population or patients with comorbidities because bowel preparations significantly alter the internal fluid and electrolyte balance. If further assessment or treatment is needed after any outpatient procedure, the patient may be admitted to the hospital.

Specific nursing interventions for each test are provided later in this chapter. General nursing interventions for the patient who is undergoing a GI diagnostic evaluation include:

- Establishing the nursing diagnosis
- Providing needed information about the test and the activities required of the patient
- Providing instructions about postprocedure care and activity restrictions
- Providing health information and procedural teaching to patients and significant others
- Helping the patient cope with discomfort and alleviating anxiety

- Informing the physician or nurse practitioner of known medical conditions or abnormal laboratory values that may affect the procedure
- Assessing for adequate hydration before, during, and immediately after the procedure, and providing education about maintenance of hydration

## Stool Tests

Basic examination of the stool includes inspecting the specimen for consistency, color, and occult (not visible) blood. Additional studies, including fecal urobilinogen, fecal fat, nitrogen, *Clostridium difficile,* fecal leukocytes, calculation of stool osmolar gap, parasites, pathogens, food residues, and other substances, require laboratory evaluation.

Stool samples are usually collected on a random basis unless a quantitative study (eg, fecal fat, urobilinogen) is to be performed. Random specimens should be sent promptly to the laboratory for analysis; however, the quantitative 24- to 72-hour collections must be kept refrigerated until transported to the laboratory. Some stool collections require the patient to follow a specific diet or refrain from taking certain medications before the collection. Thorough and accurate patient education regarding a specific stool study prior to collection greatly increases the accuracy of study results.

Fecal occult blood testing (FOBT) is one of the most commonly performed stool tests. It can be useful in initial screening for several disorders, although it is used most frequently in early cancer detection programs. FOBT can be performed at the bedside, in the laboratory, or at home.

Probably the most widely used in-office or at-home occult blood test is the Hemoccult II. It is inexpensive, noninvasive, and carries minimal risk to the patient. However, it should not be performed when there is hemorrhoidal bleeding. In addition, red meats, aspirin, nonsteroidal anti-inflammatory drugs, turnips, and horseradish should be avoided for 72 hours prior to the study, because they may cause a false-positive result. Also, ingestion of vitamin C from supplements or foods can cause a false-negative result. Therefore, a careful assessment of the patient's diet and medication regimen is essential to avoid incorrect interpretation of results. A small amount of the specimen is applied to the guaiac-impregnated paper slide. If the test is performed at home, the patient mails the slide to the physician in an envelope provided for that purpose. Other occult blood tests that may yield more specific and more sensitive readings include Hematest II SENSA and HemoQuant.

Immunologic tests are more specific to human hemoglobin and decrease the problem of dietary interference. Hemoporphyrin assays detect the broadest range of blood derivatives, but a strict dietary protocol is essential. Immunochemical tests that use antihuman antibodies extremely sensitive to human hemoglobin are also available.

## Breath Tests

The hydrogen breath test was developed to evaluate carbohydrate absorption, in addition to aiding in the diagnosis of bacterial overgrowth in the intestine and short bowel syndrome. This test determines the amount of hydrogen expelled in the breath after it has been produced in the colon (on contact of galactose with fermenting bacteria) and absorbed into the blood.

Urea breath tests detect the presence of *Helicobacter pylori,* the bacteria that can live in the mucosal lining of the stomach and cause peptic ulcer disease. After the patient ingests a capsule of carbon-labeled urea, a breath sample is obtained 10 to 20 minutes later. Because *H. pylori* metabolizes urea rapidly, the labeled carbon is absorbed quickly; it can then be measured as carbon dioxide in the expired breath to determine whether *H. pylori* is present. The patient is instructed to avoid antibiotics or loperamide (Pepto Bismol) for 1 month before the test; sucralfate (Carafate) and omeprazole (Prilosec) for 1 week before the test; and cimetidine (Tagamet), famotidine (Pepcid), and ranitidine (Zantac) for 24 hours before urea breath testing. *H. pylori* also can be detected by assessing serum antibody levels.

## Abdominal Ultrasonography

Ultrasonography is a noninvasive diagnostic technique in which high-frequency sound waves are passed into internal body structures and the ultrasonic echoes are recorded on an oscilloscope as they strike tissues of different densities. It is particularly useful in the detection of an enlarged gallbladder or pancreas, the presence of gallstones, an enlarged ovary, an ectopic pregnancy, or appendicitis. Most recently this technique has proven useful in diagnosing acute colonic diverticulitis.

Advantages of abdominal ultrasonography include an absence of ionizing radiation, no noticeable side effects, relatively low cost, and almost immediate results. A disadvantage is that it cannot be used to examine structures that lie behind bony tissue because bone prevents sound waves from traveling into deeper structures. Gas and fluid in the abdomen or air in the lungs also prevent transmission of ultrasound. An ultrasound has no dangers; there have been no substantiated ill effects of ultrasound documented in studies in either humans or animals. However, some patients, typically pregnant women, have concerns regarding the energy emitted by the probe.

Endoscopic ultrasonography (EUS) is a specialized enteroscopic procedure that aids in the diagnosis of GI disorders by providing direct imaging of a target area. A small high-frequency ultrasonic transducer is mounted at the tip of the fiberoptic scope, which displays an image that enables tumor staging and visualization of marginal structures. This procedure delivers results with higher-quality resolution and definition in comparison with regular ultrasound imaging. EUS may be used for evaluating submucosal lesions, specifically determining their location and depth of penetration. In addition, EUS may aid in the evaluation of Barrett's esophagus, portal hypertension, chronic pancreatitis, suspected pancreatic neoplasm, biliary tract disease, and changes in the bowel wall that occur in ulcerative colitis. Intestinal gas, bone, and thick layers of adipose tissue (all of which hamper conventional ultrasonography) are not problems when EUS is used.

### Nursing Interventions

The patient is instructed to fast for 8 to 12 hours before the test to decrease the amount of gas in the bowel. If gallbladder studies are being performed, the patient should eat a fat-free meal the evening before the test. If barium studies are to be performed, they should be scheduled after ultrasonography; otherwise, the barium could interfere with the transmission of the sound waves.

## DNA Testing

Researchers have refined methods for genetics risk assessment, preclinical diagnosis, and prenatal diagnosis to identify people who are at risk for certain GI disorders (eg, gastric cancer, lactose deficiency, inflammatory bowel disease, colon cancer). In some cases, DNA testing allows physicians to prevent (or minimize) disease, by intervening before its onset, and to improve therapy; however, it is imperative to educate all genetics counselors routinely, given the exponential growth of genetics information (Beery & Hern, 2004). People who are identified as at risk of certain GI disorders may choose to undergo genetic counseling to learn about the disease, to understand options for preventing and treating the disease, and to receive support in coping with the situation. There are ethical and legal issues involved in genetic testing, and there are legal protections for patients against discrimination (Lowrey, 2004). For instance, false-positive results can create unnecessary worry, alarm, and further testing, typically at the expense of the patient and the family, with potential effects on health-related quality of life (McGovern, Gross, Krueger, et al., 2004). The nurse considers the questions, "How will the results—whether positive or negative—affect the patient? Do I have the resources to help the patient with the outcome?" Family members may receive genetic test results in different ways depending on the following: (1) how people at risk understand and communicate test results, (2) the dynamics of family relationships and communication, (3) familial obligations, and (4) the biologic meaning of family (Hamilton, Bowers, & Williams, 2004). The effects on the person doing the disclosing, the family members receiving the information, and most importantly the perceptions of the person tested are important factors in the testing and counseling process.

---

## GENETICS IN NURSING PRACTICE
### Digestive and Gastrointestinal Disorders

Several digestive and gastrointestinal disorders are associated with genetic abnormalities. Some examples are:
- Cleft lip and/or palate
- Familial adenomatous polyposis
- Hereditary nonpolyposis colorectal cancer (HNPCC)
- Hirschsprung disease (aganglionic megacolon)
- Inflammatory bowel disease (eg, Crohn's disease)
- Pyloric stenosis

### NURSING ASSESSMENTS
#### Family History Assessment
- Careful family history assessment for other family members with a similar condition (eg, cleft lip/palate, pyloric stenosis)
- Assess for other family members in several generations with early-onset colorectal cancer
- Inquire about other family members with inflammatory bowel disease
- Assess family history for other cancers (eg, endometrial, ovarian, renal)

#### Patient Assessment
Assess for presence of other clinical symptoms:
- With clefting—congenital heart defect, mental retardation, other birth defects suggestive of a genetic syndrome
- With familial adenomatous polyposis—congenital hypertrophy of retinal pigment epithelium (CHRPE)

### MANAGEMENT ISSUES SPECIFIC TO GENETICS
- Inquire whether any affected family member has had DNA mutation testing
- If indicated, refer for further genetic counseling and evaluation so that family members can discuss inheritance, risk to other family members, availability of genetics testing, and gene-based interventions
- Offer appropriate genetics information and resources
- Assess patients' understanding of genetics information
- Provide support to families with newly diagnosed genetic digestive disorders
- Participate in management and coordination of care for patients with genetic conditions and for those who are predisposed to develop or pass on a genetic condition

### GENETICS RESOURCES
American Cancer Society—offers general information about cancer and support resources for families, http:/www.cancer.org

Gene Clinics—a listing of common genetic disorders with up-to-date clinical summaries and genetics counseling and testing information, http://www.geneclinics.org

Genetic Alliance—a directory of support groups for patients and families with genetic conditions, http://www.geneticalliance.org

National Cancer Institute—current information about cancer research, treatment, resources for health providers, individuals, and families, http://www.nci.nih.gov

National Organization of Rare Disorders—a directory of support groups and information for patients and families with rare genetic disorders, http://www.rarediseases.org

Online Mendelian Inheritance in Man (OMIM)—a complete listing of inherited genetic conditions, http://www.ncbi.nlm.nih.gov/omim/stats/html

## Imaging Studies

Numerous minimally invasive and noninvasive imaging studies, including x-ray and contrast studies, computed tomography (CT), three-dimensional CT, magnetic resonance imaging (MRI), positron emission tomography (PET), and scintigraphy (radionuclide imaging), are available today. Advances in technology are made daily.

### Upper Gastrointestinal Tract Study

An upper GI study delineates the entire GI tract after the introduction of a contrast agent. A radiopaque liquid (eg, barium sulfate) is commonly used; however, thin barium, Hypaque, and at times water are used due to their low associated risks. The GI series enables the examiner to detect or exclude anatomic or functional derangement of the upper GI organs or sphincters. It also aids in the diagnosis of ulcers, varices, tumors, regional enteritis, and malabsorption syndromes. The procedure may be extended to examine the duodenum and small bowel (small bowel follow-through). As the barium descends into the stomach, the position, patency, and caliber of the esophagus are visualized, enabling the examiner to detect or exclude any anatomic or functional derangement of that organ. Fluoroscopic examination next extends to the stomach as its lumen fills with barium, allowing observation of stomach motility, thickness of the gastric wall, the mucosal pattern, patency of the pyloric valve, and the anatomy of the duodenum. Multiple x-ray films are obtained during the procedure, and additional images may be taken at intervals for up to 24 hours to evaluate the rate of gastric emptying. Small bowel x-rays taken while the barium is passing through that area allow for observation of the motility of the small bowel. Obstructions, ileitis, and diverticula can be detected if present.

Variations of the upper GI study include double-contrast studies and enteroclysis. The double-contrast method of examining the upper GI tract involves administration of a thick barium suspension to outline the stomach and esophageal wall, after which tablets that release carbon dioxide in the presence of water are administered. This technique has the advantage of showing the esophagus and stomach in finer detail, permitting signs of early superficial neoplasms to be noted.

Enteroclysis is a very detailed, double-contrast study of the entire small intestine that involves the continuous infusion, through a duodenal tube, of 500 to 1000 mL of a thin barium sulfate suspension; after this, methylcellulose is infused through the tube. The barium and methylcellulose fill the intestinal loops and are observed continuously by fluoroscopy and viewed at frequent intervals as they progress through the jejunum and the ileum. This process (even with normal motility) can take up to 6 hours and can be quite uncomfortable for the patient. The procedure aids in the diagnosis of partial small-bowel obstructions or diverticula.

#### NURSING INTERVENTIONS

Education regarding dietary changes prior to the study should include a clear liquid diet, with nothing by mouth (NPO) from midnight the night before the study; however, each physician may prefer a specific bowel preparation for specific studies. When a patient with insulin-dependent diabetes is NPO, his or her insulin requirements will need to be adjusted accordingly. Smoking, chewing gum, and using mints can stimulate gastric motility, so the nurse advises against these practices. Typically, oral medications are withheld on the morning of the study and resumed that evening, but each patient's medication regimen should be evaluated on an individual basis.

Follow-up care is provided after the upper GI procedure to ensure that the patient has eliminated most of the ingested barium. Fluids may be increased to facilitate evacuation of stool and barium.

### Lower Gastrointestinal Tract Study

Visualization of the lower GI tract is obtained after rectal installation of barium. The barium enema can be used to detect the presence of polyps, tumors, or other lesions of the large intestine and demonstrate any anatomic abnormalities or malfunctioning of the bowel. After proper preparation and evacuation of the entire colon, each portion of the colon may be readily observed. The procedure usually takes about 15 to 30 minutes, during which time x-ray images are obtained.

Other means for visualizing the colon include double-contrast studies and a water-soluble contrast study. A double-contrast or air-contrast barium enema involves the instillation of a thicker barium solution, followed by the instillation of air. The patient may feel some cramping or discomfort during this process. This test provides a contrast between the air-filled lumen and the barium-coated mucosa, allowing easier detection of smaller lesions.

If active inflammatory disease, fistulas, or perforation of the colon is suspected, a water-soluble iodinated contrast agent (eg, Gastrografin) can be used. The procedure is the same as for a barium enema, but the patient must be assessed for allergy to iodine or contrast agent. The contrast agent is eliminated readily after the procedure, so there is no need for postprocedure laxatives. Some diarrhea may occur in a few patients until the contrast agent has been totally eliminated.

#### NURSING INTERVENTIONS

Preparation of the patient includes emptying and cleansing the lower bowel. This often necessitates a low-residue diet 1 to 2 days before the test (the preparation required by different radiology departments may vary); a clear liquid diet and a laxative the evening before; NPO after midnight; and cleansing enemas until returns are clear the following morning. The nurse makes sure that barium enemas are scheduled before any upper GI studies. If the patient has active inflammatory disease of the colon, enemas are contraindicated. Barium enemas also are contraindicated in patients with signs of perforation or obstruction; instead, a water-soluble contrast study may be performed. Active GI bleeding may prohibit the use of laxatives and enemas.

Postprocedural patient education includes information about increasing fluid intake; evaluating bowel movements for evacuation of barium; and noting increased number of bowel movements, because barium, due to its high osmolarity, may draw fluid into the bowel, thus increasing the intraluminal contents and resulting in greater output.

## Computed Tomography

CT provides cross-sectional images of abdominal organs and structures. Multiple x-ray images are taken from numerous angles, digitized in a computer, reconstructed, and then viewed on a computer monitor. As the sensitivity and specificity of CT have increased tremendously in the past 5 years, so has the frequency with which the study is performed. CT is a valuable tool for detecting and localizing many inflammatory conditions in the colon, such as appendicitis, diverticulitis, regional enteritis, and ulcerative colitis, as well as evaluating the abdomen for diseases of the liver, spleen, kidney, pancreas, and pelvic organs, and structural abnormalities of the abdominal wall. Because the adequacy of detail in the test depends on the presence of fat, this diagnostic tool is not useful for very thin, cachectic patients. The procedure is completely painless, but radiation doses are considerable. New continuous-motion (helical or spiral), three-dimensional CT that provides very detailed pictures of the GI organs and vasculature has been developed.

**NURSING INTERVENTIONS**

CT may be performed with or without oral or intravenous (IV) contrast, but the enhancement of the study is far superior with the administration of a contrast agent. Any allergies to contrast agents, iodine, or shellfish, the patient's current serum creatinine level, and urine human chorionic gonadotropin must be determined before administration of a contrast agent. Patients allergic to the contrast agent may be premedicated with IV prednisone 24 hours, 12 hours, and 1 hour before the scan.

In addition, renal protective measures include the administration of IV sodium bicarbonate 1 hour before and 6 hours after IV contrast and oral acetylcysteine (Mucomyst) before or after the study. Both sodium bicarbonate and Mucomyst are free radical scavengers that sequester the contrast byproducts that are destructive to renal cells.

## Magnetic Resonance Imaging

MRI is used in gastroenterology to supplement ultrasonography and CT. This noninvasive technique uses magnetic fields and radio waves to produce an image of the area being studied. The use of oral contrast agents to enhance the image has increased the application of this technique for the diagnosis of GI diseases. It is useful in evaluating abdominal soft tissues as well as blood vessels, abscesses, fistulas, neoplasms, and other sources of bleeding.

The physiologic artifacts of heartbeat, respiration, and peristalsis may create a less-than-clear image; however, newer, fast-imaging MRI techniques help eliminate these physiologic motion artifacts. MRIs are not totally safe for all people. Any ferromagnetic objects (metals that contain iron) can be attracted to the magnet and cause injury. Items that can be problematic or dangerous include jewelry, pacemakers, dental implants, paperclips, pens, keys, IV poles, clips on patient gowns, and oxygen tanks. MRI is contraindicated for patients with permanent pacemakers, artificial heart valves and defibrillators, implanted insulin pumps, or implanted transcutaneous electrical nerve stimulation devices, because the magnetic field could cause malfunction. MRI is also contraindicated for patients with internal metal devices (eg, aneurysm clips) or intraocular metallic fragments. Foil-backed skin patches (eg, NicoDerm, nitroglycerine [Transderm-Nitro], scopolamine [Transderm-Scop], clonidine [Catapres-TTS]) should be removed before an MRI because of the risk of burns; however, the patient's physician should be consulted before the patch is removed to determine whether an alternate form of the medication should be provided.

**NURSING INTERVENTIONS**

Prestudy patient education includes NPO status 6 to 8 hours before the study and removal of all jewelry and other metals. The patient and family are informed that the study may take 60 to 90 minutes; during this time, the technician will instruct the patient to take deep breaths at specific intervals. The close-fitting scanners used in many MRI facilities may induce feelings of claustrophobia, and the machine will make a knocking sound during the procedure. Patients may choose to wear a headset and listen to music or to wear a blindfold during the procedure. Open MRIs that are less close-fitting eliminate the claustrophobia that many patients experience.

## Positron Emission Tomography (PET)

PET scans produce images of the body by detecting the radiation emitted from radioactive substances. The radioactive substances are injected into the body IV and are usually tagged with a radioactive atom, such as carbon-11, fluorine-18, oxygen-15, or nitrogen-13. The atoms decay quickly, do not harm the body, have lower radiation levels than a typical x-ray or CT scan, and are eliminated in the urine or feces. The scanner essentially "captures" where the radioactive substances are in the body, transmits information to a scanner, and produces a scan with "hot spots" for evaluation by the radiologist or oncologist.

## Scintigraphy

Scintigraphy (radionuclide testing) relies on the use of radioactive isotopes (ie, technetium, iodine, and indium) to reveal displaced anatomic structures, changes in organ size, and the presence of neoplasms or other focal lesions, such as cysts or abscesses. Scintigraphic scanning is also used to measure the uptake of tagged red blood cells and leukocytes. Tagging of red blood cells and leukocytes by injection of a radionuclide is performed to define areas of inflammation, abscess, blood loss, or neoplasm. A sample of blood is removed, mixed with a radioactive substance, and reinjected into the patient. Abnormal concentrations of blood cells are then detected at 24- and 48-hour intervals. Tagged red cell studies are useful in determining the source of internal bleeding when all other studies have returned a negative result.

## Gastrointestinal Motility Studies

Radionuclide testing also is used to assess gastric emptying and colonic transit time. During gastric emptying studies, the liquid and solid components of a meal (typically scrambled eggs) are tagged with radionuclide markers. After ingestion of the meal, the patient is positioned under a scintiscanner, which measures the rate of passage of the radioactive substance from the stomach. This is useful in diagnosing disorders of gastric motility, diabetic gastroparesis, and dumping syndrome.

Colonic transit studies are used to evaluate colonic motility and obstructive defecation syndromes. This is usually an outpatient study. The patient is given a capsule containing 20 radionuclide markers and instructed to follow a regular diet and normal daily activities. Abdominal x-rays are taken every 24 hours until all markers are passed. This process usually takes 4 to 5 days, but in the presence of severe constipation it may take as long as 10 days. Patients with chronic diarrhea may be evaluated at 8-hour intervals. The amount of time that it takes for the radioactive material to move through the colon indicates colonic motility.

## Endoscopic Procedures

Endoscopic procedures used in GI tract assessment include fibroscopy/esophagogastroduodenoscopy (EGD), small-bowel enteroscopy, colonoscopy, sigmoidoscopy, proctoscopy, anoscopy, and endoscopy through an ostomy.

### Upper Gastrointestinal Fibroscopy/ Esophagogastroduodenoscopy

**Fibroscopy** of the upper GI tract allows direct visualization of the esophageal, gastric, and duodenal mucosa through a lighted endoscope (gastroscope) (Fig. 34-6). EGD is especially valuable when esophageal, gastric, or duodenal abnormalities or inflammatory, neoplastic, or infectious processes are suspected. This procedure also can be used to evaluate esophageal and gastric motility and to collect secretions and tissue specimens for further analysis.

In esophagogastroduodenoscopy (EGD), the gastroenterologist views the GI tract through a viewing lens and can take still or video photographs through the scope to document findings. Electronic video endoscopes also are available that attach directly to a video processor, converting the electronic signals into pictures on a television screen. This allows larger and continuous viewing capabilities, as well as the simultaneous recording of the procedure.

Recently, PillCam ESO, a pill-sized instrument equipped with two cameras, has become available. Each camera takes seven photographs per second and transmits them wirelessly to a nearby storage device (Eliakim, Sharma, & Yassin, 2005). This technique is gaining popularity with patients and practitioners alike as a comfortable, convenient alternative to endoscopy. Two major drawbacks to this method of endoscopy are that it evaluates only the esophagus and that it may become lodged in a previously anastomosed section of bowel and require further endoscopic or surgical intervention for removal.

Side-viewing flexible scopes are used to visualize the common bile duct and the pancreatic and hepatic ducts through the ampulla of Vater in the duodenum. This procedure, called endoscopic retrograde cholangiopancreatography (ERCP), uses the endoscope in combination with x-ray techniques to view the ductal structures of the biliary tract (Hibberts & Barnes, 2003). ERCP is helpful in evaluating jaundice, pancreatitis, pancreatic tumors, common bile duct stones, and biliary tract disease. ERCP is described further in Chapter 40.

Upper GI fibroscopy also can be a therapeutic procedure when it is combined with other procedures. Therapeutic endoscopy can be used to remove common bile duct stones, dilate strictures, and treat gastric bleeding and esophageal varices. Laser-compatible scopes can be used to provide laser therapy for upper GI neoplasms. Sclerosing solutions can be injected through the scope in an attempt to control upper GI bleeding.

After the patient is sedated, the endoscope is lubricated with a water-soluble lubricant and passed smoothly and slowly along the back of the mouth and down into the esophagus. The gastroenterologist views the gastric wall and the sphincters, and then advances the endoscope into the duodenum for further examination. Biopsy forceps to obtain tissue specimens or cytology brushes to obtain cells for microscopic study can be passed through the scope. The procedure usually takes about 30 minutes.

The patient may experience nausea, gagging, or choking. Use of topical anesthetics and moderate sedation makes it important to monitor and maintain the patient's oral airway during and after the procedure. Finger or ear oximeters are

**FIGURE 34-6.** Patient undergoing gastroscopy.

used to monitor oxygen saturation, and supplemental oxygen may be administered if needed. Precautions must be taken to protect the scope, because the fiberoptic bundles can be broken if the scope is bent at an acute angle. The patient wears a mouth guard to keep from biting the scope.

**NURSING INTERVENTIONS**

Studies indicate that preoperative or preprocedure patient education is a cost-effective intervention in enhancing patient cooperation and satisfaction during ERCP (Ratanalert, Soontrapornchai, & Ovartlarnporn, 2002; vanVliet, Grypdonck, vanZuuren, et al., 2004). The patient should be NPO for 8 hours prior to the examination. Before the introduction of the endoscope, the patient is given a local anesthetic gargle or spray. Midazolam (Versed), a sedative that provides moderate sedation and relieves anxiety during the procedure, may be administered at the initiation of the study. Atropine may be administered to reduce secretions, and glucagon may be administered to relax smooth muscle. The patient is positioned in the left lateral position to facilitate clearance of pulmonary secretions and provide smooth entry of the scope.

After gastroscopy, assessment includes level of consciousness, vital signs, oxygen saturation, pain level, and monitoring for signs of perforation (ie, pain, bleeding, unusual difficulty swallowing, and rapidly elevated temperature). After the patient's gag reflex has returned, lozenges, saline gargle, and oral analgesics may be offered to relieve minor throat discomfort. Patients who were sedated for the procedure must remain in bed until fully alert. After moderate sedation, the patient must be transported home with a family member or friend if the procedure was performed on an outpatient basis. Someone should stay with the patient until the morning after the procedure. One study found that 69% of discharged patients could not recite postprocedure instructions to a nurse the morning following the procedure (Gall & Bull, 2003). For this reason, discharge instructions are provided to the person accompanying the patient home, as well as to the patient. In addition, many endoscopy suites have a program in which a nurse telephones the patient the morning after the procedure to find out if the patient has any concerns or questions related to the procedure.

## Fiberoptic Colonoscopy

Historically, direct visualization of the bowel was the only means to evaluate the colon, but virtual colonoscopy (also known as CT colonography) has brought a more patient-friendly approach to this study. First described by Vining in 1994, virtual colonoscopy provides a computer-simulated endoluminal perspective of the air-filled distended colon using conventional spiral or helical CT scanning (Fletcher, Booya, & Johnson, 2005).

Direct visual inspection of the large intestine (anus, rectum, sigmoid, transcending and ascending colon) is possible by means of a flexible fiberoptic colonoscope (Fig. 34-7). These scopes have the same capabilities as those used for EGD but are larger in diameter and longer. Still and video recordings can be used to document the procedure and findings.

This procedure is used commonly as a diagnostic aid and screening device. It is most frequently used for cancer screening (Chart 34-2) and for surveillance in patients with previous colon cancer or polyps. In addition, tissue biopsies can be obtained as needed, and polyps can be removed and evaluated. Other uses of colonoscopy include the evaluation of patients with diarrhea of unknown cause, occult bleeding, or anemia; further study of abnormalities detected on barium enema; and diagnosis, clarification, and determination of the extent of inflammatory or other bowel disease.

Therapeutically, the procedure can be used to remove all visible polyps with a special snare and cautery through the colonoscope. Many colon cancers begin with adenomatous polyps of the colon; therefore, one goal of colonoscopic polypectomy is early detection and prevention of colorectal cancer. This procedure also can be used to treat

**FIGURE 34-7.** Colonoscopy. The flexible scope is passed through the rectum and sigmoid colon into the descending, transverse, and ascending colon.

## CHART 34-2

### Health Promotion

**Guidelines for Colon and Rectal Cancer Screening**

Beginning at age 50, both men and women should follow one of these five testing schedules:

- Yearly fecal occult blood test (FOBT)* or fecal immunochemical test (FIT)
- Flexible sigmoidoscopy every 5 years
- Yearly FOBT* or FIT, plus flexible sigmoidoscopy every 5 years†
- Double-contrast barium enema every 5 years
- Colonoscopy every 10 years

All positive tests should be followed up with colonoscopy.

People should talk to their doctor about starting colorectal cancer screening earlier and/or undergoing screening more often if they have any of the following colorectal cancer risk factors:

- A personal history of colorectal cancer or adenomatous polyps
- A strong family history of colorectal cancer or polyps (cancer or polyps in a first-degree relative younger than 60 or in two first-degree relatives of any age)‡
- A personal history of chronic inflammatory bowel disease
- A family history of an hereditary colorectal cancer syndrome (familial adenomatous polyposis or hereditary non-polyposis colon cancer)

---

*For FOBT, the take-home multiple sample method should be used.
†The combination of yearly FOBT or FIT flexible sigmoidoscopy every 5 years is preferred over either of these options alone.
‡A first-degree relative is defined as a parent, sibling, or child.
Reprinted by the permission of The American Cancer Society, Inc. from www.cancer.org. All rights reserved.

---

areas of bleeding or stricture. Use of bipolar and unipolar coagulators, use of heater probes, and injections of sclerosing agents or vasoconstrictors are all possible during this procedure. Laser-compatible scopes provide laser therapy for bleeding lesions or colonic neoplasms. Bowel decompression (removal of intestinal contents to prevent gas and fluid from distending the coils of the intestine) can also be completed during the procedure.

Colonoscopy is performed while the patient is lying on the left side with the legs drawn up toward the chest. The patient's position may be changed during the test to facilitate advancement of the scope. Biopsy forceps or a cytology brush may be passed through the scope to obtain specimens for histology and cytology examinations. Complications during and after the procedure can include cardiac dysrhythmias and respiratory depression resulting from the medications administered, vasovagal reactions, and circulatory overload or hypotension resulting from overhydration or underhydration during bowel preparation. Therefore, it is important to monitor the patient's cardiac and respiratory function and oxygen saturation continuously, with supplemental oxygen used as necessary. Typically the procedure takes about 1 hour, and postprocedure discomfort results from instillation of air to expand the colon and insertion and movement of the scope during the procedure.

### NURSING INTERVENTIONS

The success of the procedure depends on how well the colon is prepared. Adequate colon cleansing provides optimal visualization and decreases the time needed for the procedure. Cleansing of the colon can be accomplished in various ways. The physician may prescribe a laxative for two nights before the examination and a Fleet's or saline enema until the return is clear the morning of the test. However, more commonly, polyethylene glycol electrolyte lavage solutions (Go-LYTELY, CoLyte, and Nu-Lytely) are used as intestinal lavages for effective cleansing of the bowel. The patient maintains a clear liquid diet starting at noon the day before the procedure. Then the patient ingests the lavage solution orally at intervals over 3 to 4 hours. Surprisingly, patient compliance with this oral portion of the bowel prep is the same for the use of flavored and unflavored lavage solutions (Hayes, Buffum, & Fuller, 2003). If necessary, the nurse can give the solution through a feeding tube if the patient cannot swallow. Patients with a colostomy can receive this same bowel preparation. The use of lavage solutions is contraindicated in patients with intestinal obstruction or inflammatory bowel disease.

With the use of lavage solutions, bowel cleansing is fast (rectal effluent is clear in about 4 hours) and is tolerated fairly well by most patients. Side effects of the electrolyte solutions include nausea, bloating, cramps or abdominal fullness, fluid and electrolyte imbalance, and hypothermia (patients are often told to drink the preparation as cold as possible to make it more palatable). The side effects are especially problematic for elderly patients, and sometimes they have difficulty ingesting the required volume of solution. Monitoring elderly patients after a bowel prep is especially important because their physiologic ability to compensate for fluid loss is diminished. Many elderly people take multiple medications each day; therefore, the nurse's knowledge of their daily medication regimen can prompt assessment for and prevention of potential problems and early detection of physiologic changes.

Additional nursing actions include the following:

- Advise the patient with diabetes to consult with his or her physician about medication adjustment to prevent hyperglycemia or hypoglycemia resulting from the dietary modifications required in preparing for the test.
- Instruct all patients, especially the elderly, to maintain adequate fluid, electrolyte, and caloric intake while undergoing bowel cleansing.

Special precautions must be taken for some patients. Implantable defibrillators and pacemakers are at high risk of malfunction if electrosurgical procedures (ie, polypectomy) are performed in conjunction with colonoscopy. A cardiologist should be consulted before the test is performed, and the defibrillator should be turned off. These patients require careful cardiac monitoring during the procedure.

Colonoscopy cannot be performed if there is a suspected or documented colon perforation, acute severe diverticulitis, or fulminant colitis. Patients with prosthetic heart valves or a history of endocarditis require prophylactic antibiotics before the procedure.

Informed consent is obtained by the practitioner before the patient is sedated. Before the examination, an opioid analgesic or sedative (eg, midazolam) is administered to provide moderate sedation and relieve anxiety during the procedure. Glucagon may be administered, if needed, to relax the colonic musculature and to reduce spasm during the test. Elderly or debilitated patients may require a reduced dosage of the analgesic or sedative to decrease the risks of oversedation and cardiopulmonary complications.

During the procedure, the nurse monitors for changes in the patient's oxygen saturation, vital signs, color and temperature of the skin, level of consciousness, abdominal distention, vagal response, and pain intensity. After the procedure, patients who were sedated are maintained on bed rest until fully alert. Some patients have abdominal cramps caused by increased peristalsis stimulated by the air insufflated into the bowel during the procedure.

Immediately after the test, the nurse observes the patient for signs and symptoms of bowel perforation (eg, rectal bleeding, abdominal pain or distention, fever, focal peritoneal signs). If midazolam was used, the nurse explains its amnesic effects. It is important to provide written instructions, because the patient may be unable to recall verbal information. If the procedure is performed on an outpatient basis, someone must transport the patient home. After a therapeutic procedure, the nurse instructs the patient to report any bleeding to the physician.

## Anoscopy, Proctoscopy, and Sigmoidoscopy

Endoscopic examination of the anus, rectum, and sigmoid and descending colon is used to evaluate chronic diarrhea, fecal incontinence, ischemic colitis, and lower GI hemorrhage and to observe for ulceration, fissures, abscesses, tumors, polyps, or other pathologic processes.

Flexible scopes have largely replaced the rigid scopes used in the past for routine examinations. The flexible fiberoptic sigmoidoscope (Fig. 34-8) permits the colon to be examined up to 40 to 50 cm (16 to 20 inches) from the anus, much more than the 25 cm (10 inches) that can be visualized with the rigid sigmoidoscope. It has many of the same capabilities as the scopes used for the upper GI study, including the use of still or video images to document findings.

For flexible scope procedures, the patient assumes a comfortable position on the left side with the right leg bent and placed anteriorly. It is important to keep the patient informed throughout the examination and to explain the sensations associated with the examination. Biopsies and polypectomies can be performed during this procedure. Biopsy is performed with small biting forceps introduced through the endoscope; one or more small pieces of tissue may be removed. If rectal or sigmoid polyps are present, they may be removed with a wire snare, which is used to grasp the pedicle, or stalk. An electrocoagulating current is then used to sever the polyp and prevent bleeding. It is extremely important that all excised tissue be placed immediately in moist gauze or in an appropriate receptacle, labeled correctly, and delivered without delay to the pathology laboratory for examination.

**FIGURE 34-8.** Flexible fiberoptic sigmoidoscopy. The flexible scope is advanced past the proximal sigmoid and then into the descending colon.

### NURSING INTERVENTIONS

These examinations require only limited bowel preparation, including a warm tap water or Fleet's enema until returns are clear. Soap-suds and tap water enemas that were used in the past produced significantly greater returns, but patients were more uncomfortable. In addition, rectal biopsies showed surface epithelium loss after soap-suds and tap water enemas but not after Fleet's enema. Dietary restrictions usually are not necessary, and sedation usually is not required. During the procedure, the nurse monitors vital signs, skin color and temperature, pain tolerance, and vagal response. After the procedure, the nurse monitors the patient for rectal bleeding and signs of intestinal perforation (ie, fever, rectal drainage, abdominal distention, and pain). On completion of the examination, the patient can resume his or her regular activities and diet.

## Small-Bowel Enteroscopy

Technology for the use of the small-caliber transnasal endoscope to allow direct inspection of the wall of the small intestine continues to improve. Two methods are being used at this time: the "push" and the "pull" endoscope methods. The "pull" endoscope is very long and flexible and has a balloon at its tip. When inflated, the balloon tip advances the scope by peristalsis through the small intestine. Metoclopramide (Reglan) may be administered IV to assist passage, and the procedure may take up to 10 hours to complete. The patient may stay in the recovery area or go home during this period. Once the scope has entered the distal ileum, the balloon is deflated and the tube is retracted slowly while the endoscopist examines the intestinal wall. "Push" endoscopes have been designed to be smaller in caliber and longer in length, while still allowing the use of biopsy forceps and probes. These two methods are especially useful in the evaluation of patients who have continued bleeding even after extensive diagnostic testing has identified no other problem area. They can also be used when biopsy of the small bowel is needed to diagnose malabsorption syndromes.

### Endoscopy Through Ostomy

Endoscopy using a flexible endoscope through an ostomy stoma is useful for visualizing a segment of the small or large intestine and may be indicated to evaluate the anastomosis for recurrent disease, or to visualize and treat bleeding in a segment of the bowel. Nursing interventions are similar to those for other endoscopic procedures.

## Manometry and Electrophysiologic Studies

Manometry and electrophysiologic studies are methods for evaluating patients with GI motility disorders. The manometry test measures changes in intraluminal pressures and the coordination of muscle activity in the GI tract with the pressures recorded manually, on a physiograph, or on a computer.

Esophageal manometry is used to detect motility disorders of the esophagus and the upper and lower esophageal sphincter. Also known as esophageal motility studies, these studies are very helpful in the diagnosis of achalasia, diffuse esophageal spasm, scleroderma, and other esophageal motor disorders. The patient must refrain from eating or drinking for 8 to 12 hours before the test. Medications that could have a direct affect on motility (eg, calcium channel blockers, anticholinergic agents, sedatives) are withheld for 24 to 48 hours. A pressure-sensitive catheter is inserted through the nose and is connected to a transducer and a video recorder. The patient then swallows small amounts of water while the resultant pressure changes are recorded. Evaluation of a patient for gastroesophageal reflux disease (GERD) typically includes esophageal manometry.

Gastroduodenal, small intestine, and colonic manometry procedures are used to evaluate delayed gastric emptying and gastric and intestinal motility disorders such as irritable bowel syndrome or atonic colon. This is often an ambulatory outpatient procedure lasting 24 to 72 hours. Anorectal manometry measures the resting tone of the internal anal sphincter and the contractibility of the external anal sphincter. It is helpful in evaluating patients with chronic constipation or fecal incontinence and is useful in biofeedback for the treatment of fecal incontinence. It can be performed in conjunction with rectal sensory functioning tests. Phospho-Soda or a saline cleansing enema is administered 1 hour before the test, and positioning for the test is either the prone or the lateral position.

Rectal sensory function studies are used to evaluate rectal sensory function and neuropathy. A catheter and balloon are passed into the rectum, with increasing balloon inflation until the patient feels distention. Then the tone and pressure of the rectum and anal sphincter are measured. The results are especially helpful in the evaluation of patients with chronic constipation, diarrhea, or incontinence.

Electrogastrography, an electrophysiologic study, also may be performed to assess gastric motility disturbances and can be useful in detecting motor or nerve dysfunction in the stomach. Electrodes are placed over the abdomen, and gastric electrical activity is recorded for up to 24 hours. Patients may exhibit rapid, slow, or irregular waveform activity.

### Defecography

Defecography measures anorectal function and is performed with very thick barium paste instilled into the rectum. Fluoroscopy is used to assess the function of the rectum and anal sphincter while the patient attempts to expel the barium. The test requires no preparation.

## Gastric Analysis, Gastric Acid Stimulation Test, and pH Monitoring

Analysis of the gastric juice yields information about the secretory activity of the gastric mucosa and the presence or degree of gastric retention in patients thought to have pyloric or duodenal obstruction. It is also useful for diagnosing Zollinger-Ellison syndrome, or atrophic gastritis.

The patient is NPO for 8 to 12 hours before the procedure. Any medications that affect gastric secretions are withheld for 24 to 48 hours before the test. Smoking is not allowed on the morning of the test, because it increases gastric secretions. A small nasogastric tube with a catheter tip marked at various points is inserted through the nose. When the tube is at a point slightly less than 50 cm (21 inches), it should be within the stomach, lying along the greater curvature. Once in place, the tube is secured to the patient's cheek and the patient is placed in a semireclining position. The entire stomach contents are aspirated by gentle suction into a syringe, and gastric samples are collected every 15 minutes for the next hour.

The gastric acid stimulation test usually is performed in conjunction with gastric analysis. Histamine or pentagastrin is administered subcutaneously to stimulate gastric secretions. It is important to inform the patient that this injection may produce a flushed feeling. The nurse monitors the patient's blood pressure and pulse frequently to detect hypotension. Gastric specimens are collected after the injection every 15 minutes for 1 hour and are labeled to indicate the time of specimen collection after histamine injection. The volume and pH of the specimen are measured; in certain instances, cytologic study by the Papanicolaou technique may be used to determine the presence or absence of malignant cells.

Important diagnostic information to be gained from gastric analysis includes the ability of the mucosa to secrete HCl. This ability is altered in various disease states, including:

- Pernicious anemia—patients with this disease secrete no acid under basal conditions or after stimulation
- Severe chronic atrophic gastritis or gastric cancer—patients with these diseases secrete little or no acid
- Peptic ulcer—patients with this disease secrete some acid
- Duodenal ulcers—patients with this disease usually secrete an excess amount of acid

Esophageal reflux of gastric acid may be diagnosed by ambulatory pH monitoring. The patient is NPO for 6 hours before the test, and all medications affecting gastric secretions are withheld for 24 to 36 hours before the test. A probe that measures pH is inserted through the nose and into position about 5 inches above the lower esophageal sphincter. It is connected to an external recording device and is worn for 24 hours while the patient continues his or her normal daily activities. The end result is a computer analysis and graphic display of the results. This test allows for the direct correlation between chest pain and reflux episodes (Wolfe, 2000).

A Bernstein test may be performed to evaluate complaints of acid-related chest or epigastric pain. HCl is instilled through a small feeding tube positioned in the esophagus to try to elicit the reported chest pain. Resultant signs and symptoms are compared with the patient's usual symptoms. However, since the advent of ambulatory pH monitoring, this previously popular evaluation tool is used infrequently (Wolfe, 2000).

## Laparoscopy (Peritoneoscopy)

With the tremendous advances in minimally invasive surgery, diagnostic laparoscopy is efficient, cost-effective, and useful in the diagnosis of GI disease. After creating a pneumoperitoneum (injecting carbon dioxide into the peritoneal cavity, to separate the intestines from the pelvic organs), a small incision is made lateral to the umbilicus, allowing for the insertion of the fiberoptic laparoscope. This permits direct visualization of the organs and structures within the abdomen, permitting visualization and identification of any growths, anomalies, and inflammatory processes. In addition, biopsy samples can be taken from the structures and organs as necessary. This procedure can be used to evaluate peritoneal disease, chronic abdominal pain, abdominal masses, and gallbladder and liver disease. However, laparoscopy has not become an important diagnostic modality in patients with acute abdominal pain, because less invasive tools (ie, CT and MRI) are readily available. Laparoscopy usually requires general anesthesia and sometimes requires that the stomach and bowel be decompressed. Gas (usually carbon dioxide) is insufflated into the peritoneal cavity to create a working space for visualization. One of the benefits of this procedure is that after visualization of a problem, excision (eg, removal of the gallbladder) can then be performed at the same time, if appropriate.

## Pathophysiologic and Psychological Considerations

Abnormalities of the GI tract are numerous and represent every type of major pathology that can affect other organ systems, including bleeding, perforation, obstruction, inflammation, and cancer. Congenital, inflammatory, infectious, traumatic, and neoplastic lesions have been encountered in every portion, and at every site, along the length of the GI tract. As with all other organ systems, the GI tract is subject to circulatory disturbances, faulty nervous system control, and aging.

Apart from the many organic diseases to which the GI tract is susceptible, many extrinsic factors can interfere with its normal function and produce symptoms. Stress and anxiety, for example, often find their chief expression in indigestion, anorexia, or motor disturbances of the intestines, sometimes producing constipation or diarrhea. In addition to the state of mental health, physical factors such as fatigue and an inadequate or abruptly changed dietary intake can markedly affect the GI tract. When assessing and instructing the patient, the nurse should consider the variety of mental and physical factors that affect the function of the GI tract.

GI diagnostic studies can confirm, rule out, stage, or diagnose disease. It is well documented that receiving a diagnosis of a serious condition (e.g., cancer) brings psychological distress, an emotional burden, a feeling of loss of personal control, and a threat to survival and self-image (Costelloe, 2004). Time should be allotted after the diagnosis for discussion with the patient, in addition to offering resource materials for information.

## Critical Thinking Exercises

1. You are caring for a 45-year-old man who presents to the emergency department complaining of a 12-hour history of mid-epigastric pain. He denies nausea and vomiting and states that the pain worsens when he moves. He is lying flat on his back with his knees flexed, appearing hesitant to move. On palpation, his abdomen is firm and rigid with rebound tenderness in the mid-epigastrium. Bowel sounds are absent. What laboratory tests would you expect to be ordered? He is scheduled for an abdominal x-ray, a CT scan, and a sonogram of the abdomen. What are the purposes of these diagnostic studies, and what preparation is needed for these tests? What preprocedure teaching is needed?

2. **ebp** You are working in an endoscopy suite and are often assigned to care for patients who are scheduled to have screening fiberoptic colonoscopy. There are a variety of ways that cleansing of the colon can be accomplished prior to colonoscopy, with various periods of time for food and fluid restriction; laxatives; enemas; and electrolyte lavage solutions. You have found that the preparation prescribed varies from physician to physician. What is the evidence base that supports the use of each of the preparations? Discuss the strength of the evidence for the effectiveness of each of the preparations. Identify the criteria used to evaluate the strength of the evidence.

## REFERENCES AND SELECTED READINGS

Bickley, L. S., & Szilagyi, P. G. (2003). *Bates' guide to physical examination and history taking* (8th ed.). Philadelphia: Lippincott Williams & Wilkins.

Eliopoulos, C. (2001). *Gerontological nursing* (5th ed.). Philadelphia: Lippincott Williams & Wilkins.

Kirsner, J. (Ed.). (2000). *Inflammatory bowel disease* (5th ed.). Philadelphia: W. B. Saunders.

Levine, M. (Ed.). (2000). *Double contrast gastrointestinal radiology*. Philadelphia: W. B. Saunders.

Ogilvie, J., Norwitz, J., & Kalloo, A. (2002). *Johns Hopkins manual for gastrointestinal endoscopy nursing*. Thorofare, NJ: Slack Incorporated.

Porth, C. M. (2005). *Pathophysiology. Concepts of altered health states*. Philadelphia: Lippincott Williams & Wilkins.

Society of Gastroenterologic Nursing and Associates. (2003). *Core curriculum* (3rd ed.). St. Louis: Mosby.

Wolfe, M. M. (Ed) (2000). *Therapy of digestive disorders*. Philadelphia: W. B. Saunders.

## JOURNALS

*Asterisks indicate nursing research articles.

Beery, T. A., & Hern, M. J. (2004). Genetic practice, education, and research: An overview for advanced practice nurses. *Clinical Nurse Specialist, 18*(3), 126–132.

Costelloe, M. N. (2004). The needs of recently diagnosed cancer patients. *Nursing Standard, 19*(13), 42–44.

Delgados-Aros, S., Locke, R., Camilleri, M., et al. (2004). Obesity is associated with increased risk of gastrointestinal symptoms: A population-based study. *American Journal of Gastroenterology, 99*(9), 1801.

Eliakim, R., Sharma, V. K., & Yassin, K. (2005). A prospective study of the diagnostic accuracy of PillCam ESO esophageal capsule endoscopy versus conventional upper endoscopy in patients with chronic gastroesophageal reflux diseases. *Journal of Clinical Gastroenterology, 39*(7), 572–578.

Fletcher, J. G., Booya, F., & Johnson, C. D. (2005). CT colonography: Unraveling the twists and turns. *Current Opinion in Gastroenterology, 21*(1), 90–98.

*Gall, S., & Bull, J. (2003). Discharging patients with no one at home. *Gastroenterology Nursing, 27*(3), 111–114.

Gavaghan, M. (1999). Anatomy and physiology of the esophagus. *AORN Journal, 69*(2), 370–374.

*Hamilton, R. J., Bowers, B. J., & Williams, J. K. (2004). Disclosing genetic test results to family members. *Journal of Nursing Scholarship, 37*(1), 18–24.

*Hayes, A., Buffum, M., & Fuller, D. (2003). Bowel preparation comparison: Flavored versus unflavored Colyte. *Gastroenterology Nursing, 26*(3), 106–109.

Hibberts, F., & Barnes, E. (2003). Use of ERCP. *Nursing Times, 99*(20), 26–37.

Lowrey, K. M. (2004). Legal and ethical issues in cancer genetics nursing. *Seminars in Oncology Nursing, 20*(3), 203–208.

McGovern, P. M., Gross, C. R., Krueger, R. A., et al. (2004). False-positive cancer screens and health-related quality of life. *Cancer Nursing, 27*(5), 347–352.

Prather, F. M. (2002). Gastrointestinal motility problems in the elderly patient. *Gastroenterology, 122*(6), 688–700.

*Ratanalert, S., Soontrapornchai, P., & Ovartlarnporn, B. (2002). Preoperative education improves quality of patient care for endoscopic retrograde cholangiopancreatography. *Gastroenterology Nursing, 26*(1), 21–25.

VanVliet, M., Grypdonck, M., VanZuuren, F., et al. (2004). Preparing patients for gastrointestinal endoscopy: The influence of information in medical situations. *Patient Education and Counseling, 52*(1), 23–30.

CHAPTER 35

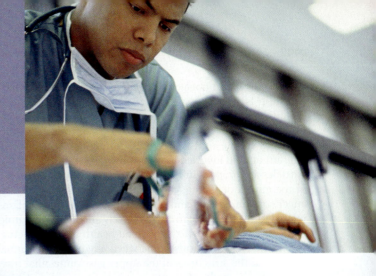

# Management of Patients With Oral and Esophageal Disorders

## Learning Objectives

*On completion of this chapter, the learner will be able to:*

1. Use the nursing process as a framework for care of patients with conditions of the oral cavity.
2. Describe the relationship of dental hygiene and dental problems to nutrition.
3. Describe the nursing management of patients with abnormalities of the lips, gums, teeth, mouth, and salivary glands.
4. Use the nursing process as a framework for care of patients with cancer of the oral cavity.
5. Identify the physical and psychosocial long-term needs of patients with oral cancer.
6. Use the nursing process as a framework for care of patients undergoing neck dissection.
7. Use the nursing process as a framework for care of patients with various conditions of the esophagus.
8. Describe the various conditions of the esophagus and their clinical manifestations and management.

Because digestion normally begins in the mouth, adequate nutrition is related to good dental health and the general condition of the mouth. Any discomfort or adverse condition in the oral cavity can affect a person's nutritional status. Changes in the oral cavity may influence the type and amount of food ingested as well as the degree to which food particles are properly mixed with salivary enzymes. Disease of the mouth or tongue can interfere with speech and thus affect communication and self-image. Esophageal problems related to swallowing can also adversely affect food and fluid intake, thereby jeopardizing general health and well-being. Given the close relationship between adequate nutritional intake and the structures of the upper gastrointestinal tract (lips, mouth, teeth, pharynx, esophagus), health teaching can help prevent disorders associated with these structures.

Oral health is a very important component of a person's physical and psychological sense of well-being. Severe periodontal disease affects approximately 14% of adults 45 to 64 years of age and 23% of adults 65 to 74 years of age (U.S. Department of Health and Human Services, 2000). Table 35-1 reviews common abnormalities of the oral cavity, their possible causes, and nursing management.

## Disorders of the Teeth

### Dental Plaque and Caries

Tooth decay is an erosive process that begins with the action of bacteria on fermentable carbohydrates in the mouth, which produces acids that dissolve tooth enamel. Although tooth enamel is the hardest substance in the human body, a recent study found that both regular and diet versions of popular soft drinks caused dental erosion by directly attacking the enamel. Soft drink consumption has increased sharply in the United States. In 1947, the average person drank about one hundred 12-ounce soft drinks per year, or two per week. Fifty years later, that number climbed to 600 annually, or two per day (von Fraunhofer & Rogers, 2004).

The extent of damage to the teeth depends on the following:

- The presence of dental plaque. Dental plaque is a gluey, gelatin-like substance that adheres to the teeth. The initial action that causes damage to a tooth occurs under dental plaque.
- The strength of the acids and the ability of the saliva to neutralize them
- The length of time the acids are in contact with the teeth
- The susceptibility of the teeth to decay

Dental decay begins with a small hole, usually in a fissure (a break in the tooth's enamel) or in an area that is hard to clean. Left unchecked, the decay extends into the dentin. Because dentin is not as hard as enamel, decay progresses more rapidly and in time reaches the pulp of the tooth. When the blood, lymph vessels, and nerves are exposed, they become infected and an abscess may form, either within the tooth or at the tip of the root. Soreness and pain usually occur with an abscess. As the infection continues, the patient's face may swell, and there may be pulsating pain.

Dentists can determine the extent of damage and the type of treatment needed using x-ray studies. Treatment for dental caries includes fillings, dental implants, and extraction, if necessary. In general, dental decay is associated with young people, but older adults are subject to decay as well, particularly from drug-induced or age-related oral dryness (Chart 35-1).

### Prevention

Measures used to prevent and control dental caries include practicing effective mouth care, reducing the intake of starches and sugars (refined carbohydrates), applying fluoride to the teeth or drinking fluoridated water, refraining from smoking, controlling diabetes, and using pit and fissure sealants (Chart 35-2).

### Mouth Care

Healthy teeth must be conscientiously and effectively cleaned on a daily basis. Brushing and flossing are particularly

## Glossary

**achalasia:** absent or ineffective peristalsis (wavelike contraction) of the distal esophagus accompanied by failure of the esophageal sphincter to relax in response to swallowing
**dysphagia:** difficulty swallowing
**dysplasia:** abnormal change in cells
**esophagogastroduodenoscopy (EGD):** passage of a fiberoptic tube through the mouth and throat into the digestive tract for visualization of the esophagus, stomach, and small intestine; biopsies can be performed
**gastroesophageal reflux:** back-flow of gastric or duodenal contents into the esophagus
**hernia:** protrusion of an organ or part of an organ through the wall of the cavity that normally contains it
**lithotripsy:** use of shock waves to break up or disintegrate stones

**odynophagia:** pain on swallowing
**parotitis:** inflammation of the parotid gland
**pyrosis:** heartburn
**periapical abscess:** abscessed tooth
**sialadenitis:** inflammation of the salivary glands
**stomatitis:** inflammation of the oral mucosa
**temporomandibular disorders:** a group of conditions that cause pain or dysfunction of the temporomandibular joint (TMJ) and surrounding structures
**vagotomy syndrome:** dumping syndrome; gastrointestinal symptoms, such as diarrhea and abdominal cramping, resulting from rapid gastric emptying
**xerostomia:** dry mouth

## TABLE 35-1  Disorders of the Lips, Mouth, and Gums

| Condition | Signs and Symptoms | Possible Causes and sequelae | Nursing Considerations |
|---|---|---|---|
| **Abnormalities of the Lips** | | | |
| Actinic cheilitis | Irritation of lips associated with scaling, crusty, fissure; white overgrowth of horny layer of epidermis (hyperkeratosis) Considered a premalignant squamous cell skin cancer | Exposure to sun; more common in fair-skinned people and in those whose occupations involve sun exposure, such as farmers May lead to squamous cell cancer | Teach patient importance of protecting lips from the sun by using protective ointment such as sun block Instruct patient to have a periodic checkup by physician |
| Herpes simplex 1 (cold sore or fever blister) | Symptoms may be delayed up to 20 days after exposure; singular or clustered painful vesicles that may rupture | An opportunistic infection; frequently seen in immunosuppressed patients; very contagious May recur with menstruation, fever, or sun exposure | Use acyclovir (Zovirax) ointment or systemic medications as prescribed Administer analgesics as prescribed Instruct patient to avoid irritating foods |
| Chancre | Reddened circumscribed lesion that ulcerates and becomes crusted | Primary lesion of syphilis; very contagious | Comfort measures: cold soaks to lip, mouth care Administer antibiotics as prescribed Instruct patient regarding contagion |
| Contact dermatitis | Red area or rash; itching | Allergic reaction to lipstick, cosmetic ointments, or toothpaste | Instruct patient to avoid possible causes Administer corticosteroids as prescribed |
| **Abnormalities of the Mouth** | | | |
| Leukoplakia | White patches; may be hyperkeratotic; usually in buccal mucosa; usually painless | Fewer than 2% are malignant, but may progress to cancer Common among tobacco users | Instruct patient to see a physician if leukoplakia persists longer than 2 weeks Eliminate risk factors, such as tobacco |
| Hairy leukoplakia | White patches with rough hair-like projections; typically found on lateral border of the tongue | Possibly viral; smoking and use of tobacco Often seen in people who are HIV positive | Instruct patient to see a physician if condition persists longer than 2 weeks |
| Lichen planus | White papules at the intersection of a network of interlacing lesions; usually ulcerated and painful | Recurrences are common May lead to a malignant process Unknown cause | Apply topical corticosteroids such as fluocinolone acetonide oral base gel Avoid foods that irritate Administer corticosteroids systemically or intralesionally as prescribed Instruct the patient of need for follow-up if condition is chronic |
| Candidiasis (moniliasis/thrush) | Cheesy white plaque that looks like milk curds; when rubbed off, it leaves an erythematous and often bleeding base | *Candida albicans* fungus; predisposing factors include diabetes, antibiotic therapy, and immunosuppression | Antifungal medications such as nystatin (Mycostatin), amphotericin B, clotrimazole, or ketoconazole may be prescribed; these may be taken in pill form or as a suspension; when used as a suspension, instruct the patient to swish vigorously for at least 1 minute and then swallow |
| Aphthous stomatitis (canker sore) | Shallow ulcer with a white or yellow center and red border; seen on the inner side of the lip and cheek or on the tongue; it begins with a burning or tingling sensation and slight swelling; painful; usually lasts 7–10 days and heals without a scar | Associated with emotional or mental stress, fatigue, hormonal factors, minor trauma (such as biting), allergies, acidic foods and juices, and dietary deficiencies Associated with HIV infection May recur | Instruct the patient in comfort measures, such as saline rinses, and a soft or bland diet Antibiotics or corticosteroids may be prescribed |

*continued >*

## TABLE 35-1  Disorders of the Lips, Mouth, and Gums (Continued)

| Condition | Signs and Symptoms | Possible Causes and sequelae | Nursing Considerations |
|---|---|---|---|
| Nicotine stomatitis (smoker's patch) | Two stages—begins as a red stomatitis; over time the tongue and mouth become covered with a creamy, thick, white mucous membrane, which may slough, leaving a beefy red base | Chronic irritation by tobacco | Cessation of tobacco use; if condition exists for longer than 2 weeks a physician should be consulted and a biopsy may be needed |
| Krythoplakia | Red patch on the oral mucous membrane | Nonspecific inflammation; more frequently seen in the elderly | |
| Kaposi's sarcoma | Appears first on the oral mucosa as a red, purple, or blue lesion; may be singular or multiple; may be flat or raised | HIV infection | Instruct patient regarding side effects of planned treatment |
| Stomatitis | Mild redness (erythema) and edema; if severe, painful ulcerations, bleeding, and secondary infection | Chemotherapy; radiation therapy; severe drug allergy; myelosuppression (bone marrow depression) | Prophylactic mouth care, including brushing, flossing, and rinsing, for any patient receiving chemotherapy or radiation therapy<br>Teach patient proper oral hygiene, including the use of a soft-bristled toothbrush and nonabrasive toothpaste; for painful ulcers, oral swabs with sponge-like applicators can be used in place of a toothbrush; avoid alcohol-based mouth rinses and hot or spicy foods<br>Apply topical anti-inflammatory, antibiotic, and anesthetic agents as prescribed |
| **Abnormalities of the Gums** | | | |
| Gingivitis | Painful, inflamed, swollen gums; usually the gums bleed in response to light contact | Poor oral hygiene: food debris, bacterial plaque, and calculus (tartar) accumulate; the gums may also swell in response to normal processes such as puberty and pregnancy | Teach patient proper oral hygiene; see Chart 35-2 |
| Necrotizing gingivitis (trench mouth) | Gray-white pseudomembranous ulcerations affecting the edges of the gums, mucosa of the mouth, tonsils, and pharynx; foul breath; painful, bleeding gums; swallowing and talking are painful | Poor oral hygiene; bacterial infection, inadequate rest, overwork, emotional stress, smoking, and poor nutrition may contribute to development | Teach patient proper oral hygiene; see Chart 35-2<br>Irrigate with 2% to 3% hydrogen peroxide or normal saline solution<br>Avoid irritants such as smoking and spicy foods |
| Herpetic gingivostomatitis | Burning sensation with the appearance of small vesicles 24–48 hours later; vesicles may rupture, forming sore, shallow ulcers covered with a gray membrane | Herpes simplex virus; occurs most frequently in people who are immunosuppressed; may occur in other infectious processes such as streptococcal pneumonia, meningococcal meningitis, and malaria | Apply topical anesthetics as prescribed; may need opioids if pain is severe<br>Saline or 2% to 3% hydrogen peroxide irrigations<br>Antiviral agents such as acyclovir may be prescribed |
| Periodontitis | Little discomfort at onset; may have bleeding, infection, gum recession, and loosening of teeth; later in the disease tooth loss may occur | May result from untreated gingivitis<br>Poor or inadequate dental hygiene and inadequate diet contribute to development | Instruct patient in proper oral hygiene<br>Instruct patient to consult a dentist |

## CHART 35-1

### Gerontologic Considerations

### Oral Conditions in the Older Adult

Many medications taken by the elderly cause dry mouth, which is uncomfortable, impairs communication, and increases the risk of oral infection. These medications include the following:
- Diuretics
- Antihypertensive medications
- Anti-inflammatory agents
- Antidepressant medications

Poor dentition can exacerbate problems of aging, such as:
- Decreased food intake
- Loss of appetite
- Social isolation
- Increased susceptibility to systemic infection (from periodontal disease)
- Trauma to the oral cavity secondary to thinner, less vascular oral mucous membranes

---

effective in mechanically breaking up the bacterial plaque that collects around teeth.

Normal mastication (chewing) and the normal flow of saliva also aid greatly in keeping the teeth clean. Because many ill patients do not eat adequate amounts of food, they produce less saliva, which in turn reduces this natural tooth cleaning process. The nurse may need to assume the responsibility for brushing the patient's teeth. Merely wiping the patient's mouth and teeth with a swab is ineffective. The most effective method is mechanical cleansing (brushing). If brushing is impossible, it is better to wipe the teeth with a gauze pad, then have the patient swish an antiseptic mouthwash several times before expectorating into an emesis basin. A soft-bristled toothbrush is more effective than a sponge or foam stick. To prevent drying, the lips may be coated with a water-soluble gel.

### Diet

Dental caries may be prevented by decreasing the amount of sugar and starch in the diet. Patients who snack should be encouraged to choose less cariogenic alternatives, such as fruits, vegetables, nuts, cheeses, or plain yogurt. In addition, frequent brushing, especially after meals, is necessary. Flossing should be performed daily.

### Fluoridation

Fluoridation of public water supplies has been found to decrease dental caries. Some areas of the country have natural fluoridation; other communities have added fluoride to public water supplies. Fluoridation may be achieved also by having a dentist apply a concentrated gel or solution to the teeth; adding fluoride to home water supplies; using fluoridated toothpaste or mouth rinse; or using sodium fluoride tablets, drops, or lozenges.

### Pit and Fissure Sealants

The occlusal surfaces of the teeth have pits and fissures, areas that are prone to caries. Some dentists apply a special coating to fill and seal these areas from potential exposure to cariogenic processes. These sealants can last 5 to 10 years, depending on how dry the tooth surface is prior to application.

## Dentoalveolar Abscess or Periapical Abscess

**Periapical abscess**, more commonly referred to as an abscessed tooth, involves a collection of pus in the apical dental periosteum (fibrous membrane supporting the tooth structure) and the tissue surrounding the apex of the tooth (where it is suspended in the jaw bone). The abscess may be acute or chronic. Acute periapical abscess is usually secondary to a suppurative pulpitis (a pus-producing inflammation of the dental pulp) that arises from an infection extending from dental caries. The infection of the dental pulp extends through the apical foramen of the tooth to form an abscess around the apex.

Chronic dentoalveolar abscess is a slowly progressive infectious process. In contrast to the acute form, a fully formed abscess may occur without the patient's knowledge. The infection eventually leads to a "blind dental abscess," which is actually a periapical granuloma. It may enlarge to as much as 1 cm in diameter. It is often discovered on x-ray films and is treated by extraction or root canal therapy, often with apicectomy (excision of the apex of the tooth root).

### Clinical Manifestations

The abscess produces a dull, gnawing, continuous pain, often with a surrounding cellulitis and edema of the adjacent facial structures, and mobility of the involved tooth. The

## CHART 35-2

### Health Promotion

### Preventive Oral Hygiene

- Brush teeth using a soft toothbrush at least two times daily. Hold toothbrush at a 45-degree angle between the brush and the gums and teeth. A small brush is better than a large brush. Gums and tongue surface should be brushed.
- Floss at least once daily.
- Use an antiplaque mouth rinse.
- Visit a dentist at least every 6 months, or when you have a chipped tooth, a lost filling, an oral sore that persists longer than 2 weeks, or a toothache.
- Avoid alcohol and tobacco products, including smokeless tobacco.
- Maintain adequate nutrition and avoid sweets.
- Replace toothbrush at first signs of wear, usually every 2 months.

gum opposite the apex of the tooth is usually swollen on the cheek side. Swelling and cellulitis of the facial structures may make it difficult for the patient to open the mouth. There may also be a systemic reaction, fever, and malaise.

## Management

In the early stages of an infection, a dentist or oral surgeon may perform a needle aspiration or drill an opening into the pulp chamber to relieve pressure and pain and to provide drainage. Usually, the infection will have progressed to a periapical abscess. Drainage is provided by an incision through the gingiva down to the jawbone. Pus (purulent material) escapes under pressure. This procedure may be performed in the dentist's office, an outpatient surgery center, or a same-day surgery department. After the inflammatory reaction has subsided, the tooth may be extracted or root canal therapy performed. Antibiotics may be prescribed.

## Nursing Management

The nurse assesses the patient for bleeding after treatment and instructs the patient to use a warm saline or warm water mouth rinse to keep the area clean. The patient is also instructed to take antibiotics and analgesics as prescribed, to advance from a liquid diet to a soft diet as tolerated, and to keep follow-up appointments.

# *Malocclusion*

Malocclusion is a misalignment of the teeth of the upper and lower dental arcs when the jaws are closed. Malocclusion can be inherited or acquired (from thumb-sucking, trauma, or some medical conditions). Malocclusion makes the teeth difficult to clean and can lead to decay, gum disease, and excess wear on supporting bone and gum tissues. About 50% of the population has some form of malocclusion. Correction of malocclusion requires an orthodontist, a patient who is motivated and cooperative, and adequate time. Most treatments begin when the patient has shed the last primary tooth and the last permanent successor has erupted, usually at about 12 or 13 years of age, but treatment may occur in adulthood. Preventive orthodontics may be started in children as early as 5 years of age if malocclusion is diagnosed early. The need for teeth straightening in adolescents is reduced if preventive orthodontics is started with the primary teeth.

## Management

People with malocclusion have an obviously misaligned bite or crooked, crowded, widely spaced, or protruding teeth. To realign the teeth, the orthodontist gradually forces the teeth into a new location by using wires or plastic bands (braces). These devices may be unattractive, but this psychological burden must be overcome if good results are to be achieved. In the final phase of treatment, a retaining device is worn for several hours each day to support the tissues as they adjust to the new alignment of the teeth.

## Nursing Management

The patient must practice meticulous oral hygiene, and the nurse encourages the patient to continue this important part of the treatment. An adolescent or adult undergoing orthodontic correction who is admitted to the hospital for some other problem may have to be reminded to continue wearing the retainer (if it does not interfere with the problem requiring hospitalization).

# Disorders of the Jaw

Abnormal conditions affecting the mandible (jaw) and of the temporomandibular joint (which connects the mandible to the temporal bone at the side of the head in front of the ear) include congenital malformation, fracture, chronic dislocation, cancer, and syndromes characterized by pain and limited motion. Temporomandibular disorders and jaw surgery (a treatment common in many structural abnormalities or cancer of the jaw) are presented in this section.

# *Temporomandibular Disorders*

**Temporomandibular disorders** are categorized as follows (U.S. Department of Health and Human Services, 2000):

- Myofascial pain—a discomfort in the muscles controlling jaw function and in neck and shoulder muscles
- Internal derangement of the joint—a dislocated jaw, a displaced disc, or an injured condyle
- Degenerative joint disease—rheumatoid arthritis or osteoarthritis in the jaw joint

Diagnosis and treatment of temporomandibular disorders remain somewhat ambiguous, but the condition is thought to affect about 10 million people in the United States. Misalignment of the joints in the jaw and other problems associated with the ligaments and muscles of mastication are thought to result in tissue damage and muscle tenderness. Suggested causes include arthritis of the jaw, head injury, trauma or injury to the jaw or joint, stress, and malocclusion (although research does not support malocclusion as a cause).

## Clinical Manifestations

Patients have pain ranging from a dull ache to throbbing, debilitating pain that can radiate to the ears, teeth, neck muscles, and facial sinuses. They often have restricted jaw motion and locking of the jaw. There also may be a sudden change in the way the upper and lower teeth fit together. The patient may hear clicking and grating noises, and chewing and swallowing may be difficult. Symptoms such as headaches, earaches, dizziness, and hearing problems may sometimes be related to temporomandibular disorders (National Institute of Dental & Craniofacial Research, 2004).

## Assessment and Diagnostic Findings

Diagnosis is based on the patient's report of pain, limitations in range of motion, dysphagia, difficulty chewing, difficulty with speech, or hearing difficulties. Magnetic resonance imaging, x-ray studies, and an arthrogram may be performed.

## Management

Although some practitioners think the role of stress in temporomandibular joint disorders is overrated, patient education in stress management may be helpful (to reduce grinding and clenching of teeth). The patient may also benefit from range-of-motion exercises. Pain management measures may include nonsteroidal anti-inflammatory drugs (NSAIDs), with the possible addition of opioids, muscle relaxants, or mild antidepressants. Occasionally, intra-oral orthotics (a plastic guard worn over the upper and lower teeth) may be worn to reposition the condyle head in the joint space to a more normal position, which in turn relieves the stress and pressure on the tissues of the joint. This allows the tissues to heal. Conservative and reversible treatment is recommended. If irreversible surgical options are recommended, the patient is encouraged to seek a second opinion.

## Jaw Disorders Requiring Surgical Management

Correction of mandibular structural abnormalities may require surgery involving repositioning or reconstruction of the jaw. Simple fractures of the mandible without displacement, resulting from a blow on the chin, and planned surgical interventions, as in the correction of long or short jaw syndrome, may require treatment by these means. Jaw reconstruction may be necessary in the aftermath of trauma from a severe injury or cancer, both of which can cause tissue and bone loss.

Mandibular fractures are usually closed fractures. Rigid plate fixation (insertion of metal plates and screws into the bone to approximate and stabilize the bone) is the current treatment of choice in many cases of mandibular fracture and in some mandibular reconstructive surgery procedures. Bone grafting may be performed to replace structural defects using bones from the patient's own ilium, ribs, or cranial sites. Rib tissue may also be harvested from cadaver donors.

## Nursing Management

The patient who has had rigid fixation should be instructed not to chew food in the first 1 to 4 weeks after surgery. A liquid diet is recommended, and dietary counseling should be obtained to ensure optimal caloric and protein intake.

## Promoting Home and Community-Based Care

The patient needs specific guidelines for mouth care and feeding. Any irritated areas in the mouth should be reported to the physician. The importance of keeping scheduled appointments to assess the stability of the fixation appliance is emphasized.

Consultation with a dietitian may be indicated so that the patient and family can learn about foods that are high in essential nutrients and ways in which these foods can be prepared so that they can be consumed through a straw or spoon while remaining palatable. Nutritional supplements may be recommended.

# Disorders of the Salivary Glands

The salivary glands consist of the parotid glands, one on each side of the face below the ear; the submandibular and sublingual glands, both in the floor of the mouth; and the buccal gland, beneath the lips. About 1200 mL of saliva are produced daily and swallowed. The glands' primary functions are lubrication, protection against harmful bacteria, and digestion.

## Parotitis

**Parotitis** (inflammation of the parotid gland) is the most common inflammatory condition of the salivary glands, although inflammation can occur in the other salivary glands as well. Mumps (epidemic parotitis), a communicable disease caused by viral infection and most commonly affecting children, is an inflammation of a salivary gland, usually the parotid.

Elderly, acutely ill, or debilitated people with decreased salivary flow from general dehydration or medications are at high risk for parotitis. The infecting organisms travel from the mouth through the salivary duct. The organism is usually *Staphylococcus aureus* (except in mumps). The onset of this complication is sudden, with an exacerbation of both the fever and the symptoms of the primary condition. The gland swells and becomes tense and tender. The patient feels pain in the ear, and swollen glands interfere with swallowing. The swelling increases rapidly, and the overlying skin soon becomes red and shiny.

Medical management includes maintaining adequate nutritional and fluid intake, good oral hygiene, and discontinuing medications (eg, tranquilizers, diuretics) that can diminish salivation. Antibiotic therapy is necessary, and analgesics may be prescribed to control pain. If antibiotic therapy is not effective, the gland may need to be drained by a surgical procedure known as parotidectomy. This procedure may be necessary to treat chronic parotitis. The patient is advised to have any necessary dental work performed prior to surgery.

## Sialadenitis

**Sialadenitis** (inflammation of the salivary glands) may be caused by dehydration, radiation therapy, stress, malnutrition, salivary gland calculi (stones), or improper oral hygiene. The inflammation is associated with infection by *S. aureus*, *Streptococcus viridans,* or pneumococci. In hospitalized or institutionalized patients, the infecting organism may be methicillin-resistant *S. aureus* (MRSA). Symptoms include pain, swelling, and purulent discharge. Antibiotics are used to treat infections. Massage, hydration, warm compresses, and corticosteroids frequently cure the problem. Chronic sialadenitis with uncontrolled pain is treated by surgical drainage of the gland or excision of the gland and its duct.

## Salivary Calculus (Sialolithiasis)

Sialolithiasis, or salivary calculi (stones), usually occurs in the submandibular gland. Salivary gland ultrasonography or sialography (x-ray studies filmed after the injection of a radiopaque substance into the duct) may be required to demonstrate obstruction of the duct by stenosis. Salivary calculi are formed mainly from calcium phosphate. If located within the gland, the calculi are irregular and vary in diameter from 3 to 30 mm. Calculi in the duct are small and oval.

Calculi within the salivary gland itself cause no symptoms unless infection arises; however, a calculus that obstructs the gland's duct causes sudden, local, and often colicky pain, which is abruptly relieved by a gush of saliva. This characteristic symptom is often disclosed in the patient's health history. On physical assessment, the gland is swollen and quite tender, the stone itself can be palpable, and its shadow may be seen on x-ray films.

The calculus can be extracted fairly easily from the duct in the mouth. Sometimes, enlargement of the ductal orifice permits the stone to pass spontaneously. Occasionally **lithotripsy**, a procedure that uses shock waves to disintegrate the stone, may be used instead of surgical extraction for parotid stones and smaller submandibular stones. Lithotripsy requires no anesthesia, sedation, or analgesia. Side effects can include local hemorrhage and swelling. Surgery may be necessary to remove the gland if symptoms and calculi recur repeatedly.

## Neoplasms

Although they are uncommon, neoplasms (tumors or growths) of almost any type may develop in the salivary gland. Tumors occur more often in the parotid gland. The incidence of salivary gland tumors is similar in men and women. Risk factors include prior exposure to radiation to the head and neck. Diagnosis is based on the health history and physical examination and the results of fine-needle aspiration biopsy.

Management of salivary gland tumors may involve partial excision of the gland, along with the tumor and a wide margin of surrounding tissue. Dissection is carefully performed to preserve the seventh cranial nerve (facial nerve), although it may not be possible to do so if the tumor is extensive. If the tumor is malignant, radiation therapy may follow surgery. Radiation therapy alone may be a treatment choice for tumors that are thought to be localized or if there is risk of facial nerve damage from surgical intervention. Chemotherapy is usually used for palliative purposes. Local recurrences are common, and the recurrent tumors usually are more aggressive than the original. Patients with salivary gland tumors have an increased incidence of second primary cancers (Bull, 2001).

## Cancer of the Oral Cavity

Cancers of the oral cavity, which can occur in any part of the mouth or throat, are curable if discovered early. If the cancer is detected before it has spread to the lymph nodes, the 5-year survival rate is approximately 80% (American Cancer Society, 2005). Oral cancers are often associated with the use of alcohol and tobacco, which if used together have a synergistic carcinogenic effect. About 95% of oral cancers occur in people older than 40 years of age, but the incidence is increasing in men younger than 30 years because of the use of smokeless tobacco, especially snuff (Centers for Disease Control and Prevention, 2004). Men are more likely to use smokeless tobacco than women, and Caucasian men have the highest percentage of smokeless tobacco use, at 18% (American Cancer Society, 2005).

Cancer of the oral cavity affects men more often than women; however, the incidence of oral cancer in women is increasing, possibly because they use tobacco and alcohol more frequently than they did in the past. Cancers of the oral cavity and oropharynx occur more often in African Americans than in Caucasians.

Approximately 30,000 new cases of oral cavity and oropharyngeal cancer occur annually in the United States (American Cancer Society, 2005). For the past 20 years, the number of new cases has been decreasing; it has decreased by 5% per year for the past 2 years. In addition, since the late 1970s, the death rate has been decreasing. Eighty-one percent of patients with cancer of the oral cavity and oropharynx survive at least 1 year after diagnosis. Regardless of the stage of cancer at diagnosis, the 5-year relative survival rate is 56% and the 10-year survival rate is 41%.

Chronic irritation by a warm pipe stem or prolonged exposure to the sun and wind may predispose a person to lip cancer. Predisposing factors for other oral cancers are exposure to tobacco (including smokeless tobacco), ingestion of alcohol, dietary deficiency, and ingestion of smoked meats.

### Pathophysiology

Malignancies of the oral cavity are usually squamous cell cancers. Any area of the oropharynx can be a site of malignant growths, but the lips, the lateral aspects of the tongue, and the floor of the mouth are most commonly affected.

### Clinical Manifestations

Many oral cancers produce few or no symptoms in the early stages. Later, the most frequent symptom is a painless sore or mass that will not heal. A typical lesion in oral cancer is a painless indurated (hardened) ulcer with raised edges. Tissue from any ulcer of the oral cavity that does not heal in 2 weeks should be examined through biopsy. As the cancer progresses, the patient may complain of tenderness; difficulty in chewing, swallowing, or speaking; coughing of blood-tinged sputum; or enlarged cervical lymph nodes.

### Assessment and Diagnostic Findings

Diagnostic evaluation consists of an oral examination as well as an assessment of the cervical lymph nodes to detect possible metastases. Biopsies are performed on suspicious lesions (those that have not healed in 2 weeks). High-risk areas include the buccal mucosa and gingiva in people who use snuff or smoke cigars or pipes. For those who smoke cigarettes and drink alcohol, high-risk areas include the floor of the mouth, the ventrolateral tongue, and the soft palate complex (soft palate, anterior and posterior tonsillar area, uvula, and the area behind the molar and tongue junction).

## Medical Management

Management varies with the nature of the lesion, the preference of the physician, and patient choice. Surgical resection, radiation therapy, chemotherapy, or a combination of these therapies may be effective.

In cancer of the lip, small lesions are usually excised liberally. Radiation therapy may be more appropriate for larger lesions involving more than one third of the lip because of superior cosmetic results. The choice depends on the extent of the lesion and what is necessary to cure the patient while preserving the best appearance. Tumors larger than 4 cm often recur.

In cancer of the tongue, treatment with radiation therapy and chemotherapy may preserve organ function and maintain quality of life. A combination of radioactive interstitial implants (surgical implantation of a radioactive source into the tissue adjacent to or at the tumor site) and external beam radiation may be used. Surgical procedures include hemiglossectomy (surgical removal of half of the tongue) and total glossectomy (removal of the tongue).

Often cancer of the oral cavity has metastasized through the extensive lymphatic channel in the neck region (Fig. 35-1), requiring a neck dissection and reconstructive surgery of the oral cavity. A common reconstructive technique involves use of a radial forearm free flap (a thin layer of skin from the forearm along with the radial artery).

## Nursing Management

The nurse assesses the patient's nutritional status preoperatively, and a dietary consultation may be necessary. The patient may require enteral (through the gastrointestinal tract) or parenteral (intravenous [IV]) feedings before and after surgery to maintain adequate nutrition. If a radial graft is to be performed, an Allen test on the donor arm must be performed to ensure that the ulnar artery is patent and can provide blood flow to the hand after removal of the radial artery. The Allen test is performed by asking the patient to make a fist and then manually compressing the ulnar artery. The patient is then asked to open the hand into a relaxed, slightly flexed position. The palm will be pale. Pressure on the ulnar artery is released. If the ulnar artery is patent, the palm will flush within about 3 to 5 seconds.

Postoperatively, the nurse assesses for a patent airway. The patient may be unable to manage oral secretions, making suctioning necessary. If grafting was part of the surgery, suctioning must be performed with care to prevent damage to the graft. The graft is assessed postoperatively for viability. Although color should be assessed (white may indicate arterial occlusion, and blue mottling may indicate venous congestion), it can be difficult to assess the graft by looking into the mouth. A Doppler ultrasound device may be used to locate the radial pulse at the graft site and to assess graft perfusion.

## ◄▼► Nursing Process

### The Patient With Conditions of the Oral Cavity

#### Assessment

Obtaining a health history allows the nurse to determine the patient's learning needs concerning preventive oral hygiene and to identify symptoms requiring medical evaluation. The history addresses the patient's normal brushing and flossing routine; frequency of dental visits; awareness of any lesions or irritated areas in the mouth, tongue, or throat; recent history of sore throat or bloody sputum; discomfort caused by certain foods; daily food intake; use of alcohol and tobacco, including smokeless chewing tobacco; and the need to wear dentures or a partial plate. For more information about dentures, see Chart 35-3.

A careful physical assessment follows the health history. Both the internal and the external structures of the mouth and throat are inspected and palpated. Dentures and partial plates are removed to ensure a thorough inspection of the mouth. In general, the examination can be accomplished by using a bright light source (penlight) and a tongue depressor. Gloves are worn to palpate the tongue and any abnormalities.

#### Lips

The examination begins with inspection of the lips for moisture, hydration, color, texture, symmetry, and

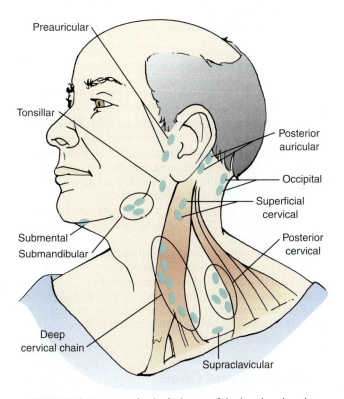

**FIGURE 35-1.** Lymphatic drainage of the head and neck.

### CHART 35-3 · Health Promotion

**Denture Care**

- Brush dentures twice a day.
- Remove dentures at night and soak them in water or a denture product. (Never put dentures in hot water, because they may warp.)
- Rinse mouth with warm salt water in the morning, after meals, and at bedtime.
- Clean well under partial dentures, where food particles tend to get caught.
- Consume nonsticky foods that have been cut into small pieces; chew slowly.
- See dentist regularly to assess and adjust fit.

**FIGURE 35-2.** Structures of the mouth, including the tongue and palate.

the presence of ulcerations or fissures. The lips should be moist, pink, smooth, and symmetric. The patient is instructed to open the mouth wide; a tongue blade is then inserted to expose the buccal mucosa for an assessment of color and lesions. Stensen's duct of each parotid gland is visible as a small red dot in the buccal mucosa next to the upper molars.

### Gums

The gums are inspected for inflammation, bleeding, retraction, and discoloration. The odor of the breath is also noted. The hard palate is examined for color and shape.

### Tongue

The dorsum (back) of the tongue is inspected for texture, color, and lesions. A thin white coat and large, vallate papillae in a "V" formation on the distal portion of the dorsum of the tongue are normal findings. The patient is instructed to protrude the tongue and move it laterally. This provides the examiner with an opportunity to estimate the tongue's size as well as its symmetry and strength (to assess the integrity of the 12th cranial nerve [hypoglossal]).

Further inspection of the ventral surface of the tongue and the floor of the mouth is accomplished by asking the patient to touch the roof of the mouth with the tip of the tongue. Any lesions of the mucosa or any abnormalities involving the frenulum or superficial veins on the undersurface of the tongue are assessed for location, size, color, and pain. This is a common area for oral cancer, which presents as a white or red plaque, an indurated ulcer, or a warty growth.

A tongue blade is used to depress the tongue for adequate visualization of the pharynx. It is pressed firmly beyond the midpoint of the tongue; proper placement avoids a gagging response. The patient is told to tip the head back, open the mouth wide, take a deep breath, and say "ah." Often this flattens the posterior tongue and briefly allows a full view of the tonsils, uvula, and posterior pharynx (Fig. 35-2). These structures are inspected for color, symmetry, and evidence of exudate, ulceration, or enlargement. Normally, the uvula and soft palate rise symmetrically with a deep inspiration or "ah"; this indicates an intact vagus nerve (10th cranial nerve).

A complete assessment of the oral cavity is essential because many disorders, such as cancer, diabetes, and immunosuppressive conditions resulting from medication therapy or acquired immunodeficiency syndrome (AIDS), may be manifested by changes in the oral cavity, including stomatitis. The neck is examined for enlarged lymph nodes (adenopathy).

### Nursing Diagnoses

Based on all the assessment data, major nursing diagnoses may include the following:

- Impaired oral mucous membrane related to a pathologic condition, infection, or chemical or mechanical trauma (eg, medications, ill-fitting dentures)
- Imbalanced nutrition, less than body requirements, related to inability to ingest adequate nutrients secondary to oral or dental conditions
- Disturbed body image related to a physical change in appearance resulting from a disease condition or its treatment
- Fear of pain and social isolation related to disease or change in physical appearance
- Pain related to oral lesion or treatment
- Impaired verbal communication related to treatment
- Risk for infection related to disease or treatment
- Deficient knowledge about disease process and treatment plan

### Planning and Goals

The major goals for the patient may include improved condition of the oral mucous membrane, improved nutritional intake, attainment of a positive self-image, relief of pain, identification of alternative communication methods, prevention of infection, and understanding of the disease and its treatment.

## Nursing Interventions

### Promoting Mouth Care

The nurse instructs the patient in the importance and techniques of preventive mouth care. If a patient cannot tolerate brushing or flossing, an irrigating solution of 1 teaspoon of baking soda to 8 ounces of warm water, half-strength hydrogen peroxide, or normal saline solution is recommended. The nurse reinforces the need to perform oral care and provides such care to patients who cannot provide it for themselves.

If a bacterial or fungal infection is present, the nurse administers the appropriate medications and instructs the patient in how to administer the medications at home. The nurse monitors the patient's physical and psychological response to treatment.

**Xerostomia,** dryness of the mouth, is a frequent sequela of oral cancer, particularly when the salivary glands have been exposed to radiation or major surgery. It is also seen in patients who are receiving psychopharmacologic agents, patients with human immunodeficiency virus (HIV) infection, and patients who cannot close the mouth and as a result become mouth-breathers. To minimize this problem, the patient is advised to avoid dry, bulky, and irritating foods and fluids, as well as alcohol and tobacco. The patient is also encouraged to increase intake of fluids (when not contraindicated) and to use a humidifier during sleep. The use of synthetic saliva, a moisturizing antibacterial gel such as Oral Balance, or a saliva production stimulant such as Salagen may be helpful.

**Stomatitis,** or mucositis, which involves inflammation and breakdown of the oral mucosa, is often a side effect of chemotherapy or radiation therapy. Prophylactic mouth care is started when the patient begins receiving treatment; however, mucositis may become so severe that a break in treatment is necessary. If a patient receiving radiation therapy has poor dentition, extraction of the teeth before radiation treatment in the oral cavity is often initiated to prevent infection. Many radiation therapy centers recommend the use of fluoride treatments for patients receiving radiation to the head and neck. (See Chapter 16 for more information about stomatitis.)

### Ensuring Adequate Food and Fluid Intake

The patient's weight, age, and level of activity are recorded to determine whether nutritional intake is adequate. A daily calorie count may be necessary to determine the exact quantity of food and fluid ingested. The frequency and pattern of eating are recorded to determine whether any psychosocial or physiologic factors are affecting ingestion. Based on the disorder and the patient's preferences, the nurse recommends changes in the consistency of foods and the frequency of eating. Consultation with a dietitian may be helpful. The goal is to help the patient attain and maintain desirable body weight and level of energy, as well as to promote the healing of tissue.

### Supporting a Positive Self-Image

A patient who has a disfiguring oral condition or has undergone disfiguring surgery may experience an alteration in self-image. The patient is encouraged to verbalize the perceived change in body appearance and to realistically discuss actual changes or losses. The nurse offers support while the patient verbalizes fears and negative feelings (withdrawal, depression, anger). The nurse listens attentively and determines the patient's needs and individualizes the plan of care. The patient's strengths, achievements, and positive attributes are reinforced.

The nurse should determine the patient's anxieties concerning relationships with others. Referral to support groups, a psychiatric liaison nurse, a social worker, or a spiritual advisor may be useful in helping the patient to cope with anxieties and fears. The patient's progress toward development of positive self-esteem is documented. The nurse should be alert to signs of grieving and should document emotional changes. By providing acceptance and support, the nurse encourages the patient to verbalize feelings.

### Minimizing Pain and Discomfort

Oral lesions can be painful. Strategies to reduce pain and discomfort include avoiding foods that are spicy, hot, or hard (eg, pretzels, nuts). The patient is instructed about mouth care. It may be necessary to provide the patient with an analgesic such as viscous lidocaine (Xylocaine Viscous 2%) or opioids, as prescribed. The nurse can reduce the patient's fear of pain by providing information about pain control methods.

### Promoting Effective Communication

Verbal communication may be impaired by radical surgery for oral cancer. It is therefore vital to assess the patient's ability to communicate in writing before surgery. Pen and paper are provided postoperatively to patients who can use them to communicate. A communication board with commonly used words or pictures is obtained preoperatively and given after surgery to patients who cannot write so that they may point to needed items. A speech therapist is also consulted postoperatively.

### Preventing Infection

Leukopenia (a decrease in white blood cells) may result from radiation, chemotherapy, AIDS, and some medications used to treat HIV infection. Leukopenia reduces defense mechanisms, increasing the risk for infections. Malnutrition, which is also common among these patients, may further decrease resistance to infection. If the patient has diabetes, the risk for infection is further increased.

Laboratory results should be evaluated frequently and the patient's temperature checked every 4 to 8 hours for an elevation that may indicate infection. Visitors who might transmit microorganisms are prohibited if the patient's immunologic system is depressed. Sensitive skin tissues are protected from trauma to maintain skin integrity and prevent infection. Aseptic technique is necessary when changing dressings. Desquamation (shedding of the epidermis) is a reaction to radiation therapy that causes dryness and itching and can lead to a break in skin integrity and subsequent infection.

As previously described, adequate nutrition is helpful in preventing infection. Signs of wound infection (redness, swelling, drainage, tenderness) are reported to the physician. Antibiotics may be prescribed prophylactically.

### Promoting Home and Community-Based Care

#### TEACHING PATIENTS SELF-CARE

The patient who is recovering from treatment of an oral condition is instructed about mouth care, nutrition, prevention of infection, and signs and symptoms of complications (Chart 35-4). Methods of preparing nutritious foods that are seasoned according to the patient's preference and at the preferred temperature are explained. For some patients, it may be more convenient to use commercial baby foods than to prepare liquid and soft diets. The patient who cannot take foods orally may receive enteral or parenteral nutrition; the administration of these feedings is explained and demonstrated to the patient and the caregiver.

For patients with cancer, instructions are provided in the use and care of any dentures. The importance of keeping dressings clean and the need for conscientious oral hygiene are emphasized.

#### CONTINUING CARE

The need for ongoing care in the home depends on the patient's condition. The patient, the family members or others responsible for home care, the nurse, and other health care professionals (eg, speech therapist, nutritionist, psychologist) work together to prepare an individual plan of care.

If suctioning of the mouth or tracheostomy tube is required, the necessary equipment is obtained and the patient and caregivers are taught how to use it. Considerations include the control of odors and humidification of the home to keep secretions moist. The patient and caregivers are taught how to assess for obstruction, hemorrhage, and infection and what actions to take if they occur. The home care nurse may provide physical care, monitor for changes in the patient's physical status (eg, skin integrity, nutritional status, respiratory function), and assess the adequacy of pain control measures. The nurse also assesses the patient's and family's ability to manage incisions, drains, and feeding tubes and the use of recommended strategies for communication. The ability of the patient and family to accept physical, psychological, and role changes is assessed and addressed.

Follow-up visits to the physician are important to monitor the patient's condition and to determine the need for modifications in treatment and general care. The nurse reinforces instructions in an effort to promote the patient's self-care and comfort.

Because patients and their family members and health care providers tend to focus on the most obvious needs and issues, the nurse reminds the patient and family about the importance of continuing health promotion and screening practices. Patients who have not been involved in these practices in the past are educated about their importance and are referred to appropriate health care providers.

## Evaluation

### Expected Patient Outcomes

Expected patient outcomes may include:

1. Shows evidence of intact oral mucous membranes
   a. Is free of pain and discomfort in the oral cavity
   b. Has no visible alteration in membrane integrity
   c. Identifies and avoids foods that are irritating (eg, nuts, pretzels, spicy foods)
   d. Describes measures that are necessary for preventive mouth care

---

**CHART 35-4**

### HOME CARE CHECKLIST • The Patient With an Oral Condition

| At the completion of the home care instruction, the patient or caregiver will be able to: | Patient | Caregiver |
|---|---|---|
| • Demonstrate use of suction equipment if indicated. | ✓ | ✓ |
| • State rationale for humidification. | ✓ | ✓ |
| • Identify foods necessary to meet caloric needs and dietary needs (ie, change in consistency, seasoning limitations, supplements). | ✓ | ✓ |
| • Demonstrate effective oral hygiene. | ✓ | ✓ |
| • Demonstrate care of incision. | ✓ | ✓ |
| • State when next medical/dental follow-up appointment will be scheduled. | ✓ | ✓ |

    e. Complies with medication regimen
    f. Limits or avoids use of alcohol and tobacco (including smokeless tobacco)
 2. Attains and maintains desirable body weight
 3. Has a positive self-image
    a. Verbalizes anxieties
    b. Is able to accept change in appearance and modify self-concept accordingly
 4. Attains an acceptable level of comfort
    a. Verbalizes that pain is absent or under control
    b. Avoids foods and liquids that cause discomfort
    c. Adheres to medication regimen
 5. Has decreased fears related to pain, isolation, and the inability to cope
    a. Accepts that pain will be managed if not eliminated
    b. Freely expresses fears and concerns
 6. Is free of infection
    a. Exhibits normal laboratory values
    b. Is afebrile
    c. Performs oral hygiene after every meal and at bedtime
 7. Acquires information about disease process and course of treatment

# Neck Dissection

Malignancies of the head and neck include those of the oral cavity, oropharynx, hypopharynx, nasopharynx, nasal cavity, paranasal sinus, and larynx (Fig. 35-3). (Laryngeal cancer is presented in Chapter 22.) These cancers account for fewer than 5% of all cancers. Depending on the location and stage, treatment may consist of radiation therapy, chemotherapy, surgery, or a combination of these modalities. Deaths from malignancies of the head and neck are primarily attributable to local-regional metastasis to the cervical lymph nodes in the neck. This often occurs by way of the lymphatics before the primary lesion has been treated. This local-regional metastasis is not amenable to surgical resection and responds poorly to chemotherapy and radiation therapy.

A radical neck dissection involves removal of all cervical lymph nodes from the mandible to the clavicle and removal of the sternocleidomastoid muscle, internal jugular vein, and spinal accessory muscle on one side of the neck. The associated complications include shoulder drop and poor cosmesis (visible neck depression). Modified radical neck dissection, which preserves one or more of the nonlymphatic structures, is used more often. A selective neck dissection (in comparison to a radical dissection) preserves one or more of the lymph node groups, the internal jugular vein, the sternocleidomastoid muscle, and the spinal accessory nerve (Fig. 35-4).

Reconstructive techniques may be performed with a variety of grafts. A cutaneous flap (skin and subcutaneous tissue), such as the deltopectoral flap, may be used. A myocutaneous flap (subcutaneous tissue, muscle and skin) is a more frequently used graft; the pectoralis major muscle is usually used. For large grafts, a microvascular free flap may be used. This involves the transfer of muscle, skin, or bone with an artery and vein to the area of reconstruction, using microinstrumentation. Areas used for a free flap include the scapula, the radial area of the forearm, or the fibula. The fibula, which provides a larger bone area, may be used if mandibular reconstruction is involved.

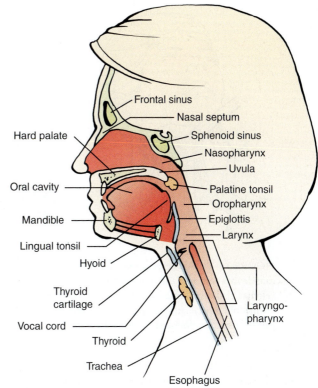

**FIGURE 35-3.** Anatomy of the head and neck.

# Nursing Process

## The Patient Undergoing a Neck Dissection

### Assessment

Preoperatively, the patient's physical and psychological preparation for major surgery is assessed, along with his or her knowledge of the preoperative and postoperative procedures. Postoperatively, the patient is assessed for complications such as altered respiratory status, wound infection, and hemorrhage. As healing occurs, neck range of motion is assessed to determine whether there has been a decrease in range of motion due to nerve or muscle damage.

### Diagnosis

#### Nursing Diagnoses

Based on all the assessment data, major nursing diagnoses may include the following:

- Deficient knowledge about preoperative and postoperative procedures

**FIGURE 35-4.** (**A**) A classic radical neck dissection in which the sternocleidomastoid and smaller muscles are removed. All tissue is removed, from the ramus of the jaw to the clavicle. The jugular vein has also been removed. (**B**) The selective neck dissection is similar but preserves the sternocleidomastoid muscle, internal jugular vein, and spinal accessory nerve. The wound is closed (**C**), and portable suction drainage tubes are in place.

- Ineffective airway clearance related to obstruction by mucus, hemorrhage, or edema
- Acute pain related to surgical incision
- Risk for infection related to surgical intervention secondary to decreased nutritional status, or immunosuppression from chemotherapy or radiation therapy
- Impaired tissue integrity secondary to surgery and grafting
- Imbalanced nutrition, less than body requirements, related to disease process or treatment
- Situational low self-esteem related to diagnosis or prognosis
- Impaired verbal communication secondary to surgical resection
- Impaired physical mobility secondary to nerve injury

### Collaborative Problems/ Potential Complications

Potential postoperative complications that may develop include the following:
- Hemorrhage
- Chyle fistula
- Nerve injury

## Planning and Goals

The major goals for the patient include participation in the treatment plan, maintenance of respiratory status, attainment of comfort, absence of infection, viability of the graft, maintenance of adequate intake of food and fluids, effective coping strategies, effective communication, maintenance of shoulder and neck motion, and absence of complications.

## Nursing Interventions
### Providing Preoperative Patient Education

Before surgery, the patient should be informed about the nature and extent of the surgery, and what the postoperative period will be like. The patient is encouraged to ask questions and to express concerns about the upcoming surgery and the expected results. During this exchange, the nurse has an opportunity to assess the patient's coping abilities, answer questions, and develop a plan for offering assistance. A sense of mutual understanding and rapport make the postoperative experience less traumatic for the patient. The patient's expressions of concern, anxieties, and fears guide the nurse in providing support postoperatively.

### Providing General Postoperative Care

The general postoperative nursing interventions are similar to those presented in Chapter 20. For the patient who has had extensive neck surgery, specific postoperative interventions include maintenance of a patent airway and continuous assessment of respiratory status, wound care and oral hygiene, maintenance of adequate nutrition, and observation for hemorrhage or nerve injury.

### Maintaining the Airway

After the endotracheal tube or airway has been removed and the effects of the anesthesia have worn off, the patient may be placed in Fowler's position to facilitate breathing and promote comfort. This position also increases lymphatic and venous drainage, facilitates swallowing, and decreases venous pressure on the skin flaps.

In the immediate postoperative period, the nurse assesses for stridor (coarse, high-pitched sound on inspiration) by listening frequently over the trachea with a stethoscope. This finding must be reported immediately because it indicates obstruction of the airway. Signs of respiratory distress, such as dyspnea, cyanosis, changes in mental status, and changes in vital signs, are assessed because they may suggest edema, hemorrhage, inadequate oxygenation, or inadequate drainage.

Pneumonia may occur in the postoperative phase if pulmonary secretions are not removed. To aid in the removal of secretions, coughing and deep breathing are encouraged. The patient should assume a sitting position, with the nurse supporting the neck so that the patient can bring up excessive secretions. If this is ineffective, the patient's respiratory tract may have to be suctioned. Care is taken to protect the suture lines during suctioning. If a tracheostomy tube is in place, suctioning is performed through the tube. The patient may also be instructed on use of Yankauer suction (tonsil tip suction) to remove oral secretions. Temperature should not be taken orally.

### Relieving Pain

Pain and the patient's fear of pain are assessed and managed. Patients with head and neck cancer often report less pain than patients with other types of cancer; however, the nurse needs to be aware that each person's pain experience is individual. The nurse administers analgesics as prescribed and assesses their effectiveness.

### Providing Wound Care

Wound drainage tubes are usually inserted during surgery to prevent the collection of fluid subcutaneously. The drainage tubes are connected to a portable suction device (eg, Jackson-Pratt), and the container is emptied periodically. Between 80 and 120 mL of serosanguineous secretions may drain over the first 24 hours. Excessive drainage may be indicative of a chyle fistula or hemorrhage (see later discussion). If dressings are present, they may need to be reinforced periodically. Dressings are observed for evidence of hemorrhage and constriction, which impairs respiration and perfusion of the graft. A graft, if present, is assessed for color and temperature, and for the presence of a pulse if applicable, to determine viability. The graft should be pale pink and warm to the touch. The surgical incisions are also assessed for infection, which is reported immediately. Prophylactic antibiotics may be prescribed.

### Maintaining Adequate Nutrition

Nutritional status is assessed preoperatively; early intervention to correct nutritional imbalances may decrease the risk of postoperative complications. Frequently, nutrition is less than optimal because of inadequate intake, and the patient often requires enteral or parenteral supplements preoperatively and postoperatively to attain and maintain a positive nitrogen balance. Supplements (eg, Ensure, Sustacal) that are nutritionally dense may help reestablish a positive nitrogen balance. They may be taken enterally by mouth, by nasogastric feeding tube, or by gastrostomy feeding tube. (See the Plan of Nursing Care in Chart 35-5 for further discussion.)

The patient who can chew may take food by mouth; the level of the patient's chewing ability determines whether some diet modification (eg, soft, puréed, or liquid foods) is necessary. Food preferences should also be discussed with the patient. Oral care before eating may enhance the patient's appetite, and oral care after eating is important to prevent infection and dental caries. Most patients can maintain and gain weight.

### Supporting Coping Measures

Preoperatively, information about the planned surgery is given to the patient and family. Postoperatively, psychological nursing interventions are aimed at supporting the patient who has had a change in body image or who has major concerns regarding the prognosis. The patient may have difficulty communicating and may be concerned about his or her ability to breathe and swallow normally. The nurse supports the patient's family and friends in encouraging and reassuring the patient that adjusting to the results of this surgery will take time.

The person who has had extensive neck surgery often is sensitive about his or her appearance. This can occur when the operative area is covered by bulky dressings, when the incision line is visible, or later after healing has occurred and the appearance of the neck and possibly the lower face has been significantly altered. If the nurse accepts the patient's appearance and expresses a positive, optimistic attitude, the patient is more likely to be encouraged. The patient also needs an opportunity to express concerns regarding the success of the surgery and the prognosis. The American Cancer Society may be a resource to provide a volunteer to meet with the patient either preoperatively or postoperatively.

People with cancer of the head and neck frequently have used alcohol or tobacco before surgery; postoperatively, the patient is encouraged to abstain from these substances. Alternative methods of coping need to be explored. A referral to Alcoholics Anonymous may be appropriate.

### Promoting Effective Communication

If a laryngectomy was performed, the nurse explores other methods of communicating with the patient and obtains a consultation with a speech/language therapist. Alternatives to verbal communication may include use of a pencil and paper or pointing to needed items on a picture pad. Alternative speech techniques, such as an electrolarynx (a mechanical device held against the neck) or esophageal speech, may be taught by a speech/language therapist.

*(text continues on page 1159)*

**CHART 35-5**

## Plan of Nursing Care: The Patient Who Has Undergone Neck Dissection

**Nursing Diagnosis:** Ineffective airway clearance related to obstruction secondary to edema, hemorrhage, or inadequate wound drainage
**Goal:** Maintenance of normal respiratory function

| NURSING INTERVENTIONS | RATIONALE | EXPECTED OUTCOMES |
|---|---|---|
| 1. Place the patient in Fowler's position. | 1. Fowler's position facilitates expansion of the lungs because the diaphragm is pulled downward and the abdominal viscera are pulled away from the lungs. Breathing is promoted. This position also increases lymphatic and venous drainage, and decreases venous pressure on the graft. Regurgitation and aspiration of stomach contents are prevented postoperatively. | • Achieves a normal respiratory rate<br>• Breathes comfortably<br>• Avoids use of accessory muscles of respiration<br>• Maintains vital signs within patient's normal range<br>• Shows evidence of normal breath sounds<br>• Coughs effectively<br>• Maintains a patent airway<br>• Does not develop a mucus plug |
| 2. Monitor vital signs according to postoperative routine. | 2. Edema, hemorrhage, or inadequate drainage will alter heart rate and respirations. Tachypnea and restlessness may indicate respiratory distress. | |
| 3. Auscultate breath sounds as needed. In the immediate postoperative period, place the stethoscope over the trachea to assess for stridor. | 3. Abnormal breath sounds may indicate ineffective ventilation, decreased perfusion, and fluid accumulation. Stridor, a harsh, high-pitched sound primarily heard on inspiration, indicates airway obstruction. | |
| 4. Encourage deep breathing and coughing. Place the patient in a sitting position and support the neck area with both hands. | 4. Deep breathing before coughing promotes expansion of the airways and a more forceful cough. The coughing mechanism assists airway cilia with removal of secretions. Splinting the incision during coughing reduces strain and promotes the expulsion of secretions by allowing deeper inspirations. | |
| 5. Suction the airway as needed using sterile technique and a soft catheter. | 5. Suctioning assists in removal of secretions that the patient may be unable to cough up, thereby assisting with maintaining a patent airway. | |
| 6. Provide humidified air or oxygen if the patient has a tracheostomy. | 6. Keeps secretions thin. | |

## CHART 35-5 Plan of Nursing Care: The Patient Who Has Undergone Neck Dissection (Continued)

**Nursing Diagnosis:** Risk for infection
**Goal:** Absence of infection

| NURSING INTERVENTIONS | RATIONALE | EXPECTED OUTCOMES |
|---|---|---|
| 1. Instruct the patient in preoperative and postoperative oral hygiene using slightly alkaline solutions such as 8 oz of water mixed with 1 teaspoon of baking soda, or normal saline solution, every 4 hours. | 1. Oral care decreases oral bacteria, thereby decreasing the risk of bacterial infection postoperatively. Hydrogen peroxide should not be used, because it may break down fresh granulation tissue. | • Patient performs oral hygiene preoperatively and postoperatively every 4 hours<br>• Mouth remains clean<br>• Wound drains less than 200 mL of serosanguineous drainage on the first postoperative day<br>• No hematoma at skin graft<br>• Serosanguineous drainage is within normal limits<br>• Dressing remains intact with no constriction of airway or blood flow<br>• Wound and surrounding skin remain clean and free of infection<br>• Patient is afebrile with normal respirations and a normal heart rate<br>• Patient is alert and aware of surroundings |
| 2. Monitor wound suction drainage. | 2. Suction drainage negates the need for pressure dressings because the skin flaps are pulled down tightly. Drainage should be 80–120 mL of serosanguineous secretions for the first 24 hours; then the secretions should decrease daily. Continuous bloody drainage indicates small vessel oozing. | |
| 3. Note drainage quantity and odor. | 3. Purulent, malodorous drainage indicates an infection. Drainage greater than 300 mL in the first 24 hours is considered abnormal. | |
| 4. Assess condition of dressing and reinforce pressure dressings as needed. Assess for any possible constrictions that would affect respirations or decrease blood flow to graft. | 4. If portable wound suction is not used, pressure dressings may be applied to obliterate dead spaces and provide immobilization. These dressings are reinforced, not changed, as needed. | |
| 5. Use aseptic technique to cleanse skin around the drains; change the dressings as ordered by surgeon (usually the second through fifth postoperative days). | 5. Aseptic technique prevents wound contamination. Sterile saline effectively cleans the skin around the drains. | |
| 6. Monitor vital signs. Assess for symptoms of infection: chills, diaphoresis, altered level of consciousness. | 6. An elevated temperature, tachypnea, and tachycardia may indicate an infection. | |

**Nursing Diagnosis:** Impaired skin integrity
**Goal:** Maintenance of intact skin and viability of graft

| NURSING INTERVENTIONS | RATIONALE | EXPECTED OUTCOMES |
|---|---|---|
| 1. Assess condition of graft for viability. | 1. Cyanotic, cool graft indicates possible necrosis. Pale graft indicates arterial thrombosis; purple graft indicates venous congestion. | • Graft is pale pink in color and warm to touch<br>• Tissue blanches to gentle touch |

*continued >*

## CHART 35-5

### Plan of Nursing Care: The Patient Who Has Undergone Neck Dissection (Continued)

| NURSING INTERVENTIONS | RATIONALE | EXPECTED OUTCOMES |
|---|---|---|
| 2. Assess wound for signs and symptoms of infection. | 2. Infected wound interferes with healing and threatens the viability of the graft. | • Graft has pulse via Doppler ultrasound<br>• Patient does not have wound infection |

**Nursing Diagnosis:** Imbalanced nutrition, less than body requirements, related to anorexia and dysphagia
**Goal:** Attainment/maintenance of adequate nutrition

| NURSING INTERVENTIONS | RATIONALE | EXPECTED OUTCOMES |
|---|---|---|
| 1. Assess nutritional status preoperatively, consult with dietitian.<br>2. Administer tube feedings as prescribed. Keep head of bed elevated during feeding to prevent aspiration. Monitor for signs of tracheoesophageal fistula (feeding in tracheal secretions).<br>3. Provide oral hygiene before and after meals.<br>4. Assist with oral intake:<br>  a. Offer easily chewed foods; mash or blenderize if necessary.<br>  b. Suggest that the head be tilted to the unaffected side when swallowing.<br>  c. Inquire whether privacy is desired when eating.<br>  d. Provide altered eating utensils as needed. | 1. Poor nutritional status preoperatively impairs wound healing and increases potential for infection.<br>2. A nasogastric tube may be in place for several days to administer enteral feedings.<br>3. Oral hygiene enhances appetite.<br>4. Soft-textured foods facilitate swallowing. Passage of food may be tolerated better when the head is tilted to the unaffected side. Self-feeding difficulties may cause embarrassment and interfere with intake. | • Does not have weight loss greater than 10% of body weight. (If weight loss is greater than 10%, supplements are given to maintain/increase weight and obtain positive nitrogen balance.)<br>• Tolerates tube feedings<br>• No signs of aspiration<br>• No sign of fistula<br>• Expresses a desire for food<br>• Swallows food easily<br>• Is comfortable eating alone or with others |

**Nursing Diagnosis:** Situational low self-esteem and body image related to changes in appearance and alterations in communication
**Goal:** Attainment of positive self-image

| NURSING INTERVENTIONS | RATIONALE | EXPECTED OUTCOMES |
|---|---|---|
| 1. Assist the patient to communicate effectively:<br>  a. Provide materials for writing messages.<br>  b. Make certain that the call bell is readily accessible. | 1. Temporary hoarseness is common after neck surgery. A tracheostomy may be performed, and verbal communication may not be possible. Communication with head movement may be impossible because of incisional pain and need to maintain position of | • Recognizes that hoarseness is temporary<br>• Develops alternative forms of communication<br>• Willingly conveys fears and concerns<br>• Accepts prognosis with realistic limitations |

## CHART 35-5

### Plan of Nursing Care: The Patient Who Has Undergone Neck Dissection (Continued)

| NURSING INTERVENTIONS | RATIONALE | EXPECTED OUTCOMES |
|---|---|---|
| c. Develop nonverbal ways to communicate (eg, finger-tapping, sign language, sign board).<br>d. Consult speech/language therapist.<br>2. Encourage verbalization of fears:<br>  a. Provide time to listen.<br>  b. Project a positive, optimistic attitude.<br>  c. Reinforce reality.<br>  d. Collaborate with family members to elicit their support and encouragement.<br>  e. Consult support groups such as New Voice Club through the American Cancer Society.<br>3. Observe for facial paralysis.<br>4. Observe for excessive drooling.<br>5. Check for normal shoulder position and function.<br>6. Provide information on clothing/cosmetics to deemphasize physical defects (offer information on "Look Good, Feel Better" program through American Cancer Society). | neck for graft. A speech/language therapist may assist with other forms of communication, such as esophageal speech or electrolarynx.<br>2. Listening conveys acceptance and encourages further verbalization. An optimistic approach conveys interest and hope. Honesty will promote a trusting relationship. This includes confirming cosmetic and functional limitations. Family members or significant others can provide valuable support to the patient.<br>3. Injury to facial nerve will cause lower facial paralysis.<br>4. Damage to the hypoglossal nerve will result in excessive drooling and decreased ability to swallow.<br>5. Damage to the spinal accessory nerve will result in drooping of the shoulder. Rehabilitation exercises are begun after the incision is healed.<br>6. Physical appearance may be enhanced through use of cosmetics or clothing. | • Accepts support as offered<br>• Absence of facial paralysis<br>• Absence of drooling and dysphagia<br>• Maintains normal shoulder function<br>• Verbalizes methods to enhance physical appearance |

### Maintaining Physical Mobility

Excision of muscles and nerves results in weakness at the shoulder that can cause shoulder drop, a forward curvature of the shoulder. Many problems can be avoided with a conscientious exercise program. These exercises are usually begun after the drains have been removed and the neck incision is sufficiently healed. The purpose of the exercises depicted in Figure 35-5 is to promote maximal shoulder function and neck motion after surgery. Physical therapists and occupational therapists can assist patients in performing these exercises.

### Monitoring and Managing Potential Complications

#### HEMORRHAGE

Hemorrhage may occur from carotid artery rupture as a result of necrosis of the graft or damage to the artery itself from tumor or infection. The following measures are indicated:

- Vital signs are assessed. Tachycardia, tachypnea, and hypotension may indicate hemorrhage and impending hypovolemic shock.
- The patient is instructed to avoid the Valsalva maneuver to prevent stress on the graft and carotid artery.

**FIGURE 35-5.** Three rehabilitation exercises after head and neck surgery. The objective is to regain maximum shoulder function and neck motion after neck surgery. From *Exercise for radical neck surgery patients.* Head and Neck Service, Department of Surgery, Memorial Hospital, New York, NY.

- Signs of impending rupture, such as high epigastric pain or discomfort, are reported.
- Dressings and wound drainage are observed for excessive bleeding.
- If hemorrhage occurs, assistance is summoned immediately.
- Hemorrhage requires the continuous application of pressure to the bleeding site or major associated vessel.
- Although some advocate placing the patient in the modified Trendelenburg position to maintain blood pressure, others recommend that the head of the patient's bed be elevated to maintain airway patency and prevent aspiration.
- A controlled, calm manner allays the patient's anxiety.
- The surgeon is notified immediately, because a vascular or ligature tear requires surgical intervention.

### CHYLE FISTULA

A chyle fistula (milk-like drainage from the thoracic duct into the thoracic cavity) may develop as a result of damage to the thoracic duct during surgery. The diagnosis is made if there is excess drainage that has a 3% fat content and a specific gravity of 1.012 or greater. Treatment of a small leak (500 mL or less) includes application of a pressure dressing and a diet of medium-chain fatty acids or parenteral nutrition. Surgical intervention to repair the damaged duct is necessary for larger leaks.

### NERVE INJURY

Nerve injury can occur if the cervical plexus or spinal accessory nerves are severed during surgery. Because lower facial paralysis may occur as a result of injury to the facial nerve, this complication is observed for and reported. Likewise, if the superior laryngeal nerve is damaged, the patient may have difficulty swallowing liquids and food because of the partial lack of sensation of the glottis. Speech therapy may be indicated to assist with the problems related to nerve injury.

## Promoting Home and Community-Based Care

**TEACHING PATIENTS SELF-CARE**

The patient and caregiver require instructions about management of the wound, the dressing, and any drains that remain in place. Patients who require oral suctioning or who have a tracheostomy may be very anxious about their care at home; the transition to home can be eased if the caregiver is given several opportunities to demonstrate the ability to meet the patient's needs (Chart 35-6). The patient and caregiver are also instructed about possible complications such as bleeding and respiratory distress and when to notify the health care provider of signs and symptoms of these complications.

If the patient cannot take food by mouth, detailed instructions and demonstration of enteral or parenteral feedings will be required. Education in techniques of effective oral hygiene is also important.

**CONTINUING CARE**

A referral for home care nursing may be necessary in the early period after discharge. The nurse assesses healing, ensures that feedings are being administered properly, and monitors for any complications. The home care nurse assesses the patient's adjustment to changes in physical appearance and status, and ability to communicate and to eat normally. Physical and speech therapy also may be continued at home.

The patient is given information regarding local support groups such as "I Can Cope" or "New Voice Club," if indicated. The local chapter of the American Cancer Society may be contacted for information and equipment needed for the patient.

## Evaluation

### Expected Patient Outcomes

Expected patient outcomes may include:

1. Discusses expected course of treatment
2. Demonstrates good respiratory exchange
    a. Lungs are clear to auscultation
    b. Breathes easily with no shortness of breath
    c. Demonstrates ability to use suction effectively
3. Remains free of infection
    a. Maintains normal laboratory values
    b. Is afebrile
4. Graft is pink and warm to touch
5. Maintains adequate intake of foods and fluids
    a. Accepts altered route of feeding
    b. Is well hydrated
    c. Maintains or gains weight
6. Demonstrates ability to cope
    a. Discusses emotional responses to the diagnosis
    b. Attends support group meetings
7. Verbalizes comfort
8. Attains maximal mobility
    a. Adheres to physical therapy exercises
    b. Attains maximal range of motion
9. Exhibits no complications
    a. Vital signs stable
    b. No excessive bleeding or discharge
    c. Able to move muscles of lower face

The Plan of Nursing Care in Chart 35-5 presents an overview of the care of a patient undergoing a neck dissection.

---

**CHART 35-6**

### HOME CARE CHECKLIST • Recovering From Neck Surgery

| At the completion of the home care instruction, the patient or caregiver will be able to: | Patient | Caregiver |
|---|---|---|
| • Demonstrate use of suction equipment. | ✓ | ✓ |
| • State rationale for humidification. | ✓ | ✓ |
| • State dietary modifications needed to meet caloric needs. | ✓ | ✓ |
| • Demonstrate enteral or parenteral feeding techniques. | ✓ | ✓ |
| • Demonstrate care of incision and drains. | ✓ | ✓ |
| • Identify signs and symptoms (eg, bleeding, respiratory distress, drainage) to be reported to health care provider. | ✓ | ✓ |
| • State when next checkup is needed. | ✓ | ✓ |
| • Demonstrate exercises. | ✓ | |
| • Identify available support groups. | ✓ | ✓ |

# Disorders of the Esophagus

The esophagus is a mucus-lined, muscular tube that carries food from the mouth to the stomach. It begins at the base of the pharynx and ends about 4 cm below the diaphragm. Its ability to transport food and fluid is facilitated by two sphincters. The upper esophageal sphincter, also called the hypopharyngeal sphincter, is located at the junction of the pharynx and the esophagus. The lower esophageal sphincter, also called the gastroesophageal sphincter or cardiac sphincter, is located at the junction of the esophagus and the stomach. An incompetent lower esophageal sphincter allows reflux (backward flow) of gastric contents. There is no serosal layer of the esophagus; therefore, if surgery is necessary, it is more difficult to perform suturing or anastomosis.

Disorders of the esophagus include motility disorders (achalasia, diffuse spasm), hiatal hernias, diverticula, perforation, foreign bodies, chemical burns, gastroesophageal reflux disease, Barrett's esophagus, benign tumors, and carcinoma. **Dysphagia** (difficulty swallowing), the most common symptom of esophageal disease, may vary from an uncomfortable feeling that a bolus of food is caught in the upper esophagus to acute pain on swallowing (**odynophagia**). Obstruction of food (solid and soft) and even liquids may occur anywhere along the esophagus. Often the patient can indicate that the problem is located in the upper, middle, or lower third of the esophagus.

## Achalasia

**Achalasia** is absent or ineffective peristalsis of the distal esophagus, accompanied by failure of the esophageal sphincter to relax in response to swallowing. Narrowing of the esophagus just above the stomach results in a gradually increasing dilation of the esophagus in the upper chest. Achalasia may progress slowly and occurs most often in people 40 years or older.

### Clinical Manifestations

The primary symptom is difficulty in swallowing both liquids and solids. The patient has a sensation of food sticking in the lower portion of the esophagus. As the condition progresses, food is commonly regurgitated either spontaneously or intentionally by the patient to relieve the discomfort produced by prolonged distention of the esophagus by food that will not pass into the stomach. The patient may also report chest pain and heartburn (**pyrosis**) that may or may not be associated with eating. Secondary pulmonary complications may result from aspiration of gastric contents.

### Assessment and Diagnostic Findings

X-ray studies show esophageal dilation above the narrowing at the gastroesophageal junction. Barium swallow, CT of the chest, and endoscopy may be used for diagnosis; however, manometry, a process in which the esophageal pressure is measured by a radiologist or gastroenterologist, confirms the diagnosis.

### Management

The patient is instructed to eat slowly and to drink fluids with meals. As a temporary measure, calcium channel blockers and nitrates have been used to decrease esophageal pressure and improve swallowing. Injection of botulinum toxin (Botox) to quadrants of the esophagus via endoscopy has been helpful because it inhibits the contraction of smooth muscle. Periodic injections are required to maintain remission.

Achalasia may be treated conservatively by pneumatic dilation to stretch the narrowed area of the esophagus (Fig. 35-6). Pneumatic dilation has a high success rate. Although perforation is a potential complication, its incidence is low. The procedure can be painful; therefore, moderate sedation in the form of an analgesic or tranquilizer, or both, is administered for the treatment. The patient is monitored for perforation. Abdominal tenderness and fever may indicate perforation (see later discussion).

Achalasia may be treated surgically by esophagomyotomy. The procedure usually is performed laparoscopically, either with a complete lower esophageal sphincter myotomy and an antireflux procedure, or without an antireflux procedure. The esophageal muscle fibers are separated to relieve the lower esophageal stricture.

## Diffuse Spasm

Diffuse spasm is a motor disorder of the esophagus. The cause is unknown, but stress may be a factor. It is more common in women and usually manifests in middle age.

### Clinical Manifestations

Diffuse spasm is characterized by difficulty (dysphagia) or pain (odynophagia) on swallowing and by chest pain similar to that of coronary artery spasm.

### Assessment and Diagnostic Findings

Esophageal manometry, which measures the motility of the esophagus and the pressure within the esophagus, indicates that simultaneous contractions of the esophagus occur irregularly. Diagnostic x-ray studies after ingestion of barium show separate areas of spasm.

### Management

Conservative therapy includes administration of sedatives and long-acting nitrates to relieve pain. Calcium channel blockers (eg, nifedipine [Procardia], verapamil [Calan]) have also been used to manage diffuse spasm. Small, frequent feedings and a soft diet are usually recommended to decrease the esophageal pressure and irritation that lead to spasm. Dilation performed by bougienage (use of progressively sized flexible dilators), pneumatic dilation, or esophagomyotomy may be necessary if the pain becomes intolerable.

If none of the conservative approaches is successful in managing symptoms, surgery may be considered. An esophageal Heller myotomy by a minimally invasive ap-

**FIGURE 35-6.** Treatment of achalasia by pneumatic dilation. (**A–C**) The dilator is passed, guided by a previously inserted guide wire. (**D**) When the balloon is in proper position, it is distended by pressure sufficient to dilate the narrowed area of the esophagus.

proach is considered first and has shown positive results. If an open surgical approach is required, then a transhiatal esophagectomy is performed (see discussion in Cancer of the Esophagus).

## Hiatal Hernia

In the condition known as hiatus (or hiatal) **hernia**, the opening in the diaphragm through which the esophagus passes becomes enlarged, and part of the upper stomach tends to move up into the lower portion of the thorax. Hiatal hernia occurs more often in women than in men. There are two types of hiatal hernias: sliding and paraesophageal. Sliding, or type I, hiatal hernia occurs when the upper stomach and the gastroesophageal junction are displaced upward and slide in and out of the thorax (Fig. 35-7A). About 90% of patients with esophageal hiatal hernia have a sliding hernia. A paraesophageal hernia occurs when all or part of the stomach pushes through the diaphragm beside the esophagus (see Fig. 35-7B). Paraesophageal hernias are further classified as types II, III, or

**FIGURE 35-7.** (**A**) Sliding esophageal hernia. The upper stomach and gastroesophageal junction have moved upward and slide in and out of the thorax. (**B**) Paraesophageal hernia. All or part of the stomach pushes through the diaphragm next to the gastroesophageal junction.

IV, depending on the extent of herniation, with type IV having the greatest herniation.

## Clinical Manifestations

The patient with a sliding hernia may have heartburn, regurgitation, and dysphagia, but at least 50% of patients are asymptomatic. Sliding hiatal hernia is often implicated in reflux. The patient with a paraesophageal hernia usually feels a sense of fullness after eating or chest pain, or there may be no symptoms. Reflux usually does not occur, because the gastroesophageal sphincter is intact. Hemorrhage, obstruction, and strangulation can occur with any type of hernia.

## Assessment and Diagnostic Findings

Diagnosis is confirmed by x-ray studies, barium swallow, and fluoroscopy.

## Management

Management for an axial hernia includes frequent, small feedings that can pass easily through the esophagus. The patient is advised not to recline for 1 hour after eating, to prevent reflux or movement of the hernia, and to elevate the head of the bed on 4- to 8-inch (10- to 20-cm) blocks to prevent the hernia from sliding upward. Surgery is indicated in about 15% of patients. Medical and surgical management of a paraesophageal hernia is similar to that for gastroesophageal reflux; however, people with paraesophageal hernias may require emergency surgery to correct torsion (twisting) of the stomach or other body organ that leads to restriction of blood flow to that area.

# Diverticulum

A diverticulum is an outpouching of mucosa and submucosa that protrudes through a weak portion of the musculature. Diverticula may occur in one of the three areas of the esophagus—the pharyngoesophageal or upper area of the esophagus, the midesophageal area, or the epiphrenic or lower area of the esophagus—or they may occur along the border of the esophagus intramurally.

The most common type of diverticulum, which is found three times more frequently in men than in women, is Zenker's diverticulum (also known as pharyngoesophageal pulsion diverticulum or a pharyngeal pouch). It occurs posteriorly through the cricopharyngeal muscle in the midline of the neck. It is usually seen in people older than 60 years. Other types of diverticula include midesophageal, epiphrenic, and intramural diverticula.

Midesophageal diverticula are uncommon. Symptoms are less acute, and usually the condition does not require surgery. Epiphrenic diverticula are usually larger diverticula in the lower esophagus just above the diaphragm. They may be related to the improper functioning of the lower esophageal sphincter or to motor disorders of the esophagus. Intramural diverticulosis is the occurrence of numerous small diverticula associated with a stricture in the upper esophagus.

## Clinical Manifestations

Symptoms experienced by the patient with a pharyngoesophageal pulsion diverticulum include difficulty swallowing, fullness in the neck, belching, regurgitation of undigested food, and gurgling noises after eating. The diverticulum, or pouch, becomes filled with food or liquid. When the patient assumes a recumbent position, undigested food is regurgitated, and coughing may be caused by irritation of the trachea. Halitosis and a sour taste in the mouth are also common because of the decomposition of food retained in the diverticulum.

Symptoms produced by midesophageal diverticula are less acute. One third of patients with epiphrenic diverticula are asymptomatic, and the remaining two thirds report dysphagia and chest pain. Dysphagia is the most common symptom of patients with intramural diverticulosis.

## Assessment and Diagnostic Findings

A barium swallow may determine the exact nature and location of a diverticulum. Manometric studies are often performed for patients with epiphrenic diverticula to rule out a motor disorder. Esophagoscopy usually is contraindicated because of the danger of perforation of the diverticulum, with resulting mediastinitis (inflammation of the organs and tissues that separate the lungs). Blind insertion of a nasogastric tube should be avoided.

## Management

Because pharyngoesophageal pulsion diverticulum is progressive, the only means of cure is surgical removal of the diverticulum. During surgery, care is taken to avoid trauma to the common carotid artery and internal jugular veins. The sac is dissected free and amputated flush with the esophageal wall. In addition to a diverticulectomy, a myotomy of the cricopharyngeal muscle is often performed to relieve spasticity of the musculature, which otherwise seems to contribute to a continuation of the previous symptoms. A nasogastric tube may be inserted at the time of surgery. Postoperatively, the surgical incision must be observed for evidence of leakage from the esophagus and a developing fistula. Food and fluids are withheld until x-ray studies show no leakage at the surgical site. The diet begins with liquids and is progressed as tolerated.

Surgery is indicated for epiphrenic and midesophageal diverticula only if the symptoms are troublesome and becoming worse. Treatment consists of a diverticulectomy and long myotomy. Intramural diverticula usually regress after the esophageal stricture is dilated.

# Perforation

The esophagus is a common site of injury. Perforation may result from stab or bullet wounds of the neck or chest, trauma from a motor vehicle crash, caustic injury from a chemical burn, or inadvertent puncture by a surgical instrument during examination or dilation such as endoscopy.

## Clinical Manifestations

The patient has persistent pain followed by dysphagia. Infection, fever, leukocytosis, and severe hypotension may be noted. In some instances, signs of pneumothorax are observed.

## Assessment and Diagnostic Findings

X-ray studies and fluoroscopy by either a barium swallow or esophagram are used to identify the site of the injury.

## Management

Because of the high risk of infection, broad-spectrum antibiotic therapy is initiated. If the perforation is small enough and without symptoms, medical intervention may not be necessary. Nothing is given by mouth; nutritional needs are met by parenteral or enteral nutrition. The type of nutritional support depends on the location of the injury. The enteral or parenteral nutrition lasts for at least 1 month to give the esophagus a chance to heal. A repeat barium swallow study is performed, and the involved area is reevaluated. If there is no evidence of perforation, foods are reintroduced, beginning with liquids and then slowly progressing to solids as tolerated.

Surgery may be necessary to close the wound; in such cases, postoperative nutritional support becomes a primary concern. Depending on the incision site and the nature of surgery, the postoperative nursing management is similar to that for patients who have had thoracic or abdominal surgery.

## Foreign Bodies

Many swallowed foreign bodies pass through the gastrointestinal tract without the need for medical intervention. However, some swallowed foreign bodies (eg, dentures, fish bones, pins, small batteries, items containing mercury or lead) may injure the esophagus or obstruct its lumen and must be removed. Pain and dysphagia may be present, and dyspnea may occur as a result of pressure on the trachea. The foreign body may be identified by x-ray. Perforation may have occurred (see earlier discussion).

Glucagon, because of its relaxing effect on the esophageal muscle, may be injected intramuscularly. An endoscope (with a covered hood or overtube) may be used to remove the impacted food or object from the esophagus. A mixture consisting of sodium bicarbonate and tartaric acid may be prescribed to increase intraluminal pressure by the formation of a gas. Caution must be used with this treatment because there is risk of perforation.

## Chemical Burns

Chemical burns of the esophagus occur most often when a patient, either intentionally or unintentionally, swallows a strong acid or base (eg, lye). This patient is emotionally distraught as well as in acute physical pain. Chemical burns of the esophagus may also be caused by undissolved medications in the esophagus. This occurs more frequently in the elderly than it does among the general adult population. A chemical burn may also occur after swallowing of a battery, which may release a caustic alkaline. An acute chemical burn of the esophagus may be accompanied by severe burns of the lips, mouth, and pharynx, with pain on swallowing. There may be difficulty in breathing due to either edema of the throat or a collection of mucus in the pharynx.

The patient, who may be profoundly toxic, febrile, and in shock, is treated immediately for shock, pain, and respiratory distress. Esophagoscopy and barium swallow are performed as soon as possible to determine the extent and severity of damage. The patient is given nothing by mouth, and IV fluids are administered. A nasogastric tube may be inserted by the physician. Vomiting and gastric lavage are avoided to prevent further exposure of the esophagus to the caustic agent. The use of corticosteroids to reduce inflammation and minimize subsequent scarring and stricture formation is of questionable value. Prophylactic antibiotics should be prescribed only if there is documented infection (Hostetler, 2004).

After the acute phase has subsided, the patient may need nutritional support via enteral or parenteral feedings. The patient may require further treatment to prevent or manage strictures of the esophagus. Dilation by bougienage may be sufficient but may need to be repeated periodically. (In bougienage, cylindrical rubber tubes of different sizes, called bougies, are advanced into the esophagus via the oral cavity. Progressively larger bougies are used to dilate the esophagus. The procedure usually is performed in the endoscopy suite or clinic by the gastroenterologist.) For strictures that do not respond to dilation, surgical management is necessary. Reconstruction may be accomplished by esophagectomy and colon interposition to replace the portion of esophagus removed.

## Gastroesophageal Reflux Disease

Some degree of **gastroesophageal reflux** (back-flow of gastric or duodenal contents into the esophagus) is normal in both adults and children. Excessive reflux may occur because of an incompetent lower esophageal sphincter, pyloric stenosis, or a motility disorder. The incidence of reflux seems to increase with aging.

## Clinical Manifestations

Symptoms of gastroesophageal reflux disease (GERD) may include pyrosis (burning sensation in the esophagus), dyspepsia (indigestion), regurgitation, dysphagia or odynophagia (pain on swallowing), hypersalivation, and esophagitis. The symptoms may mimic those of a heart attack. The patient's history aids in obtaining an accurate diagnosis.

## Assessment and Diagnostic Findings

Diagnostic testing may include an endoscopy or barium swallow to evaluate damage to the esophageal mucosa. Ambulatory 12- to 36-hour esophageal pH monitoring is used to evaluate the degree of acid reflux. Bilirubin monitoring (Bilitec) is used to measure bile reflux patterns. Exposure to bile can cause mucosal damage.

### Management

Management begins with teaching the patient to avoid situations that decrease lower esophageal sphincter pressure or cause esophageal irritation. The patient is instructed to eat a low-fat diet; to avoid caffeine, tobacco, beer, milk, foods containing peppermint or spearmint, and carbonated beverages; to avoid eating or drinking 2 hours before bedtime; to maintain normal body weight; to avoid tight-fitting clothes; to elevate the head of the bed on 6- to 8-inch (15- to 20-cm) blocks; and to elevate the upper body on pillows. If reflux persists, the patient may be given antacids or $H_2$ receptor antagonists, such as famotidine (Pepcid), nizatidine (Axid), or ranitidine (Zantac). Proton pump inhibitors (medications that decrease the release of gastric acid, such as lansoprazole [Prevacid], rabeprazole [AciPhex], esomeprazole [Nexium]) may be used; however, these products may increase intragastric bacterial growth and the risk for infection. In addition, the patient may receive prokinetic agents, which accelerate gastric emptying. These agents include bethanechol (Urecholine), domperidone (Motilium), and metoclopramide (Reglan). Metoclopramide can have extrapyramidal side effects that are increased in certain neuromuscular disorders, such as Parkinson's disease. These patients should be carefully monitored.

If medical management is unsuccessful, surgical intervention may be necessary. Surgical management involves a Nissen fundoplication (wrapping of a portion of the gastric fundus around the sphincter area of the esophagus). A Nissen fundoplication can be performed by the open method or by laparoscopy.

## Barrett's Esophagus

Barrett's esophagus is a condition in which the lining of the esophageal mucosa is altered. It typically occurs in association with GERD; indeed, longstanding untreated GERD may lead to Barrett's esophagus. Reflux eventually causes changes in the cells lining the lower esophagus. The cells that are laid to cover the exposed area are no longer squamous in origin. These precancerous cells initiate the healing process and can be a precursor to esophageal cancer.

### Clinical Manifestations

The patient complains of symptoms of GERD, notably frequent heartburn. The patient may also complain of symptoms related to peptic ulcers or esophageal stricture, or both.

### Assessment and Diagnostic Findings

An **esophagogastroduodenoscopy (EGD)** is performed. This usually reveals an esophageal lining that is red rather than pink. Biopsies are performed, and high-grade **dysplasia** (HGD) is evidenced by the squamous mucosa of the esophagus replaced by columnar epithelium that resembles that of the stomach or intestines (Porth, 2005).

### Management

Monitoring varies depending on the extent of cell changes. Some physicians recommend a repeat EGD in 6 to 12 months if there are minor cell changes.

Photodynamic therapy (PDT) may be an alternative for the patient who is considered an operative risk (eg, 70 years or older, significant cardiac risk). PDT is a type of laser thermal ablation of the esophageal mucosa that is used to destroy the metaplastic cells once the patient has received a photosensitizing agent, such as Photofrin. Early studies suggest that this therapy shows promise for the patient with early-stage disease; however, it is not recommended for the patient with late-stage disease accompanied by nodal disease (Overholt, Panjehpour, & Teffetellar, 1995). There have been no long-term follow-up studies of patients who have undergone ablation therapy. Therefore, PDT should be reserved for patients who are not surgical candidates for prophylactic esophagectomy.

Research suggests that prophylactic transhiatal esophagectomy is a recommended therapy for patients with Barrett's esophagus and HGD. Patients with Barrett's esophagus and HGD who have had prophylactic esophagectomy have shown a significant reduction in invasive adenocarcinoma following the procedure. A significant number of these patients who did not have a preoperative diagnosis of cancer have been found to have invasive adenocarcinoma during surgery. Furthermore, researchers have found that only patients with dysplasia develop invasive adenocarcinoma and that persistent HGD is a reliable histopathologic marker for the subsequent development of adenocarcinoma (Heitmiller et al., 1996). These results suggest that esophageal surgery was the best option for patients with Barrett's esophagus with HGD. Updated results continue to support the performance of a prophylactic esophagectomy in the presence of HGD. Five-year survival was 88%, and Barrett's esophagus with HGD continues to be an indication for prophylactic esophagectomy (Tseng, Wu, Yeo, et al., 2003).

## Benign Tumors of the Esophagus

Benign tumors can arise anywhere along the esophagus. The most common lesion is a leiomyoma (tumor of the smooth muscle), which can occlude the lumen of the esophagus. Most benign tumors are asymptomatic and are distinguished from cancerous lesions by a biopsy. Small lesions are excised during esophagoscopy; lesions that occur within the wall of the esophagus may require treatment via a thoracotomy.

## Cancer of the Esophagus

In the United States, carcinoma of the esophagus occurs more than three times as often in men as in women. It is seen more frequently in African Americans than in Caucasians and usually occurs in the fifth or sixth decade of life. Cancer of the esophagus has a much higher incidence (10 to 100 times higher) in other parts of the world, including China and northern Iran (American Cancer Society, 2005).

Chronic irritation is a risk factor for esophageal cancer. In the United States, cancer of the esophagus has been associated with ingestion of alcohol and the use of tobacco.

There seems to be an association between GERD and adenocarcinoma of the esophagus. People with Barrett's esophagus (which is caused by chronic irritation of the mucous membranes due to reflux of gastric and duodenal contents) have a higher incidence of esophageal cancer (Stein et al., 1999).

## Pathophysiology

Esophageal cancer can be of two cell types: adenocarcinoma and squamous cell carcinoma. The rate of adenocarcinoma is rapidly increasing in the United States as well as in other Western countries. It is found primarily in the distal esophagus and gastroesophageal junction (Quinn & Reedy, 1999).

Risk factors for adenocarcinoma of the esophagus include GERD. GERD may progress to Barrett's esophagus that can be either low-grade or high-grade dysplasia (see section on Barrett esophagus for more details).

Risk factors for squamous cell carcinoma of the esophagus include chronic ingestion of hot liquids or foods, nutritional deficiencies, poor oral hygiene, exposure to nitrosamines in the environment or food, cigarette smoking or chronic alcohol exposure (especially in Western cultures), and some esophageal medical conditions such as caustic injury.

Tumor cells of adenocarcinoma and of squamous cell carcinoma may spread beneath the esophageal mucosa or directly into, through, and beyond the muscle layers into the lymphatics. In the latter stages, obstruction of the esophagus is noted, with possible perforation into the mediastinum and erosion into the great vessels.

## Clinical Manifestations

Many patients have an advanced ulcerated lesion of the esophagus before symptoms are manifested. Symptoms include dysphagia, initially with solid foods and eventually with liquids; a sensation of a mass in the throat; painful swallowing; substernal pain or fullness; and, later, regurgitation of undigested food with foul breath and hiccups. The patient first becomes aware of intermittent and increasing difficulty in swallowing. As the tumor grows and the obstruction becomes nearly complete, even liquids cannot pass into the stomach. Regurgitation of food and saliva occurs, hemorrhage may take place, and progressive loss of weight and strength occurs from starvation. Later symptoms include substernal pain, persistent hiccup, respiratory difficulty, and foul breath.

The delay between the onset of early symptoms and the time when the patient seeks medical advice is often 12 to 18 months. Any person having swallowing difficulties should be encouraged to consult a physician immediately.

## Assessment and Diagnostic Findings

Currently, diagnosis is confirmed most often by EGD with biopsy and brushings. The biopsy can be used to determine the presence of disease and cell differentiation. At presentation, most patients have moderately differentiated tumors.

Several imaging techniques may provide useful diagnostic information. CT of the chest and abdomen is beneficial for detecting any metastatic disease, especially of the lungs, liver, and kidney. Positron emission tomography (PET) may help detect metastasis with more sensitivity than CT. Endoscopic ultrasound is used to determine whether the cancer has spread to the lymph nodes and other mediastinal structures; it can also determine the size and invasiveness of the tumor. Exploratory laparoscopy is the best method for finding positive lymph nodes in patients with distal lesions.

Future diagnostic techniques that may serve as predictors for dysplastic progression in patients with Barrett's esophagus involve molecular markers. The usefulness of molecular markers in treating esophageal cancer is being researched. Research also includes the development of medications that target the pathways of various molecular markers (Lau, Moore, Brooks, et al., 2002).

## Medical Management

If esophageal cancer is detected at an early stage, treatment goals may be directed toward cure; however, it is often detected in late stages, making relief of symptoms the only reasonable goal of therapy. Treatment may include surgery, radiation, chemotherapy, or a combination of these modalities, depending on the type of cell, the extent of the disease, and the patient's condition. A standard treatment plan for a person who is newly diagnosed with esophageal cancer includes the following: preoperative combination chemotherapy/radiation therapy for 4 to 6 weeks; followed by a period of no medical intervention for 4 weeks; and, lastly, surgical resection of the esophagus.

Standard surgical management includes a total resection of the esophagus (esophagectomy) with removal of the tumor plus a wide tumor-free margin of the esophagus and the lymph nodes in the area. The surgical approach may be through the thorax or the abdomen, depending on the location of the tumor. When tumors occur in the cervical or upper thoracic area, esophageal continuity may be maintained by a free jejunal graft transfer, in which the tumor is removed and the area is replaced with a portion of the jejunum (Fig. 35-8). A segment of the colon may be used, or the stomach can be elevated into the chest and the proximal section of the esophagus anastomosed to the stomach.

Tumors of the lower thoracic esophagus are more amenable to surgery than are tumors located higher in the esophagus. Gastrointestinal tract integrity is maintained by anastomosing the lower esophagus to the stomach (Fig. 35-9).

Surgical resection of the esophagus has a relatively high mortality rate because of infection, pulmonary complications, or leakage through the anastomosis. Postoperatively, the patient has a nasogastric tube in place that should not be manipulated. The patient is given nothing by mouth until x-ray studies confirm that the anastomosis is free from an esophageal leak, there is no obstruction, and there is no evidence of pulmonary aspiration.

Palliative treatment may be necessary to keep the esophagus open, to assist with nutrition, and to control saliva. Palliation may be accomplished with dilation of the esophagus, laser therapy, placement of an endoprosthesis (stent), radiation, or chemotherapy.

**FIGURE 35-8.** Esophageal reconstruction with free jejunal transfer. A portion of the jejunum is grafted between the esophagus and pharynx to replace the abnormal portion of the esophagus. The vascular structures are also anastomosed. A portion of the graft may be externalized through the neck wound to evaluate graft viability.

## Nursing Management

Intervention is directed toward improving the patient's nutritional and physical status in preparation for surgery, radiation therapy, or chemotherapy. A program to promote weight gain based on a high-calorie and high-protein diet, in liquid or soft form, is provided if adequate food can be taken by mouth. If this is not possible, parenteral or enteral nutrition is initiated. Nutritional status is monitored throughout treatment. The patient is informed about the nature of the postoperative equipment that will be used, including that required for closed chest drainage, nasogastric suction, parenteral fluid therapy, and gastric intubation.

Immediate postoperative care is similar to that provided for patients undergoing thoracic surgery. It is not uncommon for patients to be placed in an intensive care unit or stepdown unit. After recovering from the effects of anesthesia, the patient is placed in a low Fowler's position, and later in a Fowler's position, to help prevent reflux of gastric secretions. The patient is observed carefully for regurgitation and dyspnea. A common postoperative complication is aspiration pneumonia. Therefore, the patient is placed on a vigorous pulmonary plan of care that includes incentive spirometry, sitting up in a chair, and, if necessary, nebulizer treatments. Chest physiotherapy is avoided due to the risk for aspiration. The patient's temperature is monitored to detect any elevation that may indicate aspiration or seepage of fluid through the operative site into the mediastinum, which would indicate an esophageal leak. Drainage from the cervical neck wound, usually saliva, is evidence of an early esophageal leak. Typically, no treatment other than nothing by mouth and parenteral or enteral support is warranted.

Cardiac complications include atrial fibrillation, which occurs due to irritation of the vagus nerve at the time of surgery. Typical medical management includes digitalization or beta blockade, depending on the patient's response. Rarely, cardioversion may be used.

During surgery, a nasogastric tube is inserted and taped in place. It is connected to low intermittent suction. The nasogastric tube is not manipulated; if displacement occurs, it is not replaced, because damage to the anastomosis may occur. The nasogastric tube is removed 5 to 7 days after surgery; before the patient is allowed to eat, a barium swallow is performed to assess for any anastomotic leak.

Once feeding begins, the nurse encourages the patient to swallow small sips of water. Eventually, the diet is advanced as tolerated to a soft, mechanical diet. When the patient can increase his or her food and fluid intake to an adequate amount, parenteral fluids are discontinued. After each meal, the patient remains upright for at least 2 hours to allow the food to move through the gastrointestinal tract. It is a challenge to encourage the patient to eat, because the appetite

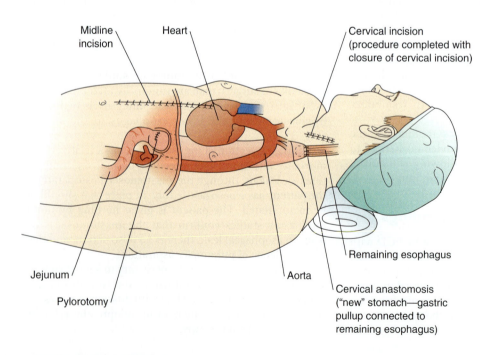

**FIGURE 35-9.** Transhiatal esophagectomy: surgical removal of tumor of the lower esophagus with anastomosis of the remaining esophagus to the stomach. Redrawn with permission from *Operative Techniques in Thoracic and Cardiovascular Surgery, 4*(3), 263 © 1999 Elsevier Inc.

is usually poor. Family involvement and home-cooked favorite foods may help the patient to eat. Antacids may help patients with gastric distress. Metoclopramide (Reglan) is useful in promoting gastric motility.

If chemotherapy and radiation are part of the therapy, the patient's appetite will be further depressed, and esophagitis may occur, causing pain when food is eaten. Liquid supplements may be more easily tolerated. However, supplements such as Boost and Ensure should be avoided because they promote the **vagotomy syndrome** (dumping syndrome), which can occur with each meal or approximately 20 minutes to 2 hours after eating. The vagotomy syndrome occurs due to interruption of vagal nerve fibers, which in turn causes an alteration in the storage function of the stomach and the pyloric emptying mechanism. As a result, large amounts of osmotically active solids and liquids rapidly "dump" into the duodenum. The patient experiences severe abdominal cramping, followed by a liquid bowel movement that may or may not be associated with diaphoresis, rapid heart rate or rapid respirations, or both. It can be quite disabling but typically resolves without incident, and the patient is left feeling extremely tired. The vagotomy syndrome is common following esophageal surgery, but as the patient's recovery progresses and the patient begins to eat in the fashion described previously, the frequency and severity of episodes decrease.

Often, in either the preoperative or the postoperative period, an obstructed or nearly obstructed esophagus causes difficulty with excess saliva, and drooling becomes a problem. Oral suction may be used if the patient cannot handle oral secretions, or a wick-type gauze may be placed at the corner of the mouth to direct secretions to a dressing or emesis basin. The possibility that the patient may aspirate saliva into the tracheobronchial tree and develop pneumonia is of great concern.

When the patient is ready to go home, the family is instructed about how to promote nutrition, what observations to make, what measures to take if complications occur, how to keep the patient comfortable, and how to obtain needed physical and emotional support.

## ◀◀▶▶ Nursing Process

## The Patient With a Condition of the Esophagus

### Assessment

Emergency conditions of the esophagus (perforation, chemical burns) usually occur in the home or away from medical help and require emergency medical care. The patient is treated for shock and respiratory distress and transported as quickly as possible to a health care facility. Foreign bodies in the esophagus do not pose an immediate threat to life unless pressure is exerted on the trachea, resulting in dyspnea or interfering with respiration, or unless there is leakage of caustic alkali from a battery or exposure to another corrosive agent. Educating the public to prevent inadvertent swallowing of foreign bodies or corrosive agents is a major health goal.

For nonemergency symptoms, a complete health history may reveal the nature of the esophageal disorder. The nurse asks about the patient's appetite. Has it remained the same, increased, or decreased? Is there any discomfort with swallowing? If so, does it occur only with certain foods? Is it associated with pain? Does a change in position affect the discomfort? The patient is asked to describe the pain. Does anything aggravate it? Are there any other symptoms that occur regularly, such as regurgitation, nocturnal regurgitation, eructation (belching), heartburn, substernal pressure, a sensation that food is sticking in the throat, a feeling of fullness after eating a small amount of food, nausea, vomiting, or weight loss? Are the symptoms aggravated by emotional upset? If the patient reports any of these symptoms, the nurse asks about when they occur, their relationship to eating, and factors that relieve or aggravate them (eg, position change, belching, antacids, vomiting).

This history also includes questions about past or present causative factors, such as infections and chemical, mechanical, or physical irritants; alcohol and tobacco use; and the amount of daily food intake. The nurse determines whether the patient appears emaciated and auscultates the patient's chest to assess for pulmonary complications.

### Nursing Diagnosis

Based on the assessment data, the nursing diagnoses may include the following:

- Imbalanced nutrition, less than body requirements, related to difficulty swallowing
- Risk for aspiration related to difficulty swallowing or to tube feeding
- Acute pain related to difficulty swallowing, ingestion of an abrasive agent, tumor, or frequent episodes of gastric reflux
- Deficient knowledge about the esophageal disorder, diagnostic studies, medical management, surgical intervention, and rehabilitation

### Planning and Goals

The major goals for the patient may include attainment of adequate nutritional intake, avoidance of respiratory compromise from aspiration, relief of pain, and increased knowledge level.

### Nursing Interventions

#### Encouraging Adequate Nutritional Intake

The patient is encouraged to eat slowly and to chew all food thoroughly so that it can pass easily into the stomach. Small, frequent feedings of nonirritating foods are recommended to promote digestion and to prevent tissue irritation. Sometimes liquid swallowed with food helps the food pass through the esophagus, but usually liquids should be consumed between meals. Food should be prepared in an appealing manner to help stimulate the appetite. Irritants such as tobacco and alcohol should be avoided. A baseline weight is obtained, and daily weights are recorded. The patient's intake of nutrients is assessed.

### Decreasing Risk of Aspiration

The patient who has difficulty swallowing or difficulty handling secretions should be kept in at least a semi-Fowler's position to decrease the risk of aspiration. The patient is instructed in the use of oral suction to decrease the risk of aspiration further.

### Relieving Pain

Small, frequent feedings (six to eight per day) are recommended because large quantities of food overload the stomach and promote gastric reflux. The patient is advised to avoid any activities that increase pain and to remain upright for 1 to 4 hours after each meal to prevent reflux. The head of the bed should be placed on 4- to 8-inch (10- to 20-cm) blocks. Eating before bedtime is discouraged.

The patient is advised that excessive use of over-the-counter antacids can cause rebound acidity. Antacid use should be directed by the primary care provider, who can recommend the daily, safe dose needed to neutralize gastric juices and prevent esophageal irritation. $H_2$ antagonists are administered as prescribed to decrease gastric acid irritation.

### Providing Patient Education

The patient is prepared physically and psychologically for diagnostic tests, treatments, and possible surgery. The principal nursing interventions include reassuring the patient and explaining the procedures and their purposes. Some disorders of the esophagus evolve over time, whereas others are the result of trauma (eg, chemical burns, perforation). In instances of trauma, the emotional and physical preparation for treatment is more difficult because of the short time available and the circumstances of the injury. Treatment interventions must be evaluated continually, and the patient is given sufficient information to participate in care and diagnostic tests. If endoscopic diagnostic methods are used, the patient is instructed regarding the moderate sedation that will be used during the procedure. If outpatient procedures are performed with the use of moderate sedation, the patient is instructed to have someone available to drive him or her home after the procedure. If surgery is required, immediate and long-term evaluation is similar to that for a patient undergoing thoracic surgery.

### Promoting Home and Community-Based Care

**TEACHING PATIENTS SELF-CARE**

The self-care required of the patient depends on the nature of the disorder and on the surgery or treatment measures used (eg, diet, positioning, medications). If an ongoing condition exists, the nurse helps the patient plan for needed physical and psychological adjustments and for follow-up care (Chart 35-7).

Special equipment, such as suction or enteral or parenteral feeding devices, may be required. The patient may need assistance in planning meals, using medications as prescribed, and resuming activities. Education about nutritional requirements and how to measure the adequacy of nutrition is important. Elderly and debilitated patients in particular often need assistance and education about ways they can adjust to their limitations and resume activities that are important to them.

---

**CHART 35-7**

## HOME CARE CHECKLIST • The Patient With an Esophageal Condition

| At the completion of the home care instruction, the patient or caregiver will be able to: | Patient | Caregiver |
|---|:---:|:---:|
| • Demonstrate use of suction equipment. | ✔ | ✔ |
| • State dietary modifications needed to meet caloric needs. | ✔ | ✔ |
| • Demonstrate enteral or parenteral feeding techniques. | ✔ | ✔ |
| • Demonstrate care of incision if indicated. | ✔ | ✔ |
| • Identify signs and symptoms (eg, difficulty swallowing, pain, respiratory distress) to be reported to health care provider. | ✔ | ✔ |
| • State when next checkup is needed. | ✔ | ✔ |
| • Identify available support groups. | ✔ | ✔ |

## CONTINUING CARE

Patients with chronic esophageal conditions require an individualized approach to their management at home. Foods may need to be prepared in a special way (blenderized foods, soft foods), and the patient may need to eat more frequently (eg, six to eight small servings per day). The medication schedule is adjusted to the patient's daily activities as much as possible. Analgesic medications and antacids can usually be taken as needed every 3 to 4 hours.

Postoperative home health care focuses on nutritional support, management of pain, and respiratory function. Some patients are discharged from the hospital with enteral feeding by means of a gastrostomy or jejunostomy tube or parenteral nutrition. The patient and caregiver need specific instructions regarding management of the equipment and treatments. Home care visits by a nurse may be necessary to assess the patient and the caregiver's ability to provide the necessary care. (See Chapter 36 for more information about parenteral nutrition and management of the patient with a gastrostomy.) For some patients, a multidisciplinary team that includes a dietitian, a social worker, and family members is helpful. Hospice care and consideration of end-of-life issues are appropriate for some patients.

## Evaluation

### Expected Patient Outcomes

Expected patient outcomes may include:

1. Achieves an adequate nutritional intake
   a. Eats small, frequent meals
   b. Drinks small sips of water with small servings of food
   c. Avoids irritants (alcohol, tobacco, very hot beverages)
   d. Maintains desired weight
2. Does not aspirate or develop pneumonia
   a. Maintains upright position during feeding
   b. Uses oral suction equipment effectively
3. Is free of pain or able to control pain within a tolerable level
   a. Avoids large meals and irritating foods
   b. Takes medications as prescribed and with adequate fluids (at least 4 ounces), and remains upright for at least 10 minutes after taking medications
   c. Maintains an upright position after meals for 1 to 4 hours
   d. Reports that there is less eructation and chest pain
4. Increases knowledge level of esophageal condition, treatment, and prognosis
   a. States cause of condition
   b. Discusses rationale for medical or surgical management and diet or medication regimen
   c. Describes treatment program
   d. Practices preventive measures so injuries are avoided

## Critical Thinking Exercises

1. You are interviewing a man in the medical clinic. During the medical history, the patient describes his symptoms: weight loss, vague chest pain, and occasional trouble swallowing solid foods only. Explain what other questions you might ask this patient to rule out the presence of an esophageal mass and to determine what diagnostic tests would be most helpful. What instructions would you provide about preparation for these tests?

2. You are the night shift nurse in the intensive care unit and have been assigned a new postoperative patient who has undergone a radical neck dissection. Which form of nutritional support would you most likely see being used, and why? What nursing measures would be used to facilitate breathing and promote comfort? Describe the potential complications of radical neck dissection and the assessment parameters that are used to detect the earliest signs and symptoms of these complications.

3. **ebp** An elderly woman is brought to the emergency department by the rescue squad. Her daughter found her on the kitchen floor. A bottle of cleaning fluid with a poison label was open next to the kitchen sink. On admission the patient was in respiratory distress. Burns were observed around her mouth. What emergency care would be provided for this patient to prevent further trauma to the gastrointestinal and respiratory tracts? Identify the evidence that supports this care and evaluate the strength of the evidence.

## REFERENCES AND SELECTED READINGS

### BOOKS

American Cancer Society (2005). *Cancer Facts and Figures*. Atlanta, GA: Author.

Bickley, L. S., & Szilagyi, P. G. (2005). *Bates' guide to physical examination and history taking* (9th ed.). Philadelphia: Lippincott Williams & Wilkins.

Brandt, L. J. (Ed.). (1999). *Clinical practice of gastroenterology* (Vols. I & II). Philadelphia: Churchill-Livingstone.

Castell, D. O., & Richter, J. E. (2003). *The esophagus* (4th ed.). Philadelphia: Lippincott Williams & Wilkins.

DeVita, V. T., Hellman, S., & Rosenberg, S. A. (Eds.). (2005). *Cancer: Principles and practice of oncology* (7th ed.). Philadelphia: Lippincott Williams & Wilkins.

Fonseca, R. J. (Ed.). (2000). *Oral and maxillofacial surgery*. Philadelphia: W. B. Saunders.

Garber, T. M. (Ed.). (2000). *Orthodontics: Current principles and techniques*. St. Louis: Mosby.

Harris, N. O., & Garcia-Godoy, F. (2003). *Primary preventive dentistry* (6th ed.). Norwalk, CT: Appleton & Lange.

Harrison, L. B., Sessions, R. B., Hong, W. K., et al. (2004). *Head and neck cancer: A multidisciplinary approach* (2nd ed.). Philadelphia: Lippincott Williams & Wilkins.

McEvoy, G. R. (Ed.). (2004). *American Hospital Formulary Service.* Bethesda, MD: American Society of Health-System Pharmacists.

Murray, J. (1999). *Manual of dysphagia assessment in adults.* San Diego: Singular Publishing.

National Institute of Dental & Craniofacial Research (2004). *Temporomandibular disorders.* Bethesda, MD: National Institutes of Health.

Pappas, T. N., Eubanks, S., & Chekan, E. G. (1999). *Atlas of laparoscopic surgery* (2nd ed.). Norwalk, CT: Appleton & Lange.

Porth, C. M. (2005). *Pathophysiology: Concepts of altered health states* (7th ed.). Philadelphia: Lippincott Williams & Wilkins.

Proffit, W. R., & Fields, H. W. (2000). *Contemporary orthodontics.* St. Louis: Mosby.

U.S. Department of Health and Human Services. (2000). *Oral health in America: A report of the Surgeon General. Executive summary.* Rockville, MD: National Institutes of Dental and Craniofacial Research, National Institutes of Health.

Yamada, T., Alpers, D. H., Laine, L., et al. (2003). *Textbook of gastroenterology* (4th ed., Vols. I & II). Philadelphia: Lippincott Williams & Wilkins.

## JOURNALS

### Conditions and Cancer of the Oral Cavity

Bova, R., Ian, C., & Coman, W. (2004). Total glossectomy: Is it justified? *Australian and New Zealand Journal of Surgery, 74*(3), 134–138.

Brown, L. G., Wall, T. P., & Lazar, V. (2002). Trends in caries among adults 18 to 45 years old. *Journal of the American Dental Association, 133*(7), 827–834.

Bull, P. D. (2001). Salivary gland stones: Diagnosis and treatment. *Hospital Medicine, 62*(7), 396–399.

Capaccio, P., Ottaviani, F., Manzo, R., et al. (2004). Extracorporeal lithotripsy for salivary calculi: A long-term clinical experience. *Laryngoscope, 114*(6), 1069–1073.

Centers for Disease Prevention and Control. (2004). Oral cancer: Deadly to ignore. Fact sheet. Available at: http://www.cdc.gov/OralHealth/factsheet/oc-facts.htm. Accessed June 8, 2006.

Jemal, A., Taylor, M., Ward, E., et al. (2005). Cancer statistics, 2005. *CA Cancer Journal for Clinicians, 55*(1), 10–30.

McQuone, S. J. (1999). Acute viral and bacterial infections of the salivary glands. *Otolaryngology Clinics of North America, 32*(5), 793–811.

Moynihan, P., & Petersen, P. E. (2004). Diet, nutrition and the prevention of dental diseases. *Public Health Nutrition, 7*(1), 201–226.

Rice, D. H. (1999). Chronic inflammatory disorders of the salivary glands. *Otolaryngology Clinics of North America, 32*(5), 813–818.

Rice, D. H. (1999). Noninflammatory, non-neoplastic disorders of the salivary gland. *Otolaryngology Clinics of North America, 32*(5), 835–843.

Sessons, D. G., et al. (2000). Analysis of treatment results for floor-of-mouth cancer. *Laryngoscope, 110*(10 Pt. 1), 1764–1772.

Von Fraunhofer, J. Q., & Rogers, M. M. (2004). Dissolution of dental enamel in soft drinks. *General Dentistry, 15*(4), 308–312.

Wright, E. F. (2000). Referred craniofacial pain patterns in patients with temporomandibular disorder. *Journal of the American Dental Association, 131*(9), 1307–1315.

### Conditions and Treatment of the Esophagus

Farshad, A., Modlin, I., Kidd, M., et al. (2004). Surgical treatment of achalasia: Current status and controversies. *Digestive Surgery, 21*(1), 165–176.

Fitzgerald, R. C. (2005). Genetics and prevention of esophageal adenocarcinoma. *Recent Results of Cancer Research, 155*(1), 35–46.

Hage, M., Siersema, P. D., vanDekken, H., et al. (2004). Esophageal cancer incidence and mortality in patients with long-segment Barrett's esophagus after a mean follow-up of 12.7 years. *Scandinavian Journal of Gastroenterology, 39*(12), 1175–1179.

Heitmiller, R. F., Redmond, M., & Hamilton, S. R. (1996). Barrett's esophagus with high grade dysplasia: An indication for prophylactic esophagectomy. *Annals of Surgery, 224*(1), 66–71.

Hemminger, L. L. (2002). Photodynamic therapy for Barrett's esophagus and high-grade dysplasia: Results of a patient satisfaction survey. *Gastroenterology Nursing, 25*(4), 139–141.

Hostetler, M. A. (2004). Chemical burns. Available at: http://www.emedicine.com/ped/topic2735.htm. Accessed June 5, 2006.

Lau, C. L., Moore, M. B., Brooks, K. R., et al. (2002). Molecular staging of lung and esophageal cancer. *Surgical Clinics of North America, 82*(3), 497–523.

May, A., Gossner, L., Pech, O., et al. (2002). Intraepithelial high-grade neoplasia and early adenocarcinoma in short-segment Barrett's esophagus (SSBE): Curative treatment using local endoscopic treatment techniques. *Endoscopy, 34*(4), 604–610.

Overholt, B. F., Panjehpour, M., & Teffetellar, E. (1995). Photodynamic therapy for treatment of early adenocarcinoma in Barrett's esophagus. *Gastrointestinal Endoscopy, 49*(1), 73–76.

Para, M. (2002). Epidemiology of esophageal cancer, especially adenocarcinoma of the esophagus and esophagogastric junction. *Recent Results in Cancer Research, 155,* 1–14.

Quinn, K. L., & Reedy, A. (1999). Esophageal cancer: Therapeutic approaches and nursing care. *Seminars in Oncology Nursing, 15*(1), 17–25.

Qureshi, W. (2002). Gastrointestinal uses of botulinum toxin. *Journal of Clinical Gastroenterology, 34*(2), 126–128.

Shenfine, J., McNamee, P., Steer, N., et al. (2005). A pragmatic randomised controlled trial of the cost-effectiveness of palliative therapies for patients with inoperable esophageal cancer. *Health Technology Assessment, 9*(5), 1–136.

Sifrim, D., Castell, D., Dent, J., et al. (2004). Gastro-oesophageal reflux monitoring: Review and consensus report on detection and definitions of acid, non-acid, and gas reflux. *Gut, 53*(7), 1024–1031.

Stein, H. J., Kauer, W. K. H., Feussoner, H., et al. (1999). Bile acids as components of the duodenogastric refluate: Detection, relationship to bilirubin, mechanism of injury, and clinical relevance. *Hepatogastroenterology, 46,* 66–73.

Tseng, E. E., Wu, T. T., Yeo, C. J., et al. (2003). Barrett's esophagus with high-grade dysplasia: Surgical results and long-term outcome—an update. *Journal of Gastrointestinal Surgery, 7*(2), 164–171.

Watson, D. (2004). Laparoscopic treatment of gastro-oesophageal reflux disease. *Best Practice & Research Clinical Gastroenterology, 18*(1), 19–35.

Wolfsen, H. (2005). Present status of photodynamic therapy for high-grade dysplasia in Barrett's esophagus. *Journal of Clinical Gastroenterology, 39*(3), 189–202.

### Conditions and Treatment of the Head and Neck

ElGhani, F., van den Brekel, M. W., DeGoede, C. J., et al. (2002). Shoulder function and patient well-being after various types of neck dissections. *Clinical Otolaryngology, 27*(5), 403–408.

Garden, A. S., Harris, J., Vokes, E. E., et al. (2004). Preliminary results of radiation therapy oncology group 97-03: A randomized phase II trial of concurrent radiation and chemotherapy for advanced squamous cell carcinomas of the head and neck. *Journal of Clinical Oncology, 22*(7), 2856–2864.

Girling, D. J. (2004). Surgical resection with or without preoperative chemotherapy in oesophageal cancer: A randomised controlled trial. *Lancet.* March 10, 2005. Available at: http://www.thelancet.com/search/search.isa. Accessed June 5, 2006.

Pre-operative chemotherapy appears to improve survival in esophageal cancer. (2004). Cancer Consultants.com. Available at: http://patient.cancerconsultants.com/esophageal_cancer_news.aspx?id=17597. Accessed June 2, 2006.

Robbins, K. D., Clayman, G., Levine, P. A., et al. (2002). Neck dissection classification update: Revisions proposed by the American Head and Neck Society and the American Academy of Otolaryngology-Head and Neck Surgery. *Archives of Otolaryngology Head and Neck Surgery, 128*(7), 751–758.

Terrell, J. E., Ronis, D. L., Fowler, K. E., et al. (2004). Clinical predictors of quality of life in patients with head and neck cancer. *Archives of Otolaryngology Head Neck Surgery, 130*(1), 401–408.

## RESOURCES

American Cancer Society, 1599 Clifton Rd. NE, Atlanta, GA 30329; 1-800-ACS-2345; http://www.cancer.org. Accessed June 2, 2006.

American Dental Association, 211 E. Chicago Ave., Chicago, IL 60611; 312-440-2806; http://www.ada.org. Accessed June 2, 2006.

Centers for Disease Control and Prevention, 1600 Clifton Rd., Atlanta, GA 30333; 404-639-7000; http://www.cdc.gov/health. Accessed June 2, 2006.

National Institute of Dental and Craniofacial Research, National Institutes of Health, 900 Rockville Pike, Bethesda, MD 20892; 301-496-4261; http://www.nidr.nih.gov. Accessed June 2, 2006.

# CHAPTER 36

# Gastrointestinal Intubation and Special Nutritional Modalities

## Learning Objectives

*On completion of this chapter, the learner will be able to:*

1. Describe the purposes and types of gastrointestinal intubation.
2. Discuss nursing management of the patient who has a nasogastric or nasoenteric tube.
3. Use the nursing process as a framework for care of the patient receiving an enteral feeding.
4. Explain the preoperative and postoperative care of the patient with a gastrostomy.
5. Use the nursing process as a framework for care of the patient with a gastrostomy.
6. Identify the purposes and uses of parenteral nutrition.
7. Use the nursing process as a framework for care of the patient receiving parenteral nutrition.
8. Describe the nursing measures used to prevent complications from parenteral nutrition.

# CHAPTER 36 • Gastrointestinal Intubation and Special Nutritional Modalities

This chapter presents several topics related to gastrointestinal (GI) intubation. Nursing management topics relate to managing the care of patients with **nasogastric (NG)** and nasoenteric tubes and gastrostomies, providing tube feedings, and teaching points concerning home health care and nutritional therapy. In addition, parenteral nutrition is presented, including general indications for this nutritional modality and nursing care of patients receiving these support measures.

## Gastrointestinal Intubation

GI intubation is the insertion of a flexible tube into the stomach beyond the pylorus into the **duodenum** (the first section of the small intestine) or the **jejunum** (the second section of the small intestine). The tube may be inserted through the mouth, the nose, or the abdominal wall. The tubes are of various lengths, depending on their intended use. GI intubation may be performed for the following reasons:

- To decompress the stomach and remove gas and fluid
- To lavage the stomach and remove ingested toxins
- To diagnose disorders of GI motility and other disorders
- To administer medications and feedings
- To treat an obstruction
- To compress a bleeding site
- To aspirate gastric contents for analysis

A variety of tubes are used for decompression, aspiration, and **lavage**. Orogastric tubes are large-bore tubes with wide proximal outlets for removal of gastric contents; they are primarily used in emergency departments or in intensive care settings (see Chapter 71). The Sengstaken-Blakemore tube is a type of NG tube used to treat bleeding esophageal varices (see Chapter 39). Various other tubes are used to administer feedings and medications. The tubes are made of various materials (rubber, polyurethane, silicone); polyurethane catheters are more resistant to deterioration (Sartori, Trevisani, Neilsen, et al., 2003). They also vary in length (90 cm to 3 m [3 to 10 ft]), in size (6 to 18 French [Fr]), in purpose, and in placement in the GI tract (stomach, duodenum, jejunum) (Table 36-1). Any solution administered through a tube is poured through a syringe or delivered by a drip mechanism by gravity or regulated by an electric pump. **Aspiration** (suctioning) to remove gas and fluids is accomplished with the use of a syringe, an electric suction machine, or a wall suction outlet.

### Gastric Tubes

An NG tube is introduced through the nose into the stomach, often before or during surgery. Commonly used gastric tubes include the Levin tube and the gastric sump tube. Gastric tubes are used in adults primarily to remove fluid and gas from the upper GI tract; this is called **decompression**. They are occasionally used for the short-term (3 to 4 weeks) administration of medications or feedings.

## Glossary

**antireflux valve:** valve that prevents return or backward flow of fluid

**aspiration:** removal of substance by suction; breathing of fluids or foods into the trachea and lungs

**bolus:** a feeding administered into the stomach in large amounts and at designated intervals

**central venous access device (CVAD):** a device designed and used for long-term administration of medications and fluids into central veins

**cyclic feeding:** periodic feeding/infusion given over a short period (8 to 12 hours)

**decompression (intestinal):** removal of intestinal contents to prevent gas and fluid from distending the coils of the intestine

**dumping syndrome:** rapid emptying of the stomach contents into the small intestine; characterized by sweating and weakness

**duodenum:** the first part of the small intestine, which connects with the pylorus of the stomach and extends to the jejunum

**gastrostomy:** surgical creation of an opening into the stomach for the purpose of administering foods and fluids

**intravenous fat emulsion (IVFE, Intralipids):** an oil-in-water emulsion of oils, egg phospholipids, and glycerin

**jejunum:** second portion of the small intestine, extending from the duodenum to the ileum

**lavage:** flushing of the stomach via the gastric tube with water or other fluids to clear it

**low-profile gastrostomy device (LPGD, G-button):** an enteral feeding access device that is flush with the skin and is used for long-term feeding

**nasoduodenal tube:** tube inserted through the nose into the beginning of the small intestine (duodenum)

**nasogastric (NG) tube:** tube inserted through the nose into the stomach

**nasojejunal tube:** tube inserted through the nose into the second portion of the small intestine (jejunum)

**osmolality:** ionic concentration of fluid

**osmosis:** passage of solvent through a semipermeable membrane; the solvent, usually water, passes through the membrane from a region of low concentration of solute to that of a higher concentration of solute

**parenteral nutrition (PN):** method of supplying nutrients to the body by an intravenous route

**percutaneous endoscopic gastrostomy (PEG):** an endoscopic procedure for inserting a feeding tube into the stomach in order to provide long-term nutritional support

**peristalsis:** wavelike movement that occurs involuntarily in the alimentary canal

**pH:** the degree of acidity or alkalinity of a substance or solution

**peripherally inserted central catheter (PICC):** a device used for intermediate-term intravenous therapy

**stoma:** artificially created opening between a body cavity (eg, intestine) and the body surface

**total nutrient admixture (TNA):** an admixture of lipid emulsions, proteins, carbohydrates, electrolytes, vitamins, trace minerals, and water

### TABLE 36-1 Nasogastric and Nasoenteric Feeding Tubes

| Tube Type | Length (cm) | Size (French) | Lumen | Other Characteristics |
|---|---|---|---|---|
| **Nasogastric Tubes** | | | | |
| Levin (plastic or rubber) | 125 | 14–18 | Single | Circular markings at intervals along the tube serve as guidelines for insertion |
| Gastric sump or Salem (plastic) | 120 | 12–18 | Double | Smaller lumen acts as a vent |
| Moss | 90 | 12–16 | Triple | Contains both a gastric decompression lumen and a duodenal lumen for postoperative feedings |
| Sengstaken-Blakemore (rubber) | | | Triple | Two lumens are used to inflate the gastric and esophageal balloons, and one tube is reserved for suction or drainage |
| **Nasoenteric Feeding Tubes** | | | | |
| Dobbhoff or EnteraFlo (polyurethane or silicone rubber) | 160–175 | 8–12 | Single | Tungsten-weighted tip, radiopaque, stylet |

## Levin Tube

The Levin tube has a single lumen (the hollow part of the tube), ranges from 14 to 18 Fr in size, and is made of plastic or rubber with openings near its tip. It is 125 cm (50 in) long. Circular markings at specific points on the tube serve as guides for insertion. A marking is made on the tube to indicate the midpoint. The tube is advanced cautiously until this marking reaches the patient's nostril, suggesting that the tube is in the stomach. Placement is checked by observing the characteristics of the aspirate and by testing the **pH** (which varies according to the source of the aspirate). Visualizing the tube's placement on x-ray is the only definitive way to verify its location. The Levin tube is connected to low intermittent suction (30 to 40 mm Hg). Intermittent suction is used to avoid erosion or tearing of the stomach lining, which can result from constant adherence of the tube's lumen to the mucosal lining of the stomach.

## Gastric Sump

The gastric sump (Salem) tube is a radiopaque, clear plastic, double-lumen NG tube used to decompress the stomach and keep it empty. It is 120 cm (48 in) long and is passed into the stomach in the same way as the Levin tube. The inner, smaller tube vents the larger suction-drainage tube to the atmosphere by means of an opening at the distal end of the tube. The sump tube can protect gastric suture lines because, when used properly, it maintains the force of suction at the drainage openings, or outlets, at less than 25 mm Hg, the level of capillary fragility. The small vent tube (known as the blue pigtail or port) controls this action. Gastric sump tubes are connected to low continuous suction. The suction lumen is irrigated as prescribed to maintain patency.

To prevent reflux of gastric contents through the vent lumen (blue pigtail), the vent lumen is kept above the patient's waist; otherwise it will act as a siphon. A one-way **antireflux valve** seated in the blue pigtail can prevent the reflux of gastric contents out the vent lumen (Fig. 36-1). The valve is removed after irrigation of the suction lumen, and 20 mL of air is injected to reestablish a buffer of air between the gastric contents and the valve.

## Enteric Tubes

Nasoenteric tubes are used for feeding. Feeding tubes placed in the duodenum are 160 cm (60 in) long and called **nasoduodenal tubes**; feeding tubes placed in the jejunum (the portion of the small intestine distal to the duodenum) are 175 cm (66 in) long. They can be inserted before or dur-

**FIGURE 36-1.** Gastric sump tube (Salem) equipped with a one-way valve that allows air to enter and can prevent reflux of gastric contents. The antireflux valve is designed with a pressure-activated air buffer (PAAB). The buffer is activated (1) and the valve closes (2) when pressure from gastric contents enters the tubing. Argyle Silicone Salem Sump Tube with preattached Argyle Salem Sump Anti-Reflux Valve courtesy of Sherwood Medical, St. Louis, Missouri.

ing surgery, by interventional radiologists assisted by fluoroscopy, or at the bedside. If the tube is inserted at the bedside, placement is verified by x-ray study. After insertion, the tip of the tube is initially placed in the stomach; it usually takes 24 hours for the tube to pass through the stomach and into the intestines by **peristalsis**. Surgically placed enteric tubes are inserted directly into the jejunum.

Polyurethane or silicone rubber feeding tubes have narrow diameters (6 to 12 Fr) and tungsten tips (rather than mercury-filled bags), and some have a water-activated lubricant that makes it easier to insert the tube. The tubing may kink when a stylet is not used, particularly if the patient is uncooperative or unable to swallow. Feeding tubes with a stylet are inserted with caution in patients predisposed to esophageal puncture, such as patients who are elderly or frail or who have thin tissues. These tubes are advanced in the same way as an NG tube (ie, with the patient in Fowler's position). If this is not possible, the patient is placed on the right side.

## Nursing Management

Nursing interventions include the following:

- Explaining to the patient the purpose of the tube and the procedure required for inserting and advancing it
- Describing the sensations to be expected during tube insertion
- Inserting the NG tube and assisting with insertion of the nasoenteric tube
- Confirming the placement of the NG tube
- Advancing the nasoenteric tube
- Monitoring the patient and maintaining tube function
- Providing oral and nasal hygiene and care
- Monitoring for potential complications
- Removing the tube

### Preparing the Patient

Before the patient is intubated, the nurse explains the purpose of the tube; this information may assist the patient to be cooperative and tolerant of what is often an unpleasant procedure. The general activities related to inserting the tube are then reviewed, including the fact that the patient may have to breathe through the mouth and that the procedure may cause gagging until the tube has passed the area of the gag reflex.

### Inserting the Tube

Before inserting the tube, the nurse determines the length of tubing that will be needed to reach the stomach or the small intestine. A mark is made on the tube to indicate the desired length. This length is determined by (1) measuring the distance from the tip of the nose to the earlobe and from the earlobe to the xiphoid process, and (2) adding 6 inches for NG placement or 8 to 10 inches for intestinal placement (Fig. 36-2).

While the tube is being inserted, the patient usually sits upright with a towel or some type of protective barrier spread bib-fashion over the chest. Tissue wipes are made

1. Mark the nasogastric tube at a point 50 cm from the distal tip; call this point 'A'.

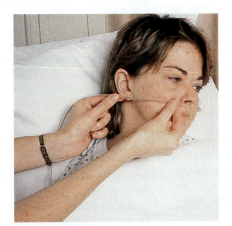

Measuring distance from nostril to tip of earlobe.

Measuring distance from earlobe to tip of xiphoid process.

2. Have the patient sit in a neutral position with head facing forward. Place the distal tip of the tubing at the tip of the patient's nose (N); extend tube to the tragus (tip) of the ear (E), and then extend the tube straight down to the tip of the xiphoid (X). Mark this point 'B' on the tubing.

**FIGURE 36-2.** Measuring length of nasogastric tube for placement into stomach.

3. To locate point C on the tube, find the midpoint between points A and B. The nasogastric tube is passed to point C to ensure optimum placement in the stomach.

available. Privacy and adequate light are provided. The physician may swab the nostril and spray the oropharynx with tetracaine/benzocaine (Cetacaine) to numb the nasal passage and suppress the gag reflex. This makes the entire procedure more tolerable. Having the patient gargle with a liquid anesthetic or hold ice chips in the mouth for a few minutes can have a similar effect. Encouraging the patient to breathe through the mouth or to pant often helps, as does swallowing water, if permitted.

A polyurethane tube may need to be warmed to make it more pliable. To make the tube easier to insert, it should be lubricated with a water-soluble lubricant unless it has a dry coating (called hydromer), which, when moistened, provides its own lubrication. The nurse wears gloves during the procedure.

The patient is placed in Fowler's position, and the nostrils are inspected for any obstruction. The more patent nostril is selected for use. The tip of the patient's nose is tilted, and the tube is aligned to enter the nostril. When the tube reaches the nasopharynx, the patient is instructed to lower the head slightly and to begin to swallow as the tube is advanced. The patient may also sip water through a straw to facilitate advancement of the tube. The oropharynx is inspected to ensure that the tube has not coiled in the pharynx or mouth.

## *Confirming Placement*

To ensure patient safety, it is essential to confirm that the tube has been placed correctly: the tube may be inadvertently inserted in the lungs, and this may go undetected in high-risk patients (eg, those with decreased levels of consciousness, confused mental states, poor or absent cough and gag reflexes, or agitation during insertion). The presence of an endotracheal tube or the recent removal of an endotracheal tube also increases the risk of inadvertent placement of the tube in the lung (Metheny, 1998). Initially, an x-ray study should be used to confirm tube placement. However, each time liquids or medications are administered, and once a shift for continuous feedings, the tube must be checked to ensure that it remains properly placed. The traditional recommendation has been to inject air through the tube while auscultating the epigastric area with a stethoscope to detect air insufflation. However, studies indicate that this auscultatory method is not absolutely accurate in determining whether the tube has been inserted into the stomach, intestines, or respiratory tract (Metheny, McSweeney, Wehrle, et al., 1990). Instead of the auscultation method, a combination of three methods is recommended:

- Measurement of tube length
- Visual assessment of aspirate
- pH measurement of aspirate

After the tube is inserted, the exposed portion of the tube is measured and the length is documented. The nurse measures the exposed tube length every shift and compares it with the original measurement. An increase in the length of exposed tube may indicate dislodgement, or a leaking or ruptured balloon if the tube has a balloon.

Visual assessment of the color of the aspirate may help identify tube placement. Gastric aspirate is most frequently cloudy and green, tan or off-white, or bloody or brown. Intestinal aspirate is primarily clear and yellow to bile-colored. Pleural fluid is usually pale yellow and serous, and tracheobronchial secretions are usually tan or off-white mucus. The appearance of the aspirate may be helpful in distinguishing between gastric and intestinal placement but is of little value in ruling out respiratory placement. Visual inspection is less helpful when the patient is receiving continuous tube feedings, because the gastric or intestinal aspirate often looks like the formula being used for the feeding (Metheny & Titler, 2001).

Determining the pH of the tube aspirate is a more accurate method of confirming tube placement than maintaining tube length or visually assessing tube aspirate. The pH method can also be used to monitor the advancement of the tube into the small intestine. The pH of gastric aspirate is acidic (1 to 5). The pH of intestinal aspirate is approximately 6 or higher, and the pH of respiratory aspirate is more alkaline (7 or greater). pH testing is best suited for distinguishing between gastric and intestinal placement. A pH sensor enteral tube that does not require fluid aspirate to obtain pH values is available and can be useful in distinguishing gastric from small intestinal placement of the tube. The pH method is less helpful with continuous feedings, because tube feedings have a pH value of 6.6 and neutralize the GI pH (Metheny & Titler, 2001).

Ensuring bedside placement of postpyloric feeding tubes into the duodenum can be a challenge. If a gastroenterologist inserts the feeding tube using fiberoptic endoscopy, appropriate confirmation is ensured. However, this method of placement is relatively costly. Other placement methods are less invasive and less costly. For instance, external magnets can sometimes be used to help guide a postpyloric feeding tube that has a magnet inserted in the tip. Metoclopramide (Reglan), a prokinetic agent, is administered intravenously (IV) and facilitates GI peristalsis, thereby encouraging movement of the feeding tube into the duodenum. Insufflating (eg, administering) 100 to 500 mL of air into the feeding tube once its placement in the stomach is confirmed may also be a useful method of ensuring eventual postpyloric placement. Findings from research suggest that the air insufflation method results in quicker postpyloric placement, particularly among patients who also receive opioid agents (Lenart & Polissar, 2003). Typical guidelines for all of these bedside methods require that the patient be placed on his or her right side.

Using gastric aspiration to verify the correct placement of the NG tube may be a problem because of the characteristic properties and diameter of the tubes. Aspiration may be performed more easily with polyurethane tubes and tubes with a size 10 Fr diameter or larger. If it is difficult to aspirate fluid from small-bore or large-bore feeding tubes, 20 mL of air is injected through the tube with a large syringe (30 to 60 mL), and then the plunger is pulled back. If this is ineffective, another 20 mL of air is injected, the large syringe is replaced with a smaller one (10 mL), and aspiration is attempted. The patient's position is changed and aspiration is again attempted. If these measures are unsuccessful, the physician is notified.

## NURSING RESEARCH PROFILE

### Postpyloric Placement of Enteral Feeding Tubes

Lenart, S., & Polissar, N. (2003). Comparison of 2 methods for postpyloric placement of enteral feeding tubes. *American Journal of Critical Care, 12*(4), 357–360.

#### Purpose
Multiple bedside techniques are used to facilitate placement of postpyloric enteral tubes. A study was conducted to determine which of two techniques, prokinetic metoclopramide (Reglan) or gastric insufflation of air, was superior in ensuring placement of these feeding tubes beyond the gastric pylorus.

#### Design
Sixty patients from cardiac care and intensive care units were prospectively randomized to two groups. Patients with basilar skull or facial fractures, esophageal varices or tears, pyloric stenosis, and ileus or recent gastrointestinal surgery were excluded. Patients in group 1 received metoclopramide 10 mg 10 minutes prior to feeding tube insertion into the stomach. Patients in group 2 had 350 mL of air insufflated via syringe through the tube immediately after tube placement into the stomach. Patients in both groups were placed on their right sides to facilitate migration of the tubes beyond the pylorus into the small bowel. Abdominal x-ray studies were used to confirm tube tip location in the duodenum.

#### Findings
Demographic and clinical data did not vary significantly between groups. Overall, success of tube placement was significantly greater in patients who had air insufflation than in those who received metoclopramide. Moreover, patients who were receiving opioids achieved better placement success than with metoclopramide.

#### Nursing Implications
Both metoclopramide administration and air insufflation are performed by the nurse at the bedside when prescribed. Although endoscopically assisted and fluoroscopically guided insertions of postpyloric feeding tubes are fairly common practices in critical care units, these procedures are more costly than bedside placement procedures in terms of time and manpower resources. Verifying an effective bedside technique facilitates more successful placement and earlier nutrition support. The results of this study suggest that there is decreased financial cost and clinical risk when air insufflation, rather than metoclopramide administration, is used to facilitate postpyloric tube placement. In addition, the possible effects of opioids should be considered when attempting to place postpyloric tubes using either air insufflation or metoclopramide.

---

Cola and cranberry juice have historically been recommended as effective, noninvasive means of declogging tubes, but evidence indicates that a mixture of pancreatic enzymes and water is superior in restoring the patency of feeding tubes (Keithley & Swanson, 2004). However, correct placement of the NG tube must be confirmed before any mixture is injected to declog the tube.

### Securing the Tube

After the correct position of the tip of the tube has been confirmed, the NG tube is secured to the nose (Fig. 36-3). A liquid skin barrier should be applied to the skin where the NG tube will be secured. The prepared area is covered with a strip of hypoallergenic tape or Op-Site, and the tube is then placed over the tape and secured with a second piece of tape. Instead of tape, a feeding tube attachment device (Hollister) can be used to secure the tube. This device adheres to the nose and uses an adjustable clip to hold the tube in place (Fig. 36-4).

### Monitoring the Patient and Maintaining Tube Function

If the NG tube is used for decompression, it is attached to suction. If it is used for enteral nutrition, the end of the tube is plugged between feedings. The nurse confirms tube placement by measuring tube length and comparing the length to the baseline before any fluids or medications are instilled and once a shift for continuous feedings. Displacement of the tube may be caused by tension on the tube (when the patient moves around in the bed or room), coughing, tracheal or nasotracheal suctioning, or airway intubation. If the NG tube is removed inadvertently in a patient who has undergone esophageal or gastric surgery, it is usually replaced under fluoroscopy by the physician to avoid trauma to the suture line.

It is important to keep an accurate record of all fluid intake, feedings, and irrigation. To maintain patency, the tube is irrigated every 4 to 6 hours with water or normal saline to avoid electrolyte loss through gastric drainage. The nurse records the amount, color, and type of all drainage every 8 hours.

When double- or triple-lumen tubes are used, each lumen is labeled according to its intended use: aspiration, feeding, or balloon inflation. To avoid tension on the tube, the portion of the tube from the nose to the drainage unit is fixed in position, either with a safety pin or with adhesive tape loops that are pinned to the patient's pajamas or gown. The tube must be looped loosely to prevent tension and dislodgement (see Fig. 36-3).

**FIGURE 36-3.** Securing nasogastric (NG) tubes. (**A**) The NG tube is secured to the nose with tape to prevent injury to the nasopharyngeal passages. (**B,C**) The tubing is secured to the patient's gown with either an elastic band or tape attached to a safety pin to prevent tension on the line during movement of the patient.

## Providing Oral and Nasal Hygiene

Regular and conscientious oral and nasal hygiene is a vital part of patient care, because the tube causes discomfort and pressure and may be in place for several days. Moistened cotton-tipped swabs can be used to clean the nose, followed by cleansing with a water-soluble lubricant. Frequent mouth care is comforting for the patient. The nasal tape is changed every 2 to 3 days, and the nose is inspected for skin irritation. If the nasal and pharyngeal mucosa are excessively dry, steam or cool vapor inhalations may be beneficial. Throat lozenges, an ice collar, chewing gum, or sucking on hard candies (if permitted) and limiting talking also assist in relieving patient discomfort. These activities keep the mucous membranes moist and help prevent inflammation of the parotid glands.

## Monitoring and Managing Potential Complications

Patients with NG or nasoenteric intubation are susceptible to a variety of problems, including fluid volume deficit, pulmonary complications, and tube-related irritations. These potential complications require careful ongoing assessment.

Symptoms of fluid volume deficit include dry skin and mucous membranes, decreased urinary output, lethargy, and increased heart rate. Assessment of fluid volume deficit involves maintaining an accurate record of intake and output. This includes measuring NG drainage, fluid instilled by irrigation of the NG tube, water taken by mouth, vomitus, water administered with tube feedings, and IV fluids. Laboratory values, particularly blood urea nitrogen and creatinine, are monitored. The nurse assesses 24-hour fluid balance and reports negative fluid balance, increased NG output, interruption of IV therapy, or any other disturbance in fluid intake or output.

Pulmonary complications from NG intubation occur because coughing and clearing of the pharynx are impaired, because gas buildup can irritate the phrenic nerve, and because tubes may become dislodged, retracting the distal end above the esophagogastric sphincter (which places the pa-

**FIGURE 36-4.** Feeding tube attachment device. Courtesy of Hollister, Incorporated.

tient at risk for **aspiration**, or breathing fluids or foods into the trachea and lungs). Medications (eg, antacids, simethicone [Gaviscon], and metoclopramide [Reglan]) can be administered to decrease potential problems. Signs and symptoms of complications include coughing during the administration of foods or medications, difficulty clearing the airway, tachypnea, and fever. Assessment includes regular auscultation of lung sounds and routine assessment of vital signs. It is important to encourage the patient to cough and to take deep breaths regularly. The nurse also carefully confirms the proper placement of the tube by assessing tube length before instilling any fluids or medications.

Irritation of the mucous membranes is a common complication of NG intubation. The nostrils, oral mucosa, esophagus, and trachea are susceptible to irritation and necrosis. Visible areas are inspected frequently, and the adequacy of hydration is assessed. When providing oral hygiene, the nurse carefully inspects the mucous membranes for signs of irritation or excessive dryness. The nurse palpates the area around the parotid glands to detect any tenderness or enlarged nodes, indicating parotitis, and observes for any irritation or necrosis at the insertion site (eg, nares) or of the mucous membranes. In addition, it is important to assess the patient for esophagitis and tracheitis; symptoms include sore throat and hoarseness.

### Removing the Tube

Before removing a tube, the nurse may intermittently clamp and unclamp it for a trial period of several hours to ensure that the patient does not experience nausea, vomiting, or distention. Before the tube is removed, it is flushed with 10 mL of water or normal saline to ensure that it is free of debris and away from the gastric lining; then the balloon (if present) is deflated. Gloves are worn to remove the tube. The tube is withdrawn gently and slowly for 15 to 20 cm (6 to 8 in) until the tip reaches the esophagus; the remainder is withdrawn rapidly from the nostril. If the tube does not come out easily, force should not be used, and the problem should be reported to the physician. As the tube is withdrawn, it is concealed in a towel to prevent secretions from soiling the patient or nurse. After the tube is removed, the nurse provides oral hygiene.

## Tube Feedings With Nasogastric and Nasoenteric Devices

Tube feedings are given to meet nutritional requirements when oral intake is inadequate or not possible and the GI tract is functioning normally. Tube feedings have several advantages over parenteral nutrition: they are low in cost, safe, well tolerated by the patient, and easy to use both in extended care facilities and in the patient's home. Tube feedings have other advantages:

- They preserve GI integrity by delivery of nutrients and medications intraluminally.
- They preserve the normal sequence of intestinal and hepatic metabolism.
- They maintain fat metabolism and lipoprotein synthesis.
- They maintain normal insulin/glucagon ratios.

Tube feedings are delivered to the stomach (in the case of NG intubation or gastrostomy) or to the distal duodenum or proximal jejunum (in the case of nasoduodenal or **nasojejunal tube** feeding). Nasoduodenal or nasojejunal feeding is indicated when the esophagus and stomach need to be bypassed or when the patient is at risk for aspiration. For long-term feedings (longer than 4 weeks), gastrostomy or jejunostomy tubes are preferred for administration of medications or food. The numerous conditions requiring enteral nutrition are summarized in Table 36-2.

### Osmosis and Osmolality

Osmolality is an important consideration for patients receiving tube feedings through the duodenum or jejunum because feeding formulas with a high osmolality may lead to undesirable effects, such as dumping syndrome (described below).

Fluid balance is maintained by **osmosis**, the process by which water moves through membranes from a dilute solution of lower **osmolality** (ionic concentration) to a more concentrated solution of higher osmolality until both solutions are of nearly equal osmolality. The osmolality of normal body fluids is approximately 300 mOsm/kg. The body attempts to keep the osmolality of the contents of the stomach and intestines at approximately this level.

Highly concentrated solutions and certain foods can upset the normal fluid balance in the body. Individual

### TABLE 36-2 Conditions Requiring Enteral Therapy

| Condition or Need | Examples |
|---|---|
| Preoperative bowel preparation | — |
| Gastrointestinal problems | Fistula, short-bowel syndrome, mild pancreatitis, Crohn's disease, ulcerative colitis, nonspecific maldigestion or malabsorption |
| Cancer therapy | Radiation, chemotherapy |
| Convalescent care | Surgery, injury, severe illness |
| Coma, semi-consciousness* | Stroke, head injury, neurologic disorder, neoplasm |
| Hypermetabolic conditions | Burns, trauma, multiple fractures, sepsis, AIDS, organ transplantation |
| Alcoholism, chronic depression, anorexia nervosa* | Chronic illness, psychiatric or neurologic disorder |
| Debilitation* | Disease or injury |
| Maxillofacial or cervical surgery | Disease or injury |
| Oropharyngeal or esophageal paralysis* | Disease or injury, neoplasm, inflammation, trauma, respiratory failure |

*Because some of these patients are at risk for regurgitating or vomiting and aspirating administered formula, each condition must be considered individually.

amino acids and carbohydrates are small particles that have great osmotic effect. Proteins are extremely large particles and therefore have less osmotic effect. Fats are not water-soluble and do not enter into a solution in water; thus, they have no osmotic effect. Electrolytes, such as sodium and potassium, are comparatively small particles; they have a great effect on osmolality and consequently on the patient's ability to tolerate a given solution.

When a concentrated solution of high osmolality is taken in large amounts, water moves to the stomach and intestines from fluid surrounding the organs and the vascular compartment. The patient has a feeling of fullness, nausea, and diarrhea; this causes dehydration, hypotension, and tachycardia, collectively termed the **dumping syndrome**. It is generally believed that starting with a more dilute commercial formula and increasing the concentration over several days may alleviate this problem. However, there is a lack of research data supporting the dilution of formula with water to relieve dumping syndrome (Parrish, 2003). Patients vary in the degree to which they tolerate the effects of high osmolality; usually debilitated patients are less tolerant. The nurse needs to be knowledgeable about the osmolality of the patient's formula and needs to observe for and take steps to prevent undesired effects.

## Tube Feeding Formulas

The choice of formula to be delivered by tube feeding is influenced by the status of the GI tract and the nutritional needs of the patient. The formula characteristics that are considered prior to selection include the chemical composition of the nutrient source (protein, carbohydrates, fat), caloric density, osmolality, residue, bacteriologic safety, vitamins, minerals, and cost.

Various major formula types for tube feedings are available commercially. Blenderized formulas can be made by the patient's family or obtained in a ready-to-use form that is carefully prepared according to directions. Commercially prepared polymeric formulas (formulas with high molecular weight) are composed of protein, carbohydrates, and fats in a high-molecular-weight form (eg, Boost Plus, TwoCal HN, Isosource). Chemically defined formulas (eg, Peptomen 1.5 or Vivonex) contain predigested and easy-to-absorb nutrients. Modular products contain only one major nutrient, such as protein (Beneprotein). Disease-specific formulas are available for various conditions. For patients with renal failure, a formula such as Nepro that is high in calories and low in electrolytes is ideal because it is formulated to maintain electrolyte and fluid balance. For patients with severe chronic obstructive pulmonary disease, a formula such as Pulmocare may be selected because it is high in fat and low in carbohydrates, has a high density (1.5 calories/mL) that helps maintain fluid restriction, and reduces carbon dioxide production. Fiber is added to some formulas (eg, Jevity) to decrease the occurrence of diarrhea in some at-risk patients. Some feedings are given as supplements, and others are designed to meet the patient's total nutritional needs. Dietitians collaborate with physicians and nurses to determine the best formula for the individual patient.

> **NURSING ALERT**
>
> Commercial formulas frequently present problems because the composition is fixed and some patients cannot tolerate certain ingredients, such as sodium, protein, or potassium. Modular products may be substituted, and the critical constituents of sodium, potassium, and fat can be added. Attention is given to including all essential minerals and vitamins. Total intake of calories, nutrients, and fluids must be assessed when there is a reduction in total intake or excessive dilution of feedings.

## Tube Feeding Administration Methods

Many patients do not tolerate NG and nasoenteric tube feedings well. Often a medium- or fine-bore Silastic nasoenteric tube is better tolerated than a plastic or rubber tube. The finer-bore tube requires a finely dispersed formula to ensure that the tube remains patent. For long-term tube feeding therapy, a gastrostomy or jejunostomy tube is often used (see later discussion).

The tube feeding method chosen depends on the location of the tube in the GI tract, patient tolerance, convenience, and cost. Intermittent bolus feedings are administered into the stomach (usually by gastrostomy tube) in large amounts at designated intervals and may be given four to eight times per day. The intermittent gravity drip, another method for administering tube feedings into the stomach, is commonly used when the patient is at home. In this instance, the tube feeding is administered over 30 minutes at designated intervals. Both of these tube feeding methods are practical and inexpensive. However, the feedings delivered at variable rates may be poorly tolerated and time-consuming.

The continuous infusion method is used when feedings are administered into the small intestine. This method is preferred for patients who are at risk for aspiration or who tolerate tube feedings poorly (Shang, Geiger, Sturm, et al., 2004). The feedings are given continuously at a constant rate by means of a pump. This method decreases abdominal distention, gastric residuals, and the risk of aspiration. However, pumps are expensive, and they allow the patient less flexibility than intermittent feedings.

An alternative to the continuous infusion method is **cyclic feeding**. The infusion is given at a faster rate over a shorter time (usually 8 to 12 hours). Feedings may be infused at night to avoid interrupting the patient's lifestyle. Cyclic continuous infusions may be appropriate for patients who are being weaned from tube feedings to an oral diet, as supplements for patients who cannot eat enough, and for patients at home who need daytime hours free from the pump.

Tube feeding solutions vary in terms of required preparation, consistency, and the number of calories and vitamins they contain. The choice of solution depends on the size and location of the tube in the GI tract, the patient's nutrient needs, the type of nutritional supplement, the method of delivery, and the convenience for the patient at home. A wide variety of containers, feeding tubes and catheters, delivery systems, and pumps are available for use with tube feedings.

## Nursing Process

### The Patient Receiving a Tube Feeding

#### Assessment

A preliminary assessment of the patient who requires a tube feeding includes several considerations:

- What is the patient's nutritional status, as judged by current physical appearance, dietary history, and history of recent weight loss?
- Are there any existing chronic illnesses or factors that will increase metabolic demands on the body (eg, surgical stress, fever)?
- What is the patient's hydration status? Are fluid requirements (ie, 30 to 40 mL/kg body weight) being met?
- Is the patient's digestive tract functioning?
- Are the patient's kidneys functioning normally? What are the patient's electrolyte levels?
- What medications and other therapies is the patient receiving that may affect nutritional intake and function of the digestive system?
- Does the dietary prescription fulfill the patient's needs?

In addition, a more elaborate assessment is performed for patients who require extensive nutritional therapy. A team that includes the nurse, advanced practice nurse, physician, and dietitian conducts this assessment. In addition to the history and physical examination (which includes anthropometric measurements), a nutritional assessment is performed. This consists of recording any weight change; determining albumin, prealbumin, and transferrin levels; measuring total lymphocyte count; and evaluating muscle function. (See Chapter 5 for a detailed description of nutritional assessment.)

#### Diagnosis

##### Nursing Diagnoses

Based on the assessment data, the major nursing diagnoses may include the following:

- Imbalanced nutrition, less than body requirements, related to inadequate intake of nutrients
- Risk for diarrhea related to the dumping syndrome or to tube feeding intolerance
- Risk for ineffective airway clearance related to aspiration of tube feeding
- Risk for deficient fluid volume related to hypertonic dehydration
- Risk for ineffective coping related to discomfort imposed by the presence of the NG or nasoenteric tube
- Risk for ineffective therapeutic regimen management
- Deficient knowledge about home tube feeding regimen

##### Collaborative Problems/ Potential Complications

Complications of NG and nasoenteric tube feeding therapy are classified into three types—GI, mechanical, and metabolic. Table 36-3 summarizes complications, possible causes, and appropriate interventions.

#### Planning and Goals

The major goals for the patient may include nutritional balance, normal bowel elimination pattern, reduced risk of aspiration, adequate hydration, individual coping, knowledge and skill in self-care, and prevention of complications.

#### Nursing Interventions

##### Maintaining Feeding Equipment and Nutritional Balance

The temperature and volume of the feeding, the flow rate, and the patient's total fluid intake are important factors to be considered when tube feedings are administered. The schedule of tube feedings, including the correct quantity and frequency, is maintained. The nurse must carefully monitor the drip rate and avoid administering fluids too rapidly.

Feedings are administered by gravity (drip), bolus, or continuous controlled pump (mL/hour). Gravity feedings are placed above the level of the stomach, with the speed of administration determined by gravity. **Bolus** feedings are given in large volumes (300 to 400 mL every 4 to 6 hours). Continuous feeding is the preferred method; delivery of the feeding in small amounts over long periods reduces the incidence of aspiration, distention, nausea, vomiting, and diarrhea. Continuous administration rates vary depending on the caloric density of the formula and the energy needs of the patient. The overall goal is to achieve positive nitrogen balance and weight maintenance or gain without producing abdominal cramps and diarrhea. If the feeding is intermittent, 200 to 350 mL is given over a span of 10 to 15 minutes.

Enteral pumps are mechanical devices that control the delivery rate of feeding formula (Fig. 36-5). Pumps allow for a constant flow rate and can infuse a viscous formula through a small-diameter feeding tube. These pumps are relatively heavy and must be attached to an IV pole. For home use, there are portable lightweight enteral pumps available that weigh about 4 pounds and are easy to handle.

Residual gastric content is measured before each intermittent feeding and every 4 to 8 hours during

## TABLE 36-3    Complications of Enteral Therapy

| Complications | Causes | Selected Nursing Interventions | |
|---|---|---|---|
| | | *Treatment* | *Prevention* |
| **Gastrointestinal** | | | |
| Diarrhea (most common) | Hyperosmolar feedings<br>Rapid infusion/bolus feedings<br>Bacteria-contaminated feedings<br>Lactase deficiency<br>Medications/antibiotic therapy<br>Decreased serum osmolality level<br>Food allergies<br>Cold formula | Assess fluid balance and electrolyte levels; report findings<br>Implement changes in tube feeding formula or rate | Assess rate of infusion and temperature of formula<br>Replace formula every 4 hours; change tube feeding container and tubing daily |
| Nausea/vomiting | Change in formula or rate<br>Hyperosmolar formula<br>Inadequate gastric emptying | Review medications | Check residuals; if ≥200 mL for NG or >100 mL for gastrostomy, continue feeding and recheck; report if residual is still high |
| Gas/bloating/cramping | Air in tube | Notify physician if persistent | Keep tubing free of air |
| Dumping syndrome | Bolus feedings/rapid rate<br>Cold formula | Check fiber and water content; report findings<br>Check rate and temperature of formula | Avoid rapid infusion of feeding<br>Administer feeding at or near room temperature |
| Constipation | High milk (lactose) content<br>Lack of fiber<br>Inadequate fluid intake/dehydration<br>Opioid use | Check fiber and water content; report findings | Administer adequate amount of hydration as flushes |
| **Mechanical** | | | |
| Aspiration pneumonia | Improper tube placement<br>Vomiting with aspiration of tube feeding<br>Flat in bed<br>Use of large tube | Assess respiratory status and notify physician | Implement reliable method for checking small-bore enteral tube placement (ie, measuring length of exposed tube)<br>Keep head of bed elevated 30 degrees continuously |
| Tube displacement | Excessive coughing/vomitus<br>Tension on the tube or unsecured tube<br>Tracheal suctioning<br>Airway intubation | Stop feeding and notify physician | Check tube placement before administering feeding |
| Tube obstruction | Inadequate flushing/formula rate | Follow policy for declogging feeding tubes | Obtain liquid medications when possible |
| Residue | Inadequate crushing of medications and flushing after administration | | Flush tube and crush medications adequately |
| Nasopharyngeal irritation | Tube position/improper taping<br>Use of large tubes | Assess nasopharyngeal mucous membranes every 4 hours | Tape tube to prevent pressure on nares |
| **Metabolic** | | | |
| Hyperglycemia | Glucose intolerance<br>High carbohydrate content of the feeding | Check blood glucose levels periodically<br>Request dietary consult to reevaluate choice of feeding product | |
| Dehydration and azotemia (excessive urea in the blood) | Hyperosmolar feedings with insufficient fluid intake | Report signs and symptoms of dehydration<br>Implement changes in tube feeding formula, rate, or ratio to water | Provide adequate hydration through flushes |

**FIGURE 36-5.** Nasoenteric tube feeding by continuous controlled pump. The head of the bed should be elevated to prevent aspiration.

continuous feedings. (This aspirated fluid is readministered to the patient.) In a recent systematic review of the literature, it was found that there was little correlation between residual volumes and tube feeding tolerance (Keithley & Swanson, 2004). Although a residual volume of 200 mL or greater is generally considered a cause for concern in patients at high risk for aspiration, feedings do not necessarily need to be withheld in all patients. Tube feedings may be continued with close monitoring of gastric residual volume, x-ray study results, and the patient's physical status. If excessive residual volumes (eg, more than 200 mL) occur twice, the nurse notifies the physician.

Maintaining tube function is an ongoing responsibility of the nurse, patient, or primary caregiver. To ensure patency and to decrease the chance of bacterial growth, crusting, or occlusion of the tube, at least 30 to 50 mL of water or normal saline is administered in each of the following instances:

- Before and after each dose of medication and each tube feeding
- After checking for gastric residuals and gastric pH
- Every 4 to 6 hours with continuous feedings
- If the tube feeding is discontinued or interrupted for any reason
- When the tube is not being used, twice-daily administration is recommended.

Any water or normal saline used to irrigate these tubes must be recorded as fluid intake. One study has shown that tap water may injure the small bowel and supports the practice of flushing postpyloric nasoduodenal or jejunostomy tubes with normal saline (Schloerb, Wood, Casillan, et al., 2004).

### Providing Medications By Tube

When different types of medications are administered, each type is given separately, using a bolus method that is compatible with the medication's preparation (Table 36-4). The tube is flushed with 30 to 50 mL of water after each dose, and this fluid is recorded as intake. If a liquid form of a medication is not available

**TABLE 36-4  Preparing Medication for Delivery by Feeding Tube**

| Medication Form | Preparation |
| --- | --- |
| Liquid | None |
| Simple compressed tablets | Crush and dissolve in water |
| Buccal or sublingual tablets | Administer as prescribed |
| Soft gelatin capsules filled with liquid | Make an opening in capsule and squeeze out contents |
| Enteric-coated tablets | Do not crush; change in form is required |
| Timed-release tablets | Do not crush tablets because doing so may release too much drug too quickly (overdose); check with pharmacist for alternative formulation |
| Timed-release capsules or sustained-release capsules | Some can be opened and contents added to tube-feeding formula; *always* check with pharmacist before doing this |

and the medication can be crushed, it must first be reduced to a fine powder or the tube will become clogged. Devices are available that crush and dissolve tablets with water (Fig. 36-6). Medications are not mixed with each other or with the feeding formula. When small-bore feeding tubes for continuous infusion are irrigated after medication administration, a 30-mL or larger syringe is used, because the pressure generated by smaller syringes could rupture the tube. Administering medications through postpyloric enteric tubes may adversely affect their absorption; therefore, this should be avoided if possible.

### Maintaining Feeding Regimens and Delivery Systems

Tube feeding formula is delivered to patients by either an open or a closed system. The open system comes as a liquid or as a powder and may be mixed with water. The feeding container (which is hung on a pole) and the tubing used with the open system are changed—usually every 24 to 72 hours. To avoid bacterial contamination, the amount of feeding formula in the bag should never exceed what should be infused in a 4-hour period.

Closed delivery systems use a prefilled, sterile container that is spiked with enteral tubing. The bag holding the feeding formula for the closed system can be hung safely for 24 to 48 hours.

The tube feeding regimen must be assessed frequently to evaluate its effectiveness and avoid complications (Chart 36-1).

### Maintaining Normal Bowel Elimination Pattern

Patients receiving NG or nasoenteric tube feedings commonly have diarrhea (watery stools occurring

> **CHART 36-1**
>
> ### Assessing for Tube Feeding Regimens
>
> - Assess tube placement, patient's position (head of bed elevated 30 to 45 degrees), and formula flow rate.
> - Determine the patient's ability to tolerate the formula. Observe for fullness, bloating, distention, urticaria, nausea, vomiting, and stool pattern and character.
> - Check clinical responses, as noted in laboratory findings (blood urea nitrogen, serum protein, prealbumin, electrolytes, renal function, hemoglobin, hematocrit).
> - Observe for signs of dehydration (dry mucous membranes, thirst, decreased urine output).
> - Record the amount of formula actually taken in by the patient.
> - Report an elevated blood glucose level, decreased urinary output, sudden weight gain, and periorbital or dependent edema.
> - Replace any formula administered by an open system every 4 hours with fresh formula. Formula should be at room temperature or cool (not cold).
> - Change tube feeding container and tubing every 24 to 72 hours.
> - Assess residual volume before each feeding or, in the case of continuous feedings, every 4 hours. Return the aspirate to the stomach.
> - Monitor intake and output.
> - Weigh the patient twice weekly.
> - Consult the dietitian regularly.

three or more times in 24 hours). Pasty, unformed stool is expected with enteral therapy, because many formulas have little or no residue. The dumping syndrome also leads to diarrhea; however, to confirm dumping syndrome as the cause of diarrhea, other possible causes must be excluded, such as:

- Contaminated formula
- Malnutrition—A decrease in the intestinal absorptive area resulting from malnutrition can cause diarrhea
- Medication therapy—Antibiotics, such as clindamycin (Cleocin); antiarrhythmics, such as quinidine (Quinaglute) and propranolol (Inderal); and aminophylline (Phyllocontin), theophylline (Theobid), and digitalis (digoxin [Lanoxin]) have been found to increase the frequency of diarrhea in some patients. Elixir-based medications often contain sorbitol, which can act as a cathartic (Dickerson et al., 2003).

**FIGURE 36-6.** The Pill Crusher™ Syringe (from Welcon, Inc.) crushes medications to a fine powder and then allows them to be administered to patients with feeding tubes. The Pill Crusher™ is also used to irrigate the feeding tube and assists in hydrating the patient. Courtesy of Welcon, Inc., Fort Worth, TX (www.welcon.com).

- *Clostridium difficile* colitis infection—This infection can result in significant diarrhea, especially in hospitalized patients (Carroll, 2003).

The dumping syndrome results from rapid distention of the jejunum when hypertonic solutions are administered rapidly (over 10 to 20 minutes). Foods high in carbohydrates and electrolytes draw extracellular fluid from the vascular system into the jejunum so that dilution and absorption can occur. Measures for managing the GI symptoms (diarrhea, nausea) associated with the dumping syndrome are presented in Chart 36-2.

### Reducing the Risk for Aspiration

Aspiration pneumonia occurs when stomach contents or enteral feedings are regurgitated and aspirated, or when an NG tube is improperly positioned and feedings are instilled into the pharynx or the trachea. Feeding patients through nasoenteric tubes placed beyond the pylorus has helped decrease the frequency of regurgitation and aspiration.

**To prevent aspiration, the nurse must verify the correct tube placement before every feeding, each time medications are administered, and once every shift if the tube feeding is continuous.**

Feedings and medications should always be administered with the patient in the proper position to prevent regurgitation. The semi-Fowler's position is necessary for an NG feeding, with the patient's head elevated at least 30 to 45 degrees to reduce the risk for reflux and pulmonary aspiration. This position is maintained at least 1 hour after completion of an intermittent tube feeding and is maintained at all times for patients receiving continuous tube feedings. Another prevention strategy is to monitor the residual volume and notify the physician and stop the feedings if the residual volume is excessive, as discussed previously.

**If aspiration is suspected, the feeding is stopped immediately, the pharynx and trachea are suctioned, and the patient is placed on the right side with the head of the bed down. The physician is notified immediately.**

### Maintaining Adequate Hydration

The nurse carefully monitors hydration because in many cases the patient cannot communicate the need for water. Water is given every 4 to 6 hours and after feedings to prevent hypertonic dehydration. At the beginning of administration, the feeding is given in continuous drip administration. This gradual administration allows assessment of residual volume and helps the patient develop tolerance, especially for hyperosmolar solutions. Key nursing interventions include observing for signs of dehydration (eg, dry mucous membranes, thirst, decreased urine output); administering water routinely and as needed; and monitoring intake, output, residual volume, and fluid balance (24-hour intake versus output).

### Promoting Coping Ability

The psychosocial goal of nursing care is to support and encourage the patient to accept physical changes and to convey hope that daily progressive improvement is possible. If the patient is having difficulty adjusting to the treatment, the nurse intervenes by encouraging self-care (eg, recording daily weight and intake and output), within the parameters of the patient's activity level. In addition, the nurse reinforces an optimistic approach by identifying indicators of progress (daily weight trends, electrolyte balance, absence of nausea and diarrhea).

### Promoting Home and Community-Based Care

#### TEACHING PATIENTS SELF-CARE

Patients who require long-term tube feedings in the home care setting have conditions such as obstruction of the upper GI tract, malabsorption syndrome, surgery of the GI tract or of the head or neck region, or decreased level of consciousness. For a patient to be considered for tube feeding at home, the following

---

**CHART 36-2**

## Preventing Symptoms of Dumping Syndrome

The following strategies may help prevent some of the uncomfortable symptoms of dumping syndrome related to tube feeding:

- Slow the formula instillation rate to provide time for carbohydrates and electrolytes to be diluted.
- Administer feedings at room temperature, because temperature extremes stimulate peristalsis.
- Administer feeding by continuous drip (if tolerated) rather than by bolus, to prevent sudden distention of the intestine.
- Advise the patient to remain in semi-Fowler's position for 1 hour after the feeding; this position prolongs intestinal transit time by decreasing the effect of gravity.
- Instill the minimal amount of water needed to flush the tubing before and after a feeding, because fluid given with a feeding increases intestinal transit time.

criteria should be met (Ireton-Jones, DeLegge, Epperson, et al., 2003):

- The patient should be medically stable and should have successfully completed a tube feeding trial (tolerated 70% of feeding).
- The patient must be capable of self-care or have a caregiver willing to assume the responsibility.
- The patient or caregiver must have access to supplies and interest in learning how to administer tube feedings at home.

Preparation of the patient for home administration of enteral feedings begins while the patient is still hospitalized. Ideally, the nurse teaches while administering the feedings so that the patient and/or caregiver can observe the mechanics of the procedure, participate in the procedure, ask questions, and express any concerns. Before discharge, the nurse provides information about the equipment needed, formula purchase and storage, and administration of the feedings (frequency, quantity, rate of instillation).

Family members who will be active in the patient's home care are encouraged to participate in all teaching sessions. Available printed information about the equipment, the formula, and the procedure is reviewed. The nurse encourages the patient and caregiver to learn the basic process with the supervision of the nurse. Arrangements are made for the caregiver to obtain the equipment and formula and have it ready for use before the patient's discharge.

**CONTINUING CARE**

Referral to a home care agency is important so that a nurse can supervise and provide support during the first feeding at home. Additional visits will depend on the skill and comfort of the patient or caregiver in administering the feedings. During all visits, the nurse monitors the patient's physical status (weight, vital signs, activity level) and the ability of the patient and family to administer the tube feedings correctly. In addition, the nurse assesses for any complications (dumping syndrome, nausea or vomiting, weight loss, lethargy, confusion, excessive thirst). The patient or caregiver is encouraged to keep a diary to record times and amounts of feedings and any symptoms that occur. The nurse can review the diary with the patient and caregiver during home visits.

## Evaluation

### Expected Patient Outcomes

Expected patient outcomes may include:

1. Attains or maintains nutritional balance
    a. Has a positive nitrogen balance
    b. Maintains laboratory values within normal limits (ie, blood urea nitrogen, hemoglobin, hematocrit, prealbumin, serum protein)
    c. Attains or maintains hydration of body tissue
    d. Attains or maintains desired body weight
2. Is free of episodes of diarrhea
    a. Has fewer than three watery stools a day
    b. Does not have a bowel movement after a bolus feeding
    c. Reports no intestinal cramping
    d. Has normal bowel sounds
3. Avoids aspiration
    a. Lungs are clear to auscultation
    b. Exhibits normal heart rate and respiratory rate
4. Attains or maintains hydration of body tissue
    a. Has a balanced fluid intake and output every 24 hours
    b. Does not have dry skin or dry mucous membranes
5. Copes effectively with tube feeding regimen
6. Demonstrates skill in managing tube feeding regimen
7. Experiences no complications
    a. Has no GI disturbances
    b. Tube remains intact and patent for duration of therapy
    c. Maintains metabolic balance within normal limits

# Gastrostomy

A **gastrostomy** is a surgical procedure in which an opening is created into the stomach for the purpose of administering foods and fluids via a feeding tube. In some instances, a gastrostomy is preferred for prolonged enteral nutrition support (longer than 4 weeks) (Roche, 2003). Gastrostomy is also preferred over NG feedings in the patient who is comatose because the gastroesophageal sphincter remains intact. Regurgitation and aspiration are less likely to occur with a gastrostomy than with NG feedings.

Different types of feeding gastrostomies may be used, including the Stamm (temporary and permanent), Janeway (permanent), and percutaneous endoscopic gastrostomy (temporary) systems. The Stamm and Janeway gastrostomies require either an upper abdominal midline incision or a left upper quadrant transverse incision. The Stamm procedure requires the use of concentric purse-string sutures to secure the tube to the anterior gastric wall. To create the gastrostomy, an exit wound is created in the left upper abdomen. The Janeway procedure necessitates the creation of a tunnel (called a gastric tube) that is brought out through the abdomen to form a permanent **stoma**.

Insertion of a **percutaneous endoscopic gastrostomy (PEG)** requires the services of two physicians (or a physician and a nurse with specialty skills). After administering a local anesthetic, one physician inserts a cannula into the stomach through an abdominal incision and then threads a nonabsorbable suture through the cannula; the second physician inserts an endoscope via the patient's upper GI tract and uses the endoscopic snare to grasp the end of the suture and guide it up through the patient's mouth. The suture is knotted to the dilator tip at the end of the PEG tube. The endoscopist then advances the dilator tip through the patient's mouth while the first physician pulls the suture through the cannula site. The attached PEG tube is guided down the esophagus, into the stomach, and out through the abdominal in-

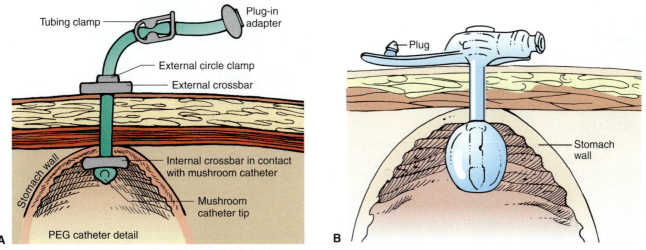

**FIGURE 36-7.** (**A**) A detail of the abdomen and the percutaneous endoscopic gastrostomy (PEG) tube, showing catheter fixation. (**B**) A detail of the abdomen and the nonobturated low-profile gastrostomy device (LPGD), showing balloon fixation.

cision (Fig. 36-7A). The mushroom catheter tip and internal crossbar secure the tube against the stomach wall. An external crossbar or bumper keeps the catheter in place. A tubing adaptor is in place between feedings, and a clamp or plug is used to close or open the tubing. If an endoscope cannot be passed through the esophagus, then the gastrostomy can be performed under x-ray guidance through the abdominal wall (Neef, Crowder, McIvor, et al., 2003).

The initial PEG device can be removed and replaced once the tract is well established (10 to 14 days after insertion). Replacement of the PEG device is indicated to provide long-term nutritional support, to replace a clogged or migrated tube, or to enhance patient comfort. The PEG replacement device should be fitted securely to the stoma to prevent leakage of gastric acid and is maintained in place through traction between the internal and anchoring devices.

An alternative to the PEG device is a **low-profile gastrostomy device (LPGD)** (see Fig. 36-7B). The LPGD may be inserted 3 to 6 months after initial gastrostomy tube placement. These devices are inserted flush with the skin; they eliminate the possibility of tube migration and obstruction and have antireflux valves to prevent gastric reflux. Two types of devices may be used—obturated or nonobturated. The obturated devices (G-button) have a dome tip that acts as an internal stabilizer. Only a physician may obturate (insert a tube that is larger than the actual stoma). The nonobturated device (MIC KEY) has an external skin disk and is inserted into the stoma without force; a balloon is inflated to secure placement. A nurse in the home setting may insert these nonobturated devices. The drawbacks of both types of LPGDs are the inability to assess residual volumes (one-way valve) and the need for a special adaptor to connect the device to the feeding container.

Reflux from stomach feedings can result in aspiration pneumonia. Therefore, patients at risk for aspiration pneumonia are not ideal candidates for a gastrostomy. A jejunostomy is preferred, or jejunal feeding through a nasojejunal tube may be recommended.

## Nursing Process

### The Patient With a Gastrostomy

#### Assessment

The focus of the preoperative assessment is to determine the patient's ability both to understand and cope with the impending surgical experience. The nurse assesses the patient's ability to adjust to a change in body image and to participate in self-care, along with the patient's and the family's psychological status. There are multiple medical and ethical issues that the patient, the caregivers, and the physician should discuss together (Angus & Burakoff, 2003) (Chart 36-3).

The purpose of the operative procedure is explained so that the patient has a better understanding of the expected postoperative course. The patient needs to know that the purpose of the procedure is to bypass the mouth and esophagus so that liquid feedings can be administered directly into the stomach by means of a rubber or plastic tube or a prosthesis. If the prosthesis is to be permanent, the patient should be made aware of this. Psychologically, this is often difficult for the patient to accept. If the procedure is being performed to relieve discomfort, prolonged vomiting, debilitation, or an inability to eat, the patient may find it more acceptable.

The nurse evaluates the patient's skin condition and determines whether a delay in healing at the tube insertion site may be anticipated because of a systemic disorder (eg, diabetes mellitus, ascites, cancer).

In the postoperative period, the patient's fluid and nutritional needs are assessed to ensure proper intake of food and fluids. The nurse inspects the tube for proper maintenance and the incision for signs of infection. At the same time, the nurse evaluates the patient's response to the change in body image and his

## CHART 36-3

### Ethics and Related Issues

### Is It Ethical to Withhold or Withdraw Nutrition and Hydration?

**SITUATION**

It is generally agreed that patients (or their designated decision makers) can refuse life-saving treatment, particularly if the means of treatment are extraordinary (eg, ventilators, dialysis machines, extracorporeal oxygenators). Extraordinary means include medications, treatments, and procedures that can be obtained only at excessive cost, pain, or inconvenience and offer no reasonable hope of benefit. Nutrition and hydration therapy, however, are perceived as ordinary means by many.

Ordinary means are those medications, treatments, and procedures that offer a reasonable hope of benefit and can be obtained without excessive expense, pain, or inconvenience. Additionally, withdrawing or withholding nutrition and hydration can in and of itself cause death. Thus, some have argued that nutrition and hydration should always be provided to every patient, regardless of the patient's preference or condition.

**DILEMMA**

The patient's desire to have nutrition or hydration withdrawn or withheld may conflict with the reluctance of others to harm the patient by withdrawing the food and water needed for survival (autonomy versus nonmaleficence).

**DISCUSSION**

Answer the following questions using as an example a patient in a persistent vegetative state (ie, unable to express his or her wishes).

- What arguments would you offer *against* the withholding and withdrawing of nutrition and hydration?
- What arguments would you offer *in favor of* withholding and withdrawing of nutrition and hydration?
- Are foods and fluids always "ordinary means," or are there instances in which they might be considered "extraordinary"? Support your answer.
- What are some of the religious, cultural, and financial issues that can complicate family and caregiver decisions?
- Should an attempt be made to involve critically ill or sedated patients in their own end-of-life decisions when their death is clearly imminent? How does one balance the issues of patient autonomy versus beneficence in this situation?

---

or her understanding of the feeding methods. Interventions are identified to help the patient cope with the tube and learn self-care measures.

## Diagnosis

### Nursing Diagnoses

Based on the assessment data, the major nursing diagnoses in the postoperative period may include the following:

- Imbalanced nutrition, less than body requirements, related to enteral feeding problems
- Risk for infection related to presence of wound and tube
- Risk for impaired skin integrity at tube insertion site
- Ineffective coping related to inability to eat normally
- Disturbed body image related to presence of tube
- Risk for ineffective therapeutic regimen management related to knowledge deficit about home care and the feeding procedure

### Collaborative Problems/ Potential Complications

Potential complications that may develop include the following (Roche, 2003):

- Wound infection, cellulitis, leakage, and abdominal wall abscess
- GI bleeding
- Premature removal of the tube
- Aspiration
- Constipation or diarrhea

## Planning and Goals

The major goals for the patient may include attaining an optimal level of nutrition, preventing infection, maintaining skin integrity, enhancing coping, adjusting to changes in body image, acquiring knowledge of and skill in self-care, and preventing complications.

## Nursing Interventions

### Meeting Nutritional Needs

The first fluid nourishment is administered soon after surgery and usually consists of tap water and 10% dextrose. At first, only 30 to 60 mL (1 to 2 oz) is given at one time, but the amount administered is increased gradually. By the second day, 180 to 240 mL (6 to 8 oz) may be given at one time, provided it is tolerated and no leakage of fluid occurs around the tube. Water and enteral feeding can be infused after 24 hours for a permanent gastrostomy.

Blenderized foods can be added gradually to clear liquids until a full diet is achieved. Powdered feedings that are easily liquefied are commercially available. The patient who receives blenderized tube feedings typically is not forced to give up usual dietary patterns, which may prove to be psychologically more acceptable. In addition, near-normal bowel function is promoted because the fiber and residue are similar to those of a normal diet.

### Providing Tube Care and Preventing Infection

A small dressing can be applied over the tube insertion site, and the gastrostomy tube can be held in place by a thin strip of adhesive tape that is first placed around the tube and then firmly attached to the abdomen. The dressing protects the skin around the incision from seepage of gastric acid and spillage of feedings (Fig. 36-8).

The nurse verifies the tube's placement, assesses residuals, and gently manipulates the tube or stabilizing disk once daily to prevent skin breakdown. Some gastrostomy tubes have balloons that are inflated with water to anchor the tube in the stomach. Balloon integrity is checked weekly by deflating and reinflating the balloon using a Luer-tip syringe.

### Providing Skin Care

The skin surrounding a gastrostomy requires special care because it may become irritated from the enzymatic action of gastric juices that leak around the tube. Left untreated, the skin becomes macerated, red, raw, and painful. The nurse washes the area around the tube with soap and water daily, removes any encrustation with saline solution, rinses the area well with water, and pats it dry. A long-term gastrostomy may require a special dressing or stabilization device to protect the skin around the tube from gastric secretions and to help secure the tube in place (see Fig. 36-8).

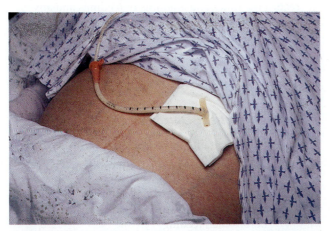

**FIGURE 36-8.** Protection at the gastrostomy site. A PEG tube may be protected by a dressing that allows access to the tube but covers the exit site. Typically, the tube is stabilized with tape over the dressing. From Craven, R., & Hirnle, C. (2006). *Fundamentals of nursing: Human health and function* (5th ed.). Philadelphia: Lippincott Williams & Wilkins.

Skin at the exit site is evaluated daily for signs of breakdown, irritation, excoriation, and the presence of drainage or gastric leakage. The nurse encourages the patient and family members to participate in this evaluation and in hygiene activities. If skin problems do occur, an enterostomal therapist or wound ostomy continence nurse can be of assistance.

### Enhancing Body Image

The patient with a gastrostomy has experienced a major assault to body image. Eating, a physiologic and social function, can no longer be taken for granted. The patient is also aware that gastrostomy as a therapeutic intervention is performed only in the presence of a major, chronic, or perhaps terminal illness.

Calm discussion of the purposes and routines of gastrostomy feeding can help keep the patient from feeling overwhelmed. Talking with a person who has had a gastrostomy can also help the patient accept the expected changes. Adjusting to a change in body image takes time and requires family support and acceptance. Evaluating the existing family support system is necessary.

### Monitoring and Managing Potential Complications

During the postoperative course, the nurse monitors the patient for potential complications. The most common complications are wound infection and other wound problems, including cellulitis at the exit site and abscesses in the abdominal wall. Because many patients who receive tube feedings are debilitated and have compromised nutritional status, any signs of infection are promptly reported to the physician so that appropriate therapy can be instituted.

Bleeding from the insertion site in the stomach may also occur. The nurse closely monitors the patient's vital signs and observes all drainage from the operative site, vomitus, and stool for evidence of bleeding. Any signs of bleeding are reported promptly.

Premature removal of the tube, whether it is done inadvertently by the patient or by the caregiver, is another complication. If the tube is removed prematurely, the skin is cleansed and a sterile dressing is applied; the nurse immediately notifies the physician. The tract will close within 4 to 6 hours if the tube is not replaced promptly.

### Promoting Home and Community-Based Care

#### TEACHING PATIENTS SELF-CARE
The patient who is to receive gastrostomy tube feedings in the home setting must be capable of, and responsible for, administering the tube feedings or have a caregiver who can do so. There must also be the physical, financial, and social resources to maintain care.

The nurse assesses the patient's level of knowledge, interest in learning about the tube feeding, and ability to understand and apply the information before providing detailed instructions about how to prepare the formula and manage the tube feeding. Written materials for patients and caregivers are designed to outline the care instructions. To facilitate self-care, the nurse encourages the patient to participate in the tube feedings during hospitalization and to establish as normal a routine as possible.

Demonstration of the tube feeding begins by showing the patient how to check for residual gastric contents before the feeding. The patient then learns how to check and maintain the patency of the tube by administering room-temperature water before and after the feeding. This establishes patency before the feeding and then clears the tube of food particles, which could decompose if allowed to remain in the tube. All feedings are given at room temperature or near body temperature.

For a bolus feeding, the nurse shows the patient how to introduce the liquid into the catheter by using a funnel or the barrel of a syringe. The receptacle is tilted to allow air to escape while the liquid is being instilled initially. As the funnel or syringe fills with liquid, the feeding is allowed to flow into the stomach by gravity by holding the barrel or syringe perpendicular to the abdomen (Fig. 36-9). Raising or lowering the receptacle to no higher than 45 cm (18 in) above the abdominal wall regulates the rate of flow.

A bolus feeding of 300 to 500 mL usually is given for each meal and requires 10 to 15 minutes to complete. The amount is often determined by the patient's reaction. If the patient feels full, it may be desirable to give smaller amounts more frequently.

The patient and caregiver must understand that keeping the head of the bed elevated a minimum of 45 degrees for at least 1 hour after feeding facilitates digestion and decreases the risk of aspiration. Any obstruction requires that the feeding be stopped and the physician notified.

The patient or caregiver is instructed to flush the tube with 30 to 50 mL of water after each bolus or medication administration and to also flush the tube daily to keep it patent. Adaptors are available that can be secured to the end of the tube to create a "Y" site for ease of flushing or medication delivery. The flushing equipment is cleaned with warm, soapy water and rinsed after each use.

The patient and caregiver are made aware that the tube is marked at skin level to provide the patient with a baseline for later comparison. They are advised to monitor the tube's length and to notify the physician or home care nurse if the segment of the tube outside the body becomes shorter or longer.

If the patient is to use an intermittent or continuous-pressure feeding pump at home, instruction in the use of the particular type of pump is essential. Most feeding pumps have built-in alarms that signal when the bag is empty, when the battery is low, or when the tube is occluded. The patient and caregiver need to be aware of these alarms and how to troubleshoot the pump.

### CONTINUING CARE

Referral to a home care agency is important to ensure initial supervision and support for the patient and caregiver. The home care nurse assesses the patient's status and progress and evaluates the techniques used in administering the tube feeding. Further instruction and supervision in the home setting may be required to help the patient and caregiver adapt to a physical environment and equipment that are different from the hospital setting. The nurse also reviews with the patient and caregiver complications to report (eg, dumping syndrome, nausea and vomiting, infection of the skin at the insertion site of the tube).

The home care nurse assists the patient and family in establishing as normal a routine as possible. The patient or caregiver is encouraged to keep a diary to record the times and amounts of feedings and any symptoms that occur. The nurse reviews the diary during home visits. In addition, the patient or caregiver must be taught how to replace the tube.

## Evaluation

### Expected Patient Outcomes

Expected patient outcomes may include the following:

1. Achieves an adequate intake of nutrients
   a. Tolerates quantity and frequency of tube feedings
   b. Has 100 mL or less of residual gastric content before each feeding
   c. Has no diarrhea
   d. Maintains or gains weight
   e. Has normal electrolyte values
2. Is free from infection and skin breakdown
   a. Is afebrile
   b. Has no drainage from the incision

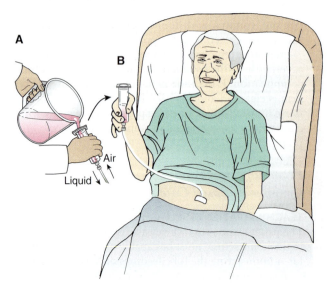

**FIGURE 36-9.** Bolus gastrostomy feeding by gravity. **(A)** Feeding is instilled at an angle so that air does not enter the stomach. **(B)** Syringe is raised perpendicular to the abdomen so that feeding can enter by gravity.

    c. Demonstrates intact skin surrounding the exit site
    d. Inspects exit site daily
 3. Adjusts to change in body image
    a. Is able to discuss expected changes
    b. Verbalizes concerns
 4. Demonstrates skill in managing feeding regimen
    a. Helps prepare prescribed formula or blenderized feeding
    b. Handles equipment competently
    c. Helps administer the feeding or does so independently
    d. Demonstrates how to maintain tube patency
    e. Cleans tubing as needed
    f. Keeps an accurate record of intake
    g. If indicated, can remove and reinsert the tube as appropriate and needed for feedings
 5. Avoids complications
    a. Exhibits adequate wound healing
    b. Has no abnormal bleeding from puncture site
    c. Tube remains intact for the duration of therapy

# Parenteral Nutrition

**Parenteral nutrition** (PN) is a method of providing nutrients to the body by an IV route. The nutrients are a very complex admixture containing proteins, carbohydrates, fats, electrolytes, vitamins, trace minerals, and sterile water in a single container. The goals of PN are to improve nutritional status, establish a positive nitrogen balance, maintain muscle mass, promote weight maintenance or gain, and enhance the healing process.

## Establishing Positive Nitrogen Balance

When a patient's intake of protein and nutrients is significantly less than that required by the body to meet energy expenditures, a state of negative nitrogen balance results. In response, the body begins to convert the protein found in muscles into carbohydrates to be used to meet energy needs. The result is muscle wasting, weight loss, fatigue, and, if left uncorrected, death. The goal for patients receiving nutrition support is to achieve positive nitrogen balance (Huckleberry, 2004).

The average postoperative adult patient requires approximately 1500 calories per day to keep the body from using its own store of protein. Traditional IV fluids do not provide sufficient calories or nitrogen to meet the body's daily requirements. PN solutions, which supply nutrients such as dextrose, amino acids, electrolytes, vitamins, minerals, and fat emulsions, provide enough calories and nitrogen to meet the patient's daily nutritional needs. In general, PN usually provides 25 to 35 kcal/kg of ideal body weight and 1.0 to 1.5 g of protein/kg of ideal body weight.

The patient with fever, trauma, burns, major surgery, or hypermetabolic disease requires additional daily calories. The volume of fluid necessary to provide these calories would surpass fluid tolerance and lead to pulmonary edema or heart failure. To provide the required calories in a small volume, it is necessary to increase the concentration of nutrients and use a route of administration (ie, a large, high-flow vein such as the subclavian) that rapidly dilutes incoming nutrients to the proper levels of body tolerance.

When highly concentrated dextrose is administered, caloric requirements are satisfied and the body uses amino acids for protein synthesis rather than for energy. Additional potassium is added to the solution to maintain proper electrolyte balance and to transport glucose and amino acids across cell membranes. To prevent deficiencies and fulfill requirements for tissue synthesis, other elements, such as calcium, phosphorus, magnesium, and sodium chloride, are added.

## Clinical Indications

The indications for PN include a 10% deficit in body weight (compared with pre-illness weight), an inability to take oral food or fluids within 7 days after surgery, and hypercatabolic situations such as major infection with fever. Enteral nutrition should be considered before parenteral support since it assists in maintaining gut mucosal integrity (Huckleberry, 2004). In both the home and hospital setting, PN is indicated in the following situations:

- The patient's intake is insufficient to maintain an anabolic state (eg, severe burns, malnutrition, short bowel syndrome, acquired immunodeficiency syndrome [AIDS], sepsis, cancer).
- The patient's ability to ingest food orally or by tube is impaired (eg, paralytic ileus, Crohn's disease with obstruction, post-radiation enteritis, severe hyperemesis gravidarum in pregnancy).
- The patient is unwilling or unable to ingest adequate nutrients (eg, anorexia nervosa, postoperative elderly patients).
- The underlying medical condition precludes being fed orally or by tube (eg, acute pancreatitis, high enterocutaneous fistula).
- Preoperative and postoperative nutritional needs are prolonged (eg, extensive bowel surgery).

## Formulas

A total of 2 to 3 L of solution is administered over a 24-hour period using a filter (1.2-micron particulate filter). Before administration, the PN infusion must be inspected for clarity and any precipitate. The label is compared with the physician's order, noting the expiration date. **Intravenous fat emulsions** (IVFEs, Intralipids) may be infused simultaneously with PN through a Y-connector close to the infusion site and should not be filtered. Before administration, the IVFE is inspected for frothiness, separation, or oily appearance. If any of these are present, the solution is not used. Usually 500 mL of a 10% emulsion or 250 mL of 20% emulsion is administered over 6 to 12 hours, one to three times a week. IVFEs can provide up to 30% of the total daily calorie intake.

IVFEs can be admixed with other components of PN to create a "three-in-one formulation" commonly called a **total nutrient admixture** (TNA). All the parenteral nutrient components are mixed in one container and administered to the patient over a 24-hour period. A special final filter (1.5-micron filter) is used with this solution. Before administration, the solution is observed for oil droplets that have separated from the solution, forming a noticeable layer ("cracking of lipid emulsion"); such a solution should be discarded. Advantages of the TNA over PN are cost savings in preparation and equipment, decreased risk of catheter or nutrient contamination, decreased pharmacy preparation time, less nursing time, and increased patient convenience and satisfaction. Ideally, the pharmacist, nutritionist, and physician collaborate to determine the specific formula needed.

## Initiating Therapy

PN solutions are initiated slowly and advanced gradually each day to the desired rate as the patient's fluid and glucose tolerance permits. The patient's laboratory test results and response to PN therapy are monitored on an ongoing basis by the physician and licensed nutrition provider. Standing orders are initiated for weighing the patient; monitoring intake, output, and blood glucose; and baseline and periodic monitoring of complete blood count, platelet count, and chemistry panel, including serum carbon dioxide, magnesium, phosphorus, triglycerides, and prealbumin. A 24-hour urine nitrogen determination may be performed for analysis of nitrogen balance. In most hospitals, the physician prescribes PN solutions on a daily standard PN order form. The formulation of the PN solutions is calculated carefully each day to meet the complete nutritional needs of the individual patient.

## Administration Methods

Various vascular access devices are used to administer PN solutions in clinical practice. PN may be administered through either peripheral or central IV lines, depending on the patient's condition and the anticipated length of therapy.

### Peripheral Method

To supplement oral intake when complete bowel rest is not indicated and NG or nasoenteric suction is not required, a peripheral parenteral nutrition (PPN) formula may be prescribed. PPN is administered through a peripheral vein; this is possible because the solution is less hypertonic than PN solution. PPN formulas are not nutritionally complete: there is typically less dextrose content. Dextrose concentrations of more than 10% should not be administered through peripheral veins because they irritate the intima (innermost walls) of small veins, causing chemical phlebitis. Lipids are administered simultaneously to buffer the PPN and to protect the peripheral vein from irritation. The usual length of therapy using PPN is 5 to 7 days (Correia, Guimaraes, de Mattos, et al., 2004).

### Central Method

Because PN solutions have five or six times the solute concentration of blood (and exert an osmotic pressure of about 2000 mOsm/L), they are injurious to the intima of peripheral veins. Therefore, to prevent phlebitis and other venous complications, these solutions are administered into the vascular system through a catheter inserted into a high-flow, large blood vessel (the subclavian vein). Concentrated solutions are then very rapidly diluted to isotonic levels by the blood in this vessel.

Four types of **central venous access devices (CVADs)** are available—nontunneled (or percutaneous) central catheters, peripherally inserted central catheters, tunneled catheters, and implanted ports. Whenever one of these catheters is inserted, catheter tip placement should be confirmed by x-ray studies before PN therapy is initiated. The optimal position is the midproximal third of the superior vena cava at the junction of the right atrium (see Chapter 16).

#### NONTUNNELED CENTRAL CATHETERS

Nontunneled central catheters are used for short-term (less than 6 weeks) IV therapy in acute care, long-term care, and home care settings. The physician inserts these catheters. Examples of nontunneled central catheters are Vas Cath, percutaneous subclavian Arrow, and Hohn catheters. The subclavian vein is the most common vessel used, because the subclavian area provides a stable insertion site to which the catheter can be anchored, allows the patient freedom of movement, and provides easy access to the dressing site. The jugular vein should only be used as a last resort and then only for 1 to 2 days. Single-, double-, and triple-lumen central catheters are available for central lines, but the Centers for Disease Control and Prevention (CDC) recommends that single-lumen catheters be used for TNA whenever practicable (CDC, 2002). To ensure accessibility in a patient with limited IV access, a triple-lumen subclavian catheter can be used, because it offers three ports for various uses (Fig. 36-10). The 16-gauge distal lumen can be used to infuse blood or other viscous fluids. The 18-gauge middle lumen is reserved for PN infusion. The 18-gauge proximal port can be used for administration of blood or medications. A port not being used for fluid administration can be used for obtaining blood specimens if indicated.

If a single-lumen central catheter is used for administering PN, various restrictions apply. Blood cannot be drawn from the catheter and transfusions of blood products cannot be given through the main line, because red blood cells may coat the lumen of the catheter, thereby reducing the flow of the nutritional solution. Medications also cannot be administered through it, because the medication may be incompatible with the components of the nutritional solution (insulin is an exception). If medications must be given, they must be infused through a separate peripheral IV line, not by piggyback into the PN line.

**Insertion.** The procedure is explained so that the patient understands the importance of not touching the catheter insertion site and is aware of what to expect during the insertion procedure. The patient is placed supine in the Trendelenburg position (to produce dilation of neck and shoulder vessels, which makes entry easier and prevents air embolus). The area is shaved if necessary, and the skin is prepared with acetone and alcohol to remove surface oils. Final skin preparation includes cleaning with tincture of 2% iodine or chlorhexidine. To afford maximal accuracy in the placement of the catheter, the patient is instructed to turn the head away from the site of venipuncture and to remain motionless while the catheter is inserted and the wound is dressed. The preferred insertion route is the subclavian vein,

**FIGURE 36-10.** Subclavian triple-lumen catheter used for parenteral nutrition and other adjunctive therapy. **(A)** The catheter is threaded through the subclavian vein into the vena cava. **(B)** Each lumen is an avenue for solution administration. The lumens are secured with threaded needleless adapters or Luer-Lok–type caps when the device is not in use.

which leads into the superior vena cava. The external jugular route can be used, but usually only in emergency situations. Because a nontunneled central catheter is always a potential source of serious infection, the insertion site should be changed every 4 to 6 weeks, or as recommended by the latest CDC guidelines.

Full-length sterile drapes are applied. Procaine or lidocaine is injected to anesthetize the skin and underlying tissues. The target area is the inferior border at the midpoint of the clavicle. A large-bore needle on a syringe is inserted and moved parallel to and beneath the clavicle until it enters the vein. The syringe is then detached and a radiopaque wire is inserted through the needle into the vein. The catheter is then advanced over the wire, the needle is withdrawn, and the hub of the catheter is attached to the IV tubing. Until the syringe is detached from the needle and the catheter is inserted, the patient may be asked to perform the Valsalva maneuver. (To do this, the patient is instructed to take a deep breath, hold it, and bear down with mouth closed. Compression of the abdomen may also accomplish the maneuver.) The Valsalva maneuver is performed to produce a positive phase in central venous pressure, thereby lessening the possibility of air being drawn into the circulatory system (air embolism). The physician sutures the catheter to the skin to avoid inadvertent removal.

The catheter insertion site is swabbed with either tincture of 2% iodine or a chlorhexidine solution. A gauze or transparent dressing is applied using strict sterile technique (CDC, 2002). An isotonic IV solution, such as dextrose 5% in water (D5W), is administered to keep the vein patent.

The position of the tip of the catheter is checked with x-ray or fluoroscopy to confirm its location in the superior vena cava and to rule out a pneumothorax resulting from inadvertent puncture of the pleura. Once the catheter's position is confirmed, the prescribed PN solution is started. The initial rate of infusion is usually 50 mL/hour, and the rate is gradually increased to the maintenance rate or predetermined dose (eg, 100 to 125 mL/hour). An infusion pump is always used for administration of PN.

An injection site cap is attached to the end of each central catheter lumen, creating a closed system. IV infusion tubing is connected to the insertion site cap of the central catheter with a threaded needleless adapter or Luer-Lok device. Each lumen is labeled according to location (proximal, middle, distal). To ensure patency, all lumens are flushed with a diluted heparin flush initially, daily when not in use, after each intermittent infusion, after blood drawing, and whenever an infusion is disconnected. Force is never used to flush the catheter. If resistance is met, aspiration may restore lumen patency; if this is not effective, the physician is notified. Low-dose tissue plasminogen activator (alteplase) may be prescribed to dissolve a clot or fibrin sheath. If attempts to clear the lumen are ineffective, the lumen is labeled as "clotted off" and not used again.

### PERIPHERALLY INSERTED CENTRAL CATHETERS

Peripherally inserted central catheters (PICCs) are used for intermediate-term (several days to months) IV therapy in the hospital, long-term care, or home setting. These catheters may be inserted at the bedside or in the outpatient setting by a specially trained nurse (Philpot & Griffiths, 2003). The basilic or cephalic vein is accessed through the antecubital space, and the catheter is threaded to a designated location, depending on the type of solution to be infused (superior vena cava for PN). Taking of blood pressure and blood specimens from the extremity with the PICC is avoided (see Chapter 14 and Chapter 16, Fig. 16-6).

### TUNNELED CENTRAL CATHETERS

Tunneled central catheters are for long-term use and may remain in place for many years. These catheters are cuffed and can have single or double lumens; examples are the Hickman, Groshong, and Permacath. These catheters are inserted surgically. They are threaded under the skin (reducing the risk of ascending infection) to the subclavian vein, and the distal end of the catheter is advanced into the superior vena cava.

### IMPLANTED PORTS

Implanted ports are also used for long-term home IV therapy; examples include the Port-A-Cath, Mediport, Hickman Port, and P.A.S. Port. Instead of exiting from the skin, as do the Hickman and Groshong catheters, the end of the catheter is attached to a small chamber that is placed in a subcutaneous pocket, either on the anterior chest wall or on the forearm. The subcutaneous port requires minimal care and allows the patient complete freedom of activity. Implanted ports are more expensive than the external catheters, and access requires passing a special non-coring needle (Huber-tipped) through the skin into the chamber to initiate IV therapy (see Chapter 16). Taking of blood pressure and blood specimens from the extremity with the port system should be avoided.

## Discontinuing Parenteral Nutrition

The PN solution is discontinued gradually to allow the patient to adjust to decreased levels of glucose. If the PN solution is abruptly terminated, isotonic dextrose is administered for 1 to 2 hours to protect against rebound hypoglycemia. Providing oral carbohydrates shortens the tapering time. Specific symptoms of rebound hypoglycemia include weakness, faintness, sweating, shakiness, feeling cold, confusion, and increased heart rate. Once all IV therapy is completed, the nurse (with a physician's order) removes the nontunneled central venous catheter or PICC and applies an occlusive dressing to the exit site. Tunneled catheters and implanted ports are removed only by the physician.

In cases of serious illness when death is imminent, some patients or families may request that PN be discontinued. This situation poses many ethical questions, some of which are discussed in Chart 36-3.

### ◀▼▶ Nursing Process

## The Patient Receiving Parenteral Nutrition

### Assessment

The nurse assists in identifying patients who may be candidates for PN. Indicators include any significant weight loss (10% or more of usual weight), a decrease in oral food intake for more than 1 week, any significant sign of protein loss (serum albumin levels less than 3.2 g/dL [32 g/L], muscle wasting, decreased tissue healing, or abnormal urea nitrogen excretion), and persistent vomiting and diarrhea. The nurse carefully monitors the patient's hydration status, electrolyte levels, and calorie intake.

## Diagnosis

### Nursing Diagnoses

Based on the assessment data, the major nursing diagnoses may include the following:

- Imbalanced nutrition, less than body requirements, related to inadequate oral intake of nutrients
- Risk for infection related to contamination of the central catheter site or infusion line
- Risk for excess or deficient fluid volume related to altered infusion rate
- Risk for immobility related to fear that the catheter will become dislodged or occluded
- Risk for ineffective therapeutic regimen management related to knowledge deficit about home PN therapy

### Collaborative Problems/ Potential Complications

The most common complications are pneumothorax, air embolism, a clotted or displaced catheter, sepsis, hyperglycemia, rebound hypoglycemia, and fluid overload. These problems and the associated collaborative interventions are described in Table 36-5.

## Planning and Goals

The major goals for the patient may include optimal level of nutrition, absence of infection, adequate fluid volume, optimal level of activity (within individual limitations), knowledge of and skill in self-care, and absence of complications.

## Nursing Interventions

### Maintaining Optimal Nutrition

A continuous, uniform infusion of PN solution over a 24-hour period is desired. However, in some cases (eg, home care patients), cyclic PN may be appropriate. With cyclic PN, there is a set time during a 24-hour period when PN is infused and a set time when it is not. The time periods for infusion are sufficient to meet the patient's nutritional and pharmacologic needs. Ideally, cyclic PN is infused over a 10- to 15-hour period during the night.

The patient is weighed daily (this may be decreased to two or three times per week) at the same time of the day under the same conditions for accurate comparison. Under the PN regimen (without additional energy expenditure), satisfactory weight maintenance

## TABLE 36-5　Complications of Parental Nutrition

| Complications | Cause | Nursing Actions and Collaborative Interventions | |
|---|---|---|---|
| | | Treatment | Prevention |
| Pneumothorax | Improper catheter placement and inadvertent puncture of the pleura | Place patient in Fowler's position. Offer reassurance. Monitor vital signs. Prepare for thoracentesis or chest tube insertion. | Assist patient to remain still in Trendelenburg position during catheter insertion. |
| Air embolism | Disconnected tubing | Replace tubing immediately and notify physician. | Tape all tubing connection sites securely. |
| | Cap missing from port | Replace cap and notify physician. | |
| | Blocked segment of vascular system | Turn patient on left side and place in the head-low position. Notify physician. | |
| Clotted catheter line | Inadequate/infrequent heparin flushes | On *rare* occasions, flush with thrombolytic declotting medication as prescribed. | Administer heparin flush in unused lines twice a day. |
| | Disruption of infusion | | Monitor infusion rate hourly and inspect the integrity of the line. |
| Catheter displacement and contamination | Excessive movement, possibly with a nonsecured catheter | Stop the infusion and notify the physician. | Tape all tubing connection sites. Avoid interrupting the main line or piggybacking other lines. |
| | Separation of tubing and contamination | | |
| Sepsis | Separation of dressings | Reinforce or change dressing quickly using aseptic technique. | Maintain sterile technique when changing tubing, dressing, or total nutrient admixture bag. |
| | Contaminated solution | Discard. Notify pharmacist. | |
| | Infection at insertion site of catheter | Notify physician. Monitor vital signs every 4 hours. | |
| Hyperglycemia | Glucose intolerance | Notify physician; addition of insulin to PN solution may be prescribed. | Monitor glucose levels (blood and urine). Monitor urine output. Observe for stupor, confusion, or lethargy. |
| Fluid overload | Fluid infusing rapidly | Decrease infusion rate. Monitor vital signs. Notify physician. Treat respiratory distress by sitting patient upright and administering oxygen as needed, if prescribed. | Use infusion pump. Verify correct infusion rate ordered. |
| Rebound hypoglycemia | Feedings stopped too abruptly | Monitor for symptoms (weakness, tremors, diaphoresis, headache, hunger, and apprehension); notify physician. | Gradually wean patient from PN. |

or gain is usually achieved. It is important to keep accurate intake and output records and calculations of fluid balance. A calorie count is kept of any oral nutrients. Trace elements (copper, zinc, chromium, manganese, and selenium) are included in PN solutions and are individualized for each patient. The PN solutions are prescribed daily by the physician on a standard PN order form based on laboratory results and patient tolerance.

### Preventing Infection

The high glucose content of PN solutions makes these solutions ideal culture media for bacterial and fungal growth, and CVADs provide a port of entry. Gram-negative cocci and gram-negative bacilli, including *Staphylococcus aureus*, *S. epidermidis*, and *Klebsiella pneumoniae*, are the most common infectious organisms (Alberti, Brun-Buisson, Burchardi, et al., 2002). Other infectious organisms can be fungal, including *Candida albicans*. Meticulous technique is essential to prevent infection.

The primary sources of microorganisms for catheter-related infections are the skin and the catheter hub. The catheter site is covered with an occlusive gauze dressing that is usually changed every other day. Alternatively, a transparent dressing may be used and changed weekly. The CDC (2002) recommends changing CVAD dressings only if they are damp, bloody, loose, or soiled. The dressings are changed using sterile technique. The nurse and patient wear masks during dressing changes to reduce the possibility of airborne contamination. The area is checked for leakage; bloody or purulent drainage; a kinked catheter; and skin reactions such as inflammation, redness, swelling, or tenderness. The nurse wears sterile gloves and cleanses the area with tincture of 2% iodine or a chlorhexidine solution on a sterile gauze. The site is cleaned thoroughly using a circular motion from the site outward to approximately 3 inches; this procedure is repeated two times. Then the same cleaning procedure is performed, using 2 × 2-inch gauze pads moistened with sterile water or saline solution (alcohol is used to remove iodine). Next the catheter ports are cleaned from the exit site to the distal end with an alcohol wipe. The insertion site is covered with an occlusive gauze pad or transparent dressing centered over the area.

The advantages of using a transparent dressing instead of a gauze pad are that it allows frequent examination of the catheter site without changing the dressing, it adheres well, and it is more comfortable for the patient. When an extension set is used with a central catheter, it is considered an extension of the catheter itself. It is not routinely changed with dressing or tubing changes. The connection (hub) between the catheter and extension tubing is secured with adhesive tape to prevent separation and exposure to air. Mainline IV tubing and filters are changed every 72 to 96 hours, and all connections are taped securely to avoid breaks in the integrity of the system (CDC, 2002). The dressing and tubing are labeled with the date, time of insertion, time of dressing change, and initials of the person who carried out the procedure; this information is also documented in the patient's medical record.

The catheter is another major source of colonization and infection. Studies have been conducted on the use of catheters with antiseptic coatings, antimicrobial coatings, and impregnated antimicrobial cuffs with varying conclusions (Bong, Kite, Wilco, et al., 2003). Prophylactic antibiotic therapy, antibiotic locks, use of antithrombolytics, various exit-site dressings, and the use of various disinfectants for cleansing catheter exit sites have also been proposed (Peterson, 2003).

### Maintaining Fluid Balance

An infusion pump is necessary for PN to maintain an accurate rate of administration. A designated rate is set in milliliters per hour, and the rate is checked every 3 to 4 hours. An alarm signals a problem. The infusion rate should not be increased or decreased to compensate for fluids that have infused too quickly or too slowly. If the solution runs out, 10% dextrose and water is infused until the next PN solution is available from the pharmacy.

If the rate is too rapid, hyperosmolar diuresis occurs. Excess glucose is excreted by the renal tubules, pulling large volumes of water into the tubules via osmosis, resulting in higher-than-normal urine output and intravascular fluid volume deficit. If the hyperosmolar diuresis is severe enough, it can cause dehydration of brain cells resulting in intractable seizures, coma, and death. Symptoms of rapid hypertonic fluid intake include headache, nausea, fever, chills, and increasing lethargy.

If the flow rate is too slow, the patient does not receive the maximal benefit of calories and nitrogen. Intake and output are recorded every 8 hours so that fluid imbalance can be readily detected. The patient is weighed two or three times a week; ideally, the patient shows neither weight loss nor significant weight gain. The nurse assesses for signs of dehydration (eg, thirst, decreased skin turgor, decreased central venous pressure) and reports these findings to the physician immediately. It is essential to monitor blood glucose levels, because hyperglycemia can cause diuresis and excessive fluid loss.

### Encouraging Activity

Activities and ambulation are encouraged when the patient is physically able. With a catheter in the subclavian vein, the patient is free to move the extremities, and activity should be encouraged to maintain good muscle tone. If applicable, the teaching and exercise program initiated in the occupational and physical therapy departments is reinforced.

### Promoting Home and Community-Based Care

#### TEACHING PATIENTS SELF-CARE

Successful home PN requires teaching the patient and family specialized skills using an intensive training program and follow-up supervision in the home. This is best accomplished through a team effort (Ireton-Jones et al., 2003). The financial costs of such programs, although high, are less than those incurred in a hospital. Initiation of a home program may be the only way the patient can be discharged from the hospital (Evans, Steinhart, Cohen, et al., 2003).

Ideal candidates for home PN are patients who have a reasonable life expectancy after return home, have a limited number of illnesses other than the one that has resulted in the need for PN, and are highly motivated and fairly self-sufficient. In addition, ability to learn, availability of family interest and support, adequate finances, and the physical plan of the home are factors that must be assessed when the decision about home PN is made (Chart 36-4).

Home health care agencies sponsoring home PN programs have developed teaching brochures and videos for every aspect of treatment, including catheter and dressing care, use of an infusion pump, administration of fat emulsions, and instillation of heparin flushes (Smith, Curtas, Kleinbeck, et al., 2003). Teaching begins in the hospital and continues in the home or in an ambulatory infusion center. If the patient or assisting family member has a disability (motor or sensory deficit, vision or hearing loss), alternate formats of educational materials are needed to ensure adequate preparation and self-management.

### CONTINUING CARE

The home care nurse should be aware that the typical patient needs several instruction sessions for assessment of learning and reinforcement. For more information about home patient education, see Charts 36-5 and 36-6. Special considerations for elderly patients who go home with nutrition support are presented in Chart 36-7.

---

**CHART 36-4**

## Discharge Planning: Home Assessment for Nutrition Support

The following aspects of the home setting must be assessed before making a decision that a patient can return home with parenteral nutrition:

- **Water:** necessary for hand washing and cleaning of work areas
- **Electricity:** reliable power source is needed to provide proper lighting and charging of pumps
- **Refrigeration:** must be adequate for accommodation of several bags of total nutrient admixture solution
- **Telephone:** necessary for contacting home health personnel, arranging for prompt delivery of supplies, and for emergency purposes
- **Environment:**
  - Should be free of rodents and insects
  - Should have storage that is not accessible to pets and small children
  - Should be assessed for stairs, carpets, and inaccessible areas, which can limit mobility with infusion pumps if the patient has a disability
  - Should be assessed for bathroom access

Adapted from Ireton-Jones, C., DeLegge, M., Epperson, L., et al. (2003). Management of the home parenteral nutrition patient. *Nutrition in Clinical Practice, 18*(4), 310–317.

---

**CHART 36-5**

## Teaching Patients About Home Parenteral Nutrition

An effective home care teaching program prepares the patient to manage the appropriate form of PN: how to store solutions, set up the infusion, flush the line with heparin, change the dressings, and troubleshoot for problems. The most common complication is sepsis. Strict aseptic technique is taught for hand hygiene, handling equipment, changing the dressing, and preparing the solution.

### Troubleshooting Mechanical Difficulties

Mechanical problems usually arise from technical complications in the infusion pump or catheter site. The patient needs to know how to measure the length of the external portion of the catheter; this measurement is used as a comparison if the line is pulled or if dislodgement is suspected. The patient also needs to know how to recognize catheter problems (eg, leakage, loose cap, blood clot, dislodgement) and should receive a list of instructions explaining what to do for each problem.

### Recognizing Metabolic Complications

The patient is given a list of signs and symptoms that indicate metabolic complications (neuropathies, mentation changes, diarrhea, nausea, skin changes, decreased urine output) and directions on how to contact the home health care nurse or physician if any of these complications occurs. The patient is instructed to have routine serum chemistry and hematology tests as well.

### Obtaining Psychosocial Support

The psychosocial aspects of home PN are as important as the physiologic and technical concerns. Patients must cope with the loss of eating and with changes in lifestyle brought on by sleep disturbances (frequent urination during infusions, usually two or three times during the night).

Major psychosocial reactions include depression, anger, withdrawal, anxiety, and impaired self-image. A successful home PN program depends on the patient's and family's motivation, emotional stability, and technical competence. Patients and families need to know which support groups are available in the community to help them cope with the transition and to minimize disruption of lifestyle.

---

## Evaluation

### Expected Patient Outcomes

Expected patient outcomes may include the following:

1. Attains or maintains nutritional balance
2. Is free of infection at the catheter site
    a. Is afebrile

## CHART 36-6

### HOME CARE CHECKLIST • The Patient Receiving Parenteral Nutrition

| At the completion of the home care instruction, the patient or caregiver will be able to: | Patient | Caregiver |
|---|---|---|
| • Discuss goal and purpose of PN therapy. | ✔ | ✔ |
| • Discuss basic components of PN solution. | ✔ | ✔ |
| • List emergency phone numbers. | ✔ | ✔ |
| • Demonstrate how to handle PN solutions and medications correctly. | ✔ | ✔ |
| • Demonstrate how to operate infusion pump. | ✔ | ✔ |
| • Demonstrate how to prime tubing and filter. | ✔ | ✔ |
| • Demonstrate how to connect and disconnect PN infusion. | ✔ | ✔ |
| • Demonstrate how to perform catheter dressing changes. | ✔ | ✔ |
| • Demonstrate how to heparinize central line. | ✔ | ✔ |
| • Identify possible PN complications and interventions. | ✔ | ✔ |

## CHART 36-7

### Gerontologic Considerations

**Home Parenteral and Enteral Nutrition**

Age-related conditions that affect home nutrition support goals include the following:

- **Arthritis:** possible decreased hand dexterity and fine motor coordination
- **Sensory impairment:** inability to hear pump alarms; vision loss may affect ability to see pump menus or fill syringes
- **Constipation:** decreased overall bowel tone, which can cause intolerance of enteral feedings; increasing water flushes and assessing fiber needs may help
- **Dehydration:** decreased sensation of thirst, which may require close clinical management of fluid needs
- **Obesity:** decreased basal metabolic rate increases tendency toward weight gain; may require a reduction in overall kilocalorie intake to compensate
- **Diabetes mellitus:** increased insulin resistance, which makes glucose control during parenteral nutrition infusion more challenging
- **Depression/dementia:** mood and memory disorders, which may present as low motivation to learn and adhere to the nutrition support regimen
- **Multiple medications:** conversion to an appropriate intravenous or enteral route, if possible, is required

Adapted from White, J., Brewer, D., Stockton, M., et al. (2003). Nutrition in chronic disease management in the elderly. *Nutrition in Clinical Practice, 18*(1), 3–11.

b. Has no purulent drainage from the catheter insertion site
c. Has intact IV access
3. Is hydrated, as evidenced by good skin turgor
4. Achieves an optimal level of activity, within limitations
5. Demonstrates skill in managing PN regimen
6. Prevents complications
   a. Maintains proper catheter and equipment function
   b. Has no symptoms of sepsis
   c. Maintains metabolic balance within normal limits
   d. Shows improved and stabilized nutritional status

## Critical Thinking Exercises

**1** You prepare to administer a patient's scheduled bolus enteral tube feeding, and he states that he feels too full for another feeding. It has been 4 hours since his last feeding. His stomach is somewhat distended but he has bowel sounds. What are some of the causes of abdominal fullness and distention? How would current medications and patterns of elimination affect these signs and symptoms? Whom should you consult?

**2** **ebp** A patient who is receiving gastrostomy tube feedings is to be discharged from the hospital to return home within the next few days. The patient has many questions regarding the equipment that he will need. What is the strength of the evidence that leads you to espouse the advantages of a simple bolus regimen of tube feeding versus around-the-clock pump feeding? For this ambulatory patient, what is the evidence base that assists you in advising him to select an optimal regimen of administration?

**3** A patient has just been diagnosed with small bowel strictures from Crohn's disease and requires preoperative total nutrient admixture (TNA) for at least 1 week. The patient does not want a central access catheter placed and prefers to continue with simple IV fluids. What can you tell her about the nutritional advantages of TNA when compared with simple hydration fluids? With strict adherence to protocols for IV line management and dressing care, what complications can be avoided?

**4** **ebp** You are preparing to administer a gravity bolus enteral tube feeding to a patient assigned to your care on a general medicine inpatient unit. You find the patient lying on his side in the bed with the tape no longer around the tube but still adhered to his outer nares. Before proceeding with the feeding, what is the strength of the evidence you will consider when you determine optimal positioning of this patient to prevent complications such as regurgitation and aspiration? What is the evidence base that guides you in determining appropriate placement of the feeding tube?

## REFERENCES AND SELECTED READINGS

### BOOKS

Buchman, A. (2004). *Practical nutrition support techniques* (2nd ed.). Thorofare, NJ: Slack International.

Gottschlich, M., Fuhrman, M., & Hammond, K., et al. (Eds.). (2000). *The science and practice of nutrition support: A case-based core curriculum.* American Society of Parenteral and Enteral Nutrition (ASPEN). Dubuque, Iowa: Kendall/Hunt.

Josephson, D. (2003). *Intravenous infusion therapy for nurses* (2nd ed.). Clifton Park, NY: Delmar Thomas Learning.

Latifi, R., & Dudrick, S. (2003). *The biology and practice of nutritional support* (2nd ed.). Georgetown, TX: Landes Bioscience.

Rolandelli, R., Bankhead, R., Boulatta, J., et al. (Eds.). (2004). *Clinical nutrition: Enteral and tube feeding* (4th ed.). Philadelphia: W. B. Saunders.

Worthington, P. (2004). *Practical aspects of nutritional support: An advanced practice guide.* Philadelphia: W. B. Saunders.

Yamada, T., & Alpers, D. H. (Eds.). (2003). *Textbook of gastroenterology* (4th ed.). Philadelphia: Lippincott Williams & Wilkins.

### JOURNALS

*Asterisks indicate nursing research articles.

#### Gastrostomies, Nasogastric and Nasoenteric Intubation and Feeding

Angus, F., & Burakoff, R. (2003). The percutaneous endoscopic gastrostomy tube. Medical and ethical issues in placement. *American Journal of Gastroenterology, 98*(2), 272–277.

Carroll, D. (2003). Moxifloxacin-induced *Clostridium difficile*-associated diarrhea. *Pharmacotherapy, 23*(11), 1517–1519.

Dickerson, R., Tidwell, A., & Brown, R. (2003). Adverse effects from inappropriate medication administration via a jejunostomy tube. *Nutrition in Clinical Practice, 18*(5), 402–405.

Keithley, J., & Swanson, B. (2004). Enteral nutrition: An update on practice recommendations. *MedSurg Nursing, 13*(2), 131–134.

*Lenart, S., & Polissar, N. (2003). Comparison of two methods for post-pyloric placement of enteral feeding tubes. *American Journal of Critical Care, 12*(4), 357–360.

Metheny, N. A. (1998). Detection of improperly positioned feeding tubes. *Journal of Health Care Risk Management, 18*(3), 37–45.

*Metheny, N. A., Dettenmeier, P., Hampton, K., et al. (1990). Determinant of inadvertent respiratory placement of small-bore feeding tubes. A report of 10 cases. *Heart and Lung, 19*(6), 631–638.

*Metheny, N. A., McSweeney, M., Wehrle, M. A., et al. (1990). Effectiveness of the auscultatory method in predicting feeding tube location. *Nursing Research, 39*(5), 282–287.

*Metheny, N. A., Smith, L., Stewart, B. J., et al. (2000). Development of a reliable and valid bedside test for bilirubin and its utility for predicting feeding tube location. *Nursing Research, 49*(6), 302–309.

*Metheny, N. A., Stewart, B. J., Smith, L., et al. (1999). pH and concentration of bilirubin in feeding tube aspirates as predictors of tube placement. *Nursing Research, 48*(3), 189–197.

Metheny, N. A., & Titler, M. G. (2001). Assessing placement of feeding tubes. *American Journal of Nursing, 101*(5), 36–46.

Neef, M., Crowder, V., McIvor, N., et al. (2003). Comparison of the use of endoscopic and radiological gastrostomy in a single head and neck cancer unit. *Australian and New Zealand Journal of Surgery, 73*(1), 590–593.

Parrish, C. (2003). Enteral feeding: The art and the science. *Nutrition in Clinical Practice, 18*(1), 76–84.

Roche, V. (2003). Percutaneous endoscopic gastrostomy: Clinical care of PEG tubes in older adults. *Geriatrics, 58*(11), 22–29.

Sartori, S., Trevisani, L., Neilsen, I., et al. (2003). Longevity of silicone and polyurethane catheters in long-term enteral feeding via percutaneous endoscopic gastrostomy. *Alimentary Pharmacology and Therapeutics, 17*(6), 853–856.

Schloerb, P., Wood, J., Casillan, A., et al. (2004). Bowel necrosis caused by water in jejunal feeding, (2004). *Journal of Parenteral and Enteral Nutrition, 28*(1), 27–29.

Shang, E., Geiger, N., Sturm, J., et al. (2004). Pump-assisted enteral nutrition can prevent aspiration in bedridden endoscopic gastrostomy patients. *Journal of Parenteral and Enteral Nutrition, 28*(3), 180–183.

Tonelli, M. (2005). Waking the dying: Must we always attempt to involve critically ill patients in end-of-life decisions? *Chest, 127*(2), 637–642.

White, J., Brewer, D., Stockton, M., et al. (2003). Nutrition in chronic disease management in the elderly. *Nutrition in Clinical Practice, 18*(1), 3–11.

#### Parenteral Nutrition

Alberti, C., Brun-Buisson, C., Burchardi, H., et al. (2002). Epidemiology of sepsis and infection in ICU patients from an international multi-centre cohort study. *Intensive Care Medicine, 28*(4), 108–121.

American Society of Parenteral and Enteral Nutrition (ASPEN). (1998). Special report: Safe practices for parenteral nutrition formulas. Available at: http://www.nutritioncare.org. Accessed June 13, 2006.

Bong, J., Kite, P., Wilco, M., et al. (2003). Prevention of catheter-related bloodstream infection by silver iontophoretic central venous catheters: A randomized controlled trial. *Journal of Clinical Pathology, 56*(10), 731–735.

Centers for Disease Control and Prevention (2002). Guidelines for the prevention of intravascular catheter-related infections. *Morbidity and Mortality Weekly Report,* 51 (RR-10), 1–36.

Correia, M., Guimaraes, J., de Mattos, L., et al. (2004). Peripheral parenteral nutrition: An option for patients with an indication for short-term parenteral nutrition. *Nutricion Hospitalaria, 19*(1), 14–18.

Evans, J., Steinhart, A., Cohen, Z., et al. (2003). Home total parenteral nutrition: An alternative to early surgery for complicated inflammatory bowel disease. *Journal of Gastrointestinal Surgery, 7*(4), 562–566.

Huckleberry, Y. (2004). Nutritional support and the surgical patient. *American Journal of Health System Pharmacy, 61*(7), 671–682.

Ireton-Jones, C., DeLegge, M., Epperson, L., et al. (2003). Management of the home parenteral nutrition patient. *Nutrition in Clinical Practice, 18*(4), 310–317.

Peterson, K. (2003). Central line sepsis. *Clinical Journal in Oncology Nursing, 7*(2), 218–221.

Philpot, P., & Griffiths, V. (2003). The peripherally-inserted central catheter. *Nursing Standard, 17*(44), 39–46.

Smith, C., Curtas, S., Kleinbeck, S., et al. (2003). Clinical trial of interactive and videotaped educational interventions reduce infection, reactive depression and rehospitalizations for sepsis in patients on home parenteral nutrition. *Journal of Parenteral and Enteral Nutrition, 27*(2), 137–145.

Teitelbaum, D., Guenter, P., Howel, W., et al. (2005). Definition of terms, style and conventions used in A.S.P.E.N. guidelines and standards. *Nutrition in Clinical Practice, 20*(2), 281–285.

## RESOURCES

American Cancer Society, 1599 Clifton Rd. N.E., Atlanta, GA 30329; 1-404-320-3333; http://www.cancer.org. Accessed June 3, 2006.

American Society for Clinical Nutrition, 9650 Rockville Pike, Bethesda, MD 20814; http://www.ascn.org. Accessed June 3, 2006.

American Society for Gastrointestinal Endoscopy, 13 Elm St., Manchester, MA 01944; http://www.asge.org. Accessed June 3, 2006.

American Society for Parenteral and Enteral Nutrition (ASPEN), 8630 Fenton St., #412, Silver Spring, MD 20910-3805; http://www.nutritioncare.org. Accessed June 3, 2006.

Oley Foundation for Home Parenteral and Enteral Nutrition, 214 Hun Memorial, A-23, New Scotland Ave., Albany, NY 12208; http://www.iffgd.org/oley.html. Accessed June 3, 2006.

Society of Gastroenterology Nurses & Associates, Inc., 140 North Michigan Ave., Chicago, IL, 60611; 800-245-7462; in Illinois, 312-321-5165; http://www.sgna.org. Accessed June 3, 2006.

# CHAPTER 37

# Management of Patients With Gastric and Duodenal Disorders

## Learning Objectives

*On completion of this chapter, the learner will be able to:*

1. Compare the etiology, clinical manifestations, and management of acute gastritis, chronic gastritis, and peptic ulcer.
2. Use the nursing process as a framework for care of patients with gastritis.
3. Use the nursing process as a framework for care of patients with peptic ulcer.
4. Describe the dietary, pharmacologic, and surgical treatment of peptic ulcer.
5. Describe the nursing management of patients who undergo surgical procedures to treat obesity.
6. Use the nursing process as a framework for care of patients with gastric cancer.
7. Use the nursing process as a framework for care of patients undergoing gastric surgery.
8. Identify the complications of gastric surgery and their prevention and management.
9. Describe the home health care needs of the patient who has had gastric surgery.

A person's nutritional status depends not only on the type and amount of intake but also on the functioning of the gastric and intestinal portions of the gastrointestinal (GI) system. This chapter describes disorders of the stomach and duodenum, their treatment, and related nursing care.

# Gastritis

**Gastritis** (inflammation of the **gastric** or stomach mucosa) is a common GI problem. Gastritis may be acute, lasting several hours to a few days, or chronic, resulting from repeated exposure to irritating agents or recurring episodes of acute gastritis.

Acute gastritis is often caused by dietary indiscretion—the person eats food that is irritating, too highly seasoned, or contaminated with disease-causing microorganisms. Other causes of acute gastritis include overuse of aspirin and other nonsteroidal anti-inflammatory drugs (NSAIDs), excessive alcohol intake, bile reflux, and radiation therapy. A more severe form of acute gastritis is caused by the ingestion of strong acid or alkali, which may cause the mucosa to become gangrenous or to perforate. Scarring can occur, resulting in **pyloric stenosis** or obstruction. Acute gastritis also may develop in acute illnesses, especially when the patient has had major traumatic injuries; burns; severe infection; hepatic, renal, or respiratory failure; or major surgery. Gastritis may be the first sign of an acute systemic infection.

Chronic gastritis and prolonged inflammation of the stomach may be caused either by benign or malignant ulcers of the stomach or by the bacteria *Helicobacter pylori* (*H. pylori*). Chronic gastritis is sometimes associated with autoimmune diseases such as pernicious anemia; dietary factors such as caffeine; the use of medications such as NSAIDs, bisphosphonate (eg, alendronate [Fosamax], or risedronate [Actonel]); alcohol; smoking; or chronic reflux of pancreatic secretions and bile into the stomach.

## Pathophysiology

In gastritis, the gastric mucous membrane becomes edematous and hyperemic (congested with fluid and blood) and undergoes superficial erosion (Fig. 37-1). It secretes a scanty amount of gastric juice, containing very little acid but much mucus. Superficial ulceration may occur and can lead to hemorrhage.

## Clinical Manifestations

The patient with acute gastritis may have a rapid onset of symptoms, such as abdominal discomfort, headache, lassitude, nausea, anorexia, vomiting, and hiccupping, which can last from a few hours to a few days. The patient with chronic gastritis may complain of anorexia, heartburn after eating, belching, a sour taste in the mouth, or nausea and vomiting. Some patients may have only mild epigastric discomfort or report intolerance to spicy or fatty foods or slight pain that is relieved by eating. Patients with chronic gastritis from vitamin deficiency usually have evidence of malabsorption of vitamin $B_{12}$ caused by the production of antibodies that interfere with the binding of vitamin $B_{12}$ to intrinsic factor. However, some patients with chronic gastritis have no symptoms.

# Glossary

**achlorhydria:** lack of hydrochloric acid in digestive secretions of the stomach

**antrectomy:** removal of the pyloric (antrum) portion of the stomach with anastomosis (surgical connection) to the duodenum (gastroduodenostomy or Billroth I) or anastomosis to the jejunum (gastrojejunostomy or Billroth II)

**bariatric:** term that comes from two Greek words meaning "weight" and "treatment"

**dumping syndrome:** physiologic response to rapid emptying of gastric contents into the jejunum, manifested by nausea, weakness, sweating, palpitations, syncope, and possibly diarrhea; occurs in patients who have had partial gastrectomy and gastrojejunostomy

**duodenum:** first portion of the small intestine, between the stomach and the jejunum

**enteroclysis:** fluoroscopic x-ray of the small intestine; a tube is placed from the nose or mouth through the esophagus and the stomach to the duodenum, a barium-based liquid contrast material is infused through the tube, and x-rays are taken as it travels through the duodenum

**gastric:** refers to the stomach

**gastric outlet obstruction (GOO):** any condition that mechanically impedes normal gastric emptying; there is obstruction of the channel of the pylorus and duodenum through which the stomach empties

**gastritis:** inflammation of the stomach

**hematemesis:** vomiting of blood

**ligament of Treitz:** suspensory ligament of the duodenum; important anatomic landmark used to divide the gastrointestinal tract into an upper and a lower portion

**melena:** tarry or black stools; indicative of blood in stools

**morbid obesity:** more than twice ideal body weight, 100 pounds or more over ideal body weight, or body mass index (BMI) exceeding 30 kg/m$^2$

**omentum:** fold of the peritoneum that surrounds the stomach and other organs of the abdomen

**peritoneum:** thin membrane that lines the inside of the wall of the abdomen and covers all the abdominal organs

**pyloroplasty:** surgical procedure to increase the opening of the pyloric orifice

**pylorus:** opening between the stomach and the duodenum

**pyrosis:** heartburn

**serosa:** thin membrane that forms the outer layer of the stomach

**stenosis:** narrowing or tightening of an opening or passage in the body

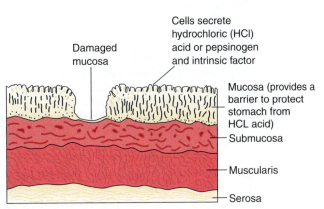

**FIGURE 37-1.** Endoscopic view of erosive gastritis (*left*). Damage from irritants (*right*) results in increased intracellular pH, impaired enzyme function, disrupted cellular structures, ischemia, vascular stasis, and tissue death. Reproduced with permission from Porth, C. (2005). *Pathophysiology: Concepts of altered health states* (7th ed.). Philadelphia: Lippincott Williams & Wilkins. © 2005, Lippincott Williams & Wilkins.

## Assessment and Diagnostic Findings

Gastritis is sometimes associated with **achlorhydria** or hypochlorhydria (absence or low levels of hydrochloric acid [HCl]) or with hyperchlorhydria (high levels of HCl). Diagnosis can be determined by an upper GI x-ray series or endoscopy and histologic examination of a tissue specimen obtained by biopsy. Diagnostic measures for detecting *H. pylori* infection may be used and are discussed in the section on peptic ulcers.

## Medical Management

The gastric mucosa is capable of repairing itself after a bout of gastritis. As a rule, the patient recovers in about 1 day, although the appetite may be diminished for an additional 2 or 3 days. Acute gastritis is also managed by instructing the patient to refrain from alcohol and food until symptoms subside. When the patient can take nourishment by mouth, a nonirritating diet is recommended. If the symptoms persist, intravenous (IV) fluids may need to be administered. If bleeding is present, management is similar to the procedures used to control upper GI tract hemorrhage discussed later in this chapter.

If gastritis is caused by ingestion of strong acids or alkalis, emergency treatment consists of diluting and neutralizing the offending agent. To neutralize acids, common antacids (eg, aluminum hydroxide) are used; to neutralize an alkali, diluted lemon juice or diluted vinegar is used. If corrosion is extensive or severe, emetics and lavage are avoided because of the danger of perforation and damage to the esophagus.

Therapy is supportive and may include nasogastric (NG) intubation, analgesic agents and sedatives, antacids, and IV fluids. Fiberoptic endoscopy may be necessary. In extreme cases, emergency surgery may be required to remove gangrenous or perforated tissue. A gastric resection or a gastrojejunostomy (anastomosis of jejunum to stomach to detour around the pylorus) may be necessary to treat pyloric obstruction, a narrowing of the pyloric orifice that cannot be relieved by medical management.

Chronic gastritis is managed by modifying the patient's diet, promoting rest, reducing stress, recommending avoidance of alcohol and NSAIDs, and initiating pharmacotherapy. *H. pylori* may be treated with selected drug combinations (Table 37-1).

## ◄▼► Nursing Process

### The Patient With Gastritis

#### Assessment

When obtaining the history, the nurse asks about the patient's presenting signs and symptoms. Does the patient have heartburn, indigestion, nausea, or vomiting? Do the symptoms occur at any specific time of the day, before or after meals, after ingesting spicy or irritating foods, or after the ingestion of certain drugs or alcohol? Has there been recent weight gain or loss? Are the

## TABLE 37-1 Pharmacotherapy for Peptic Ulcer Disease and Gastritis

| Pharmacologic Agent | Major Action | Nursing Considerations |
|---|---|---|
| **Antibiotics** | | |
| Amoxicillin (Amoxil) | A bactericidal antibiotic that assists with eradicating *H. pylori* bacteria in the gastric mucosa | • May cause diarrhea<br>• Should not be used in patients allergic to penicillin |
| Clarithromycin (Biaxin) | Exerts bactericidal effects to eradicate *H. pylori* bacteria in the gastric mucosa | • May cause GI upset, headache, altered taste<br>• Many drug–drug interactions (eg, cisapride, colchicine, lovastatin, warfarin [Coumadin]) |
| Metronidazole (Flagyl) | A synthetic antibacterial and antiprotozoal agent that assists with eradicating *H. pylori* bacteria in the gastric mucosa when administered with other antibiotics and proton pump inhibitors | • Should be administered with meals to decrease GI upset; may cause anorexia and metallic taste<br>• Patient should avoid alcohol; Flagyl increases blood-thinning effects of warfarin (Coumadin) |
| Tetracycline | Exerts bacteriostatic effects to eradicate *H. pylori* bacteria in the gastric mucosa | • May cause photosensitivity reaction; warn patient to use sunscreen<br>• May cause GI upset<br>• Must be used with caution in patients with renal or hepatic impairment<br>• Milk or dairy products may reduce effectiveness |
| **Antidiarrheal** | | |
| Bismuth subsalicylate (Pepto-Bismol) | Suppresses *H. pylori* bacteria in the gastric mucosa and assists with healing of mucosal ulcers | • Given concurrently with antibiotics to eradicate *H. pylori* infection<br>• Should be taken on empty stomach |
| **Histamine-2 ($H_2$) receptor antagonists** | | |
| Cimetidine (Tagamet) | Decreases amount of HCl produced by stomach by blocking action of histamine on histamine receptors of parietal cells in the stomach | • Least expensive of $H_2$ receptor antagonists<br>• May cause confusion, agitation, or coma in the elderly or those with renal or hepatic insufficiency<br>• Long-term use may cause diarrhea, dizziness, gynecomastia<br>• Many drug–drug interactions (eg, amiodarone, amitriptyline, benzodiazepines, metoprolol, nifedipine, phenytoin, warfarin [Coumadin]) |
| Famotidine (Pepcid) | Same as for cimetidine | • Best choice for critically ill patient, because it is known to have the least risk of drug–drug interactions; does not alter liver metabolism<br>• Prolonged half-life in patients with renal insufficiency<br>• Short-term relief for GERD |
| Nizatidine (Axid) | Same as for cimetidine | • Used for treatment of ulcers and GERD<br>• Prolonged half-life in patients with renal insufficiency<br>• May cause headache, dizziness, diarrhea, nausea/vomiting, GI upset as well as urticaria |
| Ranitidine (Zantac) | Same as for cimetidine | • Prolonged half-life in patients with renal and hepatic insufficiency<br>• Causes fewer side effects than cimetidine<br>• May cause headache, dizziness, constipation, nausea and vomiting, or abdominal discomfort |
| **Proton pump inhibitors of gastric acid (PPIs)** | | |
| Esomeprazole (Nexium) | Decreases gastric acid secretion by slowing the hydrogen-potassium adenosine triphosphatase ($H^+$, $K^+$-ATPase) pump on the surface of the parietal cells of the stomach | • Used mainly for treatment of duodenal ulcer disease and *H. pylori* infection<br>• A delayed-release capsule that is to be swallowed whole and taken before meals |
| Lansoprazole (Prevacid) | Decreases gastric acid secretion by slowing the $H^+$, $K^+$-ATPase pump on the surface of the parietal cells | • A delayed-release capsule that is to be swallowed whole and taken before meals |

### TABLE 37-1 Pharmacotherapy for Peptic Ulcer Disease and Gastritis (Continued)

| Pharmacologic Agent | Major Action | Nursing Considerations |
|---|---|---|
| Omeprazole (Prilosec) | Decreases gastric acid secretion by slowing the $H^+$, $K^+$-ATPase pump on the surface of the parietal cells | • A delayed-release capsule that is to be swallowed whole and taken before meals<br>• May cause diarrhea, nausea, constipation, abdominal pain, vomiting, headache, or dizziness |
| Pantoprazole (Protonix) | Decreases gastric acid secretion by slowing the $H^+$, $K^+$-ATPase pump on the surface of the parietal cells | • A delayed-release capsule that is to be swallowed whole and taken before meals<br>• May cause diarrhea and hyperglycemia, headache, abdominal pain, and abnormal liver function tests |
| Rabeprazole (AcipHex) | Decreases gastric acid secretion by slowing the $H^+$, $K^+$-ATPase pump on the surface of the parietal cells | • A delayed-release tablet to be swallowed whole<br>• May cause abdominal pain, diarrhea, nausea, and headache<br>• Drug–drug interactions with digoxin, iron, and warfarin (Coumadin) |
| **Prostaglandin $E_1$ analog**<br>Misoprostol (Cytotec) | Synthetic prostaglandin; protects the gastric mucosa from agents that cause ulcers; also increases mucous production and bicarbonate levels | • Used to prevent ulceration in patients using NSAIDs<br>• Administer with food<br>• May cause diarrhea and cramping (including uterine cramping) |
| Sucralfate (Carafate) | Creates a viscous substance in the presence of gastric acid that forms a protective barrier, binding to the surface of the ulcer, and prevents digestion by pepsin | • Used mainly for the treatment of duodenal ulcers<br>• Should be taken without food but with water<br>• Other medications should be taken 2 hours before or after this medication<br>• May cause constipation or nausea |

GI, gastrointestinal; NSAID, nonsteroidal anti-inflammatory drug; GERD, gastroesophageal reflux disease.

symptoms related to anxiety, stress, allergies, eating or drinking too much, or eating too quickly? How are the symptoms relieved? Is there a history of previous gastric disease or surgery? A diet history plus a 72-hour dietary recall (a list of everything the patient has eaten and drunk in the past 72 hours) may be helpful.

A thorough history is important because it helps the nurse identify whether known dietary excesses or other indiscretions are associated with the current symptoms, whether others in the patient's environment have similar symptoms, whether the patient is vomiting blood, and whether any known caustic element has been ingested. The nurse also identifies the duration of the current symptoms, any methods used by the patient to treat these symptoms, and whether the methods are effective.

Signs to note during the physical examination include abdominal tenderness, dehydration, and evidence of any systemic disorder that might be responsible for the symptoms of gastritis.

## Nursing Diagnoses

Based on the assessment data, the patient's major nursing diagnoses may include the following:

- Anxiety related to treatment
- Imbalanced nutrition, less than body requirements, related to inadequate intake of nutrients
- Risk for imbalanced fluid volume related to insufficient fluid intake and excessive fluid loss subsequent to vomiting
- Deficient knowledge about dietary management and disease process
- Acute pain related to irritated stomach mucosa

## Planning and Goals

The major goals for the patient may include reduced anxiety, avoidance of irritating foods, adequate intake of nutrients, maintenance of fluid balance, increased awareness of dietary management, and relief of pain.

## Nursing Interventions

### Reducing Anxiety

If the patient has ingested acids or alkalis, emergency measures may be necessary. The nurse offers supportive therapy to the patient and family during treatment and after the ingested acid or alkali has been neutralized or diluted. In some cases, the nurse may need to prepare the patient for additional diagnostic studies (endoscopies) or surgery. The patient may be anxious because of pain and planned treatment modalities. The nurse uses a calm approach to assess the patient and to answer all questions as completely as possible. It is important to explain all procedures and treatments based on the patient's level of understanding.

### Promoting Optimal Nutrition

For acute gastritis, the nurse provides physical and emotional support and helps the patient manage the symptoms, which may include nausea, vomiting, heartburn, and fatigue. The patient should take no foods or fluids by mouth—possibly for a few days—until the acute symptoms subside, thus allowing the gastric mucosa to heal. If IV therapy is necessary, the nurse monitors fluid intake and output along with serum electrolyte values. After the symptoms subside, the nurse may offer the patient ice chips followed by clear liquids. Introducing solid food as soon as possible may provide adequate oral nutrition, decrease the need for IV therapy, and minimize irritation to the gastric mucosa. As food is introduced, the nurse evaluates and reports any symptoms that suggest a repeat episode of gastritis.

The nurse discourages the intake of caffeinated beverages, because caffeine is a central nervous system stimulant that increases gastric activity and pepsin secretion. It also is important to discourage alcohol use. Discouraging cigarette smoking is important because nicotine reduces the secretion of pancreatic bicarbonate, which inhibits the neutralization of gastric acid in the duodenum (Wu & Cho, 2004). When appropriate, the nurse initiates and refers the patient for alcohol counseling and smoking cessation programs.

### Promoting Fluid Balance

Daily fluid intake and output are monitored to detect early signs of dehydration (minimal urine output of 30 mL/hour, minimal intake of 1.5 L/day). If food and oral fluids are withheld, IV fluids (3 L/day) usually are prescribed and a record of fluid intake plus caloric value (1 L of 5% dextrose in water = 170 calories of carbohydrate) needs to be maintained. Electrolyte values (sodium, potassium, chloride) are assessed every 24 hours to detect any imbalance.

The nurse must always be alert for any indicators of hemorrhagic gastritis, which include **hematemesis** (vomiting of blood), tachycardia, and hypotension. If these occur, the physician is notified and the patient's vital signs are monitored as the patient's condition warrants. Guidelines for managing upper GI tract bleeding are discussed later in this chapter.

### Relieving Pain

Measures to help relieve pain include instructing the patient to avoid foods and beverages that may be irritating to the gastric mucosa and instructing the patient about the correct use of medications to relieve chronic gastritis. The nurse must regularly assess the patient's level of pain and the extent of comfort attained from the use of medications and avoidance of irritating substances.

### Promoting Home and Community-Based Care

#### TEACHING PATIENTS SELF-CARE

The nurse evaluates the patient's knowledge about gastritis and develops an individualized teaching plan that includes information about stress management, diet, and medications (Chart 37-1). Dietary instructions take into account the patient's daily caloric needs, food preferences, and pattern of eating. The nurse and patient review foods and other substances to be avoided (eg, spicy, irritating, or highly seasoned foods; caffeine; nicotine; alcohol). Consultation with a dietitian may be recommended.

Providing information about prescribed antibiotics, bismuth salts, medications to decrease gastric secretion, and medications to protect mucosal cells from gastric secretions may help the patient to better understand why these medications assist in recovery and prevent recurrence. The importance of completing the medication regimen as prescribed to eradicate *H. pylori* infection must be reinforced to the patient and any caregivers.

#### CONTINUING CARE

The nurse reinforces previous teaching and conducts ongoing assessment of the patient's symptoms and progress. Patients with pernicious anemia need information about lifelong vitamin $B_{12}$ injections; the nurse may instruct a family member or caregiver how to administer the injections or make arrangements for the patient to receive the injections from a health care provider. Finally, the nurse emphasizes the

---

### CHART 37-1

## HOME CARE CHECKLIST • The Patient With Gastritis

| At the completion of the home care instruction, the patient or caregiver will be able to: | Patient | Caregiver |
| --- | :---: | :---: |
| • Identify foods and other substances that may cause gastritis. | ✔ | ✔ |
| • Report inability to ingest adequate solids and liquids. | ✔ | ✔ |
| • Describe medication regimen. | ✔ | ✔ |
| • State need for vitamin $B_{12}$ injections if patient has pernicious anemia. | ✔ | ✔ |
| • State schedule of follow-up appointments with health care provider. | ✔ | ✔ |

importance of keeping follow-up appointments with health care providers.

## Evaluation

### Expected Patient Outcomes

Expected patient outcomes may include the following:

1. Exhibits low level of anxiety
2. Avoids eating irritating foods or drinking caffeinated beverages or alcohol
3. Maintains fluid balance
   a. Has oral fluid intake of at least 1.5 L daily
   b. Drinks six to eight glasses of water daily
   c. Has urinary output of approximately 1 L daily
   d. Displays adequate skin turgor
4. Adheres to medical regimen
   a. Selects nonirritating foods and beverages
   b. Takes medications as prescribed
5. Maintains appropriate weight
6. Reports less pain

**FIGURE 37-2.** Deep peptic ulcer. Reproduced with permission from Porth, C. (2005). *Pathophysiology: Concepts of altered health states* (7th ed.). Philadelphia: Lippincott Williams & Wilkins. © 2005, Lippincott Williams & Wilkins.

# Peptic Ulcer Disease

A peptic ulcer may be referred to as a gastric, duodenal, or esophageal ulcer, depending on its location. A person who has a peptic ulcer has peptic ulcer disease. A peptic ulcer is an excavation (hollowed-out area) that forms in the mucosal wall of the stomach, in the **pylorus** (the opening between the stomach and duodenum), in the **duodenum** (the first part of small intestine), or in the esophagus. Erosion of a circumscribed area of mucous membrane is the cause (Fig. 37-2). This erosion may extend as deeply as the muscle layers or through the muscle to the **peritoneum**.

Peptic ulcers are more likely to be in the duodenum than in the stomach. As a rule they occur alone, but they may occur in multiples. Chronic gastric ulcers tend to occur in the lesser curvature of the stomach, near the pylorus. Table 37-2 compares the features of gastric and duodenal ulcers. Esophageal ulcers occur as a result of the backward flow of HCl from the stomach into the esophagus (gastroesophageal reflux disease [GERD]).

Peptic ulcer disease occurs with the greatest frequency in people between 40 and 60 years of age. It is relatively uncommon in women of childbearing age, but it has been observed in children and even in infants. After menopause, the incidence of peptic ulcers in women is almost equal to that in men. Peptic ulcers in the body of the stomach can occur without excessive acid secretion.

In the past, stress and anxiety were thought to be causes of ulcers, but research has documented that peptic ulcers result from infection with the gram-negative bacteria *H. pylori*, which may be acquired through ingestion of food and water. Person-to-person transmission of the bacteria also occurs through close contact and exposure to emesis. Although *H. pylori* infection is common in the United States, most infected people do not develop ulcers. It is not known why *H. pylori* infection does not cause ulcers in all people, but most likely the predisposition to ulcer formation depends on certain factors, such as the type of *H. pylori* and other as yet unknown factors (Moss & Sood, 2003).

In addition, excessive secretion of HCl in the stomach may contribute to the formation of peptic ulcers, and stress may be associated with its increased secretion. The ingestion of milk and caffeinated beverages, smoking, and alcohol also may increase HCl secretion. Stress and eating spicy foods may make peptic ulcers worse.

Familial tendency also may be a significant predisposing factor. People with blood type O are more susceptible to peptic ulcers than are those with blood type A, B, or AB; this is another genetic link. There also is an association between peptic ulcers and chronic pulmonary disease or chronic renal disease. Other predisposing factors associated with peptic ulcer include chronic use of NSAIDs, alcohol ingestion, and excessive smoking.

Peptic ulcers are found in rare cases in patients with tumors that cause secretion of excessive amounts of the hormone gastrin. The Zollinger-Ellison syndrome (ZES) consists of severe peptic ulcers, extreme gastric hyperacidity, and gastrin-secreting benign or malignant tumors of the pancreas.

## Pathophysiology

Peptic ulcers occur mainly in the gastroduodenal mucosa because this tissue cannot withstand the digestive action of

| TABLE 37-2 | Comparison of Duodenal and Gastric Ulcers |
|---|---|
| **Duodenal Ulcer** | **Gastric Ulcer** |
| **Incidence** | |
| Age 30–60 | Usually 50 and over |
| Male: female = 2–3:1 | Male: female = 1:1 |
| 80% of peptic ulcers are duodenal | 15% of peptic ulcers are gastric |
| **Signs, Symptoms, and Clinical Findings** | |
| Hypersecretion of stomach acid (HCl) | Normal—hyposecretion of stomach acid (HCl) |
| May have weight gain | Weight loss may occur |
| Pain occurs 2–3 hours after a meal; often awakened 1–2 AM; ingestion of food relieves pain | Pain occurs ½ to 1 hour after a meal; rarely occurs at night; may be relieved by vomiting; ingestion of food does not help, sometimes increases pain |
| Vomiting uncommon | Vomiting common |
| Hemorrhage less likely than with gastric ulcer, but if present, melena more common than hematemesis | Hemorrhage more likely to occur than with duodenal ulcer; hematemesis more common than melena |
| More likely to perforate than gastric ulcers | |
| **Malignancy Possibility** | |
| Rare | Occasionally |
| **Risk Factors** | |
| *H. pylori*, alcohol, smoking, cirrhosis, stress | *H. pylori*, gastritis, alcohol, smoking, use of NSAIDs, stress |

gastric acid (HCl) and pepsin. The erosion is caused by the increased concentration or activity of acid-pepsin, or by decreased resistance of the mucosa. A damaged mucosa cannot secrete enough mucus to act as a barrier against HCl. The use of NSAIDs inhibits the secretion of mucus that protects the mucosa. Patients with duodenal ulcer disease secrete more acid than normal, whereas patients with gastric ulcer tend to secrete normal or decreased levels of acid. Damage to the gastroduodenal mucosa allows for decreased resistance to bacteria, and thus infection from *H. pylori* bacteria may occur.

ZES is suspected when a patient has several peptic ulcers or an ulcer that is resistant to standard medical therapy. It is identified by the following: hypersecretion of gastric juice, duodenal ulcers, and gastrinomas (islet cell tumors) in the pancreas. Ninety percent of tumors are found in the "gastric triangle," which encompasses the cystic and common bile ducts, the second and third portions of the duodenum, and the junction of the head and body of the pancreas. Approximately one third of gastrinomas are malignant. Diarrhea and steatorrhea (unabsorbed fat in the stool) may be evident. The patient may have coexisting parathyroid adenomas or hyperplasia and may therefore exhibit signs of hypercalcemia. The most common symptom is epigastric pain. *H. pylori* is not a risk factor for ZES.

*Stress ulcer* is the term given to the acute mucosal ulceration of the duodenal or gastric area that occurs after physiologically stressful events, such as burns, shock, severe sepsis, and multiple organ traumas. These ulcers, which are clinically different from peptic ulcers, are most common in ventilator-dependent patients after trauma or surgery. Fiberoptic endoscopy within 24 hours of trauma or surgery reveals shallow erosions of the stomach wall; by 72 hours, multiple gastric erosions are observed. As the stressful condition continues, the ulcers spread. When the patient recovers, the lesions are reversed. This pattern is typical of stress ulceration.

Differences of opinion exist as to the actual cause of mucosal ulceration in stress ulcers. Usually, the ulceration is preceded by shock; this leads to decreased gastric mucosal blood flow and to reflux of duodenal contents into the stomach. In addition, large quantities of pepsin are released. The combination of ischemia, acid, and pepsin creates an ideal climate for ulceration.

Stress ulcers should be distinguished from Cushing's ulcers and Curling's ulcers, two other types of gastric ulcers. Cushing's ulcers are common in patients with head injury and brain trauma. They may occur in the esophagus, stomach, or duodenum and are usually deeper and more penetrating than stress ulcers. Curling's ulcer is frequently observed about 72 hours after extensive burns and involves the antrum of the stomach or the duodenum.

## Clinical Manifestations

Symptoms of an ulcer may last for a few days, weeks, or months and may disappear only to reappear, often without an identifiable cause. Many people with ulcers have no symptoms, and perforation or hemorrhage may occur in 20% to 30% of patients who had no preceding manifestations.

As a rule, the patient with an ulcer complains of dull, gnawing pain or a burning sensation in the midepigastrium or in the back. It is believed that the pain occurs when the increased acid content of the stomach and duodenum erodes the lesion and stimulates the exposed nerve endings. Another theory suggests that contact of the lesion with acid stimulates a local reflex mechanism that initiates contraction of the adjacent smooth muscle. Pain is usually relieved by eating, because food neutralizes the acid, or by taking alkali; however, once the stomach has emptied or the alkali's effect has decreased, the pain returns. Sharply localized tenderness can be elicited by applying gentle pressure to the epigastrium at or slightly to the right of the midline.

Other symptoms include **pyrosis** (heartburn), vomiting, constipation or diarrhea, and bleeding. Pyrosis is a burning sensation in the esophagus and stomach that moves up to the mouth. Heartburn is often accompanied by sour eructation, or burping, which is common when the patient's stomach is empty.

Although vomiting is rare in uncomplicated duodenal ulcer, it may be a symptom of a complication of an ulcer. It results from obstruction of the pyloric orifice, caused by either muscular spasm of the pylorus or mechanical obstruction from scarring or acute swelling of the inflamed mucous membrane adjacent to the ulcer. Vomiting may or may not be preceded by nausea; usually it follows a bout of severe pain and bloating, which is relieved by ejection of the gastric contents. Emesis often contains undigested food eaten many hours earlier. Constipation or diarrhea may occur, probably as a result of diet and medications.

Fifteen percent of patients with peptic ulcer experience bleeding. Patients may present with GI bleeding as evidenced by the passage of **melena** (tarry stools). A small portion of patients who bleed from an acute ulcer have only very mild symptoms or none at all (Yamada & Alpers, 2003).

## Assessment and Diagnostic Findings

A physical examination may reveal pain, epigastric tenderness, or abdominal distention. A barium study of the upper GI tract may show an ulcer; however, endoscopy is the preferred diagnostic procedure because it allows direct visualization of inflammatory changes, ulcers, and lesions. Through endoscopy, a biopsy of the gastric mucosa and of any suspicious lesions can be obtained. Endoscopy may reveal lesions that, because of their size or location, are not evident on x-ray studies.

Stools may be tested periodically until they are negative for occult blood. Gastric secretory studies are of value in diagnosing achlorhydria and ZES. H. pylori infection may be determined by endoscopy and histologic examination of a tissue specimen obtained by biopsy, or a rapid urease test of the biopsy specimen. Other less invasive diagnostic measures for detecting H. pylori include serologic testing for antibodies against the H. pylori antigen, stool antigen test, and urea breath test.

## Medical Management

Once the diagnosis is established, the patient is informed that the condition can be controlled. Recurrence may develop; however, peptic ulcers treated with antibiotics to eradicate H. pylori have a lower recurrence rate than those not treated with antibiotics. The goals are to eradicate H. pylori and to manage gastric acidity. Methods used include medications, lifestyle changes, and surgical intervention.

### Pharmacologic Therapy

Currently, the most commonly used therapy for peptic ulcers is a combination of antibiotics, proton pump inhibitors, and bismuth salts that suppress or eradicate H. pylori.

Recommended therapy for 10 to 14 days includes triple therapy with two antibiotics (eg, metronidazole [Flagyl] or amoxicillin [Amoxil] and clarithromycin [Biaxin]) plus a proton pump inhibitor (eg, lansoprazole [Prevacid] or omeprazole [Prilosec]), or quadruple therapy with two antibiotics (metronidazole [Flagyl] and tetracycline) plus a proton pump inhibitor and bismuth salts (Pepto-Bismol). Research is being conducted to develop a vaccine against H. pylori (Sutton & Doidge, 2003).

Histamine-2 ($H_2$) receptor antagonists and proton pump inhibitors are used to treat NSAID-induced ulcers and other ulcers not associated with H. pylori infection. Table 37-3 provides information about the drug regimens used

### TABLE 37-3 Drug Regimens for Peptic Ulcer Disease

| Indications | Drug Regimen | Comments |
|---|---|---|
| Ulcer healing | **$H_2$ receptor antagonists**<br>Ranitidine 150 mg bid or 300 mg at bedtime<br>Cimetidine 400 mg bid or 800 mg at bedtime<br>Famotidine 20 mg bid or 40 mg at bedtime<br>Nizatidine 150 mg bid or 300 mg at bedtime | Should be used for 6 weeks for duodenal ulcer; 8 weeks for gastric ulcer |
| | **Proton pump inhibitors (PPIs)**<br>Omeprazole 20 mg daily<br>Lansoprazole 30 mg daily<br>Rabeprazole 20 mg daily<br>Pantoprazole 40 mg daily<br>Esomeprazole 40 mg daily | Should be used for 4 weeks for duodenal ulcer and 6 weeks for gastric ulcer<br>Healing occurs in 90% of patients who are compliant with therapy |
| Initial *Helicobacter pylori* therapy | **First-line therapy:**<br>PPI twice a day plus clarithromycin 500 mg twice a day plus amoxicillin 1000 mg twice a day *or* metronidazole 500 mg twice a day for 10–14 days | Efficacy of therapy is approximately 85% |
| | **Second-line therapy:**<br>Pepto-Bismol 2 tabs four times a day plus tetracycline 250 mg four times a day plus metronidazole 250 mg four times a day (optional: add PPI daily) for 14 days | QID dosing may decrease compliance |
| Therapy for retreatment of *H. pylori* therapy failure | Repeat first-line therapy, substitute metronidazole for amoxicillin (or vice versa) for 14 days; may add Pepto-Bismol.<br>Add second-line *H. pylori* therapy. | Efficacy of retreatment not known; success of more than 2 courses of treatment is very low |
| Prophylactic therapy for NSAID ulcers | Peptic ulcer healing doses of PPIs (above)<br>Misoprostol 200 mcg twice a day | Prevents recurrent ulceration in approximately 80%–90% of patients |

NSAID, nonsteroidal anti-inflammatory drug

for peptic ulcer disease. (Table 37-1 presents details about medications that can be used to treat peptic ulcer disease.)

The patient is advised to adhere to and complete the medication regimen to ensure complete healing of the ulcer. Because most patients become symptom-free within a week, it is a nursing responsibility to stress to the patient the importance of following the prescribed regimen so that the healing process can continue uninterrupted and the return of chronic ulcer symptoms can be prevented. Rest, sedatives, and tranquilizers may be added for the patient's comfort and are prescribed as needed. Maintenance dosages of $H_2$ receptor antagonists are usually recommended for 1 year.

For patients with ZES, hypersecretion of acid may be controlled with high doses of $H_2$ receptor antagonists. These patients may require twice the normal dose, and dosages usually need to be increased with prolonged use. Octreotide (Sandostatin), a medication that suppresses gastrin levels, also may be prescribed.

Patients at risk for stress ulcers (eg, patients with head injury or extensive burns) may be treated prophylactically with IV $H_2$ receptor antagonists and cytoprotective agents (eg, misoprostol, sucralfate) because of the risk for upper GI tract hemorrhage.

### Stress Reduction and Rest

Reducing environmental stress requires physical and psychological modifications on the patient's part as well as the aid and cooperation of family members and significant others. The nurse assists the patient to identify situations that are stressful or exhausting. A rushed lifestyle and an irregular schedule may aggravate symptoms and interfere with regular meals taken in relaxed settings along with the regular administration of medications. The patient may benefit from regular rest periods during the day, at least during the acute phase of the disease. Biofeedback, hypnosis, behavior modification, massage, or acupuncture may be helpful.

### Smoking Cessation

Studies have shown that smoking decreases the secretion of bicarbonate from the pancreas into the duodenum, resulting in increased acidity of the duodenum. Research indicates that continued smoking may significantly inhibit ulcer repair (Konturek, Bielanski, Plenka, et al., 2003). Therefore, the patient is strongly encouraged to stop smoking. Smoking cessation support groups and other smoking cessation approaches should be offered to patients.

### Dietary Modification

The intent of dietary modification for patients with peptic ulcers is to avoid oversecretion of acid and hypermotility in the GI tract. These can be minimized by avoiding extremes of temperature of food and beverage and overstimulation from consumption of meat extracts, alcohol, coffee (including decaffeinated coffee, which also stimulates acid secretion) and other caffeinated beverages, and diets rich in milk and cream (which stimulate acid secretion). In addition, an effort is made to neutralize acid by eating three regular meals a day. Small, frequent feedings are not necessary as long as an antacid or a histamine blocker is taken. Diet compatibility becomes an individual matter: the patient eats foods that are tolerated and avoids those that produce pain.

### Surgical Management

The introduction of antibiotics to eradicate *H. pylori* and of $H_2$ receptor antagonists as treatment for ulcers has greatly reduced the need for surgical intervention. However, surgery is usually recommended for patients with intractable ulcers (those that fail to heal after 12 to 16 weeks of medical treatment), life-threatening hemorrhage, perforation, or obstruction and for those with ZES not responding to medications (Yamada & Alpers, 2003). Surgical procedures include vagotomy, with or without pyloroplasty, and the Billroth I and Billroth II procedures (Table 37-4; see also the section on gastric surgery later in this chapter).

Patients who require surgery may have had a long illness. They may be discouraged and have had interruptions in their work role and pressures in their family life that affect their outlook on surgery and resolution of their disease.

### Follow-up Care

Recurrence of peptic ulcer disease within 1 year may be prevented with the prophylactic use of $H_2$-receptor antagonists taken at a reduced dose. Not all patients require maintenance therapy; it may be prescribed only for those with two or three recurrences per year, those who have had a complication such as bleeding or gastric outlet obstruction, or those who are candidates for gastric surgery but for whom it poses too high a risk. The likelihood of recurrence is reduced if the patient avoids smoking, coffee (including decaffeinated coffee) and other caffeinated beverages, alcohol, and ulcerogenic medications (eg, NSAIDs).

## ▶▶▶ Nursing Process

### The Patient With Peptic Ulcer Disease

#### Assessment

The nurse asks the patient to describe the pain and the methods used to relieve it (eg, food, antacids). The patient usually describes peptic ulcer pain as burning or gnawing; it occurs about 2 hours after a meal and frequently awakens the patient between midnight and 3 AM. Taking antacids, eating, or vomiting often relieves the pain. If the patient reports a recent history of vomiting, the nurse determines how often emesis has occurred and notes important characteristics of the vomitus: Is it bright red, does it resemble coffee grounds, or is there undigested food from previous meals? Has the patient noted any bloody or tarry stools?

The nurse also asks the patient to list his or her usual food intake for a 72-hour period and to

## TABLE 37-4  Surgical Procedures for Peptic Ulcer Disease

| Operation | Description | Comments |
|---|---|---|
| Vagotomy | Severing of the vagus nerve. Decreases gastric acid by diminishing cholinergic stimulation to the parietal cells, making them less responsive to gastrin. May be performed via open surgical approach, laparoscopy, or thoracoscopy | May be performed to reduce gastric acid secretion. A drainage type of procedure (see pyloroplasty) is usually performed to assist with gastric emptying (because there is total denervation of the stomach). Some patients experience problems with feeling of fullness, dumping syndrome, diarrhea, and gastritis. |
| Truncal vagotomy | Severs the right and left vagus nerves as they enter the stomach at the distal part of the esophagus | This type of vagotomy is most commonly used to decrease acid secretions and reduce gastric and intestinal motility. Recurrence rate of ulcer is 10%–15%. |
| Selective vagotomy | Severs vagal innervation to the stomach but maintains innervation to the rest of the abdominal organs | |
| Proximal (parietal cell) gastric vagotomy without drainage | Denervates acid-secreting parietal cells but preserves vagal innervation to the gastric antrum and pylorus | No dumping syndrome. No need for drainage procedure. Recurrence rate of ulcer is 10%–15%. |
| Pyloroplasty | A surgical procedure in which a longitudinal incision is made into the pylorus and transversely sutured closed to enlarge the outlet and relax the muscle | Usually accompanies truncal and selective vagotomies, which produce delayed gastric emptying due to decreased innervation. |

*continued >*

## TABLE 37-4 Surgical Procedures for Peptic Ulcer Disease (Continued)

| Operation | Description | Comments |
|---|---|---|
| **Antrectomy**<br>Billroth I (Gastroduodenostomy) | Removal of the lower portion of the antrum of the stomach (which contains the cells that secrete gastrin) as well as a small portion of the duodenum and pylorus. The remaining segment is anastomosed to the duodenum (Billroth I) | May be performed in conjunction with a truncal vagotomy. The patient may have problems with feeling of fullness, dumping syndrome, and diarrhea. Recurrence rate of ulcer is <1%. |
| Billroth II (Gastrojejunostomy) | Removal of lower portion (antrum) of stomach with anastomosis to jejunum. Dotted lines show portion removed (antrectomy). A duodenal stump remains and is oversewn. | Dumping syndrome, anemia, malabsorption, weight loss. Recurrence rate of ulcer is 10%–15%. |

describe food habits (eg, speed of eating, regularity of meals, preference for spicy foods, use of seasonings, use of caffeinated beverages and decaffeinated coffee). Lifestyle and other habits are a concern as well. Does the patient use irritating substances? For example, does he or she smoke cigarettes? If yes, how many? Does the patient ingest alcohol? If yes, how much and how often? Are NSAIDs used? The nurse inquires about the patient's level of anxiety and his or her perception of current stressors. How does the patient express anger or cope with stressful situations? Is the patient experiencing occupational stress or problems within the family? Is there a family history of ulcer disease?

The nurse assesses the patient's vital signs and reports tachycardia and hypotension, which may indicate anemia from GI bleeding. The stool is tested for occult blood, and a physical examination, including palpation of the abdomen for localized tenderness, is performed.

## Diagnosis

### Nursing Diagnoses

Based on the assessment data, the patient's nursing diagnoses may include the following:

- Acute pain related to the effect of gastric acid secretion on damaged tissue
- Anxiety related to an acute illness
- Imbalanced nutrition related to changes in diet
- Deficient knowledge about prevention of symptoms and management of the condition

## Collaborative Problems/Potential Complications

Potential complications may include the following:

- Hemorrhage
- Perforation
- Penetration
- Pyloric obstruction (gastric outlet obstruction)

## Planning and Goals

The goals for the patient may include relief of pain, reduced anxiety, maintenance of nutritional requirements, knowledge about the management and prevention of ulcer recurrence, and absence of complications.

## Nursing Interventions

### Relieving Pain

Pain relief can be achieved with prescribed medications. The patient should avoid aspirin, foods and beverages that contain caffeine, and decaffeinated coffee. In addition, meals should be eaten at regularly paced intervals in a relaxed setting. Some patients benefit from learning relaxation techniques to help manage stress and pain.

### Reducing Anxiety

The nurse assesses the patient's level of anxiety. Patients with peptic ulcers are usually anxious, but their anxiety is not always obvious. Appropriate information is provided at the patient's level of understanding, all questions are answered, and the patient is encouraged to express fears openly. Explaining diagnostic tests and administering medications as scheduled also help to reduce anxiety. The nurse interacts with the patient in a relaxed manner, helps identify stressors, and explains various coping techniques and relaxation methods, such as biofeedback, hypnosis, or behavior modification. The patient's family is also encouraged to participate in care and to provide emotional support.

### Maintaining Optimal Nutritional Status

The nurse assesses the patient for malnutrition and weight loss. After recovery from an acute phase of peptic ulcer disease, the patient is advised about the importance of complying with the medication regimen and dietary restrictions.

### Monitoring and Managing Potential Complications

#### HEMORRHAGE

Gastritis and hemorrhage from peptic ulcer are the two most common causes of upper GI tract bleeding (which may also occur with esophageal varices, as discussed in Chapter 39). Hemorrhage, the most common complication, occurs in 10% to 20% of patients with peptic ulcers. Bleeding may be manifested by hematemesis or melena (Yamada & Alpers, 2003). The vomited blood can be bright red, or it can have a dark "coffee grounds" appearance from the oxidation of hemoglobin to methemoglobin. When the hemorrhage is large (2000 to 3000 mL), most of the blood is vomited. Because large quantities of blood may be lost quickly, immediate correction of blood loss may be required to prevent hemorrhagic shock. When the hemorrhage is small, much or all of the blood is passed in the stools, which appear tarry black because of the digested hemoglobin. Management depends on the amount of blood lost and the rate of bleeding.

The nurse assesses the patient for faintness or dizziness and nausea, which may precede or accompany bleeding. It is important to monitor vital signs frequently and to evaluate the patient for tachycardia, hypotension, and tachypnea. Other nursing interventions include monitoring the hemoglobin and hematocrit, testing the stool for gross or occult blood, and recording hourly urinary output to detect anuria or oliguria (absence of or decreased urine production).

Many times the bleeding from a peptic ulcer stops spontaneously; however, the incidence of recurrent bleeding is high. Because bleeding can be fatal, the cause and severity of the hemorrhage must be identified quickly and the blood loss treated to prevent hemorrhagic shock. Management of upper GI tract bleeding consists of quickly estimating the amount of blood lost and the rate of bleeding, rapidly replacing the blood that has been lost, stopping the bleeding, stabilizing the patient, and diagnosing and treating the cause. Related nursing and collaborative interventions include the following:

- Inserting a peripheral IV line for the infusion of saline or lactated Ringer's solution and blood products. The nurse may need to assist with the placement of a central venous catheter for rapid infusion of large amounts of blood and fluids as well as hemodynamic monitoring. Blood component therapy is initiated if there are signs of shock (eg, tachycardia, sweating, coldness of the extremities).
- Monitoring the hemoglobin and hematocrit to assist in evaluating blood loss
- Inserting an NG tube to distinguish fresh blood from "coffee grounds" material, to aid in the removal of clots and acid, to prevent nausea and vomiting, and to provide a means of monitoring further bleeding
- Administering an NG lavage of saline solution. The temperature of the solution (cold or room temperature) is a topic of controversy (Yamada & Alpers, 2003).
- Inserting an indwelling urinary catheter and monitoring urinary output
- Monitoring vital signs and oxygen saturation and administering oxygen therapy
- Placing the patient in the recumbent position with the legs elevated to prevent hypotension, or placing the patient on the left side to prevent aspiration from vomiting
- Treating hemorrhagic shock (described in Chapter 15)

If bleeding cannot be managed by the measures described, other treatment modalities may be used. Transendoscopic coagulation by laser, heat probe, medication, a sclerosing agent, or a combination of these therapies can halt bleeding and avoid surgical intervention. There is debate regarding how soon endoscopy should be performed. Some clinicians believe endoscopy should be performed within the first 24 hours after hemorrhage has been stabilized. Others believe endoscopy may be performed during acute bleeding, as long as the esophageal or gastric area can be visualized (blood may decrease visibility) (Yamada & Alpers, 2003).

For patients who are unable to undergo surgery, selective embolization may be used. This procedure involves forcing emboli of autologous blood clots with or without Gelfoam (absorbable gelatin sponge) through a catheter in the artery to a point above the bleeding lesion. This procedure is performed by an interventional radiologist.

Rebleeding may occur and often warrants surgical intervention. The nurse monitors the patient carefully so that bleeding can be detected quickly. Signs of bleeding include tachycardia, tachypnea, hypotension, mental confusion, thirst, and oliguria. If bleeding recurs within 48 hours after medical therapy has begun, or if more than 6 to 10 units of blood are required within 24 hours to maintain blood volume, the patient is likely to require surgery. Some physicians recommend surgical intervention if a patient hemorrhages three times. Other criteria for surgery are the patient's age (massive hemorrhaging is three times more likely to be fatal in those older than 60 years of age), a history of chronic duodenal ulcer, and a coincidental gastric ulcer. The area of the ulcer is removed or the bleeding vessels are ligated. Many patients also undergo procedures (eg, vagotomy and pyloroplasty, gastrectomy) aimed at controlling the underlying cause of the ulcers (see Table 37-4).

### PERFORATION AND PENETRATION

Perforation is the erosion of the ulcer through the gastric **serosa** into the peritoneal cavity without warning. It is an abdominal catastrophe and requires immediate surgery. Penetration is erosion of the ulcer through the gastric serosa into adjacent structures such as the pancreas, biliary tract, or gastrohepatic **omentum**. Symptoms of penetration include back and epigastric pain not relieved by medications that were effective in the past. Like perforation, penetration usually requires surgical intervention.

Signs and symptoms of perforation include the following:

- Sudden, severe upper abdominal pain (persisting and increasing in intensity); pain may be referred to the shoulders, especially the right shoulder, because of irritation of the phrenic nerve in the diaphragm
- Vomiting and collapse (fainting)
- Extremely tender and rigid (boardlike) abdomen
- Hypotension and tachycardia, indicating shock

Because chemical peritonitis develops within a few hours after perforation and is followed by bacterial peritonitis, the perforation must be closed as quickly as possible and the abdominal cavity lavaged of stomach or intestinal contents. In select patients, it may be safe and advisable to perform surgery to treat the ulcer disease in addition to suturing the perforation.

Postoperatively, the stomach contents are drained by means of an NG tube. The nurse monitors fluid and electrolyte balance and assesses the patient for localized infection or peritonitis (increased temperature, abdominal pain, paralytic ileus, increased or absent bowel sounds, abdominal distention). Antibiotic therapy is administered parenterally as prescribed.

### PYLORIC OBSTRUCTION

Pyloric obstruction, also called **gastric outlet obstruction** (GOO), occurs when the area distal to the pyloric sphincter becomes scarred and stenosed from spasm or edema or from scar tissue that forms when an ulcer alternately heals and breaks down. The patient may have nausea and vomiting, constipation, epigastric fullness, anorexia, and, later, weight loss.

In treating the patient with pyloric obstruction, the first consideration is to insert an NG tube to decompress the stomach. Confirmation that obstruction is the cause of the discomfort is accomplished by assessing the amount of fluid aspirated from the NG tube. A residual of more than 400 mL strongly suggests obstruction. Usually an upper GI study or endoscopy is performed to confirm pyloric obstruction. Decompression of the stomach and management of extracellular fluid volume and electrolyte balances may improve the patient's condition and avert the need for surgical intervention. A balloon dilation of the pylorus via endoscopy may be beneficial. If the obstruction is unrelieved by medical management, surgery (in the form of a vagotomy and **antrectomy** or gastrojejunostomy and vagotomy) may be required.

## Promoting Home and Community-Based Care

### TEACHING PATIENTS SELF-CARE

The nurse instructs the patient about the factors that will relieve and those that will aggravate the condition (Chart 37-2). The nurse reviews information about medications to be taken at home, including name, dosage, frequency, and possible side effects, stressing the importance of continuing to take medications even after signs and symptoms have decreased or subsided. The nurse instructs the patient to avoid certain medications and foods that exacerbate symptoms as well as substances that have acid-producing potential (eg, alcohol; caffeinated and decaffeinated beverages such as coffee, tea, and colas). It is important to counsel the patient to eat meals at regular times and in a relaxed setting, and to avoid overeating. If relevant, the nurse also informs the patient about the irritant effects of smoking on the ulcer and provides information about smoking cessation programs.

## CHART 37-2

### HOME CARE CHECKLIST • The Patient With Peptic Ulcer Disease

| At the completion of the home care instruction, the patient or caregiver will be able to: | Patient | Caregiver |
|---|---|---|
| • State the medication regimen and importance of complying with medication schedule. | ✔ | ✔ |
| • State dietary restrictions and foods that may exacerbate condition (caffeinated and decaffeinated products, milk). | ✔ | ✔ |
| • Identify smoking cessation groups. | ✔ | |
| • Identify methods to reduce stress. | ✔ | ✔ |
| • State signs and symptoms of complications:<br>Hemorrhage—cool skin, confusion, increased heart rate, labored breathing, blood in stool<br>Penetration and perforation—severe abdominal pain, rigid and tender abdomen, vomiting, elevated temperature, increased heart rate<br>Pyloric obstruction—nausea and vomiting, distended abdomen, abdominal pain | ✔ | ✔ |
| • State need for follow-up medical care. | ✔ | ✔ |

> **NURSING ALERT**
>
> The nurse reviews with the patient and family the signs and symptoms of complications to be reported. These complications include hemorrhage (cool skin, confusion, increased heart rate, labored breathing, and blood in the stool), penetration and perforation (severe abdominal pain, rigid and tender abdomen, vomiting, elevated temperature, and increased heart rate), and pyloric obstruction (nausea, vomiting, distended abdomen, and abdominal pain).

**CONTINUING CARE**

The nurse reinforces the importance of follow-up care for approximately 1 year, the need to report recurrence of symptoms, and the need for treating possible problems that occur after surgery, such as intolerance to dairy products and sweet foods. The nurse also reminds the patient and family of the importance of participating in health promotion activities and recommended health screening.

## Evaluation

### Expected Patient Outcomes

Expected patient outcomes may include the following:

1. Reports freedom from pain between meals
2. Reports feeling less anxiety
3. Complies with therapeutic regimen
   a. Avoids irritating foods and beverages
   b. Eats regularly scheduled meals
   c. Takes medications as prescribed
   d. Uses coping mechanisms to deal with stress
4. Maintains weight
5. Exhibits no complications

# Morbid Obesity

**Morbid obesity** is a term applied to people who are more than two times their ideal body weight or whose body mass index (BMI) exceeds 30 kg/m$^2$ (see Chapter 5). Another definition of morbid obesity is body weight that is more than 100 pounds greater than the ideal body weight (Blackwood, 2004). In the United States, where morbid obesity is a rapidly growing problem, approximately 65% of the people are overweight (O'Brien, Dixon, & Brown, 2004).

Patients with morbid obesity are at higher risk for health complications, such as diabetes, heart disease, stroke, hypertension, gallbladder disease, osteoarthritis, sleep apnea and other breathing problems, and some forms of cancer (uterine, breast, colorectal, kidney, and gallbladder). They frequently suffer from low self-esteem, impaired body image, and depression.

## Medical Management

Conservative management of obesity consists of placing the person on a weight loss diet in conjunction with behavioral modification and exercise; however, dietary and behavioral approaches to obesity have had limited success. Depression may be a contributing factor to weight gain, and treatment of the depression with an antidepressant may be helpful (Appolinario, Bueno, & Coutinho, 2004; Rosmond, 2004).

### Pharmacologic Management

Several medications are approved for obesity, including sibutramine HCl (Meridia) and orlistat (Xenical). Sibutramine decreases appetite by inhibiting the reuptake of serotonin and norepinephrine. Orlistat reduces caloric intake by binding to gastric and pancreatic lipase to prevent digestion of fats. Both medications require a prescription from a licensed health care provider. Sibutramine may increase blood pressure and should not be taken by people with a history of coronary artery disease, angina pectoris, dysrhythmias, or kidney disease; by those taking antidepressants or monoamine oxidase inhibitors; or by pregnant or nursing women. Other side effects of sibutramine may include dry mouth, insomnia, headache, diaphoresis, and increased heart rate. Side effects of orlistat may include increased frequency of bowel movements, gas with oily discharge, decreased food absorption, decreased bile flow, and decreased absorption of some vitamins. A multivitamin is usually recommended for patients taking orlistat. Orlistat should not be taken by pregnant or nursing women.

Unfortunately, these medications rarely result in loss of more than 10% of total body weight (Arterburn, Crane, & Veenstra, 2004). Furthermore, studies are needed to evaluate their long-term efficacy and risks.

## Surgical Management

**Bariatric** surgery, or surgery for morbid obesity, is performed only after other nonsurgical attempts at weight control have failed. Bariatric surgical procedures work by (1) restricting a patient's ability to eat (restrictive procedure), (2) interfering with ingested nutrient absorption (malabsorptive procedures), or both. Different bariatric surgical procedures entail different lifestyle modifications, and patients must be well informed about the specific lifestyle changes, eating habits, and bowel habits that may result from a particular procedure. Recent studies have shown that the average weight loss after bariatric surgery in the majority of patients is approximately 61% of previous body weight; comorbid conditions such as diabetes mellitus, hypertension, and sleep apnea resolve; and dyslipidemia improves (Buchwald, Avidor, Braunwald, et al., 2004). Although controversial, bariatric surgery has been extended to carefully selected adolescents because of its results in adults (Rosemurgy, 2003).

Patient selection is critical, and the preliminary process may necessitate 6 to 12 months of counseling, education, and evaluation by a multidisciplinary team, including social workers, dietitians, a nurse counselor, psychologist or psychiatrist, as well as a surgeon (Chart 37-3). Because bariatric surgery involves such a drastic change in the functioning of the digestive system, patients need extensive counseling before and after the surgery. Guidelines have been developed to assist physicians and nurses in the care of patients having bariatric surgery (AORN Bariatric Surgery Guideline, 2004). After bariatric surgery, all patients require lifelong monitoring of weight loss, comorbidities, metabolic and nutritional status, and dietary and activity behaviors because they are at risk for developing malnutrition or weight gain (Ferraro, 2004). Women of childbearing age who have bariatric surgery are advised to use contraceptives for approximately 2 years after surgery to avoid pregnancy until their weight stabilizes.

The first surgical procedure used to treat morbid obesity was jejunoileal bypass. This procedure, which resulted in significant complications, has been largely replaced by gastric restriction procedures. Roux-en-Y gastric bypass, gastric banding, vertical-banded gastroplasty, and biliopancreatic diversion with duodenal switch are the current procedures of choice. These procedures may be performed by laparoscopy or by an open surgical technique.

The Roux-en-Y gastric bypass is recommended for long-term weight loss. It is a combined restrictive and malabsorptive procedure. In this procedure, a small pouch (20 to 30 mL) is isolated from the rest of the stomach by a horizontal row of staples across the fundus of the stomach. The jejunum is divided distal to the **ligament of Treitz**. The distal end of the jejunum is anastomosed to the new pouch and the other open end of the jejunum is reanastomosed to the lower jejunum (Fig. 37-3A).

Gastric banding and vertical-banded gastroplasty are restrictive procedures. Gastric banding uses a prosthetic device to restrict oral intake by creating a small pouch of 10 to 15 mL at the fundus of the stomach. This small gastric pouch then empties through the narrow outlet to the remainder of the stomach. During laparoscopic adjustable gastric banding, a silicone band is placed around the upper stomach, and the band is connected by a catheter to a subcutaneous reservoir into which saline solution can be injected to adjust the diameter of the band (see Fig. 37-3B). Vertical-banded gastroplasty involves placement of a vertical row of staples along the lesser curvature of the stomach, creating a new, small (10 to 15 mL) gastric pouch (see Fig. 37-3C).

Biliopancreatic diversion with duodenal switch combines gastric restriction with intestinal malabsorption. Half of the stomach is removed to create a small pouch that can hold about 60 mL. The entire jejunum is excluded from the rest of the GI tract to create a shorter small intestine to absorb fewer calories. The duodenum is disconnected, and the end is closed. The small bowel (ileum) is divided approximately 300 cm above the ileocecal junction, and the

---

**CHART 37-3**

### Factors Considered in the Selection of Patients for Bariatric Surgery

- Body weight
  - Body weight ≥ 45 kg/m² or 100% above ideal weight
  - BMI > 40 kg/m²
  - BMI > 35 kg/m² with medical comorbidities (eg, severe sleep apnea, hypertension, cardiomyopathy related to obesity, severe diabetes mellitus; serious musculoskeletal or neurologic disorders)
- Long-standing history of obesity
- Failure of multiple nonsurgical attempts to lose weight
- Absence of endocrine disorders that cause morbid obesity
- Psychological stability
  - Absence of alcohol and drug use
  - Understanding of how surgery causes weight loss
  - Realization that surgery itself does not guarantee good results
  - Ability to comply with dietary and behavioral changes as recommended by the weight management team

Source: National Institutes of Health Publication No. 98-4083, 1998: *Society of American Gastrointestinal Endoscopic Surgeons (SAGES) guidelines for laparoscopic and conventional surgical treatment of morbid obesity*, May 2000; and American Society for Bariatric Surgery, 2001.

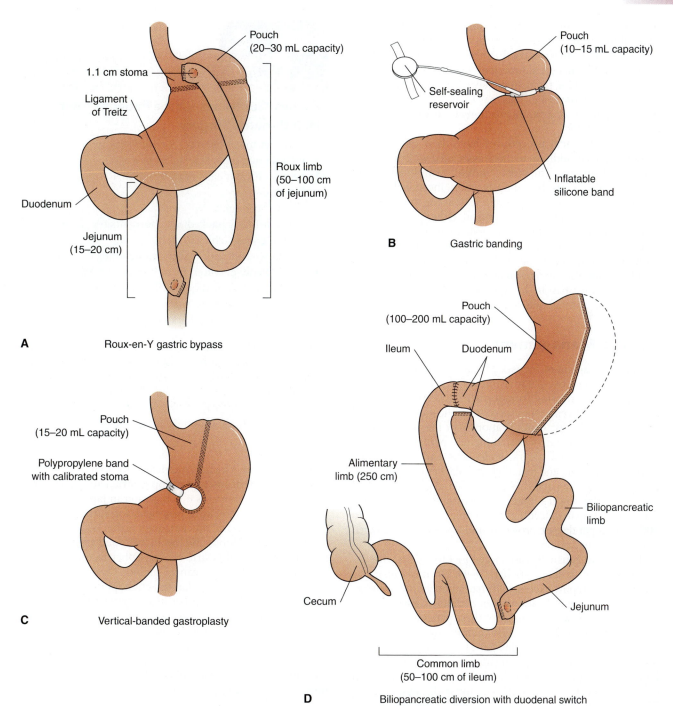

**FIGURE 37-3.** Surgical procedures for morbid obesity. (**A**) Roux-en-Y gastric bypass. A horizontal row of staples across the fundus of the stomach creates a pouch with a capacity of 20 to 30 mL. The jejunum is divided distal to the ligament of Trietz and the distal end is anastomosed to the new pouch. The proximal segment is anastomosed to the jejunum. (**B**) Gastric banding. A prosthetic device is used to restrict oral intake by creating a small pouch of 10 to 15 mL that empties through the narrow outlet into the remainder of the stomach. (**C**) Vertical-banded gastroplasty. A vertical row of staples along the lesser curvature of the stomach creates a new, smaller stomach pouch of 10 to 15 mL. (**D**) Biliopancreatic diversion with duodenal switch. Half of the stomach is removed, leaving a small area that holds about 60 mL. The entire jejunum is excluded from the rest of the GI tract. The duodenum is disconnected and sealed off. The ileum is divided above the ileocecal junction and the distal end of the jejunum is anastomosed to the first portion of the duodenum. The distal end of the biliopancreatic limb is anastomosed to the ileum.

distal end of the ileum is anastomosed to the first portion of the duodenum. The distal end of the jejunum (biliopancreatic limb) is anastomosed to the ileum 50 to 100 cm proximal to the ileocecal junction (see Fig. 37-3D).

After weight loss, the patient may need surgical intervention for body contouring. This may include lipoplasty to remove fat deposits or a panniculectomy to remove excess abdominal skinfolds.

Bariatric surgical procedures have their own unique complications in addition to those associated with any major abdominal surgery. The most common complications are bleeding, blood clots, bowel obstruction, incisional or ventral hernias, and infection from a leak at the anastomosis. Prevention of complications is critical. Other postoperative problems that may occur include nausea, usually as a result of overfilling the stomach pouch or improper chewing; dumping syndrome associated with the consumption of simple sugars; and changes in bowel function, including diarrhea and constipation. Long-term complications that are related to nutritional deficiency may occur.

## Nursing Management

Nursing management focuses on care of the patient after surgery. General postoperative nursing care is similar to that for a patient recovering from a gastric resection, but with great attention given to the risks of complications associated with morbid obesity. Complications that may occur in the immediate postoperative period include peritonitis, stomal obstruction, stomal ulcers, atelectasis and pneumonia, thromboembolism, and metabolic imbalances resulting from prolonged vomiting and diarrhea or altered gastrointestinal function. After bowel sounds have returned and oral intake is resumed, six small feedings consisting of a total of 600 to 800 calories per day are provided, and fluids are encouraged to prevent dehydration.

The patient is usually discharged in 4 to 5 days with detailed dietary instructions (Chart 37-4). The nurse instructs the patient to report excessive thirst or concentrated urine, both of which are indications of dehydration. Psychosocial interventions are also essential for these patients. Efforts are directed at helping them modify their eating behaviors and cope with changes in body image. The nurse explains that noncompliance by eating too much or too fast or eating high-calorie liquids and soft foods results in vomiting and painful esophageal distention. The nurse discusses dietary instructions before discharge and emphasizes the importance of routine follow-up outpatient appointments. Long-term side effects may include increased risk of gallstones, nutritional deficiencies, and potential to regain weight.

## Gastric Cancer

The incidence of gastric or stomach cancer continues to decrease in the United States; however, it still accounts for almost 12,000 deaths annually (American Cancer Society, 2005). The typical patient with gastric cancer is between 40 and 70 years of age, but gastric cancer can occur in people younger than 40 years of age. Men have a higher incidence of gastric cancer than women. Native Americans, Hispanic Americans, and African Americans are twice as likely as Caucasian Americans to develop gastric cancer. The incidence of gastric cancer is much greater in Japan, which has instituted mass screening programs for earlier diagnosis. Diet appears to be a significant factor: a diet high in smoked, salted, or pickled foods and low in fruits and vegetables may increase the risk of gastric cancer. Other factors related to the incidence of gastric cancer include chronic inflammation of the stomach, *H. pylori* infection, pernicious anemia, smoking, achlorhydria, gastric ulcers, previous subtotal gastrectomy (more than 20 years ago), and genetics. The prognosis is generally poor: the diagnosis is usually made late because most patients are asymptomatic during the early stages of the disease. Most cases of gastric cancer are discovered only after local invasion has advanced or metastases are present (Layke & Lopez, 2004).

### Pathophysiology

Most gastric cancers are adenocarcinomas; they can occur anywhere in the stomach. The tumor infiltrates the surrounding mucosa, penetrating the wall of the stomach and adjacent organs and structures. The liver, pancreas, esophagus, and duodenum are often affected at the time of diagnosis. Metastasis through lymph to the peritoneal cavity occurs later in the disease.

### Clinical Manifestations

Symptoms of early disease, such as pain relieved by antacids, resemble those of benign ulcers and are seldom definitive,

### CHART 37-4

### Patient Education

**Dietary Guidelines for the Patient Who Has Had Bariatric Surgery**

- Eat three meals per day (containing protein and fiber).
- Include two protein snacks per day.
- Restrict total meal size to less than 1 cup.
- Eat slowly.
- Chew thoroughly.
- Eat only foods packed with nutrients (eg, peanut butter, cheese, chicken, fish, beans).
- Do not eat and drink at the same time.
- Drink plenty of water, from 90 minutes after each meal to 15 minutes before the next meal.
- Avoid liquid calories, such as alcoholic beverages, fruit drinks, and regular soda (cola).
- Walk for at least 30 minutes per day.

From Favretti, F., O'Brien, P. E., & Dixon, J. B. (2002). Patient management after LAP-BAND placement. *American Journal of Surgery, 184*(6B), 38S–41S, and Ferraro, D. R. (2003). Laparoscopic adjustable gastric banding for morbid obesity. *AORN Journal, 77*(5), 923–940.

because most gastric tumors begin on the lesser curvature of the stomach, where they cause little disturbance of gastric function. Symptoms of progressive disease include dyspepsia (indigestion), early satiety, weight loss, abdominal pain just above the umbilicus, loss or decrease in appetite, bloating after meals, nausea and vomiting, and symptoms similar to those of peptic ulcer disease.

## Assessment and Diagnostic Findings

Usually the physical examination is not helpful in detecting the cancer because most early gastric tumors are not palpable. Advanced gastric cancer may be palpable as a mass. Ascites and hepatomegaly (enlarged liver) may be apparent if the cancer cells have metastasized to the liver. Palpable nodules around the umbilicus, called Sister Mary Joseph's nodule, are a sign of a GI malignancy, usually a gastric cancer. Esophagogastroduodenoscopy for biopsy and cytologic washings is the diagnostic study of choice, and a barium x-ray examination of the upper GI tract may also be performed. Endoscopic ultrasound is an important tool to assess tumor depth and any lymph node involvement. Computed tomography (CT) completes the diagnostic studies, particularly to assess for surgical resectability of the tumor before surgery is scheduled. CT of the chest, abdomen, and pelvis is valuable in staging gastric cancer because it determines the existence of metastases.

## Medical Management

There is no successful treatment for gastric carcinoma except removal of the tumor. If the tumor can be removed while it is still localized to the stomach, the patient may be cured. If the tumor has spread beyond the area that can be excised, cure is less likely. In many patients, effective palliation to prevent discomfort caused by obstruction or dysphagia may be obtained by resection of the tumor (see Gastric Surgery). A diagnostic laparoscopy may be the initial surgical approach to evaluate the gastric tumor, obtain tissue for pathologic diagnosis, and detect metastasis. The patient with a tumor that is deemed resectable would undergo an open surgical procedure to resect the tumor and appropriate lymph nodes. The patient with an unresectable tumor and advanced disease would undergo chemotherapy. Palliative rather than radical surgery may be performed if there is metastasis to other vital organs, such as the liver.

A total gastrectomy may be performed for a resectable cancer in the midportion or body of the stomach. The entire stomach is removed along with duodenum, the section of esophagus attached to the stomach, supporting mesentery, and lymph nodes. Reconstruction of the GI tract is performed by anastomosing the end of the jejunum to the end of the esophagus, a procedure called an esophagojejunostomy.

A radical subtotal gastrectomy is performed for a resectable tumor in the middle and distal portions of the stomach. A Billroth I or Billroth II operation (see Table 37-4) is performed. The Billroth I involves a limited resection and offers a lower cure rate than the Billroth II. The Billroth II procedure is a wider resection that involves removing approximately 75% of the stomach and decreases the possibility of lymph node spread or metastatic recurrence.

A proximal subtotal gastrectomy may be performed for a resectable tumor located in the proximal portion of the stomach or cardia. A total gastrectomy or an esophagogastrectomy is usually performed in place of this procedure to achieve a more extensive resection. A palliative surgical procedure may be required for patients with gastric cancer to achieve a better quality of life.

Common problems of advanced gastric cancer that often require surgery include pyloric obstruction, bleeding, and severe pain. Gastric perforation is an emergency situation requiring surgical intervention. A gastric resection may be the most effective palliative procedure for advanced gastric cancer. Palliative procedures such as gastric or esophageal bypass, gastrostomy, or jejunostomy may temporarily alleviate symptoms such as nausea and vomiting.

If surgical treatment does not offer cure, treatment with chemotherapy may offer further control of the disease or palliation. Commonly used single-agent chemotherapeutic medications include 5-fluorouracil (5-FU), cisplatin, doxorubicin (Adriamycin), etoposide, and mitomycin-C. For improved response rates it is more common to administer combination therapy, primarily 5-FU–based therapy, with other agents. Studies are being conducted to assess the use of chemotherapy before surgery. Radiation therapy is mainly used for palliation in patients with obstruction, GI bleeding secondary to tumor, and significant pain. Assessment of tumor markers (blood analysis for antigens indicative of cancer) such as carcinoembryonic antigen (CEA), carbohydrate antigen (CA 19-9), and CA 50 may help determine the effectiveness of treatment. If these values were elevated before treatment, they should decrease if the tumor is responding to the treatment (Mihmanli, Dilege, Demir, et al., 2004).

## Nursing Process

### The Patient With Gastric Cancer

#### Assessment

The nurse obtains a dietary history from the patient, focusing on recent nutritional intake and status. Has the patient lost weight? If so, how much and over what period of time? Can the patient tolerate a full diet? If not, what foods can he or she eat? What other changes in eating habits have occurred? Does the patient have an appetite? Does the patient feel full after eating a small amount of food? Is the patient in pain? Do foods, antacids, or medications relieve the pain, make no difference, or worsen the pain? Is there a history of infection with *H. pylori*? Other health information to obtain includes the patient's smoking and alcohol history and family history (eg, any first- or second-degree relatives with gastric or other cancer). A psychosocial assessment, including questions about social support, individual and family coping skills, and financial resources, helps the nurse plan for care in acute and community settings.

After the interview, the nurse performs a complete physical examination, carefully assesses the patient's abdomen for tenderness or masses, as well as palpates and percusses the abdomen to detect ascites.

## Nursing Diagnosis

Based on the assessment data, the patient's major nursing diagnoses may include the following:

- Anxiety related to the disease and anticipated treatment
- Imbalanced nutrition, less than body requirements, related to early satiety or anorexia
- Pain related to tumor mass
- Anticipatory grieving related to the diagnosis of cancer
- Deficient knowledge regarding self-care activities

## Planning and Goals

The major goals for the patient may include reduced anxiety, optimal nutrition, relief of pain, and adjustment to the diagnosis and anticipated lifestyle changes.

## Nursing Interventions

### Reducing Anxiety

A relaxed, nonthreatening atmosphere is provided so the patient can express fears, concerns, and possibly anger about the diagnosis and prognosis. The nurse encourages the family or significant other to support the patient, offering reassurance and supporting positive coping measures. The nurse advises the patient about any procedures and treatments so that the patient knows what to expect. The nurse also may suggest talking with a support person (eg, social worker, spiritual advisor), if the patient desires.

### Promoting Optimal Nutrition

The nurse encourages the patient to eat small, frequent portions of nonirritating foods to decrease gastric irritation. Food supplements should be high in calories, as well as vitamins A and C and iron, to enhance tissue repair. If the patient is unable to eat adequately prior to surgery to meet nutritional requirements, parenteral nutrition may be necessary. Because the patient may develop dumping syndrome when enteral feeding resumes after gastric resection, the nurse explains ways to prevent and manage it (six small feedings daily that are low in carbohydrates and sugar; fluids between meals rather than with meals) and informs the patient that symptoms often resolve after several months. If a total gastrectomy is performed, injection of vitamin $B_{12}$ will be required for life, because dietary vitamin $B_{12}$ is absorbed in the stomach. The nurse monitors the IV therapy and nutritional status and records intake, output, and daily weights to ensure that the patient is maintaining or gaining weight. The nurse assesses for signs of dehydration (thirst, dry mucous membranes, poor skin turgor, tachycardia, decreased urine output) and reviews the results of daily laboratory studies to note any metabolic abnormalities (sodium, potassium, glucose, blood urea nitrogen). Antiemetics are administered as prescribed.

### Relieving Pain

The nurse administers analgesics as prescribed. A continuous IV infusion of an opioid may be necessary for postoperative or severe pain. The nurse routinely assesses the frequency, intensity, and duration of the pain to determine the effectiveness of the analgesic. The nurse works with the patient to help manage pain by suggesting nonpharmacologic methods for pain relief, such as position changes, imagery, distraction, relaxation exercises (using relaxation audiotapes), backrubs, massage, and periods of rest and relaxation.

### Providing Psychosocial Support

The nurse helps the patient express fears, concerns, and grief about the diagnosis. It is important to answer the patient's questions honestly and to encourage the patient to participate in treatment decisions. Some patients mourn the loss of a body part and perceive their surgery as a type of mutilation. Some express disbelief and need time and support to accept the diagnosis.

The nurse offers emotional support and involves family members and significant others whenever possible. This includes recognizing mood swings and defense mechanisms (eg, denial, rationalization, displacement, regression) and reassuring the patient, family members, and significant others that emotional responses are normal and expected. The services of clergy, psychiatric clinical nurse specialists, psychologists, social workers, and psychiatrists are made available, if needed. The nurse projects an empathetic attitude and spends time with the patient. Many patients may begin to participate in self-care activities after they have acknowledged their loss.

### Promoting Home and Community-Based Care

#### TEACHING PATIENTS SELF-CARE

Self-care activities depend on the type of treatments used—surgery, chemotherapy, radiation, or palliative care. Patient and family teaching will include information about diet and nutrition, treatment regimens, activity and lifestyle changes, pain management, and possible complications (Chart 37-5). Consultation with a dietitian is essential to determine how the patient's nutritional needs can best be met at home. The nurse teaches the patient or caregiver about administration of enteral or parenteral nutrition. If chemotherapy or radiation is prescribed, the nurse provides explanations to the patient and family about what to expect, including the length of treatments, the expected side effects (eg, nausea, vomiting, anorexia, fatigue, neutropenia), and the need for transportation

## CHART 37-5

### HOME CARE CHECKLIST • The Patient With Gastric Cancer

At the completion of the home care instruction, the patient or caregiver will be able to:

| | Patient | Caregiver |
|---|:---:|:---:|
| • Demonstrate safe management of enteral or parenteral feedings, if applicable. | ✔ | ✔ |
| • Describe dietary restrictions. | ✔ | ✔ |
| • Identify potential side effects of chemotherapy or radiation therapy, if applicable | ✔ | ✔ |
| • Identify signs and symptoms of wound infection. | ✔ | ✔ |
| • State signs and symptoms of obstruction or perforation. | ✔ | ✔ |
| • Describe follow-up needs. | ✔ | ✔ |
| • Make decisions about end-of-life care as appropriate. | ✔ | ✔ |

to appointments for treatment. Psychological counseling may also be helpful.

**CONTINUING CARE**

The need for ongoing care in the home depends on the patient's condition and treatment. The home care nurse reinforces nutritional counseling and supervises the administration of any enteral or parenteral feedings; the patient or caregiver must become skillful in administering the feedings and in detecting and preventing untoward effects or complications related to the feedings (see Chapter 36 to review management of enteral and parenteral feedings). The nurse teaches the patient or a caregiver to record the patient's daily intake, output, and weight and explains strategies to manage pain, nausea, vomiting, or other symptoms. The nurse also teaches the patient or caregiver to recognize and report signs and symptoms of complications that require immediate attention, such as bleeding, obstruction, perforation, or any symptoms that become progressively worse. It is important to explain the chemotherapy or radiation therapy regimen. The patient and family or significant other need to understand the care that will be needed during and after treatments (see Chapter 16). Because the prognosis for gastric cancer is poor, the nurse may need to assist the patient, the family, or significant other with decisions regarding end-of-life care and make referrals as warranted.

## Evaluation

### Expected Patient Outcomes

Expected patient outcomes may include the following:

1. Reports less anxiety
   a. Expresses fears and concerns about surgery
   b. Seeks emotional support
2. Attains optimal nutrition
   a. Eats small, frequent meals high in calories, iron, and vitamins A and C
   b. Complies with enteral or parenteral nutrition as needed
3. Has decreased pain
4. Performs self-care activities and adjusts to lifestyle changes
   a. Resumes normal activities within 3 months
   b. Alternates periods of rest and activity
   c. Manages enteral feedings
5. Prepares for the dying process
   a. Acknowledges disease process
   b. Reports control of symptoms
   c. Verbalizes fears and concerns about dying; involves family/caregiver in discussions
   d. Completes advance directives, and other appropriate documents

## Gastric Surgery

Gastric surgery may be performed on patients with peptic ulcers who have life-threatening hemorrhage, obstruction, perforation, or penetration or whose condition does not respond to medication. It also may be indicated for patients with gastric cancer or trauma. Surgical procedures include a vagotomy and **pyloroplasty** (transecting nerves that stimulate acid secretion and opening the pylorus), a partial gastrectomy, or a total gastrectomy (see Table 37-4).

### ▶▶ Nursing Process

## The Patient Undergoing Gastric Surgery

### Assessment

Before surgery, the nurse assesses the patient's and family's knowledge of preoperative and postoperative surgical routines and the rationale for surgery. The nurse also assesses the patient's nutritional status: Has the patient lost weight? How much? Over how much time? Does the patient have nausea and vomiting? Has the patient had hematemesis? The nurse assesses for the presence of bowel sounds and palpates the abdomen to detect masses or tenderness.

After surgery, the nurse assesses the patient for complications secondary to the surgical intervention, such as hemorrhage, infection, abdominal distention, atelectasis, or impaired nutritional status (see Chapters 20 and 25).

## Diagnosis

### Nursing Diagnoses

Based on the assessment data, the patient's major nursing diagnoses may include the following:

- Anxiety related to surgical intervention
- Acute pain related to surgical incision
- Deficient knowledge about surgical procedure and postoperative course
- Imbalanced nutrition, less than body requirements, related to poor nutrition before surgery and altered GI system after surgery

### Collaborative Problems/ Potential Complications

In addition to the complications to which all postoperative patients are subject, the patient undergoing gastric surgery is at increased risk for:

- Hemorrhage
- Dietary deficiencies
- Bile reflux
- Dumping syndrome

## Planning and Goals

The major goals for the patient undergoing gastric surgery may include reduced anxiety, increased knowledge and understanding about the surgical procedure and postoperative course, optimal nutrition and management of the complications that can interfere with nutrition, relief of pain, avoidance of hemorrhage and steatorrhea, and enhanced self-care skills at home. General postoperative care guidelines for the patient who has received general anesthesia, as discussed in Chapter 20, should be followed.

## Nursing Interventions

### Reducing Anxiety

An important part of the preoperative nursing care involves allaying the patient's fears and anxieties about the impending surgery and its implications. The nurse encourages the patient to verbalize fears and concerns and answers the patient's and family's questions. If the patient has an acute obstruction, a perforated bowel, or an active GI hemorrhage, adequate psychological preparation may not be possible. In this event, the nurse caring for the patient after surgery should anticipate the concerns, fears, and questions that are likely to surface and should be available for support and further explanations.

### Relieving Pain

After surgery, analgesics may be administered as prescribed to relieve pain and discomfort. It is important to provide adequate pain relief so the patient can perform pulmonary care activities (deep breathing and coughing) and leg exercises, turn from side to side, and ambulate. The nurse assesses the effectiveness of analgesic intervention and consults with other members of the health care team if pain is not adequately controlled. Positioning the patient in Fowler's position promotes comfort and allows emptying of the stomach after gastric surgery.

The nurse maintains functioning of the NG tube to prevent distention and secures the tube to prevent dislocation, which may result in increased pain and tension on the suture line. Normally, the amount of NG drainage after a total gastrectomy is minimal, as there is no reservoir where secretions can collect.

### Increasing Knowledge

The nurse explains routine preoperative and postoperative procedures to the patient, which include preoperative medications, NG intubation, IV fluids, abdominal dressings, the possible need for a feeding tube, pain management, and pulmonary care. These explanations need to be reinforced after surgery, especially if the patient had emergency surgery.

### Resuming Enteral Intake

The patient's nutritional status is evaluated before surgery. If surgery is performed for gastric cancer, the patient is often malnourished and may require preoperative enteral or, more often, parenteral nutrition (see Chapter 36). After surgery, parenteral nutrition may be continued to meet caloric needs, to replace fluids lost through drainage and vomiting, and to support the patient metabolically until oral intake is adequate.

After the return of bowel sounds and removal of the NG tube, the nurse may give fluids, followed by food in small portions. Foods are gradually added until the patient is able to eat six small meals a day and drink 120 mL of fluid between meals. The key to increasing the dietary content is to offer food and fluids gradually as tolerated and to recognize that each patient's tolerance is different.

### Recognizing Obstacles to Adequate Nutrition

#### DYSPHAGIA AND GASTRIC RETENTION
Dysphagia may occur in patients who have had a truncal vagotomy, a surgical procedure that may result in trauma to the lower esophagus. Gastric retention may be evidenced by abdominal distention, nau-

## NURSING RESEARCH PROFILE

### Assessment of Life After Gastric Surgery

Hicks, F. D., & Spector, N. M. (2004). The Life After Gastric Surgery Index—Conceptual basis and initial psychometric assessment. *Gastroenterology Nursing, 27*(2), 50–54.

**Purpose**
The purpose of this methodological study was to better understand the influence of postoperative symptoms on a person's life. The researchers developed the Life After Gastric Surgery Index (LAGSI) to assist health care providers in assessing the frequency, intensity, or bothersomeness of symptoms that may occur after gastrointestinal surgery.

**Design**
Initial development and testing of the LAGSI was undertaken to estimate the tool's reliability and validity. In the first version, only a scale that assessed the frequency of symptoms made up the survey, and it was administered to a sample of 27 people who had either a total gastrectomy or a Roux-en-Y procedure. In the second version, severity and bothersomeness dimensions were added to the scale, and it was administered to 36 people participating in a study examining life satisfaction and health-related quality of life after gastroesophageal surgery for cancer. A total of 92 LAGSI surveys were then mailed to subjects identified from a cancer data bank of a Midwestern medical center. Thirty-six of the indexes were returned (39% return rate). Participants also completed the Gastrointestinal Quality of Life Index (GQLI), an instrument designed to measure disease-specific aspects of quality of life in persons with general gastrointestinal conditions, and the Cantril Life Satisfaction Ladder, an instrument designed to measure general life satisfaction. The following psychometric analyses were conducted: estimation of internal consistency reliability (Cronbach's alpha) of each of the scales, and determination of inter-item, item-to-item, and scale-to-scale correlations. Validity was examined by correlating the scores on the LAGSI with those of the GQLI and with the Cantril Life Satisfaction Ladder.

**Findings**
Internal consistency reliability for the LAGSI was determined to be acceptable for a new tool, at 0.87 for the frequency scale and 0.90 for both the severity scale and the bothersomeness scale. Likewise, the validity of the tool was determined to be acceptable, with positive correlations with the GQLI and the Cantril Life Satisfaction Ladder. The LAGSI shares common characteristics with these other valid and reliable tools, and it also appears to measure different underlying constructs, namely frequency, severity, and bothersomeness. However, sample sizes were small, and further study is needed.

**Nursing Implications**
The LASGI is only one page in length, is easily understandable, and is easily administered and scored. The instrument allows for multidimensional assessment of significant gastrointestinal symptoms in patients who have undergone gastric surgery. This assessment could help understand the symptoms that patients are experiencing and how these symptoms are affecting their quality of life. This could in turn suggest nursing interventions that would be most appropriate and helpful for patients.

---

sea, and vomiting. Regurgitation may also occur if the patient has eaten too much or too quickly. It also may indicate that edema along the suture line is preventing fluids and food from moving into the intestinal tract. If gastric retention occurs, it may be necessary to reinstate NPO status and NG suction; pressure must be low in the remaining portion of the stomach to avoid disrupting the sutures.

### BILE REFLUX
Bile reflux gastritis and esophagitis may occur with the removal of the pylorus, which acts as a barrier to the reflux of duodenal contents. Burning epigastric pain and vomiting of bilious material manifest this condition. Eating or vomiting does not relieve the situation. Agents that bind with bile acid, such as cholestyramine (Questran), may be helpful. Aluminum hydroxide gel (an antacid) and metoclopramide hydrochloride (Reglan) have been used with limited success.

### DUMPING SYNDROME
**Dumping syndrome** is an unpleasant set of vasomotor and GI symptoms that sometimes occur in patients who have had gastric surgery or a form of vagotomy. It may be the mechanical result of surgery in which a small gastric remnant is connected to the jejunum through a large opening. Foods high in carbohydrates and electrolytes must be diluted in the jejunum before absorption can take place, but the passage of food from the stomach remnant into the jejunum is too rapid to allow this to happen. The hypertonic intestinal contents draw extracellular fluid from the circulating blood volume into the jejunum to dilute the high concentration of electrolytes and sugars. The ingestion of fluid at mealtime is another factor that causes the stomach contents to empty rapidly into the jejunum.

Early symptoms include a sensation of fullness, weakness, faintness, dizziness, palpitations, diaphoresis, cramping pains, and diarrhea. These symptoms resolve once the intestine has been evacuated. Later, there is a rapid elevation of blood glucose, followed by increased insulin secretion. This results in a reactive hypoglycemia, which also is unpleasant for the patient. Vasomotor symptoms that occur 10 to 90 minutes after eating are pallor, perspiration, palpitations, headache, and feelings of warmth, dizziness, and even drowsiness. Anorexia may also be a result of the dumping syndrome, as the person may be reluctant to eat.

Steatorrhea also may occur in the patient with gastric surgery. It is partially the result of rapid gastric emptying, which prevents adequate mixing with pancreatic and biliary secretions. In mild cases, reducing the intake of fat and administering an antimotility medication (eg, loperamide [Imodium]) may control steatorrhea.

**VITAMIN AND MINERAL DEFICIENCIES**

Other dietary deficiencies that the nurse should be aware of include malabsorption of organic iron, which may require supplementation with oral or parenteral iron, and a low serum level of vitamin $B_{12}$, which may require supplementation by the intramuscular route. Total gastrectomy results in lack of intrinsic factor, a gastric secretion required for the absorption of vitamin $B_{12}$ from the GI tract. Unless this vitamin is supplied by parenteral injection after gastrectomy, the patient inevitably will suffer vitamin $B_{12}$ deficiency, which eventually leads to a condition identical to pernicious anemia. All manifestations of pernicious anemia, including macrocytic anemia and combined system disease (neurologic disorders of the central and peripheral nervous systems), may be expected to develop within a period of 5 years or less; they progress in severity thereafter and, in the absence of therapy, are fatal. This complication is avoided by the regular monthly intramuscular injection of vitamin $B_{12}$. This regimen should be started without delay after gastrectomy. Weight loss is a common long-term problem because the patient experiences early fullness, which suppresses the appetite.

## Teaching Dietary Self-Management

Because the patient may experience any of the described conditions affecting nutrition, nursing intervention includes proper dietary instruction. The following teaching points are emphasized:

- To delay stomach emptying and dumping syndrome, the patient should assume a low Fowler's position during mealtime, and after the meal the patient should lie down for 20 to 30 minutes.
- Antispasmodics, as prescribed, also may aid in delaying the emptying of the stomach.
- Fluid intake with meals is discouraged; instead, fluids may be consumed up to 1 hour before or 1 hour after mealtime.
- Meals should contain more dry items than liquid items.
- The patient can eat fat as tolerated but should keep carbohydrate intake low and avoid concentrated sources of carbohydrates.
- The patient should eat smaller but more frequent meals.
- Dietary supplements of vitamins and medium-chain triglycerides and injections of vitamin $B_{12}$ and iron may be prescribed.

The nurse also gives instructions regarding enteral or parenteral supplementation if it is needed.

## Monitoring and Managing Potential Complications

Occasionally hemorrhage complicates gastric surgery. The patient has the usual signs of rapid blood loss and shock (see Chapter 15) and may vomit considerable amounts of bright-red blood. The nurse assesses NG drainage for type and amount; some bloody drainage for the first 12 hours is expected, but excessive bleeding should be reported. The nurse also assesses the abdominal dressing for bleeding. Because this situation is upsetting to the patient and family, the nurse should remain calm. The nurse performs emergency measures, such as NG lavage and administration of blood and blood products, along with vigilant hemodynamic monitoring.

## Promoting Home and Community-Based Care

**TEACHING PATIENTS SELF-CARE**

Patient teaching is based on the assessment of the patient's physical and psychological readiness to participate in self-care. The nurse provides information about nutrition, enteral or parenteral nutrition if required, nutritional supplements, pain management, and the symptoms of dumping syndrome and measures to prevent or minimize these symptoms (Chart 37-6). It is important to emphasize the continued need for vitamin $B_{12}$ injections.

**CONTINUING CARE**

The patient and caregivers benefit from a team approach to discharge planning. The team members include the patient and caregiver along with the nurse, physician, dietitian, and social worker. Written or video instructions about meals, activities, medications, and follow-up care are helpful. After the patient is discharged from the hospital, the home care nurse helps with the transition to home by supervising the administration of any enteral or parenteral feedings, emphasizing information about detection and prevention of untoward effects or complications related to feedings. Information about community support groups and end-of-life care is provided to the patient, family, or significant other when indicated.

## Evaluation

### Expected Patient Outcomes

Expected patient outcomes may include:

1. Reports decreased anxiety; expresses fears and concerns about surgery

## CHART 37-6

### HOME CARE CHECKLIST • The Patient With Gastric Resection

At the completion of the home care instruction, the patient or caregiver will be able to:

| | Patient | Caregiver |
|---|:---:|:---:|
| • Demonstrate enteral or parenteral feedings as applicable. | ✔ | ✔ |
| • State necessary dietary changes. | ✔ | ✔ |
| • Use nutritional supplements as appropriate. | ✔ | |
| • Relieve pain with pharmacologic or nonpharmacologic interventions. | ✔ | ✔ |
| • Identify available support groups. | ✔ | ✔ |
| • Explain medication regimen. | ✔ | ✔ |
| • Identify the need for continued vitamin $B_{12}$ injections. | ✔ | ✔ |
| • Identify signs and symptoms of complications. | ✔ | ✔ |
| • State schedule of follow-up appointments. | ✔ | ✔ |

2. Demonstrates knowledge regarding postoperative course by discussing the surgical procedure and postoperative course
3. Attains optimal nutrition
   a. Maintains a reasonable weight
   b. Does not have excessive diarrhea
   c. Tolerates six small meals a day
   d. Does not experience dysphagia, gastric retention, bile reflux, dumping syndrome, or vitamin and mineral deficiencies
4. Attains optimal level of comfort
5. Exhibits no complications

# Duodenal Tumors

Tumors of the duodenum are uncommon and are usually benign and asymptomatic. They are most often discovered at autopsy. Malignant tumors are more likely to cause specific signs and symptoms leading to diagnosis. Unfortunately, malignant tumors are often not discovered until they have metastasized to distant sites. Benign tumors may place patients at an increased risk for malignancy. The relative rarity of tumors of the duodenum and the nonspecific nature of their manifestations complicate their diagnosis and treatment.

## Clinical Manifestations

Duodenal tumors often present insidiously with vague, nonspecific symptoms. Most benign tumors are discovered incidentally on an x-ray study, during surgery, or at autopsy. When the patient is symptomatic, benign tumors often present with intermittent pain. The next most common presentation is occult bleeding. Malignant tumors often result in symptoms that lead to their diagnosis, although these symptoms may reflect advanced disease. Most patients have sustained weight loss and are malnourished at diagnosis. Bleeding and pain are common. Perforation of the bowel occurs in approximately 10% of patients (Kummar, Ciesielski, & Fogarasi, 2002).

## Assessment and Diagnostic Findings

An upper GI x-ray series with small bowel follow-through using oral water-insoluble contrast with frequent and detailed x-rays to follow the contrast through the small bowel is the traditional approach to diagnosis. A more sensitive examination is an **enteroclysis**, in which a nasogastric tube is advanced into the small bowel to a position above the area in question; the area is then studied by single-contrast and double-contrast techniques. Abdominal CT is used to determine the extent of disease outside the lumen of the duodenum.

## Management

Benign tumors of the duodenum include adenomas, lipomas, hemangiomas, and hamartomas (a focal malformation that resembles a neoplasm, but unlike a neoplasm does not result in compression of adjacent tissue). These tumors may be treated endoscopically by excision/resection or electrocautery if the patient is symptomatic. Routine surveillance may be recommended to assess for malignant transformation.

The most common primary malignant tumor of the duodenum is adenocarcinoma; the second and third portions of the duodenum are most often involved. These tumors may present with bleeding or duodenal obstruction. If the tumor is located at the ampulla of Vater, obstructive jaundice is likely. Other rare malignant tumors of the duodenum include carcinoid tumors, lymphoma, and gastrointestinal stromal tumors. Specialized abdominal surgery may be required to remove these rare tumors. Chemotherapy and radiation therapy may also be part of the treatment regimen.

The nursing process related to the care of the patient with a duodenal tumor is similar to that of the patient with gastric cancer. Each patient requires specialized care, astute assessment for complications, prompt interventions, and individualized teaching for self-care.

## Critical Thinking Exercises

1. A 45-year-old woman with a history of rheumatoid arthritis and gastritis related to her medication is admitted with abdominal discomfort, headache, lassitude, and nausea and vomiting. What questions should you ask the patient? What signs should be noted during the physical examination? What diagnostic studies should you anticipate for this patient? Describe your nursing interventions, including teaching. How would you modify teaching for this patient if she does not understand English?

2. **ebp** A 27-year-old morbidly obese woman has tried conservative medical management (weight loss diet, behavior modification, exercise, medications for obesity) of her weight condition. She is scheduled for a vertical-banded gastroplasty. Describe the dietary modifications along with nutritional needs for this patient during the immediate postoperative period, after discharge from the hospital, and for long-term maintenance. What is the evidence base that supports the use of specific dietary modifications to meet her nutritional needs after surgical procedures to treat obesity? Describe the strength of this evidence and identify the criteria used to evaluate the strength of the evidence that supports the appropriateness of the dietary modifications.

3. You are caring for a 60-year-old man who has been diagnosed with gastric cancer and is scheduled for a total gastrectomy. The patient has been reluctant to discuss his diagnosis and proposed surgery. What should you do to prepare your patient for this surgery, both physically and emotionally? What nutritional needs do you anticipate for this patient preoperatively, immediately postoperatively, and after discharge from the hospital?

4. A 54-year-old business executive has been admitted with the diagnosis of peptic ulcer disease. As you enter his room, he is vomiting bright-red blood. What are the nursing interventions for managing and monitoring this complication? If the bleeding cannot be controlled, what invasive measures may need to be performed? How would you prepare your patient for these? What other complications may occur with a peptic ulcer and how should they be managed? What teaching interventions are warranted for this patient?

## REFERENCES AND SELECTED READINGS

### BOOKS

American Cancer Society. (2005). *Cancer facts and figures*. Atlanta: Author.
Cameron, J. L. (Ed.). (2004). *Current surgical therapy*. Philadelphia: Elsevier Mosby.
Cotton, P., & Williams, C. (2003). *Practical gastrointestinal endoscopy*. Massachusetts: Blackwell Publishing Ltd.
DeVita, V. T., Hellman, S., & Rosenberg, S. A. (Eds.). (2004). *Cancer: Principles and practice of oncology* (7th ed.). Philadelphia: Lippincott Williams & Wilkins.
Friedman, S. L., McQuaid, K. R., & Grendell, J. H. (Eds.). (2003). *Current diagnosis and treatment in gastroenterology*. New York: McGraw-Hill.
McEvoy, G. R. (Ed.). (2004). *American Hospital Formulary drug information service*. Bethesda, MD: American Society of Health-System Pharmacists.
Macfadyen, B. V., Arrequi, M. E., Eubanks, S., et al. (Eds.). (2003). *Laparoscopic surgery of the abdomen*. New York: Springer.
National Institutes of Health. (2000). *The practical guide: Identification, evaluation and treatment of overweight and obesity in adults*. Bethesda, MD: National Institutes of Health, National Heart, Lung and Blood Institute and North American Association for the Study of Obesity; 2000. NIH publication 00-4084.
Shelton, B. K., Ziegfeld, C. R., & Olsen, M. M. (Eds.). (2004). *The Sidney Kimmel Comprehensive Cancer Center at Johns Hopkins manual of cancer nursing*. Philadelphia: Lippincott Williams & Wilkins.
U.S. Department of Health and Human Services. (2001). *The Surgeon General's call to action to prevent and decrease overweight and obesity*. Rockville, MD: Author.
Yamada, T., & Alpers, D. H. (2003). *Textbook of gastroenterology*. Philadelphia: Lippincott Williams & Wilkins.
Yarbro, C. H., Frogge, M. H., Goodman, M., et al. (Eds.). (2005). *Cancer nursing: Principles and practice*. Boston: Jones & Bartlett.

### JOURNALS

*Asterisks indicate nursing research articles.

#### Gastric Cancer

Asao, T., Kuwano, H., & Mochiki, E. (2004). Laparoscopic surgery update for gastrointestinal malignancy. *Journal of Gastroenterology, 39*(4), 309–318.
Ba-Ssalamah, A., Prokop, M., Uffmann, M., et al. (2003). Dedicated multidetector CT of the stomach: Spectrum of diseases. *RadioGraphics, 23*(3), 625–644.
Enzinger, P. C., & Mayer, R. J. (2004). Gastrointestinal cancer in older patients. *Seminars in Oncology, 31*(2), 206–219.
Genta, R. M. (2003). The gastritis connection: Prevention and early detection of gastric neoplasms. *Journal of Clinical Gastroenterology, 36*(Suppl. 1), S44–S49.
Gonzalez, C. A., Sala, N., & Capella, G. (2002). Genetic susceptibility and gastric cancer risk. *International Journal of Cancer, 100*(3), 249–260.
Hicks, F. D., & Spector, N. M. (2004). The life after gastric surgery index—Conceptual basis and initial psychometric assessment. *Gastroenterology Nursing, 27*(2), 50–54.
Jemal, A., Murray, T., Ward, E. et al. (2005). Cancer statistics, 2005. *CA: A Cancer Journal for Clinicians, 55*(1), 10–30.
Kelley, J. R., & Duggan, J. M. (2003). Gastric cancer epidemiology and risk factors. *Journal of Clinical Epidemiology, 56*, 1–9.
Layke, J. C., & Lopez, P. P. (2004). Gastric cancer: Diagnosis and treatment options. *American Family Physician, 69*(5), 1133–1146.
Louhimo, J., Kokkola, A., Alfthan, H., et al. (2004). Preoperative hCG beta and CA 72-4 are prognostic factors in gastric cancer. *International Journal of Cancer, 111*(6), 929–933.
Macdonald, J. S. (2004). Treatment of localized gastric cancer. *Seminars in Oncology, 31*(4), 566–573.
Macdonald, J. S. (2004). Clinical overview: Adjuvant therapy of gastrointestinal cancer. *Cancer Chemotherapy and Pharmacology, 54*(Suppl 1), S4–S11.
Mihmanli, M., Dilege, E., Demir, U., et al. (2004). The use of tumor markers as predictors of prognosis in gastric cancer. *Hepatogastroenterology, 51*(9), 1544–1547.
Moreto, M. (2003). Diagnosis of esophagogastric tumors. *Endoscopy, 35*(1), 36–42.

Suerbaum, S., & Michetti, P. (2002). Medical progress: *Helicobacter pylori* infection. *New England Journal of Medicine, 347*(15), 1175–1186.

Ushijima, T., & Sasako, M. (2004). Focus on gastric cancer. *Cancer Cell, 5*(2), 121–125.

Wong, B. C., Lam, S. K., Wong, W. M., et al. (2004). Helicobacter pylori eradication to prevent gastric cancer in a high-risk region of China: A randomized controlled study. *Journal of the American Medical Association, 291*(2), 187–194.

Yasui, W., Oue, N., Ito, R., et al. (2004). Search for new biomarkers of gastric cancer through serial analysis of gene expression and its clinical implications. *Cancer Science, 95*(5), 385–392.

## Morbid Obesity

Abir, F., & Bell, R. (2004). Assessment and management of the obese patient. *Critical Care Medicine, 32*(Suppl)(4), S87–S91.

American Society for Bariatric Surgery. (2001). Rationale for the surgical treatment of morbid obesity. Available at: http://www.asbs.org/html/rationale/rationale.html. Accessed June 29, 2006.

AORN Bariatric Surgery Guideline. (2004). *AORN Journal, 79*(5), 1026–1052.

Appolinario, J. C., Bueno, J. R., & Coutinho, W. (2004). Psychotropic drugs in the treatment of obesity: What promise? *CNS Drugs, 18*(10), 629–651.

Arterburn, D. E., Crane, P. K., & Veenstra, D. L. (2004). The efficacy and safety of sibutramine for weight loss: A systematic review. *Archives of Internal Medicine, 163*(9), 994–1003.

Baltasar, A., Bou, R., Bengochea, M., et al. (2001). Duodenal switch: An effective therapy for morbid obesity: Intermediate results. *Obesity Surgery, 11*(1), 54–58.

Blackwood, H. S. (2004). Obesity: A rapidly expanding challenge. *Nursing Management, 35*(5), 27–36.

Brody, F. (2004). Minimally invasive surgery for morbid obesity. *Cleveland Clinic Journal of Medicine, 71*(4), 289–298.

Brolin, R. E. (2002). Bariatric surgery and long-term control of morbid obesity. *Journal of the American Medical Association, 288*(22), 2793–2796.

Buchwald, H., Avidor, Y., Braunwald, E., et al. (2004). Bariatric surgery: A systematic review and meta-analysis. *Journal of the American Medical Association, 292*(14), 1724–1737.

Chapman, A. E., Kiroff, G., Game, P., et al. (2004). Laparoscopic adjustable gastric banding in the treatment of obesity: A systematic literature review. *Surgery, 135*(3), 326–351.

Choban, P. S., Jackson, B., Poplawski, S., et al. (2002). Bariatric surgery for morbid obesity: Why, who, when, how, where, and what? *Cleveland Clinic Journal of Medicine, 69*(11), 897–903.

Collene, A. L., & Hertzler, S. (2003). Metabolic outcomes of gastric bypass. *Nutrition in Clinical Practice, 18*(2), 136–139.

Cottam, D. R., Mattar, S. G., & Schauer, P. R. (2003). Laparoscopic era of operations for morbid obesity. *Archives of Surgery, 13*(4), 367–375.

Damcott, C. M., Sack, P., & Shuldiner, A. R. (2003). The genetics of obesity. *Endocrinology and Metabolism Clinics of North America, 32*(4), 761–786.

Davidson, J. E., Kruse, M. W., Cox, D. H., et al. (2003). Critical care of the morbidly obese. *Critical Care Nurse Quarterly, 26*(2), 105–116.

Deitel, M., & Shikora, S. (2002). The development of the surgical treatment of morbid obesity. *Journal of the American College of Nutrition, 21*(5), 365–371.

Dressel, A., Kuhn, J. A., & McCarty, T. M. (2004). Laparoscopic Roux-en-Y gastric bypass in morbidly obese patients. *American Journal of Surgery, 187*(2), 230–232.

Elliot, K. (2003). Nutritional considerations after bariatric surgery. *Critical Care Nursing Quarterly, 26*(2), 133–138.

Favretti, F., O'Brien, P. E., & Dixon, J. B. (2002). Patient management after LAP-BAND placement. *American Journal of Surgery, 184*(6B), 38S–41S.

Ferraro, D. R. (2003). Laparoscopic adjustable gastric banding for morbid obesity. *AORN Journal, 77*(5), 923–940.

Ferraro, D. R. (2004). Preparing patients for bariatric surgery: The clinical considerations. *Clinician Reviews, 14*(1), 58–63.

Ferraro, D. R. (2004). Management of the bariatric surgery patient: Lifelong postoperative care. *Clinician Reviews, 14*(2), 74–79.

Fobi, M. A. (2004). Surgical treatment of obesity: A review. *Journal of National Medical Association, 96*(1), 61–75.

Herron, D. M. (2004). The surgical management of severe obesity. *Mount Sinai Journal of Medicine, 71*(1), 63–71.

Hurst, S., Blanco, K., Boyle, D., et al. (2004). Bariatric implications of critical care nursing. *Dimensions of Critical Care Nursing, 23*(2), 76–83.

Jacob, B. P., & Gagner, M. (2003). New developments in gastric bypass procedures and physiologic mechanisms. *Surgical Technology International, 11*, 119–126.

Jones, K. B. (2004). Bariatric surgery—where do we go from here? *International Surgery, 89*(1), 51–57.

Kim, J., Tarnoff, M., & Shikora, S. (2003). Surgical treatment for extreme obesity: evolution of a rapidly growing field. *Nutrition in Clinical Practice, 18*(2), 109–123.

Lamvu, G., Zolnoun, D., Boggess, J., et al. (2004). Obesity: Physiologic changes and challenges during laparoscopy. *American Journal of Obstetrics and Gynecology, 191*(2), 669–674.

Livingston, E. H., & Fink, A. S. (2003). Quality of life: Cost and future of bariatric surgery. *Archives of Surgery, 138*(4), 383–388.

McGohan, L. D., & Caflisch, A. J. (2004). Bariatric surgery. *Journal of Continuing Education in Nursing, 35*(5), 198–199.

Miller, K., & Hell, E. (2003). Laparoscopic surgical concepts of morbid obesity. *Archives of Surgery, 388*(6), 375–384.

Nguyen, N., Goldman, C., Rosenquist, C., et al. (2001). Laparoscopic versus open gastric bypass: A randomized study of outcomes, quality of life, and costs. *Annals of Surgery, 234*(3), 279–899.

O'Brien, P. E., Dixon, J. B., & Brown, W. (2004). Obesity is a surgical disease: Overview of obesity and bariatric surgery. *Australia and New Zealand Journal of Surgery, 74*(4), 200–204.

O'Donnell, K. (2004). Bariatric surgery: Nutritional concerns on the weigh down. *Practical Gastroenterology, 28*(2), 33–46.

Padwal, R., Li, S. K., & Lau, D. C. (2004). Long-term pharmacology for obesity and overweight. *Cochrane Database of Systematic Reviews, 3*, CD004094.

Raftopoulos, I., Ercole, J., Udekwu, A. O., et al. (2005). Outcomes of Roux-en-Y gastric bypass stratified by a body mass index of 70 kg/m$^2$: A comparative analysis of 825 procedures. *Journal of Gastrointestinal Surgery, 9*(1), 44–52.

Rosmond, R. (2004). Obesity and depression: Same disease, different name? *Medical Hypotheses, 62*(6), 976–979.

Rosemurgy, A. S. (2003). What's new in surgery: Gastrointestinal conditions. *Journal of the American College of Surgeons, 197*(5), 792–801.

Sammons, D. (2002). Roux-en-Y gastric bypass. *American Journal of Nursing, 102*(10), 24A–24D.

Schauer, P. R., Ilramuddin, S., Gourash, W., et al. (2000). Outcomes after laparoscopic Roux-en-Y gastric bypass for morbid obesity. *Annals of Surgery, 232*(4), 515–529.

Sjostrom, L., Lindroos, A. K., Petonen, M., et al. (2004). Lifestyle, diabetes, and cardiovascular risk factors 10 years after bariatric surgery. *New England Journal of Medicine, 351*(26), 2683–2693.

Sogg, S., & Mori, D. L. (2004). The Boston interview for gastric bypass: Determining the psychological suitability of surgical candidates. *Obesity Surgery, 14*(3), 370–380.

Ukleja, A., & Stone, R. L. (2004). Medical and gastroenterologic management of the post-bariatric surgery patient. *Journal of Clinical Gastroenterology, 38*(4), 312–321.

Woodward, B. G. (2003). Bariatric surgery options. *Critical Care Nurse Quarterly, 26*(2), 89–100.

## Peptic Ulcers and Gastritis

Aihara, T., Nakamura, E., & Amagase, K. (2003). Pharmacological control of gastric acid secretion for the treatment of acid-related peptic disease: Past, present, and future. *Pharmacology & Therapeutics, 98*(1), 109–127.

Allen, M. E., Kopp, B. J., & Erstad, B. L. (2004). Stress ulcer prophylaxis in the postoperative period. *American Journal of Health System-Pharmacy, 61*(6), 588–596.

Basset, C., Holton, J., Gatta, L., et al. (2004). *Helicobacter pylori* infection: Anything new we should know? *Alimentary Pharmacology & Therapeutics, 20*(Suppl 2), 31–41.

Dore, M. P., & Graham, D. Y. (2004). Ulcers and gastritis. *Endoscopy, 36*(1), 42–47.

Der, G. (2003). An overview of proton pump inhibitors. *Gastroenterology Nursing, 26*(5), 1182–1190.

Ford, A., Delaney, B., Forman, D., et al. (2003). Eradication therapy for peptic ulcer disease in *Helicobacter pylori*-positive patients. *Cochrane Database System Review,* 4:CD003840.

Garnett, W. R. (2003). History of acid suppression: Focus on the hospital setting. *Pharmacotherapy, 23*(10), 56S–60S.

Gene, E., Calvet X., Azagra, R., et al. (2003). Triple vs. quadruple therapy for treating *Helicobacter pylori* infection: A meta-analysis. *Alimentary Pharmacology & Therapeutics, 17*(9), 1137–1143.

Goto, H. (2003). *Helicobacter pylori* and gastric diseases. *Nagoya Journal of Medical Science, 66*(3-4), 77–85.

Greenwald, D. A. (2004). Aging, the gastrointestinal tract, and risk of acid-related disease. *American Journal of Medicine, 117*(Suppl 5A), 8S–13S.

Hawkey, C. J., & Langman, M. J. S. (2002). Non-steroidal anti-inflammatory drugs: Overall risks and management. Complementary roles for COX-2 inhibitors and proton pump inhibitors. *Gut, 52*(4), 600–608.

Hellstrom, P. M., & Vitols, S. (2004). The choice of proton pump inhibitor: Does it matter? *Basic & Clinical Pharmacology & Toxicology, 94*(3), 106–111.

Hirschowitz, B. I. (2003). Usual and unusual causes of duodenal ulcer. *Digestive and Liver Disease, 35*(8), 519–522.

Holtmann, G., & Howden, C. W. (2004). Management of peptic ulcer bleeding: The roles of proton pump inhibitors and *Helicobacter pylori* eradication. *Alimentary Pharmacology & Therapeutics, 19*(Suppl 1), 66–70.

Horton, K. M., & Fishman, E. K. (2003). Current role of CT in imaging of the stomach. *Radiographics, 23*(1), 75–87.

Konturek, S. J., Bielanski, W., Plenka, M., et al. (2003). *Helicobacter pylori* nonsteroidal anti-inflammatory drugs and smoking in risk pattern of gastroduodenal ulcers. *Scandanavian Journal of Gastroenterology, 38*(9), 923–930.

Laine, L. (2003). Gastrointestinal effects of NSAIDs and coxibs. *Journal of Pain and Symptom Management, 25*(2), 32–40.

Laine, L. (2003). The role of proton pump inhibitors in NSAID-associated gastropathy and upper gastrointestinal symptoms. *Reviews in Gastroenterological Disorders, 3*(Suppl 4), S30.

Lehman, F., Hildebrand, P., & Beglinger, C. (2003). New molecular targets for treatment of peptic ulcer disease. *Drugs, 63*(17), 1785–1797.

Meurer, L. N., & Bower, D. J. (2002). Management of *Helicobacter pylori* infection. *American Family Physician, 65*(7), 1327–1336.

Moss, S. F., & Sood, S. (2003). *Helicobacter pylori*. Current Opinions in *Infectious Disease, 16,* 445–451.

Mukherjee, D., Nissen, S. E., & Topol, E. J. (2001). Risk of cardiovascular events associated with selective COX-2 inhibitors. *Journal of the American Medical Association, 286*(8), 954–959.

Robinson, M., & Horn, J. (2004). Clinical pharmacology of proton pump inhibitors: What the practicing physician needs to know. *Drugs, 63*(24), 2739–2754.

Scheiman, J. M. (2003). Gastroduodenal safety of cyclooxygenase-2 inhibitors. *Current Pharmaceutical Design,* (27), 2197–2206.

Sharma, P., & Vakil, N. (2003). *Helicobacter pylori* and reflux disease. *Alimentary Pharmacology & Therapeutics, 17*(3), 297–305.

Spirt, M. J. (2004). Stress-related mucosal disease: Risk factors and prophylactic therapy. *Clinical Therapeutics, 26*(2), 197–213.

Suerbaum, S., & Michetti, P. (2002). *Helicobacter pylori*. New England *Journal of Medicine, 347,* 1175–1186.

Sung, J. J. (2003). The role of acid suppression in the management and prevention of gastrointestinal hemorrhage associated with gastroduodenal ulcers. *Gastroenterology Clinics of North America, 32*(3 Suppl), S11–S23.

Sutton, P., & Doidge, C. (2003). *Helicobacter pylori* vaccines spiral into the new millennium. *Digestive and Liver Disease, 35*(10), 675–687.

Thomopoulos, K. C., Vagenas, K. A., & Vagianos, E. C. (2004). Changes in etiology and clinical outcome of acute upper gastrointestinal bleeding during the last 15 years. *European Journal of Gastroenterology and Hepatology, 16*(2), 177–182.

Tytgat, G. (2000). *Helicobacter pylori*: Past, present and future. *Journal of Gastroenterology and Hepatology, 15*(Suppl.), G30–G33.

Van Rensburg, O. (2004). *Helicobacter pylori* in peptic ulcer disease. *Journal of the South African Dental Association, 59*(8), 334–335.

Wolfe, M. M. (2003). Risk factors associated with the development of gastroduodenal ulcers due to the use of NSAIDs. *International Journal of Clinical Practice Supplement,* (135), 32–37.

Wu, W. K. K., & Cho, C. H. (2004). The pharmacological actions of nicotine on the gastrointestinal tract. *Journal of Pharmacological Sciences, 94*(4), 348–358.

### *Duodenal Tumors*

Kummar, S., Ciesielski, T. E., & Fogarasi, M. (2002). Management of small bowel adenocarcinoma. *Oncology, 16*(10), 1364–1370.

Wei, C., Chiang, J., Lin, W., et al. (2003). Tumor and tumor-like lesions of the duodenum: CT and barium imaging features. *Journal of Clinical Imaging, 27*(2), 89–96.

## RESOURCES

American Cancer Society, 1599 Clifton Rd., N.E., Atlanta, GA 30329; 1-800-ACS-2345; http://www.cancer.org. Accessed June 29, 2006.

American Gastroenterological Association, 4930 Del Ray Avenue, Bethesda, MD 20814; 301-654-2005l; http://www.gastro.org. Accessed June 29, 2006.

Cancer Source, 263 Summer St., Boston, MA 02210-1506; http://www.cancerSource.com. Accessed June 29, 2006.

Agency for Healthcare Research and Quality, 540 Gaither Road, Rockville, MD 20850; 301-427-1364; http://www.ahrq.gov. Accessed June 29, 2006.

American Society for Bariatric Surgery, 100 SW 75th Street, Suite 201, Gainesville, FL 32607; 352-331-4900; http://www.asbs.org. Accessed June 29, 2006.

Centers for Disease Control and Prevention, 1600 Clifton Rd., Atlanta, GA 30333; 404-639-3311; http://www.cdc.gov/nchs/products/pubs/pubd/hestats/obese/obese99.htm. Accessed June 29, 2006.

National Comprehensive Cancer Network (NCCN) Clinical Practice Guidelines, 5000 Old York Road, Suite 250, Jenkintown, PA 19046; 215-690-0300; http://www.nccn.org. Accessed June 29, 2006.

National Digestive Diseases Information Clearinghouse (NDDIC), 2 Information Way, Bethesda, MD 20892; 1-800-891-5389; http://digestive.niddk.nih.gov/ (NDDIC is a service of the National Institute of Diabetes and Digestive and Kidney Diseases [NIDDK]). Accessed June 29, 2006.

Obesity Law and Advocacy Center, 1392 East Palomar Street, Suite 403-233, Chula Vista, CA 91913; 619-656-5251; http://www.obesitylaw.com. Accessed June 29, 2006.

Society of American Gastrointestinal Endoscopic Surgeons (SAGES), 11300 West Olympic Boulevard, Suite 600, Los Angeles, CA 90064; 310-437-0544; http://www.sages.org/sg_pub30.html. Accessed June 29, 2006.

Weight loss surgery information: http://weightlossurgeryinfo.com. Accessed June 29, 2006.

# CHAPTER 38

# Management of Patients With Intestinal and Rectal Disorders

## Learning Objectives

*On completion of this chapter, the learner will be able to:*

1. Identify the health care learning needs of patients with constipation or diarrhea.
2. Compare the conditions of malabsorption with regard to their pathophysiology, clinical manifestations, and management.
3. Use the nursing process as a framework for care of patients with diverticulitis.
4. Compare regional enteritis and ulcerative colitis with regard to their pathophysiology; clinical manifestations; diagnostic evaluation; and medical, surgical, and nursing management.
5. Use the nursing process as a framework for care of the patient with inflammatory bowel disease.
6. Describe the responsibilities of the nurse in meeting the needs of the patient with an ileostomy.
7. Describe the various types of intestinal obstructions and their management.
8. Use the nursing process as a framework for care of the patient with cancer of the colon or rectum.
9. Use the nursing process as a framework for care of the patient with an anorectal condition.

At least 60 million people in the United States are diagnosed with some type of disease of the gastrointestinal (GI) tract. These diseases account for more than 45 million office visits and approximately 14 million hospital admissions annually. GI diseases cost the American public more than $100 billion each year and account for approximately 9% of all deaths each year (National Institutes of Health [NIH], 2005). The types of diseases and disorders that affect the lower GI tract are many and varied.

In all age groups, a fast-paced lifestyle, high levels of stress, irregular eating habits, insufficient intake of fiber and water, and lack of daily exercise contribute to GI disorders. There is a growing understanding of the biopsychosocial implications of GI disease. Nurses can have an impact on these GI disorders by identifying behavior patterns that put patients at risk, by educating the public about prevention and management, and by helping those affected to improve their condition and prevent complications.

# Abnormalities of Fecal Elimination

Changes in patterns of fecal elimination are symptoms of functional disorders or diseases of the GI tract. The most common changes seen are constipation, diarrhea, and fecal incontinence. The nurse should be aware of the causes and therapeutic management of these disorders and of nursing management techniques. Education is important for patients with these conditions.

## Constipation

**Constipation** is an abnormal infrequency or irregularity of defecation, abnormal hardening of stools that makes their passage difficult and sometimes painful, a decrease in stool volume, or retention of stool in the rectum for a prolonged period. Any variation from normal habits may be considered a problem. It is estimated that 4.5 million Americans are clinically constipated at any time and that women and adults older than 65 years are disproportionately constipated (Stessman, 2003).

Constipation can be caused by certain medications (ie, tranquilizers, anticholinergics, antidepressants, antihypertensives, bile acid sequestrants, opioids, aluminum-based antacids, iron preparations); rectal or anal disorders (eg, hemorrhoids, fissures); obstruction (eg, bowel tumors); metabolic, neurologic, and neuromuscular conditions (eg, diabetes mellitus, Hirschsprung's disease, Parkinson's disease, multiple sclerosis); endocrine disorders (eg, hypothyroidism, pheochromocytoma); lead poisoning; and connective tissue disorders (eg, scleroderma, systemic lupus erythematosus). Constipation is a major problem for patients

## Glossary

**abscess:** localized collection of purulent material surrounded by inflamed tissues, typically associated with signs of infection

**borborygmus:** rumbling noise caused by the movement of gas through the intestines

**colostomy:** surgical opening into the colon by means of a stoma to allow drainage of bowel contents; one type of fecal diversion

**constipation:** subjectively described infrequency or irregularity of defecation, with or without an abnormal hardening of feces that makes their passage difficult and sometimes painful, with or without a decrease in fecal volume

**diverticulitis:** inflammation of a diverticulum from obstruction (by fecal matter), resulting in abscess formation

**diverticulosis:** presence of several diverticula in the intestine; common in middle age

**diverticulum:** saclike outpouching of the lining of the bowel protruding through the muscle of the intestinal wall, usually caused by high intraluminal pressure

**enterostomal therapist:** nurse specially educated in the appropriate use of fecal and urinary diversions; guides patients, their families, surgeons, and nurses by recommending appropriate use of skin, wound, ostomy, and continence products; often referred to as a wound-ostomy-continence nurse (WOCN)

**fecal incontinence:** involuntary passage of feces

**fissure:** normal or abnormal fold, groove, or crack in body tissue

**fistula:** anatomically abnormal tract that arises between two internal organs or between an internal organ and the body surface

**hemorrhoids:** dilated portions of the anal veins; can occur internal or external to the anal sphincter

**ileostomy:** surgical opening into the ileum by means of a stoma to allow drainage of bowel contents; one type of fecal diversion

**inflammatory bowel disease (IBD):** group of chronic disorders (most common are ulcerative colitis and regional enteritis [Crohn's disease]) that result in inflammation or ulceration (or both) of the bowel lining; associated with abdominal pain, diarrhea, fever, and weight loss

**irritable bowel syndrome (IBS):** functional disorder that affects frequency of defecation and consistency of stool; associated with crampy abdominal pain and bloating

**Kock pouch:** type of continent ileal reservoir created surgically by making an internal pouch with a portion of the ileum and placing a nipple valve flush with the stoma

**malabsorption:** impaired transport across the mucosa

**peritonitis:** inflammation of the lining of the abdominal cavity, usually as a result of a bacterial infection of an area in the gastrointestinal tract with leakage of contents into the abdominal cavity

**steatorrhea:** excess of fatty wastes in the feces or the urine

**tenesmus:** ineffective and sometimes painful straining to eliminate either feces or urine

**Valsalva maneuver:** forcible exhalation against a closed glottis followed by a rise in intrathoracic pressure and subsequent possible dramatic rise in arterial pressure; may occur during straining at stool taking opioids for pain. Diseases of the colon commonly associated with constipation include irritable bowel syndrome and diverticular disease. Constipation can also occur with an acute disease process in the abdomen (eg, appendicitis).

Other causes of constipation may include weakness, immobility, debility, fatigue, and an inability to increase intraabdominal pressure to facilitate the passage of stools, as may occur in patients with emphysema, for instance. Many people develop constipation because they do not take the time to defecate or they ignore the urge to defecate. Constipation is also a result of dietary habits (ie, low consumption of fiber and inadequate fluid intake), lack of regular exercise, and a stress-filled life.

Perceived constipation can also be a problem. This subjective problem occurs when a person's bowel elimination pattern is not consistent with what he or she perceives as normal. Chronic laxative use may contribute to this problem and is a major health concern in the United States.

## Pathophysiology

The pathophysiology of constipation is poorly understood, but it is thought to include interference with one of three major functions of the colon: mucosal transport (ie, mucosal secretions facilitate the movement of colon contents), myoelectric activity (ie, mixing of the rectal mass and propulsive actions), or the processes of defecation. Any of the causative factors previously identified can interfere with any of these three processes.

The urge to defecate is stimulated normally by rectal distention, which initiates a series of four actions: stimulation of the inhibitory rectoanal reflex, relaxation of the internal sphincter muscle, relaxation of the external sphincter muscle and muscles in the pelvic region, and increased intraabdominal pressure. Interference with any of these processes can lead to constipation.

If all organic causes are eliminated, idiopathic constipation is diagnosed. When the urge to defecate is ignored, the rectal mucous membrane and musculature become insensitive to the presence of fecal masses, and consequently a stronger stimulus is required to produce the necessary peristaltic rush for defecation. The initial effect of fecal retention is to produce irritability of the colon, which at this stage frequently goes into spasm, especially after meals, giving rise to colicky midabdominal or low abdominal pains. After several years of this process, the colon loses muscular tone and becomes essentially unresponsive to normal stimuli. Atony or decreased muscle tone occurs with aging. This also leads to constipation because the stool is retained for longer periods.

## Clinical Manifestations

Clinical manifestations of constipation include fewer than three bowel movements per week; abdominal distention; pain and pressure; decreased appetite; headache; fatigue; indigestion; a sensation of incomplete evacuation; straining at stool; and the elimination of small-volume, lumpy, hard, dry stools.

## Assessment and Diagnostic Findings

Chronic constipation is usually considered idiopathic, but secondary causes should be excluded. In patients with severe, intractable constipation, further diagnostic testing is needed (Stessman, 2003). The diagnosis of constipation is based on the patient's history, physical examination, possibly the results of a barium enema or sigmoidoscopy, and stool testing for occult blood. These tests are used to determine whether this symptom results from spasm or narrowing of the bowel. Anorectal manometry (ie, pressure studies) may be performed to determine malfunction of the sphincter. Defecography and colonic transit studies can also assist in the diagnosis (see Chapter 34).

## Complications

Complications of constipation include hypertension, fecal impaction, **hemorrhoids** (dilated portions of anal veins), **fissures** (tissue folds), and megacolon. Increased arterial pressure can occur with defecation. Straining at stool, which results in the **Valsalva maneuver** (ie, forcibly exhaling with the glottis closed), has a striking effect on arterial blood pressure. During active straining, the flow of venous blood in the chest is temporarily impeded because of increased intrathoracic pressure. This pressure tends to collapse the large veins in the chest. The atria and the ventricles receive less blood, and consequently less blood is ejected by the left ventricle. Cardiac output is decreased, and there is a transient drop in arterial pressure. Almost immediately after this period of hypotension, an increase in arterial pressure occurs; the pressure is elevated momentarily to a point far exceeding the original level (ie, rebound phenomenon). In patients with hypertension, this compensatory reaction may be exaggerated greatly, and the peak pressure attained may be dangerously high—sufficient to rupture a major artery in the brain or elsewhere.

Fecal impaction occurs when an accumulated mass of dry feces cannot be expelled. The mass may be palpable on digital examination, may produce pressure on the colonic mucosa that results in ulcer formation, and frequently causes seepage of liquid stools.

Hemorrhoids and anal fissures can develop as a result of constipation. Hemorrhoids develop as a result of perianal vascular congestion caused by straining. Anal fissures may result from the passage of the hard stool through the anus, tearing the lining of the anal canal.

Megacolon is a dilated and atonic colon caused by a fecal mass that obstructs the passage of colon contents. Symptoms include constipation, liquid fecal incontinence, and abdominal distention. Megacolon can lead to perforation of the bowel.

### Gerontologic Considerations

Physician visits for constipation are more common in people 65 years and older (Stessman, 2003). The most common complaint they voice is the need to strain at stool. People who have loose-fitting dentures or have lost their teeth have difficulty chewing and frequently choose soft, processed foods that are low in fiber. Older adults tend to have decreased food intake, reduced mobility, and weak abdominal and pelvic muscles, and they are more likely to have multiple chronic illnesses requiring medications (eg, calcium channel blockers, bile acid sequestrants, opioids) that often cause constipation. Low-fiber convenience foods are widely used by people who have lost interest in eating. Some older people reduce their fluid intake if they are not eating regular meals. Depression, weakness, or prolonged bed rest also contribute to constipation by decreasing intestinal motility and anal sphincter tone. Nerve impulses are dulled, and there is a decreased urge to defecate. Many older people overuse laxatives in an attempt to have a daily bowel movement and become dependent on them.

## Medical Management

Treatment is aimed at the underlying cause of constipation and includes education, bowel habit training, increased fiber and fluid intake, and judicious use of laxatives. Management may also include discontinuing laxative abuse. Routine exercise to strengthen abdominal muscles is encouraged. Biofeedback is a technique that can be used to help patients learn to relax the sphincter mechanism to expel stool (Stessman, 2003). Daily dietary intake of 6 to 12 teaspoonfuls of unprocessed bran is recommended, especially for the treatment of constipation in the elderly. If laxative use is necessary, one of the following may be prescribed: bulk-forming agents, saline and osmotic agents, lubricants, stimulants, or fecal softeners. The physiologic action and patient education information related to these laxatives are given in Table 38-1. Enemas and rectal suppositories are generally not recommended for treating constipation; they should be reserved for the treatment of impaction. If long-term laxative use is necessary, a bulk-forming agent may be prescribed in combination with an osmotic laxative.

Specific medications may be prescribed to enhance colonic transit by increasing propulsive motor activity. These may include cholinergic agents (eg, bethanechol [Urecholine]), cholinesterase inhibitors (eg, neostigmine [Prostigmin]), or prokinetic agents (eg, metoclopramide [Reglan]).

## Nursing Management

The nurse elicits information about the onset and duration of constipation, current and past elimination patterns, the

### TABLE 38-1 Laxatives: Classification, Agent, Action, and Patient Education

| Classification | Sample Agent | Action | Patient Education |
| --- | --- | --- | --- |
| Bulk forming | Psyllium hydrophilic mucilloid (Metamucil) | Polysaccharides and cellulose derivatives mix with intestinal fluids, swell, and stimulate peristalsis. | Take with 8 oz water and follow with 8 oz water; do not take dry. Report abdominal distention or unusual amount of flatulence. |
| Saline agent | Magnesium hydroxide (Milk of Magnesia) | Nonabsorbable magnesium ions alter stool consistency by drawing water into the intestines by osmosis; peristalsis is stimulated. Action occurs within 2 h. | The liquid preparation is more effective than the tablet form. Only short-term use is recommended because of toxicity (CNS or neuromuscular depression, electrolyte imbalance). Magnesium laxatives should not be taken by patients with renal insufficiency. |
| Lubricant | Mineral oil | Nonabsorbable hydrocarbons soften fecal matter by lubricating the intestinal mucosa; the passage of stool is facilitated. Action occurs within 6–8 h. | Do not take with meals, because mineral oils can impair the absorption of fat-soluble vitamins and delay gastric emptying. Swallow carefully, because drops of oil that gain access to the pharynx can produce a lipid pneumonia. |
| Stimulant | Bisacodyl (Dulcolax) | Irritates the colon epithelium by stimulating sensory nerve endings and increasing mucosal secretions. Action occurs within 6–8 h. | Catharsis may cause fluid and electrolyte imbalance, especially in the elderly. Tablets should be swallowed, not crushed or chewed. Avoid milk or antacids within 1 hour of taking the medication, because the enteric coating may dissolve prematurely. |
| Fecal softener | Dioctyl sodium sulfosuccinate (Colace) | Hydrates the stool by its surfactant action on the colonic epithelium (increases the wetting efficiency of intestinal water); aqueous and fatty substances are mixed. Does not exert a laxative action. | Can be used safely by patients who should avoid straining (cardiac patients, patients with anorectal disorders) |
| Osmotic agent | Polyethylene glycol and electrolytes (Colyte) | Cleanses colon rapidly and induces diarrhea | This is a large-volume product. It takes time to consume it safely. It can cause considerable nausea and bloating. |

patient's expectation of normal bowel elimination, and lifestyle information (eg, exercise and activity level, occupation, food and fluid intake, and stress level) during the health history interview. Past medical and surgical history, current medications, and laxative and enema use are important, as is information about the sensation of rectal pressure or fullness, abdominal pain, excessive straining at defecation, and flatulence.

Patient education and health promotion are important functions of the nurse (Chart 38-1). After the health history is obtained, the nurse sets specific goals for teaching. Goals for the patient include restoring or maintaining a regular pattern of elimination by responding to the urge to defecate, ensuring adequate intake of fluids and high-fiber foods, learning about methods to avoid constipation, relieving anxiety about bowel elimination patterns, and avoiding complications.

## Diarrhea

Diarrhea is an increased frequency of bowel movements (more than three per day), an increased amount of stool (more than 200 g per day), and altered consistency (ie, looseness) of stool. It is usually associated with urgency, perianal discomfort, incontinence, or a combination of these factors. Any condition that causes increased intestinal secretions, decreased mucosal absorption, or altered motility can produce diarrhea. Irritable bowel syndrome, inflammatory bowel disease, and lactose intolerance are frequently the underlying disease processes that cause diarrhea.

Diarrhea can be acute or chronic. Acute diarrhea is most often associated with infection and is usually self-limiting; chronic diarrhea persists for a longer period and may return sporadically. Diarrhea can be caused by certain medications (eg, thyroid hormone replacement, stool softeners and laxatives, antibiotics, chemotherapy, magnesium-based antacids), certain tube-feeding formulas, metabolic and endocrine disorders (eg, diabetes, Addison's disease, thyrotoxicosis), and viral or bacterial infectious processes (eg, dysentery, shigellosis, food poisoning). Other disease processes associated with diarrhea include nutritional and malabsorptive disorders (eg, celiac disease), anal sphincter defect, Zollinger-Ellison syndrome, paralytic ileus, intestinal obstruction, and acquired immunodeficiency syndrome (AIDS).

### Pathophysiology

Types of diarrhea include secretory, osmotic, and mixed diarrhea. Secretory diarrhea is usually high-volume diarrhea and is caused by increased production and secretion of water and electrolytes by the intestinal mucosa into the intestinal lumen. Osmotic diarrhea occurs when water is pulled into the intestines by the osmotic pressure of unabsorbed particles, slowing the reabsorption of water. Mixed diarrhea is caused by increased peristalsis (usually from inflammatory bowel disease) and a combination of increased secretion and decreased absorption in the bowel. The pathophysiology of diarrhea related to infection is discussed in Chapter 70.

### Clinical Manifestations

In addition to the increased frequency and fluid content of stools, the patient usually has abdominal cramps, distention, intestinal rumbling (ie, **borborygmus**), anorexia, and thirst. Painful spasmodic contractions of the anus and ineffective straining (ie, **tenesmus**) may occur with defecation. Other symptoms depend on the cause and severity of the diarrhea but are related to dehydration and to fluid and electrolyte imbalances.

Watery stools are characteristic of disorders of the small bowel, whereas loose, semisolid stools are associated more often with disorders of the large bowel. Voluminous, greasy stools suggest intestinal malabsorption, and the presence of mucus and pus in the stools suggests inflammatory enteritis or colitis. Oil droplets on the toilet water are almost always diagnostic of pancreatic insufficiency. Nocturnal diarrhea may be a manifestation of diabetic neuropathy.

### Assessment and Diagnostic Findings

When the cause of the diarrhea is not obvious, the following diagnostic tests may be performed: complete blood cell count; serum chemistries; urinalysis; routine stool examination; and stool examinations for infectious or parasitic organisms, bacterial toxins, blood, fat, and electrolytes. Endoscopy or barium enema may assist in identifying the cause.

---

**CHART 38-1**

### Health Promotion

**Preventing Constipation**

- Describe the physiology of defecation.
- Emphasize the importance of responding to the urge to defecate.
- Discuss normal variations in patterns of defecation.
- Teach how to establish a bowel routine, and explain that having a regular time for defecation (eg, best time is after breakfast) may aid in initiating the reflex.
- Provide dietary information; suggest eating high-residue, high-fiber foods, adding bran daily (must be introduced gradually), and increasing fluid intake (unless contraindicated).
- Explain how an exercise regimen, increased ambulation, and abdominal muscle toning will increase muscle strength and help propel colon contents.
- Describe abdominal toning exercises (contracting abdominal muscles 4 times daily and leg-to-chest lifts 10 to 20 times each day).
- Explain that the normal position (semisquatting) maximizes use of abdominal muscles and force of gravity.

## Complications

Complications of diarrhea include the potential for cardiac dysrhythmias because of significant fluid and electrolyte loss (especially loss of potassium). Urinary output of less than 30 mL per hour for 2 to 3 consecutive hours, muscle weakness, paresthesia, hypotension, anorexia, and drowsiness with a potassium level of less than 3.5 mEq/L (3.5 mmol/L) must be reported.

> **NURSING ALERT**
>
> Decreased potassium levels cause cardiac dysrhythmias (ie, atrial and ventricular tachycardia, ventricular fibrillation, premature ventricular contractions) that can lead to death.

### Gerontologic Considerations

Elderly patients can become dehydrated quickly and develop low potassium levels (ie, hypokalemia) as a result of diarrhea. The nurse observes for clinical manifestations of muscle weakness, dysrhythmias, or decreased peristaltic motility that may lead to paralytic ileus. The older patient taking digitalis (eg, digoxin [Lanoxin]) must be aware of how quickly dehydration and hypokalemia can occur with diarrhea. The nurse teaches the patient to recognize the symptoms of hypokalemia because low levels of potassium intensify the action of digitalis, leading to digitalis toxicity.

## Medical Management

Primary management is directed at controlling symptoms, preventing complications, and eliminating or treating the underlying disease. Certain medications (eg, antibiotics, anti-inflammatory agents) may be used to reduce the severity of the diarrhea and treat the underlying disease.

## Nursing Management

The nurse's role includes assessing and monitoring the characteristics and pattern of diarrhea. A health history should address the patient's medication therapy, medical and surgical history, and dietary patterns and intake. Reports of recent exposure to an acute illness or recent travel to another geographic area are important. Assessment includes abdominal auscultation and palpation for abdominal tenderness. Inspection of the abdomen, mucous membranes, and skin is important to determine hydration status. Stool samples are obtained for testing.

During an episode of acute diarrhea, the nurse encourages bed rest and intake of liquids and foods low in bulk until the acute attack subsides. When the patient is able to tolerate food intake, the nurse recommends a bland diet of semisolid and solid foods. The patient should avoid caffeine, carbonated beverages, and very hot and very cold foods, because they stimulate intestinal motility. It may be necessary to restrict milk products, fat, whole-grain products, fresh fruits, and vegetables for several days. The nurse administers antidiarrheal medications such as diphenoxylate (Lomotil) or loperamide (Imodium) as prescribed. Intravenous (IV) fluid therapy may be necessary for rapid rehydration in some patients, especially in elderly patients and in patients with preexisting GI conditions (eg, inflammatory bowel disease). It is important to monitor serum electrolyte levels closely. The nurse immediately reports evidence of dysrhythmias or a change in a patient's level of consciousness.

The perianal area may become excoriated because diarrheal stool contains digestive enzymes that can irritate the skin. The patient should follow a perianal skin care routine to decrease irritation and excoriation (see Chapter 56). The skin of an older person is very sensitive because of decreased turgor and reduced subcutaneous fat layers.

# Fecal Incontinence

**Fecal incontinence** describes the involuntary passage of stool from the rectum. Factors that influence fecal continence include the ability of the rectum to sense and accommodate stool, the amount and consistency of stool, the integrity of the anal sphincters and musculature, and rectal motility.

## Pathophysiology

Fecal incontinence can result from trauma (eg, after surgical procedures involving the rectum), neurologic disorders (eg, stroke, multiple sclerosis, diabetic neuropathy, dementia), inflammation, infection, chemotherapy, radiation treatment, fecal impaction, pelvic floor relaxation, laxative abuse, medications, or advancing age (ie, weakness or loss of anal or rectal muscle tone). It is an embarrassing and socially incapacitating problem that requires a many-tiered approach to treatment and much adaptation on the patient's part.

## Clinical Manifestations

Patients may have minor soiling, occasional urgency and loss of control, or complete incontinence. Patients may also experience poor control of flatus, diarrhea, or constipation.

## Assessment and Diagnostic Findings

Diagnostic studies are necessary because the treatment of fecal incontinence depends on the cause. A rectal examination and other endoscopic examinations such as a flexible sigmoidoscopy are performed to rule out tumors, inflammation, or fissures. X-ray studies such as barium enema, computed tomography (CT), anorectal manometry, and transit studies may be helpful in identifying alterations in intestinal mucosa and muscle tone or in detecting other structural or functional problems.

## Medical Management

Although there is no known cause or cure for fecal incontinence, specific management techniques can help the patient achieve a better quality of life. If fecal incontinence is related to diarrhea, the incontinence may disappear when diarrhea is successfully treated. Fecal incontinence is frequently a symptom of a fecal impaction. After the impaction is removed and the rectum is cleansed, normal functioning of the anorectal area can resume. If the fecal incontinence is related to a more permanent condition, other treatments are initiated. Biofeedback therapy can be of assistance if the problem is decreased sensory awareness or sphincter control. Bowel training programs can also be effective. Surgical procedures include surgical reconstruction, sphincter repair, or fecal diversion.

## Nursing Management

The nurse obtains a thorough health history, including information about previous surgical procedures, chronic illnesses, dietary patterns, bowel habits and problems, and current medication regimen. The nurse also completes an examination of the rectal area.

The nurse initiates a bowel-training program that involves setting a schedule to establish bowel regularity. The goal is to help the patient achieve fecal continence. If this is not possible, the goal should be to manage the problem so the person can have predictable, planned elimination. Sometimes, it is necessary to use suppositories to stimulate the anal reflex. After the patient has achieved a regular schedule, the suppository can be discontinued. Biofeedback can be used in conjunction with these therapies to help the patient improve sphincter contractility and rectal sensitivity.

Fecal incontinence can also cause problems with perineal skin integrity. Maintaining skin integrity is a priority, especially in the debilitated or elderly patient. Incontinence briefs, although helpful in containing the fecal material, allow for increased skin contact with the feces and may cause excoriation of the skin. The nurse encourages and teaches meticulous skin hygiene.

Continence sometimes cannot be achieved, and the nurse assists the patient and family to accept and cope with this chronic situation. The patient can use fecal incontinence devices, which include external collection devices and internal drainage systems. External devices are special pouches that are drainable. They are attached to a synthetic adhesive skin barrier specially designed to conform to the buttocks. Internal drainage systems can be used to eliminate fecal skin contact and are especially useful when there is extensive excoriation or skin breakdown. A large catheter is inserted into the rectum and is connected to a drainage system.

## Irritable Bowel Syndrome

**Irritable bowel syndrome** (IBS) is one of the most common GI conditions. Approximately 12% of adults in the United States report classic symptoms of IBS (Mertz, 2003). It occurs more commonly in women than in men, and the cause remains unknown (Motzer, Hertig, Jarrett, et al., 2003). Although no anatomic or biochemical abnormalities have been found that account for the common symptoms, various factors are associated with the syndrome: heredity, psychological stress or conditions such as depression and anxiety, a diet high in fat and stimulating or irritating foods, alcohol consumption, and smoking. The diagnosis is made only after tests confirm the absence of structural or other disorders.

## Pathophysiology

IBS results from a functional disorder of intestinal motility. The change in motility may be related to neuroendocrine dysregulation, infection or irritation, or a vascular or metabolic disturbance. The peristaltic waves are affected at specific segments of the intestine and in the intensity with which they propel the fecal matter forward. There is no evidence of inflammation or tissue changes in the intestinal mucosa.

## Clinical Manifestations

There is a wide variability in symptom presentation. Symptoms range in intensity and duration from mild and infrequent to severe and continuous. The primary symptom is an alteration in bowel patterns—constipation, diarrhea, or a combination of both. Pain, bloating, and abdominal distention often accompany changes in bowel pattern. The abdominal pain is sometimes precipitated by eating and is frequently relieved by defecation.

## Assessment and Diagnostic Findings

A definite diagnosis of IBS requires tests that confirm the absence of structural or other disorders. Stool studies, contrast x-ray studies, and proctoscopy may be performed to rule out other colon diseases. Barium enema and colonoscopy may reveal spasm, distention, or mucus accumulation in the intestine (Fig. 38-1). Manometry and electromyography

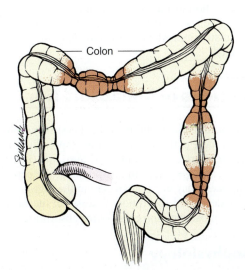

**FIGURE 38-1.** In irritable bowel syndrome (IBS), the spastic contractions of the bowel can be seen on x-ray contrast studies.

(EMG) are used to study intraluminal pressure changes generated by spasticity.

## Medical Management

The goals of treatment are relieving abdominal pain, controlling the diarrhea or constipation, and reducing stress. Restriction and then gradual reintroduction of foods that are possibly irritating may help determine what types of food are acting as irritants (eg, beans, caffeinated products, fried foods, alcohol, spicy foods). A high-fiber diet is prescribed to help control the diarrhea and constipation. Exercise can assist in reducing anxiety and increasing intestinal motility. Patients often find it helpful to participate in a stress reduction or behavior modification program. Hydrophilic colloids (ie, bulk) and antidiarrheal agents (eg, loperamide [Imodium]) may be given to control the diarrhea and fecal urgency. Antidepressants can assist in treating underlying anxiety and depression. Anticholinergics (eg, propantheline [Pro-Banthine]) may be taken to decrease smooth muscle spasm, decreasing cramping and constipation.

Tegaserod (Zelnorm) may be prescribed to treat women with IBS whose chief complaint is chronic constipation. Tegaserod increases the effects of serotonin in the intestines, thereby increasing intestinal motility. The most commonly reported side effect of this medication is diarrhea, which typically subsides after the first week of treatment. Research has shown that some women with IBS who take tegaserod develop diarrhea with hypovolemia and hypotension (Aschenbrenner, 2004). Thus, women who take tegaserod must be taught to discontinue the drug and contact their primary health care provider if they develop severe diarrhea, particularly if it is accompanied by dizziness or orthostasis.

## Nursing Management

The nurse's role is to provide patient and family education. The nurse emphasizes teaching and reinforces good dietary habits. Patients are encouraged to eat at regular times and to chew food slowly and thoroughly. They should understand that although adequate fluid intake is necessary, fluid should not be taken with meals because this results in abdominal distention. Alcohol use and cigarette smoking are discouraged.

# Conditions of Malabsorption

**Malabsorption** is the inability of the digestive system to absorb one or more of the major vitamins (especially A and $B_{12}$), minerals (ie, iron and calcium), and nutrients (ie, carbohydrates, fats, and proteins). Interruptions in the complex digestive process may occur anywhere in the digestive system and cause decreased absorption. Diseases of the small intestine are the most common cause of malabsorption.

## Pathophysiology

The conditions that cause malabsorption can be grouped into the following categories:

- Mucosal (transport) disorders causing generalized malabsorption (eg, celiac sprue, regional enteritis, radiation enteritis)
- Infectious diseases causing generalized malabsorption (eg, small bowel bacterial overgrowth, tropical sprue, Whipple's disease)
- Luminal disorders causing malabsorption (eg, bile acid deficiency, Zollinger-Ellison syndrome, pancreatic insufficiency)
- Postoperative malabsorption (eg, after gastric or intestinal resection)
- Disorders that cause malabsorption of specific nutrients (eg, disaccharidase deficiency leading to lactose intolerance)

Table 38-2 lists the clinical and pathologic aspects of malabsorptive diseases.

## Clinical Manifestations

The hallmarks of malabsorption syndrome from any cause are diarrhea or frequent, loose, bulky, foul-smelling stools that have increased fat content and are often grayish. Patients often have associated abdominal distention, pain, increased flatus, weakness, weight loss, and a decreased sense of well-being. The chief result of malabsorption is malnutrition, manifested by weight loss and other signs of vitamin and mineral deficiency (eg, easy bruising, osteoporosis, anemia). Patients with a malabsorption syndrome, if untreated, become weak and emaciated because of starvation and dehydration. Failure to absorb the fat-soluble vitamins A, D, and K causes a corresponding avitaminosis.

## Assessment and Diagnostic Findings

Several diagnostic tests may be prescribed, including stool studies for quantitative and qualitative fat analysis, lactose tolerance tests, D-xylose absorption tests, and Schilling tests. The hydrogen breath test that is used to evaluate carbohydrate absorption (see Chapter 34) is performed if carbohydrate malabsorption is suspected. Endoscopy with biopsy of the mucosa is the best diagnostic tool. Biopsy of the small intestine is performed to assay enzyme activity or to identify infection or destruction of mucosa. Ultrasound studies, CT scans, and x-ray findings can reveal pancreatic or intestinal tumors that may be the cause. A complete blood cell count is used to detect anemia. Pancreatic function tests can assist in the diagnosis of specific disorders.

## Medical Management

Intervention is aimed at avoiding dietary substances that aggravate malabsorption and at supplementing nutrients that have been lost. Common supplements are water-soluble vitamins (eg, $B_{12}$, folic acid), fat-soluble vitamins (ie, A, D, and K), and minerals (eg, calcium, iron). Primary disease states may be managed surgically or nonsurgically. Dietary therapy is aimed at reducing gluten intake in patients with celiac sprue. Folic acid supplements are prescribed for patients with tropical sprue. Antibiotics (eg, tetracycline [Tetracap, Tetracyn], ampicillin [Polycillin]) are sometimes

## NURSING RESEARCH PROFILE

### Quality of Life in Women with Irritable Bowel Syndrome

Motzer, S. A., Hertig, V., Jarrett, M., et al. (2003). Sense of coherence and quality of life in women with and without irritable bowel syndrome. *Nursing Research, 52*(5), 329–337.

**Purpose**

Irritable bowel syndrome (IBS) disproportionately affects women, and its onset occurs most commonly during adolescence or early adulthood. It is thought that IBS symptoms are negatively associated with feelings of confidence that life is manageable and meaningful, which is referred to as a sense of coherence (SOC). It is also believed that IBS has detrimental effects on quality of life (QOL) because of its chronic, relapsing nature, its refractoriness to effective treatment, and its associated psychological distress. The aims of this study were to compare the SOC and QOL in women with and without IBS and to examine the relationships between IBS and SOC, QOL, and psychological distress.

**Design**

The sample consisted of 342 women participants between 18 and 49 years of age, 235 of whom self-reported IBS and 89 of whom did not report IBS or similar gastrointestinal (GI) symptoms. Participants completed several surveys, including the following:
- Antonovsky's SOC Questionnaire, to measure SOC
- Flanagan's Modified Quality of Life Scale (MQOLS), to measure QOL
- Bowel Disease Questionnaire (BDQ), to measure GI symptoms
- Global Severity Index (GSI) and the subscales for depression, anxiety, and somatization from Derogatis's Symptom Checklist-90-R, to measure general and select psychological symptoms

Independent sample *t* tests were analyzed to determine whether there was a difference in SOC, QOL, GI symptoms, and psychological symptoms between women with and without IBS. Pearson's correlation coefficients were also analyzed to identify the relationships among these variables of interest.

**Findings**

Women with IBS reported significantly lower SOC and QOL than women without IBS. In addition, women with IBS reported significantly more global distress, somatization with and without GI symptoms, depression, and anxiety than did women without IBS. Low SOC and low QOL were both correlated with increased feelings of global distress, depression, anxiety, somatization without GI symptoms, and the GI symptom of alternating constipation and diarrhea.

**Nursing Implications**

Findings from this study confirm that women with IBS report a decreased SOC and QOL compared with women without IBS. Moreover, women with IBS report having more psychological symptoms of global distress, somatization, depression, and anxiety than women without IBS. It remains unknown whether symptoms of IBS cause psychological distress or whether psychological distress exacerbates symptoms of the syndrome. Nursing interventions targeted at enhancing SOC and QOL should be developed to determine whether they improve the psychological distress associated with IBS.

---

needed in the treatment of tropical sprue and bacterial overgrowth syndromes. Antidiarrheal agents may be used to decrease intestinal spasms. Parenteral fluids may be necessary to treat dehydration.

### Gerontologic Considerations

The older patient may have more subtle symptoms of malabsorption that may be extraintestinal, including fatigue and confusion. Medical management may include the administration of corticosteroids, which may cause a host of adverse effects such as hypertension, hypokalemia, and confusion. Antibiotics may reduce vitamin K–producing intestinal flora, resulting in a prolonged prothrombin time (PT) and international normalized ratio (INR) if the patient is concurrently taking warfarin (Coumadin). Urinary retention, altered mental status, or glaucoma may occur as adverse effects of anticholinergic drug therapy in older people.

### Nursing Management

The nurse provides patient and family education regarding diet and the use of nutritional supplements (Chart 38-2). It is important to monitor patients with diarrhea for fluid and electrolyte imbalances. The nurse conducts ongoing assessments to determine whether the clinical manifestations related to the nutritional deficits have abated. Patient education includes information about the risk of osteoporosis related to malabsorption of calcium.

## Acute Inflammatory Intestinal Disorders

Any part of the lower GI tract is susceptible to acute inflammation caused by bacterial, viral, or fungal infection. Two such conditions are appendicitis and diverticulitis,

### TABLE 38-2  Characteristics of Diseases of Malabsorption

| Diseases/Disorders | Physiologic Pathology | Clinical Features |
|---|---|---|
| Gastric resection with gastrojejunostomy | Decreased pancreatic stimulation because of duodenal bypass; poor mixing of food, bile, pancreatic enzymes; decreased intrinsic factor | Weight loss, moderate steatorrhea, anemia (combination of iron deficiency, vitamin $B_{12}$ malabsorption, folate deficiency) |
| Pancreatic insufficiency (chronic pancreatitis, pancreatic carcinoma, pancreatic resection, cystic fibrosis) | Reduced intraluminal pancreatic enzyme activity, with maldigestion of lipids and proteins | History of abdominal pain followed by weight loss; marked steatorrhea, azotorrhea (excess of nitrogenous matter in the feces or urine); also frequent glucose intolerance (70% in pancreatic insufficiency) |
| Ileal dysfunction (resection or disease) | Loss of ileal absorbing surface leads to reduced bile-salt pool size and reduced vitamin $B_{12}$ absorption; bile in colon inhibits fluid absorption | Diarrhea, weight loss with steatorrhea, especially when greater than 100 cm resection, decreased vitamin $B_{12}$ absorption |
| Stasis syndromes (surgical strictures, blind loops, enteric fistulas, multiple jejunal diverticula, scleroderma) | Overgrowth of intraluminal intestinal bacteria, especially anaerobic organisms, to greater than $10^6$/mL results in deconjugation of bile salts, leading to decreased effective bile-salt pool size, also bacterial utilization of vitamin $B_{12}$ | Weight loss, steatorrhea; low vitamin $B_{12}$ absorption; may have low D-xylose absorption |
| Zollinger-Ellison syndrome | Hyperacidity in duodenum inactivates pancreatic enzymes | Ulcer diathesis, steatorrhea |
| Lactose intolerance | Deficiency of intestinal lactase results in high concentration of intraluminal lactose with osmotic diarrhea | Varied degrees of diarrhea and cramps after ingestion of lactose-containing foods; positive lactose intolerance test, decreased intestinal lactase |
| Celiac disease (gluten enteropathy) | Toxic response to a gluten fraction by surface epithelium results in destruction of absorbing surface | Weight loss, diarrhea, bloating, anemia (low iron, folate), osteomalacia, steatorrhea, azotorrhea, low D-xylose absorption; folate and iron malabsorption |
| Tropical sprue | Unknown toxic factor results in mucosal inflammation, partial villous atrophy | Weight loss, diarrhea, anemia (low folate, vitamin $B_{12}$); steatorrhea; low D-xylose absorption, low vitamin $B_{12}$ absorption |
| Whipple's disease | Bacterial invasion of intestinal mucosa | Arthritis, hyperpigmentation, lymphadenopathy, serous effusions, fever, weight loss, steatorrhea, azotorrhea |
| Certain parasitic diseases (giardiasis, strongyloidiasis, coccidiosis, capillariasis) | Damage to or invasion of surface mucosa | Diarrhea, weight loss; steatorrhea; organism may be seen on jejunal biopsy or recovered in stool |
| Immunoglobulinopathy | Decreased local intestinal defenses, lymphoid hyperplasia, lymphopenia | Frequent association with *Giardia*: hypogammaglobulinemia or isolated IgA deficiency |

both of which may lead to **peritonitis**, an inflammation of the lining of the abdominal cavity.

## Appendicitis

The appendix is a small, finger-like appendage about 10 cm (4 in) long that is attached to the cecum just below the ileocecal valve. The appendix fills with food and empties regularly into the cecum. Because it empties inefficiently and its lumen is small, the appendix is prone to obstruction and is particularly vulnerable to infection (ie, appendicitis).

Appendicitis, the most common cause of acute abdomen in the United States, is the most common reason for emergency abdominal surgery. Although it can occur at any age, it more commonly occurs between the ages of 10 and 30 years (NIH, 2005).

## Pathophysiology

The appendix becomes inflamed and edematous as a result of becoming kinked or occluded by a fecalith (ie, hardened mass of stool), tumor, or foreign body. The inflammatory process increases intraluminal pressure, initiating a progressively severe, generalized or periumbilical pain that becomes localized to the right lower quadrant of the abdomen within a few hours. Eventually, the inflamed appendix fills with pus.

## CHART 38-2

### Patient Education

**Managing Lactose Intolerance**

- Deficiency of lactase, a digestive enzyme essential for the absorption of lactose from the intestines, results in an intolerance to milk.
- Elimination of milk and milk substances can prevent symptoms.
- Many processed foods have fillers, such as dried milk, added to them.
- Pretreatment of foods with lactase preparations (eg, LactAid drops) before ingestion can reduce symptoms.
- Ingestion of lactase enzyme tablets with the first bite of food can reduce symptoms.
- Most people can tolerate 1 to 2 cups of milk or milk products daily without major problems; they are best tolerated if ingested in small amounts during the day.
- Lactase activity of yogurt with "active cultures" helps the digestion of lactose within the intestine better than lactase preparations do.
- Milk and milk products are rich sources of calcium and vitamin D; elimination of milk from the diet may result in calcium and vitamin D deficiencies; decreased intake without supplements can lead to osteoporosis.

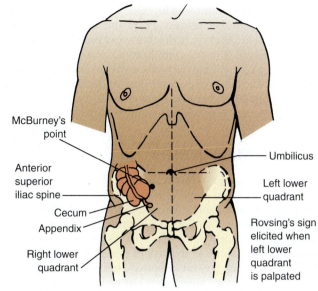

**FIGURE 38-2.** When the appendix is inflamed, tenderness can be noted in the right lower quadrant at McBurney's point, which is between the umbilicus and the anterior superior iliac spine. Rovsing's sign is pain felt in the right lower quadrant after the left lower quadrant has been palpated.

## Clinical Manifestations

Vague epigastric or periumbilical pain progresses to right lower quadrant pain and is usually accompanied by a low-grade fever and nausea and sometimes by vomiting. Loss of appetite is common. In up to 50% of presenting cases, local tenderness is elicited at McBurney's point when pressure is applied (Fig. 38-2). Rebound tenderness (ie, production or intensification of pain when pressure is released) may be present. The extent of tenderness and muscle spasm and the existence of constipation or diarrhea depend not so much on the severity of the appendiceal infection as on the location of the appendix. If the appendix curls around behind the cecum, pain and tenderness may be felt in the lumbar region. If its tip is in the pelvis, these signs may be elicited only on rectal examination. Pain on defecation suggests that the tip of the appendix is resting against the rectum; pain on urination suggests that the tip is near the bladder or impinges on the ureter. Some rigidity of the lower portion of the right rectus muscle may occur. Rovsing's sign may be elicited by palpating the left lower quadrant; this paradoxically causes pain to be felt in the right lower quadrant (see Fig. 38-2). If the appendix has ruptured, the pain becomes more diffuse; abdominal distention develops as a result of paralytic ileus, and the patient's condition worsens.

Constipation can also occur with an acute process such as appendicitis. Laxatives administered in this instance may result in perforation of the inflamed appendix. In general, a laxative or cathartic should never be given when a person has fever, nausea, or pain.

## Assessment and Diagnostic Findings

Diagnosis is based on results of a complete physical examination and on laboratory findings and imaging studies. The complete blood cell count demonstrates an elevated white blood cell count with an elevation of the neutrophils. Abdominal x-ray films, ultrasound studies, and CT scans may reveal a right lower quadrant density or localized distention of the bowel. A diagnostic laparoscopy may be used to rule out acute appendicitis in equivocal cases.

## Complications

The major complication of appendicitis is perforation of the appendix, which can lead to peritonitis, **abscess** formation (collection of purulent material), or portal pylephlebitis, which is septic thrombosis of the portal vein caused by vegetative emboli that arise from septic intestines. Perforation generally occurs 24 hours after the onset of pain. Symptoms include a fever of 37.7°C (100°F) or greater, a toxic appearance, and continued abdominal pain or tenderness.

## Gerontologic Considerations

Acute appendicitis is uncommon in the elderly population. When it does occur, classic signs and symptoms are altered and may vary greatly. Pain may be absent or minimal. Symptoms may be vague, suggesting bowel obstruction or another process. Fever and leukocytosis may not be present. As a result, diagnosis and prompt treatment may be delayed, causing complications and mortality. The patient may have no symptoms until the appendix ruptures. The incidence of perforated appendix is higher in the elderly population because many of these patients do not seek health care as quickly as younger patients.

## Medical Management

Immediate surgery is typically indicated if appendicitis is diagnosed. To correct or prevent fluid and electrolyte imbalance, dehydration, and sepsis, antibiotics and IV fluids are administered until surgery is performed. Appendectomy (ie, surgical removal of the appendix) is performed as soon as possible to decrease the risk of perforation. It may be performed using general or spinal anesthesia with a low abdominal incision (laparotomy) or by laparoscopy. Both laparotomy and laparoscopy are safe and effective in the treatment of appendicitis with perforation. However, recovery after laparoscopic surgery is generally quicker.

When perforation of the appendix occurs, an abscess may form. If this occurs, the patient may be initially treated with antibiotics, and the surgeon may place a drain in the abscess. After the abscess is drained and there is no further evidence of infection, an appendectomy is then typically performed.

## Nursing Management

Goals include relieving pain, preventing fluid volume deficit, reducing anxiety, eliminating infection due to the potential or actual disruption of the GI tract, maintaining skin integrity, and attaining optimal nutrition.

The nurse prepares the patient for surgery, which includes an IV infusion to replace fluid loss and promote adequate renal function and antibiotic therapy to prevent infection. If there is evidence or likelihood of paralytic ileus, a nasogastric tube is inserted. An enema is not administered because it can lead to perforation.

After surgery, the nurse places the patient in a high-Fowler position. This position reduces the tension on the incision and abdominal organs, helping to reduce pain. An opioid, usually morphine sulfate, is prescribed to relieve pain. When tolerated, oral fluids are administered. Any patient who was dehydrated before surgery receives IV fluids. Food is provided as desired and tolerated on the day of surgery when normal bowel sounds are present.

The patient may be discharged on the day of surgery if the temperature is within normal limits, there is no undue discomfort in the operative area, and the appendectomy was uncomplicated. Discharge teaching for the patient and family is imperative. The nurse instructs the patient to make an appointment to have the surgeon remove the sutures between the fifth and seventh days after surgery. Incision care and activity guidelines are discussed; normal activity can usually be resumed within 2 to 4 weeks.

If there is a possibility of peritonitis, a drain is left in place at the area of the incision. Patients at risk for this complication may be kept in the hospital for several days and are monitored carefully for signs of intestinal obstruction or secondary hemorrhage. Secondary abscesses may form in the pelvis, under the diaphragm, or in the liver, causing elevation of the temperature, pulse rate, and white blood cell count.

When the patient is ready for discharge, the nurse teaches the patient and family to care for the incision and perform dressing changes and irrigations as prescribed. A home care nurse may be needed to assist with this care and to monitor the patient for complications and wound healing. Other complications of appendectomy are listed in Table 38-3.

## Diverticular Disease

A **diverticulum** is a saclike herniation of the lining of the bowel that extends through a defect in the muscle layer. Diverticula may occur anywhere in the small intestine or colon but most commonly occur in the sigmoid colon (at least 95%) (Beitz, 2004).

**Diverticulosis** exists when multiple diverticula are present without inflammation or symptoms. Diverticular disease of the colon is very common in developed countries, and its prevalence increases with age: more than 50% of Americans older than 80 years have diverticulosis (Beitz, 2004). A low intake of dietary fiber is considered a predisposing factor, but the exact cause has not been identified. Most patients with diverticular disease are asymptomatic, so its exact prevalence is unknown.

| TABLE 38-3 | Potential Complications and Nursing Interventions After Appendectomy |
|---|---|
| **Complication** | **Nursing Interventions** |
| Peritonitis | Observe for abdominal tenderness, fever, vomiting, abdominal rigidity, and tachycardia. |
| | Employ constant nasogastric suction. |
| | Correct dehydration as prescribed. |
| | Administer antibiotic agents as prescribed. |
| Pelvic abscess | Evaluate for anorexia, chills, fever, and diaphoresis. |
| | Observe for diarrhea, which may indicate pelvic abscess. |
| | Prepare patient for rectal examination. |
| | Prepare patient for surgical drainage procedure. |
| Subphrenic abscess (abscess under the diaphragm) | Assess patient for chills, fever, and diaphoresis. |
| | Prepare for x-ray examination. |
| | Prepare for surgical drainage of abscess. |
| Ileus (paralytic and mechanical) | Assess for bowel sounds. |
| | Employ nasogastric intubation and suction. |
| | Replace fluids and electrolytes by intravenous route as prescribed. |
| | Prepare for surgery, if diagnosis of mechanical ileus is established. |

**Diverticulitis** results when food and bacteria retained in a diverticulum produce infection and inflammation that can impede drainage and lead to perforation or abscess formation. At least 10% of patients with diverticulosis have diverticulitis at some point. A congenital predisposition is suspected when the disorder occurs in those younger than 40 years. Diverticulitis may occur as an acute attack or may persist as a continuing, smoldering infection. The symptoms manifested generally result from complications: abscess, **fistula** (abnormal tract) formation, obstruction, perforation, peritonitis, and hemorrhage.

## Pathophysiology

Diverticula form when the mucosa and submucosal layers of the colon herniate through the muscular wall because of high intraluminal pressure, low volume in the colon (ie, fiber-deficient contents), and decreased muscle strength in the colon wall (ie, muscular hypertrophy from hardened fecal masses). Bowel contents can accumulate in the diverticulum and decompose, causing inflammation and infection. The diverticulum can also become obstructed and then inflamed if the obstruction continues. The inflammation of the weakened colonic wall of the diverticulum can cause it to perforate, giving rise to irritability and spasticity of the colon (ie, diverticulitis). In addition, abscesses develop and may eventually perforate, leading to peritonitis and erosion of the arterial blood vessels, resulting in bleeding.

## Clinical Manifestations

Chronic constipation often precedes the development of diverticulosis by many years. Frequently, no problematic symptoms occur with diverticulosis. Signs and symptoms of diverticulosis are relatively mild and include bowel irregularity with intervals of diarrhea, nausea and anorexia, and bloating or abdominal distention. With repeated local inflammation of the diverticula, the large bowel may narrow with fibrotic strictures, leading to cramps, narrow stools, and increased constipation or at times intestinal obstruction. Weakness, fatigue, and anorexia are common symptoms. With diverticulitis, the patient reports an acute onset of mild to severe pain in the lower left quadrant, accompanied by nausea, vomiting, fever, chills, and leukocytosis. The condition, if untreated, can lead to septicemia.

## Assessment and Diagnostic Findings

Diverticulosis is typically diagnosed by colonoscopy, which permits visualization of the extent of diverticular disease and allows the clinician to biopsy tissue to rule out other diseases as needed. Until recently, barium enema had been the preferred diagnostic test, but it is now used less frequently than colonoscopy. If there are symptoms of peritoneal irritation when the diagnosis is diverticulitis, barium enema is contraindicated because of the potential for perforation.

CT is the diagnostic test of choice if the suspected diagnosis is diverticulitis; it can also reveal abscesses. Abdominal x-rays may demonstrate free air under the diaphragm if a perforation has occurred from the diverticulitis. Laboratory tests that assist in diagnosis include a complete blood cell count, revealing an elevated white blood cell count, and elevated erythrocyte sedimentation rate (ESR).

## Complications

Complications of diverticulitis include peritonitis, abscess formation, and bleeding. If an abscess develops, the associated findings are tenderness, a palpable mass, fever, and leukocytosis. An inflamed diverticulum that perforates results in abdominal pain localized over the involved segment, usually the sigmoid; local abscess or peritonitis follows. Abdominal pain, a rigid board-like abdomen, loss of bowel sounds, and signs and symptoms of shock occur with peritonitis. Noninflamed or slightly inflamed diverticula may erode areas adjacent to arterial branches, causing massive rectal bleeding.

### Gerontologic Considerations

The incidence of diverticular disease increases with age because of degeneration and structural changes in the circular muscle layers of the colon and because of cellular hypertrophy. The symptoms are less pronounced in the elderly than in other adults. The elderly may not have abdominal pain until infection occurs. They may delay reporting symptoms because they fear surgery or are afraid that they may have cancer. Blood in the stool is overlooked frequently, especially in the elderly, because of a failure to examine the stool or the inability to see changes if vision is impaired.

## Medical Management

### Dietary and Medication Management

Diverticulitis can usually be treated on an outpatient basis with diet and medication. When symptoms occur, rest, analgesics, and antispasmodics are recommended. Initially, the diet is clear liquid until the inflammation subsides; then a high-fiber, low-fat diet is recommended. This type of diet helps increase stool volume, decrease colonic transit time, and reduce intraluminal pressure. Antibiotics are prescribed for 7 to 10 days. A bulk-forming laxative also is prescribed.

In acute cases of diverticulitis with significant symptoms, hospitalization is required. Hospitalization is often indicated for those who are elderly, immunocompromised, or taking corticosteroids. Withholding oral intake, administering IV fluids, and instituting nasogastric suctioning if vomiting or distention occurs are used to rest the bowel. Broad-spectrum antibiotics are prescribed for 7 to 10 days. An opioid (eg, meperidine [Demerol]) is prescribed for pain relief. Morphine is contraindicated because it can increase intraluminal pressure in the colon, exacerbating symptoms. Oral intake is increased as symptoms subside. A low-fiber diet may be necessary until signs of infection decrease.

Antispasmodics such as propantheline bromide (Pro-Banthine) and oxyphencyclimine (Daricon) may be prescribed. Often it is not possible for patients to consume the 20 to 30 g of daily fiber that is recommended. Normal stools can be achieved by supplementing dietary fiber by using bulk preparations (psyllium [Metamucil]) or stool softeners (docusate [Colace]), by instilling warm oil into the rectum, or by inserting an evacuant suppository (bisacodyl [Dulcolax]). Such a prophylactic plan can reduce the bacterial flora of the bowel, diminish the bulk of the stool, and soften the fecal mass so that it moves more easily through the area of inflammatory obstruction.

### Surgical Management

Although acute diverticulitis usually subsides with medical management, immediate surgical intervention is necessary if complications (eg, perforation, peritonitis, hemorrhage, obstruction) occur. In cases of abscess formation without peritonitis, hemorrhage, or obstruction, CT-guided percutaneous drainage may be performed to drain the abscess, and IV antibiotics are administered. After the abscess is drained and the acute episode of inflammation has subsided (after approximately 6 weeks), surgery may be recommended to prevent repeated episodes. Two types of surgery are typically considered either to treat acute complications or prevent further episodes of inflammation:

- One-stage resection, in which the inflamed area is removed and a primary end-to-end anastomosis is completed
- Multiple-stage procedures for complications such as obstruction or perforation (Fig. 38-3)

The type of surgery performed depends on the extent of complications found during surgery. When possible, the area of diverticulitis is resected and the remaining bowel is joined end-to-end (ie, primary resection and end-to-end anastomosis). This is performed through traditional surgical or laparoscopically assisted colectomy. A two-stage resection may be performed in which the diseased colon is resected (as in a one-stage procedure) but no anastomosis is performed; both ends of the bowel are brought out onto the abdomen as stomas. This "double-barrel" temporary colostomy is then reanastomosed in a later procedure. Fecal diversion procedures are discussed later in this chapter.

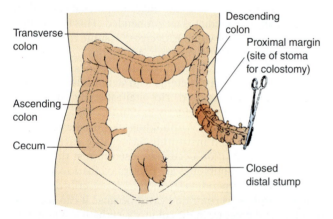

**FIGURE 38-3.** The Hartmann procedure for diverticulitis: primary resection for diverticulitis of the colon. The affected segment (*clamp attached*) has been divided at its distal end. In a primary anastomosis, the proximal margin (*dotted line*) is transected and the bowel attached end-to-end. In a two-stage procedure, a colostomy is constructed at the proximal margin with the distal stump oversewn (Hartmann procedure, as shown) or brought to the outer surface as a mucous fistula. The second stage consists of colostomy takedown and anastomosis.

## Nursing Process

## The Patient With Diverticulitis

### Assessment

During the health history, the nurse asks the patient about the onset and duration of pain and about past and present elimination patterns. The nurse reviews dietary habits to determine fiber intake and asks the patient about straining at stool, history of constipation with periods of diarrhea, tenesmus, abdominal bloating, and distention.

Assessment includes auscultation for the presence and character of bowel sounds and palpation for lower left quadrant pain, tenderness, or firm mass. The stool is inspected for pus, mucus, or blood. Temperature, pulse, and blood pressure are monitored for abnormal variations.

### Diagnosis

#### Nursing Diagnoses

Based on the assessment data, the nursing diagnoses may include the following:

- Constipation related to narrowing of the colon from thickened muscular segments and strictures
- Acute pain related to inflammation and infection

#### Collaborative Problems/ Potential Complications

Potential complications that may develop include the following:

- Peritonitis
- Abscess formation
- Bleeding

### Planning and Goals

The major goals for the patient may include attainment and maintenance of normal elimination patterns, pain relief, and absence of complications.

### Nursing Interventions

#### Maintaining Normal Elimination Patterns

The nurse recommends a fluid intake of 2 L per day (within limits of the patient's cardiac and renal reserve) and suggests foods that are soft but have increased fiber, such as prepared cereals or soft-cooked vegetables, to increase the bulk of the stool and facilitate peristalsis, thereby promoting defecation. An individualized exercise program is encouraged to improve abdominal muscle tone. It is important to review the patient's daily routine to establish a schedule for meals and a set time for defecation and to assist in identifying habits that may have suppressed the urge to defecate. The nurse encourages daily intake of bulk laxatives such as psyllium (Metamucil), which helps propel feces through the colon. Stool softeners are administered as prescribed to decrease straining at stool, which decreases intestinal pressure. Oil retention enemas may be prescribed to soften the stool, making it easier to pass.

### Relieving Pain

Opioid analgesics (eg, meperidine [Demerol]) to relieve the pain of diverticulitis and antispasmodic agents to decrease intestinal spasm are administered as prescribed. The nurse records the intensity, duration, and location of pain to determine whether the inflammatory process worsens or subsides.

### Monitoring and Managing Potential Complications

The major nursing focus is to prevent complications by identifying patients at risk and managing their symptoms as needed. The nurse assesses for the following signs and symptoms of perforation:

- Increased abdominal pain and tenderness accompanied by abdominal rigidity
- Elevated white blood cell count
- Elevated ESR
- Increased temperature
- Tachycardia
- Hypotension

Perforation is a surgical emergency. The clinical manifestations of perforation and peritonitis and the care of the patient with peritonitis are presented in the next section. The nurse monitors vital signs and urine output and administers IV fluids to replace volume loss as needed.

### Promoting Home and Community-Based Care

Because patients and their family members and health care providers tend to focus on the most obvious needs and issues, the nurse reminds the patient and family about the importance of continuing health promotion and screening practices. The nurse educates patients who have not been involved in these practices in the past about their importance and refers the patients to appropriate health care providers.

## Evaluation

### Expected Patient Outcomes

Expected patient outcomes may include the following:

1. Attains a normal pattern of elimination
    a. Reports less abdominal cramping and pain
    b. Reports the passage of soft, formed stool without pain
    c. Adds unprocessed bran to foods
    d. Drinks at least 10 glasses of fluid each day (if fluid intake is tolerated)
    e. Exercises daily
2. Reports decreased pain
    a. Requests analgesics as needed
    b. Adheres to a low-fiber diet during acute episodes
3. Recovers without complications
    a. Is afebrile
    b. Has normal blood pressure
    c. Has a soft, nontender abdomen with normal bowel sounds
    d. Maintains adequate urine output
    e. Has no blood in the stool

## Peritonitis

Peritonitis is inflammation of the peritoneum, the serous membrane lining the abdominal cavity and covering the viscera. Usually, it is a result of bacterial infection; the organisms come from diseases of the GI tract or, in women, from the internal reproductive organs. Peritonitis can also result from external sources such as injury or trauma (eg, gunshot wound, stab wound) or an inflammation that extends from an organ outside the peritoneal area, such as the kidney. The most common bacteria implicated are *Escherichia coli*, *Klebsiella*, *Proteus*, and *Pseudomonas*. Inflammation and paralytic ileus are the direct effects of the infection. Other common causes of peritonitis are appendicitis, perforated ulcer, diverticulitis, and bowel perforation (Fig. 38-4). Peritonitis may also be associated with abdominal surgical procedures and peritoneal dialysis.

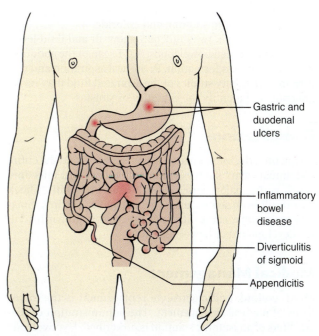

**FIGURE 38-4.** Common GI causes of peritonitis.

## Pathophysiology

Peritonitis is caused by leakage of contents from abdominal organs into the abdominal cavity, usually as a result of inflammation, infection, ischemia, trauma, or tumor perforation. Bacterial proliferation occurs. Edema of the tissues results, and exudation of fluid develops in a short time. Fluid in the peritoneal cavity becomes turbid with increasing amounts of protein, white blood cells, cellular debris, and blood. The immediate response of the intestinal tract is hypermotility, soon followed by paralytic ileus with an accumulation of air and fluid in the bowel.

## Clinical Manifestations

Symptoms depend on the location and extent of the inflammation. The early clinical manifestations of peritonitis frequently are the symptoms of the disorder causing the condition. At first, a diffuse type of pain is felt. The pain tends to become constant, localized, and more intense near the site of the inflammation. Movement usually aggravates it. The affected area of the abdomen becomes extremely tender and distended, and the muscles become rigid. Rebound tenderness and paralytic ileus may be present. Diminished perception of pain in peritonitis can occur in people receiving corticosteroids or analgesics. Patients with diabetes who have symptoms of advanced neuropathy and patients with cirrhosis who have signs of ascites may not experience pain during an acute bacterial episode. Usually, nausea and vomiting occur and peristalsis is diminished. A temperature of 100° to 101°F (37.8° to 38.3°C) can be expected, along with an increased pulse rate.

## Assessment and Diagnostic Findings

The white blood cell count is almost always elevated. The hemoglobin and hematocrit levels may be low if blood loss has occurred. Serum electrolyte studies may reveal altered levels of potassium, sodium, and chloride.

An abdominal x-ray study may show air and fluid levels as well as distended bowel loops. A CT scan of the abdomen may show abscess formation. Peritoneal aspiration and culture and sensitivity studies of the aspirated fluid may reveal infection and identify the causative organisms.

## Complications

Frequently, the inflammation is not localized, and the entire abdominal cavity shows evidence of widespread infection. Sepsis is the major cause of death from peritonitis. Shock may result from septicemia or hypovolemia. The inflammatory process may cause intestinal obstruction, primarily from the development of bowel adhesions.

## Medical Management

Fluid, colloid, and electrolyte replacement is the major focus of medical management. The administration of several liters of an isotonic solution is prescribed. Hypovolemia occurs because massive amounts of fluid and electrolytes move from the intestinal lumen into the peritoneal cavity and deplete the fluid in the vascular space.

Analgesics are prescribed for pain. Antiemetics are administered as prescribed for nausea and vomiting. Intestinal intubation and suction assist in relieving abdominal distention and in promoting intestinal function. Fluid in the abdominal cavity can cause pressure that restricts expansion of the lungs and causes respiratory distress. Oxygen therapy by nasal cannula or mask generally promotes adequate oxygenation, but airway intubation and ventilatory assistance occasionally are required.

Antibiotic therapy is initiated early in the treatment of peritonitis. Large doses of a broad-spectrum antibiotic are administered IV until the specific organism causing the infection is identified and appropriate antibiotic therapy can be initiated.

Surgical objectives include removing the infected material and correcting the cause. Surgical treatment is directed toward excision (ie, appendix), resection with or without anastomosis (ie, intestine), repair (ie, perforation), and drainage (ie, abscess). With extensive sepsis, a fecal diversion may need to be created.

The two most common postoperative complications are wound evisceration and abscess formation. Any suggestion from the patient that an area of the abdomen is tender or painful or "feels as if something just gave way" must be reported. The sudden occurrence of serosanguineous wound drainage strongly suggests wound dehiscence (see Chapter 20).

## Nursing Management

Intensive care is often needed. The blood pressure is monitored by arterial line if shock is present. The central venous pressure or pulmonary artery wedge pressure and urine output are monitored frequently. In addition, ongoing assessment of pain, GI function, and fluid and electrolyte balance is important. The nurse reports the nature of the pain, its location in the abdomen, and any changes in location. Administering analgesic medication and positioning the patient for comfort are helpful in decreasing pain. The patient is placed on the side with knees flexed; this position decreases tension on the abdominal organs. Accurate recording of all intake and output and central venous pressures and/or pulmonary artery pressures assist in calculating fluid replacement. The nurse administers and closely monitors IV fluids.

Signs that indicate that peritonitis is subsiding include a decrease in temperature and pulse rate, softening of the abdomen, return of peristaltic sounds, passing of flatus, and bowel movements. The nurse increases fluid and food intake gradually and reduces parenteral fluids as prescribed. A worsening clinical condition may indicate a complication, and the nurse must prepare the patient for emergency surgery.

Drains are frequently inserted during the surgical procedure, and the nurse must observe and record the character of the drainage postoperatively. Care must be taken when moving and turning the patient to prevent the drains from being dislodged. It is also important for the nurse to prepare the patient and family for discharge by teaching the patient to care for the incision and drains if the patient will be sent home with the drains still in place. Referral for home care may be indicated for further monitoring and patient and family teaching.

# Inflammatory Bowel Disease

**Inflammatory bowel disease** (IBD) refers to two chronic inflammatory GI disorders: regional enteritis (ie, Crohn's disease) and ulcerative colitis. Both disorders have striking similarities but also several differences. Table 38-4 compares regional enteritis and ulcerative colitis.

The incidence of IBD in the United States has increased in the past century: over 30,000 new cases occur annually. People between 15 and 30 years of age are at the greatest risk of developing IBD, followed by people between 50 and 70 years of age. Women and men tend to be equally affected, and family history appears to predispose people to develop IBD, particularly if a first-degree relative has the disease. Although it was previously believed that psychological symptoms such as anxiety or depression predisposed certain people to IBD, this theory has been discarded (NIH, 2005).

Despite extensive research, the cause of IBD is still unknown. Researchers theorize that it is triggered by environmental agents such as pesticides, food additives, tobacco, and radiation (Green, Morris, & Lin, 2005; NIH, 2005). Nonsteroidal anti-inflammatory drugs (NSAIDs) have been found to exacerbate IBD. Allergies and immune

### TABLE 38-4 Comparison of Regional Enteritis and Ulcerative Colitis

| Factor | Regional Enteritis | Ulcerative Colitis |
|---|---|---|
| **Course** | Prolonged, variable | Exacerbations, remissions |
| **Pathology** | | |
| Early | Transmural thickening | Mucosal ulceration |
| Late | Deep, penetrating granulomas | Minute, mucosal ulcerations |
| **Clinical Manifestations** | | |
| Location | Ileum, ascending colon (usually) | Rectum, descending colon |
| Bleeding | Usually not, but if it occurs, tends to be mild | Common—severe |
| Perianal involvement | Common | Rare—mild |
| Fistulas | Common | Rare |
| Rectal involvement | About 20% | Almost 100% |
| Diarrhea | Less severe | Severe |
| **Diagnostic Study Findings** | | |
| Barium series | Regional, discontinuous lesions | Diffuse involvement |
| | Narrowing of colon | No narrowing of colon |
| | Thickening of bowel wall | No mucosal edema |
| | Mucosal edema | Stenosis rare |
| | Stenosis, fistulas | Shortening of colon |
| Sigmoidoscopy | May be unremarkable unless accompanied by perianal fistulas | Abnormal inflamed mucosa |
| Colonoscopy | Distinct ulcerations separated by relatively normal mucosa in ascending colon | Friable mucosa with pseudopolyps or ulcers in descending colon |
| **Therapeutic Management** | Corticosteroids, sulfonamides (sulfasalazine [Azulfidine]) | Corticosteroids, sulfonamides; sulfasalazine useful in preventing recurrence |
| | Antibiotics | Bulk hydrophilic agents |
| | Parenteral nutrition | Antibiotics |
| | Partial or complete colectomy, with ileostomy or anastomosis | Proctocolectomy, with ileostomy |
| | Rectum can be preserved in some patients | Rectum can be preserved in only a few patients "cured" by colectomy |
| | Recurrence common | |
| **Systemic Complications** | Small bowel obstruction | Toxic megacolon |
| | Right-sided hydronephrosis | Perforation |
| | Nephrolithiasis | Hemorrhage |
| | Cholelithiasis | Malignant neoplasms |
| | Arthritis | Pyelonephritis |
| | Retinitis, iritis | Nephrolithiasis |
| | Erythema nodosum | Cholangiocarcinoma |
| | | Arthritis |
| | | Retinitis, iritis |
| | | Erythema nodosum |

disorders have also been suggested as causes. Abnormal response to dietary or bacterial antigens has been studied extensively, and genetic factors also are being studied. There is a high prevalence of coexistent IBS, which complicates the overall symptom presentation.

## Types of Chronic Inflammatory Bowel Disease

### Regional Enteritis (Crohn's Disease)

Regional enteritis is usually first diagnosed in adolescents or young adults but can appear at any time of life. Histopathologic changes consistent with regional enteritis most commonly occur in the distal ileum and colon but can occur anywhere along the GI tract. The incidence of regional enteritis has risen over the past 30 years (NIH, 2005). Regional enteritis is seen more often in smokers than in nonsmokers (Colwell, Goldberg, & Carmel, 2004).

#### Pathophysiology

Regional enteritis is a subacute and chronic inflammation of the GI tract wall that extends through all layers (ie, transmural lesion). Although it can occur anywhere in the GI tract, it most commonly occurs in the distal ileum and, to a lesser degree, the ascending colon. It is characterized by periods of remission and exacerbation. The disease process begins with edema and thickening of the mucosa. Ulcers begin to appear on the inflamed mucosa. These lesions are not in continuous contact with one another and are separated by normal tissue. Hence, these clusters of ulcers tend to take on a classic "cobblestone" appearance. Fistulas, fissures, and abscesses form as the inflammation extends into the peritoneum. Granulomas occur in 50% of patients. As the disease advances, the bowel wall thickens and becomes fibrotic, and the intestinal lumen narrows. Diseased bowel loops sometimes adhere to other loops surrounding them.

#### Clinical Manifestations

The onset of symptoms is usually insidious in regional enteritis, with prominent lower right quadrant abdominal pain and diarrhea unrelieved by defecation. Scar tissue and the formation of granulomas interfere with the ability of the intestine to transport products of the upper intestinal digestion through the constricted lumen, resulting in crampy abdominal pains. There is abdominal tenderness and spasm. Because eating stimulates intestinal peristalsis, the crampy pains occur after meals. To avoid these bouts of crampy pain, the patient tends to limit food intake, reducing the amounts and types of food to such a degree that normal nutritional requirements are often not met. As a result, weight loss, malnutrition, and secondary anemia occur. Ulcers in the membranous lining of the intestine and other inflammatory changes result in a weeping, edematous intestine that continually empties an irritating discharge into the colon. Disrupted absorption causes chronic diarrhea and nutritional deficits. The result is a person who is thin and emaciated from inadequate food intake and constant fluid loss. In some patients, the inflamed intestine may perforate, leading to intra-abdominal and anal abscesses. Fever and leukocytosis occur. Chronic symptoms include diarrhea, abdominal pain, **steatorrhea** (ie, excessive fat in the feces), anorexia, weight loss, and nutritional deficiencies.

Abscesses, fistulas, and fissures are common. Manifestations may extend beyond the GI tract and commonly include joint disorders (eg, arthritis), skin lesions (eg, erythema nodosum), ocular disorders (eg, conjunctivitis), and oral ulcers. The clinical course and symptoms can vary; in some patients, periods of remission and exacerbation occur, but in others, the disease follows a fulminating course.

#### Assessment and Diagnostic Findings

A proctosigmoidoscopy is usually performed initially to determine whether the rectosigmoid area is inflamed. A stool examination is also performed; the result may be positive for occult blood and steatorrhea. The most conclusive diagnostic aid for regional enteritis is a barium study of the upper GI tract that shows the classic "string sign" on an x-ray film of the terminal ileum, indicating the constriction of a segment of intestine. Endoscopy, colonoscopy, and intestinal biopsies may be used to confirm the diagnosis. A barium enema may show ulcerations (the cobblestone appearance described earlier), fissures, and fistulas. A CT scan may show bowel wall thickening and fistula formation.

A complete blood cell count is performed to assess hematocrit and hemoglobin levels (usually decreased) as well as the white blood cell count (may be elevated). The ESR is usually elevated. Albumin and protein levels may be decreased, indicating malnutrition.

#### Complications

Complications of regional enteritis include intestinal obstruction or stricture formation, perianal disease, fluid and electrolyte imbalances, malnutrition from malabsorption, and fistula and abscess formation. The most common type of small bowel fistula caused by regional enteritis is the enterocutaneous fistula (ie, an abnormal opening between the small bowel and the skin). Abscesses can be the result of an internal fistula that results in fluid accumulation and infection. Patients with regional enteritis are also at increased risk of colon cancer.

### Ulcerative Colitis

Ulcerative colitis is a recurrent ulcerative and inflammatory disease of the mucosal and submucosal layers of the colon and rectum. The prevalence of ulcerative colitis is highest in Caucasians and people of Jewish heritage (Johnson & Chan, 2004). It is a serious disease, accompanied by systemic complications and a high mortality rate. Approximately 5% of patients with ulcerative colitis develop colon cancer (NIH, 2005).

#### Pathophysiology

Ulcerative colitis affects the superficial mucosa of the colon and is characterized by multiple ulcerations, diffuse inflammations, and desquamation or shedding of the colonic epithelium. Bleeding occurs as a result of the ulcerations.

The mucosa becomes edematous and inflamed. The lesions are contiguous, occurring one after the other. Abscesses form, and infiltrate is seen in the mucosa and submucosa, with clumps of neutrophils found in the lumens of the crypts (ie, crypt abscesses) that line the intestinal mucosa (Porth, 2005). The disease process usually begins in the rectum and spreads proximally to involve the entire colon. Eventually, the bowel narrows, shortens, and thickens because of muscular hypertrophy and fat deposits.

### Clinical Manifestations

The clinical course is usually one of exacerbations and remissions. The predominant symptoms of ulcerative colitis include diarrhea, lower left quadrant abdominal pain, intermittent tenesmus, and rectal bleeding. The bleeding may be mild or severe, and pallor, anemia, and fatigue result. The patient may have anorexia, weight loss, fever, vomiting, and dehydration, as well as cramping, the feeling of an urgent need to defecate, and the passage of 10 to 20 liquid stools each day. The disease is classified as mild, severe, or fulminant, depending on the severity of the symptoms. Hypocalcemia and anemia frequently develop. Rebound tenderness may occur in the right lower quadrant. Extra-intestinal manifestations include skin lesions (eg, erythema nodosum), eye lesions (eg, uveitis), joint abnormalities (eg, arthritis), and liver disease.

### Assessment and Diagnostic Findings

The patient should be assessed for tachycardia, hypotension, tachypnea, fever, and pallor. Other assessments address level of hydration and nutritional status. The abdomen is examined for bowel sounds, distention, and tenderness. These findings assist in determining the severity of the disease.

The stool is positive for blood, and laboratory test results reveal low hematocrit and hemoglobin levels in addition to an elevated white blood cell count, low albumin levels, and an electrolyte imbalance. Abdominal x-ray studies are useful for determining the cause of symptoms. Free air in the peritoneum and bowel dilation or obstruction should be excluded as a source of the presenting symptoms. Sigmoidoscopy or colonoscopy and barium enema are valuable in distinguishing this condition from other diseases of the colon with similar symptoms. A barium enema may show mucosal irregularities, focal strictures or fistulas, shortening of the colon, and dilation of bowel loops. Colonoscopy may reveal friable, inflamed mucosa with exudate and ulcerations. This procedure assists in defining the extent and severity of the disease. CT scanning, magnetic resonance imaging (MRI), and ultrasound studies can identify abscesses and perirectal involvement. Leukocyte scanning (see Chapter 34) is useful when severe colitis prohibits the use of colonoscopy to determine the extent of inflammation.

Careful stool examination for parasites and other microbes is performed to rule out dysentery caused by common intestinal organisms, especially *Entamoeba histolytica* and *Clostridium difficile*.

### Complications

Complications of ulcerative colitis include toxic megacolon, perforation, and bleeding as a result of ulceration, vascular engorgement, and highly vascular granulation tissue. In toxic megacolon, the inflammatory process extends into the muscularis, inhibiting its ability to contract and resulting in colonic distention. Symptoms include fever, abdominal pain and distention, vomiting, and fatigue. If the patient with toxic megacolon does not respond within 24 to 72 hours to medical management with nasogastric suction, IV fluids with electrolytes, corticosteroids, and antibiotics, surgery is required. Total colectomy is then indicated. For many patients, surgery becomes necessary to relieve the effects of the disease and to treat these serious complications; an ileostomy usually is performed. The surgical procedures involved and the care of patients with this type of fecal diversion are discussed later in this chapter.

Patients with IBD also have a significantly increased risk of osteoporotic fractures due to decreased bone mineral density. Corticosteroid therapy may also contribute to the diminished bone density.

## Medical Management of Chronic Inflammatory Bowel Disease

Medical treatment for regional enteritis and ulcerative colitis is aimed at reducing inflammation, suppressing inappropriate immune responses, providing rest for a diseased bowel so that healing may take place, improving quality of life, and preventing or minimizing complications. Most patients have long periods of well-being interspersed with short intervals of illness (Lederman & Winshall, 2004). Management depends on the disease location, severity, and complications.

### Nutritional Therapy

Oral fluids and a low-residue, high-protein, high-calorie diet with supplemental vitamin therapy and iron replacement are prescribed to meet nutritional needs, reduce inflammation, and control pain and diarrhea. Fluid and electrolyte imbalances from dehydration caused by diarrhea are corrected by IV therapy as necessary if the patient is hospitalized or by oral fluids if the patient is managed at home. Any foods that exacerbate diarrhea are avoided. Milk may contribute to diarrhea in those with lactose intolerance. Cold foods and smoking are avoided because both increase intestinal motility. Parenteral nutrition may be indicated (see Chapter 36).

### Pharmacologic Therapy

Sedatives and antidiarrheal and antiperistaltic medications are used to minimize peristalsis to rest the inflamed bowel. They are continued until the patient's stools approach normal frequency and consistency.

Aminosalicylate formulations such as sulfasalazine (Azulfidine) are often effective for mild or moderate inflammation and are used to prevent or reduce recurrences in long-term maintenance regimens. Sulfa-free aminosalicylates (eg, mesalamine [Asacol, Pentasa]) are effective in preventing and treating recurrence of inflammation.

Antibiotics (eg, metronidazole [Flagyl]) are used for secondary infections, particularly for purulent complications such as abscesses, perforation, and peritonitis.

Corticosteroids are used to treat severe and fulminant disease and can be administered orally (eg, prednisone [Deltasone]) in outpatient treatment or parenterally (eg, hydrocortisone [Solu-Cortef]) in hospitalized patients. Topical (ie, rectal administration) corticosteroids (eg, hydrocortisone enema, budesonide [Entocort]) are also widely used in the treatment of distal colon disease. When the dosage of corticosteroids is reduced or stopped, the symptoms of disease may return. If corticosteroids are continued, adverse sequelae such as hypertension, fluid retention, cataracts, hirsutism (ie, abnormal hair growth), adrenal suppression, poor wound healing, and loss of bone density may occur.

Immunomodulators (eg, azathioprine [AZA], 6-mercaptopurine [6-MP], methotrexate, cyclosporine) have been used to alter the immune response. The exact mechanism of action of these medications in treating IBD is unknown. They are used for patients with severe disease who have not responded favorably to other therapies. These medications are useful in maintenance regimens to prevent relapses. Newer biologic therapies using monoclonal antibodies are being studied, including natalizumab (Tysabri) for treating Crohn's disease (Sandborn, Colombel, Enns, et al., 2005) and infliximab (Remicade) for treating ulcerative colitis (Rutgeerts, Sandborn, Feagan, et al., 2005). Initial reports from clinical trials appear promising for both these agents (Rutgeerts et al., 2005; Sandborn et al., 2005), although the adverse effects of natalizumab may seriously limit its therapeutic usefulness.

## Surgical Management

When nonsurgical measures fail to relieve the severe symptoms of IBD, surgery may be necessary. More than 50% of all patients with regional enteritis require surgery within 5 years of diagnosis (Colwell et al., 2004). The most common indications for surgery are medically intractable disease, poor quality of life, or complications from the disease or its treatment. Recurrence of inflammation and disease after surgery in regional enteritis is inevitable. The rate of recurrence after surgery is approximately 28% in the first 5 years (Colwell et al., 2004).

A common procedure performed for strictures of the small intestines is laparoscope-guided strictureplasty, in which the blocked or narrowed sections of the intestines are widened, leaving the intestines intact. In some cases, a small bowel resection is performed and diseased segments of the small intestines are resected and the remaining portions of the intestines are anastomosed. Surgical removal of up to 50% of the small bowel usually can be tolerated. In cases of severe regional enteritis of the colon, a total colectomy and ileostomy may be the procedure of choice.

A newer surgical procedure developed for patients with severe regional enteritis is intestinal transplant. This technique is now available to children and to young and middle-aged adults who have lost intestinal function from disease. Although this procedure is not a cure, it may eventually provide improvement in quality of life for some patients. The associated technical and immunologic problems remain formidable, and the costs and mortality rates remain high.

At least 25% of patients with ulcerative colitis eventually have total colectomies (NIH, 2005). When the colon is surgically removed, the patient is considered "cured" in that extra-intestinal manifestations subside and the disease process is otherwise limited to the colon. Indications for surgery include lack of improvement and continued deterioration, profuse bleeding, perforation, continued stricture formation, and cancer. Surgical excision usually improves quality of life. Proctocolectomy with ileostomy (ie, complete excision of colon, rectum, and anus) is recommended when the rectum is severely diseased. If the rectum can be preserved, restorative proctocolectomy with ileal pouch anal anastomosis (IPAA) is the procedure of choice.

Other types of surgical procedures, known as fecal diversions, are discussed later in this chapter.

### Total Colectomy With Ileostomy

An **ileostomy**, the surgical creation of an opening into the ileum or small intestine (usually by means of an ileal stoma on the abdominal wall), is commonly performed after a total colectomy (ie, excision of the entire colon). It allows for drainage of fecal matter (ie, effluent) from the ileum to the outside of the body. The drainage is very mushy and occurs at frequent intervals. Nursing management of the patient with an ileostomy is discussed later in this chapter.

### Continent Ileostomy

Another procedure involves the creation of a continent ileal reservoir (ie, **Kock pouch**) by diverting a portion of the distal ileum to the abdominal wall and creating a stoma. This procedure eliminates the need for an external fecal collection bag. Approximately 30 cm of the distal ileum is reconstructed to form a reservoir with a nipple valve that is created by pulling a portion of the terminal ileal loop back into the ileum. GI effluent can accumulate in the pouch for several hours and then be removed by means of a catheter inserted through the nipple valve. In many patients, a total colectomy is also performed with the Kock pouch. Possible indications for a total colectomy with Kock pouch placement (rather than a restorative proctocolectomy with IPAA) include a badly diseased rectum, lack of rectal sphincter tone, or inability to achieve fecal continence post-IPAA.

The major problem with the Kock pouch is malfunction of the nipple valve. Surgical research is currently focused on developing valves that may slip less frequently than the nipple valve.

### Restorative Proctocolectomy With Ileal Pouch Anal Anastomosis

A restorative proctocolectomy with IPAA is the surgical procedure of choice in cases where the rectum can be preserved, in that it eliminates the need for a permanent ileostomy. It establishes an ileal reservoir, and anal sphincter control of elimination is retained. The procedure involves connecting a portion of the ileum to the anus (ie, ileoanal anastomosis) in conjunction with removal of the colon and the rectal mucosa (ie, total abdominal colectomy and mucosal proctectomy) (Fig. 38-5). A temporary diverting loop ileostomy is constructed at the time of surgery and closed about 3 months later.

With ileoanal anastomosis, the diseased colon and rectum are removed, voluntary defecation is maintained, and anal continence is preserved. The ileal reservoir decreases the number of bowel movements by 50%, from approximately 14 to 20 per day to 7 to 10 per day. Nighttime elimination is gradually reduced to one bowel movement. Complications of ileoanal anastomosis include irritation of the perianal skin from leakage of fecal contents, stricture formation at the anastomosis site, and small bowel obstruction.

## Nursing Management of Chronic Inflammatory Bowel Disease

Nursing management of patients with IBD may be medical, surgical, or both. Patients in the community setting or those recently diagnosed may require education about diet and medications and referral to support groups. Hospitalized patients with long-standing or severe disease also require careful monitoring, parenteral nutrition, fluid replacement, and possibly emergent surgery. The surgical procedures may involve a fecal diversion, with attendant needs for physical care, emotional support, and extensive teaching about management of the ostomy.

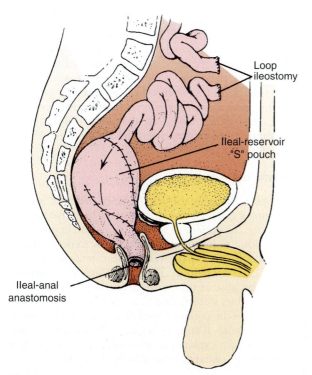

**FIGURE 38-5.** A mucosal proctectomy precedes anastomosis of the ileal reservoir. A temporary loop ileostomy diverts effluent for several months to allow healing.

# Nursing Process

## Management of the Patient With Inflammatory Bowel Disease

### Assessment

The nurse obtains a health history to identify the onset, duration, and characteristics of abdominal pain; the presence of diarrhea or fecal urgency, straining at stool (tenesmus), nausea, anorexia, or weight loss; and family history of IBD. It is important to discuss dietary patterns, including the amounts of alcohol, caffeine, and nicotine-containing products used daily and weekly. The nurse asks about patterns of bowel elimination, including character, frequency, and presence of blood, pus, fat, or mucus. It is important to note allergies and food intolerance, especially milk (lactose) intolerance. The patient may identify sleep disturbances if diarrhea or pain occurs at night.

Assessment includes auscultating the abdomen for bowel sounds and their characteristics; palpating the abdomen for distention, tenderness, or pain; and inspecting the skin for evidence of fistulas or signs of dehydration. The stool is inspected for blood and mucus.

Pain is usually localized in the right lower quadrant in regional enteritis, where hyperactive bowel sounds can be heard because of borborygmus and increased peristalsis. Abdominal tenderness is present with palpation. The most prominent symptom is intermittent pain that occurs with diarrhea but does not decrease after defecation. Pain in the periumbilical region usually indicates involvement of the terminal ileum. With ulcerative colitis, the abdomen may be distended, and rebound tenderness may be present. Rectal bleeding is a significant sign.

### Diagnosis

#### Nursing Diagnoses

Based on the assessment data, the nursing diagnoses may include the following:

- Diarrhea related to the inflammatory process
- Acute pain related to increased peristalsis and GI inflammation
- Deficient fluid volume related to anorexia, nausea, and diarrhea
- Imbalanced nutrition, less than body requirements, related to dietary restrictions, nausea, and malabsorption
- Activity intolerance related to fatigue
- Anxiety related to impending surgery
- Ineffective coping related to repeated episodes of diarrhea
- Risk for impaired skin integrity related to malnutrition and diarrhea

- Risk for ineffective therapeutic regimen management related to insufficient knowledge concerning the process and management of the disease

### Collaborative Problems/ Potential Complications

Potential complications that may develop include the following:

- Electrolyte imbalance
- Cardiac dysrhythmias related to electrolyte depletion
- GI bleeding with fluid volume loss
- Perforation of the bowel

## Planning and Goals

The major goals for the patient include attainment of normal bowel elimination patterns, relief of abdominal pain and cramping, prevention of fluid volume deficit, maintenance of optimal nutrition and weight, avoidance of fatigue, reduction of anxiety, promotion of effective coping, absence of skin breakdown, increased knowledge about the disease process and therapeutic regimen, and avoidance of complications.

## Nursing Interventions

### Maintaining Normal Elimination Patterns

The nurse determines if there is a relationship between diarrhea and certain foods, activities, or emotional stressors. Identifying precipitating factors, the frequency of bowel movements, and the character, consistency, and amount of stool passed is important. The nurse provides ready access to a bathroom, commode, or bedpan and keeps the environment clean and odor-free. It is important to administer antidiarrheal medications as prescribed, to record the frequency and consistency of stools after therapy is initiated, and to encourage bed rest to decrease peristalsis.

### Relieving Pain

The character of the pain is described as dull, burning, or crampy. It is important to ask about its onset. Does it occur before or after meals, during the night, or before elimination? Is the pattern constant or intermittent? Is it relieved with medications? The nurse administers anticholinergic medications 30 minutes before a meal as prescribed to decrease intestinal motility and administers analgesics as prescribed for pain. Position changes, local application of heat (as prescribed), diversional activities, and prevention of fatigue also are helpful for reducing pain.

### Maintaining Fluid Intake

To detect fluid volume deficit, the nurse keeps an accurate record of oral and IV fluids and maintains a record of output (ie, urine, liquid stool, vomitus, wound or fistula drainage). The nurse monitors daily weights for fluid gains or losses and assesses the patient for signs of fluid volume deficit (ie, dry skin and mucous membranes, decreased skin turgor, oliguria, exhaustion, decreased temperature, increased hematocrit, elevated urine specific gravity, and hypotension). It is important to encourage oral intake of fluids and to monitor the IV flow rate. The nurse initiates measures to decrease diarrhea (eg, dietary restrictions, stress reduction, antidiarrheal agents).

### Maintaining Optimal Nutrition

Parenteral nutrition is used when the symptoms of IBD are severe. With parenteral nutrition, the nurse maintains an accurate record of fluid intake and output as well as the patient's daily weight. The patient should gain 0.5 kg daily during parenteral nutrition therapy. Because parenteral nutrition is very high in glucose and can cause hyperglycemia, blood glucose levels are monitored every 6 hours. Once the symptoms of IBD exacerbation have diminished and the patient has gained or stabilized weight, parenteral nutrition is stopped and the patient is advanced on oral elemental feedings. Elemental feedings are high in protein and low in fat and residue. They are digested primarily in the jejunum, do not stimulate intestinal secretions, and allow the bowel to continue to rest. The nurse notes intolerance if the patient exhibits nausea, vomiting, diarrhea, or abdominal distention.

If oral foods are tolerated, small, frequent, low-residue feedings are given to avoid overdistending the stomach and stimulating peristalsis. It is important that the patient restrict activity to conserve energy, reduce peristalsis, and reduce calorie requirements.

### Promoting Rest

The nurse recommends intermittent rest periods during the day and schedules or restricts activities to conserve energy and reduce the metabolic rate. It is important to encourage activity within the limits of the patient's capacity. The nurse suggests bed rest for a patient who is febrile, has frequent diarrheal stools, or is bleeding. The patient on bed rest should perform active exercises, however, to maintain muscle tone and prevent thromboembolic complications. If the patient cannot perform these active exercises, the nurse performs passive exercises and joint range of motion. Activity restrictions are modified as needed on a day-to-day basis.

### Reducing Anxiety

Rapport can be established by being attentive and displaying a calm, confident manner. The nurse allows time for the patient to ask questions and express feelings. Careful listening and sensitivity to nonverbal indicators of anxiety (eg, restlessness, tense facial expressions) are helpful. The patient may be emotionally labile because of the consequences of the disease; the nurse tailors information about possible impending surgery to the patient's level of understanding and desire for detail. If surgery is planned, pictures and illustrations help explain the surgical procedure and help the patient visualize what a stoma looks like.

### Enhancing Coping Measures

Because the patient may feel isolated, helpless, and out of control, understanding and emotional support are essential. The patient may respond to stress in a variety of ways that may alienate others (eg, anger, denial, social self-isolation).

The nurse needs to recognize that the patient's behavior may be affected by a number of factors unrelated to inherent emotional characteristics. Any patient suffering the discomforts of frequent bowel movements and rectal soreness is anxious, discouraged, and depressed. It is important to develop a relationship with the patient that supports all attempts to cope with these stressors. It is also important to communicate that the patient's feelings are understood by encouraging the patient to talk and express his or her feelings and to discuss any concerns. Stress reduction measures that may be used include relaxation techniques, visualization, breathing exercises, and biofeedback. Professional counseling may be needed to help the patient and family manage issues associated with chronic illness and resulting disability.

### Preventing Skin Breakdown

The nurse examines the patient's skin frequently, especially the perianal skin. Perianal care, including the use of a skin barrier (eg, petroleum ointment [Vaseline]), is important after each bowel movement. The nurse gives immediate attention to reddened or irritated areas over bony prominences and uses pressure-relieving devices to prevent skin breakdown. Consultation with an **enterostomal therapist** (a nurse specially trained in the use of a variety of fecal and urinary diversions) otherwise known as wound-ostomy-continence nurse (WOCN) is often helpful.

### Monitoring and Managing Potential Complications

Serum electrolyte levels are monitored daily, and electrolyte replacements are administered as prescribed. It is important to report evidence of dysrhythmias or changes in level of consciousness immediately.

The nurse closely monitors rectal bleeding and administers blood component therapy and volume expanders as prescribed to prevent hypovolemia. It is important to monitor the blood pressure for hypotension and to obtain coagulation profiles and hemoglobin and hematocrit levels frequently. Vitamin K may be prescribed to increase clotting factors.

The nurse closely monitors the patient for indications of perforation (ie, acute increase in abdominal pain, rigid abdomen, vomiting, or hypotension) and obstruction and toxic megacolon (ie, abdominal distention, decreased or absent bowel sounds, change in mental status, fever, tachycardia, hypotension, dehydration, and electrolyte imbalances).

### Promoting Home and Community-Based Care

**TEACHING PATIENTS SELF-CARE**
The nurse assesses the patient's understanding of the disease process and his or her need for additional information about medical management (eg, medications, diet) and surgical interventions. The nurse provides information about nutritional management; a bland, low-residue, high-protein, high-calorie, and high-vitamin diet relieves symptoms and decreases diarrhea. It is important to explain the rationale for the use of corticosteroids and anti-inflammatory, antibacterial, antidiarrheal, and antispasmodic medications. The nurse emphasizes the importance of taking medications as prescribed and not abruptly discontinuing them (especially corticosteroids) to avoid development of serious medical problems (Chart 38-3). The nurse reviews ileostomy care as necessary (see Nursing Management of the Patient with an Ileostomy). Patient education information can be obtained from the National Foundation for Ileitis and Colitis.

---

**CHART 38-3**

## HOME CARE CHECKLIST • Inflammatory Bowel Disease

| At the completion of the home care instruction, the patient or caregiver will be able to: | Patient | Caregiver |
|---|:---:|:---:|
| • Verbalize an understanding of the disease process. | ✔ | ✔ |
| • Discuss nutritional management: bland, low-residue, high-protein, high-vitamin diet; identify foods to include and foods to be avoided. | ✔ | ✔ |
| • Describe medication regimen; identify medications by name, use, route, and frequency. | ✔ | ✔ |
| • Identify measures to be used to treat exacerbation of symptoms, to include rest, dietary modifications, and medications. | ✔ | ✔ |
| • Identify measures to be used to promote fluid and electrolyte balance during acute exacerbations | ✔ | ✔ |
| • Demonstrate management of parenteral nutrition therapy, if applicable; identify possible complications and interventions | ✔ | ✔ |
| • Incorporate stress reduction measures into lifestyle | ✔ | |

### CONTINUING CARE

Patients with chronic IBD are managed at home with follow-up care by their physician or through an outpatient clinic. Those whose nutritional status is compromised and who are receiving parenteral nutrition need home care nursing to ensure that their nutritional requirements are being met and that they or their caregivers can follow through with the instructions for parenteral nutrition. Patients who are medically managed need to understand that their disease can be controlled and that they can lead a healthy life between exacerbations. Control implies management based on an understanding of the disease and its treatment. Patients in the home setting need information about their medications (ie, name, dose, side effects, and frequency of administration) and need to take medications on schedule. Medication reminders such as containers that separate pills according to day and time or daily checklists are helpful.

During a flare-up, the nurse encourages the patient to rest as needed and to modify activities according to his or her energy level. Patients should limit tasks that impose strain on the lower abdominal muscles. They should sleep in a room close to the bathroom because of the frequent diarrhea (10 to 20 times per day); quick access to a toilet helps alleviate worry about having an "accident." Room deodorizers help control odors.

Dietary modifications can control but do not cure the disease; the nurse recommends a low-residue, high-protein, high-calorie diet, especially during an acute phase. It is important to encourage the patient to keep a record of the foods that irritate the bowel and to avoid them and to drink at least eight glasses of water each day.

The prolonged nature of the disease has an impact on the patient and often strains his or her family life and financial resources. Family support is vital; however, some family members may be resentful, guilty, and tired and feel unable to cope with the emotional demands of the illness and the physical demands of providing care. Some patients with IBD do not socialize for fear of being embarrassed. Many prefer to eat alone. Because they have lost control over elimination, they may fear losing control over other aspects of their lives. They need time to express their fears and frustrations. Individual and family counseling may be helpful.

## Evaluation

### Expected Patient Outcomes

Expected patient outcomes may include the following:

1. Reports a decrease in the frequency of diarrheal stools
    a. Complies with dietary restrictions; maintains bed rest
    b. Takes medications as prescribed
2. Has reduced pain
3. Maintains fluid volume balance
    a. Drinks 1 to 2 L of oral fluids daily
    b. Has normal body temperature
    c. Displays adequate skin turgor and moist mucous membranes
4. Attains optimal nutrition; tolerates small, frequent feedings without diarrhea
5. Avoids fatigue
    a. Rests periodically during the day
    b. Adheres to activity restrictions
6. Is less anxious
7. Copes successfully with diagnosis
    a. Verbalizes feelings freely
    b. Uses appropriate stress reduction behaviors
8. Maintains skin integrity
    a. Cleans perianal skin after defecation
    b. Uses lotion or ointment as skin barrier
9. Acquires an understanding of the disease process
    a. Modifies diet appropriately to decrease diarrhea
    b. Adheres to medication regimen as prescribed
10. Recovers without complications
    a. Electrolytes within normal ranges
    b. Normal sinus or baseline cardiac rhythm
    c. Maintains fluid balance
    d. Experiences no perforation or rectal bleeding

## Nursing Management of the Patient Requiring an Ileostomy

Some patients with IBD eventually require a permanent fecal diversion with creation of an ileostomy to manage symptoms and to treat or prevent complications. The Plan of Nursing Care summarizes care for the patient requiring an ostomy (Chart 38-4).

### Providing Preoperative Care

A period of preparation with intensive replacement of fluid, blood, and protein is necessary before surgery is performed. Antibiotics may be prescribed. If the patient has been taking corticosteroids, they will be continued during the surgical phase to prevent steroid-induced adrenal insufficiency. Usually, the patient is given a low-residue diet, provided in frequent, small feedings. All other preoperative measures are similar to those for general abdominal surgery. The abdomen is marked for the proper placement of the stoma by the surgeon or the enterostomal therapist. Care is taken to ensure that the stoma is conveniently placed—usually in the right lower quadrant about 2 inches below the waist, in an area away from previous scars, bony prominences, skin folds, or fistulas.

The patient must have a thorough understanding of the surgery to be performed and what to expect after surgery. Information about an ileostomy is presented to the patient by means of written materials, models, and discussion. Preoperative teaching includes management of drainage from the stoma; the nature of drainage; and the need for nasogastric intubation, parenteral fluids, and possibly perineal packing.

### Providing Postoperative Care

General abdominal surgery wound care is required. The nurse observes the stoma for color and size. It should be

*(text continues on page 1258)*

CHART 38-4

## Plan of Nursing Care: The Patient Undergoing Ostomy Surgery

**Nursing Diagnosis:** Deficient knowledge about the surgical procedure and preoperative preparation
**Goal:** Understands the surgical process and the necessary preoperative preparations

| NURSING INTERVENTIONS | RATIONALE | EXPECTED OUTCOMES |
|---|---|---|
| **Preoperative Care** <br> 1. Ascertain whether the patient has had a previous surgical experience and ask for recollections of positive and negative impressions. <br><br> 2. Determine what information the surgeon gave the patient and family and whether it was understood. Clarify and elaborate as necessary. Determine whether the stoma is permanent or temporary. Be aware of the patient's prognosis if carcinoma exists. <br> 3. Use pictures or drawings to illustrate the location and appearance of the surgical wounds (abdominal, perineal) and the stoma if the patient is receptive. <br> 4. Explain that oral/parenteral antimicrobials will be administered to cleanse the bowel preoperatively. Mechanical cleansing may also be required. <br> 5. Assist the patient during nasogastric/nasoenteric intubation. Measure drainage from the tube. | 1. Fear of a repeated negative experience increases anxiety. Talking about the experience with a nurse helps clarify misconceptions and helps the patient ventilate any repressed emotions. Positive experiences are reinforced. <br> 2. Clarification prevents misunderstandings and alleviates anxiety. <br><br><br><br><br> 3. Knowledge, for some, alleviates anxiety because fear of the unknown is decreased. Others choose not to know because it makes them more anxious. <br> 4. Antimicrobials and mechanical cleansing reduce intestinal bacterial flora. <br><br> 5. Nasoenteral intubation is used for decompression and drainage of gastrointestinal contents before surgery. | • Expresses anxieties and fears about the surgical process <br> • Projects a positive attitude toward the surgical procedure <br> • Repeats in own words information given by the surgeon <br> • Identifies normal anatomy and physiology of gastrointestinal tract and how it will be altered; can point to expected location of abdominal wound and stoma; describes stoma appearance and size <br> • Adheres to "bowel prep" regimen of antimicrobials or mechanical cleansing <br> • Tolerates the presence of nasogastric/nasoenteric tube |

**Nursing Diagnosis:** Disturbed body image
**Goal:** Attainment of a positive self-concept

| NURSING INTERVENTIONS | RATIONALE | EXPECTED OUTCOMES |
|---|---|---|
| 1. Encourage the patient to verbalize feelings about the stoma. Offer to be present when the stoma is first viewed and touched. <br><br> 2. Suggest that the spouse or significant other view the stoma. <br> 3. Offer counseling, if desired. <br> 4. Arrange for a visit with an ostomate. | 1. Free expression of feelings allows the patient the opportunity to verbalize and identify concerns. Expressed concerns can be therapeutically addressed by health care team members. <br> 2. Helps patient to overcome fears about partner's response. <br> 3. Provides opportunity for additional support. <br> 4. Ostomates can offer support and share mutual feelings and experiences. | • Freely expresses concerns and fears <br> • Accepts support <br> • Seeks help as needed <br> • States is willing to talk with an ostomate |

*continued >*

## CHART 38-4

### Plan of Nursing Care: The Patient Undergoing Ostomy Surgery (Continued)

**Nursing Diagnosis:** Anxiety related to the loss of bowel control
**Goal:** Reduction of anxiety

| NURSING INTERVENTIONS | RATIONALE | EXPECTED OUTCOMES |
|---|---|---|
| **Postoperative Care**<br>1. Provide information about expected bowel function:<br>   a. Characteristics of effluent<br>   b. Frequency of discharge<br>2. Teach the patient how to prepare the appliance for an adequate fit.<br>   a. Choose the drainage appliance that will provide a secure fit around the stoma. Measure the stoma size with a measuring guide provided by the ostomy equipment manufacturer and compare with the opening on the pouch. About 3-mm (⅛-in) clearance should be provided around the stoma.<br>   b. Remove any plastic covering that protects the appliance adhesive. *Note:* The pouch is applied by pressing the adhesive for 30 seconds to the skin or skin barrier.<br>3. Demonstrate how to change the appliance before leakage occurs. Be aware that the elderly person may have diminished vision and difficulty handling equipment.<br>4. When appropriate, demonstrate how to irrigate the colostomy (usually on the 4th–5th day). Recommend that irrigation be performed at a consistent time, depending on the type of colostomy. | 1. Emotional adjustment is facilitated if adequate information is provided at the level of the learner.<br><br>2. Adequate fit is necessary for successful use of the appliance.<br><br>   a. The appliance opening should be larger than the stoma for an adequate fit. Available brands come in different sizes to fit the stoma. Adjustments are made as necessary.<br><br><br><br><br><br>   b. The appliance is ready to apply directly to the skin or skin protector.<br><br><br><br>3. Manipulation of the appliance is a learned motor skill that requires practice and positive reinforcement.<br><br>4. Colostomy irrigation is used to regulate the passage of fecal material; alternatively the bowel can be allowed to evacuate naturally. | • Expresses interest in learning about altered bowel function<br>• Handles equipment correctly<br>• Changes the appliance unassisted<br>• Irrigates colostomy successfully<br>• Progresses toward a regular schedule of elimination |

**Nursing Diagnosis:** Risk for impaired skin integrity related to irritation of the peristomal skin by the effluent
**Goal:** Maintenance of skin integrity

| NURSING INTERVENTIONS | RATIONALE | EXPECTED OUTCOMES |
|---|---|---|
| 1. Provide information about signs and symptoms of irritated or inflamed skin. Use pictures if possible. | 1. Peristomal skin should be slightly pink without abrasions and similar to that of the entire abdomen. | • Describes appearance of healthy skin<br>• Correctly cleanses the skin<br>• Successfully applies a skin barrier |

### CHART 38-4

## Plan of Nursing Care: The Patient Undergoing Ostomy Surgery (Continued)

| NURSING INTERVENTIONS | RATIONALE | EXPECTED OUTCOMES |
|---|---|---|
| 2. Teach patient how to cleanse the peristomal skin gently. | 2. Mild friction with warm water and a gentle soap cleanses the skin and minimizes irritation and possible abrasions. Patting the skin dry prevents tissue trauma. | • Gently removes the drainage appliance without skin damage |
| 3. Demonstrate how to apply a skin barrier (powder, gel, paste, wafer). | 3. Skin barriers protect the peristomal skin from enzymes and bacteria. | • Demonstrates intact skin around the colostomy stoma |
| 4. Demonstrate how to remove the pouch. | 4. Gently separate adhesive from the skin to avoid irritation. Never pull! | |

**Nursing Diagnosis:** Potential imbalanced nutrition, less than body requirements, related to avoidance of foods that may cause GI discomfort
**Goal:** Achievement of an optimal nutritional intake

| NURSING INTERVENTIONS | RATIONALE | EXPECTED OUTCOMES |
|---|---|---|
| 1. Conduct a complete nutritional assessment to identify any foods that may increase peristalsis by irritating the bowel. | 1. Patients react differently to certain foods because of individual sensitivity. | • Modifies diet to avoid offensive foods yet maintains adequate nutritional intake |
| 2. Advise the patient to avoid food products with a cellulose or hemicellulose base (nuts, seeds). | 2. Cellulose food products are the nondigestible residue of plant foods. They hold water, provide bulk, and stimulate elimination. | • Avoids cellulose-based foods such as peanuts |
| 3. Recommend moderation in intake of certain irritating fruits such as prunes, grapes, and bananas. | 3. These fruits tend to increase the quantity of effluent. | • Modifies intake of certain fruits |

**Nursing Diagnosis:** Sexual dysfunction related to altered body image
**Goal:** Attainment of satisfactory sexual performance

| NURSING INTERVENTIONS | RATIONALE | EXPECTED OUTCOMES |
|---|---|---|
| 1. Encourage the patient to verbalize concerns and fears. The sexual partner is welcomed to participate in the discussion. | 1. Expressed needs help the therapist develop a plan of care. | • Expresses fears and concerns |
| 2. Recommend alternative sexual positions. | 2. Avoid patient embarrassment with the visual appearance of the stoma. Avoid peristomal skin irritation secondary to friction. | • Discusses alternative sexual positions |
| 3. Seek assistance from a sexual therapist, enterostomal therapist, or advanced practice nurse. | 3. Some patients need professional sexual counseling. | • Accepts services of a professional counselor |

*continued >*

### CHART 38-4

## Plan of Nursing Care — The Patient Undergoing Ostomy Surgery (Continued)

**Nursing Diagnosis:** Risk for deficient fluid volume related to anorexia and vomiting and increased loss of fluids and electrolytes from GI tract
**Goal:** Attainment of fluid balance

| NURSING INTERVENTIONS | RATIONALE | EXPECTED OUTCOMES |
|---|---|---|
| 1. Estimate fluid intake and output: | 1. Provides indication of fluid balance. | • Maintains fluid balance |
|    a. Strict intake and output |    a. An early indicator of fluid imbalance is a daily, significant difference between intake and output. The average person ingests (food, fluids) and loses (urine, feces, lungs) about 2 L of fluid every 24 h. | |
|    b. Daily weights |    b. A gain/loss of 1 L of fluid is reflected in a body weight change of 2.2 lb. | |
| 2. Assess serum and urinary values of sodium and potassium. | 2. Sodium is the major electrolyte regulating water balance. Vomiting results in decreased urinary and serum sodium levels. Urinary sodium values, in contrast to serum values, reflect early, sensitive changes in sodium balance. Sodium works in conjunction with potassium, which is also decreased with vomiting. A significant deficiency in potassium is associated with a decrease in intracellular potassium bicarbonate, which leads to acidosis and compensatory hyperventilation. | • Maintains normal serum and urinary values for sodium and potassium |
| 3. Observe and record skin turgor and the appearance of the tongue. | 3. Adequate hydration is reflected by the skin's ability to return to its normal shape after being grasped between the fingers. *Note:* In the older person, it is normal for the return to be delayed. Changes in the mucous membrane covering the tongue are accurate and early indicators of hydration status. | • Normal skin turgor<br>• Surface of tongue is pink, with a moist mucous membrane |

---

pink to bright red and shiny. Typically, a temporary plastic bag with an adhesive facing is placed over the ileostomy in the operating room and firmly pressed onto the surrounding skin. The nurse monitors the ileostomy for fecal drainage, which should begin about 72 hours after surgery. The drainage is a continuous liquid from the small intestine because the stoma does not have a controlling sphincter. The contents drain into the plastic bag and are thus kept from coming into contact with the skin. They are collected and measured when the bag becomes full. If a continent ileal reservoir was created, as described for the Kock pouch, continuous drainage is provided by an indwelling reservoir catheter for 2 to 3 weeks after surgery. This allows the suture lines to heal.

As with other patients undergoing abdominal surgery, the nurse encourages those with an ileostomy to engage in early ambulation. It is important to administer prescribed pain medications as required.

Because these patients lose much fluid in the early postoperative period, an accurate record of fluid intake, urinary output, and fecal discharge is necessary to help gauge the fluid needs of the patient. There may be 1000 to 2000 mL of fluid lost each day in addition to expected fluid loss through urine, perspiration, respiration, and other sources. With this loss, sodium and potassium are depleted. The nurse monitors laboratory values and administers electrolyte replacements as prescribed. Fluids are administered IV for 4 to 5 days to replace lost fluids.

Nasogastric suction is also a part of immediate postoperative care, with the tube requiring frequent irrigation, as prescribed. The purpose of nasogastric suction is to prevent a buildup of gastric contents. After the tube is removed, the nurse offers sips of clear liquids and gradually progresses the diet. It is important to report nausea and abdominal distention, which may indicate intestinal obstruction, immediately.

By the end of the first week, rectal packing is removed. Because this procedure may be uncomfortable, the nurse may administer an analgesic an hour before its removal. After the packing is removed, the perineum is irrigated two or three times daily until full healing takes place.

### PROVIDING EMOTIONAL SUPPORT

The patient may think that everyone is aware of the ileostomy and may view the stoma as a mutilation compared with other abdominal incisions that heal and are hidden. Because there is loss of a body part and a major change in anatomy and function, the patient often goes through the various phases of grieving—shock, disbelief, denial, rejection, anger, and restitution. Nursing support through these phases is important, and understanding of the patient's emotional outlook in each instance should determine the approach taken. For example, teaching may be ineffective until the patient is ready to learn. Concern about body image may lead to questions related to family relationships, sexual function, and, for women, the ability to become pregnant and to deliver a baby normally. Patients need to know that someone understands and cares about them. A calm, nonjudgmental attitude exhibited by the nurse aids in gaining the patient's confidence. It is important to recognize the dependency needs of these patients. Their prolonged illness can make them irritable, anxious, and depressed. The nurse can coordinate patient care through meetings attended by consultants such as the physician, psychologist, psychiatrist, social worker, enterostomal therapist, and dietitian. The team approach is important in facilitating the often complex care of the patient.

Conversely, a surgical procedure to create an ileostomy can produce dramatic positive changes in patients who have suffered from IBD for several years. After the discomfort of the disease has decreased and the patient learns how to take care of the ileostomy, he or she often develops a more positive outlook. Until the patient progresses to this phase, an empathetic and tolerant approach by the nurse plays an important part in recovery. The sooner the patient masters the physical care of the ileostomy, the sooner he or she will psychologically accept it.

Support from other people with ostomies is also helpful. The United Ostomy Association is dedicated to the rehabilitation of people with ostomies. This organization gives patients useful information about living with an ostomy through an educational program of literature, lectures, and exhibits. Local associations offer visiting services by qualified members who provide hope and rehabilitation services to patients with new ostomies. Hospitals and other health care agencies may have an enterostomal therapist on staff who can serve as a valuable resource person for the patient with an ileostomy.

### MANAGING SKIN AND STOMA CARE

The patient with a traditional ileostomy cannot establish regular bowel habits because the contents of the ileum are fluid and are discharged continuously. The patient must wear a pouch at all times. Stomal size and pouch size vary initially; the stoma should be rechecked 3 weeks after surgery, when the edema has subsided. The final size and type of appliance is selected in 3 months, after the patient's weight has stabilized and the stoma shrinks to a stable shape.

The location and length of the stoma are significant in the management of the ileostomy by the patient. The surgeon positions the stoma as close to the midline as possible and at a location where even an obese patient with a protruding abdomen can care for it easily. Usually, the ileostomy stoma is about 2.5 cm (1 in) long, which makes it convenient for the attachment of an appliance.

Skin excoriation around the stoma can be a persistent problem. Peristomal skin integrity may be compromised by several factors, such as an allergic reaction to the ostomy appliance, skin barrier, or paste; chemical irritation from the effluent; mechanical injury from the removal of the appliance; and infection. If irritation and yeast growth occur, nystatin powder (Mycostatin) is dusted lightly on the peristomal skin.

### CHANGING AN APPLIANCE

A regular schedule for changing the pouch before leakage occurs must be established for those with a traditional ileostomy. The patient can be taught to change the pouch in a manner similar to that described in Chart 38-5.

The amount of time a person can keep the appliance sealed to the body surface depends on the location of the stoma and on body structure. The usual wearing time is 5 to 7 days. The appliance is emptied every 4 to 6 hours, or at the same time the patient empties the bladder. An emptying spout at the bottom of the appliance is closed with a special clip made for this purpose.

Most pouches are disposable and odor-proof. Foods such as spinach and parsley act as deodorizers in the intestinal tract; foods that cause odors include cabbage, onions, and fish. Bismuth subcarbonate tablets, which may be prescribed and taken orally three or four times each day, are effective in reducing odor. Oral diphenoxylate (Lomotil) can also be prescribed to diminish intestinal motility, thereby thickening the stool and assisting in odor control.

### IRRIGATING A CONTINENT ILEOSTOMY

For a continent ileostomy (ie, Kock pouch), the nurse teaches the patient to drain the pouch, as described in Chart 38-6. A catheter is inserted into the reservoir to drain

## CHART 38-5 Guidelines for Changing an Ileostomy Appliance

Changing an ileostomy appliance is necessary to prevent leakage (the bag is usually changed every 5 to 7 days), to allow for examination of the skin around the stoma, and to assist in controlling odor if this becomes a problem. The appliance should be changed at any time that the patient complains of burning or itching under the disk or pain in the area of the stoma; routine changes should be performed early in the morning before breakfast or 2 to 4 hours after a meal, when the bowel is least active.

### NURSING ACTION

1. Promote patient comfort and involvement in the procedure.
   a. Have the patient assume a relaxed position.
   b. Provide privacy.
   c. Explain details of the procedure.
   d. Expose the ileostomy area; remove the ileostomy belt (if worn).
2. Remove the appliance.
   a. Have the patient sit on the toilet or on a chair facing the toilet. A patient who prefers to stand should face the toilet.
   b. The appliance (pouch) can be removed by gently pushing the skin away from the adhesive.

### RATIONALE

1. Providing a relaxed atmosphere and adequate explanations help the patient to become an active participant in the procedure.

2. These positions facilitate disposal or drainage.

3. Cleanse the skin:
   a. Wash the skin gently with a soft cloth moistened with tepid water and mild soap; the patient may prefer to bathe before putting on a clean appliance.

3. The patient may shower with or without the pouch.
   a. Micropore or waterproof tape applied to the sides of the faceplate will keep it secure during bathing.

# CHAPTER 38 • Management of Patients With Intestinal and Rectal Disorders

## CHART 38-5 Guidelines for Changing an Ileostomy Appliance, continued

| NURSING ACTION | RATIONALE |
|---|---|
| b. Rinse and dry the skin thoroughly after cleansing.<br>4. Apply appliance (when there is *no* skin irritation):<br>   a. An appropriate skin barrier is applied to the peristomal skin before the appliance is applied.<br>   b. Remove cover from adherent surface of disk of disposable plastic appliance and apply directly to the skin.<br>   c. Press firmly in place for 30 seconds to ensure adherence. | b. Moisture or soap residue will interfere with appliance adhesion.<br>4. Many appliances have a built-in skin barrier. The skin should be thoroughly dried before applying the appliance.<br><br>Pressing the appliance into place. Courtesy of Convatec, a Squibb Company. |
| 5. Apply appliance (when there is skin irritation):<br>   a. Cleanse the skin thoroughly but gently; pat dry.<br>   b. Apply Kenalog spray; blot excess moisture with a cotton pledget and dust lightly with nystatin (Mycostatin) powder.<br><br>                     OR<br><br>Apply as an alternative a wafer of Stomahesive (Squibb), which is commercially available. The stomal opening should be cut the same size as the stoma; use a cutting guide (supplied with Stomahesive). The wafer is applied directly to the skin.<br>   c. Another alternative is to moisten a karaya gum washer and apply when it is tacky. If the skin is moist, karaya powder may be applied first and any excess dusted off gently.<br>   d. The pouch is then applied to the treated skin. | 5.<br>   a. To remove debris<br>   b. The corticosteroid preparation (Kenalog) helps to decrease inflammation. The antifungal agent (nystatin) treats those types of infections that are common around stomas. A prescription is required for either medication.<br><br>Stomahesive is a substance that facilitates healing of excoriated skin. It adheres well even to moist, irritated skin.<br><br>   c. Karaya also facilitates skin healing. Tackiness promotes adherence.<br><br>   d. This will allow skin to heal while the appliance is in place. |
| 6. Check the pouch bottom for closure; use the rubber band or clip provided. | 6. Proper closure controls leakage. |

the fluid. The length of time between drainage periods is gradually increased until the reservoir needs to be drained only every 4 to 6 hours and irrigated once each day. A pouch is not necessary; instead, most patients wear a small dressing over the opening.

When the fecal discharge is thick, water can be injected through the catheter to loosen and soften it. The consistency of the effluent is affected by food intake. At first, drainage is only 60 to 80 mL, but as time goes on, the amount increases significantly. The internal Kock pouch stretches, eventually accommodating 500 to 1000 mL. The patient learns to use the sensation of pressure in the pouch as a gauge to determine how often the pouch should be drained.

## CHART 38-6 Guidelines for Draining a Continent Ileostomy (Kock Pouch)

A continent ileostomy is the surgical creation of a pouch of small intestine that can serve as an internal receptacle for fecal discharge; a nipple valve is constructed at the outlet. Postoperatively, a catheter extends from the stoma and is attached to a closed drainage suction system. To ensure patency of the catheter, 10 to 20 mL of normal saline is instilled gently into the pouch usually every 3 hours; return flow is not aspirated but is allowed to drain by gravity.

After approximately 2 weeks, when the healing process has progressed to the point at which the catheter is removed from the stoma, the patient is taught to drain the pouch. The equipment required includes a catheter, tissues, water-soluble lubricant, gauze squares, a syringe, irrigating solution in a bowl, and an emesis or receiving basin.

The following procedure is used to drain the pouch; the patient is helped to participate in this procedure to learn to perform it unassisted.

| NURSING ACTION | RATIONALE |
|---|---|
| 1. Lubricate the catheter and gently insert it about 5 cm (2 in), at which point some resistance may be felt at the valve or nipple. | 1. When gentle pressure is used, the catheter usually will enter the pouch. |
| 2. If there is much resistance, fill a syringe with 20 mL of air or water and inject it through the catheter, while still exerting some pressure on the catheter. | 2. This will permit the catheter to enter the pouch. |
| 3. Place the other end of the catheter in a drainage basin held below the level of the stoma. Later this process can be carried out at the toilet with drainage delivered into the toilet bowl. | 3. Gravity facilitates drainage. Drainage may include flatus as well as effluent. |
| 4. After drainage, the catheter is removed and the area around the stoma is gently washed with warm water. Pat dry and apply an absorbent pad over the stoma. Fasten the pad with hypoallergenic tape. | 4. The entire procedure requires about 5 to 10 min; at first it is performed every 3 h. The time between procedures is gradually lengthened to three times daily. |

### MANAGING DIETARY AND FLUID NEEDS

A low-residue diet is followed for the first 6 to 8 weeks. Strained fruits and vegetables are given. These foods are important sources of vitamins A and C. Later, there are few dietary restrictions, except for avoiding foods that are high in fiber or hard-to-digest kernels, such as celery, popcorn, corn, poppy seeds, caraway seeds, and coconut. Foods are reintroduced one at a time. The nurse assesses the patient's tolerance for these foods and reminds him or her to chew food thoroughly.

Fluids may be a problem during the summer, when fluid lost through perspiration adds to the fluid loss through the ileostomy. Fluids such as Gatorade are helpful in maintaining electrolyte balance. If the fecal discharge is too watery, fibrous foods (eg, whole-grain cereals, fresh fruit skins, beans, corn, nuts) are restricted. If the effluent is excessively dry, salt intake is increased. Increased intake of water or fluid does not increase the effluent, because excess water is excreted in the urine.

### PREVENTING COMPLICATIONS

Monitoring for complications is an ongoing activity for the patient with an ileostomy. Peristomal skin irritation, which results from leakage of effluent, is the most common complication of an ileostomy. A drainable pouching system that does not fit well is often the cause. Components of the drainable pouching system include the pouch, a solid skin barrier, and adhesive. The enterostomal therapist typically recommends the appropriate drainable pouching system. The solid skin barrier is the component of this system that is most important in ensuring healthy peristomal skin. Solid skin barriers are typically shaped as rectangular or elliptical wafers and are composed of polymers and hydrocolloids. They protect the skin around the stoma from effluent from the stoma and provide a stable interface between the stoma and the pouch.

Other common complications include diarrhea, stomal stenosis, urinary calculi, and cholelithiasis. Even in the presence of a properly fitted drainable pouching system, diarrhea can be problematic. Diarrhea, manifested by very irritating effluent that rapidly fills the pouch (every hour or sooner), can quickly lead to dehydration and electrolyte losses. Supplemental water, sodium, and potassium are administered to prevent hypovolemia and hypokalemia. Antidiarrheal agents are administered. Stenosis is caused by circular scar tissue that forms at the stoma site. The scar tissue must be surgically released. Urinary calculi may occur in patients with ileostomies and are at least partly attributed to dehydration from decreased fluid intake. Intense lower abdominal pain that radiates to the legs, hematuria, and signs of dehydration indicate that the urine should be strained. Fluid intake is encouraged. Sometimes, small stones are passed during urination; otherwise, treatment is necessary to crush or remove the calculi (see Chapter 45).

Cholelithiasis (ie, gallstones) occurs more commonly in patients with an ileostomy than in the general population because of changes in the absorption of bile acids that occur postoperatively. Spasm of the gallbladder causes severe upper right abdominal pain that can radiate to the back and right shoulder (see Chapter 40).

### PROMOTING HOME AND COMMUNITY-BASED CARE

**Teaching Patients Self-Care.** The spouse and family should be familiar with the adjustments that will be necessary when the patient returns home. They need to know why it is necessary for the patient to occupy the bathroom for 10 minutes or more at certain times of the day and why certain equipment is needed. Their understanding is necessary to reduce tension; a relaxed patient tends to have fewer problems. Visits from an enterostomal therapist may be arranged to ensure that the patient is progressing as expected and to provide additional guidance and teaching as needed.

**Continuing Care.** The patient needs to know the commercial name of the drainable pouching system to be used so that he or she can obtain a ready supply and should know how to obtain other supplies. The names and contact information of a local enterostomal therapist and local self-help groups are often helpful. Any restrictions on driving or working also need to be reviewed. The nurse teaches the patient about common postoperative complications and how to recognize and report them (Chart 38-7).

# Intestinal Obstruction

Intestinal obstruction exists when blockage prevents the normal flow of intestinal contents through the intestinal tract. Two types of processes can impede this flow:

- *Mechanical obstruction:* An intraluminal obstruction or a mural obstruction from pressure on the intestinal wall occurs. Examples are intussusception, polypoid tumors and neoplasms, stenosis, strictures, adhesions, hernias, and abscesses.
- *Functional obstruction:* The intestinal musculature cannot propel the contents along the bowel. Examples are amyloidosis, muscular dystrophy, endocrine disorders such as diabetes mellitus, or neurologic disorders such as Parkinson's disease. The blockage also can be temporary and the result of the manipulation of the bowel during surgery.

The obstruction can be partial or complete. Its severity depends on the region of bowel affected, the degree to which the lumen is occluded, and especially the degree to which the vascular supply to the bowel wall is disturbed.

Most bowel obstructions occur in the small intestine. Adhesions are the most common cause of small bowel obstruction, followed by hernias and neoplasms. Other causes include intussusception, volvulus (ie, twisting of the bowel), and paralytic ileus. Most obstructions in the large bowel occur in the sigmoid colon. The most common causes are carcinoma, diverticulitis, inflammatory bowel disorders, and benign tumors. Table 38-5 and Figure 38-6 list mechanical causes of obstruction and describe how they occur.

## Small Bowel Obstruction

### Pathophysiology

Intestinal contents, fluid, and gas accumulate above the intestinal obstruction. The abdominal distention and retention of fluid reduce the absorption of fluids and stimulate more gastric secretion. With increasing distention, pressure within the intestinal lumen increases, causing a decrease in venous and arteriolar capillary pressure. This causes edema, congestion, necrosis, and eventual rupture or perforation of the intestinal wall, with resultant peritonitis.

Reflux vomiting may be caused by abdominal distention. Vomiting results in loss of hydrogen ions and potassium from the stomach, leading to reduction of chlorides

---

**CHART 38-7**

### HOME CARE CHECKLIST • Managing Ostomy Care

| At the completion of the home care instruction, the patient or caregiver will be able to: | Patient | Caregiver |
|---|---|---|
| • Demonstrate ostomy care, including wound cleansing, irrigation, and appliance changing. | ✔ | ✔ |
| • Describe the importance of maintaining peristomal skin integrity. | ✔ | ✔ |
| • Identify sources for obtaining additional dressing and appliance supplies. | ✔ | ✔ |
| • Identify dietary restrictions (foods that can cause diarrhea and constipation). | ✔ | ✔ |
| • Identify measures to be used to promote fluid and electrolyte balance | ✔ | ✔ |
| • Describe medication regimen: identify medications by name, use, route, and frequency. | ✔ | ✔ |
| • Describe potential complications and necessary actions to be taken if complications occur. | ✔ | ✔ |
| • Identify how to contact enterostomal therapist or home health nurse. | ✔ | ✔ |

## TABLE 38-5  Mechanical Causes of Intestinal Obstruction

| Cause | Course of Events | Result |
|---|---|---|
| Adhesions | Loops of intestine become adherent to areas that heal slowly or scar after abdominal surgery. | After surgery, adhesions produce a kinking of an intestinal loop. |
| Intussusception | One part of the intestine slips into another part located below it (like a telescope shortening). | The intestinal lumen becomes narrowed. |
| Volvulus | Bowel twists and turns on itself. | Intestinal lumen becomes obstructed. Gas and fluid accumulate in the trapped bowel. |
| Hernia | Protrusion of intestine through a weakened area in the abdominal muscle or wall. | Intestinal flow may be completely obstructed. Blood flow to the area may be obstructed as well. |
| Tumor | A tumor that exists within the wall of the intestine extends into the intestinal lumen, or a tumor outside the intestine causes pressure on the wall of the intestine. | Intestinal lumen becomes partially obstructed; if the tumor is not removed, complete obstruction results. |

and potassium in the blood and to metabolic alkalosis. Dehydration and acidosis develop from loss of water and sodium. With acute fluid losses, hypovolemic shock may occur.

## Clinical Manifestations

The initial symptom is usually crampy pain that is wavelike and colicky. The patient may pass blood and mucus but no fecal matter and no flatus. Vomiting occurs. If the obstruction is complete, the peristaltic waves initially become extremely vigorous and eventually assume a reverse direction, with the intestinal contents propelled toward the mouth instead of toward the rectum. If the obstruction is in the ileum, fecal vomiting takes place. First, the patient vomits the stomach contents, then the bile-stained contents of the duodenum and the jejunum, and finally, with each paroxysm of pain, the darker, fecal-like contents of the ileum. The signs of dehydration become evident: intense thirst, drowsiness, generalized malaise, aching, and a parched tongue and mucous membranes. The abdomen becomes distended. The lower the obstruction is in the GI tract, the more marked the abdominal distention. If the obstruction continues uncorrected, hypovolemic shock occurs from dehydration and loss of plasma volume.

## Assessment and Diagnostic Findings

Diagnosis is based on the symptoms described previously and on imaging studies. Abdominal x-ray and CT findings include abnormal quantities of gas, fluid, or both in the intestines. Laboratory studies (ie, electrolyte studies and a complete blood cell count) reveal a picture of dehydration, loss of plasma volume, and possible infection.

**FIGURE 38-6.** Three causes of intestinal obstruction. (**A**) Intussusception invagination or shortening of the colon caused by the movement of one segment of bowel into another. (**B**) Volvulus of the sigmoid colon; the twist is counterclockwise in most cases. Note the edematous bowel. (**C**) Hernia (inguinal). The sac of the hernia is a continuation of the peritoneum of the abdomen. The hernial contents are intestine, omentum, or other abdominal contents that pass through the hernial opening into the hernial sac.

## Medical Management

Decompression of the bowel through a nasogastric tube (see Chapter 36) is successful in most cases. When the bowel is completely obstructed, the possibility of strangulation warrants surgical intervention. Before surgery, IV therapy is necessary to replace the depleted water, sodium, chloride, and potassium.

The surgical treatment of intestinal obstruction depends largely on the cause of the obstruction. In the most common causes of obstruction, such as hernia and adhesions, the surgical procedure involves repairing the hernia or dividing the adhesion to which the intestine is attached. In some instances, the portion of affected bowel may be removed and an anastomosis performed. The complexity of the surgical procedure for intestinal obstruction depends on the duration of the obstruction and the condition of the intestine.

## Nursing Management

Nursing management of the nonsurgical patient with a small bowel obstruction includes maintaining the function of the nasogastric tube, assessing and measuring the nasogastric output, assessing for fluid and electrolyte imbalance, monitoring nutritional status, and assessing improvement (eg, return of normal bowel sounds, decreased abdominal distention, subjective improvement in abdominal pain and tenderness, passage of flatus or stool). The nurse reports discrepancies in intake and output, worsening of pain or abdominal distention, and increased nasogastric output. If the patient's condition does not improve, the nurse prepares him or her for surgery. The exact nature of the surgery depends on the cause of the obstruction. Nursing care of the patient after surgical repair of a small bowel obstruction is similar to that for other abdominal surgeries (see Chapter 20).

## *Large Bowel Obstruction*

### Pathophysiology

As in small bowel obstruction, large bowel obstruction results in an accumulation of intestinal contents, fluid, and gas proximal to the obstruction. Obstruction in the large bowel can lead to severe distention and perforation unless some gas and fluid can flow back through the ileal valve. Large bowel obstruction, even if complete, may be undramatic if the blood supply to the colon is not disturbed. However, if the blood supply is cut off, intestinal strangulation and necrosis (ie, tissue death) occur; this condition is life threatening. In the large intestine, dehydration occurs more slowly than in the small intestine because the colon can absorb its fluid contents and can distend to a size considerably beyond its normal full capacity.

Adenocarcinoid tumors account for the majority of large bowel obstructions. Most tumors occur beyond the splenic flexure, making them accessible with a flexible sigmoidoscope.

### Clinical Manifestations

Large bowel obstruction differs clinically from small bowel obstruction in that the symptoms develop and progress relatively slowly. In patients with obstruction in the sigmoid colon or the rectum, constipation may be the only symptom for months. The shape of the stool is altered as it passes the obstruction that is gradually increasing in size. Blood in the stool may result in iron deficiency anemia. The patient may experience weakness, weight loss, and anorexia. Eventually, the abdomen becomes markedly distended, loops of large bowel become visibly outlined through the abdominal wall, and the patient has crampy lower abdominal pain. Finally, fecal vomiting develops. Symptoms of shock may occur.

### Assessment and Diagnostic Findings

Diagnosis is based on symptoms and on imaging studies. Abdominal x-ray and abdominal CT or MRI findings reveal a distended colon and pinpoint the site of the obstruction. Barium studies are contraindicated.

### Medical Management

Restoration of intravascular volume, correction of electrolyte abnormalities, and nasogastric aspiration and decompression are instituted immediately. A colonoscopy may be performed to untwist and decompress the bowel. A cecostomy, in which a surgical opening is made into the cecum, may be performed in patients who are poor surgical risks and urgently need relief from the obstruction. The procedure provides an outlet for releasing gas and a small amount of drainage. A rectal tube may be used to decompress an area that is lower in the bowel. However, the usual treatment is surgical resection to remove the obstructing lesion. A temporary or permanent colostomy may be necessary. An ileoanal anastomosis may be performed if it is necessary to remove the entire large bowel.

### Nursing Management

The nurse's role is to monitor the patient for symptoms that indicate that the intestinal obstruction is worsening and to provide emotional support and comfort. The nurse administers IV fluids and electrolytes as prescribed. If the patient's condition does not respond to nonsurgical treatment, the nurse prepares the patient for surgery. This preparation includes preoperative teaching as the patient's condition indicates. After surgery, general abdominal wound care and routine postoperative nursing care are provided.

## *Colorectal Cancer*

Tumors of the colon and rectum are relatively common; the colorectal area (the colon and rectum combined) is now the third most common site of new cancer cases and deaths in the United States. Colorectal cancer is a disease of Western cultures. Almost 150,000 new cases and 56,000 deaths from colorectal cancer occur annually (American Cancer Society [ACS], 2006).

The incidence increases with age (the incidence is highest in people older than 85 years) and is higher in people with a family history of colon cancer and those with IBD or polyps. The exact cause of colon and rectal cancer is still unknown, but risk factors have been identified (Chart 38-8).

Improved screening strategies have helped reduce the number of deaths from colon cancer in recent years. Of the approximately 150,000 people diagnosed each year, fewer than half that number die annually (ACS, 2006). Early diagnosis and prompt treatment could save almost three of every four people. If the disease is detected and treated at an early stage, the 5-year survival rate is 90%; however, only 34% of colorectal cancers are detected at an early stage (ACS, 2006). Survival rates after late diagnosis are very low. Most people are asymptomatic for long periods and seek health care only when they notice a change in bowel habits or rectal bleeding. Prevention and early screening are key to detection and reduction of mortality rates.

## Pathophysiology

Cancer of the colon and rectum is predominantly (95%) adenocarcinoma (ie, arising from the epithelial lining of the intestine) (ACS, 2006). It may start as a benign polyp but may become malignant, invade and destroy normal tissues, and extend into surrounding structures. Cancer cells may migrate away from the primary tumor and spread to other parts of the body (most often to the liver).

## Clinical Manifestations

The symptoms are greatly determined by the location of the cancer, the stage of the disease, and the function of the intestinal segment in which it is located. The most common presenting symptom is a change in bowel habits. The passage of blood in the stools is the second most common symptom. Symptoms may also include unexplained anemia, anorexia, weight loss, and fatigue.

The symptoms most commonly associated with right-sided lesions are dull abdominal pain and melena (ie, black, tarry stools). The symptoms most commonly associated with left-sided lesions are those associated with obstruction (ie, abdominal pain and cramping, narrowing stools, constipation, distention), as well as bright-red blood in the stool. Symptoms associated with rectal lesions are tenesmus (ie, ineffective, painful straining at stool), rectal pain, the feeling of incomplete evacuation after a bowel movement, alternating constipation and diarrhea, and bloody stool.

## Assessment and Diagnostic Findings

Along with an abdominal and rectal examination, the most important diagnostic procedures for cancer of the colon are fecal occult blood testing, barium enema, proctosigmoidoscopy, and colonoscopy (see Chapter 34). The majority of colorectal cancer cases can be identified by colonoscopy with biopsy or cytology smears.

Carcinoembryonic antigen (CEA) studies may also be performed. Although CEA may not be a highly reliable indicator in diagnosing colon cancer because not all lesions secrete CEA, studies show that CEA levels are reliable prognostic predictors. With complete excision of the tumor, the elevated levels of CEA should return to normal within 48 hours. Elevations of CEA at a later date suggest recurrence.

## Complications

Tumor growth may cause partial or complete bowel obstruction. Extension of the tumor and ulceration into the surrounding blood vessels result in hemorrhage. Perforation, abscess formation, peritonitis, sepsis, and shock may occur.

### Gerontologic Considerations

The incidence of carcinoma of the colon and rectum increases with age. These cancers are considered common malignancies in advanced age. In men, only the incidence of prostate cancer and lung cancer exceeds that of colorectal cancer. In women, only the incidence of breast cancer exceeds that of colorectal cancer. Symptoms are often insidious. Patients with colorectal cancer usually report fatigue, which is caused primarily by iron deficiency anemia. In early stages, minor changes in bowel patterns and occasional bleeding may occur. The later symptoms most commonly reported by the elderly are abdominal pain, obstruction, tenesmus, and rectal bleeding.

Colon cancer in the elderly has been closely associated with dietary carcinogens. Lack of fiber is a major causative factor because the passage of feces through the intestinal tract is prolonged, which extends exposure to possible carcinogens. Excess dietary fat, high alcohol consumption, and smoking all increase the incidence of colorectal tumors. Physical activity and dietary folate have protective effects (Varricchio, Ades, Hinds, et al., 2004).

## Medical Management

The patient with symptoms of intestinal obstruction is treated with IV fluids and nasogastric suction. If there has been significant bleeding, blood component therapy may be required.

Treatment for colorectal cancer depends on the stage of the disease (Chart 38-9) and consists of surgery to remove the tumor, supportive therapy, and adjuvant therapy. Patients

---

**CHART 38-8**

### ⚠ Risk Factors for Colorectal Cancer

- Increasing age
- Family history of colon cancer or polyps
- Previous colon cancer or adenomatous polyps
- History of inflammatory bowel disease
- High-fat, high-protein (with high intake of beef), low-fiber diet
- Genital cancer (eg, endometrial cancer, ovarian cancer) or breast cancer (in women)

## CHART 38-9

### Staging of Colorectal Cancer: Dukes' Classification—Modified Staging System

**Class A:** Tumor limited to muscular mucosa and submucosa
**Class $B_1$:** Tumor extends into mucosa
**Class $B_2$:** Tumor extends through entire bowel wall into serosa or pericolic fat, no nodal involvement
**Class $C_1$:** Positive nodes, tumor is limited to bowel wall
**Class $C_2$:** Positive nodes, tumor extends through entire bowel wall
**Class D:** Advanced and metastasis to liver, lung, or bone

Another staging system, the TNM (tumor, nodal involvement, metastasis) classification, may be used to describe the anatomic extent of the primary tumor, depending on:

- Size, invasion depth, and surface spread
- Extent of nodal involvement
- Presence or absence of metastasis

---

Rudy, D. R., & Zdon, M. J. (2000). Update on colorectal cancer. *American Family Physician*, 61(6), 1759–1774.

---

who receive some form of adjuvant therapy, which may include chemotherapy, radiation therapy, immunotherapy, or multimodality therapy, typically demonstrate delays in tumor recurrence and increases in survival time.

### Adjuvant Therapy

The standard adjuvant therapy administered to patients with Dukes' class C colon cancer is the 5-fluorouracil plus levamisole regimen. Patients with Dukes' class B or C rectal cancer are given 5-fluorouracil and high doses of pelvic irradiation. Mitomycin is also used. Radiation therapy is used before, during, and after surgery to shrink the tumor, to achieve better results from surgery, and to reduce the risk of recurrence. For inoperative or unresectable tumors, radiation is used to provide significant relief from symptoms. Intracavitary and implantable devices are used to deliver radiation to the site. The response to adjuvant therapy varies.

### Surgical Management

Surgery is the primary treatment for most colon and rectal cancers. It may be curative or palliative. Advances in surgical techniques can enable the patient with cancer to have sphincter-saving devices that restore continuity of the GI tract. The type of surgery recommended depends on the location and size of the tumor. Cancers limited to one site can be removed through the colonoscope. Laparoscopic colotomy with polypectomy minimizes the extent of surgery needed in some cases. A laparoscope is used as a guide in making an incision into the colon; the tumor mass is then excised. Use of the neodymium/yttrium-aluminum-garnet (Nd:YAG) laser has proved effective with some lesions as well. Bowel resection is indicated for most class A lesions and all class B and C lesions. Surgery is sometimes recommended for class D colon cancer, but the goal of surgery in this instance is palliative; if the tumor has spread and involves surrounding vital structures, it is considered nonresectable.

Surgical procedures include the following:

- Segmental resection with anastomosis (ie, removal of the tumor and portions of the bowel on either side of the growth, as well as the blood vessels and lymphatic nodes) (Fig. 38-7)
- Abdominoperineal resection with permanent sigmoid colostomy (ie, removal of the tumor and a portion of the sigmoid and all of the rectum and anal sphincter) (Fig. 38-8)
- Temporary colostomy followed by segmental resection and anastomosis and subsequent reanastomosis of the colostomy, allowing initial bowel decompression and bowel preparation before resection
- Permanent colostomy or ileostomy for palliation of unresectable obstructing lesions
- Construction of a coloanal reservoir called a colonic J pouch, which is performed in two steps. A temporary loop ileostomy is constructed to divert intestinal flow, and the newly constructed J pouch (made from 6 to 10 cm of colon) is reattached to the anal stump. About 3 months after the initial stage, the ileostomy is reversed and intestinal continuity is restored. The anal sphincter and therefore continence are preserved.

A **colostomy** is the surgical creation of an opening (ie, stoma) into the colon. It can be created as a temporary or permanent fecal diversion. It allows the drainage or evacuation of colon contents to the outside of the body. The consistency of the drainage is related to the placement of the colostomy, which is dictated by the location of the tumor and the extent of invasion into surrounding tissues (Fig. 38-9). With improved surgical techniques, colostomies are performed in fewer than one third of patients with colorectal cancer.

### GERONTOLOGIC CONSIDERATIONS

The elderly are at increased risk of complications after surgery and may have difficulty managing colostomy care. Some elderly patients may have decreased vision, impaired hearing, and difficulty with fine motor coordination. It may be helpful for patients to handle ostomy equipment and simulate cleaning the peristomal skin and irrigating the stoma before surgery. Skin care is a major concern in older patients with a colostomy because of the skin changes that occur with aging—the epithelial and subcutaneous fatty layers become thin, and the skin is irritated easily. To prevent skin breakdown, special attention is paid to skin cleansing and the proper fit of an appliance. Arteriosclerosis causes decreased blood flow to the wound and stoma site. As a result, transport of nutrients is delayed, and healing time may be prolonged. Some patients have delayed elimination after irrigation because of decreased peristalsis and mucus production. Most patients require 6 months before they feel comfortable with their ostomy care.

**FIGURE 38-7.** Examples of areas where cancer can occur, the area that is removed, and how the anastomosis is performed (*small diagrams*).

Cecum and lower ascending colon

Descending colon and upper sigmoid

Low sigmoid and upper rectum

Rectal sigmoid resection

## Nursing Process

### The Patient With Colorectal Cancer

#### Assessment

The nurse obtains a health history about the presence of fatigue, abdominal or rectal pain (eg, location, frequency, duration, association with eating or defecation), past and present elimination patterns, and characteristics of stool (eg, color, odor, consistency, presence of blood or mucus). Additional information includes a history of IBD or colorectal polyps, a family history of colorectal disease, and current medication therapy. The nurse identifies dietary habits, including fat and fiber intake, as well as amounts of alcohol consumed and history of smoking. The nurse describes and documents a history of weight loss and feelings of weakness and fatigue.

Assessment includes auscultation of the abdomen for bowel sounds and palpation of the abdomen for areas of tenderness, distention, and solid masses. Stool specimens are inspected for character and presence of blood.

### Diagnosis

#### Nursing Diagnoses

Based on the assessment data, the major nursing diagnoses may include the following:

- Imbalanced nutrition, less than body requirements, related to nausea and anorexia
- Risk for deficient fluid volume related to vomiting and dehydration
- Anxiety related to impending surgery and the diagnosis of cancer
- Risk for ineffective therapeutic regimen management related to knowledge deficit concerning the diagnosis, the surgical procedure, and self-care after discharge
- Impaired skin integrity related to the surgical incisions (abdominal and perianal), the formation of a stoma, and frequent fecal contamination of peristomal skin
- Disturbed body image related to colostomy
- Ineffective sexuality patterns related to presence of ostomy and changes in body image and self-concept

#### Collaborative Problems/ Potential Complications

Potential complications that may develop include the following:

**FIGURE 38-8.** Abdominoperineal resection for carcinoma of the rectum. (**A**) Prior to surgery. Note tumor in rectum. (**B**) During surgery, the sigmoid is removed and the colostomy is established. The distal bowel is dissected free to a point below the pelvic peritoneum, which is sutured over the closed end of the distal sigmoid and rectum. (**C**) Perineal resection includes removal of the rectum and free portion of the sigmoid from below. A perineal drain is inserted. (**D**) The final result after healing. Note the healed perineal wound and the permanent colostomy.

- Intraperitoneal infection
- Complete large bowel obstruction
- GI bleeding
- Bowel perforation
- Peritonitis, abscess, and sepsis

## Planning and Goals

The major goals for the patient may include attainment of optimal level of nutrition; maintenance of fluid and electrolyte balance; reduction of anxiety; learning about the diagnosis, surgical procedure, and self-care after discharge; maintenance of optimal tissue healing; protection of peristomal skin; learning how to irrigate the colostomy and change the appliance; expressing feelings and concerns about the colostomy and the impact on himself or herself; and avoidance of complications.

## Nursing Interventions

### Preparing the Patient for Surgery

The patient awaiting surgery for colorectal cancer has many concerns, needs, and fears. He or she may be physically debilitated and emotionally distraught with concerns about lifestyle changes after surgery, prognosis, ability to perform in established roles, and finances. Priorities for nursing care include preparing the patient physically for surgery; providing information about postoperative care, including stoma care if a colostomy is to be created; and supporting the patient and family emotionally.

Physical preparation for surgery involves building the patient's stamina in the days preceding surgery and cleansing and sterilizing the bowel the day before surgery. If the patient's condition permits, the nurse

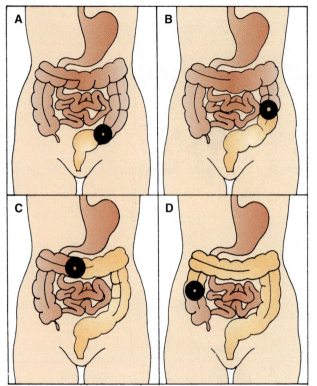

**FIGURE 38-9.** Placement of permanent colostomies. The nature of the discharge varies with the site. Shaded areas show sections of bowel removed. With a sigmoid colostomy (**A**), the feces are solid. With a descending colostomy (**B**), the feces are semimushy. With a transverse colostomy (**C**), the feces are mushy. With an ascending colostomy (**D**), the feces are fluid.

recommends a diet high in calories, protein, and carbohydrates and low in residue for several days before surgery to provide adequate nutrition and minimize cramping by decreasing excessive peristalsis. A full liquid diet may be prescribed 24 to 48 hours before surgery to decrease bulk. If the patient is hospitalized in the days preceding surgery, parenteral nutrition may be required to replace depleted nutrients, vitamins, and minerals. In some instances, parenteral nutrition is administered at home before surgery. Antibiotics such as kanamycin (Kantrex), neomycin (Mycifradin), and cephalexin (Keflex) are administered orally the day before surgery to reduce intestinal bacteria. The bowel is cleansed with laxatives, enemas, or colonic irrigations the evening before and the morning of surgery.

For the patient who is very ill and hospitalized, the nurse measures and records intake and output, including vomitus, to provide an accurate record of fluid balance. The patient's intake of oral food and fluids may be restricted to prevent vomiting. The nurse administers antiemetics as prescribed. Full or clear liquids may be tolerated, or the patient may be allowed nothing by mouth. A nasogastric tube may be inserted to drain accumulated fluids and prevent abdominal distention. The nurse monitors the abdomen for increasing distention, loss of bowel sounds, and pain or rigidity, which may indicate obstruction or perforation.

It also is important to monitor IV fluids and electrolytes. Monitoring serum electrolyte levels can detect the hypokalemia and hyponatremia that occur with GI fluid loss. The nurse observes for signs of hypovolemia (eg, tachycardia, hypotension, decreased pulse volume); assesses hydration status; and reports decreased skin turgor, dry mucous membranes, and concentrated urine.

The nurse assesses the patient's knowledge about the diagnosis, prognosis, surgical procedure, and expected level of functioning after surgery. It is important to include information about the physical preparation for surgery, the expected appearance and care of the wound, the technique of ostomy care (if applicable), dietary restrictions, pain control, and medication management in the teaching plan (see the Plan of Nursing Care in Chart 38-4). If the patient is admitted the day of surgery, the physician's office may arrange for the patient to be seen by an enterostomal therapist in the days preceding surgery. The enterostomal therapist helps determine the optimal site for the stoma and provides teaching about care. If the patient is hospitalized before the day of surgery, the enterostomal therapist is involved in the preoperative teaching. All procedures are explained in language the patient understands.

### Providing Emotional Support

Patients anticipating bowel surgery for colorectal cancer may be very anxious. They may grieve about the diagnosis, the impending surgery, and possible permanent colostomy. Patients undergoing surgery for a temporary colostomy may express fears and concerns similar to those of a person with a permanent stoma. All members of the health care team, including the enterostomal therapist, should be available for assistance and support. The nurse's role is to assess the patient's anxiety level and coping mechanisms and suggest methods for reducing anxiety, such as deep-breathing exercises and visualizing a successful recovery from surgery and cancer. Other supportive measures include providing privacy and teaching relaxation techniques to the patient. Time is set aside to listen to the patient who wishes to talk, cry, or ask questions. The nurse can arrange a meeting with a spiritual advisor if the patient desires or with the physicians if the patient wishes to discuss the treatment or prognosis. To promote patient comfort, the nurse projects a relaxed, professional, and empathetic attitude.

The patient undergoing a colostomy may find the anticipated changes in body image and lifestyle profoundly disturbing. Because the stoma is located on the abdomen, the patient may think that everyone will be aware of the ostomy. The nurse helps reduce this fear by presenting facts about the surgical procedure and the creation and management of the ostomy. If the patient is receptive, the nurse can use diagrams, photographs, and appliances to explain and clarify. Because the patient is experiencing emotional stress, the nurse may need to repeat some of the information. The nurse provides time for the patient and family to ask questions; the nurse's acceptance and understanding of the patient's concerns and feelings convey a caring, competent attitude that promotes confidence and cooperation. Consultation with an enterostomal therapist during the preoperative period can be extremely helpful, as can speaking with a person who is successfully managing a colostomy. The United Ostomy Association provides useful information about living with an ostomy through literature, lectures, and exhibits. Visiting services by qualified members and rehabilitation services for patients with new ostomies are provided.

### Providing Postoperative Care

Postoperative nursing care for patients undergoing colon resection or colostomy is similar to nursing care for any abdominal surgery patient (see Chapter 20), including pain management during the immediate postoperative period. The nurse also monitors the patient for complications such as leakage from the site of the anastomosis, prolapse of the stoma, perforation, stoma retraction, fecal impaction, skin irritation, and pulmonary complications associated with abdominal surgery. The nurse assesses the abdomen for returning peristalsis and assesses the initial stool characteristics. It is important to help patients with a colostomy out of bed on the first postoperative day and encourage them to begin participating in managing the colostomy.

### Maintaining Optimal Nutrition

The nurse teaches all patients undergoing surgery for colorectal cancer about the health benefits to be derived from consuming a healthy diet. The diet is individualized as long as it is nutritionally sound and does not cause diarrhea or constipation. The return to normal diet is rapid.

A complete nutritional assessment is important for the patient with a colostomy. The patient avoids foods that cause excessive odor and gas, including foods in the cabbage family, eggs, fish, beans, and high-cellulose products such as peanuts. It is important to determine whether the elimination of specific foods is causing any nutritional deficiency. Nonirritating foods are substituted for those that are restricted so that deficiencies are corrected. The nurse advises the patient to experiment with an irritating food several times before restricting it, because an initial sensitivity may decrease with time. The nurse can help the patient identify any foods or fluids that may be causing diarrhea, such as fruits, high-fiber foods, soda, coffee, tea, or carbonated beverages. Diphenoxylate with atropine (Lomotil) may be prescribed as needed to control the diarrhea. For constipation, prune or apple juice or a mild laxative is effective. The nurse suggests fluid intake of at least 2 L per day.

### Providing Wound Care

The nurse frequently examines the abdominal dressing during the first 24 hours after surgery to detect signs of hemorrhage. It is important to help the patient splint the abdominal incision during coughing and deep breathing to lessen tension on the edges of the incision. The nurse monitors temperature, pulse, and respiratory rate for elevations, which may indicate an infectious process. If the patient has a colostomy, the stoma is examined for swelling (slight edema from surgical manipulation is normal), color (a healthy stoma is pink or red), discharge (a small amount of oozing is normal), and bleeding (an abnormal sign).

If the malignancy has been removed using the perineal route, the perineal wound is observed for signs of hemorrhage. This wound may contain a drain or packing, which is removed gradually. Bits of tissue may slough off for a week. This process is hastened by mechanical irrigation of the wound or with sitz baths performed two or three times each day initially. The condition of the perineal wound and any bleeding, infection, or necrosis are documented.

### Monitoring and Managing Complications

The patient is observed for signs and symptoms of complications. It is important to frequently assess the abdomen, including decreasing or changing bowel sounds and increasing abdominal girth, to detect bowel obstruction. The nurse monitors vital signs for increased temperature, pulse, and respirations and for decreased blood pressure, which may indicate an intra-abdominal infectious process. It is important to report rectal bleeding immediately because it indicates hemorrhage. The nurse monitors hemoglobin and hematocrit levels and administers blood component therapy as prescribed. Any abrupt change in abdominal pain is reported promptly. Elevated white blood cell counts and temperature or symptoms of shock are reported because they may indicate sepsis. The nurse administers antibiotics as prescribed.

Pulmonary complications are always a concern with abdominal surgery; patients older than 50 years are at risk, especially if they are or have been receiving sedatives or are being maintained on bed rest for a prolonged period. Two major pulmonary complications are pneumonia and atelectasis. Frequent activity (eg, turning the patient from side to side every 2 hours), deep breathing, coughing, and early ambulation can reduce the risk for these complications. Table 38-6 lists postoperative complications.

The incidence of complications related to the colostomy is about half that of an ileostomy. Some common complications are prolapse of the stoma (usually from obesity), perforation (from improper stoma irrigation), stoma retraction, fecal impaction, and skin irritation. Leakage from an anastomotic site can occur if the remaining bowel segments are diseased or weakened. Leakage from an intestinal anastomosis causes peritonitis with abdominal distention and rigidity, temperature elevation, and signs of shock. Surgical repair is necessary.

### Removing and Applying the Colostomy Appliance

The colostomy begins to function 3 to 6 days after surgery. The nurse manages the colostomy and

### TABLE 38-6 — Potential Complications and Nursing Interventions After Intestinal Surgery

| Complication | Nursing Interventions |
|---|---|
| **General Complications** | |
| Paralytic ileus | Initiate or continue nasogastric intubation as prescribed. |
| | Prepare patient for x-ray study. |
| | Ensure adequate fluid and electrolyte replacement. |
| | Administer prescribed antibiotics if patient has symptoms of peritonitis. |
| Mechanical obstruction | Assess patient for intermittent colicky pain, nausea, and vomiting. |
| **Intra-abdominal Septic Conditions** | |
| Peritonitis | Evaluate patient for nausea, hiccups, chills, spiking fever, tachycardia. |
| | Administer antibiotics as prescribed. |
| | Prepare patient for drainage procedure. |
| | Administer parenteral fluid and electrolyte therapy as prescribed. |
| | Prepare patient for surgery if condition deteriorates. |
| Abscess formation | Administer antibiotics as prescribed. |
| | Apply warm compresses as prescribed. |
| | Prepare for surgical drainage. |
| **Surgical Wound Complications** | |
| Infection | Monitor temperature; report temperature elevation. |
| | Observe for redness, tenderness, and pain around the surgical wound. |
| | Assist in establishing local drainage. |
| | Obtain specimen of drainage material for culture and sensitivity studies. |
| Wound disruption | Observe for sudden drainage of profuse serous fluid from wound. |
| | Cover wound area with sterile towels held in place with binder. |
| | Prepare patient immediately for surgery. |
| Intraperitoneal infection and abdominal wound infection | Monitor for evidence of constant or generalized abdominal pain, rapid pulse, and elevation of temperature. |
| | Prepare for tube decompression of bowel. |
| | Administer fluids and electrolytes by IV route as prescribed. |
| | Administer antibiotics as prescribed. |
| **Anastomotic Complications** | |
| Dehiscence of anastomosis | Prepare patient for surgery. |
| Fistulas | Assist in bowel decompression. |
| | Administer parenteral fluids as prescribed to correct fluid and electrolyte deficits. |

teaches the patient about its care until the patient can take over its management. The nurse teaches skin care and how to apply and remove the drainage pouch. Care of the peristomal skin is an ongoing concern because excoriation or ulceration can develop quickly. The presence of such irritation makes adhering the ostomy appliance difficult, and adhering the ostomy appliance to irritated skin can worsen the skin condition. The effluent discharge and the degree to which it is irritating vary with the type of ostomy. With a transverse colostomy, the stool is soft and mushy and irritating to the skin. With a descending or sigmoid colostomy, the stool is fairly solid and less irritating to the skin. Other skin problems include yeast infections and allergic dermatitis.

If the patient wants to bathe or shower before putting on the clean appliance, micropore tape applied to the sides of the pouch will keep it secure during bathing. To remove the appliance, the patient assumes a comfortable sitting or standing position and gently pushes the skin down from the faceplate while pulling the pouch up and away from the stoma. Gentle pressure prevents the skin from being traumatized and any liquid fecal contents from spilling out. The nurse advises the patient to protect the peristomal skin by then washing the area gently with a moist, soft cloth and a mild soap. Soap acts as a mild abrasive agent to remove enzyme residue from fecal spillage. The patient should remove any excess skin barrier. While the skin is being cleansed, a gauze dressing can cover the stoma, or a vaginal tampon can be inserted gently to absorb excess drainage. After cleansing the skin, the patient pats the skin completely dry with a gauze pad, taking care not to rub the area. The patient can lightly dust nystatin (Mycostatin) powder on the peristomal skin if irritation or yeast growth is present.

Smoothly applying the drainage appliance for a secure fit requires practice and a well-fitting appliance. Patients can choose from a wide variety of appliances, depending on their individual needs. The stoma is measured to determine the correct size for the pouch; the pouch opening should be about 0.3 cm (1/8 in) larger than the stoma. After the skin is cleansed according to the previously described procedure, the patient applies the peristomal skin barrier (ie, wafer, paste, or powder). Mild skin irritation may require dusting the skin with karaya or Stomahesive powder before attaching the pouch. The patient removes the backing from the adherent surface of the appliance and applies pressure over the adhesive backing for approximately 30 seconds to ensure adherence over the stoma. The patient empties or changes the drainage appliance when it is one-third to one-fourth full so that the weight of its contents does not cause the appliance to separate from the adhesive disk and spill the contents. Most appliances are disposable and odor-resistant; commercially prepared deodorizers are available.

For some patients, colostomy appliances are not always necessary. As soon as the patient has learned a routine for evacuation, bags may be dispensed with, and a closed ostomy appliance or a simple dressing of disposable tissue (often covered with plastic wrap) is used, held in place by an elastic belt. Except for gas and a slight amount of mucus, nothing escapes from the colostomy opening between irrigations. Colostomy plugs that expand on insertion to prevent passage of flatus and feces are available.

### Irrigating the Colostomy

The purpose of irrigating a colostomy is to empty the colon of gas, mucus, and feces so that the patient can go about social and business activities without fear of fecal drainage. A stoma does not have voluntary muscular control and may empty at irregular intervals. Regulating the passage of fecal material is achieved by irrigating the colostomy or allowing the bowel to evacuate naturally without irrigations. The choice often depends on the person and the type of the colostomy. By irrigating the stoma at a regular time, there is less gas and retention of the irrigant. The time for irrigating the colostomy should be consistent with the schedule the person will follow after leaving the hospital. Chart 38-10 describes the irrigating procedure.

### Supporting a Positive Body Image

The patient is encouraged to verbalize feelings and concerns about altered body image and to discuss the surgery and the stoma (if one was created). A supportive environment and a supportive attitude on the nurse's part are crucial in promoting the patient's adaptation to the changes brought about by the surgery. If applicable, the patient must learn colostomy care and begin to plan for incorporating stoma care into daily life. The nurse helps the patient overcome aversion to the stoma or fear of self-injury by providing care and teaching in an open, accepting manner and by encouraging the patient to talk about his or her feelings about the stoma. The nurse's positive, supportive facial expression and other nonverbal cues help the patient develop a positive attitude toward independent stoma care.

### Discussing Sexuality Issues

The nurse encourages the patient to discuss feelings about sexuality and sexual function. Some patients may initiate questions about sexual activity directly or give indirect clues about their fears. Some may view the surgery as mutilating and a threat to their sexuality; some fear impotence. Others may express worry about odor or leakage from the pouch during sexual activity. Although the appliance presents no deterrent to sexual activity, some patients wear silk or cotton covers and smaller pouches during sex. Alternative sexual positions are recommended, as well as alternative methods of stimulation to satisfy sexual drives. The nurse assesses the patient's needs and attempts to identify specific concerns. If the nurse is uncomfortable with this or if the patient's concerns seem complex, it is appropriate for the nurse to seek assistance from an enterostomal therapist, sex counselor or therapist, or advanced practice nurse.

### Promoting Home and Community-Based Care

**TEACHING PATIENTS SELF-CARE**
Patient education and discharge planning require the combined efforts of the physician, nurse, enterostomal therapist, social worker, and dietitian. Patients are given specific information, individualized to their needs, about ostomy care and signs and symptoms of potential complications. Dietary instructions are essential to help patients identify and eliminate irritating foods that can cause diarrhea or constipation. It is important to teach patients about their prescribed medications (ie, action, purpose, and possible side and toxic effects).

The nurse reviews treatments (eg, irrigations, wound cleansing) and dressing changes and encourages the family to participate. Because the hospital stay is short, the patient may not be able to become proficient in stoma care techniques before discharge home. Many patients need referral to a home care agency and the telephone number of the local chapter of the American Cancer Society. The home care nurse goes to the home to provide further care and teaching and to assess how well the patient and family are adjusting to the colostomy. The home environment is assessed for adequacy of resources that allow the patient to manage self-care activities. A family member may assume responsibility for purchasing the equipment and supplies needed at home.

Patients need very specific directions about when to call the physician. They need to know which complications require prompt attention (ie, bleeding, abdominal distention and rigidity, diarrhea, fever, wound drainage, and disruption of suture line). If radiation therapy is planned, the possible side effects (ie, anorexia, vomiting, diarrhea, fatigue) are reviewed.

## CHART 38-10 Guidelines for Irrigating a Colostomy

A colostomy is irrigated to empty the colon of feces, gas, or mucus, cleanse the lower intestinal tract, and establish a regular pattern of evacuation so that normal life activities may be pursued. A suitable time for the irrigation is selected that is compatible with the patient's posthospital pattern of activity (preferably after a meal). Irrigation should be performed at the same time each day.

Before the procedure, the patient sits on a chair in front of the toilet or on the toilet itself. An irrigating reservoir containing 500 to 1500 mL of lukewarm tapwater is hung 45 to 50 cm (18 to 20 in) above the stoma (shoulder height when the patient is seated). The dressing or pouch is removed. The following procedure is used; the patient is helped to participate in the procedure so he or she can learn to perform it unassisted.

### NURSING ACTION

1. Apply an irrigating sleeve or sheath to the stoma. Place the end in the commode.

2. Allow some of the solution to flow through the tubing and catheter/cone.

3. Lubricate the catheter/cone and gently insert it into the stoma. Insert the catheter no more than 8 cm (3 in). Hold the shield/cone gently, but firmly, against the stoma to prevent backflow of water.

4. If the catheter does not advance easily, allow water to flow slowly while advancing catheter. *Never force the catheter!*

5. Allow tepid fluid to enter the colon slowly. If cramping occurs, clamp off the tubing and allow the patient to rest before progressing. Water should flow in over a 5- to 10-minute period.

6. Hold the shield/cone in place 10 seconds after the water has been instilled; then gently remove it.

### RATIONALE

1. This helps to control odor and splashing and allows feces and water to flow directly into the commode.

Colostomy irrigation. **(A)** Irrigating catheter has a cone attachment to prevent injury to stomal tissue. **(B)** Irrigating fluid is instilled with sleeve in place. Drainage contents empty into toilet. **(C)** The bulb syringe method can be used to stimulate fecal drainage. Note that a portion of the hard nozzle is removed and a catheter attached to minimize stomal irritation.

2. Air bubbles in the setup are released so that air is not introduced into the colon, which would cause crampy pain.

3. Lubrication permits ease of insertion of the catheter/cone.

4. A slow rate of flow helps to relax the bowel and facilitates passage of the catheter.

5. Painful cramps usually are caused by too rapid a flow or by too much solution; 300 mL of fluid may be all that is needed to stimulate evacuation. Volume may be increased with subsequent irrigations to 500, 1000, or 1500 mL as needed by the patient for effective results.

6. This minimizes or eliminates spillage of water.

## CHART 38-10  Guidelines for Irrigating a Colostomy, continued

| NURSING ACTION | RATIONALE |
|---|---|
| 7. Allow 10 to 15 minutes for most of the return; then dry the bottom of the sleeve/sheath and attach it to the top, or apply the appropriate clamp to the bottom of the sleeve. | 7. Most of the water, feces, and flatus will be expelled in 10 to 15 minutes. |
| 8. Leave the sleeve/sheath in place for 30 to 45 minutes while the patient gets up and moves around. | 8. Ambulation stimulates peristalsis and completion of the irrigation return. |
| 9. Cleanse the area with a mild soap and water; pat the area dry. | 9. Cleanliness and dryness will provide the patient with hours of comfort. |
| 10. Replace the colostomy dressing or appliance. | 10. The patient should use an appliance until the colostomy is sufficiently controlled. Then a dressing may be all that is needed. |

### CONTINUING CARE

Ongoing care of the patient with cancer and a colostomy often extends well beyond the initial hospital stay. Home care nurses manage ostomy follow-up care, manage the assessment and care of the debilitated patient, and coordinate adjuvant therapy. The home visits also provide the nurse with opportunities to assess the patient's physical and emotional status and the patient's and family's ability to carry out recommended management strategies. Visits from an enterostomal therapist are available to the patient and family as they learn to care for the ostomy and work through their feelings about it, the diagnosis of cancer, and the future. Some patients are interested in and can benefit from involvement in an ostomy support group.

## Evaluation

### Expected Patient Outcomes

Expected patient outcomes may include the following:

1. Consumes a healthy diet
   a. Avoids foods and fluids that cause diarrhea
   b. Substitutes nonirritating foods and fluids for those that are restricted
2. Maintains fluid balance
   a. Experiences no vomiting or diarrhea
   b. Experiences no signs or symptoms of dehydration
3. Feels less anxious
   a. Expresses concerns and fears freely
   b. Uses coping measures to manage stress
4. Acquires information about diagnosis, surgical procedure, preoperative preparation, and self-care after discharge
   a. Discusses the diagnosis, surgical procedure, and postoperative self-care
   b. Demonstrates techniques of ostomy care
5. Maintains clean incision, stoma, and perineal wound
6. Expresses feelings and concerns about self
   a. Gradually increases participation in stoma and peristomal skin care
   b. Discusses feelings related to changed appearance
7. Discusses sexuality in relation to ostomy and to changes in body image
8. Recovers without complications
   a. Is afebrile
   b. Regains normal bowel activity
   c. Exhibits no signs and symptoms of perforation or bleeding
   d. Identifies signs and symptoms that should be reported to health care provider

## Polyps of the Colon and Rectum

A polyp is a mass of tissue that protrudes into the lumen of the bowel. Polyps can occur anywhere in the intestinal tract and rectum. They can be classified as neoplastic (ie, adenomas and carcinomas) or non-neoplastic (ie, mucosal and hyperplastic). Non-neoplastic polyps, which are benign epithelial growths, are common in the Western world. They occur more commonly in the large intestine than in the small intestine. Although most polyps do not develop into invasive neoplasms, they must be identified and followed closely. Adenomatous polyps are more common in men. The proportion of these polyps arising in the proximal part of the colon increases with age (after 50 years of age). Prevalence rates vary from 25% to 60%, depending on age. Non-neoplastic polyps occur in 80% of the population, and their frequency increases with age. Up to two thirds of people older than 65 years are at risk for colonic adenomas (Tierney, 2004).

Clinical manifestations depend on the size of the polyp and the amount of pressure it exerts on intestinal tissue. The most common symptom is rectal bleeding. Lower abdominal pain may also occur. If the polyp is large enough, symptoms of obstruction occur. The diagnosis is based on history and digital rectal examination, barium enema studies, sigmoidoscopy, or colonoscopy.

After a polyp is identified, it should be removed. There are several methods: colonoscopy with the use of special equipment (ie, biopsy forceps and snares), laparoscopy, or colonoscopic excision with laparoscopic visualization. The latter technique enables immediate detection of potential problems and allows laparoscopic resection and repair of the major complications of perforation and bleeding that may occur with polypectomy. Microscopic examination of the polyp then identifies the type of polyp and indicates what further surgery is required, if any.

# Diseases of the Anorectum

Anorectal disorders are common, and the majority of the population will experience one at some time during their lives. Patients with anorectal disorders seek medical care primarily because of pain, rectal bleeding, or change in bowel habits. Other common complaints are protrusion of hemorrhoids, anal discharge, perianal itching, swelling, anal tenderness, stenosis, and ulceration. Constipation results from delaying defecation because of anorectal pain.

There has been a steady increase in the prevalence of sexually transmitted diseases (STDs; also called sexually transmitted infections, or STIs) in recent decades, leading to the identification of new anorectal syndromes. The prevalence of these conditions is increasing. These syndromes include venereal infections such as syphilis, gonorrhea, herpes, chlamydia, and candidiasis, and they are most commonly seen in male homosexuals who practice anorectal intercourse.

## Anorectal Abscess

An anorectal abscess is caused by obstruction of an anal gland, resulting in retrograde infection. People with regional enteritis or immunosuppressive conditions such as AIDS are particularly susceptible to these infections. Many of these abscesses result in fistulas.

An abscess may occur in a variety of spaces in and around the rectum. It often contains a quantity of foul-smelling pus and is painful. If the abscess is superficial, swelling, redness, and tenderness are observed. A deeper abscess may result in toxic symptoms, lower abdominal pain, and fever.

Palliative therapy consists of sitz baths and analgesics. However, prompt surgical treatment to incise and drain the abscess is the treatment of choice. When a deeper infection exists with the possibility of a fistula, the fistulous tract must be excised. If possible, the fistula is excised when the abscess is incised and drained, or a second procedure may be necessary to do so. The wound may be packed with gauze and allowed to heal by granulation.

## Anal Fistula

An anal fistula is a tiny, tubular, fibrous tract that extends into the anal canal from an opening located beside the anus (Fig. 38-10A). Fistulas usually result from an infection. They may also develop from trauma, fissures, or regional enteritis. Pus or stool may leak constantly from the cutaneous opening. Other symptoms may be the passage of flatus or feces from the vagina or bladder, depending on the fistula tract. Untreated fistulas may cause systemic infection with related symptoms.

Surgery is always recommended, because few fistulas heal spontaneously. A fistulectomy (ie, excision of the fistulous tract) is the recommended surgical procedure. The lower bowel is evacuated thoroughly with several prescribed enemas. The fistula is dissected out or laid open by an incision from its rectal opening to its outlet. The wound is packed with gauze.

## Anal Fissure

An anal fissure is a longitudinal tear or ulceration in the lining of the anal canal (see Fig. 38-10B). Fissures are usually caused by the trauma of passing a large, firm stool or from persistent tightening of the anal canal because of stress and

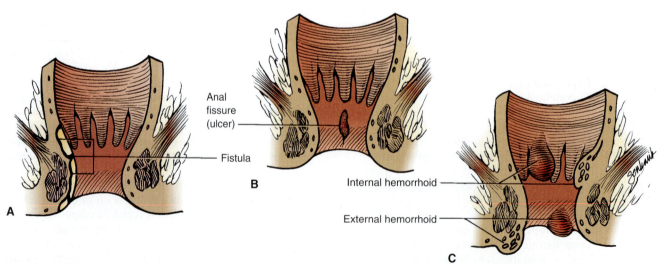

**FIGURE 38-10.** Various types of anal lesions. **(A)** Fistula. **(B)** Fissure. **(C)** External and internal hemorrhoids.

anxiety (leading to constipation). Other causes include childbirth, trauma, and overuse of laxatives.

Extremely painful defecation, burning, and bleeding characterize fissures. Bright-red blood may be seen on the toilet tissue after a bowel movement. Most of these fissures heal if treated by conservative measures, which include dietary modification with addition of fiber supplements, stool softeners and bulk agents, an increase in water intake, sitz baths, and emollient suppositories. A suppository combining an anesthetic with a corticosteroid helps relieve the discomfort. Anal dilation under anesthesia may be required.

If fissures do not respond to conservative treatment, surgery is indicated. Most surgeons consider the procedure of choice to be the lateral internal sphincterotomy with excision of the fissure.

## Hemorrhoids

Hemorrhoids are dilated portions of veins in the anal canal. They are very common: by 50 years of age, about 50% of people have hemorrhoids (NIH, 2005). Shearing of the mucosa during defecation results in the sliding of the structures in the wall of the anal canal, including the hemorrhoidal and vascular tissues. Increased pressure in the hemorrhoidal tissue due to pregnancy may initiate hemorrhoids or aggravate existing ones. Hemorrhoids are classified as one of two types: those above the internal sphincter are called internal hemorrhoids, and those appearing outside the external sphincter are called external hemorrhoids (see Fig. 38-10C).

Hemorrhoids cause itching and pain and are the most common cause of bright-red bleeding with defecation. External hemorrhoids are associated with severe pain from the inflammation and edema caused by thrombosis (ie, clotting of blood within the hemorrhoid). This may lead to ischemia of the area and eventual necrosis. Internal hemorrhoids are not usually painful until they bleed or prolapse when they become enlarged.

Hemorrhoid symptoms and discomfort can be relieved by good personal hygiene and by avoiding excessive straining during defecation. A high-residue diet that contains fruit and bran along with an increased fluid intake may be all the treatment that is necessary to promote the passage of soft, bulky stools to prevent straining. If this treatment is not successful, the addition of hydrophilic bulk-forming agents such as psyllium (Metamucil) may help. Warm compresses, sitz baths, analgesic ointments and suppositories, astringents (eg, witch hazel), and bed rest allow the engorgement to subside.

There are several types of nonsurgical treatments for hemorrhoids. Infrared photocoagulation, bipolar diathermy, and laser therapy are used to affix the mucosa to the underlying muscle. Injection of sclerosing agents is also effective for small, bleeding hemorrhoids. These procedures help prevent prolapse.

A conservative surgical treatment of internal hemorrhoids is the rubber-band ligation procedure. The hemorrhoid is visualized through the anoscope, and its proximal portion above the mucocutaneous lines is grasped with an instrument. A small rubber band is then slipped over the hemorrhoid. Tissue distal to the rubber band becomes necrotic after several days and sloughs off. Fibrosis occurs; the result is that the lower anal mucosa is drawn up and adheres to the underlying muscle. Although this treatment has been satisfactory for some patients, it has proven painful for others and may cause secondary hemorrhage. It has also been known to cause perianal infection.

Cryosurgical hemorrhoidectomy, another method for removing hemorrhoids, involves freezing the hemorrhoid for a sufficient time to cause necrosis. Although it is relatively painless, this procedure is not widely used because the discharge is very foul-smelling and wound healing is prolonged. The Nd:YAG laser is useful in excising hemorrhoids, particularly external hemorrhoidal tags. The treatment is quick and relatively painless. Hemorrhage and abscess are rare postoperative complications.

The previously described methods of treating hemorrhoids are not effective for advanced thrombosed veins, which must be treated by more extensive surgery. Hemorrhoidectomy, or surgical excision, can be performed to remove all the redundant tissue involved in the process. During surgery, the rectal sphincter is usually dilated digitally and the hemorrhoids are removed with a clamp and cautery or are ligated and then excised. After the surgical procedures are completed, a small tube may be inserted through the sphincter to permit the escape of flatus and blood; pieces of Gelfoam or Oxycel gauze may be placed over the anal wounds.

## Sexually Transmitted Anorectal Diseases

Three infectious syndromes that are related to STDs have been identified: proctitis, proctocolitis, and enteritis. Proctitis involves the rectum. It is commonly associated with recent anal-receptive intercourse with an infected partner. Symptoms include a mucopurulent discharge or bleeding, pain in the area, and diarrhea. The pathogens most frequently involved are *Neisseria gonorrhoeae, Chlamydia,* herpes simplex virus, and *Treponema pallidum.* Proctocolitis involves the rectum and lowest portion of the descending colon. Symptoms are similar to proctitis but may also include watery or bloody diarrhea, cramps, pain, and bloating. Enteritis involves more of the descending colon, and symptoms include watery, bloody diarrhea; abdominal pain; and weight loss. The most common pathogens causing enteritis are *E. histolytica, Giardia lamblia, Shigella,* and *Campylobacter.*

Sigmoidoscopy is performed to identify portions of the anorectum involved. Samples are taken with rectal swabs, and cultures are obtained to identify the pathogens involved. Antibiotics (ie, cefixime [Suprax], doxycycline [Vibramycin], and penicillin G) are the treatment of choice for bacterial infections. Acyclovir [Zovirax] is given to patients with viral infections. Antiamebic therapy (ie, metronidazole [Flagyl]) is appropriate for infections with *E. histolytica* and *G. lamblia.* Ciprofloxacin (Cipro) is effective for *Shigella.* The antibiotics erythromycin (E-Mycin) and ciprofloxacin are the treatment of choice for *Campylobacter* infection.

## Pilonidal Sinus or Cyst

A pilonidal sinus or cyst is found in the intergluteal cleft on the posterior surface of the lower sacrum (Fig. 38-11). Current theories suggest that it results from local trauma, causing the penetration of hairs into the epithelium and subcutaneous tissue. It may also be formed congenitally by

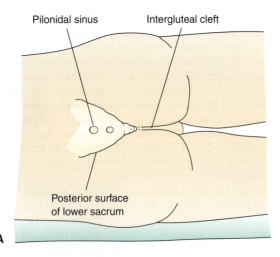

FIGURE 38-11. (A) Pilonidal sinus on lower sacrum about 5 cm (2 in) above the anus in the intergluteal cleft. (B) Hair particles emerge from the sinus tract, and localized indentations (pits) can appear on the skin near the sinus openings.

an infolding of epithelial tissue beneath the skin, which may communicate with the skin surface through one or several small sinus openings. Hair frequently is seen protruding from these openings, and this gives the cyst its name, *pilonidal* (ie, a nest of hair). The cysts rarely cause symptoms until adolescence or early adult life, when infection produces an irritating drainage or an abscess. Perspiration and friction easily irritate this area.

In the early stages of the inflammation, the infection may be controlled by antibiotic therapy, but after an abscess has formed, surgery is indicated. The abscess is incised and drained under local anesthesia. After the acute process resolves, further surgery is performed to excise the cyst and the secondary sinus tracts. The wound is allowed to heal by granulation. Gauze dressings are placed in the wound to keep its edges separated while healing occurs.

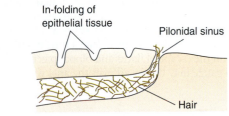

## Nursing Process

## The Patient With an Anorectal Condition

### Assessment

The nurse obtains a health history to determine the presence and characteristics of pruritus, burning, or anorectal pain. Other questions included in the medical history include the following: Do these symptoms occur during bowel movements? How long do they last? Is any abdominal pain associated with them? Does any bleeding occur from the rectum? How much? How frequently? Is it bright red? Is there any other discharge, such as mucus or pus? Other questions relate to elimination patterns and laxative use, diet history (including fiber intake), amount of exercise, activity levels, and occupation (especially one that involves prolonged sitting or standing). Assessment also includes inspection of the stool for blood or mucus and the perianal area for hemorrhoids, fissures, irritation, or purulent drainage.

### Diagnosis

#### Nursing Diagnoses

Based on the assessment data, the major nursing diagnoses may include the following:

- Constipation related to ignoring the urge to defecate because of pain during elimination
- Anxiety related to impending surgery and embarrassment
- Acute pain related to irritation, pressure, and sensitivity in the anorectal area from anorectal disease and sphincter spasms after surgery
- Urinary retention related to postoperative reflex spasm and fear of pain
- Risk for ineffective therapeutic regimen management

#### Collaborative Problems/ Potential Complications

Potential complications that may develop include the following:

- Hemorrhage

### Planning and Goals

The major goals for the patient may include adequate elimination patterns, reduction of anxiety, pain relief, promotion of urinary elimination, managing the therapeutic regimen, and absence of complications.

### Nursing Interventions

#### Relieving Constipation

The nurse encourages intake of at least 2 L of water daily to provide adequate hydration and recommends high-fiber foods to promote bulk in the stool and to make it easier to pass fecal matter through the rectum. Bulk laxatives such as psyllium (Metamucil) and stool softeners (eg, docusate [Colace]) are administered as prescribed. The patient is advised to set aside a time for bowel movements and to heed the urge to defecate as promptly as possible. It may be helpful to have the patient perform relaxation exercises before defecating to relax the abdominal and perineal muscles, which may be constricted or in spasm. Administering an analgesic before a bowel movement is beneficial.

## Reducing Anxiety

Patients facing rectal surgery may be upset and irritable because of discomfort, pain, and embarrassment. The nurse identifies specific psychosocial needs and individualizes the plan of care. The nurse maintains the patient's privacy while providing care and limits visitors, if the patient desires. Soiled dressings are removed from the room promptly to prevent unpleasant odors; room deodorizers may be needed if dressings are foul-smelling.

## Relieving Pain

During the first 24 hours after rectal surgery, painful spasms of the sphincter and perineal muscles may occur. Control of pain is a prime consideration. The patient is encouraged to assume a comfortable position. Flotation pads under the buttocks when sitting help decrease the pain, as may ice and analgesic ointments. Warm compresses may promote circulation and soothe irritated tissues. Sitz baths taken three or four times each day can relieve soreness and pain by relaxing sphincter spasm. Twenty-four hours after surgery, topical anesthetic agents may be beneficial in relieving local irritation and soreness. Medications may include topical anesthetics (ie, suppositories), astringents, antiseptics, tranquilizers, and antiemetics. Patients are more compliant and less apprehensive if they are free of pain.

Wet dressings saturated with equal parts of cold water and witch hazel help relieve edema. When wet compresses are being used continuously, petrolatum is applied around the anal area to prevent skin maceration. The patient is instructed to assume a prone position at intervals because this position reduces edema of the tissue.

## Promoting Urinary Elimination

Voiding may be a problem after surgery because of a reflex spasm of the sphincter at the outlet of the bladder and a certain amount of muscle guarding from apprehension and pain. The nurse tries all methods to encourage voluntary voiding (ie, increasing fluid intake, listening to running water, and pouring warm water over the urinary meatus) before resorting to catheterization. After rectal surgery, urinary output is closely monitored.

## Monitoring and Managing Complications

The operative site is examined frequently for rectal bleeding. The nurse assesses the patient for systemic indicators of excessive bleeding (ie, tachycardia, hypotension, restlessness, and thirst). After hemorrhoidectomy, hemorrhage may occur from the veins that were cut. If a tube has been inserted through the sphincter after surgery, blood may be visible on the dressings. If bleeding is obvious, direct pressure is applied to the area, and the physician is notified. It is important to avoid using moist heat because it encourages vessel dilation and bleeding.

## Promoting Home and Community-Based Care

### TEACHING PATIENTS SELF-CARE

Most patients with anorectal conditions are not hospitalized. Those who undergo surgical procedures to correct the condition often are discharged directly from the outpatient surgical center. If they are hospitalized, it is for a short time, usually only 24 hours. Patient teaching is essential to facilitate recovery at home.

The nurse instructs the patient to keep the perianal area as clean as possible by gently cleansing with warm water and then drying with absorbent cotton wipes. The patient should avoid rubbing the area with toilet tissue. Instructions are provided about how to take a sitz bath and how to test the temperature of the water.

### CONTINUING CARE

Sitz baths may be given in the bathtub or plastic sitz bath unit three or four times each day. Sitz baths should follow each bowel movement for 1 to 2 weeks after surgery. The nurse encourages the patient to respond quickly to the urge to defecate to prevent constipation. The diet is modified to increase fluids and fiber. Moderate exercise is encouraged, and the patient is taught about the prescribed diet, the significance of proper eating habits and exercise, and the laxatives that can be taken safely.

## Evaluation

### Expected Patient Outcomes

Expected patient outcomes may include the following:

1. Attains a normal pattern of elimination
    a. Sets aside a time for defecation, usually after a meal or at bedtime
    b. Responds to the urge to defecate and takes the time to sit on the toilet and try to defecate
    c. Uses relaxation exercises as needed
    d. Increases fluid intake to 2 L per day
    e. Adds high-fiber foods to diet
    f. Reports passage of soft, formed stools
    g. Reports decreased abdominal discomfort
2. Is less anxious
3. Has less pain
    a. Modifies body position and activities to minimize pain and discomfort
    b. Applies warmth or cold to anorectal area
    c. Takes sitz baths three or four times each day
4. Voids without difficulty
5. Adheres to the therapeutic regimen
    a. Keeps perianal area dry
    b. Eats bulk-forming foods
    c. Has a soft, formed stool on a regular basis
6. Exhibits no evidence of complications
    a. Has a clean incision
    b. Has normal vital signs
    c. Shows no signs of hemorrhage

## Critical Thinking Exercises

1. As a community health nurse you are conducting a regularly scheduled blood pressure clinic in a suburban community. In talking with an apparently well 74-year-old woman, you ask her if she has any questions regarding her health. She whispers to you that she has noticed some blood on the toilet tissue after bowel movements but has been too embarrassed to tell anyone about it. Consider what additional questions you might ask her during your initial nursing assessment. Analyze these findings, indicate what you think the possible causes may be, and explain the actions you would take and why. Explain the implications of this woman's age on likely subsequent referrals and treatments.

2. **ebp** A 22-year-old graduate student presents to the student health center of a local university with complaints of a five-day episode of watery diarrhea, lethargy, poor sleep patterns, and nervousness. She reports a recent weight loss of 15 pounds. Her social history reveals that she is preparing for her comprehensive final examinations and is very anxious about her examinations and her current health status. Her family history reveals that her father has had Crohn's disease for many years. What is the strength of the evidence that suggests her risk of having Crohn's disease? Prioritize your nursing plan and actions. What further data would be helpful? What specific nursing actions should be taken? Identify the evidence base for each aspect of your care.

3. You are the charge nurse in the emergency department of a large urban teaching hospital. A 53-year-old man presents with an acute onset of severe abdominal pain. Your physical examination of his abdomen reveals involuntary guarding and a rigid abdomen. The CT scan confirms intra-abdominal findings of purulent peritonitis. Intraperitoneal free air is evident. He is to be admitted to the hospital with an apparent perforation of diverticulitis into the peritoneal cavity. Both he and his wife are extremely upset. The operating room is put on call for an immediate surgical intervention. Identify priority nursing measures that must be initiated to meet the urgent physical needs of this man, what steps must be initiated to prepare him for surgery, and how to offer appropriate emotional support for him and his wife.

4. A 34-year-old attorney is admitted to the outpatient surgical center for drainage of an anorectal abscess. You are the admitting nurse and take his history, which includes a 6-week episode of swelling, throbbing, continuous perirectal pain accompanied by purulent drainage from his anus. He is scheduled for an incision and drainage within the next hour but asks why he must have surgery; he asks you, "Why can't I just get an antibiotic?" Considering the pathophysiologic implications of his diagnosis, what would you say to him? Make a judgment regarding essential actions you must take before he is taken to the operating room.

After your interventions, this man decided to undergo surgery. Later that afternoon, he is prepared for discharge. Design a discharge plan for him for the next 2 weeks, and include the principles of care that you will teach him so that he may understand the reasons for his home care routine.

## REFERENCES AND SELECTED READINGS

### BOOKS

American Cancer Society. (2006). *Cancer facts and figures 2006.* Atlanta, GA: Author.

Andreoli, T., Carpenter, D. J., Griggs, R. C., et al. (2003). *Cecil essentials of medicine* (6th ed.). Philadelphia: W. B. Saunders.

Chan, P. D., Safani, M., & Winkle, P. (2005). *Medicine.* Laguna Hills, CA: Current Clinical Strategies Publishing.

Colwell, J. C., Goldberg, M. T., & Carmel, J. E. (2004). *Fecal and urinary diversions: Management principles.* St. Louis, MO: Mosby.

Friedman, S., McQuaid, R., & Grendell, J. (2003). *Current diagnosis and treatment in gastroenterology.* New York: McGraw-Hill Companies.

Gilbert, D. M., Moellering, R., Eliopoulos, G., et al. (2005). *The Sanford guide to antimicrobial therapy.* Spercyville, VA: Antimicrobial Therapy.

Green, G., Morris, J., & Lin, G. (2005). *Washington manual of medical therapeutics* (31st ed.). Philadelphia: Lippincott Williams & Wilkins.

Johnson, M., & Chan, P. (2004). *Treatment guidelines for medicine and primary care, 2004.* Laguna Hills, CA: Current Clinical Strategies Publishing.

Kasper, D., Braunwald, E., Fauci, A., et al. (2004). *Harrison's principles of internal medicine* (16th ed.). New York: McGraw-Hill Professional.

Lederman, R., & Winshall, J. (2004). *Tarascon internal medicine & critical care pocketbook* (3rd ed.). Loma Linda, CA: Tarascon Publishing.

National Institutes of Health: National Institute of Diabetes and Digestive and Kidney Diseases (2005). *National digestive diseases information clearinghouse.* Bethesda, MD: National Institutes of Health.

Porth, C. (2005). *Pathophysiology: Concepts of altered health states* (7th ed.). Philadelphia: Lippincott Williams & Wilkins.

Rothrock, S. (2004). *Tarascon adult emergency handbook* (3rd ed.). Loma Linda, CA: Tarascon Publishing.

Tierney, L. (2004). *Current medical diagnosis and treatment, 2005* (44th ed.). New York: McGraw-Hill Medical.

Townsend, C., Beauchamp, D., Evers, M., et al. (2004) *Sabiston textbook of surgery: The biological basis of modern surgical practice* (17th ed.). Philadelphia: W. B. Saunders.

Varricchio, C., Ades, T., Hinds, P., et al. (2004). *A cancer sourcebook for nurses.* Atlanta, GA: American Cancer Society and Jones & Bartlett Publishers.

### JOURNALS

*Asterisk indicates nursing research article

### General

Beitz, J. (2004). Diverticulosis and diverticulitis: Spectrum of a modern malady. *Journal of Wound, Ostomy and Continence Nursing, 31*(2), 75–84.

*Gall, S., & Bull, J. (2004). Clinical risk: Discharging patients with no one at home. *Gastroenterology Nursing, 27*(3), 111–114.

*Li, H., Melnyk, B. M., & McCann, R. (2004). Review of intervention studies of families with hospitalized elderly relatives. *Journal of Nursing Scholarship, 36*(1), 54–59.

Mick, D. J., & Ackerman, M. H. (2004). Critical care nursing for older adults: Pathophysiological and functional considerations. *Nursing Clinics of North America, 39*(3), 473–493.

*Reilly, T., & Walker, G. (2004). Reasons for poor colonic preparation with inpatients. *Gastroenterology Nursing, 27*(3), 115–117.

*Scible, L., & Anwer, M. B. (2004). Detecting a small bowel tumor via wireless capsule endoscopy: A clinical case study. *Gastroenterology Nursing, 27*(3), 118–120.

Smith, C., Hellebusch, S. J., & Mandel, K. G. (2003). Patient and physician evaluation of a new bulk fiber laxative tablet. *Gastroenterology Nursing, 26*(1), 31–37.

Steffen, K. A. (2003) When your trauma patient is over 65. *Nursing, 33*(4), 53–56.

Stessman, M. (2003). Biofeedback: Its role in the treatment of chronic constipation. *Gastroenterology Nursing, 26*(6), 251–260.

*Zalon, M. (2004). Correlates of recovery among older adults after major abdominal surgery. *Nursing Research, 53*(2), 99–106.

## Cancer of the Colon and Rectum

Banks, N., & Razor, B. (2003). Preoperative stoma site assessment and marking. *American Journal of Nursing, 103*(3), 64A–64E.

Feingold, D., Addona, T., Forde, K. A., et al. (2004). Safety and reliability of tattooing colorectal neoplasm prior to laparoscopic resection. *Journal of Gastrointestinal Surgery, 8*(5), 543–546.

Lynch, H. T., Coronel, S. M., Okimoto, R., et al. (2004). A founder mutation of the *MSH2* gene and hereditary nonpolyposis colorectal cancer in the United States. *Journal of the American Medical Association, 291*(6), 718–724.

Madoff, R. D. (2004). Chemoradiotherapy for rectal cancer: When, why, and how? *New England Journal of Medicine, 351*(17), 1790–1791.

Morrin, M., & LaMont, T. (2003). Screening virtual colonoscopy: Ready for prime time? *New England Journal of Medicine, 349*(13), 2261–2264.

Rudy, D. R., & Zdon, M. J. (2000). Update on colorectal cancer. *American Family Physician, 61*(6), 1759–1774.

Sauer, R., Becker, H., Hohenberger, W., et al. (2004). Preoperative versus postoperative chemoradiotherapy for rectal cancer. *New England Journal of Medicine, 351*(17), 1731–1740.

Sargent, C., & Murphy, D. (2003). What you need to know about colorectal cancer. *Nursing, 33*(2), 36–41.

## Inflammatory Bowel Disease

Rutgeerts, P., Sandborn, W. J., Feagan, B. G., et al. (2005). Infliximab for induction and maintenance therapy for ulcerative colitis. *New England Journal of Medicine, 353*(23), 2462–2476.

Sandborn, W. J., Colombel, J. F., Enns, R., et al. (2005). Natalizumab induction and maintenance therapy for Crohn's disease. *New England Journal of Medicine, 353*(18), 1912–1925.

## Irritable Bowel Syndrome

Aschenbrenner, D. (2004). Risks have been newly associated with a drug taken for IBS: Changes to labeling of tegaserod. *American Journal of Nursing, 104*(7), 33–34.

Kupecz, D., & Berardinelli, C. (2003). Drug news: New therapy for women with irritable bowel syndrome. *Nurse Practitioner, 28*(4), 48–50.

Mertz, H. (2003). Drug therapy: Irritable bowel syndrome. *New England Journal of Medicine, 349*(22), 2136.

*Motzer, S., Hertig, V., Jarrett, M., et al. (2003). Sense of coherence and quality of life in women with and without irritable bowel syndrome. *Nursing Research, 52*(5), 329–337.

## RESOURCES

American Cancer Society, 1599 Clifton Rd., N.E., Atlanta, GA 30329; 1-800-277-2345; http://www.cancer.org. Accessed June 20, 2006.

Colon Cancer Alliance, 175 Ninth Ave., New York, NY 10011; 1-212-627-7451; http://www.ccalliance.org. Accessed June 20, 2006.

Crohn's & Colitis Foundation of America, 386 Park Avenue South, New York, NY 10016; 1-800-932-2423; http://www.ccfa.org. Accessed June 20, 2006.

International Foundation for Functional Gastrointestinal Disorders, P.O. Box 17864, Milwaukee, WI 17864; 1-888-964-2001; http://www.iffgd.org. Accessed June 20, 2006.

Medicine Online: Colon Cancer Information Library: http://www.meds.com/colon/colon.html. Accessed June 20, 2006.

National Association for Continence, P.O. Box 544, Union, SC 29379; 1-803-585-8789; http://www.nafc.org/site2/index.html. Accessed June 20, 2006.

STOP Colon/Rectal Cancer Foundation, P.O. Box 1616, Barrington, IL 60010; 1-312-782-4828; http://www.coloncancerprevention.org. Accessed June 20, 2006.

United Ostomy Association, 19772 MacArthur Blvd., Suite 200, Irvine, CA 92612; 1-800-826-0826; http://www.uoa.org. Accessed June 20, 2006.

# Index

Page numbers followed by c indicate charts; those followed by f indicate figures; those followed by t indicate tables.

## A

AAI. See Ankle-arm index
Abacavir (Ziagen), for HIV infection, 1827t
Abbreviations
　in reference ranges, 2577
　related to vision and eye health, 2043
ABCDs
　of cardiopulmonary resuscitation, 970
　in emergency assessment, 2521
　of moles, 1983, 1983c
Abciximab (ReoPro), 871
ABCs, in emergency management of burns, 2002–2003
Abdomen
　examination of
　　in cardiac patient, 805
　　for gastrointestinal function, 1127–1129, 1128f
　　in trauma victim, 2531
　quadrants of, 1127, 1128f
　referred pain in, 1126, 1126f
　regions of, 1127, 1128f
Abdominal aortic aneurysm, 998–1000, 1000f
Abdominal breathing, in pain management, 289
Abdominal distention
　postoperative, 543
　in renal surgical patient, 1553
Abdominal fluid wave, assessment of, 1294, 1294f
Abdominal injury
　blunt, 2530–2531
　emergency management of, 2530–2532
　penetrating, 2530–2531
Abdominal pain
　with appendicitis, 1241
　in colorectal cancer, 1266
　in Hodgkin's disease, 1080
Abdominal pressure, with increased intracranial pressure, nursing interventions for, 2178t
Abdominal thrust maneuver, 608, 609c
　in airway obstruction, 2523, 2523c
Abdominal ultrasonography, 1130–1131
Abducens nerve (V), 2136–2137, 2136f, 2137t, 2292f
　assessment of, 2147c
　disorders of, 2293t
Abduction, 199c, 200c, 2343c
　definition of, 198c, 2355
　after hip replacement, 2373, 2373f
Abduction pillow, for hip replacement patient, 2373, 2373f
ABI. See Ankle-brachial index

Ablation
　of cardiac arrhythmias, 853
　definition of, 823
Abnormal uterine bleeding, 1639–1640
Abortion, 1647–1650
　elective, 1648–1650
　　types of, 1648, 1649c
　habitual, 1647–1648
　spontaneous, 1647–1648
Above-elbow amputation, 2461f
Above-knee amputation, 2460, 2461f
Abrasion(s)
　corneal, 2074
　definition of, 2528c
Abscess(es)
　anorectal, 1276
　in appendicitis, 1241, 1242
　blind dental, 1145
　definition of, 1232, 1661
　dental, 1145–1146
　dentoalveolar, 1145–1146
　hepatic, 1340
　　amebic, 1340
　　pyogenic, 1340
　lactational, 1710
　lung, 650–652
　pelvic, after appendectomy, 1242, 1242t
　periapical, 1145–1146
　　definition of, 1142
　peritonsillar, 599, 600–601, 603
　prevention of, 2499c–2500c
　renal, 1571
　subphrenic, after appendectomy, 1242, 1242t
Absolute neutrophil count, 424–425, 1066, 1067c
　definition of, 1036
Absorption
　definition of, 1121
　of drugs, age-related changes in, 238, 239t
　in small intestine, 1121, 1125
Abstinence, as contraceptive measure, 1640
Abuse
　assessment for, 1622, 1622c, 2550–2551, 2550c
　domestic violence and, 1620–1622, 1621c
　elder, 249
　　assessment for, 73
　　definition of, 225
　emergency management of, 2550–2552
　risk for, assessment of, 69c, 73
　　for persons with disabilities, 178c
　sexual, childhood, 1622
　substance. See Substance abuse; specific substance

Abuse Assessment Screen-Disability, 1622, 1622c
Acantholysis, 1971
　definition of, 1945
Acarbose (Precose), 1399t, 1401
Acceptance, as stage of dying, 472t
Accommodation (visual), 2044
　definition of, 2043
Acculturation, definition of, 129
Accu-Zyme collagenase (Santyl), 1946
Acebutolol (Sectral), for hypertension, 1028t
ACE-I. See Angiotensin-converting enzyme inhibitors
ACE inhibitors. See Angiotensin-converting enzyme inhibitors
Acetabulum, fracture of, 2445–2446
Acetaminophen
　and amphotericin B therapy, 2276
　hepatitis caused by, 1317
　for low back pain, 2393
　for pharyngitis, 598
　poisoning with, emergency management of, 2548t
　therapeutic levels (conventional units and SI units), 2601t
　for viral rhinitis, 593
Acetazolamide (Diamox)
　for glaucoma, 2057, 2058t
　for sleep apnea, 605
Acetic acid, for burns, 2017
Acetohexamide (Dymelor), 1399t
Acetylcholine, 2130t
　in gastrointestinal regulation, 1124t
Acetylcholine receptors, and myasthenia gravis, 2285, 2285f
Acetylcholinesterase, and myasthenia gravis, 2285
Acetylcysteine (Mucomyst)
　for cystic fibrosis, 719
　for ventilator-dependent patient, 749
Achalasia, 1162
　definition of, 1142
Achieving Health for All, 57
Achilles tendon, rupture of, 2430–2431
Achondroplasia, genetics of, 144, 146
Acid–base balance, 334–338
　disturbances of, 334–338. See also Acidosis; Alkalosis
　compensation in, 338, 338t
　mixed, 338
　regulation of, 1497–1498
Acid–base monitoring
　gastric, ambulatory, 1138
　of gastric secretions, 1138

I-1

Acidosis
    anion gap, 335
    definition of, 301
    high anion gap, 335
    hyperchloremic, 335
    and hyperkalemia, 324
    metabolic. *See* Metabolic acidosis
    normal anion gap, 335
    renal insufficiency and, 2411
    respiratory. *See* Respiratory acidosis
    reversal of, in diabetic ketoacidosis, 1414–1415
    and wound healing, 541t
ACL. *See* Anterior cruciate ligament
Acne vulgaris, 1953–1956
    assessment of, 1954
    clinical manifestations of, 1954
    diagnosis of, 1954
    distribution of, 1940f
    medical management of, 1954–1956, 1954t
    nursing management of, 1956
    pathophysiology of, 1954
    pharmacologic therapy for
        systemic, 1954t, 1955
        topical, 1954t, 1955
    surgery for, 1955–1956
Acoustic, definition of, 2095c
Acoustic nerve, 2096, 2136–2137, 2136f, 2137t
    assessment of, 2147c
    definition of, 2095c
Acoustic neuroma, 2119–2120, 2302
Acoustic trauma, 2102
Acquired immunity, 1786–1788
    active, 1786
    passive, 1786
Acquired immunodeficiency syndrome, 1814–1852, 2505. *See also* Human immunodeficiency virus
    assessment in, 1844–1845
    causative organism of, 2476t
    complications of, 1845, 1849–1850
    confidentiality in, 1851
    continuing care for, 1850
    and cytomegalovirus retinitis, 1835–1836
    definition of, 1661
    diagnosis of, 1824–1825
    emotional concerns in, 1851–1852
    epidemiology of, 1815, 2512
    ethical considerations in, 1851, 1851c
    expected outcomes in, 1850–1851
    fungal encephalitis in, 2275–2276
    gerontologic considerations in, 248
    immigration and, 2512
    indicator conditions, 1823t, 1824
    Kaposi's sarcoma in, 1832–1833, 1832f, 1836
    and meningitis, 1835
    nurses caring for patients with, concerns of, 1851–1852
    nursing care plan for, 1838c–1844c
    nursing diagnoses related to, 1845
    nursing interventions for, 1846–1850
    nursing process with, 1837–1851
    planning and goals for, 1845
    pneumonia in, 534, 633t, 634
    risk factors for, 1816, 1816c
    stages of, 1823–1824
    stigmatization of, 1851
    transfusion-transmitted, 1104t
    in women, 1672–1673
Acromegaly, 1446, 2302
    definition of, 1440
ACTH. *See* Adrenocorticotropic hormone
Acticoat dressing, for burns, 2017, 2018t

Actin filaments, 2341
Actinic cheilitis, 1143t
Actinic keratoses, 1977
Action potential
    cardiac, 784–785, 784f
    skeletal muscle, 2341
Activated partial thromboplastin time, 808t
Activated protein C resistance, 1095, 1099, 1099t
Active acquired immunity, 1786
Active-assistive exercises, 201t
Active exercises, 201t
Active transport, definition of, 301
Activities of daily living, 169, 175, 191
    Alzheimer's disease and, 244
    capacity to perform, assessment of, 193
    casts and, 2360, 2361c
    definition of, 190
    instrumental. *See* Instrumental activities of daily living
    patient teaching about, 194, 194c
    self-care deficits in
        nursing interventions for, 194–195
        nursing process and, 193–195
Activity/exercise. *See also* Exercise(s)
    in cardiovascular disease, assessment of, 796
    in chronic obstructive pulmonary disease, tolerance of, improvement of, 697, 705c
    in Cushing's syndrome, 1482
    definition of, 46c
    diversional, with vertigo, 2117c
    in health promotion, 58
    in hypothyroidism, 1454, 1455c
    in liver disease, 1323c
    in multiple sclerosis, 2281
    after myocardial infarction, 884, 885c
    pacing of, in chronic obstructive pulmonary disease, 695
    parenteral nutrition and, 1198
    physical, in patients with COPD, nursing research on, 691
    postoperative, 537–538
        and wound healing, 541t
    in prevention of atherosclerosis, 864
    tolerance
        burns and, 2033
        in cardiomyopathy, 932
        in chronic obstructive pulmonary disease, improvement of, 697, 705c
        in chronic renal failure, 1530, 1534c
        in heart failure, 959–960
        in HIV-infected (AIDS) patients, 1846
        in rheumatic diseases, 1894
    in tuberculosis, 649
Activity theory, of aging, 227
Acupuncture, 134
Acute care settings, gerontologic considerations in, 248–249
Acute chest syndrome, of sickle cell anemia, 1057
Acute confusional state. *See* Delirium
Acute coronary syndrome, 788, 790, 874
    clinical manifestations of, 874, 874c
    definition of, 859
    in elderly, ethical considerations in, 869c
    with or without percutaneous coronary intervention, clinical pathway for, 2609f–2613f
Acute intermittent peritoneal dialysis, 1548
Acute lung injury, 361
    definition of, 625
    transfusion-related, 1110
Acute lymphocytic leukemia, 1073–1074

Acute myeloid leukemia, 1–71–1072, 1054
    chemotherapy for, 1071–1072
    clinical manifestations of, 1071
    complications of, 1071
    medical management of, 1071–1072
        complications of, 1072
    polycythemia vera and, 1065
Acute-phase reactions, in infectious disease, 2492
Acute promyelocytic leukemia, 1071
Acute radiation syndrome, 2573–2574, 2573t
    phases of, 2573, 2573t
Acute renal failure. *See* Renal failure, acute
Acute respiratory distress syndrome, 361, 557, 657–659
    assessment in, 657
    in burn victim, 2002, 2030
    causes of, 656, 657c
    clinical manifestations of, 657
    definition of, 625
    diagnosis of, 657
    medical management of, 657–658
    nursing management of, 658–659
    nutritional support in, 658
    pathogenesis of, 656, 657f
    pathophysiology of, 656–657, 657f
    pharmacologic therapy for, 658
Acute tubular necrosis
    in acute renal failure, 1522–1523
    after cardiac surgery, 893t
    definition of, 1515
Acyclovir
    for herpes infections in HIV-infected (AIDS) patients, 1836
    for herpes simplex virus encephalitis, 2274
AD. *See* Alzheimer's disease
ADA. *See* Americans With Disabilities Act of 1990
Adalimumab (Humira)
    for rheumatic diseases, 1896t
    for rheumatoid arthritis, 1908
Adaptation, 92
    definition of, 91
    Selye's theory of, 94–95
    to stress, theory of, 94–95
    stress and, 92
Adaptive device(s), 191. *See also* Assistive device(s)
    definition of, 190
    in rehabilitation, 194–195
Adaptive immunity. *See* Acquired immunity
Addiction. *See also* Substance abuse
    definition of, 259
    opioid, 284
Addiction Severity Index, 120
Addisonian crisis, 1477, 1482
    definition of, 1440
Addison's disease, 1477–1479, 1479c
    cutaneous manifestations of, 1935t
    definition of, 1440
    T-cell deficiencies and, 1806
Adduction, 199c, 200c, 2343c
    definition of, 198c, 2355
Adenine (A), 142
Adenoidectomy, 599–600
Adenoiditis, 599–600
Adenoids, anatomy of, 554
Adenomyosis, 1682
Adenosine
    adverse effects and side effects of, 811
    for atrial flutter, 832
    for atrioventricular (AV) nodal reentry tachycardia, 83
    in cardiac stress testing, 810

# INDEX

intravenous, for atrial fibrillation, 833
pharmacology of, 811
Adenosine triphosphate
  and muscle contractions, 2341
  in muscles, 2341
Adenovirus, pneumonia caused by, 629, 631t
Aδ fibers, in pain transmission, 264
ADH. See Antidiuretic hormone
Adherence
  definition of, 49
  to therapeutic regimen, 50
    chronic illness and, 168
    factors affecting, 50
    gerontologic considerations in, 50
Adhesions
  and intestinal obstruction, 1263, 1264t
  pelvic inflammatory disease and, 1671
Adjuvant chemotherapy
  for breast cancer, 1726, 1727t
  definition of, 1701
Adjuvant hormonal therapy, for breast cancer, 1729
  adverse effects and side effects of, 1729, 1729t, 1730c
Adjuvant therapy for colorectal cancer, 1267
ADLs. See Activities of daily living
Adnexa, 1615
  definition of, 1613
  palpation of, 1626
Adolescent(s)
  health promotion for, 58–59
  nutritional assessment of, 84
Adoptive cell therapy, 1113
Adrenal cortex, 1474, 1474f
Adrenalectomy, definition of, 1440
Adrenal glands
  anatomy and physiology of, 1473–1475, 1474f
  disorders of, 1475–1485
  in fluid and electrolyte balance, 306
Adrenaline, topical, for epistaxis, 605
Adrenal medulla, 1473–1474, 1474f
Adrenergic agents
  for allergic rhinitis, 1870–1872, 1872t
  for asthma, 713, 713t, 714
  as bronchodilators, 692, 693t
  for glaucoma, 2057, 2058t
  for hypertension, 1027t, 1028t
  for hypertensive crises, 1033
  for status asthmaticus, 717
β-Adrenergic receptor antagonists. See Beta-blockers
Adrenocortical insufficiency, 1477–1479, 1479c. See also Addison's disease
Adrenocorticotropic hormone, 1446, 1473, 1475
  definition of, 91, 1440
  in stress response, 94, 95
Adrenogenital syndrome, 1475
  definition of, 1440
Adriamycin. See Doxorubicin
Adult(s)
  health promotion for, 59–61, 59t
  older. See Older adults
  vaccination schedule for, 2484–2487, 2485f–2487f
Adult day care, 249
Adult-onset conditions
  inheritance of, 149–153, 151t–152t
  testing and screening for, 151t–152t
Advance directive(s), 33, 251, 457, 457c
  definition of, 225
Advanced practice nurses, 12–13, 226–227
Adynamic ileus, 2363
Aerosol(s), for wound care, 1950
Aerosol mask, for oxygen delivery, 725t, 727

Afferent arteriole, 1495f
  renal, 1494
After-death care, 469–471
Afterload, 787, 945, 946, 946f
  definition of, 781, 945
Agammaglobulinemia
  definition of, 1802
  sex-linked, 1803t, 1805–1806. See also Bruton's disease
Age. See also Older adults
  and burn injury, 1995, 1996
  and wound healing, 541t
Ageism, 228
  definition of, 225
Age-related macular degeneration, 236, 2051t, 2069–2072, 2069f, 2070f
Agglutination, 1788–1789
  definition of, 1783
Aggression, as psychiatric emergency, 2553–2554
Aging. See also Older adults
  biologic theories of, 227
  and bone mass, 2405
  and cardiovascular system, 230–232, 231t
  cognitive aspects of, 53–54, 237
  demographics of, 7, 225–226
  developmental theories of, 227
  and disability, 175
  environmental aspects of, 227–228
  and gastrointestinal system, 231t, 234
  and genitourinary system, 231t, 233–234
  health care costs of, 249–250
  and health care delivery, 7
  and integumentary system, 231t, 233
  and intervertebral disk changes, 2392
  intrinsic, 227
  and memory, 237
  and musculoskeletal system, 231t, 235–236, 2342, 2344t
  and nervous system, 232t, 236
  nursing theory of, 228
  and nutrition, 234–235
  pharmacologic aspects of, 237–238, 239t
  physical aspects of, 230–237, 231t–232t
  psychosocial aspects of, 228–230
  and reproductive system, 231t, 233
  resources and websites on, 125–126
  and respiratory system, 231t, 232–233
  and sensory changes, 232t, 236–237
  and sleep, 235
  sociologic theories of, 227–228
  theories of, 227–228
Agitation, in Alzheimer's disease patients, 244, 245
Agnogenic myeloid metaplasia, 1079–1080
Agnosia, 2210
  assessment of, 2145, 2145t
  definition of, 2129, 2206
  stroke and, 2210
  types of, 2145, 2145t
Agonist, 287
  definition of, 259
  opioid, definition of, 259
Agorithms, 9
Agranulocytes, 1040f, 1041–1042
AIDS. See Acquired immunodeficiency syndrome
AIDS dementia complex. See HIV encephalopathy
AIDS-related pain, 261c
Airborne Precautions, 2482, 2483c
Air-contrast barium enema, 1132
Air embolism, 349
  in decompression sickness, 2537
  in parenteral nutrition, 1197t

Air plethysmography, in peripheral vascular disease, 983
Air trapping
  in chronic obstructive pulmonary disease, 697
  definition of, 686
Airway
  in burn patient, 2002–2004, 2009–2015, 2010c–2011c
  in cardiopulmonary resuscitation, 970, 970f
  clearance, 735, 736c
    in chronic obstructive pulmonary disease, 697, 704c
    in HIV-infected (AIDS) patients, 1839c–1840c, 1847–1848
    in renal surgical patient, 1554, 1555c
    spinal cord injury and, 2257
    in thoracic surgical patient, 756–757, 765–766, 772c
    in tuberculosis, 649
    in ventilator-dependent patient, 749
  establishing, in airway obstruction, 2522–2525
  maintenance
    brain injury and, 2244
    in facial reconstructive surgery, 1989
    after neck dissection, 1154–1155
  management of, 735–739
    in postanesthesia care unit, 525–526, 526f
    in unconscious patient, 2166
    in ventilator-dependent patient, 749
  obstruction of
    assessment of, 2522
    clinical manifestations of, 2522
    diagnosis of, 2522
    emergency management of, 735, 736c, 2522–2526
    pathophysiology of, 2522
  patency
    with increased intracranial pressure, 2175
    in laryngectomy patient, 616–617
    in pneumonia, 640
    in upper airway infection, 602
  remodeling of, 710
  upper. See Respiratory system, upper
Airway pressure release ventilation, 744
  definition of, 723
Airway resistance, 557, 557c
Akathisia
  definition of, 2301
  in Huntington's disease, 2319–2320
Akinetic mutism, definition of, 2161, 2162
Alanine aminotransferase, serum, 1290t
Alaryngeal communication, 613–614
  definition of, 589
Albumin, 1042
  for fluid replacement in shock, 364, 367t
  and magnesium balance, 329–330
  plasma, therapy with, 1103t
  serum, 78–80, 79t, 1290t
    in chronic glomerulonephritis, 1519
    laboratory values for, 310t
    and serum calcium, 326
Albumin/globulin ratio, 1290t
Albuterol, 693t
  for anaphylactic shock, 376
  for anaphylaxis, 2538
  for ventilator-dependent patient, 749
Albuterol + ipratropium (Combivent), for ventilator-dependent patient, 749
Alcohol
  and breast cancer, 1713–1714
  consumption of, in diabetes, 1387
  and esophageal cancer, 1166, 1167
  for hand decontamination, 2481, 2481c

Alcohol (*continued*)
  intoxication, acute, emergency management of, 2544–2549
  and oral cancer, 1148
  thrombocytopenia caused by, 1087t
  use and abuse. *See also* Alcoholism
    assessment for, 70, 70c
      preoperative, 486
    as cause of disability, 192
    cellular injury caused by, 102
    and depression, 240
    by persons with disabilities, 192
    treatment programs for, 192–193
  withdrawal syndrome, emergency management of, 2549–2550
Alcoholism. *See also* Alcohol, use and abuse
  hypomagnesemia in, 329
  and pneumonia, 635
Alcohol septal ablation, 927–928
Aldosterone, 1474
  actions of, 1497
  definition of, 1493
  in fluid and electrolyte balance, 305
Aldosterone receptor blockers, for hypertension, 1026t
Aldosteronism, primary, 1484
Aldrete Score, Modified, 529, 530f
Alemtuzumab (Campath), 419t
  for acute lymphocytic leukemia, 1074
  adverse effects and side effects of, 421t
  for chronic lymphocytic leukemia, 1074
Alendronate (Fosamax)
  for osteoporosis, 2409
  for Paget's disease, 2412
Alfentanil (Alfenta), for intravenous anesthesia, 512t
Algogenic substance(s)
  definition of, 259
  in pain transmission, 264
Alkaline phosphatase
  leukocyte, laboratory values for, 2579
  serum, 1290t
    in biliary/pancreatic disease, 1349t
Alkalosis, definition of, 301
Alkylating agents
  for cancer treatment, 399t
  and immune system, 1797t
ALL. *See* Acute lymphocytic leukemia
Allele(s), 142
  definition of, 140
Allen test, before radial graft, 1149
Allergen(s), 1856
  definition of, 1856
Allergic contact dermatitis, 1877, 1877t
  latex and, 1883t
Allergic reactions. *See also* Allergy(ies)
  antigens in, 1857
  B lymphocytes in, 1857
  chemical mediators in, 1857–1859, 1858f, 1858t
  clinical manifestations of, 1861–1863
  diagnosis of, 1863–1865
  immunoglobulins and, 1857
  physiology of, 1856–1861
  T lymphocytes in, 1857
Allergic rhinitis, 589, 1869–1876
  adherence to therapeutic regimen in, 1874
  assessment in, 1870, 1873–1874
  avoidance therapy for, 1870
  causes of, 1869
  clinical manifestations of, 1870
  complications of, 1874
  continuing care for, 1876
  coping with, 1874
  diagnosis of, 1870
  expected outcomes with, 1876

  home and community-based care for, 1875–1876, 1875c
  medical management of, 1870–1873, 1871t
  nursing diagnoses related to, 1874
  nursing interventions for, 1874–1875
  nursing process with, 1873–1875
  pathophysiology of, 1869
  pharmacologic therapy for, 1870–1872, 1871t
  planning and goals for, 1874
  self-care for, 1875–1876, 1875c
Allergy(ies), 1856. *See also* Anaphylactic reaction; specific disorder
  to antivenin, 2540
  assessment for, 1861–1863, 1862c–1863c
    preoperative, 488, 489f
  and asthma, 710
  cutaneous manifestations of, 1929t
  definition of, 1856
  food. *See* Food allergy
  and immune system, 1796
  insect, 2539
  latex. *See* Latex allergy
  management of, 1874, 1875–1876, 1875c, 1876f
Alloantibody(ies), 1062
AlloDerm, 1948
  for burns, 2020t, 2022
  definition of, 1995
Allograft
  bone, 2439
    definition of, 2425
  definition of, 915
  for heart valve replacement, 924
  skin, 1986
Alloimmune hemolytic anemia, 1062
Allopurinol
  for chemotherapy patient, 402
  for gout, 1918, 1919t
  for polycythemia vera, 1065
Almotriptan, for migraine, 2201
Alopecia, 1930
  in cancer patient, 425
    nursing care plan for, 407c–408c
    nursing interventions for, 427–428
  definition of, 381, 1927
ALP. *See* Alkaline phosphatase
Alpha$_1$-antitrypsin deficiency, 688
  definition of, 686
Alpha-glucosidase inhibitor(s), 1398, 1399t, 1401
  definition of, 1376
ALS. *See* Amyotrophic lateral sclerosis
Alteplase, for venous thrombosis, 1006
Altered level of consciousness. *See also* Consciousness
  definition of, 2161
Alternative medical systems, 134. *See also* Complementary and alternative therapies
Alternative pathway, of complement system activation, 1792–1793
Alveolar cells
  type I, 556
  type II, 556
  type III, 556
Alveoli, 555f, 556
Alzheimer's disease, 243–246, 2320
  anxiety and agitation in, 244, 245
  assessment in, 244
  characteristics of, 242t–243t, 243
  clinical manifestations of, 242t, 243, 244
  cognition in, 244, 245
  communication with patients with, 245
  versus delirium, 242t–243t
  diagnosis of, 244

  early-onset, 243
  and exercise, 246
  familial, 243
    early-onset, 151t
    late-onset, 151t
  genetics of, 147, 243
  home and community-based care for, 246
  medical management of, 244
  nursing management of, 244–246
  and nutrition, 245–246
  pathophysiology of, 243–244
  and rest, 246
  risk factors for, 243
  safety of patients with, 245
  and self-care, 245
  socialization of patients with, 245
  sporadic, 243
  support groups for caregivers/families of patients, 246
Amantadine (Symmetrel)
  for fatigue, in multiple sclerosis, 2280
  for influenza, 637
  for Parkinson's disease, 2314
  for viral rhinitis, 593
Ambulation
  assessment of, 195–196
  with cane, 205–207
  with crutches, 204–205, 205f, 206c
  after ischemic stroke, 2218
  orthoses/prostheses and, 207
  paraplegia and, 2263
  parenteral nutrition and, 1198
  postoperative, 535, 537–538
    gastrointestinal benefits of, 543
  preparation for, in rehabilitation, 203–204
  promotion of, after joint replacement, 2373
  with walker, 205
Ambulatory health care, nursing in, 21
Ambulatory payment classifications, 8
Ambulatory pH monitoring, 1138
Ambulatory surgery
  definition of, 481
  nursing management of, 491
  patient teaching about, 495
  usage rates, 481
AMD. *See* Age-related macular degeneration
Amebiasis, causative organism of, 2476t
Amenorrhea, 1639
  definition of, 1613
  primary, 1639
  with prolactinoma, 2302
  secondary, 1639
American Burn Association, criteria for burn center referral, 2005
American College of Cardiology/American Heart Association, classification of heart failure, 947, 947t
American Nurses Association, 161c
  Code for Nurses, 5
  Code of Ethics, 29, 31c
  definition of nursing, 5, 29
  on nursing care, focus for, 5
  on nursing research, focus for, 5
  position statement, on assisted suicide, 451
  Social Policy Statement, 5, 29
  *Standards and Scope of Gerontological Nursing Practice*, 226
American Society of Anesthesiologists, Physical Status Classification System, 505, 506c
American Spinal Injury Association, impairment scale of, 2251, 2253c
Americans With Disabilities Act of 1990, 176–177, 191
  definition of disability, 175

# INDEX

Amiloride (Midamor), 954t
  for hypertension, 1026t
Aminocaproic acid (EACA, Amicar)
  for hemophilia, 1091
  for idiopathic thrombocytopenic purpura, 1089
  and von Willebrand's disease, 1092
Aminoglycosides
  for tuberculosis, 647
  for urinary tract infections, 1574
Aminopeptidase, source and digestive action of, 1123t
Aminophylline, 693t
  for anaphylaxis, 2538
  therapeutic levels (conventional units and SI units), 2601t
Amiodarone, 830t
  for atrial fibrillation, 833
  for atrial flutter, 832
  for atrioventricular (AV) nodal reentry tachycardia, 835
  mechanism of action of, 785
  for ventricular fibrillation, 837
  for ventricular tachycardia, 836
Amitriptyline (Elavil)
  abuse/overdose, emergency management of, 2548t
  in migraine prevention, 2200
  for Parkinson's disease, 2314
  for post-stroke pain, 2218
  for rheumatic diseases, 1894
  for rheumatoid arthritis, 1909
  therapeutic blood levels of, 2601t
AML. See Acute myeloid leukemia
Amlodipine (Norvasc), 870, 955
  for hypertension, 1029t
AMM. See Agnogenic myeloid metaplasia
Ammonia
  conversion, liver in, 1286
  plasma, 1290t
  serum, in hepatic encephalopathy, 1305
Amnion grafts, for burns, 2021
Amobarbital (Amytal), abuse/overdose, emergency management of, 2545t–2546t
Amoxicillin
  for gastritis and peptic ulcer disease, 1206t
  for pneumonia, 637
  for sinusitis, 595
Amoxicillin-clavulanate
  for pneumonia, 637
  for sinusitis, 595, 596
Amphetamine (Benzedrine), abuse/overdose, emergency management of, 2546t
Amphetamine-type drugs, abuse/overdose, emergency management of, 2546t
Amphiarthrosis joints, 2340
Amphotericin B
  adverse effects and side effects of, 2276
  for fungal encephalitis, 2276
  for meningitis, in HIV-infected (AIDS) patients, 1835
Ampicillin
  for sinusitis, 596
  for urinary tract infections, 1574
Ampicillin-sulbactam (Unasyn), for pneumonia, 637
Amprenavir (Agenerase), for HIV infection, 1827t
Ampulla, of inner ear, 2094f
Ampulla of Vater, 1121, 1346
Amputation, 2460–2469
  above-elbow, 2461f
  above-knee, 2460, 2461f
  ankle disarticulation, 2460, 2461f
  assessment with, 2462
  below-elbow, 2461f

below-knee, 2460, 2461f
and body image, 2464
for bone tumors, 2418
complications of, 2461, 2463, 2467–2468
definition of, 2371c, 2425
expected outcomes with, 2469
of foot, 2460, 2461f
grieving with, 2464
home care for, 2468–2469, 2468c
levels of, 2460–2461, 2461f
of lower extremity, in Buerger's disease, 996
medical management of, 2461–2462
and mobility, 207
mobility after, 2465–2467
nonambulatory, 2467
nursing diagnoses related to, 2462–2463
nursing interventions for, 2464–2469
nursing process with, 2462–2469
pain management for, 2464
phantom limb pain after, 2464
planning and goals for, 2464
prosthesis for, 2467
rehabilitation therapy for, 2462, 2462f
residual limb shaping after, 2464, 2465f, 2466f, 2467f
self-care after, 2465, 2468, 2468c
staged, 2461
Syme, 2460
upper extremity, 2460–2461, 2461f
and wound healing, 2464
Amrinone (Inocor), for shock, 366t, 370
Amsler grid, 2049
Amylase, 1124
  definition of, 1121, 1345
  pancreatic, 1124, 1345, 1346
  salivary, 1123
  source and digestive action of, 1123t
Amyl nitrate
  abuse/overdose, emergency management of, 2546t
  for cyanide poisoning, 2569t, 2571
Amyloid, and Alzheimer's disease, 243–244
Amyotrophic lateral sclerosis, 2320–2323
Amyotrophic Lateral Sclerosis Association, 2323
ANA. See American Nurses Association
Anagen phase, of hair growth, 1928
  definition of, 1927
Anagrelide (Agrylin)
  for polycythemia vera, 1065
  for thrombocythemia, 1086
Anakinra (Kineret)
  for rheumatic diseases, 1896t
  for rheumatoid arthritis, 1908
Anal fissure, 1276–1277, 1276f
Anal fistula, 1276, 1276f
Analgesia, 277–288. See also Pain management; Patient-controlled analgesia
  administration of
    adverse effects and side effects of, nursing management of, 288
    epidural, 285t, 287–288, 287f
      adverse effects and side effects of, 288
      home and community-based care for, 288
    gastrointestinal, 285–286, 285t
    home and community-based care for, 288
    intramuscular, 285, 285t
    intraspinal, 285t, 287–288, 287f
      adverse effects and side effects of, 288
    intrathecal, 287–288, 287f
    intravenous, 285, 285t
    oral, 285, 285t
    parenteral, 285, 285t
    preventive approach for, 278–279
    pro re nata (PRN), 278

    rectal, 285t, 286
    routes for, 285–288, 285t
    subcutaneous, 285, 285t
    topical, 285t, 286
    transdermal, 285t, 286
    transmucosal, 285t, 287
  balanced, 278
    definition of, 259
  for burn patients, 2024
  concerns and misconceptions about, 271c–272c
  in end-of-life care, 464–465
  epidural, postoperative, 535–536
  gerontologic considerations in, 277
  inadequate, 279–280, 280c, 282278
  individualized dosage of, 279–280
  for low back pain, 2393
  metabolism of, and pain management, 269
  mode of delivery, and serum analgesic level, 278, 278f
  in myocardial infarction, 877
  perioperative, 495
  for pharyngitis, 598
  in pleurisy, 652
  postoperative, 535–536
  for septic arthritis, 2416
  topical, for rheumatic diseases, 1896t
  for ventilator patient, in acute respiratory distress syndrome, 659
Anal sphincter, function of, 1125
Analysis
  in critical thinking, 25
  in nursing process, 34
Anaphylactic reaction
  causes of, 2537
  clinical manifestations of, 2538, 2538c
  emergency management of, 2537–2538
  prevention of, 2537, 2537c
Anaphylactoid (anaphylaxis-like) reaction, 1866, 1866c
Anaphylaxis, 1865–1869. See also Shock, anaphylactic
  allergic rhinitis and, 1874
  causes of, 1865–1866, 1866c
  clinical manifestations of, 1866–1867
  complement system and, 1793t
  definition of, 1856
  intraoperative, 516
  medical management of, 1868
  nursing management of, 1868–1869
  pathophysiology of, 1865–1866
  prevention of, 1867–1868
Anaplasia, 383
  definition of, 381
Anastomosis, definition of, 975
Anastrazole (Arimidex), for breast cancer, 1729
ANC. See Absolute neutrophil count
Ancestry, assessment of, in genetic assessment, 155–156
Ancylostoma duodenale
  incubation period of, 2476t
  transmission of, 2476t
Androgen(s), 1474, 1475
  and autoimmune disorders, 1796
  in cancer treatment, 399t
  definition of, 1440, 1613
  and hair growth, 1930
  in menstrual cycle, 1615
Anemia, 1039. See also Sickle cell anemia
  in acute renal failure, 1524
  aplastic, 1051–1052
    assessment in, 1052
    causes of, 1051
    clinical manifestations of, 1051
    diagnosis of, 1052

Anemia, aplastic (*continued*)
  medical management of, 1052
  thrombocytopenia in, 1087t
assessment of, 1047
autoimmune, 1045t
bleeding-related, 1045t, 1046
causes of, 1045–1046, 1046t
chemotherapy-related, 401
of chronic disease, 1051
in chronic glomerulonephritis, 1519
of chronic illness, 1045t, 1501
in chronic renal failure, 1529, 1536c–1537c
in cirrhosis, 1319
classification of, 1045, 1045t, 1046
clinical manifestations of, 1046–1047
compliance with therapy in, 1048
complications of, 1047, 1048–1049
Cooley's. *See* Thalassemia major
definition of, 1036
diagnosis of, 1047
drug-induced, 1045t
expected outcomes in, 1049
and heart failure, 1047, 1049
hemolytic, 1045t, 1046, 1055–1064
  causes of, 1046, 1046t
in Hodgkin's disease, 1080
hypoproliferative, 1045t, 1046, 1049–1055
iron deficiency, 1039, 1045t, 1049–1051
  assessment of, 1049–1050
  causes of, 1049
  clinical manifestations of, 1047, 1049
  diagnosis of, 1049–1050
  medical management of, 1050, 1050c
  nursing management of, 1050–1051
mechanical heart valve-related, 1045t
medical management of, 1047
megaloblastic, 1040, 1045t, 1052–1054
  clinical manifestations of, 1047
  complications of, 1047, 1049
  nursing management of, 1053–1054
  thrombocytopenia in, 1087t
in multiple myeloma, 1083
neurologic complications of, 1047, 1049
normochromic normocytic, 1051
nursing diagnoses related to, 1047–1048
nursing interventions for, 1048–1049
nursing process with, 1047–1049
in older persons, 1043
and pressure ulcers, 208
in renal disease, 1045t, 1051
sickle cell, 1045t
unexplained, 1501
Anencephaly, genetics of, 147t, 148
Anergy, 80, 1074
  definition of, 1036, 1815
  in Hodgkin's disease, 1080
  tuberculin skin test and, 1831
Anesthesia
  administration of, methods for, 510–511, 510t, 512t–513t
  deaths related to, 508
  definition of, 503, 508
  epidural, 511–513
  intrapleural, postoperative, 535–536
  local infiltration, 515–516
  moderate sedation with, 515
  paravertebral, 515
  potential adverse effects of, 503, 504c
    gerontologic considerations in, 503–504
  regional, 511–515
    agents for, 514t
  safety of, 508
  spinal, 511, 513–515
  types of, 508

Anesthesia awareness, 508–509
Anesthesiologist, 503
  activities of, 505
  definition of, 503
Anesthetic(s), 503. *See also* Anesthesia
  administration of, 505
  for burn patients, 2024
  definition of, 503
  inhalation, 509–511
    administration of, 510–511, 511f
    advantages and disadvantages of, 510t
  intravenous, 511, 512t–513t
    advantages and disadvantages of, 511, 512t–513t
  medications interacting with, 490t
  topical, for eye, 2085
  volatile
    advantages and disadvantages of, 510t
    gas, 510–511, 510t
    liquid, 510–511, 510t
Anesthetist, 503
  activities of, 505
  definition of, 503
Aneuploidy, 148
Aneurysm
  abdominal aortic, 998–1000, 1000f
  anastomotic, 998c
  aortic, 997
  cerebral, 2134
  characteristics of, 997f, 998
  classification of, 998c
  congenital, 998c
  definition of, 975, 2206
  dissecting, 997f
  etiologic classification of, 998c
  false, 997f
  fusiform, 997, 997f
  graft, 998c
  infectious, 998c
  inflammatory (noninfectious), 998c
  intracranial
    and hemorrhagic stroke, 2223, 2224, 2224f
    Hunt-Hess classification of, 2225, 2225t
    precautions for, 2228
    surgical management of, 2226–2227
  mechanical (haemodynamic), 998c
  mycotic, 997, 998c
  postarteriotomy, 998c
  pregnancy-related degenerative, 998c
  saccular, 997, 997f
  thoracic aortic, 997–998, 997f
  traumatic (pseudoaneurysm), 998c
  ventricular, signs and symptoms of, 790
Angelman syndrome, genetics of, 147
Anger
  in family members of emergency patient, 2520
  as stage of dying, 472t
Angina pectoris, 790, 791t, 860, 867–874
  assessment of, 793t, 868, 871–872, 871c
  clinical manifestations of, 867–868
  definition of, 859
  diagnosis of, 868
  gerontologic considerations in, 868
  hypertension and, 1023
  intractable (refractory), 867, 867c
  medical management of, 868–871
  nursing process in, 871–874
  pathophysiology of, 867
  pharmacologic therapy for, 869–870
  silent, 867, 867c
  stable, 867, 867c
  treatment of, 872
  types of, 867, 867c

unstable, 867, 867c, 875
  recognizing symptoms of, nursing research on, 868
  variant, 867, 867c
Angioedema, hereditary, 1879
Angiogenesis
  in agnogenic myeloid metaplasia, 1079
  in cancer, 385
  definition of, 1036
  in fracture healing, 2340
  in macular degeneration, 2071
  in multiple myeloma, 1084
Angiography, 814–815
  cerebral, 2154, 2181
    in head injuries, 2235
  computed tomographic, in peripheral vascular disease, 983
  fluorescein, 2049–2050
  indocyanine green, 2050
  in liver disease, 1291t
  magnetic resonance, in peripheral vascular disease, 983
  in peripheral vascular disease, 983
  pulmonary
    with pulmonary embolism, 663
    in respiratory disease, 580
  renal, 1509
Angiomas, 1978
  of brain, 2303
  cherry, 1939c
  port-wine, 1978
  spider, 1939c
    in liver disease, 1308, 1308f
  strawberry, 1978
Angioneurotic edema, 608, 1803t, 1808–1809, 1878–1879
  definition of, 1802, 1856
Angioplasty, definition of, 975
Angiotensin, vascular effects of, 978
Angiotensin-converting enzyme inhibitors, 952–953, 952t
  and acute renal failure, 1523
  for atrial fibrillation, 833
  definition of, 859
  for hypertension, 1029t
  for hypertensive crises, 1033
  for myocardial infarction, 877
  and stroke prevention, 2211
Angiotensin II, 1497
Angiotensin receptor blockers, 953
  for atrial fibrillation, 833
  for hypertension, 1029t
Angular cheilosis, 1047, 1049
  definition of, 1036
Animals, working, 219
Anion gap, 335
  reference range for, 335
  serum, 334
Anion gap acidosis, 335
Anions, 302
Ankle, sprains of, sports-related, 2426
Ankle-arm index, 981
  definition of, 975
Ankle-brachial index, 981, 982c
  definition of, 975
Ankylosing spondylitis, 1917
Ankylosis, definition of, 1887
Annuloplasty, 922, 922f
  definition of, 915
Anophthalmic ocular prosthesis, 2082, 2082f
Anorectal abscess, 1276
Anorectal disorders, 1276–1279
  nursing process for, 1278–1279
Anorectal function, assessment of, 1138

# INDEX

Anorectal manometry, 1138
Anorectal reflex, stimulation of, 217
Anorexia, 83
  in cancer patient, 400
    nursing interventions for, 428
  in heart failure, 951
  management of, 467t
  in terminal illness, 465–466
  traction and, 2370
Anorexia-cachexia syndrome, 465–466
Anoscopy, 1137
Anosmia, brain injury and, 2244
ANP. *See* Atrial natriuretic peptide
Antacids
  for gastroesophageal reflux disease, 1166
  and hypermagnesemia, 330
  and hypophosphatemia, 331
  and metabolic alkalosis, 336
  in treatment of shock, 366
Antagonist, 287
  definition of, 259
Antagonist muscles, 2342
Anterior chamber, of eye, 2044, 2045f
  definition of, 2043
Anterior cord syndrome, 2251, 2252c
Anterior cruciate ligament, 2429f
  injury to, 2430
Anthrax
  as bioterrorism threat, 2566–2568
  causative organism of, 2476t
  treatment of, 2568
  vaccine against, 2568
Antiallergy medications, ocular, 2086
Antiandrogens, in cancer treatment, 399t
Antiarrhythmic agents
  actions of, 830t
  adverse effects and side effects of, 830t
  for atrial fibrillation, 833
  for atrial flutter, 832
  for cardiogenic shock, 370
  classes of, 830t
  class I, 784
    mechanism of action of, 784–785
  class II, mechanism of action of, 785
  class III, mechanism of action of, 785
  class IV, mechanism of action of, 785
  definition of, 823
  nursing interventions for, 830t, 841
  for sinus bradycardia, 829
  for sinus tachycardia, 830–831, 830t
  for ventricular fibrillation, 837
  for ventricular tachycardia, 836
Antibiotics
  for adenoidectomy, 599
  antitumor, 399t
    cardiac toxicity of, 402
  in bronchiectasis, 709
  for cystic fibrosis, 718–719
  for gastritis, 1206t
  for gonorrhea, 2508
  and immune system, 1797t
  for infective endocarditis, 937
  for inflammatory bowel disease, 1250
  interactions with anesthetics, 490t
  for lung abscess, 651
  ocular use of, 2086
  oral, for acne vulgaris, 1954t, 1955
  for osteomyelitis, 2414
  for peritonsillar abscess, 600
  for pharyngitis, 598
  for pneumonia, 636–637
  for renal surgical patient, 1553, 1558
  for septic arthritis, 2416
  for septic shock, 374
  for sinusitis, 595

for tonsillectomy, 599
topical
  for acne vulgaris, 1954t, 1955
  for burn wounds, 2017, 2018t
  for tracheobronchitis, 628
  for urinary tract infections, 1574
  and wound healing, 541t
Antibody(ies), 1042
  in allergic reaction, 1856
  antitumor properties of, 388
  definition of, 1783, 1856, 1887
  in humoral immune response, 1786–1787, 1788–1789
  in inflammation, 1887–1888
  and passive acquired immunity, 1786
  structure of, 1788, 1790f
Antibody specificity, 1787
Anticardiolipin antibody, 1099t
Anticholinergic agents
  adverse effects and side effects of, 2314
  as bronchodilators, 692, 693t
  for Parkinson's disease, 2314
Anticholinesterase agents
  adverse effects and side effects of, 2286, 2286c
  for myasthenia gravis, 2286
Anticipatory grief. *See* Grief, anticipatory
Anticoagulants
  for angina, 870–871
  for arterial embolism, 1003
  for atrial fibrillation, 833
  contraindications to, 1006, 1006c
  for heart failure, 956
  for ischemic stroke, 2212
  patient teaching about, 1010c
  perioperative management of, 490t
  for prevention of pulmonary embolism, 663
  for pulmonary embolism, 663–665
  and stroke prevention, 2210–2211
  therapy with
    assessment of, 1007
    complications of, 1007, 1093
    monitoring of, 1007
  for thrombophlebitis, 2259
  for thrombotic disorders, 1095
  for venous thrombosis, 1006
  and wound healing, 541t
Anticonvulsant(s). *See also* Antiseizure agents
  for pain management, 285
Anti-D, for idiopathic thrombocytopenic purpura, 1089
Antidepressants
  for depression, 240
  for HIV-infected (AIDS) patients, 1836
  for Parkinson's disease, 2314
  for rheumatic diseases, 1894
  for rheumatoid arthritis, 1909
Antidiabetic agents, oral, 1398–1402, 1399t–1400t
  mechanism of action of, 1398, 1400f
Antidiuretic hormone, 1446
  in blood pressure regulation, 358
  deficiency of, 320
  definition of, 91, 1493
  in fluid and electrolyte balance, 305, 306
  in physiologic response to stress, 96
  and thirst, 306
Anti-DNA test, in rheumatic diseases, 1893t
Antiemetics
  for chemotherapy patient, 398–400
  postoperative use of, 528
Antiestrogens, in cancer treatment, 399t
Antifungal agents
  for fungal encephalitis, 2276
  ocular use of, 2086

Antigen(s), 1787
  in allergic reaction, 1856, 1857
  complete protein, 1857
  definition of, 1783, 1856, 1887
  and HIV infection, 1822
  in inflammation, 1887–1888
  low-molecular-weight substances, 1857
  recognition of, in immune response, 1788
Antigen–antibody binding, 1790
Antigen–antibody tests, 1799t
Antigenic determinant(s), 1784, 1790
  definition of, 1783
Antihemophilic factor, for transfusion, 1103, 1103t
Antihistamines, 1859
  for allergic rhinitis, 1870, 1871t
  for anaphylaxis, 2538
  definition of, 1856
  for Parkinson's disease, 2314
  for pruritus, 1952
  for sinusitis, 595
  for viral rhinitis, 592
Antihypertensive agents
  for chronic renal failure, 1530
  and stroke prevention, 2211
Anti-inflammatory agents, for cystic fibrosis, 719
Antilipid drugs. *See also* Lipid-lowering agents
  for osteoporosis, 2409
Antimalarials
  for rheumatic diseases, 1895t
  for systemic lupus erythematosus, 1911
Antimetabolites
  in cancer treatment, 399t
  and immune system, 1797t
Antineoplastic agents. *See also* Chemotherapy
  administration of, 398–402
  adverse effects and side effects of, 399t, 402
  classification of, 397–398, 399t
  combination of, 398
  dosage of, 398
  fatigue caused by, 402
  and immune system, 1797t
  investigational, 398, 400c
  toxicity of, 398–402
    cardiopulmonary, 402
    gastrointestinal, 398–400
    hematopoietic, 400–401
    neurologic, 402
    renal, 401–402
    reproductive, 402
Antinuclear antibody test, in rheumatic diseases, 1893t
Antiparkinsonian medications, 2313–2314
Antiphospholipid antibodies, thrombophilia caused by, 1099
Antiplatelet medications, for angina, 870–871
Antiprogestins, in cancer treatment, 399t
Antipsychotics, metabolism of, genetic factors affecting, 154t
Antireflux valve
  definition of, 1175
  in gastric sump tube, 1176, 1176f
Antiretroviral agents, for HIV infection, 1826, 1827t–1828t
Antiseizure agents
  adverse effects and side effects of, 2194, 2194t
  for cerebral metastases, 2307
  for chronic renal failure, 1530
  for migraine, 2201
  and osteomalacia, 2411
  perioperative management of, 490t
  preoperative use of, for intracranial surgery, 2181

Antiseizure agents (continued)
    for status epilepticus, 2198
    toxic effects of, 2194, 2194t
    for trigeminal neuralgia, 2295
Antiserum, and passive acquired immunity, 1786
Antithrombin III concentrate, 1103t
Antithrombin III deficiency, 1095, 1098–1099, 1099t
Antithymocyte globulin (Thymoglobulin), for kidney transplant recipient, 1561
Antithyroid medications, 1460–1461, 1462t
    and immune system, 1797t
Antituberculosis agents, 646–648, 647t
    adherence to therapy with, promoting, 649
    adverse effects and side effects of, 647t, 649
    dosage and administration of, 647t
    drug interactions, 647t
Antitussives, for pharyngitis, 598
Antivenin
    administration of, 2540
    allergic response to, 2540
    definition of, 2517
Antivenin Polyvalent, 2539–2540
Antiviral therapy
    ocular, 2086
    in Parkinson's disease, 2314
Antrectomy
    definition of, 1204
    in peptic ulcer disease, 1214t
Anuria, 1503, 1503t
    in acute renal failure, 1522
    definition of, 945, 1493, 1515
Anus, 1121, 1122f. See also Anorectal disorders
    examination of, 1129
Anxiety, 116
    assessment of, 116, 118c
    causes of, 116
    chest pain caused by, assessment of, 792t
    definition of, 112
    dyspnea and, 465
    intraoperative, 518–519
    management of, 116, 118c
    medical conditions causing, 116
    mitral valve prolapse and, 917
    nursing interventions for
        in acute leukemia, 1078
        in Alzheimer's disease, 245
        in angina, 872
        in anorectal disorders, 1279
        in blistering diseases, 1973
        in brain tumor patient, 2308
        in breast cancer, 1719
        in burn victim, 2012c–2013c
            pain and, 2024–2025
        with cardiac dysrhythmias, 841
        in cardiomyopathy, 932
        in diabetes mellitus, 1417–1418
        in disseminated intravascular coagulation, 1098c
        in family members of emergency patient, 2519
        in gastric cancer, 1222–1223
        in gastric surgery patient, 1224
        in gastritis, 1207
        in genital herpes, 1668
        in Guillain-Barré syndrome, 2290
        in heart failure, 961–962
        with hysterectomy, 1692–1693
        in ileostomy patient, 1256c
        in inflammatory bowel disease, 1252
        intraoperative, 518–519
        in kidney transplant recipient, 1562
        in laryngectomy patient, 618
        in mastoid surgery, 2109
        in melanoma, 1983–1984
        in myocardial infarction, 882c–883c, 884
        in peptic ulcer disease, 1214
        in prostatectomy, 1765
        in pulmonary embolism, 667
        in renal surgical patient, 1556c
        in renal-urologic testing, 1512
        in sexually transmitted disease, 2509
        in stroke patient, 2228
        in thoracic surgical patient, 757, 773c
        in toxic epidermal necrolysis or Stevens-Johnson syndrome, 1976
        traction and, 2370
        with urinary diversion, 1600, 1603–1604
        with vertigo, 2115c–2116c
        with vulvar surgery, 1686–1687
        with vulvovaginal infections, 1665
    nursing research on, 117
    pain-related, 266–267
        management of, 276
    postoperative, 544
        nursing interventions for, 528
    preoperative, 495
        nursing interventions for, 495, 499c
    resources and websites on, 126
    shock and, 361
    signs and symptoms of, 116, 118c
Anxiolytics, for burn patients, 2024–2025
AORN. See Association of PeriOperative Registered Nurses
Aorta, 975, 976f
    age-related changes in, 788t
    dissection of, 997f, 1001
Aortic aneurysm, 997
Aortic arch, pressures in, 785f
Aortic valve, 782f, 783, 915, 916f
    definition of, 915
    regurgitation, 918–919
    replacement of, 999f
    stenosis of, 919–920
Aortitis, 996
    syphilitic, 996, 2509
Aortography, 814
Aortoiliac disease, 996–997
APCs. See Ambulatory payment classifications
Aphakia, 2061
    definition of, 2043
Aphasia, 2146, 2146t
    with brain tumor, 2304
    communicating with patient with, 2221, 2221c
    definition of, 2206
    expressive
        definition of, 2206
        stroke and, 2208t, 2209
    global (mixed), stroke and, 2208t
    receptive
        definition of, 2206
        stroke and, 2208t, 2209
    stroke and, 2208t, 2209, 2220–2221
Apheresis
    therapeutic, for blood disorders, 1102
    types of, 1102, 1102t
Aphonia
    definition of, 589
    in laryngitis, 601
Aphthous stomatitis, 1143t
Apical area, examination of, 801, 801f
Apical impulse, 801
    definition of, 781
APL. See Acute promyelocytic leukemia
Aplasia
    bone marrow, 1051
    definition of, 1036
Apligraf, 1948
Apligraf CEA, for burns, 2021t
Apnea, 570
    definition of, 589
    during sleep, 604–605
Apneustic center, 562
APNs. See Advanced practice nurses
Apocrine sweat glands, 1930
Aponeuroses, 2341
Apoptosis, 385, 422, 1074, 1786
    definition of, 381, 1036, 1783
Appearance, patient's, assessment of, in cardiovascular disease, 798
Appendectomy, 1242
    complications of, 1242, 1242t
Appendicitis, 1240–1242
    gerontologic considerations in, 1241–1242
Appendix, 1121, 1122f, 1240
Appetite, stimulation of
    for HIV-infected (AIDS) patients, 1836
    in terminally ill patients, 466
Applanation tonometer, 2050
Appraisal, cognitive, of stress, 93–94
Apraclonidine, for glaucoma, 2057, 2058t
Apraxia
    constructional. See Constructional apraxia
    definition of, 2206
    stroke and, 2209
Apripetant (Emend), for chemotherapy patient, 398–400
APRV. See Airway pressure release ventilation
aPTT. See Activated partial thromboplastin time
Aquacel Ag, for burns, 2020t
Aqueous humor, 2055, 2055f
Arachnoid, 2133, 2134f, 2135–2136
Arachnoiditis, after disk surgery, 2329
Arbovirus infection, 2274
ARDS. See Acute respiratory distress syndrome
Area Agencies on Aging, 249
Areflexia, in Guillain-Barré syndrome, 2289
Arenaviruses, 2511–2512
Areola, reconstruction of, 1733
ARF. See Renal failure, acute
Argatroban, for pulmonary embolism, 665
Arginine, in wound healing, 487t
Argon laser, for skin lesions, 1991
Arm cast(s), 2355, 2356f
    care of patient with, 2362
Aromatase inhibitors
    for breast cancer, 1729
    in cancer treatment, 399t
    definition of, 1701
ART. See Assisted reproductive technology
Arterial blood gases
    in acute respiratory distress syndrome, 658
    in acute respiratory failure, 655
    assessment of, 339t, 340c
    in atelectasis, 627
    measurement of, 579
    in chronic obstructive pulmonary disease, 689
    in metabolic acidosis, 335
    in metabolic alkalosis, 336
    normal values for, 339t
    in respiratory acidosis, 337
    in respiratory alkalosis, 338
Arterial disorder(s)
    management of, 986–987
    peripheral
        assessment of, 980
        diagnostic evaluation of, 980–983
        gerontologic considerations in, 980
        nursing diagnoses related to, 987

nursing interventions for, 987–991
nursing process with, 987–992
occlusive, 992–995
planning and goals for, 987
Arterial embolization, in liver cancer, 1334
Arterial insufficiency, 978–979
in extremities, 992–995
Arterial occlusive disease
peripheral, 992–995
assessment of, 992
clinical manifestations of, 992
diagnosis of, 992
medical management of, 992
nursing management of, 994–995
pharmacologic therapy for, 992
risk factors for, 992
sites of involvement in, 993f
surgical management of, 992–994
of upper extremity, 995
Arteriole(s), 975–976
Arteriosclerosis
definition of, 975, 983–984
and foot disorders, 2401
Arteriovenous fistula
definition of, 1515
for hemodialysis, 1539, 1539f
Arteriovenous graft
definition of, 1515
for hemodialysis, 1539, 1539f
Arteriovenous malformations, and hemorrhagic stroke, 2223, 2224
Arteriovenous oxygen difference, systemic, 977
Artery(ies), 975–976, 976f
age-related changes in, 788t
repair of, 993–994, 994f
complications of, 994
home and community-based care after, 994–995
nursing management of, 994–995
Arthritis, 1887. *See also* Rheumatic diseases
gonococcal, 2509
infections and, 1919–1920
Paget's disease and, 2412
rheumatoid. *See* Rheumatoid arthritis
septic. *See* Septic arthritis
Arthrocentesis, 2351
for rheumatic diseases, 1889–1891
Arthrodesis, 2372
definition of, 2355
for rheumatoid arthritis, 1909
Arthrography, 2350
Arthroplasty, 2372
definition of, 1887, 2355, 2371c
for osteoarthritis, 1916
for rheumatoid arthritis, 1909
Arthropod-borne virus encephalitis, 2274–2275
assessment of, 2275
clinical manifestations of, 2274–2275
diagnosis of, 2275
medical management of, 2275
nursing management of, 2275
pathophysiology of, 2274
Arthroscope, 2430
definition of, 2425
Arthroscopic surgery, of knee, 2430
Arthroscopy, 2351
Articular cartilage, 2338, 2338f
degeneration of, 1888
Articular system
function of, 2338–2340
structure of, 2338–2340
Artificial blood, 2526
Artificial insemination, 1651–1652

Artificial kidney. *See* Dialyzer
Arytenoid cartilage, 554
Asbestosis, 669
definition of, 625
Ascending colon, 1122f
Ascites, 315, 1289, 1293–1298
assessment of, 1294, 1294f
in cirrhosis, 1318–1319
clinical manifestations of, 1293–1294
definition of, 945
medical management of, 1294–1295
nursing management of, 1295–1297, 1298c
pathophysiology of, 1293, 1294f
Asepsis, surgical, 505
definition of, 503
guidelines for, 507
principles of, 506–508
ASIA. *See* American Spinal Injury Association
Asparaginase, in cancer treatment, 399t
Aspartame (NutraSweet), 1388
Aspartate aminotransferase, serum, 1290t
*Aspergillus*
encephalitis caused by, 2275–2276
pneumonia caused by, 633t
Aspirate, gastric
pH testing of, in GI intubation, 1175, 1178–1179
visual assessment of, in GI intubation, 1178–1179
Aspiration (inhalation), 681–682
in amyotrophic lateral sclerosis, 2323
definition of, 1175
of foreign bodies, 608
of gastric contents, 516
pneumonia caused by, 534
in tube feedings, 1184t, 1187
postoperative, prevention of, 525–526
prevention of, 681–682
in myasthenia gravis, 2287
in tube feedings, 1187
risk factors for, 681, 681c
risk of, reduction of
in esophageal conditions, 1170
in tube feedings, 187
in septic arthritis, 2416
silent, 681
of vomitus, prevention of, 527
Aspiration (suctioning), 1175
definition of, 1175
from gastrointestinal tubes, facilitation of, 1178
Aspirin
for coronary artery disease, 870
enteric-coated, for skin ulcer healing, 1948
and immune system, 1797t
in infertility treatment, 1651c
for pharyngitis, 598
platelet defect caused by, 1089
poisoning with, emergency management of, 2547t–2548t
precautions with, 593
for rheumatic diseases, 1895t
and stroke prevention, 2210–2211
and surgical patient, 488
therapy with, in peripheral arterial disease, 992
for thrombotic complications, in polycythemia vera, 1065
for viral rhinitis, 592
Assessment. *See also specific condition*
in asthma, 711
biochemical, 78–80
in cancer management, 423–426
after cardiac surgery, 897–899
of cardiovascular function, 787–805

in chronic obstructive pulmonary disease, 689–690, 690c
cultural, 135–136, 136c
in genetic assessment, 155–156
data in, recording, 35
documentation of, 35
emergency, 2521–2522
in ethical analysis, 34c
formats for, 73–74
in gastric cancer, 1221
of gastrostomy patient, 1189–1190
genetic, 102, 154–156
cultural, social, and spiritual considerations in, 155–156
physical examination in, 155
psychosocial considerations in, 156, 157c
genetics in, 68
guidelines for, 64
health history in, 35
in home and community, 84–85, 84c
of intraoperative patient, 518
in kidney surgery, 1553
in neck dissection, 1153
nurse's role in, 64
in nursing process, 34, 35, 36c
database, recording, 35
of oral cavity, 1149–1150
of pacemaker therapy, 847, 848t
in parenteral nutrition, 1196
of people with disabilities, 72c, 178c
in peptic ulcer disease, 1211
physical, 35. *See also* Physical examination
in pneumonia, 636, 639
in postanesthia care unit, 525
postoperative
of hospitalized patient, 532–533
nursing activities in, 482c
of thoracic surgical patient, 764
preoperative, 485–491
for gastric surgery patient, 1223–1224
in thoracic surgical patient, 756
psychosocial
in genetic assessment, 156, 157c
of surgical patient, 489–490
of respiratory function, 563–578
of sexual assault victim, 2551
social, in genetic assessment, 155–156
spiritual, in genetic assessment, 155–156
of substance use, 120, 120c
in teaching-learning process, 54, 55c
technology and, 64–65
of thoracic surgery patient
postoperative, 764
preoperative, 756
in tube feeding, 1183
in tuberculosis, 645–646
in upper airway infection, 601–602
of ventilator-dependent patient, 747–748
Assist-control ventilation, 743, 743f
definition of, 723
and respiratory weaning, 752
Assisted dying, patients' requests for, nurses' response to, nursing research on, 453
Assisted reproductive technology, 1652
Assisted suicide, 450–451, 468, 2310c
definition of, 448
ethical issues in, 451, 452c
Assistive device(s), 191
definition of, 190
for foot surgery patients, 2403
after hip replacement, 2375
for ischemic stroke patients, 2218, 2219c
for orthopedic surgery patients, 2375, 2376c
in Parkinson's disease, 2317

Assistive device(s) (*continued*)
  for patient transfer, 202–203
  pressure-relieving, 210–212
  for pressure ulcers, 210–212
  in rehabilitation, 194–195
  for rheumatic diseases, 1894, 1898
  for surgical patient, nursing management of, 492
  with vertigo, 2116c
Assistive technology, 191
  definition of, 190
Assited living facilities, older adults in, 229
Association of PeriOperative Registered Nurses, 484
  recommendations for latex allergy management, 508
  recommendations for surgical attire, 506
Association of Women's Health, Obstetrical and Neonatal Nurses, 161c
Asterixis, 1305, 1306f
  definition of, 1285
Asthma, 709–718
  action plan for, 714, 715f
  allergy and, 710
  assessment findings in, 576t
  assessment in, 711
  clinical manifestations of, 711
  complications of, 711
  and COPD, 686
    differentiation of, 690
  definition of, 686
  diagnosis of, 711
  epidemiology of, 709–710
  exacerbations of, 711
    management of, 714, 715f
  exercise-induced, 711
  management of, stepwise approach for, 712t–713t
  medical management of, 711–714, 712t–713t
  pathophysiology of, 710–711, 710f
  peak flow monitoring in, 714, 716c, 716f
    patient teaching about, 714, 716c
  pharmacologic therapy for, 711–714, 712t–713t
    quick-relief medications, 712t–713t, 714
  predisposing factors for, 710
  prevention of, 711
  self-care in, patient teaching about, 714–717
Astigmatism, 2051
  definition of, 2043
Astrocytomas, 2302
Asymmetric septal hypertrophy. *See* Cardiomyopathy(ies), hypertrophic
Asystole, 837–838, 838f
Ataxia, 1807, 2142, 2146
  with brain tumor, 2304
  definition of, 1802, 2129, 2206
  in multiple sclerosis, 2279, 2280
  stroke and, 2208t
Ataxia-telangiectasia, 1803t, 1807
  definition of, 1802
Atazanavir (Reyataz), for HIV infection, 1828t
Atelectasis, 557, 625–628
  assessment findings in, 576t
  in bronchiectasis, 709
  in chronic obstructive pulmonary disease, nursing interventions for, 707c
  clinical manifestations of, 627
  definition of, 625
  lobar, 625
  management of, 627–628
  pathophysiology of, 625–627, 626f
  in pneumonia, 638, 641

  postoperative, 534, 625–626, 626f
    in hip fracture, 2449
    orthopedic surgery and, 2387
  prevention of, 627, 627c
  rib fracture and, 2459
  risk factors for, 625–626, 626f
    in thoracic surgery patient, risk factors for, 757c
  traction and, 2370
Atenolol (Tenormin), 830t, 869
  for hypertension, 1027t
Atherectomy, 886
Atheroma, definition of, 859
Atherosclerosis, 859. *See also* Arterial occlusive disease
  clinical manifestations of, 986
  coronary, 859–867
    clinical manifestations of, 860
    pathophysiology of, 859–860, 860f
    prevention of, 862–866
    risk factors for, 860–862
  definition of, 859, 975, 984
  in diabetes, 1422
  medical management of, 986–987
  pathophysiology of, 984–985, 984f
  prevention of, 985–986
  radiologic interventions for, 986–987
  risk factors for, 985
  surgical management of, 986
Athetoid movements, in hypomagnesemia, 329
Athetosis, 2142
Athlete's foot, 1960–1961, 1961t
Atmospheric pressure, 559
Atonic muscles, 2342
  definition of, 2337
Atopic dermatitis, 1877–1878
  definition of, 1856
Atopy, 1856
  definition of, 1856
Atorvastatin (Lipitor), 864–865, 865t, 986
ATP. *See* Adenosine triphosphate
Atracurium (Tacrium), 432t
Atrial fibrillation, 832–833, 833f
  with accessory pathway, 833
  acute-onset, 833
  catheter ablation therapy for, 854–855
  lone, 832
  paroxysmal, 832
  and pulmonary embolism, 662
  recurrence, prevention of, 833
  risk factors for, 832
  and stroke, 833, 2206, 2210
Atrial flutter, 832, 832f
Atrial kick, 786, 824
Atrial natriuretic peptide, 948
  and fluid balance, 307–308, 308f
  release of, 307–308
Atrioventricular (AV) block
  first-degree, 838–839
  second-degree
    type I, 839, 839f
    type II, 839–840, 839f
  third-degree, 840, 840f
Atrioventricular (AV) nodal reentry tachycardia, 834–835, 834f
  catheter ablation therapy for, 854–855
Atrioventricular (AV) node, 783–784, 784f, 824
Atrioventricular (AV) valves, 782f, 783
Atripla, for HIV infection, 1829
Atrium/atria, cardiac, 782–783, 782f
  age-related changes in, 788t
  pressures in, 785f
Atrophic vaginitis, 1663t, 1664

Atrophy, 100, 100t
  definition of, 2337
  of muscle, 2342
  skin, 1938c
Atropine
  for asystole, 838
  in cardiopulmonary resuscitation, 971, 972t
  for nerve agent exposure, 2570–2571
  ocular applications of, 2086t
  for sinus bradycardia, 829
Atropine sulfate drops, in end-of-life care, 471t
Atypical hyperplasia
  in breast, 1711
  definition of, 1701
Audiometry, 2099–2100, 2100f
AUDIT, 70
Auditory brain stem response, 2100
Aura, and migraine, 2198
Aural rehabilitation, 2120–2123
Auranofin (Ridaura), for rheumatic diseases, 1895t
Auricle, 2093, 2094f
Aurothioglucose (Solganol), for rheumatic diseases, 1895t
Auscultation
  of abdomen, 1128f, 1129
  cardiac, 802–804
    procedure for, 803–804
  in physical examination, 76–77, 77–78
  postoperative, 532–533
  thoracic/pulmonary, 574–576, 576t
    with lung abscess, 651
    in pneumonia, 636
Autoantibody(ies), 1062
Autograft
  bone, 2439
  definition of, 2425
  for burns, 2019, 2021t, 2022–2024
  cultured epithelial
    for burns, 2020t, 2023
    definition of, 1995
  definition of, 915, 1995
  for heart valve replacement, 924
  skin, 1986
Autoimmune disorders, 1796
  chronic lymphocytic leukemia and, 1074
  gerontologic considerations in, 1795
  of nervous system, 2277–2292
Autoimmune hemolytic anemia, 1062
  chronic lymphocytic leukemia and, 1074
Autoimmune thyroiditis. *See* Hashimoto's disease
Automaticity, of cardiac conduction cells, 783, 823, 854
Autonomic dysfunction, in Guillain-Barré syndrome, 2288–2289
Autonomic dysreflexia
  definition of, 2233
  signs and symptoms of, 2256
  spinal cord injury and, 2256, 2259–2260
Autonomic nervous system, 2137–2139, 2139t, 2140f. *See also* Parasympathetic nervous system; Sympathetic nervous system
  and cardiac function, 825
  definition of, 2129
Autonomic neuropathy, in diabetes, 1427
Autonomy
  definition of, 448
  of dying patient, 450
  ethical principle of, 28c
Autoregulation
  of blood pressure, 1498–1499
  definition of, 2161, 2170

Autosome(s), 141–142
    definition of, 140
Avascular necrosis, 1920
    of bone, 2439–2440
    compartment syndrome and, 2438
    definition of, 2355, 2425
    of femoral head, postoperative, in hip fracture, 2447, 2449
    fracture and, 2447, 2449
    and joint replacement, 2372
Avian flu, 2489
AVM. *See* Arteriovenous malformations
Avoidance therapy, for allergic rhinitis, 1870
Avulsion, definition of, 2528c
Awareness, of terminal illness
    closed, 449–450
    mutual pretense, 450
    open, 450
    suspected, 450
Axillary lymph nodes, dissection of, in breast cancer, 1716–1718, 1717t
    lymphedema after, 1721–1722, 1722c
    self-care after, 1723–1725, 1723c
Axon(s), 2129, 2130f
    definition of, 2129
    and diffuse axonal injury, 2236
Ayurveda, 134
5-Azacytidine, in cancer treatment, 399t
Azathioprine (Imuran)
    for idiopathic thrombocytopenic purpura, 1088
    for immune hemolytic anemia, 1062
    for myasthenia gravis, 2286
    for rheumatic diseases, 1896t
Azithromycin (Zithromax)
    for chlamydia, 1670, 2508
    for Legionnaire's disease, 2511
    for *Mycobacterium avium* complex, 1835
    for pharyngitis, 598
    for pneumonia, 636
    for sinusitis, 595
Azithromycin with rifabutin (Mycobutin), for *Mycobacterium avium* complex, 1835
Azoospermia, chemotherapy-induced, 402
Azotemia
    in acute glomerulonephritis, 1518
    in acute renal failure, 1523, 1524
    definition of, 1515
    in hypervolemia, 314
    in tube feedings, 1184t

# B

Babinski reflex (sign), 2147, 2149–2150, 2149f
    assessment of, in unconscious patient, 2165t
    definition of, 2129
Bacille Calmette-Guérin (BCG)
    for bladder cancer, 1597
    in cancer treatment, 418
    intravesical, for bladder cancer, 1597
Bacille Calmette-Guérin (BCG) vaccine, 2512
*Bacillus anthracis*, 2566
    incubation period of, 2476t
    transmission of, 2476t
Back, healthy, health promotion for, 2396c
Back pain, 1920. *See also* Low back pain
Baclofen (Lioresal)
    for spasticity, in multiple sclerosis, 2280
    for trigeminal neuralgia, 2295
Bacteremia
    definition of, 373c, 2475, 2484
    health care–associated, prevention of, 2483–2484
    prevention of, 2498c
    vascular access device-related, 2484, 2484c
Bacteria
    and cancer, 385–386
    colony-forming units, 507
    disease caused by, 102
    invasion by, immune response to, 1786–1788
    in operating room, 507
    pharyngitis caused by, 597–598
    uropathogenic, 1572
Bacterial arthritis, 1919–1920
Bacterial infections. *See also specific infection*
    phagocytic dysfunction and, 1802–1805, 1803t
    of skin, 1956–1958
Bacterial keratitis, 2076t
Bacterial vaginosis, 1626, 1626t, 1662–1664, 1663t
    in HIV-infected (AIDS) patients, 1673
Bacteriuria, 1572. *See also* Urinary tract infection(s)
    definition of, 1493, 1570
    detection of, 1506
    gerontologic considerations in, 1572
    in males, 1750
Baker tube, 1176t
Balance, 2096
    assessment of, 2146–2147
    in elderly, 236
Balanced analgesia, 278
    definition of, 259
Balanced suspension traction, 2366, 2367f
Ball-and-socket joints, 2340
Balloon sign, 2348, 2348f
Balloon tamponade
    definition of, 1285
    for esophageal varices, 1300–1301, 1301f, 1304t
Balloon valvuloplasty, 921, 921f
Ballottement, of knee, 2348, 2348f
Balneotherapy, 1948
    definition of, 1945
Band cell, 1041
    definition of, 1036
Barbiturates
    abuse/overdose, emergency management of, 2545t–2546t
    effect on metabolic demands, 2173
    in palliative sedation of terminally ill patient, 468
Bargaining, as stage of dying, 472t
Bariatric surgery, 1218–1220, 1219f
Barium enema, 1132
    air-contrast, 1132
    double-contrast, 1132
Barium swallow, 1132
    double-contrast, 1132
Baroreceptors, 562, 786
    age-related changes in, 788t
    in blood pressure regulation, 358
    definition of, 781
    in fluid and electrolyte balance, 306
Barotrauma, in ventilator-dependent patient, 751
Barrel chest, 569–570, 688, 689, 689f
Barrett's esophagus, 1166
    and esophageal cancer, 1166
Barrier protection, in Standard Precautions, 1820c
Barthel Index, 193
Bartholinitis, 1663t
Bartholin's cyst, 1677–1678
    definition of, 1661
Bartholin's gland, 1614, 1625
    cancer of, 1685–1686
Basal body temperature method, of family planning, 1646
Basal cell carcinoma
    of eyelid, 2080
    of skin, 1979–1981, 1979f
Basal ganglia, 2132, 2142
Basal metabolic rate, 1447
    definition of, 1440
Base(s), nucleotide, 141, 143f
Basilar artery, 2134
Basilar skull fracture, 2234, 2234f
Basophil(s), 1038f, 1040f, 1041
    functions of, 1037t, 1042
    laboratory values for, 2579
    in natural immunity, 1785
Basophil kallikrein, in allergic reaction, 1858t
Bath(s), therapeutic, 1948, 1949c
Battle's sign, 2235
B-cell lymphoma
    definition of, 1815
    in HIV-infected (AIDS) patients, 1832–1833
B cells (B lymphocytes), 1038f, 1039, 1042, 1784, 1787, 1792t
    in allergic reaction, 1857
    deficiencies, 1805–1806
        assessment of, 1805
        clinical manifestations of, 1805
        combined with T-cell deficiencies, 1803t, 1806–1807
            clinical manifestations of, 1807
            medical management of, 1807, 1808c
            nursing management of, 1807
            pathophysiology of, 1807
        diagnosis of, 1805
        medical management of, 1806
        pathophysiology of, 1805
    definition of, 1783, 1856
    functions of, 1037t, 1042, 1787–1788, 1788c, 1792t
    in humoral immune response, 1787
    and immunodeficiency disorders, 1803t
    in inflammation, 1887–1888
    in natural immunity, 1785–1786
    production of, 1784
BCG. *See* Bacille Calmette-Guérin (BCG)
BCG Matrix, for burn grafts, 2020t, 2021–2022
*BCR-ABL* gene, 1072–1073
Beau's lines, 1936, 1940f
Becaplermin, 1948
Beclomethasone, 1485t
Beclomethasone dipropionate (Vanceril), for laryngitis, 601
Bed
    patient positioning in, and pressure ulcers, 209f, 210
    positioning patient in, 196, 197c
    rotating, 2253, 2254f
    transfer from, 201–203, 202f, 203c
Bed rest
    for ascites, 1295
    for low back pain, 2394c
Behavior
    definition of, 46c
    health-protecting, 57
    patterns of, and heart disease, 867
Belching, 1127
Bell's palsy, 2295–2296
Below-elbow amputation, 2461f
Below-knee amputation, 2460, 2461f
Benazepril (Lotensin), 952–953, 952t
    for hypertension, 1029t
Bendroflumethazide (Naturetin), 954t
Beneficence, ethical principle of, 28c
Benign paroxysmal positional vertigo, 2119

Benign proliferative breast disease, 1711, 1713
definition of, 1701
Benign prostatic hyperplasia, 233, 1504, 1751–1752
definition of, 1740
Benson Relaxation Response, 105, 107
Benzodiazepines
for anaphylaxis, 2538
for delirium, 468
for nerve agent exposure, 2571
in palliative sedation of terminally ill patient, 468
for spasticity, in multiple sclerosis, 2280
Benzoyl peroxide, for acne vulgaris, 1954t, 1955
Benzthiazide (Exna), 954t
Bepridil (Vascor), 830t
Bereavement, 121–122, 472–473
definition of, 112, 448, 471
nursing interventions for, 122
resources and websites on, 126
stages of, 121
Bernard, Claude, 91–92
Bernstein test, 1139
Beta-blockers, 830t
adverse effects and side effects of, 869–870
for angina, 869–870
for atrial flutter, 832
for atrioventricular (AV) nodal reentry tachycardia, 835
in cluster headache prevention, 2200
for esophageal varices, 1300
for glaucoma, 2057, 2058t
for heart failure, 953
for hypertension, 1027t
for hypertensive crises, 1033
for hyperthyroidism, 1462
in migraine prevention, 2200
with sympathomimetic activity, for hypertension, 1028t
Beta-lactams, for pneumonia, 636
Betamethasone, 1485t
Betaxolol
for glaucoma, 2057, 2058t
for hypertension, 1027t
Bethanechol (Urecholine), for gastroesophageal reflux disease, 1166
Bevacizumab (Avastin), 419t
adverse effects and side effects of, 421t
Bextra. See Valdecoxib
Bias, evaluation for, in critical thinking, 25
Bicarbonate
and acid-base equilibrium, 334–335
in body fluids, 302t
deficit, 335–336
manifestations of, 1516t
in renal disorders, 1516t
excess, 336
manifestations of, 1516t
in renal disorders, 1516t
and hypochloremia, 333
imbalances of, in renal disorders, 1516t
Bigeminy, 835
Biguanides, 1398, 1399t, 1401
Bile, 1124
circulation of, 1345
formation of, 1287
source and digestive action of, 1123t
Bile acid sequestrants, 865, 865t, 986
Bile ducts, 1286
anatomy of, 1345, 1346f
Bile reflux, after gastric surgery, 1225
Biliary colic, with gallstones, 1349
Biliary drainage
in acute pancreatitis, 1360

in liver cancer, 1334
postoperative, for gallbladder surgery, 1356
Biliary system, anatomy of, 1345, 1346f
Bilirubin, 1345
excretion of, 1287
in jaundice, 1289–1293
serum, 1290t
urine, 1290t
Billroth I procedure, in peptic ulcer disease, 1214t
Billroth II procedure, in peptic ulcer disease, 1214t
Bilobectomy, of lung, 672c
Binocular vision, 2061
definition of, 2043
Bioartificial liver, 1317
Bioavailability, 1286–1287
Biobrane, 2020t, 2021, 2022f
definition of, 1995
Biochemical mediators, definition of, 356
Biocompatibility, of dialyzer, 1538
Biofeedback, for urinary incontinence, 216
Biofields, 134
Biologically based therapies, 134
Biological warfare, 2566–2569
definition of, 2559
Biologic dressings, for burns, 2019–2021, 2020t
Biologic response modifiers
adverse effects and side effects of, 420–422, 421t
for cancer
home and community-based care with, 422
nursing management of, 420–422
in cancer treatment, 418–422
definition of, 381
for melanoma, 1982
nonspecific, 418
Biologic therapy, for rheumatoid arthritis, 1908
Biologic weapons, 2566–2569
Biomarkers, cardiac, 876, 876t
Biopsy
bone, 2351
bone marrow, 2351
breast, 1708–1709
brush, renal and ureteral, 1510
of cancer, 391–392
excisional, 392
incisional, 392
needle, 392
cervical, 1628–1629
cone, 1629
definition of, 381
endometrial (aspiration), 1629–1630
excisional, for breast disorders, 1709
incisional, for breast disorders, 1709
of liver, 1289, 1290t, 1292c–1293c
lung, 582–585
open, definition of, 625
lymph node, in respiratory disease, 585
musculoskeletal, 2351
pleural, 582–585
renal, 1510
sentinel lymph node, in breast cancer, 1717–1718, 1717t
of skin, 1942
synovial, 2351
Biosynthetic dressings, for burn grafts, 2020t, 2021–2022
Bioterrorism, 2566–2569
smallpox in, 2568
weapons used in, 2566–2569, 2567t
Biotinidase deficiency, genetic screening for, 150t

Biot's respiration, 570, 572t
Bi-PAP. See Ventilation, bilevel positive airway pressure
Bird flu, 2489
Bismuth salts, for gastritis, 1206t
Bismuth subsalicylate (Pepto-Bismol), for gastritis and peptic ulcer disease, 1206t
Bisoprolol, 830t
for hypertension, 1027t
Bisphosphonates, 328
for complex regional pain syndrome, 2440
in multiple myeloma, 1084
for osteoporosis, 2409
administration of, patient teaching about, 2410
for Paget's disease, 2412
Bites
poisonous, emergency management of, 2539–2540
snake, emergency management of, 2539–2540
Bitolerol (Tornalate), 693t
Bivalving, of cast, 2359, 2359c
Black lung disease, 669–670
Bladder
anatomy of, 1494f, 1495–1496
artificial sphincter for, 1581, 1583f
capacity of
anatomic, 1499
functional, 1499
compliance of, 1499
distention of, in cardiac patient, 805
drainage of, after prostatectomy, 1767
dysfunction of, after hysterectomy, 1693
emptying of, 1500
filling of, 1499
flaccid, 1584
function, assessment of, 215
infection of. See Cystitis; Urinary tract infection(s)
irrigation of, after prostatectomy, 1767, 1767f
management, paraplegia/quadriplegia and, 2263–2264
neurogenic, 1584–1589
definition of, 2233
palpation of, 1504, 1505f
percussion of, 1504
reflex, 1584
retraining of, 1582c
after urinary catheterization, 1588, 1589c
spastic, 1584
trauma to, 1595
management of, 1595
ultrasonography of, 1507–1508
urine storage in, 1499
Bladder cancer, 1596–1597
in elderly, 234
risk factors for, 1596, 1596c
Bladder control
in multiple sclerosis, 2280, 2282
in stroke patient, 2220
Bladder incontinence. See Urinary incontinence
Bladder neck obstruction, prevention and control of, in prostate cancer, 1760c
Bladder training, 216
Blast cell, 1041
definition of, 1036
Bleeding. See also Hemorrhage
abnormal, uterine, 1639–1640
in acute leukemia
management of, 1075, 1076c
precautions for, 1075, 1076c
prevention of, 1075, 1076c
in acute myeloid leukemia, 1071

# INDEX

with anticoagulant therapy, 1007
in cancer patient, 425, 432–433
  nursing management of, 414c–415c
in cardiac surgical patient, 891t
in cirrhosis, 1321
corticosteroid-induced, after kidney transplantation, 1563
in disseminated intravascular coagulation, 1093–1094, 1094c
in gastrostomy, 1191
in hemophilia, 1090–1091, 1090–1092
with hemorrhoids, 1277
heparin therapy and, 871
in liver disease, 1307, 1330c–1332c
in liver transplantation, 1338
nasal. *See* Epistaxis
in neurosurgical patient, nursing interventions for, 2188
patient at risk for, home care checklist for, 1085, 1085c
in peptic ulcer disease, 1215–1216
peritoneal dialysis and, 1547
in renal surgical patient, 1558
risk of, in hematologic disorders, 1068c
uterine
  abnormal, 1639–1640
  postmenopausal, 1640
Bleeding disorders, 1084–1092
  clinical manifestations of, 1085
  medical management of, 1085
  nursing management of, 1085, 1085c
Bleeding time, laboratory values for, 2578
Bleomycin
  in cancer treatment, 399t
  pulmonary toxicity of, 402
Blepharitis, 2076t
Blind dental abscess, 1145
Blindness, 2051–2054
  definition of, 2043
  in Guillain-Barré syndrome, 2289
  people with, interacting and communicating with, 179c–180c, 2053, 2054c
Blistering diseases, 1971–1972
  nursing process for, 1972–1974
Bloating, in tube feeding, 1184t
Blood, 1037
  artificial, 2526
  chemistry studies, in musculoskeletal assessment, 2351
  intraoperative exposure to, safety precautions for, 508
  intraoperative salvage of, 1106
  loss, in kidney surgery, assessment of, 1554
  pH of, 339t
  replacement, in hypovolemic shock, 367, 368
  in stool, 1127
  substitutes for, 2526
  for transfusion, processing of, 1106–1107
  whole, reference ranges for, 2581t–2593t
Blood agents, as terrorism threats, 2569t, 2571
Bloodborne hepatitis, causative organism of, 2476t
Bloodborne pathogens, Standard Precautions against, 1818–1819, 1820c–1821c
Blood–brain barrier, 2135
Blood cells, 1037t, 1038f, 1039–1042, 1040f
Blood chemistry, in cardiac patient, 806–808, 807t
Blood clotting, 1043, 1044f
  acquired disorders of, 1092–1102
  assessment of, in cardiac patient, 807t–808t
  laboratory analysis of, in cardiac patient, 807t–808t

Blood component therapy, 1103–1104, 1103t
Blood disorders. *See also* Hematologic disorders
  treatment of, 1102–1104. *See also* Transfusion therapy
Blood donation, 1104–1106
  autologous, 1105–1106
  complications of, 1106
  directed, 1105
  standard, 1105
Blood flow, 977
Blood gas analysis, 338, 340c
  normal values for, 339t
Blood pressure, 799. *See also* Hypertension; Hypotension
  age-related changes in, 805
  autoregulation of, 1498–1499
  classification of, 1021, 1021t
  control of, 1022, 1022f
  definition of, 1021
  factors affecting, 825
  intra-arterial monitoring of, 820, 820f
  measurement of, 799, 1030c
  monitoring of
    for dialysis patient, 1552
    for hospitalized dialysis patient, 1552
  postural changes and, 799
  regulation of, 358, 786
  screenings, 1031
Blood substitute, 1111–1112
Blood tests
  with back pain, 2393c
  for gastrointestinal disorders, 1129
  for rheumatic diseases, 1892, 1893t–1894t
Blood transfusion(s), 1103, 1103t
  acute lung injury related to, 1110
  administration of, 1107–1112
    pretransfusion assessment for, 1107c, 1108–1109, 1108c
    setting for, 1107–1108
  bacterial contamination of, 1110
  circulatory overload caused by, 1110
  complications of, 1109–1111. *See also* Transfusion reaction(s)
  disease transmission by, 1104t, 1110
    prevention of, 1104
  in emergency care, 2526
  in hemorrhage, 2526
  and HIV transmission, 1816
  in hypovolemic shock, 367, 368, 2528
  and immune system function, 1796–1797
  leukocyte-depleted products for, 1106–1107
  leukocyte-poor products for, 1106
  pharmacologic alternatives to, 1111–1112, 1112c
  postoperative, 528
  recipient
    history-taking from, 1108
    patient teaching for, 1109
    physical assessment of, 1108–1109
Blood types, 1106
  and peptic ulcer disease, 1209
Blood urea nitrogen, 305, 1507t
  in acute renal failure, 1523t, 1524
  in cardiac patient, 807t
  in chronic renal failure, 1529
  in hypovolemia, 309
  usual reference range for, 310t
Blood urea nitrogen to creatinine ratio, 1507t
  usual reference range for, 310t
Blood vessels. *See also* Vascular system; specific vessel
  alterations in, 978
  in fluid and electrolyte balance, 306
  fragility of, cutaneous manifestations of, 1929t

Blood volume, 1037
Blue pigtail, 1176
BMD. *See* Bone mineral density
Body cast, 2355
  care of patient with, 2363
Body image
  amputation and, 2464
  breast surgery and, 1719–1720
  burns and, 2033–2034
  of cancer patient, 426, 431
    nursing interventions for, 413c
  of colostomy patient, 1273
  in continuous ambulatory peritoneal dialysis, 1549
  in Cushing's syndrome, 1482
  enhancement of, in gastrostomy, 1191
  hysterectomy and, 1693
  after laryngectomy, nursing interventions for, 617
  in liver disease, 1327c
  in psoriasis, 1969
  rheumatic diseases and, 1902c, 1904
  with urinary diversion, 1605
Body lice, 1962–1963
Body mass index (BMI), 77–78, 79f, 1217, 1384
  calculation of, 77–78, 79f
  definition of, 77, 1021
Body mechanics, proper, 2394c, 2395–2397, 2395f, 2396f
Body movements
  active, preoperative teaching about, 493–495
  assessment of, 75
  asymmetry of, 75
  choreiform, 75
Body temperature. *See* Temperature (body)
Body weight. *See* Weight
Body wrap, 742
Boil(s). *See* Furuncles
Bolus, definition of, 1175
Bolus feeding(s), by gastrostomy, 1192
Bone(s)
  age-related changes in, 2342, 2344t
  avascular necrosis of, 2439–2440
    fracture and, 2447, 2449
  biopsy of, in osteomalacia, 2411
  blood supply to, 2338f, 2339, 2340
  cancellous (trabecular), 2338, 2339, 2340
    definition of, 2337
  cells of, 2338, 2338f
  cortical (compact), 2338–2339, 2338f, 2340
    definition of, 2337
  flat, 2338
  formation of, 2339, 2406
    in fracture healing, 2340
  functions of, 2338–2340
  healing of, 2340
    with fragments firmly approximated, 2340
  imaging of, 2350
  integrity of, assessment of, 2347
  irregular, 2338
  long, 2338
  maintenance of, 2339–2340
  matrix of, 2338–2339
  metabolic disorders of, 2404–2413
  in Paget's disease, 2412
  pelvic, 2444, 2444f
  remodeling of. *See* Remodeling
  resorption of, 2339
    biochemical markers of, 2352
    definition of, 2337
  short, 2338
  shortening of, fracture and, 2431

Bone(s) (continued)
    structure of, 2338–2340
    turnover, in Paget's disease, 2412
    types of, 2338
Bone conduction device(s), 2122
Bone cortex, in fracture healing, 2340
Bone cyst, 2417
Bone densitometry, 2350
Bone density, age-related changes in, 235
Bone disease, 1920
    in chronic renal failure, 1529, 1537c
    uremic, in chronic renal failure, 1529
Bone graft
    definition of, 2371c
    for nonunion of fracture, 2438–2439
    nursing management of, 2439
    problems with, 2439
Bone healing stimulator, 2439, 2439f
Bone health, perimenopausal, 1635
Bone marrow, 1784, 1784f
    anatomy of, 1037–1039
    aplasia, 1051
    aspiration of, 1045
    biopsy of, 1045
    in fracture healing, 2340
    hyperplasia of, 1052
    and lymphocytes, 1784, 1785f
    physiology of, 1037–1039
    red, 2338f, 2339
    yellow, 2338f, 2339
Bone marrow transplantation, 402–417,
        1112–1113
    for acute lymphocytic leukemia, 1074
    in acute myeloid leukemia, 1072
    allogeneic, 415, 416
    autologous, 416
    for chronic myeloid leukemia, 1073
    donors, caring for, 417
    immunosuppression for, 416
    for multiple myeloma, 1083–1084
    for myelodysplastic syndromes, 1054
    for non-Hodgkin's lymphoma, 1082
    nursing management in, 416–417
    posttransplantation care in, 417
    pretransplantation care in, 416–417
    for severe combined immunodeficiency disease, 1807
    for sickle cell anemia, 1057
    syngeneic, 416
Bone mass, loss of, aging and, 2405
Bone mineral density
    estimation of, 2350
    and osteoporosis, 2407
    osteoporosis and, 2405–2406
    in postpolio syndrome, 2331
Bone pain, 2344
    in Hodgkin's disease, 1080
    in multiple myeloma, 1083
Bone scan, 2350–2351
    for low back pain, 2393c
    in osteomyelitis, 2413
    in rheumatic diseases, 1891
Bone tumors, 2417–2421
    assessment of, 2418, 2419
    benign, 2417
    clinical manifestations of, 2418
    complications of, 2419, 2420
    continuing care for, 2420
    coping with, 2420
    diagnosis of, 2418
    expected outcomes with, 2421
    malignant, 2417
    nursing diagnoses related to, 2419
    nursing interventions for, 2419–2420
    nursing process with, 2419–2421

pathologic fractures with, prevention of,
    2419–2420
pathophysiology of, 2417–2418
patient teaching about, 2419
planning and goals for, 2419
primary, 2417
    medical management of, 2418
secondary, 2417
    medical management of, 2418–2419
self-care with, patient teaching about, 2420,
    2421c
Bony labyrinth, 2094f, 2096
Borborygmus, definition of, 1232
*Borrelia burgdorferi*
    incubation period of, 2476t
    transmission of, 2476t
Bortezomib (Velcade), 422
    for multiple myeloma, 1084
Botulinum toxin (Botox), for achalasia, 1162
Botulism
    as bioterrorism threat, 2567t
    gastrointestinal, 2567t
    inhalation, 2567t
    mortality rate for, 2567t
    treatment of, 2567t
Bougienage, for esophageal spasm, 1162
Bovine spongiform encephalopathy, 2276
Bowel elimination. *See* Elimination
Bowel function
    in hypothyroidism, 1455c–1456c
    in multiple sclerosis, 2280, 2282
    in paraplegia/quadriplegia, 2264
    postoperative, 543
    promotion of, in unconscious patient, 2168
Bowel habits, in bowel disease, 1127
Bowel incontinence. *See* Incontinence
Bowel preparation, preoperative, 496
Bowel sounds, 1129
Bowel training program(s), 217
    for paraplegia/quadriplegia, 2264
Bowen's disease, 1774
    definition of, 1740
Bowman's capsule, 1495, 1495f
Bowman's membrane, 2044, 2045f
BPH. *See* Benign prostatic hyperplasia
BPPV. *See* Benign paroxysmal positional vertigo
Brace(s), 2364
    definition of, 2355
    for humeral fracture, 2442, 2442f
    for paraplegia, 2263
Brachial plexus block, 515
Brachytherapy
    automated high-dose rate intracavitary,
        1695
    for beast cancer, 1726
    for brain tumors, 2305
    for cancer, 395
    for cervical cancer, 1684
    in coronary arteries, 886–887
    definition of, 381, 1661, 1701
Braden scale, 209
Bradycardia, after cardiac surgery, 892t
Bradykinesia
    definition of, 2301
    in Parkinson's disease, 2312, 2313
Bradykinin
    in allergic reaction, 1858t, 1859
    definition of, 1856
    in inflammation, 103
    vascular effects of, 978
Bradypnea, 570, 572t
Brain
    anatomy of, 2130–2133, 2131f, 2132f
    computed tomography of, 2162
    and health, 113–114

oncologic disorders of, 2301–2309
    in stress response, 95–97
    structures protecting, 2133, 2133f
Brain attack, 2206. *See also* Ischemic stroke;
    Stroke
Brain death, 2168–2169, 2238–2239, 2240c
    definition of, 2161
Brain injury(ies), 2235–2250. *See also* Head
    injury(ies)
    and airway maintenance, 2244
    assessment of, 2240, 2240c, 2241f,
        2242t–2243t
    and body temperature, 2244, 2245
    clinical manifestations of, 2236c
    closed, 2235
        definition of, 2233
    complications of, 2241, 2248–2249
    definition of, 2233
    expected outcomes with, 2250
    family of patient with, 2246–2248
    and fluid and electrolyte balance, 2244,
        2249
    home and community-based care for,
        2249–2250, 2250c
    and injury prevention, 2244–2245, 2245f
    management of, 2238–2239, 2239f
    mother-child relationship after, nursing
        research on, 2246
    nursing diagnoses related to, 2126–2127
    nursing interventions for, 2126–2127
    nursing outcomes with, 2126–2127
    and nutrition, 2244
    open, 2236
        definition of, 2233
    planning and goals for, 2241–2243
    self-care after, 2249
    and skin integrity, 2245
    and sleep, 2246
    supportive care for, 2238
    types of, 2236
Brain Injury Association, 2246
Brain mapping, for brain tumors, 2305, 2306f
Brain (B-type) natriuretic peptide, in cardiac
    patient, 806
Brainstem, 2130, 2133
    herniation of, brain injury and, 2248
Brain tumor(s)
    assessment with, 2307
    classification of, 2301, 2302c
    clinical manifestations of, 2303–2304
    continuing care for, 2309
    diagnosis of, 2304–2305
    expected outcomes for, 2309
    gerontologic considerations in, 2303
    home and community-based care for,
        2308–2309, 2309c
    incidence of, 2301
    localization of, 2304, 2305, 2306f
    localized symptoms of, 2304
    medical management of, 2305
    nursing diagnoses related to, 2307
    nursing interventions for, 2308–2309
    nursing management of, 2306
    nursing process with, 2307–2309
    planning and goals for, 2307–2308
    primary, 2301–2306
        epidemiology of, 2301
        incidence of, 2301
        radiation exposure and, 2301
        types of, 2301–2303, 2302c
    secondary (metastatic), 2301, 2306–2309
    self-care and, 2308
    sites of, 2303, 2303f
    surgical management of, 2305
Branch retinal vein occlusion, 2069

# INDEX

BRCA-1 and BRCA-2 genes, 152t
  and breast cancer, 1714
  definition of, 1701
  penetrance of, 146
  population screening for, 153
*BRCA-1* and *BRCA-2* genes, 386, 389
Breakthrough pain, 287
  definition of, 259
Breast(s)
  anatomy of, 1701–1702, 1702f
  areas of, 1702f
  assessment of, 1702–1705
    abnormal findings in, 1704c–1705c
    health history in, 1702
    physical examination in, 1702–1703
    in women with disabilities, 1735
  atypical hyperplasia in, 1711
  benign conditions of, 1710–1712
  biopsy of
    excisional, 1709
    incisional, 1709
    nursing management of, 1709
    percutaneous, 1708–1709
    surgical, 1709
    wire needle localization in, 1709
  cyst of, 1710–1711, 1711t
    clinical manifestations of, 1704c
  development of, Tanner stages of, 1701
  examination of, recommendations for, 1702, 1703c
  fat necrosis in, 1712
  fibroadenoma of, 1711, 1711t
    clinical manifestations of, 1704c
  inspection of, 1702–1703, 1704c–1705c
  male
    diseases of, 1735–1736
    physical assessment of, 1703–1705
  malignant conditions of, 1712–1736
  masses of, clinical manifestations of, 1704c
  pain in, 1710
  palpation of, 1703, 1705f
  peau d'orange in, 1704c
  prosthetic, 1733
  reconstructive surgery for, 1731–1733, 1732f, 1733f
  retraction signs in, 1704c
  superficial thrombophlebitis of, 1712
  tissue analysis, 1708–1709
  venous prominence in, 1704c
Breast cancer, 1712–1736
  chemoprevention of, 1714–1715
  clinical manifestations of, 1704c, 1715
  diagnosis of, 390t, 1715
  early detection of, recommendations for, 1702, 1703c
  epidemiology of, 1712
  familial occurrence of, 386
  genetics of, 152t
  genetic testing and, 1733–1734
  gerontologic considerations in, 1735
  hormonal therapy for, 1729
  infiltrating ductal, 1712
  infiltrating lobular, 1712
  inflammatory, 1712–1713
  invasive, 1712–1713
  long-term surveillance for, 1714
  lymphatic spread of, 1715, 1716f
  male, 1712, 1735–1736
  medullary, 1712
  metastasis, to bone, 2417
  metastatic, 1730–1731
  mucinous, 1712
  pregnancy and, 1734
  prevention of, 388–389, 393
    in high-risk patient, 1714–1715
  prognosis for, 1715–1716, 1716c, 1716t
  protective factors for, 1714
  quality of life after, 1734–1735
  recurrent, 1730–1731
  risk factors for, 1713–1714, 1713c
    genetic, 1714
    nongenetic, 1713–1714
  sentinel node biopsy in, 1717–1718, 1717t
  staging of, 1715, 1716t
  surgery for, 1716–1725
    nursing process with, 1718–1725
    patients and partners in, nursing interventions for, 1720, 1721c, 1722c
    postoperative sensations and, 1719
    sensory morbidity after, nursing research on, 1720
  survivorship, 1734–1735
  targeted therapy for, 1729–1730
  tubular ductal, 1712
  types of, 1712
Breast conservation treatment, 1712
  for breast cancer, 1717
  contraindications to, 1726, 1726c
  definition of, 1701
  for ductal carcinoma in situ, 1712
Breastfeeding, and acquired immunity, 1786
Breast self-examination, 1705–1706, 1707c
Breathing
  in acute pancreatitis, 1360, 1362, 1366c
  allergic rhinitis and, 1874
  assessment of, in acutely ill patient, 576–578
  in burn patient, 2002–2004
  in cardiopulmonary resuscitation, 970, 970f
  deep, preoperative teaching about, 492–493, 494c
  diaphragmatic, 697, 730c, 734
    for low back pain, 2394
    preoperative teaching about, 494c
  in hypothyroidism, 1456c–1457c
  impaired, in HIV-infected (AIDS) patients, 1843c
  improvement of, in chronic obstructive pulmonary disease, 697, 704c–705c
  with increased intracranial pressure, 2175
  patterns of, assessment of, 570, 572t
  pursed-lip, 697, 730c, 734
  in renal surgical patient, 1554, 1555c
  sounds of, at end of life, 469
  spinal cord injury and, 2257
Breathing exercises, 730c, 734
  in chronic obstructive pulmonary disease, 695
  for thoracic surgical patient, 757
    postoperative, 765
Breathing retraining, 734–735
Breath sounds, 574–576, 575t
  adventitious, 574–576, 575t
  in heart failure, 950
  in pneumonia, 636
Breath tests, in gastrointestinal assessment, 1130
Bridging technique, in pressure reduction, 210
Brimonidine, for glaucoma, 2057, 2058t
Broca's area, 2221
Bromide, therapeutic levels (conventional units and SI units), 2601t
Bromocriptine
  for infertility treatment, 1651c
  for Parkinson's disease, 2314
Bronchi, anatomy of, 555f, 556, 556f
Bronchial brushing, 585
Bronchiectasis, 701–709
  assessment in, 709
  causes of, 701
  clinical manifestations of, 709
  definition of, 686, 701
  diagnosis of, 709
  medical management of, 709
  nursing management of, 709
  pathophysiology of, 708–709
Bronchioles
  anatomy of, 556, 556f
  terminal, 556
Bronchitis. *See also* Chronic obstructive pulmonary disease
  assessment findings in, 576t
  chronic, pathophysiology of, 687, 687f
  definition of, 686
Bronchodilator(s)
  administration of, 693t
  for COPD, 692
  for cystic fibrosis, 719
  duration of action of, 693t, 711–713
  for dyspnea, 465
  metered-dose inhaler for, 692, 692f, 713
  types of, 692, 693t
  for ventilator-dependent patient, 749
Bronchodilator reversibility testing, in chronic obstructive pulmonary disease, 689
Bronchogenic carcinoma, pleural effusion with, 653
Bronchophony, 576
Bronchoplastic resection, of lung, 755c
Bronchopleural fistula, 651
  in thoracic surgical patient, 769–770
Bronchopneumonia, 534, 534f, 634, 634f
Bronchoscopy, 581–582, 581f
  complications of, 581
  definition of, 553
  diagnostic, 581
  indications for, 636
  nursing interventions for, 581–582
  therapeutic, 581
Brooke Army formula, for fluid replacement in burn patients, 2007c
Brown-Sequard syndrome, 2251, 2252c
Brown-tan skin, 1935t
Brugada syndrome, 836
Bruit(s)
  with cerebral angioma, 2303
  definition of, 975
Brush biopsy, renal and ureteral, 1510
Bruton's disease, 1803c, 1805–1806, 1806
BSE. *See* Breast self-examination
B symptoms
  in chronic lymphocytic leukemia, 1074
  in Hodgkin's disease, 1074
  in non-Hodgkin's lymphoma, 1082
B-type natriuretic peptide, 948
Bubbling, terminal, 469
Buccal gland, 1147
Buck's extension traction, 2366–2367, 2366f
  for hip fracture, 2447
Budd-Chiari syndrome, 1303
  definition of, 1285
Buerger's disease. *See* Thromboangiitis obliterans
Buffer(s), and acid-base equilibrium, 334–335
Bulbar paralysis
  in Guillain-Barré syndrome, 2289, 2290
  in myasthenia gravis, 2285
Bulbourethral gland, 1741, 1741f
Bulla, 1937c
Bullectomy, in bullous emphysema, 694
Bullous pemphigois, 1972
Bumetanide (Bumex), 954t
  for heart failure, 965
  for hypertension, 1026t
  for hypervolemia, 313
BUN. *See* Blood urea nitrogen

Bundle of His, 784, 824, 824f
Bunion. *See* Hallux valgus
Bunionectomy, 2402
Bunyaviruses, 2511–2512
Bupivacaine (Marcaine, Sensorcaine), 514t
  for postoperative analgesia, in thoracic surgical patient, 766, 767f
Bupropion (Wellbutrin)
  contraindications to, in Parkinson's disease, 2314
  for depression, 240
Bupropion SR (Zyban), for smoking cessation, 691–692, 866
Burn(s), 1994–2037
  acute renal failure in, 1523
  antibacterial agents for, topical, 2017, 2018t
  assessment of, in emergent/resuscitative phase, 2004
  and blood volume, 1999
  cardiovascular response to, 1999
  as cause of death, by age group, 1996, 1996c
  causes of, 1995
  chemical, 2543–2544
    of esophagus, 1165
  classification of, 1997–1998, 1997t
  complications of, 2030
  continuing care for, 2034–2036
  deep partial-thickness, 1997, 1997t
  depth of, 1997, 1997t
    characteristics of, 1997t
  and distributive shock, 1999, 2013c–2014c
  and edema, 1999
  electrical, 1998–1999
    complications of, 2030
  extent of, classification of, 2005c
  extent of body surface area injured by, 1997–1998
    Lund and Browder method for, 1998
    palm method for, 1998
    rule of nines for, 1997, 1998f
  and fluid and electrolyte balance, 1999–2001, 2005–2007, 2006t, 2027
  full-thickness, 1997, 1997t
  and gastrointestinal system, 2002, 2004
  gerontologic considerations in, 1996
  hemodynamic instability after, 1999
  and immune system function, 1796, 2002
  incidence of, 1995
  and infections, 2002, 2027–2028
  local and systemic responses to, 1999–2002, 2000f
  major, 2005c
  minor, 2005c
  and mobility, 2028–2029
  moderate uncomplicated, 2005c
  mortality rate for, 1995
    in older adults, 1996
  and neurologic conditions, nursing research on, 2009
  ocular, 2075
  pain management for, 2024–2025, 2028
  partial-thickness
    deep, 1997, 1997t
    superficial, 1997, 1997t
  pathophysiology of, 1999–2002, 2000f
  physiologic responses to, 1999–2002, 2000f
  prevention of, 1995, 1996c
    in older adults, 1996
  pulmonary response to, 2001–2002
  recovery after, 1996–1997
  risk factors for, 1995
  superficial partial-thickness, 1997, 1997t
  survival after, 1996–1997
  wound breakdown in, 2032t
  zones of injury in, 1998f

Burn care
  acute/intermediate phase of, 2003t, 2009–2031
    assessment in, 2026–2027
    complications of, 2027
    expected outcomes in, 2030–2031
    gerontologic considerations in, 2027
    nursing diagnoses related to, 2027
    nursing interventions in, 2027–2030
    nursing process with, 2026–2030
    planning and goals in, 2027
  débridement in. *See* Débridement
  emergent/resuscitative phase of, 2002–2003, 2003t
    medical management in, 2004–2007
    nursing care plan for, 2010c–2015c
  ethical considerations in, 2008c
  gerontologic considerations in, 2008–2009, 2019
  home and community-based care for, 2034–2036, 2035c–2036c
  nutritional support in, 2025–2026
  on-the-scene care, 2002–2003, 2003c
  pain management in. *See* Pain management
  phases of, 2003t
  rehabilitation phase of, 192, 2003t, 2031–2037
    assessment in, 2033
    complications of, 2031, 2032t
    nursing diagnoses related to, 2033
    nursing interventions in, 2033–2034
    nursing process with, 2033–2037
    planning and goals in, 2033
  wound cleaning in, 2016
  wound dressings for. *See* Dressing(s)
Burn center, transfer to, 2005
Burn pain, 261c
Burn shock, 1999, 2013c–2014c
Burr holes, in neurosurgery, 2180, 2182f
Bursa, 2341
  definition of, 2337
  neoplasms of, 1920
Bursitis, 1920, 2397
  definition of, 2392
  infections and, 1919–1920
Busulfan
  adverse effects and side effects of, 402
  in cancer treatment, 399t
    adverse effects and side effects of, 399t
  for chronic myeloid leukemia, 1073
Butorphanol, transmucosal, 287

## C

Cachexia
  in cancer patient, nursing interventions for, 428
  in HIV-infected (AIDS) patients, 1849
  in terminal illness, 465–466
CAD. *See* Coronary artery disease
Café-au-lait spot, 1929t, 1935t, 1978
CAGE Questionnaire, 70, 120
CAGE Questions Adapted to Include Drugs (CAGEAID), 70, 70c, 120
Calcification
  of cartilage, in fracture healing, 2340
  metastatic, in chronic renal failure, 1537c
Calcijex, for hyperphosphatemia, 333
Calcipotriene (Dovonex), for psoriasis, 1966, 1967
Calcitonin, 1449
  administration of, patient teaching about, 2410
  and bone health, 2339
  and calcium balance, 328

  definition of, 1440
  for osteoporosis, 2409
  for Paget's disease, 2412
Calcitriol (Rocaltrol). *See also* Vitamin D
  for hyperphosphatemia, 333
Calcium
  in acute renal failure, 1524
  in body fluids, 302t
  and bone health, 2339
  and bone strength, 2339
  in chronic glomerulonephritis, 1519
  deficiency, and osteomalacia, 2411
  deficit, 316t, 325–327
    manifestations of, 1516t
    in renal disorders, 1516t
  dietary sources of, 327
  excess, 317t, 327–328
    manifestations of, 1516t
    in renal disorders, 1516t
  homeostasis, control of, 2339
  imbalances of
    in chronic renal failure, 1529
    in renal disorders, 1516t
  intake, for Paget's disease, 2412
  intravenous, for hypocalcemia, 327
  ionized, laboratory values for, 310t
  and ischemic stroke, 2207
  in malignant hyperthermia, 517
  in muscle contraction, 2341
  recommended intake of, 2406
  serum
    calculation of, 326
    in cardiac patient, 807t
    in hypercalcemia, 317t, 328
    in hypocalcemia, 316t
    ionized, 325, 326
    laboratory values for, 310t
    reference range for, 325
    serum albumin and, 326
    significance of, 325
  supplementation, for osteoporosis, 2408
Calcium acetate (PhosLo), for chronic renal failure, 1529–1530
Calcium alginate dressings, 1948
Calcium binders, for chronic renal failure, 1529–1530
Calcium carbonate (Os-Cal), for chronic renal failure, 1529–1530
Calcium-channel blockers, 830t
  for angina, 870
  for atrial fibrillation, 833
  for cerebral vasospasm, 2226
  for heart failure, 955
  for hypertension, 1029t
  mechanism of action of, 785
  in migraine prevention, 2200
  for scleroderma, 1912
Calcium chloride, 324, 327
Calcium gluconate, 327
  for hyperkalemia, 324
  for hypermagnesemia, 331
Calcivirus, and diarrheal disease, 2501–2502
Calculi. *See* Stones (calculi)
Calendar method, of family planning, 1646
Callus
  definition of, 2337
  of foot, 2401
  in fracture healing, 2340
Calories
  dietary distribution of, in diabetes, 1385–1386
  requirements for, in diabetes, 1385
*Campylobacter*
  and diarrheal diseases, 2501
  incubation period of, 2476t
  transmission of, 2476t

**INDEX**

*Campylobacter jejuni,* and Guillain-Barré syndrome, 2288
Canaliculi
  bile, 1286
  in bones, 2339
Canavan disease
  carrier testing for, 150t, 156
  genetics of, 147t
  genetic testing in, 149, 150t
Cancellous (trabecular) bone, 2338–2339, 2340
  definition of, 2337
Cancer. *See also* Oncology nursing; *specific neoplasm*
  advanced, management of, 437
  angiogenesis in, 385
  assessment in, 423–426
  bacteria and, 385–386
  bladder. *See* Bladder cancer
  bone. *See* Bone tumors
  bone marrow transplantation for, 402–417
  brachytherapy for, 395
  of breast. *See* Breast cancer
  cardiac tamponade in, 439t–440t
  cervical. *See* Cervical cancer; Pap smear
  chemicals and, 386
  chemotherapy for, 397–402
  collaborative problems in, 426
  colorectal. *See* Colorectal cancer
  continuing care in, 434
  definition of, 381
  and depression, 468
  detection of, 390t, 391t
  diagnosis of, 389–391, 390t, 391t
  diet and, 386
  disseminated intravascular coagulation in, 440t–441t
  drugs for, unproven and unconventional, 423
  endometrial, 1685, 1685c
  epidemiology of, 381–383
  of esophagus, 1166–1169
  etiology of, 385–387
  expected outcomes in, 435
  of fallopian tubes, 1689
  familial predispositions to, 386
  and febrile neutropenia, emergency department management of, nursing research on, 1070
  female reproductive, 1682–1683
  gene therapy for, 422
  genetics of, 384, 386, 387
  of gums, 1148–1149
  gynecologic, 1682–1683
    radiation therapy for, 395
  of head and neck, 1153–1161
  hematogenous spread of, 385
  in HIV-infected (AIDS) patients, 1832–1833
  hormonal agents and, 386–387
  hypercalcemia in, 327–328, 438t
  hypercoagulable state caused by, 1099–1100, 1099t
  hyperthermia (thermal therapy) for, 417–418
  and immune system, 1796
  immune system in, 387–388
  incidence of, by site and sex, 381, 382f
  infectious disease-related, prevention of, 2500c
  laryngeal, 608–614
  of lips, 1148–1149
  of liver, 1333–1336
  of lung. *See* Lung cancer
  lymphatic spread of, 385
  management of, 391–423

  metabolic and dietary regimens for, unproven and unconventional, 423
  metastasis of, 384–385
    mechanisms of, 385
  monoclonal antibody therapy for, 418, 419t
  mortality rate for
    racial differences in, 381–383
    by site and sex, 381, 382f
  mystical and spiritual therapies for, unproven and unconventional, 423
  neutropenia in, and prevention of infection, nursing research on, 1809
  nursing care plan for, 403–415
  nursing diagnoses related to, 426
  nursing interventions for, 426–434
  nursing process with, 423–434
  of oral cavity, 1148–1149
  ovarian. *See* Ovarian cancer
  pain in. *See* Pain, cancer-related
  pain management in, 411c–412c, 429–430, 437, 464–465
  pancreatic, 1369–1370
  pathophysiology of, 383–388
  patient with, nursing care plan for, 403c–415c
  penile. *See* Penile cancer
  pericardial effusion in, 439t–440t
  photodynamic therapy for, 422
  physical agents and, 386
  potential complications in, 426
  prevention of
    patient teaching about, 389c
    primary, 388
    secondary, 388–389, 389c, 390t
  prostate. *See* Prostate cancer
  radiation therapy for, 394–397
    caregivers in, protection of, 395, 397
    dosage of, 395
    external, 395
    internal, 395
    nursing management in, 396–397
    oral mucosa in, 395–397
    palliative, 394
    radiosensitizers for, 394–395
    skin protection in, 396–397
    toxicity of, 395–396
  retinoid therapy for, 420
  risk factors for, 389c
  screening for, 388–389
  self-care in, patient teaching about, 434
  skin. *See* Skin cancer
  spinal cord compression in, 438t–439t
  superior vena cava syndrome in, 438t
  surgery for, 391–394
    diagnostic, 391–392
    nursing management in, 393–394
    palliative, 393, 394c
    as primary treatment, 392–393
    prophylactic, 393
    reconstructive, 393
    salvage, 393
  syndrome of inappropriate antidiuretic hormone secretion in, 441t
  testicular. *See* Testicular cancer
  tissue invasion by, 384–385
  of tongue, 1148–1149
  treatment of
    in advanced disease, 437
    age-related concerns in, 436–437, 436t
    complications of, nursing interventions for, 431–433
    emergencies in, 438t–442t
    gerontologic considerations in, 436–437, 436t
    hospice in, 437

    machines and devices for, unproven and unconventional, 423
    mystical and spiritual approaches for, 423
    nursing interventions in, 426–434–364
    patients' need for information about, nursing research on, 396
    planning and goals in, 426
    tumor lysis syndrome in, 442t
    unproven and unconventional therapy for, 422–423
  of urinary tract, 1563–1565
  uterine. *See* Uterine cancer
  vaccines against, 420
  vaginal. *See* Vaginal cancer
  viruses and, 385–386
  vulvar. *See* Vulvar cancer
Cancer nursing. *See* Oncology nursing
Cancer rehabilitation, 434–436
  assessment for, 434, 434c
  exercise in, nursing research on, 435
Cancer-related check-ups, 390t
Candesartan (Atacand), for hypertension, 1029t
*Candida albicans,* encephalitis caused by, 2275–2276
Candidiasis
  chronic mucocutaneous. *See* Chronic mucocutaneous candidiasis
  definition of, 1661, 1815
  in HIV-infected (AIDS) patients, 1672
    treatment of, 1836
  oral, 1143t
    in HIV-infected (AIDS) patients, 1832
  vulvovaginal, 1626, 1626t, 1662, 1663t
Cane
  ambulation with, 205–207
  for stroke patient, 2218
Canine companion programs, 219
Canine teeth, 1150f
Canker sore, 1143t
Cannabinoids, abuse/overdose, emergency management of, 2546t–2547t
Cannon, Walter, 92
Cannula, nasal, for oxygen administration, 725t, 726
Cantor tube, 1176, 1176t
CAPD. *See* Continuous ambulatory peritoneal dialysis
Capecitabine (Xeloda), in cancer treatment, 399t
Capillariasis, malabsorption in, 1240t
Capillary(ies), 975, 976f
  anatomy of, 976
Capillary filtration, 977–978
Capillary refill time, assessment of, 804
Capnography, 360
Capreomycin, for tuberculosis, 647
Capsaicin (Zostrix)
  for osteoarthritis, 1916
  for rheumatic diseases, 1896t
Captopril (Capoten), 952–953, 952t
  for hypertension, 1029t
  for hypertensive crises, 1033
Capture, in pacemaker therapy, 846
Caput medusae, 1319
Carbachol, for glaucoma, 2057, 2058t
Carbamates, as terrorism threat, 2570–2571
Carbamazepine (Tegretol)
  adverse effects and side effects of, 2194t, 2295
  therapeutic blood levels of, 2601t
  toxic effects of, 2194t
  for trigeminal neuralgia, 2295
Carbidopa (Sinemet), for Parkinson's disease, 2314

Carbohydrate(s)
　absorption of, evaluation of, 1130
　in acute renal failure, 1526
　for burn patient, 2025
　dietary, in diabetes, 1385–1386
　digestion of, 1125
　　enzymes for, 1123t
　metabolism of, endocrine control of, 1346–1347
　in wound healing, 487t
Carbon dioxide ($CO_2$)
　and acid-base equilibrium, 334–335
　in blood, laboratory values for, 310t
　sublingual monitoring of, 360
　transport of, 561–562
Carbon dioxide laser, for skin lesions, 1991–1992
Carbonic acid
　and acid-base equilibrium, 334–335
　deficit, 337–338
　excess, 336–337
Carbonic anhydrase inhibitors
　for glaucoma, 2057, 2058t
　for metabolic alkalosis, 336
Carbon monoxide poisoning, 2541–2543
　blood levels in, 2601t
　and skin color, 1935t
Carboplatin
　in cancer treatment, 399t
　for ovarian cancer, 1691
Carboxyhemoglobin, 2001, 2541
　definition of, 1995, 2517
Carbuncles, 1957–1958
　definition of, 1945
Carcinogen(s), 385, 388
Carcinogenesis, 385
　definition of, 381
　immune system failure and, 388
　initiation of, 385
　progression of, 385
　promotion of, 385
Cardiac arrest, 969–972
　clinical manifestations of, 969–970
　emergency management of, 970–972
Cardiac catheterization
　applications of, 813
　definition of, 781
　hemostasis after, 814
　left heart, 814–815
　nursing interventions in, 815
　nursing responsibilities after, 815
　nursing responsibilities before, 815
　patient teaching about, 815c
　procedure for, 813–814
　with pulmonary hypertension, 660
　right heart, 814
　self-care after, patient teaching about, 815c
Cardiac conduction surgery, 854–855
Cardiac conduction system, 783–785
　abnormalities in, ECG findings in, 838–840
　age-related changes in, 788t
　automaticity in, 783, 823, 854
　conductivity in, 783
　definition of, 781
　excitability in, 783
　normal, 824–825, 824f
　physiology of, 783–784
Cardiac cycle, 786, 824–825
Cardiac dysrhythmia(s). See Dysrhythmia(s), cardiac
Cardiac enzyme analysis, 805
Cardiac failure. See Heart failure
Cardiac function, definition of, 46c
Cardiac hemodynamics, 945–946

　assessment of
　　invasive, 946
　　noninvasive, 946
Cardiac muscle, 783
Cardiac output, 786, 945
　assessment of, 798
　after cardiac surgery, 891t, 898, 900, 904c–905c
　in cardiomyopathy, 931–932
　and cerebral perfusion, 2173
　definition of, 781, 945, 1021
　factors affecting, 798
　in myocardial infarction, 882c
　and oxygen transport, 561
　postoperative, 536–537
Cardiac rehabilitation, 192, 877–879
　phases of, 878–879
Cardiac resynchronization therapy
　definition of, 945
　in heart failure, 957
Cardiac sphincter, 1121, 1162
Cardiac status, after cardiac surgery, 897
Cardiac stress test(ing), 810–811
　definition of, 781
　exercise, 810
　mental, 810
　nursing interventions in, 810–811
　pharmacologic, 810–811
Cardiac tamponade, 670, 941, 968–969, 969c
　in cancer patient, 439t–440t
　in cardiac surgical patient, 891t
　in trauma patient, 675
Cardiogenic shock, 965–968, 966f
　hemodynamic monitoring in, 369
　laboratory monitoring in, 369
　pharmacologic therapy for, 369–370
　vasoactive agents for, 369–370
Cardiomyopathy(ies), 925–933, 948
　arrhythmogenic right ventricular, 925, 927
　clinical manifestations of, 927
　congestive. See Cardiomyopathy(ies), dilated
　definition of, 915
　diagnosis of, 927
　dilated, 925–926, 926f
　hemochromatosis and, 1063
　hypertrophic, 925, 926, 926f
　ischemic, 925
　medical management of, 927–930
　nursing process with, 930–933
　pathophysiology of, 925–927, 926f
　restrictive/constrictive, 925, 926–927, 926f
　surgical management of, 928–930
　unclassified, 925, 927
Cardiopulmonary bypass, 888–890, 889f, 920–921
　in cardiogenic shock, 371
Cardiopulmonary resuscitation, 970–972
　for asystole, 838
　family presence during, nursing research on, 971
　medications used in, 971, 972t
　for ventricular fibrillation, 837
Cardiopulmonary system, chemotherapy and, 402
Cardiovascular disease, 152t
　chest radiography in, 808
　clinical manifestations of, 790–792
　diagnostic evaluation in, 805–816
　elimination in, assessment of, 796
　in end-stage renal disease, 1527, 1536c–1537c
　fluoroscopy in, 808
　genetics of, 789
　health history in, 788–790

　　health perception and management in, assessment of, 792–793, 793t–794t
　　hemodialysis and, 1547–1548, 1551
　　hypertension and, risk factors for, 1022, 1023c
　　laboratory testing in, 805–808
　　nutrition in, assessment of, 795–796
　　prevention of, 798
　　risk factors for, 796c, 798
Cardiovascular system
　age-related changes in, 230–232, 231t, 787, 788t, 805
　assessment of, 787–805
　　preoperative, 487–488
　brain injury and, 2242t–2243t
　in burn victim, 1999
　chronic renal failure and, 1527, 1528c, 1536c–1537c
　function, assessment of, 780–820
　immune dysfunction and, 1794c
　management of, in postanesthesia care, 526–528
　perimenopausal considerations in, 1635
Cardioversion
　for atrial flutter, 832
　definition of, 823
　electrical, 843–844
　　for atrioventricular (AV) nodal reentry tachycardia, 83
　for ventricular tachycardia, 836
Care/cure dichotomy, 449
Caregivers
　adult children as, 230
　coping with death and dying, 473–474
　of dementia/Alzheimer's disease patients, 246
　of stroke patient, 2223
Care mapping, 9
Caring, as foundation of nursing, 29
Carmustine
　for cerebral metastases, 2307
　in cancer treatment, 399t
　pulmonary toxicity of, 402
Carotenemia, and skin color, 1935t
Carotid artery(ies), internal, 2134
Carotid blood flow, noninvasive studies of, 2155
Carotid endarterectomy
　complications of, nursing interventions for, 2215, 2215t
　for ischemic stroke, 2214, 2214f
　nursing management of, 2214–2215, 2215t
Carotid sinus massage, 835, 835f
Carotid stenting, 2214
Carpal tunnel syndrome, 2398
Carrier(s)
　definition of, 2475
　of gene mutations, 146
　　definition of, 140
　　testing for, 149, 150t
Cartilage
　age-related changes in, 2344t
　articular, 2338, 2338f
　　degeneration of, 1888
　definition of, 2337
　in fracture healing, 2340
　hyaline, 2341
　malignant tumors of, 2417
Carvedilol (Coreg), 953
　for hypertension, 1028t
Case management, 9, 10, 2602
Case manager(s), nurses as, 12
Cast(s), 2355–2363
　application of, 2358c
　arm, 2355
　　care of patient with, 2362

# INDEX

bivalving of, 2359, 2359c
body, 2355
    care of patient with, 2363
complications of, 2359–2360
continuing care for, 2360–2362
definition of, 2355
and disuse syndrome, 2360
expected outcomes with, 2362
fiberglass, 2355–2356
gauntlet, 2355
hip spica, 2355
home and community-based care for, 2360–2362, 2361c
leg, 2355
    care of patient with, 2362–2363
long-arm, 2355
    pressure areas in, 2356f
long-leg, 2355
    pressure areas in, 2356f
materials for, 2355–2356
and mobility, 2357
nonplaster, 2355–2356
pain management with, 2357
patients in
    assessment of, 2356
    complications of, 2357
    nursing diagnoses related to, 2356
    nursing interventions for, 2357–2362
    nursing process for, 2356–2362
    planning and goals for, 2357
patient teaching about, 2357
plaster, 2356
pressure areas in, 2356f
removal of, 2360–2362, 2361c
short-arm, 2355
short-leg, 2355
shoulder spica, 2355
and skin care, 2357
spica, care of patient with, 2363
thumb spica, 2355
types of, 2355
walking, 2355
Cast syndrome, 2363
    definition of, 2355
Cataracts, 2051t, 2059–2063, 2059f
    clinical manifestations of, 2060
    in diabetes, 1423t
    diagnosis of, 2060
    extracapsular extraction of, 2061
    intracapsular extraction of, 2061
    medical management of, 2061–2063
    nursing management of, 2063
    pathophysiology of, 2060
    phacoemulsification for, 2061
    risk factors for, 2060, 2060c
    surgical management of, 2061–2063
        complications of, 2061, 2062t
Catastrophic reactions, 245
Catecholamines. *See also* Epinephrine; Norepinephrine
    definition of, 91
    in stress response, 94, 95
Catechol-*O*-methyltransferase inhibitors, for Parkinson's disease, 2314
Catheter(ization)
    external, for urinary incontinence, 216
    implanted device for, 398, 401f
    indwelling, for urinary incontinence, 216
    intermittent self-, for urinary incontinence, 216
    intraotologic, 2113
    pleural, 654
    right atrial, 301f, 398, 401f
    site of, caring for, in hospitalized dialysis patient, 1552
    urinary
        in burn victim, 2004, 2007–2008
        indwelling, 1585
            infections and, 1586
        infections with
            manifestations of, 1586, 1587f
            pathophysiology of, 1586, 1587f
            prevention of, 1586, 1588c
        nursing research on, 1576
        obstructed, after prostatectomy, 1767, 1767f
        paraplegia/quadriplegia and, 2263–2264
        postoperative, 543
        prostatectomy and, 1767, 1767f
        removal of, after prostatectomy, 1767
        suprapubic, 1584, 1585–1586, 1586f
        trauma in, minimizing, 1586–1588
        UTI prevention with, 1575
    vascular
        in burn victim, 2007–2008, 2015
        clotted, in parenteral nutrition, 1197t
        displacement of, in parenteral nutrition, 1197t
        double-lumen, 1194–1195
        for hemodialysis, 1539, 1539f
        nontunnelled, 1194–1195
        peripherally inserted (PICC), 429, 429f, 1175, 1195–1196
        single-lumen, 1194–1195
        triple-lumen, 1194–1195
        tunnelled, 1194–1195
    venous. *See* Venipuncture
Catheter ablation therapy, for cardiac dysrhythmias, 854–855
Catheter embolism, 348–349
Cations, 302
Cauda equina, 2135
Causalgia, 261c
Causative organism, of infection, 2475, 2476t–2477t
CAVH. *See* Continuous arteriovenous hemofiltration
CAVHD. *See* Continuous arteriovenous hemodialysis
CBC. *See* Complete blood count
CC-5013, for multiple myeloma, 1084
CCPD. *See* Continuous cyclic peritoneal dialysis
CCR5
    definition of, 1815
    and HIV-1, 1823
CD52 antigen, in chronic lymphocytic leukemia, 1074
CDC. *See* Centers for Disease Control and Prevention
CD4/CD8 ratio, for HIV diagnosis, 1825t
CD4 cell count
    in HIV-infected (AIDS) patients, 1823t, 1824
    and skin disorders, 1941
CD4 cells, and HIV, 1821–1823
Cecal reservoir, for urinary diversion, 1603
Cecum, 1121, 1122f
Cefamandole (Mandol), for pneumonia, 637
Cefixime (Suprax), for gonorrhea, 2508
Cefotaxime (Claforan), for pneumonia, 637
Cefpodoxime (Vantin)
    for pneumonia, 636
    for sinusitis, 596
Cefprozil (Cefzil), for sinusitis, 595
Ceftriaxone
    for gonorrhea, 2508
    and immune system, 1797t
    for pneumonia, 637
Cefuroxime
    and immune system, 1797t
    for pneumonia, 636–637
Cefuroxime axetil, for sinusitis, 595, 596
Celecoxib
    in pain management, 284
    for rheumatic diseases, 1895t
Celiac axis arteriography, 1290t
    in biliary/pancreatic disease, 1349t
Celiac disease, malabsorption in, 1240t
Celiac plexus, 2139, 2140f
Cell(s)
    adaptation to stressors, 100, 100t
    in continuum of function and structure, 99, 99f
    division of, 142–143
    energy metabolism in, 357
    growth of, patterns of, 100, 100t
    healing of
        by regeneration, 104
        by replacement, 104
    in inflammation, 104
    injury to, 101–103
    labile, 104
    malignant, characteristics of, 384, 384t
    permanent, 104
    proliferation of, patterns of, 383
    regeneration of, 104
    response to infection, 2479, 2479f
    response to injury, 104
    shock and, 357
    stable, 104
Cell cycle, 397, 397f
    chemotherapy and, 397, 397f
Cell kill, chemotherapy and, 397, 397f
Cellular hypersensitivity. *See* Delayed-type hypersensitivity
Cellular immune response, 1787, 1788c, 1790–1792, 1792t
    assessment of, tests for, 1799t
    definition of, 1783
    natural killer cells in, 1792, 1792t
    null lymphocytes in, 1792, 1792t
    T cells in, 1790–1792, 1792t
Cellular immunity, 1042
Cellular layer, of skin, 1928f
Cellulitis, 1017
Center(s), neurologic, 2129, 2132
Centers for Disease Control and Prevention
    definition of, 2475
    guidelines and summaries published by, 2480
    and infection control and prevention, 2480
    Internet site of, 2480
Centers for Medicare and Medicaid Services, standards on use of restraints, 31
Central alpha agonists, for hypertension, 1027t
Central cord syndrome, 2251, 2252c
Central incisor(s), 1150f
Central nervous system, 2130–2136, 2161. *See also* Brain; Cranial nerve(s)
Central retinal artery occlusion, 2069
Central retinal vein occlusion, 2068–2069
Central venous access device(s). *See also* Catheter(ization), vascular
    definition of, 1175
    dressing changes for, 1198
    types of, 1194–1195
Central venous pressure monitoring, 816–818
    nursing interventions in, 818
Cephalosporins, for urinary tract infections, 1574
Cerebellar signs, 2142
Cerebellum, 2130, 2131f, 2133, 2142
Cerebral aneurysm. *See* Aneurysm, intracranial

Cerebral angiography, 2154, 2181
  in head injuries, 2235
Cerebral blood flow, decreased
  hemorrhagic stroke and, 2225–2226
  increased intracranial pressure and, 2169–2170
Cerebral circulation, 2134–2135, 2135f
  impaired, after cardiac surgery, 899
Cerebral cortex, 2131, 2131f
  functional topography of, 2132–2133, 2132f
Cerebral dominance, 2131–2132
Cerebral edema
  brain injury and, 2248
  decreasing, 2173
  definition of, 2170
  in diabetes mellitus, 1418
  with increased intracranial pressure, 2170
  interventions for, 2178t
  in neurosurgical patient
    management of, 2182
    nursing interventions for, 2184c–2185c
Cerebral function, assessment of, 2145–2146
Cerebral perfusion
  hemorrhagic stroke and, 2227–2228
  with increased intracranial pressure, 2175–2178
  maintenance of, in neurosurgical patient, 2183–2186
  in neurosurgical patient, nursing interventions for, 2183–2186
Cerebral perfusion pressure, 2170
  decreased, brain injury and, 2248
  maintaining, 2173
Cerebrospinal fluid, 2133–2134
  analysis, in herpes simplex virus encephalitis, 2274
  analysis of, 2156–2158
    with brain tumor, 2305
  composition of, 2133–2134
  drainage, in increased intracranial pressure, 2173–2174
  leakage of
    with basilar skull fracture, 2234, 2234f
    head injury and, 2234, 2234f, 2235
    nasal, 607
    in neurosurgical patient, nursing interventions for, 2185c
  production of, 2133
  reference ranges for, 2600t
Cerebrovascular accident, 2134. See also Ischemic stroke
Cerebrovascular disease, 2205–2230
  definition of, 2206
  in diabetes, 1421–1422
  signs and symptoms of, 790
Cerebrum, 2130–2133, 2131f, 2132f
Cerebyx. See Fosphenytoin
Certified registered nurse anesthetist, 505
Cerumen, 2093
  definition of, 2095c
  impaction of, 2104
Ceruminous glands, 1930
Cervical cancer, 1625, 1682–1685
  detection of, 390t
  epidemiology of, 1682
  in HIV-infected (AIDS) patients, 1835
  invasive, 1684–1685
  precursor lesion, 1684
  preinvasive, 1684
  prevention of, 420
  risk factors for, 1682, 1683c
  surgery for, 1684–1685, 1684c
Cervical cap, 1645
Cervical collar, 2253, 2254f, 2326, 2328c

Cervical discectomy, nursing process with, 2326–2329
Cervical spine
  fractures of, management of, 2254
  immobilization, for spinal cord injury, 2251
  injury to, assessment of, 2349
Cervicitis, 1663t, 1669–1670
Cervix, uterine, 1614, 1615f
  biopsy of, 1628–1629
  cancer of. See Cervical cancer; Pap smear
  definition of, 1613
  inspection of, 1625
  palpation of, 1626
Cetirizine (Zyrtec), 1871t
  for sinusitis, 595
Cetuximab (Erbitux), 419t
  adverse effects and side effects of, 421t
C fibers, in pain transmission, 264–265
CGMS. See Continuous glucose monitoring system
Chadwick's sign, 1625
Chalazion, 2076t
Chancre, 1672
  definition of, 1661
  on lips, 1143t
Chancroid, causative organism of, 2476t
Chandelier sign, 1626
  definition of, 1613
Charcot-Marie-Tooth disease, and pes cavus, 2402
Charleston pouch, 1602
  definition of, 1570
Charting, 35. See also Documentation
Cheilitis
  actinic, 1143t
  definition of, 1945
Chelation therapy, for iron excess, 1055
Chemical(s)
  burns caused by, 2543–2544
    esophageal, 1165
  as carcinogens, 386
  characteristics of, 2569–2570
  exposure to, limiting, 2570
  latency of, 2570
  persistence of, 2569
  toxicity of, 2569–2570
  vesicant, 2569t, 2570
  volatility of, 2569
Chemical barriers, in natural immunity, 1786
Chemical burns, emergency management of, 2003c
Chemical face peeling, 1988
Chemical mediators, in allergic reaction, 1857–1859, 1858f, 1858t
  primary mediators, 1858, 1858t
  secondary mediators, 1857, 1858t
Chemical warfare
  agents used in, 2569, 2569t
  definition of, 2559, 2569
Chemolysis, for urolithiasis, 1593
Chemoreceptors, 562
  in blood pressure regulation, 358
Chemoreceptor trigger zone, 398
Chemosis, 2074
  definition of, 2043
Chemosurgery, for cancer, 393
Chemotaxis, complement system and, 1793t
Chemotherapy, 397–402
  for acute lymphocytic leukemia, 1073–1074
  for acute myeloid leukemia, 1071–1072
  administration of, 398–402
    home care checklist for, 400c
    nursing management of, 402, 416c
    safety in, 398, 402, 416c

agents for. See also Antineoplastic agents
  administration of, 398–402
  classification of, 397–398
  dosage of, 398
  extravasation of, 398
  investigational, 398, 400c
  toxicity of, 398–402
for bladder cancer, 1597
bleeding risk in, nursing management of, 402, 414c–415c
for bone tumors, 2418
for breast cancer, 1726–1729
caregivers in, protection of, 402
for cerebral metastases, 2307
for chronic lymphocytic leukemia, 1074–1075
for chronic myeloid leukemia, 1073
definition of, 381
fluid and electrolyte status in
  assessment of, 402
  nursing management of, 402
for gastric cancer, 1221
gerontologic considerations in, 436–437, 436t
and hair, 1930
for HIV/AIDS-related neoplasia, 1836
for Hodgkin's disease, 1081, 1081c
hypercoagulable state caused by, 1099t
for idiopathic thrombocytopenic purpura, 1088
and immune system function, 1796
infection risk in, 402
  nursing management of, 402, 403c–404c
for Kaposi's sarcoma, 1836
for liver cancer, 1334
for lung cancer, 672–673
for melanoma, 1982
for multiple myeloma, 1083–1084
for non-Hodgkin's lymphoma, 1082
for ovarian cancer, 1691
for prostate cancer, 1760–1761
for thrombocythemia, 1086
thrombocytopenia caused by, 1087t
toxicity of, 398–402
  gastrointestinal, 398–400
  neurologic, 402
Chenodeoxycholic acid, for gallstones, 1351
Cherry angioma, 1939c
Chest. See also Thorax
  barrel, 569–570, 688, 689, 689f
  configuration of, 569–570
  funnel, 570
  pigeon, 570
  trauma to, 675–681
    blunt, 675–678
    penetrating, 675, 678–682
  tumors of, 670–675
Chest compressions, in cardiopulmonary resuscitation, 970–971, 971f
Chest cuirass, 742
Chest drainage, postoperative, for thoracic surgical patient, 758–764, 758t, 759c–761c
Chest drainage system(s), 758–764, 758t, 759c–761c
  definition of, 723
  dry suction, 762, 763
  dry suction water seal, 758t
  dry suction with one-way valve, 758t, 763–764, 764f
  management of, 758–764, 759c–761c
  water seal, 758t, 762, 763
Chest pain. See also Angina pectoris
  assessment of, 790–792, 791t–792t
  cardiac, 860

# INDEX

in cardiovascular disease, assessment of, 793t
clinical significance of, 567
with esophageal spasm, 1162
in lung cancer, 671
pleuritic, 567
with pulmonary embolism, 662
management of, 666
relief measures for, 567–568
in respiratory disease, 567–568
Chest percussion, 731–734, 733c, 801–802
definition of, 723
Chest physiotherapy, 731–735
activities of, 42c
in bronchiectasis, 709
in chronic obstructive pulmonary disease, 697
for cor pulmonale, 661
definition of, 42c, 723
at home, patient teaching about, 734–735
in pneumonia, 640
in thoracic surgery patient, 765–766
Chest tube(s). See also Chest drainage system(s)
large-bore, 761–762
placement of, 761
for pneumothorax, 679–680
removal of, pain control for, nursing research on, 768
small-bore, 761
for trauma patient, 678
Chest wall
dysfunction of, and acute respiratory failure, 655–656
in emphysema, 689, 689f, 690f
normal characteristics of, 689, 689f
resection, 672c
Chest x-ray
in cardiovascular disease, 808
with pulmonary embolism, 663
in respiratory disease, 580
Chewing, 1123
Cheyne-Stokes respiration, 570, 572t
in cardiac patient, 804
CHF. See Congestive heart failure
Chickenpox
causative organism of, 2476t
vaccine against, 2488
Chief complaint, in health history, 66
Child(ren)
and burns, 1995, 1996
functional ability of, assessment of, 193
health promotion for, 58–59
leading health problems of, 21
school health programs for, 21–22
Child abuse, mandatory reporting of, 2551
Childbearing, by Black women with and without HIV infection, nursing research on, 1819
Child-Pugh classification, of severity of liver disease, 1318, 1318t
Chiropractic, 134
Chlamydia, 1669–1670
in HIV-infected (AIDS) patients, 1672
*Chlamydia inguinale*
incubation period of, 2476t
transmission of, 2476t
*Chlamydia pneumoniae* pneumonia, 631t
*Chlamydia trachomatis*, 2507–2508
infection, 2507–2508
assessment in, 2507
clinical manifestations of, 2507
co-infection in gonorrhea, 2507–2508
complications of, 2507
diagnosis of, 2507

medical management of, 2507–2508
nursing management of, 2508
patient teaching about, 2508
prevention of, 2508
Chlorambucil
in cancer treatment, 399t
for chronic lymphocytic leukemia, 1074
Chloramphenicol (Chloromycetin), and immune system, 1797t
Chlordiazepoxide
abuse/overdose, emergency management of, 2547t
therapeutic blood levels of, 2601t
Chlorhexidine gluconate, 2484
Chloride
in body fluids, 302t
deficit, 317t, 333–334
excess, 317t, 334
food sources of, 334
serum
in hyperchloremia, 317t, 334
in hypochloremia, 317t
laboratory values for, 310t
reference range for, 333
significance of, 333
urinary
laboratory values for, 310t
in metabolic alkalosis, 336
Chloride shift, 333
Chlorine, as terrorism threat, 2569t, 2571
Chloroquine (Aralen), for rheumatic diseases, 1895t
Chlorothiazide (Diuril), 954t
for hypertension, 1026t
Chlorpheniramine (Chlor-Trimeton), 1871t
Chlorpromazine (Thorazine), interactions with anesthetics, 490t
Chlorpropamide, 1399t
for diabetes insipidus, 1448
Chlorthalidone (Hygroton), 954t
for hypertension, 1026t
Choking
abdominal thrust maneuver for, 608, 609c
management of, 608, 609c
Cholangiography, 1290t
in biliary/pancreatic disease, 1349t
percutaneous transhepatic, 1351
Cholecystectomy, 1351, 1354
definition of, 1345, 1347c
laparoscopic, 1351, 1353–1354, 1353f
definition of, 1345, 1347c
self-care after, 1357, 1357c
laser, definition of, 1347c
mini-, 1354
Cholecystitis, 1347
acalculous, 1347
calculous, 1347
definition of, 1345, 1347c
Cholecystography, 1290t, 1349t, 1350
Cholecystojejunostomy, definition of, 1345
Cholecystokinin, in gastrointestinal regulation, 1124t
Cholecystokinin-pancreozymin (CCK-PZ), 1345–1347
definition of, 1345
Cholecystostomy
definition of, 1345, 1347c
percutaneous, 1354–1355
surgical, 1354
Choledochoduodenostomy, definition of, 1347c
Choledochojejunostomy, definition of, 1347c
Choledocholithiasis, definition of, 1345, 1347c
Choledocholithotomy, definition of, 1347c

Choledochostomy, 1354
definition of, 1345
Choledochotomy, definition of, 1347c
Cholelithiasis, 1347–1355, 1348f
assessment of, 1349–1351
clinical manifestations of, 1349
definition of, 1345, 1347c
diagnosis of, 1349–1351, 1349t
ileostomy and, 1263
lithotripsy for, 1352–1353
medical management of, 1351–1355
nonsurgical stone removal in, 1352–1353, 1352f, 1353f
nutritional therapy in, 1351
pathophysiology of, 1348
pharmacologic therapy for, 1351
risk factors for, 1348, 1348c
stone removal by instrumentation in, 1352, 1352f
supportive therapy in, 1351
surgical management of, 1353–1355, 1353f
gerontologic considerations in, 1355
Cholera, 2502
causative organism of, 2476t
Cholescintigraphy, 1350
Cholesteatoma, 2107–2108
definition of, 2093
Cholesterol, serum, 861, 985, 1290t
in biliary/pancreatic disease, 1349t
control of, 862–865, 863f, 864t, 865t
Cholestyramine, 865, 865t, 986
Cholinergics, for glaucoma, 2057, 2058t
Choline salicylate (Arthropan), for rheumatic diseases, 1895t
Chondroitin, for osteoarthritis, 1916
Chondrolysis, 1920
Chondrosarcoma, 2417
Chordae tendineae, 782f, 783
Chordoplasty, 923
definition of, 915
Chorea, 2142
definition of, 2301
in Huntington's disease, 2319
Choriocarcinoma, definition of, 1661
Chorionic gonadotropin, for infertility treatment, 1651c
Choroid, 2044, 2045, 2045f
Choroid plexus, 2133
Chromosome(s), 141–142, 143f
abnormalities of, 384
definition of, 140
examination of, 148–149
extra, 148
missing, 148
rearrangements of, balanced, 148
Chronic illness, 166–174
and adherence to therapeutic regime, 168
adjustment to, factors affecting, 166
age and, 167
care for
goals of, 171–172
home and community-based, 172–174
outcomes evaluation in, 172
plan of, 172
in special populations, 174
causes of, 166–167
characteristics of, 166–168
continuing care in, 174
costs of, 167, 167t
cultural considerations in, 174
deaths from, 166
definition of, 166–167
in developing countries, 167
and disability, 166
epidemiology of, 166

Chronic illness (*continued*)
　ethical considerations in, 168
　and family life, 168
　follow-up in, 172
　goals of care in, establishing, 171–172
　and health care, 6, 8, 16
　health education in, 49–50
　and immune system function, 1796
　lifestyle and, 167
　management of, 168–169
　　costs of, 168
　　problems of, 168–169
　nursing interventions for, 172
　　effectiveness of, evaluation of, 172
　nursing management of, 169–174
　obesity and, 167
　overweight and, 167
　patient with, characteristics of, 170c
　phases of, 168, 169, 170t, 171t
　　acute, 171t
　　comeback, 171t
　　crisis, 171t
　　downward, 171t
　　dying, 171t
　　pretrajectory, 171t
　　problems in, identification of, 170–171
　　stable, 171t
　　trajectory, 170–171
　　trajectory onset, 171t
　　unstable, 171t
　physical inactivity and, 167
　prevalence of, 167
　　global, 167
　and quality of life, 168–169
　risk factors for, 167
　self-care in, patient teaching about, 172–174
　self-management in, patient's perspective on, 173c
　smoking and, 167
　trajectory model of, 169, 171t
　types of, 167
Chronic lymphocytic leukemia, 1062–1063, 1074–1075
　thrombocytopenia in, 1087t
Chronic mucocutaneous candidiasis, 1803t, 1806
Chronic myeloid leukemia, 1072–1073
　blast crisis in, 1073
Chronic obstructive pulmonary disease, 686–701
　assessment in, 689–690, 690c, 696, 696c
　and asthma, 686
　　differentiation of, 690
　atelectasis in, 707c
　classification of, by lung function, 690t
　clinical manifestations of, 689
　complications of, 690–691, 697, 698–699
　coping in, 706c
　cor pulmonale in, 660–661
　definition of, 686
　diagnosis of, 689–690
　dyspnea-anxiety-dyspnea cycle in, nursing research on, 567
　exacerbation of, management of, 693
　expected outcomes in, 700–701
　fatigue in, nursing research on, 691
　gas exchange in, improvement of, 702c–703c
　goals in, 697
　hospitalized patients with, psychological distress and quality of life in, nursing research on, 701
　medical management of, 690–695
　mortality rate for, 686
　nursing care plan for, 702c–708c
　nursing diagnoses related to, 696, 702c–708c
　nursing interventions in, 697–700, 702c–708c
　nursing process in, 696–701
　oxygen therapy in, 694, 695
　pathophysiology of, 686–688
　pharmacologic therapy for, 692–693
　physical activity in, nursing research on, 691
　pneumonia in, 635, 636
　posture in, 689, 690f
　pulmonary hypertension in, 659
　pulmonary rehabilitation in, 694–695
　respiratory failure in, 655–656
　risk factors for, 688, 688c
　risk for, reduction of, 691–692
　self-care in, 705c, 706c
　signs and symptoms of, 563
　stages of, 690, 690t
　surgical management of, 694
　symptoms in, patients' descriptions of, nursing research on, 566
Chronic renal failure. *See* Renal failure, chronic
Chronotropy, 825
　definition of, 823
Chvostek's sign, 326, 329
　definition of, 1440
Chyle fistula, after neck dissection, 1160
Chyme, 1124, 1125
　definition of, 1121
Cicatrix, 1938c
Cidofovir (Vistide), for cytomegalovirus retinitis, 2084
Cigarette smoking. *See* Smoking
Cilia, 553
　definition of, 553
Ciliary body, 2044
Cilostazol (Pletal), in peripheral arterial disease, 992
Cimetidine, 1206t, 1859
　for metabolic alkalosis, 336
Ciprofloxacin (Cipro)
　for gonorrhea, 2508
　for pneumonia, 637
　for urinary tract infections, 1574
Ciprozil, for sinusitis, 596
Circle of Willis, 2134, 2135f
Circulating nurse, 503
　activities of, 504–505
　definition of, 503
Circulation
　in burn patient, 2002–2003
　in cardiopulmonary resuscitation, 970–971, 971f
　maintenance of, after arterial repair, 994
　peripheral arterial, improving, 987, 990
　pulmonary, 557–558, 975, 976f
　systemic, 975, 976f
Circulator. *See* Circulating nurse
Circulatory impairment
　in patient in cast, 2357–2359, 2359f
　in skin traction, 2367–2368
Circulatory system, age-related changes in, 1795t
Circumcision, 1741, 1775
　definition of, 1740
Circumduction, 2343c
Cirrhosis, hepatic, 1318–1322
　alcoholic, 1318
　assessment of, 1318, 1319–1320, 1319c
　biliary, 1318
　clinical manifestations of, 1318–1319
　compensated, 1318, 1319c
　decompensated, 1318, 1319c
　definition of, 1285
　diagnosis of, 1319–1320
　medical management of, 1320
　nursing process with, 1320–1322
　pathophysiology of, 1318
　postnecrotic, 1318
　severity of, classification of, 1318, 1318t
Cisatracurium (Nimbex), 512t
CISM. *See* Critical incident stress management
Cisplatin
　in cancer treatment, 399t
　　adverse effects and side effects of, 399t
　neural toxicity of, 402
　renal toxicity of, 401–402
CJD. *See* Creutzfeldt-Jakob disease
Clarithromycin (Biaxin)
　for gastritis and peptic ulcer disease, 1206t
　for Legionnaire's disease, 2511
　for *Mycobacterium avium* complex, 1835
　for pharyngitis, 598
　for pneumonia, 636
　for sinusitis, 595, 596
Classic pathway, of complement system activation, 1792
Clavicle, fracture of, 2440, 2441f
　range-of-motion exercises for, 2441f
Clavicular strap, 2440, 2441f
Clawfoot. *See* Pes cavus
Clearance, renal, 1499
　definition of, 1493
Cleft lip and/or palate, genetics of, 147t
Click(s), definition of, 803
Client. *See also* Patient
　definition of, 5
Clindamycin
　for bacterial vaginosis, 1663–1664
　for pneumonia, 637
Clinical guidelines, 9
Clinical nurse specialist, 12
Clinical pathways, 9
　elements of, 2603–2604, 2603f
　formats for, 2606, 2607f–2613f
　interventional categories in, 2603f, 2604
　outcomes in, 2603f, 2604
　patient population in, 2603–2604, 2603f
　time frames in, 2603f, 2604
　understanding, 2602–2613
　use of, nurses' role in, 2604
　and variance record, 2604, 2605f
Clinical trials, investigational antineoplastic agents and, 400c
Clinicians, attitudes toward death, 449–450
Clitoris, 1614, 1614f
CLL. *See* Chronic lymphocytic leukemia
Clofazimine, for tuberculosis, 647
Clofibrate (Atromid-S), 865, 865t, 1448
Clomiphene citrate (Clomid, Serophene), for ovulation induction, 1650–1651, 1651c
Clonazepam (Klonopin)
　adverse effects and side effects of, 2194t
　toxic effects of, 2194t
Clonidine (Catapres)
　for atrial fibrillation, 833
　for atrial flutter, 832
　for hot flashes, 1635
　for hypertension, 1027t
　for hypertensive crises, 1033
　for smoking cessation, 692
Clonidine patch (Catapres TTs), for hypertension, 1027t
Clonus, 2148, 2349
　definition of, 2129, 2337

# INDEX

Clopidogrel (Plavix)
　for coronary artery disease, 870
　in peripheral arterial disease, 992
　and stroke prevention, 2211
Closed awareness, of terminal status, 449–450
Closed fracture, 2431
　home care for, 2434c
　nursing management of, 2434, 2434c
Closed reduction, for hip fracture, 2447
*Clostridium botulinum,* 2567t
*Clostridium difficile*
　health care–associated infection potential of, 2482
　incubation period of, 2476t
　transmission of, 2476t
*Clostridium tetani*
　incubation period of, 2477t
　transmission of, 2477t
Clothing
　protective, in Standard Precautions, 1820c
　for stroke patients, 2218–2219
Clotrimazole
　for burns, 2017
　for candidiasis, 1662
　　in HIV-infected (AIDS) patients, 1836
Clotting factors, 1042
Clubbing
　of digits, 568, 568f, 804
　　in bronchiectasis, 709
　of nails, 1936, 1940f
CML. *See* Chronic myeloid leukemia
CMV. *See* Cytomegalovirus
CNS. *See* Central nervous system
Coagulation. *See* Blood clotting
Coal workers' pneumoconiosis, 669–670
Cocaine
　abuse/overdose, emergency management of, 2545t
　topical, for epistaxis, 605
Co-carcinogens, 385
*Coccidioides immitis,* encephalitis caused by, 2275–2276
Coccidiosis, malabsorption in, 1240t
Coccyx, 2136
　fracture of, 2445
Cochlea, 2094–2096, 2094f
　definition of, 2095c
Cochlear duct, 2094f
Cochlear implant, 2122–2123, 2123f
Codeine
　abuse/overdose, emergency management of, 2545t
　pharmacology of, 283t
　for pharyngitis, 598
　for septic arthritis, 2416
Code of Ethics, American Nurses Association, 29, 31c
Cognition
　age-related changes in, 53–54
　in Alzheimer's disease, 244, 245
　brain injury and, 2245–2246
　in cardiovascular disease, assessment of, 797
　in Huntington's disease, 2319
　in hypothyroidism, 1454
　impaired, and pressure ulcers, 208
　in liver disease, 1332c
　in multiple sclerosis, 2282
　of persons with disabilities, assessment of, 178c
　in pneumonia, 641
　Rancho Los Amigos Scale of, 2246, 2247t–2248t
　stroke and, 2209t, 2210, 2220
Cognitive appraisal, of stress, 93–94

Cognitive disability, people with, interacting and communicating with, 181c
Cognitive rehabilitation, 2245
Cogwheeling, in Parkinson's disease, 2313
Coitus interruptus, 1646
Colchicine, for gout, 1918, 1919t
Cold sore(s), 592, 592c, 1143t
Cold therapy
　after foot surgery, 2403
　for low back pain, 2393
　for pain management, with casts, 2357
　postoperative, for hand/wrist surgery, 2399
　for rheumatic diseases, 1894
Colectomy, prophylactic, 393
Colesevelam (Welchol), 865t
Colestipol (Colestid), 865t, 986
Colitis, granulomatous. *See* Regional enteritis
Collaborative care, in home health care, 17
Collaborative practice, 13, 13f
Collaborative problems, 34, 36c, 37–39, 40f
　and nursing diagnoses, differentiation of, 39, 40f
Collagen, definition of, 1995
Collar bone. *See* Clavicle
Collateral circulation, 984–985, 985f
Collecting ducts, renal, 1495f
Collecting tubule(s), 1491–1495, 1495f
Colles' fracture, 2427, 2443–2444
Colloids, 312t
　for anaphylaxis, 2538
　definition of, 356
　for fluid replacement in shock, 364, 367, 367t
Colon. *See also* Large intestine
　function of, 1125
Colonic J pouch, 1267
Colonic manometry, 1138
Colonic motility, testing of, 1134
Colonic transit studies, 1134
Colonization, 2479
　definition of, 2475
Colonoscopy, 1135–1137, 1135f
　bowel cleansing for, nursing research on, 309–310
　flexible fiberoptic, 1135, 1135f
Colony-forming units, bacterial, 507
Colony-stimulating factor(s), in cancer treatment, 401
Color blindness, genetics of, 147t
Colorectal cancer, 1265–1275
　adjuvant therapy for, 1267
　clinical manifestations of, 1266
　complications of, 1266
　detection of, 390t
　diagnosis of, 1266
　epidemiology of, 1265–1266
　familial occurrence of, 386
　gerontologic considerations in, 1266
　medical management of, 1266–1267
　nursing process with, 1268–1275
　pathophysiology of, 1266
　prophylactic surgery for, 393
　risk factors for, 1265–1266, 1266c
　staging of, 1266–1267, 1267c
　surgical management of, 1267, 1268f, 1269f, 1270f
　　gerontologic considerations in, 1267
　　postoperative care in, 1271
　　preparing patient for, 1269–1270
Color fundus photography, 2049
Color vision testing, 2049
Colostomy, 1267, 1270f
　appliance
　　applying, 1271–1273
　　removal of, 1271–1273

　complications of, 1271, 1272t
　definition of, 1232
　for diverticulitis, 1244, 1244f
　irrigating, 1273, 1274c–1275c
　nutrition/nutritional support for, 1271
　self-care after, 1273
　wound care after, 1271
Colporrhaphy, 1675
　definition of, 1661
Colposcopy, 1628–1629
Coma
　arousal from, 2168
　definition of, 2161, 2162
　hepatic, 1304–1307
　myxedema, 1453–1454, 1457c–1458c
Combination therapy, for HIV, 1826–1829, 1827t–1828t
Combitube, in emergency, 2524–2525, 2525f
Combivir, for HIV infection, 1827t
Comedones, 1953–1954
　definition of, 1945
　extraction of, 1956
Comfort
　definition of, 46c
　promotion of
　　in hypothyroidism, 1454
　　in liver disease, 1327c–1328c
　　in upper airway infection, 602
　　with venous thrombosis, 1008
　spinal cord injuries and, 2258, 2259c
Comminuted fracture, 2431
Commissure, 921
Commissurotomy, 920
　closed, 921, 921f
　definition of, 915
　open, 921–922
Common bile duct, 1121, 1122f, 1286
　anatomy of, 1345, 1346f
Common cold. *See* Rhinitis, viral
Common variable immunodeficiency, 1803t, 1805–1806
　clinical manifestations of, 1805
　diagnosis of, 1805
　medical management of, 1806
Communication
　alaryngeal, 613–614
　　definition of, 589
　Alzheimer's disease patients and, 244, 245
　cross-cultural, 130–131, 131c
　definition of, 46c
　disabilities and, 177, 178c, 179c–181c, 182, 182f
　in end-of-life care, 457–459
　after facial reconstructive surgery, 1990
　with families, in emergency operations plan, 2562–2563
　in Guillain-Barré syndrome, 2290
　after head and neck surgery, nursing research on, 613
　hearing loss and, 2103, 2104c
　after laryngectomy, 613–614, 617
　　nursing interventions for, 617
　after mastoid surgery, 2109
　with media, in emergency operations plan, 2562
　in multiple sclerosis, 2282
　after neck dissection, 1155, 1158c–1159c
　in oral cavity conditions, 1151
　in Parkinson's disease, 2317
　stroke and, 2208t, 2209, 2220–2221
　therapeutic, 35, 37t
　in upper airway infection, 602
　for ventilator-dependent patient, 750
Community
　definition of, 49

Community (continued)
  with identified health problem
    nursing diagnoses related to, 2–3
    nursing interventions for, 2–3
    nursing outcomes for, 2–3
  infection prevention in, 2484–2489
Community-based nursing, 11–12, 16–18. *See also* Home health care nursing
  challenges of, 18
  in chronic illness, 172–174
  concepts of, 16
  cultural considerations in, 16
  focus of, 16, 17f
  forms of, 16, 17f
  genetics in, 68
  and hospital-based nursing, comparison of, 18
  prevention in, 16–17
  settings for, 16, 21–22
  skills needed for, 16
Community nurse-managed centers, 22
Community nursing centers, 12
Community-oriented/public health nursing, 11–12
Community resources, for patients
  identification of, 18–19
  referrals to, 19
Community services, for emergency patient, 2520
Community wellness, 49–50
Compact bone. *See* Cortical (compact) bone
Compartment(s), anatomic, 2436, 2437f
Compartment syndrome, 2357–2359, 2359f
  acute, 2436
    clinical manifestations of, 2436
  arm cast and, 2362
  assessment of, 2436–2437
  burns and, 2014c
  casts and, 2359
  chronic, 2436
  crush, 2436
  diagnosis of, 2436–2437
  elbow fractures and, 2443
  fractures and, 2436–2438, 2443, 2459
  management of, 2438
  pain caused by, 2357
  pathophysiology of, 2349
  tibial fracture and, 2459
Competence (mental), 252
Complement. *See* Complement system and complement
Complementary and alternative therapies, 112–113, 112c, 134. *See also* Folk healers
  definition of, 96
  for HIV/AIDS patients, 1837
  in pain management, 290
  for prostate cancer, 1761
  in rehabilitation, 219
  use of, screening for, 71
Complement system and complement, 1792–1793
  activation of
    alternative pathway, 1792–1793
    classic pathway, 1792
    lectin pathway, 1792–1793
  assessment of, tests for, 1799t
  deficiencies of, 1807–1809
  definition of, 1783, 1792, 1887
  and immune response, 1787, 1787f, 1793t
  and immunodeficiency disorders, 1803t
  in rheumatic disease, 1889–1891
  serum levels, in rheumatic diseases, 1893t
Complete blood count, 1044, 1047
  in cardiac patient, 808t

Complete blood count with differential, in diagnosis of allergic disorder, 1863
Complete fracture, 2431
Complete protein antigens, 1857
Complete spinal cord lesion, 2251
  definition of, 2233
Complex regional pain syndrome, 261c
  in burn patient, 2032t
  fracture and, 2440
Compliance
  lung, 557
  with therapy, in sexually transmitted disease, 2509
  ventricular, 945
    definition of, 945
Complications. *See also specific diagnosis*
  intraoperative, 516–518
    management of, 520–521
    monitoring for, 520–521
    respiratory, 516
  postoperative, in hospitalized patient, 532, 533f
  in postoperative phase, 544–546
    in older persons, 546–548
  of surgery, risk factors for, 485–486, 486c
Compression fracture, osteoporosis and, 2404
Compression garments, 198
Compression stockings
  application of, with venous thrombosis, 1008–1009
  gerontologic considerations with, 1008
  for orthostatic hypotension, 2259
Compression syndrome, 1920
Computed tomographic angiography, in peripheral vascular disease, 983
Computed tomography
  abdominal, 1133
    nursing interventions in, 1133
    in trauma victim, 2532
  in biliary/pancreatic disease, 1349t
  of brain, 2162
  of brain tumor, 2304
  in cancer detection, 391t
  in cardiac patient, 812–813
  cranial, 2180–2181
  in degenerative disk disease, 2325
  in gastrointestinal assessment, 1133
  in head injuries, 2235
  helical, 1133
  of hepatobiliary system, 1289
  in laryngeal cancer, 610
  in liver disease, 1291t
  in low back pain, 2393c
  of musculoskeletal system, 2350
  of nervous system, 2152
  nursing interventions in, 812–813
  pelvic, in females, 1631
  in peripheral vascular disease, 983
  of pulmonary embolism, 663
  in respiratory disease, 580
  of spinal cord injury, 2251
  spiral, 1133
  of stroke, 2210
  of urinary tract, 1508
  in UTI diagnosis, 1574
Concept map(s), 2614–2630
  for abdominal surgery patient, 2618f
  for activity intolerance, 2620f
  for acute pain, 2618f, 2626f
  for alcoholism and dysfunctional family processes, 2628f
  for anticipatory grieving, 2624f
  for anxiety, 2616f
  for aspiration, 2619f
  for chronic pain, 2617f, 2620f

  for community with identified health problem, 2615f
  for complications of diabetes, 2622f
  for decisonal conflict, 2624f
  for decreased cardiac output, 2630f
  for deficient fluid volume, 2621f, 2630f
  for disturbed tactile sensory perception, 2622f
  for disturbed visual sensory perception, 2627f
  for fear accompanied by somatic complaints unsubstantiated by physical findings, 2616f
  for hemorrhage, 2630f
  for hemothorax, 2630f
  for immunosuppressed patient with history of oral infections, 2625f
  for impaired cough reflex, 2619f
  for impaired gas exchange, 2618f, 2619f, 2630f
  for impaired physical mobility, 2618f, 2629f
  for impaired skin integrity, 2626f
  for increased cranial pressure, 2628f
  for ineffective airway clearance, 2618f, 2619f
  for ineffective breathing pattern, 2619f, 2630f
  for ineffective coping, 2616f
  for ineffective therapeutic regimen management, 2622f, 2625f
  for ineffective tissue perfusion, 2620f, 2622f
  for infection, 2623f, 2625f, 2626f
  for intermittent claudication with ulceration, 2620f
  for multiple trauma, 2630f
  for nausea, vomiting, and diarrhea, 2621f
  for risk for disuse syndrome, 2629f
  for risk for imblanced nutrition, 2626f
  for risk for injury, 2627f, 2628f
  for risk for shock, 2630f
  for stress urinary incontinence, 2623f
  for thermal injury, 2626f
  for unilateral neglect, 2627f
  for urinary retention, 2623f
  for vision impairment, 2627f
Conchae, anatomy of, 553, 554f
Concussion
  cerebral, 2236
  definition of, 2233
Condom
  female, 1645, 1645f
    and HIV prevention, 1817
  male, 1646
    correct use of, 1818c
    and HIV prevention, 1817, 1818c
Condom catheters. *See* External catheters
Condoms, and prevention of sexually transmitted disease, 2509
Conduction
  definition of, 823
  heat loss by, 1931
Conductive hearing loss. *See* Hearing loss, conductive
Conductive keratoplasty, 2067
Conductivity, of cardiac conduction cells, 783
Condylomata, 1666
  definition of, 1661
Cone biopsy, cervical, 1629
Cones, 2046
  definition of, 2043
Confidentiality
  ethical principle of, 28c, 31
  of genetic information, 158–159
  of HIV-infected (AIDS) patients, 1851
Confusion
  in pneumonia, 641

postoperative
  in older adults, 547
  in older persons, 529
Congenital heart disease, genetics of, 147t
Congenital infections, of sexually transmitted disease, 2509
Congestive heart failure, 946. *See also* Heart failure
  in acute glomerulonephritis, 1518
  burns and, 2030
  in chronic renal failure, 1527
  definition of, 945
Conization, 1684
  definition of, 1661
Conjunctiva, 2044, 2045f
  benign tumors of, 2080
  bulbar, 2044
  malignant tumors of, 2081
  palpebral, 2044
  retraction of, in toxic epidermal necrolysis or Stevens-Johnson syndrome, 1976
Conjunctivitis, 2076–2079
  allergic, 2078, 2079
  bacterial, 2077, 2078
  inclusion, 2077
  microbial, 2077–2078
  toxic, 2078, 2079
  viral, 2077–2078, 2078–2079, 2078c
Consanguinity, 155
Consciousness
  altered level of
    assessment of, 2163–2164, 2164f, 2165t–2166t
    causes of, 2162
    clinical manifestations of, 2162
    complications of, 2163, 2164, 2169
    definition of, 2161, 2162
    diagnosis of, 2162
    expected outcomes with, 2169
    with increased intracranial pressure, 2170
    medical management of, 2163
    nursing diagnoses related to, 2164
    nursing interventions for, 2166–2169
    nursing process with, 2163–2169
    pathophysiology of, 2162
    planning and goals for, 2164–2166
  level of, brain injuries and, 2240, 2243
Consensus formula, for fluid replacement in burn patients, 2007c
Consent, for emergency treatment, documentation of, 2518
Consolidation
  definition of, 625
  in pneumonia, 629, 636
  pulmonary, assessment findings in, 576t
Constancy principle, 92
Constipation, 215, 1127, 1232–1235, 1278
  with appendicitis, 1241
  causes of, 1232–1233
  clinical manifestations of, 1233
  in colorectal cancer, 1266
  definition of, 1232
  and diverticulosis, 1243
  gerontologic considerations in, 234, 1233–1234
  idiopathic, 1233
  medical management of, 1234, 1234t
  nursing management of, 1234–1235
  opioid-related, 282
  in orthopedic surgery patient, 2387
  osteoporosis and, 2410
  pathophysiology of, 1233
  perceived versus actual, 1233
  postoperative, 543

prevention of, 218, 1235, 1235c
  in stroke patient, 2220
  traction and, 2370
  in tube feeding, 1184t
Constructional apraxia, 1305, 1306f
  definition of, 1285
Contact dermatitis, 1877, 1877t, 1964–1965
  allergic, 1877, 1877t
    latex and, 1883t
  clinical manifestations of, 1964
  distribution of, 1940f
  irritant, 1877, 1877t
    latex and, 1883t
  of lips, 1143t
  medical management of, 1964–1965
  photoallergic, 1877, 1877t
  phototoxic, 1877, 1877t
  prevention of, 1964, 1965c
Contact Precautions, 2482, 2483c
Continent ileal urinary reservoir, 1602
Continent urinary diversion(s). *See* Urinary diversion
Continuing care, in upper airway infection, 603
Continuity theory, of aging, 227
Continuous ambulatory peritoneal dialysis, 1546, 1546f, 1548–1551
  continuing care in, 1550–1551
  definition of, 1515
  suitability for, assessment of, 1549c
Continuous arteriovenous hemodialysis, 1544
Continuous arteriovenous hemofiltration, 1544
Continuous cyclic peritoneal dialysis, 1548, 1551
  definition of, 1515
Continuous glucose monitoring system, 1390–1391, 1391f
  definition of, 1376
Continuous infusion method, of tube feeding, 1182
Continuous passive motion (CPM) device, 2382f
  definition of, 2355
  after knee replacement, 2376
Continuous positive airway pressure, 743, 743f
  definition of, 723
  with oxygen therapy, 724–725
  and respiratory weaning, 752
Continuous quality improvement (CQI), 9
Continuous renal replacement therapies, 1542–1545, 1543f
  for acute renal failure, 1525
  definition of, 1515
Continuous subcutaneous insulin infusion, 1397–1398, 1397f
  definition of, 1376
Continuous venovenous hemodialysis, 1544–1545, 1544f
  definition of, 1515
Continuous venovenous hemofiltration, 1544, 1544f
  definition of, 1515
Contraception, 1640–1647
  combined methods for, 1642, 1643c
  emergency, 1646–1647
    for sexual assault victim, 2552
  hormonal methods, 1641–1644
    contraindications to, 1642
    FDA-approved, 1643, 1643c
  mechanical barriers for, 1644–1646
  oral contraceptives for. *See* Oral contraceptives
  postcoital, 1647

Contraceptive(s). *See also* Oral contraceptives
  injectable, 1644
  transdermal, 1643
  vaginal, 1644
Contraceptive sponge, 1645
Contractility, cardiac/myocardial, 787, 869, 945
  definition of, 781, 859, 945
  factors affecting, 825
Contraction, of skeletal muscle, 2341–2342, 2343c
Contractures, 2348
  with amputation, 2461, 2465–2466
  burn and, 2032t
  burns and, 2019, 2026, 2034
  definition of, 1995, 2337, 2392
  Dupuytren's, 2399, 2399f
  joint, nursing interventions for, 195–196
  in multiple sclerosis, 2281
  paraplegia/quadriplegia and, 2263
  spinal cord injury and, 2257
  Volkmann's, 2362
Contrast agents
  iodine in, allergic reaction to, 983
  urologic testing with, 1508
    patient care during, 1508, 1508c
Contrast phlebography, in peripheral vascular disease, 83
Contrast-sensitivity testing, 2052
Contrecoup contusion, pulmonary, 677
Control, of cancer, 391
  definition of, 381
Controlled ventilation, 743, 743f
  definition of, 723
Contusion(s), 2425
  cerebral, 2236
  definition of, 2233, 2425, 2528c
  renal, 1565–1566, 1565f
  sports-related, 2426–2427
  treatment of, 2425
Conus medullaris, 2135
Convection, heat loss by, 1931
Cooley's anemia. *See* Thalassemia major
Coomb's test, 1062
Coordination, assessment of, 2146–2147
COPD. *See* Chronic obstructive pulmonary disease
Coping
  with anticipation of death, 471, 472t
  assessment of, 34
  with bone tumors, 2420
  breast surgery and, 1720
  in burn victim, 2029, 2034
  in cardiovascular disease, assessment of, 797
  in chronic obstructive pulmonary disease, 696, 698, 706c
  with death and dying, by professional caregivers, 473–474
  definition of, 46c, 91, 92, 94
  with disabilities, 219c
  emotion-focused, 94
  enhancement of
    in family, 115–116
    nursing interventions for, 105, 106c
  with enteral therapy, 1187
  factors affecting, 114
  family
    in brain injury, 2246–2248
    in recovery from stroke, 2221–2222
    with hip fracture, 2452c–2453c
  with HIV/AIDS, for health care providers, 1851–1852
  in HIV-infected (AIDS) patients, 1849
  in hyperthyroidism, 1464
  in hypothyroidism, 1454

Coping (continued)
  with implanted cardiac device, 851
  inappropriate, in response to stress, 97
  in inflammatory bowel disease, 1252–1253
  with low vision/blindness, 2053
  in multiple sclerosis, 2283
  after neck dissection, 1155
  nursing research on, 117
  in older persons, 228
  paraplegia/quadriplegia and, 2264
  in Parkinson's disease, 2317
  problem-focused, 94
  in prostate cancer, 1755c
  in rheumatic diseases, 1902c, 1904
  in sickle cell crisis, 1059–1060
  strategies for, for surgical patient, 495
  with stress, 94
  stress and, 92, 94
  surgery for breast cancer and, 1719
  for ventilator-dependent patient, 750
  with vertigo, 2116c–2117c
Coping mechanism, denial as, 450
Copper
  serum level, in Hodgkin's disease, 1080
  in wound healing, 487t
Cordotomy, in pain management, 291, 291f
Core needle biopsy, of breast, 1708
Corn, of foot, 2401
Cornea, 2044, 2045f
  abrasions of, 2074
  care for, in myasthenia gravis, 2288
  disorders of, 2064–2067
  integrity of, maintenance of, for unconscious patient, 2167
  nursing interventions for, in toxic epidermal necrolysis or Stevens-Johnson syndrome, 1976
  surgeries for, 2064–2065
Corneal dystrophies, 2064
Corneal transplantation, 2065, 2065c
Coronary arteriography, 814
Coronary artery(ies)
  anatomy of, 783, 860, 861f
  brachytherapy in, 886, 886f
  revascularization of, 888–890
  stent/stenting for, 886, 886f
Coronary artery bypass graft, 862, 888–890
  alternative techniques for, 890, 890f
  candidates for, 888
  complications of, 890, 891t–894t
  definition of, 859
  indications for, 888
  off-pump, 890, 890f
  recovery after, in women, nursing research on, 903
  traditional, 888–890, 889f
  vessels used for, 888, 888f, 889f
Coronary artery disease, 790, 859–885, 948. See also Angina pectoris; Atherosclerosis, coronary; Myocardial infarct/infarction
  hypertension and, 1023
  risk factors for, 796c, 806, 860–862, 861c, 862c
Coronary vein(s), anatomy of, 783
Coronavirus, pneumonia caused by, 629, 631t
Corpak tube, 1176t
Cor pulmonale, 660–661
  causes of, 660
  clinical manifestations of, 661
  definition of, 625, 660
  medical management of, 661
  nursing management of, 661
  pathophysiology of, 661
  with pulmonary hypertension, 660

Corpus callosum, 2131, 2131f, 2132f
Corpus luteum, 1615
  definition of, 1613
Corrosive poison, definition of, 2517
Cortical (compact) bone, 2338–2339, 2338f, 2340
Corticobulbar tract, 2135f, 2136
Corticospinal tracts, 2135f, 2136
Corticosteroid(s)
  adverse effects and side effects of, 1064c, 1484–1485, 1486t
  for allergic rhinitis, 1872
  for anaphylaxis, 1872, 2538
  for asthma, 713
  in cancer treatment, 399t
  for cerebral metastases, 2307
  for chronic lymphocytic leukemia, 1074
  complications of, after kidney transplantation, 1563
  concentrated fluorinated, 1950, 1950t
  for COPD, 692–693
  for cystic fibrosis, 719
  definition of, 1440
  for dermatologic problems, 1485
  dosage of, 1485
  for dyspnea, 465
  for epicondylitis, 2429
  for gout, 1918
  for immune hemolytic anemia, 1062
  and immune system, 1797t
  for inflammatory bowel disease, 1250
  interactions with anesthetics, 490t
  for kidney transplant recipient, 1561, 1563
  management of, perioperative, 488
  for myasthenia gravis, 2286
  ocular therapy with, 2086
  for ophthalmologic disorders, 1485
  for polymyositis, 1913
  preparations of, 1484, 1485t
  for rheumatic diseases, 1896t
  for rotator cuff tears, 2429
  for spinal cord injury, 2254
  for status asthmaticus, 717
  for systemic lupus erythematosus, 1911
  tapering of, 1485–1486
  therapeutic uses of, 1485
  therapy with, 1484–1486
    complications of, 1064c
  topical, 1950, 1950t
    for pruritus, 1952
    for psoriasis, 1966–1967, 1966t
  and wound healing, 541t
Corticotropin. See Adrenocorticotropic hormone
Corticotropin-releasing hormone, 1473
Cortisol, 1473
  and bone health, 2339
  in fluid and electrolyte balance, 306
  and immune system function, 1796
Cortisone, 1485t
Corynebacterium parvum, 418
Costochondritis, 1920
  chest pain caused by, assessment of, 792t
Costovertebral angle, 1504, 1504f
Cotton-wool spots, 2048
  in hypertension, 1023
Cough(ing)
  in asthma, 711
  in bronchiectasis, 709
  in cardiac patient, 804
  in chronic obstructive pulmonary disease, 689
  clinical significance of, 564–565
  effective
    technique for, 731, 733c, 757
    in thoracic surgery patient, 765–766

  in heart failure, 950
  in Hodgkin's disease, 1080
  huff, 697, 757
  incisional pain during, minimizing, 766, 767f
  after laryngectomy, 616–617
  in lung cancer, 671
  in pneumonia, 640
  postoperative, 534
  preoperative teaching about, 492–493, 494c, 757
  in respiratory disease, 564–565
  rib fracture and, 2459
  spinal cord injury and, 2257
  and wound healing, 541t
Cough reflex, impaired
  nursing diagnoses related to, 550–551
  nursing interventions for, 550–551
  nursing outcomes for, 550–551
Countertraction, 2365–2366
Cowper's gland, 1741, 1741f
COX-2 inhibitors
  and immune system, 1797t
  for osteoarthritis, 1915
  for rheumatic diseases, 1895t
  for rheumatoid arthritis, 1908
Coxsackievirus
  incubation period of, 2476t
  transmission of, 2476t
CPAP. See Continuous positive airway pressure
CPM device. See Continuous passive motion device
CPT. See Chest physiotherapy
Crab lice, 1962–1963
Crackles, 575, 575t
  in cardiac patient, 805
  definition of, 553
  in heart failure, 950
Cramping, intestinal, in tube feeding, 1184t
Cranberry juice, in UTI prevention, 1575
Cranial arteritis, 2198–2199, 2199
  clinical manifestations of, 2200
  medical management of, 2201
  nursing management of, 2201
Cranial nerve(s), 2130, 2133, 2136–2137, 2136f, 2137t, 2292f
  assessment of, 2146, 2147c
  disorders of, 2292–2296, 2293t–2294t
  in Guillain-Barré syndrome, 2289
  involvement with brain tumor, 2304
Craniectomy, 2180
  definition of, 2161
Craniostomy, 2180
Craniotomy, 2180
  for brain tumor, 2304
  definition of, 2161
  infratentorial, 181t, 2180–2183
  supratentorial, 181t, 2180–2183
C-reactive protein
  in cardiac patient, 806
  in coronary artery disease, 868
  serum levels, in rheumatic diseases, 1893t
Creams, for wound care, 1949
Creatine kinase, 876, 876t
  analysis of, in cardiac patient, 805
  definition of, 859
  isoenzymes of, 876, 876t
Creatinine, 1499
  in cardiac patient, 807t
  definition of, 1493
  serum, 305, 1507t
    in acute renal failure, 1523t, 1524
    in chronic renal failure, 1529
    laboratory values for, 310t
    in rheumatic diseases, 1893t

# INDEX

Creatinine clearance, 1507, 1507t
   test of, 1507t
Creatinine/height index, 80
Crepitus, 2348
   definition of, 2337, 2425
   fracture and, 2431
   subcutaneous, 676
CREST syndrome, 1912
Cretinism, 1450
   definition of, 1440
Creutzfeldt-Jakob disease, 2276–2277
   assessment in, 2277
   clinical manifestations of, 2276–2277
   diagnosis of, 2277
   medical management of, 2277
   new-variant, 2276–2277
   nursing management of, 2277
   pathophysiology of, 2276
   prevention of, 2277
   risk factors for, 2276
   transfusion-transmitted, 1104t
CRH. See Corticotropin-releasing hormone
Cricohyoidopexy, 612
Cricoid cartilage, 554
Cricothyroidotomy, 2525
   definition of, 2517
Critical incident stress management, 2564
Critical thinking
   characteristics of, 25
   components of, 25
   definition of, 25
   exercises, 26
   in nursing practice, 26–27, 26c
   process of, 26–27, 26c
   questions addressed in, 26c
   research and, 26–27
   skills needed in, 25
Crohn's disease. See Regional enteritis
Cromolyn sodium
   for allergic rhinitis, 1872
   for asthma, 713, 713t
Cross-cultural nursing care, 129. See also Transcultural nursing
   assessment in, 135–136, 136c
Cross-reactivity, 1790
Crotalidae Polyvalent Immune Fab Antivenin, 2540
CRPS. See Complex regional pain syndrome
CRRT. See Continuous renal replacement therapies
Crush injury
   acute renal failure in, 1523
   emergency management of, 2532–2533
Crust, 1938c
Crutches
   ambulation with, 204–205, 205f, 206c
      assessment of, 195–196
   fit of, 204
   gait with, 204–205, 206c
   for paraplegia, 2263
Crutch paralysis, 204
Cruzan, Nancy, 33
Cryoablation
   definition of, 1285
   in liver cancer, 1335
Cryomyolysis, laparoscopic, 1679
Cryoprecipitate, for transfusion, 1103t
Cryosurgery
   for acne, 1955
   for cancer, 393
   for hemorrhoids, 1277
   in liver cancer, 1335
   of prostate, 1761
      definition of, 1740
   for skin cancer, 1980

Cryotherapy
   cervical, 1629
   definition of, 1661
Cryptococcal meningitis, in HIV-infected (AIDS) patients, 1833
Cryptococcosis, causative organism of, 2476t
Cryptococcus neoformans
   encephalitis caused by, 2275–2276
   in HIV-infected (AIDS) patients, 1833
   incubation period of, 2476t
   transmission of, 2476t
Cryptorchidism, 1770
   definition of, 1740
Cryptosporidiosis, causative organism of, 2476t
Cryptosporidium
   incubation period of, 2476t
   transmission of, 2476t
Crystalloids
   for anaphylaxis, 2538
   definition of, 356
   for fluid replacement in shock, 364, 367, 367t
Crystalluria, detection of, 1506
Crystal meth, abuse/overdose, emergency management of, 2546t
CSF. See Cerebrospinal fluid
CT. See Computed tomography
Cultural blindness, definition of, 129
Cultural care diversity and universality, 130f
Cultural considerations
   in chronic illness, 174
   in communication, 130–131, 131c
   in emergency operations plan, 2563c
   with health history, 65–66
   in medication administration, 133–134
   in nutritional assessment, 81
   in pain management, 267–268
Cultural diversity, 7
   definition of, 128
Cultural imposition, definition of, 129
Culturally competent nursing care, 128, 129–130
Culturally congruent nursing care, 129–130
Cultural nursing assessment, 135–136, 136c
Cultural taboos, definition of, 129
Culture. See also Transcultural nursing
   and biologic variations, 133–134
   definition of, 7, 128
   and diet, 133, 133c
   and end-of-life care, 459–461
   and eye contact, 132
   and food intake, 81
   and formulation of teaching plan, 51, 51c
   and genetic assessment, 155–156
   and health care delivery, 7–8
   and holidays, 133
   and learning readiness, 51
   and menstruation, 1632
   of nurse, 136
   and pain, 267–268
   patient characteristics mediated by, 131–134
   and personal space and distance, 132
   physiologic effects of, 133–134
   of surgical patient, 490–491, 495
   and terminal illness, 456–457
   and time, 132
   and touch, 132–133
Culture care accommodation, 129
Culture care restructuring (repatterning), 129
Cultured epithelial autograft
   for burns, 2020t, 2023
   definition of, 1995
Cure, of cancer, 391
   definition of, 381

Curling's ulcers, 1210
   in burn victim, 2002, 2015c
Curreiri formula, for nutritional support, 2025
Cushing's disease, 2302–2303
Cushing's response, 2170
   definition of, 2161
Cushing's syndrome, 1446, 1479–1481
   clinical manifestations of, 1480, 1480c
   definition of, 1440
   and hair, 1930
   medical management of, 1481
   nursing process with, 1481–1484, 1483c
Cushing's triad, 2170
   definition of, 2161
Cushing's ulcers, 1210
Cut, definition of, 2528c
Cutaneous flap, for head and neck reconstruction, 1153
Cutaneous stimulation, in pain management, 288–289
Cutaneous ureterostomy, 1598f
Cutaneous urinary diversions. See Urinary diversion
CVID. See Common variable immunodeficiency
CVVH. See Continuous venovenous hemofiltration
CVVHD. See Continuous venovenous hemodialysis
Cyanide
   exposure to, management of, 2569t, 2571
   as terrorism threat, 2569t, 2571
Cyanogen chloride
   exposure to, management of, 2571
   as terrorism threat, 2571
Cyanohemoglobin, production of, in cyanide poisoning, 2571
Cyanosis, 1933, 1934, 1934f, 1935t
   assessment of, 568
   in asthma, 711
   central, 627, 798
      definition of, 625
      in pneumonia, 636
   definition of, 568
   peripheral, 798
Cyclic 3',5'-adenosine monophosphate, as second messenger, 1441
Cyclic continuous infusions, of tube feedings, 1183
Cyclic feeding, 1182
   definition of, 1175
Cyclooxygenase (COX), 284
Cyclopentolate, ocular applications of, 2086t
Cyclophosphamide
   in cancer treatment, 399t
      adverse effects and side effects of, 399t
   for chronic lymphocytic leukemia, 1074
   for idiopathic thrombocytopenic purpura, 1088
   for immune hemolytic anemia, 1062
   and immune system, 1797t
   for myasthenia gravis, 2286
   for rheumatic diseases, 1896t
   for rheumatoid arthritis, 1909
Cycloplegics, 2085, 2086t
Cycloserine, for tuberculosis, 647
Cyclosporine (Neoral)
   adverse effects and side effects of, 1561
   and immune system, 1797t
   for kidney transplant recipient, 1561
   for myasthenia gravis, 2286
   for psoriasis, 1966t, 1967
   for rheumatic diseases, 1896t
   for rheumatoid arthritis, 1909

Cylindruria, detection of, 1506
Cyst(s)
    bone, 2417
    breast, 1710–1711, 1711t
    epidermal, 1977
    epidermoid, 1977
    ovarian, 1678–1679
    pancreatic, 1369
    pilar, 1977
    pilonidal, 1277–1278
    sebaceous, 1977
    skin, 1937c
    of skin, 1977
    synovial, 1920
    trichilemmal, 1977
    vulvar, 1677–1678
Cystectomy
    for bladder cancer, 1596–1597
    definition of, 1570
Cystic duct, 1286
    anatomy of, 1345, 1346f
Cystic fibrosis, 141, 718–719
    carrier testing for, 150t, 156
    clinical manifestations of
        nonpulmonary, 718
        pulmonary, 718
    genetics of, 146, 147, 147t, 718
    genetic testing in, 150t
    nursing management of, 719
    pathophysiology of, 718
    and pneumonia, 635
    screening for, 150t
Cystitis, 1570
    definition of, 1570
    interstitial. *See* Interstitial cystitis
    in males, 1750
    signs and symptoms of, 1572
Cystocele, 1505, 1624, 1674–1675, 1674f
    definition of, 1613, 1661
Cystography, 1509
Cystolitholapaxy, for urolithiasis, 1593
Cystosarcoma phyllodes, 1711
Cystoscopy, 1509–1510, 1509f
    for urolithiasis, 1591–1593, 1592f
Cystostomy, for urolithiasis, 1593
Cytarabine
    for acute myeloid leukemia, 1071–1072
    for cancer treatment, 399t
Cytochrome P450, variations, clinical effects of, 153–154, 154t
Cytokines. *See also* Biochemical mediators
    actions of, 1791t
    in cancer treatment, 418–420
        adverse effects and side effects of, 421t
    in cellular immune response, 1791, 1791t
    definition of, 381, 1036, 1783, 1887
    and HIV infection, 1822
    and myelopoiesis, 1041
    in rheumatoid arthritis, 1908
    and wasting syndrome, 1832
Cytolysis, complement system and, 1793t
Cytomegalovirus, 1667
    blood testing for, 1106
    and cancer, 385
    definition of, 1815
    gene products, and HIV infection, 1822
    and Guillain-Barré syndrome, 2288
    incubation period of, 2476t
    infection
        in HIV-infected (AIDS) patients, 1833
        with long-term PRBC therapy, 1111t
    pneumonia caused by, 629, 631t
    retinitis caused by, 2083–2084
        in HIV-infected (AIDS) patients, 1835–1836

transfusion-transmitted, 1104t
transmission of, 2476t
Cytophilic antibody, action of, 1791t
Cytosine (C), 141
Cytotoxic agents
    definition of, 1945
    and immune system, 1797t
    for myasthenia gravis, 2286
Cytotoxic factor, action of, 1791t
Cytotoxic (type II) hypersensitivity, 1859–1860, 1860f
Cytotoxic T cells, 1787, 1791, 1792t
    definition of, 1783
    functions of, 1787–1788

## D

Dacarbazine, in cancer treatment, 399t
Dactinomycin
    in cancer treatment, 399t
    and immune system, 1797t
Dakin's solution, for burns, 2017
Danazol (Cyclomen, Danocrine), for immune hemolytic anemia, 1062
Dantrolene (Dantrium)
    for malignant hyperthermia, 517
    for spasticity, in multiple sclerosis, 2280
Darbopoetin alfa (Aranesp), 1051
    in breast cancer treatment, 1728
Darvon. *See* Propoxyphene
DASH, and prevention of hypertension, 1025, 1025t
Daunomycin, for chronic myeloid leukemia, 1073
Daunorubicin
    for acute myeloid leukemia, 1071
    in cancer treatment, 399t
        adverse effects and side effects of, 399t
Day care, adult, 249
D & C. *See* Dilation and curettage
DCIS. *See* Ductal carcinoma in situ
DDAVP. *See* Desmopressin
D-dimer
    definition of, 1036
    in disseminated intravascular coagulation, 1093
D-dimer assay, with pulmonary embolism, 663
D & E. *See* Dilation and evacuation
Dead space
    physiologic, 556
        definition of, 553
    in surgical wound, 538
    and ventilation-perfusion ratio, 559, 559c
Deaf-blind persons, interacting and communicating with, 180c
Deafness, definition of, 2093
Deaf persons, interacting and communicating with, 180c
Death
    anxiety about, nursing interventions for, in disseminated intravascular coagulation, 1098c
    causes of, among older adults, 226, 226t
    pronouncement (determination) of, 469
Death and dying, 122, 468–473. *See also* End-of-life care
    and after-death care, 469–471
    anticipation of, coping with, 471, 472t
    approaching, signs of, 469, 470c
    chronic illness and, 171t
    clinicians' attitudes toward, 449–450
    context for, 448–449
    denial of, 450

patient close to
    nursing care of, 468–473
    physiologic changes in, 469, 470c
    professional caregivers' coping with, 473–474
    sociocultural context of, 449–452
Death vigil, 469
Débridement
    autolytic, 1946
    for burns, 2018–2019
        mechanical, 2019
        natural, 2019
        surgical, 2019
    definition of, 1945, 1995, 2425
    enzymatic, 1946
    for open fracture, 2434
    for pressure ulcers, 214
    for rotator cuff tear, 2429
Debriefing
    definition of, 2564
    emergency, 2564
Decerebration (decerebrate posturing), 2142, 2164, 2164f, 2166t
    definition of, 2161
Decibel, 2100
Decisional conflict
    nursing diagnoses related to, 1610–1611
    nursing interventions for, 1610–1611
    nursing outcomes for, 1610–1611
Decision-making
    in end-of-life care, 461, 462f
    surgery for breast cancer and, 1719
Decompression, intestinal
    definition of, 1175
    tubes for, 1176
Decompression sickness, 2537
Deconditioning, in acute leukemia, nursing interventions for, 1077
Decongestants
    adrenergic, 1870–1872, 1872t
    precautions with, 593
    for sinusitis, 595
    for viral rhinitis, 592–593
Decontamination, 2565
    definition of, 2559
    for nerve agent exposure, 2570
    after radiation exposure, 2572–2573
    of skin, 2543–2544
Decortication (decorticate posturing), 2142, 2164, 2164f, 2166t
    definition of, 2161
Deep brain stimulation
    for epilepsy, 2195
    in pain management, 291
    for Parkinson's disease, 2315, 2315f
Deep-breathing
    postoperative, 534
    preoperative teaching about, 492–493, 494c
Deep vein thrombosis, 1004–1010
    cerebral metastases and, 2307
    clinical manifestations of, 1005
    fracture and, 2438, 2448
    hip fracture and, 2456c–2457c
    with hysterectomy, 1693
    in orthopedic surgery patient, 2375, 2385, 2387
    pathophysiology of, 1004–1005
    postoperative
        prevention of, 545
        risk factors for, 544, 544c
    prevention of, 1006
        after hip replacement, 2375
    with prostatectomy, 1766
    and pulmonary embolism, 662
    in renal surgical patient, 1559

risk factors for, 1004c
signs and symptoms of, 545
spinal cord injury and, 2256, 2259
total hip replacement and, 2375, 2380c
in unconscious patient, 2169
in vulvar surgical patient, 1687
Defecation, 1125
Defecography, 1138
Defibrillation, 842–844, 842f, 843f
definition of, 823
multifunction pads for, 842, 843f
for ventricular fibrillation, 837
for ventricular tachycardia, 836
Deformity, fracture and, 2431
Defusing, in critical incident stress management, 2564
Degenerative disk disease, 2324–2325
clinical manifestations of, 2325
diagnosis of, 2325
pathophysiology of, 2324–2325
Degenerative joint disease, 1914–1917
and temporomandibular disorders, 1146
Dehiscence, wound, 546, 546f
definition of, 524
Dehydration
diarrheal diseases and, 2503
during gastrointestinal intubation, 1180
in infectious disease, prevention of, 2499c
mild, 2503
moderate, 2503
in older persons, hip fracture and, 2447
rehydration therapy for, 2503
severe, 2503
in tube feedings, 1184t
Delavirdine (Rescriptor), for HIV infection, 1827t
Delayed-type hypersensitivity, 1791, 1860–1861, 1861f
Delayed union, of fracture, 2438–2439
definition of, 2425
Delirium
definition of, 225, 2129
versus dementia, 241–243, 242t–243t
gerontologic considerations in, 240–243
management of, 243
postcardiotomy, 900–901, 908c–909c
postoperative, 546–547, 547c
in terminally ill patients, 468
Delirium tremens
emergency management of, 2549–2550
postoperative, 486
Demand oxygen delivery systems, 727
Dementia, 243–246. See also Alzheimer's disease
Alzheimer's type, 243–246
anxiety and agitation in, 245
assessment of, 244
caregivers of people with, intervention for, nursing research on, 2322
causes of, 242t, 243
clinical manifestations of, 244
cognition in, 244, 245
communication with patients with, 244, 245
definition of, 225, 2301
versus delirium, 241–243, 242t–243t
versus depression, 239–240
diagnosis of, 244
diagnostic criteria for, 243
home and community-based care for, 246
in Huntington's disease, 2319
and intimacy needs, 245
medical management of, 244
multi-infarct, 242t–243t, 246
nursing management of, 244–246

and nutrition, 245–246
in Parkinson's disease, 2313
pathophysiology of, 243–244
prevalence of, 243
safety of patients with, 245
and self-care, 245
socialization of patients with, 245
symptoms of, 242t–243t, 243
vascular, 242t–243t, 246
Demerol. See Meperidine
Demographics, and health care delivery, 7, 16
Demyelination
in Guillain-Barré syndrome, 2288
in multiple sclerosis, 2278, 2278f, 2281, 2281f
Dendrite(s), 2129, 2130f
definition of, 2129
Dendritic cells, in natural immunity, 1785
Dengue fever, immigration and, 2512
Denial
in family members of emergency patient, 2519
as stage of dying, 472t
of terminal illness, 450
Dental abscess, 1145–1146
blind, 1145
Dental caries, 1142–1145
prevention of, 1142–1145, 1145c
treatment for, 1142
Dental decay. See Dental caries; Tooth decay
Dental plaque, 1142–1145
Dentoalveolar abscess, 1145–1146
chronic, 1145
Denture care, 1149, 1150c
Deoxyribonucleic acid (DNA), 141, 143f. See also Gene(s)
definition of, 140
of HIV, 1821
mutations of. See Gene(s), mutations of
radiation and, 394
recombinant, 1793
Department of Homeland Security, 2559
Dependence, opioid, definition of, 259
Depolarization, 784, 784f, 824
definition of, 781, 823
on ECG, 826, 827f
Depo-Provera, 1644
Depression, 118–120
definition of, 112, 225
diagnostic criteria for, 118, 119c
disability and, 178c
gerontologic considerations in, 238–240
versus grief, 122
in HIV-infected (AIDS) patients, 1833
treatment of, 1836
in laryngectomy patient, 615
in melanoma, 1983–1984
nursing interventions for, 118–120
in older persons, treatment of, 240
pain and, 266–267
in Parkinson's disease, 2313
as psychiatric emergency, 2554–2555
resources and websites on, 126
risk factors for, 118, 119c
signs and symptoms of, 118
somatic complaints in, 118
as stage of dying, 472t
in stroke patient, 2222
in terminally ill patients, 468
Dermabrasion, 1988–1989
for acne, 1955
Dermagraf, 1948
Dermal substitutes, for burn grafts, 2020t, 2022, 2023f
Dermatitis, 1948, 1949

atopic, 1877–1878
contact, 1877, 1877t
distribution of, 1940f
of lips, 1143t
definition of, 1945
exfoliative, 1970–1971
seborrheic. See Seborrheic dermatitis
Dermatitis herpetiformis, 1972
Dermatitis medicamentosa, 1878
Dermatofibroma, 1978
Dermatologic problems, 1944–1992. See also Skin conditions
of foot, 2401
Dermatomes, 2137, 2138f
Dermatoses
definition of, 1927, 1936, 1945
infectious, 1956–1964
noninfectious inflammatory, 1965–1968
Dermis, 1927, 1928, 1928f
definition of, 1995
Dermis-epidermis junction, 1930
Dermoid cysts, 1678–1679
conjunctival, 2080
definition of, 1661
orbital, 2080
Dermolipoma, of conjunctiva, 2080
DES. See Diethylstilbestrol
Descemet's membrane, 2044, 2045f
Descending colon, 1122f
Desflurane (Suprane), 510t
Desipramine (Norpramin), for depression, in HIV-infected (AIDS) patients, 1836
Desloratidine (Clarinex), 1871t
Desmopressin (DDAVP), 1448
for diabetes insipidus, 320
for hemophilia, 1091
and von Willebrand's disease, 1092
Desquamation, 1152
Detoxification
for ingested poison, 2541
for inhaled poison, 2543
Detrusor hyperactivity with impaired contractility, 247
Detrusor instability, 247
Detrusor muscle, in micturition, 1500
Developmental stages, adult, 115, 115c
Developmental theories, of aging, 227
Deviation
radial, 200c
ulnar, 200c
DEXA. See Dual-energy x-ray absorptiometry
Dexamethasone, 1485t
for appetite stimulation, 466
for idiopathic thrombocytopenic purpura, 1088
Dextran
for fluid replacement in shock, 367t
in normal saline, 312t
Dextroamphetamine (Dexedrine), abuse/overdose, emergency management of, 2546t
Dextromethorphan
for pharyngitis, 598
precautions with, 593
Dextrose, in peripheral parenteral nutrition, 1193
Dextrose (5%), in water ($D_5W$), 311t
Diabetes Control and Complications Trial (DCCT), 1383, 1393–1396
Diabetes insipidus, 1446, 1447–1448, 2180
brain injury and, 2244
definition of, 1440
hypernatremia in, 320
medical management of, 320
nursing management of, 320–321

Diabetes mellitus
  adult-onset. *See* Diabetes mellitus, type 2
  alcohol consumption in, 1387
  assessment in, 1382, 1383c
  associated with other syndromes or conditions, 1379t
    nursing process with, 1202–1205
  blood glucose monitoring in, 1389–1391
  and blood pressure, 1023
  caloric requirements in, 1385
  cardiac involvement in, 861, 862f
  classification of, 1377–1378, 1379t–1380t
  clinical manifestations of, 1382
  complications of, 1378, 1383
    acute, 1410–1416
    long-term, 1421–1429
    macrovascular, 1421–1422
    microvascular, 1422–1427
    nursing diagnoses related to, 1282–1283
    nursing interventions for, 1282–1283
    nursing outcomes for, 1282–1283
    ocular, 1422, 1423t
  costs of, 1377
  definition of, 1376
  diagnostic criteria for, 1382, 1382c
  epidemiology of, 1377
  exercise in, 1388–1389, 1388c
  foot and leg problems in, 1427–1428, 1428f, 2401
  foot care in, 1419, 1419c, 1427–1429, 1429f
  genetics of, 147, 147t
  gerontologic considerations in, 1382–1383, 1432–1433
  gestational. *See* Gestational diabetes mellitus
  glucose control in, 1383–1384
    perioperative, 1429, 1430c
  and heart disease, 866
  hemochromatosis and, 1063
  hospitalized patient with, 1429–1432
    diet for, 1431–1432
    hyperglycemia in, 1430–1431
    hypoglycemia in, 1431
  and immune system function, 1796
  insulin-dependent. *See* Diabetes mellitus, type 1
  juvenile. *See* Diabetes mellitus, type 1
  management of, 1383–1402. *See also* Insulin therapy
    components of, 1384, 1384f
    gerontologic considerations in, 1389, 1389c
    perioperative, 488
    sick day rules for, 1413, 1414c
  meal planning in, 1384–1387
  metabolic syndrome in, 861, 862f
  newly diagnosed, nursing process in, 1416–1421
  non–insulin-dependent. *See* Diabetes mellitus, type 2
  nurse-directed care for, in minority population, nursing research on, 1378
  nursing management of, 1402–1410
  nutritional management of
    caloric distribution in, 1385–1386
    exchange lists for, 1386–1387, 1386t
    food classification systems for, 1386–1387
    Food Guide Pyramid and, 1387
    food labels and, 1387, 1388
    glycemic index and, 1387
    for hospitalized patient, 1431–1432
    patient teaching about, 1384–1387
  nutritional therapy in, 1384–1388
  ocular involvement in, 2083. *See also* Retinopathy, diabetic
  pathophysiology of, 1378–1382
  patient teaching about, 1402–1404
    continuing education in, 1404
    for experienced patients, 1406
    implementation of, 1406–1410
    in-depth, 1404
    methods for, 1404
    and readiness to learn, 1404
    survival information in, 1403–1404
    teaching plan for, 1402–1404
    via telemedicine versus in person, nursing research on, 1403
  perioperative management of, 1429, 1430c
  and pes cavus, 2402
  pharmacologic therapy for, 1391–1402. *See also* Insulin therapy
  and pressure ulcers, 208
  risk factors for, 1377, 1377c
  as secondary diagnosis (associated with other syndromes or conditions), 1379t
    nursing process with, 1433–1435
  self-care in
    for hospitalized patient, 1429–1430
    nursing interventions for, 1418–1419, 1419c
  skin disorders in, 1941
  type 1, 1377–1378, 1379t
    definition of, 1376
    pathophysiology of, 1380
  type 2, 151t, 1377–1378, 1379t
    definition of, 1376
    pathogenesis of, 1381, 1381f
    pathophysiology of, 1381
    population screening for, 153
    prevention of, 1381, 1381c
Diabetic dermopathy, 1941
Diabetic ketoacidosis, 1376, 1412–1415, 1418
  definition of, 1376
  and hyperglycemic hyperosmolar nonketotic syndrome, comparison of, 1415t
  pathophysiology of, 1412, 1413f
  prevention of, 1413, 1414c
Diagnosis
  of life-threatening illness, patient and family receiving, nursing interventions for, 458
  nursing. *See* Nursing diagnoses
  in nursing process, 34, 35–39, 36c
  withholding information about from patient, ethical considerations in, 31–32
Diagnosis-related groups, 8, 16
*Diagnostic and Statistical Manual of Mental Disorders,* 114
  diagnostic criteria, for depression, 118, 119c
Diagnostic studies, 2577–2601
Dialysate
  definition of, 1515, 1538
  leakage of, in peritoneal dialysis, 1547
Dialysis, 1531–1537, 1531–1552. *See also* Hemodialysis; Peritoneal dialysis
  for acute renal failure, 1525
  catheter site care for, 1552
  chronic, 1537
  for chronic glomerulonephritis, 1519
  for chronic renal failure, 1530
  high-flux, 1538–1539
  hospitalized patient on, nursing interventions for, 1551–1552
  indications for, 1537
  intravenous therapy during, nursing interventions for, 1551
  before kidney transplantation, 1537
  maintenance, 1537
  medication administration during, 1552
  psychological support for patient on, 1552
  vascular access for, nursing interventions for, 1551
Dialyzer, 1537–1539
  definition of, 1515
Diaphragm (contraceptive), 1644
Diaphragm (muscle), 1122f
Diaphragmatic breathing
  for low back pain, 2394
  preoperative teaching about, 494c
Diaphragmatic excursion, 573–574
Diaphragmatic hiatus, 1121
Diaphragmatic pacing, for spinal cord injury, 2254
Diaphragm sellae, 2133
Diaphysis, 2338, 2338f
  definition of, 2337
DIAPPERS mnemonic, 1580c
Diarrhea/diarrheal diseases, 1127, 2492–2504
  acute, 1235
  assessment in, 1235, 2502–2503
  bacteremia in, 2504
  bacterial, causes of, 2476t
  calcivirus and, 2501–2502
  *Camplyobacter* and, 2501
  causes of, 1235, 2501–2502
  in chemotherapy patient, 400
  chronic, 1235
  clinical manifestations of, 1235
  in colorectal cancer, 1266
  complications of, 1236, 2503, 2504
  definition of, 1235
  dehydration in, 2503
  diagnosis of, 1235
  drug-induced, 1235
  *Escherichia coli* and, 2501
  expected outcomes in, 2504
  gerontologic considerations in, 1236
  *Giardia lamblia* and, 2502
  in HIV-infected (AIDS) patients, 1831–1832, 1846
    nursing interventions for, 1838c
    treatment of, 1836
  and hypovolemic shock, 2504
  medical management of, 1236
  norovirus and, 2501–2502
  nursing diagnoses related to, 1118–1119, 2503
  nursing interventions for, 1118–1119
    in HIV-infected (AIDS) patients, 1838c
  nursing interventions in, 2503–2504
  nursing management of, 1236
  nursing outcomes with, 1118–1119
  nursing process for, 2502–2504
  pathophysiology of, 1235
  patient teaching about, 2503–2504
  planning and goals for, 2503
  prevention of, 2503–2504
  rehydration therapy in, 2503
  *Salmonella* and, 2501
  *Shigella* and, 2501
  transmission of, 2492
    prevention of, 2503–2504
  in tube feedings, 1184t, 1186
  *Vibrio cholerae* and, 2502
Diarthrodial joints, definition of, 1887
Diarthrosis joints, 2340, 2341
Diastole, 781, 785, 786, 802–803, 802f, 824–825
  definition of, 781
Diazepam (Valium)
  abuse/overdose, emergency management of, 2547t

## INDEX

interactions with anesthetics, 490t
for intravenous anesthesia, 513t
metabolism of, genetic factors affecting, 154t
for nerve agent exposure, 2571
for status epilepticus, 2198
therapeutic blood levels of, 2601t
DIC. *See* Disseminated intravascular coagulation
Diclofenac (Voltaren), for rheumatic diseases, 1895t
Didanosine (Videx, Videx EC), for HIV infection, 1827t
Dietary Approaches to Stop Hypertension (DASH) Diet, 1025, 1025t
Dietary practices, culture and, 133, 133c
Diet/dietary therapy. *See also* Nutrition/nutritional support
  in acute glomerulonephritis, 1518
  in acute renal failure, 1525–1526
  for ascites, 1294
  assessment of, 80–83
  and bone health, 2339
  and cancer, 386
  in cancer treatment, 423
  for chronic glomerulonephritis, 1519
  in chronic renal failure, 1530
  clear liquid, in diabetes mellitus, for hospitalized patient, 1431–1432
  culture and, 133, 133c
  in gastroesophageal reflux disease, 1166
  gerontologic considerations in, 234–235
  hemodialysis and, 1540–1541
  in hypertension, 1031
  low-fat, 985
  and lung cancer, 671
  for Ménière's disease, 2113, 2113c
  in nephrotic syndrome, 1521
  in prevention of atherosclerosis, 863–864, 864t
  and prevention of hypertension, 1025, 1025t
  in prevention of tooth decay, 1145
  religion and, 133, 133c
  for ulcer patient, 1212
Diethylstilbestrol, and cancer, 386
Differential, 424
Differentiation, definition of, 1036
Diffuse axonal injury, 2236
Diffuse connective tissue diseases, 1906–1914
  systemic nature of, 1888
Diffuse idiopathic skeletal hyperostosis (DISH), 1920
Diffusion, 303, 303f, 557–558
  definition of, 301, 553, 1515
  in hemodialysis, 1537
Diflusinal (Dolobid), for rheumatic diseases, 1895t
diGeorge syndrome. *See* Thymic hypoplasia
Digestion/digestive function, 1122–1125, 1125
  age-related changes in, 1139
  assessment of, 1126–1129
  definition of, 1121
  diagnostic assessment of, 1129–1139
  genetic factors affecting, 1131
  pathophysiologic considerations in, 1139
  psychological considerations in, 1139
  regulatory substances of, 1124t
  waste products of, 1125
Digestive enzymes
  actions of, 1123t
  sources of, 1123t
Digestive function. *See* Digestion/digestive function

Digestive secretions
  actions of, 1123t
  sources of, 1123t
Digestive system, functions of, 1122–1125
Digitalis, 954–955. *See also* Digoxin
  for atrioventricular (AV) nodal reentry tachycardia, 835
  toxicity of, 324
    calcium and, 328
Digital rectal examination, 1504, 1742, 1743, 1744f, 1753
Digoxin. *See also* Digitalis
  for atrial fibrillation, 833
  for atrial flutter, 832
  reversal of, 956c
  therapeutic blood levels of, 2601t
  toxicity of, 956c, 957
  use of, 956c
Dihydropyridines, for hypertension, 1029t
Dilation, esophageal
  for achalasia, 1162, 1163f
  for esophageal spasm, 1162
Dilation and curettage, 1630
Dilation and evacuation (D & E), 1648, 1649c
Diltiazem, 830t, 870, 955
  for atrial fibrillation, 833
  for atrial flutter, 832
  for atrioventricular (AV) nodal reentry tachycardia, 83
  for hypertension, 1029t
  long-acting (Cardizem LA), for hypertension, 1029t
  mechanism of action of, 785
Dilutional hyponatremia, 315, 1448
  definition of, 1440
Dimenhydrinate (Dramamine), 2112
  postoperative use of, 528
Dipeptidase, source and digestive action of, 1123t
Diphenhydramine, 1859, 1871t
  and amphotericin B therapy, 2276
  for anaphylactic shock, 376
  for Parkinson's disease, 2314
  for pruritus, 1952
  for sinusitis, 595
Dipivefrin, for glaucoma, 2057, 2058t
Diploid cell(s), 143
  definition of, 140
Diplopia, 2143
  with brain tumor, 2304
  definition of, 2043
  in multiple sclerosis, 2279, 2282
  in myasthenia gravis, 2285, 2288
  stroke and, 2208t
Dipyridamole (Persantin)
  in cardiac stress testing, 810–811
  for peripheral arterial disease, 992
  and stroke prevention, 2211
Disability(ies)
  and access to health care, 177–183
  acquired, 175
  and activities of daily living, 175
  age-associated, 175
  among older persons, 191, 191c, 226, 250–251
  assessment of people with, 72c
  biopsychosocial model of, 176, 177c
  categories of, 175
  characteristics of, 175–176
  chronic illness and, 166
  coping with, 219c
  definition of, 166, 174–175, 190
  and depression, 178c
  developmental, 175
  versus disabling disorders, 162

and fatigue, 218–219
gerontologic considerations in, 184, 191, 191c
and health care, 8
  barriers in, 182
  federal legislation addressing, 176–177
interface model of, 176, 177c
learning, 175
limitations imposed by, helping patients accept, 195
medical model of, 176, 177c
in medical-surgical nursing practice, 184–185
models of, 176, 177c
older adults with, concerns of, 191, 191c
patients' reactions to, 191
"people-first" language and, 184
people with
  communicating with, 177, 178c, 179c–181c
  complementary therapies for, 219
  continuing care for, 185, 221–222
  federal assistance programs for, 182–183
  health care for, barriers to, 178c, 182
  home and community-based care for, 185
  hospitalization of, nursing considerations in, 183
  independence versus dependence of, 179c
  insurance coverage for, 179c
  interacting with, 177, 179c–181c
  nursing care of, 183–185
  pain assessment in, 275
  patient teaching for, 52–53, 53t, 179c
people with, caring for
  in disaster, 2563c
  in disasters, 2563
physical or mental, in patient profile, 69c, 71
prevalence of, 175, 191
rehabilitation model of, 176, 177c
self-care in, patient teaching about, 185
sensory, 175
severe
  definition of, 191
  prevalence of, 191
and sexuality issues, 218
social model of, 176, 177c
speech/language, 175
in surgical patient, nursing management of, 492
temporary, 175
types of, 175
women with
  assessment of, 1622–1623, 1623c
  breast health of, 1735
  health issues of, 1622–1623
  predicting risk of osteoporosis in, nursing research on, 2407
Disarticulation, definition of, 2425
Disaster(s)
  at risk populations in, caring for, 2563
  levels of, 2559c
  natural, 2565–2566
  psychological responses to, 2564
  victims of
    behavioral issues in, nursing interventions for, 2564
    identification of, 2561
    triage of, 2521, 2561–2562
Disaster management, 2559
Disaster Medical Assistance Teams, 2560
Disaster Mortuary Response Teams, 2560
Disaster response plans, nurse's role in, 2563–2564

Discectomy
  cervical, nursing process with, 2326–2329
  in degenerative disk disease, 2325
  with fusion, 2325
Discharge planning
  for emergency patient, 2520
  for home care, 18
Discoloration, fracture and, 2431
Discomfort, management of. See also Pain management
  in hospitalized dialysis patient, 1552
  with prostatectomy, 1765
  with vulvovaginal infection, 1665
Disease(s). See also Illness
  changing patterns of, and health care, 7–8
  chronic, and health care, 8
  definition of, 92
  maladaptation and, 97
  stress and, 93, 97–98
Disease-modifying antirheumatic drugs (DMARDs), for rheumatoid arthritis, 1908–1909
Disequilibrium, 247
Disinfection
  for calcivirus, 2502
  of skin, 2484
Dislocation, of joint, 2426
  definition of, 2425
  sports-related, 2426–2427
Disopyramide (Norpace), 830t
  for atrial fibrillation, 833
Dissection
  definition of, 975
  vascular, in percutaneous transluminal angioplasty, 986
Disseminated intravascular coagulation, 1087t, 1093–1095, 1096c–1098c
  bleeding in, 1093–1094, 1094c
  in cancer patient, 440t–441t
  clinical manifestations of, 1093, 1094c
  complications of, 1095
  fracture and, 2438
  intraoperative, 517–518
  laboratory findings in, 1093, 1093t
  medical management of, 1093–1094
  nursing care plan for, 1096c–1098c
  nursing diagnoses related to, 1095, 1096c–1098c
  nursing interventions for, 1096c–1098c
  nursing process with, 1094–1095, 1096c–1098c
  pathophysiology of, 1093
  risk factors for, 1094
  thrombosis in, 1095
    treatment of, 1093–1094
Dissolution therapy
  definition of, 1345
  for gallstones, 1352
Distal convoluted tubule, 1495f
Distraction, in pain management, 289
Distribution, of drugs, age-related changes in, 238, 239t
Distributive justice, 28c
Disuse syndrome
  casts and, 2360
  in paraplegia/quadriplegia, prevention of, 2263
Diuresis, 1497
  for acute renal failure, 1525
  hyperosmolar, in parenteral nutrition, 1198
  osmotic, 303
Diuretics
  adverse effects and side effects of, 953
  for ascites, 1294–1295
  and calcium balance, 327
  for cardiogenic shock, 370, 966
  for cerebral edema, 2173
  for heart failure, 953, 954t, 955c, 965
  for hypermagnesemia, 331
  for hypertension, 1026t
  for hypervolemia, 313–314
  and hypokalemia, 321
  interactions with anesthetics, 490t
  loop, for hypertension, 1026t
  and potassium balance, 313–314, 321, 325
  potassium-sparing, 325
    for hypertension, 1026t
  thiazide
    for hypertension, 1026t
    and stroke prevention, 2211
Divalproex (Valproate), in migraine prevention, 2200
Diversion therapy, for low back pain, 2394
Diverticular disease, 1242–1244
  gerontologic considerations in, 1243
Diverticulitis, 1243
  definition of, 1232
  nursing process in, 1244–1245
  surgical management of, 1244, 1244f
Diverticulosis, definition of, 1232, 1242
Diverticulum
  definition of, 1232, 1242
  esophageal, 1164
  pharyngoesophageal pulsion, 1164
  Zenker's, 1164
Diving medicine, 2537
Dizziness, 2112, 2143
  in cardiovascular disease, assessment of, 790, 794t
  definition of, 2093
  in older persons, 247
DKA. See Diabetic ketoacidosis
DNA. See Deoxyribonucleic acid
DNA binding test, in rheumatic diseases, 1893t
DNA testing, in gastrointestinal assessment, 1131
DNR (do-not-resuscitate) orders, ethical considerations with, 32, 518c
Dobbhoff tube, 1176t
Dobutamine (Dobutrex)
  and cardiac output, 2173
  in cardiac stress testing, 811
  for cardiogenic shock, 966
  for heart failure, 955, 965
  for shock, 366t, 370
Docetaxel, for cancer treatment, 399t
Documentation
  of abdominal examination, 1127
  of assessment, 35
  of assessment data, 35, 64
  of burn wound, 2004
  of forensic evidence, 2529–2530
  of outcomes, 43
  of preoperative checklist, 497, 497f, 498f
Dofetilide (Tikosyn), 830t
Dolasetron, for chemotherapy patient, 398
Domestic violence, 1620–1622, 1621c. See also Abuse
Dominant, definition of, 140, 145
Domperidone (Motilium), for gastroesophageal reflux disease, 1166
Donepezil (Aricept)
  for Alzheimer's disease, 244
  for vascular dementia, 246
Donor lymphocyte infusion, 1113
Donor site
  definition of, 1995
  for skin graft, care of, 2024
Do-not-resuscitate orders, ethical considerations with, 32, 518c
Door-to-balloon time, 877
Dopamine, 2130t
  for anaphylaxis, 2538
  for cardiogenic shock, 366t, 370, 966
Dopamine agonists, for Parkinson's disease, 2314
Doppler ultrasound
  flow studies
    in peripheral vascular disease, 982f
  in vascular disease, 980–982
  transcranial, 2155, 2181
Dornase alfa (Pulmozyme), for cystic fibrosis, 719
Dorsal position. See Supine position
Dorsiflexion, 200c
  definition of, 198c
Dorzolamide, for glaucoma, 2057, 2058t
Dose-dense chemotherapy
  for breast cancer, 1727
  definition of, 1701
Double-contrast barium enema, 1132
Double-contrast study, of upper gastrointestinal tract, 1132
Double effect
  ethical principle of, 28c
  principle of, 32
Douche, 1665
  definition of, 1661
Down syndrome, 143
  diagnosis of, 150t
  genetics of, 148
  prenatal diagnosis of, 148–149, 150t
Doxazosin (Cardura), for hypertension, 1028t
Doxepin
  abuse/overdose, emergency management of, 2548t
  for pruritus, 1952
  therapeutic blood levels of, 2601t
Doxorubicin (Adriamycin)
  in cancer treatment, 399t
    adverse effects and side effects of, 399t
  for chronic lymphocytic leukemia, 1074
Doxycycline
  for chlamydia, 1670, 2508
  for pneumonia, 636, 637
  for syphilis, 2506
Drain(s), wound, 538, 538f
Drainage implants/shunts, for glaucoma, 2058
DRE. See Digital rectal examination
Dressing(s)
  active, 1945–1946
  for amputation, 2461–2462, 2464, 2465f, 2466f
  for burns, 2017–2018
    biologic, 2019–2021, 2020t
    biosynthetic, 2020t, 2021–2022
    changing, 2017–2018
    occlusive, 2017
    synthetic, 2020t, 2021–2022
  categories of, 1946–1948, 1947t
  categorization of, 1946
  changes, 1946
    in parenteral nutrition, 1198
  evolution of, 1946
  foam, 1948
  functions of, 1946–1948, 1947t
  interactive, 1945–1946
  moisture-retentive, 1947–1948
  nursing management of, 540, 1950–1951
  occlusive, 1946–1947
    for psoriasis, 1967
  passive, 1945
  practice with, 1946

selection of, 1946
wet, 1947
and wound healing, 541t
DRG. See Diagnosis-related groups
Drinker respirator tank, 742
drip mnemonic, 247
Driving, by older persons, 236
Dromotropy, 825
definition of, 823
Dronabinol (Marinol)
for appetite stimulation, 466
for HIV-infected (AIDS) patients, 1836
Droplet Precautions, 2482, 2483c
Drop rate, in intravenous therapy, 345–346
Drotrecogin alfa (Xigris), for septic shock, 374
Drowning, 2536–2537
Drug(s). See also Medication(s)
abuse of. See Substance abuse
administration of, culturally competent, 133–134
anaphylactic reaction to, 2537–2538
aplastic anemia caused by, 1051
cellular injury caused by, 102
extensive metabolizers of, 153
with hemolytic effects, in glucose-6-phosphate dehydrogenase (G6PD) deficiency, 1061
hepatitis caused by, 1316–1317
intermediate metabolizers of, 153
metabolism of
genetic factors affecting, 153–154
liver in, 1286–1287
and pain management, 269
and osteoporosis, 2405
overdose, emergency management of, 2545t–2548t
and platelet function, 1089, 1090c
poor metabolizers of, 153
therapeutic levels (conventional units and SI units), 2601t
toxic blood levels of, 2601t
ultrarapid metabolizers of, 153
use and abuse, assessment for, 70c
Drug resistance
multidrug, 647
primary, 647
secondary (acquired), 647
in tuberculosis, 647
Drusen, 2048, 2069, 2069f
Dry eye syndrome, 2075–2076
Dry mouth, 1151
Dual-energy x-ray absorptiometry, in osteoporosis, 2407, 2449
Dubos, Rene Jules, 92
Duchenne muscular dystrophy, genetics of, 144, 146, 147t
Ductal carcinoma in situ, 1712
definition of, 1701
Dullness, on percussion, 76
Duloxetine (Cymbalta), for diabetic neuropathy, 1427
Dumping syndrome
definition of, 1175, 1204, 1225
after gastric surgery, 1225–1226
in tube feeding, 1184t, 1186–1187
confirmation of, 1186–1187
prevention of, 1187c
Duodenal tumors, 1227
Duodenal ulcers, 1209–1217, 1210t. See also Peptic ulcer disease
Duodenum, 1121, 1122f
definition of, 1175, 1204
feeding tubes in, 1175
function of, 1124
DuoDerm, for burn grafts, 2022

Dupuytren's contracture, 2399, 2399f
Durable medical power of attorney, 457
Durable power of attorney, 251
definition of, 225
for health care, 33
Duragesic. See Fentanyl
Dura mater, 2133, 2134f, 2135–2136
DVT. See Deep vein thrombosis
Dwarfism, 1446
definition of, 1440
Dying. See Death and dying
Dying person(s), bill of rights for, 451c
Dynamic cardiomyoplasty, 928
Dynamic orthoses, 207
Dysarthria
definition of, 2206
stroke and, 2208t, 2209
Dysautonomia, 917
Dyschezia, with endometriosis, 1680
Dysfibrinogenemia, 1099t
Dyskinesia
definition of, 2301
in Guillain-Barré syndrome, 2288
in Parkinson's disease, 2314
Dyslipidemia
definition of, 1021
and hypertension, 1022
Dysmenorrhea, 1617, 1638–1639
definition of, 1613
Dyspareunia, 1617, 1640
definition of, 1613
Dysphagia, 1162
in achalasia, 1162
definition of, 589, 1142, 2129
in elderly, 234
esophageal cancer and, 1167
with esophageal spasm, 1162
after gastric surgery, 1224–1225
ischemic stroke and, 2220
in laryngeal cancer, 610
with peritonsillar abscess, 600
stroke and, 2208t
Dysphasia, stroke and, 2209
Dysphonia
definition of, 2301
myasthenia gravis and, 2285
in Parkinson's disease, 2313
Dysplasia, 100, 100t, 383
in Barrett's esophagus, 1166
of blood cells, 1054
cervical
in HIV-infected (AIDS) patients, 1672
HPV and, 1666
definition of, 91, 381, 1036, 1142, 1661
Dysplastic nevus syndrome, 1981
Dyspnea, 563–564
assessment of, 75
in asthma, 711
in cardiovascular disease, assessment of, 790, 793t
in chronic obstructive pulmonary disease, 689
clinical significance of, 563–564
definition of, 553, 563
on exertion, 950
definition of, 945
in heart failure, 950–951
in laryngeal cancer, 610
in lung cancer, 671
nursing interventions for, 673
with pulmonary embolism, 662
relief measures for, 564
in terminal illness, 465
assessment of, 465
nursing interventions for, 465, 466c

Dyspnea-anxiety-dyspnea cycle, in COPD, nursing research on, 567
Dysreflexia, autonomic
definition of, 2233
spinal cord injury and, 2259–2260
Dysrhythmia(s), cardiac, 790, 800, 823–842
ablation of, 853
adjunctive therapies for, 842–855
assessment for, 840–841
atrial, 831–833
in cardiogenic shock, 369, 370
catheter ablation therapy for, 854–855
classification of
by mechanisms of formation or conduction, 823c
by site of origin, 823c
complications of, 841
continuing care for, 841–842
definition of, 823
electrophysiologic testing with, 851–854
expected outcomes with, 842
foci of, mapping of, 853
hemochromatosis and, 1063
home and community-based care for, 841–842
incidence of, factors affecting, 825
junctional, 833–835
management of. See Antiarrhythmic agents
monitoring with, 841
nursing diagnoses related to, 841
nursing interventions for, 841–842
nursing process with, 840–842
patient teaching about, 841
planning and goals with, 841
postoperative, 528, 768
sinus node, 828–831
after thoracic surgery, 768
types of, 828–840
ventricular, 835–836
Dysuria, 1503, 1503t, 1742
definition of, 1493, 1570
in urinary tract infections, 1572

# E

Ear(s). See also Balance; Equilibrium; Hearing
anatomy of, 2093–2096, 2094f
assessment of, 2096–2099
diagnostic evaluation of, 2099–2101
functions of, 2096
infection of, 599
inner
anatomy of, 2094–2096, 2094f
conditions of, 2112–2120
definition of, 2095c
perfusion, for Ménière's disease, 2113
middle
anatomy of, 2094, 2094f
conditions of, 2106–2108
definition of, 2095c
effusion, 2107
definition of, 2093
endoscopy of, 2101
infection of, 599
masses of, 2111–2112
perfusion, for Ménière's disease, 2113
otoscopic examination of, 2098, 2098f
Eardrum. See Tympanic membrane
Eating disorder(s), resources and websites on, 126
EBCT. See Electron-beam computed tomography
Ebola virus, 2511–2512
incubation period of, 2476t
transmission of, 2476t

Ecchymosis, 798, 1929t, 1939c
  in acute myeloid leukemia, 1071
  definition of, 1036, 2528c
Eccrine sweat glands, 1930
ECF-A. *See* Eosinophil chemotactic factor of anaphylaxis
Echocardiography, 811–812, 951
  in myocardial infarction, 876
  with pulmonary hypertension, 660
Economics, and health care, 8
Ecstasy (drug), abuse/overdose, emergency management of, 2545t–2546t
Ectopic pregnancy, 1653–1657
  clinical manifestations of, 1653–1654
  diagnosis of, 1654
  nursing process with, 1654–1656
  pelvic inflammatory disease and, 1671
  pharmacologic treatment of, 1654
  sexually transmitted disease and, 2509
  sites of, 1653, 1653f
  surgical treatment of, 1654
Eczema herpeticum, 1960
ED. *See* Emergency department; Erectile dysfunction
Edatrexate, for cancer treatment, 399t
Edema, 979, 1505. *See also* Cerebral edema; Lymphedema; Pulmonary edema
  in acute glomerulonephritis, 1517
  angioneurotic. *See* Angioneurotic edema
  burns and, 1999
  in cardiovascular disease, assessment of, 793t
  causes of, 314–315
  in chronic glomerulonephritis, 1519
  in chronic renal failure, 1529
  in cirrhosis, 1319
  definition of, 2355
  fracture and, 2431
  with fractures, 2357
  in heart failure, 951, 951f
  laryngeal, 608
  in liver disease, 1307
  management of, 314–315
  in nephrotic syndrome, 1520–1521
  pain caused by, in patient in cast, 2357
  patient teaching about, 315
  peripheral, 804
  pitting, 951, 951f
  and pressure ulcers, 208
  prevention of, 314–315
  and wound healing, 541t
Edrophonium chloride (Tensilon), in myasthenia gravis diagnosis, 2285
Education
  of nurses, 12
  patient. *See* Patient teaching
  in prevention of injury, 2530
EEG. *See* Electroencephalography
Efavirenz (Sustiva), for HIV infection, 1827t
Effector stage, of immune response, 1788, 1789f
Effusion. *See also* Pericardial effusion; Pleural effusions
  joint
    assessment for, 2348, 2348f
    definition of, 2337
  middle ear, 2107
EGD. *See* Esophagogastroduodenoscopy
Egophony, in pneumonia, 636
EIA. *See* Enzyme immunoassay
Ejaculation, disorders of, 1746–1750
Ejection fraction, 787, 947
  definition of, 781, 945
EKC. *See* Epidemic keratoconjunctivitis
ELAD (extracorporeal liver assist devices), 1317

Elastic stockings, 198
Elbow
  fracture of, 2443
  tennis, 2427
Elder abuse, 249
  assessment for, 73
  definition of, 225
Elderly. *See* Older adults
Elder neglect, 249
Electrical bone stimulation, 2439
  nursing management of, 2439
Electrical burn(s), 1998–1999
  complications of, 2030
Electrical shock
  injury caused by, 102
  ventricular fibrillation caused by, 836
Electrical stimulation, in pain management, 291
Electric larynx, 614
Electrocardiography, 808–810, 868
  analysis of, 825–828
    for pacemaker malfunction, 847, 848, 850, 850f
  complexes of, 826–827
  conduction abnormalities seen on, 838–840
  continuous ambulatory monitoring with, 809–810
  continuous monitoring with, 808–810
  in cor pulmonale, 661
  electrical activity shown on, 824f, 825
  electrode placement for, 824f, 825, 826f
  graph of, 826–827, 827f
  hardwire monitoring system for, 809, 809f
  in hypercalcemia, 328
  in hyperkalemia, 322f, 324
  in hypermagnesemia, 331
  in hypocalcemia, 326
  in hypokalemia, 322, 322f
  in hypomagnesemia, 330
  interpretation of, 826–828, 828c
  intervals of, 826–827, 827f
  12-lead, 808, 825
  15-lead, 808
  18-lead, 808
  leads for, 824f
  in myocardial infarction, 874, 875, 875f, 876f
  obtaining, 825
  with pulmonary embolism, 663
  with pulmonary hypertension, 660
  segments of, 826–827, 827f
  signal-averaged, 809
  telemetry for, 809
  transtelephonic monitoring with, 810
  waveforms of, 826–827, 827f
  wireless mobile monitoring, 810
Electroconvulsive therapy, for depression, in HIV-infected (AIDS) patients, 1836
Electroencephalography, 2155
  with brain tumor, 2304
  in epilepsy, 2193
  in hepatobiliary disease, 1305
  in herpes simplex virus encephalitis, 2274
  in liver disease, 1291t
Electrohydraulic lithotripsy, for urolithiasis, 1593
Electrolytes
  in acute renal failure, 1525–1526, 1535c
  in body fluids, 301–302, 302t
  excretion of, regulation of, 1497
  gains and losses of, routes of, 304
  imbalances of, 315–334, 316t–317t
    in renal disorders, 1515–1517, 1516t
  serum, in cardiac patient, 807t
Electromyography, 2155–2156, 2199, 2351
  in low back pain, 2393c

Electron-beam computed tomography, in cardiac patient, 812–813
Electronystagmography, 2100
Electrophysiologic testing
  cardiac, 851–854
  in cardiac patient, 816
  nursing interventions in, 816
Electrosurgery
  for cancer, 393
  for skin cancer, 1980
Elephantiasis, 1016–1017
Elimination
  assessment of, 215
  definition of, 46c, 1121
  in HIV-infected (AIDS) patients, 1846
  in inflammatory bowel disease, 1252
  maintenance of, in tube feedings, 1186–1187
  osteoporosis and, 2410
  in Parkinson's disease, 2317
  process of, 1125
  spinal cord injuries and, 2258
  in stroke patient, 2220
Elimination patterns
  altered
    interventions for, 216–218, 1252
    nursing process for, 215–218
  assessment of, 215
  gerontologic considerations for, 215c
ELISA. *See* Enzyme-linked immunosorbent assay
Embolectomy, 1000
Embolism. *See also* Pulmonary embolism; Thromboembolism
  air, in parenteral nutrition, 1197t
  arterial, 1001–1003
  types of, 662
Emergency care. *See also* Environmental emergencies; Psychiatric emergencies
  ABCD method in, 2521
  for burn victim, 2002–2003, 2003c
  for fractures, 2431–2432
  primary survey in, 2521
  secondary survey in, 2522
  for spinal cord injuries, 2251–2253
  triage in, 2520–2521
Emergency department
  gerontologic considerations in, 2520
  health risks in, limiting exposure to, 2518
  infection control in, 2518
  patients in, characteristics of, 2517, 2517c
  precautions in, 2518
  triage in, 2520–2521
  violence in, 2518–2519, 2553–2554
  visits to, facts about, 2517, 2517c
Emergency management, 2517
  federal agencies for, 2559–2560
  state and local agencies in, 2560
Emergency nursing, 2516–2555
  assessment in, 2521–2522
  and community services, 2520
  and continuum of care, 2520
  discharge planning in, 2520
  family-focused interventions in, 2519–2520
  gerontologic considerations in, 2520
  holistic care in, 2519–2520
  interventions in, 2521–2522
  issues in, 2518–2520
  patient-focused inteventions in, 2519
  principles of, 2520–2522
  scope and practice of, 2517–2520
  triage in, 2520–2521
Emergency operations plan(s), 2560
  behavioral issues and, 2564
  communication with families in, 2562–2563
  components of, 2560–2561

cultural considerations in, 2563, 2563c
documentation of patient information in, 2561
ethical, considerations in, 2563–2564
initiation of, 2561–2564
internal problems in, management of, 2562
nursing in, 2563–2564
patient identification in, 2561
triage in, 2561–2562
Emergency preparedness
federal agencies' responses in, 2559–2560
hospital plans for, 2560
local agencies' responses in, 2560
state agencies for, 2560
Emergency treatment, of pulmonary embolism, 664–665
Emergent patients, 2520
definition of, 2517
Emerging infectious diseases, 2509–2512
definition of, 2475
Emesis, 1127
EMG. See Electromyography
EMLA cream, 281
for postoperative analgesia, in thoracic surgical patient, 766
Emmetropia, 2050–2051, 2050f
definition of, 2043
Emotion(s)
brain injury and, 2243t
in Huntington's disease, 2319–2320
ischemic stroke and, 2209t, 2210
in multiple sclerosis, 2282
in older persons, 248–249
stress and, 94
Emotional, definition of, 46c
Emotional considerations, in HIV-infected (AIDS) patients, 1851
Emotional distress, 114–115
Emotional health, 114–115
Emotional status, assessment of, 2145
Emotional support
for colorectal cancer patient, 1270–1271
for ileostomy patient, 1259
Emphysema. See also Chronic obstructive pulmonary disease
assessment findings in, 576t
barrel chest in, 569–570
bullous, bullectomy in, 694
centrilobular (centroacinar), 687f, 688
clinical manifestations of, 689, 689f, 690f
definition of, 686
lung transplantation in, 694
panlobular (panacinar), 687f, 688
pathophysiology of, 687–688, 687f
subcutaneous, 670–681
Empyema, 638, 654–655
definition of, 625
loculated, 654
Emtricitabine (Emtriva), for HIV infection, 1827t
Enalapril (Vasotec), 952–953, 952t
for hypertension, 1029t
Enalaprilat (Vasotec IV), 952–953, 952t
for hypertension, 1029t
for hypertensive crises, 1033
Encephalitis
fungal, 2275–2276
herpes simplex virus, 2274
Encephalopathy. See also Progressive multifocal leukoencephalopathy
hepatic. See Hepatic encephalopathy
HIV, 1833, 1834c
definition of, 1815
hypertensive, in acute glomerulonephritis, 1518

Endarterectomy. See also Carotid endarterectomy
aortoiliac, 994f
in peripheral arterial disease, 994f
Endocarditis
management of, 2500c
prevention of, 2500c
rheumatic, 933–935
Endocardium, 782, 782f
Endocervicitis, 1669–1670
definition of, 1661
Endochondral ossification, 2339
Endochondroma, 2417
Endocrine, definition of, 1345, 1440
Endocrine disorders
clinical manifestations of, 1442
health history in, 1442
and rheumatic diseases, 1917
Endocrine functions, of pancreas, 1345–1347
Endocrine system
anatomy and physiology of, 1441–1442, 1442f
assessment of, 1442–1444
preoperative, 488
diagnostic evaluation of, 1444–1445
glands of, 1441, 1442f
health history concerning, 1442
in HIV-infected (AIDS) patients, 1834
physical assessment of, 1442–1444
End-of-life care, 447–474
after-death care in, 469–471
in amyotrophic lateral sclerosis, 2323
beliefs, preferences, and practices, assessment of, 460, 460c
for brain tumor patient, 2309
care/cure dichotomy and, 449
communication in, 457–459
cultural sensitivity in, 459–461
decision making in, 461, 462f
difficult questions in, nurse's response to, 458–459
discussing, 458–459, 459t
dying in, 468–473
hemodialysis and, nursing research on, 1542
hope in, 462–463
hospice care in, 452–456
hydration in, 466–467, 467t
nursing and, 448–452
nursing care in, 456–468
nutrition in, 466–467, 467t
pain management in, 464–465
palliative care in, 452–454
palliative sedation in, 468
preferences for
assessment of, 459–461
methods of stating, 457, 457c
principles of, 448–449
psychosocial issues in, 456–457
sociocultural context of, 449–452
for spinal cord tumor patient, 2310, 2310c
spiritual care in, 461–462
technology and, 449
End-of-life issues, 28, 122
in cystic fibrosis, 719
pain management as, 271c–272c
Endolymphatic hydrops, 2112
definition of, 2093
Endolymphatic sac decompression, for Ménière's disease, 2113
Endometrial ablation, 1631
definition of, 1613
Endometrial biopsy, 1629–1630
Endometrial cancer, 1685, 1685c
etiology of, 386
Endometrial hyperplasia, 1682

Endometriosis, 1626, 1680–1682
definition of, 1613, 1661
women's views of, nursing research on, 1680
Endometritis, and pelvic inflammatory disease, 1670
Endometrium
definition of, 1613
in menstrual cycle, 1615, 1616f
Endorphin(s), 2130t
definition of, 259
and pain transmission, 265
in stress response, 96
Endoscopic retrograde cholangiopancreatography, 1291t, 1349t, 1350, 1350f
definition of, 1345
Endoscopy
in cancer detection, 391t
esophageal, 1290t
of esophageal varices, 1299
of female reproductive system, 1630–1631
gastrointestinal
definition of, 1121
through ostomy, 1138
in gastrointestinal assessment, 1134–1138
of middle ear, 2101
musculoskeletal, 2351
in respiratory disease, 581–582
of upper gastrointestinal tract, 1134–1135, 1134f
urologic, 1509–1510, 1509f
Endosteum, 2338f, 2339
definition of, 2337
Endothelin, vascular effects of, 978
Endotracheal catheter, nasal, 510, 511f
Endotracheal intubation, 735–738
in cardiopulmonary resuscitation, 970
complications of, prevention of, 737–738
definition of, 723
in emergency patient, 2524, 2525f
nursing management of, 737c
oral, 510, 511f
prolonged, nursing management of, 682
Endotracheal tube
cuff, management of, 735
removal of, 737c
suctioning of, 735, 739, 741c
Endovascular repair
of abdominal aortic aneurysm, 1000, 1000f
nursing management of, 1000
End-stage renal disease, 1527–1537
in acute glomerulonephritis, 1518
definition of, 1515
dialysis for, indications for, 1537
stages of, 1527, 1527c
Enema
barium, 1132
preoperative, 496
retention, for hyperkalemia in acute renal failure, 1525
Energy, conservation, in pneumonia, 640
Energy therapies, 134
Enflurane (Ethrane), 510t
Enfuvirtide (T-20, Fuzeon), for HIV infection, 1826–1828, 1828t
Enkephalins, 2130t
definition of, 259
and pain transmission, 265
Enoxaparin (Lovenox), for deep vein thrombosis prevention, 2375
Entacapone (Comtan), for Parkinson's disease, 2314
*Entamoeba histolytica*
incubation period of, 2476t
liver abscess caused by, 1340
transmission of, 2476t

EnteraFlo tube, 1176t
Enteral nutrition. *See also* Tube feeding(s)
  for brain injury patients, 2244
  complications of, 1184t
  conditions requiring, 1181t
  in diabetes mellitus, for hospitalized patient, 1431–1432
  after gastric surgery, 1224
Enteral pumps, 1183
Enterobacteriaceae, pneumonia caused by, 629, 633–634
*Enterobacter* pneumonia, 629, 634
*Enterobius vermicularis*
  incubation period of, 2477t
  transmission of, 2477t
Enterocele, 1505, 1674–1675, 1674f
Enteroclysis, 1132
*Enterococcus*, vancomycin-resistant, 2475
  health care–associated infection potential of, 2482–2483
Enterohepatic circulation, 1287
Enteroscopy, small-bowel, 1137–1138
Enterostomal therapist, definition of, 1232, 1345
Enterotoxigenic *Escherichia coli*, 2501
Entropion, 2077
Enucleation, 2082–2083
  definition of, 2043
Enuresis, 1503, 1503t
Envenomation
  definition of, 2517
  insect, 2539
  snake, 2539–2540
    emergency management of, 2539–2540
    signs and symptoms of, 2539
Environment
  cultural, 69c, 70
  interpersonal, 69c, 70
  and lung cancer, 671
  in patient profile, 69c
  physical, 70
  spiritual, 69c, 70
Environmental control, in Standard Precautions, 1820c
Environmental domain, definition of, 46c
Environmental emergencies, 2533–2540
Enzyme immunoassay
  definition of, 1815
  for HIV diagnosis, 1825, 1825t
Enzyme-linked immunosorbent assay
  definition of, 1815
  for HIV diagnosis, 1825
Enzymes
  cardiac, analysis of, 805
  digestive, 1123t
  pancreatic, 1124
EOP. *See* Emergency operations plan
Eosinophil(s), 1038f, 1040f, 1041
  in allergic reaction, 1859
  definition of, 1856
  functions of, 1037t, 1042
  laboratory values for, 2579
  in natural immunity, 1785
  and phagocytic immune response, 1786
Eosinophil chemotactic factor of anaphylaxis, in allergic reaction, 1858t, 1859
Eosinophil count, in diagnosis of allergic disorder, 1864
Epicardium, 782, 782f
Epicel, 1948
Epidemic keratoconjunctivitis, 2077–2078
Epidemiology of Diabetes Interventions and Complications (EDIC), 1383–1384
Epidermis, 1927, 1928, 1928f
  definition of, 1995

Epidermopoiesis, 1967
  definition of, 1945
Epididymitis, 1769
  definition of, 1740
Epidural hematoma, 2236–2237, 2237f
Epidural monitor, 2172
  definition of, 2161
Epigastric area, examination of, 801, 801f
Epiglottis, 554, 555f, 1153f
Epilepsy, 2191–2197. *See also* Seizures; Status epilepticus
  assessment in, 2191–2193, 2195
  clinical manifestations of, 2191
  complications of, 2195, 2196
  continuing care in, 2196–2197
  coping in, improving, 2196
  definition of, 2161, 2191
  diagnosis of, 2191–2193
  epidemiology of, 2191
  expected outcomes in, 2197
  gerontologic considerations in, 2193
  home and community-based care in, 2196–2197, 2197c
  injury prevention in, 2195
  medical management of, 2193–2195
  nursing diagnoses related to, 2195
  nursing interventions for, 2195–2197
  nursing process with, 2195–2197
  pathophysiology of, 2191
  patient and family education about, 2196
  pharmacologic therapy for, 2193–2194, 2194t
  planning and goals for, 2195
  prevention of, 2193
  primary, 2191
  secondary, 2191
  self-care in, 2196, 2197c
  surgical management of, 2194–2195
  in women, 2193
Epilepsy Foundation of America, 2196
Epimysium, 2341
  definition of, 2337
Epinephrine
  for anaphylaxis, 376, 1868, 1869c, 2538
  for anaphylaxis in home IV antibiotic therapy, nursing research on, 1867
  for cardiogenic shock, 370, 966
  in cardiopulmonary resuscitation, 971, 972t
  for glaucoma, 2057, 2058t
  intravenous, for asystole, 838
  self-administration of, 1869c
  in stress response, 95
  in treatment of shock, 366t, 370, 376
  vascular effects of, 978
  for ventricular fibrillation, 837
EpiPen, 1868, 1868f
EpiPen Jr., 1868, 1868f
Epiphysis, 2338, 2338f
  definition of, 2337
Epispadias, 1774
Epistaxis, 605–606
  definition of, 589
  medical management of, 605–606
  with nasal fractures, 607
  nursing management of, 606
  prevention of, 606
  risk factors for, 605c
Epitope(s), 1784
  in allergic reaction, 1857
  definition of, 1783, 1856
Eplerenone (Inspra), for hypertension, 1026t
Epoetin alfa (Epogen, Procrit), 1051
  in breast cancer treatment, 1728
Eprosartan (Tevetan), for hypertension, 1029t
Epstein-Barr virus, 1667
  and cancer, 385

gene products, and HIV infection, 1822
  and Guillain-Barré syndrome, 2288
  and Hodgkin's disease, 1080
  incubation period of, 2477t
  transmission of, 2477t
Eptifibatide (Integrelin), 871
Epzicom, for HIV infection, 1827t
Equilibrium, 2096
Equilibrium radionuclide angiocardiography, 812
Erb's point, 801, 801f
ERCP. *See* Endoscopic retrograde cholangiopancreatography
Erectile dysfunction, 233, 1744–1746. *See also* Impotence
  assessment of, 1745, 1746f
  definition of, 1740
  diagnosis of, 1744, 1745
  drugs causing, 1745, 1745c
  medical management of, 1745–1746, 1746f, 1747t–1748t, 1748c–1749c
Ergotamine
  in cluster headache prevention, 2200
  for migraine, 2201
Erikson, Erick, developmental theory of, 227
ERNA. *See* Equilibrium radionuclide angiocardiography
Erosion, of skin, 1938c
Erthromelalgia, 1920
Erythema, 1933, 1935t
  definition of, 1856, 1927
  in skin test, 1864
Erythroblasts, 1039
Erythrocytapheresis, 1102, 1102t
Erythrocyte(s). *See* Red blood cell(s)
Erythrocyte sedimentation rate
  definition of, 1036
  in Hodgkin's disease, 1080
  laboratory values for, 2579
  in rheumatic diseases, 1893t
Erythroid cells, 1051
  definition of, 1036
Erythromelalgia, 1086
  in polycythemia vera, 1065
Erythromycin
  and immune system, 1797t
  interactions with anesthetics, 490t
  for Legionnaires' disease, 2511
Erythropoiesis, 1039–1041
  definition of, 1036
Erythropoietin, 1039
  adverse effects and side effects of, 421t
  as alternative to blood transfusion, 1112c
  in breast cancer treatment, 1728
  in cancer treatment, 401, 420
  definition of, 1036
  recombinant (Epogen), 1051
    for chronic renal failure, 1530
  renal disease and, 1051
Eschar, 2001
  definition of, 1995
Escharotomy, 2001
  definition of, 1995
*Escherichia coli*
  and diarrheal diseases, 2501
  enterotoxigenic, 2501
  0157:H7, 2501
  and osteomyelitis, 2413
  pneumonia, 629, 633–634
  in urinary tract infections, 1571, 1572
Esmolol (Brevibloc), 830t
Esomeprazole (Nexium), for gastroesophageal reflux disease, 1166
Esophageal banding therapy, for esophageal varices, 1302, 1302f, 1304t

## INDEX

Esophageal disorders
  continuing care for, 1171
  expected outcomes with, 1171
  nursing diagnoses related to, 1169
  nursing interventions in, 1169–1171
Esophageal manometry, 1138
Esophageal pain, assessment of, 792t
Esophageal reflux, diagnosis of, 1138
Esophageal speech, 613–614
Esophageal sphincter, 1162
Esophageal varices, 1298–1304
  balloon tamponade for, 1300–1301, 1301f, 1304t
  banding therapy for, 1302, 1302f, 1304t
  bleeding, management of, 1304t
  clinical manifestations of, 1299
  diagnosis of, 1299
  endoscopic sclerotherapy for, 1301–1302, 1301f, 1304t
  esophageal devascularization and transection for, 1303, 1304t
  medical management of, 1299–1303, 1304t
  nursing management of, 1303, 1304t
  pathophysiology of, 1298–1299, 1298f
  pharmacologic therapy for, 1300, 1304t
  surgical management of, 1302–1303, 1303f, 1304t
Esophagectomy
  in Barrett's esophagus, 1166
  for cancer of esophagus, 1167, 1168f
Esophagitis, bile reflux, after gastric surgery, 1225
Esophagogastric junction, 1121
Esophagogastroduodenoscopy, 1134–1135
  in Barrett's esophagus, 1166
  definition of, 1142
Esophagomyotomy, for achalasia, 1162
Esophagoscopy, 1290t
Esophagus, 1122f
  age-related changes of, 1125, 1126c
  anatomy of, 1121
  barium study of, 1290t
  Barrett's, 1166
    and esophageal cancer, 1166
  benign tumors of, 1166
  cancer of, 1166–1169
    nursing management of, 1168–1169
  definition of, 1121
  diffuse spasm of, 1162–1163
  disorders of, 1162–1171
    nursing process for, 1169–1171
  foreign body in, 1165
  motility of, evaluation of, 1138
  perforation of, 1164–1165
  reconstruction of, 1167, 1168f
ESR. *See* Erythrocyte sedimentation rate
ESRD. *See* End-stage renal disease
Estrogen(s)
  and autoimmune disorders, 1796
  and bone health, 2405
  and bone mass, 2405
  in cancer treatment, 399t
  cardiovascular effects of, 787
  definition of, 1613
  and HIV transmission, 1818
  in menstrual cycle, 1615
  for osteoporosis, 2409
  skeletal effects of, 2339–2340
Estrogen and progesterone receptor assay
  in breast cancer, 1729
  definition of, 1701
ESWL. *See* Extracorporeal shock wave lithotripsy
Etanercept (Enbrel)
  for rheumatic diseases, 1896t
  for rheumatoid arthritis, 1908

ETEC. *See* Enterotoxigenic *Escherichia coli*
Ethacrynic acid (Edecril), 954t
Ethambutol (Myambutol), for tuberculosis, 647–648, 647t
Ethanol, blood levels of, 2601t
Ethical analysis, steps in, 33, 34c
Ethics
  and acute coronary syndrome in elderly, 869c
  applied, 27
  and assisted suicide, 451, 452c, 2310c
  and chronic illness, 168
  decision making in, 33
  in disaster care, 2563–2564
  and do-not-resuscitate orders, 518c
  in end-of-life care, 28
  and genetic testing, 158, 160–161
  gerontologic considerations in, 251–252, 251c
  HIV status and, 1851, 1851c
  in liver transplantation, 1338, 1339c
  versus morality, 27–28
  nursing, code of, 29, 31c
  in nursing care, 27–34
  and pain management, 271c–272c
  preventive, 33
  principles of, 27, 28c
  and right to refuse treatment, 615c
  theories of, 27
  of withholding/withdrawing food and hydration, 1190c
Ethics committees, 33
Ethionamide, for tuberculosis, 647
Ethnic culture, 128
Ethnicity, assessment of, in genetic assessment, 155–156
Ethosuximide (Zarontin)
  adverse effects and side effects of, 2194t
  toxic effects of, 2194t
Etidronate (Didronel), 328
  for Paget's disease, 2412
Etodolac (Lodine), for rheumatic diseases, 1895t
Etomidate (Amidate), for intravenous anesthesia, 513t
Etoposide
  for acute myeloid leukemia, 1071
  for cancer treatment, 399t
Eupnea, 572t
Eustachian tube, 2094f
  definition of, 2095c
Euthanasia, 468. *See also* Assisted suicide
  definition of, 448
Euthyroid, definition of, 1440
Evaluation
  in critical thinking, 25
  in ethical analysis, 34c
  in nursing process, 34, 36c, 42–43
  preoperative, 499, 499c
  in teaching-learning process, 55c, 56
Evans formula, for fluid replacement in burn patients, 2007c
Eversion, 201c, 2343c
  definition of, 198c
Evidence-based practice, 8–9
Evisceration, 546, 546f
  definition of, 524
  intraocular, 2082
    definition of, 2043
Evoked potentials, studies of, 2156
Ewing's sarcoma, 2417
Excision, definition of, 1995
Excitability, of cardiac conduction cells, 783
Excretion, of drugs, age-related changes in, 238, 239t

Exemestane (Aromasin), fro breast cancer, 1729
Exenatide (Byetta), 1402
Exenteration, orbital, 2082
  definition of, 2043
Exercise(s)
  active, 198, 201t
  active-assistive, 198, 201t
  Alzheimer's disease and, 246
  arm and shoulder, after thoracic surgery, 767, 769c, 774c
  benefits of, for elderly, 235–236
  and bone formation, 2406, 2408
  and bone health, 2339
  after breast surgery, 1723–1725, 1724c
  in cancer rehabilitation, nursing research on, 435
  in cardiovascular disease, assessment of, 796
  in chronic obstructive pulmonary disease, 695
  in diabetes, 1388–1389, 1388c
  in HIV-infected (AIDS) patients, nursing research on, 1847
  and hypertension, 1031
  isometric, 198, 201t
  for low back pain, 2394c
  in multiple sclerosis, 2281
  muscle-setting, 198, 201t
  after neck dissection, 1159, 1160f
  and osteoporosis, 2410
  paraplegia/quadriplegia and, 2262
  passive, 198, 201t
  perimenopausal, 1636
  postoperative, 537–538
    with amputation, 2466
    preoperative teaching about, 494c, 495
  range-of-motion, 196–198, 198c, 199c–201c
    terminology used in, 198c
  resistive, 198, 201t
  for rheumatic diseases, 1898
  in rheumatic diseases, 1894, 1897t
  and skeletal traction, 2369
  therapeutic, 198, 201t
  with venous thrombosis, 1009–1010
Exercise stress test, 810
Exercise testing, in peripheral vascular disease, 982
Exfoliative dermatitis, 1970–1971
Exocrine, definition of, 1345, 1440
Exocrine functions, of pancreas, 1345–1347
Exophthalmos
  definition of, 1440
  in hyperthyroidism, 1459
Exostoses, 2105–2106
  definition of, 2093
Expiratory reserve volume, 558t
Explanation, in critical thinking, 25
Expressive aphasia
  definition of, 2206
  stroke and, 2208t, 2209
Extended care facilities, for people with disabilities, 219, 222
Extension, 200c, 201c, 2343c
  definition of, 198c
External, definition of, 198c
External auditory canal, 2093, 2094f
  definition of, 2095c
  examination of, 2098, 2098f
  inflammation of. *See* Otitis externa
External catheters, for urinary incontinence, 216
External ear
  anatomy of, 2093, 2094f

External ear (continued)
  conditions of, 2104–2106
  definition of, 2095c
  foreign bodies in, 2104–2105
  gapping ear puncture in, 2106
  inspection of, 2096–2098
  masses of, 2105–2106
External fixator, 2364–2365, 2364f
  definition of, 2355
  for femoral shaft fracture, 2449, 2458
  patient teaching about, 2365, 2365c
  self-care with, 2365, 2365c
External otitis, 2105. See also Otitis externa
  acute, 2107t
  malignant, 2105
External rotation, 199c
Extracellular fluid, 301–302
  components of, 301–302, 302t
  electrolytes in, 301–302, 302t
  expansion of, 313–315
Extracorporeal liver assist devices, 1317
Extracorporeal membrane oxygenation, 929
Extracorporeal shock wave lithotripsy
  for gallstones, 1353
  for urolithiasis, 1591–1593, 1592f
Extradural hematoma. See Epidural hematoma
Extraocular movements, 2048
Extraocular muscle(s), 2044, 2044f
Extraocular muscle palsy, in diabetes, 1423t
Extrapyramidal system, 2140
Extravasation
  of chemotherapy agents, 398
  definition of, 381
  with intravenous therapy, 350
Extremity(ies)
  circulatory insufficiency of, 978–979
  girth of, measurement of, 2349
  inspection of, in cardiovascular disease, 804
  lower
    amputation of, 2460, 2461f
      in Buerger's disease, 996
    venous thrombosis in, 1004–1005
    shortening of, fracture and, 2431
  upper
    amputation of, 2460–2461, 2461f
      in farmers, nursing research on, 2463
    arterial occlusive disease of, 995
    musculoskeletal problems of, 2397–2399
    venous thrombosis in, 1004–1005
Extubation, 752
  nursing management of, 737c
Eye(s). See also Ocular
  age-related changes in, 236, 2051, 2051t
  anatomy and physiology of, 2043–2046, 2044f, 2045f
  assessment of, 2046–2048
  in diabetes, 1422, 1423t
  disorders of
    diagnosis of, 2048–2050
    genetics of, 2047
  external examination of, 2048
  foreign bodies in, 2073, 2074
  hypertension and, 2084
  infections of, 2075–2080, 2076t
  inflammation of, 2075–2080
  injuries to, prevention of, 2072, 2072c
  medication administration in, 2084–2087, 2088c
  topical anesthetics for, 2085
  tumors of, 2080–2081
Eyeball
  contusions of, 2074
  penetrating injuries of, 2074
Eye contact, culture and, 132

Eyelids
  benign tumors of, 2080
  malignant tumors of, 2080–2081
Eye movement, assessment of, in unconscious patient, 2165t
Eye patches, 2073, 2074f
Eye protection, in Standard Precautions, 1820c

# F

Fab fragment, of antibody molecule, 1788, 1790f
Face lift, 1990–1991
Face shields, in Standard Precautions, 1820c
Faces Pain Scale, Revised, 274, 274f
Face tents, for oxygen delivery, 725t, 727
Facial nerve (VII), 2094–2096, 2094f, 2136–2137, 2136f, 2137t, 2292f
  assessment of, 2147c
  and Bell's palsy, 2295–2296
  disorders of, 2293c
  distribution of, 2295, 2296f
  neuroma of, 2112
Facial reconstructive surgery, 1989–1990
Facial symmetry, assessment of, in unconscious patient, 2165t
Factor V assay, laboratory values for, 2578
Factor VII assay, laboratory values for, 2578
Factor IX assay, laboratory values for, 2578
Factor X assay, laboratory values for, 2578
Factor IX complex, 1103t
Factor VIII concentrate, 1103–1104, 1103t
Factor IX concentrate, 1103–1104, 1103t
Factor V Leiden mutation, 1095, 1099, 1099t
Factor V Leiden thrombophilia, 151t
  diagnosis of, 152
Faith
  definition of, 112
  religious, 123
Faith healing, 135
Fall(s)
  by older persons, 247
  prevention of, 2410
  in vertigo, 2114c
Fallopian tubes, 1615, 1615f
  cancer of, 1689
Falx cerebelli, 2133
Falx cerebri, 2133
Famciclovir, for herpes infections, in HIV-infected (AIDS) patients, 1836
Family
  in after-death care, 469–471
  of brain-injury patient, 2246–2248
  of brain tumor patient, nursing interventions for, 2308
  of burn patient, nursing interventions for, 2004–2005, 2012c–2013c, 2029–2030
  caring for, in disaster, 2562–2563
  chronic illness and, 168
  codependent members of, caring for, 120
  coping in, after facial reconstructive surgery, 1990
  death vigil of, 469
  definition of, 112
  of dementia/Alzheimer's disease patient, 246
  of emergency patient, nursing interventions for, 2519–2520
  genetic inheritance patterns in, 145
  involvement of
    in end-of-life care, 465
    in rehabilitation, 192, 219, 221
  of ischemic stroke patient
    coping in, 2221–2222
    nursing interventions for, 2223

of older persons persons, role in care, 230
presence during cardiopulmonary resuscitation, nursing research on, 971
of surgical patient
  emotional support for, 544
  nursing interventions for, 499
of terminally ill patients
  communication with, 458
  denial by, 450
of unconscious patient, nursing interventions for, 2168–2169
Family functioning
  and health, 115
  nursing interventions for, 115–116
Family history
  genetic, 154–155, 155c
  in health history, 67
Family planning, natural, 1646
Family tree, 67, 67f
Family violence, emergency management of, 2550–2552
Famotidine (Pepcid), 1206t
  for gastroesophageal reflux disease, 1166
Farsightedness. See Hyperopia
Fascia, 2341
  definition of, 2337
Fasciculations, 2349
  definition of, 2337
Fasciculi, 2341
Fasciotomy
  for compartment syndrome, 2359, 2438
  after crush injury, 2533
  definition of, 1995, 2355, 2371c, 2517
FAST (Focused Assessment for Sonographic Examination of the Trauma Patient), 2532
Fasting, preoperative, 496
Fasting plasma glucose. See also Impaired fasting glucose
  definition of, 1376
Fat(s). See also Lipid(s)
  dietary
    and breast cancer, 1713
    in diabetes, 1386
    digestion of, 1123t, 1125
    in wound healing, 487t
  metabolism of, liver in, 1286
  trans, 82
Fat embolism, in orthopedic surgery patient, 2385
Fat embolism syndrome, fracture and, 2435–2436
  clinical manifestations of, 2435–2436
  management of, 2436
  prevention of, 2436
Fat emulsions, in parenteral nutrition, 1193
Fatigue
  in acute leukemia, nursing interventions for, 1077
  in anemia, management of, 1048
  cancer-related, 425–426
    nursing interventions for, 430–431
    sources of, 430, 430c
  in cardiovascular disease, assessment of, 790, 794t
  chemotherapy-related, 402
    nursing management of, 411c
  in chronic obstructive pulmonary disease, nursing research on, 691
  disability and, 218–219
  in hepatitis C, nursing research on, 1316
  in multiple sclerosis, 2279, 2280
  in liver disease, 1323c
  in lung cancer, nursing interventions for, 673

# INDEX

in rehabilitation, 218–219
rheumatic diseases and, 1898–1903, 1899c–1900c
Fat redistribution syndrome, in HIV-infected (AIDS) patients, 1826
Fatty acids, and immune system function, 1795
Fatty liver, 1286
Fc fragment, of antibody molecule, 1788, 1790f
Fear(s)
accompanied by somatic complaints unsubstantiated by physical findings
nursing diagnoses related to, 88–89
nursing interventions for, 88–89
nursing outcomes for, 88–89
in cardiac surgical patient, 895–896
in Guillain-Barré syndrome, 2290
after neck dissection, 1159c
preoperative, nursing interventions for, 495, 499c
in renal surgical patient, 1556c
in renal-urologic testing, 1512
Febrile response, in older persons, 248
Fecal elimination. See also Elimination
abnormalities of, 1232–1238. See also Constipation; Diarrhea/diarrheal diseases
in diverticulitis, 1244–1245
in irritable bowel syndrome, 1237–1238
Fecal impaction, 1233
Fecal incontinence. See Incontinence, fecal
Fecal occult blood testing, 1130
Feces, 1125. See also Stool
Federal Emergency Management Agency, 2560
Feedback
definition of, 49
and learning, 52
negative
in control of steady state, 99
definition of, 91
positive
in control of steady state, 100
definition of, 91
Feeding, cyclic, definition of, 1175
Feeding gastrostomy. See Gastrostomy
Feeding pump(s)
for gastrointestinal intubation, 1183
in gastrostomy, 1192
Feeding tube(s), 1175–1176, 1175–1177. See also Nasoenteric tube(s); Nasogastric (NG) tube(s)
definition of, 1175
displacement of, 1184t
location of, assessment of, 1178–1179
maintaining, 1183–1184
obstruction of, 1184t
placement of
assessment of, nursing research on, 1179
confirmation of, 1178–1179
providing medications by, 1185–1186, 1186f
refusal of, by elderly person, 251c
residue in, 1184t
Felbamate (Felbatol)
adverse effects and side effects of, 2194t
toxic effects of, 2194t
Felodipine (Plendil), 955
for hypertension, 1029t
Female condom, and HIV prevention, 1817
Female genital mutilation, 1620
Female reproductive system
age-related changes in, 231t, 233, 1616, 1617t
anatomy of, 1614–1615, 1614f

assessment of, 1616–1627
gerontologic considerations in, 1623
diagnostic testing for, 1627–1631
disorders of, genetic aspects of, 1619
function of, 1615–1616
in HIV-infected (AIDS) patients, 1834–1835
internal structures of, 1614–1615, 1615f
physical examination of, 1623–1627
Femur
fractures of, 2446–2449
types of, 2458f
neck of, fracture of, 2458f
proximal, regions of, 2446, 2446f
shaft of, fracture of, 2449–2458, 2458f
Fenofibrate (Tricor), 865, 865t
Fenoldopam mesylate (Corlopam)
for hypertension, 1028t
for hypertensive crises, 1033
Fentanyl
abuse/overdose, emergency management of, 2545t
for anesthesia, intravenous, 512t
for burn victim, 2024
transdermal, 286, 286c
transmucosal, 287
Ferritin, 1039
Fetor hepaticus, definition of, 1285
Fever, 103
with appendicitis, 1241
in burn victim, 2002, 2015
definition of, 75
with increased intracranial pressure, management of, 2174
in infectious disease, nursing interventions for, 2492, 2497c
in lung cancer, 671
in older persons, 248
in pneumonia, 636
in septic shock, 375
in unconscious patient, management of, 2167
in upper respiratory infection, 603
Fever blister, 1143t. See also Cold sore(s)
Fexofenadine (Allegra), 1871t
for pruritus, 1952
for sinusitis, 595
FGM. See Female genital mutilation
Fiber, dietary, 864
in diabetes, 1386
insoluble, 1386
soluble, 864, 1386
Fiberglass casts, 2355–2356
Fiberoptic monitor, 2172
definition of, 2161
Fibrates, 865, 865t
Fibric acids, 865, 865t, 986
Fibrin, 1042
definition of, 1036
Fibrin degradation products, 1043
laboratory values for, 2578
Fibrinogen, 1037, 1042
definition of, 1036
laboratory values for, 2578
Fibrinolysin, laboratory values for, 2578
Fibrinolysis, 1037, 1043
definition of, 1036
Fibrinolytic, definition of, 1945
Fibrinolytic action, 1948
Fibrocystic breast changes, 1711
definition of, 1701
Fibroid tumors, 1679, 1679f
definition of, 1661
Fibroma, musculoskeletal, 2417
Fibromyalgia, 1919
pain of, 261c

Fibrosarcoma, 2417
Fibroscopy, definition of, 1121
Fibrositis. See Fibromyalgia
Fibula, fracture of, 2459
Fidelity, ethical principle of, 28c
Fight-or-flight response, 94, 95, 97, 2137, 2138
Figure-of-eight bandage, 2440, 2441f
Filgrastim
for acute myeloid leukemia, 1071
adverse effects and side effects of, 421t
as alternative to blood transfusion, 1112c
in breast cancer treatment, 1728
Filoviruses, 2511–2512
Filtering procedures, for glaucoma, 2058
Filtration, of body fluids, 303
Fine-needle aspiration
of breast, 1708
definition of, 625, 1701
in lung cancer diagnosis, 672
of thyroid, 1451
Finger(s)
clubbing of, 568, 568f, 804
in bronchiectasis, 709
positioning of, in stroke recovery, 2217
Fingerprints, 1928
Finger sweep, of patient's mouth, 2523c
First-pass effect, 1287
FISH. See Fluorescent in situ hybridization
Fissure, 1938c
anal, 1233, 1276–1277, 1276f
definition of, 1232
Fissure sealants, in prevention of tooth decay, 1145
Fistula
anal, 1276, 1276f
arteriovenous, definition of, 1515
definition of, 1232, 1661, 1673
vaginal, 1673–1674, 1673f
Fixation, for hip fracture, 2447, 2447f
complications of, 2448–2449
Flaccid muscle, 2141–2142, 2342
definition of, 2129, 2337
Flaccid posturing, 2142
Flail chest, 676–677, 677f
rib fracture and, 2460
Flank approach, in renal surgery, 1553f
Flaps, 1987–1988
free, 1988
Flat bones, 2338
Flatfoot. See Pes planus
Flatness, on percussion, 76
Flatulence, 1127
Flaviviruses, 2511–2512
Flecainide (Tambocor), 830t
for atrial fibrillation, 833
for atrial flutter, 832
Flexible fiberoptic sigmoidoscopy, 1135, 1135f, 1137, 1137f
Flexion, 199c, 200c, 201c, 2343c
definition of, 198c
palmar, definition of, 198c
plantar, definition of, 198c
Flora
normal, 2479
definition of, 2475
transient, 2481
definition of, 2475
Fluconazole (Diflucan)
adverse effects and side effects of, 2276
for candidiasis, 1662
in HIV-infected (AIDS) patients, 1836
for fungal encephalitis, 2276
for meningitis, in HIV-infected (AIDS) patients, 1835

Flucytosine
  for fungal encephalitis, 2276
  for meningitis, in HIV-infected (AIDS) patients, 1835
Fludarabine (Fludara)
  in cancer treatment, 399t
  for chronic lymphocytic leukemia, 1074
Fluid(s)
  intake and output of, 302
  intake of, for urolithiasis, 1591, 1594
  restriction of, for cerebral edema, 2173
Fluid(s) (body)
  amount of, 301–302
  balance of
    in acute renal failure, 1525
    osmosis and, 180
    in parenteral nutrition, 1198
    in renal disorders, 1515–1517, 1516t
    in renal surgical patient, 1557c–1558c, 1558–1559
    tube feedings and, 1180
  capillary filtration of, 977–978
  composition of, 301–302
  deficits in, during gastrointestinal intubation, 1180
  electrolytes in, 301–302, 302t
  extracellular, 301–302, 302t
    expansion of, 313–315
  filtration of, 303
  gains and losses of, routes of, 304
  homeostatic mechanisms for, 305–308
    gerontologic considerations in, 308
  intracellular, 301–302, 302t
  intraoperative exposure to, safety precautions for, 508
  intravascular, 301
  osmolality of, 304
  overload
    in cardiac surgical patient, 891t
    in diabetes mellitus, 1418
    with intravenous therapy, 349
    in parenteral nutrition, 1197t
    in renal disorders, 1515–1517, 1516t
    in renal surgical patient, 1559
  reabsorption of, 977–978
  regulation of, 302–304, 305–308
    gerontologic considerations in, 308
  skin and, 1931
  third spacing of, 301–302
  tonicity of, 302
  transcellular, 301
Fluid and electrolyte balance
  in acute pancreatitis, 1367c
  in biochemical assessment, 80
  in blistering diseases, 1973
  brain injury and, 2244, 2249
  burns and, 2005–2007, 2006t, 2011c, 2015, 2015t, 2027
  after cardiac surgery, 893t, 897, 899, 900, 906c–908c
  definition of, 46c
  in diabetes mellitus, 1417
  in diabetic ketoacidosis, 1414
  in heart failure, 960–961
  hemodialysis and, 1540–1541
  in HIV-infected (AIDS) patients, 1836–1837, 1844c, 1845
  in ileostomy patient, 1258c, 1262
  in inflammatory bowel disease, 1252
  in myocardial infarction, 881c
  with prostatectomy, 1765
  in toxic epidermal necrolysis or Stevens-Johnson syndrome, 1975
  vertigo and, 2115c
Fluid challenge test, 312

Fluid management and replacement
  in acute leukemia, 1077–1078
  in acute renal failure, 1525–1526
  in acute respiratory distress syndrome, 658
  for burn patients, 2005–2007, 2006t, 2007c, 2011c, 2015, 2027
  in cardiovascular disease, 319
  in chloride imbalance, 334
  in chronic renal failure, 1530, 1532c
  complications of, 365
    in shock, 365
  in disseminated intravascular coagulation, 1096c
  during gastrointestinal intubation, 1180
  in hemorrhage, 2526
  in hypercalcemia, 328
  in hypernatremia, 320
  in hypovolemia, 310–312, 311t–312t
  in hypovolemic shock, 2528
  with increased intracranial pressure, 2178–2179
  intravenous, solutions for, types of, 339–341
  after laryngectomy, nursing interventions for, 617
  for metabolic alkalosis, 336
  in oral cavity conditions, 1151
  parenteral, 339–341
  in parenteral nutrition, 1198
  in pneumonia, 640
  postoperative, 537
    in neurosurgical patient, 2184c, 2187
  preoperative, 486, 496
  in shock, 364–365, 367t, 368, 371
    complications of, 365
  in thoracic surgical patient, 767, 774c
  traction and, 2371
  in unconscious patient, 2166–2167
  in upper airway infection, 603
Fluid volume
  after cardiac surgery, 893t, 899
  deficits in, 309–313, 316t. See also Hypovolemia
    manifestations of, 1516t
    in renal disorders, 1515–1517, 1516t
    in renal surgical patient, 1558–1559
  in disseminated intravascular coagulation, 1097c
  disturbances of, 309–313
  excess, 313–315, 316t. See also Hypervolemia
    in acute renal failure, 1525
    in chronic renal failure, 1530
    in cirrhosis, 1322
    manifestations of, 1516t
    in renal disorders, 1516t
    in renal surgical patient, 1558–1559
    in liver disease, 1328c
Flunarizine, in migraine prevention, 2200
Fluorescein angiography, 2049–2050
Fluorescent in situ hybridization, 149
Fluorescent treponemal antibody absorption test, for syphilis, 2506
Fluoridation, in prevention of tooth decay, 1145
Fluoroquinolones
  and immune system, 1797t
  for pneumonia, 636, 637
  for urinary tract infections, 1574
Fluoroscopy
  in cancer detection, 391t
  in cardiovascular disease, 808
  in respiratory disease, 580
5-Fluorouracil
  in cancer treatment, 399t
  and immune system, 1797t

Fluoxetine (Prozac)
  contraindications to, in Parkinson's disease, 2314
  for depression, in HIV-infected (AIDS) patients, 1836
  for fatigue, in multiple sclerosis, 2280
Flurbiprofen (Ansaid), for rheumatic diseases, 1895t
Fluvastatin, 986
  as lipid-lowering agent, 865t
FNA. See Fine-needle aspiration
Folic acid
  deficiency of, 1040, 1045t, 1052–1054, 1095–1098
    clinical manifestations of, 1053
    diagnosis of, 1053
    in liver disease, 1307
    medical management of, 1053
    pathophysiology of, 1052
  and erythropoiesis, 1040
Folk healers, 135
Follicle-stimulating hormone, 1445–1446, 1615–1616
  definition of, 1613
Folliculitis, 1957–1958
  in HIV-infected (AIDS) patients, 1834
Follitropin alpha (Gonal-F), for ovulation induction, 1651c
Follitropin beta (Follistim), for ovulation induction, 1651c
Food. See also Diet/dietary therapy; Nutrition/nutritional support
  cultural meanings associated with, 133, 133c
  in end-of-life care, ethical issues with, 32–33
  intake of
    cultural and religious factors affecting, 81
    Food Guide Pyramid for, 81, 82f
    24-hour recall of, 81
    in oral cavity conditions, 1151
    religious considerations and, 81
Food allergy, 1879–1880, 1880c
Foodborne hepatitis, causative organism of, 2476t
Food Guide Pyramid, 81, 82f
  and meal planning in diabetes, 1387
Food labels, and meal planning in diabetes, 1387, 1388
Food poisoning, 2544, 2544c
Food record, 81
Foot
  amputation of, 2460, 2461f
  diabetic, 2401
  musculoskeletal disorders of, 2400–2404, 2402f
Foot care, in diabetes, 1419, 1419c, 1427–1429, 1429f
Footdrop, 2367
  prevention of, 196
Foot surgery
  assessment in, 2402–2403
  expected outcomes in, 2403–2404
  home care after, 2403
  nursing diagnoses related to, 2403
  nursing interventions for, 2403
  nursing process with, 2402–2404
  planning and goals for, 2403
  self-care after, 2403, 2404c
Foramen of Monro, 2179–2180, 2180f
Foraminotomy, 2325
Forced end expiratory flow, 578t
Forced expiratory flow, 578t
Forced expiratory volume, 578t
  in 1 second ($FEV_1$), 578t
  as percentage of forced vital capacity ($FEV_1/FVC\%$), 578t

# INDEX

Forced midexpiratory flow, 578t
Forced vital capacity, 578t
Foreign bodies
  aspiration of, 608
  in external ear, 2104–2105
  in eye, 2073, 2074
  intraocular, 2074–2075
  swallowing of, and esophageal injury or obstruction, 1165
  and wound healing, 541t
Forensic evidence
  in sexual assault, collection of, 2552
  in trauma, collection of, 2529–2530
Formoterol (Foradil), 693t
  for asthma, 713t
Formula(s), for tube feeding, 1182
Fornix, 1614
  definition of, 1613
Fosamprenavir (Lexiva), for HIV infection, 1828t
Foscarnet (Foscavir)
  adverse effects and side effects of, 1836
  for cytomegalovirus retinitis, 1836, 2084
Fosinopril (Monopril), 952–953, 952t
  for hypertension, 1029t
Fosphenytoin
  blood levels of, 2601t
  preoperative use of, for intracranial surgery, 2181
  for status epilepticus, 2198
4 point gait, 206c
FPG. See Fasting plasma glucose
Fraction of inspired oxygen, 724
  definition of, 723
Fracture(s), 2431–2460
  of acetabulum, 2445–2446
  avascular necrosis of bone and, 2439–2440
  casts for, 2355
  cervical, management of, 2254
  of clavicle, 2440, 2441f
    range-of-motion exercises for, 2441f
  clinical manifestations of, 2431
  closed, 2431
    home care for, 2434c
    nursing management of, 2434, 2434c
  of coccyx, 2445
  comminuted, 2431
  and compartment syndrome, 2436–2438
  complete, 2431
  and complex regional pain syndrome, 2440
  complications of
    delayed, 2435, 2438–2440
    early, 2435–2438
  definition of, 2355, 2425, 2431
  delayed union of, 2438–2439
  of elbow, 2443
  emergency management of, 2431–2432, 2533
  external fixator for, in femoral shaft fracture, 2449, 2458
  external fixators for, 2364–2365, 2364f
  and fat embolism syndrome, 2435–2436
  of femoral shaft, 2449, 2458f
  of fibula, 2459
  of hand, 2444
  healing of, 2340
    complications in, 2435–2440
    factors affecting, 2435, 2435c
    and heterotopic ossification, 2440
  of hip, 2446–2449
    gerontologic considerations in, 2450c–2458c
  of humeral neck, 2441–2442, 2442f
  of humeral shaft, 2442, 2442f
  incomplete, 2431
  and infection, 2438
  internal fixation for, 2433, 2433f
    devices for, reaction to, 2440
    in femoral shaft fracture, 2449
    in hip fracture, 2447, 2447f
    in nonunion, 2438
  and joint replacement, 2372
  of knee, 2458–2459
  maintaining and restoring function after, 2433–2434
  malunion of
    in clavicular fracture, 2440
    definition of, 2425
  mandibular, 1147
  medical management of, 2433–2434
  nasal, 607–608
  nonunion of, 2438–2439
    definition of, 2425
  nursing interventions for, 2410
  nursing management of, 2434–2435
  open, 2431
    emergency management of, 2432
    nursing management of, 2434–2435
  orbital, 2073
  osteoporotic, 2404, 2409–2411
    assessment of, 2409
    expected outcomes for, 2410–2411
    nursing diagnoses related to, 2409
    nursing interventions for, 2410
    nursing process for, 2409–2411
    planning and goals for, 2410
  Paget's disease and, 2412
  pathologic, with bone tumors, 2419–2420
  of pelvis, 2444–2449
  of phalanx, 2444
  of radial head, 2443
  of radial shaft, 2443
  reduction of, 2433
    closed, 2091, 2433
      for hip fracture, 2447
    definition of, 2425
    for hip fracture, 2447
    open, 2433, 2433f
      in hip fracture, 2447, 2447f
  of rib, 2459–2460
    flail chest with, 676–677, 677f
    in trauma patient, 676
  and shock, 2435
  of skull, 2234, 2234f, 2235
  sports-related, 2426–2427
  sternal, in trauma patient, 676
  of thoracolumbar spine, 1460
  of tibia, 2459
  types of, 2431
  of ulnar shaft, 2443
  of wrist, 2443–2444
Fragile X syndrome
  diagnosis of, 150t
  genetics of, 144
Frail elder(s), 246
*Francisella tularensis*, 2567t
Frank-Starling law, 787
Free jejunal graft transfer, for esophageal reconstruction, 1167, 1168f
Freon, abuse/overdose, emergency management of, 2546t
Frequency
  of sound, 77, 2100
  urinary, 1503, 1503t
    definition of, 1493, 1570
    in urinary tract infections, 1572
Fresh-frozen plasma, transfusion of, 1108c
Friction, and pressure ulcers, 208–209, 209f, 213
Friction rubs, 575–576, 575t
  cardiac, 803
definition of, 625
with lung abscess, 651
Frontal lobe, 2131, 2131f
Frontal sinus, 1153f
Frostbite, 2534–2535
Frusemide (Lasix), for lymphedema, 1017
FSH. See Follicle-stimulating hormone
FTA-ABS. See Fluorescent treponemal antibody absorption test
FUDR, in cancer treatment, 399t
Fulminant hepatic failure, 1317
  definition of, 1285
Functional abilities, assessment of, 193
  in elderly, 227
Functional consequences theory, of aging, 228
Functional domain, definition of, 46c
Functional incontinence, 215
Functional Independence Measure(tm), 193, 2218
Functional residual capacity, 558t
Fundoplication, for gastroesophageal reflux disease, 1166
Fundus, of uterus, 1614–1615, 1615f
  definition of, 1613
Funerals, planning of, 472
Fungal encephalitis, 2275–2276
  assessment of, 2275
  diagnosis of, 2275
  medical management of, 2275–2276
  nursing management of, 2276
Fungal infections. See also specific infection
  phagocytic dysfunction and, 1802–1805, 1803t
  of skin, 1960–1962, 1961t
Fungemia
  definition of, 2475, 2484
  health care–associated, prevention of, 2483–2484
  vascular access device-related, 2484, 2484c
Funnel chest, 570
Furosemide (Lasix), 953, 954t
  for ascites, 1294–1295
  and calcium balance, 328
  for heart failure, 965
  for hypertension, 1026t
  for hypervolemia, 313
  for lymphedema, 1017
Furuncles, 1957–1958
  definition of, 1945
Fusion inhibitors, for HIV infection, 1826–1828, 1828t

## G

Gabapentin
  adverse effects and side effects of, 2194t
  for hot flashes, 1635
  for migraine, 2201
  toxic effects of, 2194t
  for trigeminal neuralgia, 2295
Gait
  assessment of, 2347
  with brain tumor, 2304
  in burn patient, 2032t
  with crutches, 204–205, 206c
  in elderly, 236
  in Huntington's disease, 2319
  in Parkinson's disease, 2313
  shuffling, 2347
  steppage, 2347
Galactography, 1706
  definition of, 1701
Galactorrhea, with prolactinoma, 2302
Galactosemia
  genetics of, 147t
  screening for, 150t

Galantamine hydrobromide (Reminyl), for
    Alzheimer's disease, 244
Gallbladder, 1122f
    anatomy of, 1345, 1346f
    disorders of, 1347–1355
        surgery for, nursing process for,
            1355–1358
Gallium scan, 580–581
Gallop(s), 802–803
    definition of, 802
Gallstones. See Cholelithiasis
Gamete intrafallopian transfer, 1652
Gamma-aminobutyric acid, 2130t
Gamma glutamyltransferase
    in biliary/pancreatic disease, 1349t
    serum, 1290t
Gamma glutamyltranspeptidase, 1290t
    in biliary/pancreatic disease, 1349t
Gamma-hydroxybutyrate, abuse/overdose,
    emergency management of,
    2545t–2546t
Ganciclovir
    for cytomegalovirus retinitis, 1835, 2084
    for pneumonia, 637
Ganglion, 1920, 2398
Gangrene, 1012f
    surgical management of, 996
Gapping ear puncture, 2106
Gardnerella vaginalis, 1662–1664, 1663t
Gargle(s), for pharyngitis, 598
Gas(es)
    intestinal, 1125, 1127
    in tube feeding, 1184t
    partial pressure of, 559c, 560
Gas exchange
    burns and, 2010c
    after cardiac surgery, 906c
    impaired, after cardiac surgery, 893t, 899,
        900
    in neurosurgical patient, nursing interven-
        tions for, 2186
    pulmonary, 557, 663
        in chronic obstructive pulmonary dis-
            ease, 697
        genetic factors affecting, 564
        partial pressure in, 560, 561f
    in thoracic surgical patient, 765, 771c
    in ventilator-dependent patient, 749
Gasoline, abuse/overdose, emergency manage-
    ment of, 2546t
Gastric, definition of, 1204
Gastric acid, secretion of, and peptic ulcer dis-
    ease, 1209–1210
Gastric acid stimulation test, 1138–1139
Gastric analysis, 1138–1139
Gastric artery, 1121
Gastric aspirate, and feeding tube placement,
    1178–1179
Gastric banding, laparoscopic, 1218
Gastric bypass surgery, 1218–1220, 1219f
Gastric cancer, 1220–1223
    assessment in, 1221
    clinical manifestations of, 1220–1221
    continuing care in, 1223
    diagnosis of, 1221
    expected outcomes in, 1223
    familial occurrence of, 386
    medical management of, 1221
    nursing diagnoses related to, 1222
    nursing interventions for, 1222–1223
    nursing process with, 1223–1227
    pathophysiology of, 1220
    patient teaching about, 1222–1223, 1223c
    pernicious anemia and, 1053, 1054
    surgical management of, 1221

Gastric content, residual, measurement of, in
    tube feedings, 1183–1184
Gastric emptying
    assessment of, 1133–1134
    delayed, identification of, 682
Gastric lavage, 2541, 2542c–2543c
Gastric motility
    evaluation of, 1138
    regulators of, 1124t
Gastric resection with gastrojejunostomy,
    malabsorption in, 1240t
Gastric retention, after gastric surgery,
    1224–1225
Gastric secretions, 1123, 1123t
Gastric sump tube, 1175–1176, 1176f
Gastric surgery, 1223–1227
    complications of, 1224–1226
    continuing care after, 1226
    dietary self-management after, patient
        teaching about, 1226, 1227c
    expected outcomes in, 1226–1227
    nursing diagnoses related to, 1224
    nursing interventions for, 1224–1226
    nursing process with, 1223–1227
    patient teaching about, 1226
    planning and goals for, 1224
    preoperative assessment for, 1223–1224
Gastric tonometry, 360
Gastric ulcers, 1209–1217, 1210t. See also
    Peptic ulcer disease
Gastrin, in gastrointestinal regulation, 1124t
Gastritis, 1204–1208
    acute, 1204
    assessment in, 1205–1207
    bile reflux, after gastric surgery, 1225
    chronic, 1204
    clinical manifestations of, 1204
    definition of, 1204
    diagnosis of, 1204
    expected outcomes in, 1208–1209
    medical management of, 1205–1207,
        1206t–1207t
    nursing diagnoses related to, 1207
    nursing interventions for, 1207–1208
    nursing process with, 1205–1208
    pathophysiology of, 1204, 1205f
    planning and goals for, 1207
Gastroduodenal manometry, 1138
Gastroduodenostomy, in peptic ulcer disease,
    1214t
Gastroesophageal reflux, 1162
    definition of, 1142
    gastrostomy and, 1189
Gastroesophageal reflux disease, 1165–1166,
    1209
    and esophageal cancer, 1167
Gastroesophageal sphincter, 1162. See also
    Lower esophageal sphincter
Gastrointestinal function
    age-related changes in, 1125, 1126c, 1139
    assessment of, 1126–1129
    in burn victim, 2002, 2004
    diagnostic assessment of, 1129–1139
    genetic factors affecting, 1131
    pathophysiologic considerations in, 1139
    postoperative management of, 542–543
    psychological considerations in, 1139
    regulatory substances of, 1124t
Gastrointestinal intubation. See also Tube
    feeding(s)
    complications of, 1180–1181
    instruction for patient before, 1177
    maintaining tube function in, 1179
    monitoring patient with, 1179
    nasal hygiene in, 1179

oral hygiene in, 1179
securing tube in, 1177, 1180f
tube insertion in, 1177–1178
tube placement in, confirmation of,
    1178–1179
    nursing research on, 1179
tube removal in, 1181
Gastrointestinal motility studies, 1133–1134
Gastrointestinal tract
    age-related changes in, 231t, 234, 1125,
        1126c, 1139, 1795t
    anatomy of, 1121–1122, 1122f
    blood supply of, 1121–1122, 1123f
    brain injury and, 2242t
    chemotherapy and, 398–400
    chronic renal failure and, 1528, 1528c
    digestive enzymes and secretions of, 1123t
    dysfunction of
        clinical manifestations of, 1126–1127
        health history for, 1126–1127
    in fluid and electrolyte balance, 304
    in HIV-infected (AIDS) patients, 1831–1832
    immune dysfunction and, 1794c
    inflammation of. See also Inflammatory
        bowel disease
    innervation of, 1122
    lower, imaging of, 1132
        nursing interventions in, 1132
    magnesium loss from, 329
    organs and associated structures of, 1122f
    physical assessment of, 1127–1129, 1128f
    regulatory substances of, 1124t
    in shock, 362
    in tube feeding, 1184t
    upper, imaging of, 1132
        nursing interventions in, 1132
Gastrointestinal ulcers, in kidney transplant
    recipient, 1563
Gastrojejunostomy
    gastric resection with, malabsorption in,
        1240t
    in peptic ulcer disease, 1212, 1214t
Gastroplasty, vertical banded, 1218–1220,
    1219f
Gastroscopy, 1134–1135, 1134f
Gastrostomy, 1188–1193
    complications of, 1190, 1191
    continuing care in, 1192
    contraindications to, 1189
    definition of, 1175, 1188
    gastroesophageal reflux and, 1189
    Janeway, 1188
    nursing diagnoses related to, 1190
    nursing process with, 1189–1193
    percutaneous endoscopic, 1188–1189,
        1189f
    Stamm, 1188
    tube care in, 1191
    types of, 1188–1189
Gate control theory, of pain, 266, 267f, 291
Gatifloxacin (Tequin), for pneumonia, 636
Gaucher's disease, genetics of, 146
Gauntlet cast, 2355
Gaze, cardinal directions of, 2048
G-button. See Low-profile gastrostomy device
GB virus-C, 1315
G-CSF. See Granulocyte colony-stimulating
    factor
GDM. See Gestational diabetes mellitus
Gefitinib (Iressa), 422
Gels, for wound care, 1949
Gemcitabine, in cancer treatment, 399t
Gemfibrozil (Lopid), 986
Gemtuzumab ozogamicin (Mylotarg), 418, 419t
    adverse effects and side effects of, 421t

# INDEX

Gender differences
  in cardiac structure and function, 787
  in heart, 787
  in heart disease, 866–867
  in oral cancer, 1148
  in pain, 268–269
Gene(s), 141–145. *See also* Deoxyribonucleic acid (DNA)
  mutations of, 140, 143–145, 144f
    acquired, 144, 145f
    carriers of, 140, 146
      testing for, 149, 150t
    deletion, 144
    duplication, 144
    germline (inherited), 144, 144f
    insertion, 144
    penetrance of, 140, 146
    somatic, 144, 145f
    spontaneous, 144
    translocation, 144
  suicide, 422
General adaptation syndrome, 94–95
General anesthesia, 508–511
  stages of
    I (beginning), 509
    II (excitement), 509
    III (surgical anesthesia), 509
    IV (medullary depression), 509
Gene therapy, 1793
  for cancer, 422
  for cystic fibrosis, 719
  for ovarian cancer, 1691
Genetic counseling, 156–160
  components of, 157, 158c
  confidentiality in, 158–159
  ethical considerations in, 158, 160–161
  follow-up, 160
  information in, communication of, to patient, 160
  informed consent for, 159
  patients' rights in, respect for, 158–159
  preparation for, 159–160
  services for, 157
  support for patient in, 160
Genetic counselling
  issues in, across lifespan, 157, 159c
  nursing role in, 157–158
Genetic disorders, 102
Genetic engineering
  definition of, 1783
  and immunology, 1793
Genetic evaluation. *See* Assessment, genetic; Genetic testing
Genetic profile(s), 153–154
Genetic referral
  background information for, 159
  indications for, 156c
Genetics, 139–161. *See also* Inheritance
  advances in, and health care, 8
  and assessment, 154–156–157
  of cancer, 384, 386
  of cardiovascular disease, 789
  clinical applications of, 149–154
  definition of, 140
  diagnostic, 102
  of female reproductive disorders, 1619
  of gastrointestinal disorders, 1131
  of hearing loss, 2101
  of Huntington's disease, 2319
  of lung cancer, 671
  of melanoma, 1981
  of metabolic disorders, 1444
  and musculoskeletal system, 2345
  of neurologic disorders, 2144
  in nursing practice, 68, 141
    applications of, 154–160

  of peptic ulcer disease, 1209
  and perioperative nursing, 493
  resources on, for nurses, 161c
  and respiratory function, 564
  of skin disorders, 1933
  of urinary tract disorders, 1501, 1502
Genetic screening, 149, 150t
  for adult-onset conditions, 151t–152t
  family history in, 154–155, 155c
Genetic testing, 102, 149. *See also* Prenatal screening
  for adult-onset conditions, 151t–152t
  current uses of, 149, 150t
  diagnostic, 150t
  ethical considerations in, 158, 160–161
  follow-up for, 160
  for non-disease genes, 153–154
  nursing interventions for, 153
  predisposition, 140, 152t, 153
  prenatal, 150t
  preparation for, 159–160
  presymptomatic, 140, 150t, 151t–152t, 152
  results of
    communication of, to patient, 160
    confidentiality of, 158–159
  services for, 157
  susceptibility, 150t
Genetic variation, 145
Genitalia, external, female, 1614, 1614f
Genitourinary pain, 1501–1503, 1502t, 1512c
Genitourinary system
  brain injury and, 2242t
  female, age-related changes in, 231t, 233
  immune dysfunction and, 1794c
  male
    age-related changes in, 231t, 233–234
    infections of, 1750
Genitourinary trauma, 1595–1597, 2532
Genogram, 67, 67f
Genome, 140
  definition of, 140
Genomic medicine, 140
Genomics, 141
  definition of, 140
Genotype, 141
  definition of, 140
Gentamicin, therapeutic blood levels of, 2601t
Gentamicin sulfate, for burns, 2017
Gentamicin sulfate (Garamycin), and immune system, 1797t
Geriatric Depression Scale, 241c
Geriatric nursing. *See* Gerontologic/geriatric nursing
Geriatrics, definition of, 225
Gerontologic considerations. *See* Older adults
Gerontologic/geriatric nursing, 226
  definition of, 225
Gerontology, 226
  definition of, 225
Gestational diabetes mellitus, 1379t
  definition of, 1376
  management of, 1382
  pathophysiology of, 1382
  risk factors for, 1382
GFR. *See* Glomerular filtration rate
GH. *See* Growth hormone
Ghon tubercle, 644, 650
GHRH. *See* Growth hormone-releasing hormone
Giant cell tumors, of bone, 2417
*Giardia lamblia*
  CVID and, 1805
  and diarrhoeal diseases, 2502
Giardiasis, malabsorption in, 1240t
GIFT. *See* Gamete intrafallopian transfer

Gigantism, 1446
Gigantomastia, 1712
Gingiva. *See* Gums
Gingivitis, 1144t
  necrotizing, 1144t
Gingivostomatitis, herpetic, 1144t
Glands, of skin, 1930
Glare testing, 2052
Glasgow Coma Scale, 2162, 2240, 2240c, 2243
Glatiramer acetate (Copaxone), for multiple sclerosis, 2280
Glaucoma, 2051, 2054–2059
  angle-closure, 2056, 2056t
  classification of, 2056, 2056t
  clinical manifestations of, 2056
  in diabetes, 1423t
  diagnosis of, 2056–2057
  medical management of, 2057–2058
  nursing management of, 2059
  open-angle, 2056, 2056t
  pathophysiology of, 2055, 2055f
  pharmacologic therapy for, 2057, 2058t, 2085–2086
  primary, 2056
  risk factors for, 2055, 2055c
  secondary, 2056
  stages of, 2055, 2055c
  surgical management of, 2057–2058
  visual field defects in, progression of, 2057, 2057f
Gliding joints, 2341
Glimepiride (Amaryl), 1399t
Gliomas, 2302
Glipizide (Glucatrol), 1399t
Globe, malignant tumor of, 2081
Globulins, 1042
  serum, 1290t
Glomerular disease(s), primary, 1517–1521
Glomerular filtration, 1496, 1496f
Glomerular filtration rate, 1499
  in chronic renal failure, 1527, 1527c, 1528–1529
  definition of, 1021, 1493
Glomerulonephritis
  acute, 1517–1521
    complications of, 1518
    continuing care in, 1518
    pathophysiology of, 1517, 1517f
  chronic, 1518–1520
    continuing care in, 1520
    definition of, 1515, 1517
    postinfectious, 1517
    rapidly progressive, 1518
Glomerulus, 1494–1495, 1495f
  definition of, 1493
Glomus jugulare, 2111
Glomus tympanicum, 2111
Glossectomy, 1149
Glossopharyngeal nerve (IX), 2136–2137, 2136f, 2137t, 2292f
  assessment of, 2147c
  disorders of, 2293t
Glottis, 554
Gloves
  in infection control and prevention, 2481
  in Standard Precautions, 1820c
Glucagon
  action of, 1346
  secretion of, 1346
Glucocorticoid(s), 1474–1475
  definition of, 91, 1440
  in stress response, 95
Gluconeogenesis, 1380
  definition of, 91
  in stress response, 95

I-43

Glucosamine, for osteoarthritis, 1916
Glucose
    blood level of. *See also* Continuous glucose monitoring system; Fasting plasma glucose; Impaired fasting glucose; Impaired glucose tolerance; Self-monitoring of blood glucose
        in cardiac patient, 807t
        laboratory values for, 310t
    metabolism of
        abnormalities of, in liver disease, 1307–1308
        endocrine control of, 1346–1347
        liver in, 1286
    in water ($D_5W$), 339
Glucose-6-phosphate dehydrogenase (G6PD) deficiency, 1061–1062
Glutamate, and ischemic stroke, 2207
Gluteal-strengthening exercises, 203
Glyburide (Micronase), 1399t
Glycemic index, 1385, 1387
Glycogen, in muscles, 2341
Glycogenolysis, 1380
Glycopyrrolate (Robinul), in end-of-life care, 471t
Glycosuria, detection of, 1505
GM-CSF. *See* Granulocyte-macrophage colony-stimulating factor
GnRH. *See* Gonadotropin-releasing hormone
Goiter, 1450
    definition of, 1440
    diffuse, 1450, 1450t
    endemic (iodine-deficient), 1466–1467
    nodular, 1467
Gold-containing compounds, for rheumatic diseases, 1895t
Gold sodium thiomalate (Myochrysine), for rheumatic diseases, 1895t
Gonadotropin-releasing hormone, 1616
Goniometer, 2348
Gonococcal arthritis, 2509
Gonococcal meningitis, 2509
Gonorrhea, 1669–1670, 2507–2508
    assessment in, 2507
    causative organism of, 2476t
    clinical manifestations of, 2507
    complications of, 2507
    diagnosis of, 2507
    medical management of, 2508
    nursing management of, 2508
    pathophysiology of, 1670–1671, 1671f
    and pelvic inflammatory disease, 1670–1672
Gout, 1918–1919
    joint involvement in, 2348
    medical management of, 1918, 1919t
    nodules in, 2348
Gouty arthritis, 1918
Gowns, in Standard Precautions, 1820c
GpIIb/IIIa agents, 871
Graafian follicle, 1615
    definition of, 1613
Grading, of tumors, 390–391
    definition of, 381
Graft(s)
    arteriovenous
        definition of, 1515
        for hemodialysis, 1539, 1539f
    assessment of
        after neck dissection, 1155
        after oral cancer surgery, 1149
    for head and neck reconstruction, 1153
    jejunal, in esophageal reconstruction, 1167, 1168f
    in neck dissection, nursing interventions for, 1156c–1157c
    for oral cancer, 1149

Graft-versus-disease effect
    in bone marrow transplant recipient, 416
    definition of, 381
Graft-versus-host disease, 1113
    in acute myeloid leukemia, 1072
    in bone marrow transplant recipient, 416
    definition of, 381
    transfusion-related, 1104t
        prevention of, 1106–1107
Gram-negative bacteria, enteric, pneumonia caused by, risk factors for, 637c
Gram-negative sepsis, with urinary tract infections, 1575
Granisetron, for chemotherapy patient, 398
Granular leucocytes, in natural immunity, 1785
Granulex, 1946
Granulocyte(s), 1040f, 1041
    definition of, 1036
    in natural immunity, 1785
    and phagocytic immune response, 1786
    for transfusion, 1103t
Granulocyte colony-stimulating factor
    for acute myeloid leukemia, 1071
    adverse effects and side effects of, 421t
    as alternative to blood transfusion, 1112c
    in breast cancer treatment, 1727–1728
    in cancer treatment, 401, 420
    for phagocytic dysfunction, 1805
Granulocyte-macrophage colony-stimulating factor
    for acute myeloid leukemia, 1071
    adverse effects and side effects of, 421t
    as alternative to blood transfusion, 1112c
    in cancer treatment, 401, 420
    for phagocytic dysfunction, 1805
Granulocytopenia
    in cancer patient, 424
    definition of, 1036
Granuloma(s)
    periapical, 1145
    in sarcoidosis, 667
    in tuberculosis, 644
Granulomatous colitis. *See* Regional enteritis
Graves' disease, 1459–1465
    definition of, 1440
Gravity drip, in tube feeding, 1182
Gray matter, 2131, 2134f, 2135–2136
Great vessels, pressures in, 785f
Grief, 121–122, 471–473
    in acute leukemia, 1078
    amputation and, 2464
    anticipatory, 471, 473c
        in cancer patient, nursing management of, 412c–413c, 431
        nursing diagnoses related to, 1610–1611
        nursing interventions for, 1610–1611
        nursing outcomes for, 1610–1611
    assessment for, 121, 122c
    in cancer patient and family, nursing interventions for, 412c–413c, 431
    complicated, 473
    definition of, 112, 448, 471
    versus depression, 122
    in ectopic pregnancy, 1655
    in family members of emergency patient, 2520
    in HIV-infected (AIDS) patients, 1849
    nursing interventions for, 121–122, 473c
    signs and symptoms of, 121, 122c
    stages of, 121
    uncomplicated, 471–473
Griess nitrite reduction test, in UTI diagnosis, 1574
Growth and development, definition of, 46c

Growth factor(s), 1948
    as alternative to blood transfusion, 1112c
    in breast cancer treatment, 1727–1729, 1728c
    and cancer treatment, 422
Growth hormone, 1446
    skeletal effects of, 2339
Guanfacine (Tenex), for hypertension, 1027t
Guanine (G), 141
Guardianship, of older persons, 252
Guided imagery
    definition of, 91, 107
    for low back pain, 2394
    in pain management, 289–290
    relaxation with, 107
Guide dogs, 2054
Guillain-Barré syndrome, 2288–2292
    assessment in, 2289
    clinical manifestations of, 2288–2289
    complications of, 2289–2291
    continuing care for, 2291–2292
    diagnosis of, 2289
    expected outcomes in, 2292
    home and community-based care for, 2291–2292, 2291c
    medical management of, 2289
    Miller-Fisher variant of, 2289
    nursing diagnoses related to, 2289
    nursing interventions for, 2290–2291
    nursing process with, 2289–2292
    and pain, 261c–262c
    pathophysiology of, 2288
    planning and goals for, 2290
    self-care in, 2291
Guilt, in family members of emergency patient, 2519
Gums, 1150f
    cancer of, 1148–1149
    disorders of, 1144t
    inflammation of. *See* Gingivitis
    inspection of, 1150
Gunshot wound, thoracic, 678
Gynecomastia, 1705, 1735
    definition of, 1701
Gyri, 2131, 2131f

# H

Habilitation, 190
    definition of, 190
Habit retraining, 1582c
Habit training, for urinary incontinence, 216
*Haemophilus ducreyi*
    incubation period of, 2476t
    transmission of, 2476t
*Haemophilus influenzae*
    and Guillain-Barré syndrome, 2288
    pneumonia, 629, 630t, 634, 635
Hair
    aging and, 1932
    assessment of, 1936
    color of, 1930, 1936
    distribution of, 1936–1939
    functions of, 1930
    growth of, 1928
    loss of, 1939. *See also* Alopecia
        in cancer patient, 425
    texture of, 1936
Hair follicle, 1928, 1928f
Hair shaft, 1928f
Hairy leukoplakia, 1143t
HAIs. *See* Health care–associated infection
Hallucinations, in Parkinson's disease, 2313
Hallucinogens, abuse/overdose, emergency management of, 2546t–2547t

# INDEX

Hallux valgus, 2401–2402, 2402f
Haloperidol
　for delirium, 468
　for postoperative confusion in older patients, 547
Halothane, 510t
　hepatitis caused by, 1317
Halo traction, 2254–2255, 2255f
　comfort measures for, 2258, 2259c
Halo vest
　definition of, 2233
　in traction, 2254–2255, 2255f
Hammer toe, 2401, 2402f
Hand(s)
　decontamination of, in infection control and prevention, 2481, 2481c
　fracture of, 2444
　hygiene for, in infection control and prevention, 2480–2481, 2481c
　positioning of, in stroke recovery, 2217
Handedness, 2131–2132
Handicap, definition of, 174
Handwashing
　in infection control and prevention, 2480–2481, 2481c
　in Standard Precautions, 1820c
Hand/wrist surgery
　assessment in, 2399
　expected outcomes in, 2400
　home and community-based care after, 2400, 2400c
　nursing diagnoses related to, 2399
　nursing interventions for, 2399–2400
　nursing process for, 2399–2400
　planning and goals for, 2399
Hantavirus pulmonary syndrome, 2511
　incubation period of, 2476t
　transmission of, 2476t
Haploid cell(s), 143
　definition of, 140
Hapten, 1857l
　definition of, 1856
Hardiness, 94
Hard palate, 1150f, 1153f
Hare traction, 2533
　definition of, 2517
Harris-Benedict equation, for nutritional support, 2025
Hartmann procedure, for diverticulitis, 1244, 1244f
Hashimoto's disease, 1452, 1466
　definition of, 1440
Haversian canal, 2339
Haversian remodeling, 2340
Haversian system, 2339
Havighurst's developmental tasks of aging, 227
Hay fever. See Allergic rhinitis
HbS gene, 1056
Headache, 2198–2202. See also Migraine headache
　assessment of, 2199
　with brain tumor, 2304
　classification of, 2198, 2198c
　clinical manifestations of, 2200
　cluster, 2198, 2199
　　clinical manifestations of, 2200
　　medical management of, 2201
　　nursing management of, 2201
　　prevention of, 2200
　continuing care for, 2201
　diagnostic evaluation of, 2199
　International Headache Society Classification of, 2198, 2198c
　nursing management of, 2201

　other primary types of, 2198
　pathophysiology of, 2199
　post-lumbar puncture, 2158
　prevention of, 2200
　primary, 2198
　　definition of, 2161
　secondary, 2198–2199
　　definition of, 2161
　spinal anesthesia and, 515
　tension-type, 2198, 2199
　　clinical manifestations of, 2200
　　nursing management of, 2201
Head and neck
　anatomy of, 1153f
　malignancies of, 1153–1161
Headgear, for surgery, 506
Head injury(ies), 2233–2235. See also Brain injury(ies)
　assessment of, 2235
　clinical manifestations of, 2235
　definition of, 2233
　diagnosis of, 2235
　epidemiology of, 2233
　gerontologic considerations in, 2235
　medical management of, 2235
　pathophysiology of, 2234, 2234f
　prevention of, 2233c
Head lice, 1962–1963
Head-tilt-chin-lift maneuver, 2523
Healing, 104. See Wound healing
Health. See also Mental health
　brain and, 113–114
　definition of, 6, 57
　determinants of, 57
　family functioning and, 115
　of nation, indicators of, 56c
　positive, predictors of, nursing research on, 71
　and wellness, 6, 57
Health belief model, of health promotion, 57
Health care
　changes in, 5–6, 16
　community-based, need for, 16
　delivery, alternative systems for, 9–10
　durable power of attorney for, 33
　financing of, 16
　focus of, in 21st century, 6
　for people with disabilities
　　access to, 177–183, 178c
　　barriers to, 178c, 182
　　federal legislation addressing, 176–177
　　strategies to ensure quality of, 178c–179c
　primary, 11
　regulation of, 16
　reimbursement for, 8
Health care–associated infection, 2480–2484
　bloodstream, prevention of, 2483–2484
　definition of, 2475
　organisms in, 2482–2483
Health care costs, 2602
　of aging, 249–250
Health care delivery, factors affecting, 7–10
Health care providers, HIV transmission to, 1818–1819
　postexposure prophylaxis for, 1819, 1821c, 2505, 2506t
　Standard Precautions for, 1818–1819, 1820c–1821c
Health care system, definition of, 46c
Health care workers, HIV transmission risk and, 2505, 2506t
Health disparities, 136
Health education. See also Patient teaching
　definition of, 49
　in nursing practice, 49–50
　purpose of, 49–50

Health history, 35. See also Patient profile
　for allergic assessment, 1861–1863, 1862c–1863c
　biographical data in, 66
　of blood donor, 1104–1105
　in cardiovascular disease, 788–790
　chief complaint in, 66
　components of, 65
　content of, 66–73
　cultural considerations with, 65–66
　ethical considerations with, 64
　family history in, 67
　formats for, 65
　in immune system assessment, 1794–1798
　informant for, 65
　in integumentary system assessment, 1932
　for musculoskeletal system assessment, 2342–2346
　　assessment data in, 2344–2346
　　initial interview in, 2344
　obtaining, 65–73
　of older adult, 65c
　past history in, 66–67
　patient profile in, 67–73, 69c
　present health concern or illness in, 66
　in respiratory disease, 563
　review of systems in, 67
　urologic, 1500–1504
Health–illness continuum, 6
Health maintenance organizations, 9–10
Health promotion, 56–58
　for adolescents, 58–59
　for children, 58–59
　components of, 57–58
　definition of, 6, 49, 56–57
　for elderly, nursing research on, 60
　genetics in, 68
　gerontologic considerations in, 60–61
　after hip fracture, 2449, 2457c–2458c
　immunizations in, 59t
　for low back pain, 2396c
　models of, 57
　after myocardial infarction, 884, 885c
　nursing implications of, 61
　in orthopedic surgery patient
　　postoperative, 2386
　　preoperative, 2383–2384
　over life span, 58–61
　for people with disabilities, 179c, 183–184
　screening in, 58, 59–60, 59t
　strategies for, 6
　variables affecting, 57
　for young and middle-aged adults, 59–60
Health-protecting behavior, 57
Health risk appraisal, 107
Health risk questionnaires, 105, 105c
*Healthy People 2000*, 56
*Healthy People 2010*, 56, 113, 113c
　and health care for people with disabilities, 176
Hearing, 2096. See also Ear(s)
　age-related changes in, 232t, 236–237
　diagnostic evaluation of, 2099–2101
　evaluation of, 2098–2099, 2099f
　after mastoid surgery, 2109
Hearing aids, 2120–2122
　care of, 2121, 2122t
　problems with, 2121, 2121c
　types of, 2121, 2121t
Hearing device(s)
　bone conduction, 2122
　implanted, 2122–2123
　semi-implantable, 2122
Hearing guide dogs, 2123

Hearing loss, 2101–2104
  assessment for, 2102, 2102c
  aural rehabilitation for, 2120–2123
  clinical manifestations of, 2102
  conductive, 2101–2102
    management of, 2120, 2120f
  definition of, 2093
  functional (psychogenic), 2102
  genetics of, 2101
  gerontologic considerations in, 2103
  medical management of, 2103
  mixed, 2102
  noise-induced, 2102
  nursing management of, 2103
  people with, interacting and communicating with, 180c, 2103, 2104c
  prevention of, 2102–2103
  risk factors for, 2102–2103, 2103c
  sensorineural, 2102
    definition of, 2093
  severity of, 2100, 2100t
Heart. See also Cardiac; Cardiomyopathy(ies)
  age-related changes in, 787, 788t
  anatomy of, 782–783
  auscultation of, 802–804
  chambers of, 782–783, 782f
    pressures in, 785, 785f, 786
  in chronic glomerulonephritis, 1519
  conduction abnormalities of, 838–840
  electrical conduction in
    abnormal. See Dysrhythmia(s)
    normal, 824–825, 824f
  filling volumes and pressures, assessment of, 798
  in fluid and electrolyte balance, 306
  gender differences in, 787
  in hypercalcemia, 328
  in hyperkalemia, 324
  in hypermagnesemia, 331
  in hypocalcemia, 326
  in hypokalemia, 322, 322f
  in hypomagnesemia, 330
  inspection of, 800–801
  palpation of, 800–801
  physiology of, 783–787
  pumping action of, 781
    assessment of, 798
    failure of, 978
  in shock, 361–362
  valves of, 783
    age-related changes in, 788t
Heart attack. See Myocardial infarct/infarction
Heart block, 838–840. See also Atrioventricular (AV) block
Heartburn. See Pyrosis
Heart disease
  aging and, 230–232
  gender differences in, 866–867
  hypertension and, 1023
  infectious, 933–941
  pulmonary. See Cor pulmonale
  risk factors for, 796c
Heart failure, 946–965, 978
  acute, 964–965
  in acute glomerulonephritis, 1518
  anemia and, 1047, 1049
  assessment in, 950, 950c
  burns and, 2030
  after cardiac surgery, 892t
  chronic, 947–964
  in chronic renal failure, 1527, 1529
  classification of, 947
  clinical manifestations of, 950–951
  complications of, 957–958
  definition of, 945
  diagnosis of, 951
  diastolic, 947
    definition of, 945
    medications for, 955–956
  etiology of, 948–949
  with exfoliative dermatitis, 1971
  gerontologic considerations in, 958
  hypertension and, 1023
  left-sided, 916f, 950–951
    definition of, 945
  medical management of, 952–957
  nursing management of, 957–958
  nursing process with, 958–964
  pathophysiology of, 947–948, 949f
  pharmacologic therapy for, 952–957
  readiness for behavioral change in, nursing research on, 960
  right-sided, 950, 951
    definition of, 945
    with pulmonary hypertension, 659–660
    signs and symptoms of, 660
  signs and symptoms of, 790
  systolic, 947
    definition of, 945
Heart murmur(s)
  characteristics of, 803c
  definition of, 781, 803
Heart rate, 945
  control of, 784, 786
    for atrial fibrillation, 833
  factors affecting, 825
  in heart failure, 951
  ventricular, determination of, on ECG, 827–828, 827f
Heart rhythm
  abnormalities of. See Dysrhythmia(s), cardiac
  determination of, on ECG, 828, 828c
Heart sounds, 802–803, 802f. See also Heart murmur(s)
  age-related changes in, 805
  clicks, 803
  gallops, 802–803, 802f
  interpretation of, 804
  normal, 802, 802f
    definition of, 781
  snaps, 803
Heart transplantation
  for cardiomyopathy, 928–929
  in heart failure, 957
  orthotopic, 928–929, 929f
    definition of, 915
  women's perspective after, nursing research on, 930
Heart valve(s). See also Valvular heart disease
  prosthetic, 923–924, 923f, 924f
  repair of, 920–923
    nursing management of, 924–925
  replacement of, 923–924
    nursing management of, 924–925
Heat, in muscle contractions, 2341
Heat stroke, 2533–2534
  gerontologic considerations in, 2533–2534
  prevention of, 2533, 2534c
Heat therapy
  for low back pain, 2393
  in pain management, 289
  in peripheral vascular disease, 987
  for rheumatic diseases, 1894, 1898
Height
  assessment of, 78
  loss of
    aging and, 2404, 2405f
    osteoporosis and, 2404, 2405f
  osteoporosis and, 78
Heimlich maneuver, in airway obstruction, 2523, 2523c

*Helicobacter pylori* infection, 1204
  diagnosis of, 1130, 1204
  and gastric cancer, 386
  medical management of, 1206t
  in peptic ulcer disease, 1209
Helper T cells, 1791
  definition of, 1783
Hemangiomas
  of eyelid, 2080
  orbital, 2080
Hemarthrosis, 2351
  arthrocentesis and, 1889
  definition of, 1887
Hematemesis, 1127
  definition of, 1204
  with esophageal varices, 1299
  in peptic ulcer disease, 1215–1216
Hematocrit, 305, 1044
  in cardiac patient, 808t
  definition of, 1036
  laboratory values for, 2579
  in rheumatic diseases, 1893t
  usual reference range for, 310t
Hematologic disorders, 1035–1113
  assessment of, 1043–1045
  bleeding in, risk of, 1068c
  infection in, risk of, 1066, 1067, 1068c
  laboratory studies of, 1044
  therapies for, 1102–1104
Hematologic system
  anatomy of, 1037–1043
  assessment of, 1043–1045
  chronic renal failure and, 1528c
  diagnostic findings in, 1043–1045
  gerontologic considerations in, 1043
  laboratory studies of, 2578t–2580t
  pathophysiology of, 1045–1102
  physiology of, 1037–1043
Hematology, reference ranges for, 2578t–2580t
Hematoma, 804
  after breast surgery, 1722–1723
  carotid endarterectomy and, 2215t
  definition of, 2528c
  epidural, 2236–2237, 2237f
  in fracture healing, 2340
  intracerebral, 2236–2237, 2237f, 2238
  with intravenous therapy, 351
  postoperative, 545
  subdural, 2236–2237, 2237f
Hematopoiesis, 1037, 1038f, 1067
  definition of, 1036
  extramedullary, 1039, 1067
  in metastatic bone disease, 2418
Hematopoietic growth factors, in cancer treatment, 420, 421t
Hematoporphyrin, for bladder cancer, 1597
Hematuria, 1503, 1503t, 1742
  in acute glomerulonephritis, 1517
  clinical significance of, 1506
  definition of, 1493
  detection of, 1506
  in renal trauma, 1565
  in urinary tract infections, 1572, 1574
Hemianopsia, definition of, 2206
Hemiarthroplasty
  definition of, 2371c
  for hip fracture, 2447
Hemiglossectomy, 1149
Hemilaminectomy, 2325
Hemilaryngectomy, for laryngeal cancer, 611
Hemiparesis
  with brain tumor, 2304
  definition of, 2206
  spastic, 2347
  stroke and, 2208t, 2209

# INDEX

Hemiplegia, 2141
  definition of, 2206
  nursing interventions for, 2216–2217
  stroke and, 2208t, 2209
Hemiplegia-associated shoulder pain, 261c
Hemisphere(s), cerebral, 2130–2133, 2131f, 2132f
  functions of, 95
Hemlock Society, 451
Hemoccult test, 1130
Hemochromatosis, 1063–1064
  hereditary, 151t
    population screening for, 153
Hemodialysis, 1537–1542, 1538f
  for acute renal failure, 1525
  complications of, 1540, 1551
  continuing care in, 1542
  definition of, 1515
  and end-of-life treatment, nursing research on, 1542
  fluid therapy with, 1540–1541
  at home, 1541–1542
  for hypervolemia, 314
  before kidney transplantation, 1561
  nursing management of, 1540–1542
  nutritional therapy in, 1551–1552
  nutrition during, 1540–1541
  pharmacologic therapy in, 1540
  vascular access for, 1539, 1539f
Hemodilution, 1106
Hemodynamic monitoring, 786, 816–820
  in cardiogenic shock, 369
  definition of, 781
  in hypertensive crises, 1033
Hemodynamics, cardiac, 785–786, 785f
Hemoglobin, 1039
  $A_2$, laboratory values for, 2578
  A1C, 1391
    definition of, 1376
  in acute renal failure, 1523
  $A_{1c}$, 1391
    definition of, 1376
  in cardiac patient, 808t
  definition of, 1036
  in diagnosis of anemia, 1501
  F, laboratory values for, 2579
  glycated, 1391
    definition of, 1376
  glycosylated, 1391
    in cardiac patient, 807t
    definition of, 1376
  laboratory values for, 2579
  oxygen saturation of ($SpO_2$), measurement of, 579
  in oxygen transport, 560
  S, 143–144, 1055, 1056
Hemolysis, 1045t, 1046
  definition of, 1036
Hemophilia, 1090–1091
  genetics of, 146, 147t
Hemopneumothorax, 679
Hemoptysis
  in bronchiectasis, 709
  in cardiac patient, 804
  causes of, 568
  definition of, 553, 563, 625
  diagnostic evaluation of, 568
  in lung cancer, 671
Hemorrhage. *See also* Bleeding
  after adenoidectomy, 600
  amputation and, 2461, 2467–2468
  in cancer patient, 432–433
  after cardiac surgery, 893t
  in cirrhosis, 1321
  classification of, 527, 528t
  control of, pressure points for, 2526–2527, 2527f

in ectopic pregnancy, 1654
emergency management of, 2526–2527
external, control of, 2526–2527, 2527f
fluid replacement in, 2526
hip fracture and, 2454c
with hysterectomy, 1693
internal
  control of, 2527
  emergency management of, 2532
intracerebral, 2238. *See* Intracerebral hemorrhage
after laryngectomy, nursing interventions for, 618
in liver disease, 1330c–1332c
in multiple trauma, 2472–2473
after neck dissection, 1155, 1159–1160
pelvic fracture and, 2444
postoperative, 527–528
in prostate cancer, 1760c
with prostatectomy, 1766
subarachnoid. *See* Subarachnoid hemorrhage
after thoracic surgery, 769
after tonsillectomy, 600
after total hip replacement, 2378c–2379c
in trauma patient, 675
in vulvar surgical patient, 1688
and wound healing, 541t
Hemorrhagic fevers, viral, 2511–2512
Hemorrhagic stroke, 2134, 2223–2230
  assessment in, 2225, 2225t, 2227
  causes of, 2207t
  with cerebral angioma, 2303
  and cerebral hypoxia, 2225–2226
  clinical manifestations of, 2208t–2209t, 2224
  complications of, 2225–2226, 2227, 2228–2229
  continuing care for, 2229, 2229c
  and decreased cerebral blood flow, 2225–2226
  delf-care after, 2229
  diagnosis of, 2225, 2225t
  DNR orders in, ethical considerations for, 2225c
  expected outcomes in, 2230
  home and community-based care for, 2229, 2229c
  and hydrocephalus, 2228
  and hypertension, 2226
  and increased intracranial pressure, 2226
  medical management of, 2226–2227
  nursing diagnoses related to, 2227
  nursing interventions for, 2227–2228
  nursing process for, 2227–2230
  pathophysiology of, 2223–2224
  planning and goals for, 2227
  prevention of, 2225
  prognosis for, 2224
  and rebleeding, 2228
  risk factors for, 2223
  and seizures, 2228
  surgical management of, 2226–2227
  and vasospasm, 2226, 2228
Hemorrhoidectomy, 1277
Hemorrhoids, 1233, 1276f, 1277
  definition of, 1232
Hemosiderin, 1063
  definition of, 1036
Hemostasis, 1037, 1043, 1044f, 1084–1085
  definition of, 301, 1036
  primary, 1043, 1044f
  secondary, 1043, 1044f
Hemothorax, 557, 679
  atelectasis with, 626
  definition of, 625

rib fracture and, 2460
in thoracic surgical patient, 761
in trauma patient, 675
Hemovac drain, 538, 538f
Heparin
  in allergic reaction, 1858t
  for atrial fibrillation, 833
  bleeding precautions with, 871
  for coronary artery disease, 870–871
  for deep vein thrombosis prevention, 2375
  in infertility treatment, 1651c
  low-molecular-weight
    subcutaneous administration of, 871
    for thrombotic disorders, 1100
    for venous thrombosis, 1006
  for pulmonary embolism, 663, 665
  therapy with
    complications of, 1007
    in disseminated intravascular coagulation, 1093–1094
  thrombocytopenia caused by, 1100
  for thrombophlebitis, 2259
  toxicity of, 1093
  unfractionated
    intravenous, 870–871
    for thrombotic disorders, 1100
    for venous thrombosis, 1006
Hepatic artery, 1285
Hepatic duct, 1286
Hepatic encephalopathy, 1289, 1304–1307, 1322
  assessment of, 1305
  clinical manifestations of, 1305
  definition of, 1285
  diagnosis of, 1305
  medical management of, 1305–1306
  nursing management of, 1306–1307
  nutritional management of, 1306, 1307c
  stages of, 1305, 1305t
Hepatitis
  bloodborne, causative organism of, 2476t
  chronic active, 1920
  drug-induced, 1316–1317
  foodborne, causative organism of, 2476t
  nonviral, 1315–1317
  toxic, 1316
  viral, 1308–1315
    epidemiology of, 1310t
    and HIV infection, 1822
    outcomes in, 1310t
    signs and symptoms of, 1310t
    terminology for, 1308, 1309c
Hepatitis A, 1308–1312, 1310t
  incubation period of, 1310t, 2476t
  management of, 1311, 1311c
  prevention of, 1309–1311, 1311c
  transmission of, 1310t, 2476t
Hepatitis B, 1310t, 1312–1314
  blood testing for, 1106
  and cancer, 385–386
  clinical manifestations of, 1310t, 1312
  diagnosis of, 1312–1313
  incubation period of, 1310t, 2476t
  medical management of, 1314
  nursing management of, 1314
  prevention of, 1313
  risk factors for, 1312, 1312c
  transfusion-transmitted, 1104t
    with long-term PRBC therapy, 1111t
  transmission of, 2476t
  vaccine against, 1313
Hepatitis B immune globulin (HBIG), 1313–1314
Hepatitis C, 1310t, 1314–1315
  blood testing for, 1106
  and cancer, 386

Hepatitis C (continued)
  fatigue in, nursing research on, 1316
  incubation period of, 1310t, 2476t
  risk factors for, 1314–1315, 1315c
  transfusion-transmitted, 1104t
    with long-term PRBC therapy, 1111t
  transmission of, 1310t, 2476t
Hepatitis D, 1310t, 1315
  incubation period of, 1310t, 2476t
  transmission of, 1310t, 2476t
Hepatitis E, 1310t, 1315
  incubation period of, 1310t, 2476t
  transmission of, 1310t, 2476t
Hepatitis G, 1315
  incubation period of, 2476t
  transmission of, 2476t
Hepatobiliary system, age-related changes in, 1287, 1287c
Hepatocellular carcinoma, 1333–1336
  hemochromatosis and, 1063
Hepatocytes, 1285
Hepatojugular reflux, in cardiac patient, 805
Herbal therapy, 134
  for cancer, 423
  and surgical patient, 488–489
Herbert's pits, 2077
Hereditary angioedema, 1879
Hereditary breast/ovarian cancer, 152t, 156
  genetics of, 146, 147t
  genetic testing in, 150t
  susceptibility testing, 150t
Hereditary hemochromatosis, 1063–1064
Hereditary hyperbilirubinemia, 1293
Hereditary nonpolyposis colorectal cancer, 152t
  genetics of, 147t
  genetic testing in, 150t
  susceptibility testing, 150t
Hereditary spherocytosis, 1062
Hering-Breuer reflex, 562
Hernia(s)
  definition of, 1142
  hiatal, 1163–1164
  and intestinal obstruction, 1263, 1264f, 1264t
  paraesophageal, 1163–1164, 1163f
  sliding esophageal, 1163–1164, 1163f
Herniation
  of brain, 2170, 2170f
  brainstem, brain injury and, 2248
  definition of, 2161
Heroin, abuse/overdose, emergency management of, 2545t
Herpangina, causative organism of, 2476t
Herpes, orolabial, 592, 592c
Herpes genitalis, 1667
Herpes labialis, 592, 592c
Herpes simplex, 1959–1960
  cold sores caused by, 592, 592c
  definition of, 589
  encephalitis caused by, 2274
    assessment of, 2274
    clinical manifestations of, 2274
    diagnosis of, 2274
    medical management of, 2274
    nursing management of, 2274
    pathophysiology of, 2274
  gene products, and HIV infection, 1822
  genital, 1667, 1959–1960
    nursing process for, 1667–1669
    prevention of, 1668
    spread of, prevention of, 1668
  HSV-1, 1143t, 1667, 1959–1960
    and encephalitis, 2274
  HSV-2, 1667, 1959–1960, 2274
    and cancer, 385

incubation period of, 2476t
infection, in HIV-infected (AIDS) patients, treatment of, 1836
keratitis, 2076t
neonatal, 1960
orolabial, 1959–1960
transmission of, 2476t
types of, 1959–1960
Herpes zoster, 1958–1959, 1958f
  distribution of, 1940f
  in Hodgkin's disease, 1074
Herpetic gingivostomatitis, 1144t
Herpetic whitlow, 1960
Hesitancy, urinary, 1503, 1503t
Hetastarch, for fluid replacement in shock, 367t
Heterograft
  for burns, 2019–2021, 2020t
  definition of, 915, 1995
  for heart valve replacement, 924
Heterotopic ossification, 2440
  in burn patient, 2032t
  definition of, 2355
HFE gene, 1063, 1064
HHNS. See Hyperglycemic hyperosmolar nonketotic syndrome
Hiatal hernia, 1163–1164, 1163f
  chest pain caused by, assessment of, 792t
Hiccups, postoperative, 542
HIE syndrome. See Hyperimmunoglobulinemia E syndrome
High-density lipoproteins
  and cardiac risk, 806
  definition of, 859, 1021
  serum levels, 863, 1290t
High-frequency chest wall oscillation vest, 731–734, 733
High linear transfer radiation, 395
Highly active antiretroviral therapy, 1826, 2084
Hinge joints, 2340
Hip
  external rotation of, prevention of, 196
  fracture of, 2446–2449
    clinical manifestations of, 2446
    complications of, 2448–2449, 2454c–2457c
    coping with, 2452c–2453c
    extracapsular, 2446, 2446f
    gerontologic considerations in, 2446–2447
    health promotion after, 2449
    internal fixation of, 2447, 2447f
    intracapsular, 2446, 2446f
    medical management of, 2447
    nursing care plan for, 2450c–2458c
    pain with, 2446
    positioning after, 2448
    postoperative nursing management for, 2447–2449
    strengthening exercises after, 2448
    surgery for, 2447, 2447f
Hip protectors, 2405
Hip replacement, 2372f
  total, 2373–2375
    complications of, 2373–2375, 2378c–2381c
    continuing care for, 2375
    and deep vein thrombosis, 2380c
    and hemorrhage, 2378c–2379c
    home and community-based care for, 2375, 2376c
    and infection, 2381c
    mobility after, 2378c

and neurovascular dysfunction, 2379c
nursing care plan for, 2377c–2381c
nursing interventions for, 2373–2375
pain management for, 2377c
prosthesis dislocation in, 2373–2374, 2373f, 2374c, 2380c
self-care after, 2381c
wound drainage after, 2374
Hip spica cast, 2355
Hirsutism, 1930
  definition of, 1927
Histamine
  in allergic reaction, 1858–1859, 1858t
  definition of, 1856
  in gastrointestinal regulation, 1124t
  in humoral immune response, 1789
  in inflammation, 103
Histamine ($H_1$) antagonists, 1870, 1871t
Histamine ($H_2$) antagonists, 1870, 1871t
  for gastritis and peptic ulcer disease, 1206t
  for metabolic alkalosis, 336
Histamine-1 ($H_1$) receptors, 1858–1859
Histamine-2 ($H_2$) receptors, 1859
Histiocyte(s), 1043
  definition of, 1036
  in natural immunity, 1785
*Histoplasma capsulatum*
  encephalitis caused by, 2275–2276
  incubation period of, 2476t
  transmission of, 2476t
Histoplasmosis
  causative organism of, 2476t
  incubation period of, 2476t
  transmission of, 2476t
HIV. See Human immunodeficiency virus
HIV encephalopathy, 1833, 1834c
  definition of, 1815
Hives. See Urticaria
HMG-CoA reductase inhibitors, 864–865, 865t
  for osteoporosis, 2409
  and stroke prevention, 2211
HMOs. See Health maintenance organizations
Hoarseness, in laryngeal cancer, 609–610
Hodgkin's disease, 1080–1081
  cause of, 1080
  clinical manifestations of, 1080
  diagnosis of, 1080–1081
  epidemiology of, 1080
  Epstein-Barr virus and, 1080
  medical management of, 1081
    long-term complications of, 1081, 1081c
  prognosis for, 1080
  subgroups of, 1080
Holiday heart syndrome, 832
Holidays, culture and, 133
Holistic care, 17
Holistic health, 112–113
  definition of, 112
Homans' sign, 1005
Homatropine, ocular applications of, 2086t
Home, assessment of, 84–85, 84c
Home and community-based care
  in acute glomerulonephritis, 1518
  in acute leukemia, 1078–1079
  for allergic rhinitis, 1875–1876, 1875c
  for Alzheimer's disease, 246
  for amputation, 2468–2469, 2468c
  assessment in, 84–85, 84c
  in asthma, 714–717
  for bone tumors, 2420, 2421c
  for brain injuries, 2249–2250, 2250c
  for brain tumor patient, 2308–2309, 2309c
  and breathing retraining, 734–735
  for burns, 2034–2036, 2035c–2036c

with cardiac dysrhythmia, 841–842
after cardiac surgery, 902–903
in cardiomyopathy, 932–933
for casts, 2360–2362, 2361c
and chest physiotherapy, 734–735
for chronic glomerulonephritis, 1519–1520
in chronic illness, 172–174
in chronic obstructive pulmonary disease, 700
in chronic renal failure, 1531
for closed fracture, 2434c
for continuous ambulatory peritoneal dialysis patient, 1549–1550, 1550c
for cor pulmonale, 661
for dementia, 246
with enteral therapy, 1188
and epidural analgesia, 288
for esophageal conditions, 1170–1171, 1170c
for foot surgery patients, 2403, 2404c
for fractures, 2434c
after gastric surgery, 1226
for gastrostomy, 1192
for Guillain-Barré syndrome, 2291–2292, 2291c
for hand/wrist surgery patients, 2400, 2400c
for headache, 2201
for hemodialysis, 1541–1542, 1543c
for HIV-infected (AIDS) patients, 1850
in Huntington's disease, 2320
for hypertension, 1031–1032
in hypothyroidism, 1454–1459, 1458c
for immunodeficiency, 1810–1812, 1811c
with implanted cardiac device, 851
in inflammatory bowel disease, 1253–1254, 1253c
after intracranial surgery, 2188
for intravenous therapy, 351–352
for kidney transplant recipient, 1563
for laryngectomy patient, 618–620, 619c
after mastoid surgery, 2110, 2110c
with mechanical ventilation, 746–747
for multiple sclerosis, 2283, 2284c
after myocardial infarction, 884, 885c
after neck dissection, 1161, 1161c
in oral cavity conditions, 1152, 1152c
for orthopedic surgery patient, postoperative, 2387–2388
for osteomyelitis, 2415, 2416c
for osteoporosis, 2408c
and oxygen therapy, 728–729, 728c
for paraplegia/quadriplegia, 2265–2266
and parenteral nutrition, 1198, 1200t
in Parkinson's disease, 2317–2318, 2318c
in peptic ulcer disease, 1216–1217, 1217c
in peripheral vascular disease, 991, 994–995
for peritoneal dialysis, 1549–1550, 1550c
for persons with disabilities, 185
for postoperative patient, 548
for psoriasis, 1969–1970, 1970c
in rehabilitation, 219–222, 220c–221c
for renal cancer patient, 1564–1565
for renal surgical patient, 1559
in rheumatic diseases, 1904–1906, 1905c
safety precautions in, 18, 19, 20c
for shock, 377–378
in sickle cell anemia, 1059
for spinal cord injuries, 2260–2261
for stroke patient, 2222–2223, 2229, 2229c
after thoracic surgery, 769–770, 770c, 774c–775c
for total hip replacement, 2375, 2376c
transfers in, 203

for urinary diversions, 1600–1602, 1606–1607
for urinary tract infections, 1576
in urolithiasis, 1594
for venous thrombosis, 1010
Home care, discharge planning for, 18
Home health care nursing, 11–12
Home health nursing, 17f
Homeless persons, care for, 22
Home management, in multiple sclerosis, 2283
Homeopathic medicine, 134
  definition of, 112
Homeostasis, 92, 99
  definition of, 91, 301
Home visit
  closing/ending, 21
  conducting, 19–21
  documentation of, 20
  future, determining need for, 20–21, 20c
  initial (first), 19–20
  need for, assessment of, 20–21, 20c
  preparation for, 19
  safety precautions in, 19, 20c
Homicide, forensic evidence in, collection of, 2529–2530
Homocysteine, in cardiac patient, 806–808
Homocystinuria, genetic screening for, 150t
Homograft
  for burns, 2019–2021, 2020t
  definition of, 915, 1995
  for heart valve replacement, 924
Homonymous hemianopsia, 2220
  with brain tumor, 2304
  nursing diagnoses related to, 2040–2041
  nursing interventions for, 2040–2041
  nursing outcomes for, 2040–2041
  stroke and, 2208t, 2209
Hookworm disease, causative organism of, 2476t
Hope, in end-of-life care, 462–463
Hordeolum, 2076t
Hormone(s). *See also specific hormone*
  actions of, 1441–1442, 1443t
  and bone health, 2339
  and cancer, 386–387
  for cancer treatment, 399t
  classification of, 1441–1442
  in contraception, 1641–1644
  definition of, 1440
  function of, 1441
  gastrointestinal, 1124t
  peptide, 1441–1442
  protein, 1441–1442
  regulation of, 1441
  sources of, 1443t
  steroid, 1441–1442
Hormone therapy
  for acne vulgaris, 1954t, 1955
  adverse effects and side effects of, 2409
  and heart disease, 866–867
  for menopause, 1634–1635
  for osteoporosis, 2408–2409
  for prostate cancer, 1754–1760
Horny layer, of skin, 1928f
Horseback riding, therapeutic, 219
Hospice, definition of, 448
Hospice care, 452–456. *See also* End-of-life care
  for brain tumor patient, 2309
  for cancer patient, 437
  continuous care in, 456
  definition of, 250
  eligibility criteria for, 455, 455c
  general inpatient care in, 456

historical perspective on, 454
inpatient respite care in, 456
Medicare coverage of, 455–456
for older persons, 250
principles of, 454–455
routine home care level of, 456, 456c
in United States, 455
Hospice nursing, 17
Hospital(s)
  emergency preparedness plans in, 2560
  infection prevention in, 2480–2484
Host
  definition of, 2475
  of infectious organism, 2475
  response to infection, 2479, 2479f
  susceptible, 2478–2479
Hot/cold theory of health and illness, 135
Hot flashes, in menopause, therapy for, 1635
Howship's lacunae, 2339
HPS. *See* Hantavirus pulmonary syndrome
HPV. *See* Human papillomavirus
Huber needles, 401f
Huff coughing, 697, 757
Human B-lymphotrophic virus, 1667
Human Genome Project, 102, 141
  definition of, 140
Human herpesvirus (HHV), 6, 2477t
Human immunodeficiency virus, 2505, 2506t. *See also* Acquired immunodeficiency syndrome
  blood testing for, 1106
  co-infection in gonorrhea, 2508
  encephalopathy caused by. *See* HIV encephalopathy
  glycoproteins of, 1821, 1822f
  and Guillain-Barré syndrome, 2288
  and health care providers
    postexposure prophylaxis for, 1819, 1821c, 2505, 2506t
    Standard Precautions for, 1818–1819, 1820c–1821c
  HIV-1
    definition of, 1815
    life cycle of, 1821, 1822f
    structure of, 1821, 1822f
    subtypes of, 1822
    transmission of, 1816
  HIV-2
    definition of, 1815
    transmission of, 1816
  infection, 1750
    assessment in, 1824–1825
    asymptomatic, 1823t, 1824
    and childbearing by Black women, nursing research on, 1819
    classification of, 1823–1824, 1823t
    clinical manifestations of, 1830–1835
    complications of, 1843c–1844c, 2509
    confidentiality in, 1851
    continuing care for, 1850
    cutaneous signs of, 1941
    and depression, 1833
    diagnosis of, 1824–1825
    emotional concerns in, 1851–1852
    endocrine manifestations of, 1834
    epidemiology of, 1815–1816, 2512
    ethics and, 1851, 1851c
    expected outcomes with, 1850–1851
    gastrointestinal manifestations of, 1831–1832
    gerontologic considerations in, 248, 1816–1817
    gynecologic manifestations of, 1834–1835
    home and community-based care for, 1850

Human immunodeficiency virus, infection (*continued*)
  incubation period of, 2476t
  integumentary system in, 1834
  and Kaposi's sarcoma, 386. *See also* Kaposi's sarcoma
  medical management, 1835–1837
  medication reactions in, 1844c, 1849–1850
  mental status in, 1846–1847
  neurologic manifestations of, 1833, 1845
  and nutrition, 1840c–1841c, 1844–1845
  nutrition therapy in, 1836–1837
  oncologic manifestations of, 1832–1833
  pathophysiology of, 1819–1823
  pneumonia in, 633t, 634
  postexposure prophylaxis for, 1819, 1821c, 2505, 2506t
  prevention of, 1817–1818, 1819, 1821c
  primary, 1823t, 1824
  respiratory manifestations of, 1831, 1845, 1849
  risk factors for, 1816, 1816c
  risks to health care workers, 2505, 2506t
  self-care for, 1850
  stages of, 1823–1824
  symptomatic, 1823t, 1824
  testing for, 1824–1825
    home-based kits for, 1825
    patient reactions to, 1825, 1825c
    reporting of results, 1825, 1825c
  tests for, 1799t
  and toxic epidermal necrolysis or Stevens-Johnson syndrome, 1974
  transmission of, 1816, 2476t
    to health care providers, 1818–1819
    risk to health care workers, 2505, 2506t
  treatment of, 1826–1830, 1827t–1828t
    adherence to regimens in, 1826, 1829c
    adverse effects and side effects of, 1826, 1827t–1828t
    combination therapy for, 1826–1829, 1827t–1828t
    complementary and alternative modalities, 1837
    drug resistance in, 1829–1830
    immunomodulator therapy for, 1830
    interruption of, 1830
    reinstitution of, CD4 cell count and, 1830
    supportive care in, 1837
    viral load test for, 1825, 1825t
  in women, 1672–1673, 1834–1835
  testing for, in sexual assault victim, 2552–2553
  transfusion-transmitted, 1104t
  vaccination against, 1830
Human immunodeficiency virus antibody tests, 1824–1825
Human leukocyte antigen(s)
  HLA-B27, in rheumatic diseases, 1894t
  in multiple sclerosis, 2277–2278
Human papillomavirus, 1977–1978
  and cancer, 385, 1685–1686
  definition of, 1815
  epidemiology of, 1666
  in HIV-infected (AIDS) patients, 1672, 1834–1835
  infection, pathophysiology of, 1666
  and penile cancer, 1774
  vaccine against, 420, 1666
Human T-cell lymphotropic virus
  blood testing for, 1106
  and cancer, 386
  transfusion-transmitted, 1104t

Humerus
  neck of, fracture of, 2441–2442, 2442f
  shaft of, fracture of, 2442, 2442f
Humoral immune response, 1042, 1786–1788, 1787–1788
  antigen–antibody binding in, 1790
  assessment of, tests for, 1799t
  definition of, 1783
Hunt-Hess classification, 2225, 2225t
Huntington's disease, 151t, 2319–2323
  continuing care in, 2320
  diagnosis of, 152
  genetics of, 144, 147t
  genetic testing in, 150t
  home and community-based care in, 2320
  nursing care plan for, 2321c
  nursing diagnoses related to, 2321c
  nursing interventions for, 2321c
  nursing process in, 2321c
  presymptomatic testing for, 150t, 152
Hyaline cartilage, malignant tumors of, 2417
Hyaluronic acid (Hyalgan, Synvisc), for osteoarthritis, 1916
Hybridomas, 418
Hydatidiform mole, definition of, 1661
Hydradenitis suppurativa, 1952–1953
Hydralazine (Apresoline), 953
  for hypertension, 1028t
Hydration. *See also* Fluid management and replacement
  in end-of-life care, 466–467, 467t
    ethical issues with, 32–33
  after laryngectomy, nursing interventions for, 617
  maintenance of, in tube feedings, 1187
  withdrawal of, ethics of, 1190c
Hydrocele, 1743–1744, 1773
  definition of, 1740
Hydrocephalus, hemorrhagic stroke and, 2228
Hydrochloric acid, 1121, 1123
  in gastric analysis, 1138–1139
  source and digestive function of, 1123t
Hydrochlorothiazide, 954t
  for hypertension, 1026t
  for hypervolemia, 313
  interactions with anesthetics, 490t
Hydrocodone
  pharmacology of, 283t
  for pharyngitis, 598
Hydrocolloids, 1948
Hydrocortisone, 1474, 1485t
  for rheumatic diseases, 1896t
Hydroflumethazide (Diucardin, Saluron), 954t
Hydrogels, 1947
Hydrogen breath test, 1130
Hydrophilic, definition of, 1945
Hydrophilic surface, 1948
Hydrophobic, definition of, 1945
Hydrophobic backing, 1948
Hydrops, endolymphatic, definition of, 2093
Hydrostatic pressure, 302
  definition of, 301
Hydrostatic therapy, for bladder cancer, 1597
Hydrotherapy, definition of, 1995
Hydroxychloroquine (Plaquenil)
  for polymyositis, 1913
  for rheumatic diseases, 1895t
Hydroxycobalamin, for cyanide poisoning, 2569t, 2571
Hydroxyurea
  in cancer treatment, 399t
  for chronic myeloid leukemia, 1073
  for polycythemia vera, 1065
  for psoriasis, 1966t, 1967
  for sickle cell anemia, 1057
  for thrombocythemia, 1086

Hydroxyzine, 1871t
  postoperative use of, 528
  for pruritus, 1952
Hygiene
  in diabetes mellitus, for hospitalized patient, 1432
  hand, in infection control and prevention, 2480–2481, 2481c
  after laryngectomy, patient teaching about, 619–620
  for nails, in infection control and prevention, 2481
Hygiene therapy, for acne vulgaris, 1954–1955
Hygroscopic, definition of, 1945
Hygroscopic agents, 1949
Hymen, 1624
  definition of, 1613
Hyoid, 1153f
Hyoscyamine (Levsin), in end-of-life care, 471t
Hyperaldosteronism, and potassium balance, 321
Hyperbaric oxygen therapy, 727–728
Hyperbilirubinemia, hereditary, 1293
Hypercalcemia, 317t, 327–328
  and bone tumor metastasis, 2418
  bone tumors and, 2420
  in cancer patient, 439t
  after cardiac surgery, 908c
  medical management of, 328
  in multiple myeloma, 1083
  nursing management of, 328
  symptoms of, 2420
Hypercalcemic crisis, 328
Hypercapnia, 337
  with increased intracranial pressure, interventions for, 2178t
  sleep apnea and, 605
Hyperchloremia, 317t, 334
Hypercholesterolemia, familial, 152t
  genetics of, 147t
Hypercoagulable states, 1095, 1099t
Hyperemia
  conjunctival, 2077, 2077f
  definition of, 2043
  and skin color, 1935t
Hyperextension, 200c
Hyperglycemia
  after cardiac surgery, 908c
  definition of, 1376
  in diabetes, 1376
  in diabetes mellitus, 1418
  enteral nutrition and, 1184t
  in hospitalized patient with diabetes, 1430–1431
  morning, in insulin therapy, 1396, 1397t
  in parenteral nutrition, 1197t
  perioperative, 488
Hyperglycemic hyperosmolar nonketotic syndrome, 1376, 1415–1416
  definition of, 1376
  and diabetic ketoacidosis, comparison of, 1415t
Hyperhomocystinemia, 1095–1098, 1099t
Hyperimmunoglobulinemia E (HIE) syndrome, 1803t, 1804
Hyperinsulinism, 1372
Hyperkalemia, 316t, 323–325
  in acute myeloid leukemia treatment, 1072
  in acute renal failure, 1524
    treatment of, 1525
  assessment of, 324
  after cardiac surgery, 907c–908c
  in chronic glomerulonephritis, 1519
  in chronic renal failure, 1529, 1535c
    prevention of, 1530

clinical manifestations of, 324
correction of, 325
diagnosis of, 324
diuretic-induced, 314
in hypovolemia, 309
medical management of, 324
and metabolic acidosis, 335
nursing management of, 324–325
prevention of, 325
in respiratory acidosis, 337
Hyperlipidemia, 152t
Hypermagnesemia, 317t, 330–331
Hypermetabolism, in burn victim, 2002, 2025–2026
Hypernatremia, 316t, 319–321
assessment of, 320
correction of, 321
diagnosis of, 320
in hypovolemia, 309
nursing management of, 320–321
prevention of, 320
Hyperopia, 2050f, 2051
Hyperopia, definition of, 2043
Hyperosmolar diuresis, in parenteral nutrition, 1198
Hyperparathyroidism, 1470–1472, 1472c
and osteomalacia, 2411
Hyperperfusion syndrome, carotid endarterectomy and, 2215t
Hyperphosphatemia, 317t, 332–333
and hypocalcemia, 325
Hyperpigmentation, 1934
definition of, 1927
Hyperplasia, 100, 100t, 383
definition of, 91, 381, 1036
endometrial, 1682
Hyperpnea, 570
Hyperreflexia, autonomic. *See* Dysreflexia, autonomic
Hyperresonance, 76
Hypersensitivity, 1859–1861, 1860f
anaphylactic (type I), 1859, 1860f
cytotoxic (type II), 1859–1860, 1860f
definition of, 1856
delayed-type (type IV), 1791, 1860–1861, 1861f
immune complex (type III), 1860, 1861f
tests for, 1799t
Hypertension, 232, 786, 1020–1033
in acute glomerulonephritis, 1517–1518
assessment of, 1023, 1023c, 1025–1030
in cardiac surgical patient, 891t
carotid endarterectomy and, 2215t
causes of, 1021, 1023
in chronic renal failure, 1527, 1529, 1536c
classification of, 1021, 1021t
clinical manifestations of, 1023
complications of, 1030–1031, 1032
management of, 1030–1031
consequences of, 1022
continuing care for, 1032
definition of, 781, 1021
diagnosis of, 1030–1031
diagnostic evaluation of, 1023, 1023c
as disease, 1022
dyslipidemia and, 1022
epidemiology of, 1021
expected outcomes in, 1033
follow-up care for, 1032, 1032t
genetics of, 147, 147t
gerontologic considerations in, 1023, 1025, 1031
hemorrhagic stroke and, 2226
home and community-based care for, 1031–1032

lifestyle modification therapy for, 1031
management of, lifestyle modifications for, 1024–1025, 1025t
medical management of, 866, 1024–1025, 1024f, 1026t–1029t
monotherapy for, gerontologic considerations in, 1031
nursing diagnoses related to, 1030
nursing interventions for, 1031–1033
nursing process for, 1025–1033
ocular changes in, 2084
pathophysiology of, 986, 1022–1023, 1024f
pharmacologic therapy for, 1025, 1026t–1029t
planning and goals for, 1031
portal. *See* Portal hypertension
postoperative, 528
prevention of, lifestyle modifications for, 1024–1025, 1025t
primary, 1021
definition of, 1021
pulmonary, 948
rebound, 1031
definition of, 1021
as risk factor for atherosclerosis, 1022
risk factors for, 1023, 1023c
secondary, 1021
definition of, 1021
self-care for, 1031
as sign, 1022
stage 1, 1021, 1021t
stage 2, 1021, 1021t
systemic, 948
systolic, 1021
treatment of, 1024–1025, 1024f
algorithm for, 1024f
hypotension related to, 1032
Hypertensive crises, 1033
Hypertensive emergency, 1033
definition of, 1021
Hypertensive encephalopathy, in acute glomerulonephritis, 1518
Hypertensive urgency, 1033
definition of, 1021
Hyperthermia
in burn victim, 2002
therapeutic, for cancer, 417–418
Hyperthyroidism, 1450, 1459–1465
assessment in, 1459–1460
clinical manifestations of, 1459
diagnosis of, 1459–1460
epidemiology of, 1459
gerontologic considerations in, 1463
medical management of, 1460–1462
nursing process for, 1463–1465
pharmacologic therapy for, 1460–1462, 1462t
surgical management of, 1462
Hypertonic solution(s), 312t, 339–341
definition of, 301
Hypertrophic scar
in burn patient, 2032t
definition of, 1995
prevention of, 2026, 2031–2033
Hypertrophy, 100, 100t
definition of, 2337
of muscle, 2342
Hyperuricemia
gout and, 1918
in hypervolemia, 314
Hyperventilation, 570, 572t
in increased intracranial pressure, 2173–2174
and respiratory alkalosis, 337
Hyperviscosity, in multiple myeloma, 1083, 1084

Hypervolemia, 313–315, 316t
assessment of, 313
clinical manifestations of, 313
diagnosis of, 313
edema in, 314–315
medical management of, 313–314
nursing management of, 314–315
pathophysiology of, 313
prevention of, 314
Hyphae, 1662
definition of, 1661
Hyphema, 2074
definition of, 2043
Hypnosis, in pain management, 290
Hypnotics. *See also* Sedative-hypnotics
Hypoalbuminemia, in chronic glomerulonephritis, 1519
Hypocalcemia, 316t, 325–327
in acute myeloid leukemia treatment, 1072
after cardiac surgery, 908c
drug-induced, 325l–326
medical management of, 327, 1806
nursing management of, 327
T-cell deficiencies and, 1806
Hypochloremia, 317t, 333–334
Hypochromia
definition of, 1036
in thalassemia, 1061
Hypogammaglobulinemia, 1805–1806
definition of, 1802
Hypoglossal nerve (XII), 2136–2137, 2136f, 2137f, 2292f
assessment of, 2147c
disorders of, 2294t
Hypoglycemia
definition of, 1376
in diabetes, 1383, 1410–1412, 1418
assessment of, 1411
clinical manifestations of, 1410–1411
diagnosis of, 1411
emergency management of, 1411–1412
gerontologic considerations in, 1410
management of, 1411–1412
patient teaching about, 1411, 1412
in hospitalized patient with diabetes, 1431
in liver disease, 1308
perioperative, 488
rebound, in parenteral nutrition discontinuation, 1196, 1197t
Hypoglycemic unawareness, 1427
Hypogonadism, hemochromatosis and, 1063
Hypokalemia, 316t, 321–323
after cardiac surgery, 907c
in diabetes mellitus, 1418
diuretic-induced, 313–314
drug-induced, 321
in hypovolemia, 309
medical management of, 322
and metabolic alkalosis, 336
nursing management of, 322–323
prevention of, 322–323
Hypokinesia
in Huntington's disease, 2320
in Parkinson's disease, 2313
Hypomagnesemia, 317t, 329–330
after cardiac surgery, 908c
drug-induced, 329
medical management of, 330
nursing management of, 330
Hyponatremia, 315–318, 316t
assessment of, 318
after cardiac surgery, 908c
cellular effects of, 318, 318f
detection of, 319
diagnosis of, 318

Hyponatremia (continued)
  dilutional, 315, 1440, 1448
  diuretic-induced, 314
  and hypochloremia, 333
  in hypovolemia, 309
  nursing management of, 319
  in older persons, 319
Hypoparathyroidism, 1472–1473, 1474c
  and hypocalcemia, 325
  T-cell deficiencies and, 1806
Hypopharyngeal obstruction, management of, 525, 526f
Hypopharyngeal sphincter, 1162. *See also* Upper esophageal sphincter
Hypophosphatemia, 317t, 331–332
  medical management of, 333
  nursing management of, 333
  prevention of, 333
Hypophysectomy, 1447
  definition of, 1440
Hypopigmentation, 1934
  definition of, 1927
Hypopituitarism, 1446, 1447
Hypoplasia, thymic, 1803t, 1806
  definition of, 1802
Hypopyon, 2079
  definition of, 2043
Hyporeflexia, in Guillain-Barré syndrome, 2288
Hypospadias, 1774
Hypotension, 786
  in acute respiratory distress syndrome, 658
  carotid endarterectomy and, 2215t
  definition of, 373c, 781
  in elderly, 232
  hypertension treatment and, 1032
  management of, in postanesthesia care, 526–527
  orthostatic (postural)
    postoperative, 537
    spinal cord injury and, 2259
  postoperative, 526–527, 527
Hypothalamic-pituitary axis, in physiologic response to stress, 95–96, 96f
Hypothalamus, 2131f, 2132, 2137–2138
  functions of, 95
  in stress response, 95–96
Hypothermia, 2535–2536
  in blistering diseases, 1973
  after cardiac surgery, 902
  in cardiac surgical patient, 891t
  induced, after cardiac arrest, 837
  and intracranial pressure, 2173
  intraoperative, 517
  prevention of, in toxic epidermal necrolysis or Stevens-Johnson syndrome, 1976
Hypothyroidism, 1452–1459
  causes of, 1452, 1452c
  clinical manifestations of, 1453
  continuing care for, 1458–1459
  gerontologic considerations in, 1459
  and hair, 1930
  hemochromatosis and, 1063
  home and community-based care in, 1454–1459, 1458c
  medical management of, 1453–1454
  nursing care plan for, 1455c–1458c
  nursing management of, 1454–1459
Hypotonic solution(s), 311t, 339
  definition of, 301
Hypoventilation, 572t
  oxygen-induced, 725
  risk factors for, 577c
Hypovolemia, 309–313, 316t
  in acute respiratory distress syndrome, 658

assessment for, 312
in cardiac surgical patient, 891t
correction of, 313
diarrheal diseases and, 2504
gerontologic considerations in, 309–310
medical management of, 310–312, 311t–312t, 313
and metabolic alkalosis, 337
nursing management of, 312–313
prevention of, 313
  in acute pancreatitis, 1367c
  and wound healing, 541t
Hypovolemic shock, in orthopedic surgery patient, 2386–2387
Hypoxemia, 724
  in acute respiratory distress syndrome, 658
  in atelectasis, 627
  in bronchoscopy, 581
  clinical manifestations of, 724
  definition of, 553, 723
  episodic, 534
  in pneumonia, 636
  postoperative, 534
  in sleep apnea, 605
  subacute, 534
Hypoxia, 724
  anemic, 724c
  causes of, 101
  cellular injury caused by, 101
  cellular response to, 99
  cerebral
    in carbon monoxide poisoning, 2541–2543
    hemorrhagic stroke and, 2225–2226
  circulatory, 724c
  clinical manifestations of, 724
  cyanosis in, 568
  definition of, 91, 553, 723
  histotoxic, 724c
  hypoxemic, 724c
  with increased intracranial pressure, interventions for, 2178t
  intraoperative, 516
  after laryngectomy, nursing interventions for, 618
  myocardial, in carbon monoxide poisoning, 2541–2543
  types of, 724, 724c
  and wound healing, 541t
Hysterectomy, 1675, 1679, 1691–1694
  definition of, 1661
  laparoscopically assisted, 1692
  nursing process with, 1692–1694
  postoperative management of, 1692
  preoperative management of, 1692
  radical, 1692
  subtotal, 1692
  supracervical, 1692
  total, 1692
Hysterosalpingography, 1631
Hysteroscopy, 1631
  definition of, 1613
  for fibroid tumors, 1679

# I

Ibandronate (Boniva), for osteoporosis, 2409
Ibritumomab, adverse effects and side effects of, 421t
Ibritumomab-tiuxetan (Zevalin), 418, 419t
Ibuprofen
  contraindications to, 956
  and immune system, 1797t
  for low back pain, 2393
  mechanism of action of, 284

in pain management, 284
precautions with, 593
for rheumatic diseases, 1895t
for viral rhinitis, 592, 593
Ibutilide (Corvert), 830t
  for atrial fibrillation, 833
ICCE. *See* Intracapsular cataract extraction
Ice collar, for pharyngitis, 598
Ice therapy, in pain management, 289
ICP. *See* Intracranial pressure
Idarubicin
  for acute myeloid leukemia, 1071
  in cancer treatment, 399t
Ideal body weight, calculation of, 79c
Idiopathic hypertrophic subaortic stenosis. *See* Cardiomyopathy(ies), hypertrophic
Idiopathic thrombocytopenic purpura, 1087t, 1088–1089
  chronic lymphocytic leukemia and, 1074
Idioventricular rhythm, 837, 837f, 840f
IFG. *See* Impaired fasting glucose
Ifosfamide, in cancer treatment, 399t
  adverse effects and side effects of, 399t
IGT. *See* Impaired glucose tolerance
Ileal conduit (ileal loop), 1598–1602, 1598f
  definition of, 1570
Ileal dysfunction, malabsorption in, 1240t
Ileocecal valve, 1121
  function of, 1125
Ileostomy
  appliance, changing, 1259, 1260c–1261c
  complications of, 1262–1263
  continent, 1250
    irrigating/draining, 1259–1261, 1262c
  definition of, 1232
  nursing care plan for, 1255c–1258c
  nursing management of patient requiring, 1254–1263
  postoperative phase of, nursing management of, 1254–1263
  preoperative phase of, nursing management of, 1254
  self-care for, 1263, 1263c
  total colectomy with, 1250
Ileum, 1121
Ileus
  adynamic, 2363
  mechanical, after appendectomy, 1242, 1242t
  paralytic
    after appendectomy, 1242, 1242t
    in burn victim, 2002, 2004, 2014c
    spinal fracture and, 2460
    vertebral collapse and, 2410
Ilizarov external fixator, 2365
Illness. *See also* Disease(s)
  causes of
    biomedical (scientific) view of, 134
    magico-religious view of, 135
    naturalistic (holistic) view of, 135
  chronic. *See* Chronic illness
  stress and, 93, 97–98
  terminal. *See* Death and dying; Terminal illness
  trajectory (course) of, 169, 171t
Imaging
  in cancer detection, 391t
  gastrointestinal, 1132–1134
  in respiratory disease, 580
  of trauma patient, 62
Imatinib mesylate (Gleevec), for chronic myeloid leukemia, 1073
Imipramine
  abuse/overdose, emergency management of, 2548t

for depression, in HIV-infected (AIDS) patients, 1836
therapeutic blood levels of, 2601t
Immigration
and acquired immunodeficiency syndrome, 2512
and infectious diseases, 2512
and tuberculosis, 2512
and vector-borne disease, 2512, 2513f
Immobility
of joints, 1889
and pressure ulcers, 208
Immobilization
for epicondylitis, 2429
for fractures, 2433
for joint dislocation, 2426
for sprains and strains, 2426
Immune, definition of, 2475
Immune complex (type III) hypersensitivity, 1860, 1861f
Immune function
assessment of, 1794, 1794c
gerontologic considerations in, 1794–1795, 1795t
Immune globulins
and passive acquired immunity, 1786
for transfusion, 1103–1104, 1103t
Immune hemolytic anemia, 1062–1063
Immune reconstitution syndrome, in HIV-infected (AIDS) patients, 1831
Immune response
to cancer cells, 388
cellular, 1787–1788, 1788c, 1790–1792, 1792t
definition of, 1783
natural killer cells in, 1792
null lymphocytes in, 1792
T cells in, 1791
complement-mediated, 1787f
complement system and, 1792–1793
disordered, 102
effector stage of, 1788, 1789f
humoral, 1786–1788
antigen–antibody binding in, 1790
definition of, 1783
to infection, 102
and inflammation, 1887–1888
phagocytic, 1786
definition of, 1783
proliferation stage of, 1787, 1789f
recognition stage of, 1787, 1789f
response stage of, 1787–1788, 1789f
skin and, 1931
Immune system
age-related changes in, 1794–1795, 1795t
allergy and, 1796
alterations of, in burn victim, 2002
anatomy of, 1784, 1784f
antitumor activity of, 388
assessment of, 1782–1800, 1794–1798, 1794c
health history in, 1794–1798
physical examination in, 1798
preoperative, 488
cancer and, 387–388, 1796
cells of, development of, 1784, 1785f
diagnostic evaluation of, 1799, 1799c
disorders of, 1783, 1783t, 1796
autoimmunity. See Autoimmune disorders
signs and symptoms of, 1794c
failure, and carcinogenesis, 388
functions of, 1786–1788
immunization and, 1795–1796
infections and, 1795–1796
medications and, 1797t

nutrition and, 1795
psychoneuroimmunologic factors and, 1798
response to invasion, 1786–1788
in stress response, 96–97
Immunity, 2478–2479
acquired, 1786–1788
adaptive. See Acquired immunity
definition of, 1783
Immunization(s), 59t. See also Vaccine(s)
and acquired immunity, 1786
in chronic obstructive pulmonary disease, 693, 698
and immune system, 1795–1796
Immunocompromised host(s), 1809. See also Acquired immunodeficiency syndrome
definition of, 1802
pneumonia in, 634
Immunoconjugate therapy, for cancer, 418
Immunodeficiency, 1786, 1801–1812
and cancer risk, 388
continuing care for, 1810–1812
home and community-based care for, 1810–1812, 1811c
infection prevention in, 1810, 1811c
nursing management of, 1809–1812
primary, 1802–1809, 1803t
warning signs of, 1804c
secondary, 1802, 1809
self-care in, 1810, 1811c
Immunodiagnostic tests, reference ranges for, 2594t–2595t
Immunofluorescence, 1942
Immunogen. See Antigen(s)
Immunoglobulin(s), 1042
definition of, 1856
electrophoresis, in rheumatic diseases, 1893t
functions of, 1857
in humoral immune response, 1789
IgA, 1789, 1790c, 1857
deficiency of, 1803t
IgD, 1789, 1790c, 1857
IgE, 1789, 1790c, 1856, 1857
in allergic reaction, 1858f
total serum level, in diagnosis of allergic disorder, 1864
IgG, 1789, 1790c, 1857
deficiency of, 1803t
IgM, 1789, 1790c, 1857
production of, 1857
types of, 1789
Immunoglobulinopathy, malabsorption in, 1240t
Immunology
advances in, 1793
genetic engineering and, 1793
Immunomodulators
for HIV infection, 1830
for inflammatory bowel disease, 1250
for rheumatic diseases, 1896t
Immunopathology, definition of, 1783
Immunoregulation, 1786
definition of, 1783
Immunosenescence, 1794–1795
Immunosuppression
in bone marrow transplant recipient, 416
in burn victim, 2002
and cancer risk, 387–388
for idiopathic thrombocytopenic purpura, 1088
for immune hemolytic anemia, 1062
after kidney transplantation, 1561
potential infection with, 1561–1562, 1562c
in liver transplantation, 1336

and oral infections
nursing diagnoses related to, 1780–1781
nursing interventions for, 1780–1781
nursing outcomes for, 1780–1781
perioperative management of, 488
for polymyositis, 1913
for rheumatic diseases, 1896t
for systemic lupus erythematosus, 1911
and wound healing, 541t
Immunotherapy
active, and cancer treatment, 422
adoptive, and cancer treatment, 422
for allergic rhinitis, 1872–1873, 1873c
in liver cancer, 1334
for melanoma, 1982
Impaction. See Fecal impaction
Impaired fasting glucose, 1378
definition of, 1376
Impaired glucose tolerance, 1378, 1379t
definition of, 1376
Impairment, 190
definition of, 166, 174, 190
Impetigo, 1956–1957, 1957f
causative organism of, 2476t
Impingement syndrome, 2398, 2398c
Implantable cardioverter defibrillator, 849–850, 849f
definition of, 823, 945
in heart failure, 957
home care instruction for, 852c
Implanted ports
for intravenous therapy, 1194–1195
for parenteral nutrition, 1196
Implementation
in ethical analysis, 34c
in nursing process, 34, 36c, 41–42
in teaching-earning process, 55c
in teaching-learning process, 55–56
Impotence. See also Erectile dysfunction
drug-induced, 797
hemochromatosis and, 1063
Imprinting, 147
IMV. See Intermittent mandatory ventilation
Incentive spirometer
flow type, 729
volume type, 729
Incentive spirometry, 729–730
assisting patients with, 729c
definition of, 723
postoperative, 534
preoperative teaching about, 492–493
for thoracic surgical patient, 765
Incest, 1622
Incident Command System, 2560
Incisor(s)
central, 1150f
lateral, 1150f
Incomplete fracture, 2431
Incomplete spinal cord lesion, 2251
definition of, 2233
Incontinence
fecal, 217–218
assessment of, 215
clinical manifestations of, 1236
definition of, 1232, 1236
diagnosis of, 1236
medical management of, 1237
nursing interventions for, 217–218
nursing management of, 1237
pathophysiology of, 1236
postoperative, in hip fracture, 2449, 2452c
total, 215
urinary. See Urinary incontinence
Incontinence pads/briefs, for urinary incontinence, 216–217

Incubation period
 definition of, 2475
 of infectious diseases, 2475
Incus, 2094, 2095f
 definition of, 2095c
Indapamide (Lozol), for hypertension, 1026t
Independence
 functional, assessment of, 193
 of people with disabilities, 179c
Indiana pouch, 1599f, 1602
Indigestion, 1126–1127
Indinavir (Crixivan), for HIV infection, 1828t
Indocyanine green angiography, 2050
Indomethacin (Indocin)
 and immune system, 1797t
 for rheumatic diseases, 1895t
Induration
 definition of, 625
 in tuberculin skin test, 645
Indwelling catheters, for urinary incontinence, 216
Infarction, definition of, 2206
Infection(s), 102. *See also* Infectious disease(s); Superinfection
 amputation and, 2461, 2468
 and arthritis, 1919–1920
 in blistering diseases, 1973
 bone tumors and, 2420
 of breast, 1710
 after breast surgery, 1723
 bronchopulmonary, in chronic obstructive pulmonary disease, 698
 burns and, 2027–2028
 in cancer patient, 423–425
  nursing interventions for, 431, 432
  prevention of, 402, 403c–404c
  risk factors for, 423–424, 424t
 cardiac involvement in, 933–941
 after cardiac surgery, 894t
 causative organism of, 2478
 cellular response to, 2479, 2479f
 chain of, 2475–2479
  health care interventions and, 2478f
 in cirrhosis, 1319
 colonization in, 2479
 congenital, in sexually transmitted disease, 2509
 cutaneous manifestations of, 1929t
 CVID and, 1805
 definition of, 373c, 2475, 2479
 elements of, 2475–2477
 foot surgery and, 2403
 fractures and, 2434–2435, 2438, 2449
 genitourinary, in males, 1750
 gerontologic considerations in, 248
 hand/wrist surgery and, 2400
 health care–associated, 2480–2484
  definition of, 2475
 hip replacement and, 2375, 2381c
 in HIV-infected (AIDS) patients
  nursing interventions for, 1838c–1839c
  treatment of, 1835–1836
 host response to, 2479, 2479f
 hypophosphatemia and, 332
 and immune system function, 1795–1796
 versus inflammation, 103
 intravenous therapy and, 349
 after laryngectomy, nursing interventions for, 618
 in liver transplant recipient, 1338
 of lower respiratory tract, 628–652
 musculoskeletal, 2413–2417
 nosocomial, 2480
  definition of, 2475
 nursing interventions for, in HIV-infected (AIDS) patients, 1838c–1839c
 open fractures and, 2434–2435
 opportunistic
  definition of, 1815
  in HIV-infected (AIDS) patients, 1843c, 1849
 oral, in immunosuppressed patient
  nursing diagnoses related to, 1780–1781
  nursing interventions for, 1780–1781
  nursing outcomes for, 1780–1781
 orthopedic surgery and, 2375, 2387
 paraplegia/quadriplegia and, 2265
 patient at risk of, nursing management of, 1067, 1068c
 pelvic, 1670–1672
 phagocytic dysfunction and, 1802–1805, 1803t
 postoperative
  in hip fracture, 2449
  in neurosurgical patient, nursing interventions for, 2185c, 2187–2188
 and pressure ulcers, 209
 prevention and control of, 2480–2489. *See also* Asepsis, surgical
  in acne, 1956
  in acute renal failure, 1526
  in burn victim, 2015–2016
  for cancer patient, 402, 403c–404c
  in community, 2484–2489
  in community-based nursing, 18
  in Cushing's syndrome, 1482
  for dialysis patient, 1552
  in emergency department, 2518
  in gastrostomy, 1191
  after hip replacement, 2375
  in HIV-infected (AIDS) patients, 1838c–1839c, 1846
  in home health care nursing, 18
  in hospital, 2480–2484
  in hospitalized dialysis patient, 1552
  in hospitalized neutropenic cancer patients, nursing research on, 1809
  in immunodeficiency, 1810, 1811c
  with implanted cardiac device, 851
  with increased intracranial pressure, 2179
  in joint replacement, 2372–2373, 2375, 2381c
  after kidney transplantation, 1561–1562, 1562c
  in liver disease, 1329c
  in mastoid surgery, 2109
  after neck dissection, 1156c
  in oral cavity conditions, 1151–1152
  organizations involved in, 2480
  with pacemaker implantation, 852c, 853c
  in parenteral nutrition, 1197–1198
  in prostate cancer, 1760c
  in renal surgical patient, 1558
  in sickle cell crisis, 1059
  in ventilator-dependent patient, 749–750, 751
 primary, definition of, 1815
 process of, 2475–2480
 with prostatectomy, 1766
 respiratory, 628–652
  in bronchiectasis, 709
  in cystic fibrosis, 718–719
 risk of
  in acute lymphocytic leukemia, 1074
  in acute myeloid leukemia treatment, 1072
  in chronic lymphocytic leukemia, 1074
  in hematologic disorders, 1068c
  in multiple myeloma, 1084
  in neutropenia, 1066
 in sickle cell crisis, management of, 1059
 skin. *See* Skin infection(s)
 of surgical wound, 545–546
 thrombocytopenia in, 1087t
 transmission routes, 2478
 urinary catheter-related
  manifestations of, 1586, 1587f
  pathophysiology of, 1586, 1587f
  prevention and control of, 1586, 1588c
 of urinary tract. *See* Urinary tract infection(s)
 after vulvar surgery, 1687
 vulvovaginal, 1661–1666
  nursing process for, 1664–1666
  reinfection, prevention of, 1665
  risk factors for, 1662, 1662c
  spread of, prevention of, 1665
Infectious agents
 definition of, 91
 disease caused by, 102
Infectious arthritis. *See* Septic arthritis
Infectious disease(s), 2479–2480, 2812–2851. *See also* Infection(s); *specific disease*
 assessment in, 2490–2491
 complications of, 2491, 2492
 complications of, prevention of, 2498c–2500c
 definition of, 2475, 2479
 emerging, 2509–2512
  definition of, 2475
 expected outcomes in, 2492
 immigration and, 2512
 incubation period of, definition of, 2475
 versus infection, 2479
 nursing care plan for, 2493c–2500c
 nursing care process for, 2490–2492
 nursing diagnoses related to, 2491
 nursing interventions for, 2491–2492
 patient teaching about, 2492, 2497c
 planning and goals for, 2491
 prevention and control of
  equipment care and, 2490
  in family members, 2490
  in household members, 2490
  patient teaching about, 2490
 prevention and control of, in home care setting, 2489–2490, 2489c
 transmission of, prevention of, 2491–2492, 2493c–2496c
 travel and, 2512
Infective endocarditis, 933, 935–938
 clinical manifestations of, 936
 complications of, 937
 diagnosis of, 936
 medical management of, 937
 nursing management of, 937–938
 pathophysiology of, 935–936
 pharmacologic therapy for, 937
 prevention of, 936–937
 risk factors for, 935, 935c
 surgical management of, 937
Inference, in critical thinking, 25
Infertility, 1650–1652
 infectious disease-related, prevention of, 2500c
 male factor, 1650
 ovarian factors in, 1650
 ovulation factors in, 1650
 primary, 1650
 secondary, 1650
 semen factors in, 1650
 sexually transmitted disease and, 2509
 tubal factors in, 1650
 uterine factors in, 1650
Infiltration, with intravenous therapy, 350, 350c

# INDEX

Infiltration anesthesia, 515–516
Inflammation, 103–104
  acute, 103–104
  in asthma, 710, 710f
  cardinal signs of, 103
  chemical mediators of, 103
  chronic, 104
  in chronic obstructive pulmonary disease, 686–687
  definition of, 91, 103
  in fracture healing, 2340
  versus infection, 103
  intestinal. See also Inflammatory bowel disease
    acute, 1239–1247
  in natural immunity, 1786
  physiology of, 03f, 103
  in rheumatic diseases, 1887–1888
  subacute, 104
  systemic response to, 103, 103f
  types of, 103–104
Inflammatory bowel disease, 1247–1254. See also Regional enteritis; Ulcerative colitis
  assessment in, 1251
  cancer, 1247–1248
  complications of, 1252, 1253
  definition of, 1232, 1247
  epidemiology of, 1247
  home and community-based care in, 1253–1254, 1253c
  medical management of, 1247t, 1249–1251
  nursing diagnoses related to, 1251–1252
  nursing interventions for, 1252–1254
  nursing management of, 1251
  nursing process in, 1251–1254
  nutritional therapy in, 1249
  pharmacologic therapy for, 1249–1250
  planning and goals for, 1252
  self-care in, 1253, 1253c
  surgical management of, 1250–1251, 1251f
Inflammatory response. See Inflammation
Infliximab (Remicade)
  for inflammatory bowel disease, 1250
  for rheumatic diseases, 1896t
  for rheumatoid arthritis, 1908
Influenza
  avian, 2489
  causative organism of, 2476t
  epidemics of, 2488
  gerontologic considerations in, 248
  incubation period of, 2476t
  pandemic of, 2488–2489
  pneumonia caused by, 629, 631t
  transmission of, 2476t
Influenza vaccine, 248, 2488
  in chronic obstructive pulmonary disease, 693, 698
  and Guillain-Barré syndrome, 2288
  recommendations for, 2488
Informed consent
  definition of, 481
  for genetic counselling, 159
  for surgery, 484–485
  valid, criteria for, 484, 485c
Infusion drip pyelography, 1508–1509
Infusion sets, and nosocomial infections, 2484
Ingestion, 1122
  definition of, 1121
Ingrown toenail, 2401
INH. See Isoniazid
Inhalant(s), abuse/overdose, emergency management of, 2546t
Inhalation injury, 2001–2002
Inheritance. See also Genetics
  of adult-onset conditions, 151t–152t

autosomal dominant, 145–146, 145f, 147t
autosomal recessive, 145, 146, 147f, 147t, 148f
mendelian, 145
multifactorial, 147t, 148f
patterns of, in families, 145
X-linked, 145, 146, 147t, 148f
recessive, 147t, 148f
Inhibited response, by pacemaker, 823
Injection, definition of, 2043
Injection drug use, and HIV infection, 1816c, 1817–1818
Injury(ies)
  accidental, in health care, prevention of, 1820c–1821c
  brain, 2235–2250
  causes of, 101, 101f
    chemical, 102
    nutritional, 101
    physical, 101–102
  cellular, 101–103
  definition of, 101
  head, 2233–2235
  immune-mediated, 102
  and immune system function, 1796
  intraoperative, prevention of, 520
  multiple, management of, 2530, 2531f
  musculoskeletal, assessment of, 2349–2350
  in nursing personnel, prevention of, 2427–2429
  occupation-related, musculoskeletal, 2427–2429
  ocular, prevention of, 2072, 2072c
  in older adults, restraints and, 247
  perioperative, prevention of, 520
  postoperative, prevention of, 544
  prevention of, 2530
    in brain injury patients, 2244–2245, 2245f
    in cirrhosis, 1321
    in Cushing's syndrome, 1481–1482
    in liver disease, 1325c–1326c, 1332c
    after mastoid surgery, 2109
    in multiple sclerosis patients, 2282
    in osteoporosis, 2410
    with vertigo, 2114c
  renal, 1565–1566, 1565f
  sports-related, 2426–2427
Innate immunity. See Natural immunity
  delayed mechanisms of, 1785
  immediate mechanisms of, 1785
Inner ear. See Ear(s), inner
Inotropic receptors, 2130
Inotropy, 825
  definition of, 823
INR. See International Normalized Ratio
Insect(s)
  stinging
    anaphylactic reaction to, 2537–2538
    limiting exposure to, 2539c
  stings/bites
    and anaphylaxis, 1868
    emergency management of, 2539, 2539c
Insensible perspiration, 1931
Insight, in critical thinking, 25
Inspection, in physical examination, 74–75
Inspiratory capacity, 558t
Inspiratory force, in acutely ill patient, 578
Inspiratory muscle training, in chronic obstructive pulmonary disease, 695
Inspiratory reserve volume, 558t
Instrumental activities of daily living, 169, 175, 191
  capacity to perform, assessment of, 193
  definition of, 190

Insulin. See also Hyperinsulinism; Insulin therapy
  actions of, 1346, 1376
  continuous subcutaneous infusion of. See Continuous subcutaneous insulin infusion
  definition of, 1376
  inhaled, 1393
  interactions with anesthetics, 490t
  intermediate-acting, 1392, 1392t
  long-acting, 1392, 1392t
  and potassium balance, 321, 324
  rapid-acting, 1392, 1392t
  secretion of, 1346, 1378–1382
    by pancreatic islet tumor, 1372
  short-acting, 1392, 1392t
  source of, 1393
  storage of, patient teaching about, 1406
  very long-acting, 1392, 1392t
Insulin Aspart (NovoRapid), 1392t
Insulin-dependent diabetes mellitus. See Diabetes mellitus, type 1
Insulin glargine (Lantus), 1392t
Insulin jet injector, 1397
Insulin Lente (Humulin N, Iletin II Lente, Iletin II NPH, Novolin L, Novolin N), 1392t
Insulin Lispro (Humalog), 1392t
Insulin neutral protamine Hagedorn (NPH), 1392t
Insulinoma, 1372
Insulin pen, 1396–1397
Insulin pump, 1383, 1397–1398, 1397f. See also Continuous subcutaneous insulin infusion
Insulin Regular (Humalog R, Novolin R, Ilelin II Regular), 1392t
Insulin resistance, in insulin therapy, 1396
Insulin therapy, 1391–1393
  for acute renal failure, 1525
  allergic reactions to
    local, 1396
    systemic, 1396
  alternative delivery methods for, 1396–1398
  continuing care in, 1410
  hypoglycemia in, 1410–1412
  injection preparation in, 1406
  injection sites for, 1407–1408, 1408f
  insulin delivery in
    alternative methods of, 1396–1398
    implantable, 1398
    inhalant, 1393, 1398
  insulin preparations for, 1391–1393, 1392t
    complications of, 1396
    conventional regimen for, 1393, 1394t–1395t
    inhaled, 1393, 1398
    intensive regimen for, 1393–1396, 1394t–1395t
    regimens for, 1393–1396, 1394t–1395t
    species (source) of, 1393
    time course of action of, 1392–1393, 1392t
  insulin resistance in, 1396
  lipodystrophy caused by, 1396
  misconceptions about, 1404, 1405t
  mixing insulins for, 1406
  morning hyperglycemia in, 1396, 1397t
  needle disposal in, 1408
  needle insertion in, 1408
  patient teaching about
    effectiveness of, evaluation of, 1408, 1409c
    problems with, 1408–1410
  perioperative, 1429, 1430c

Insulin therapy (continued)
  regimens for
    conventional, 1393, 1394t–1395t
    intensive, 1393–1396, 1394t–1395t
  self-administration of, patient teaching about, 1406–1410, 1407c
  self-care in, 1408–1410
  skin preparation for, 1408
  syringe for
    disposal of, 1408
    selection of, 1406, 1407f
  withdrawing insulin for, 1406–1407
Insulin Ultralente, 1392t
Integra
  for burns, 2020t, 2022, 2023f
  definition of, 1995
Integumentary system, 1926–1942. *See also* Hair; Nails; Skin
  age-related changes in, 231t, 233, 1795t
  anatomy and physiology of, 1927–1932
  assessment of
    health history in, 1932
    physical examination in, 1932–1940
  brain injury and, 2242t
  chronic renal failure and, 1528c
  diagnostic evaluation of, 1941–1942
  in HIV-infected (AIDS) patients, 1834
Intellectual disability, people with, interacting and communicating with, 181c
Intellectual function, assessment of, 2145
Intelligence, age-related changes in, 237
Intensity, of sound, 77
Intensive care, in acute pancreatitis, 1360
Intercultural nursing, 129. *See* Transcultural nursing
Interdisciplinary collaboration, 17, 452
  definition of, 448
Interferon(s), 1791, 1791t
  action of, 1791t
  alpha-
    definition of, 1815
    for Kaposi's sarcoma, 1836
  antitumor properties of, 388
  beta-1a, for multiple sclerosis, 2280
  beta-1b, for multiple sclerosis, 2280
  in cancer treatment, 419–420
    adverse effects and side effects of, 421t
  definition of, 1783
  in immune response, 1793
  and natural immunity, 1786
Interferon-alfa (Roferon-A), for chronic myeloid leukemia, 1073
Interferon alfa-2b (Intron-A), for pruritus, in polycythemia vera, 1065
Interferon-alfa-2b (Intron-A), for thrombocythemia, 1086
Interleukin(s)
  action of, 1791t
  in cancer treatment, 420
    adverse effects and side effects of, 421t
  in cellular immune response, 1791, 1791t
  IL-1
    action of, 1791t
    and wasting syndrome, 1832
  IL-2
    action of, 1791t
    for renal cell carcinoma, 1564
  IL-11, in cancer treatment, 420
Intermittent claudication, 979, 992
  definition of, 975
  nursing diagnoses related to, 778–779
  nursing interventions for, 778–779
  nursing outcomes with, 778–779
Intermittent mandatory ventilation, definition of, 723

Intermittent pneumatic compression device, use of, 1008–1009
Intermittent positive-pressure breathing, 730–731
  ventilator for, 742
Intermittent self-catheterization, 1588–1589
  for urinary incontinence, 216
Internal, definition of, 198c
Internal auditory canal, definition of, 2095c
Internal capsule, 2132
Internal fixation
  definition of, 2371c
  for fracture, 2433, 2433f
    in femoral shaft fracture, 2449
    in hip fracture, 2447, 2447f
    in nonunion, 2438
    reaction to devices used in, 2440
  open reduction and. *See* Open reduction with internal fixation
Internal mammary artery(ies), grafts, in coronary artery bypass grafting, 888, 889f
Internal rotation, 199c
International Headache Society, classification of headache, 2198, 2198c
International Normalized Ratio, 814
  in cardiac patient, 808t
  definition of, 781, 975
  laboratory values for, 2578
International nursing, 129
International Society of Nurses in Genetics, 161c
  position statements of, 160, 161c
Internet, access, for visually impaired persons, 2052, 2053t
Interpretation, in critical thinking, 25
Interstitial cystitis, definition of, 1570
Interstitial fluid, 301
Interstitial nephritis, 1524, 1571
  definition of, 1515
Intervertebral disk(s). *See also* Degenerative disc disease
  age-related changes in, 2392
  anatomy of, 2324, 2325f
  cervical, herniation of, 2326
  degeneration of, 2392
  lumbar, herniation of, 2329–2331
  ruptured, 2324, 2325f
  surgery on. *See also* Discectomy
    complications of, 2327, 2329–2330
Interviewing
  in health assessment, 64
  for health history, 35
  in nutritional assessment, 81–83
Intestinal aspirate, and feeding tube placement, 1178–1179
Intestinal decompression, definition of, 1175
Intestinal disorders
  acute inflammatory. *See also* Inflammatory bowel disease
  inflammatory. *See also* Inflammatory bowel disease
    acute, 1239–1247
Intestinal gas(es), 1125, 1127
Intestinal motility, evaluation of, 1138
Intestinal obstruction
  causes of, 1263, 1264f, 1264t
  functional, 1263
  mechanical, 1263, 1264f, 1264t
Intestinal peristalsis, 1124–1125
Intestinal villi, 1125
Intima, vascular, 976
Intimacy needs, of Alzheimer's disease patients, 245
Intra-abdominal pressure, with increased intracranial pressure, nursing interventions for, 2178t

Intra-aortic balloon pump, for cardiogenic shock, 370, 371, 966–967, 967f
Intra-arterial blood pressure monitoring, 820, 820f
Intracardiogram, 854
Intracellular fluid, 301–302
  electrolytes in, 301–302, 302t
Intracerebral hematoma, 2236–2237, 2237f, 2238
Intracerebral hemorrhage, 2238
  carotid endarterectomy and, 2215t
  and hemorrhagic stroke, 2223, 2224
Intracranial hemorrhage, 2236–2237, 2237f
  in neurosurgical patient, nursing interventions for, 2185c
Intracranial pressure
  definition of, 2161
  determinants of, 2169
  increased, 2161, 2169–2180, 2248, 2249c
    assessment in, 2175
    assessment of, 2171
    brain injury and, 2236, 2243
    with brain tumor, 2302, 2303–2304
    cerebral response to, 2169, 2170, 2170f
    clinical manifestations of, 2170–2171
    complications of, 2171, 2175, 2179–2180
    diagnosis of, 2171
    early indications of, detection of, 2179
    expected outcomes with, 2180
    in fungal encephalitis, 2275–2276
    head injury and, 2234
    hemorrhagic stroke and, 2226
    interventions for, 2175, 2178t
    ischemic stroke and, 2212
    later indications of, detection of, 2179
    medical management of, 2171–2174
    neurologic assessment with, 2175, 2176f–2177f
    in neurosurgical patient, nursing interventions for, 2188
    nursing diagnoses related to, 2175
    nursing interventions for, 2175–2180
    nursing process with, 2175–2180
    pathophysiology of, 2169–2170
    planning and goals for, 2175
    secondary complications of, monitoring for, 2180
    treatment of, 2238
  monitoring, in neurosurgical patient, 2183, 2188
  monitoring of, 2171–2173, 2172f, 2179–2180, 2180f
  in neurosurgical patient, monitoring, 2183
  waveforms, 2172–2173, 2173f
Intracranial surgery, 2180–2190
  complications of, nursing interventions for, 2184c–2185c, 2187–2188
  continuing care after, 2188
  expected outcomes for, 2185c, 2188–2189
  nursing process with, 2183–2189
  postoperative phase of, 2182–2183
    assessment in, 2183
    complications of, 2183
    nursing diagnoses related to, 2183
    nursing interventions for, 2183–2188, 2184c–2185c
    nursing management of, 2184c–2185c
    planning and goals for, 2183
  preoperative phase of, 2180–2182
    medical management in, 2180–2181
    nursing management in, 2181–2182
  self-care after, 2188
  surrogate consent for, ethical considerations in, 2182, 2182c
Intracytoplasmic sperm injection, 1652

# INDEX

Intradermal skin testing, for allergic disorders, 1864, 1864f, 1865f
Intramembranous ossification, 2339
Intraocular lens implant, 2061–2063
  nursing management of, 2063, 2064c
  phakic, 2066
Intraocular pressure, 2044, 2055
Intraoperative phase, 482c, 483–484
  definition of, 481
  expected outcomes in, 521
  gerontologic considerations in, 503–504
  nursing activities in, 482c, 483–484
  nursing care in, 504
  patient advocacy in, 520
  patient in, 503–504
  potential complications in, 516–518
    management of, 520–521
    monitoring for, 520–521
  "surgical or preprocedure pause" in, 505
  surgical procedure and site verification in, 505
  "time-out" in, 505
Intraperitoneal injury, emergency management of, 2532
Intrapleural anesthesia, postoperative, 535–536
Intrathoracic pressure, nursing interventions for, with increased intracranial pressure, 2178t
Intrauterine device, 1644
  and HIV transmission, 1818
  postcoital insertion of, 1647
Intravenous immunoglobulin(s), 1103t, 1104
  for ataxia-telangiectasia, 1807
  for B-cell deficiencies, 1806
  for Guillain-Barré syndrome, 2289
  home infusion of, management of, 1810–1812, 1811c
  for idiopathic thrombocytopenic purpura, 1088
  nursing management of, 1807, 1808c
  for T-cell deficiencies, 1806
  for toxic epidermal necrolysis or Stevens-Johnson syndrome, 1974
Intravenous pyelography, 1508–1509
Intravenous (IV) therapy. See also Venipuncture
  blood clots in, 351
  continuing care in, 352
  discontinuation of, 348–349
  drop rate in, calculation of, 345–346
  electronic infusion devices for, 348
  flow in
    factors affecting, 345
    monitoring, 345–348
  at home, 351–352
  local complications of, management of, 350–351
  for lung abscess, 651
  maintaining, 345
  needleless delivery systems for, 342–343, 343f
  nursing management of, 341–352
  obstruction in, 351
  patient teaching about, 343
  peripherally inserted ceentral catheter for, 343, 344t–345t
  peripheral-midline catheter access lines for, 343, 344t–345t
  postoperative, in thoracic surgical patient, 767
  precautions with, for hospitalized dialysis patient, 1551
  preparation for, 341
  procedure for, 345, 346c–348c
  self-care in, patient teaching about, 351–352
  skin preparation for, 345
  systemic complications of, management of, 349
Intravenous urography, 1508–1509
  for ureteral trauma, 1595
  in UTI diagnosis, 1574
Intrinsic aging, 227
Intrinsic factor, 1040, 1052, 1121, 1123–1124
Intrinsic factor antibody test, 1053
Introitus, vaginal, 1614, 1614f
  definition of, 1613
Intubation. See also Endotracheal intubation
  emergency, 2524, 2525f
  gastrointestinal. See Gastrointestinal intubation
Intussusception, and intestinal obstruction, 1263, 1264f, 1264t
Inversion, 201c, 2343c
  definition of, 198c
In vitro fertilization (IVF), 1652
Involucrum, 2413
  definition of, 2392
Iodine, in contrast agents, allergic reaction to, 983
Iodism, 1462
IOFB. See Intraocular foreign bodies
IOP. See Intraocular pressure
IORT. See Intraoperative radiation therapy
Ipratropium, 693t
  for asthma, 714
  for ventilator-dependent patient, 749
Irbesartan (Avapro), for hypertension, 1029t
Irinotecan, in cancer treatment, 399t
Iris, 2044
Iron
  in blood, 1039
  body stores of, 1039
  deficiency of, 1039. See also Anemia
  dietary sources of, 1050
  excess, chelation therapy for, 1055
  in hereditary hemochromatosis, 1063–1064
  metabolism of, 1039
  overload, with long-term PRBC therapy, 1111, 1111t
  and pressure ulcer healing, 212–213
  storage of, in liver, 1286
  supplements, 1050–1051, 1050c
Iron lung, 742
Irregular bones, 2338
Irrigants, ocular, 2086–2087
Irrigation
  definition of, 1175
  of wound
    with open fracture, 2434
    in sequestrectomy, 2414
Irritable bowel syndrome
  clinical manifestations of, 1237, 1237f
  definition of, 1232
  diagnosis of, 1237–1238, 1237f
  epidemiology of, 1237
  medical management of, 1238
  nursing management of, 1238
  pathophysiology of, 1237, 1237f
  women with, quality of life in, nursing research on, 1239
Irritant contact dermatitis, 1877, 1877t
  latex and, 1883t
Ischemia, 101. See also Myocardial ischemia
  definition of, 859, 975
  gastrointestinal, in shock, 362, 366
Ischemic cascade, in stroke, 2207, 2207f
Ischemic stroke
  ambulation after, 2218
  assessment in, 2210, 2215–2216
  carotid endarterectomy for, 2214–2215, 2214f
  causes of, 2206, 2207t
  clinical manifestations of, 2207–2210
  and communication, 2220–2221
  complications of, 2212–2215, 2214, 2216
  continuing care after, 2222–2223
  coping with, by family members, 2221–2222
  diagnosis of, 2210
  and emotions, 2210
  exercise program after, 2217–2218
  home and community-based care after, 2222–2223
  left versus right hemisphere, 2209t, 2221
  medical management of, 2212–2214
    monitoring in, 2212–2214
  and motor deficits, 2217–2218
  nursing diagnoses related to, 2216
  pain after, 2218, 2219
  pathophysiology of, 2207, 2207f
  and perceptual disturbances, 2219–2220
  prevention of, 2210
  recovery from
    assistive devices for, 2218, 2219c
    expected outcomes in, 2223
    nursing interventions in, 2216–2223
    nursing process for, 2215–2223
    planning and goals in, 2216
  self-care after, 2222
  and sensory deficits, 2219–2220
  and sexual dysfunction, 2222
  surgical prevention of, 2214–2215
  thrombolytic therapy for, 2211–2212
  types of, 2206, 2207t
Isiadipine (Dynacirc CR), for hypertension, 1029t
Islet cell transplantation, 1398
  definition of, 1376
Islets of Langerhans, 1346, 1378–1382
  tumors of, 1372
ISO. See International Organization for Standardization
Isoetharine (Bronkosol), for ventilator-dependent patient, 749
Isoflurane (Forane), 510t
Isolation, social, of HIV/AIDS patients, 1842c–1843c, 1848–1849
Isometric contractions, 2341–2342
  definition of, 2337
Isometric exercises, 201t
ISONG. See International Society of Nurses in Genetics
Isoniazid
  adverse effects and side effects of, 647t, 649
  dosage and administration of, 647t
  drug interactions with, 647t
  preventive therapy with, 648
  for tuberculosis, 647–648, 647t
Isoniazid + rifampin (Rifamate)
  dosage and administration of, 647t
  for tuberculosis, 647–648, 647t
Isonizid + pyrazinamide + rifampin (Rifater), for tuberculosis, 647
Isoproterenol (Isuprel)
  for anaphylaxis, 2538
  for ventilator-dependent patient, 749
  for ventricular tachycardia, 836
Isosorbide, 953
  for esophageal varices, 1300
Isotonic contractions, 2341–2342
  definition of, 2337
Isotonic solution(s), 311t, 339
  definition of, 301

Itching. *See* Pruritus
IUD. *See* Intrauterine device
IVF. *See* In vitro fertilisation; In vitro fertilization
IVIG. *See* Intravenous immunoglobulin(s)

## J

Jackson-Pratt drain, 538, 538f
Janeway gastrostomy, 1188
Japanese encephalitis serogroup, 2274
Jaundice, 1289–1293, 1933, 1934f, 1935t
   with gallstones, 1349
   hemolytic, 1291
   hepatocellular, 1291
   in Hodgkin's disease, 1080
   obstructive, 1291–1293
Jaw
   disorders of, 1146–1147
   fractures of, 1147
Jaw-thrust maneuver, 2524
JCAHO. *See* Joint Commission on Accreditation of Healthcare Organizations
Jejunal graft, for esophageal reconstruction, 1167, 1168f
Jejunum, 1121, 1175
   feeding tubes in, 1176
   tube feeding into, 1176
Jevity, 1182
JNC 7, 1021
   definition of, 1021
Job syndrome. *See* Hyperimmunoglobulinemia E syndrome
Jock itch, 1961t, 1962. *See* Tinea cruris
Joint(s), 2340–2341
   age-related changes in, 2344t
   ball-and-socket, 2340
   contractures. *See also* Contractures
      with amputation, 2461
      nursing interventions for, 195–196
   definition of, 2337
   deformity of, prevention of, in stroke patient, 2216–2218
   degeneration of, 1888, 1889f
   diarthrodial, definition of, 1887
   dislocation of, 2348, 2426
      medical management of, 2426
      nursing management of, 2426
      sports-related, 2426–2427
   function of, assessment of, 2347–2349
   gliding, 2341
   hinge, 2340
   immobility of, 1889
   inflammation of, 1887–1888, 1888f
   instability of, in burn patient, 2032t
   integrity of, maintenance of, for unconscious patient, 2167
   loose bodies in, 2397
   lubrication of, 1888
   mechanical stress on, 1888
   mobility of, maintenance of, during rehabilitation, 196–198, 198c, 199c–201c
   motion of, assessment of, 2348
   neoplasms of, 1920
   nodules in, 2348
   pivot, 2341
   range of motion, assessment of, 2347–2348
   range-of-motion exercises for, 196–198, 198c, 199c–201c
      terminology used in, 198c
   and rheumatic diseases. *See* Rheumatic diseases
   saddle, 2341
   septic arthritis of, 2416–2417
   size of, 2348–2349
   subluxation of, 2348
   supporting structures of, disruption of, 2348
   synovial, 2341
      definition of, 1887
   types of, 2340–2341
Joint arthroplasty/replacement, 2372–2373, 2372f
   components for, 2372
   definition of, 2371c
   nursing interventions for, 2372–2373
Joint capsule, 2341
   definition of, 2337
Joint Commission on Accreditation of Healthcare Organizations
   and continuous quality improvement, 9
   and quality assurance, 8–9
   standards on use of restraints, 31
Joint effusion, 1888
   definition of, 1887
Joint National Committee on Prevention, Detection, Evaluation, and Treatment of High Blood Pressure. *See* JNC VII
Journal writing, for people with disabilities, 219
J point, 875, 876f
J pouch, colonic, 1267
Jugular vein(s), pulsations of, 800
Jugular venous bulb, oxygen saturation in, monitoring, 2173
Jugular venous distention, 946, 951
Junctional rhythm, 834, 834f
Junctional tachycardia, nonparoxysmal, 834
Justice
   distributive, 28c
   ethical principle of, 28c
   retributive, 28c

## K

Kaposi, Moritz, 1832
Kaposi's sarcoma
   classic, 1985
   clinical manifestations of, 1929t
   definition of, 1815
   endemic (African), 1985
   in HIV-infected (AIDS) patients, 1832–1833, 1832f, 1985
      treatment of, 1836
   immunosuppression-associated, 1985
   oral lesion of, 1144t
   pain management for, 1848
Kegel exercises. *See* Pelvic muscle exercise
Keloids, 1938c, 1978
   burns and, 2026
Keratin, 1927, 1930
   definition of, 1927
Keratitis
   bacterial, 2076t
   herpes simplex, 2076t
Keratoconjunctivitis, in toxic epidermal necrolysis or Stevens-Johnson syndrome, 1974, 1976
Keratoconjunctivitis sicca, 2075–2076. *See* Dry eye syndrome
Keratoconus, 2064
   definition of, 2043
Keratopathy, bullous, definition of, 2043
Keratoplasty, 2065
Ketamine
   abuse/overdose, emergency management of, 2546t–2547t
   for intravenous anesthesia, 513t
Ketoacidosis. *See* Diabetic ketoacidosis
Ketoconazole (Nizoral), for candidiasis, in HIV-infected (AIDS) patients, 1836
Ketones/ketone bodies, 1286. *See also* Diabetic ketoacidosis
   definition of, 1376
   testing for, in diabetes, 1391
Ketonuria, detection of, 1505
Ketoprofen (Orudis, Oruvail), for rheumatic diseases, 1895t
Kevorkian, Jack, 451
Kidney(s). *See also* Renal
   and acid-base equilibrium, 335, 338, 338t
   in acute glomerulonephritis, 1517–1518
   age-related changes in, 1516–1517
   anatomy of, 1493–1495, 1494f, 1495f
   artificial. *See* Dialyzer
   assessment of
      after cardiac surgery, 897
      preoperative, 488
   biopsy of, 1510
   in blood pressure regulation, 358
   in burn victim, 2002
   cancer of, 1563–1565
      assessment in, 1563
      chemotherapy for, 1564
      clinical manifestations of, 1563
      continuing care in, 1564–1565
      diagnosis of, 1563
      in elderly, 234
      medical management of, 1564
      nursing management of, 1564–1565
      renal artery embolization for, 1564
      risk factors for, 1563, 1563c
      surgical management of, 1564
   chemotherapy and, 401–402
   failure. *See* Renal failure
   in fluid and electrolyte balance, 304
   function of, 305
      age-related changes in, 308
      tests of, 1507, 1507t
   functions of, 1493, 1493c
   and hypertension, 1023
   inflammation of. *See* Interstitial nephritis; Pyelonephritis
   in multiple myeloma, 1083
   palpation of, 1504, 1504f
   in potassium balance, 321
   in shock, 362
   stones in. *See also* Urolithiasis
      assessment for, 1593
      complications of, 1593, 1594
      nursing diagnoses related to, 1593
      nursing interventions for, 1594
      nursing process for, 1593–1595
      planning and goals for, 1594
      prevention of, 1591, 1591c
   trauma to, management of, 1565–1566
   tumors of, 1563–1565
Kidney disease, 1514–1566
   anemia in, 1045t, 1051
   end-stage. *See* End-stage renal disease
   fluid and electrolyte imbalances in, 1515–1517, 1516t
   gerontologic considerations in, 1500–1501, 1516–1517
   risk factors for, 1500, 1501t
Kidney surgery, 1552–1560
   complications of, 1553, 1554, 1558–1559
   continuing care in, 1559
   expected outcomes with, 1559–1560
   home and community-based care for, 1559
   incisional approaches for, 1553, 1553f
   nursing care plan for, 1555c–1558c
   nursing diagnoses related to, 1554, 1555c–1558c

# INDEX

nursing process with, 1553–1560
patient positioning for, 1553, 1553f
perioperative considerations in, 1552–1553, 1553
postoperative management of, 1553, 1554, 1555c–1558c, 1558–1559
Kidney transplantation, 1560–1563
complications of, 1562–1563
continuing care after, 1563
dialysis and, 1560, 1561
graft rejection in, 1561, 1562c
home and community-based care after, 1563
immunosuppressive therapy for, 1561
infection control and prevention after, 1561–1562, 1562c
numbers of, 1560
organ donation in, 1560, 1560c
postoperative management of, 1561–1563
preoperative management of, 1560–1561
surgical procedure for, 1560, 1561f
Killer T cells. See Cytotoxic T cells
Kinins, in inflammation, 103
*Klebsiella pneumoniae* pneumonia, 632t
Knee
anatomy of, 2429f
anterior and posterior cruciate ligament injury to, 2430
balloon sign in, 2348, 2348f
ballottement of, 2348, 2348f
disarticulation of, 2460, 2461f
effusion (fluid) in, assessment for, 2348, 2348f
fractures of, 2458–2459
hinge joints of, 2341f
ligaments of, 2429f
medial or lateral collateral ligament injury to, 2429–2430
meniscal injuries of, 2430
sports-related, 2427
Knee replacement, 2372f
total, 2375–2376
nursing interventions for, 2375–2376
Knowledge, definition of, 46c
Kock pouch, 1250, 1599f, 1602. See Ileostomy, continent
definition of, 1232, 1570
irrigating/draining, 1259–1261, 1262c
Korsakoff's syndrome, 2227
definition of, 2206
in liver disease, 1307
*k-ras*, 385
Krythoplakia, 1144t
KS. See Kaposi's sarcoma
Kübler-Ross, Elizabeth, 450, 454, 456, 462
on death and dying, 449
on stages of dying, 471, 472t
KUB study, 1507, 1631
Kupffer cells, 1287
Kyphoscoliosis, 570, 805
Kyphosis, 2342, 2347, 2347f
aging and, 2404
definition of, 2337
progressive, 2404

## L

Labetalol, 830t
for hypertension, 1028t, 2226
Labia majora, 1614, 1614f
Labia minora, 1614, 1614f
Labor, induction of, for elective abortion, 1648, 1649c
Laboratory monitoring, in cardiogenic shock, 369

Labyrinthitis, 2118–2119
definition of, 2093
Laceration
definition of, 2528c
renal, 1565–1566, 1565f
Lacrimal gland, 2044
Lactase, source and digestive action of, 1123t
Lactate dehydrogenase
analysis of, in cardiac patient, 805
in biliary/pancreatic disease, 1349t
serum, 1290t
Lactated Ringer's solution, 311t, 339
for fluid replacement in shock, 367t
Lactational abscess, 1710
Lactic acid, in muscles, 2341
Lactobacilli, 1661–1662
definition of, 1661
Lactose intolerance, malabsorption in, 1240t
Lactulose (Cephulac), for hepatic encephalopathy, 1305–1306
Lacunae, 2339
Lamellae, 2339
definition of, 2337
Laminar airflow, 507
Laminectomy, 2325
partial, 2325
Laminotomy, 2325
Lamivudine (3TC, Epivir), for HIV infection, 1827t
Lamotrigine (Lamictal)
adverse effects and side effects of, 2194t
medication errors with, 2194
for post-stroke pain, 2218
toxic effects of, 2194t
Langerhans cells, 1928, 1931
definition of, 1927
Language
nursing, unified framework for, 43–45, 46c
"people-first," 184
Language ability, assessment of, 2146
Language barriers, overcoming, 130–131, 131c
Lansoprazole (Prevacid), 1206t
for gastroesophageal reflux disease, 1166
Laparoscope, 1675
definition of, 1661
Laparoscopic cholecystectomy, 1351, 1353–1354, 1353f
definition of, 1345, 1347c
self-care after, 1357, 1357c
Laparoscopy
in biliary/pancreatic disease, 1349t
in endometriosis, 1681
of female reproductive system, 1630–1631, 1630f
in gastrointestinal assessment, 1139
of hepatobiliary system, 1289, 1290t
Large intestine, 1122f
age-related changes in, 1125, 1126c
anatomy of, 1121, 1123f
blood supply of, 1123f
definition of, 1121
function of, 1125
motility of
evaluation of, 1138
testing of, 1134
obstruction of, 1265
peristalsis of, 1125
secretions of, 1125
Laryngeal mask airway, 505, 511f
Laryngectomy
airflow after, 611, 612f
assessment for, 614
communication after, 613–614
nursing interventions for, 617

complications of, 615
nursing interventions for, 617–618
continuing care after, 620
definition of, 589, 610
expected outcomes for, 620
home care after, 618–620, 619c
for laryngeal cancer, 611–612, 612f
partial, 611
supraglottic, 611
nursing diagnoses related to, 614–615
nursing interventions for, 615–620, 1155
nursing process in, 614–620
preoperative patient teaching for, 615
speech therapy after, 612–614
supracricoid, 612
supracricoid partial, 612
total, 611–612, 612f
Laryngectomy tube, nursing management of, 616–617
Laryngitis, 601
definition of, 589
Laryngopharynx, 554, 555f
Laryngoscopy, in laryngeal cancer, 610
Larynx
anatomy of, 554, 555f
cancer of, 608–614
assessment of, 610
clinical manifestations of, 609–610
diagnosis of, 610
epidemiology of, 608
glottic, 609
medical management of, 610–614
prognosis for, 610
radiation therapy for, 612
recurrence of, 610
risk factors for, 608–609, 609c
subglottic, 609
supraglottic, 609
surgical management of, 610–612
TNM scoring system for, 610
edema of, 608
electric, 614
obstruction of, 608
risk factors for, 608t
Laser
argon, for skin lesions, 1991
carbon dioxide, for skin lesions, 1991–1992
pulse-dye, for skin lesions, 1992
Laser-assisted in situ keratomileusis, 2065, 2066, 2066f
Laser cholecystectomy, definition of, 1347c
Laser hyperthermia, in liver cancer, 1334
Laser iridotomy, for glaucoma, 2058
Laserskin, 1948
Laser therapy
for cancer, 393
cervical, 1629
for cutaneous lesions, 1991–1992
for low back pain, 2393
for psoriasis, 1968
safety precautions in, 508
Laser trabeculoplasty, for glaucoma, 2057
Laser vision correction, 2065, 2066
LASIK. See Laser-assisted in situ keratomileusis
Lassa fever, causative organism of, 2476t
Lassa virus
incubation period of, 2476t
transmission of, 2476t
Last Acts Campaign, Palliative Care Task Force, principles of end-of-life care, 448–449
Latanoprost, for glaucoma, 2057, 2058t
Latency
definition of, 2475
in syphilis, 2505

Lateral collateral ligament, 2429f
  injury to, 2429–2430
Lateral cord syndrome, 2251, 2252c
Lateral horn, 2136
Lateral incisor(s), 1150f
Lateral position. See Sidelying position
Latex
  products containing, 1882t
  reactions to, types of, 1883t
Latex allergy, 1881–1884, 1883t, 2538–2539
  assessment for, 488, 489f
  precautions with, 508
Latex gloves, 2481
Latissimus dorsi muscle wrap, for cardiomyopathy, 928
Laxative(s), 1234, 1234t, 1243
  and hypermagnesemia, 330
  for opioid-related constipation, 282
  precautions with, 1241
  preoperative, 496
LCIS. See Lobular carcinoma in situ
LDL. See Low-density lipoproteins
Leaflet repair, 922–923, 922f
  definition of, 915
Learning
  age-related changes in, 237
  definition of, 49, 50
  health education and, 50–51
Learning environment, 52
Learning readiness, 51–52
  definition of, 49
Leber congenital amaurosis, 2081c
LEEP. See Loop electrosurgical excision procedure
Left heart catheterization, 814–815
Left shift, 1041
  definition of, 1036
Left ventricular area, examination of, 801, 801f
Left ventricular hypertrophy, in hypertension, 1022
Left ventricular outflow tract surgery, 928
Legal issues, involving older persons, 251–252
Leg bags, for urinary incontinence, 216
Leg cast(s), 2355, 2356f
  care of patient with, 2362–2363
Leg exercises, preoperative teaching about, 494c
*Legionella pneumophila*, 25102511
  incubation period of, 2476t
  pneumonia, 629, 630t
  transmission of, 2476t
Legionnaires' disease, 629, 630t, 25102511
  assessment in, 2511
  causative organism of, 2476t
  clinical manifestations of, 2511
  diagnosis of, 2511
  medical management of, 2511
  pathophysiology of, 2510
  risk factors for, 2510–2511
Legislation, in prevention of injury, 2530
Leg ulcers. See Ulcer(s), leg (lower extremity)
Leininger, Madeleine, 128, 129, 130f
Leiomyomas, uterine, 1679, 1679f
Lenalidomide, for multiple myeloma, 1084
Lens, of eye, 2044
  in diabetes, 1423t
  replacement of, for cataracts, 2061–2063
Lepirudin (Refludan), for pulmonary embolism, 665
Lesbian health care, 1633c
Letrozole (Femara), for breast cancer, 1729
Leukapheresis, 1102, 1102t
Leukemia(s), 1047, 1067–1079
  acute, 1071
    assessment in, 1075

complications of, 1075
continuing care in, 1078–1079
expected outcomes in, 1079
nursing diagnoses related to, 1075
nursing interventions for, 1075–1079
nursing process with, 1075–1079
thrombocytopenia in, 1087t
  chronic, 1071
  classification of, 1071
  definition of, 1036
  pathophysiology of, 1067
Leukocyte(s)
  granular, in natural immunity, 1785
  in inflammation, 103
  laboratory assessment of, 1799t
  in natural immunity, 1785
  nongranular, in natural immunity, 1785
  tagging of, in gastrointestinal assessment, 1133
Leukocytosis, 1067–1079
Leukopenia, 1066
  in cancer patient, 396, 401, 424
  chemotherapy-related, 401
  definition of, 1036
  in older persons, 1043
  in oral cavity conditions, 1151–1152
  radiation therapy and, 396
Leukoplakia, 1143t
Leukorrhea, 1664
Leukotriene(s)
  in allergic reaction, 1858t, 1859
  definition of, 1856, 1887
  in inflammation, 1888
Leukotriene modifiers (inhibitors), for asthma, 713, 713t
Leustatin, in cancer treatment, 399t
Levalbuterol (Xopenax), 693t
Levetiracetam (Keppra)
  adverse effects and side effects of, 2194t
  toxic effects of, 2194t
Levin tube, 1176, 1176t
Levodopa (Larodopa), for Parkinson's disease, 2314
Levofloxacin (Levaquin)
  for Legionnaires' disease, 2511
  for pneumonia, 636, 637
  for sinusitis, 595, 596
  for urinary tract infections, 1574
Levothyroxine
  for hypothyroidism, 1453–1454
  perioperative management of, 490t
Lewisite, as terrorism threat, 2569t, 2570
LH. See Luteinizing hormone
Libido, decreased, hemochromatosis and, 1063
Lice, infestation of, 1962–1963
Lichenification, 1938c, 1948
  definition of, 1927, 1945
Lichen planus, of mouth, 1143t
Lichen sclerosus, definition of, 1661
LICOX, 2173, 2174f
Lidocaine, 514t, 830t
  mechanism of action of, 784–785
  for postoperative analgesia, in thoracic surgical patient, 766, 767f
  therapeutic blood levels of, 2601t
  for ventricular fibrillation, 837
Lidocaine patch (Lidoderm), 281
Life-change units, 93
Life events scales, 93
Life expectancy
  definition of, 225
  trends in, 225, 225f
Lifespan, 227
  definition of, 225

Lifestyle
  and chronic illness, 167
  healthy, promotion of, 105
  and immune function, 1797
  and immune system function, 1797
  modification of, in COPD, 698
  neurologic impairment and, 2146
  in patient profile, 69c, 70–71
  vertigo and, 2114c–2115c
Life support, ethical considerations with, 32
Life-threatening illness, diagnosis, patient and family receiving, nursing interventions for, 458
Lifting, proper technique for, 2396, 2396c, 2396f
Ligament(s), 2341
  age-related changes in, 2344t
  definition of, 2337
Limbic system, functions of, 95
Limb-sparing procedures, for bone tumors, 2418
Limbus, 2044
  definition of, 2043
Linezolid, for pneumonia, 637
Lingual tonsil, 1153f
Liniments, 1949
  definition of, 1945
Lip(s), 1150f
  cancer of, 1148–1149
  disorders of, 1143t
  inspection of, 1149–1150
Lipase, 1124, 1346
  definition of, 1121, 1345
  source and digestive action of, 1123t
Lipid(s). See also Fat(s)
  in peripheral parenteral nutrition, 1193
  and stratum corneum, 1930
Lipid emulsions, in parenteral nutrition, 1193
Lipid-lowering agents, 864–865, 865t, 986
Lipid profile, in cardiac patient, 806
Lipoatrophy, facial, in HIV-infected (AIDS) patients, 1826, 1829f
Lipodystrophy
  in HIV-infected (AIDS) patients, 1826
  in insulin therapy, 1396
Lipoprotein(s)
  and atherosclerosis, 862–863, 863f
  measurement of, in cardiac patient, 806
Lipoprotein(a), 861–862
Liposarcoma, 2417
Liposomal therapy
  definition of, 1661
  for ovarian cancer, 1691
Lisinopril, 952–953, 952t
  for hypertension, 1029t
Listening, effective, 458
*Listeria monocytogenes*
  incubation period of, 2476t
  transmission of, 2476t
Listeriosis, causative organism of, 2476t
Lithium
  in cluster headache prevention, 2200
  hyponatremia and, 319
  therapeutic blood levels of, 2601t
Lithotomy position
  for pelvic examination, 1624
  supine, for pelvic examination, 1624
Lithotripsy
  definition of, 1142, 1345, 1347c
  electrohydraulic, for urolithiasis, 1593
  intracorporeal, for gallstones, 1352–1353
  for sialolithiasis, 1148
Liver, 1122f
  abscess of, 1340
  age-related changes in, 1287, 1287c

## INDEX

anatomy of, 1285–1286, 1285f–1286f, 1345, 1346f
assessment of, preoperative, 488
bioartificial, 1317
biopsy of, 1289, 1290t, 1292c–1293c
blood supply to, 1285
cancer of, 1333–1336
disease, and wound healing, 541t
enlargement of, in cirrhosis, 1318
functions of, 1286–1287
in glucose metabolism, 1380
in heart failure, 951
palpation of, 1288, 1288f
physical examination of, 1288, 1288f
in shock, 362
Liver disease, 1284–1341. *See also* Fulminant hepatic failure
assessment in, 1287–1288
coagulation disorder of, 1092
diagnosis of, 1288–1289, 1290t–1291t, 1292c–1293c
health history in, 1287–1288
manifestations of, 1289–1308
nursing care plan for, 1323c–1332c
physical examination in, 1288, 1288f
severity of, classification of, 1318, 1318t
Liver failure, after cardiac surgery, 894t
Liver function tests, 1288–1289, 1290t–1291t
Liver scan, 1290t
Liver transplantation, 1336–1340
ethical considerations in, 1338, 1339c
graft rejection in, 1338
in liver cancer, 1335
orthotopic, 1336–1340
definition of, 1285
Living arrangements, for older persons, 228–230
Living will, 251, 457, 457c
Lobectomy
in bronchiectasis, 709
hepatic, in liver cancer, 1335
of lung, 672c, 755c
Lobular carcinoma in situ, 1711
definition of, 1701
Lobules, hepatic, 1285, 1286f
LOC. *See* Consciousness, level of
Local adaptation syndrome, 95
Local anesthesia/anesthetics, 514t. *See also* Regional anesthesia
for analgesia
intraspinal administration of, 281
topical application of, 281
for conduction blocks, 515
epidural administration of, 281
for epidural anesthesia, 511–513
eutectic mixture of, 281
infiltration, 515–516
for postoperative analgesia, in thoracic surgical patient, 766
for regional anesthesia, 511–515, 514t
for spinal anesthesia, 511, 513–515
Locked-in syndrome, definition of, 2161, 2162
Logrolling technique, 2330, 2330f
Lomustine
for cerebral metastases, 2307
in cancer treatment, 399t
Long-arm cast, 2355, 2356f
Long bones, 2338
Long-leg cast, 2355, 2356f
Long-term care facilities, palliative care in, 454
Long tubes, 1176–1177
Loop diuretics, 953, 954t, 955c
for hypertension, 1026t

Loop electrosurgical excision procedure, 1629, 1684
definition of, 1661
Loop of Henle, 1495f
Loose bodies, in joints, 2397
Lopinavir + ritonavir (Kaletra), for HIV infection, 1828t
Loratadine (Alavert, Claritin), 1871t
Lorazepam (Ativan)
abuse/overdose, emergency management of, 2547t
for burn patients, 2025
for postoperative confusion, in older adults, 547
precautions with, 468
for status epilepticus, 2198
Lordosis, 2347, 2347f
definition of, 2337
Losartan (Cozaar), for hypertension, 1029t
Loss, 121–122
patient with difficult health care choices involving
nursing diagnoses related to, 1610–1611
nursing interventions for, 1610–1611
nursing outcomes for, 1610–1611
Loss of function, fracture and, 2431
Lost Chord Club. *See* Laryngectomee Association of NSW
Lotions, for wound care, 1948–1949
Lovastatin (Mevacor), 865t, 986
Low back neurosis, 2397
Low back pain, 2000–2002
acute, 2392–2397
assessment of, 2392, 2393
clinical manifestations of, 2392
diagnosis of, 2392, 2393c
expected outcomes with, 2397
management strategies for, 2394c
medical management of, 2393
nursing diagnoses related to, 2394
nursing process with, 2393–2397
pathophysiology of, 2392
planning and goals for, 2394
causes of, 2392
chronic, 2392
health promotion for, 2396c
with lumbar disk herniation, 2329
and mobility, 2394–2395
nursing interventions for, 2394–2397
patient teaching about, 2394c
weight reduction for, 2397
Low-density lipoproteins, 861
and cardiac risk, 806
definition of, 859, 1021
elevated levels of, 152t
serum levels, 862–863, 1290t
Lower esophageal sphincter, 1162
anatomy of, 1121
function of, 1123
Lower motor neurons, 2140–2141
lesions, 2141–2142, 2141t
Low-molecular-weight substances, 1857
Low-profile gastrostomy device (LPGD, G-button), 1189, 1189f
definition of, 1175
Low vision, 2051–2054
activities affected by, 2052, 2052t
aids in, 2052, 2052t
assessment of, 2052
diagnosis of, 2052
medical management of, 2052–2053
nursing management of, 2053–2054
people with, interacting and communicating with, 179c–180c, 2053, 2054c
Lubricants, ocular, 2086–2087

Lubrication, of joints, 1888
Lucentis (ranibizumab), 2071
Lugol's solution, for hyperthyroidism, 1462
Lumbar approach, in renal surgery, 1553f
Lumbar puncture, 2156–2158, 2157c
complications of, 2158
headache after, 2158
Lund and Browder method, of estimating burn extent, 1998
Lung(s). *See also* Pulmonary
abscess in, 650–652
clinical manifestations of, 651
diagnosis of, 651
medical management of, 651
microbiology of, 651
nursing management of, 651–652
pathophysiology of, 651
prevention of, 651
risk factors for, 650–651
and acid-base equilibrium, 335, 338, 338t
age-related changes in, 232–233, 562t
anatomy of, 555–556, 555f
assessment of, in cardiovascular disease, 804–805
biopsy of, 582–585
open
definition of, 625
in sarcoidosis, 667
transbronchial, 585
in sarcoidosis, 667
in burn victim, 2001–2002
compliance, 557
contusion of, in trauma patient, 677–678
in fluid and electrolyte balance, 304, 306
lobes of, 555–556, 556f, 571c
parenchyma, dysfunction of, and acute respiratory failure, 655–656
resection of, types of, 672, 672c
in shock, 361
transplantation of
for cystic fibrosis, 719
in emphysema, 694
Lung cancer, 670–674
adenocarcinoma, 670
asbestos and, 669
assessment in, 671–672
bronchoalveolar cell, 670
chemotherapy for, 672–673
classification of, 670
clinical manifestations of, 671
nursing research on, 674
diagnosis of, 671–672
diet and, 671
epidemiology of, 670
familial occurrence of, 386
genetics of, 671
gerontologic considerations in, 673–674
large cell, 670
medical management of, 672–673
metastases of, 671
metastasis, to bone, 2417
mortality rate for, 670
non-small cell, 670
nursing management of, 673
palliative therapy for, 673
pathophysiology of, 670
radiation therapy for, 672
risk factors for, 670–671
small cell, 670
smoking and, 670–671
squamous cell, 670
staging of, 670
surgery for, 672, 672c
treatment-related complications in, 673
Lung capacities, 557, 558t

Lung disease. *See also* Chronic obstructive pulmonary disease
  obstructive, in silicosis, 669
  occupational, 668–670
  restrictive, 669
    definition of, 625
    in silicosis, 669
Lung scans, in respiratory disease, 580–581
Lung volume reduction surgery, 755c
  in chronic obstructive pulmonary disease, 694
Lung volumes, 557, 558t
Lupus anticoagulant, 1099t
Lupus erythematosus. *See also* Systemic lupus erythematosus
Luteal phase, of menstrual cycle, 1616
  definition of, 1613
Luteinizing hormone, 1615–1616
  definition of, 1613
Luteinizing hormone-releasing hormone analogs, in cancer treatment, 399t
Lyme disease, causative organism of, 2476t
Lymph, 301
Lymphangiography, in peripheral vascular disease, 983
Lymphatic system, 975
  alterations in, 978
  anatomy of, 976–977
  disorders of, management of, 1016–1017
Lymphedema, 1016–1017
  after breast surgery, 1721–1722, 1722c
  definition of, 1701
Lymph node(s), 1784, 1784f, 1787
  biopsy of, 391–392
  of head and neck. *See also* Neck dissection
    metastases to, 1153
    oral cancer and, 1149, 1149f
  in Hodgkin's disease, 1080
  scalene, biopsy of, 585
  thoracic, biopsy of, 585
Lymphocyte(s), 1037, 1040f, 1042
  definition of, 1036
  functions of, 1037t, 1042
  in immune response, 1787–1788, 1792t
  laboratory assessment of, 1799t
  laboratory values for, 2580
  in natural immunity, 1785–1786
  null
    in cellular immune response, 1792, 1792t
    definition of, 1783
  production of, 1784, 1785f
  for transfusion, 1103t
Lymphocyte blastogenic factor, action of, 1791t
Lymphocytopenia, in burn victim, 2002
Lymphocytosis, in chronic lymphocytic leukemia, 1074
Lymphogranuloma venereum, causative organism of, 2476t
Lymphoid, definition of, 1036
Lymphoid tissues, 1784, 1784f
Lymphokines, 388, 1857
  in cellular immune response, 1791
  definition of, 1783, 1856
Lymphoma(s), 1067, 1080–1082
  AIDS-related, treatment of, 1836
  B-cell, 1815
    in HIV-infected (AIDS) patients, 1832–1833
  thrombocytopenia in, 1087t
Lymphopenia, 1066, 1067
Lymphoscintigraphy, in peripheral vascular disease, 983
Lymphotoxin, action of, 1791t

Lysergic acid diethylamide, abuse/overdose, emergency management of, 2546t–2547t
Lysis, definition of, 1036

# M

MAC. *See* Mycobacterium avium complex
Macrocytosis, definition of, 1036
Macrolides
  and immune system, 1797t
  for pneumonia, 636, 637
  for sinusitis, 595, 596
Macromastia, 1712
Macrophage(s), 1042
  definition of, 1036, 1815
  functions of, 1042, 1043
  and immune response, 1787
  and natural immunity, 1785
  and phagocytic immune response, 1786
  tissue, 1043
Macrophage activation factor, action of, 1791t
Macrophage aggregation factor, action of, 1791t
Macrophage chemotactic factor, action of, 1791t
Macrovascular diseases, diabetes and, 1421–1422
Macugen (pegaptanib sodium), 2071
Macula, 2046
Macular degeneration, 2051, 2051t, 2069–2072, 2069f, 2070f
  age-related, 236
  medical management of, 2070–2071, 2071f
  nursing management of, 2071
Macular translocation, for macular degeneration, 2072
Macule, 1937c
Mafenide acetate (Sulfamylon), for burns, 2017, 2018t
Magnesium
  for atrial fibrillation, 833
  for atrial flutter, 832
  in body fluids, 302t
  in cardiopulmonary resuscitation, 971, 972t
  deficit, 317t, 329–330
    manifestations of, 1516t
    in renal disorders, 1516t
  dietary, 330
  excess, 317t, 330–331
    manifestations of, 1516t
    in renal disorders, 1516t
  imbalances of, in renal disorders, 1516t
  serum
    in cardiac patient, 807t
    diuretics and, 314
    in hypermagnesemia, 317t, 331
    in hypomagnesemia, 317t, 329
    laboratory values for, 310t
    reference range for, 329
    significance of, 329
  for ventricular fibrillation, 837
  for ventricular tachycardia, 836
  in wound healing, 487t
Magnesium sulfate, 330
Magnetic resonance angiography, in peripheral vascular disease, 983
Magnetic resonance imaging, 2153–2154, 2153f, 2181
  in biliary/pancreatic disease, 1349t
  of brain tumor, 2304, 2305f
  breast biopsy guided by, 1709
  of breasts, 1708
  in cancer detection, 391t
  in cardiac patient, 813

  in degenerative disk disease, 2325
  in epilepsy, 2193
  in fungal encephalitis, 2275
  in gastrointestinal assessment, 1133
  of head injuries, 2234
  of hepatobiliary system, 1289
  in herpes simplex virus encephalitis, 2274
  in laryngeal cancer, 610
  in liver disease, 1291t
  for low back pain, 2393c
  of musculoskeletal system, 2350
  nursing interventions in, 813
  pelvic, in females, 1631
  in respiratory disease, 580
  safety precautions in, 2350
  of spinal cord injury, 2251
  of urinary tract, 1508
Mainz reservoir, for urinary diversion, 1603
Malabsorption
  in cancer patient, nursing interventions for, 428–429
  causes of, 1238, 1240t
  clinical manifestations of, 1238, 1240t
  definition of, 1232, 1238
  diagnosis of, 1238
  gerontologic considerations in, 1239
  medical management of, 1238–1239
  nursing management of, 1239
  pathophysiology of, 1238, 1240t
Maladaptation, and diseases, 97–98
Malaria
  causative organism of, 2476t
  immigration and, 2512, 2513f
Malathion, as terrorism threat, 2570
Male pattern baldness, 1939, 1941f
Male reproductive system
  age-related changes in, 231t, 233, 1742, 1742t
  anatomy and physiology of, 1740–1741, 1741f
  assessment of, 1742–1745
  gerontologic considerations in, 1742
  physical examination of, 1743–1744
Malignancy, gynecologic, 1682–1683
Malignant, definition of, 381
Malignant external otitis, 2105
Malignant hyperthermia
  clinical manifestations of, 517
  definition of, 517
  medical management of, 517
  mortality rate for, 517
  nursing management of, 517
  pathophysiology of, 517
Malignant melanoma. *See* Melanoma
Malignant neoplasm(s), 383–388, 383t, 384t
Malleus, 2094, 2095f
  definition of, 2095c
Malnutrition, 83
  in elderly, 78c, 234–235
  gerontologic considerations in, 2447
  in HIV/AIDS patients, 1836–1837
  in tuberculosis, 649
Malocclusion, 1146
Maltase, source and digestive action of, 1123t
Maltreatment
  assessment for, 2550–2551, 2550c
  emergency management of, 2550–2552
Malunion
  of clavicular fracture, 2440
  definition of, 2425
Mamillary bodies, 2132
Mammary duct, malignancy of. *See* Paget's disease
Mammography, 1706, 1708f
Mammoplasty
  augmentation, 1731

definition of, 1701
  reduction, 1731
Managed care, 9–10
Mandible, 1153f
  disorders of, 1146–1147
  fractures of, 1147
Mannitol
  for cerebral metastases, 2307
  for increased intracranial pressure, 2226
Manometry, 1138
  esophageal, 1162
Mantoux test, 645, 646f
Manual traction, 2366
Marburg hemorrhagic fever, 2477t
Marburg virus, 2511–2512
  incubation period of, 2477t
  transmission of, 2477t
Marfan syndrome, 2081c
  genetics of, 144, 147t
Marijuana, abuse/overdose, emergency management of, 2546t–2547t
Marriage, and multiple sclerosis, nursing research on, 2284
Marshall-Boney maneuver, 1505
Mask(s). See also Oxygen mask
  in Standard Precautions, 1820c
  for surgical personnel, 506
Massage, 134
  for low back pain, 2393
  in pain management, 288–289
Mass casualty incident. See also Disaster(s)
  definition of, 2559
MAST, 71
Mastalgia, 1710
  definition of, 1701
Mast cell(s)
  in allergic reaction, 1857, 1858f
  definition of, 1036, 1856
Mast cell stabilizers, for allergic rhinitis, 1872
Mastectomy
  modified radical, 1716
    definition of, 1701
  prophylactic, 393, 1715
    definition of, 1701
  reconstructive procedures after, 1731–1733, 1732f, 1733f
  total, 1716–1717
    definition of, 1701
Mastitis, 1710
  clinical manifestations of, 1705c
  definition of, 1701
Mastoidectomy, 2108
Mastoid surgery, nursing process for, 2108–2110
Mastopexy, 1731
Material safety data sheet, 2565
  definition of, 2559
Matrix, definition of, 1887
Maximal voluntary ventilation (MVV), 578t
Maze procedure, 854
McBurney's point, 1241, 1241f
MDA, abuse/overdose, emergency management of, 2546t
MDEA (Eve), abuse/overdose, emergency management of, 2546t
MDI. See Metered-dose inhaler
MDMA (Ecstasy, Adam), abuse/overdose, emergency management of, 2546t
Mean arterial pressure, 358, 358c
Mean corpuscular hemoglobin, laboratory values for, 2578
Mean corpuscular hemoglobin concentration, laboratory values for, 2579
Mean corpuscular volume, 1047
  laboratory values for, 2578

Measles, mumps, and rubella (MMR) vaccine, 2487–2488
  adverse effects and side effects of, 2488
Mechanical stress, and articular cartilage degeneration, 1888
Mechanical ventilation, 739–754
  in acute respiratory distress syndrome, 658–659
  barotrauma caused by, 751
  cardiac function during, 750–751
  complications of, 748, 750–751
  continuing care with, 747
  for cor pulmonale, 661
  expected outcomes for, 751
  extended, postoperative, risk factors for, nursing research on, 527
  in Guillain-Barré syndrome, 2290
  for HIV-infected (AIDS) patients, 1849
  home care with, 746–747
  indications for, 742, 742c
  and intracranial pressure, 2178
  modes of, 743–744, 743f
  nursing diagnoses related to, 748
  nursing process for, 747–751
  nutritional support during, 754
  paralysis for, 658–659
  patient receiving
    assessment of, 747–748
    goals for, 748
    nursing interventions for, 749–751
  pneumonia prevention with, nursing research on, 746
  pneumothorax caused by, 751
  postoperative, for thoracic surgical patient, 758
  problems with, 745–746, 745t
  and respiratory acidosis, 337
  weaning from, 751–754
    nursing interventions for, 753c
Mechanical ventilator(s), 742–743
  adjusting, 744, 744c
  bucking, 746
  care for, patient and family teaching about, 747, 748c
  classification of, 742–743
  definition of, 723
  home use of, criteria for, 747, 747c
  initial settings for, 744, 744c
  malfunctions of, 745–746, 745t
  monitoring, 744–745
  negative-pressure, 742
  operation of, 744, 744c
  positive-pressure, 742–743, 743f
  pressure-cycled, 742
  time-cycled, 742
  volume-cycled, 742, 743f
Mechlorethamine HCl (Mustargen), and immune system, 1797t
Meclizine (Antivert), 2112, 2113
Meclofenamate (Meclomen), for rheumatic diseases, 1895t
Media, vascular, 976
Medial collateral ligament, 2429f
  injury to, 2429–2430
Median nerve function, assessment of, 2346c
Mediastinoscopy, 585
Mediastinum, 555
  chest tube placement in, 761
  tumors of, 674–675
Medicaid, 17, 249–250
  for people with disabilities, 183
Medical nutrition therapy, definition of, 1376
Medicare, 8, 17–18, 249–250
  and nursing home care for elderly, 229
  for people with diabilities, 182–183

Medicare Hospice Benefit, 453, 455–456
  definition of, 448
Medication(s). See also Drug(s)
  and acute renal failure, 1523
  for acute renal failure, 1525
  administration of
    by feeding tube, 1185–1186, 1185t, 1186f
    in hospitalized dialysis patient, 1552
  adverse effects and side effects of, in HIV-infected (AIDS) patients, 1844c, 1849–1850
  for chronic renal failure, 1529–1530
  dispensers, for older adults, 238, 240f
  gerontologic considerations with, 237–238, 239t
  and immune system, 1797t
  and immune system function, 1796–1797, 1797t
  nutritional effects of, 83
    in elderly, 78c
  perioperative management of, 488–489, 490t
  preanesthetic, administration of, 496–497
  self-administration of, by older persons, 238
  and wound healing, 541t
Medication history, preoperative, 488–489
Medium tubes, 1176
Medroxyprogesterone acetate (Provera), for sleep apnea, 605
Medulla oblongata, 2131f, 2133, 2140
Megacolon, 1233
Megakaryocytes, 1042
Megestrol acetate (Megace), for appetite stimulation, 466
  in HIV-infected (AIDS) patients, 1836
Meglitinides, 1398–1401, 1399t–1400t
Meiosis, 142–143
  definition of, 140
Melanin
  definition of, 1927
  and hair color, 1930
  and skin color, 1927
Melanocytes, 1927
  definition of, 1927
Melanocyte-stimulating hormone, 1927–1928
Melanoma, 1981–1984
  acral-lentiginous, 1981, 1982
  assessment of, 1982
  clinical manifestations of, 1981–1982, 1982f
  conjunctival, 2081
  diagnosis of, 1982
  epidemiology of, 1981
  of eyelid, 2080
  genetics of, 1981
  immunotherapy for, 1982
  lentigo-maligna, 1981
  medical management of, 1982
  metastatic, 1984
    treatment of, 1982
  nodular, 1981, 1982, 1982f
  nursing process for, 1983–1984
  prevention of, 1984
  prognosis for, 1982, 1984
  risk factors for, 1981, 1981c
  satellite lesions with, 1983
  self-examination for, 1984, 1985c
  sites of, 1983
  superficial spreading, 1981, 1982f
  vulvar, 1685–1686
Melanoptysis, 670
MELD. See Model of End Stage Liver Disease
Melena, 1127
  in colorectal cancer, 1266
  definition of, 1204
  with esophageal varices, 1299
  in peptic ulcer disease, 1215

Meloxicam (Mobic), for rheumatic diseases, 1895t
Melphalan, in cancer treatment, 399t
Memantadine (Namenda), for Alzheimer's disease, 244
Membranous labyrinth, 2094f, 2096
Memory
 age-related changes and, 237
 loss of, Alzheimer's disease and, 244
Memory cells, 1788, 1792t
 in cellular immune response, 1791, 1792t
 definition of, 1783
Men. See also Gender differences; Male
 heart disease in, 866–867
 older, perceptions of health care needs, nursing research on, 1743
Menarche, 1617, 1632
 definition of, 1613
Ménière's disease, 2112–2113
 atypical, 2112
 cochlear, 2112
 dietary therapy for, 2113, 2113c
 vestibular, 2112
Meninges, 2133, 2134f, 2135–2136
Meningiomas, 2302
Meningitis
 cryptococcal, in HIV-infected (AIDS) patients, 1833
  treatment of, 1835
 gonococcal, 2509
 in HIV-infected (AIDS) patients, treatment of, 1835
 meningococcal, causative organism of, 2477t
 upper airway infection and, 603
Meningococcal meningitis, causative organism of, 2477t
Meniscectomy, 2430
 definition of, 2371c
Meniscus
 definition of, 2425
 injury to, 2430
  sports-related, 2427
Menopause, 233, 1616, 1633–1636
 and bone mass, 2405
 definition of, 1613
 hormone therapy for, 1634–1635
 nursing management of, 1636, 1637c
Menorrhagia, 1639
 with fibroid tumors, 1679
Menotropin (Repronex, Pergonal), for ovulation induction, 1651c
Menstrual cycle, 1615–1616, 1616f
 hormonal changes in, 1615–1616, 1617t
Menstrual disorders, 1636–1640
Menstruation, 1616, 1616f, 1632
 cultural considerations and, 1632
 definition of, 1613
 retrograde, with endometriosis, 1681
Mental disorder(s)
 characteristics of, 114, 114c
 definition of, 112
 gerontologic considerations in, 238–246
 risk factors for, 114–115
Mental function, in hypovolemia, 313
Mental health, 113
 characteristics of, 114, 114c
 definition of, 112
 national policy on, 113
 problems, risk factors for, 114–115
Mental status. See also Neurologic status
 age-related changes in, 2151
 assessment of, 2145
  in elderly, 240
  postoperative, 533

changes in, in Parkinson's disease, 2313
 in cirrhosis, 1319
 gerontologic considerations with, 236
 in HIV-infected (AIDS) patients, assessment of, 1846–1847
 in liver disease, 1328c–1329c
 in shock, 362
Meperidine, abuse/overdose, emergency management of, 2545t
Meperidine (Demerol), pharmacology of, 283t
6-Mercaptopurine
 in cancer treatment, 399t
 and immune system, 1797t
Merkel cells, 1928
 definition of, 1927
Meropenem (Merrem), for pneumonia, 637
Mescaline, abuse/overdose, emergency management of, 2546t–2547t
Mesenteric arteries, 1121, 1123f
Metabolic acidosis, 335–336
 acute, 335–336
 in acute renal failure, 1524
 chronic, 335–336
 in chronic glomerulonephritis, 1519
 in chronic renal failure, 1529
 compensation in, 338, 338t
Metabolic alkalosis, 336
 compensation in, 338, 338t
 and hypokalemia, 321, 322
Metabolic bone disorders, 2404–2413
Metabolic demands, with increased intracranial pressure, reducing, 2174
Metabolic disorders
 genetics of, 1444
 and rheumatic diseases, 1917
Metabolic rate
 in acute renal failure, 1526
 definition of, 91
 in physiologic response to stress, 95–96
 in stress response, 95
Metabolic syndrome, 861, 862f
 definition of, 859
Metabolism
 abnormalities of, in liver disease, 1307–1308
 aerobic, 357
 anaerobic, 357
 brain injury and, 2242t
 in burn victim, 2002, 2025–2026
 of drugs, age-related changes in, 238, 239t
 with increased intracranial pressure, 2174
Metacognition, 25
Meta-ethics, 27
Metaplasia, 100, 100t, 383
 definition of, 91, 381
Metaproterenol, 693t
 for ventilator-dependent patient, 749
Metastasis, 384–385
 to brain, 2306–2309
 definition of, 381
 to liver, 1333
 mechanisms of, 385
 of renal cancer, 1564–1565
 to skin, 1984
Metastatic bone disease, 2417. See also Bone tumors
 blastic, 2417
 lytic, 2417
 medical management of, 2418–2419
 polyostotic, 2417
Metastatic calcifications, in chronic renal failure, 1537c
Metatarsal, fracture of, 2427
Metered-dose inhaler, 692, 692f, 713
 definition of, 686
 patient teaching about, 698, 699c

Metformin, 1399t, 1401
 for infertility treatment, 1651c
Metformin with glyburide (Glucovance), 1399t
Methadone, abuse/overdose, emergency management of, 2545t
Methamphetamine (Desoxyn), abuse/overdose, emergency management of, 2546t
Methanol, toxic blood levels of, 2601t
Methazolamide, for glaucoma, 2057, 2058t
Methemoglobin, in cyanide poisoning, 2571
Methicillin-resistant *Staphylococcus aureus*
 definition of, 2475
 health care–associated infection potential of, 2482
Methimazole (Tapazole), for hyperthyroidism, 1460–1461, 1462t
Methotrexate
 in cancer treatment, 399t
  adverse effects and side effects of, 399t
 for elective abortion, 1648, 1649c
 and immune system, 1797t
 for psoriasis, 1966t, 1967
 renal toxicity of, 401–402
 for rheumatic diseases, 1896t
 for rheumatoid arthritis, 1908, 1909
 toxic blood levels of, 2601t
Methyclothiazide (Enduron), 954t
 for hypertension, 1026t
Methyldopa (Aldomet), for hypertension, 1027t
Methylenedioxymethamphetamine. See MDMA
Methylphenidate (Ritalin), for HIV-infected (AIDS) patients, 1836
Methylprednisolone, 1485t
 for asthma, 713t
 for multiple sclerosis, 2280
 for spinal cord injury, 2254
Methylsalicylate, for osteoarthritis, 1916
Methylxanthines
 for asthma, 713, 713t
 as bronchodilators, 692, 693t
Methysergide (Sansert), in cluster headache prevention, 2200
Metoclopramide
 for chemotherapy patient, 398
 for gastroesophageal reflux disease, 1166
 postoperative use of, 528
Metocurine (Metubine), 513t
Metolazone, 953, 954t
 for heart failure, 965
 for hypertension, 1026t
 for hypervolemia, 313
Metoprolol, 830t, 869, 953
 extended-release (Toprol XL), for hypertension, 1027t
 for hypertension, 1027t
 mechanism of action of, 785
Metro Medical Response Teams Systems, 2560
Metronidazole
 for bacterial vaginosis, 1663
 for gastritis and peptic ulcer disease, 1206t
 for *Giardia lamblia* infections, 1806, 2502
 for trichomoniasis, 1664
Metrorrhagia, 1639–1640
 with fibroid tumors, 1679
Mexiletine (Mexitil), 830t
Meyer, Adolph, 93
Michigan Alcohol Screening Test (MAST), 120
Miconazole
 for burns, 2017
 for candidiasis, 1662
Microbicide, 1817

# INDEX

Microbiology laboratory report, 2479–2480
Microcirculation, 975
Microcytosis
  definition of, 1036
  in thalassemia, 1061
Microdialysis, 2173
  definition of, 2161
Micrographia
  definition of, 2301
  in Parkinson's disease, 2313
Microhemagglutination test, for syphilis, 2506
*Microsporum* spp.
  incubation period of, 2477t
  transmission of, 2477t
Microsurgery, with cervical disk herniation, 2326
Microtrauma injury, 2398
Microvascular free flap, for head and neck reconstruction, 1153
Micturition, 1495, 1500, 1578. *See also* Voiding
  changes in, 1503, 1503t
  definition of, 1493, 1570
Midaxillary line, 571c
Midazolam (Versed)
  abuse/overdose, emergency management of, 2547t
  for burn patients, 2025
  for gastrointestinal endoscopy, 1135, 1137
  for intravenous anesthesia, 513t
Midbrain, 2131f, 2133
Midclavicular line, 571c
Middle ear. *See* Ear(s), middle
Midsternal line, 571c
Mifepristone, 1648, 1649c
Miglitol (Glyset), 1399t, 1401
Migraine headache, 2198, 2198c
  aura phase of, 2198, 2200
  clinical manifestations of, 2200
  definition of, 2161
  headache phase of, 2200
  home care for, 2201, 2202c
  medical management of, 2200–2201
  nursing management of, 2201
  pathophysiology of, 2199
  prevention of, 2200
  prodrome phase of, 2200
  recovery phase of, 2200
Migration inhibitory factor, action of, 1791t
Milia, 1988, 2080
Miliaria, 1951
Milk-alkali syndrome, 327
Miller-Fisher variant, of Guillain-Barré syndrome, 2289
Milliequivalents (mEq), 302
Milrinone (Primacor)
  for cardiogenic shock, 370, 966
  for heart failure, 955, 965
  in treatment of shock, 366t
Mineral deficiency, after gastric surgery, 1226
Mineralocorticoids, 1474, 1475
  definition of, 1440
Mini-cholecystectomy, 1354
Mini-Mental State Examination, 240c
Mini-nebulizer therapy, 730
Minitransplant, of hematopoietic cells, 1113
Minor category, in triage, 2521
Minority(ies)
  cultural context of, 129
  definition of, 129
  and health disparities, 136
Minoxidil (Loniten), for hypertension, 1028t
Minute ventilation, in acutely ill patient, 577
Miotics, 2057, 2058t
  definition of, 2043

Mirtazapine (Remeron), for depression, 240
Misoprostol, 1207t
  for elective abortion, 1648, 1649c
Mithramycin, and calcium balance, 328
Mitogen(s), and HIV infection, 1822
Mitogenic, definition of, 1945
Mitogenic activity, 1948
Mitomycin
  in cancer treatment, 399t
  renal toxicity of, 401–402
Mitonoxantrone (Novantrone), for acute myeloid leukemia, 1071
Mitosis, 142–143, 384
  definition of, 140
Mitotic spindle poisons, for cancer treatment, 399t
Mitoxantrone
  in cancer treatment, 399t
  for multiple sclerosis, 2280
Mitral (bicuspid) valve, 782f, 783, 915, 916f
  definition of, 915
  prolapse of, 915–917
  regurgitation, 917–918
  stenosis, 918
Mivacurium (Mivacron), 512t
MMR vaccine. *See* Measles, mumps, and rubella vaccine
Mobility
  after amputation, 2465–2467
  assistance with, in rehabilitation, 195–207
  burns and, 2028–2029
  after cervical discectomy, 2327
  in elderly, 236
  foot surgery and, 2403
  in Guillain-Barré syndrome, 2290
  after hip fracture, 2449, 2451c
  impaired, in older persons, 246
  improvement of
    with leg ulcers, 1014
    in Parkinson's disease, 2316
  improving, for patient in cast, 2357
  independent, promotion of, 198–204, 207
  with leg ulcers, 1014
  limitations of, people with, interacting and communicating with, 179c–180c
  with low vision/blindness, 2053
  maintenance of, after neck dissection, 1159, 1160f
  in multiple sclerosis, 2281–2282
  in orthopedic surgery patient
    postoperative, 2386
    preoperative, 2384
  in osteoarthritis, nursing research on, 1916
  osteomyelitis and, 2415
  paraplegia/quadriplegia and, 2262–2263
  physical
    assessment of, 195–196
    impaired
      musculoskeletal complications of, prevention of, 196, 197f
      nursing process for, 195–207
      positioning of person with, 196, 197f, 198
  postoperative
    promoting, 493–495
    in thoracic surgical patient, 767, 774c
  and pressure ulcer prevention, 212
  promotion of, for ventilator-dependent patient, 750
  in prostate cancer, 1759c
  rheumatic diseases and, 1900c–1901c, 1903–1904
  spinal cord injury and, 2257
  in stroke patient, 2216–2218
  after total hip replacement, 2378c

Modafinil (Provigil), for sleep apnea, 605
Model of End Stage Liver Disease, 1336, 1338
Mode of entry, of infectious organism, 2475
Mode of exit, of infectious organism, 2475, 2478
Moderate sedation, 515
  definition of, 503
Moexipril (Univasc), 952–953, 952t
  for hypertension, 1029t
Mohs' micrographic surgery
  for penile cancer, 1775
  for skin cancer, 1979–1980
Moisture, and pressure ulcers, 209
Molar(s), 1150f
  six-year, 1150f
Moles, 1978
  ABCDs of, 1983, 1983c
Molluscum contagiosum, 2080
  in HIV-infected (AIDS) patients, 1834
Mondor disease, 1712
Moniliasis, of mouth, 1143t
Monitored anesthesia care, 515
  definition of, 503
Monitoring
  with barbiturate therapy, 2173
  with cardiac dysrhythmia, 841
  of hypothermia patient, 2535
  of intracranial pressure, 2179–2180, 2180f
  intraoperative, nursing management of, 482c
  microdialysis for, 2173
  of oxygen saturation in jugular venous bulb, 2173
  with pharmacologic paralysis, 2173
Monoamine oxidase inhibitors
  interactions with anesthetics, 490t
  for Parkinson's disease, 2314
Monoamine oxidase inhibitors (MAOIs), drug interactions with, 593
Monoarticular disease, 1887
Monoclonal antibody(ies), therapy with, for inflammatory bowel disease, 1250
Monoclonal antibody(ies) (MAb), for idiopathic thrombocytopenic purpura, 1088
Monoclonal antibody(ies)
  in cancer treatment, 418, 419t
    adverse effects and side effects of, 421t
  production of, 418, 419f
Monoclonal protein, in multiple myeloma, 1083
Monocyte(s), 1038f, 1040f, 1041–1042, 1042–1043
  definition of, 1036, 1815
  functions of, 1037t, 1042
  laboratory values for, 2580
  in natural immunity, 1785
Monofilament test, 1428, 1429f
Mononeuropathy, 2297
  in burn patient, 2032t
Mononucleosis, causative organism of, 2477t
Monosomy, 143
  definition of, 140
Monotherapy
  definition of, 1021
  for hypertension, 1031
Monro-Kellie hypothesis, 2169
  definition of, 2161
Montelukast (Singulair), for asthma, 713, 713t
Moral dilemmas, 27–29
Moral distress, 27–28
Morality, versus ethics, 27–28
Moral problems, 27–28
Moral situations, 27–29
Moral uncertainty, 27

**I-66 INDEX**

*Morbidity and Mortality Weekly Report,* 2480
Morphine
  abuse/overdose, emergency management of, 2545t
  for burn victim, 2024
  for cardiogenic shock, 369
  in heart failure, 965
  intranasal, 287
  for intravenous anesthesia, 512t
  pharmacology of, 283t
  for postoperative analgesia, in thoracic surgical patient, 766
  transmucosal, 287
Mortality, of end-stage renal disease, 1527
Morton's neuroma, 2402, 2402f
Mosquitoes, and infectious disease, 2512
Mosquitos, and viral encephalitis, 2274
Motility
  colonic, testing of, 1134
  gastric, testing of, 1133
Motion sickness, 2112
Motor cortex, 2139–2142, 2141f
Motor function, 2139–2142
  age-related changes in, 2151
  assessment of, 2145–2146
  brain injury and, 2243
  with brain tumor, 2304
  stroke and, 2208t
Motor system, examination of, 2146–2147
Mourning, 471–473
  definition of, 448, 471
  nursing interventions for, 473c
  uncomplicated, 471–473
Mouth, 1122f. *See also* Oral cavity
  age-related changes in, 1125, 1126c, 1145c
  anatomy of, 1121, 1150f
  cancer of, 1148–1149
    gender difference in, 1148
  definition of, 1121
  disorders of, 1143t–1144t
  dry, 1151
  examination of, 1127
  inspection of, 1149–1150
  physical examination of, 569, 570f
Mouth care
  for patient with gastrointestinal intubation, 1179
  in prevention of tooth decay, 1142–1145
  promotion of, 1151
  for unconscious patient, 2167
Movement(s)
  coordination of, 2142
  muscle contractions producing, 2342, 2343c
M protein, in multiple myeloma, 1083
MRI. *See* Magnetic resonance imaging
MRSA. *See* Methicillin-resistant *Staphylococcus aureus*
MS. *See* Multiple sclerosis
MS Contin, for burn patients, 2024
MSDS. *See* Material safety data sheet
Mucocutaneous candidiasis, chronic. *See* Chronic mucocutaneous candidiasis
Mucolytic agents
  adverse effects and side effects of, 749
  for cystic fibrosis, 718–719
  for ventilator-dependent patient, 749
Mucopurulent cervicitis, definition of, 1661
Mucositis
  in acute leukemia, nursing interventions for, 1077
  in chemotherapy patient, 400
  oral, 1151
Mucous membranes
  integrity of, in toxic epidermal necrolysis or Stevens-Johnson syndrome, 1975

irritation of, during gastrointestinal intubation, 1180
MUGA. *See* Multiple-gated acquisition scanning
Multicultural nursing, 129. *See* Cultural considerations; Transcultural nursing
Multiculturism, in United States, 128–129
Multidisciplinary action plans (MAPs), 9
Multidisciplinary care, 452
Multidrug resistance, in tuberculosis, 647, 649
Multi-infarct dementia, characteristics of, 242t–243t
Multimononeuropathy, in burn patient, 2032t
Multiple endocrine neoplasia, 152t
Multiple-gated acquisition scanning, 812
Multiple myeloma, 1067, 1082–1084, 2417
  clinical manifestations of, 1083
  diagnosis of, 1083
  gerontologic considerations in, 1083, 1084
  medical management of, 1083–1084
  nursing management of, 1084
  pathophysiology of, 1083
Multiple organ dysfunction syndrome, 376–377
  clinical manifestations of, 377
  medical management of, 377
  nursing management of, 377
  pathophysiology of, 377
  prevention of, 377
Multiple organ dysfunction syndrome (MODS)
  communication about, 377
  definition of, 373, 373c
Multiple sclerosis, 2277–2285
  assessment in, 2280, 2281
  causes of, 2277
  clinical manifestations of, 2278–2279
  continuing care for, 2283
  course of, 2278, 2279f
  diagnosis of, 2280
  disease-modifying therapies for, 2280
  epidemiology of, 2277
  expected outcomes in, 2283–2285
  genetics of, 2277–2278
  gerontologic considerations in, 2279–2280
  home and community-based care for, 2283, 2284c
  medical management of, 2280
  nursing diagnoses related to, 2281
  nursing interventions for, 2281–2283
  nursing process in, 2281–2285
  pathophysiology of, 2278, 2278f
  pharmacologic therapy for, 2280
  planning and goals for, 2281
  primary-progressive, 2278, 2279f
  progressive-relapsing, 2278, 2279f
  relapsing-remitting, 2278, 2279f
  secondary-progressive, 2278, 2279f
  self-care in, 2283, 2284c
  symptom management in, 2280
  and trigeminal neuralgia, 2294
  types of, 2278, 2279f
  and vision, 2143
Multiple sclerosis (MS)
  exacerbations of, 2279
  remissions of, 2279
Multivitamins, and pressure ulcer healing, 213, 213t
Mumps, 1147
Muscle(s). *See also* Skeletal muscle
  actions of, 2342, 2343c
  age-related changes in, 2342, 2344t
  antagonist, 2342
  atrophy of, 2342
  contractions of
    isometric, 2341–2342

    isotonic, 2341–2342
    in skeletal (striated) muscle, 2341–2342
    types of, 2341–2342
  disuse of, 2342
  exercise of, 2342
  fatigue, 2341
  glycogen in, 2341
  hypertrophy of, 2342
  prime mover, 2342
  repair of, 2342
  size of, assessment of, 2349
  strengthening of
    for ambulation, 203
    in elderly, 235–236
    during rehabilitation, 196–198, 199c–201c
  strength of, assessment of, 2146, 2148f, 2349
  synergist, 2342
Muscle cell/fiber, 2341
Muscle relaxant(s). *See* Neuromuscular blocking drugs
Muscle relaxation, progressive, 107
Muscle setting exercises, 201t, 203
Muscle-setting exercises, 201t, 2342, 2360, 2360f. *See also* Isometric exercises
Muscle spindles, 2342
Muscle tone (tonus), 2342
  assessment of, 2349
Muscular dystrophy, 2323–2324
Musculoskeletal disorders
  chest pain caused by, assessment of, 792t
  in nurses, nursing research on, 2428
  nursing implications of, 2352
Musculoskeletal system
  age-related changes in, 231t, 235–236, 2342, 2344t
  altered sensations in, 2345–2346
  anatomy of, 2337–2338
  arthrocentesis of, 2351
  arthrography of, 2350
  arthroscopy of, 2351
  assessment of, 2342–2350
    health history in, 2342–2346
    nursing implications of, 2352
    physical, 2346–2350
  biopsy of, 2351
  brain injury and, 2242t
  chronic renal failure and, 1528c
  computed tomography of, 2350
  disorders of
    in foot, 2400–2404, 2402f
    infectious, 2413–2417
    in upper extremity, 2397–2399
  electromyography of, 2351
  endoscopic studies of, 2351
  genetic influences on, 2345
  gerontologic considerations and, 2342, 2344t
  health history for, 2342–2346
    assessment data in, 2344–2346
    initial interview in, 2344
  imaging of, 2350
    nursing interventions for, 2350
  immune dysfunction and, 1794c
  injury, assessment of, 2349–2350
  laboratory studies of, 2351–2352
  magnetic resonance imaging of, 2350
  medical illness and
    nursing diagnoses related to, 2334–2335
    nursing interventions for, 2334–2335
    nursing outcomes with, 2334–2335
  nuclear studies of, 2350–2351
  pain in, 2344–2345
  physical assessment of, 2346–2350, 2346c

physiology of, 2337–2338
radiographic studies of, 2350
trauma to, 2424–2470
sports-related, 2426–2427
Music therapy, in pain management, 290
Mutation(s). *See* Gene(s), mutations of
Mutation, definition of, 140
Mutual pretense awareness, of terminal status, 450
MVI Plan. *See* Multiple Victim Incident Plan
Myasthenia gravis, 2285–2288
assessment of, 2285–2286
clinical manifestations of, 2285
complications of, 2287
diagnosis of, 2285–2286
medical management of, 2286
nursing management of, 2287–2288
pathophysiology of, 2285, 2285f
pharmacologic therapy for, 2286
plasmapheresis for, 2287
surgical management of, 2287
Myasthenic crisis, 2288
Mycobacterial disease, causative organisms of, 2477t
*Mycobacterium avium* complex, 643, 2477t
definition of, 1815
in HIV-infected (AIDS) patients, 1831
treatment of, 1835
*Mycobacterium bovis,* 643
*Mycobacterium fortuitum,* 2477t
*Mycobacterium gordonae,* 2477t
*Mycobacterium kansasii,* 2477t
*Mycobacterium tuberculosis,* 643
drug resistance in, 647
incubation period of, 2477t
pneumonia, 633t
portal of entry, 2479
transmission of, 2477t, 2478
Mycophenolate (CellCept), for kidney transplant recipient, 1561
*Mycoplasma pneumoniae*
and Guillain-Barré syndrome, 2288
incubation period of, 2477t
pneumonia, 629, 631t
transmission of, 2477t
Mydriatics, 2085, 2086t
definition of, 2043
Myelin, 2281, 2281f
Myelodysplastic syndrome(s), 1047
polycythemia vera and, 1065
Myelodysplastic syndromes, 1054–1055
thrombocytopenia in, 1087t
Myelography/myelogram, 2154–2155
Myeloid, definition of, 1036
Myeloid metaplasia with myelofibrosis, polycythemia vera and, 1065
Myelopathy, vascular, in HIV-infected (AIDS) patients, 1833
Myelopoiesis, 1041
definition of, 1036
Myeloproliferative disorders, 1099t
Myelosuppression
chemotherapy-related, 400–401
definition of, 381
Myocardial infarct/infarction, 860, 874–885
assessment in, 874–876, 879
biomarkers in, 876, 876t
cardiac enzyme analysis in, 805
cardiac rehabilitation after, 877–879
clinical manifestations of, 874, 874c
complications of, 879, 884
definition of, 859
in diabetes, 1421
diagnosis of, 874–876
health promotion after, 884, 885c

history-taking in, 875
hypertension and, 1022, 1023
intraoperative, in cardiac surgery, 892t
medical management of, 876–877, 877c
non–ST-segment elevation, 874, 875
nursing care plan for, 880c–883c
nursing process for, 879–885
pathophysiology of, 874
pharmacologic therapy for, 876–877, 877c
postoperative, in cardiac surgical patient, 892t
signs and symptoms of, 790–792, 791t
ST-segment elevation, 874, 875
symptoms of, in women, nursing research on, 795
types of, 874
Myocardial ischemia, 783, 860. *See also* Angina pectoris
clinical manifestations of, 867–868
definition of, 781
signs and symptoms of, 790
silent, 867, 867c
Myocardial perfusion imaging, 812
Myocarditis, 933, 938
clinical manifestations of, 938
diagnosis of, 938
management of, 938
prevention of, 938
Myocardium, 782, 782f, 783
contractility of. *See* Contractility, myocardial
definition of, 781
Myocutaneous flap, for head and neck reconstruction, 1153
Myofibrils, 2341
Myoglobin
in acute renal failure, 1523
in cardiac patient, 805–806
in myocardial infarction, 876, 876t
Myoglobulin, in muscle contractions, 2342
Myolysis, laparoscopic, for fibroid tumors, 1679
Myomas, uterine, 1679, 1679f
Myomectomy, 1679
definition of, 1661
laparoscopic, for fibroid tumors, 1679
Myopia, 2050f, 2051
definition of, 2043
Myosin filaments, 2341
Myositis ossificans, 2440
Myotonic dystrophy
diagnosis of, 150t
genetics of, 144
genetic testing in, 150t
presymptomatic testing for, 150t
Myringoplasty, 2108
Myringotomy, 2106–2107
definition of, 2093
Myxedema, 1452–1453, 1457c–1458c
definition of, 1440
Myxedema coma, 1453–1454, 1457c–1458c

## N

Nabumetone (Relafen), for rheumatic diseases, 1895t
NACI. *See* National Advisory Committee on Immunization
Nadir, definition of, 381
Nadolol (Corgard)
for esophageal varices, 1300, 1304t
for hypertension, 1027t
Nafcillin (Unipen), for pneumonia, 637
Naglitinide (Starlix), 1400t
Nails, 1930
anatomy of, 1930

artificial, 2481
ban on, in OR, 506
assessment of, 1936
clubbing of, 1936, 1940f
disorders of, 1940f
growth of, 1930
hygiene for, in infection control and prevention, 2481
of OR personnel, 506
pitting of, 1940f
NANDA. *See* North American Nursing Diagnosis Association
Naphazoline hydrochloride, for allergic rhinitis, 1872t
Naproxen, precautions with, 593
Naproxen (Aleve, Anaprox, Naprosyn), for rheumatic diseases, 1895t
Naproxen (Naprosyn), in cluster headache prevention, 2200
Naratriptan (Amerge), for migraine, 2201
Narcotic(s). *See* Opioid(s)
abuse/overdose, emergency management of, 2545t
Nares, anterior, 553
NARIC. *See* National Rehabilitation Information Center
Nasal hygiene, during gastrointestinal intubation, 1177
Nasal septum, 1153f
deviation of, 606–607
NASBA. *See* Nucleic acid sequence-based amplification
Nasoduodenal tube, definition of, 1175
Nasoenteric tube(s)
for decompression, 1176, 1176t
for feeding, 1176–1177, 1176t
feeding with, 1176–1182
insertion of, 1177–1178
long, 1176
maintaining, 1179
medium-length, 1176
oral and nasal hygiene and, 1179
patient teaching about, 1177
placement of, assessment of, 1177–1178, 1178–1179
residue in, 1184t
securing, 1180f
Nasoenteric tube feedings. *See* Tube feeding(s)
Nasogastric (NG) intubation, nursing interventions for, in acute pancreatitis, 1365c
Nasogastric (NG) tube(s), 1175–1176, 1176t
complications of, 1180–1181
definition of, 1175
feeding with, 1176–1182
insertion of, 1177–1178
maintaining, 1179
measurement of, 1177, 1177f
monitoring patient with, 1180
oral and nasal hygiene and, 1179
patient teaching about, 1177
placement of, assessment of, 681–682, 1177–1178, 1178–1179
removal of, 1181
residue in, 1184t
securing, 1180f
Nasogastric (NG) tube feedings. *See* Tube feeding(s)
Nasojejunal tube, definition of, 1175
Nasopharyngeal irritation, in tube feedings, 1184t
Nasopharynx, 554, 555f, 1153f
Nasotracheal suction, in thoracic surgery patient, 765, 766c

NASPE-BPEG code, 845–846
   for implantable cardioverter defibrillator, 849
Nataliizumab (Tysabri), for inflammatory bowel disease, 1250
National Disaster Medical System, 2560
National Guard Civil Strike Teams, 2560
National Headache Foundation, 2201
National Institutes of Health Stroke Scale (NIHSS), 2212, 2213t–2214t
National Medical Response Teams for Weapons of Mass Destruction, 2560
National Pain Care Policy Act, 259
Natriuretic peptides, 948
Natural disasters, 2565–2566
Natural immunity, 1784–1786
   chemical barriers in, 1786
   disorders of, 1786
   inflammatory response in, 1786
   physical barriers in, 1786
   white blood cells in, 1785–1786
Natural killer (NK) cells
   antitumor properties of, 388
   in cellular immune response, 1792, 1792t
   definition of, 1783
Natural methods, of contraception, 1646
Naturopathic medicine, 134
Nausea and vomiting. *See also* Vomiting
   with appendicitis, 1241
   in cancer patient, nursing management of, 408c–409c
   chemotherapy and, 398–400
   enteral nutrition and, 1184t
   in gastrointestinal disease, 1127
   intraoperative, 516
   management of, in HIV-infected (AIDS) patients, 1848
   nursing diagnoses related to, 1118–1119
   nursing interventions for, 1118–1119
   nursing outcomes with, 1118–1119
   opioid-related, 282
   postoperative, 542
      management of, 526, 528
NCCAM. *See* National Center for Complementary and Alternative Medicine
NCEA. *See* National Center on Elder Abuse
NCI. *See* National Cancer Institute
NCNZ. *See* Nursing Council of New Zealand
Near-drowning, 2536–2537
Nearsightedness. *See* Myopia
Near-syncope, 247
*Necator americanus*
   incubation period of, 2476t
   transmission of, 2476t
Neck
   anatomy of, 1153f
   assessment of, in unconscious patient, 2165t
   malignancies of, 1153
Neck dissection, 1153–1161
   anatomical considerations in, 1153f, 1154f
   complications of, 1154, 1159–1161
   continuing care after, 1161
   expected outcomes with, 1161
   home and community-based care after, 1161, 1161c
   modified radical, 1153
   nursing care plan for, 1156c–1159c
   nursing diagnoses related to, 1153–1154
   nursing interventions for, 1154–1159
   nursing process with, 1153–1161
   radical, 1153, 1154f
   selective, 1153, 1154f
Neck pain, 1920

Necrotizing gingivitis, 1144t
Nedocromil, for asthma, 713t
Nedocromil (Tilade), for asthma, 713
Need(s)
   Maslow's hierarchy of, 5, 5f
   of patients, 5, 5f
Needle biopsy, 392
Needle exchange programs, for HIV prevention, 1818
Needlestick, prevention of, 1820c–1821c
Needlestick injuries, HIV transmission and, 2505
Needlesticks, prevention of, 2481
Needlestick Safety and Prevention Act, 342
Nefazodone (Serzone), for depression, 240
Negative feedback, 1473
   in control of steady state, 99
   definition of, 91, 1440
Negative-pressure devices, for erectile dysfunction, 1746, 1748t
Neglect
   assessment for, 2550–2551, 2550c
   elder, 249
   emergency management of, 2550–2552
*Neisseria gonorrhoeae*, 2507
   and arthritis, 1919–1920
   incubation period of, 2476t
   transmission of, 2476t
*Neisseria meningitidis*
   incubation period of, 2477t
   transmission of, 2477t
Nelfinavir (Viracept), for HIV infection, 1828t
Nembutal. *See* Pentobarbital
Neoadjuvant chemotherapy, definition of, 1701
Neoplasia, 383
   definition of, 381
Neoplasm(s). *See also* Tumor(s)
   benign, 383, 383c
      characteristics of, 384t
      by tissue type, 383t
   of joints, tendons, or bursae, 1920
   malignant, 383–388, 383c. *See also* Cancer; *specific neoplasm*
      characteristics of, 384t
      by tissue type, 383t
   of salivary glands, 1148
Neovascularization, 2049–2050
   definition of, 2043
Nephrectomy
   partial, for renal tumor, 1564
   radical, for renal tumor, 1564
   for urolithiasis, 1593
Nephroblastoma, familial occurrence of, 386
Nephrolithiasis, 1589–1595
   assessment of, 1590–1591
   clinical manifestations of, 1590
   diagnosis of, 1590–1591
   prevention of, 1591, 1591c
   risk factors for, 1590
Nephrolithotomy, percutaneous, 1593
Nephron, 1494–1495, 1495f
   definition of, 1493
Nephron-sparing surgery, for renal tumor, 1564
Nephropathy
   definition of, 1376
   diabetic, 1383, 1425–1426
Nephrosclerosis, 1521
   definition of, 1515
Nephrostomy, 1598f
Nephrotic syndrome, 1099t, 1520–1521
   complications of, 1521
   pathogenesis of, 1520, 1520f
Nephrotoxicity, and acute renal failure, 1523, 1524–1525

Nephroureterectomy, laparoscopic, for renal tumor, 1564
Nepro, 1182
Nerve agents
   exposure to, treatment of, 2569t, 2570–2571
   as terrorism threats, 2569t, 2570–2571
Nerve block(s), 515
Nerve conduction studies, 2156
   for low back pain, 2393c
Nerve damage, skin traction and, 2367
Nerve entrapment, in burn patient, 2032t
Nerve injury, after neck dissection, 1160–1161
Nerve pressure
   in patient in cast, 2357–2359, 2359f
   in skin traction, 2367
Nervous system. *See also* Autonomic nervous system; Central nervous system; Peripheral nervous system
   age-related changes in, 232t, 236, 2150–2152
   anatomy and physiology of, 2129–2143
   brain injury and, 2242t
   cells of, 2129, 2130f
   chemotherapy and, 402
   chronic renal failure and, 1528, 1528c
   disorders of. *See* Neurologic dysfunction
Nesiritide, for heart failure, 965
Nesiritide (Natrecor), for heart failure, 955
Neteglide (Starlix), 1400t
Neural transplantation, for Parkinson's disease, 2315
Neural tube defects
   genetics of, 147–148, 147t
   prenatal diagnosis of, 150t
Neurocognition, definition of, 46c
Neurodegenerative disorder(s), 2311–2331
   definition of, 2301
Neurofibroma, plantar, 2402, 2402f
Neurofibromatosis, 1978
   cutaneous manifestations of, 1929t
   genetics of, 147t
   malignant, familial occurrence of, 386
   type 1, genetics of, 144
Neurogenic bladder, 1584–1589
   definition of, 1570, 2233
Neurogenic incontinence. *See* Reflex incontinence
Neurogenic shock, spinal cord injury and, 2255–2256
Neuroglia, 2131
Neuroglial cells, 2129
Neuroimaging
   in fungal encephalitis, 2275
   in herpes simplex virus encephalitis, 2274
Neurokinin-1 receptor antagonists, for chemotherapy patient, 398
Neuroleptics, atypical, for Alzheimer's disease, 244
Neurologic assessment, 2128–2158
   after cardiac surgery, 897, 899
   health history in, 2143
   with increased intracranial pressure, 2175, 2176f–2177f
   physical examination in, 2144–2150
Neurologic disorders/dysfunction
   and burns, nursing research on, 2009
   after cardiac surgery, 893t
   clinical manifestations of, 2143–2144
   genetics of, 2144
   and rehabilitation, 192
Neurologic function
   age-related changes in, 1795t
   assessment of, 2128–2158
   brain injuries and, 2240, 2240c, 2241f, 2243–2244

# INDEX

Neurologic status, in HIV-infected (AIDS) patients, 1845
Neurologic system. *See* Nervous system
Neurologic trauma, 2232–2266–1943, 2240, 2240c, 2241f, 2243–2244
Neuroma
  acoustic. *See* Acoustic neuroma
  Morton's, 2402, 2402f
Neuromatrix, 266
Neuromodulation, in pain management, 291
Neuromuscular blocking drugs, 511
  depolarizing, 512t
  nondepolarizing
    intermediate onset and duration, 512t
    longer onset and duration, 513t
  for ventilator patient, in acute respiratory distress syndrome, 658–659
Neuron(s), 2129, 2130f
Neuropathy
  in burn patient, 2032t
  chemotherapy-induced, 402
  definition of, 1376
  diabetic, 1383, 1426–1427, 2151
  peripheral. *See* Peripheral neuropathy
  in HIV-infected (AIDS) patients, 1833
  postherpetic, 2151
Neuroprotectants, 2207
Neuroregulators, of gastrointestinal tract, 1124t
Neuroscience nursing, 2161–2162
Neurosensory system, immune dysfunction and, 1794c
Neurosignature, 266
Neurostimulation, in pain management, 291–292
Neurosyphilis, 2509
Neurotransmitters, 2129–2130, 2130f
Neurovascular disorders, 1920
Neurovascular status
  assessment of, 2349, 2349c
  casts and, 2356, 2357–2359, 2359f
  definition of, 2355
  femoral shaft fracture and, 2449
  hand/wrist surgery and, 2399
  hip fracture and, 2448, 2455c–2456c
  musculoskeletal disorders and, 2349, 2349c
  nursing interventions for, for patient in cast, 2357–2359
  in orthopedic surgery patient
    postoperative, 2386
    preoperative, 2383
  skeletal traction and, 2368
  skin traction and, 2367
  after total hip replacement, 2379c
Neutropenia, 1066–1067
  in aplastic anemia, 1051
  assessment in, 1069c
  in cancer, and prevention of infection, nursing research on, 1809
  in cancer patient, 425
    treatment of, 420
  causes of, 1066, 1066c
  definition of, 381, 1036
  diagnosis of, 1069c
  expected outcomes in, 1070c
  febrile, in cancer patient, emergency department management of, nursing research on, 1070
  nursing diagnoses related to, 1069c
  nursing interventions for, 1069c–1070c
  precautions in, 1067, 1069c–1070c
Neutrophil(s), 1038f, 1041
  definition of, 1036
  functions of, 1037, 1037t, 1041f, 1042
  laboratory values for, 2579

  in natural immunity, 1785
  and phagocytic dysfunction, 1802
  polymorphonuclear, 1041
  segmented, 1041
Nevi
  conjunctival, 2080
  dysplastic, 1981
  of eyelid, 2080
  and melanoma, 1981
  pigmented, 1978
Nevirapine (Viramune), for HIV infection, 1827t
Newborn screening, 149
New-variant Creutzfeldt-Jakob disease, 2276–2277
New York Heart Association, classification of heart failure, 947, 947t
Nezelof's syndrome, 1803t
NG tube. *See* Nasogastric (NG) tube
Niacin, 986
Niacin (Niacor, Niaspan), 864–865, 865t
NIC. *See* Nursing Interventions Classification
Nicardipine (Cardene)
  for hypertension, 1029t, 2226
  for hypertensive emergency, 1033
Nicotine patch, 866
Nicotine stomatitis, 1144t
Nicotinic acid, 864–865, 865t, 986
  extended-release, 865t
  immediate-release, 865t
  sustained-release, 865t
NIDRR. *See* National Institute on Disability and Rehabilitation Research
Nifedipine (Adalat, Procardia), 955
Nifedipine (Procardia), for cerebral vasospasm, 2226
Nifedipine long-acting (Procardia XL, Adalat CC), for hypertension, 1029t
NIHSS. *See* National Institutes of Health Stroke Scale
Nimodipine (Nimotop), for cerebral vasospasm, 2226
Nipple(s)
  discharge from, 1710
  fissures in, 1710
  inversion of, 1704c
Nipple, reconstruction of, 1733
Nisoldipine (Sular), for hypertension, 1029t
Nitrates
  for esophageal varices, 1300
  mechanism of action of, 869
Nitric oxide, vascular effects of, 978
Nitrofurantoin (Macrodantin, Furadantin), for urinary tract infections, 1574
Nitrofurazone (Furacin), for burns, 2017
Nitrogen, partial pressure of, 560
Nitrogen balance, 83
  in liver disease, 1323c–1324c
  negative, and pressure ulcers, 208
  positive, with parenteral nutrition, 1193
Nitrogen mustard
  in cancer treatment, 399t
  as terrorism threat, 2569t, 2570
Nitroglycerin
  for angina, 869, 872
  mechanism of action of, 869
  self-administration of, 869, 870c
Nitroglycerin (Nitro-Bid IV, Tridil)
  for hypertension, 1028t
  for hypertensive emergency, 1033
Nitroglycerin (Tridil), for cardiogenic shock, 370, 966
Nitroglycerine (Tridil), for shock, 366t
Nitroprusside (Nipride), in treatment of shock, 366t

Nitroprusside (Nitropress), for hypertension, 2226
Nitrosureas, for cancer treatment, 399t
Nitrous oxide, 510t
  for burn patients, 2024
Nizantidine (Axid), 1206t
  for gastroesophageal reflux disease, 1166
NK cells. *See* Natural killer cells
NNRTIs. *See* Non-nucleoside reverse transcriptase inhibitors
NOC. *See* Nursing Outcomes Classification
Nociception, 265, 265f
  definition of, 259
Nociceptor(s), 264
  definition of, 259
Nocturia, 1499, 1503, 1503t
  definition of, 1493, 1570, 1740
  in heart failure, 796, 951
  in hypertension, 1023
  in urinary tract infections, 1572
Nocturnal penile tumescence tests, 1744
Nodal cells, cardiac, 783
Nodules, 1929t, 1937c
Noise, hearing loss caused by, 2102
Nondihydropyridines, for hypertension, 1029t
Nondisjunction, 143
  definition of, 140
Nongranular leukocytes, in natural immunity, 1785
Non-Hodgkin's lymphoma, 1081–1082
  clinical manifestations of, 1081–1082
  diagnosis of, 1082
  epidemiology of, 1081
  medical management of, 1082
  nursing management of, 1082
Non–insulin-dependent diabetes mellitus. *See* Diabetes mellitus, type 2
Nonmaleficence, ethical principle of, 28c
Non-nociceptor(s), 265, 265f
  definition of, 259
Non-nociceptors, 265f, 266
Non-nucleoside reverse transcriptase inhibitors, for HIV infection, 1826, 1827t
Nonoliguria, in acute renal failure, 1522
Nonoxynol-9, 1645–1646, 1673, 1750, 1817
Nonsteroidal anti-inflammatory drugs
  and acute renal failure, 1523
  adverse effects and side effects of, 285
  for complex regional pain syndrome, 2440
  contraindications to, 956
  for epicondylitis, 2429
  for gout, 1918
  and immune system, 1797t
  mechanism of action of, 284
  ocular therapy with, 2086
  for osteoarthritis, 1915
  in pain management, 284–285
  and peptic ulcer disease, 1212
  platelet defect caused by, 1089
  for rheumatic diseases, 1894, 1895t
  for rheumatoid arthritis, 1908
  for rotator cuff tears, 2429
  for septic arthritis, 2416
  for systemic lupus erythematosus, 1911
  for urolithiasis, 1591, 1594
Nonsteroidal anti-inflammatory drugs (NSAIDs), for viral rhinitis, 592, 593
Non-sulfonylurea insulin secretagogues, 1398, 1400t, 1401
Nontunneled central catheter(s), 1194–1195
Nontunnelled central catheter(s), insertion of, 1194–1195
Nonunion, of fracture, 2438–2439
  definition of, 2425

Nonunion, of fracture (continued)
　medical management of, 2438–2439
　nursing management of, 2439
Nonurgent patients, 2521
　definition of, 2517
NORD. See National Organization for Rare Disorders, Inc.
Norepinephrine, 2130t
　in gastrointestinal regulation, 1124t
　in physiologic response to stress, 95
　vascular effects of, 978
Norepinephrine (Levophed)
　for cardiogenic shock, 370
　for shock, 366t
Norepinephrine bitartrate (Levophed), and cardiac output, 2173
Normal flora, 2479
Normochromic, definition of, 1036
Normocytic, definition of, 1036
Norovirus
　and diarrheal disease, 2501–2502
　incubation period of, 2477t
　transmission of, 2477t
North American Nursing Diagnosis Association
　diagnoses
　　for community with identified health problem, 2–3
　　for patient with fear and somatic complaints, 88–89
　nursing diagnoses approved by, 36, 38c–39c
　taxonomy used by, in unified Taxonomy of Nursing Practice, 43–45, 46c
　Unitary Person Framework for health history, 73
North American Society of Pacing and Electrophysiology. See also NASPE-BPEG code
Norton scale, 209
Nortriptyline, abuse/overdose, emergency management of, 2548t
Nortriptyline (Aventyl), for smoking cessation, 692
Norwalk-like virus. See Norovirus
Nose
　anatomy of, 553, 554f
　fractures of, 607–608
　obstruction of, 606–607
　packing, to control bleeding in epistaxis, 605–606, 606f
　physical examination of, 568–569
　vascular anatomy of, 605
Nosebleed. See Epistaxis
Nosocomial, definition of, 625
Nosocomial infection, 2480
　definition of, 2475
Nostrils, 553
Nothing by mouth, for diabetic hospitalized patient, 1431
Novocain. See Procaine
Noxious stimuli, response to, assessment of, in unconscious patient, 2165t, 2166t
NPCPA. See National Pain Care Policy Act
NPH insulin. See Insulin neutral protamine Hagedorn; Insulin neutral protamine Hagedorn (NPH)
NRTIs. See Nucleoside reverse transcriptase inhibitors
NSAIDs. See Nonsteroidal anti-inflammatory drugs
N-Terface, for burn grafts, 2022
Nuchal rigidity, 595
　definition of, 589
Nuclear imaging
　in cancer detection, 391t
　in cardiovascular disease, 12
　in gastrointestinal assessment, 1133
　of urinary tract, 1508
Nuclear radiation exposure, 2571–2574
Nuclear warfare, 2571
　definition of, 2559
Nucleic acid amplification testing, 1106
Nucleoli, 384
Nucleoside reverse transcriptase inhibitors, for HIV infection, 1826, 1827t
Nucleotide, 141
　definition of, 140
Null lymphocytes
　in cellular immune response, 1792
　definition of, 1783
Nurse(s)
　advanced practice, 12–13
　advocacy role of, for intraoperative patient, 520
　attitudes, experiences, and assumptions of, 142c
　leadership role of, 10
　musculoskeletal problems in, nursing research on, 2428
　occupation-related injuries in, prevention of, 2427–2429
　practitioner role of, 10
　research role of, 10–11
　roles of, 10–11
　specialization by, 12–13
Nurse practice acts, 12–13
Nurse practitioner(s), 12
Nursing
　caring as foundation of, 29
　changes in, 6
　in collaborative practice, 13, 13f
　community-based, 11–12, 18. See also Home health care nursing
　　and hospital-based nursing, comparison of, 18
　　need for, 16
　community-oriented/public health, 11–12
　cultural considerations in, 7
　cultural diversity and, 7
　cultural diversity of, 136
　definition of, 5, 29
　and end-of-life care, 448–452
　expanded roles in, 12–13
　functions of, 13
　in intraoperative phase, 504–505
　occupational health, 21
　primary, 11
　transcultural, 128–137
Nursing care
　delivery of, models of, 11–12
　ethical, 27–34
　individualized plan of, example of, 43c–45c
　refusal to provide (denial of), 32
Nursing care plan(s)
　for acute pancreatitis, 1364c–1367c
　for cancer patient, 403c–415c
　for chronic renal failure, 1532c–1537c
　for disseminated intravascular coagulation, 1096c–1098c
　for emergent/resuscitative phase of burn care, 2010c–2015c
　example of, 43c–45c
　for hip fracture, 2450c–2458c
　for HIV-infected (AIDS) patients, 1838–1844, 1838c–1844c
　for hypothyroidism, 1455c–1458c
　for kidney surgery, 1555c–1558c
　for liver disease, 1323c–1332c
　for myocardial infarction, 880c–883c
　for neck dissection, 1156c–1159c
　for pain management, 294c
　for peripheral vascular disease, 987
　for postoperative care of cardiac surgical patient, 904c–911c
　for prostate cancer, 1755c–1760c
　revision of, 43
　for rheumatic disease, 1899c–1903c
　for thoracotomy patient, 771c–775c
　for total hip replacement, 2377c–2381c
　for vertigo, 2114c–2118c
Nursing diagnoses, 34. See also specific disorder
　characteristics of, 36
　choosing, 36–37
　and collaborative problems, differentiation of, 39, 40f
　for fear accompanied by somatic complaints unsubstantiated by physical findings, 88–89
　for intraoperative patient, 518
　NANDA-approved, 36, 38c–39c
　in nursing process, 36c
　perioperative, 478–479
　postoperative, for hospitalized patient, 533–534
　selection of, 35–36
　stress-related, 104
　taxonomy of, 36
　in teaching-earning process, 55c
　in teaching-learning process, 54
Nursing history. See Health history
Nursing home(s)
　costs of, funding for, 229
　levels of care in, 229–230
　older adults in, 229–230
Nursing interventions, 41–42, 42c. See also specific disorder
　for fear accompanied by somatic complaints unsubstantiated by physical findings, 88–89
　implementation of, 41–42
　in life-threatening illness, 458
　for patient and family receiving diagnosis of life-threatening illness, 458
　perioperative, 478–479
　for respiratory weaning, 753c
　tobacco-related, research on, 642
　for unconscious patient, 2166–2169
Nursing Interventions Classification, 41, 42c
　application of, for patient with fear and somatic complaints, 88–89
　for community with identified health problem, 2–3
　taxonomy used by, in unified Taxonomy of Nursing Practice, 43–45, 46c
Nursing language, unified framework for, 43–45, 46c
Nursing outcomes. See Nursing Outcomes Classification; Outcomes
　for fear accompanied by somatic complaints unsubstantiated by physical findings, 88–89
Nursing Outcomes Classification
　for community with identified health problem, 2–3
　for patient with fear and somatic complaints, 88–89
　taxonomy used by, in unified Taxonomy of Nursing Practice, 43–45, 46c
Nursing process, 35f. See also specific disorder
　for hospitalized postoperative patient, 532–548
　intraoperative, 518–521
　in patient teaching, 54–56, 55c

steps in, 34–35, 36c
using, 35–45
Nursing research, 10–11
  on anxiety and coping behaviors, 117
  on assessment of feeding tube placement, 1179
  on bowel cleansing for colonoscopy, 309–310
  on burns and neurologic conditions, 2009
  on cancer and febrile neutropenia, emergency department management of, 1070
  on childbearing by Black women with and without HIV infection, 1819
  on communication after head and neck surgery, 613
  on device for measuring pupil size and reactivity, 2163
  on diabetes education via telemedicine versus in person, 1403
  on dyspnea-anxiety-dyspnea cycle in COPD, 567
  on endometriosis, 1680
  on epinephrine for anaphylaxis in home IV antibiotic therapy, 1867
  on exercise and cancer rehabilitation, 435
  on exercise in HIV-infected (AIDS) patients, 1847
  on family presence during cardiopulmonary resuscitation, 971
  on fatigue in hepatitis C, 1316
  on fatigue in patients with COPD, 691
  on health promotion for elderly, 60
  on hemodialysis and end-of-life care, 1542
  in infection prevention in hospitalized neutropenic cancer patients, 1809
  on intervention for caregivers of people with dementia, 2322
  on life with urinary catheter, 1576
  on living with rheumatoid arthritis, 1910
  on marriage and multiple sclerosis, 2284
  on mother-child relationship after brain injury, 2246
  on musculoskeletal problems in nurses, 2428
  on nurse-directed care for diabetes in minority population, 1378
  on nutritional health in older adults, 235
  on older men's perceptions of health care needs, 1743
  on oral care in ventilator-dependent patient, 746
  on osteoarthritis, 1916
  on pain assessment, 273
  on pain control for chest tube removal, 768
  on pain in stroke patient, 2218, 2219
  on patient and caregiver congruence in assessment of symptoms at end of life, 464
  on patients' descriptions of respiratory symptoms, 566
  on patients' need for information about cancer treatment, 396
  on patients' requests for assisted dying, and nurses' responses, 453
  on patient teaching about stroke risk, 2211
  on perimenopausal health information, 1634
  on physical activity in patients with COPD, 691
  on pneumonia prevention, in ventilator-dependent patient, 746
  on predicting risk of osteoporosis, in women with disabilities, 2407
  on predictors of positive health, 71
  on preoperative education in rural population, 2383
  on preoperative skin testing of surgical materials, 509
  on psychological distress and quality of life in hospitalized patients with chronic obstructive pulmonary disease (COPD), 701
  on psychoneuroimmunology, 1798
  on quality of life in women with irritable bowel syndrome, 1239
  on readiness for behavioral change in heart failure, 960
  on recovery after coronary artery bypass graft, in women, 903
  on risk for extended postoperative mechanical ventilation, 527
  on sensory morbidity after breast surgery, 1720
  on symptoms of lung cancer, 674
  on symptoms of myocardial infarction in women, 795
  on testicular self-examination, 1772
  on thyroid cancer and quality of life, 1469
  on tobacco-related nursing interventions, 642
  on total joint arthroplasty/replacement, 2383
  on upper extremity amputation in farmers, 2463
  on urinary management after spinal cord injury, 217
  on women's perspectives after heart transplantation, 930
Nursing-Sensitive Outcomes Classification (NOC), 40, 41c
Nutrients
  absorption of, 1125
  deficiencies of, in liver disease, 1289
Nutrition
  and bone health, 2339
  definition of, 46c
Nutritional assessment, 75, 77–84. See also Body mass index (BMI)
  of adolescents, 84
  biochemical assessment in, 78–80
  clinical examination in, 80, 80t
  dietary data in, 80–83
  dietary interview in, 81–83
  in older adult, 78c
  preoperative, 486
Nutritional deficiency, 101
  risk factors for, 83, 83t
Nutritional imbalance
  cellular injury caused by, 101
  definition of, 101
  injuries caused by, 101
Nutritional status
  analysis of, 83–84
  of elderly, 78c
  factors affecting, 83, 83t
  physical signs of, 80, 80t
Nutrition labels, and meal planning in diabetes, 1387, 1388
Nutrition/nutritional support. See also Diet/dietary therapy; Medical nutrition therapy
  for acne vulgaris, 1954–1955
  in acute leukemia, 1077
  in acute pancreatitis, 1362, 1365c–1366c
  in acute renal failure, 1525–1526
  in acute respiratory distress syndrome, 658
  Alzheimer's disease and, 245–246
  in anemia, management of, 1048
  artificial, in terminally ill patients, 466–467
  assessment of, 75
  bone tumors and, 2420
  brain injury and, 2242t, 2244, 2249
  for brain tumor patient, 2308
  for burn patients, 2025–2026, 2028
  for cancer patient, 425, 428–429
    nursing management of, 409c–410c
  in chronic obstructive pulmonary disease, 695–696
  in chronic renal failure, 1530, 1532c–1533c
  in cirrhosis, 1321
  for colostomy patient, 1271
  definition of, 49
  in diabetes mellitus, 1384–1388, 1417
    for hospitalized patient, 1431–1432
  in end-of-life care, 466–467, 467t
  in esophageal conditions, 1169–1170
  in facial reconstructive surgery, 1989–1990
  in gastric cancer, 1222
  in gastritis, 1207–1208
  gerontologic considerations in, 234–235
  in Guillain-Barré syndrome, 2290
  in health promotion, 58
  in heart failure, 957
  in hemodialysis, 1540–1541, 1551–1552
  in hepatic encephalopathy, 1306, 1307c
  in HIV-infected (AIDS) patients, 1836–1837, 1840c–1841c, 1848
  and hypertension, 1025, 1025t
  in hypertension, 1031
  in hyperthyroidism, 1463–1464
  in hypervolemia, 314
  hypomagnesemia and, 329
  in ileostomy patient, 1257c, 1262
  and immune system, 1795
  in inflammatory bowel disease, 1249, 1252
  after laryngectomy, nursing interventions for, 617
  in liver disease, 1323c–1324c
  after neck dissection, 1155, 1158c
  in older adults, nursing research on, 235
  in oral cavity conditions, 1151
  in osteomalacia, 2411
  and osteoporosis, 2406
  in parenteral nutrition, 1196–1197
  in Parkinson's disease, 2317
  in peptic ulcer disease, 1212, 1215
  perimenopausal, 1636
  in peripheral vascular disease, 990–991
  for pharyngitis, 598
  in pneumonia, 640–641
  postoperative, 543
    for gallbladder surgery, 1356
    for older persons, 547
  preoperative, management of, 496
  and pressure ulcer healing, 212–213, 213t
  and pressure ulcers, 208
  promotion of, with leg ulcers, 1014
  in prostate cancer, 1757c–1758c
  for rheumatoid arthritis, 1909
  in septic shock, 374–375
  in shock, 365–366
  for stroke patient, 2220
  for thoracotomy patient, 767
  in tube feeding, 1183–1184
  in tuberculosis, 649
  for unconscious patient, 2166–2167
  for ventilator-dependent patient, 754
  for weight reduction, low back pain and, 2397
  withdrawal of, ethics of, 1190c
  and wound healing, 486, 487t, 541t
Nutrition/nutritional therapy, for urinary diversion, 1604
NuvaRing, 1644

Nystagmus, 2048, 2112, 2143
  definition of, 2043, 2093
Nystatin (Mycostatin), for candidiasis, 1662
NZORD. See New Zealand Organisation for Rare Disorders

# O

OA. See Osteoarthritis
OASIS. See Outcome and Assessment Information Set
Obesity
  body mass index (BMI) in, 78
  and breast cancer, 1713
  and cancer, 386
  and chronic illness, 167
  and diabetes, 1384, 1388
  and health care, 8
  injury caused by, 101
  and low back pain, 2393, 2397
  morbid, 1217–1220
    definition of, 1204, 1217
    medical management of, 1217–1218
    nursing management of, 1220
    surgical management of, 1218–1220, 1219f
  and pressure ulcers, 208
  in surgical patient, nursing management of, 491
Occipital lobe, 2131, 2131f
Occlusive dressings, for burns, 2017
Occupational exposure, and lung cancer, 671
Occupational health nursing, 21, 668
Occupational Safety and Health Administration, 21
  definition of, 2559
Occupational therapy, for stroke patient, 2222
Occupation-related injuries, musculoskeletal, 2427–2429
Octreotide, for diarrhea, in HIV-infected (AIDS) patients, 1836
Ocular burns, 2075
Ocular history, 2046, 2048c
Ocular medication, 2084–2087, 2088c
Ocular prostheses, 2082, 2082f, 2083
Ocular trauma, 2073–2075
Oculomotor nerve (III), 2044, 2136–2137, 2136f, 2137t, 2292f
  assessment of, 2147c
OD, definition of, 2043
Odynophagia, 1162
  definition of, 1142
  with esophageal spasm, 1162
Oedema. See also Cerebral edema; Lymphedema; Pulmonary edema
Office of Emergency Management, 2560
Ofloxacin (Floxin), for gonorrhea, 2508
OHSS. See Ovarian hyperstimulation syndrome
OI. See Opportunistic infections
Ointments, for wound care, 1949–1950
Older adults, 224–252. See also Aging; Gerontologic considerations; Women, older
  abdominal aortic aneurysm in, 999
  abuse and neglect of, 249
  acquired immunodeficiency syndrome in, 248
  in acute care settings, 248–249
  acute pancreatitis in, 1358
  acute renal failure in, 1527
  adherence to therapeutic regimes, 50
  age-related changes in, 230–237
  alcohol abuse in, 240
  analgesia in, 277
  anemia in, 1043
  angina pectoris in, 868
  appendicitis in, 1241–1242
  back pain in, 2392
  brain tumors in, 2303
  burn injury in, 2008–2009, 2019
  cancer treatment in, 436–437, 436t
  cardiac structure and function in, 787, 788t
  cardiovascular assessment in, 805
  cardiovascular system in, 230–232, 231t, 805
  care of, family involvement in, 230
  causes of death among, 226, 226t
  chronic illnesses among, 226
  cognition in, 237
  colorectal cancer in, 1266, 1267
  compression stockings for, 1008
  constipation in, 234, 1233–1234
  coping strategies for, 228
  dehydration in, 2447
  delirium in, 240–243
  dementia in, 243–246
  demographics of, 7, 225–226, 225f
  denture care for, 1149, 1150c
  depression in, 238–240
  diabetes in, 1382–1383, 1389, 1389c, 1432–1433
    and hypoglycemia, 1410
  diarrhea in, 1236
  digestive function in, 1125, 1126c, 1139
  with disability, 184, 191, 191c
    concerns of, 191, 191c
  diverticular disease in, 1243
  dizziness in, 247
  drug abuse in, 240
  elimination patterns in, 215c
  emergency care for, 2520
  emotions in, 248–249
  epilepsy in, 2193
  ethical considerations for, 251–252, 251c
  falls in, 247
  febrile response in, 248
  fluid and electrolyte balance in, 308
  frail, 246
  gallstones in, surgical management of, 1355
  gastrointestinal function in, 215c, 231t, 234, 1125, 1126c, 1139
  genitourinary system in, 231t, 233–234
  head injuries in, 2235
  health assessment in, 65c
  health promotion for, 60–61
  health status of, 226
  hearing in, 232t, 236–237
  hearing loss in, 2103
  heart failure in, 958
  heat stroke in, 2533–2534
  hematologic system in, 1043
  hepatobiliary system in, 1287, 1287c
  hip fracture in, 2446–2447
    nursing care plan for, 2450c–2458c
  HIV infection in, 1816–1817
  home health care for, 17–18, 17f, 250
  in hypertension, 1023, 1025, 1031
  hyperthyroidism in, 1463
  hyponatremia in, 319
  hypothyroidism in, 1459
  hypovolemia in, 309–310
  immune function in, 1794–1795, 1795t
  impaired mobility in, 246
  infection susceptibility in, 248
  integumentary system in, 231t, 233
  learning in, 237
  legal, 251–252
  leukopenia in, 1043
  living arrangements for, 228–230
  lung cancer in, 673–674
  malabsorption in, 1239
  malnutrition in, 2447
  memory in, 237
  mental health problems in, 238–246
  multiple myeloma in, 1083, 1084
  multiple sclerosis in, 2279–2280
  musculoskeletal system in, 231t, 235–236, 2342, 2344t
  nervous system in, 232t, 236, 2150–2152
  nutritional assessment in, 78c
  nutrition in, 78c, 234–235
  oral problems in, 1145c
  osteomalacia in, 2411
  osteoporosis in, 2404, 2405, 2405f, 2410
  Paget's disease in, 2412–2413
  pain in, 268
  pain management in, 268, 277
  pain response in, 248
  pancreatic function in, 1347
  patient teaching for, 53–54
  perioperative risk in, 503–504
  pharmacology in, 237–238, 239t, 277
  pneumonia in, 638
  postoperative care for, 528–529
  postoperative complications in, 546–548
  in preoperative period, nursing management of, 491
  pressure ulcers in, 209
  pruritus in, 1951
  reproductive system in, 231t, 233
  respiratory function in, 231t, 232–233, 562–563, 562t, 728
  rheumatic disease in, 1892
  scabies in, 1964
  sensory system in, 236–237
  septic arthritis in, 2416–2417
  shock in, recognition of, 359–361, 361c
  skin in, 1931–1932, 1932c
  sleep in, 235
  smell perception in, 232t, 237
  social services for, 249
  sociologic considerations for, 227–228
  special senses in, 232t
  stress in, 228
  systemic response in, 249
  taste sensation in, 232t, 237
  thrombangiitis obliterans in, 996
  tuberculosis in, 646
  urinary function in, 1500–1501, 1503–1504
  urinary incontinence in, 247–248
  vascular disorders in, 978, 979
  vision in, 232t, 236
Older Americans Act, 249
Olfaction, 553
Olfactory nerve (I), 2130, 2136–2137, 2136f, 2137t, 2292f
  assessment of, 2147c
  disorders of, 2293t
Oligodendrogliomas, 2302
Oliguria, 1503, 1503t
  in acute renal failure, 1522
  definition of, 945, 1493
  in heart failure, 950
Olmesartan (Benicar), for hypertension, 1029t
Omeprazole (Prilosec, Losec), 1206t
OMIM. See Online Medelian Inheritance in Man; Online Mendelian Inheritance in Man
Onchocryptosis, 2401
Oncogenes, 385
Oncologic emergencies, 438t–442t
Oncology, definition of, 381
Oncology nursing
  areas of responsibility in, 381, 382c
  definition of, 381

Oncology Nursing Society, 161c
OncoScint, 418
Oncotic pressure, 303
Ondansetron, 398
Ondansetron (Zofran), postoperative therapy with, 528
*On Death and Dying* (Kübler-Ross), 449
Onychomycosis, 1961t, 1962
Oocyte(s), 143
Oophorectomy
   definition of, 1661
   in endometriosis, 1681
   prophylactic, 393
Oophoritis, and pelvic inflammatory disease, 1670
Open awareness, of terminal status, 450
Open fracture, 2431
   emergency management of, 2433
   nursing management of, 2434–2435
Open reduction, 2371c
   of fractures, 2433, 2433f
   with internal fixation, 2371
      definition of, 2355
Operating room
   asepsis in. *See* Asepsis, surgical
   attire in, 506
   environmental controls in, 507
   environment of, 505–508
   restricted zone in, 503, 506
   safety in, 508
   semirestricted zone in, 503, 506
   sterile field in, 507
   unrestricted zone in, 503, 506
   ventilation of, 507
Ophthalmology, issues in, 2087
Ophthalmoscopy
   direct, 2048
   indirect, 2049
Opioid(s), 260
   addiction to, 259, 284
   administration of, 281. *See also* Analgesia, administration of
   adverse effects and side effects of, 288
   administration routes for, 281
   adverse effects and side effects of, 281–284
      risk factors for, 282–284
   agonists, 287
      definition of, 259
   antagonists, 287
      definition of, 259
   for burn patients, 2024
   constipation with, 282
   definition of, 259
   delivery route for, and analgesia, 278, 278f
   dependence, definition of, 259
   dosage and administration of, 279–280, 282, 283t
   drug interactions with, 284
   for dyspnea, 465
   in end-of-life care, 464–465
   equianalgesic doses of, 282, 283t
   gerontologic considerations with, 277
   inadequate dose of, 282
   for intravenous anesthesia, 512t
   nausea and vomiting with, 282
   pharmacology of
      age-related changes in, 277
      genetics of, 269
   for postoperative pain relief, 535
   postoperative therapy with, 528
   PRN range orders for, 279, 279c
   pruritus with, 282
   respiratory depression with, 281–282
   sedation with, 281–282
   tolerance, 262c
   tolerance of, 259, 284
   toxicity of, 282
   for urolithiasis, 1591, 1594
Opioid receptors, 265, 265t
Opium, abuse/overdose, emergency management of, 2545t
Opportunistic infections
   definition of, 1815
   in HIV-infected (AIDS) patients, 1843c, 1849
Opposition, 200c
   definition of, 198c
Oprelvekin, adverse effects and side effects of, 421t
Op-Site, for burn grafts, 2022
Opsonization, 1789, 1793t
   complement system and, 1793t
   definition of, 1783
Optical coherence tomography, 2049
Optic chiasm, 2046, 2046f, 2132
Optic disc, 2046
Optic nerve (II), 2043–2044, 2046, 2046f, 2130, 2136–2137, 2136f, 2137t, 2292f
   assessment of, 2147c
   disorders of, 2293t
Oral candidiasis, in HIV-infected (AIDS) patients, 1832
Oral cavity, 1122f, 1153f. *See also* Mouth
   age-related changes in, 1125, 1126c, 1145c
   anatomy of, 1150f
   cancer of, 1148–1149
      clinical manifestations of, 1148
      diagnosis of, 1148–1149
      epidemiology of, 1148
      gender difference in, 1148
      medical management of, 1149
      nursing management of, 1149
      pathophysiology of, 1148
      risk factors for, 1148
   conditions of
      continuing care in, 1152
      expected outcomes with, 1152–1153
      nursing diagnoses related to, 1150
      nursing interventions in, 1151–1152
      nursing process for, 1149–1153
      patient teaching about, 1152, 1152c
      planning and goals for, 1150–1151
   discomfort in, in blistering diseases, nursing interventions for, 1973
   infections of, in immunosuppressed patient
      nursing diagnoses related to, 1780–1781
      nursing interventions for, 1780–1781
      nursing outcomes for, 1780–1781
   inspection of, 1149–1150
Oral contraceptives, 1642, 1642c, 1643, 1643c
   benefits and risks of, 1641–1642, 1643c
   and HIV transmission, 1818
   postcoital use of, 1647
Oral hygiene
   in acute leukemia, 1077
   in cancer patient, 397, 426–427
   during gastrointestinal intubation, 1179
   in HIV-infected (AIDS) patients, 1848
   in prevention of tooth decay, 1142–1145, 1145c
   promotion of, 1151
   in ventilator-dependent patient, nursing research on, 746
Oral mucosa, nursing interventions for, in disseminated intravascular coagulation, 1097c
Oral rehydration solution, 2503
OraQuick Rapid HIV-1 Antibody Test, for HIV diagnosis, 1825
OraSure, for HIV diagnosis, 1825
Orbit, surgeries of, 2081–2082
Orbital cellulitis, 2079–2080
Orbital fractures, 2073
Orbital trauma, 2072–2073
Orbital tumors
   benign, 2080
   malignant, 2080
Orchiectomy, 1754–1760
   definition of, 1740
Orchitis, 1769
   definition of, 1740
Ordre des infirmières et infirmiers du Québec, contact information for, 42
Oregon, Death With Dignity Act, 451
Organ donation, 2239
Organ donors, for kidney transplantation, 1560, 1560c
Organic acids, in body fluids, 302t
Organism, causative, of infection, 2475
Organ of Corti, 2096
   definition of, 2095c
Organophosphates, as terrorism threat, 2569t, 2570–2571
Organ transplantation, immune response in, 1796
Orientation, definition of, 225
Orientation status, in older person with hip fracture, 2453c–2454c
ORIF. *See* Open reduction, with internal fixation
Orlistat (Xenical), 1217
Orogastric tube, 1175
Oropharyngeal airway, insertion of, 2524, 2524f
Oropharyngeal catheter, for oxygen administration, 725t, 726
Oropharynx, 554, 555f, 1153f
Orphenadrine citrate (Banflex), for Parkinson's disease, 2314
ORS. *See* Oral rehydration solution
Ortho Evra, 1643
Orthopedic rehabilitation, 192
Orthopedic surgery, 2371–2388
   assessment for
      postoperative, 2384–2385
      preoperative, 2376–2382
   complications of, postoperative, 2385, 2386–2387
   continuing care after, 2387–2388
   expected outcomes in
      postoperative, 2388
      preoperative, 2384
   home and community-based care after, 2387–2388, 2388c
   nursing diagnoses related to
      postoperative, 2385
      preoperative, 2382
   nursing interventions for
      postoperative, 2385–2388
      preoperative, 2373, 2382–2384
   nursing process for
      postoperative, 2384–2388
      preoperative, 2376–2384
   planning and goals for
      postoperative, 2385
      preoperative, 2382
   preoperative patient teaching about, in rural population, nursing research on, 2383
   types of, 2371, 2371c
Orthopnea
   definition of, 553, 625, 945
   in pneumonia, 636
Orthopnoea
   causes of, 563
   definition of, 563

Orthoses. *See also* Braces
  and mobility, 207
  types of, 207
Orthostatic hypotension. *See* Hypotension
Orthotopic transplantation
  cardiac, 928–929, 929f
    definition of, 915
  of liver, 1336–1340
    definition of, 1285
OS, definition of, 2043
OSHA. *See* Occupational Safety and Health Administration
OSHA. *See* Occupational Safety and Health Administration
Osmolality, 302–303, 304
  of body fluids, 304
  definition of, 301, 1175
  serum, 304
    in hypernatremia, 320
    laboratory values for, 310t
  in tube feedings, 1181–1182
  of urine, 304, 1497, 1506, 1507, 1507t
    in acute renal failure, 1523t
    laboratory values for, 310t
Osmolarity, 1497
  definition of, 301
Osmoles, 303
Osmolite HN, 1182
Osmoreceptors, in fluid and electrolyte balance, 306
Osmosis, 302–303, 303f
  definition of, 301, 1175, 1515
  in hemodialysis, 1538
  and tube feedings, 1181–1182
Osmotic diuresis, 303
  for cerebral metastases, 2307
Osmotic pressure, 303
Ossicles, 2094, 2095f
  definition of, 2095c
Ossiculoplasty, 2108
  definition of, 2093
Ossification, 2339
  definition of, 2337
  endochondral, 2339
  heterotopic, 2355, 2440
  intramembranous, 2339
Osteitis deformans. *See* Paget's disease
Osteoarthritis, 1914–1917, 2342, 2372
  assessment of, 1915
  clinical manifestations of, 1914–1915
  definition of, 2337
  diagnosis of, 1915
  genetics of, 147, 147t
  gerontologic considerations in, 1892
  joint involvement in, 2348
  medical management of, 1915–1916
  nodules in, 2348
  nursing management of, 1916–1917
  pathophysiology of, 1914, 1915f
  pharmacologic therapy for, 1915–1916
  risk factors for, 1914, 1915c
  surgical management of, 1916
  and temporomandibular disorders, 1146–1147
Osteoblast(s), in Paget's disease, 2412
Osteoblasts, 2338
  definition of, 2337
  estrogen and, 2340
Osteochondroma, 2417
Osteoclast(s), 2338–2339
  definition of, 2337
  estrogen and, 2340
  in Paget's disease, 2412
Osteoclastomas, 2417
Osteoconduction, 2438
Osteocyte(s), 2338–2339, 2338f
  definition of, 2337

Osteodystrophy, renal, in chronic renal failure, 1529
Osteogenesis, 2339, 2438
  definition of, 2337
Osteogenic sarcoma, 2417
Osteoid, 2339
  definition of, 2337
  in osteomalacia, 2411
Osteoid osteoma, 2417
Osteoinduction, 2438
Osteolysis, 1920
Osteomalacia, 1920, 2411
  assessment of, 2411
  diagnosis of, 2411
  gerontologic considerations in, 2409
  medical management of, 2411
  pathophysiology of, 2411
Osteomyelitis, 2373, 2413–2416
  assessment of, 2413, 2414
  bone tumors and, 2420
  chronic, 2413
  clinical manifestations of, 2413
  continuing care in, 2415
  definition of, 2355
  diagnosis of, 2413
  expected outcomes in, 2415–2416
  expected patient outcomes in, 2415–2416
  home and community-based care for, 2415
  infectious process in, management of, 2415
  medical management of, 2414
  nursing diagnoses related to, 2414
  nursing interventions for, 2415
  nursing process with, 2414–2416
  pathophysiology of, 2413
  pharmacologic treatment of, 2414
  planning and goals for, 2415
  prevention of, 2413–2414
  skeletal traction and, 2368–2369
Osteon, 2339
  definition of, 2337
  in fracture healing, 2340
Osteonecrosis, 1920
Osteopathy, 134
Osteophytes
  definition of, 1887
  formation of, 1888
Osteoporosis, 1635, 1920, 2342, 2404–2411
  assessment of, 2406–2407
  definition of, 1613, 2337
  diagnosis of, 2406–2407
  in elderly, 235
  fractures caused by, 2404, 2409–2411
    assessment of, 2409
    expected outcomes for, 2410–2411
    nursing diagnoses related to, 2409
    nursing interventions for, 2410
  gerontologic considerations in, 2404, 2405, 2405f, 2410
  height changes with, 78
  and height loss, 2404, 2405f
  home care checklist for, 2408c
  home care for, 2408c
  and hypocalcemia, 325
  with internal fixation for fractures, 2440
  medical management of, 2408–2409
  nursing interventions for, 2410
  nursing management of, 327
  nursing process for, 2409–2411
  pathophysiology of, 2405, 2406f
  patient teaching about, 2410
  pharmacologic treatment of, 2408–2409
  planning and goals for, 2410
  in postpolio syndrome, 2331
  prevention of, 2406, 2406c
  risk factors for, 2405–2406, 2406c, 2406f
  risk of, in women with disabilities, nursing research on, 2407

  screening for, 2449
  secondary, 2405, 2406
Osteosarcoma, 2417
Osteotomy, 2373
  definition of, 2355
  for osteoarthritis, 1916
Ostomy surgery. *See also* Colostomy; Ileostomy
Otalgia, definition of, 2093
Otic capsule, 2094
Otitis externa, 2105, 2105c
  definition of, 2093
  malignant, 2105
Otitis media
  acute, 2106–2107, 2107t
    definition of, 2093
  chronic, 2107–2108
    definition of, 2093
  serous, 2107
  in upper airway infection, 603
Otorrhea, 2106
  cerebrospinal fluid (CSF), 2235
  definition of, 2093
Otosclerosis, 2110–2111
  definition of, 2093
  genetics of, 146
Otoscopy, 2098, 2098f
Ototoxicity, 2119
  drugs/substances causing, 2118, 2118c, 2119
Ottawa decision rules, for knee fractures, 2459
OU, definition of, 2043
Outcome markers, 9
Outcomes. *See also specific condition*
  documentation of, 43
  expected
    identification of, 40
    postoperative, 548
    preoperative, 499, 499c
    for surgery, 521
  perioperative, 478–479
Oval window, 2094, 2094f
  definition of, 2095c
Ovarian cancer, 1689–1691
  epidemiology of, 1682
  familial occurrence of, 386
  recurrence of, 1691
  stages of, 1690, 1690c
  surgical treatment of, 1690–1691
Ovarian cysts, 1678–1679
Ovarian hyperstimulation syndrome, 1651
Ovary(ies)
  anatomy of, 1615, 1615f
  definition of, 1613
Overnutrition, 101
Overuse injury, 2398, 2398c
Overweight. *See also* Obesity
  body mass index (BMI) in, 78
Oviducts. *See* Fallopian tubes
Ovulation, 1615
  definition of, 1613
  induction of, medications for, 1650, 1651c
Ovulation detection methods, of contraception, 1646
Oxacarbazepine (Trileptal)
  adverse effects and side effects of, 2194t
  toxic effects of, 2194t
Oxaliplatin, in cancer treatment, 399t
Oxaprozin (DayPro), for rheumatic diseases, 1895t
Oxazepam (Serax), abuse/overdose, emergency management of, 2547t
Oxitropium bromide (Oxivent), 693t
Oxycodone, pharmacology of, 283t
Oxycodone (OxyContin), for burn patients, 2024

# INDEX

OxyContin. *See* Oxycodone
  abuse/overdose, emergency management of, 2545t
Oxygen. *See also* Fraction of inspired oxygen
  in anesthesia, 510t
  consumption, by tissues, 976
  partial pressure of, 560
    arterial, in atelectasis, 627
  toxicity of, 724–725
Oxygenation
  brain injury and, 2248–2249
  in burn patient, 2010c
  cerebral, monitoring of, 2171–2173
  maintenance of, with increased intracranial pressure, 2174
  tissue, and wound healing, 541t
Oxygen catheter, transtracheal, 725t, 726, 727
Oxygen deficit, and wound healing, 541t
Oxygen mask
  aerosol, 725t
  non-rebreathing, 725t, 726–727, 726f
  partial rebreathing, 725t, 726, 726f
  simple, 725t, 726
  Venturi, 725t, 726, 726f, 727
Oxygen therapy, 723–729. *See also* Hyperbaric oxygen therapy
  in acute respiratory distress syndrome, 658
  administration of, 725–728, 725t, 726f, 727f
  for angina, 871
  in cardiogenic shock, 369
  in cardiopulmonary resuscitation, 971, 972t
  in chronic obstructive pulmonary disease, 694, 695
  complications of, 724–725
  continuing care for, 728–729
  for cor pulmonale, 661
  for cystic fibrosis, 718–719
  for decompression sickness, 2537
  fire safety with, 725
  gerontologic considerations in, 728
  in heart failure, 957, 964–965
  high-flow systems for, 725t, 726
  home care and, 728–729, 728c
  in hypovolemic shock, 368
  indications for, 724
  infection control with, 725
  low-flow systems for, 725t, 726
  patient teaching about, 728, 728c
  in pneumonia, 640
  precautions with, 724–725
  for pulmonary embolism, 665, 667
  in sleep apnea, 605
  for status asthmaticus, 717
  weaning from, 754
Oxygen transport, 557
Oxyhemoglobin, 560, 1039
  definition of, 1036
Oxyhemoglobin dissociation curve, 560–561, 561c
Oxymetazoline hydrochloride, for allergic rhinitis, 1872t
Oxypentifylline, for peripheral arterial disease, 992
Oxytocin, 1446
  definition of, 1440

## P

PAAB. *See* Pressure activated air buffer
Pacemaker
  atrial-ventricular, 927
  biventricular, 927
  ventricular, 784, 927
Pacemaker(s), electronic
  design of, 844–845
  electrodes of, 844–845
    dislodgement of, 847
  electromagnetic interference with, 847–848, 852c, 853c
  function
    functions of, 845–846
    NASPE-BPEG code for, 845–846
  generator for, 844–845
    functions of, 845–846
  implantation of, infection prevention after, 851, 852c, 853c
  inhibited response by, 823
  leads, 844–845
  malfunction of, 850, 850f
    assessment of, 847, 848t
  permanent, 844
  safety considerations with, 847–848, 852c, 853c
  surveillance of, 848–849
  temporary, 844
  triggered response by, 823
  types of, 844–845
Pacemaker syndrome, 847
Pacemaker therapy, 844–849
  assessment of, 850
  for atrial fibrillation, 833
  biventricular, 844
    synchronized, 847
  capture in, 846
    loss of, 850, 850f
  complications of, 847–848, 850
  emotional responses to, 851
  expected outcomes with, 851
  fixed (asynchronous), 846, 847f
  implanted transvenous, 845, 845f
  loss of sensing in, 850, 850f
  nursing diagnoses related to, 850
  nursing interventions for, 851, 853c
  nursing process and, 850–851
  on-demand, 846, 846f
  patient teaching about, 851, 852c
  planning and goals for, 850
  self-care in, patient teaching about, 851, 852c
  transcutaneous, 845, 845f
Pacific people. *See* Indigenous people
Packed red blood cells
  for transfusion, 1103t
  transfusion of, administration of, 1107c
  transfusions of, in emergency care, 2526
Paclitaxel, for cancer treatment, 399t
Paclitaxel (Taxol), for ovarian cancer, 1691
PACU. *See* Postanesthia care unit
PAF. *See* Platelet-activating factor
Paget disease, of breast, 1705c, 1713
  definition of, 1701
Paget's disease, 2412–2413
  assessment of, 2412
  of bone, 1920
  clinical manifestations of, 2412
  complications of, 2412
  diagnosis of, 2412
  gerontologic considerations in, 2412–2413
  medical management of, 2412
  pharmacologic treatment of, 2412
Pain, 2143
  abdominal
    with appendicitis, 1241
    in colorectal cancer, 1266
    in Hodgkin's disease, 1080
  acute, 260, 2143
    harmful effects of, 263–264
  age and, 268
  aggravating factors and, 270–272
  alleviating factors and, 270–272
  anxiety and, 266–267
    management of, 276
  assessment of, 259, 270–276
    guidelines for, 274–275
    instruments for, 273–275
    nursing research on, 273
    in patients with disabilities, 275
    postoperative, 533
  breakthrough, 287
    definition of, 259
  breast, 1710
  burn, 261c
  in burn victim, and anxiety, 2024–2025
  cancer-related, 260, 262
    in advanced disease, 437
    assessment of, 425
    depression and, 267
    management of, 262, 262f, 429–430
    nursing management of, 411c–412c
    sources of, 429, 430t
  characteristics of, 270–273
  chronic, 2143
  chronic (noncancer), 260
    harmful effects of, 264
  chronic (nonmalignant)
    depression and, 267
    nursing diagnoses related to, 256–257
    nursing interventions for, 256–257
    nursing outcomes for, 256–257
  in circulatory insufficiency, 979
  classification of
    by duration, 260
    by etiology, 260, 262–263
    by location, 262
  concerns and misconceptions about, 271c–272c, 272c
  control of. *See* Pain management
  culture and, 267–268
  definition of, 259–260
  denial of, 260
  with dentoalveolar abscess, 1145–1146
  and depression, 468
  depression and, 266–267
  in ectopic pregnancy, 1653–1654
  at end of life, 271c–272c
  esophageal, assessment of, 792t
  factors affecting, 266–270
  as fifth vital sign, 259–260
  fracture and, 2446
  with gallstones, 1349
  in gastrointestinal disease, 1126, 1126f
  gate control theory of, 266, 267f, 291
  gender and, 268–269
  genitourinary, 1501–1503, 1502t, 1512c
  gerontologic considerations in, 248
  Guillain-Barré syndrome and, 261c–262c
  harmful effects of, 263–264
  hip fracture and, 2446
  incisional, minimization, during coughing, 766, 767f
  in inflammation, 103
  intensity of, 270
    scales of, 270, 272f, 273, 274f
  location of, 270
  in multiple sclerosis, 2279
  musculoskeletal, assessment of, 2344–2345
  myofascial, in temporomandibular disorders, 1146–1147
  in Paget's disease, 2412
  past experience and, 266
  pathophysiology of, 264–270
  pelvic, chronic, 1682
  in peptic ulcer disease, 1210
  perception of, age-related changes in, 2151
  persistent, 260, 2143
  personal meaning of, 270
  phantom limb, 266
  pleuritic, 652

Pain (continued)
  quality of, 270
  reassessment of, during pain management, 293–295
  rectal, in colorectal cancer, 1266
  referred
    abdominal, 1126, 1126f
    definition of, 259
  sensitization and, 276
  severe, 261c–262c
  shoulder, hemiplegia-associated, 261c
  in sickle cell anemia, and substance abuse, 1059
  of sickle cell anemia, 261c
  in stroke patient, 2218, 2219
  subjective character of, 260
  in temporomandibular disorders, 1146
  in thoracic surgical patient, 772c–773c
  in thrombangiitis obliterans, 996
  timing of, 270
  transmisiion of, pathways for, surgical interruption of, 291–292
  transmission of, 264–266
    central nervous system in, 265, 265f
    descending control system and, 265–266
    peripheral nervous system and, 264–265
  types of, 260–263
  in urinary tract infections, 1572, 1575
Pain behavior(s), 272–273
Pain Care Bill of Rights, 259, 260c
Pain management, 258–295
  in acute leukemia, 1077
  in acute pancreatitis, 1360, 1361, 1364c–1365c
  alternative and complementary approaches for, 288–290
  alternative therapies in, 290
  for amputation, 2464
  in angina, 872
  in anorectal disorders, 1279
  for bone tumors, 2419
  for breast surgery, 1719
  for burns, 2012c, 2024–2025, 2028
  for cancer patient, 262, 262f, 263f, 411c–412c, 429–430, 437
  after cardiac surgery, 897, 901, 909c
  in cardiogenic shock, 369
  for casts, 2357
  with cerebral metastases, 2307
  with cervical disk herniation, 2326, 2327
  for chest tube removal, nursing research on, 768
  in complex regional pain syndrome, 2440
  concerns and misconceptions about, 271c–272c, 272c
  continuing care in, 292–293
  cultural considerations in, 267–268
  cutaneous stimulation in, 288–289
  for dialysis patient, 1552
  in diverticulitis, 1245
  in ectopic pregnancy, 1655
  in end-of-life care, 271c–272c
    ethical issues in, 32
  in esophageal conditions, 1170
  in facial reconstructive surgery, 1989
  after foot surgery, 2403
  in gastric cancer, 1222
  after gastric surgery, 1224
  genetics and, 269
  for genital herpes, 1668
  gerontologic considerations in, 268, 277
  goals for, identification of, 275–276
  for hand/wrist surgery, 2399
  in headache, 2201
  heat therapy in, 289
  for hip fracture, 2450c–2451c
  in HIV-infected (AIDS) patients, 1848
  at home, 292, 293c
  home and community-based care for, 292–293
  for hysterectomy, 1693
  ice therapy in, 289
  inadequate, 279–280, 280c, 282
  in inflammatory bowel disease, 1252
  in liver disease, 1327c–1328c
  for low back pain, 2393
  massage in, 288–289
  in mastoid surgery, 2109
  in melanoma, 1983
  for metastatic bone disease, 2419
  in multiple myeloma, 1083–1084
  in myocardial infarction, 880c–881c, 883–884
  after neck dissection, 1155
  neurologic approach to, 290–292
  neurostimulation in, 291–292
  neurosurgical approach to, 290–292
  in neurosurgical patient, 2182
  nonpharmacologic interventions for, 288–290
  nurse-patient relationship in, 276
  nurse's role in, 275–276
  nursing care plan for, 294c
  in oral cavity conditions, 1151–1152
  in orthopedic surgery
    postoperative, 2385–2386
    preoperative, 2382–2383
  for osteoarthritis, 1916
  for osteomyelitis, 2415
  in osteoporosis, 2410
  outcomes, 295, 295c
  patient teaching in, 276
  in peptic ulcer disease, 1215
  in pericarditis, 939–941
  perioperative, 495
  in peripheral vascular disease, 990
  pharmacogenetics and, 269
  pharmacologic interventions for, 276–285
  physical care in, 276
  postoperative, 528, 533, 535–536
    in cervical discectomy, 2327
    in foot surgery, 2403
    for gallbladder surgery, 1356
    in gastric surgery, 1224
    in hand/wrist surgery, 2399
    in neck dissection, 1155
    in neurosurgical patient, 2182
    in older adults, 547
    in thoracic surgery, 758, 766–767
  premedication assessment in, 277
  preventive approach for, 278–279
  PRN range orders for, 279, 279c
  in prostate cancer, 1758c–1759c
  with prostatectomy, 1766
  in renal surgical patient, 1554, 1555c
  for rheumatic diseases, 1894, 1895t–1897t, 1898, 1899c
  for septic arthritis, 2416
  in septic arthritis, 2416
  in sickle cell anemia, 1058
  in sickle cell crisis, 1059
  for spinal cord tumor, 2310–2311
  standards for, 259
  strategies for, 276–290
    evaluation of, 293–295
  subcutaneous system for, 536, 536f
  in temporomandibular disorders, 1147
  in terminal illness, 464–465
  for thoracic surgical patient, 758, 766–767
  in thoracic surgical patient, 772c–773c
  in total hip replacement, 2377c
  in toxic epidermal necrolysis or Stevens-Johnson syndrome, 1976
  in trigeminal neuralgia, 2295
  untested therapies in, 290
  with urinary diversion, 1605
  in urinary tract infection, 1575
  in urolithiasis, 1591, 1594
  with vulvar surgery, 1687
Pain management programs, 192
Pain receptors. See Nociceptors
Pain sensation, assessment of, 2150
Pain syndromes, 261c–262c
Pain threshold, definition of, 259
Pain tolerance, definition of, 259
Palate
  hard, 1150f, 1153f
  soft, 1150f
Palatine tonsil, 1150f, 1153f
Palindromic rheumatism, 1920
Palliation
  of cancer, 391
    of esophagus, 1167
    radiation therapy for, 394
    surgical techniques for, 393, 394c
  definition of, 381
Palliative care
  definition of, 448, 452
  goal setting in, 461, 463c
  in hospital setting, 454
  in long-term care facilities, 454
  services included in, 452
Palliative sedation
  definition of, 448
  in end-of-life care, 468
Pallidotomy, for Parkinson's disease, 2315
Pallor, 798, 1933, 1935t
  in systemic disease, 1929t
Palmar erythema, in liver disease, 1308
Palmar flexion, definition of, 198c
Palm method, of estimating burn extent, 1998
Palonosetron, for chemotherapy patient, 398
Palpation
  of abdomen, 1128f, 1129
  of heart, 800–801, 802f
  in physical examination, 75–76, 76f
  thoracic, 570–573
Palpitations, assessment of, 790, 794t
Pamidronate (Aredia), 328
  for complex regional pain syndrome, 2440
  in multiple myeloma, 1084
Pancreas, 1122f
  age-related changes in, 1347
  anatomy of, 1345–1346, 1346f
  cancer of, 1369–1370
  disorders of, 1358–1360
  endocrine, 1345–1347
  enzyme secretion by, 1124
  exocrine, 1345–1347
  head of, tumors of, 1370–1372
  secretions of, 1124
Pancreatic cyst(s), 1369
Pancreatic disease, and rheumatic diseases, 1920
Pancreatic duct, 1122f
Pancreatic insufficiency, malabsorption in, 1240t
Pancreatic islet tumors, 1372
  ulcerogenic, 1372
Pancreatic lipase, source and digestive action of, 1123t
Pancreaticoduodenectomy, 1368–1369, 1371, 1371f
Pancreaticojejunostomy, 1368–1369
  definition of, 1345

Pancreatitis
  acute, 1358–1363
    gerontologic considerations in, 1358
    nursing care plan for, 1364c–1367c
    nursing process in, 1360–1363
    severity of, criteria for predicting, 1359, 1359c
  chronic, 1363–1369
  definition of, 1345, 1358
  epidemiology of, 1358
  and hypocalcemia, 325
  risk factors for, 1358
Pancuronium (Pavulon), 513t
Pancytopenia, 1052
  definition of, 1036
Pandemic
  definition of, 2488
  influenza, 2488–2489
Panhypoglobulinemia, 1805–1806
  definition of, 1802
Panhypopituitarism, 1446
Panic disorders, chest pain caused by, assessment of, 792t
Pannus, 1887, 1888f
  definition of, 1887
p24 antigen test, 1816
  definition of, 1815
Papillary muscles, 782f, 783
Papilledema, 2084
  with brain tumor, 2304
  definition of, 2043, 2301
  in hypertension, 1023
Papillomas, conjunctival, 2080
Pap smear, 1625–1626, 1627–1628, 1628f, 1629c
PapSure, 1626
Papule, 1937c
Para-aminosalicylate sodium, for tuberculosis, 647
Paracentesis, for ascites, 1295, 1296c–1297c
Paraesophageal hernia, 1163–1164, 1163f
Parainfluenza, pneumonia caused by, 629, 631t
Paralysis, 2141, 2342
  compartment syndrome and, 2437
  definition of, 2337
  for mechanical ventilation, in acute respiratory distress syndrome, 658–659
  pharmacologic, effect on metabolic demands, 2173
  spinal cord injury and, 2251
Paralytic ileus
  after appendectomy, 1242, 1242t
  in burn victim, 2002, 2004, 2014c
  spinal fracture and, 2460
Paraplegia, 2141
  assessment in, 2261–2262
  complications of, 2262
  continuing care for, 2265–2266
  definition of, 2233
  expected outcomes in, 2266
  home and community-based care for, 2265–2266
  nursing diagnoses related to, 2262
  nursing interventions for, 2262–2265
  nursing process for, 2261–2266
  planning and goals for, 2262
  self-care for, 2265
  spinal cord injury and, 2251, 2261–2262
Parasitic disease
  malabsorption in, 1240t
  of skin, 1962–1964
Parasympathetic nervous system, 2137, 2139, 2139t
  and cardiac function, 825
  definition of, 2129

Parathormone, 1470
  and bone health, 2339, 2405
  in chronic renal failure, 1529
Parathyroid disorders, 1470–1473
  pathophysiology of, 1470
Parathyroid glands, anatomy and physiology of, 1470, 1470f
Parathyroid hormone
  and bone loss, 2405
  and bone strength, 2339
  and calcium balance, 325, 328
  in fluid and electrolyte balance, 306
  and phosphorus balance, 333
Paravertebral anesthesia, 515
Paregoric, abuse/overdose, emergency management of, 2545t
Parenteral fluid therapy, 338–352
Parenteral nutrition, 1193–1200
  administration, methods for, 1194–1195
  for brain injury patients, 2244
  for burn patient, 2025–2026
  for cancer patient, 429, 429f
  complications of, 1197, 1197t
  definition of, 1175, 1193
  in diabetes mellitus, for hospitalized patient, 1432
  discontinuation of, 1190c
  discontinuing, 1196
  ethical issues with, 1190c
  expected outcomes with, 1199–1200
  formulas for, 1193
  goals of, 1193
  at home, 1198–1199, 1199c, 1200t
  inications for, 1193
  initiation of, 1194
  nursing diagnoses related to, 1196
  nursing interventions in, 1196–1197
  nursing process with, 1196–1200
Paresthesia, 1049, 2345–2346
  with cervical disk herniation, 2326
  compartment syndrome and, 2437
  definition of, 2301, 2337
  in Guillain-Barré syndrome, 2288
  stroke and, 2208t
Paricalcitol (Zemplar), for hyperphosphatemia, 333
Parietal lobe, 2131, 2131f
Parish nursing, 17
Parkinson's disease, 2311–2319
  assessment in, 2316
  assistive devices in, 2317
  clinical manifestations of, 2312–2313
  continuing care in, 2318
  epidemiology of, 2311
  expected outcomes in, 2318–2319
  falls in, 2313
  medical management of, 2313–2314
  nursing diagnoses related to, 2316
  nursing interventions in, 2316–2318
  nursing process in, 2316–2319
  on-off syndrome in, 2314
  pathophysiology of, 2311–2312, 2312f
  surgical management of, 2315
Parkland/Baxter formula, for fluid replacement in burn patients, 2007c
Paronychia, 1936, 1940f
Parotid glands, 1122f, 1147
Parotitis, 1147
  definition of, 1142
Paroxetine (Paxil)
  for hot flashes, 1635
  for rheumatoid arthritis, 1909
Paroxetine (Paxtine), for depression, 240
Paroxysmal (dysrhythmia), 832
  definition of, 823

Paroxysmal nocturnal dyspnea, 950
  definition of, 945
Paroxysmal nocturnal hemoglobinuria, 1099t, 1803t, 1808–1809
Paroxysmal supraventricular tachycardia, 835
Pars flaccida, 2094, 2095f
Pars plana vitrectomy, 2068
Pars tensa, 2094, 2095f
Partial pressure, of gas, 559–560, 559c
  in pulmonary gas exchange, 560, 561f
Partial thromboplastin time, 2578t
Partial thromboplastin time (PTT)
  in cardiac patient, 808t
  laboratory values for, 2578
Particle-beam radiation therapy, 395
PARU. See Postanesthetic recovery unit
Passive acquired immunity, 1786
Passive exercises, 201t
Pastes, for wound care, 1949
Patch, 1937c
Patched cecal reservoir, for urinary diversion, 1603
Patch testing, 1942
Paternalism, ethical principle of, 28c
Pathogens, invasion by, immune response to, 1786–1788
Pathophysiology, 91
Patient(s)
  culturally mediated characteristics of, 131–134
  definition of, 5
  needs of, 5, 5f
  terminally ill
    communication with, 457–459
    denial by, 450
  unconscious. See also Consciousness, altered level of
Patient autonomy, in terminal illness, 450
Patient care equipment, in Standard Precautions, 1820c
Patient Care Partnership, 29, 29c–30c
Patient-controlled analgesia
  administration of, 280–281
  for burn victim, 2024
  definition of, 259
  postoperative, 535
    in orthopedic surgery, 2386
  for thoracic surgical patient, 766–767
Patient education. See Health education; Patient teaching
  genetics in, 68
  nursing process in, 55c
Patient Evaluation Conference System, 193
Patient knowledge, of HIV/AIDS, 1841c–1842c, 1845
Patient profile
  education in, 69, 69c
  environment in, 69–70, 69c
  family relationships in, 69c, 70
  in health history, 67–73, 69c
  life history in, 69c
  lifestyle in, 69c, 70–71
  occupation in, 69, 69c
  past life events related to health in, 68–69, 69c
  physical or mental disability in, 69c, 71
  risk for abuse in, 69c
  self-concept in, 69c, 71
  sexuality in, 69c, 71–73
  stress and coping response in, 69c
  stress and coping responses in, 73
  support system in, 70
Patient Self-Determination Act, 32, 33, 252
Patient teaching. See also Health education
  about activities of daily living, 194, 194c
  about acute glomerulonephritis, 1518

Patient teaching (continued)
  about adenoidectomy, 600
  about angina, 872–873, 873c
  about anticoagulants, 1010c
  about arm and shoulder exercises, after thoracic surgery, 767, 769c, 774c
  about asthma, 714–717
  about bleeding, 1085, 1085c
  about bone tumors, 2419, 2420
  about brain tumor, 2308, 2309c
  about breathing exercises, 730c
  about cardiac catheterization, 815c
  about cardiac dysrhythmia, 841
  about casts, 2357
  about chest physiotherapy, 734–735
  about chronic glomerulonephritis, 1519–1520
  about chronic illness, 172–174
  about chronic obstructive pulmonary disease, 700
  about chronic renal failure, 1531, 1533c–1534c
  about condom use, 1818
  about continuous ambulatory peritoneal dialysis, 1549–1550
  about cor pulmonale, 661
  about cutaneous urinary diversions, 1600–1602, 1601c
  about diabetes mellitus, 1402–1404. *See also* Diabetes education
  about diarrhea/diarrheal diseases, 2503–2504
  about dietary self-management after gastric surgery, 1226, 1227c
  about edema, 315
  about epilepsy, 2196
  about epistaxis, 606
  about esophageal conditions, 1170, 1170c
  about external fixator, 2365, 2365c
  about foot and leg care in peripheral vascular disease, 991c, 994–995
  about gastric cancer, 1222–1223, 1223c
  about gastric surgery, 1226, 1227c
  about genital herpes, 1668
  about glaucoma, 2059, 2059c
  about gonorrhea, 2508
  about hemodialysis, 1541, 1549–1550
  about hemotologic disorders, 1068c
  about Huntington's disease, 2320
  about hypertension, 1031
  about hypothyroidism, 1456c
  about ileostomy, 1255c
  about implantable cardioverter defibrillator, 852c
  about implanted cardiac device, 851
  about infectious disease, 2497c
  about infectious diseases, 2492
  about intravenous (IV) therapy, 343
  about iron supplements, 1050c
  about kidney transplantation, 1563
  about laryngectomy, 618–620
  about low back pain, 2394c
  about metered-dose inhaler, 698, 699c
  about neck dissection, 1161, 1161c
  about neutropenia, 1068c
  about oral cavity conditions, 1152, 1152c
  about osteoporosis, 2410
  about ostomy care, after urinary diversion surgery, 1606–1607
  about oxygen therapy, 728, 728c
  about pacemaker therapy, 851, 852c
  about pain management, 276, 292, 293c
  about parenteral nutrition, 1198–1199, 1199c, 1200t
  about Parkinson's disease, 2317–2318, 2318c
  about peptic ulcer disease, 1216–1217, 1217c
  about pneumonia, 641
  about preventive oral hygiene, 1145c
  about prostate cancer, 1756c–1757c
  about prostatectomy, 1765
  about pulmonary embolism, 667
  about renal cancer, 1564
  about rheumatic diseases, 1904–1905
  about rhinitis, 591
  about risk of infection in hemotologic disorders, 1068c
  about self-care
    in acute leukemia, 1078
    after neck dissection, 1161, 1161c
    in osteomyelitis, 2415, 2416c
    for postoperative phase, 529, 531c
    in postoperative phase, 548
  about sexually transmitted infections, 2508–2509
  about shoulder healing, 2398c
  about sickle cell anemia, 105
  about sinusitis, 597
  about skin cancer prevention, 1980, 1980c, 1981
  about stress management, 105–107, 107
  about stroke risk, nursing research on, 2211
  about surgery for breast cancer, 1718
  about syphilis, 2507, 2507c
  about tonsillectomy, 600
  about transfusion reactions, 1109
  about tube feedings, 1188
  about tuberculosis, 650
  about upper airway infection, 603
  about urinary diversion, 1604
  about urolithiasis, 1594
  about urologic testing, 1510, 1511c
  about viral rhinitis, 593
  about wound care, 540, 542c
  gerontologic considerations in, 2152
  after hip replacement, 2375
  nursing process in, 54–56
  preoperative, 492–495
    for laryngectomy, 615
    in neck dissection, 1154
    in rural population, nursing research on, 2383
  in prevention of injury, 2530
  in pulmonary rehabilitation, 695
  for renal surgical patient, 1559
  for thoracic surgical patient, 757, 769–770, 770c, 774c–775c
PAV. *See* Proportional assist ventilation
PCA. *See* Patient-controlled analgesia
PCL. *See* Posterior cruciate ligament
PCP. *See* Phencyclidine; *Pneumocystis carinii*, pneumonia
PCR. *See* Polymerase chain reaction
PCV regimen, for cerebral metastases, 2307
PDT. *See* Photodynamic therapy
PE. *See* Pulmonary embolism
Peau d'orange, 1704c
PECS. *See* Patient Evaluation Conference System
Pediatric rehabilitation programs, 192
Pediculosis, 1962–1963, 2477t
Pediculosis capitis, 1962–1963
Pediculosis corporis, 1963
Pediculosis pubis, 1963
*Pediculus humanus capitis,* 1962–1963
  incubation period of, 2477t
  transmission of, 2477t
*Pediculus humanus corporis,* 1962–1963
Pedigree, 145
  definition of, 140

PEEP. *See* Positive end-expiratory pressure
Peer review organizations, 8
PEG. *See* Percutaneous endoscopic gastrostomy
Pegfilgrastim, in breast cancer treatment, 1728
Pelvic examination, 1623–1627
  bimanual palpation in, 1626–1627, 1626f
  gerontologic considerations in, 1627
  patient teaching about, 1624, 1624c
  positioning for, 1624
Pelvic exenteration
  for cervical cancer, 1685
  definition of, 1661
Pelvic floor exercises. *See* Pelvic muscle exercise
Pelvic fracture, 2444–2449
  stable, 2445, 2445f
  unstable, 2445, 2446f
Pelvic inflammatory disease, 1670–1672, 2507
  *Chlamydia* and, 1669
  definition of, 1661
  in HIV-infected (AIDS) patients, 1672–1673
  pathophysiology of, 1670–1671, 1671f
  sexually transmitted disease and, 2509
Pelvic muscle exercise (PME, Kegel exercises), 1582c, 1674, 1675c
  for urinary incontinence, 216, 247
Pelvic organ prolapse, 1505, 1674–1675
Pelvic pain, chronic, 1682
Pelvic peritoneoscopy, 1630–1631, 1630f
Pelvis
  anatomy of, 2444, 2444f
  bones of, 2444, 2444f
Pemoline (Cylert), for fatigue, in multiple sclerosis, 2280
Pemphigus, 1091f, 1971–1972
Penbutolol (Levatrol), for hypertension, 1028t
Penetrance, 146
  definition of, 140
  incomplete, 146
Penicillamine (Cuprimine, Depen), for rheumatic diseases, 1895t
Penicillin
  and immune system, 1797t
  for pharyngitis, 598
Penicillin G benzathine, for syphilis, 2506
Penile cancer, 1774–1775
Penile cancer, definition of, 1740
Penile implants, 1746, 1748t
Penile injection therapy, 1747t
Penile suppository, 1747t
Penis, 1741, 1741f
  cancer of, 1774–1775
  conditions affecting, 1774–1775
  definition of, 1740
Penrose drain, 538, 538f
Pentamidine (Pentacarinat, Pentam 300, NebuPent), for *Pneumocystis jiroveci* pneumonia, 1835
Pentobarbital (Nembutal)
  effect on metabolic demands, 2173
  emergency management of, 2545t–2546t
Pentostatin, in cancer treatment, 399t
Pentoxifylline (Trental)
  for peripheral arterial disease, 992
  for skin ulcer healing, 1948
Penumbra region, 2207
  definition of, 2206
"People-first" language, 184
PEP. *See* Post-exposure prophylaxis
Pep pills, abuse/overdose, emergency management of, 2546t
Pepsin, 1123
  definition of, 1121
  source and digestive action of, 1123t

# INDEX

Peptic ulcer disease, 1209–1217
  assessment in, 1212–1213
  clinical manifestations of, 1210–1211
  complications of, 1215–1216
  diagnosis of, 1211
  epidemiology of, 1209
  expected outcomes in, 1217
  follow-up care for, 1212
  genetics of, 1209
  hemorrhage in, 1215–1216
  medical management of, 1206t–1207t, 1211–1212
  nursing diagnoses related to, 1214
  nursing interventions for, 1215–1216
  nursing process with, 1212–1217
  pathophysiology of, 1209–1210, 1209f
  patient teaching about, 1216–1217, 1217c
  perforation in, 1216
  pharmacologic therapy for, 1211–1212
  predisposing factors for, 1209
  pyloric obstruction in, 1216
  surgical management of, 1212, 1213t–1214t
Perception
  assessment of, 2145
  after cardiac surgery, 900–901, 908c–909c
  in cardiovascular disease, assessment of, 797
Perceptual disturbances
  ischemic stroke and, 2219–2220
  spinal cord injuries and, 2257–2258
  stroke and, 2209
Perchlorethylene, abuse/overdose, emergency management of, 2546t
Percussion
  of abdomen, 1128f, 1129
  of chest, 801–802
  in physical examination, 76, 76f
  thoracic, 573–574, 574f, 574t
  of thorax, 576t
Percutaneous balloon microcompression, of trigeminal nerve, 2295
Percutaneous coronary intervention, 862, 885–888
  definition of, 859
  emergent, 877
Percutaneous endoscopic gastrostomy, 1188–1189, 1189f
  definition of, 1175
  protection of, 1191f
Percutaneous needle biopsy, of lung, 585
Percutaneous nephrolithotomy, for urolithiasis, 1591–1593, 1592f
Percutaneous radiofrequency thermal coagulation, of trigeminal nerve, 2295
Percutaneous transluminal angioplasty, 986
Percutaneous transluminal coronary angioplasty, 868, 885–886, 886f
  complications of, 887, 887t
  definition of, 859
  postprocedure care for, 887–888
Percutaneous vertebroplasty/kyphoplasty, for osteoporotic fractures, 2409
Perforation, of esophagus, 1164–1165
Pergolide (Permax), for Parkinson's disease, 2314
Periapical abscess, 1145–1146
  definition of, 1142
Periapical granuloma, 1145
Pericardial effusion, 670, 941, 968–969
  atelectasis with, 626
  in cancer patient, 439t–440t
  in chronic renal failure, 1535c–1536c
Pericardial friction rub, 803
Pericardial space, 782, 782f
Pericardial tamponade, in chronic renal failure, 1535c–1536c

Pericardiocentesis, 968–969
  definition of, 945
Pericardiotomy, 969
  definition of, 945
Pericarditis, 933, 939–941
  causes of, 939, 939c
  in chronic renal failure, 1527, 1529, 1535c–1536c
  clinical manifestations of, 939
  diagnosis of, 939
  friction rub in, 803
  medical management of, 939–940
  nursing process with, 940–941
  signs and symptoms of, 791t
Pericardium, 782
Periconception health care, 1652–1653
Perilymph, 2096
Perimenopause, 1632–1633
  definition of, 1613
  health information in, nursing research on, 1634
Perimetry testing, 2050
  automated, 2050
  manual, 2050
Perindopril (Accon), for hypertension, 1029t
Perineorrhaphy, 1675
  definition of, 1661
Perineum, examination of, 1129
Periodontitis, 1144t
Perioperative and perianesthesia nursing
  activities in, 481–484, 482c–483c
  genetic considerations in, 493
  patient-focused model for, 484, 484f
Perioperative phase
  definition of, 481
  nursing diagnoses related to, 478–479
  nursing interventions for, 478–479
  nursing outcomes for, 478–479
Periosteum, 2338f, 2339
  definition of, 2337
  in fracture healing, 2340
Peripheral arterial insufficiency, in diabetes, 1422
Peripheral arterial insufficiency of extremities, nursing process with, 987–992
Peripheral blood smear, 1044
Peripheral blood stem cell transplantation, 1112–1113
  for acute lymphocytic leukemia, 1074
  in acute myeloid leukemia, 1072
  for chronic myeloid leukemia, 1073
  for multiple myeloma, 1083–1084
  for non-Hodgkin's lymphoma, 1082
Peripheral edema, 804
Peripherally inserted central catheter(s), 1195–1196
  definition of, 1175
Peripheral nervous system, 2136–2137
  assessment of, 2346, 2346c
  disorders of, 2296–2297. See also Peripheral neuropathy
  skin traction and, 2367
Peripheral neuropathy
  in burn patient, 2032t
  in chronic glomerulonephritis, 1519
  chronic renal failure and, 1528
  definition of, 1815, 2296
  in diabetes, 1426–1427, 2296
  in HIV-infected (AIDS) patients, 1833
  pain management for, 1848
Peripheral neurovascular dysfunction
  hip fracture and, 2455c–2456c
  indicators of, 2349, 2349c
Peripheral parenteral nutrition, 1194
Peripheral vascular disease
  and foot disorders, 2401

  nursing process with, 987–992
  self-care in, patient teaching about, 991, 991c, 994–995
Peripheral vascular status, after cardiac surgery, 897
Peripheral vasculature, regulation of, 978
Peripheral vision, loss of, stroke and, 2208t
Peristalsis
  definition of, 1175
  of large intestine, 1125
  of small intestine, 1124–1125
  of stomach, 1124
  after surgery, 1177
Peritoneal catheter(ization), insertion of, 1546, 1546f
Peritoneal dialysis, 1545–1551
  acute intermittent. See Acute intermittent peritoneal dialysis
  for acute renal failure, 1525
  complications of, 1547–1548
  continuous ambulatory. See Continuous ambulatory peritoneal dialysis
  continuous cyclic. See Continuous cyclic peritoneal dialysis
  definition of, 1515
  home and community-based care for, 1549–1550, 1550c
  leakage in, 1547
  procedure for, 1545–1547
Peritoneal lavage, diagnostic
  definition of, 2517
  in trauma victim, 2532
Peritoneoscopy, in gastrointestinal assessment, 1139
Peritoneovenous shunt, for ascites, 1295
Peritonitis
  after appendectomy, 1242, 1242t
  in appendicitis, 1241, 1242
  causes of, 1245, 1245f
  in cirrhosis, 1319
  clinical manifestations of, 1246
  complications of, 1246
  in continuous ambulatory peritoneal dialysis, 1548
  definition of, 1245, 1515
  diagnosis of, 1246
  medical management of, 1246
  nursing management of, 1246–1247
  pathophysiology of, 1246
  peritoneal dialysis and, 1547
  with urinary diversion, 1606
Peritonsillar abscess, 603
Periurethral bulking, for urinary incontinence, 1581
Permeability factor, action of, 1791t
Pernicious anemia, B-cell deficiencies and, 1805–1806
Peroneal artery, 981, 981f
Peroneal nerve, function of, assessment of, 2346c, 2367
Persistent vegetative state, definition of, 2161, 2162
Personality
  changes in
    with brain tumor, 2304
    in Huntington's disease, 2319
  changes in, Alzheimer's disease and, 244
  and response to stress, 97
  type A, 97
    and heart disease, 867
Personal protective equipment, 2565
  categories of, 2565
  definition of, 2559
Personal space, 132
Person-environment fit theory, of aging, 227

Perspiration, insensible, 1931
Pes cavus, 2402, 2402f
Pes planus, 2402
Pessaries, 1627, 1674, 1675f
PET. *See* Positron emission tomography
Petechiae, 1085, 1939c
　in acute myeloid leukemia, 1071
　definition of, 1036, 1927
PET fusion, in cancer detection, 391t
Pet therapy, 219
Peyronie's disease, 1775
　definition of, 1740
p53 gene, 385
pH
　definition of, 1175
　gastric, monitoring of, ambulatory, 1138
　testing, in GI intubation placement, 1178
Phacoemulsification, for cataracts, 2061
Phagocytic cells
　assessment of, tests for, 1799t
　and immunodeficiency disorders, 1803t
　and natural immunity, 1785
　in natural immunity, 1785
Phagocytic dysfunction, 1802–1805, 1803t
　assessment of, 1804
　clinical manifestations of, 1802–1804
　diagnosis of, 1804, 1804c
　medical management of, 1804–1805
　pathophysiology of, 1802
Phagocytic immune response, 1786
　definition of, 1783
Phagocytosis, 103, 1041, 1041f
　definition of, 1036
　in inflammation, 1887–1888
Phakic intraocular lenses, 2066
Phalanx, fracture of, 2444
Phantom limb pain, 266, 2461, 2464
　definition of, 2425
Pharmacogenetics, 153–154
　and pain management, 269
Pharmacokinetics, aging and, 238, 239t, 277
Pharmacological function, definition of, 46c
Pharmacology, aging and, 237–238, 239t, 277
Pharyngeal lipase, source and digestive action of, 1123t
Pharyngeal pouch, 1164
Pharyngitis
　acute, 597–598
　　clinical manifestations of, 597, 597f
　　complications of, 597
　　diagnosis of, 597–598
　　medical management of, 598
　　nursing managament of, 598
　　pathophysiology of, 597, 597f
　atrophic, 598
　chronic, 598–599
　chronic granular, 598
　definition of, 589
　hypertrophic, 598
　nursing interventions for, 602–603
　streptococcal, and acute glomerulonephritis, 1517, 1517f
Pharyngoesophageal pulsion diverticulum, 1164
Pharynx, 1122f
　age-related changes in, 1125, 1126c
　anatomy of, 554
　cancer of, 1148–1149
　inspection of, 1150
　physical examination of, 569, 570f
Phenazopyridine (Pyridium), for urinary tract infections, 1574
Phencyclidine (PCP, angel dust), abuse/overdose, emergency management of, 2546t–2547t

Phenelzine sulfate (Nardil), interactions with anesthetics, 490t
Phenindamine hydrochloride (Neo-Synephrine), for Parkinson's disease, 2314
Phenobarbital (Luminal)
　adverse effects and side effects of, 2194t
　for status epilepticus, 2198
　toxic effects of, 2194t
Phenobarbital, therapeutic blood levels of, 2601t
Phenothiazines, interactions with anesthetics, 490t
Phenotype, 141
　definition of, 140
Phenylalanine derivatives, 1398, 1399t–1400t, 1401
Phenylbutazone, and immune system, 1797t
Phenylephrine (Neo-Synephrine)
　for cardiogenic shock, 370
　ocular applications of, 2086t
　in treatment of shock, 366t
Phenylephrine, topical, for epistaxis, 605
Phenylephrine hydrochloride, for allergic rhinitis, 1872t
Phenylketonuria, 141
　genetics of, 146, 147t
　screening for, 150t
Phenytoin
　metabolism of, genetic factors affecting, 154t
　therapeutic blood levels of, 2601t
Phenytoin (Dilantin)
　adverse effects and side effects of, 2194, 2194t
　contraindications to, subarachnoid hemorrhage and, 2228
　preoperative use of, for intracranial surgery, 2181
　for status epilepticus, 2198
　for trigeminal neuralgia, 2295
Pheochromocytoma, 1475–1477
　definition of, 1440
　familial occurrence of, 386
Philadelphia chromosome, 1073
Phimosis, 1774
　definition of, 1740
Phlebitis
　grades of, 351, 351c
　with intravenous therapy, 350–351
Phlebostatic axis, 817, 817f
Phlebostatic level, 817, 817f
Phlebothrombosis, 1004–1010
Phlebotomy
　in hemochromatosis, 1063
　therapeutic, 1102–1103
Phosgene, as terrorism threat, 2569t, 2570, 2571
Phosphate
　in body fluids, 302t
　for hypercalcemia, 328
Phosphodiesterase-5 inhibitors, 1745, 1747t, 1748c–1749c
Phosphorus
　in acute renal failure, 1524
　deficit, 317t, 331–332
　　manifestations of, 1516t
　　in renal disorders, 1516t
　dietary, 332
　excess, 317t, 332–333
　　manifestations of, 1516t
　　in renal disorders, 1516t
　imbalance of, in chronic renal failure, 1529
　imbalances of, in renal disorders, 1516t
　intravenous, 332

　radioactive, for polycythemia vera, 1065
　serum
　　in chronic glomerulonephritis, 1519
　　in hyperphosphatemia, 317t, 332
　　in hypophosphatemia, 317t, 332
　　laboratory values for, 310t
　　reference range for, 331
　　significance of, 331
Phosphorus binders, for chronic renal failure, 1529–1530
Photoablation, for cancer, 393
Photoaging, 1932
Photoallergic contact dermatitis, 1877, 1877t
Photochemotherapy, for psoriasis, 1966t, 1967–1968
Photocoagulation
　for cancer, 393
　for hemorrhoids, 1277
Photodynamic therapy
　in Barrett's esophagus, 1166
　for bladder cancer, 1597
　for cancer, 422
　for macular degeneration, 2070–2071, 2071f
Photographs, clinical, of skin, 1942
Photophobia, 2079
　definition of, 2043, 2129
Photorefractive keratectomy, 2065, 2066
Phototherapeutic keratectomy, 2064–2065
Phototoxic contact dermatitis, 1877, 1877t
*Phthirus pubis*, 1962–1963
　incubation period of, 2477t
　transmission of, 2477t
Physical abuse. *See* Abuse
Physical barriers, in natural immunity, 1786
Physical conditioning, in chronic obstructive pulmonary disease, 695
Physical examination, 35, 74–77
　auscultation in, 77–78, 77f
　in cardiovascular disease, 798–805
　ethical considerations with, 64
　of female reproductive system, 1623–1627
　in genetic assessment, 155
　in immune system assessment, 1798
　inspection in, 74–75
　of integumentary system, 1932–1940
　of lower respiratory tract, 569–576
　of musculoskeletal system, 2346–2350, 2346c
　nursing implications of, 104
　in nutritional assessment, 80, 80t
　palpation in, 75–76, 76f
　percussion in, 76, 76f
　of sexual assault victim, 2552
　of trauma patient, 62
　of upper respiratory tract, 568–569, 569f, 570f
Physical fitness
　definition of, 49
　in health promotion, 58
Physical mobility. *See* Mobility
Physical regulation, definition of, 46c
Physical therapy, for rotator cuff tear, 2429
Physician-assisted suicide. *See* Assisted suicide
Physiological domain, definition of, 46c
Physiologic dead space, 556
　definition of, 553
Pia mater, 2133, 2134f, 2135–2136
Pica, 1047
PICC. *See* Peripherally inserted central catheter(s)
Pick-up walker, 205
PID. *See* Pelvic inflammatory disease
Pigskin grafts, for burns, 2021
PillCam ESO, 1134

# INDEX

Pill Crusher Syringe, 1186f
Pilocarpine, for glaucoma, 2057, 2058t
Pilonidal cyst, 1277–1278
Pilonidal sinus, 1277–1278, 1278f
Pindolol, for hypertension, 1028t
Pinna, definition of, 2095c
Pinworm, causative organisms of, 2477t
Pioglitazone (Actos), 1400t, 1401
Pirbuterol (Maxair), 693t
　for ventilator-dependent patient, 749
PIRO method, definition of, 373c
Piroxicam (Feldene), for rheumatic diseases, 1895t
Pitch, of sound, 77, 2100
Pit sealants, in prevention of tooth decay, 1145
Pitting, of nails, 1940f
Pituitary adenomas, 2302–2303
　hormonal effects of, 2302–2303
　pressure effects of, 2302
Pituitary disorders, 1446–1448
　pathophysiology of, 1446
Pituitary gland, 2132
　anatomy of, 1445–1446, 1445f, 2303
　anterior
　　anatomy of, 1445–1446, 1445f
　　pathophysiology of, 1446
　in fluid and electrolyte balance, 306
　posterior
　　anatomy of, 1445f, 1446
　　pathophysiology of, 1446
　removal of. See Hypophysectomy
　tumors of, 1446–1447
Pivot joints, 2341
Pizotyline, in migraine prevention, 2200
PL 101-336. See Americans With Disabilities Act of 1990
Placebo(s), administration of, ethical considerations in, 269, 269c
Placebo effect, 269
　definition of, 259
Placebos, use of, ethical considerations in, 31
Plague
　as bioterrorism threat, 2567t
　bubonic, 2567t
　mortality rate for, 2567t
　pneumonic, 2567t
　primary septicemic, 2567t
　transmission of, 2567t
　treatment of, 2567t
Plan B, 1673
Planning
　in ethical analysis, 34c
　in nursing process, 34, 36c, 39–41
　　assigning priorities in, 40
　　expected outcome in, establishing, 40
　　goals in, establishing, 40
　　nursing actions in, determining, 40–41
　in teaching-learning process, 54–55, 55c
Plant alkaloids
　adverse effects and side effects of, 399t
　for cancer treatment, 399t
Plantar digital neuroma, 2402
Plantar fasciitis, 2401
Plantar flexion, definition of, 198c
Plaque
　atherosclerotic. See Atheroma
　neuritic, in Alzheimer's disease, 243–244
　of skin, 1929t, 1937c
Plasma, 301, 1042
　definition of, 1036
　pH of
　　homeostatic mechanisms for, 334
　　reference range for, 334
　reference ranges for, 2581t–2593t
　for transfusion, 1103, 1103t

Plasma cells, 1037t, 1042
Plasmapheresis, 1102, 1102t
　definition of, 1945
　for Guillain-Barré syndrome, 2289
　for myasthenia gravis, 2287
　for pemphigus, 1972
Plasma proteins, 1042
Plasmin, 1043
Plasminogen, 1043
　definition of, 1036
Plasmodium falciparum
　incubation period of, 2476t
　transmission of, 2476t
Plasmodium malariae
　incubation period of, 2476t
　transmission of, 2476t
Plasmodium ovale
　incubation period of, 2476t
　transmission of, 2476t
Plasmodium vivax
　incubation period of, 2476t
　transmission of, 2476t
Plaster casts, 2356
Plastic reconstructive surgery, 1985–1991
Platelet(s)
　in cardiac patient, 807t
　disorders of, cutaneous manifestations of, 1929t
　in immune response, 1793
　transfusions of, in emergency care, 2526
Platelet-activating factor, in allergic reaction, 1858t, 1859
Platelet count, laboratory values for, 2580
Platelet growth factor, adverse effects and side effects of, 421t
Platelet pheresis, 1102, 1102t
Platelets, 1038f, 1040f
　consumption of, increased, 1087, 1087t
　defects, 1089. See also Thrombocytopaenia; Thrombocytopenia
　definition of, 1036
　destruction of, increased, 1087, 1087t
　functions of, 1037, 1037t, 1042
　　medications and substances affecting, 1089, 1090c
　production of, 1042
　　decreased, 1087, 1087t
　　increased, 1085–1086
　sequestration of, 1087, 1087t
　for transfusion, 1103t
　　random, 1103t
　　single donor, 1103t
　transfusion of, 1108c
　transfusions, for idiopathic thrombocytopenic purpura, 1089
Platform posturography, 2100
Pleura, 555, 555f
　biopsy of, 582–585
Pleural effusions, 557, 570, 652–654
　assessment findings in, 576t
　atelectasis with, 626
　definition of, 625
　malignant, 653–654
　parapneumonic, 638
　pathophysiology of, 653, 653f
　in pneumonia, 638, 641
Pleural fluid, 761
Pleural friction rub
　definition of, 625
　with lung abscess, 651
Pleural space, 626
　chest tube placement in, 761
　definition of, 625
Pleurectomy, for pleural effusion, 654
Pleurisy, 652

Pleurodesis, for pleural effusion, 653
Pleuroperitoneal shunt, for pleural effusion, 654
Plicamycin, in cancer treatment, 399t
Plicamycin (Mithracin), for Paget's disease, 2412
PLISSIT model, 1619, 1742–1743
PME. See Pelvic muscle exercise
PML. See Progressive multifocal leukoencephalopathy
PMMA. See Polymethyl methacrylate
PMNs. See Polymorphonuclear leucocytes
PMS. See Premenstrual syndrome
PNDS. See Perioperative Nursing Data Set
Pneumatic dilation, esophageal
　for achalasia, 1162, 1163f
　for esophageal spasm, 1162
Pneumatic retinopexy, 2068
Pneumococcal vaccine, 248
　in chronic obstructive pulmonary disease, 693, 698
　indications for, 635
Pneumoconiosis, 668–670
　coal workers', 669–670
　definition of, 668
　prevention of, 668
Pneumocystis carinii, pneumonia, 633t
Pneumocystis jiroveci, pneumonia
　B-cell deficiencies and, 1805
　incubation period of, 2477t
　transmission of, 2477t
Pneumocystis jiroveci pneumonia
　definition of, 1815
　in HIV-infected (AIDS) patients, 1831
　treatment of, 1835
Pneumonectomy, 672c, 755c
　in bronchiectasis, 709
Pneumonia, 628–643
　aspiration, 634, 681–682
　　enteral nutrition and, 1184t
　　in tube feedings, 1187
　assessment in, 636, 639
　atelectasis in, 638, 641
　bacterial, 629–631, 630t–631t
　　medical management of, 636–638
　bronchial, 634, 634f
　in bronchiectasis, 709
　chest pain in, 791t
　chlamydial, 631t
　classification of, 629, 630t–631t
　clinical manifestations of, 636
　cognitive status in, 641
　community-acquired, 629, 630t–631t
　　medical management of, 636–638, 639f
　　risk factors for, 637c
　complications of, 638–639, 640
　　monitoring and managing, 641
　continuing care in, 642–643
　diagnosis of, 636
　Enterobacter, 634
　Enterobacteriaceae, 629, 633–634
　epidemiology of, 629
　Escherichia coli, 629, 633–634
　expected patient outcomes in, 643
　fungal, 633t, 634
　gerontologic considerations in, 248, 638
　Haemophilus influenzae, 629, 630t, 634, 635
　hospital-acquired, 629–634, 632t
　　medical management of, 637
　　microbiology of, 629–631
　　prevention of, 634–635, 635t
　in immunocompromised host, 633t, 634
　Klebsiella, 533, 632t, 633, 636
　Legionella, 629, 630t
　lobar, 533, 533f, 634, 634f

Pneumonia (continued)
    medical management of, 636–638, 639f
        continuing symptoms after initiation of, 641
    microbiology of, 629
    mortality caused by, 628
    *Mycobacterium tuberculosis*, 533, 533f, 633t.
        See also Tuberculosis, pulmonary
    mycoplasma, 629, 631t
    mycoplasmal, causative organisms of, 2477t
    nosocomial, 629–634
    nursing diagnoses related to, 639–640
    nursing interventions in, 640–643
    nursing process in, 639–643
    in orthopedic surgery patient, 2387
    pathophysiology of, 533, 533f, 634f
    patient teaching about, 641
    planning and goals in, 640
    pleural effusions in, 638, 641, 652–653
    pneumococcal, 629, 630t, 635–636
        causative organism of, 2477t
        risk factors for, 637c
    *Pneumocystis*, 533, 533f
    *Pneumocystis carinii*, 633t
    *Pneumocystis jiroveci*
        definition of, 1815
        in HIV-infected (AIDS) patients, 1831
            treatment of, 1835
    postoperative, 534
        in hip fracture, 2449
        in older persons, 547
    prevention of, 634–635, 634–636, 635t
    *Proteus*, 633
    pseudomonal, 629, 632t, 633–634
        medical management of, 636–638
    in renal surgical patient, 1558
    respiratory failure in, 638, 641
    rib fracture and, 2459
    risk factors for, 634–636, 635t
    self-care in, patient teaching about, 641
    *Serratia*, 633
    shock in, 638, 641
    staphylococcal, 629–631, 632t
    streptococcal, 629, 630t, 635–636
    superinfection in, 639, 641
    in thoracic surgery patient, risk factors for, 757c
    traction and, 2370
    ventilator-associated, 629–634
        in burn patient, 2009
        prevention of, nursing research on, 746
    viral, 629, 631t
Pneumonitis, aspiration, 681–682
Pneumotaxic center, 562
Pneumothorax, 557, 570, 678–679
    atelectasis with, 626
    in chronic obstructive pulmonary disease, 698–699, 707c
        nursing interventions for, 698–699
    clinical manifestations of, 576t, 679
    definition of, 625, 723
    open, 679–680, 680f
    in parenteral nutrition, 1197t
    rib fracture and, 2460
    simple (spontaneous), 679
    tension, 679–680, 680f
    in thoracic surgical patient, 761, 768
    traumatic, 62, 679
    in ventilator-dependent patient, 751
Pneumo-wrap, 742
PNH. See Paroxysmal nocturnal hemoglobinuria
PNS. See Peripheral nervous system
POF. See Premature ovarian failure
Poikilocytosis, 1052
    definition of, 1036

Point of maximal impulse, 571c, 783, 801, 801f, 802f
Poison(s)
    corrosive, 2541
        definition of, 2517
    definition of, 2540
    ingested (swallowed), emergency management of, 2541, 2542c–2543c
    inhaled, emergency management of, 2543
    skin contamination with, 2543–2544
Poisoning, 102
    emergency management of, 2540–2544
Pollinosis. See Allergic rhinitis
Polyarticular disease, 1887
Polycystic kidney disease, end-stage renal disease in, 1527
Polycystic ovary syndrome, 1678–1679
Polycythemia
    definition of, 686
    in emphysema, 688
    and skin color, 1935t
Polycythemia(s), 1064–1066
    definition of, 1036, 1064
    secondary, 1066
Polycythemia vera, 1065–1066
Polydipsia
    in diabetic ketoacidosis, 1412
    psychogenic, 315
PolyHeme, 2526
Polymerase chain reaction
    definition of, 1815
    in herpes simplex virus encephalitis, 2274
Polymorphism(s), 142, 145
    definition of, 140
    testing for, 153
Polymorphonuclear leukocytes, in natural immunity, 1785
Polymorphonuclear neutrophils, 1041
Polymyalgia rheumatica, 1913–1914
Polymyositis, 1913
Polyp(s)
    cervical, 1625
        definition of, 1613
    colorectal, 1275–1276
    endometrial, definition of, 1613
    nasal, 606–607
Polypharmacy, 237
    definition of, 225
    in older persons, 78c, 102
Polythiazide (Renese), 954t
Polyuria, 1503, 1503t
    in diabetic ketoacidosis, 1412
Pons, 2131f, 2133
Poor metabolizers, and pain management, 269
Populations, definition of, 46c
Population screening, 153
    definition of, 140
Portal hypertension, 1289, 1293
    definition of, 1285
Portal obstruction, in cirrhosis, 1318–1319
Portal of entry, of infections, 2479
Portal pressure, measurement of, 1290t
    with esophageal varices, 1299
Portal pylephlebitis, in appendicitis, 1241
Portal systemic shunts, for esophageal varices, 1302–1303, 1303f, 1304t
Portal vein, 1121, 1285
    septic thrombosis of, in appendicitis, 1241
Port-wine angiomas, 1978
Positioning, patient, for gastrointestinal intubation, 1177
Positioning injury, intraoperative, nursing interventions for, 519–520
Position/positioning, patient
    in bed, 196, 197c

    for colonoscopy, 1136
    dorsal recumbant, 519–520, 519f
    for gastrointestinal tube insertion, 1177
    in heart failure, 965
    hip fracture surgery and, 2448
    hip replacement and, 2373–2374, 2373f, 2374c
    with increased intracranial pressure, 2175
    for kidney surgery, 1553, 1553f
    lateral (Sims), 519f, 520
    lithotomy, 519f, 520
    for low back pain, 2393
    after lumbar disk surgery, 2330
    postoperative, 524
        preoperative teaching about, 494c
    for pressure reduction, 210
    prone (on abdomen), 196, 197f
    in rehabilitation for impaired physical mobility, 196, 197f, 198
    side-lying (lateral), 196, 197f
    of spinal cord injury patients, 2258
    in stroke recovery, 2216–2217, 2217f, 2228
    supine (dorsal), 196, 197f
    after thoracic surgery, 757–758, 765
    Trendelenburg, 519f, 520
    with venous thrombosis, 1009–1010
Position (postural) sense, 2133, 2150
    definition of, 2129
Positive end-expiratory pressure, 743f
    in acute respiratory distress syndrome, 658
    definition of, 723
    and intracranial pressure, 2178
    with oxygen therapy, 724–725
Positive feedback
    in control of steady state, 100
    definition of, 91
Positron emission tomography, 2130, 2152–2153, 2162
    of brain tumor, 2304
    in cancer detection, 391t
    in cardiac patient, 813
    in laryngeal cancer, 610
    of lung, 581
    nursing interventions in, 813
Postanesthetic recovery unit, patient transfer to, nursing management of, 482c
Postanesthia care unit, 524–531
    admission to, 524–525
        anesthesia provider-to-nurse report for, 525
    care record for, 529, 530f
    definition of, 524
    discharge from, 529
    environment of, 524
    nursing management in, 525–529
    patient transfer to, 524–525
    phase I, 524
        definition of, 524
    phase II, 524
        definition of, 524
    phase III, 524
        definition of, 524
Posterior chamber, of eye, 2045, 2045f
    definition of, 2043
Posterior cruciate ligament, 2429f
    injury to, 2430
Postinfarction syndrome, after renal artery embolization, 1564
Postmastectomy pain syndrome, 261c
Postoperative phase
    acute respiratory failure in, 656
    with adenoidectomy, 600
    continuing care in, 530–531, 548
    definition of, 481
    expected outcomes in, 548

gerontologic considerations in, 528–529
hospitalised patient in
  nursing interventions for, 534–548
  respiratory complications in, prevention of, 534–535
hospitalized patient in, 531–532
  nursing diagnoses for, 533–534
  nursing interventions for, 531–532, 532c
  nursing management of, 531–532
  nursing process and, 532–548
  planning and goals for, 534
  potential complications in, 532, 533f
in neck dissection, 1154
nursing activities in, 482c–483c, 484
nursing diagnoses related to, 478–479
nursing interventions in, 478–479
nursing outcomes for, 478–479
potential complications in, 544–546
  in older persons, 546–548
  with tonsillectomy, 600
Postpolio syndrome, 2331
Post-streptococcal glomerulonephritis, 1517, 1517f
Post-traumatic seizures, 2249
Posttraumatic stress disorder, 116–118
  acute, 117
  chronic, 117
  definition of, 112
  delayed, 117
  indicators of, 119c
  nursing implications of, 117
  as psychiatric emergency, 2554
  resources and websites on, 126
Postural drainage, 731, 732f
  in bronchiectasis, 709
  definition of, 723
Postural (orthostatic) hypotension, 799
  definition of, 781
Posture
  assessment of, 75, 2347, 2347f
  in Parkinson's disease, 2313
  proper, 2394c, 2395–2397, 2395f, 2396f
Potassium
  in body fluids, 302t, 303
  deficit, 316t, 321–323
    manifestations of, 1516t
    in renal disorders, 1516t
  dietary, 322
  excess, 316t, 323–325
    in acute renal failure, 1524
      treatment of, 1525
    manifestations of, 1516t
    in renal disorders, 1516t
  excretion of, regulation of, 1497
  imbalances of, in renal disorders, 1516t
  intravenous, administration of, 322, 323, 325
  replacement, for hypokalemia, 322, 323
  restriction of, in acute renal failure, 1526
  serum
    in cardiac patient, 807t
    diuretics and, 321
    in hyperkalemia, 316t
    in hypokalemia, 316t
    in hypovolemia, 309
    laboratory values for, 310t
    reference range for, 321
  significance of, 321
  supplements, precautions with, 323
  urinary, laboratory values for, 310t
Potassium iodide, for hyperthyroidism, 1462
Potassium-sparing diuretics, 953, 954t
  for hypertension, 1026t
Poverty, and disability, 175
Povidone-iodine (Betadine), for burns, 2017

Powders, for wound care, 1949
Powerlessness
  in cardiomyopathy, 932
  in heart failure, 962
  nursing interventions for, with vertigo, 2118c
Power of attorney, durable medical, 457c
Power of attorney for health care, 33
PPD test. *See* Mantoux test; Purified protein derivative test
PPE. *See* Personal protective equipment
PP interval
  definition of, 823
  on ECG, 827, 827f
PPN. *See* Peripheral parenteral nutrition
PPS. *See* Prospective Payment System; Prospective payment system
Pralidoxime, for nerve agent exposure, 2571
Pramipexole (Mirapex), for Parkinson's disease, 2314
Pramlintide (Symlin), 1402
Pravastatin (Pravachol), 986
Prazosin hydrochloride (Minipress), for hypertension, 1028t
Preadmission testing, 481, 482c
Prealbumin, serum, 78–80, 79t
Precautions
  Airborne, 2482, 2483c
  Contact, 2482, 2483c
  Droplet, 2482, 2483c
  isolation, 2480–2482
  Standard, 1818–1819, 1820c–1821c, 2475, 2480–2482, 2483c
  Transmission-Based, 2475, 2480, 2482
Preconception health care, 1652–1653
Precordium, 801f
  examination of, 801, 801f
Prediabetes, 1378, 1379t–1380t
  definition of, 1376
Predisposition testing, 152t, 153
  definition of, 140
Prednisolone, 1485t
  for asthma, 713t
  for rheumatic diseases, 1896t
Prednisone, 1485t
  for asthma, 713t
  for idiopathic thrombocytopenic purpura, 1088
  and immune system, 1797t
  for rheumatic diseases, 1896t
Prednisone (Deltasone), interactions with anesthetics, 490t
Preferred provider organizations, 9–10
Pregnancy
  and breast cancer, 1734
  ectopic. *See* Ectopic pregnancy
  and epilepsy, 2193
  and HIV transmission, 1816
  multiple gestation. *See* Multiple gestation
Pregnancy loss, chromosomal abnormalities and, 148–149
Prehypertension, 1021, 1021t
  definition of, 1021
Preload, 786, 869, 945, 946f
  definition of, 781, 945
Premature atrial complex, 831–832, 831f
Premature ejaculation, 1746–1750
Premature junctional complex, 833–834
Premature ventricular complex, 835, 836f
Premenstrual syndrome, 1636–1638, 1638c
Premolars, 1150f
Prenatal screening, 149, 150t
  definition of, 140
Preoperative checklist, 497, 497f, 498f
Preoperative phase
  definition of, 481

expected outcomes in, 499, 499c
family needs in, 499
immediate preoperative nursing interventions in, 496–499
in neck dissection, 1154
nursing activities in, 481–483, 482c–483c
nursing interventions in, 492–499
patient transport to presurgical area in, 497–499
special considerations in, 491–492
Prepuce, excision of. *See* Circumcision
Presbycusis, 237
  definition of, 225, 2093
Presbyopia, 236, 2051t
  definition of, 225
Pressure, for control of hemorrhage, 2526–2527, 2527f
Pressure activated air buffer, 1176f
Pressure garments, for burn patient, 2032, 2032f
Pressure support ventilation, 743f, 744
  definition of, 723
Pressure ulcer(s)
  areas susceptible to, 208, 208f
  assessment for, 208–210
  casts and, 2357, 2360
  débridement of, 214
  definition of, 190
  gerontologic considerations with, 209
  healing of, 213–214
  hip fracture and, 2449, 2457c
  immobility and, 208
  nursing diagnoses related to, 210
  nursing interventions for, 210–214
  orthoses and, 207
  pain caused by, in patient in cast, 2357
  pressure-relieving devices for, 210–212
  recurrence of, prevention of, 214
  in rehabilitation, 207–215
  risk factors for, 208–209, 209, 210c
  severity/stages of, assessment of, 209–210, 211c
  traction and, 2370
Presymptomatic genetic testing, 150t, 152
Presymptomatic testing, 151t–152t
  definition of, 140
Prevastatin (Pravachol), 865t
Prevention. *See also* Health promotion
  activities for, over life cycle, 59t
  in community-based nursing, 16–17
  for people with disabilities, 179c, 183–184
  primary, 16, 861
    definition of, 859
  secondary, 16–17, 861
    definition of, 859
Preventive ethics, 33
Preventive health care. *See also* Health promotion; Patient teaching
  by community-based nurses, 17
Priapism, 1775
  definition of, 1740
  in sickle cell anemia, 1059
Prilocaine, for postoperative analgesia, in thoracic surgical patient, 766
Primary health care, 11
Primary hypertension. *See* Hypertension, primary
Primary infection, definition of, 1815
Primary intention healing, 104
  definition of, 91
Primary nursing, 11
Prime mover (muscle), 2342
Primidone (Mysoline)
  adverse effects and side effects of, 2194t
  toxic effects of, 2194t

Primidone, therapeutic blood levels of, 2601t
PR interval
    definition of, 823
    on ECG, 826, 827f
Prion, 2276
Privacy, in emergency treatment, 2518
PRK. See Photorefractive keratectomy
Proarrhythmic, definition of, 823
Probenecid (Benemid), for gout, 1918, 1919t
Probucol, 986
Procainamide (Pronestyl), 830t
    for ventricular tachycardia, 836
Procaine (Novocain), contraindications to, in myasthenia gravis, 2286
Procaine (Novocaine), 514t
Procarbazine, in cancer treatment, 399t
Prochlorperazine (Compazine), postoperative use of, 528
Proctoscopy, 1137
Progesterone, 1615
    definition of, 1613
    for infertility treatment, 1651c
Progestin, in cancer treatment, 399t
Progressive multifocal leukoencephalopathy
    definition of, 1815
    in HIV-infected (AIDS) patients, 1833
Progressive muscle relaxation, 107
Prokinetic agents, for gastroesophageal reflux disease, 1166
Prolactin, 1446
Prolactinomas, 2302–2303
Prolapse
    definition of, 915
    mitral valve, 915–917
Proliferation inhibitor factor, action of, 1791t
Proliferation stage, of immune response, 1787, 1789f
Proliferative phase, of menstrual cycle, 1616
    definition of, 1613
Promethazine (Phenergan), postoperative use of, 528
Pronation, 199c, 2343c
    definition of, 198c
Prone position, 196, 197c
Propafenone (Rhythmol), 830t
    for atrial fibrillation, 833
    for atrial flutter, 832
    mechanism of action of, 784–785
Propane, abuse/overdose, emergency management of, 2546t
*Propionibacterium acnes*, 1954
Propofol (Diprivan)
    effect on metabolic demands, 2173
    for intravenous anesthesia, 513t
Proportional assist ventilation, 744
    definition of, 723
    and respiratory weaning, 752
Propoxyphene, pharmacology of, 283t
Propranolol (Inderal)
    for esophageal varices, 1300, 1304t
    for hypertension, 1027t
    long-acting (inderal LA), for hypertension, 1027t
Propranolol (Inderal, Innopran), 830t
Propranolol, therapeutic blood levels of, 2601t
Proprioception, 2133, 2150
Proptosis, 2073
    definition of, 2043
Propylthiouracil, 1460–1461, 1462t
Propylthiouracil (Propacil, PTU), and immune system, 1797t
PROs. See Peer review organizations
Prosorba, for rheumatoid arthritis, 1909
Prospective payment system, 8
Prostaglandin(s)

in allergic reaction, 1858t, 1859
definition of, 259, 1856, 1887
in inflammation, 103, 1888
in pain transmission, 264
secretion of, 1499
vascular effects of, 978
Prostaglandin analogs, for glaucoma, 2057, 2058t
Prostate cancer, 234, 1752–1761
    assessment in, 1753–1754
    chemotherapy for, 1760–1761
    clinical manifestations of, 1753
    complementary and alternative therapies for, 1761
    complications of, 1754, 1760c
    definition of, 1740
    detection of, 390t
    diagnosis of, 1753–1754
    epidemiology of, 1752–1753
    familial occurrence of, 386
    hormone therapy for, 1754–1760
    medical management of, 1754–1761
    metastases, 1761
    nursing care plan for, 1755c–1760c
    prevention of, 1761
    radiation therapy for, 1754
    risk factors for, 1753
    screening for, 1744
    surgery for, 1754
Prostatectomy, 1754, 1761–1769
    complications of, 1764, 1765, 1766–1767
    laparoscopic radical, 1754, 1762t, 1763
    nursing process with, 1764–1769, 1768c
    perineal, 1761–1763, 1762t, 1763f
    retropubic, 1762t, 1763, 1763f
    suprapubic, 1761, 1762t, 1763f
Prostate fluid analysis, 1744
Prostate gland, 1741, 1741f
    definition of, 1740
    disorders of, 1750–1769
    enlarged, 1751–1752. See also Benign prostatic hyperplasia
    inflammation of. See Prostatitis
Prostate-specific antigen, 1753
    definition of, 1740
    laboratory evaluation of, 1744
Prostate-specific antigen (PSA), 1504
Prostate tissue analysis, 1744
Prostatism, definition of, 1740
Prostatitis, 1570, 1750–1751
    definition of, 1570, 1740
Prostheses
    for amputation, 2468
    for hip replacement, 2373–2374, 2373f
    and mobility, 207
Prosthetic heart valves, 923–924, 923f, 924f
    mechanical, 924
    tissue (biologic), 924
Protease inhibitors
    definition of, 1815
    for HIV infection, 1826–1828, 1827t–1828t
Protein(s)
    for burn patient, 2025
    deficiency of
        manifestations of, 1516t
        and pressure ulcers, 208
        in renal disorders, 1516t
    dietary, and pressure ulcer healing, 212–213, 213t
    digestion of, 1125
        enzymes and secretions for, 1123t
    imbalances of, in renal disorders, 1516t
    and immune system function, 1795
    metabolism of, liver in, 1286
    in peripheral parenteral nutrition, 1194

restriction of
    in acute glomerulonephritis, 1518
    in acute renal failure, 1526
    serum, 78–80, 1290t
        electrophoresis of, 1290t
    in wound healing, 487t
Protein A immunoadsorption column (Prosorba Column), for rheumatoid arthritis, 1909
Proteinate, in body fluids, 302t
Protein C
    activated, resistance, 1095, 1099, 1099t
    deficiency, 1095, 1099, 1099t
    recombinant human activated, for septic shock, 374
Protein S deficiency, 1095, 1099, 1099t
Proteinuria, 1496, 1503, 1503t
    in acute glomerulonephritis, 1518
    causes of, 1506
    clinical significance of, 1506
    definition of, 1493
    detection of, 1505
    in nephrotic syndrome, 1521
Proteomics, of ovarian cancer, 1691
*Proteus*
    and osteomyelitis, 2413
    pneumonia, 629, 633
Prothrombin time, 1290t
    laboratory values for, 2578
Prothrombin time (PT), in cardiac patient, 808f
Proton pump inhibitors
    for gastritis, 1206t
    for gastroesophageal reflux disease, 1166
Proto-oncogenes, 385
Protraction, 2343c
Protriptyline (Triptil), for sleep apnea, 605
Provirus
    definition of, 1815
    of HIV, 1821, 1822
Provocative testing, for allergic disorders, 1865
Proximal convoluted tubule, 1495f
Proxy directive, 457
Pruritus, 1933, 1951–1952
    causes of, 1951, 1951t
    in chronic renal failure, 1528
    gerontologic considerations in, 1951
    in Hodgkin's disease, 1080
    in liver disease, 1308
    medical management of, 1951–1952
    medications causing, 1951
    nursing management of, 1952
    opioid-induced, 282
    pathophysiology of, 1951
    perianal, 1952
    perineal, 1627, 1952
    pharmacologic therapy for, 1952
    in polycythemia vera, 1065–1066
    in systemic disease, 1929t
    systemic disorders associated with, 1951, 1951t
    vulvar, 1686
PSA. See Prostate-specific antigen
PSA test. See Prostate-specific antigen test
PSDA. See Patient Self-Determination Act
Pseudo-Cushing's syndrome, HIV treatment and, 1826
Pseudoephedrine hydrochloride, for allergic rhinitis, 1872t
Pseudofolliculitis barbae, 1957
Pseudohyperkalemia, 323
*Pseudomonas*, and osteomyelitis, 2413
*Pseudomonas aeruginosa*, pneumonia, 629–634, 632t

# INDEX

medical management of, 636–638
risk factors for, 637c
Pseudopodia, 1864
Psilocybin, abuse/overdose, emergency management of, 2546t–2547t
Psoriasis, 1965–1968
  and arthritis, 1966
  assessment of, 1966
  clinical manifestations of, 1965–1966, 1965f
  complications of, 1966
  cutaneous manifestations of, 1929t
  diagnosis of, 1966
  epidemiology of, 1965
  erythrodermic, 1966
  guttate, 1965
  home and community-based care for, 1969–1970, 1970c
  intralesional agents for, 1966t, 1967
  laser therapy for, 1968
  medical management of, 1966–1968, 1966t
  nursing process for, 1968–1970
  pathophysiology of, 1965
  pharmacologic therapy for, 1966–1968, 1966t
  photochemotherapy for, 1966t, 1967–1968
  systemic therapy for, 1966t, 1967
  topical therapy for, 1966–1967, 1966t
Psoriatic arthritis, 1917, 1966
  nursing interventions for, 1969
PSV. *See* Pressure support ventilation
Psychedelic-type drugs, abuse/overdose, emergency management of, 2546t–2547t
Psychiatric disability, people with, interacting and communicating with, 181c
Psychiatric emergencies, 2553–2555
  depression as, 2554–2555
  overactive patients as, 2553
  posttraumatic stress disorder as, 2554
  suicidality as, 2555
  underactive patients as, 2554–2555
  violent patient as, 2553–2554
Psychobiology, 113
Psychological abuse. *See* Abuse
Psychological support
  in acute renal failure, 1526–1527
  in heart failure, 965
  for hospitalized dialysis patient, 1552
  for kidney transplant recipient, 1562
  in lung cancer, 673
Psychoneuroimmunology, 97, 113, 1798
  and immune system function, 1798
  nursing research on, 1798
Psychosis, in Huntington's disease, 2319–2320
Psychosocial assessment, of cardiac surgical patient, 894–895
Psychosocial domain, definition of, 46c
Psychosocial status
  of cancer patient, 426
  of surgical patient, 489–490
Psychosocial support, in gastric cancer, 1222
PT. *See* Prothrombin time
PTH. *See* Parathyroid hormone
PTK. *See* Phototherapeutic keratectomy
Ptosis, 2048
  definition of, 2043
  in myasthenia gravis, 2288
  myasthenia gravis and, 2285
PTSD. *See* Posttraumatic stress disorder
PTT. *See* Partial thromboplastin time
PTU. *See* Propylthiouracil
Ptyalin, 1123
  source and digestive action of, 1123t
Puberty, 1615
Pubic lice, 1962–1963
Public health nurses, 17

Public health nursing. *See* Community health-public health nursing
Pull-up exercises, 204
Pulmocare, 1182
Pulmonary agents, as terrorism threat, 2569t, 2571
Pulmonary angiography
  with pulmonary embolism, 663
  in respiratory disease, 580
Pulmonary artery catheter, 818–820, 818f, 819f
Pulmonary artery pressure monitoring, 818–820, 818f
Pulmonary capillary wedge pressure, 978
Pulmonary complications, hip fracture and, 2448, 2455c
Pulmonary contusion, in trauma patient, 677–678
Pulmonary disorders, chest pain with, 791t
Pulmonary edema, 557, 655, 964–965
  in acute glomerulonephritis, 1518
  assessment findings in, 576t
  burns and, 2030
  in chronic renal failure, 1527
  definition of, 625, 655, 945
  flash, 655
  noncardiogenic, 361
  re-expansion, 655
  after thoracic surgery, 769
Pulmonary effusion(s), in Hodgkin's disease, 1080
Pulmonary embolism, 662–667, 967, 968f
  cerebral metastases and, 2307
  chest pain with, 791t
  clinical manifestations of, 662–663
  complications of, monitoring for, 667
  continuing care for, 667
  definition of, 625, 662
  diagnosis of, 663
  emergency treatment of, 664–665
  fracture and, 2438
  medical management of, 664–666
  nursing management of, 666–667
  pathophysiology of, 662
  patient teaching about, 667
  pharmacologic therapy for, 665
  postoperative, risk factors for, 544c
  potential for, assessment of, 666
  prevention of, 663, 664c
  recurrent, prevention of, 663, 664c
  risk factors for, 662, 662c, 1004c
  spinal cord injury and, 2259
  surgical management of, 665–666
    postoperative care for, 667
Pulmonary fibrosis, 557
  chemotherapy-related, 401
Pulmonary function, in facial reconstructive surgery, 1989
Pulmonary function tests, 578–579, 578t
  in chronic obstructive pulmonary disease, 689
  with pulmonary hypertension, 660
Pulmonary hypertension, 659–660
  causes of, 659c
  in chronic obstructive pulmonary disease, 699, 708c
    nursing interventions for, 699
  due to known cause, 659, 659c
  medical management of, 660
  primary (idiopathic), 659
  in sickle cell anemia, 1057
Pulmonary perfusion, 557–558. *See also* Ventilation-perfusion ratios
  definition of, 553
Pulmonary rehabilitation, 192
  applications of, 694–695

  in chronic obstructive pulmonary disease, 694–695
  nursing management of, 695–696
  patient teaching in, 695
Pulmonary system
  acute renal failure and, 1526
  age-related changes in, 1795t
  chronic renal failure and, 1528c
Pulmonary vascular resistance, 787
  definition of, 781
Pulmonic area, examination of, 801, 801f
Pulmonic valve, 782f, 783, 915
  definition of, 915
Pulpitis, suppurative, 1145
Pulse(s)
  absent, 800
  arterial, assessment of, 800
  bounding, 800
  collapsing, 800
  configuration (contour) of, assessment of, 800
  diminished, 800
  in heart failure, 951
  normal, 800
  peripheral, assessment of, 980, 980f
  quality (amplitude) of, assessment of, 800
  rate, assessment of, 799–800
  rhythm of, assessment of, 800
  in thrombangiitis obliterans, 996
  vessel quality and, 800
  water hammer, 800
Pulse-dye laser, for skin lesions, 1992
Pulseless electrical activity, 837, 838, 969
  definition of, 945
Pulse oximetry, 579, 579f, 980f
  in atelectasis, 627
  in chronic obstructive pulmonary disease, 698
  postoperative, 534
  in thoracic surgical patient, 765
Pulse pressure, 799
  assessment of, 799
PULSES profile, 193
Pulsus paradoxus, 968
  definition of, 945
  in hemodialysis, 1551
Pupil(s)
  assessment of, in unconscious patient, 2165t
  brain injury and, 2244
  reactivity of, 2048
    brain injury and, 2244
  size of
    brain injury and, 2244
    device for measuring, nursing research on, 2163
Pupillary block glaucoma. *See* Glaucoma, angle-closure
Purkinje cells, 783–784
Purkinje fibers, 784, 824, 824f
Purpura, 1929t
Purulent, definition of, 625
Push-up exercises, 203
Pustule, 1937c
PUVA. *See* Psoralen medication combined with ultraviolet-A
  for psoriasis, 1966t, 1967–1968, 1969
P wave
  definition of, 823
  on ECG, 826, 827f
Pyelography, 1631
Pyelolithotomy, for urolithiasis, 1593
Pyelonephritis, 1571
  acute, 1577–1578
  chronic, 1578

Pyelonephritis (*continued*)
  definition of, 1570
  signs and symptoms of, 1572
  treatment of, 1574
Pyloric obstruction, in peptic ulcer disease, 1216
Pyloric sphincter, 1121
Pyloroplasty, definition of, 1204
Pylorus, definition of, 1204
Pyodermas, 1956–1964
  definition of, 1945
Pyramidal tract, 2140
Pyrazinamide, for tuberculosis, 647–648, 647t
  adverse effects and side effects of, 647t
  dosage and administration of, 647t
  drug interactions with, 647t
Pyridostigmine bromide (Mestinon), for myasthenia gravis, 2286
Pyridoxine, deficiency of, in liver disease, 1307
Pyrogens, endogenous, 103
Pyrosis
  in achalasia, 1162
  definition of, 1142, 1204
Pyuria
  definition of, 1493, 1570
  detection of, 1506
  in urinary tract infections, 1574

# Q

Qi gong, 134
QRS complex
  definition of, 823
  on ECG, 826, 827f
QT interval
  definition of, 823
  on ECG, 826, 827f
Quad cane, 205–207
Quadriceps-setting exercises, 203
Quadrigeminy, 835, 836f
Quality, of sound, 77
Quality assurance, 8–9
Quality of care, 8–9
Quality of life
  after breast cancer, 1734–1735
  chronic illness and, 168–169
  in hospitalized patients with COPD, nursing research on, 701
  thyroid cancer and, nursing research on, 1469
  in women with irritable bowel syndrome, nursing research on, 1239
QuantiFERON-TB Gold test, 646
Queckenstedt's test, 2156
Quinacrine hydrochloride (Atabrine), for *Giardia lamblia* infestation, 1806
Quinapril (Accupril), 952–953, 952t
  for hypertension, 1029t
Quinethazone (Hydromox), 954t
Quinidine, 830t
  mechanism of action of, 784–785
  therapeutic blood levels of, 2601t
Quinolones
  for sinusitis, 595, 596
  for tuberculosis, 647
Q wave, on ECG, 826, 827f, 875, 875f

# R

RA. *See* Rheumatoid arthritis
Rabeprazole (Aciphex), 1206t
  for gastroesophageal reflux disease, 1166
Rabies virus
  incubation period of, 2477t
  transmission of, 2477t

rad (unit), 2572
Radial deviation, 200c
Radial forearm free flap, for cancer of oral cavity, 1149
Radial nerve, function of, assessment of, 2346c
Radiation
  alpha particles in, 2572
  beta-, 2572
  gamma-, 2572
  half-life of, 2572
  heat loss by, 1931
  injury caused by, 102
  ionizing, effects on DNA, 394
  safety considerations for, 1695
  types of, 2572
Radiation exposure
  acute radiation syndrome caused by, 2573–2574, 2573t
  and breast cancer, 1713
  and cancer, 386
  contamination in, 2572
  decontamination after, 2572–2573
  dermatologic effects of, 2574
  detection of, 2572
  external, 2572
  factors affecting, 2572
  gastrointestinal effects of, 2573
  hematopoietic effects of, 2573
  incorporation of radioactive material in, 2572
  measurement of, 2572
  neurologic effects of, 2573–2574
  phases of, 2573, 2573t
  secondary injury from, 2574
  sources of, 2572
  survival after, 2574
  survivors
    improbable, 2574
    possible, 2574
    probable, 2574
  as terrorism threat, 2571–2574
  and thyroid cancer, 1467, 1468c
  triage after, 2574
Radiation therapy
  adverse effects and side effects of, 1696, 1726
  for bladder cancer, 1597
  for breast cancer, 1726
  for cancer, 394–397
  for cervical cancer, 1684
  definition of, 381
  dosage of, 395
  external, 395, 1694
  in gynecologic malignancy, 395, 1694–1696
  and immune system function, 1796
  internal (intracavitary), 395, 1685f, 1694–1695
  intraoperative, 1694
    for beast cancer, 1726
  for Kaposi's sarcoma, 1836
  for laryngeal cancer, 612
  for liver cancer, 1334
  for lung cancer, 672
  for metastatic bone disease, 2419
  in multiple myeloma, 1083
  nursing interventions for, 1695–1696
  particle-beam, 395
  for prostate cancer, 1754
  for skin cancer, 1980
  skin integrity in, nursing care plan for, 405c
  toxicity of, 395–396
Radiculopathy, 1920, 2392
  definition of, 2301, 2392
  in degenerative disk disease, 2324–2325

Radioactive iodine therapy, 1460
Radioactive iodine uptake test, 1451
Radioallergosorbent test, for allergic disorders, 1865
Radiography
  abdominal, 1290t
    in biliary/pancreatic disease, 1349
  for low back pain, 2393c
  of musculoskeletal system, 2350
  in rheumatic diseases, 1891
Radioimmunoassay, 1444
  definition of, 1440
Radioimmunoconjugates, in cancer detection, 391t
Radioimmunodetection, 418
Radioisotope(s), 12
  definition of, 781
Radionuclide imaging, in biliary/pancreatic disease, 1350
Radius
  head of, fracture of, 2443
  shaft of, fracture of, 2443
Radon gas, 386
  and lung cancer, 671
Rales. *See* Crackles
Raloxifene (Evista)
  in breast cancer prevention, 1714–1715
  for osteoporosis, 2409
Ramipril (Altace), 952–953, 952t
  for hypertension, 1029t
Rancho Los Amigos Scale, of cognitive function, 2246, 2247t–2248t
Range of motion
  assessment of, 2347–2348
  terminology for, 198c
Range-of-motion exercises, 196–198 198c, 199c–201c
  postoperative, with amputation, 2466
  terminology used in, 198c
Ranitidine (Zantac), 1206t, 1859
  for gastroesophageal reflux disease, 1166
RANKL, 2340
Rape, 1622. *See also* Sexual assault
  definition of, 2551
Rape trauma syndrome, 2551
Rapidly progressive glomerulonephritis, 1518
Rapid plasma reagin circle card test, for syphilis, 2506
Rash, 1933
RAST. *See* Radioallergosorbent test
Rationality, in critical thinking, 25
Raynaud's disease, 1003–1004
Raynaud's phenomenon, 1003, 1920
RBC. *See* Red blood cell(s)
Reaction time, in older persons, 236
Reactive arthritis, 1917
Reappraisal, cognitive, of stress, 94
Rebound hypertension, 1031
  definition of, 1021
Rebound hypoglycemia, in parenteral nutrition discontinuation, 1196, 1197t
Rebound tenderness, of abdomen, 1129, 1241, 1241f
Recent Life Changes Questionnaire, 93
Receptive aphasia
  definition of, 2206
  stroke and, 2209
Receptor(s)
  direct, 2130
  excitatory, 2130
  indirect, 2130
  inhibitory, 2130
  inotropic, 2130
Recessive, definition of, 140, 145

# INDEX

Recognition stage, of immune response, 1787, 1789f
Recombinant DNA, 1793
Reconstructive surgery, 484
  for breasts, 1731–1733, 1732f, 1733f
  of esophagus, 1167, 1168f
  facial, 1989–1990
  in neck dissection, 1153
  for rheumatoid arthritis, 1909
Rectal sensory functioning, assessment of, 1138
Rectocele, 1505, 1624, 1674–1675, 1674f
  definition of, 1613, 1661
Rectum, 1121, 1122f
  cancer of. See Colorectal cancer
  examination of, 1129
  palpation of, in women, 1626–1627
Red blood cell(s), 1038f, 1039–1041, 1040f
  definition of, 1036
  destruction of, 1040–1041, 1055
    increased, 1045t, 1046
  functions of, 1037, 1037t
  in immune response, 1793
  laboratory values for, 2578
  life span of, 1040
  loss of, 1045t, 1046
  nucleated, 1039
    definition of, 1036
  packed
    long-term therapy with, complications of, 1111, 1111t
    transfusion of, 1107c
  production of
    decreased, 1045t, 1046
    regulation of, 1499
  in sickle cell disease, 1055–1056, 1055f
  tagging of, in gastrointestinal assessment, 1133
  for transfusion, 1103t
  transfusion, for sickle cell anemia, 1057–1058
Red blood cell count, in rheumatic diseases, 1893t
Red blood cell indices, laboratory values for, 2578–2579
Red cell distribution width, 1047
Red pulp, of spleen, 1784
Reed-Sternberg cell, 1080
Reference ranges
  abbreviations used in, 2577
  for cerebrospinal fluid, 2600t
  for drug levels, 2601t
  for hematology, 2578t–2580t
  for immunodiagnostic tests, 2594t–2595t
  miscellaneous, 2601t
  for serum, plasma, and whole blood chemistries, 2581t–2593t
  for urine chemistry, 2596t–2599t
Referrals, in community, 19
Referred pain
  abdominal, 1126, 1126f
  definition of, 259
Reflex(es), 2141
  abdominal, 2147, 2148–2149
  ankle, 2147, 2148, 2149f
  biceps, 2147, 2148, 2149f
  brachioradialis, 2147, 2148
  corneal, 2148–2149
    assessment of, in unconscious patient, 2165t
  cough, absent, and aspiration, 681
  cremasteric, 2148–2149
  cutaneous, 2147
  deep tendon, 2147
    assessment of, in unconscious patient, 2165t

definition of, 2129
  examination of, 2147–2150, 2149f, 2150c
  gag, 2148–2149
    absent, and aspiration, 681
  glottic, absent, and aspiration, 681
  grading, 2148
  laryngeal, absent, and aspiration, 681
  patellar, 2147, 2148, 2149f
  pathologic, assessment of, in unconscious patient, 2165t
  perianal, 2148–2149
  plantar, 2147, 2148–2149
  superficial, 2147, 2148–2149
  swallowing, 2148–2149
  triceps, 2147, 2148, 2149f
Reflex incontinence, 215
Reflexology, 134
Reflex sympathetic dystrophy, 261c. See also Complex regional pain syndrome
Reflux esophagitis, chest pain caused by, assessment of, 792t
Refraction, definition of, 2043
Refractive surgeries, 2065–2067
Refractory period, in cardiac conduction, 785
Refusal to provide care, 32
Regional anesthesia, agents for, 514t
Regional enteritis, 1247t. See also Inflammatory bowel disease
  clinical manifestations of, 1247t, 1248
  complications of, 1247t, 1248
  diagnosis of, 1247t, 1248
  medical management of, 1247t
  pathophysiology of, 1247t, 1248
Registered nurse first assistant, 505
Regranex gel, 1948
Regurgitation
  definition of, 915
  valvular, 915
Rehabilitation, 189–222
  activities of daily living in, 194, 194c
  and altered elimination patterns, 215–218
  for amputation, 2462
  assessment of functional abilities in, 193
  aural, 2120–2123
  cardiac, 877–879
  cognitive, 2245
  complementary therapies in, 219
  continuing care in, 221–222
  definition of, 190
  ethical considerations in, 190, 190c
  family involvement in, 219, 221
  and fatigue, 218–219
  goal of, 190
  home and community-based care in, 219–222, 220c–221c
  for impaired physical mobility, positioning in, 196, 197f, 198
  for knee injury, 2430
  mobility assistance in, 195–207
  positioning in, 198
  right to, 190, 190c
  sexuality issues in, 218
  skin integrity in, 207–215
  specialty programs for, 192–193
  in stroke recovery programs, 192
  and substance abuse, 192–193
  for traumatic brain injury, 192
Rehabilitation Act of 1973, 176
Rehabilitation team, 191–192
Rehydration therapy
  in diabetic ketoacidosis, 1414
  in diarrhea/diarrheal diseases, 2503
Reimbursement
  for health care, 8, 16
  for home health care, 17

Reinforcement
  definition of, 49
  and learning, 52
Reiter's syndrome, 1917
Relaxation
  with guided imagery, 107
  muscle, progressive, 107
  in pain management, 289
  techniques for, teaching, 105–107
Relaxation exercises, 219
  for low back pain, 2394
Religion, 122–123
  and diet, 133, 133c
  and end-of-life care, 461–462
  of surgical patient, 495
rem (unit), 2572
Remifentanil (Ultiva), for intravenous anesthesia, 512t
Remodeling, 2339
  of bone, 2405
  definition of, 2337
  in fracture healing, 2340
Remorse, in family members of emergency patient, 2519
REM sleep. See Rapid eye movement sleep
Renal angiography, 1509
Renal artery, 1494
  embolization of, in renal cancer treatment, 1564
  injury to, 1565–1566
Renal cell carcinoma, 1563–1565
Renal clearance, 1499
  definition of, 1493
Renal colic, in renal trauma, 1565
Renal concentration tests, 1507, 1507t
Renal cortex, 1494, 1494f
Renal failure, 1521–1537
  acute, 1522–1527
    assessment of, 1523–1524
    burns and, 2014c
    causes of, 1522–1523, 1522c
    classification of, 1522–1523, 1522c, 1523t
    clinical manifestations of, 1523, 1523t
    diagnosis of, 152301524
    diuresis period of, 1523
    gerontologic considerations in, 1527
    initiation period of, 1523
    intrarenal causes of, 1522c, 1523, 1523t
    medical management of, 1525–1526
    nonoliguric form of, 1523
    nursing management of, 1526–1527
    oliguria period of, 1523
    pahses of, 1523
    pathophysiology of, 1522–1523, 1522c, 1523t
    phases of, 1523
    postrenal causes of, 1522c, 1523, 1523t
    prerenal causes of, 1522, 1522c, 1523t
    prevention of, 1524–1525, 1524c
    recovery period of, 1523
  in shock, 362
  after cardiac surgery, 893t
  chronic, 1527–1537. See also End-stage renal disease
    assessment of, 1528–1529
    causes of, 1527
    clinical manifestations of, 1527–1528, 1528c
    complications of, 1529, 1535c–1537c
    continuing care in, 1531
    diagnosis of, 1528–1529
    epidemiology of, 1527
    nursing diagnoses related to, 1530, 1532c–1537c

Renal failure, chronic (*continued*)
    nursing interventions in, 1532c–1537c
    pathophysiology of, 1527
    stages of, 1527, 1527c
    hypermagnesemia in, 330
    hypocalcemia in, 325
    and immune system function, 1796
    osteomalacia and, 2411
    and wound healing, 541t
Renal function, postoperative, in cardiac surgical patient, 910c
Renal function tests, 1507, 1507t
Renal glycosuria, 1496
    definition of, 1493
Renal medulla, 1494, 1494f
Renal osteodystrophy, in chronic renal failure, 1529
Renal parenchyma, 1494
Renal pedicle injury, 1565–1566, 1565f
Renal pelvis, 1494
    inflammation of. *See* Pyelonephritis
Renal perfusion, postoperative, in cardiac surgical patient, 910c
Renal surgery. *See* Kidney surgery; Nephrostomy
Renal vein(s), injury to, 1565–1566
Renin-angiotensin-aldosterone system, in fluid and electrolyte balance, 306
Renin-angiotensin system, 1497, 1498f
    in blood pressure regulation, 358
Repaglinide (Prandin), 1400t, 1401
Repolarization, 784, 784f, 824
    definition of, 781, 823
    on ECG, 826, 827f
Reproduction, definition of, 46c
Reproductive history, in cardiovascular disease, 797
Reproductive system. *See also* Female reproductive system; Male reproductive system
    age-related changes in, 231t, 233
    chemotherapy and, 402
    chronic renal failure and, 1528c
RES. *See* Reticuloendothelial system
Research. *See also* Nursing research
    and critical thinking, 26–27
    nurses' role in, 10–11
Reserpine (Serpasil), for hypertension, 1027t
Reservoir, 2478
    definition of, 2475
    of infection, 2475
Residual gastric content, measurement of, in tube feedings, 1183–1184
Residual limb shaping, 2464, 2465f, 2466f, 2467
Residual urine, 1500, 1570, 1581
Residual volume, 558t
Resistance (R)
    hemodynamic, 978
    peripheral vascular, 978
Resistance vessels, 976
Resistive exercises, 201t
Resonance, 76
Resorption, of bones, 2339
    definition of, 2337
Resource model, of preventive health behavior, 57
Respect for persons, ethical principle of, 28c
Respiration, 557
    Biot's, 570, 572t
    Cheyne-Stokes, 570, 572t
    definition of, 553
    expiratory phase of, 555
    inspiratory phase of, 555
    in myasthenia gravis, 2288

nursing interventions for, after neck dissection, 1156c
    spinal cord injury and, 2257
Respiratory acidosis, 336–337
    compensation in, 338, 338t
Respiratory alkalosis, 337–338
    compensation in, 338, 338t
Respiratory aspirate, and feeding tube placement, 1178
Respiratory depression
    intraoperative, 516
    opioid-related, 281–282
    postoperative, 533
        nursing interventions for, 534
Respiratory disease
    assessment findings in, 576t
    diagnostic evaluation in, 578–585
    psychosocial factors related to, 563, 565c
    risk factors for, 563, 563c
    signs and symptoms of, 563
Respiratory distress, after laryngectomy, nursing interventions for, 618
Respiratory drive, decreased, and acute respiratory failure, 655–656
Respiratory excursion, 570–572, 572f
Respiratory failure
    acute, 655–656
        burns and, 2013c, 2030
        definition of, 655
        postoperative, 656
    in bronchiectasis, 709
    in burn victim, 2002, 2013c
    chronic, 655
    in chronic obstructive pulmonary disease, 690–691, 708c
        nursing interventions for, 698–699
    in Guillain-Barré syndrome, 2290
    in HIV-infected (AIDS) patients, 1849
    in pneumonia, 638, 641
    with pulmonary contusion, 677–678
Respiratory function, 556–563. *See also* Respiratory depression
    in acutely ill patient, assessment of, 576–578
    in acute pancreatitis, 1360, 1362, 1366c
    assessment of, 552–585, 563–578
        postoperative, 532–533
        preoperative, 486–487
        in unconscious patient, 2165t
    after cardiac surgery, 897
    definition of, 46c
    after gallbladder surgery, 1356
    genetic influences in, 564
    in hypothyroidism, 1456c–1457c
    in liver disease, 1330c
    in myocardial infarction, 881c, 884
    in older persons, 562–563, 728
    psychosocial factors related to, 563, 565c
Respiratory rate, assessment of, 570, 572t
Respiratory syncytial virus
    incubation period of, 2477t
    transmission of, 2477t
Respiratory system
    age-related changes in, 231t, 232–233, 562, 728
    brain injury and, 2242t
    complications in
        from gastrointestinal intubation, 1181
        intraoperative, 516
        postoperative, 532–533, 534–535, 547
    in Guillain-Barré syndrome, 2290
    in HIV-infected (AIDS) patients, 1831, 1845, 1849
    immune dysfunction and, 1794c
    lower, 554–556. *See also* Lung(s)

    anatomy of, 554–556, 555f
    disorders of, 624–670
    physical examination of, 569–576
    spinal cord injury and, 2251, 2256
    upper, 553–554
        anatomy of, 555f
        disorders of, 589–601
            in elderly, 590
        infection of. *See also* Rhinitis; Sinusitis
            assessment of, 601–602
            complications of, 602, 603
            expected outcomes in, 603–604
            management of, 594c
            nursing care plan for, 601–604
            nursing diagnoses related to, 602
            nursing interventions for, 602–603
            patient teaching about, 603
            prevention of, 594c, 603
        obstruction of, during sleep, 604–605
        physical examination of, 568–569, 569f, 570f
Respiratory therapy. *See also* Airway, management of; Mechanical ventilation
    noninvasive, 723–725
    for spinal cord injury, 2254
Respiratory weaning, 751–754
    criteria for, 751–752
    definition of, 723
    methods for, 752–754
    nursing interventions during, 753c
    patient preparation for, 752
Response stage, of immune response, 1787–1788, 1789f
Rest
    in Alzheimer's disease, 246
    after cardiac surgery, 901
    in cardiovascular disease, assessment of, 796–797
    in cirrhosis, 1321
    in Cushing's syndrome, 1482
    in inflammatory bowel disease, 1252
    in multiple sclerosis, 2281
    in pneumonia, 640
Restlessness, postoperative, 533
Restorative proctocolectomy with ileal pouch anal anastomosis, 1250–1251, 1251f
Rest pain, 979
    definition of, 975
Restraints
    and injury, in older adults, 247
    management of, 2549
    precautions with, 2553, 2554
    use of, ethical considerations in, 31
Restricted zone, 506
    definition of, 503
Restrictive lung disease, definition of, 625
Resuscitation
    bag and mask, 736c
    definition of, 2517
    in hypovolemic shock, 2528
    as triage category, 2521
Retention enema, for hyperkalemia in acute renal failure, 1525
Reteplase (t-PA, Retavase), 1003
    for venous thrombosis, 1006
Rete ridges, 1928
    definition of, 1927
Reticular activating system, 95
Reticulocyte(s), 1036, 1039
Reticulocyte count, laboratory values for, 2579
Reticuloendothelial system, 1036, 1042–1043
    definition of, 1036
Retina, 2045f, 2046. *See also* Retinopathy
    in chronic glomerulonephritis, 1519

disorders of, 2067–2072
  sensory, 2046, 2067
  vascular disorders of, 2068–2069
Retinal detachment, 2067–2068, 2067f
  exudative, 2067
  traction, 2067
Retinal pigment epithelium, 2046, 2067
Retinal vessels, 2046
Retinitis, cytomegalovirus, 2083–2084
  in HIV-infected (AIDS) patients, treatment of, 1835–1836
Retinitis pigmentosa, 2053
Retinoblastoma, 2081, 2081c
  familial occurrence of, 386
  genetics of, 146
Retinoic acid, adverse effects and side effects of, 421t
Retinoid(s)
  in cancer treatment, 420
    adverse effects and side effects of, 421t
  oral
    for acne vulgaris, 1954t, 1955
    for psoriasis, 1966t, 1967
Retinol-binding protein, serum, 80
Retinopathy
  definition of, 1376
  diabetic, 1383, 1422–1425, 1423t, 1424f, 2051, 2083
    background, 1422, 1423t
    preproliferative, 1422, 1423t
    proliferative, 1422, 1423t
Retirement communities, 229
Retraction, 2343c
Retraining, of bladder. See Bladder, retraining
Retributive justice, 28c
Retrograde ejaculation, 1746–1750
Retrograde pyelography, 1509
Retrovirus
  definition of, 1815
  HIV as, 1821
Reverse transcriptase, 1821
  definition of, 1815
Review of systems, in health history, 67
Revlimid, for multiple myeloma, 1084
Rewarming, 2535–2536
  active core, 2535–2536
  in frostbite, 2535
  in hypothermia, 2535–2536
  passive external, 2536
  supportive care during, 2536
RF. See Rheumatoid factor
Rhabdomyoma, 2417
Rhabdomyosarcoma, 2417
  of orbit, 2080
Rh antigen, 1106
Rheumatic diseases, 1886–1920
  activity level and, 1894
  assessment of, 1889–1892, 1890c–1891c, 1897
  blood tests for, 1892, 1893t–1894t
  classification of, 1887
  clinical manifestations of, 1889
  complications of, 1903c, 1904
  continuing care for, 1905–1906
  degeneration in, 1888, 1889f
  diagnosis of, 1889–1892, 1890c–1891c
  drug-related, 1920
  exercise and, 1894, 1897t, 1898
  expected outcomes in, 1906
  gerontologic considerations in, 1892
  home and community-based care for, 1904–1906, 1905c
  inflammation in, 1887–1888
  medical management of, 1894
  metabolic and endocrine disorders associated with, 1917

nursing care plan for, 1899c–1903c
nursing diagnoses related to, 1897–1898
nursing interventions for, 1898–1904
nursing process with, 1897–1906
pain management in, 1894, 1895t–1897t
pathophysiology of, 1887–1889
pharmacologic therapy for, 1894, 1895t–1897t
planning and goals for, 1894t
treatment of, gerontologic considerations in, 1892
Rheumatic endocarditis, 933–935
Rheumatic fever, 933, 933c
  cross-reactivity in, 1790
Rheumatism
  extra-articular, 1920
  palindromic, 1920
Rheumatoid arthritis, 1906–1909, 1907f, 1908f
  advanced, unremitting, 1909
  clinical manifestations of, 1907, 1908f
  early-stage, 1908
  and foot disorders, 2401
  gerontologic considerations in, 1892
  joint deformity in, 2348, 2349f
  joint involvement in, 2348–2349, 2349f
  living with, nursing research on, 1910
  medical management of, 1908–1909
  moderate, erosive, 1909
  nursing management of, 1909
  nutrition therapy for, 1909
  pathophysiology of, 1906, 1907f
  persistent, erosive, 1909
  and temporomandibular disorders, 1146–1147
Rheumatoid factor, in rheumatic diseases, 1894t
Rheumatoid nodules, 1907
Rhinitis, 589–591
  allergic. See Allergic rhinitis
  causes of, 589, 590t
  clinical manifestations of, 590–591
  definition of, 589, 1856
  drug-induced, 589
  medical management of, 591
  nonallergic, 589
  nursing management of, 591
  pathophysiology of, 589–590, 590f
  pharmacologic therapy for, 591
  viral, 591–593
    causative agents, 591, 592f
    clinical manifestations of, 592
    medical management of, 592–593
    nursing management of, 593
    prevention of, 593, 594c
    seasonal incidence of, 591, 592f
Rhinitis medicamentosa, 1875, 1876f
Rhinorrhea, 590, 2106
  cerebrospinal fluid (CSF), 2235
  definition of, 589
Rhizotomy, in pain management, 291, 292f
Rhythm methods of contraception, 1646
Rhytidectomy, 1990–1991
Rib(s), fractures of, 2459–2460
  flail chest with, 676–677, 677f
  in trauma patient, 676
Riboflavin, deficiency of, in liver disease, 1307
RICE (Rest, Ice, Compression, Elevation), 2425, 2426, 2427, 2429, 2430
Rickettsia rickettsii
  incubation period of, 2477t
  transmission of, 2477t
Rifabutin (Mycobutin), for tuberculosis, 647, 647t
  adverse effects and side effects of, 647t

dosage and administration of, 647t
drug interactions with, 647t
Rifampin
  adverse effects and side effects of, 647t, 649
  dosage and administration of, 647t
  drug interactions with, 647t, 649
  for tuberculosis, 647–648, 647t
Rifapentine (Priftin), for tuberculosis, 647–648, 647t
Right heart catheterization, 814
Rights, of dying patient, 451c
Right to Know law, 668
Right to refuse treatment, 615c
Right ventricular area, examination of, 801, 801f
Rigidity, 2146
  definition of, 2129
  in Huntington's disease, 2320
  in Parkinson's disease, 2313
Riluzole (Rilutek), for amyotrophic lateral sclerosis, 2322–2323
Rimantadine
  for influenza, 637
  for viral rhinitis, 593
Ringworm, 1960–1962, 1961t. See Tinea
  causative organisms of, 2477t
Rinne test, 2099, 2099f, 2099t
Risedronate (Actonel), for osteoporosis, 2409
Risk management, definition of, 46c
Ritonavir (Norvir), for HIV infection, 1828t
Rituximab (Rituxan), 419t
  adverse effects and side effects of, 421t
  for chronic lymphocytic leukemia, 1074
Rivastigmine (Exelon), for Alzheimer's disease, 244
Rizatriptan (Maxalt), for migraine, 2201
RK. See Radial keratotomy
RNFA. See Registered nurse first assistant
Rocky Mountain spotted fever, causative organism of, 2477t
Rocuronium (Zemuron), 512t
Rods, 2046
  definition of, 2043
Rofecoxib, in pain management, 284
Rohypnol (roofies, date rape drug), abuse/overdose, emergency management of, 2547t
Roles/relationships
  in cardiovascular disease, assessment of, 797
  definition of, 46c
Rolling walker, 205
Romberg test, 2147
  definition of, 2129
Ropinirole hydrochloride (Requip), for Parkinson's disease, 2314
Roseola infantum, causative organism of, 2477t
Rosiglitizone (Avandia), 1400t, 1401
Rosuvastatin (Crestor), 865t
Rotation, 2343c
  definition of, 198c
  external, 199c
  internal, 199c
Rotator cuff
  definition of, 2425
  tear, 2429
Rotavirus
  gastroenteritis caused by, 2477t
  incubation period of, 2477t
  transmission of, 2477t
Roto Rest bed, 2254f
Round window, 2094, 2094f
  definition of, 2095c
Rovsing's sign, 1241, 1241f

RPE. *See* Retinal pigment epithelium
RPR-CT. *See* Rapid plasma reagin circle card test
RR interval, on ECG, 827, 827f
RT-PCR. *See* Reverse transcriptase polymerase chain reaction
RU 486. *See* Mifepristone
Rubber-band ligation, for hemorrhoids, 1277
Rubella virus
 incubation period of, 2477t
 transmission of, 2477t
Rubor, 980
 definition of, 975
 in thrombangiitis obliterans, 996
Rule of nines, 1997, 1998f
 definition of, 1995
Running traction, 2366
Rupture, renal, 1565, 1565f

# S

Saccule, 2094f
Sacrum, 2136
Saddle joints, 2341
Safer sex, 1672, 1817c, 2505
Safety
 of Alzheimer's disease patients, 245
 of caregivers, in radiation therapy, 395, 397
 in chemotherapy administration, 398, 402, 416c
 in emergency department, 2518–2519
 in home health care, 19, 20c
 intraoperative, 520
  latex allergy and, 508
  nursing management of, 482c
 after laryngectomy, patient teaching about, 619–620
 in laser surgery, 508
 in liver disease, 1332c
 in magnetic resonance imaging, 2153–2154
 nurse's, in home visit, 19, 20c
 in operating room, 508
 in ophthalmology, 2087
 patient, preoperative management of, 496, 496c
 for postoperative patient, 544
 in preoperative area, 499
 in prevention of injury, 2530
 promotion of, in shock, 361
 radiation, nursing considerations for, 1695
 in shock, promoting, 361
 during transfers, 203
 of unconscious patient, 2166
 in vesicant administration, 398, 402, 416c
St. Christopher's Hospice, 454
St. Louis encephalitis, 2274–2275
Salem sump tube, 1176
Salem tube, 1176, 1176f
Salicylates
 poisoning with, emergency management of, 2547t–2548t
 for rheumatic diseases, 1894, 1895t
 therapeutic blood levels of, 2601t
 toxic blood levels of, 2601t
Saline (solution)
 half-strength, 311t
 hypertonic, 312t
  for fluid replacement
   in burn patients, 2007c
   in shock, 367t
 normal, 311t, 339
  for fluid replacement in shock, 367t
Saline irrigation, for sinusitis, 595
Saliva, 1123, 1123t
Salivary amylase, 1123
 source and digestive action of, 1123t

Salivary calculi, 1158
Salivary glands, 1122f, 1147
 disorders of, 1147–1148
 inflammation of, 1147
Salmeterol, 693t
 for asthma, 713t
 for ventilator-dependent patient, 749
Salmeterol/fluticasone (Seretide), for asthma, 713t
*Salmonella* diarrhea, 2501
 incubation period of, 2476t
 transmission of, 2476t
Salpingitis, 1670
 definition of, 1661
Salpingo-oophorectomy
 definition of, 1661
 in endometriosis, 1681
Salsalate (Disalcid), for rheumatic diseases, 1895t
Salt substitutes, potassium in, 325
Sanctity of life, ethical principle of, 28c
SANE. *See* Sexual assault nurse examiner
Saphenous vein(s), grafts, in coronary artery bypass grafting, 888, 888f, 889f
Saquinavir (Invirase, Fortovase), for HIV infection, 1828t
Sarcoidosis, 667–668, 1920
 assessment in, 667
 diagnosis of, 667
 epidemiology of, 667
 medical management of, 668
 pathophysiology of, 667
 pulmonary involvement in, 667
Sarcomas, 2417
 vulvar, 1685–1686
Sarcomeres, 2341
Sarcoplasmic reticulum, 2341
*Sarcoptes scabei*
 incubation period of, 2477t
 transmission of, 2477t
Sargramostim (Leukine)
 for acute myeloid leukemia, 1071
 adverse effects and side effects of, 421t
 as alternative to blood transfusion, 1112c
Sarin, as terrorism threat, 2569t, 2570–2571
SARS. *See* Severe acute respiratory syndrome
SARS-associated coronavirus
 incubation period of, 2477t
 transmission of, 2477t
Saturated solution of potassium iodide (SSKI), for hyperthyroidism, 1462
Saunders, Cicely, 454
Saw palmetto, for benign prostatic hyperplasia, 1752
Scabies, 1963–1964
 assessment of, 1964
 causative organism of, 2477t
 clinical manifestations of, 1963
 diagnosis of, 1964
 distribution of, 1940f
 gerontologic considerations in, 1964
 medical management of, 1964
 nursing management of, 1964
Scala tympani, 2096
Scalded skin syndrome, 1974
Scale, 1929t, 1938c
Scalp injury, 2234
Scapular line, 571c
Scars, 1938c
 assessment of, 799
 burns and, 2026, 2031–2033
 hypertrophic, 2026
  in burn patient, 2032t
  prevention of, 2026, 2031–2033
 prevention of, in acne, 1956

Schiavo, Terri, 33
Schilling test, 1053
School health programs, 21–22
School nurse(s), 17, 22
SCI. *See* Spinal cord injuries
Sciatica, 2329, 2392
 definition of, 2301, 2392
SCID. *See* Severe combined immunodeficiency disease
Scintigraphy, in gastrointestinal assessment, 1133
Sclera, 2044, 2045f
Scleral buckle, 2067–2068, 2068f
Scleral shells, 2082, 2082f
Scleroderma, 1912–1913
 assessment of, 1912
 clinical manifestations of, 1912
 diagnosis of, 1912
 medical management of, 1912
 nursing management of, 1913
 pathophysiology of, 1912
 pharmacologic therapy for, 1912
Sclerotherapy
 definition of, 1285
 endoscopic, for esophageal varices, 1301–1302, 1301f, 1304t
 in liver cancer, 1334
 for varicose veins, 1015
Scoliosis, 2347, 2347f
 definition of, 2337
Scopolamine
 in end-of-life care, 471t
 ocular applications of, 2086t
 postoperative use of, 528
Scoring system, postoperative, 520f, 529
Scotomas, 2050
 definition of, 2043
Scout. *See* Circulating nurse
Screening
 for alcohol or drug abuse, 70, 70c
 genetic, 150t, 152
  for adult-onset conditions, 151t–152t
 in health promotion, 58, 59–60, 59t
Scrotum, 1741, 1741f
Scrub attire, 506
Scrub role
 activities of, 505
 definition of, 503
Sealants, in prevention of tooth decay, 1145
Sebaceous glands, 1928f, 1930
 definition of, 1927
Seborrheic dermatitis, 1953
 clinical manifestations of, 1953
 distribution of, 1940f
 dry form of, 1953
 in HIV-infected (AIDS) patients, 1834
 medical management of, 1953
 nursing management of, 1953
 oily form of, 1953
Seborrheic keratoses, 1977
Sebum, 1930
 definition of, 1927
Secobarbital (Seconal), abuse/overdose, emergency management of, 2545t–2546t
Secondary conditions or disorders, 183
 assessment for, 178c
 definition of, 166
Secondary hypertension. *See* Hypertension, secondary
Secondary injury, definition of, 2233
Secondary intention healing, 104
 definition of, 91
Secretin, 1346
 definition of, 1345
 in gastrointestinal regulation, 1124t

# INDEX

Secretory phase, of menstrual cycle, 1616
  definition of, 1613
Sedation
  moderate, 515
    definition of, 503
  opioid-related, 281–282
  palliative
    definition of, 448
    in end-of-life care, 468
Sedatives, nonbarbiturate, abuse/overdose, emergency management of, 2547t
Seeing-Eye dogs, 2054
Segmentation contractions, of small intestine, 1124–1125
Segmentectomy
  of lung, 672c, 755c
  pulmonary, in bronchiectasis, 709
Seizures, 2143, 2190–2191. See also Epilepsy
  absence, 2191
  aura in, 2192c
  brain injury and, 2249
  with brain tumor, 2304
  causes of, 2190
  in chronic renal failure, 1530
  complex partial, 2190c, 2191
  definition of, 2161, 2190
  fear of, reducing, 2195–2196
  generalized, 2190, 2190c, 2191
  after head injury, 2238
  hemorrhagic stroke and, 2228
  in hypocalcemia, 326
  in hypomagnesemia, 329
  injury prevention in, 2195
  International Classification of, 2190, 2190c
  Jacksonian, 2304
  nursing management after, 2191, 2192c
  nursing management during, 2190–2191, 2192c
  partial, 2190, 2190c
  postoperative
    in neurosurgical patient
      nursing interventions for, 2185c, 2188
      prevention of, 2182
    prevention of, in intracranial surgery, 2181
  post-traumatic, 2249
Selective estrogen receptor modulators
  for breast cancer, 1729
  for osteoporosis, 2409
Selective serotonin reuptake inhibitors (SSRIs)
  contraindications to, in Parkinson's disease, 2314
  for depression, 240
  metabolism of, genetic factors affecting, 154t
Selegiline (Eldepryl), for Parkinson's disease, 2314
Self-care. See also Patient teaching
  for acne, 1956
  in acute leukemia, patient teaching about, 1078
  after acute pancreatitis, 1362–1363
  for allergic rhinitis, 1875–1876, 1875c
  Alzheimer's disease and, 245
  after amputation, 2465, 2468, 2468c
  for angina, 872–873, 873c
  in anorectal disorders, 1279
  with bone tumors, 2420, 2421c
  in brain-injury patient, 2249
  for brain tumor patient, 2308
  after breast surgery, 1723–1725, 1723c
  for burn patient, 2034
  with cardiac dysrhythmia, 841
  after cardiac surgery, 902, 911c
  in cardiomyopathy, 932
  casts and, 2360, 2361c
  for chlamydia infection, 1670
  in chronic obstructive pulmonary disease, 695, 700, 705c, 706c
    enhancement of, 698
  for colostomy patient, 1273
  in coronary artery disease, 872–873
  definition of, 46c
  dementia and, 245
  in diabetes mellitus, 1418–1419, 1419c
  after ectopic pregnancy, 1655
  after foot surgery, 2403, 2404c
  after gallbladder surgery, 1357, 1357c
  for genital herpes, 1668, 1669t
  for glaucoma, 2059, 2059c
  for Guillain-Barré syndrome, 2291
  hand/wrist surgery and, 2399–2400, 2400c
  for headache, 2201
  in heart failure, 962, 963c
  after hip replacement, 2375, 2381c
  for HIV-infected (AIDS) patients, 1850
  in Huntington's disease, 2320
  for hypertension, 1031
  in hyperthyroidism, 1464–1465, 1465c
  in hypothyroidism, 1454–1458
  after hysterectomy, 1694
  for ileostomy patient, 1263, 1263c
  in immunodeficiency, 1810, 1811c
  with implanted cardiac device, 851
  in inflammatory bowel disease, 1253, 1253c
  after intracranial surgery, 2188
  after laparoscopic cholecystectomy, 1357, 1357c
  after mastoid surgery, 2110, 2110c
  after myocardial infarction, 884, 885c
  for orthopedic surgery patient, postoperative, 2387
  in osteomyelitis, 2415, 2416c
    patient teaching about, 2415, 2416c
  for paraplegia/quadriplegia, 2265–2266
  in Parkinson's disease, 2316–2317, 2317–2318, 2318c
  in pelvic inflammatory disease, 1671, 1672c
  postoperative, patient teaching about, 548
  after prostatectomy, 1767–1768, 1768c
  in psoriasis, 1969–1970
  rehabilitation and, 193–195, 194c
  for renal surgical patient, 1559
  in rheumatic diseases, 1901c–1902c, 1904
  for skin cancer, 1980–1981
  for spinal cord-injured patient, 2260
  for staphylococcal skin infections, 1958
  for stroke patient, 2218–2219, 2222, 2229
  in toxic epidermal necrolysis or Stevens-Johnson syndrome, 1976
  with vertigo, 2117c
  for vulvar surgical patient, 1688
Self-catheterization, intermittent, for urinary incontinence, 216
Self-concept
  burns and, 2033–2034
  in cardiovascular disease, 797
  after facial reconstructive surgery, 1990
  after ileostomy, 1255c
  in patient profile, 69c, 71
  in psoriasis, 1969
Self-esteem
  bone tumors and, 2420
  of cancer patient, 413c
  in chronic renal failure, 1530, 1535c
  in hyperthyroidism, 1464
  after laryngectomy, 617
  in liver disease, 1327c
  low back pain and, 2397
  in orthopedic surgery patient
    postoperative, 2386
    preoperative, 2384
Self-help devices. See Assistive devices/technology
Self-image
  in disfiguring oral conditions, 1151
  after neck dissection, 1158c–1159c
  in neurosurgical patient, 2186–2187
Self-injury, protection from, in brain-injured patient, 2244–2245, 2245f
Self-monitoring of blood glucose, 1389–1390
  definition of, 1376
Self-perception
  in cardiovascular disease, assessment of, 797
  definition of, 46c
Self-regulation, in critical thinking, 25
Self-responsibility
  definition of, 49l
  in health promotion, 58
Selye, Hans, 94–95, 97
Semicircular canals, 2094–2096, 2094f
  definition of, 2095c
Semi-implantable hearing device, 2122
Semilunar valves, 782f, 783
Seminal vesicles, 1741, 1741f
Semirestricted zone, 506
  definition of, 503
Semustine, in cancer treatment, 399t
Sengstaken-Blakemore tube, 1175, 1176t
Sensation, skin and, 1930–1931
Sensation/perception, definition of, 46c
Senses, age-related changes in, 232t, 236–237
Sensitivity, in communication with terminally ill patients, 457–459
Sensitization
  definition of, 259
  and pain, 276
Sensorineural hearing loss. See Hearing loss, sensorineural
Sensory alterations, 2144
  age-related, 2151
  with brain tumor, 2304
  after cardiac surgery, 900–901, 908c–909c
  after mastoid surgery, 2109
  spinal cord injuries and, 2257–2258
  stroke and, 2209–2210, 2219–2220
Sensory deprivation, 236
  in neurosurgical patient, nursing interventions for, 2186
  in stroke patient, 2228
Sensory function, 2142–2143
Sensory loss, 236, 2142–2143
Sensory perception
  altered, amputation and, 2464
  disturbed, in neurosurgical patient, nursing interventions for, 2184c
  and pressure ulcer prevention, 212
  pressure ulcers and, 208
Sensory stimulation, for unconscious patient, 2168
Sensory system, examination of, 2150
Sentinel lymph node
  biopsy, in breast cancer, 1717–1718, 1717t
  definition of, 1701
Sepsis
  in blistering diseases, 1973
  burns and, 2030
  in burn victim, 2002
  definition of, 373c
  gram-negative, with urinary tract infections, 1575
  paraplegia/quadriplegia and, 2265
  in parenteral nutrition, 1197t
  prevention of, 2498c

Sepsis (continued)
  severe, definition of, 373c
  in toxic epidermal necrolysis or Stevens-Johnson syndrome, 1974, 1976
  upper airway infection and, 603
  wound. See Wound, surgical, infection of; Wound(s), infections of
  and wound healing, 541t
Septal repair, 925
Septic arthritis, 2416–2417
  assessment of, 2416
  clinical manifestations of, 2416
  diagnosis of, 2416
  gerontologic considerations in, 2416–2417
  management of, 2416–2417
Septicemia
  intravenous therapy and, 349
  prevention of, 2498c
Septic shock, prevention of, 2498c
Septoplasty, 607
Sequestrectomy, 2414
Sequestrum, 2413
  definition of, 2392
Serax. See Oxazepam
SERMs. See Selective oestrogen receptor modulators
Seroma, after breast surgery, 1722–1723
Serotonin, 2130t
  in allergic reaction, 1858t, 1859
  definition of, 1856
  vascular effects of, 978
Serotonin antagonists
  for chemotherapy patient, 398
  in migraine prevention, 2200
*Serratia*, pneumonia, 629, 633
Sertraline (Zoloft), for rheumatoid arthritis, 1909
Serum, 1042
  definition of, 1036
  laboratory studies of, in musculoskeletal assessment, 2351–2352
  osmolality of, 304
    in hypernatremia, 320
    usual reference range for, 310t
Serum chemistry, reference ranges for, 2581t–2593t
Serum sickness, 1880
Service dogs
  for blind, 2054
  for hearing-impaired persons, 2123
Sevelamer hydrochloride (Renagel), for chronic renal failure, 1529
Severe acute respiratory syndrome, 643, 2510
  as bioterrorism threat, 2569
  causative organism of, 2477t
  clinical manifestations of, 2569
  treatment of, 2569
Severe combined immunodeficiency disease, 1803t, 1807
  definition of, 1802
  genetics of, 146
Sevin, as terrorism threat, 2570
Sevoflurane (Ultrane), 510t
Sex chromosomes, 142, 143f, 146
Sex hormones
  adrenal, 1474, 1475. See also Androgen(s)
  and autoimmune disorders, 1796
  and hair growth, 1930
Sex-linked agammaglobulinemia. See Bruton's disease
Sexual abuse. See also Abuse
  childhood, 1622
Sexual activity, physiologic demands during, 797
Sexual assault, 1622

definition of, 2551
emergency management of, 2551–2553
and sexually transmitted disease, 2552–2553
victim of
  emergency contraception for, 2552
  follow-up care for, 2553
  forensic examination of, 2552
  physical examination of, 2552
  psychological response in, 2551
  services for, 2553
  specimen collection from, 2552
  STD prevention measures for, 2552
Sexual assault nurse examiner, 2551
Sexual function/sexuality issues
  in Alzheimer's disease, 245
  assessment of, 69c, 71–73
  breast surgery and, 1720–1721
  for cancer patient, 431
  in cardiovascular disease, assessment of, 797
  of colostomy patient, 1273
  in continuous ambulatory peritoneal dialysis, 1549
  definition of, 46c
  in diabetes, 1427
  disability and, 218
  for elderly, 233
  hypertension treatment and, 1031
  in ileostomy patient, 1257c
  male
    disorders of, 1744–1750
    tests of, 1744
  in multiple sclerosis, 2283
  paraplegia/quadriplegia and, 2264
  in prostate cancer, 1758c
  after prostatectomy, 1767
  in stroke patient, 2222
  after urinary diversion surgery, 1605
  with vulvar surgery, 1687
Sexual history
  female, 1618–1620
  in sexually transmitted disease assessment, 2508
Sexually transmitted disease, 2504–2509. See also specific disease
  anorectal involvement in, 1277
  assessment in, 2508
  co-infections in, 2505, 2508
  complications of, 2508, 2509
  conditions classified as, 2504, 2504t
  congenital, 2509
  epidemiology of, 2504
  expected outcomes in, 2509
  health history in, 2508
  and immune system function, 1795–1796
  in males, 1750
  nursing diagnoses related to, 2508
  nursing interventions for, 2508–2509
  nursing process with, 2508–2509
  patient teaching about, 2508–2509
  planning and goals for, 2508
  prevention of, 1645, 1646, 2504–2505, 2508–2509
    education about, 2504–2505
    in sexual assault victim, 2552–2553
  risk factors for, 2504t
  significance of, 2505
  tests for, in UTI diagnosis, 1574
  transmission routes for, 2504t
Sexual partners, in sexually transmitted disease, 2508
Shear, and pressure ulcers, 208–209, 209f, 213
Sheehan's syndrome, 1446. See Postpartum pituitary necrosis
Shift to the left, 1041
  definition of, 1036

*Shigella* diarrhea, 2501
  incubation period of, 2476t
  transmission of, 2476t
Shingles. See also Herpes zoster
  distribution of, 1940f
Shock
  anaphylactic, 356, 372, 376
    medical management of, 376
    nursing management of, 376
    risk factors for, 372c
  anxiety in, reducing, 361, 371
  blood pressure in, 360
  burns and, 1999, 2013c–2014c
  cardiogenic, 356, 368–371, 965–968, 966f
    clinical manifestations of, 369
    coronary versus non-coronary, 368
    first-line treatment of, 369
    fluid replacement in, 371
    hemodynamic monitoring in, 369, 371
    mechanical assist devices for, 370–371
    medical management of, 369–371
    nursing management of, 371
    oxygenation in, 369
    pain control in, 369
    pathophysiology of, 368–369, 369f
    postoperative, 527
    prevention of, 371
    risk factors for, 368
    safety and comfort in, enhancing, 371
  cellular effects of, 357, 357f
  circulatory (distributive), 356, 371–372. See also Shock, anaphylactic; Shock, neurogenic; Shock, septic
    burns and, 1999, 2013c–2014c
    pathophysiology of, 371–372, 372f, 373–374
    types of, 372
  classification of, 356–357
  compensatory stage of, 358–361
    clinical findings in, 359, 359f, 359t
    compensatory stage of, medical management of, 359
    nursing management of, 359–361
    tissue perfusion in, monitoring, 360–361
  conditions precipitating, 356–358
  continuing care for, 378
  definition of, 356, 527
  in elderly, recognition of, 359–361, 361c
  electrical, injury caused by, 102
  fluid redistribution in, 367–368
  fluid replacement in, 364–365, 367t, 368
    complications of, 365
  fracture and, 2435, 2444
  hemorrhagic, and wound healing, 541t
  home and community-based care for, 377–378
  hypovolemic, 312, 356, 366–368, 2527–2528
    blood replacement in, 367, 368, 2528
    diarrheal diseases and, 2504
    emergency management of, 2528
    fluid redistribution in, 367–368, 368f
    fluid replacement in, 367, 367t, 368, 2528
    medical management of, 366–368
    nursing management of, 368, 2528
    in orthopedic surgery patient, 2386–2387
    oxygen therapy in, 368
    pathophysiology of, 366, 367f
    pharmacologic therapy for, 368
    postoperative, 527
    risk factors for, 366, 366c
    signs and symptoms of, 2526, 2526c
    underlying cause of, treatment of, 366–367

# INDEX

irreversible stage of, 363–364
  clinical findings in, 359t, 363
  medical management of, 363
  nursing management of, 363–364
management of
  general strategies for, 364–366
  in postanesthesia care, 527
medical management of, 365, 366t
in multiple trauma, 2472–2473
neurogenic, 356, 372, 375–376, 2255–2256
  medical management of, 375
  nursing management of, 375–376
  postoperative, 527
  risk factors for, 372c
nutritional support in, 365–366
pathophysiology of, 357–358
patient positioning in, 367, 368f
pelvic fracture and, 2444
in pneumonia, 638, 641
postoperative, management of, 527
prevention of, in acute pancreatitis, 1367c
progressive stage of, 361–363
  assessment in, 361–362
  cardiovascular effects of, 361–362
  clinical findings in, 359t, 361–362
  complications of, prevention of, 363
  family members of patient with, supporting, 363
  gastrointestinal effects of, 362
  hematologic effects of, 362
  hepatic effects of, 362
  medical management of, 362
  neurologic effects of, 362
  nursing management of, 362–363
  pathophysiology of, 361
  renal effects of, 362
  respiratory effects of, 361
  rest and comfort in, promoting, 352
pulse pressure in, 360
self-care in, patient teaching about, 377–378
septic, 356, 372–375. *See also* Toxic shock syndrome
  in cancer patient, 432
  definition of, 373c
  hyperdynamic phase of, 374
  hypodynamic phase of, 374
  medical management of, 374–375
  microbiology of, 373
  nursing management of, 375
  nutritional support in, 374–375
  pharmacologic therapy for, 374
  risk factors for, 372, 372c
significance of, 356
signs of, 527
and skin color, 1935t
spinal, 2255–2256
stages of, 358–364
after thoracic surgery, 769
in trauma patient, 62
traumatic, 356
treatment of, 2435
vascular response to, 357–358
vasoactive agents in, 365
Shock lung, 361
Shoes, for surgical personnel, 506
Short-arm cast, 2355
Short bones, 2338
Short-leg cast, 2355
Short tubes, 1175–1176
Shoulder
  adduction, ischemic stroke and, 2217
  healing of, patient education about, 2398c
  pain in, in stroke patient, 2218
  range-of-motion exercises for, 2440, 2441f
Shoulder pain, hemiplegia-associated, 261c

Shoulder spica cast, 2355
Shunt(s), respiratory, and ventilation-perfusion ratio, 558, 559c
SIADH. *See* Syndrome of inappropriate antidiuretic hormone
Sialadenitis, 1147
  definition of, 1142
Sialolithiasis, 1148
Sibutramine HCl (Meridia), 1217
Sickle cell anemia, 1055–1058
  acute chest syndrome of, 1057
  carrier testing for, 150t, 156
  clinical manifestations of, 1056–1057
  complications of, 1056–1057, 1056t, 1058, 1059
  diagnosis of, 1057
  expected outcomes in, 1060–1061
  genetics of, 143–144, 146, 147t
  genetic testing in, 150t
  medical management of, 1057–1058
  pain of, 261c
  pharmacologic therapy for, 1057
  prognosis for, 1057
  red blood cells in, 1055f
  screening for, 150t
  supportive therapy for, 1058
  transfusion therapy for, 1057–1058
Sickle cell beta-thalassemia, 1056
Sickle cell crisis, 1055–1056
  aplastic, 1056
  assessment in, 1059
  complications of, 1059
  nursing diagnoses related to, 1059
  nursing interventions for, 1059–1060
  nursing process with, 1058–1061
  sequestration, 1056
  sickle crisis type, 1056
Sickle cell hemoglobin C disease, 1056
Sickle cell hemoglobin D disease, 1056
Sickle cell trait, 1056
Side-lying position, 196, 197c
Sigmoid colon, 1121, 1122f
Sigmoidoscopy, 1137, 1137f
  flexible fiberoptic, 1137, 1137f
Sildenafil, (Viagra), 1745, 1747t, 1748c–1749c
Silent unit, 559c
Silicosis, 668–669
Silver nitrate, for burns, 2017, 2018t
Silver sulfadiazine (Silvadene), for burns, 2017, 2018t
Simmonds' disease. *See* Panhypopituitarism
SIMV. *See* Synchronized intermittent mandatory ventilation
Simvastatin (Zocor), 864–865, 865t, 986
  and stroke prevention, 2211
Sinex long-lasting. *See* Oxymetazoline hydrochloride
Single nucleotide polymorphisms, 145
Single-photon emission computed tomography, 2130, 2153, 2162
  in cardiac assessment, 812
  in epilepsy, 2193
Sin Nombre virus, 2511
  incubation period of, 2476t
  transmission of, 2476t
Sinoatrial node, 783–784, 784f, 785, 786, 824
  definition of, 781
Sinography, in intraperitoneal injury, 2532
Sinus(es)
  frontal, 1153f
  paranasal
    anatomy of, 553, 554f
    infection of. *See* Sinusitis
    physical examination of, 568–569, 569f, 595
  sphenoid, 1153f

Sinus arrhythmia(s), 831, 831f
Sinus bradycardia, 828–829, 829f
Sinusitis
  acute, 593–595
    assessment in, 595
    causative organisms in, 593
    clinical manifestations of, 593–595
    complications of, 595
    diagnosis of, 595
    medical management of, 595
  chronic, 595–597
    assessment in, 596
    clinical manifestations of, 596
    complications of, 596
    diagnosis of, 596
    medical management of, 596
    nursing management of, 598
    pathophysiology of, 596
    surgical management of, 596–597
  definition of, 589
  nursing interventions for, 602–603
  pathophysiology of, 590f, 593, 596
  self-care in, patient teaching about, 595, 598
  in upper airway infection, 603
Sinus node dysrhythmias, 828–831
Sinusoidal harmonic acceleration, 2100–2101
Sinusoids, hepatic, 1285, 1286f
Sinus rhythm
  definition of, 823
  ECG criteria for, 828
  normal, 828, 829f
Sinus tachycardia, 829–831, 829f
Sirolimus (Rapamune), for kidney transplant recipient, 1561
Sitting, with crutches, 205
Six-year molar, 1150f
SJS. *See* Stevens-Johnson syndrome
Skeletal fractures, reduction, for spinal cord injury, 2254–2255, 2255f
Skeletal muscle
  actions of, 2342
  anatomy of, 2341
  contraction of, 2341–2342, 2343c
  disuse of, 2342
  functions of, 2341–2342, 2343c
  repair of, 2342
  structure of, 2341–2342
  tone of, 2342
Skeletal system
  function of, 2340–2341
  structure of, 2340–2341
Skeletal tongs, 2254
Skeletal traction, 2366, 2368–2369
  and exercise, 2369
  neurovascular status in, 2368
  nursing interventions for, 2368–2369
  pin site care in, 2368–2369
  positioning with, 2368
  skin breakdown in, 2368–2369
  for spinal cord injury, 2254
Skin. *See also* Integumentary system
  abrasions of, healing of, for patient in cast, 2357
  age-related changes in, 1931–1932, 1932c
  anatomy of, 1927–1930, 1928f
  appearance of
    assessment of, 1932–1933
    changes in, in arterial disease, 979–980
  artificial, in burn care, 2020t, 2022
  biopsy of, 1942
  breakdown
    amputation and, 2461, 2468
    hip fracture and, 2448–2449
    skeletal traction and, 2368
    skin traction and, 2367

Skin (continued)
  chemical burns of, 2543–2544
  chronic renal failure and, 1528, 1528c
  in circulatory insufficiency, 979–980
  clinical photographs of, 1942
  color of, 1932
    in carbon monoxide poisoning, 2541
    changes in, 1934, 1935t
    in Raynaud's disease, 1004
  cysts of, 1977
  dark, assessment of, 1934, 1935t
  decontamination of, 2543–2544
  diagnostic evaluation of, 1941–1942
  discomfort in, in blistering diseases, 1973
  disinfection of, 2484
  disorders of. See Skin conditions
  in fluid and electrolyte balance, 304, 304t, 1931
  gerontologic considerations in, 1931–1932, 1932c
  hygiene, and pressure ulcer healing, 213
  immune dysfunction and, 1794c
  and immune response, 1931
  inspection of, in cardiovascular disease, 798–799
  lesions of. See also Skin conditions
    aging and, 1931–1932, 1932c
    anatomic distribution of, 1936
    annular, 1940f
    arciform, 1940f
    assessment of, 1934–1936
    configurations of, 1940f
    confluent, 1940f
    discrete, 1940f
    grouped, 1940f
    laser treatment of, 1991–1992
    linear, 1940f
    patterns of, 1936
    primary, 1934, 1937c
    secondary, 1934–1936, 1938c
    ulcerated, 1929t
    zosteriform, 1940f
  malignancies of, 428
  moistness of, 798
  musculoskeletal disorders and, 2349
  after neck dissection, 1156c–1157c
  in oral cavity conditions, 1152
  preoperative preparation of, 496
  protection of, 1945
  protective function of, 1930
  secretory disorders of, 1952–1956
  self-examination of, 1984, 1985c
  and sensation, 1930–1931
  substitutes, 1948
  in systemic disease, 1929t
  in systemic lupus erythematosus, 1910, 1911f
  temperature of, 798
    changes in, in arterial disease, 979–980
  and temperature regulation, 1931
  thickening/hardening of, in systemic disease, 1929t
  tumors of, 1937c, 1977–1982
    metastatic, 1984
  turgor of, 1936
    assessment of, 312, 798
    in older persons, 310, 312
  ulcerations of, 1977
  and vitamin production, 1931
  and water balance, 1931
  wounds
    coverage of, 1986–1988
    flaps for, 1987–1988
    grafts for, 1986–1987
Skin cancer, 1978–1982
  basal cell. See Basal cell carcinoma
  melanoma. See Melanoma
  prevention of, 1980, 1980c, 1981, 1984
  risk factors for, 1978, 1978c
  self-examination for, 1984, 1985c
  squamous cell. See Squamous cell carcinoma
Skin care
  in acute pancreatitis, 1362
  in acute renal failure, 1526
  for cancer patient, 425
  in cirrhosis, 1321
  in Cushing's syndrome, 1482
  with cutaneous urinary diversions, 1600
  in disseminated intravascular coagulation, 1097c
  in gastrostomy, 1191, 1191f
  in ileostomy patient, 1256c–1257c, 1259
  in inflammatory bowel disease, 1253
  in liver disease, 1324c
  perianal, in diarrhea, 1236
  perineal, with fecal incontinence, 1237
  postoperative, for gallbladder surgery, 1356
  with skin conditions, 1945
  with urinary diversion, 1605
  with vulvar surgery, 1687
Skin conditions, 1944–1992
  anatomic distribution of, 1940f
  assessment for, 1934c
  blistering, 1971–1972
  in cancer patient, 425
  genetics of, 1933
  inflammatory process in, reversing, 1945
  intralesional therapy for, 1950
  laser treatment of, 1991–1992
  medical management of, 1948–1950
  nursing management of, 1950–1951
  parasitic, 1962–1964
  pharmacologic therapy for, 1948–1950
  psychosocial considerations in, 1939–1940
  secondary infection in, prevention of, 1945
  skin care with, 1945
  systemic medications for, 1950
  wound care for, 1945–1951
Skin disorders. See Skin conditions
Skin grafts, 1986–1987
  allograft, 1986
  application of, 1987
  autograft, 1986
  in burn care, 2021t, 2022–2024
  donor site for, 1986, 1987f
    care of, 1986–1987
  full-thickness, 1986, 1986f
  split-thickness, 1986, 1986f
  xenograft, 1986
Skin infection(s)
  bacterial, 1956–1958
  in blistering diseases, 1973
  in diabetes, 1941
  fungal (mycotic), 1960–1962, 1961t
  viral, 1958–1960
Skin integrity
  in blistering diseases, 1973
  brain injury and, 2245
  burns and, 2028
  casts and, 2357
  in disseminated intravascular coagulation, 1097c
  in HIV/AIDS patients, 1845, 1846
  with leg ulcers, restoration of, 1014
  maintenance of, for unconscious patient, 2167
  paraplegia/quadriplegia and, 2263
  in psoriasis, 1969
  in rehabilitation, 207–215
  spinal cord injuries and, 2258
  in stroke patient, 2221
  in toxic epidermal necrolysis or Stevens-Johnson syndrome, 1975
Skin reactive factor, action of, 1791t
Skin scrapings, 1942
Skin tests, for allergic disorders, 1864, 1864f, 1865f
  interpretation of, 1864, 1865f
  types of, 1864
Skin traction, 2366–2368
  complications of, 2367
  nursing interventions for, 2367–2368
Skull
  bones of, 2133, 2133f
  fracture of, 2234, 2234f, 2235
  in Paget's disease, 2412
  sutures of, 2133, 2133f
SLE. See Systemic lupus erythematosus
Sleep
  age-related changes in, 235
  brain injuries and, 2246
  in cardiovascular disease, assessment of, 796–797
  in Parkinson's disease, 2313
  in rheumatic diseases, 1903
  upper airway obstruction during, 604–605
Sleep apnea, 235, 604–605
  central, 604
  mixed, 604
  obstructive, 604
    assessment for, 604c
    causes of, 604
    clinical manifestations of, 604–605
    definition of, 604
    medical management of, 605
    risk factors for, 604
Sleep/rest, definition of, 46c
Sleeve resection, of lung, 672c, 755c
Sliding board, 202
Sliding esophageal hernia, 1163–1164, 1163f
Sling
  with arm cast, 2362
  definition of, 2355
  for humeral fracture, 2442, 2442f
Slit-lamp examination, 2049
Slow code, 32
Slow-reacting substance, in humoral immune response, 1789
Slow-reacting substance of anaphylaxis. See Leukotriene(s)
Small-bowel enteroscopy, 1137–1138
Small intestine, 1122f
  age-related changes in, 1125, 1126c
  anatomy of, 1121
  contractions of, 1124–1125
  definition of, 1121
  function of, 1124–1125
  manometry in, 1138
  motility of, evaluation of, 1138
  obstruction of, 1263–1265
  secretions of, 1123t, 1124–1125, 1124t
Smallpox
  as bioterrorism threat, 2568
  causative organism of, 2477t
  clinical manifestations of, 2567tf, 2568
  hemorrhagic, 2568
  treatment of, 2568
  vaccination against, 2568
SMAST, 70
SMBG. See Self-monitoring of blood glucose
Smell perception, age-related changes in, 232t, 237, 2151
Smoker's patch, 1144t
Smoking
  and breast cancer, 1714

# INDEX

and cancer, 386
  of lung, 670–671
and cardiovascular disease, 985
cessation, 866
  in bronchiectasis, 709
  in cardiovascular disease, 798
  in chronic obstructive pulmonary disease, 698
  in COPD, 691–692
  for cor pulmonale, 661
  preoperative, 487
  promotion of, 697
  strategy for, 691–692
  for ulcer patient, 1212
and chronic illness, 167
and chronic obstructive pulmonary disease, 688
and esophageal cancer, 1166, 1167
and hypertension, 1022, 1031
nursing interventions, research on, 642
and oral cancer, 1148
passive (second-hand), and cancer, of lung, 671
respiratory effects of, 642
Smooth muscle, vascular, 976
Snake bite, emergency management of, 2539–2540
Snap(s), definition of, 803
Snellen chart, 2047
SNPs. See Single nucleotide polymorphisms
Social isolation, of HIV-infected (AIDS) patients, 1842c–1843c, 1848–1849
Socialization, of Alzheimer's disease patients, 245
Social learning theory, and health promotion, 57
Social orientation, and genetic assessment, 155–156
Social Security Disability Insurance, 182–183
Social services, for older adults, 249
Social support
  appraisal of, 107
  definition of, 107
  enhancing, in stress management, 107–108
Societal participation, definition of, 174
Sociologic theories, of aging, 227–228
Sodium
  in body fluids, 302t, 303, 319–320
  deficit, 315–318, 316t
    manifestations of, 1516t
    in renal disorders, 1516t
  dietary, 960, 961c
  excess, 316t, 319–321
    manifestations of, 1516t
    in renal disorders, 1516t
  excretion of, regulation of, 1497, 1498f
  imbalances of, in renal disorders, 1516t
  replacement of, in hyponatremia, 318
  restriction of
    in acute glomerulonephritis, 1518
    in heart failure, 960
  retention of, in chronic renal failure, 1529
  serum
    in cardiac patient, 807t
    in hypernatremia, 316t, 319316
    in hyponatremia, 315, 316t, 318
    in hypovolemia, 309
    laboratory values for, 310t
  significance of, 315, 319–320
  urinary, 305
    laboratory values for, 310t
Sodium bicarbonate
  for acute renal failure, 1525
  in cardiopulmonary resuscitation, 971, 972t
  for hyperkalemia, 324
  for malignant hyperthermia, 517

Sodium chloride
  for fluid replacement in shock, 367t
  for hypercalcemia, 328
  for hypermagnesemia, 331
  for metabolic alkalosis, 336
Sodium methohexital (Brevital), for intravenous anesthesia, 513t
Sodium nitrite, for cyanide poisoning, 2569t, 2571
Sodium nitroprusside
  for cardiogenic shock, 966
  for hypertension, 1028t
  for hypertensive emergency, 1033
Sodium polystyrene sulfonate (Kayexalate), for acute renal failure, 1525
Sodium-potassium pump, 303
Sodium salicylate, for rheumatic diseases, 1895t
Sodium thiocyanate, for cyanide poisoning, 2569t
Sodium thiosulfate, for cyanide poisoning, 2571
Soft palate, 1150f
Solutions, and nosocomial infections, 2484
Soman, as terrorism threat, 2569t, 2570–2571
Somatostatin, 1836
  action of, 1346
Somatostatin/octreotide (Sandostatin), for esophageal varices, 1300, 1304t
Somatotropin. See Growth hormone
Sorbitol, for acute renal failure, 1525
Sore throat. See also Pharyngitis; Tonsillitis
  and acute glomerulonephritis, 1517
Sotalol, 830t
  for atrial fibrillation, 833
  mechanism of action of, 785
  for ventricular tachycardia, 836
Sound
  conduction and transmission of, 2096, 2097f
  frequency of, 2100
  intensity of, 2100
  pitch of, 2100
Sound(s)
  body
    auscultation of, 77–78, 77f
    frequency of, 77
    intensity of, 77
    palpation of, 76
    quality of, 77
  breath. See Breath sounds
  heart. See Heart sounds
Spasticity, 75, 2146
  in amyotrophic lateral sclerosis, 2323
  definition of, 2129
  in multiple sclerosis, 2279, 2280, 2281
  paraplegia/quadriplegia and, 2264–2265
Spastic muscle, 2342
  definition of, 2337
Spatial orientation, low vision/blindness and, 2053
Specific gravity
  definition of, 1493
  of urine, 304, 313, 1497, 1506, 1507, 1507t
    in acute renal failure, 1523, 1523t
    in hypovolemia, 309
    usual reference range for, 310t
SPECT. See Single-photon emission computed tomography
Speculum examination, 1625–1626, 1625f
Speech
  assessment of, 75
  disturbances
    with brain tumor, 2304

people with, interacting and communicating with, 180c–181c
stroke and, 2221
esophageal, 613–614
in Huntington's disease, 2319
Speech therapy, after laryngectomy, 612–614
Speed, abuse/overdose, emergency management of, 2546t
Sperm, 143
Spermatogenesis, 1741
  definition of, 1740
Sperm banking, 1774
Spermicides, 1645–1646
Sphenoid sinus, 1153f
Sphincter of Oddi, 1286, 1345, 1346
  function of, 1124
Spica cast(s), 2355
  care of patient with, 2363
Spica wrap, 2448–2449, 2448f
Spider angiomas, 1939c
  in liver disease, 1308, 1308f
Spina bifida, genetics of, 147t, 148
Spinal accessory nerve (XI), 2136–2137, 2136f, 2137t, 2292f
  assessment of, 2147c
  disorders of, 2294t
Spinal anesthesia, 511, 513–515
  complications of, 514–515
Spinal cord
  anatomy of, 2135–2136
  compression, in cancer patient, 438t–439t
  oncologic disorders of, 2309–2311
  stimulation of, in pain management, 291
  tumors of, 2309–2311
    complications of, 2311
    continuing care with, 2311
    diagnosis of, 2310
    extramedullary-extradural, 2309
    extramedullary-intradural, 2309
    home and community-based care for, 2311
    intramedullary, 2309
    medical management of, 2310
    nursing management of, 2310–2311
    self-care with, 2311
    surgical management of, 2310
    types of, 2309
Spinal cord injury(ies), 2250–2266
  assessment of, 2251, 2256
  clinical manifestations of, 2251, 2252c
  complications of, 2257, 2259–2260
    acute, management of, 2255–2256
    long-term, medical management of, 2261
  continuing care for, 2260–2261
  definition of, 2233
  diagnosis of, 2251
  emergency management of, 2251–2253
  epidemiology of, 2250–2251
  expected outcomes with, 2261
  home and community-based care for, 2260–2261
  level of, and functional abilities, 2251, 2253t
  management of, in acute phase, 2254–2255
  nursing diagnoses related to, 2256–2257
  nursing interventions for, 2257–2261
  nursing process for, 2256–2261
  pathophysiology of, 2251
  pharmacologic therapy for, 2254
  planning and goals for, 2257
  prevention of, 2233c, 2251
  primary, 2251
  and rehabilitation, 192
  respiratory therapy for, 2254
  risk factors for, 2251
  secondary, 2251

Spinal cord injury(ies) (continued)
    self-care after, 2260
    skeletal fracture reduction and traction for, 2254–2255, 2255f
    surgical management of, 2255
    urinary management after, nursing research on, 217
    vertebral involvement in, 2251
Spinal cord lesion
    anterior cord syndrome with, 2251, 2252c
    central cord syndrome with, 2251, 2252c
    complete, 2251
        definition of, 2233
    incomplete, 2251
        definition of, 2233
    lateral cord syndrome with, 2251, 2252c
Spinal fracture, 1460
Spinal manipulation, for low back pain, 2393
Spinal nerves, 2137, 2137f
Spinal shock, 2255–2256
Spinal stenosis, 1920
Spinal tap. See Lumbar puncture
Spinal tracts, 2135f, 2136
Spine
    curvature of, 2347, 2347f
    inspection of, 2347, 2347f
Spinocerebellar tracts, 2135f, 2136
Spinothalamic tracts, 2135f, 2136
SPIRIT (mnemonic), 461–462
Spirituality (and spiritual distress), 122–123
    in acute leukemia, 1078
    definition of, 448
    and end-of-life care, 461–462
    and genetic assessment, 155–156
    and surgical experience, 490–491, 495
Spirometry
    applications of, 689
    in chronic obstructive pulmonary disease, 689, 690t
    definition of, 686
Spironolactone (Aldactone), 953, 954t
    for hypertension, 1026t
Splash exposure, prevention of, 2481–2482
Splash injuries, to eye, 2074
Spleen, 1043, 1122f, 1784, 1784f
Splenectomy
    for blood disorders, 1102
    for idiopathic thrombocytopenic purpura, 1088
    for immune hemolytic anemia, 1062
    therapeutic, 1102
Splenoportogram, 1290t
Splints, 2364
    definition of, 2355
    for fractures, 2433, 2533
    for humeral fracture, 2442
    for rheumatic diseases, 1898
Spondyloarthropathies, 1917
Spondylosis, 2326
    definition of, 2301
Spoon nails, 1940f
Sports-related injuries, 2426–2427
    prevention of, 2427
Sprain, 2425–2426
    definition of, 2425
    sports-related, 2426–2427
    treatment of, 2426
Spray(s), for wound care, 1950
Spray exposure, prevention of, 2481–2482
Sputum
    in bronchiectasis, 709
    in chronic obstructive pulmonary disease, 689
    in lung cancer, 671
    in pneumonia, 636

production of
    clinical significance of, 565
    relief measures for, 565–567
    in respiratory disease, 565–567
purulent, 636, 651
specimen collection, 579–580, 636
studies of, 579–580
Squamous cell carcinoma
    of eyelid, 2080
    of skin, 1979–1981, 1979f
    vulvar, 1685–1686
SSKI. See Saturated solution of potassium iodide
SSRIs. See Selective serotonin reuptake inhibitors
Stab wound
    definition of, 2528c
    thoracic, 678
Stadol. See Butorphanol
Staged amputation, 2461
Staging, of tumor(s), 390–391, 392c
    definition of, 381
Stairs, climbing/descending
    with cane, 207
    with crutches, 205
Stamm gastrostomy, 1188
Standard Precautions, 1818–1819, 1820c–1821c, 2480–2482, 2483c
Standing, with crutches, 205
Stapedectomy, 2111, 2111f
Stapes, 2094, 2095f
    definition of, 2095c
Staphylococci, skin infections caused by, 1957–1958
Staphylococcus aureus
    and arthritis, 1919–1920
    impetigo caused by
        incubation period of, 2476t
        transmission of, 2476t
    methicillin-resistant, 2475
        health care–associated infection potential of, 2482
        pneumonia, antibiotics for, 637
        pneumonia caused by, 629, 633
    methicillin-sensitive
        pneumonia, antibiotics for, 637
        pneumonia caused by, 629
    and osteomyelitis, 2413
    in parotitis, 1147
    pneumonia, 629–634, 632t
    pneumonia caused by, 633
    and septic arthritis, 2416
    transmission of, 2478
    vancomycin-resistant, 2475
        health care–associated infection potential of, 2482
Staphylokinase, for venous thrombosis, 1006
START. See Simple Triage & Rapid Treatment
Starvation, differentiation from anorexia and cachexia, 466
Stasis dermatitis, in diabetes, 1941
Stasis syndromes, malabsorption in, 1240t
Static orthoses, 207
Statins, 864–865, 865t, 986
    for osteoporosis, 2409
    and stroke prevention, 2211
Status asthmaticus, 711, 717–718
    assessment in, 717
    clinical manifestations of, 717
    diagnosis of, 717
    medical management of, 717–718
    nursing management of, 718
    pathophysiology of, 717
Status epilepticus, 2197–2198
    definition of, 2161, 2197

medical management of, 2197–2198
nursing management of, 2198
postoperative, in neurosurgical patient, 2188
Stavudine (Zerit), for HIV infection, 1827t
STD. See Sexually transmitted disease
Steady state, 91–92
    control of, 99–100
    definition of, 91
    stressors and, 92–93
Steapsin, source and digestive action of, 1123t
Steatorrhea
    definition of, 1232, 1345
    after gastric surgery, 1226
Stem cell(s), 1038f, 1039
    definition of, 1036, 1783
    differentiation of, 1038f, 1039
    embryonic, 1793
    harvest of, 1102, 1102t
    and immunology, 1793
    and lymphocytes, 1784, 1785f
    lymphoid, 1038f, 1039
    myeloid, 1038f, 1039
    pluripotent, 1793
Stem cell transplantation, 1793
    for severe combined immunodeficiency disease, 1807
Stenosis
    definition of, 915, 975
    valvular, 915
    vascular, 980
Stent(s)
    coronary artery, 886, 886f
    definition of, 859
    peripheral vascular, 986, 986f
Stent-grafts, peripheral vascular, 986
Stereotactic biopsy
    of breast, 1708–1709
    definition of, 1701
Stereotactic radiosurgery, for cancer, 393
Stereotactic surgery
    for brain tumors, 2305
    for Parkinson's disease, 2315, 2315f
Sterility
    chemotherapy-induced, 402
    pelvic inflammatory disease and, 1671
Sterilization
    female, 1640–1646
    male, 1641, 1641c
    reversal of, 1774
Sternum, fractures of, in trauma patient, 676
Steroid hormone(s), 1441–1442
Stethoscope, 78
Stevens-Johnson syndrome, 1974–1975
    nursing process for, 1975–1977
STI. See Sexually transmitted infection(s)
Stings, poisonous, emergency management of, 2539
Stoma, definition of, 1175
Stoma care
    with cutaneous urinary diversions, 1600
    in ileostomy patient, 1256c–1257c, 1259
    after laryngectomy, patient teaching about, 618–620
    with urinary diversion, 1606
Stomach, 1122f. See also Gastric
    age-related changes in, 1125, 1126c
    anatomy of, 1121
    cancer of. See Gastric cancer
    definition of, 1121
    function of, 1123–1124
    motility of
        regulators of, 1124t
        testing of, 1133
    secretions of, 1123, 1123t

# INDEX

Stomatitis, 1144t, 1151
  in acute leukemia, 1077
  aphthous, 1143t
  in cancer patient, nursing management of, 405c–407c, 426–427
  in chemotherapy patient, 400
  definition of, 381, 1142
  nicotine, 1144t
  severe, in cancer patient, nursing management of, 406c–407c
Stones (calculi)
  calcium, 1591
  cystine, 1591
  gallbladder. See Cholelithiasis
  oxalate, 1591
  salivary, 1148, 1158
  uric acid, 1591
  in urinary tract. See Urolithiasis
Stool
  blood in, 1127
  characteristics of, 1127, 1127t
  color of
    with gallstones, 1349
    substances altering, 1127, 1127t
Stool softeners, for opioid-related constipation, 282
Stool tests, for gastrointestinal disorders, 1130
Stopcock caps, and nosocomial infections, 2484
Strabismus, definition of, 2043
Straight traction, 2366
Strain, 2425–2426
  definition of, 2425
  sports-related, 2426–2427
  treatment of, 2426
Straining, and wound healing, 541t
Stratum corneum, 1930
Strawberry angiomas, 1978
Strep throat, 597–598
  and acute glomerulonephritis, 1517, 1517f
  immune response to, 1787
*Streptococcus pneumoniae*
  drug-resistant, pneumonia caused by
    medical management of, 637
    risk factors for, 637c
  incubation period of, 2477t
  pneumonia, 629, 630t
    risk factors for, 637c
  transmission of, 2477t
*Streptococcus pyogenes*, antibodies against, and cross-reactivity, 1790
Streptokinase, for venous thrombosis, 1006
Streptomycin, and immune system, 1797t
Streptozocin, in cancer treatment, 399t
Stress
  with acute pain, 307–308
  and adaptation, 92
  assessment for, 73, 98
  at cellular level, 99, 99f
  cognitive appraisal of, 93–94
  definition of, 91, 92
  and disease, 93, 97–98
  and emotional distress, 114–115
  and function, 91
  in hospitalized patient with diabetes, 1432
  indicators of, 98, 114c
  laboratory findings in, 98
  mediators of, 93
  metabolic effects of, 95–96
  nursing diagnoses related to, 104
  in older persons, 228
  response to
    immunologic, 96–97
    maladaptive, 97–98
    physiologic, 94–97
    psychological, 93–94
  tolerance, in cardiovascular disease, assessment of, 797
Stress and coping response, in patient profile, 69c
Stress fractures, sports-related, 2427
Stress incontinence, 215
Stress management
  definition of, 49l
  in health promotion, 58
  nurse's role in, 98–99
  nursing interventions in, 104–108
  patient teaching about, 105–107, 107
  progressive muscle relaxation for, 107
  social support and, 107–108
  support and therapy groups for, 108
  for ulcer patient, 1212
Stressor(s)
  definition of, 92–93
  duration of, 93
  physical, 93
  physiologic, 93
  psychosocial, 93
  types of, 92–93
Stress ulcers, 1209
  medical management of, 1212
  pathophysiology of, 1210
  in shock, 362, 366
Stretching, for injury prevention, 2427
Striae, definition of, 1945
Stridor, after neck dissection, 1155
Stroke. See also Hemorrhagic stroke; Ischemic stroke
  acute ischemic, clinical pathway for, 2607f–2608f
  atrial fibrillation and, 833
  after cardiac surgery, 893t
  cardiogenic embolic, 2206, 2207t
  clinical manifestations of, 2207–2210
  and cognitive deficits, 2209t
  cryptogenic, 2206, 2207t
  disability caused by, 2206
  economic effects of, 2206
  and emotional deficits, 2209t
  epidemiology of, 2206
  hypertension and, 1023
  large artery thrombotic, 2206, 2207t
  and motor deficits, 2208t, 2209
  neurologic deficits of, 2207–2210, 2208t–2209t
  prevention of, patient teaching about, nursing research on, 2211
  rehabilitation after, 192
  and sensory deficits, 2208t
  small penetrating artery thrombotic, 2206, 2207t
  and verbal deficits, 2208t
  and visual field deficits, 2208t
Stroke volume, 786, 945
  control of, 786–787
  definition of, 781, 945
Strongyloidiasis, malabsorption in, 1240t
ST segment, 875, 875f, 876f
  definition of, 823
  on ECG, 826
Study to Understand Prognoses and Preferences for Outcomes and Risks of Treatment, 454
Stye, 2076t
Subacute care, for older persons, 230
Subarachnoid hemorrhage
  and hemorrhagic stroke, 2223, 2224
  Hunt-Hess classification of, 2225, 2225t
Subarachnoid screw or bolt, 2172
  definition of, 2161

Subchondral bone
  definition of, 1887
  thinning of, 1888
Subclavian catheter, triple-lumen, 1194
Subculture(s)
  definition of, 128
  and nursing, 128–129
  in United States, 128–129
Subcutaneous tissue, 1927, 1928, 1928f
  aging and, 1931
Subdural hematoma, 2236–2237, 2237f
  acute, 2237
  chronic, 2237–2238
  subacute, 2237
Sublingual gland, 1122f, 1147
Subluxation, 2426
  definition of, 2425
Submandibular gland, 1122f, 1147
Submucosal resection
  definition of, 589
  of deviated nasal septum, 607
Substance abuse, 113
  assessment for, 70, 70c, 120–121, 120c
    preoperative, 486
  and codependent family members, 120
  definition of, 112
  disability and, 192
  in elderly, 240
  emergency management of, 2544–2550, 2545t–2548t
  and HIV infection, 1816c, 1817–1818
  nursing interventions for, 120–121
  pain in sickle cell anemia and, 1059
  rehabilitation programs for, 192–193
  resources and websites on, 126
Succinylcholine (Anectine, Quelicin), 512t
Sucralfate (Sulcrate), 1207t
Sucralose (Splenda), 1388
Sucrase, source and digestive action of, 1123t
Suctioning. See also Aspiration (suctioning)
  nasotracheal, in thoracic surgery patient, 765, 766c
  after neck dissection, 1155
  of tracheal tube, 735, 739, 741c
Sudden cardiac death, 860
  definition of, 859
Sudden death, coping with, helping family members with, 2519, 2519c
Sudomotor neuropathy, in diabetes, 1427
Sufentanil
  for intravenous anesthesia, 512t
  transmucosal, 287
Suicide, 118, 120
  assisted. See Assisted suicide
  attempted, as psychiatric emergency, 2555
  forensic evidence in, collection of, 2529–2530
  in Huntington's disease, 2319, 2320
  intent, as psychiatric emergency, 2555
  risk factors for, 120, 120c
Suicide gene, 422
Suicide rate, in United States, 120
Sulfasalazine (Azulfidine), for rheumatic diseases, 1895t
Sulfate, in body fluids, 302t
Sulfmethemoglobin, in cyanide poisoning, 2571
Sulfonylureas, 1398–1401, 1399t–1400t
  definition of, 1376
Sulfur mustard, as terrorism threat, 2569t, 2570
Sulindac (Clinoril), for rheumatic diseases, 1895t
Sumatriptan (Imitrex), for migraine, 2201
  adverse effects and side effects of, 2201
  contraindications to, 2201

Sump tube(s), 1175–1176
Sundowning, definition of, 225
Sun exposure, and skin cancer, 1978–1979, 1984
Sunlight, and cancer, 386
Superinfection, in pneumonia, 639, 641
Superior mesenteric artery syndrome, with cast, 2363
Superior vena cava, pressures in, 785f
Superior vena cava syndrome, in cancer patient, 438t
Supination, 199c, 2343c
   definition of, 198c
Supine position, 196, 197c
Support, psychological
   in acute renal failure, 1526–1527
   for dialysis patient, 1541, 1552
Support groups, for stress management, 108
Supportive care, for HIV/AIDS patients, 1837
Support system
   in cardiovascular disease, assessment of, 797
   enhancing, in stress management, 107–108
   in patient profile, 70
   for people with disabilities, 219, 221
Suppository, in bowel training, 217
Suppressor T cells
   in cellular immune response, 1791, 1792t
   definition of, 1783
Suppurative pulpitis, 1145
Suprapubic catheter(ization), 1584, 1585–1586, 1586f
   definition of, 1570
Supraventricular tachycardia, 835
   definition of, 823
Surgeon, 505
Surgery
   for acne vulgaris, 1955–1956
   in acute pancreatitis, 1360, 1361f
   ambulatory
     nursing management of, 491
     patient teaching about, 495
   for appendicitis, 1242
   for bladder cancer, 1596–1597
   for brain tumors, 2305
   for breast cancer, 1716–1725
     nursing process with, 1718–1725
   for cancer, 391–394
   cardiac
     complications of, 890, 891t–894t, 895–896, 899
       assessment for, 898–899
     expected outcomes with, 903, 904c–911c
     home and community-based care after, 902–903
     intraoperative nursing management of, 896–897
     nursing management of, 924–925
     postoperative phase
       nursing care plan for, 904c–911c
       nursing process in, 897–911, 898f
     preoperative phase, nursing process for, 890–896
     self-care after, 902, 911c
   cardiac conduction, 854–855
   for cervical cancer, 1684–1685, 1684c
   for cervical disk herniation, 2326
   for chemical burns of esophagus, 1165
   in chronic pancreatitis, 1368–1369
   classification of, by urgency, 484, 485t
   for colorectal cancer, 1267, 1268f, 1269f, 1270f
   complications of, risk factors for, 485–486, 486c
   consent for, 484–485
   continuing care after, 530–531
   cosmetic, 484
   curative, 484
   dermatologic, 1985–1991
   diagnostic, 484
   for diverticular disease, 1244, 1244f
   elective, 484, 485t
   emergency, nursing management of, 492
   emergent, 484, 485t
   for epilepsy, 2194–2195
   for esophageal varices, 1302–1303, 1303f, 1304t
   expected outcomes in, 521
   for gallbladder disease, 1353–1355, 1353f
     nursing process for, 1355–1358
   for glaucoma, 2057–2058
   home and community-based care after, 529–531
   for hyperthyroidism, 1462
   and immune system function, 1796
   for inflammatory bowel disease, 1250–1251, 1251f
   intracranial, 2180–2190
   kidney, 1552–1560
   for laryngeal cancer, 610–612
   in liver cancer, 1334–1335
   for liver transplantation, 1336–1338, 1337f
   mastoid, nursing process for, 2108–2110
   for Ménière's disease, 2113
   for neurogenic bladder, 1585
   optional, 484, 485t
   orbital, 2081–2082
   outpatient (same-day), 481
     definition of, 481
   for ovarian cancer, 1690–1691
   palliative, 484
   for Parkinson's disease, 2315
   in peptic ulcer disease, 1212, 1213t–1214t
   for peritonsillar abscess, 601
   for pituitary tumors, 1447
   plastic reconstructive, 1985–1991
   potential adverse effects of, 503, 504c
     gerontologic considerations in, 503–504
   preoperative assessment for, 485–491
   of prostate, 1761–1769
     complications of, 1764
   for prostate cancer, 1754
   reconstructive, 484
     for breasts, 1731–1733, 1732f, 1733f
     of esophagus, 1167, 1168f
     in neck dissection, 1153
   in renal trauma, 1566
   for renal tumor, 1564
   reparative, 484
   required, 484, 485t
   for rheumatoid arthritis, 1909
   for rotator cuff tears, 2429
   same-day, 481
     definition of, 481
   self-care after, patient teaching for, 529, 531c
   short stay, 481
     definition of, 481
   for skin cancer, 1979–1980
   team for, 503–505
   technology for, advances in, 481
   for temporomandibular disorders, 1147
   for tonsillitis, 599–600
   urgent, 484, 485t
   urinary diversion. See Urinary diversion
   for urolithiasis, 1593
   valid consent for, 484, 485c
   vulvar, nursing process for, 1686–1688
Surgical biopsy, definition of, 1701
Surgical environment, 505–508
   health hazards in, 508

Susceptibility testing, 153
Susceptible, definition of, 2475
Susceptible host, 2475, 2478–2479
Suspected awareness, of terminal status, 450
Suspensions, 1949
   definition of, 1945
Sutures, of skull, 2133, 2133f
Swallowing, 1123
   in amyotrophic lateral sclerosis, 2323
   difficulty in. See also Dysphagia
     esophageal cancer and, 1167
   of foreign bodies, 1165
   nursing interventions for, in multiple sclerosis, 2282
   pain on. See Odynophagia
   in Parkinson's disease, 2317
Swallowing reflex, assessment of, in unconscious patient, 2165t
Sweat, 1931, 1952
Sweat chloride test, 718
Sweat glands, 1928f, 1930
   apocrine, 1930
   eccrine, 1930
Sweeteners, artificial, for diabetic patient, 1387–1388
Swelling, fracture and, 2431
Swing-through gait, 206c
Swing-to gait, 206c
Syme amputation, 2460, 2461f
Sympathetic-adrenal-medullary response, to stress, 95, 96f, 97t
Sympathetic nervous system, 2137–2139, 2139f
   age-related changes in, 788t
   and cardiac function, 825
   definition of, 2129
   in physiologic response to stress, 95, 96f, 97t
   vascular effects of, 978
Sympathetic ophthalmia, 2074
   definition of, 2043
Sympathetic syndromes, 2139
Sympathomimetics, in treatment of shock, 366t
Symptothermal method, of ovulatory timing, 1646
Synarthrosis joints, 2340
Synchronized intermittent mandatory ventilation, 743f, 744
   definition of, 723
   and respiratory weaning, 752
Syncope, in cardiovascular disease, assessment of, 790, 794t
Syndrome of inappropriate antidiuretic hormone secretion, 315–318, 1448, 2180
   brain injury and, 2244
   in cancer patient, 441t
   definition of, 1440
   medical management of, 318
   monitoring for, 2180
   postoperative, in neurosurgical patient, 2187
Synergist muscles, 2342
Synovectomy, for rheumatoid arthritis, 1909
Synovial joints
   definition of, 1887
   inflammation of, 1888f
   movement of, 1887
Synovitis, villonodular, 1920
Synovium, 2341
   definition of, 2337
Synthetic dressings, for burn grafts, 2020t, 2021–2022, 2022f
Syphilis, 2505–2507
   assessment in, 2505–2506

## INDEX

causative organism of, 2477t
co-infection in gonorrhea, 2508
cutaneous manifestations of, 1929t
diagnosis of, 2505–2506
in HIV-infected (AIDS) patients, 1672
latency in, 2505
medical management of, 2506–2507, 2507c
nursing management of, 2507
patient teaching about, 2507, 2507c
and pes cavus, 2402
prevention of, 2507, 2507c
primary, 2505
secondary, 2505
stages of, 2505
tertiary, 2505
Syphilitic aortitis, 996, 2509
Systemic diseases, cutaneous manifestations of, 1929t
Systemic inflammatory response syndrome, 374
definition of, 356, 373c
Systemic lupus erythematosus, 1909–1912
assessment of, 1911
clinical manifestations of, 1909–1911
diagnosis of, 1911
medical management of, 1911
nursing management of, 1911–1912
pathophysiology of, 1909
pharmacologic therapy for, 1911
systemic manifestations of, 1910–1911
thrombocytopenia in, 1087t
Systemic response, in older adults, 249
Systemic sclerosis. See Scleroderma
Systemic vascular resistance, 787
definition of, 781
Systole, 781, 785, 786, 802–803, 802f, 824
atrial, 786
definition of, 781
Systolic hypertension, 1021

## T

Tabun, as terrorism threat, 2570–2571
Tachycardia, in malignant hyperthermia, 517
Tachydysrhythmias, after cardiac surgery, 892t
Tachypnea, 570, 572t
in cardiac patient, 804
in heart failure, 951
with pulmonary embolism, 662
Tacrolimus (Prograf), for kidney transplant recipient, 1561
Tactile fremitus, 76, 572–573, 573f, 576t
Tactile sensation, 2150
age-related changes in, 2151
Tactiloe fremitus, in pneumonia, 636
Tadalafil (Cialis), 1745, 1747t, 1748c–1749c
T'ai chi, 186
Tail of Spence, 1702f
Takayasu's disease, 996
Tamm-Horsfall protein, 1506
Tamoxifen, 388
in breast cancer prevention, 1714–1715
Targeted therapy(ies)
for breast cancer, 1729–1730
in cancer treatment, 418
definition of, 381
Taste perception, age-related changes in, 232t, 237, 2151
tau protein, and Alzheimer's disease, 244
Taxanes
adverse effects and side effects of, 399t
for cancer treatment, 399t
Taxonomy, nursing, unified framework for, 43–45, 46c

Tay-Sachs disease
carrier testing for, 150t, 156
genetics of, 147t
genetic testing in, 149, 150t
screening for, 150t
Tazarotene (Tazorac), for psoriasis, 1966t, 1967
TBG. See Thyroxine-binding globulin
T-cell deficiencies, 1806
assessment of, 1806
clinical manifestations of, 1805–1806
combined with B-cell deficiencies, 1803t, 1806–1807
clinical manifestations of, 1807
medical management of, 1807, 1808c
nursing management of, 1807
pathophysiology of, 1806–1807
diagnosis of, 1806
medical management of, 1806
pathophysiology of, 1805–1806
T cells (T lymphocytes), 1038f, 1039, 1042, 1784, 1787, 1792t
in allergic reaction, 1857
antitumor activity of, 388
CD4, and HIV, 1821–1823
CD8, 1822
in cellular immune response, 1790–1792, 1792t
cytotoxic, 1787–1788, 1791, 1792t
definition of, 1783
definition of, 1783, 1856
functions of, 1037t, 1042, 1787–1788, 1788c
helper, 1791, 1792t
definition of, 1783
in immune response, 1791
and immunodeficiency disorders, 1803t
in inflammation, 1887–1888
in natural immunity, 1785–1786
production of, 1784
suppressor
and carcinogenesis, 388
in cellular immune response, 1791, 1792t
definition of, 1783
Teaching. See also Patient teaching
aids for, 52
definition of, 49l, 50
as function of nursing practice, 49
gerontologic considerations in, 53–54
nursing process in, 54–56, 55c
for people with disabilities, 52–53, 53t
techniques for, 52–53
Tears, 2044
Technetium-99m, for cardiac imaging, 12
Technetium-99m sestamibi (Cardiolite), for cardiac imaging, 812
Technology
advances in, and health care, 8, 16
in assessment, 64–65
and end-of-life care, 449
and surgery, 481
surgical, 481
Teeth, 1150f
cleaning of, in prevention of tooth decay, 1142–1145
disorders of, 1142–1146
Tegaderm, for burn grafts, 2022
Telangiectasia, 1807, 1936, 1939c
definition of, 1802
Tele-health, 16
Telemetry
definition of, 781
for ECG monitoring, 809
Telmisartan (Micardis), for hypertension, 1029t
Telogen phase, of hair growth, 1928

Temperature (body)
brain injury and, 2244, 2245
burns and, 2002, 2011c–2012c, 2015
after cardiac surgery, 902, 910c–911c
in hyperthyroidism, 1464
in hypothyroidism, 1455c
and intracranial pressure, 2173
intraoperative, 517
in liver disease, 1329c
in malignant hyperthermia, 517
normal, 75
in older adults, 248
postoperative, 540–542
regulation of
age-related changes in, 2151
in neurosurgical patient, nursing interventions for, 2186
skin and, 1931
of unconscious patient, 2167
Temperature, environmental, extremes of
avoiding, in COPD, 698
injury caused by, 101–102
Temporal bone, definition of, 2095c
Temporal lobe, 2131, 2131f
Temporomandibular disorders, 1146–1147
definition of, 1142
TEN. See Toxic epidermal necrolysis
Tendinitis, 2397
Achilles, 2427
definition of, 2392, 2425
of elbow, 2427
epicondylar, 2427
infrapatellar, 2427
sports-related, 2427
Tendon(s), 2341
definition of, 2337
neoplasms of, 1920
Tendon transfer, definition of, 2371c
Tenesmus
in colorectal cancer, 1266
definition of, 1232
Teniposide, for cancer treatment, 399t
Tennis elbow, 2427, 2429
Tenofovir (Viread), for HIV infection, 1827t
Tenorrhaphy, for rheumatoid arthritis, 1909
Tenosynovitis, infections and, 1919–1920
TENS. See Transcutaneous electrical nerve stimulation
Tension pneumothorax, 679–680, 680f
definition of, 625
Tentorium cerebelli, 2133
Terazosin (Hytrin), for hypertension, 1028t
Terbutaline (Brethine, Brethaire, Bricanyl), for ventilator-dependent patient, 749
Terconazole (Terazol), for candidiasis, 1662
Teriparatide (Forteo), for osteoporosis, 2409
Terminal bubbling, 469
Terminal illness. See also Death and dying; End-of-life care
awareness of
closed, 449–450
mutual pretense, 450
open, 450
suspected, 450
definition of, 448
delirium in, 468
denial of, 450
depression in, 468
dyspnea in, 465, 466c
hydration in, 466–467, 467t
nursing care in, 456–468
nutrition in, 466–467, 467t
pain in, 464–465
physiologic responses to, management of, 463–468, 463c

Terminal illness (*continued*)
  psychosocial issues in, 456–457
  sociocultural context of, 449–452
  symptoms associated with, 463–468, 463c
    assessment of, patient and caregiver congruence in, nursing research on, 464
Terminally ill patient, communication with, 457–459
Terrorism, 2559
  awareness of, 2564–2565
  biological weapons of, 2566–2569, 2567t
  chemical weapons of, 2569–2571, 2569t
  nuclear materials in, 2571–2574
  preparedness for, 2564–2565
  pulmonary agents in, 2569t, 2571
  recognition of, 2564–2565
Testes, 1741, 1741f
  definition of, 1740
  examination of, 1743–1744
Testicular cancer, 1770–1773
  clinical manifestations of, 1770
  definition of, 1740
  diagnosis of, 1770
  germinal, 1770
  medical management of, 1770–1772
  nongerminal, 1770
  nursing management of, 1772–1773
  risk factors for, 1770
  secondary, 1770
Testicular self-examination, 1744, 1770, 1771c
  nursing research on, 1772
Testosterone
  definition of, 1740
  secretion of, 1741
  skeletal effects of, 2339–2340
Tetanus
  causative organism of, 2477t
  prophylaxis, in burn victim, 2004
Tetany
  in hypocalcemia, 26
  in hypomagnesemia, 329
  T-cell deficiencies and, 1806
Tetracaine (Pontocaine), 514t
Tetracycline (Novotetra), for gastritis and peptic ulcer disease, 1206t
Tetrahydrocannabinol, for nausea/vomiting suppression, 1836
Tetrahydrozoline hydrochloride, for allergic rhinitis, 1872t
Tetraplegia, 2141
  assessment in, 2261–2262
  complications of, 2262
  continuing care for, 2265–2266
  definition of, 2162, 2233
  expected outcomes in, 2266
  in Guillain-Barré syndrome, 2288
  home and community-based care for, 2265–2266
  in locked-in syndrome, 2162
  nursing diagnoses related to, 2262
  nursing interventions for, 2262–2265
  nursing process for, 2261–2266
  planning and goals for, 2262
  self-care for, 2265–2266
  spinal cord injury and, 2251
Tg. *See* Thyroglobulin
Thalamotomy, for Parkinson's disease, 2315
Thalamus, 2131f, 2132, 2142–2143
Thalassemia, 1061
  alpha-, 1061
  beta-, 1061
  carrier testing, 150t
  genetic testing in, 150t
  screening for, 150t

Thalassemia major, 1061
Thalidomide (Thalomid)
  adverse effects and side effects of, 1084
  therapy with, in multiple myeloma, 1084
Thallium-201, for cardiac imaging, 12
THC. *See* Tetrahydrocannabinol
Theophylline, 693t
  for asthma, 713
  therapeutic levels (conventional units and SI units), 2601t
Therapeutic communication, techniques of, 35, 37t
Therapeutic exercises, 198, 201t
Therapeutic Lifestyle Changes (TLC) diet, 863, 864t
Therapeutic regimen
  adherence to, 50
    gerontologic considerations in, 50
  definition of, 49
Therapy group(s), for stress management, 108
Thermal injury. *See also* Burn(s)
  nursing diagnoses related to, 1924–1925
  nursing interventions for, 1924–1925
  nursing outcomes with, 1924–1925
Thiamine deficiency, in liver disease, 1307
Thiazide diuretics, 953, 954t, 955c
  for hypertension, 1026t
Thiazolidinediones, 1398, 1399t–1400t, 1401
  definition of, 1376
6-Thioguanine, in cancer treatment, 399t
Thiopental
  for intravenous anesthesia, 513t
  metabolic effects of, 2173
Thiotepa, in cancer treatment, 399t
Thirst
  antidiuretic hormone and, 306
  in hypernatremia, 320
Thoracentesis, 582, 583c–584c, 628
  definition of, 625
  emergency, 670
  for empyema, 654
  for pleural effusion, 653
Thoracic aortic aneurysm, 997–998, 999f
Thoracic surgery
  anxiety about, 757
  cardiopulmonary complications of, 768–769
    prevention of, 761c
  complications of, 764, 767–769
  expected outcomes after, 770
  nursing diagnoses related to, 764, 771c–775c
  nursing interventions for, 765–770
  nursing process and, 764–775
  patient undergoing
    airway clearance in, 756–757, 765–766, 772c
    arm and shoulder exercises for, 767, 774c
    assessment of, 756, 764
    fluid volume in, 767, 774c
    goals for, 764–765
    nutritional support for, 767
    patient teaching for, 757
    postoperative management of, 757–775
    turning, procedure for, 765
  self-care after, patient teaching about, 769–770, 770c, 774c–775c
  types of, 754, 755c–756c
Thoracoabdominal approach, in renal surgery, 1553f
Thoracolumbar spine, fracture of, 1460
Thoracoscopy, 582, 582f
  video, 756c
Thoracostomy, tube, for empyema, 654
Thoracotomy, 754. *See also* Thoracic surgery

  definition of, 723
  emergency, 670
  expected outcomes after, 770
  nursing care plan for, 771c–775c
  open chest drainage via, for empyema, 654
  pain relief after, 766–767
  patient teaching about, 769–770, 770c
Thorax. *See also* Chest
  anatomic landmarks for, 569, 571c
  palpation of, 570–573
  percussion of, 573–574, 574f, 574t
  physical examination of, 569–573
Thought content, assessment of, 2145
Thought processes
  in Cushing's syndrome, 1482
  in HIV-infected (AIDS) patients, 1846–1847
  in hypothyroidism, 1457c
3 point gait, 206c
Thrills, 76, 801
Throat
  sore. *See* Pharyngitis; Tonsillitis
  strep. *See* Strep throat
Throat culture, 679
Thrombangiitis obliterans, 995–996
Thrombi, prevention of, 666
Thrombin, 1043
  definition of, 1036
Thrombocyte(s). *See also* Platelets
  definition of, 1036
Thrombocythemia, primary (essential), 1085–1086
Thrombocytopenia, 1087–1088
  with anticoagulant therapy, 1007–1008
  in aplastic anemia, 1051
  in cancer patient, 396, 401
    treatment of, 420
  causes of, 1087, 1087t
  chemotherapy-related, 401
  definition of, 381, 1036
  heparin-induced, 871, 1100
  management of, 1087, 1087t
  radiation therapy and, 396
Thrombocytosis
  definition of, 1036
  secondary (reactive), 1086–1087
Thromboembolism, 967
  cerebral metastases and, 2307
  prevention of, 663, 664c
  venous
    fracture and, 2438
    in orthopedic surgery patient, 2385, 2387
    traction and, 2371
Thrombolytic therapy
  for arterial embolism, 1003
  definition of, 859
  in myocardial infarction, 876–877, 878c
  nursing management of, 665, 666
  for pulmonary embolism, 665
    monitoring, 666
  for stroke, 2211–2212
    administration of, 2212
    adverse effects and side effects of, 2212
    dosage of, 2212
  for venous thrombosis, 1006
Thrombophilia, 1095, 1099t
  acquired, 1095, 1099–1102, 1099t
  inherited disorders with, 1095, 1099t
Thrombophlebitis, 1004–1010
  with intravenous therapy, 351
  spinal cord injury and, 2259
  superficial, of breast, 1712
Thrombopoiesis, 1085
Thrombopoietin, 1042
  as alternative to blood transfusion, 1112c

# INDEX

Thrombosis, 1037
  arterial, 1001–1003
  cancer-related, 1099–1100
  in disseminated intravascular coagulation, 1093–1094, 1094c, 1097c–1098c
  in polycythemia vera, 1065
  venous, 1004–1010
    causes of, 662, 662c
Thrombotic disorders, 1095, 1099t
  medical management of, 1095, 1100
  nursing management of, 1100–1102
  pharmacologic therapy for, 1095, 1100
Thrush, of mouth, 1143t
Thumb spica cast, 2355
Thymic hypoplasia, 1803t, 1806
  definition of, 1802
Thymine (T), 141
Thymus gland
  in myasthenia gravis, 2285
  and T cells, 1788, 1790
  transplantation of, 1807
Thyrocalcitonin. See Calcitonin
Thyroglobulin, serum, 1452
Thyroid antibodies, 1451
Thyroid-binding globulin, 1042
Thyroid cancer, 1467–1470, 1467t
  and quality of life, nursing research on, 1469
  radiation exposure and, 1467, 1468c
Thyroid cartilage, 554, 1153f
Thyroid disorders, 1452–1470
  diagnosis of, 1450–1452
  laboratory diagnosis of, 1450–1451
  pathophysiology of, 1450
Thyroidectomy
  definition of, 1440
  subtotal, 1462
Thyroid gland, 1153f
  anatomy and physiology of, 1448–1449, 1449f
  assessment of, 1450–1452
    preoperative, 488
  fine-needle aspiration biopsy of, 1451
  physical examination of, 1450, 1450t
  tumors of, 1466–1470
Thyroid hormone(s), 1448–1449. See also Thyroxine; Triiodothyronine
  and bone health, 2339
  function of, 1449
  oversecretion of. See Hyperthyroidism
  regulation of, 1449
  synthesis of, 1449
  therapy with, perioperative management of, 490t
  undersecretion of. See Hypothyroidism
Thyroiditis, 1466
  acute, 1466
  chronic, 1466
  definition of, 1440
  subacute, 1466
Thyroid nodule(s), 1450, 1450t
Thyroid scan, 1451–1452
Thyroid-stimulating hormone, 1446, 1449
  definition of, 1440
  serum, 1444, 1451
Thyroid storm, definition of, 1440
Thyroid tests, 1451–1452
  medications affecting, 1452, 1452c
Thyrotoxic crisis. See Thyroid storm
Thyrotoxicosis, 1459–1460
  definition of, 1440
Thyrotropin-releasing hormone, 1449
Thyroxine ($T_4$), 1448–1449
  definition of, 1440
  serum, 1451
  serum free, 1451

TIA. See Transient ischemic attack(s)
Tiagabine (Gabitril)
  adverse effects and side effects of, 2194t
  toxic effects of, 2194t
Tibia, fracture of, 2459
Tibial nerve, function of, assessment of, 2346c, 2367
Tic(s), 2146
Ticarcillin-clavulanate (Timentin), for pneumonia, 637
Tic douloureux. See Trigeminal neuralgia
Ticlopidine (Ticlid)
  for coronary artery disease, 870
  for peripheral arterial disease, 992
  and stroke prevention, 2211
Tidal volume, 558t
  in acutely ill patient, 577
Tilt table, 198
Time, attitudes toward, culture and, 132
Timolol
  for glaucoma, 2057, 2058t
  for hypertension, 1027t
Tinea, definition of, 1945
Tinea capitis, 1961–1962, 1961t
Tinea corporis, 1961, 1961f, 1961t
Tinea cruris, 1961t, 1962
Tinea pedis, 1960–1961, 1961t
Tinea unguium, 1961t, 1962
Tinel's sign, 2398, 2398f
Tinnitus, 2118
  with brain tumor, 2304
  definition of, 2093
Tiotropium (Spiriva), for ventilator-dependent patient, 749
Tirofiban (Aggrastat), 871
Tissue(s)
  biopsy, in rheumatic diseases, 1891
  blood flow to, 977
  circulatory needs of, 977. See also Tissue perfusion
  handling of, and wound healing, 541t
  metabolic requirements of, 977
  oxygenation, in burn patient, 2010c
  oxygen consumption by, 977
Tissue expander with permanent implant, definition of, 1701
Tissue integrity
  definition of, 46c
  maintaining
    in cancer patient, 427
    in peripheral vascular disease, 990–991
Tissue perfusion
  in anemia, management of, 1048
  after cardiac surgery, 901–902
  in disseminated intravascular coagulation, 1097c–1098c
  foot surgery and, 2403
  in myocardial infarction, 882c, 884
  and pressure ulcers, 208, 212
Tissue plasminogen activator, 1003
  adverse effects and side effects of, 2212
  criteria for therapy with, 2212, 2212c
  dosage and administration of, 2212
  recombinant, for ischemic stroke, 2211–2212
  for stroke, 2207, 2211–2212
Tissue typing, in rheumatic diseases, 1894t
Tizanidine (Zanaflex), for spasticity, in multiple sclerosis, 2280
TMP-SMZ. See Trimethoprim-sulfamethoxazole
TNF. See Tumor necrosis factor
TNM staging system, 390, 392c
Tobacco
  and cancer, 386

  and cancer of oral cavity, 1148
  and esophageal cancer, 1166, 1167
  and heart disease, 866
  and urinary tract cancers, 1596
Tobacco-related nursing interventions, research on, 642
Tocainide (Tonocard), 830t
Toenail, ingrown, 2401
Tolazamide (Tolinase), 1399t
Tolbutamide (Orinase), 1399t
  metabolism of, genetic factors affecting, 154t
Tolcapone (Tasmar), for Parkinson's disease, 2314
Tolerance
  opioid, 284
    definition of, 259
  pain, 429
    definition of, 259
Tolmetin sodium (Tolectin), for rheumatic diseases, 1895t
Toluene, abuse/overdose, emergency management of, 2546t
Tone, of muscle, 2146, 2342
  assessment of, 2349
  definition of, 2129, 2337
Tongue, 1150f, 1153f
  cancer of, 1148–1149
  inspection of, 1150
  turgor of, assessment of, 312
Tonicity, 302
  definition of, 301
Tonometry, 2050
Tono-Pen, 2050
Tonsil(s). See also Peritonsillar abscess
  anatomy of, 554, 599
  inspection of, 1150
  lingual, 1153f
  palatine, 1150f, 1153f
Tonsillectomy, 599–600
  with peritonsillar abscess, 601
Tonsillitis, 599–600
  definition of, 589
Tonus, 2342
  definition of, 2337
Tooth. See also Teeth
  abscessed, 1145–1146
Tooth decay, 1142–1145
Tophi
  definition of, 1887
  gout and, 1918
Topical preparation(s), 1948, 1949t
Topiramate (Topamax)
  adverse effects and side effects of, 2194t
  for migraine, 2201
  toxic effects of, 2194t
Topoisomerase I inhibitors, for cancer treatment, 399t
Topotecan
  in cancer treatment, 399t
  for cerebral metastases, 2307
Torres Strait Islanders. See Indigenous people
Torsades de pointes
  in hypocalcemia, 326
  treatment of, 836
Torsemide (Demadex), 954t
  for hypertension, 1026t
  for hypervolemia, 313
Tortoise shell, 742
Tositumomab (Bexxar), 418, 419t
  adverse effects and side effects of, 421t
Total artificial heart, 929
  definition of, 915
Total hip replacement, 2373–2375, 2373f
Total incontinence, 215

Total joint arthroplasty/replacement, definition of, 2371c
Total knee replacement, 2375–2376
Total lung capacity, 558t
Total nutrient admixture, definition of, 1175
Touch, culture and, 132–133
Tourniquet, for control of hemorrhage, 2527
Toxic anterior segment syndrome, 2063
Toxic epidermal necrolysis, 1974–1975
　nursing process for, 1975–1977
Toxic shock syndrome, definition of, 1661
Toxin(s)
　aplastic anemia caused by, 1051
　chemical injury caused by, 102
Toxoplasmosis, in HIV-infected (AIDS) patients, 1833
t-PA. See Tissue plasminogen activator
T-piece, for oxygen delivery, 725t, 727, 727f, 752
TP interval, on ECG, 826, 827f
　definition of, 823
Trabeculae, 2339
　definition of, 2337
Trabecular bone. See Cancellous (trabecular) bone
Trabeculectomy, for glaucoma, 2058
Trace elements, and immune system function, 1795
Trachea, 1122f
　anatomy of, 554
　obstruction of, 608
　physical examination of, 569
Tracheobronchitis, acute, 628
Tracheoesophageal puncture, 614, 614f
Tracheostomy, 735, 738–739
　care for, patient teaching about, 619
　complications of, 738–739, 739c
　nursing management of, 739, 740c–741c
Tracheostomy button, 754
Tracheostomy collar, 725t, 727, 727f
Tracheostomy tube, 738–739, 738f
　complications with, 738–739, 739c
　cuff, management of, 739
　definition of, 723
　self-care for, patient teaching about, 739
　suctioning of, 739, 741c
　weaning from, 754
Tracheotomy, 738–739
　definition of, 723
Trachoma, 2077
　definition of, 2043
Traction, 2365–2371
　and anxiety, 2370
　assessment of patient in, 2369
　balanced suspension, 2366, 2367f
　Buck's extension, 2366–2367, 2366f
　complications of, 2367, 2369–2371
　definition of, 2355
　effective
　　ensuring, 2367, 2368
　　principles of, 2365–2366
　expected outcomes with, 2371
　for fracture reduction, 2433
　halo, 2254–2255, 2255f, 2258, 2259c
　for hip fracture, 2447, 2449
　manual, 2366
　and mobility, 2370
　nursing diagnoses related to, 2369
　nursing interventions for, 2370–2371
　nursing process for, 2369–2371
　patient teaching about, 2370
　planning and goals for, 2370
　running, 2366
　and self-care, 2370
　skeletal, 2366
　　for spinal cord injury, 2254–2255, 2255f
　skin, 2366–2368
　straight, 2366
　types of, 2366
　vectors of force in, 2365, 2366f
Tramadol, pharmacology of, 283t
TRAM flap. See Transverse rectus abdominis myocutaneous flap
Trandolapril (Mavik), 952–953, 952t
　for hypertension, 1029t
Tranquilizers, interactions with anesthetics, 490t
Transbronchial, definition of, 625
Transbronchial lung biopsy, 585
　in sarcoidosis, 667
Transcatheter bronchial brushing, 585
Transcellular fluid, 301
Transcranial Doppler, 2155
Transcription, 143
　definition of, 140
Transcultural nursing, 128–137
　definition of, 129
Transcultural nursing care, future of, 136–137
Transcutaneous electrical nerve stimulation, in pain management, 289
TransCyte, for burn grafts, 2022
Transection, definition of, 2233
Transesophageal echocardiography, 811–812
　nursing interventions in, 811–812
Trans fats, 82
Transfer, assisting patient with, 201–203, 203c
Transfer board, 202
Transferrin, 1039, 1042
　serum, 80
Transfusion reaction(s), 1109–1111
　acute hemolytic, 1109
　acute renal failure in, 1523
　allergic, 1109–1110
　delayed hemolytic, 1110
　febrile nonhemolytic, 1109
　hemolytic, 1062–1063
　with long-term PRBC therapy, 1111t
　nursing management of, 1111
　patient teaching about, 1109
　prevention of, 1106–1107
Transfusion therapy, 1103–1104, 1103t. See also Blood transfusion(s)
　complications of, 1057
　long-term, complications of, 1111, 1111t
　for sickle cell anemia, 1057–1058
Transient ischemic attack(s). See also Ischemic stroke
　carotid endarterectomy for, 2214
　definition of, 2210
　diagnosis of, 2210
　hypertension and, 1023
Transjugular intrahepatic portosystemic shunt, 1295, 1297f
　for esophageal varices, 1302, 1304t
Transmission, route of, of infectious organism, 2475
Transmission-Based Precautions, 2480, 2482
Transnational nursing, 129
Transrectal electrical stimulation, for urinary incontinence, 1583c
Transrectal ultrasound
　in males, 1753–1754
　of prostate, 1744
　in UTI diagnosis, 1574
Transsacral (caudal) block, 515
Transsphenoidal approach, 181t, 2180, 2189–2190
　for brain tumor, 2304
　complications of, 2189
　definition of, 2161, 2180
　postoperative phase of
　　medical management of, 2189
　　nursing management of, 2189–2190
　preoperative phase of
　　medical management in, 2189
　　nursing management in, 2189
Transurethral fulguration, for bladder cancer, 1596–1597
Transurethral incision of prostate, 1752, 1762t, 1763, 1763f
Transurethral resection, for bladder cancer, 1596–1597
Transurethral resection of prostate, 1746, 1761, 1762t, 1763f
　definition of, 1740
Transurethral resection syndrome, 1761, 1764c
Transvaginal electrical stimulation, for urinary incontinence, 1583c
Transverse colon, 1122f
Transverse rectus abdominis myocutaneous flap (TRAM flap), 1732–1733, 1733f
　definition of, 1701
Trapeze
　with body casts, 2363
　definition of, 2355
Trastuzumab (Herceptin), 419t
　adverse effects and side effects of, 421t
Trauma. See also Posttraumatic stress disorder
　acoustic, 2102
　bladder, 1595
　　management of, 1595
　blunt, abdominal, 2530–2531
　chest, 675–681
　crush injuries in, 2532–2533
　definition of, 2529
　emergency care for, 2529–2533
　forensic evidence in, collection of, 2529–2530
　fractures in, 2533
　genitourinary, 1595–1597
　　medical management of, 1595
　incidence of, 2529
　injury prevention and, 2530
　intra-abdominal injuries in, 2530–2531
　mechanical, injury caused by, 102
　mortality rate for, 2529
　multiple
　　assessment in, 2530
　　diagnosis in, 2530
　　management of, 2530, 2531f
　　nursing diagnoses related to, 2472–2473
　　nursing interventions for, 2472–2473
　　nursing outcomes with, 2472–2473
　musculoskeletal, assessment of, 2349–2350
　neurologic, 2232–2266–1943, 2240, 2240c, 2241f, 2243–2244
　ocular, 2073–2075
　orbital, 2072–2073
　and pelvic fracture, 2444–2449
　penetrating, abdominal, 2530–2531
　and post-traumatic seizures, 2249
　prevention and control of
　　in ventilator-dependent patient, 749–750
　　with vertigo, 2116c
　pulmonary contusion in, 677–678
　renal, management of, 1565–1566
　and rheumatic disorders, 1920
　to scalp, 2234
　ureteral, 1595
　urethral, 1595
　　management of, 1595
Traumatic brain injury, and rehabilitation, 192
Travel, and infectious diseases, 2512
Travellers, vaccinations for, 2487

# INDEX

Travel vision, 2051
Tremor(s), 75, 2142, 2146
　in Parkinson's disease, 2312
Trench mouth, 1144t
*Treponema pallidum*, 2505
　incubation period of, 2477t
　transmission of, 2477t
$T_3$ resin uptake test, 1451
Tretinoin. *See* Vitamin A
TRH. *See* Thyrotropin-releasing hormone
Triage
　categories of, 2562, 2562t
　data collection in, 2521
　definition of, 2517
　of disaster victims, 2521, 2561–2562
　in emergency care, 2520–2521
　field, 2521
　five-level system for, 2521
　history-taking in, 2521
　in mass casualty incident, 2561–2562
　routine, 2521
Triamcinolone, 1485t
Triamterene (Dyrenium), 954t
　for hypertension, 1026t
Trichiasis, 2077
*Trichinella spiralis*
　incubation period of, 2477t
　transmission of, 2477t
Trichinosis, causative organism of, 2477t
Trichlorethylene, abuse/overdose, emergency management of, 2546t
Trichlormethiazide (Metahydrin, Naqua), 954t
Trichomoniasis, 1626, 1626t, 1663t, 1664
　in HIV-infected (AIDS) patients, 1673
*Trichophyton*, and tinea unguium, 1962
Tricuspid area, examination of, 801, 801f
Tricuspid valve, 782f, 783, 915, 916f
　definition of, 915
Tricyclic antidepressants
　abuse/overdose, emergency management of, 2548t
　for depression, 240
　metabolism of, genetic factors affecting, 154t
　for pain management, 285
　for pruritus, 1952
Trigeminal nerve (VI), 2044, 2136–2137, 2136f, 2137t, 2292f
　assessment of, 2147c
　branches of, distribution of, 2292
　disorders of, 2293t
　microvascular decompression of, 2295
Trigeminal neuralgia, 2292–2295
　medical management of, 2295
　pharmacologic therapy for, 2295
　surgical management of, 2295
Trigeminy, 835
Triggered response, by pacemaker, 823
Triglycerides, 806
　digestion of, enzymes for, 1123t
　serum levels of, management of, 863
Triiodothyronine ($T_3$), 1448–1449
　definition of, 1440
　serum, 1451
Trimethoprim-sulfamethoxazole
　for *Pneumocystis jiroveci* pneumonia, 1835
　therapy with, in HIV-infected (AIDS) patients, 1835
　　adverse effects and side effects of, 1835
　　indications for, 1835
　for urinary tract infections, 1574
Trinucleotide repeat, 144
Triple-H therapy, for cerebral vasospasm, 2226

Triple-lumen subclavian catheter, 1194
Tripod position, 75
　for crutch stance, 204, 205f
Triptans, for migraine, 2201
Trisomy, 143
　definition of, 140
Trisomy 13, 148
Trisomy 18, 148
　screening for, 150t
Trisomy 21. *See* Down syndrome
Trizivir, for HIV infection, 1827t
Trochlear nerve (IV), 2044, 2136–2137, 2136f, 2137t, 2292f
　assessment of, 2147c
Tropical sprue, malabsorption in, 1240t
Tropicamide, ocular applications of, 2086t
Troponin
　definition of, 859
　in myocardial infarction, 805–806, 876, 876t
Troponin I, in cardiac patient, 805–806, 876, 876t
Troponin T, in cardiac patient, 805–806, 876, 876t
Trousseau's sign, 326, 326f, 329
　definition of, 1440
TRUS. *See* Transrectal ultrasound; Transurethral resection, of the prostate
Trust, in nurse-patient relationship, 31–32
Truvada, for HIV infection, 1827t
*Trychophyton* spp.
　incubation period of, 2477t
　transmission of, 2477t
Trypsin, 1124, 1346
　definition of, 1121, 1345
　source and digestive action of, 1123t
TSE. *See* Testicular self-examination; Transmissible spongiform encephalopathies
TSH. *See* Thyroid-stimulating hormone
TSS. *See* Toxic shock syndrome
Tubal ligation, 1640–1641, 1641c
Tubal pregnancy. *See* Ectopic pregnancy
Tube(s)
　aspirate from, pH testing of, to confirm tube placement, 1175, 1178
　gastric sump, 1175–1176, 1176, 1176f, 1176t
　gastrointestinal
　　blue pigtail, 1176
　　insertion of, 1177–1178
　　Levin, 1175–1176
　　long, 1176
　　measurement of, 1177f
　　medium, 1176
　　placement of, confirmation of, 1178
　　Salem, 1176, 1176f
　　securing, 1178, 1180f
　　Sengstaken-Blakemore, 1175
　　short, 1175–1176
　　sump, 1175–1176
　　types of, 1175–1177, 1176t
　nasoduodenal, definition of, 1175
　nasoenteric, 1177
　　for decompression, 1176–1177, 1176t, 1177
　　for feeding, 1176–1177, 1176t
　　long, 1176–1177
　　medium-length, 1176–1177
　nasogastric, 1175–1176, 1176t
　　definition of, 1175
　nasojejunal, definition of, 1175
　orogastric, 1175
Tube feeding(s). *See also* Enteral nutrition
　administration methods for, 1182–1183

　for brain injury patients, 2244
　complications of, 1183, 1184t
　continuing care in, 1188
　delivery systems for, 1186
　expected outcomes with, 1188
　gastrostomy and, comparison of, 1188
　nasoenteric, 1176–1182
　nasogastric, 1176–1182
　nursing diagnoses related to, 1183
　nursing interventions for, 1183–1188
　nursing process for, 1183–1188
　nutritional balance in, 1183–1184
　refusal of, by elderly person, 251c
　regimens, assessment of, 1186c
　regimens for, 1186, 1187c
Tube feeding formula(s), 1182
　delivery systems for, 1186
Tube feeding syndrome, 1184t
Tuberculin skin test, 645, 646f, 2512
Tuberculosis, 643–650
　adult-type, 644
　assessment in, 645–646
　causative organism of, 643, 2477t
　classification of, 646
　clinical manifestations of, 644
　complications of, 649–650
　continuing care in, 650
　epidemiology of, 643, 2512
　expected outcomes in, 650
　extrapulmonary, 644, 650
　follow-up for, 650
　gerontologic considerations in, 248, 646
　in HIV-infected (AIDS) patients, 643, 645–646, 1831, 1833
　　tuberculin skin test results in, 645–646
　immigration and, 2512
　malnutrition in, 649
　miliary, 650
　multidrug resistance in, 649
　nursing process in, 648–650
　planning and goals in, 649
　prevention of, 648
　pulmonary, 643–650
　　clinical manifestations of, 644
　　medical management of, 647t
　　　adherence to, promoting, 649
　　　adverse effects and side effects of, 647t, 649
　　pathophysiology of, 644
　reactivation, 644
　risk factors for, 643, 644c
　self-care in, patient teaching about, 650
　with silicosis, 669
　spread of, 650
　transmission of, 644
　　in health care settings, prevention of, 644, 645c
　vaccine against, 648
*d*-Tubocurarine, 513t
Tubular reabsorption, 1496–1497, 1496f
　definition of, 1493
Tubular secretion, 1496–1497, 1496f
　definition of, 1493
TUIP. *See* Transurethral incision of prostate
Tularemia
　as bioterrorism threat, 2567t
　mortality rate for, 2567t
　treatment of, 2567t
Tumor(s). *See also* Brain tumor(s); Neoplasm(s); *specific tumor*
　benign, 383
　　characteristics of, 384t
　　nomenclature for, 383t
　of skin, 1977–1978
　of external ear, 2106

Tumor(s) (continued)
  of head of pancreas, 1370–1372
  and intestinal obstruction, 1263, 1264t
  of liver
    metastatic, 1333
    primary, 1333
  malignant, 383
    characteristics of, 384t
    nomenclature for, 383t
    of skin, 1978–1982
  ocular, 2080–2081
  orbital, 2080–2081
  pancreatic islet, 1372
  pituitary, 1446–1447
  renal, 1563–1565
  of skin, 1937c, 1977–1982
  testicular, 1770
  thyroid, 1466–1470
  ulcerogenic, 1372
  uterine, benign, 1679
Tumor-associated antigens, 388
Tumor cell antigens, 388
Tumor lysis syndrome, 442t
  in acute myeloid leukemia treatment, 1072
Tumor markers, identification of, in cancer detection, 391t
Tumor necrosis factor, 1791, 1791t
  alpha, action of, 1791t
  beta, action of, 1791t
  in rheumatoid arthritis, 1908
  and wasting syndrome, 1832
Tumor-specific antigen, 384
  definition of, 381
Tumor suppressor gene(s), 385
Tunnelled central catheter(s), 1196
TUR. See Transurethral resection of the prostate
Turbinate bones
  anatomy of, 553, 554f
  hypertrophy of, 606–607
Turgor
  of skin, 1936
    assessment of, 312, 798
      in older persons, 310, 312
  of tongue, assessment of, 312
Turner syndrome, 143, 148
TURP. See Transurethral resection of the prostate
TWAR agent. See Chlamydia pneumoniae
T wave, on ECG, 826, 827f
  definition of, 823
TWEAK, 70
2 point gait, 206c
Tympanic membrane, 2094, 2094c, 2095f
  definition of, 2095c
  perforation of, 2106
Tympanogram, 2100
Tympanoplasty, 2106, 2108
  definition of, 2093
Tympanotomy, 2106–2107
Tympany, 76
Type 1 diabetes. See Diabetes mellitus, type 1
Type 2 diabetes. See Diabetes mellitus, type 2
Tzanck smear, 1942

## U

Ulcer(s)
  Curling's, 1210
    in burn victim, 2002, 2015c
  Cushing's, 1210
  duodenal, 1209–1217, 1210t
  esophageal, 1209
  of foot, in diabetes, 1941
  gastric, 1209–1217, 1210t
  gastrointestinal. See also Peptic ulcer disease
    in neurosurgical patient, nursing interventions for, 2185c
  genital
    in HIV-infected (AIDS) patients, 1673
    in males, 1750
  leg (lower extremity), 804, 1011–1012
    arterial, 1011–1012, 1012f
    assessment of, 1012, 1013
    clinical manifestations of, 1011–1012
    complications of, 1013
    débridement of, 1012–1013
    in diabetes, 1427–1428, 1941
    diagnosis of, 1012
    expected outcomes with, 1014
    home and community-based care for, 1014
    medical management of, 1012–1013
    nursing diagnoses related to, 1013
    nursing interventions for, 1013–1014
    nursing process with, 1013–1014
    pathophysiology of, 1011
    pharmacologic therapy for, 1012
    planning and goals for, 1013
    in sickle cell anemia, 1059
    stimulated healing of, 1013
    topical therapy for, 1013
    venous, 1012
    wound dressing for, 1013
  pressure. See Pressure ulcers
  skin, 1929t, 1938c, 1977
  stress, 1209
    medical management of, 1212
    pathophysiology of, 1210
    in shock, 362, 366
  venous, with chronic venous insufficiency, 1011
Ulcerative colitis, 1247t. See also Inflammatory bowel disease
  clinical manifestations of, 1247t, 1249
  complications of, 1247t, 1249
  diagnosis of, 1247t, 1249
  epidemiology of, 1248
  medical management of, 1247t
  pathophysiology of, 1247t, 1248–1249
Ulnar deviation, 200c
Ulnar nerve, function of, assessment of, 2346c
Ulnar shaft, fracture of, 2443
Ultrafiltration
  definition of, 1515
  in hemodialysis, 1538
Ultram. See Tramadol
Ultrasonography
  abdominal, 1130–1131, 1507
    in biliary/pancreatic disease, 1349–1350, 1349t
    in gastrointestinal assessment, 1130–1131
    nursing interventions in, 1130–1131
    in trauma victim, 2532
  bladder, 1507–1508
  breast biopsy guided by, 1709
  of breasts, 1706–1708
  in cancer detection, 391t
  continuous-wave, in peripheral vascular disease, 981, 981f
  definition of, 1701
  duplex
    colour flow techniques, in peripheral vascular disease, 982, 982f
    definition of, 975
    in peripheral vascular disease, 982
  of eye, 2049
  FAST (Focused Assessment for Sonographic Examination of the Trauma Patient), 2532
  in females, 1631
  of hepatobiliary system, 1289
  in liver disease, 1291t
  of prostate, 1744
  quantitative, in osteoporosis, 2407
  in UTI diagnosis, 1574
Ultraviolet-A light therapy, for psoriasis, 1966t, 1967–1968
Ultraviolet-B light therapy, for psoriasis, 1966t, 1968
Ultraviolet radiation
  and cancer, 386
  for osteomalacia, 2411
Unconscious patient. See Consciousness, altered level of
Undernutrition, 101
Uniform Determination of Brain Death Act, 2239
United Kingdom Prospective Diabetes Study Group, 1383–1384, 1393
United Organ Sharing Network, 1338
United States
  causes of death in, 226, 226t
  health goals for, 56
  health indicators used in, 56c
  life expectancy in, 225, 225f
  multiculturalism in, 128–129
  population demographics in, 7, 16
  subcultures in, 128–129
  suicide rate in, 118
Unrestricted zone, 506
  definition of, 503
Upper esophageal sphincter, 1162
Upper extremity, amputation of, 2461, 2461f
  in farmers, nursing research on, 2463
Upper gastrointestinal endoscopy, 1134–1135
  nursing interventions in, 1135
Upper motor neurons, 2140–2141
  lesions, 2141, 2141t
Uppers, abuse/overdose, emergency management of, 2546t
Urban Search and Rescue Teams, 2560
Urea, serum, 305
Urea breath tests, 1130
Urea nitrogen. See also Blood urea nitrogen
  definition of, 1493
Uremia
  in acute glomerulonephritis, 1518
  in chronic renal failure, 1528, 1529
  definition of, 1515
  in dialysis patient, nursing interventions for, 1551
  and immune system function, 1796
  and skin color, 1935t
Uremic bone disease, in chronic renal failure, 1529
Uremic frost, in chronic renal failure, 1528
Ureter(s)
  anatomy of, 1494f, 1495–1496
  trauma to, 1595
Ureterolithotomy, for urolithiasis, 1593
Ureteropelvic junction, 1495
Ureteroscopy, for urolithiasis, 1591–1593, 1592f
Ureterosigmoidostomy, 1599f, 1602–1603
  definition of, 1570
Ureterostomy, cutaneous, 1598f
Ureterovesical junction, 1495
Ureterovesical reflux, 1571, 1572f
  definition of, 1570
  and pyelonephritis, 1577
Urethra
  anatomy of, 1495–1496
  inflammation of. See Urethritis
  male, 1741, 1741f
    stricture of, 1775

# INDEX

trauma to, 1595
  management of, 1595
  in urinary catheterization, 1586–1588
Urethritis, 1570
  definition of, 1570
  in males, 1750
Urethrocele, 1505
Urethrovesical reflux, 1571, 1572f
  definition of, 1570
Urge incontinence, 215, 247
Urgency, urinary, 1503, 1503t
Urgent patients, 2520–2521
  definition of, 2517
Uric acid, serum, in rheumatic diseases, 1893t
Uricosuric agents, for gout, 1918
Urinalysis, 1505–1506, 1506t, 1507t
  in chronic glomerulonephritis, 1519
Urinary casts
  in chronic glomerulonephritis, 1519
  definition of, 1515
Urinary catheter(ization). See Catheter(ization), urinary
Urinary continence, promotion of, strategies for, 1583c
Urinary diversion, 1597–1607
  complications of, 1605–1606
  continent, 1598
    definition of, 1570
    types of, 1599f
  continuing care after, 1607
  cutaneous, 1597–1602, 1598f
    continuing care with, 1601–1602
    ostomy appliance in
      changing of, 1600, 1601c
      cleaning, 1601
      deodorizing, 1601
      management of, 1600–1602
      selection of, 1600
    types of, 1598f
  expected outcomes of, 1607
  nursing process with, 1603–1607
  postoperative phase of, nursing process for, 1604–1607
  preoperative phase of, nursing process for, 1603–1604
  stoma care with, 1606
Urinary drainage, in renal surgical patient, 1554–1558, 1556c–1557c
Urinary elimination
  in anorectal disorders, 1279
  impaired, hip fracture and, 2452c
  in prostate cancer, 1755c–1756c
  in renal surgical patient, 1554–1558, 1556c–1557c
  spinal cord injuries and, 2258
Urinary incontinence, 215, 1503, 1503t, 1578–1589
  assessment of, 1580
  behavioral therapy for, 1581, 1582c–1583c
  definition of, 225, 1493, 1570
  diagnosis of, 1580
  epidemiology of, 1578–1579
  functional, 215, 1579–1580
    definition of, 1570
  gerontologic considerations in, 233, 247–248, 1580
  iatrogenic, 1580
    definition of, 1570
  medical management of, 1580–1581
  mixed, 1580
  nursing management of, 216–217, 1581
  overflow, 1579
    definition of, 1570
  pharmacologic therapy for, 1581

postoperative
  in older adults, 547
  in older persons, 547
reflex, 215, 1579
  definition of, 1570
risk factors for, 1579, 1580c
stress, 215, 1579
  definition of, 1570
  nursing diagnoses related to, 1490–1491
  nursing interventions for, 1490–1491
  nursing outcomes for, 1490–1491
  risk factors for, 1500
in stroke patient, 2220
surgical management of, 1581
transient, 1580
treatment for, 247
types of, 1579–1580
urge, 215, 247, 1579
  definition of, 1570
in urinary tract infections, 1572
Urinary retention, 1581–1584
  nursing diagnoses related to, 1490–1491
  nursing management of, 1490–1491, 1584
  nursing outcomes for, 1490–1491
  in orthopedic surgery patient, 2387
  pathophysiology of, 1583
  postoperative, 543
Urinary sediment, in acute renal failure, 1523t, 1524
Urinary sphincter, artificial, 1581, 1583f
Urinary stasis, traction and, 2370–2371
Urinary system, age-related changes in, 1795t
Urinary tract
  age-related changes in, 1500, 1503–1504
  anatomy of, 1493–1496
  bacterial invasion of, 1571
  cancers of, 1563–1565
  diagnostic evaluation of, 1505–1513
    nursing care plan for, 1511c–1512c
    nursing diagnoses related to, 1510
    nursing implications of, 1510–1513
    patient teaching about, 1510, 1511c
  disorders of
    gastrointestinal symptoms in, 1503
    genetic aspects of, 1501
    gerontologic considerations in, 1503–1504
    risk factors for, 1500, 1501t
  function, monitoring of, after kidney transplantation, 1561
  imaging of, 1507–1509
  lower, phsyiology of, 1496–1500
  physical examination of, 1504–1505, 1504f, 1505f
  physiology of, 1496f
  stones in. See Urolithiasis
  upper, phsyiology of, 1496–1500
Urinary tract infection(s), 1570–1578
  catheter-related, 1586
  classification of, 1570, 1570c
  clinical manifestations of, 1572
  complicated, 1570, 1570c, 1571
    clinical manifestations of, 1572
  epidemiology of, 1571
  gerontologic considerations in, 1572
  lower, 1570, 1570c, 1571–1577
    assessment of, 1573–1574, 1575
    clinical manifestations of, 1572
    complications of, 1575–1576
    diagnosis of, 1573–1574
    expected outcomes in, 1576–1577
    gerontologic considerations in, 1572–1573, 1573c
    medical management of, 1574–1575
    nursing diagnoses related to, 1575

nursing interventions for, 1575–1576
nursing process with, 1575–1577
pathophysiology of, 1571–1572
patient teaching about, 1576, 1577c
pharmacologic therapy for, 1574–1575
planning and goals for, 1575
recurrence, prevention of, 1576, 1577c
in multiple sclerosis, 2280
paraplegia/quadriplegia and, 2263
recurrence of, prevention of, 1576, 1577c
risk factors for, 1571, 1571c
routes of, 1572
traction and, 2370–2371
uncomplicated, 1570, 1570c, 1571
upper, 1570, 1570c, 1577–1578. See also Pyelonephritis
  clinical manifestations of, 1577–1578
and urolithiasis, 1594
Urine
  in acute glomerulonephritis, 1517
  color of, 1505, 1506t
    with gallstones, 1349
  cultures, in UTI diagnosis, 1573–1574
  formation of, 1496–1497, 1496f
  glucose in, testing for, 1391
  laboratory studies of, in musculoskeletal assessment, 2351–2352
  leakage of, 1505
  osmolality of, 304, 1497, 1506, 1507, 1507t
    in acute renal failure, 1523t
    usual reference range for, 310t
  output of, in acute renal failure, 1523–1524, 1523t
  pH of, usual reference range for, 310t
  residual, 1500, 1581
    definition of, 1570
  retention of, 1500
    prevention of, in unconscious patient, 2167–2168
  specific gravity of, 304, 313, 1497, 1506, 1507, 1507t
    in acute renal failure, 1523, 1523t
    in hypovolemia, 309
    usual reference range for, 310t
  storage of, 1499
Urine chemistry, reference ranges for, 2596t–2599t
Urobilinogen
  fecal, 1290t
  urine, 1290t
Urofollitropin (Bravelle), for ovulation induction, 1651c
Urography, intravenous, for ureteral trauma, 1595
Urokinase, for venous thrombosis, 1006
Urolithiasis, 1589–1595
  assessment of, 1590–1591
  clinical manifestations of, 1590
  continuing care in, 1594
  diagnosis of, 1590–1591
  expected outcomes with, 1595
  medical management of, 1591–1592
  in neurogenic bladder, 1585
  pathophysiology of, 1589–1590, 1590f
  prevention of, 1591, 1591c
  risk factors for, 1590
  surgical management of, 1591–1592
Uromodulin, 1506
Urosepsis, 1575
  definition of, 1570
Ursodeoxycholic acid, for gallstones, 1351
Urticaria, 1878–1879, 1929t
  definition of, 1856
Uterine artery, embolization of, 1679

Uterine cancer, 1685
  epidemiology of, 1682
  risk factors for, 1685, 1685c
Uterine prolapse, 1624, 1627, 1675–1677, 1676f
  definition of, 1613
Uterotubography, 1631
Uterus
  anatomy of, 1614–1615
  benign tumors of, 1679
  palpation of, 1626, 1626f
  positions of, 1675, 1676f
UTI. See Urinary tract infection(s)
Uvea, 2044
Uveitis, 2079
Uvula, 1150f, 1153f
  inspection of, 1150
U wave
  definition of, 823
  on ECG, 826

## V

Vaccination programs, 2484–2488
Vaccine(s). See also Immunization(s)
  and acquired immunity, 1786
  for adults, 2484–2487, 2485f–2487f
  adverse reactions to, 2484
    reporting, 2488
  anthrax, 2568
  cancer, 420
    allogeneic, 420
    autologous, 420
    prophylactic, 420
    therapeutic, 420
  in chronic obstructive pulmonary disease, 693, 698
  contraindications to, 2488
  human immunodeficiency virus, 1830
  influenza, 248, 2488
    in chronic obstructive pulmonary disease, 693, 698
    and Guillain-Barré syndrome, 2288
  information about, sources of, 2487
  Internet resources on, 2487
  live, contraindications to, 2488
  for older adults, 248
  pneumococcal, 248
    in chronic obstructive pulmonary disease, 693, 698
  recommendations for, 2487
  smallpox, 2568
  tuberculosis, 648
Vacuum aspiration, 1648, 1649c
VAD. See Vascular access device
Vagal maneuvers, for atrioventricular (AV) nodal reentry tachycardia, 835
Vagina
  age-related changes in, 1664
  anatomy of, 1614
  cancer of, 1689
  fistulas of, 1673–1674, 1673f
  palpation of, 1626–1627
  pH of, 1661–1662
Vaginal cancer, 1689
  epidemiology of, 1682
Vaginal cone retention exercises, for urinary incontinence, 1582c
Vaginal discharge, 1626, 1626t
Vaginal vault, definition of, 1661
Vaginitis, 1662, 1663t
  definition of, 1661
Vagotomy, in peptic ulcer disease, 1213t
Vagotomy syndrome, 1169
  definition of, 1142

Vagus nerve (X), 2136–2137, 2136f, 2137t, 2139, 2292f
  assessment of, 2147c
  disorders of, 2294t
Valacyclovir
  for herpes simplex virus encephalitis, 2274
  for HIV-related herpes infections, 1836
Valdecoxib, in pain management, 284
Valid consent, 484, 485c
Valproate (Depakote, Depakene)
  adverse effects and side effects of, 2194t
  toxic effects of, 2194t
Valproic acid, therapeutic blood levels of, 2601t
Valsalva maneuver
  and blood pressure, 1233
  cardiovascular effects of, 796
  definition of, 1232
  and intracranial pressure, 2178
  and wound healing, 541t
Valsartan (Diovan), 953
  for hypertension, 1029t
Values/beliefs, definition of, 46c
Valve(s)
  cardiac. See Heart valve(s)
  vascular, 976
  venous, incompetent, 1011f
Valve replacement, definition of, 915
Valvular heart disease, 915–920, 916f, 948
  nursing management of, 920
  signs and symptoms of, 790–792
Valvuloplasty, 920–923, 921f
  definition of, 915
  nursing management of, 924–925
Vancomycin
  and immune system, 1797t
  for pneumonia, 637
  therapeutic blood levels of, peak and trough, 2601t
Vancomycin-resistant *Enterococcus*, 2475
  health care–associated infection potential of, 2482–2483
Vancomycin-resistant *Staphylococcus aureus*, 2475
  health care–associated infection potential of, 2482
Vardenafil (Levitra), 1745, 1747t, 1748c–1749c
Variable expression, 145–146
  definition of, 140
Variance record, clinical pathway and, 2603f, 2604
Variceal banding, 1302, 1302f, 1304t
  definition of, 1285
Varicella, 1667
  incubation period of, 2476t
  transmission of, 2476t
Varicella vaccine, 2484
Varices, 1289. See also Esophageal varices
  gastrointestinal, in cirrhosis, 1319
Varicocele, 1505, 1773
  definition of, 1740
Varicose veins, 1014–1016
  medical management of, 1015
Variola, 2568. See also Smallpox
  incubation period of, 2477t
  transmission of, 2477t
Vascular access device
  bacteremia related to, 2484, 2484c
  fungemia related to, 2484, 2484c
  for hemodialysis, 1539, 1539f
  implanted, 398, 401f
Vascular compression, prevention of, in peripheral vascular disease, 987, 990
Vascular dementia. See Multi-infarct dementia

Vascular endothelial growth factor, in macular degeneration, 2071
Vascular myelopathy, in HIV-infected (AIDS) patients, 1833
Vascular system
  age-related changes in, 979
  alterations in, 978
  anatomy of, 975–976
  function of, 977–978
  pathophysiology of, 978–979
  resistance in, 978
Vasculature, peripheral, assessment of, 804. See also Pulse(s)
Vas deferens, 1741, 1741f
Vasectomy, 1773–1774, 1773f
  definition of, 1740
  nursing management of, 1774
Vasoactive agents
  for asystole, 838
  for cardiogenic shock, 369–370
  in treatment of shock, 365, 366t
  for ventricular fibrillation, 837
Vasoactive substances, in humoral immune response, 1789
Vasoconstriction
  definition of, 91
  in response to stress, 95
  sympathetic, 978
Vasoconstrictor(s), 978
  topical, for epistaxis, 605
  in treatment of shock, 366t
Vasodilation, promotion of, in peripheral vascular disease, 987, 990
Vasodilator(s), 978
  for cardiogenic shock, 966
  for hypertension, 1028t
  for hypertensive crises, 1033
  in treatment of shock, 366t
Vasopressin, 1446
  for cardiogenic shock, 370
  in cardiopulmonary resuscitation, 971, 972t
  definition of, 1440
  for esophageal varices, 1300, 1304t
  intravenous, for asystole, 838
  for shock, 366t
  for ventricular fibrillation, 837
Vasopressor(s)
  for anaphylaxis, 2538
  for cardiogenic shock, 966
  for orthostatic hypotension, 2259
Vasospasm, hemorrhagic stroke and, 2228
Vasovagal effect, 790
Vasovagal response, 887
Vasovasostomy, 1774
VDRL. See Venereal Disease Research Laboratory test
Vector-borne diseases, immigration and, 2512, 2513f
Vecuronium (Norcuron), 512t
Vein(s), 820, 820f, 976. See also Varicose veins
  anatomy of, 976
  cerebral, 2134–2135
  deep, thrombosis of. See Deep vein thrombosis
  superficial, thrombosis of, clinical manifestations of, 1005
Vena caval filter, 665–666, 666f
Venereal Disease Research Laboratory test
  in rheumatic diseases, 1893t
  for syphilis, 2506
Venipuncture
  cannulas for, 342–343
  devices for, 342–343
  and needleless delivery systems, 342–343, 343f

procedure for, 345, 346c–348c
site for, 341–342, 341f
preparation of, 345
Venlafaxine (Effexor)
for depression, 240
for hot flashes, 1635
Venodilating agent, 787
definition of, 781
Venom immunotherapy, 1868
Venous disorder(s), management of, 1006–1007
Venous insufficiency, chronic, 1010–1011
Venous return, impaired, with increased intracranial pressure, nursing interventions for, 2178t
Venous star, 1939c
Venous stasis. See also Thromboembolism, venous
postoperative, prevention of, 537
prevention of, 198
and pulmonary embolism, 662, 662c
and skin color, 1935t
traction and, 2371
Venous thrombosis, 1004–1010
assessment of, 1005–1006
clinical manifestations of, 1005
diagnosis of, 1005–1006
home and community-based care for, 1010
medical management of, 1006–1007
in neurosurgical patient, nursing interventions for, 2185c
nursing management of, 1007–1010
prevention of, 1006
surgical management of, 1007
Ventilation, 553, 557. See also Mechanical ventilation
air pressure variances and, 557
in airway obstruction, 2525–2526
airway resistance and, 557
bilevel positive airway pressure (bi-PAP), 743
brain injury and, 2248–2249
definition of, 553
in Guillain-Barré syndrome, 2290
mechanics of, 557
for myasthenia gravis, 2287
neurologic control of, 562
positive-pressure, noninvasive, 742–743
and respiratory acidosis, 336–337
Ventilation-perfusion imbalance, 557–559
Ventilation-perfusion ratio, 556, 558–559, 559c
definition of, 625
Ventilation-perfusion scan, 580–581
with pulmonary embolism, 663
with pulmonary hypertension, 660
Ventilator(s). See Mechanical ventilator(s)
Ventricle(s)
cardiac, 782–783, 782f
age-related changes in, 788t
function of, tests of, 812
wall motion of, test of, 812
cerebral, 2133
Ventricular assist devices, 929, 931f
in cardiogenic shock, 370–371
definition of, 915
electromagnetic, 929
pneumatic, 929
Ventricular asystole, 837–838, 838f
Ventricular escape rhythm. See Idioventricular rhythm
Ventricular fibrillation, 836–837, 837f
Ventricular tachycardia, 835–836, 836f
catheter ablation therapy for, 854–855
definition of, 823

Ventriculostomy, definition of, 2161
Venule(s), 976
anatomy of, 976
Veracity, ethical principle of, 28c
Verapamil, 830t, 955
and atrial fibrillation, 833
for atrioventricular (AV) nodal reentry tachycardia, 83
for cerebral vasospasm, 2226
for hypertension, 1029t
immediate release, for hypertension, 1029t
long-acting, for hypertension, 1029t
mechanism of action of, 785
Vermiform appendix, 1121, 1122f
Verrucae, 1977–1978
Vertebrae, 2136
fractures of, osteoporosis and, 2409–2411
Vertebral artery(ies), 2134
Vertebral line, 571c
Vertebra prominens, 571c
Vertebroplasty, in multiple myeloma, 1083
Vertical banded gastroplasty, 1218–1220, 1219f
Vertigo, 247, 2112, 2143. See also Ménière's disease
benign paroxysmal positional, 2119
with brain tumor, 2304
definition of, 2093, 2129
nursing care plan for, 2114c–2118c
surgical management of, 2113
Vesicant(s)
definition of, 381
extravasation of, 398
as terrorism threats, 2569t
Vesicle, 1937c
Vesicostomy, 1598f
Vesicoureteral reflux, 1495, 1571, 1572f
definition of, 1570
and pyelonephritis, 1577
Vestibular gland. See Bartholin's gland
Vestibular nerve section, for Ménière's disease, 2113
Vestibulitis, definition of, 1661
Vestibulocochlear nerve (VIII), 2094–2096, 2094f, 2292f
definition of, 2095c
disorders of, 2293t
Vestibulospinal tracts, 2135f, 2136
Veterinary Medical Assistance Teams, 2560
Vibration, chest, 731–734, 733c
definition of, 723
Vibration sense, assessment of, 2150
Vibrio cholerae
and diarrheal diseases, 2502
incubation period of, 2476t
transmission of, 2476t
Video thoracoscopy, 756c
Villi, intestinal, 1125
Villonodular synovitis, 1920
Vinblastine, for cancer treatment, 399t
Vincristine
for cancer treatment, 399t
adverse effects and side effects of, 399t
for chronic lymphocytic leukemia, 1074
for idiopathic thrombocytopenic purpura, 1088
Vindesine, for cancer treatment, 399t
Vinorelbine, for cancer treatment, 399t
Violence
domestic, 1620–1622, 1621c
in emergency department, 2518–2519, 2553–2554
family, emergency management of, 2550–2552
as psychiatric emergency, 2553–2554

Vioxx. See Rofecoxib
Viral hemorrhagic fevers, 2511–2512
Viral infection. See also specific infection
of skin, 1958–1960
Viral load test
definition of, 1815
for HIV diagnosis, 1825, 1825t
Viral set point
definition of, 1815
of HIV, 1824
Virkon-S, for calcivirus, 2502
Virulence
definition of, 2475
of Escherichia coli, 2501
Virus(es)
and cancer, 385–386
disease caused by, 102
gene products, and HIV infection, 1822
invasion by, immune response to, 1786–1788
pharyngitis caused by, 597–598
rhinitis caused by. See Rhinitis, viral
Visceral injury, in electrical burns, 2030
Viscosupplementation, for osteoarthritis, 1916
Vision
age-related changes in, 232t, 236, 2151
changes in, with brain tumor, 2304
count fingers (CF), 2047–2048
disorders of, 2143
diagnosis of, 2048–2050
genetics of, 2047
hand motion (HM), 2048, 2051
impaired, 2050–2054
nursing diagnoses related to, 2040–2041
nursing interventions for, 2040–2041
nursing outcomes with, 2040–2041
light perception (LP), 2048
loss of. See also Blindness; Low vision
people with, interacting and communicating with, 179c–180c
myasthenia gravis and, 2285, 2288
no light perception (NLP), 2048
nursing interventions for, in multiple sclerosis, 2282
refractive errors and, 2050–2051, 2050f
stroke and, 2208t, 2219–2220
travel, 2051
Visual acuity, 2046, 2047–2048
Visual analogue scales, for pain assessment, 272f, 273, 274f
Visual field(s), defects, with brain tumor, 2304
Visual pathway, 2046, 2046f
Vital capacity, 558t
in acutely ill patient, 577–578
Vital signs
assessment of, 75
brain injury and, 2243
monitoring, in hypothyroidism, 1454
Vitamin(s)
deficiency of
in cirrhosis, 1319
with gallstones, 1349
after gastric surgery, 1226
in liver disease, 1307
for hot flashes, 1635
and immune system function, 1795
production of, 1931
storage of, in liver, 1286
Vitamin A
deficiency of, in liver disease, 1307
and pressure ulcer healing, 213, 213t
in wound healing, 487t
Vitamin $B_6$, deficiency of, 1095–1098

Vitamin B$_{12}$
  absorption of, 1123–1124
  for cyanide poisoning, 2571
  deficiency of, 1040, 1045t, 1052–1054, 1095–1098
    clinical manifestations of, 1047, 1053
    diagnosis of, 1053
    medical management of, 1053
    pathophysiology of, 1052
  and erythropoiesis, 1040
Vitamin B complex, in wound healing, 487t
Vitamin C
  deficiency of, in liver disease, 1307
  and pressure ulcer healing, 213, 213t
  in wound healing, 487t
Vitamin D (calcitriol), 1931
  and bone health, 2339, 2406
  deficiency of, and osteomalacia, 2411
  for hypocalcemia, 327
  for Paget's disease, 2412–2413
  recommended intake of, 2406
  synthesis of, 1499
Vitamin K, 1286
  deficiency of, 1092
    in liver disease, 1307
  for warfarin toxicity, 1093
  in wound healing, 487t
Vitiligo, 1934
  definition of, 1927
Vitreous humor, 2045, 2045f
  definition of, 2043
Vocal cords, 554, 1153f
Vocal resonance, 576
Voice
  in laryngeal cancer, 609–610
  resting, in laryngitis, 601
Voice box. See Larynx
Voice sounds, 576
Voiding. See also Micturition
  changes in, 1503, 1503t
  postoperative, 543
  prompted, 1582c
  timed, 1582c
Voiding cystourethrography, 1509
Volkmann's canals, 2338f, 2339
Volkmann's contractures, 2362, 2443, 2443c
Volumetric pump, 348
Volvulus, and intestinal obstruction, 1263, 1264f, 1264t
Vomiting. See also Nausea and vomiting
  with brain tumor, 2304
  enteral nutrition and, 1184t
  in gastrointestinal disease, 1127
  induced, in poisoning, 2541
  and wound healing, 541t
Vomitus, 1127
von Recklinghausen's disease, 1978
  cutaneous manifestations of, 1929t
von Willebrand factor, 1092
von Willebrand's disease, 1092
Voodoo, 135
VRSA. See Vancomycin-resistant Staphylococcus aureus
Vulva, 1614, 1614f
  cancer of, 1685–1686
  inspection of, 1626
Vulvar cancer, 1685–1686
  epidemiology of, 1682
Vulvar cysts, 1677–1678
Vulvar dystrophy, 1678
  definition of, 1661
Vulvar vestibulitis, 1677
Vulvectomy, 1686
  definition of, 1661
Vulvitis, 1677
  definition of, 1661

Vulvodynia, 1677
  definition of, 1661
  dysesthetic, 1677
VX, as terrorism threat, 2570–2571

# W

Waist circumference, 78
Walker, ambulation with, 205
Walking cast, 2355
Warfarin (Coumadin)
  agents that interact with, 1100, 1101c
  for atrial fibrillation, 833
  drug interactions with, 1100, 1101c
  inhibition of, agents causing, 1100, 1101c
  metabolism of, genetic factors affecting, 154t
  perioperative management of, 490t
  potentiation of, agents causing, 1100, 1101c
  for pulmonary embolism, 665
  and stroke prevention, 2210
  for stroke prevention, with atrial fibrillation, 833
  for thrombotic disorders, 1100
  toxicity of, 1093
Warts, 1977–1978
  anogenital, in HIV-infected (AIDS) patients, 1672
  genital, 1666
    in males, 1750
Waste products
  of digestion, 1125
  excretion of, 1499
Wasting syndrome
  definition of, 1815
  in HIV-infected (AIDS) patients, 1832, 1844c, 1849
Water
  excretion of, regulation of, 1497
  intake
    and pressure ulcer healing, 213, 213t
    restriction of, in hyponatremia, 318–319
    retention of, in chronic renal failure, 1529
    in wound healing, 487t
Water balance, skin and, 1931
Water flush(es), for feeding tubes, 1185
Water intoxication, 315
Water loss
  insensible, 304
  lungs and, 304
  skin and, 304
Wavefront technology, 2051
WBC. See White blood cell(s)
Weakness, 2144
  in amyotrophic lateral sclerosis, 2323
  in Guillain-Barré syndrome, 2288–2289
  in myasthenia gravis, 2285
Weapons of mass destruction, 2559
  definition of, 2559
Weber test, 2098, 2099f, 2099t
Wedge resection, of lung, 672c, 755c
WeeFIM, 193
Weight
  assessment of, 75
  body
    assessment of, 77–78
    changes in, fluid imbalance and, 1505
    gain, in cardiovascular disease, assessment of, 793t
    loss
      in burn patient, 2025–2026
      in diabetes, 1384, 1388
      reduction, for low back pain, 2397
Wellness, 6, 57. See also Health
  definition of, 6, 49, 57
  promotion of, as function of nursing practice, 49

Western blot assay
  definition of, 1815
  for HIV diagnosis, 1825, 1825t
West Nile virus, 2510
  encephalitis caused by, 2274–2275
  incubation period of, 2477t
  transmission of, 2477t
Wheal(s), 1937c
  urticarial, 1864
Wheelchair
  and pressure ulcers, 210, 212f
  for stroke patient, 2218
  transfer to, 201–203, 202f, 203c
  use after amputation, 2467
Wheezes/wheezing, 563, 568, 575, 575t, 576
  in asthma, 711
  in cardiac patient, 805
  definition of, 553
  in respiratory disease, 568
Whiff test, 1665
Whipple's disease, malabsorption in, 1240t
Whispered pectoriloquy, 576
  in pneumonia, 636
Whisper test, 2098
White blood cell(s), 1040f, 1041–1042
  definition of, 1036
  functions of, 1037, 1037t, 1042
  laboratory values for, 2579
White blood cell (WBC) count. See also Neutropenia
  in cancer patient, 424
  in cardiac patient, 808t
  in rheumatic diseases, 1893t
White matter, 2131, 2134f, 2135–2136
White pulp, of spleen, 1784
Whitlow, herpetic, 1960
WHO. See World Health Organization
Whole blood, 1103t
Wick catheter, 2437–2438, 2438f
Will, living, 251, 457, 457c
Window period
  definition of, 1815
  of HIV infection, 1816
Windpipe. See Trachea
Wiskott-Aldrich syndrome, 1803t, 1807
  definition of, 1802
  genetics of, 147t
Withdrawal method, of contraception, 1646
WMDs. See Weapons of mass destruction
Wolff-Parkinson-White syndrome
  catheter ablation therapy for, 854–855
  ECG findings in, 854, 855f
Women. See also Female; Gender differences
  and disability, 175
  health counseling for, 1616, 1618c
  health history in, 1616–1623
  health screening for, 1616, 1618c
  heart disease in, 866–867
  heart transplantation in, nursing research on, 930
  HIV infection (AIDS) in, 1834–1835
  with irritable bowel syndrome, quality of life in, nursing research on, 1239
  older
    breast cancer in, 1735
    gynecologic concerns in, 1623
    pelvic examination in, 1627
    vaginal physiology in, 1664
  osteoporosis in, 2405
  periconception health care for, 1652–1653
  preconception health care for, 1652–1653
  recovery after coronary artery bypass graft, nursing research on, 903
  sexual history in, 1618–1620
  symptoms of myocardial infarction in, nursing research on, 795

Women's health, role of nurses in, 1613–1614
Wood's light, 1942
  definition of, 1927
Working animals, 219
Workplace
  health-promotion activities in, 60
  occupational health nursing in, 21
World Health Organization (WHO)
  classification of functioning, disability, and health, 174
  definition of health, 6
  and infection control and prevention, 2480
Wound(s)
  assessment of, 799
  burn. See also Wound care
    grafting for, 2019–2024, 2020t
    cleansing of, 2529
    drainage of, after hip replacement, 2374
    emergency care for, 2528–2529
    infections of, 545–546
      bone tumors and, 2420
      postoperative, 2413
    irrigation of
      with open fracture, 2434
      in sequestrectomy, 2414
    patterned, definition of, 2528c
    primary closure of, 2529
      delayed, 2529
    stressors for, and wound healing, 541t
  surgical. See also Dressing(s)
    breakdown, after laryngectomy, nursing interventions for, 618
    care for, patient teaching about, 540, 542c
    classification of, by degree of contamination, 545, 545t
    clean, 545t
    clean-contaminated, 545t
    contaminated, 545t
    dehiscence of, 546, 546f
    dirty, 545t
    drains for, 538, 538f
    evisceration, 546, 546f
    healing of. See Wound healing
    infection of, 538, 545–546
  types of, 2528, 2528c
Wound care
  advances in, 1948
  burns and, 2016
  for colostomy patient, 1271
  five rules of, 1946
  in gastrostomy, 1191
  after neck dissection, 1155
  in parenteral nutrition, 1198
  products for, 1946, 1946c
  for skin conditions, 1945–1951
Wound care specialist, definition of, 1570
Wound dressings. See Dressing(s)
Wound healing
  amputation and, 2464
  in burns
    disorders of, 2026
    failure of, 2026
  delayed, bone tumors and, 2420
  factors affecting, 540, 541t
  hip fracture and, 2452c
  after mastoid surgery, 2109
  nutrients important for, 486, 487t
  open fracture and, 2434
  phases of, 538
    inflammatory (lag, exudative), 538, 539t
    maturation (differentiation, resorptive, remodelling, plateau), 538, 539t
    proliferative (fibroblastic, connective tissue), 538, 539t
  by primary (first) intention, 104, 538–539, 539f
    definition of, 524
  by secondary (second) intention, 104, 538, 539–540, 539f
    definition of, 524
  third-intention, 538, 539f, 540
    definition of, 524
Wrist, fracture of, 2443–2444
Wrist surgery
  assessment for, 2399
  expected outcomes in, 2400
  home care after, 2400c
  nursing diagnoses related to, 2399
  nursing interventions for, 2399–2400
  nursing process with, 2399–2400
  planning and goals for, 2399

## X

Xanthelasma, 798, 2080
X chromosome, 142, 143f
  mutations of, 146
Xenograft
  as bridge to liver transplantation, 1317
  for burns, 2020t, 2021
  definition of, 915, 1285
  for heart valve replacement, 924
  skin, 1986
Xerosis, definition of, 1945
Xerostomia, 1151
  definition of, 381, 589, 1142
  after radiation therapy, 612
  radiation therapy and, 395
X-linked inheritance, 145, 146, 147t, 148f
  definition of, 140
X-rays. See Radiation; Radiography
Xylometazoline hydrochloride, for allergic rhinitis, 1872t

## Y

Y chromosome, 142, 143f
*Yersinia*, diarrhea caused by
  incubation period of, 2476t
  transmission of, 2476t
*Yersinia pestis*, 2567t
Yin/yang theory, 135

## Z

Zafirlukast (Accolate), for asthma, 713, 713t
Zalcitabine (Hivid), for HIV infection, 1827t
Zenker's diverticulum, 1164
ZES. See Zollinger-Ellison syndrome
Zevalin. See Ibrituzumab-tiuxetan (Zevalin)
Zidovudine
  and cytomegalovirus retinitis, 1835–1836
  for HIV infection, 1827t
ZIFT. See Zygote intrafallopian transfer
Zileuton (Zyflo), for asthma, 713, 713t
Zinc
  precautions with, 593
  for viral rhinitis, 593
  in wound healing, 487t
Zinc sulfate, and pressure ulcer healing, 213, 213t
Zoledronic acid (Zometa), in multiple myeloma, 1084
Zollinger-Ellison syndrome, 1209, 1240t, 1372
  definition of, 1345
  diagnosis of, 1211
  medical management of, 1212
Zolmitriptan (Zomig), for migraine, 2201
Zonisamide (Zonegran, Excegran)
  adverse effects and side effects of, 2194t
  toxic effects of, 2194t
Zymase, 1946